Clinical Otology

Third Edition

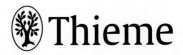

Clinical Otology
Third Edition

Gordon B. Hughes, M.D., F.A.C.S.
Professor and Head
Section of Otology and Neurotology
Head and Neck Institute
Cleveland Clinic
Cleveland, Ohio

Myles L. Pensak, M.D., F.A.C.S.
H. B. Broidy Professor and Chairman
Department of Otolaryngology–Head and Neck Surgery
Professor
Department of Neurologic Surgery
University of Cincinnati Medical Center
Cincinnati, Ohio

Thieme
New York • Stuttgart

Thieme Publishers, Inc.
333 Seventh Ave.
New York, NY 10001

Editor: Esther Gumpert
Associate Editor: J. Owen Zurhellen IV
Editorial Assistant: Judith Tomat
Vice President, Production and Electronic Publishing: Anne T. Vinnicombe
Production Editor: Print Matters, Inc.
Sales Director: Ross Lumpkin
Associate Marketing Manager: Verena Diem
Chief Financial Officer: Peter van Woerden
President: Brian D. Scanlan
Medical Illustrator: Kathleen I. Jung
Compositor: Alden Prepress Services
Printer: Everbest Printing Company, Ltd

Library of Congress Cataloging-in-Publication Data

Clinical otology / [edited by] Gordon B. Hughes, Myles L. Pensak. — 3rd ed.
       p. ; cm.
     Includes bibliographical references and index.
     ISBN 3-13-671103-3 (HC-GTV) — ISBN 1-58890-364-8 (HC-US)
      1. Ear—Diseases. 2. Otology. 3. Hearing disorders. I. Hughes, Gordon B. II. Pensak,
    Myles L.
     [DNLM: 1. Ear Diseases. 2. Ear—physiology. 3. Hearing Disorders. WV 200 C6411 2006]
    RF120.H84 2006
    617.8—dc22

                                                                        2006044663

Important note: Medical knowledge is ever-changing. As new research and clinical experience broaden our knowledge, changes in treatment and drug therapy may be required. The authors and editors of the material herein have consulted sources believed to be reliable in their efforts to provide information that is complete and in accord with the standards accepted at the time of publication. However, in view of the possibility of human error by the authors, editors, or publisher of the work herein or changes in medical knowledge, neither the authors, editors, or publisher, nor any other party who has been involved in the preparation of this work, warrants that the information contained herein is in every respect accurate or complete, and they are not responsible for any errors or omissions or for the results obtained from use of such information. Readers are encouraged to confirm the information contained herein with other sources. For example, readers are advised to check the product information sheet included in the package of each drug they plan to administer to be certain that the information contained in this publication is accurate and that changes have not been made in the recommended dose or in the contraindications for administration. This recommendation is of particular importance in connection with new or infrequently used drugs.

Some of the product names, patents, and registered designs referred to in this book are in fact registered trademarks or proprietary names even though specific reference to this fact is not always made in the text. Therefore, the appearance of a name without designation as proprietary is not to be construed as a representation by the publisher that it is in the public domain.

Printed in China

5 4 3 2 1

The Americas ISBN 1-58890-364-8
                    978-1-58890-364-8
Rest of World ISBN 3-13-671103-3
                    978-3-13-671103-3

To Myra and Gordon Jr.

Gordon B. Hughes

To Penny, Ben, Meredith, and Carly

Myles L. Pensak

To the memory of our friend and colleague John Lawrence Kemink, M.D. (September 4, 1949–June 25, 1992)

Contents

Foreword

Gordon Hughes and Myles Pensak asked me to write this foreword for their third edition of *Clinical Otology* with emphasis on my personal perspective of the many advances that have occurred in the field of otology over the past forty years. I have inserted some bias that is my responsibility entirely and not those of the authors.

I finished my otology fellowship and entered private practice in 1966. In the ensuing years the changes that have occurred in our field of medicine are astounding. Back in 1966 we had no computerized tomography (CT), magnetic resonance imaging (MRI), or positron emission tomography (PET) scans; no lasers or facial nerve monitors; no auditory brainstem response (ABR). There was no Internet, no fax machines, and no cell phones. Yet we managed to diagnose and surgically manage acoustic neuromas, glomus tympanicum tumors, and jugulare tumors as well as numerous other skull base lesions. The new diagnostic tools mentioned above did allow us, over time, to lower the mortality rates for most surgical procedures. When I started my fellowship with William F. House, the mortality rate for acoustic neuromas was 10 to 15%. Over the years with better diagnostic capability, improved anesthesia, and surgical technique, we were able to lower mortality to 0.5%.

Every generation of surgeons learns from those who precede them. We are fortunate in otology to have had the benefit of outstanding mentors. These men all had one thing in common: they unselfishly shared their knowledge and surgical expertise with anyone who was willing to visit and learn.

In 1966 there were few or no otologists practicing in academic medicine. Now almost every otolaryngology program has one or more otologist and neurotologist. Residents graduating from first-rate programs today are much better prepared to take care of the more-routine otologic problems.

While there have been exceptional advances in our field there have been some setbacks. Having practiced during the golden era of medicine, I personally find it disquieting that third-party payers have turned the practice of medicine into a business. These organizations have interrupted the centuries-old doctor-patient relationship and often interfere with physicians' patient care.

I was extremely fortunate during my years of practice to work with a group of outstanding young doctors who decided to take a fellowship at the Otology Group in Nashville, Tennessee. I learned more from them than I was able to impart. As well as surgical technique, I did try to emphasize the importance of the art of medicine. Two of my former fellows, Gordon Hughes and Myles Pensak, have edited an outstanding text on otology and neurotology that clearly articulates the most contemporary science and management paradigms available for otolaryngologists, audiologists, residents, and medical students.

This book focuses on the fundamental principles of basic science, evaluation, management, and rehabilitation of otologic-neurotologic pathologies. Each chapter is heavily referenced and has an excellent bibliographic foundation. Eiji Yanagisawa has provided splendid photographic illustrations that clearly delineate anatomy and surgical technique. The text is easy to read and presented in a straightforward manner. This third edition is an excellent follow-up on the first and second editions. Thirty-three chapters have been updated. The text encourages surgeons to hone their skills and should be in every surgeon's personal library.

Drs. Hughes and Pensak have called on 36 world-renowned surgeons and scientists to provide chapters in this edition. Twenty-four of these are new authors. The book is organized in such a manner that the busy clinician can zero in on the subject that most interests him.

I highly recommend this book. As a teacher, it is extremely rewarding to see my students succeed and produce quality scientific works.

Michael E. Glasscock III, M.D., F.A.C.S.
Dripping Springs, Texas

Preface

This new edition of *Clinical Otology* presents the current generation of technical innovations in otology and related sciences since the second edition was published in 1997. Four new chapters cover middle ear molecular biology, inner ear molecular disorders, pharmacology of otologic drugs, and cystic lesions of the petrous apex. Twenty-four new authors significantly revised and updated 33 chapters to address state-of-the-art genetic diagnosis of hereditary hearing loss, management of superior canal dehiscence and variants of benign paroxysmal positional vertigo (BPPV), evidence-based management of otitis media with effusion, T-cell initiation of autoimmune inner ear disease, middle ear and brainstem implantable hearing devices, new applications of transtympanic therapy, and many other advances.

Using the successful structure of the second edition, in which the book is divided into four sections—basic science, evaluation, management, and rehabilitation—this new edition provides a strong foundation for successful clinical practice and an exhaustive bibliography for deeper investigation into selected topics, and sets the stage for the next generation of technical innovations: molecular diagnosis and therapy; fully implantable hearing devices; endoscopic, endovascular, and robotic surgery; functional ear and brain imaging; vestibular pacemakers; genetic engineering; and more.

The two editors deeply appreciate the elegant color photography of Eiji Yanagisawa, who replaced 27 older photographs with beautiful new prints. His chapter on otologic photography and videography is superbly updated. In addition, many of Kathleen Jung's detailed drawings are re-created for this edition, and new drawings have been added. The artists' beautiful color photography and artwork visually enhance the book; the superb quality of their work speaks for itself. As for the book cover, Richard Nodar's fanciful illustration is a study in conceptual design: graphic, playful, insightful, and fun.

For most busy clinicians, writing a book chapter is laborious. Even a revised, updated chapter with contemporary references often must be completely rewritten. Virtually all 36 internationally recognized clinicians and scientists accepted our invitation to write chapters for this edition. Their contributions again create a truly state-of-the-art book. We applaud Thieme Medical Publishers for their commitment to scholarship and academic excellence in otology, and are indebted to Thieme, Eiji Yanagisawa, Kathleen Jung, and all the authors for their outstanding contributions. *Clinical Otology, Third Edition*, again provides broad clinical perspective, focused patient care strategy, and contemporary references in a highly readable, beautifully illustrated, medium-sized yet comprehensive work to enable students and practitioners alike to achieve optimal clinical practice of otology.

Contributors

Kelly S. Beaudoin, M.S.P.T.
Balance Solutions Physical Therapy Inc.
University Heights, Ohio

David K. Brown, Ph.D.
Assistant Professor
Departments of Communication Sciences and Disorders; and
    Otolaryngology–Head and Neck Surgery
University of Cincinnati Medical Center
Cincinnati Children's Hospital Medical Center
Cincinnati, Ohio

Michael C. Byrd, M.D.
Associate Staff
Head and Neck Institute
Cleveland Clinic
Cleveland, Ohio

Ryan M. Carpenter, Au.D.
Assistant Professor
Department of Otolaryngology–Head and Neck Surgery
Johns Hopkins School of Medicine
Clinical Faculty
The Listening Center at Johns Hopkins
The Johns Hopkins Hospital
Baltimore, Maryland

Daniel I. Choo, M.D.
Associate Professor
Department of Otolaryngology–Head and Neck Surgery
University of Cincinnati Medical Center
Cincinnati Children's Hospital Medical Center
Cincinnati, Ohio

Kathleen D. Coale, P.T.
Northeast Health Systems
Addison Gilbert Hospital
Gloucester, Massachusetts

Rebecca S. Cornelius, M.D.
Associate Professor
Division of Neuroradiology
University of Cincinnati Medical Center
Cincinnati, Ohio

Charles C. Della Santina, M.D., Ph.D.
Assistant Professor
Departments of Otolaryngology–Head and Neck Surgery; and
    Biomedical Engineering
Johns Hopkins School of Medicine
Baltimore, Maryland

Ronald K. de Venecia, M.D., Ph.D.
Instructor
Department of Otology and Laryngology
Harvard Medical School
Assistant
Department of Otolaryngology
Massachusetts Eye & Ear Infirmary
Boston, Massachusetts

Joni K. Doherty, M.D., Ph.D.
Assistant Professor
Department of Surgery
University of California, San Diego—School
    of Medicine
La Jolla, California

Rick A. Friedman, M.D., Ph.D.
Clinical Associate Professor
Department of Otolaryngology
University of Southern California Keck School of Medicine
Los Angeles, California

Bruce J. Gantz, M.D.
Professor
Department of Otolaryngology–Head and Neck Surgery
University of Iowa Hospitals
Iowa City, Iowa

Joel A. Goebel, M.D., F.A.C.S.
Professor and Vice Chairman
Department of Otolaryngology–Head and
    Neck Surgery
Washington University at St. Louis School
    of Medicine
St. Louis, Missouri

John H. Greinwald Jr., M.D., F.A.A.P.
Associate Professor
Departments of Otolaryngology–Head and Neck Surgery;
    and Pediatrics
University of Cincinnati Medical Center
Cincinnati Children's Hospital Medical Center
Cincinnati, Ohio

A. Julianna Gulya, M.D., F.A.C.S.
Clinical Professor
Department of Otolaryngology–Head and Neck Surgery
The George Washington University School of Medicine
    and Health Sciences
Washington, D.C.

Michelle Hernandez, M.D.
Allergy Fellow
Department of Medicine
University of California, San Diego–School
    of Medicine
La Jolla, California

Keiko Hirose, M.D.
Assistant Professor
Head and Neck Institute
Department of Neurosciences
Lerner Research Institute
Cleveland Clinic
Cleveland, Ohio

May Y. Huang, M.D.
Otologist and Neurotologist
Northwest Ear
Seattle, Washington

Gordon B. Hughes, M.D., F.A.C.S.
Professor and Head
Section of Otology and Neurotology
Head and Neck Institute
Cleveland Clinic
Cleveland, Ohio

Chandra M. Ivey, M.D.
Department of Otolaryngology–Head and
    Neck Surgery
University of Cincinnati Medical Center
Cincinnati, Ohio

Robert K. Jackler, M.D.
Sewall Professor and Chair
Department of Otolaryngology–Head and Neck Surgery
Stanford University School of Medicine
Stanford, California

Abraham Jacob, M.D.
Assistant Professor
Department of Otolaryngology–Head and Neck Surgery
The Ohio State University College of Medicine
Columbus, Ohio

Pawel J. Jastreboff, Ph.D., Sc.D., M.B.A.
Professor and Director
Tinnitus Center
Department of Otolaryngology
Emory University School of Medicine
Atlanta, Georgia

Margaret M. Jastreboff, Ph.D.
Visiting Resident Professor
Department of Audiology, Speech-Language Pathology,
    and Deaf Studies
Towson University
Towson, Maryland

Robert W. Keith, Ph.D.
Professor
Department of Otolaryngology–Head and Neck Surgery
University of Cincinnati Medical Center
Cincinnati, Ohio

William C. Kinney, M.D.
Assistant Professor
Department of Otolaryngology–Head and Neck Surgery
University of Missouri-Columbia School of Medicine
Columbia, Missouri

Brian Kung, M.D.
Assistant Professor
Jefferson Medical College at Thomas Jefferson
    University
Philadelphia, Pennsylvania
Delaware Biotechnology Institute
Newark, Delaware

John F. Kveton, M.D.
Clinical Professor
Section of Otolaryngology
Yale University School of Medicine
Department of Surgery
Yale-New Haven Hospital
New Haven, Connecticut

Paul R. Lambert, M.D., F.A.C.S.
Professor and Chair
Department of Otolaryngology–Head and Neck Surgery
Medical University of South Carolina
Charleston, South Carolina

Joung H. Lee, M.D.
Director, Neurofibromatosis and Benign Tumors
Head
Section of Skull Base Surgery
Brain Tumor and Neuro-Oncology Center
Cleveland Clinic
Cleveland, Ohio

John P. Leonetti, M.D.
Professor
Department of Otolaryngology–Head and Neck Surgery
Loyola University Chicago–Stritch School of Medicine
Maywood, Illinois

Benjamin D. Liess, M.D.
Resident Physician
Department of Otolaryngology–Head and
    Neck Surgery
University of Missouri-Columbia School of Medicine
Columbia, Missouri

David J. Lim, M.D.
Research Professor
University of Southern California Keck School
    of Medicine
Los Angeles, California
Professor Emeritus
The Ohio State University College of Medicine
Columbus, Ohio

Jerry W. Lin, M.D., Ph.D.
Resident Physician
Department of Otorhinolaryngology
Weill Medical College of Cornell University
New York, New York

Lawrence R. Lustig, M.D.
Associate Professor
Department of Otolaryngology
University of California, San Francisco—School of Medicine
Stanford, California

Sam J. Marzo, M.D.
Associate Professor
Department of Otolaryngology–Head and Neck Surgery
Loyola University Chicago–Stritch School of Medicine
Maywood, Illinois

John S. McDonald, D.D.S.
Volunteer Professor
Departments of Anesthesia and Surgery
University of Cincinnati Medical Center
Cincinnati, Ohio

Michael J. McKenna, M.D.
Professor
Department of Otology and Laryngology
Harvard Medical School
Massachusetts Eye & Ear Infirmary
Boston, Massachusetts

Edwin M. Monsell, M.D., Ph.D.
Professor
Department of Otolaryngology–Head and Neck Surgery
Wayne State University School of Medicine
Detroit, Michigan

Craig W. Newman, Ph.D.
Professor
Head
Section of Audiology
Head and Neck Institute
Cleveland Clinic
Cleveland, Ohio

John K. Niparko, M.D.
George T. Nager Professor
Department Otolaryngology—Head and Neck Surgery
Director
Division of Otology, Audiology, Neurotology, and
    Skull Base Surgery
Director
The Listening Center
Johns Hopkins University School of Medicine
Baltimore, Maryland

Myles L. Pensak, M.D., F.A.C.S.
H. B. Broidy Professor and Chairman
Department of Otolaryngology–Head and Neck Surgery
Professor
Department of Neurologic Surgery
University of Cincinnati Medical Center
Cincinnati, Ohio

Mukesh Prasad, M.D.
Assistant Professor
Department of Otorhinolaryngology
Weill Medical College of Cornell University
New York, New York

Pamela C. Roehm, M.D., Ph.D.
Assistant Professor
Department of Otolaryngology
New York University School of Medicine
New York, New York

Jay T. Rubenstein, M.D., Ph.D.
Professor
Department of Otolaryngology–Head and Neck Surgery
University of Washington School of Medicine
Seattle, Washington

Paul M. Ruggieri, M.D.
Head
Section of MRI
Cleveland Clinic
Cleveland, Ohio

Allen F. Ryan, Ph.D.
Professor
Department of Surgery
University of California, San Diego–School of Medicine
La Jolla, California

Leonard P. Rybak, M.D., Ph.D.
Division of Otolaryngology
Southern Illinois University School of Medicine
Springfield, Illinois

Sharon A. Sandridge, Ph.D.
Head
Section of Auditory Electrophysiology and
    Hearing Aids
Head and Neck Institute
Cleveland Clinic
Cleveland, Ohio

Nathan Sautter, M.D.
Resident Physician
Head and Neck Institute
Cleveland Clinic
Cleveland, Ohio

Mitchell K. Schwaber, M.D.
Consulting Staff
Department of Otolaryngology
Nashville Ear, Nose, and Throat Clinic
Nashville, Tennessee

Samuel H. Selesnick, M.D.
Professor
Department of Otorhinolaryngology
Weill Medical College of Cornell University
New York, New York

Kevin A. Shumrick, M.D.
Otolaryngologist
Cincinnati Group Health Associates
Cincinnati, Ohio

Aristides Sismanis, M.D., F.A.C.S.
Professor and Chairman
Department of Otolaryngology
Virginia Commonwealth University Medical Center
Richmond, Virginia

Eric L. Slattery, M.D.
Resident Physician
Department of Otolaryngology
Washington University at St. Louis School of Medicine
St. Louis, Missouri

C. Arturo Solares, M.D.
Fellow
Department of Otolaryngology–Head and Neck Surgery
Princess Alexandra Hospital
Brisbane, Australia
Resident Physician
Head and Neck Institute
Cleveland Clinic
Cleveland, Ohio

Baran Sumer, M.D.
Department of Otolaryngology–Head and Neck Surgery
Washington University at St. Louis School of Medicine
St. Louis, Missouri

Michael T. Teixido, M.D.
Assistant Professor
Jefferson Medical College at Thomas Jefferson University
Philadelphia, Pennsylvania
Delaware Biotechnology Institute
Newark, Delaware

Alyssa R. Terk, M.D.
Resident Physician
Section of Otolaryngology
Yale University School of Medicine
New Haven, Connecticut

Debara L. Tucci, M.D.
Associate Professor of Surgery
Division of Otolaryngology–Head and Neck Surgery
Department of Surgery
Duke University Medical Center
Durham, North Carolinsa

Vincent K. Tuohy, Ph.D.
Department of Immunology
Cleveland Clinic
Cleveland, Ohio

Stephen I. Wasserman, M.D.
Professor
Department of Medicine
University of California, San Diego–School of Medicine
La Jolla, California

Peter C. Weber, M.D.
Professor and Program Director
Director
Hearing Implant Program
Head and Neck Institute
Gamma Knife Center
Cleveland Clinic
Cleveland, Ohio

D. Bradley Welling, M.D., Ph.D.
Professor and Chair
Department of Otolaryngology–Head and Neck Surgery
The Ohio State University College of Medicine
Columbus, Ohio

Judith A. White, M.D., Ph.D.
Head and Neck Institute
Cleveland Clinic
Cleveland, Ohio

Mark D. Wilson, M.D.
Department of Otolaryngology–Head and Neck Surgery
Wayne State University School of Medicine
Division of Surgery
North Ottawa Community Hospital
Detroit, Michigan

Eiji Yanagisawa, M.D., F.A.C.S.
Clinical Professor
Section of Otolaryngology
Department of Surgery
Yale University School of Medicine
Southern New England Ear, Nose, Throat and Facial
    Plastic Surgery Group
New Haven, Connecticut

Ken Yanagisawa, M.D., F.A.C.S.
Clinical Assistant Professor
Yale University School of Medicine
Attending Otolaryngologist
Yale–New Haven Hospital and Hospital of St. Raphael
Southern New England Ear, Nose, Throat and Facial
    Plastic Surgery Group
New Haven, Connecticut

Chad A. Zender, M.D.
Resident Physician
Department of Otolaryngology–Head and
    Neck Surgery
Loyola University Chicago–Stritch School of Medicine
Maywood, Illinois

I

Basic Science

1

Anatomy and Embryology of the Ear

A. Julianna Gulya

It is incumbent upon the otologic surgeon to possess a detailed familiarity with the structure of the temporal bone and its environs. Additionally, as a number of otologic disorders are based on, or rendered more complicated by, aberrant development of the ear and temporal bone, an understanding of the normal embryologic sequences and the more common anomalies is critical to skillful otologic diagnosis and management. This chapter, in its review of the critical concepts of temporal bone anatomy and embryology, provides an important basis for better understanding the subsequent chapters. It begins with the structure of the temporal bone and the ear, followed by their development, both normal and abnormal. The interested reader is referred to *Anatomy of the Temporal Bone with Surgical Implications*[1] for details beyond the scope of this chapter.

◆ Anatomy

Pinna

The pinna is a bilaterally symmetric, cartilage-framed, cranial appendage that serves to focus and localize sound. The precise configuration of each individual pinna displays considerable variability, owing to its multicomponent embryologic origin, but there are also constant features.

The cartilaginous frame of the pinna determines its contour, and is composed of elastic cartilage. The lateral surface of the pinna is characterized by its convexities, the dominant one being the concha, which is bordered anteriorly by the tragus, superiorly and posteriorly by the anthelix and its anterior crus, and inferiorly by the antitragus. The helix, lacking in lop ears, extends superiorly and posteriorly from its crus and ends at the lobule; the Darwinian, or auricular, tubercle is a projection occasionally seen at its posterosuperior aspect. Another convexity is the triangular fossa, cradled by the two crura of the anthelix. The scaphoid fossa is the groove separating the helix and anthelix. The tragus is a nearly independent island of cartilage, connected to the main flange of the pinna by a narrow, inferiorly located, isthmus. The lobule is the fibrofatty inferior appendage of the pinna.

The skin and subcutaneous tissue recapitulate the irregularities of the cartilaginous frame; both the medial and lateral surfaces display hair, and sebaceous and sudoriferous glands, but the skin attachment differs, being loosely tethered on the medial aspect and snugly attached on the lateral.

The pinna attaches to the cranium by skin, cartilage, three extrinsic muscles, and extrinsic ligaments. The six intrinsic auricular muscles of the pinna are generally poorly represented in the human.

External Auditory Canal

The external auditory canal extends for approximately 2.5 cm; its lateral third is elastic, oriented posterosuperiorly, and is perforated anteriorly by two to three variably present fissures, the fissures of Santorini. The medial two thirds is osseus, oriented inferiorly and anteriorly (**Fig. 1–1**). The isthmus, located just medial to the junction of the bony and fibrocartilaginous canals, is the narrowest portion of the external auditory canal. Owing to the different angulations of the canal segments in the adult, the auricle must be pulled superiorly and posteriorly to allow alignment for otoscopic examination.

The skin of the osseous canal is much thinner than that of the fibrocartilaginous canal, and is lacking the usual adnexal structures, for example, hair follicles, in the subcutaneous layer. The subcutaneous layer of the fibrocartilaginous canal skin bears, in addition to hair follicles and sebaceous glands, ceruminous (modified apocrine) glands.

The sensory innervation of the pinna and the external auditory canal derives from the auriculotemporal branch of the trigeminal nerve, the greater auricular nerve of C3 origin, the auricular branch of the vagus, and twigs from the facial nerve. The auriculotemporal nerve innervates the anterior canal wall and tympanic membrane, as well as the anterior aspect of the pinna. The greater auricular nerve supplies the mastoid process and both lateral and medial aspects of the posterior pinna and tympanic membrane. The auricular branch of the vagus innervates the inferior bony canal and tympanic membrane, the posterosuperior cartilaginous canal, and the cymba concha. Branches of the facial and chorda tympani nerves innervate the posterosuperior bony external auditory canal.

Number key for Figures 1-1 to 1-5 1, external auditory canal; 2, fossa mastoidea; 3, squama; 4, mastoid tip; 5, tympanomastoid suture; 6, zygoma; 7, glenoid fossa; 8, temporal line; 9, petrotympanic fissure; 10, styloid process; 11, middle meningeal artery sulcus; 12, petrous bone; 13, internal auditory canal; 14, sigmoid sulcus; 15, superior petrosal sulcus; 16, inferior petrosal sulcus; 17, petrous apex; 18, arcuate eminence; 19, internal carotid artery foramen (internal); 20, tegmen; 21, facial hiatus; 22, stylomastoid foramen; 23, jugular fossa; 24, internal carotid artery foramen (external); 25, cochlear aqueduct; 26, endolymphatic fossette.

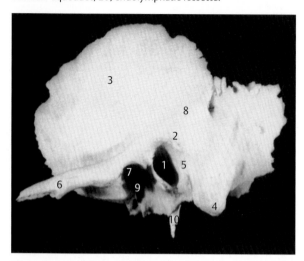

Figure 1–1 Left temporal bone, lateral view.

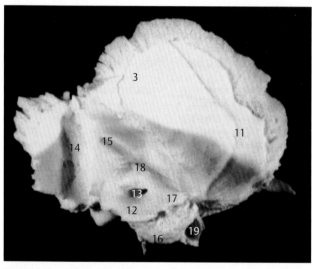

Figure 1–2 Left temporal bone, medial view.

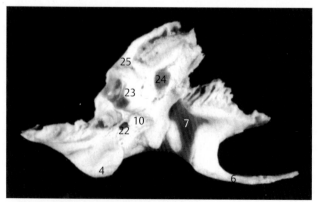

Figure 1–4 Left temporal bone, inferior view.

Temporal Bone

The tympanic bone of the osseous external auditory canal constitutes one component of the temporal bone; the petrous, squamous, and mastoid bones constitute the remaining portions, whereas the styloid process represents a separate bone (**Figs. 1–1** to **1–5**). The temporal bone articulates with the zygomatic, sphenoid, parietal, and occipital bones, and forms part of the lateral and posterior cranial fossae as well as the lateral wall and base of the skull.

The petrous portion of the temporal bone is the pyramidal core of the temporal bone and houses the inner ear. Its superior surface (**Fig. 1–3**), marked by the arcuate eminence, the tegmen of the tympanomastoid compartment, and the trigeminal impression for the fifth cranial nerve, makes up part of the floor of the middle cranial fossa. The facial hiatus, located anterior to the arcuate eminence, marks the exit of the greater superficial petrosal nerve from the geniculate ganglion. The posterior face (**Fig. 1–5**) of the petrous bone lies vertically between the superior petrosal sinus and the inferior

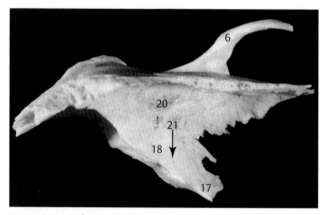

Figure 1–3 Left temporal bone, superior view.

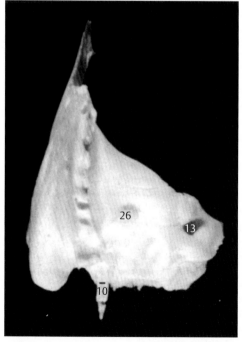

Figure 1–5 Posterior surface of temporal bone.

I Basic Science

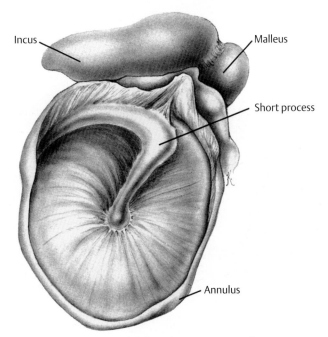

Incus

Malleus

Short process

Annulus

Figure 1–6 Lateral view of the right tympanic membrane.

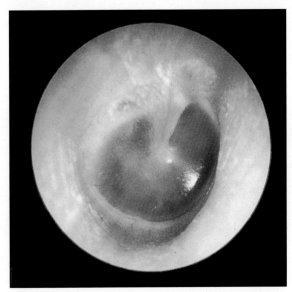

Figure 1–7 Normal right tympanic membrane.

petrosal sinus as it forms the anterolateral wall of the posterior cranial fossa. The porus of the internal auditory canal, the subarcuate fossa, and the endolymphatic fossette for the endolymphatic sac are located on the posterior face of the petrous bone. At the apex of the petrous bone, which is oriented anteromedially, the internal carotid artery exits its intrapetrous course, closely approximated by the orifice of the eustachian tube and the lesser superficial petrosal nerve. The inferior aspect (**Fig. 1–4**) of the petrous bone is highly irregular, providing attachment for several deep neck muscles, and is punctuated by the foramina for the internal carotid artery and the jugular bulb, separated by the jugulocarotid crest, housing the inferior tympanic artery and Jacobson's nerve (the tympanic branch of the ninth cranial nerve). The cranial orifice of the cochlear aqueduct opens at the medial aspect of the jugular fossa, whereas the styloid process arises posterolaterally. The stylomastoid foramen of the facial nerve arises posterior to the styloid process.

The squamous portion of the temporal bone (**Figs. 1–1** and **1–2**) forms the lateral wall of the middle cranial fossa, and articulates with the parietal bone superiorly and anteriorly with both the zygoma (by means of the zygomatic process) and the sphenoid bone. Arterial sulci mark both its lateral (the middle temporal artery) and medial (the middle meningeal artery) surfaces.

The mastoid portion of the temporal bone (**Figs. 1–1, 1–4,** and **1–5**) comprises inferiorly directed projections of both the petrous (medially) and squamous (laterally) portions, separated by Koerner's (petrosquamous) septum. Posterosuperior to the external auditory canal opening lies the spine of Henle, posterosuperior to which is the fossa mastoidea, or Macewen's triangle, which laterally overlies the mastoid antrum. The mastoid incisure accommodates the posterior belly of the digastric muscle; medial to the mastoid incisure is the temporal groove for the occipital artery. The mastoid foramen marks the passage of the mastoid emissary vein, located posteriorly on the lateral surface of the mastoid.

The tympanic portion of the temporal bone (**Fig. 1–1**) joins the mastoid at the tympanosquamous suture, and constitutes the inferior, anterior, and part of the posterior external auditory canal. The petrotympanic fissure represents the interface of the tympanic bone with the petrous bone, and is traversed by the chorda tympani nerve, the anterior tympanic artery, and the anterior process of the malleus. An inferior projection of the tympanic bone, the vaginal process, forms a sheath for the styloid bone. At the medial aspect of the tympanic bone is a groove (the annular sulcus), deficient superiorly (the notch of Rivinus), which houses the tympanic membrane annulus.

Tympanic Membrane

The tympanic membrane (**Fig. 1–6**) is an irregular cone, the apex of which is located at the umbo, corresponding to the tip of the manubrium (**Figs. 1–7** and **1–8**). In the adult, the tympanic membrane measures about 9 mm in diameter, and rests

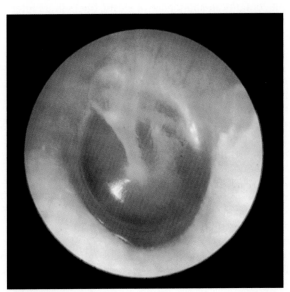

Figure 1–8 Normal left tympanic membrane.

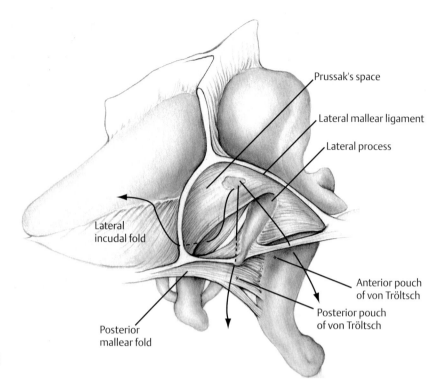

Figure 1–9 Prussak's space and environs. (Adapted from Hughes G. Cholesteatoma and the middle ear cleft: review of pathogenesis. Am J Otol 1979;1:109–114. Reprinted by permission.)

at a 140-degree angle with the superior wall of the external auditory canal. The tympanic membrane is firmly attached to the malleus at the lateral process and at the umbo; in between these two points, the plica mallearis, a flimsy fold of mucosal tissue, tethers the tympanic membrane to the malleus. The anterior and posterior tympanic striae, running from the lateral malleal process to the anterior and posterior tympanic spines, respectively, separate the superiorly located pars flaccida (Shrapnell's membrane) from the pars tensa. The pars tensa comprises three layers: a lateral epidermal layer, which is continuous with the skin of the external auditory canal; a medial mucosal layer, which is continuous with the mucosa of the middle ear; and an intermediate fibrous layer (the pars propria), consisting of outer radial and inner circular layers. The pars flaccida is also trilaminar and is thicker than the pars tensa, but contains an abundance of elastic fibers in its intermediate layer, which is irregularly organized.

Prussak's space (**Fig. 1–9**), or the superior recess of the tympanic membrane, is bordered laterally by Shrapnell's membrane, anterosuperiorly by the lateral malleal ligament, and inferiorly by the anterior and posterior malleal folds, and opens posteriorly into the epitympanum.

The fibrous annulus is the thickened periphery of the tympanic membrane and is lodged in the tympanic sulcus, both of which are deficient superiorly at the notch of Rivinus, where the tympanic membrane attaches directly to the squama.

Ossicles

The ossicular chain (**Fig. 1–10**) conveys sound from the tympanic membrane to the cochlea, and is made up of the malleus, incus, and stapes.

The malleus is the lateralmost ossicle, and consists of a manubrium (handle), head, neck, and lateral and anterior processes. The lateral process has a lateral, cartilaginous component that imperceptibly blends with, and, thus is

densely adherent to, the pars propria of the tympanic membrane. At the umbo, dense adherence is afforded by the splitting of the pars propria to encircle the tip of the manubrium. The anterior process to the petrotympanic fissure anchors the malleus, and, with the posterior incudal ligament, establishes

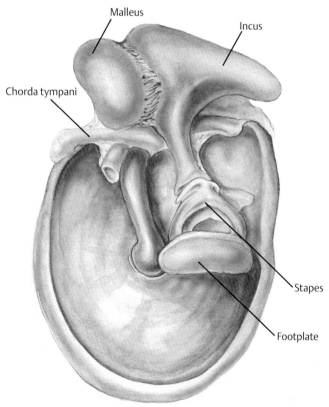

Figure 1–10 The ossicles, medial view in relation to the tympanic membrane.

the ossicular axis of rotation. The tendon of the tensor tympani muscle sweeps around the cochleariform process and attaches to the medial aspect of the neck and manubrium. Ordinarily, the medial pull of the tensor tympani muscle is opposed by the tympanic membrane; in cases of long-standing perforation, however, the tensor tympani acts unopposed, and can medially displace the manubrium, rendering myringoplasty and ossiculoplasty more difficult by contracting the middle ear space. Forcible lateralization of the malleus, or sectioning of the tendon, may be required to perform these procedures.

The incus is the largest of the ossicles and comprises a body and a short, a long, and a lenticular process. The body rests in the epitympanum with the head of the malleus, with which it articulates in a cog-type fashion. The short process of the incus occupies the incudal fossa, anchored by the posterior incudal ligament. The long process stretches inferiorly, paralleling the manubrium, to which it lies posterior, and terminates in the lenticular process, which articulates with the stapes. The long process in particular is susceptible to osteitic resorption with chronic otitis media, possibly related to its tenuous blood supply.

The medially located stapes is the smallest of the ossicles and is made up of a head, footplate, and two crura. The footplate, rimmed by the annular ligament, seals the oval window. The stapedius tendon stretches anteriorly from the pyramidal process to attach to the superior aspect of the posterior crus and the head of the stapes. When dissecting disease from the stapes, for example, cholesteatoma, it is best to work parallel to the plane of the stapedius tendon, working from posterior to anterior, so that the tendon resists displacement of the stapes.

Muscles

The tensor tympani muscle, arising from the greater wing of the sphenoid, the eustachian tube cartilage, and the walls of its semicanal, has both striated and nonstriated fibers that converge into a tendon. Innervation is derived from the trigeminal nerve.

The stapedius muscle occupies a vertical sulcus adjacent to the facial nerve, from which it derives its innervation, in the posterior wall of the tympanic cavity. Its action tilts the stapes, stretching the annular ligament and diminishing response to sound stimulation.

Middle Ear Spaces

The tympanic cavity is a sagittally oriented slit that is pneumatized by the eustachian tube, traversed by the ossicular chain, lined by mucosa, and connected posteriorly to the mastoid air cells by the antrum and aditus ad antrum. Its tegmen, or roof, serves also as the floor of the middle cranial fossa, whereas its irregularly contoured floor is dominated by the jugular bulb; in the posterior part of the floor is the root of the styloid process, from which arises the styloid eminence. Anteriorly, progressing sequentially from inferiorly, are located the internal carotid artery, the eustachian tube orifice, and the tensor tympani muscle. The tympanic membrane forms the lateral wall.

The more anatomically interesting aspects of the tympanic cavity are its posterior and medial walls. The posterior wall features the pyramidal eminence associated with the

stapedius tendon, and laterally, the chordal eminence, which is pierced by a foramen, the iter chorda posterius, traversed by the chorda tympani nerve as it enters the tympanic cavity. In between the pyramidal and chordal eminences is the facial recess, limited superiorly by the short process of the incus. Superior to the incus, the epitympanum opens into the mastoid antrum.

The medial wall (**Fig. 1–11**) is marked by three depressions of note: the sinus tympani and the oval and round window niches. The sinus tympani is delimited superiorly by the ponticulus, running between the pyramidal eminence and the promontory, inferiorly by the subiculum, which extends from the styloid eminence to the round window niche, laterally by the vertical segment of the facial nerve, and medially by the posterior semicircular canal. The sinus tympani variably extends posteriorly, but never communicates directly with the mastoid cavity, owing to different embryonic routes of pneumatization. The round window niche rests anteroinferior to the subiculum and posteroinferior to the promontory overlying the basal turn of the cochlea; the round window membrane lies in the depths of the niche; generally in the horizontal plane. The round window membrane, frequently obscured by a mucous membrane veil, has been implicated as a site of perilymph leakage; in making such as assessment, it is important to be sure that one is not being fooled by a leak through the veil. The oval window niche lies anterosuperior to the ponticulus. The cochleariform process is anterosuperior to the oval window, and is surmounted by the facial nerve in its tympanic segment.

The anterior epitympanic recess is anterior to the head of the malleus, which blocks the surgeon's view of this space, and demonstrates considerable variability in size. Cholesteatoma may extend into this region from the epitympanum, and it is important to remember that the facial nerve and geniculate ganglion may lie dehiscent in the surgical floor (medial wall) of the epitympanum.

Eustachian Tube

The eustachian tube is the mucosally lined pathway that ventilates, clears, and protects the tympanic cavity as it extends from the nasopharynx. The fibrocartilaginous portion is

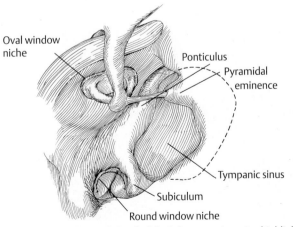

Figure 1–11 The medial wall of the left tympanic cavity, highlighting the sinus tympani, the round window niche, and the oval window niche. (Adapted from Schuknecht HF, Gulya AJ. Anatomy of the Temporal Bone with Surgical Implications. Philadelphia: Lea & Febiger, 1986:88. Reprinted by permission.)

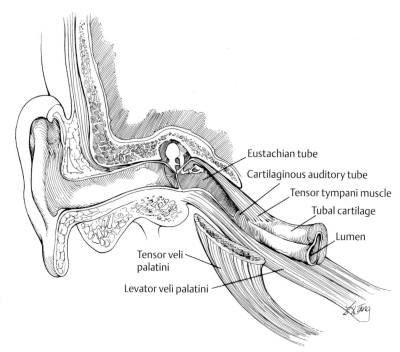

Figure 1–12 The eustachian tube and its associated muscles. (Adapted from Bluestone CD, Stool CE, eds. Pediatric Otolaryngology. Philadelphia: WB Saunders, 1990:320. Reprinted with permission.)

located anteromedially and composes two thirds of the approximately 35-mm tube; its union with the posterolateral osseous segment is marked by the isthmus (**Fig. 1–12**). The bony eustachian tube lies lateral to the internal carotid artery and is perforated by the passage of the caroticotympanic arteries. The tympanic ostium of the tube is in the anterior wall of the tympanic cavity, a few millimeters above the floor.

The fibrocartilaginous eustachian tube (**Fig. 1–13**) has a shepherd's crook cross section, with a larger medial and a smaller lateral lamella; the inferior margin of the medial

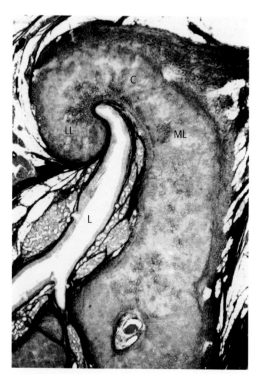

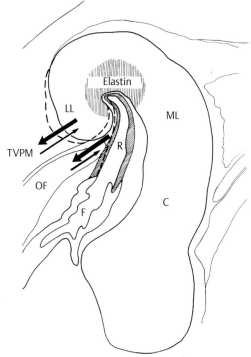

Figure 1–13 **(A)** Vertical section through the fibrocartilaginous (C) eustachian tube of an adult, illustrating the medial lamella (ML), the lateral lamella (LL), and their relation to the lumen (L). **(B)** Line drawing of fibrocartilaginous (C) eustachian tube, illustrating the hypothesized functional area. Tensor veli palatini muscle (TVPM) contraction causes lateral movement (heavy arrows) of the lateral lamella (LL) with respect to the medial lamella (ML) from its resting position (heavy outline) to its new position (dashed line). The elastin in the hinge portion mediates a return to resting position (thin arrows). (R, roof; F, floor; OF, lateral fat pad of Ostmann).

lamella has a groove for the levator palatini muscle, whereas the tensor veli palatini muscle attaches to the tip of the lateral lamella. Active opening of the upper half of the tube, which ventilates the tympanic cavity, is accomplished by contraction of the tensor veli palatini muscle.[2] The mucociliary clearance function is located in the lower half of the tube, which has an abundance of mucociliary cells. The lateral fat pad (of Ostmann) contributes to the resting closure of the tube, which protects the tympanic cavity.[2]

Middle Ear Mucosa

The tympanomastoid compartment has four types of lining cells: nonciliated with secretory granules, ciliated, intermediate, and basal.[3] The distribution of cell types varies within the middle ear and mastoid, with ciliated cells found in conjunction with secretory cells,[4,5] resulting in the formation of mucociliary tracts located on the promontory, the hypotympanum, and the epitympanum. These tracts work with the mucociliary clearance system of the eustachian tube.

Pneumatization

The degree of pneumatization of the temporal bone displays considerable variability, related to heredity, environment, nutrition, infection, and eustachian tube function. The pneumatized regions of the temporal bone are divided into five regions: the middle ear, the mastoid, the perilabyrinthine, the petrous apex, and the accessory (**Fig. 1–14**). Defined by the tympanic annulus, the tympanic region is divided into mesotympanic, epitympanic, hypotympanic, protympanic,

and posterior tympanic areas. The mastoid region can be divided into the mastoid antrum area, the central mastoid tract, and peripheral mastoid areas, for example, the tip cells. The perilabyrinthine region consists of a supra- and infralabyrinthine area, based on relation to the bony labyrinth. The petrous apex region is divided into an apical area and a peritubal area; the anterior petrous apex is pneumatized in 10 to 15% of specimens[6]; more often (80% of the time), the petrous apex is diploic, and in 7% of the cases it is sclerotic.[7] The accessory region is made up of the zygomatic, squamous, occipital, and styloid areas. Five tracts of pneumatization are recognized: the posterosuperior, running at the juncture of the posterior and middle fossa plates of the temporal bone; the posteromedial, paralleling and running inferior to the posterosuperior tract; the subarcuate, running through the arch of the superior semicircular canal; the perilabyrinthine tracts, running superior and inferior to the bony labyrinth; and the peritubal, around the eustachian tube.

Inner Ear

The bony labyrinth shelters the sensorineural and membranous structures of the inner ear, and comprises the vestibule, the semicircular canals, and the cochlea. The bone is trilaminar, with an inner, or endosteal, layer, an outer, or periosteal layer, and in between, a mixed layer of intrachondrial and endochondral bone, characterized by globuli interossei or islands of cartilage. Both the middle and endosteal layers demonstrate poor reparative capacities, and thus fractures of the labyrinth tend to heal only by the formation of fibrous tissue, with some bony repair by the periosteal layer.

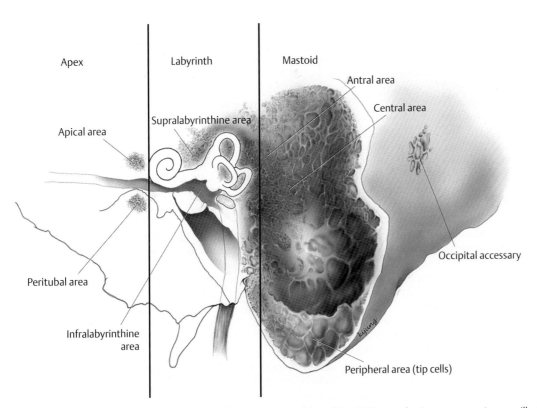

Figure 1–14 Pneumatization of the temporal bone. The mastoid, perilabyrinthine, and petrous apex regions are illustrated here. (From Nadol JB, Jr, Schuknecht HF, eds. Surgery of the Ear and Temporal Bone. New York: Raven Press, 1993. Reprinted by permission.)

The vestibule is the 4–mm central chamber of the bony labyrinth, and is dominated by depressions housing the utricule (the elliptical recess), the saccule (the spherical recess), and the basal end of the cochlear duct (the cochlear recess). The cribrose areas are perforations through which the nerve bundles gain access to the inner ear. The endolymphatic duct, housed within the bony vestibular aqueduct, originates at the posteroinferior aspect of the vestibule.

The cochlea is a 32–mm bony spiral that winds 2½ turns about its central axis, the modiolus, to a total height of 5 mm. The base of the cochlea abuts the fundus of the internal auditory canal, and is perforated (the cribrose area) for the transmission of cochlear nerve fibers. The apex, pointing anteriorly, inferiorly, and laterally, lies medial to the tensor tympani muscle. The osseous spiral lamina also winds about the modiolus, partially subdividing the cochlear canal into the scala tympani and scala vestibuli. The interscalar septum separates cochlear turns.

There are three semicircular canals: the lateral (horizontal), posterior (posterior vertical), and superior (anterior vertical). The three canals are orthogonally related to one another, measure 1 mm in diameter (expanding to 2 mm at the ampullae), and describe a 240-degree arc. Each of the three ampullae opens into the vestibule, as does the nonampullated end of the lateral canal, but the nonampullated ends of the posterior and superior canals fuse to form the crus commune, and thus open into the vestibule.

Microfissures of the bony labyrinth, or breaks in the endosteal and endochondral layers filled with fibrous tissue and acellular matrix, are commonly encountered in two locations—between the round window niche and the posterior semicircular canal ampulla, and superior and inferior to the oval window. The round window niche microfissure is uniformly present after the age of 6 years, whereas the oval-window–related microfissures are seen in about 25% of specimens, especially after the age of 40 years.[8] Their etiology remains unclear, but it is unlikely that they permit the flow of perilymph from the inner ear to the tympanic cavity.[9]

There are three fissures related to the bony labyrinth. The fistula ante fenestram is a constantly occurring evagination of the perilymphatic space that extends from the vestibule anterosuperiorly to the oval window, and in adulthood is filled with fibrous tissue and cartilage. The fossula post fenestram is a less consistently occurring evagination of the perilymphatic labyrinth that extends posterior to the oval window; it too is occupied by fibrous tissue. Hyrtl's fissure (the tympanomeningeal hiatus) is a remnant of the embryologic development of the temporal bone and its course parallels that of the cochlear aqueduct from the medial aspect of the jugular fossa to inferior to the round window niche. It has been implicated as a site for cerebrospinal fluid leakage into the middle ear.[10]

The membranous labyrinth (**Fig. 1–15**), consisting of the cochlear duct, the three semicircular ducts and their ampullae, the otolithic organs (the utricle and the saccule), and the endolymphatic duct and sac, is housed within the bony labyrinth, with the connective tissue, blood vessels, and fluid of the perilymphatic space interposed. The membranous labyrinth is filled with endolymph, with the utricular duct, saccular duct, and ductus reuniens connecting the major structures.

The cochlear duct (**Fig. 1–16**), or scala media, is an epithelial duct that spirals from the vestibular cecum in the vestibule to

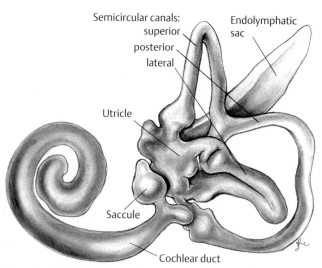

Figure 1–15 The adult membranous labyrinth as viewed from medially. (Adapted from Anson BJ, Donaldson JA. Surgical Anatomy of the Temporal Bone and Ear. Philadelphia: WB Saunders, 1983. Reprinted by permission.)

the cupular cecum at the apex of the bony cochlea. The epithelium of the floor of the cochlear duct is dominated by the organ of Corti, which rests on the basilar membrane. The inner and outer hair cells are the primary auditory receptors; in the human, there is one row of inner hair cells and three rows of outer hair cells. The hair cells are partially enveloped by the synaptic terminations of cochlear nerve fibers and are associated with several types of supporting cells. The spiral ligament is a specialized layer of periosteum in the outer wall of the bony cochlea, upon which rests the stria vascularis, a band of specialized tissue that is composed of three layers of cells and a rich capillary network. Reissner's membrane forms the anterior wall, or roof, of the cochlear duct, and extends from the spiral limbus to attach to the spiral ligament at the vestibular crest. The tectorial membrane is a gelatinous leaf that extends from the vestibular lip of the limbus to end in the border net, blanketing the organ of Corti.

The utricle is an elliptical tube that sweeps inferiorly from the elliptical recess. Its macula, oriented in the horizontal plane, is the sense organ of the utricle, containing its hair cells, and is divided into two regions by the striola. The otolithic membrane is the otoconia-studded gelatinous blanket into which the cilia of the macular hair cells project.

The saccule is a flattened sac, and its macula lies in the spherical recess inferior to the utricle, predominantly in the vertical plane. The saccule is characterized by a reinforced area, and its endolymphatic space communicates with that of the cochlea by means of the ductus reuniens.

The semicircular ducts run in the periphery of their bony canals; at the ampullae are the cristae ampullares, mounds of sensory neuroepithelium, connective tissue, and blood vessels surmounted by a gelatinous dome, the cupula.

The endolymphatic ducts run from its sinus, located in the posterolateral wall of the vestibule, to the endolymphatic sac, which lies on the posterior surface of the petrous pyramid, in a bony channel, the vestibular aqueduct. The course of the aqueduct initially parallels the crus commune, but then

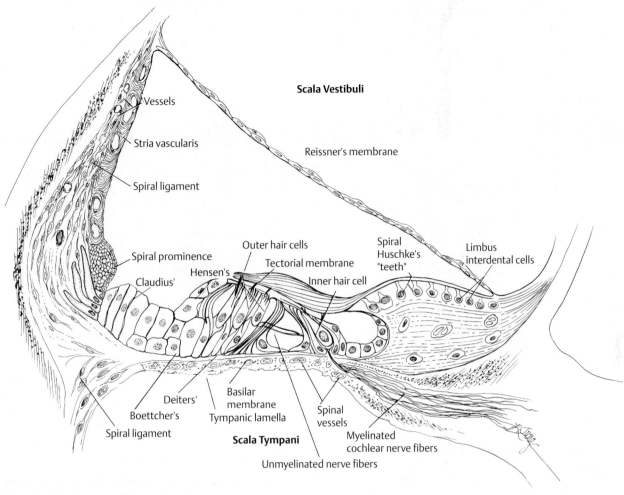

Figure 1–16 Structures of the cochlear duct.

makes a turn to parallel the posterior semicircular canal for the remainder of the course. The total length of the vestibular aqueduct has been related to peri- and infralabyrinthine pneumatization.[11]

The endolymphatic sac lies about 10 mm posterolateral to the porus of the internal auditory canal in a slight depression called the endolymphatic fossette, which is covered by the operculum. A surgical landmark for the sac is Donaldson's line, derived by extending the plane of the lateral semicircular canal perpendicular to, and bisecting, the posterior semicircular canal through to the posterior fossa dura; the sac lies inferior to this line, but in some ears with Meniere's disease it may be located more inferiorly and medial to the facial nerve.[11] The sac is believed to have both resorptive and immunologic functions.[12,13]

The utriculoendolymphatic valve (of Bast) is located in the anteroinferior wall of the utricle at the orifice of the utricular duct, and is believed to act in a passive manner to release excess endolymphatic pressure.[14]

The perilymphatic labyrinth comprises the fluid-filled spaces located between the bony labyrinth and the membranous labyrinth, including the vestibule, the scalae tympani and vestibuli, the perilymphatic spaces of the semicircular canals, and the periotic duct.

The cochlear aqueduct carries the periotic duct from its origin at the basal turn of the scala tympani to medial to the jugular fossa; as the duct parallels the inferior margin of the internal auditory canal, it is a useful landmark for the inferior limit of dissection about the internal auditory canal. The duct itself is filled with loose connective tissue, but does allow for the transmission of fluid and particles between the scala tympani and the subarachnoid space. From the surgeon's perspective, the duct is encountered during mastoidectomy when drilling medial to the jugular bulb; its penetration results in the flow of cerebrospinal fluid into the mastoid, a useful maneuver for the release of spinal fluid pressure in the course of a translabyrinthine resection of cerebellopontine angle lesions such as vestibular schwannomas. The cochlear aqueduct also marks the limit of such dissection, for further extension puts the lower cranial nerves (IX through XI) at risk, as they exit through the jugular foramen.

Internal Auditory Canal

The internal auditory canal (**Figs. 1–2** and **1–5**) is an osseous channel that is traversed by the superior and inferior vestibular, cochlear, facial, and intermediate nerves, as well as the labyrinthine artery and vein, as they course from the posterior

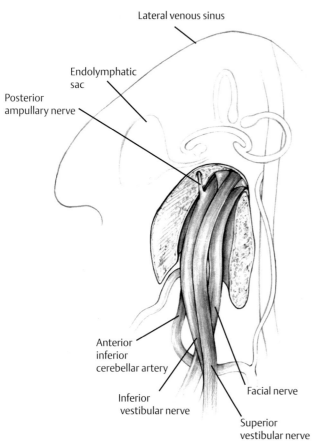

Figure 1–17 Illustration of the anatomic relationships of the nerves in the internal auditory canal, and how they rotate as they traverse the canal. (Adapted from Nadol JB, Jr, Schukneckt HF, eds. Surgery of the Ear and Temporal Bone. New York: Raven Press, 1993. Reprinted by permission.)

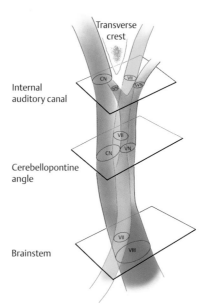

Figure 1–18 Illustration of the rotation of the nerves in the internal auditory canal. (From Nadol JB Jr., Schukneckt HF, eds. Surgery of the Ear and Temporal Bone. New York: Raven Press, 1993. Reprinted by permission.)

cranial fossa into the temporal bone. The dimensions of the canal display substantial variability, with the diameter averaging 3.7 mm and the length averaging 8 mm.[15]

The porus is the medial terminus of the canal, whereas the lateral end is called the fundus. At the fundus of the canal, the vestibular, facial, and cochlear nerves are in constant relative anatomic position determined by the falciform (horizontal) crest and the vertical (Bill's bar) crest (**Fig. 1–17**). Progressing medially in the canal, the nerves undergo a rotation and fusion,[16] which results in the facial nerve assuming a position anterior to the eighth nerve bundle, and the vestibular nerve assuming a position superior to the cochlear nerve (**Fig. 1–18**). The medial anatomic relations are used in vestibular nerve section, but are less reliable in tumor work, where considerable displacement can distort the expected anatomy.

◆ Neuroanatomy

Facial Nerve

As the nerve of the second branchial arch, the facial nerve innervates the structures derived from Reichert's cartilage. Its trunk is made up of five types of fibers: (1) special visceral efferent fibers, supplying the facial expression, stapedius, stylohyoid, and digastric (posterior belly) muscles; (2) general visceral efferent fibers to the lacrimal, nasal cavity seromucinous, submaxillary, and sublingual glands; (3) special sensory (taste) fibers from the anterior two thirds of the tongue, tonsillar fossae, and the posterior palate; (4) somatic sensory fibers from the external auditory canal and conchal region; and (5) visceral afferent fibers from the mucosa of the nose, pharynx, and palate.

There are three nuclei related to the facial nerve. The motor nucleus of the facial nerve is in the caudal pons; its superior aspect, supplying the frontalis and orbicularis oculi muscles, receives both crossed and uncrossed input from the motor cortex, whereas the inferior aspect receives only ipsilateral, uncrossed input. The superior salivatory nucleus, located dorsal to the motor nucleus, conveys parasympathetic secretory stimuli to the submaxillary, sublingual, lacrimal, nasal, and palatine glands. The nucleus of the solitary tract is in the medulla oblongata and receives the taste, proprioceptive, and cutaneous sensory fibers of the facial nerve.

The course of the facial nerve is divided into five segments (**Fig. 1–19**). The intracranial segment extends some 24 mm from the pons to the porus of the internal auditory canal; the next, or intracanalicular, segment runs in the internal auditory canal for 8 mm, joined at the fundus, where the facial nerve occupies the anterosuperior quadrant, by the nervus intermedius. The labyrinthine segment is the shortest, stretching for only 4 mm from the entrance to the fallopian canal to the geniculate ganglion. The fourth, or tympanic, segment covers approximately 13 mm in the medial wall of the tympanic cavity, superior to the cochleariform process and the oval window. At the sinus tympani, the facial nerve turns (the second genu), marking the beginning of the mastoid segment, which extends some 20 mm to the stylomastoid foramen.

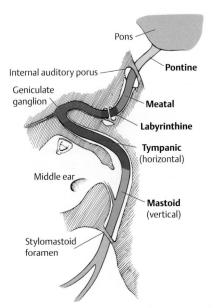

Figure 1–19   The segments of the course of the facial nerve.

Anomalous courses of the facial nerve are recognized; common among these is a course that takes the facial nerve more anterior and inferior to the oval window.[17,18] Another common anomaly involves the facial nerve bulging more posteriorly and laterally just inferior to the prominence of the lateral semicircular canal.[19] Bi- and even tri-partition of the vertical segment of the nerve can occur.

The fallopian canal demonstrates numerous gaps, or dehiscences, which render the contained facial nerve prone to injury. Baxter[20] found gaps of ≥4 mm in over half the specimens studied; the most common site, composing 66% of all dehiscences, was the tympanic segment near the oval window. Dehiscences can also occur in the medial wall of the epitympanum, superior to the geniculate ganglion, in the facial recess, and adjacent to the tensor tympani tendon. On occasion, the facial nerve can protrude through the dehiscence (**Fig. 1–20**), mimicking a middle ear mass.[21]

In the infant, the facial nerve is vulnerable to injury as it exits the stylomastoid foramen, lacking the protective cover of the mastoid process; with lateral growth of the tympanic ring and inferior growth of the mastoid process, the stylomastoid foramen becomes more secluded.

There are three branches of the facial nerve that arise in the temporal bone. The greater superficial petrosal nerve, carrying preganglionic parasympathetic and sensory fibers, originates from the anterior aspect of the geniculate ganglion and emerges onto the floor of the middle cranial fossa via the facial hiatus. The nerve to the stapedius muscle arises from the mastoid segment of the facial nerve near the pyramidal eminence.

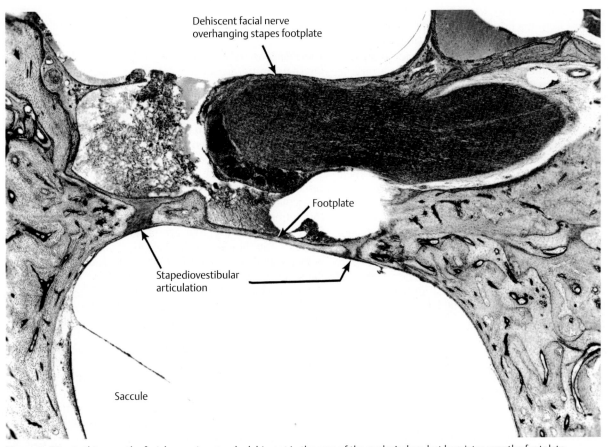

Figure 1–20   In this case, the facial nerve is not only dehiscent in the area of the oval window, but herniates over the footplate (male, 51 years). (From Gulya AJ, Schuknecht HF. Anatomy of the Temporal Bone with Surgical Implications, 2nd ed. Pearl River, NY: Pantheon Press, 1995. Reprinted with permission.)

The chorda tympani nerve composes the sensory bundle of the facial nerve, constituting some 10% of its cross-sectional area. The chorda separates from the main trunk a few millimeters superior to the stylomastoid foramen, although it may occasionally arise distal to the foramen, or as high as at the level of the lateral semicircular canal. The chorda takes a vertical course through the temporal bone, anterior and lateral to the mastoid segment of the facial nerve, and enters the tympanic cavity at the iter chorda posterius. The chorda passes lateral to the long process of the incus and medial to the malleus before exiting the tympanic cavity through the iter chorda anterius (canal of Huguier) to enter the petrotympanic (glaserian) fissure. Variations in the location of the chorda tympani nerve can occur and are of surgical significance. In addition to variations seen in its vertical segment (see above), the chorda may pass lateral, rather than medial, to the tympanic membrane, and may pass lateral, rather than medial, to the malleus.

The nervus intermedius (nerve of Wrisberg) is the sensory component of the facial nerve, and carries taste, secretory, and sensory fibers. In the internal auditory canal, the nervus intermedius runs between the superior vestibular and facial nerves, whereas in the tympanic segment it rests dorsally in the facial nerve. In the mastoid segment, the sensory bundle is found in the lateroposterior portion of the facial nerve, and finally exits anteriorly as the chorda tympani nerve.

Sensory Nerves of the Middle Ear

The tympanic branch of the glossopharyngeal (Jacobson's nerve) originates from the inferior ganglion of the ninth cranial nerve in the petrosal fossula at the jugulocarotid crest, and enters the tympanic cavity by the inferior tympanic canaliculus, accompanied by the inferior tympanic artery; it mediates referred otalgia from pharyngeal disorders. It ascends the promontory and medial tympanic cavity wall to be joined at the level of the round window by the caroticotympanic nerves (sympathetic fibers from the pericarotid plexus), forming the lesser superficial petrosal nerve. The lesser superficial petrosal nerve enters the superior tympanic canaliculus inferior to the cochleariform process, and then extends to the middle cranial fossa near, or even within, the semicanal of the tensor tympani muscle.

The auricular branch of the vagus (Arnold's nerve) consists of seventh, ninth, and tenth cranial nerve fibers. It originates in the jugular foramen and passes to the fallopian canal by passing over the dome of the jugular bulb, generally in the mastoid canaliculus. Arnold's nerve mediates herpetic involvement of the external auditory canal in herpes zoster oticus, as well as the coughing elicited by touching the skin of the external auditory canal.

Vestibular Nerves

The superior and inferior vestibular nerves occupy the posterior half of the internal auditory canal. The superior vestibular nerve innervates the superior and lateral semicircular canal cristae, the macula of the utricle, and the superior portion of the saccular macula. The inferior vestibular nerve innervates the inferior portion of the saccular macula, and, via the posterior ampullary nerve, the posterior semicircular canal. The posterior ampullary nerve separates from the inferior vestibular nerve trunk a few millimeters from the porus of the internal auditory canal and passes to the posterior canal ampulla via the singular canal.

Cochlear Nerve

The cochlear nerve originates from spiral ganglion neurons; at the fundus of the internal auditory canal, the cochlear nerve rests in the anteroinferior quadrant; traversing and rotating in the canal, the cochlear nerve enters the brain a few millimeters caudal to the root entry zone of the fifth cranial nerve.

◆ Vascular Anatomy

External Auditory Canal and Pinna

The vascular supply of the pinna arises from the external carotid artery through its posterior auricular, superficial temporal (anterior auricular branch), and occipital (mastoid branch) arteries.

The vascular supply of the external auditory canal is also based on the external carotid artery, through the posterior auricular, internal maxillary, and superficial temporal arteries.

Temporal Bone Arteries

The major artery associated with the temporal bone is the internal carotid artery. It enters the temporal bone anteromedial to the styloid process at the external carotid foramen, ascends anterior to the tympanic cavity and cochlea, and bends anteriorly (the "knee") to pass medial to the eustachian tube and inferomedial to the semicanal of the tensor tympani muscle.[22] The artery then ascends again, exiting the temporal bone at the internal carotid foramen to enter the cranium. Throughout its course in the temporal bone the internal carotid artery is encased in a bony canal, surrounded by both a vascular and neural (sympathetic) plexus; the canal wall is thin, often less than 0.5 mm,[23] and in 6% of the specimens from individuals over the age of 40 years there are dehiscences.[24] The thinness of the wall, especially when combined with erosion from chronic otitis media and cholesteatoma, mandates gentle dissection, especially in the medial wall of the eustachian tube orifice.

Anomalies of the internal carotid artery have been described,[25] such as the artery runs lateral and posterior to the vestibular line (on coronal sections, a vertical line through the lateral aspect of the vestibule) instead of medially, as is normally the case.

The anterior inferior cerebellar artery (AICA) is often encountered in the internal auditory canal as a vessel loop.[26,27] Its disruption in internal auditory canal dissection can result in hemorrhage and infarction of the labyrinth and brainstem structures.

Temporal Bone Veins

Three venous sinuses are in close anatomic relationship to the temporal bone and hence of surgical relevance: the lateral (sigmoid), the inferior petrosal, and the superior petrosal. The lateral venous sinus is the major route of drainage of the head and neck; in the posterior mastoid, it occupies an S-shaped (or sigmoid) sulcus, extending from the transverse sinus to the jugular bulb. The jugular vein and sigmoid sinus are larger on the right side than on the left in 75% of the cases.[28]

The superior petrosal sinus runs in the superior petrosal sulcus at the junction of the middle and posterior fossa dural plates; it provides venous drainage from the cavernous sinus anteriorly to the lateral venous sinus.

The inferior petrosal sinus occupies the petro-occipital suture line and provides venous drainage from the cavernous sinus to the medial aspect of the jugular bulb.

The internal jugular vein is the continuation of the sigmoid sinus, with the transition marked by the jugular bulb. The jugular bulb generally is located in the inferior mastoid, medial to the facial nerve. Its superior extent is quite variable, on occasion reaching into the middle ear, to such a degree that the round window is obstructed, causing a conductive hearing loss; in translabyrinthine surgery, a high jugular bulb can constrict the surgical field.[28]

Jugular Foramen

Traditionally, the jugular foramen has been thought to divide into an anteromedial pars nervosa, which transmits the ninth cranial nerve, and a posterolateral pars vascularis, traversed by the jugular bulb accompanied by cranial nerves X and XI. More recent studies[29-31] have pointed out the variability in anatomic relationships in this region. In 70% of the specimens studied, there was a bone or fibrous tissue septum, with cranial nerve IX passing in the anterior compartment and the tenth and eleventh nerves passing posteriorly in all but one instance. Occasionally, all three cranial nerves ran anteriorly, separated from the jugular bulb by a bony septum, whereas in 55% of the specimens three compartments separated by bony septa were found, with the ninth nerve most anteriorly located, the tenth and eleventh in the middle, and the jugular bulb most posteriorly.[31] The inferior petrosal sinus drains into the jugular bulb, in two thirds of the cases by more than one opening[31]; usually the inferior petrosal sinus passes between the ninth cranial nerve superolaterally and cranial nerves X and XI inferomedially.[31]

Middle Ear Vascular Anatomy

Three major arteries—the external carotid, the internal carotid, and the basilar—supply the middle ear and mastoid through their branches.

The inferior tympanic artery is particularly relevant, as it commonly supplies tympanic paragangliomas. It is a branch of the ascending pharyngeal artery (from the external carotid artery) and enters the tympanic cavity by the inferior tympanic canaliculus, accompanying Jacobson's nerve.

Other vessels that arise from the external carotid artery and contribute to the anastomotic network of the middle ear are the anterior tympanic artery, the deep auricular artery, the mastoid artery, the stylomastoid artery, the superficial petrosal artery, the superior tympanic artery, and the tubal artery.

Inner Ear Vascular Anatomy

The membranous labyrinth derives the majority of its blood supply from the labyrinthine artery, a branch of the AICA, which divides into the common cochlear artery and the anterior vestibular artery, the latter supplying the ampullae of the superior and lateral semicircular canals and the maculae of the utricle and saccule. The common cochlear artery divides into the main cochlear artery, which supplies predominantly the middle and apical three quarters of the cochlea, and the posterior vestibular artery. The posterior vestibular artery supplies the posterior semicircular canal ampulla, and, through its cochlear ramus, the basal cochlea.

Vascular Anatomy of the Facial Nerve

The extrinsic vasculature of the facial nerve arises from a variety of sources along its course. Intracranially, it is supplied by the AICA, whereas in its intracanalicular segment it is supplied by the labyrinthine artery. The geniculate ganglion is supplied by the superficial petrosal artery. The facial nerve in the fallopian canal is supplied by both the superficial petrosal and stylomastoid arteries.

The facial nerve also has an intrinsic network, which variably has been demonstrated to be poorest at its labyrinthine segment, as compared with its mastoid and tympanic segments.[32,33]

◆ Embryology

This section presents a synopsis of the development of the ear, emphasizing those features especially relevant to the clinical practice of otology. The discussion progresses from lateral to medial in the temporal bone. Time of onset and development, expressed in days, weeks, or months, refers to gestational growth, not postpartum growth, unless otherwise stated. The interested reader is encouraged to peruse the referenced works by Bast and Anson,[34] Anson and Donaldson,[35] Streeter,[36] and Padget,[37,38] or the reviews by Gulya and Schuknecht[1] and Gulya.[39]

External Ear

The appearance of tissue condensations of the mandibular (first branchial) and hyoid (second branchial) arches at 4 weeks' gestation marks the beginning of development of the pinna. By 6 weeks, six ridges (the hillocks of His) are distinguishable and, according to some theories, give rise to specific parts of the pinna (**Fig. 1–21**). Adult configuration is achieved by the fifth month. The development of the pinna occurs independently of that of the middle and inner ears.

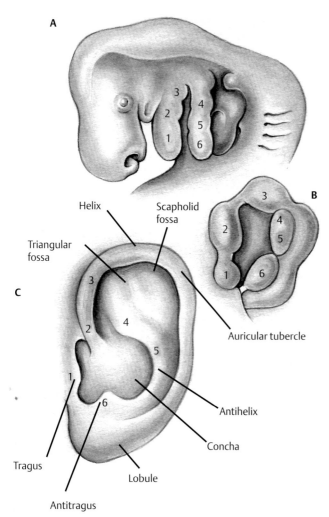

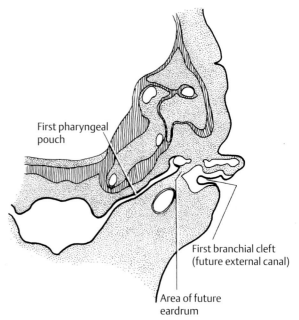

Figure 1–22 Line drawing depicting the development of the human external auditory canal.

Figure 1–21 Schematic drawing of the human ear origin from the first and second branchial arches, illustrating the development of the six hillocks, and their contribution to the final adult structure. **(A)** Approximately 6 weeks. **(B)** Approximately 7 weeks. **(C)** Adult. (Adapted from Anson BJ, Donaldson JA. Surgical Anatomy of the Temporal Bone and Ear. Philadelphia, PA: WB Saunders, 1983. Reprinted by permission.)

Temporal Bone, External Auditory Canal, Tympanic Ring, and Tympanic Membrane

During the second month, the dorsal part of the first branchial groove, the tissue of origin of the external auditory canal, progressively deepens so that its ectoderm transiently abuts the endoderm of the first pharyngeal pouch (**Fig. 1–22**). At 6 weeks, mesodermal ingrowth separates the two layers, but, beginning 2 weeks later, the inferior portion of the first branchial groove deepens again, resulting in the primary external auditory canal (the future fibrocartilaginous canal). After 9 weeks, a cord of epithelial cells at the medial aspect of the primary canal extends medially, terminating in the meatal plate. The lamina propria of the tympanic membrane arises from mesenchyme located medial to this plate; four ossification centers, the future tympanic ring, surround the lamina propria, and by 10 weeks have fused, except superiorly (the

notch of Rivinus). After the fifth month, the epithelial cell cord splits open, first at its medial aspect, resulting in the formation of the bony external auditory canal by the seventh month; the cells remaining at the medial aspect form the superficial layer of the tympanic membrane, whereas those at the periphery give rise to the epithelial lining of the bony canal. These developments occurring in the external auditory canal lag far behind those occurring in the inner, middle, and external (pinna) ears.

The squama first appears at approximately 8 weeks, and by 4 months it projects posterior to the tympanic ring, forming the roof of the external auditory canal, the squamous portion of the mastoid, and the lateral wall of the antrum. The medial portion of the mastoid develops as the periosteal layer of the bony labyrinth is invaded by air cells.

The hypotympanum develops between 22 and 32 weeks from three bony constituents: the tympanic bone, the canalicular otic capsule, and a petrosal ridge. This multicomponent structure is implicated in the predilection of this area to anomalous development, for example, the variability in bony coverage of the jugular bulb in the middle ear.

Fusion of the tympanic ring to the otic capsule (**Fig. 1–23**) begins after 8 months' gestation, a process that is not completed until after birth. Postnatal lateral growth of the tympanic ring extends the external auditory canal, alters the angulation of the tympanic membrane to the adult state, and deepens the relative position of the stylomastoid foramen.

Abnormal development of the first and second branchial arches manifests in pinna abnormalities (**Figs. 1–24** through **1-28**), whereas developmental failure of the first branchial groove results in canal atresia or stenosis (**Fig. 1–29**). Depending on the stage at which development went awry, there may be associated defects in the middle and inner ears.

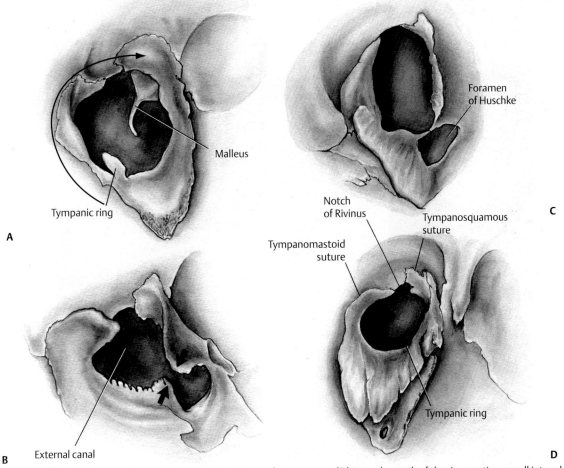

A

Malleus

Tympanic ring

B

External canal

Foramen of Huschke

Notch of Rivinus

Tympanomastoid suture

Tympanosquamous suture

C

Tympanic ring

D

Figure 1–23 **(A)** The membranous tympanic ring is incomplete superiorly at the notch of Rivinus throughout life. **(B)** Inferiorly, two bone protuberances grow toward each other. **(C)** Persistence of incomplete closure inferiorly creates a patent foramen of Huschke, which can promote spread of infection or tumor beyond the canal.

(D) Lateral growth of the ring continues well into adult life to form a more tortuous external canal. (Adapted from Anson BJ, Donaldson JA. Surgical Anatomy of the Temporal Bone and Ear. Philadelphia: WB Saunders, 1983. Reprinted by permission.)

Tympanomastoid Compartment and Eustachian Tube

The tympanomastoid compartment finds its phylogenetic heritage in the aquatic gill slit apparatus, and in the developing human first appears at 3 weeks' gestation as an outpouching of the first pharyngeal pouch (the tubotympanic recess). The endodermal tissue of the dorsal end of this pouch gives rise to the eustachian tube and tympanic cavity. The terminal end of the pouch buds into four sacci, which progressively pneumatize the tympanomastoid compartment. By 30 weeks, the tympanic cavity has essentially completed development, whereas the mastoid continues to grow throughout the second decade. At birth, the antrum approximates that of the adult, but resolution of embryonic mesenchymal tissue continues during the first postnatal year. Remnants of embryonic connective tissue are manifest as strands draped over the round and oval windows in particular.

Ossicular Chain

The first signs of ossicular development appear at 4 weeks as the upper ends of the first and second branchial arches are connected by a bridge of condensed mesenchyme that eventually gives rise to the malleus and incus (**Fig. 1–30**). The stapes arises from the second branchial arch, except for the footplate and annular ligament, both of which are of otic capsule origin.

During the ensuing 11 weeks, the ossicular chain undergoes growth and development in a cartilaginous form (enchondral bone formation). Development of the stapes involves surrounding the stapedial artery, leaving the obturator foramen as an empty ring after the artery involutes.

By 15 weeks, the ossicles have attained adult size, and ossification begins, first in the incus and last in the stapes. At the same time, the tensor tympani and stapedius muscles develop from the mesenchyme of the first and second branchial arches, respectively. The adult configuration of the malleus and incus is

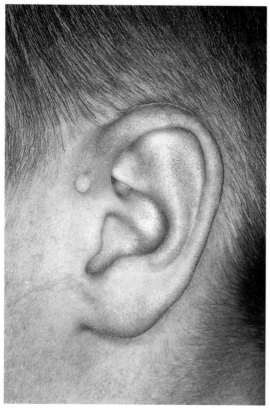

Figure 1–24   Infected preauricular cyst.

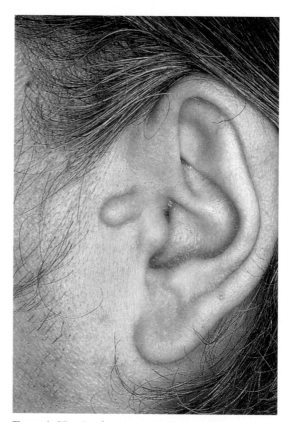

Figure 1–25   Cartilaginous auricular appendage.

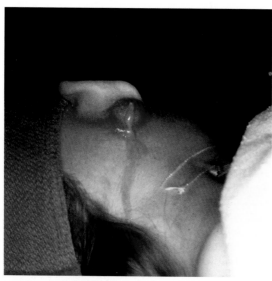

Figure 1–26   Infected first branchial arch remnant.

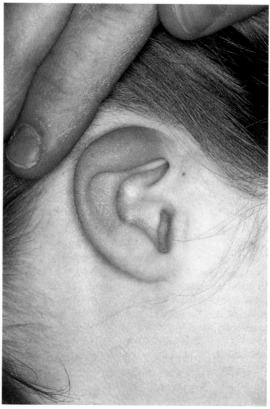

Figure 1–27   Mild microtia with stenosis of the ear canal.

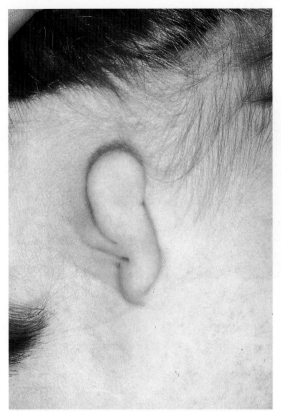

Figure 1–28 Severe microtia with atresia of the ear canal.

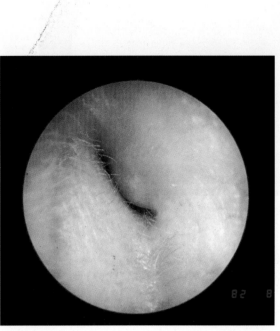

Figure 1–29 Stenosis of the ear canal, requiring a postauricular approach.

achieved by 20 weeks, whereas the stapes continues to evolve into its adult dimensions into the 32nd week. The endochondral bone of the ossicles, like that of the otic capsule, undergoes little change over the life of the individual, and demonstrates poor reparative response to trauma. Abnormal development of the ossicles results in anomaly or fusion (**Figs. 1–31** and **1–32**).

Otic Labyrinth

A plaque-like thickening of surface ectoderm dorsal to the first branchial groove, the otic placode, appears at the end of the third week. The auditory pit evolves into the otic vesicle as invagination into the underlying mesenchyme progresses; the

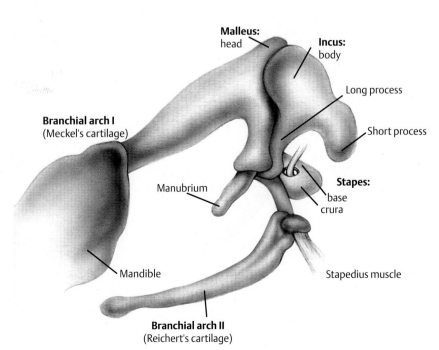

Figure 1–30 Lateral view of the ossicles as they develop from branchial arches one and two (8 to 9 weeks' gestation). (Adapted from Hanson et al. Arch Otolaryngol 1962;76:211; and from Schuknecht HF, Gulya AJ. Anatomy of the Temporal Bone with Surgical Implications. Philadelphia: WB Saunders, 1986. Reprinted by permission.)

19

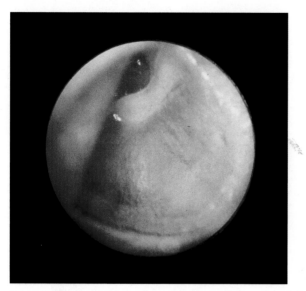

Figure 1–31 Anomalous malleus with abnormally large manubrium.

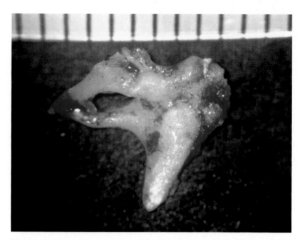

Figure 1–32 Abnormal ossicle development resulting in fusion.

otic vesicle gives rise to the otic labyrinth, whereas the mesenchyme that surrounds it becomes the bony labyrinth. Within a few days, the endolymphatic appendage can be discerned, and by the fourth week flanges that will give rise to the superior and lateral semicircular canals emerge. Three folds (I, II, and III) (**Fig. 1–33**) gradually demarcate the utricle and semicircular canals, the endolymphatic duct and sac, and the

sacculae and cochlear duct. The utriculoendolymphatic valve (of Bast) derives from fold III.

In the sixth week, the lumina of the semicircular ducts have appeared, and the cochlear duct has completed one turn. As the semicircular ducts expand in both diameter and radius of curvature, the cochlea rapidly spirals, completing 2½ turns by the eighth week. A variety of cochlear anomalies

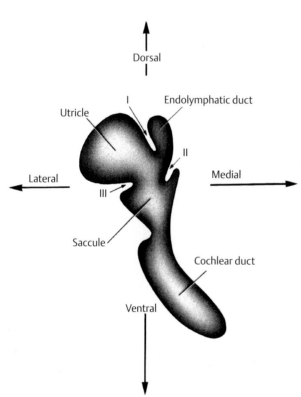

A

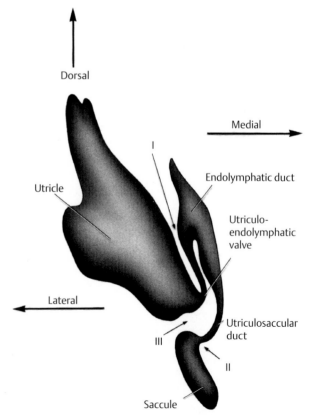

B

Figure 1–33 **(A)** Folds I, II, and III begin to indent the otic vesicle (6 to 8 weeks' gestation). **(B)** By 9 weeks, the utricle, saccule, and endolymphatic duct can be distinguished. (Adapted from Bast TH, Anson BJ. The Temporal Bone and the Ear. Springfield, IL: Charles C.

Thomas, 1949. From Schuknecht HF, Gulya AJ. Anatomy of the Temporal Bone with Surgical Implications. Philadelphia: WB Saunders, 1986. Reprinted by permission.)

are recognized (**Fig. 1–34**), reflecting varying stages at which normal development is disrupted.[40]

The otic labyrinth approximates adult configuration by the 16th week, and the sensory neuroepithelium of the semicircular canals and otolithic organs, as well as that of the cochlea, begins to differentiate. By 20 weeks, the superior semicircular duct has reached adult size, followed in sequence by the lateral and posterior canals. Continuing growth of the posterior fossa and lateral venous sinus results in an inferior and lateral bend in the course of the endolymphatic duct and sac; accordingly, the proximal endolymphatic duct is a relative anatomic constant, whereas the distal duct and sac vary in position, related to posterior fossa and lateral venous sinus development.[1] The large vestibular aqueduct syndrome[41] implicates anomalous development of this structure in profound, and perhaps progressive, sensorineural hearing loss.[42,43]

In the cochlea, the organ of Corti is differentiated to such an extent that the fetus can hear and respond to fluid-transmitted sounds[44]; by 25 weeks, the organ of Corti approaches adult configuration.

Perilymphatic Labyrinth

The first evidence of perilymphatic space formation is seen at about 8 weeks, as mesodermal tissue surrounding the otic capsule anlage retrogressively dedifferentiates into a loose, vascular reticulum, initially around the semicircular canals and vestibule, and then later about the cochlea. The perilymphatic

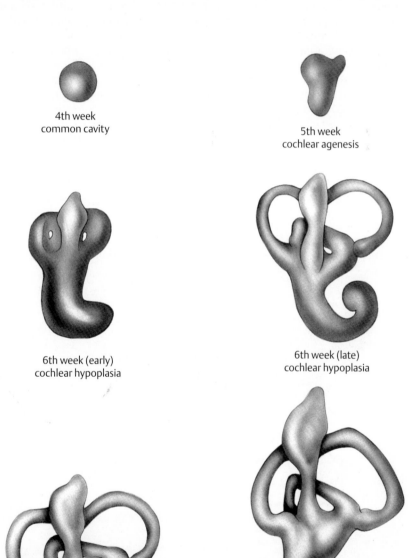

4th week
common cavity

5th week
cochlear agenesis

6th week (early)
cochlear hypoplasia

6th week (late)
cochlear hypoplasia

7th week
incomplete partition
(classic Mondini's)

8th week
normal development

Figure 1–34 Anomalies associated with disrupted otic vesicle development, based on the stage at which the interruption occurred. [From Jackler RK et al. Congenital malformations of the inner ear: a classification based on embryogenesis. Laryngoscope 1987;97(suppl 40):2–14. Reprinted by permission.]

cistern of the vestibule, appearing late in the 12th week, is the first recognizable space of the perilymphatic labyrinth, followed soon thereafter by the appearance of the scala tympani and the scala vestibuli. The canalicular portion appears later, and development is usually completed by 20 weeks.

The primordial cochlear aqueduct, traversed by the periotic duct, inferior cochlear vein, and tympanomeningeal hiatus, first appears at 7 weeks as precartilage dedifferentiates into reticulum at the medial wall of the basal turn of the cochlea, thus extending from the developing round window niche to the posterior cranial fossa, close to the ninth cranial nerve and the inferior petrosal sinus. By the ninth week, the inferior cochlear vein is distinguishable in the syncytium of the primordial cochlear aqueduct, and the floor and medial rim of the round window niche begins to emerge (**Fig. 1–35**). Completion of the cochlear aqueduct occurs by the 40th week. The tympanomeningeal hiatus may persist into adulthood (**Fig. 1–36**), representing incomplete ossification of the primordial cochlear aqueduct, and extends from the depths of the round window niche to the posterior cranial fossa at the junction of the inferior petrosal sinus and jugular bulb. A widely patent cochlear aqueduct (**Fig. 1–37**) is thought to underlie the perilymph "oozer" occasionally seen in stapes surgery.[45] Radiographic criteria of an enlarged cochlear aqueduct have been proposed as constituting, on high-resolution computed tomographic scanning, a duct that is 0.2 mm throughout its course.[46]

Otic Capsule

The otic capsule, which eventually gives rise to the petrous portion of the temporal bone, develops from the precartilage that surrounds it, beginning in the fourth week of gestation.

By the eighth week, the otic capsule emerges as a cartilaginous model, but does not begin ossification until 16 weeks when the contained membranous labyrinth has attained adult size. A total of 14 ossification centers appears, and three layers of bone can be discerned as a result of the ossification process (**Fig. 1–38**). The endosteal layer, arising from the perichondral membrane lining the inner layer of the otic capsule, undergoes little change throughout life, although it may proliferate in response to infection or trauma, even to the extent of labyrinthine obliteration. The periosteal layer evolves from the perichondrial layer surrounding the external surface of the otic capsule; the periosteal layer is capable of a good reparative response to trauma or infection, and undergoes considerable change until early adult life, both in terms of pneumatization and lamellar addition of bone, as well as remodeling, similar to periosteal bone elsewhere in the body. In between the endosteal and periosteal layers is the enchondral layer of bone, made up of intrachondral and endochondral bone. The intrachondral bone (globuli interossei) represents persistent islands of calcified cartilage; its lacunae are occupied by osteocytes, and endochondral bone is deposited on their surfaces. The enchondral layer undergoes little change throughout life, and has minimal reparative capabilities, healing by fibrous union at best.

The cochlear modiolus arises independently from membranous bone, beginning at about 20 weeks; its ossification is nearly complete by 25 weeks. The modiolus is anchored by interscalar septa, which are extensions of otic capsule bone. Scala communis, or partial absence of the interscalar septa, is a relatively common development anomaly that does not appear to interfere with cochlear function (**Fig. 1–39**). A failure of

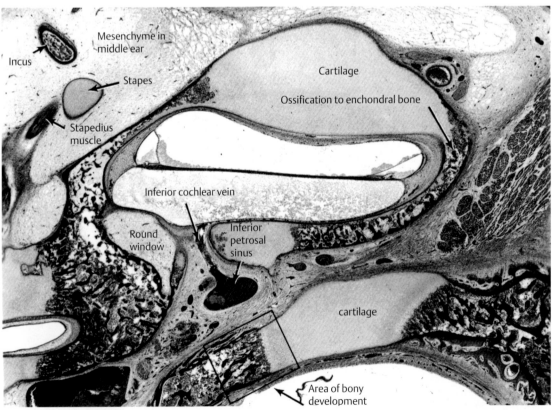

Figure 1–35 The primitive cochlear aqueduct at approximately 17 weeks. (From Gulya AJ, Schuknecht HF. Anatomy of the Temporal Bone with Surgical Implications, 2nd ed. Pearl River, NY: Pantheon Press, 1995. Reprinted by permission.)

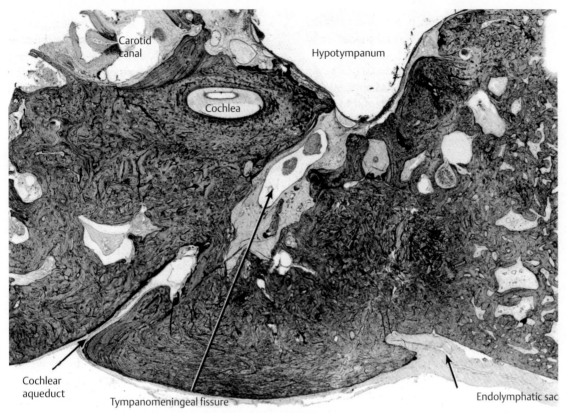

Figure 1–36 The persistent tympanomeningeal fissure is paralleled by the cochlear aqueduct (male, 44 years). (From Gulya AJ, Schuknecht HF. Anatomy of the Temporal Bone with Surgical Implications, 2nd ed. Pearl River, NY: Pantheon Press, 1995. Reprinted by permission.)

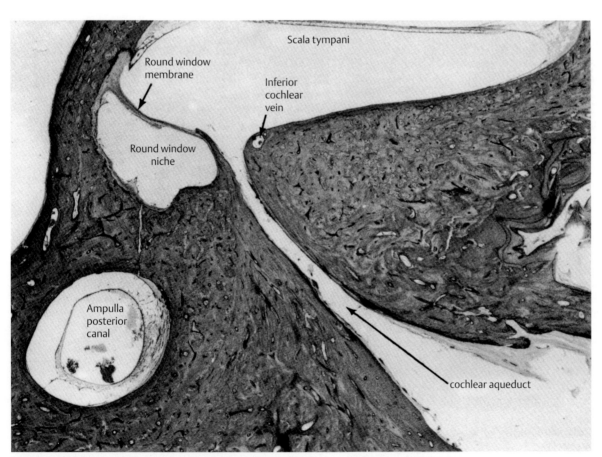

Figure 1–37 Illustration of both the widely patent cochlear aqueduct and the microfissure between the posterior semicircular canal and the round window niche (male, 67 years). (From Schuknecht HF, Seifi AE. Experimental observations on the fluid physiology of the inner ear. Ann Otol Rhinol Laryngol 1963;72:687. Reprinted by permission.)

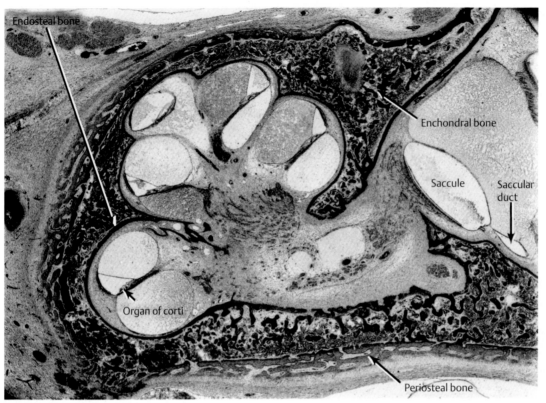

Figure 1–38 In the fetus of 16 weeks, the three layers of otic capsule bone are clearly demarcated. (From Gulya AJ, Schuknecht HF. Anatomy of the Temporal Bone with Surgical Implications, 2nd ed. Pearl River, NY: Pantheon Press, 1995. Reprinted by permission.)

development of the modiolus leaves open wide communication between the scala vestibuli of the basal turn and the subarachnoid space of the internal auditory canal (**Fig. 1–40**). This anomaly is thought to underlie the perilymph "gusher" occasionally seen in stapes surgery. X-linked mixed deafness, in which stapes fixation coexists with an abnormally wide communication between the internal auditory canal and the inner ear, has been associated with an alteration in the Xq21 band.[47]

Acoustic Nerve and Ganglion

In the fourth week, the initial steps in the development of the acoustic nerve, ganglion, and in Schwann cells involve ventral streaming, between the epithelium of the otic vesicle and its basement membrane, of cells of otic placode derivation. After passing through the basement membrane, the cells reach the area at which the acoustic ganglion forms, ventral and somewhat medial to the otic vesicle.

By the end of the fifth week, the ganglion has divided into superior and inferior segments, with the superior segment giving rise to the fibers that innervate the superior and lateral semicircular canals and the utricle, and the inferior segment giving rise to the fibers that innervate the saccular macula, posterior semicircular canal, and the cochlea.

Facial Nerve and Geniculate Ganglion

According to Gasser et al,[48] at about 4 weeks "the facial nerve primordium arises from the rhombencephalon" as a column of neutral crest cells "extends ventrally to contact

the epibranchial placode of the second arch," a thickened area of ectoderm just caudal to the dorsal aspect of the first groove. The geniculate ganglion forms at the area of contact.

By approximately 6 weeks, there is a distinguishable geniculate ganglion, and the facial crest has evenly divided into caudal and rostral segments; the caudal segment becomes the main trunk of the facial nerve, and the rostral segment becomes the chorda tympani nerve, the first branch of the facial nerve to form.

The greater superficial petrosal nerve, the second branch of the facial nerve to form, appears at the seventh week of gestation from the ventral aspect of the geniculate ganglion, and the main trunk of the facial nerve establishes its intratemporal anatomic relationship in the cartilaginous otic capsule.

The fallopian canal begins formation at the end of 20 weeks' gestation as the apical cochlear ossification center gives rise to two projections of bone that eventually are to encircle the anterior tympanic segment of the facial nerve.[49]

Arteries

The primordial vascular supply of the brain first appears in the third week as a coalescence of vascular islands. A total of six aortic arches arises sequentially from the aortic sac to run ventrally through their corresponding branchial arches into the ipsilateral dorsal aorta; not all of the arch arteries are present simultaneously, as the first and second arch arteries disappear before the more caudal arteries have developed (**Fig. 1–41**).

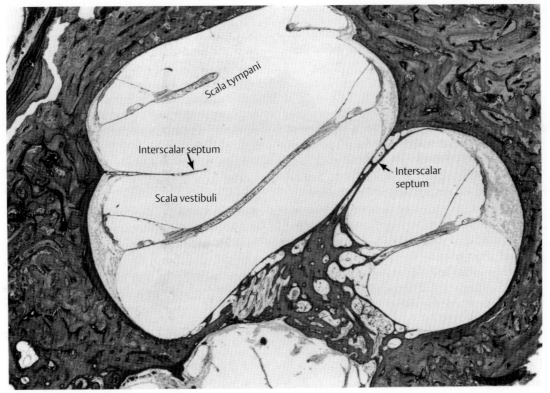

Figure 1–39 Partial absence of the interscalar septum, or scala communis, is thought to have little functional impact (female 63 years). (From Gulya AJ, Schuknecht HF. Anatomy of the Temporal Bone with Surgical Implications, 2nd ed. Pearl River, NY: Pantheon Press, 1995. Reprinted by permission.)

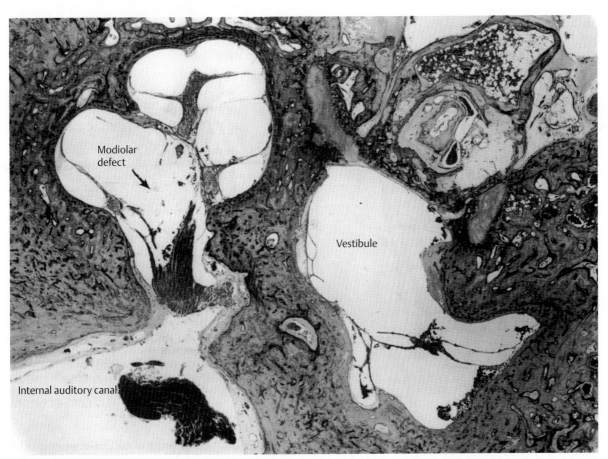

Figure 1–40 The defect of the cochlear modiolus results in a wide communication between the subarachnoid space of the internal auditory canal and the basal turn of the cochlea (2½-year-old child). (From Shi S-R. Temporal bone findings in a case of otopalatodigital syndrome. Arch Otolaryngol 1985;111:120. Reprinted by permission.)

During the fourth week, the first and second arch arteries involute, leaving behind dorsal fragments, the mandibular and hyoid arteries, respectively, and the anterior segments of the dorsal aortae evolve into the adult internal carotid arteries. In the hindbrain region, the otic vesicle and acoustic nerve are supplied by the primitive otic artery, derived from the aortae.

At 6 weeks, the stapedial artery appears as a small branch of the hyoid artery, passing through the primordial stapes. It reaches its height of development at 7 weeks, and thereafter shrinks; however, remnants of the stapedial artery are thought to play a role in the development of the caroticotympanic arteries, the anterior tympanic artery, and the superior petrosal artery. Rarely (five of 1045 temporal bones studied)[50] the stapedial artery may persist into adulthood posing an impediment to the completion of stapes operations especially. Anomalies of development of the stapedial artery, such as abnormal branching patterns, are associated with anomalies in stapes development, such as three-legged stapes. The anomalous stapedial artery is also associated with anomalous development of the internal carotid artery (**Fig. 1–42**).

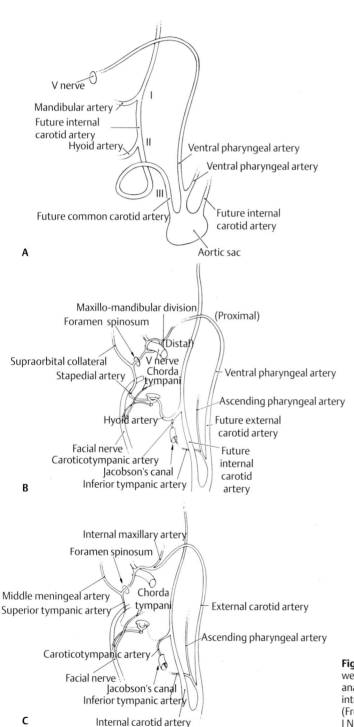

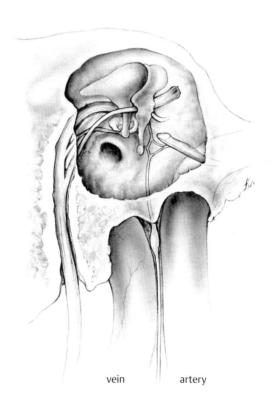

Figure 1–41 Development of the cranial arteries. **(A)** Three to 4 weeks. **(B)** Approximately 7 weeks. **(C)** Adult configuration. **(D)** The anatomic interrelations of the tympanomastoid compartment, the internal jugular vein, and the internal carotid artery in the adult. (From Moret et al. Abnormal vessels in the middle ear. J Neuroradiology 1982;9:227–236. Reprinted by permission.)

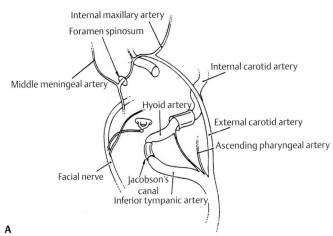

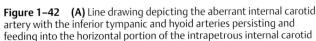

A

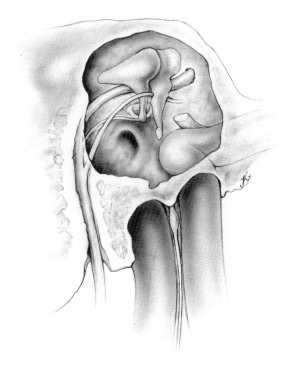

B

Figure 1–42 **(A)** Line drawing depicting the aberrant internal carotid artery with the inferior tympanic and hyoid arteries persisting and feeding into the horizontal portion of the intrapetrous internal carotid artery. **(B)** Line drawing showing the aberrant internal carotid artery in relation to the tympanic cavity. (From Moret et al. Abnormal vessels in the middle ear. J Neuradiology 1982;9:227–236. Reprinted with permission.)

By the ninth week, the adult pattern of the cranial arteries is visible.

Veins

The development of the venous system in general lags that of the arterial system. By 4 weeks, the first true drainage channel of the cervicocranial region, the primary head sinus (also known as the lateral capital vein), has appeared. The primary head sinus is in continuity with the anterior cardinal vein (the primitive internal jugular vein).

The fifth and sixth weeks of development are characterized by migration of the primary head sinus and the anterior cardinal vein to assume a lateral position with respect to the lower cranial nerves.

By approximately 8 weeks, the primary head sinus has disappeared, leaving three remaining segments: a cranial remnant, which becomes the lateral wing of the sphenoid sinus; a caudal remnant, which contributes to the veins draining the middle ear; and a segment that accompanies the facial nerve extracranially. At this same stage, the tendency for drainage to pass more on the right than on the left is first seen.

By 12 weeks, the superior petrosal sinus, the last of the major adult sinuses to become definitive, appears.

References

1. Gulya AJ, Schuknecht HF. Anatomy of the Temporal Bone with Surgical Implications, 2nd ed. Pearl River: Pantheon Press, 1995
2. Sando I, Takahashi H, Matsune S, Aoki H. Localization of function in the eustachian tube: a hypothesis. Ann Otol Rhinol Laryngol 1994;103:311–314
3. Hentzer E. Ultrastructure of the normal mucosa in the human middle ear, mastoid cavities, and eustachian tube. Ann Otol Rhinol Laryngol 1970;79:1143–1157
4. Lim DJ. Functional morphology of the lining membrane of the middle ear and eustachian tube. An overview. Ann Otol Rhinol Laryngol 1974; 83(suppl 11):5–22
5. Lim DJ. Normal and pathological mucosa of the middle ear and eustachian tube. Clin Otolaryngol 1979;4:213–234
6. Lindsay JR. Suppuration in the petrous pyramid. Ann Otol Rhinol Laryngol 1938;47:3–36
7. Chole RA. Petrous apicitis: surgical anatomy. Ann Otol Rhinol Laryngol 1985;94:251–257
8. Harada T, Sando I, Myers EN. Microfissure in the oval window area. Ann Otol Rhinol Laryngol 1981;90:174–180
9. El Shazly MAR, Linthicum FH Jr. Microfissures of the temporal bone: do they have any clinical significance? Am J Otol 1991;12:169–171
10. Gacek RR, Leipzig B. Congenital cerebrospinal fluid otorrhea. Ann Otol Rhinol Laryngol 1979;88:358–365
11. Arenberg IK, Rask-Andersen H, Wilbrand H, Stahle J. The surgical anatomy of the endolymphatic sac. Arch Otolaryngol 1977;103:1–11
12. Parker DA, Schindler RA, Amoils CP, Lustig LR, Hradek GT. Hyaluronan synthesis in the adult guinea pig endolymphatic sac. Laryngoscope 1992;102:152–156
13. Wackym PA. Histopathologic findings in Meniere's disease. Otolaryngol Head Neck Surg 1995;112:90–100
14. Schuknecht HF, Belal AA. The utriculoendolymphatic valve: its functional significance. J Laryngol Otol 1975;89:985–996
15. Perez-Olivares F, Schuknecht HF. Width of the internal auditory canal. A histological study. Ann Otol Rhinol Laryngol 1979;88:316–323
16. Silverstein H. Cochlear and vestibular gross and histologic anatomy (as seen from postauricular approach). Otolaryngol Head Neck Surg 1984;92:207–211
17. Hough JVD. Malformations and anatomical variations seen in the middle ear during the operation for mobilization of the stapes. Laryngoscope 1958;68:1337–1379
18. Hough JVD. Ossicular malformations and their correction. In: Shambaugh GE, Shea JJ, eds. Proceedings of the Shambaugh Fifth International Workshop on Middle Ear Microsurgery and Fluctuant Hearing Loss. Huntsville, AL: Strode, 1977:186–197

19. Proctor B, Nager GT. The facial canal: normal anatomy, variations and anomalies. Ann Otol Rhinol Laryngol 1982;91(suppl 87):33–61

20. Baxter A. Dehiscence of the fallopian canal: an anatomical study. J Laryngol Otol 1971;85:587–594.

21. Johnsson L-G, Kingsley TC. Herniation of the facial nerve in the middle ear. Arch Otolaryngol 1970;91:598–602

22. Leonetti JP, Smith PG, Linthicum FH. The petrous carotid artery: anatomic relationships in skull base surgery. Otolaryngol Head Neck Surg 1990;102:3–12

23. Goldman NC, Singleton GT, Holly EH. Aberrant internal carotid artery. Arch Otolaryngol 1971;94:269–273

24. Moreano EH, Paparella MM, Zelterman D, Goycoolea MV. Prevalence of carotid canal dehiscence in the human middle ear; a report of 1000 temporal bones. Laryngoscope 1994;104:612–618

25. Bold EL, Wanamaker HH, Hughes GB, et al. Magnetic resonance angiography of vascular anomalies of the middle ear. Laryngoscope 1994;104:1404–1411

26. Mazzoni A. Internal auditory canal arterial relations at the porus acusticus. Ann Otol Rhinol Laryngol 1969;78:797–814

27. Reisser C, Schuknecht HF. The anterior inferior cerebellar artery in the internal auditory canal. Laryngoscope 1991;101:761–766

28. Kennedy DW, El Sisry HH, Nager GT. The jugular bulb in otologic surgery: anatomic, clinical, and surgical considerations. Otolaryngol Head Neck Surg 1986;94:6–15

29. Kveton JF, Cooper MH. Microsurgical anatomy of the jugular foramen region. Am J Otol 1988;9:109–112

30. Schwaber MK, Netterville JL, Maciunas R. Microsurgical anatomy of the lower skull base—a morphometric analysis. Am J Otol 1990;11:401–405

31. Saleh E, Naguib M, Aristegui M, Cokkeser Y, Sanna M. Lower skull base: anatomic study with surgical implications. Ann Otol Rhinol Laryngol 1995;104:57–61

32. Balkany T, Fradis M, Jafek BW, Rucker NC. Intrinsic vasculature of the labyrinthine segment of the facial nerve- implications for site of lesion in Bell's palsy. Otolaryngol Head Neck Surg 1991;104:20–23

33. Bagger-Sjoback D, Graham MD, Thomander L. The intratemporal vascular supply of the facial nerve: a light and electron microscopic study. In: Graham MD, House WF, eds. Disorders of the Facial Nerve: Anatomy. Diagnosis and Management. New York: Raven Press, 1982:17–31

34. Bast TH, Anson BJ. The Temporal Bone and the Ear. Springfield, IL: Charles C. Thomas, 1949

35. Anson BJ, Donaldson JA. Surgical Anatomy of the Temporal Bone, 3rd ed. Philadelphia: WB Sunders, 1981

36. Streeter GL. On the development of the membranous labyrinth and the acoustic and facial nerves in the human embryo. Am J Anat 1906;6:139–165

37. Padget DH. The development of the cranial arteries in the human embryo. Contrib Embryol 1948;32:205–261

38. Padget DH. Development of the cranial venous system in man, from the viewpoint of comparative anatomy. Contrib Embryol 1957;36:79–139

39. Gulya AJ. Developmental anatomy of the ear. In: Glasscock ME III. Shambaugh GE, Johnson GD, eds. Surgery of the Ear, 4th ed. Philadelphia: WB Saunders, 1990:5–33

40. Jackler RK, Luxford WM, House WF. Congenital malformations of the inner ear: a classification based on embryogenesis. Laryngoscope 1987;97(suppl 40):2–14

41. Valvassori GE, Clemis JD. The large vestibular aqueduct syndrome. Laryngoscope 1978;88:723–728

42. Okumura T, Takahashi H, Honji I, Takagi A, Mitamura K. Sensorineural hearing loss in patients with large vestibular aqueduct. Laryngoscope 1995;105:289–293

43. Zalzal GH, Tomaski SM, Vezina LG, Bjornsti P, Grundfast KM. Enlarged vestibular aqueduct and sensorineural hearing loss in childhood. Arch Otolaryngol Head Neck Surg 1995;121:23–28

44. Smith RJH. Medical diagnosis and treatment of hearing loss in children. In: Cummings CW, Frederickson JM, Harker LA, et al. Otolaryngology Head and Neck Surgery. St Louis: CV Mosby, 1986

45. Schuknecht HF, Reisser C. The morphologic basis for perilymphatic gushers and oozers. Adv Otorhinolayngol 1988;39:1–12

46. Jackler RK, Hwang PH. Enlargement of the cochlear aqueduct: fact or fiction? Otolaryngol Head Neck Surg 1993;109:14–25

47. deKok YJM, van der Maarel SM, Bitner-Glindzicz M, et al. Association between X-linked mixed deafness and mutations in the POU domain gene POU3F4. Science 1995;267:685–688

48. Gasser RF, Shigihara S, Shimada K. Three-dimensional development of the facial nerve path through the ear region in human embryos. Ann Otol Rhinol Laryngol 1994;103:395–403

49. Spector JG, Ge X. Ossification patterns of the tympanic facial canal in the human fetus and neonate. Laryngoscope 1993;103:1052–1065

50. Moreano EH, Paparella MM, Zelterman D, Goycoolea MV. Prevalence of facial and canal dehiscence and of persistent stapedial artery in the human and middle ear: a report of 1000 temporal bones. Laryngoscope 1994;104:309–320

◆ Appendix

The following photomicrographs are horizontal and vertical selected serial sections of right human temporal bones. Each section is presented with an inset line drawing that gives the approximate level of the section with respect to the bony labyrinth. The horizontal series, seen first, is from a 5-year-old boy. The vertical series progresses from superior to inferior, starting posterolaterally and heading anteromedially; both series follow the plane of the cochlear modiolus. (From Gulya AJ, Schuknecht HF. Anatomy of the Temporal Bone with Surgical Implications. 2nd ed. Pearl River, NY: Pantheon Press, 1995. Reprinted by permission.)

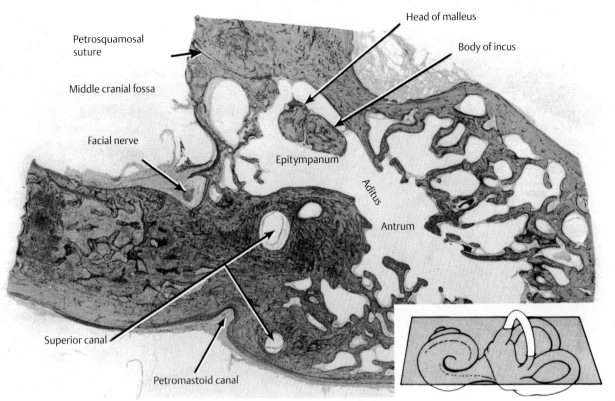

Figure 1–I This section is at the level of the superior semicircular canal. The malleus and incus are seen in the epitympanum, and the anterior epitympanic space is visible anterior to the head of the malleus. The genu of the facial nerve is dehiscent into the middle cranial fossa. Posterior to the incus, the aditus opens into the mastoid antrum.

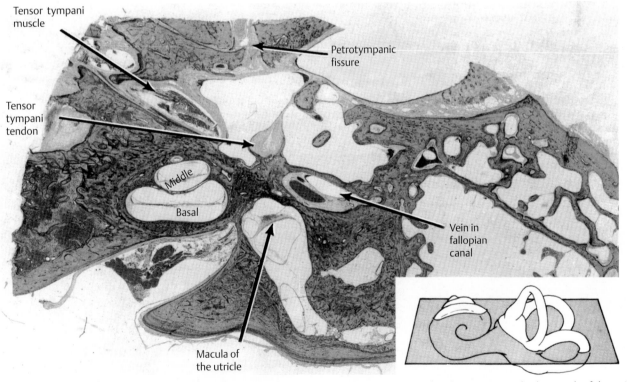

Figure 1–II This section shows the bony external and internal auditory canals, and the tensor tympani tenon crossing the tympanic cavity to attach to the malleus. The facial nerve is seen in its horizontal segment, accompanied by a large vein. Middle and basal cochlear turns are visualized anteriorly, whereas posteriorly, the macula of the utricle occupies the vestibule. Koerner's septum divides the mastoid into medial and lateral sections.

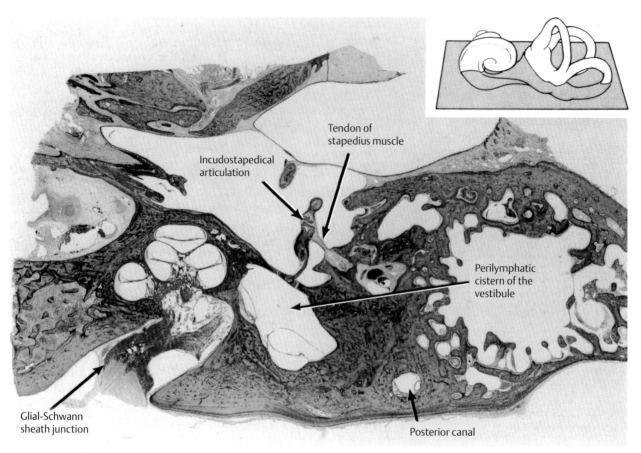

Figure 1–III The stapes and stapedius tendon are seen in this section, as are all three turns of the cochlea and the internal carotid artery and its canal anteriorly. The cochlear and inferior vestibular nerves are located in the anterior and posterior portions of the internal auditory canal, respectively. The saccule occupies the spherical recess in the vestibule.

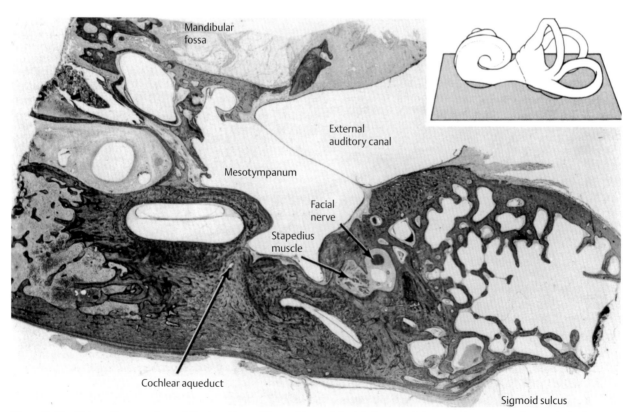

Figure 1–IV This section goes through the basal turn of the cochlea and the inferior part of the posterior semicircular canal. The facial nerve is in its mastoid (vertical) segment, accompanied by the stapedius muscle. The chorda tympani nerve is located anterolateral to the facial nerve.

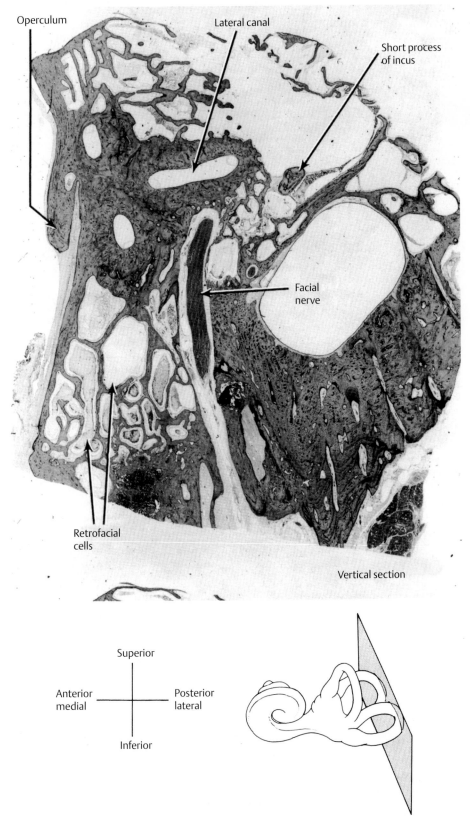

Operculum

Lateral canal

Short process
of incus

Facial
nerve

Retrofacial
cells

Vertical section

Superior

Anterior
medial

Posterior
lateral

Inferior

Figure 1–V This vertical section illustrates the facial nerve in its vertical segment, as well as the retrofacial cells and the facial recess area. The orthogonal relationship of the posterior and lateral canals is evident, extending the plane of the lateral canal through to the posterior fossa leads to the endolymphatic sac, covered by the operculum.

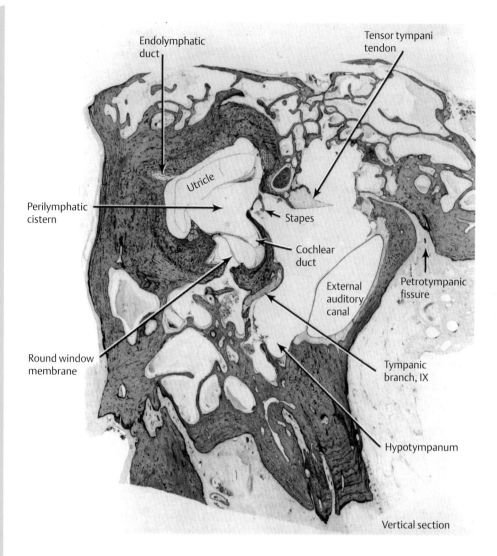

Endolymphatic duct

Tensor tympani tendon

Utricle

Perilymphatic cistern

Stapes

Cochlear duct

External auditory canal

Petrotympanic fissure

Round window membrane

Tympanic branch, IX

Hypotympanum

Vertical section

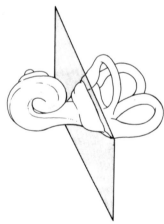

Figure 1–VI The infralabyrinthine and supralabyrinthine air cells border the vestibule, with the utricle and its macula visible superiorly. Inferiorly appears the basal turn of the cochlea, with the promontory being scaled by Jacobson's nerve. Both the round window niche and the oval window niche can be seen. The facial nerve is in its horizontal (tympanic) segment, immediately superior to the cochleariform process.

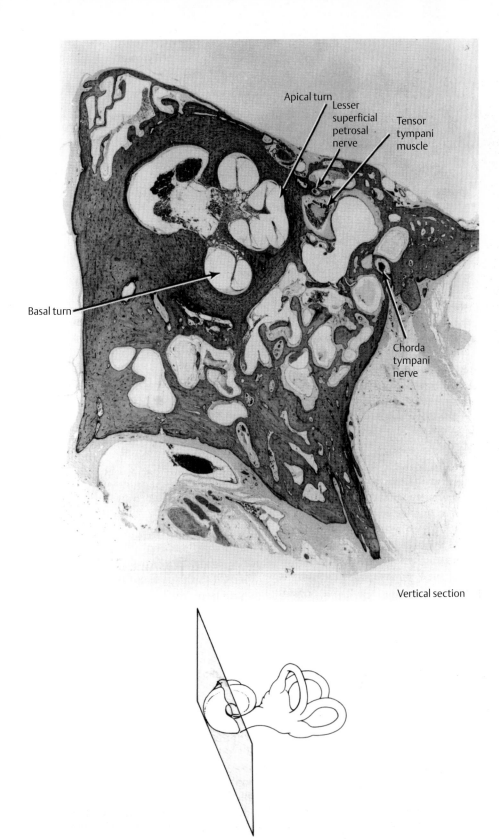

Vertical section

Figure 1–VII   All three cochlear turns are visible, as is the tensor tympani muscle, which is medial to the eustachian tube. The chorda tympani nerve is in the petrotympanic fissure.

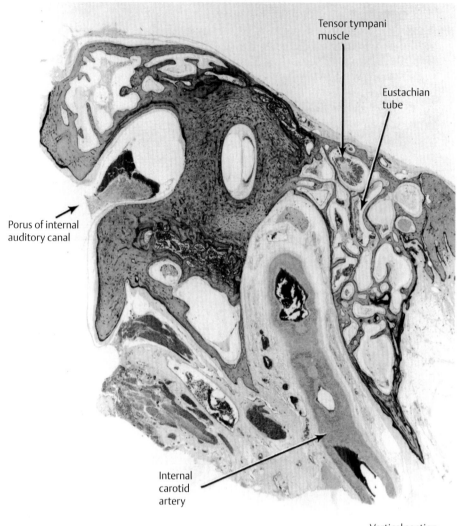

Tensor tympani muscle

Eustachian tube

Porus of internal auditory canal

Internal carotid artery

Vertical section

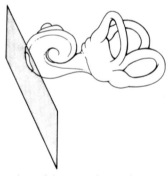

Figure 1–VIII The anatomic relationships of the internal carotid artery, the eustachian tube, and the basal turn of the cochlea are illustrated in this section.

2

Principles of Audiology and Auditory Physiology

David K. Brown and Robert W. Keith

The physiology of the auditory system is complex, and our understanding of how the system works is not yet complete. Chapter 1 discussed the anatomy of the auditory system, but a complete understanding of the auditory system also requires knowledge of the nature of sound and the function of the structures. Only with this comprehensive understanding can we have the greatest impact on patients with hearing loss.

The complex nature of the auditory system has been observed, studied, and debated since the days of George Berkeley and his tree falling in the forest, and we are still acquiring new knowledge about the auditory system. In fact, a large part of what we know was learned only since World War II, when many men returned home after the war with hearing loss. Audiology, the study of hearing, was born in the 1940s and the profession of audiology is dedicated to the detection, evaluation, and rehabilitation of patients with hearing disorders.

This chapter discusses the nature of acoustics and the way sound can be described and measured. The physiology of sound, which is the input to the auditory system, is discussed as it traverses through the outer, middle, and inner ear to the brain.

◆ Acoustics

Acoustics is the science that is concerned with the production, control, transmission, reception, and effects of sound. *Sound* is energy, mechanical radiant energy that is transmitted through pressure waves in a material medium (e.g., air, water, metal). In the case of hearing, sound is the sensation perceived by the ear. This sound energy is captured by the outer ear, transformed by the middle ear, and transduced by the inner ear. Sound is described in terms of its basic physical attributes: frequency, intensity, and time/phase of the vibration.[1] These physical attributes also have psychological correlates, which are pitch, loudness, and quality, respectively. These terms are often used interchangeably, thus leading to misunderstanding and misuse, which is especially true for frequency and intensity.

People often mistakenly refer to the pitch of a tone when they really mean its frequency and to the loudness of a tone when they mean its intensity. The pitch of a tone is perceived by the listener, whereas one can quantifiably measure the frequency of the same tone with an oscilloscope. A tone with a frequency of 1000 Hz may fluctuate in frequency by a few *hertz* (cycles per second) either up or down over a period of time, which can be measured by the oscilloscope. However, the normal-hearing listener is not able to perceive such small changes in pitch. Changes in pitch are what we detect when the frequency of a tone changes and are measured in a unit called the *mel*. There is little correlation between the two except that mels increase and decrease with frequency. For example, when we play the scale on the piano from middle C (256 Hz) to the C above middle C (512 Hz), we are moving up an octave; every time we move up an octave, the frequency doubles. However, as we move from one C to the next C the units on the mel scale do not double[2] because pitch, although highly correlated with frequency, is subjective and influenced by both the frequency and the intensity of the sound.

Loudness is the psychological correlate of intensity. Changes in the intensity of a sound may or may not result in a perceived change in loudness. Loudness is a subjective analysis of the sound by the listener. It is affected by the duration and frequency of the sounds that are present, and a unit of loudness level is the *phon*. The smallest change in a physical parameter of sound (such as frequency or intensity) that results in a perceived change (of pitch or loudness) is called a just noticeable difference (JND).

Frequency

A single-frequency sound, or pure tone, is the standard used in the assessment of auditory sensitivity (threshold). Frequency is a physical attribute of a sound and is defined as the number of cycles per unit of time. For example, if a metronome were to move back and forth 1000 times in 1 second, it would have 1000 cycles per second. One cycle, therefore, is defined as one complete event and has occurred when a particle has completed all its variations, returned to its original point of rest, and is about to begin the same variations again. Although measured in cycles per second, frequency is reported in hertz (Hz). As in the above example, the result would be a 1000-Hz tone because it completed 1000 cycles per second. A sound can be visualized in the time domain, as shown in **Fig. 2–1**, which describes tones of different frequencies.

Period refers to the amount of time it takes for one cycle to occur; therefore, period is the reciprocal of frequency (period = 1/frequency). This 1000-Hz tone would have a period of 1/1000 seconds. *Wavelength* (λ) is the distance sound travels in one period and is reported in centimeters, feet, or miles, depending on how the velocity is recorded. *Velocity* is the speed in which the sound travels from the source to a distant point and is determined by the density of the medium. Because sound is transmitted mainly through the air, the velocity would be 344 m (or 1130 feet) per second. Therefore, wavelength is the speed at which the sound travels divided by the frequency of the sound (λ = velocity/frequency). Given a 1000-Hz tone, the period and the wavelength can be computed, as shown in **Table 2–1**.

A single-frequency sound is a simple sound or pure tone. However, sounds in the real world are seldom simple and are made of more than one frequency; these are called complex sounds. If the variations of a sound are repetitive over time, the sound is periodic. Both simple (pure tones) and complex (voice) sounds may be periodic. Sounds that are not repetitive over time are aperiodic (e.g., noise).

Noise is defined as an aperiodic, complex sound. There are several types of noise, such as white noise, speech, and narrow-band noise. *White noise* is a broadband noise that is complex and aperiodic. Its name is derived from the fact that it contains all the frequencies in the audible spectrum, randomly distributed, just as white light contains all the colors of the visual spectrum. White noise is not often used in audiometry as it is too broad in its spectrum. However, the other noises, speech and narrow-band noise, are derived from this white noise with a narrower band or frequency response than white noise.

Speech noise refers to a band of noise that has had the frequencies above and below the speech frequencies (300 to 3 kHz) filtered out. Speech noise is most often used for masking during speech audiometry. *Narrow-band noise* (NBN) is actually white noise with certain frequencies (above and below a given center frequency) filtered out. The result of the filtering is a frequency range of noise smaller than broadband white noise but broad enough to effectively mask the tested frequency. NBN is most often used for masking in pure-tone testing.

Intensity

The number of times an object vibrates determines its frequency, but how far the object moves determines its intensity. Intensity or amplitude then becomes another physical attribute of sound. Intensity relates to the strength of a sound as shown in **Fig. 2–2**; the distance a mass moves from the point of rest is the amplitude of the sound. Intensity is usually measured in decibels (dB), after the renowned Alexander Graham Bell. There are five descriptors of the decibel; it is (1) a relative unit of measure, (2) a ratio, (3) logarithmic, (4) nonlinear, and (5) expressed in terms of various reference levels.[2] An often-overlooked aspect of the decibel is that it is a relative unit of measure that needs to be described with a reference or it loses its meaning. For example, dB SPL is related to sound pressure level, dB HL is related to hearing level, and dB SL is related to the sensation level, where the tone is presented at above that amount above the threshold. The use of the term dB without a referent is meaningless and should be avoided.

In the simplest terms, the decibel represents a difference between two sounds: a referent and the sound being described. The formula for dB (pressure) is dB = 20 log *R*, where *R* is the ratio between the referent and a given sound. For example, if we were discussing a sound that was the same pressure as the referent (i.e., dB = 20 log 0.0002 µPa/ 0.0002µ, where the referent is 0.0002µ), the ratio equals 1, and the log of 1 = 0. Therefore, 20 × 0 = 0 dB, and 0 dB means that there is no difference between the two sounds—our sound and its referent. It is also important to be aware that the decibel represents a logarithmic series, not an interval series. Therefore, in pressure measurements, a 20-dB step represents a 10-fold

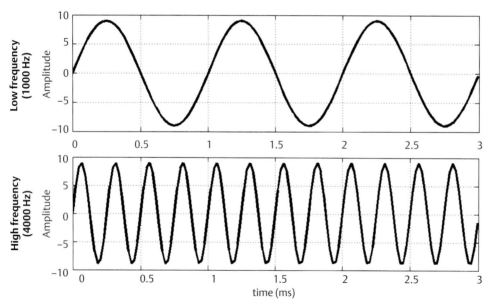

Figure 2–1 Graphs of two sine waves of different frequencies plotted over time. The top graph is a low frequency (1000 Hz) and the bottom is a higher frequency (4000 Hz) as denoted by the number of cycles in the same time window.

Table 2–1 Frequency, Period, and Wavelength of a 1000-Hz Tone

Frequency	Period	Wavelength (λ)
$\text{Frequency} = \dfrac{\text{Velocity}}{\text{Wavelength}}$	$\text{Period} = \dfrac{1}{\text{Frequency}}$	$\lambda = \dfrac{\text{Velocity}}{\text{Frequency}}$
$\text{Frequency} = \dfrac{344\,\text{m/s}}{0.344\,\text{m}}$ $= 1000\,\text{Hz}$	$\text{Period} = \dfrac{1}{1000\,\text{Hz}}$ $= 0.001\,\text{second}$ (1 millisecond)	$\lambda = \dfrac{344\,\text{m/s}}{1000\,\text{cycles/s (Hz)}}$ $\lambda = 0.344\,\text{m}$

increase (i.e., a ratio of 10:1) and a 40-dB step represents a 100-fold increase; a 60-dB step represents a 1000-fold increase, and so forth. For example, people attending a rock concert where the level of the sound is 140 dB SPL (2000 dynes/cm²) are exposed to 1000 times more pressure than they should be exposed to if the safe level is 80 dB SPL (2.0 dynes/cm²).

The basic acoustical measurement that is used for almost all acoustic measures is the sound pressure level (SPL). This measure is independent of frequency and has a referent of 0.0002 dyne/cm² (or 0.0002μ). This referent was determined in the Bell Laboratories many years ago and has stood the test of time. It remains the basic referent for all acoustic measures, but, unfortunately, very few people are able to detect a sound at 0 dB SPL. Therefore, a different system had to be set up using SPL as a referent and criteria ascertained from several studies of auditory sensitivity in humans. The American National Standards Institute (ANSI) in 1969 issued the standard for audiometric zero.

Audiometric zero is frequency-specific and indicates that auditory sensitivity in humans is poorer at lower frequencies (125 Hz) and higher frequencies (8000 Hz) than it is in the midfrequencies (500 to 4000 Hz) range as shown in **Table 2–2**. When audiometric zero is the referent, the designation is hearing level (HL); thus, when indicating a decibel measurement the method of measurement (i.e., SPL or HL) is very important. The use of dB HL instead of dB SPL allows the hearing threshold for normal individuals to be calibrated to audiometric zero across all frequencies (despite normal auditory sensitivity being better for the middle frequencies of the test range).

As previously noted, dB sensation level (SL) refers to any measurement that is above an individual's threshold. This term is both frequency-specific and individual-specific. If someone is tested at 30 dB SL, this means he or she was tested at 30 dB above his or her threshold for that particular frequency or for speech. Because the decibel is a measurement based on a referent, it is possible to move back and forth between dB SPL, dB HL, and dB SL. For example, at 250 Hz, a sound is to be presented to a patient at 35 dB SL. The patient's threshold is 40 dB HL. What is the level of presentation in dB SPL? We know from **Table 2–2** that the 0 dB HL is 25.5 dB SPL; thus the dB SPL equivalent of 35 dB SL is 100.5. Because all of the units are mathematically related, it is possible to convert from one to another.

Phase

The phase of a sound refers to the relative timing of sound waves. It is simplest to refer to the starting phase of the signal; therefore, at time zero the point of the sine wave where the signal begins will be the starting phase as shown in

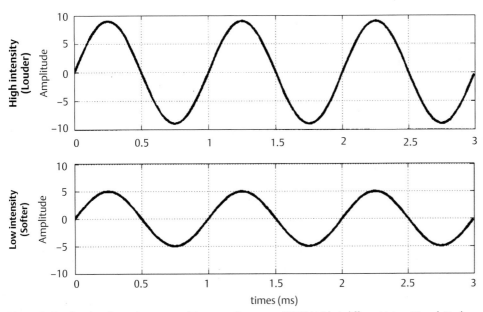

Figure 2–2 Graphs of two sine waves of the same frequency (1000 Hz) but different intensities plotted over time. The tones have the same cycles per second but differ in the amplitude of the waves.

Table 2–2 Standard Referenced Sound Pressure Levels (0.0002 dynes/cm²) for 0 dB Hearing Level as Developed for a Standard Audiometer Earphone (TDH 39) (ANSI, 1996)

Frequency (Hz)	Standard Earphone (TDH 39)
125	45.0
250	25.5
500	11.5
750	8.0
1000	7.0
1500	6.5
2000	9.0
3000	10.0
4000	9.5
6000	15.5
8000	13.0

Fig. 2–3. This will act as a referent point for other waves. Two tones of the same frequency that begin 180 degrees out of phase will cancel each other out.

In a complex sound, that is, one that has more than one frequency, the lowest frequency in that sound is called the fundamental. The fundamental frequency of a complex, periodic sound is the frequency at which the source vibrates. All frequencies above that are called overtones. Frequencies that are multiples of the fundamental are called harmonics and those that are not multiples are called aharmonics.

Resonance refers to the phenomenon whereby one body can be set into motion by the vibration of another body. If a given area has a "resonant frequency," then that frequency is amplified when it is presented in that area. In other words, there is an increase in the intensity of that signal because the surface of the area with the resonant frequency vibrates at the particular frequency that has been presented and therefore increases its intensity. The fundamental frequency of the voice is the slowest rate at which the vocal folds vibrate for a given "voiced" sound. There may be several overtones imposed by the inertial effect of the vibrating vocal folds.

Differences in the sounds that come out of the vocal mechanism are caused by changing the resonating cavities above the vocal folds. Complex sounds may be described in terms of spectra. The spectrum of a sound identifies the frequencies and the relative amplitudes of the various components of a sound.

◆ Physiology of Hearing

The anatomy of the auditory system was addressed in Chapter 1. This chapter traces the course of the auditory stimulus from its generator to the auditory cortex, as shown in **Fig. 2–4**. Although the many waystations in the auditory system all contribute to signal processing in a unique way, we highlight those areas pertinent to the practicing otologist and to those interested in the complexity of this exciting and mysterious sensory system.

The natural or usual manner by which humans detect sound is via an airborne or acoustic signal. Once the sound is generated, it travels through the air in a disturbance called a sound wave. This sound is slightly modified by the body and head, specifically the head and shoulders, which affect the frequencies below 1500 Hz by shadowing and reflection.[3] The flange and concha of the pinna collect, amplify, and direct the sound wave to the tympanic membrane by the external auditory meatus. At the tympanic membrane, several transformations of the signal occur: (1) the acoustic signal becomes mechanoacoustic; (2) it is faithfully reproduced; and (3) it is passed along to the ossicular chain, is amplified, or (under certain conditions) is attenuated.

Transmission and Natural Resonance of the External Ear

Natural resonance refers to inherent anatomic and physiologic properties of the external and middle ear that allow certain frequencies to pass more easily to the inner ear.[4] The external ear serves to enhance the sound as it travels to the cochlea and to protect the tympanic membrane.[5] The concha and ear canal increase the intensity of the sound over the frequency range

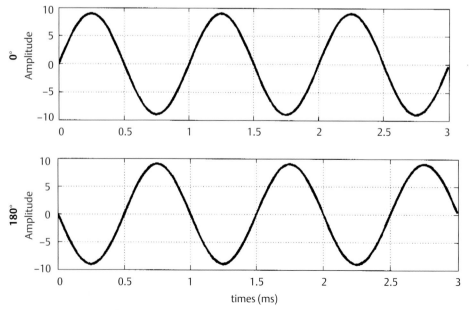

Figure 2–3 Two tones that are 180 degrees out of phase; note that the starting points for the two waves are the same, creating a mirror image.

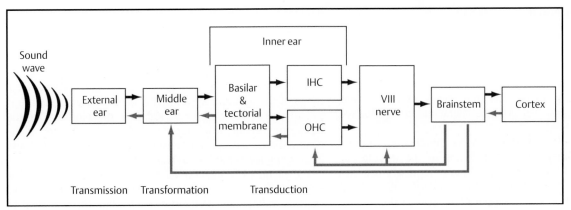

Figure 2–4 Block diagram of the auditory system. The sound leaves its generator and travels through the external, middle, and inner ear and travels to the auditory cortex. (IHC, inner hair cell; OHC, outer hair cell)

1500 to 7000 Hz by as much as 10 to 20 dB SPL using only simple resonance.[6] The natural resonance of the external auditory canal is 2700 Hz[6] in the adult, and 5300 to 7200 Hz in newborns.[7] This ear canal resonance is dependent on the size and shape of the ear canal and is inversely related to its length.

The natural resonance of the middle ear is 800 Hz. The tympanic membrane is most efficient in transmitting sounds between 800 and 1600 Hz, whereas the ossicular chain is most efficient in transmitting sounds between 500 and 2000 Hz. These structures enhance sensitivity to sound between 500 and 3000 Hz, which are approximately the frequencies that are most important in human speech.[4]

Transformation and the Middle Ear Mechanism

The middle ear system is a mechanical transformer used to help compensate for the impedance mismatch between sound traveling through air and cochlear fluid. This mismatch is caused by the much larger cochlear input impedance, which allows about 3% of the sound energy to be transmitted into the cochlea and reflects 87%.[8] The impedance matching is accomplished by the area effect of the tympanic membrane, the lever ratio of the ossicular chain, the natural resonance and efficiency of the middle ear, and the phase difference between the oval and round windows. Many of these principles were first suggested by Helmholtz,[9] and were later confirmed by Wever and Lawrence.[4]

Area Effect of the Tympanic Membrane

The adult human tympanic membrane measures approximately 90 mm^2. Of this area, approximately 55 mm^2 are functional in that primarily the lower two thirds of the membrane vibrates in response to sound. The tympanic membrane in turn is connected to the stapes footplate by way of the ossicular chain. The stapes footplate has an area of 3.2 mm^2. The hydraulic ratio created by the vibrating area of the tympanic membrane in comparison with that of the stapes footplate produces a 17:1 increase in sound energy transmission across the middle ear.

Lever Ratio of the Ossicular Chain

Tympanic membrane vibrations are transmitted by way of the malleus to the incus. The axis of rotation of the ossicular chain is from the anterior process of the malleus through the posterior (short) process of the incus. The long process of the incus and handle of the malleus move in unison; however, the malleus handle is 1.3 times longer than the long process of the incus. This difference in length produces a 1.3:1 lever ratio of the middle ear ossicles. The overall middle ear transformer ratio is the product of 1.3 × 17, or a transformer ratio of 22:1 due to the combined area effect of the drum and lever ratio of the ossicles.[4] This equates to approximately 27 dB of gain and when combined with the action of the external ear will compensate for the loss of energy due to the impedance mismatch.[10]

Phase Difference Between Oval and Round Windows

As sound energy is transmitted to the stapes footplate, fluid vibrations travel from the scala vestibuli up the cochlear partition to the helicotrema.[8,11] For most frequencies, the helicotrema acts mechanically as though it were closed. Therefore, it is incorrect to assume that displacement of the stapes causes perilymph to flow back and forth through this opening. If this in fact occurred, there would be no displacement of the cochlear partition. The helicotrema is instead involved in the static balance of fluid pressure within the cochlea.[8] The round window membrane is an elastic membrane several cell layers thick that vibrates in response to sound waves traveling through the fluid medium of the inner ear. Because impulses created at the oval window must travel through the vestibule and scala vestibuli before reaching the round window membrane, movements of the stapes footplate precede those of the round window membrane; that is, there is a phase difference between the two windows. Clinically, if the round window niche were sealed by bone or other pathologic disease, lack of membrane movements would impede the traveling fluid wave.

For the fluid system of the inner ear to transmit sound most efficiently, there must be oval window exposure and round window protection. Oval window exposure permits transmission of tympanic membrane vibrations through the ossicles to the oval window. Round window protection prevents the sound wave from striking the round window simultaneously with the oval window, thus canceling out the vibrations. Phase difference between the oval and round windows produces a minor effect in the normal ear (approximately 4 dB) but a very large effect in the diseased ear.[4]

Middle ear muscles (tensor tympani and stapedius) probably play a role in protecting the inner ear from acoustic trauma.[11] Whether they enhance audition is not known.

Sound Transmission in the Diseased Ear

Middle ear pathology may alter the normal transformation mechanism by creating stiffness of the eardrum and ossicular chain or by a mass within the middle ear cavity. Both pathologic results produce conductive hearing loss, but middle ear stiffness involves primarily low frequencies. Thus, different pathologic processes can produce characteristic conductive hearing losses.

Eustachian tube obstruction, negative middle ear pressure, and early effusion produce a stiffening of the middle ear transformation mechanism causing a low-frequency conductive hearing loss. If effusion becomes secondarily infected and progresses to the stage of suppuration, increased pressure within the middle ear cleft produces a mass effect on the transformation mechanism, resulting in a high-frequency loss in addition to the low-frequency loss. Perforations of the tympanic membrane alter the function of the middle ear transformation mechanism by decreasing the area effect of the drum and by producing abnormal phase on the oval and round windows. Perforation size is more important than its location. For example, a small central perforation may impair the area effect of the drum to produce a relatively small conductive hearing loss (e.g., 15 dB) primarily in the low frequencies, whereas a large central perforation of the tympanic membrane may produce a greater (e.g., 30 dB) conductive hearing loss. This is due not only to further loss of area effect of the drum, but also to passage of sound directly to the round window membrane where the phase effect may be altered.

When the ossicular chain is disrupted, the area effect of the drum and the lever ratio of the ossicles do not contribute to the middle ear transformation mechanism. If a large central perforation of the drum coexists with ossicular discontinuity, at least some sound energy will pass through the perforation to vibrate the stapes, causing a greater conductive hearing loss (e.g., 45 dB). If, however, the tympanic membrane is intact but the ossicular chain is disrupted, sound vibrations from the drum will not be passed to either the oval or round windows and the result will be a maximal conductive hearing loss of 60 dB.

In the office examination, the clinician should correlate audiometric findings with physical findings. A small attic perforation with cholesteatoma may preserve the larger vibrating portion of the drum, but a coexistent conductive hearing loss of 30 or 40 dB usually implies that ossicular erosion has taken place. Knowledge of the middle ear transformation mechanism often can aid the surgeon in determining the extent of disease preoperatively.

Transduction and the Inner Ear

As the vibrations reach the footplate of the stapes and enter the inner ear (the vestibule) via the oval window, they are transformed into hydroacoustic waves in the perilymph. This disturbance, called a traveling wave, enters the cochlea at its base, via the scala vestibuli, and courses its length, displacing the cochlear partition in a particular fashion. The movement within the inner ear can be described by two components: passive and active cochlear mechanics. Passive linear mechanics consist of the traveling wave and its interactions with the structures of the inner ear. A traveling wave with a certain frequency grows in amplitude as it moves apically up the cochlea until it has reached its maximum displacement at the place where the cochlea is tuned to that frequency and then rapidly dampens out.[12] The tuning of the basilar membrane is such that it vibrates according to its characteristic frequency. Thus the basal end of the basilar membrane is tuned to the high frequencies and the tuning becomes lower in frequency toward the apex. The active cochlear mechanism accounts for the high sensitivity, sharp frequency tuning, and wide dynamic range of the auditory system. This occurs because energy is provided into the system to enhance the vibration of the basilar membrane, resulting in sufficient amplification of the weak vibration to stimulate the inner hair cells (IHCs) and accounting for our ability to hear soft sounds.[13]

The cochlea is a snail-shaped, 32-mm-long structure that makes 2.75 turns in the normal postnatal temporal bone. Delicate membranes divide the cochlea into three fluid-filled chambers. The two outer chambers contain perilymph, which has an ionic composition similar to that of extracellular fluid. These two chambers communicate at the apex of the cochlea where the scala media terminates (helicotrema). The middle cochlear chamber (also called cochlear duct, scala media, and otic duct) contains endolymph, which has an ionic composition similar to that of intracellular fluid. Different ionic compositions of the fluid compartments are ideal for propagation of afferent auditory neural impulses.

With the delivery of an auditory stimulus, transduction of the mechanical traveling wave into neural activity begins with the deflection of the outer hair cells' (OHC) stereocilia. Each OHC supports about three stereocilia rows, all configured into a W pattern. The actin-filled OHC stereocilia, like the IHCs' stereocilia, are interconnected by cross-links.[14] OHC stereocilia generally number from 50 to 150 per bundle, with greater numbers appearing toward the cochlear base. OHC stereocilia have lengths ranging from 0.5 to 1 µm or greater near the lower frequency cochlear apex. Each stereocilia row is progressively graded in length as a function of its distance from the modiolus.[14] OHC stereocilia are relatively more rounded at their extremes, compared with the more flattened distal tips of the IHC stereocilia. OHC stereocilia are also thinner ($\approx$0.20 µm) relative to the wider diameters ($\approx$0.45 µm) of the IHC stereocilia.[15] The tips of the tallest OHC stereocilia appear to be embedded within the tectorial membrane, whereas by contrast the IHC stereocilia show no evidence of tectorial membrane-embedding.[16] It is therefore likely that the stereocilia of the OHCs are displaced directly by the combined displacement of the tectorial and basilar membranes. The three stereocilia rows therefore provide stiffness; the OHC subplasma membrane provides an elastic hair cell attachment (for a restorative force), and the overlying tectorial membrane provides a resonant system.[17] Indeed, the gradient of stiffness along the basilar membrane is the key factor in determining the tonotopic specificity of the basilar membrane.

There are three to five rows of OHCs (approximately 12,000 to 15,000 in humans). The cylindrically shaped mammalian OHCs have lengths ranging from 0.20 µm (near the cochlear base) to 80 µm nearer to the apex of the cochlea.[14] The OHCs are securely attached at their perinuclear region to the Deiters' cells,[15] which are capable of stretching,[18] and to the reticular lamina at the OHC apex. The OHCs exhibit a much poorer afferent innervation compared with the well-innervated IHCs,[19] yet they seem to be capable of both responding to forces, as in detecting and boosting the amplitude of the traveling wave, and generating forces as in the production of otoacoustic emissions (OAEs).[17,20] It is important to note that the existence of OAEs depends largely on the micromechanical integrity of the cochlear OHCs.[21] The current view is that OHCs serve as active, nonlinear force-generating mechanical effectors, providing a threshold boost in basilar membrane mechanics within the initial 40 dB of hearing sensitivity.[20,22]

A depolarizing current applied to the apical region of the OHCs produces a decrease in OHC length and an increase in cell width, whereas hyperpolarizing currents produce increases in cell length and decreases in cell width.[20,22]

These observed contractile properties have never been observed in IHCs or in supporting cells. As effectors, the OHCs are capable of altering the shape of the basilar membrane and reticular lamina independent of the traveling wave, changing their relative position to the tectorial membrane along select frequency regions.[23] Such actions may well serve to facilitate or damp sensitivity at select frequency bands.[24] Therefore, the OHCs are recognized as key elements in the dynamic maintenance of auditory threshold sensitivity and in frequency tuning.[25,26] All available evidence indicates that their dynamic, micromechanical nonlinear properties fall under the modulatory control of the medial efferent olivocochlear (OC) system.[27]

From cochlear base to apex, the flask-shaped mammalian IHCs (number 3000 to 3500) line up in a single row. IHCs remain constant in morphology, and each supports approximately 60 to 77 stereocilia, having lengths ranging from 1 μm (at the cochlear base) to greater than 8 μm near the cochlear apex. The IHC stereocilia are also interconnected by cross-links, and by tip-links.[14] Located at or near the distal tips of the stereocilia are the elastically gated, mechanosensitive transduction channels, numbering approximately four per stereocilium.[28-32]

These apical transduction channels prefer cations over anions.[17,20] Stereocilia deflection (1 to 100 nm) in a positive direction, toward the bundle's tall edge, produces IHC depolarization.[33] During the resting state the hair cell is exposed to a constant and random buffeting by surrounding molecules, and each apical transduction channel can randomly fluctuate from an open to a closed state. This permits a small steady flow of positively charged ions to cross into the hair cell. Only approximately 15% of the IHC transducer channels are open during the resting, or inactive state. The two principal cations, K^+ and Ca^{2+}, appear to be the major carriers of the mammalian depolarizing current across the apical IHC membrane.[17,20] At frequencies <200 Hz, the displacement of the free-standing IHC stereocilia is proportional to basilar membrane velocity, and at frequencies >200 Hz, to basilar membrane displacement.[34] A positive deflection of the stiff, actin-filled IHC stereocilia is sufficient to gate an inward flow of current through almost one hundred mechanosensitive transducer channels associated within each stereocilia bundle.

The IHCs, as shown in **Fig. 2–5**, are the primary end-organs for transmitting information to the myelinated type I dendrites of the auditory nerve.[35] The initiation of auditory signaling and hearing within the mammalian periphery is therefore highly dependent on the release of the primary excitatory neurotransmitter from within the IHCs. This afferent neurotransmitter is probably glutamate or a related excitatory amino acid.[36,37]

The central pillar of petrous bone around which the cochlea is wound is the modiolus, and in the cavity (Rosenthal's canal) created within the modiolus are the cell bodies of the neurons that compose the auditory portion of the eighth cranial nerve. Collectively, these cell bodies are called the auditory spiral

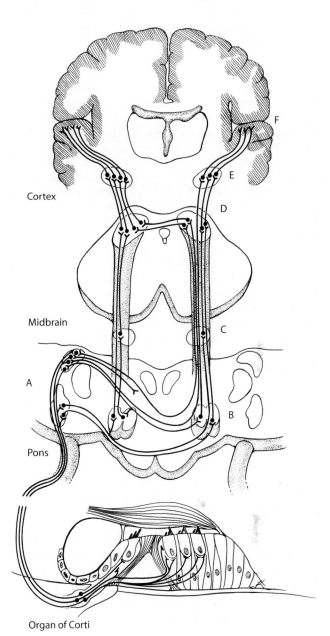

Figure 2–5 Electrical impulses beginning at the level of the cochlea traverse to the primary auditory cortex through both the ipsilateral and contralateral auditory pathways. A, cochlear nuclei; B, superior olivary complex; C, lateral lemniscus; D, inferior colliculus; E, medial geniculate body; F, auditory cortex.

ganglia. These cell bodies, totaling approximately 30,000 in humans, are of two types, and the dendrites of both types emerge from out of the osseous spiral lamina, and enter the organ of Corti. The myelinated type I neurons make up at least 90 to 95% of the total neurons used in hearing and are therefore responsible for most or all of the auditory input reaching the brain.[19] Type I afferent neurons innervate the IHCs exclusively, with approximately 7 to 10 type I neurons per IHC.

Auditory Pathways and Cortex

The mammalian auditory system also contains descending neural pathways. Although the efferent system begins at the cortex, we will discuss the system only as it arises from the superior olivocochlear region. These efferent fiber bundles originate from neurons located near the brainstem superior olivary region, and innervate the cochlea via anatomically segregated medial and lateral divisions.[38] Descending lateral efferent axons are distributed primarily within the ipsilateral cochlea and terminate directly upon the dendrites of auditory type I spiral ganglia neurons.[39] The purpose of these unmyelinated lateral efferents is not well defined, although numerous attempts have been made to clarify their role in auditory function.[40,41] Anatomic studies have demonstrated that auditory type I dendrites are segregated with respect to the number of lateral efferent terminations they receive. About 10 to 30% of the total number of type I afferents exhibit relatively high thresholds and relatively low rates of spontaneous discharge. These relatively less responsive afferents receive twice as many lateral efferent terminals, as compared with the remaining afferents that characteristically exhibit lower thresholds and higher rates of spontaneous discharge.[42] This segregated synaptic distribution has suggested that tonic input from the lateral efferents may be required to establish or maintain the distribution of spontaneous activity and sensitivity within primary auditory inputs to the brain.[43]

Centrifugal axons arising from the medial pre- and periolivary efferent nuclei terminate upon the basal and circumnuclear regions of the OHCs, bilaterally.[39] A convincing argument has been made in favor of a medial efferent system that functions to reduce primary afferent neural responses to low levels of "nonessential" auditory stimuli,[44-46] improving the response range ($\approx$3 to 8 dB) of individual auditory neurons in backgrounds of noise.[47] The resulting improvement in signal encoding then permits a greater detection of intensity changes in noise backgrounds, at relatively lower signal-to-noise ratios.

A considerable amount of evidence indicates that both efferent divisions utilize several neurotransmitters, including acetylcholine (ACh) and γ-aminobutyric acid (GABA). The lateral efferent system also utilizes neuroactive enkephalin and dynorphin opioid peptides.[36]

At the level of the organ of Corti the stimulus changes from hydroacoustic to synaptic (**Fig. 2–5**). The neural impulses leave the cochlea via the afferent neurons and coalesce to form the acoustic division of the eighth cranial nerve. The nerve enters the brainstem at the level of the pons. Here the fibers bifurcate and send collaterals to the dorsal and ventral cochlear nuclei. The central auditory system (CAS) begins at the cochlear nuclei. The CAS is responsible not only for transferring acoustic information to the brain but also for many subtle but critical functions that afford us the experience of hearing. The CAS plays a critical role in such processes as hearing in noise, localization, temporal judgments, and decoding complex acoustic stimuli.

Approximately 80% of the fibers leave the cochlear nuclei and traverse the brainstem to the contralateral superior olivary nucleus (SON) in a nerve bundle called the trapezoid body. From the SON, fibers travel up the brainstem in another pathway called the lateral lemniscus. At the nucleus of the lateral lemniscus, fibers may synapse, cross to the contralateral nucleus, or may bypass the nucleus on the way to the inferior colliculus, where the same three possibilities may occur. The next stations are the medial geniculates, and from there cortical radiations travel to the surface of the cortex (Brodmann's area 41) located at the superior aspect of the temporal lobe along the floor of the lateral cerebral fissure.

◆ Conclusion

The chapter has discussed some principles of acoustics; some terms, concepts, and definitions; and the pathway of a sound from its generator to the brain. Each section in this chapter could have been the subject of a complete text. Therefore, the interested reader should view the information contained within as a threshold and not as an end point.

References

1. Yost WA. Overview: psychoacoustics. In: Yost WA, Popper AN, Fay RR, eds. Human Psychophysics. New York: Springer-Verlag, 1993:1–12

2. Martin FN, Clark JG. Introduction to Audiology. Boston: Allyn and Bacon, 2003

3. Zwicker E, Fastl H. Psychoacoustics: Facts and Models. New York: Springer-Verlag, 1990

4. Wever EG, Lawrence M. Physiological Acoustics. Princeton, NJ: Princeton University Press, 1954

5. Peck JE. Development of hearing. Part I: Phylogeny. J Am Acad Audiol 1994;5:291–299

6. Shaw EAG. The external ear. In: Keidel WD, Neff WD, eds. Handbook of Sensory Physiology—Auditory Systems, vol 5. Berlin: Springer-Verlag, 1974:455–490

7. Kruger B. An update on the external ear resonance in infants and young children. Ear Hear 1987;8:333–336

8. Durrant JD, Lovrinic JH. Bases of Hearing Science, 3rd ed. Owings Mills, MD: William & Wilkins, 1995

9. Helmholtz H. Die Mechanick der gehorknochelchen und des trommelfells. Pfluegers Arch Ges Physiol;I:1868

10. Killion MC, Dallos P. Impedance matching by the combined effects of the outer and middle ear. J Acoust Soc Am 1979;66:599–602

11. Ferraro JA, Melnick W, Gerhardt KR. Effects of prolonged noise exposure in chinchillas with severed middle ear muscles. Am J Otolaryngol 1981;2:13–18

12. Pickles JO. An Introduction to the Physiology of Hearing, 2nd ed. New York: Academic Press, 1988

13. Ryan A, Dallos P. Effect of absence of cochlear outer hair cells on behavioural auditory threshold. Nature 1975;253:44–46

14. Harrison RV, Hunter-Duvar IM. An anatomical tour of the cochlea. In: Jahn AF, Santos-Sacchi J, eds. Physiology of the Ear. New York: Raven Press, 1988:159–171

15. Santi PA. Cochlear microanatomy and ultrastructure. In: Jahn AF, Santos-Sacchi J, eds. Physiology of the Ear. New York: Raven Press, 1988: 173–199

16. Lim DJ. Cochlear anatomy related to cochlear micromechanics. A review. J Acoust Soc Am 1980;67:1686–1695

17. Ashmore JF. The electrophysiology of hair cells. Annu Rev Physiol 1991;53:465–476

18. LePage EL. Functional role of the olivo-cochlear bundle: a motor unit control system in the mammalian cochlea. Hear Res 1989;38:177–198

19. Spoendlin HH. Neural anatomy of the inner ear. In: Jahn AF, Santos-Sacchi J, eds. Physiology of the Ear. New York: Raven Press, 1988:201–219

20. Ashmore JF. Ionic mechanisms in hair cells of the mammalian cochlea. In: Hamann W, Iggo A, eds. Progress in Brain Research, vol 74. New York: Elsevier Science, 1988:3–9

21. Probst R. Otoacoustic emissions: an overview. Adv Otorhinolaryngol 1990;44:1–91

22. Ashmore JF. A fast motile response in guinea-pig outer hair cells: the cellular basis of the cochlear amplifier. J Physiol 1987;388:323–347

23. Reuter G, Gitter AH, Thurm U, Zenner HP. High frequency radial movements of the reticular lamina induced by outer hair cell motility. Hear Res 1992;60:236–246

24. Patuzzi R, Yates GK, Johnstone BM. Outer hair cell receptor current and its effect on cochlear mechanics. In: Wilson JP, Kemp DT, eds. Cochlear Mechanisms: Structure, Function and Models. New York: Plenum Press, 1989:169–176

25. Cody AR. Acoustic lesions in the mammalian cochlea: implications for the spatial distribution of the 'active process.' Hear Res 1992;62:166–172

26. Cody AR, Russell LL. Effects of intense acoustic stimulation on the nonlinear properties of mammalian hair cells. In: Dancer AL, Salvi RH, Hamernik RP, eds. Noise-Induced Hearing Loss. St. Louis: Mosby Year Book, 1992:11–27

27. Brownell WE. Outer hair cell electromotility and otoacoustic emissions. Ear Hear 1990;11:82–92

28. Holton T, Hudspeth AJ. The transduction channel of hair cells from the bull-frog characterized by noise analysis. J Physiol 1986;375:195–227

29. Hudspeth AJ. Extracellular current flow and the site of transduction by vertebrate hair cells. J Neurosci 1982;2:1–10

30. Hudspeth AJ. The hair cells of the inner ear. They are exquisitely sensitive transducers that in human beings mediate the senses of hearing and balance. A tiny force applied to the top of the cell produces an electrical signal at the bottom. Sci Am 1983;248:54–64

31. Hudspeth AJ. The cellular basis of hearing: the biophysics of hair cells. Science 1985;230:745–752

32. Hudspeth AJ, Roberts WM, Howard J. Gating compliance, a reduction in hair-bundle stiffness associated with the gating of transduction channels in hair cells from the bullfrog's sacculus. In: Wilson JP, Kemp DT, eds. Cochlear Mechanisms: Structure, Function and Models. New York: Plenum Press, 1989:117–123

33. Roberts WM, Jacobs RA, Hudspeth AJ. Colocalization of ion channels involved in frequency selectivity and synaptic transmission at presynaptic active zones of hair cells. J Neurosci 1990;10:3664–3684

34. Russell IJ, Sellick PM. Low-frequency characteristics of intracellularly recorded receptor potentials in guinea-pig cochlear hair cells. J Physiol 1983;338:179–206

35. Santos-Sacchi J. Cochlear Physiology. In: Jahn AF, Santos-Sacchi J, eds. Physiology of the Ear. New York: Raven Press, 1988:271–293

36. Eybalin M. Neurotransmitters and neuromodulators of the mammalian cochlea. Physiol Rev 1993;73:309–373

37. Guth PS, Aubert A, Ricci AJ, Norris CH. Differential modulation of spontaneous and evoked neurotransmitter release from hair cells: some novel hypotheses. Hear Res 1991;56:69–78

38. Helfert RH, Snead CR, Altschuler RA. The ascending auditory pathways. In: Altschuler RA, Bobbin RP, Clopton BM, Hoffman D, eds. Neurobiology of Hearing: The Central Auditory System. New York: Raven Press, 1991:1–25

39. Warr WB. Organization of olivocochlear efferent systems in mammals. In: Webster DB, Popper AN, Fay RR, eds. The Mammalian Auditory Pathway: Neuroanatomy. New York: Springer-Verlag, 1992:410–448

40. Liberman MC. The olivocochlear efferent bundle and susceptibility of the inner ear to acoustic injury. J Neurophysiol 1991;65:123–132

41. Sahley TL, Nodar RH. Improvement in auditory function following pentazocine suggests a role for dynorphins in auditory sensitivity. Ear Hear 1994;15:422–431

42. Liberman MC. Morphological differences among radial afferent fibers in the cat cochlea: an electron-microscopic study of serial sections. Hear Res 1980;3:45–63

43. Liberman MC. Effects of chronic cochlear de-efferentation on auditory-nerve response. Hear Res 1990;49:209–223

44. Guinan JJ Jr, Gifford ML. Effects of electrical stimulation of efferent olivocochlear neurons on cat auditory-nerve fibers. I. Rate-level functions. Hear Res 1988;33:97–113

45. Guinan JJ Jr, Gifford ML. Effects of electrical stimulation of efferent olivocochlear neurons on cat auditory-nerve fibers. II. Spontaneous rate. Hear Res 1988;33:115–127

46. Guinan JJ Jr, Gifford ML. Effects of electrical stimulation of efferent olivocochlear neurons on cat auditory-nerve fibers. III. Tuning curves and thresholds at CF. Hear Res 1988;37:29–45

47. Winslow RL, Sachs MB. Effect of electrical stimulation of the crossed olivocochlear bundle on auditory nerve response to tones in noise. J Neurophysiol 1987;57:1002–1021

3

Vestibular Physiology

Joel A. Goebel and Baran Sumer

The vestibular portion of the inner ear is anatomically suited for two main functions: stabilization of gaze during rapid impulsive head movements and postural control in a gravitational field. To function optimally, however, labyrinthine input is combined with visual, proprioceptive, auditory, and other sensory cues within the brainstem so that resultant eye and body movements are in context with the task at hand (**Fig. 3–1**). This sensory integration is the crucial element in gaze stabilization and postural control, and the vestibular end organ serves as an internal reference frame against which all other inputs are compared.

This chapter discusses basic physiology of the semicircular canals, utricle, and saccule in isolation, and explores funda-mental elements of visual and proprioceptive mechanisms and how they interact with labyrinthine inputs. Central adaptation of the vestibulo-ocular reflex (VOR) to injury will be discussed, followed by case illustrations involving labyrinthine injury, abnormal visual or proprioceptive input, and sensory conflict.

◆ Vestibular End-Organ Physiology

The basic sensory element of the vestibular end organ for the semicircular canals and the otolithic organs is the hair cell. Hair cells are specialized sensory cells that maintain a resting

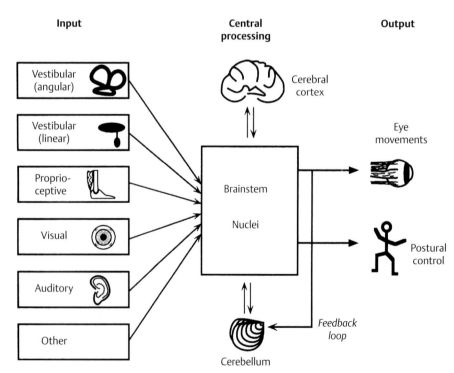

Figure 3–1 The multisensory nature of ocular motor and postural control. Sensory inputs from multiple sources are coded and compared within the brainstem, and modified by cortical and cerebellar connections, and the appropriate motor output is sent to the ocular muscles for gaze stabilization and to the antigravity muscles for postural stability. Feedback occurs to allow adaptation in the event of suboptimal ocular and postural control.

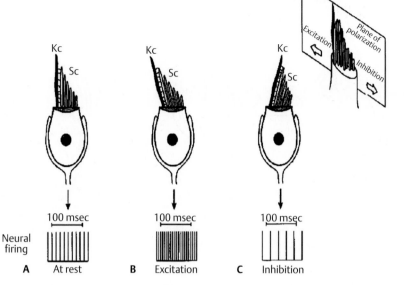

Figure 3–2 Example of a type I hair cell. The cell has a baseline firing rate at rest **(A)**, which increases with deflection of the stereocilia (Sc) toward the kinocilium (Kc) and depolarization of the cell **(B)**. Deflection of the stereocilia away from the kinocilium causes hyperpolarization and a decrease in the rate of neural firing **(C)**. (Courtesy of Kamran Barin, Ph.D.)

transmembrane potential of about –60 mV via selective permeability to cations, predominantly potassium. Each hair cell has an apical ciliary bundle made up of a single large kinocilium and multiple smaller stereocilia. The stereocilia are bound to the kinocilium of each hair cell, and all move together as a unit. When a force is applied parallel to the top of the cell deflecting the stereocilia toward the kinocilium, the hair cell is depolarized to –40 mV. Deflection of the stereocilia away from the kinocilium hyperpolarizes the cell to –64 mV. Forces perpendicular to the kinocilium-stereocilia axis have minimal effect on transmembrane potential[1] (**Fig. 3–2**).

There are two morphologically distinct types of hair cells. Type 1 hair cells have cell bodies that are globular in shape and are surrounded by calyceal nerve endings. Type 1 hair cells are concentrated toward the center of vestibular neuroepithelial structures, near the apex of the canal cristae and the striola of the otolith maculae. Their afferents have predominantly thick axons with fast conduction velocities and irregular firing rates that adapt to acceleration stimuli. Type II hair cells are columnar in shape and are contacted directly by multiple bouton synaptic endings. They are concentrated more on the periphery of the vestibular neuroepithelium. The afferents of type II hair cells tend to have thin, more slowly conducting axons with regular firing rates that tend to accurately encode prolonged acceleration stimuli. Both cell types also receive efferent synaptic contact.[2]

Semicircular Canals

Sensory Transduction

In the semicircular canals, hair cells are arranged along the crista ampullaris within the ampulla of each canal in a polarized fashion. Their cilia are embedded in the substance of the cupula, a neutrally buoyant gelatinous structure that spans the width and height of the ampulla. Angular head acceleration causes relative endolymph flow in a direction opposite to that of the head movement, which displaces the cupula. Cupular displacement in turn causes bending of the hair cell

bundle, resulting in a change in membrane potential. Due to hair cell orientation on the cristae of the horizontal canals, ampullopetal flow (toward the ampulla) causes hair cell depolarization, whereas ampullofugal flow (away from the ampulla) causes hyperpolarization. In the posterior and superior canals, the hair cells have an opposite orientation, and this pattern of excitation and inhibition is reversed (**Fig. 3–3**).

Modeling of Semicircular Canal Dynamics

Endolymph flow and cupular displacement in the semicircular canals can be described mathematically using an inverted pendulum model. Simple mechanical considerations reveal that the inertial force of the endolymph and cupula and the viscous force of the endolymph will cause a time delay between the onset of an acceleration stimulus and maximal deflection of the cupula. In addition, the elastic force of the cupula acting against the viscous force will tend to return the cupula to its resting position when acceleration ceases. Both the initial displacement and the return of the cupula to its resting position will occur with an exponential time course.

Using an inverted pendulum model, one can predict an exponential time constant for an acceleration stimulus to produce initial cupular deflection. In humans, this time constant has a value of approximately 3 ms. The duration of most natural human head movements exceeds this interval, and inertial forces are important only for the briefest of head accelerations.[3]

According to the inverted pendulum model of cupular deflection, the cupula will return toward its resting position (and hair cells will repolarize) following the end of angular acceleration with a time constant of approximately 7 seconds. That is, it takes approximately 7 seconds for the cupula to return to within 37% of its original resting position. After four time constants, the return will be nearly complete. Experimental data, however, indicate that the time course of exponential decay of the slow phase velocity of nystagmus in response to step velocity rotations is consistent with a time

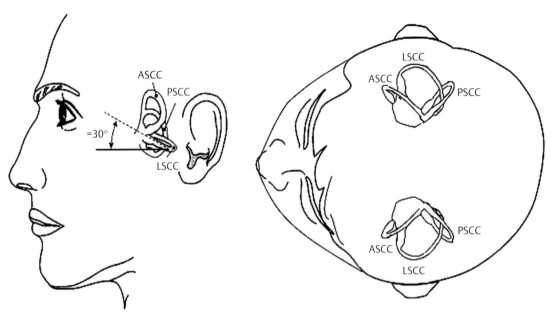

Figure 3–3 Orientation of semicircular canals. The lateral semicircular canals lie in the same horizontal plane. The right superior (anterior) canal lies parallel to the left posterior canal and the left superior (anterior) canal lies parallel to the right posterior canal. LSCC, lateral semicircular canal; ASCC, anterior (superior) semicircular canal; PSCC, posterior semicircular canal. (Courtesy of Kamran Barin, Ph.D.)

I Basic Science

constant of approximately 12 to 15 seconds, about twice as long as necessary for the return of the cupula to a resting position. This difference is accounted for by central nervous system perseveration of the vestibular afferent signal, a phenomenon that has been called velocity storage. It is believed to involve commissural connections between the vestibular nuclei and cerebellar projections. The system is charged by head acceleration and discharges over an interval after the acceleration has ceased. The main purpose of velocity storage appears to be to perseverate low-frequency (low-acceleration) vestibular input, effectively extending the dynamic range of the system.[4]

During sinusoidal head rotation, time constants derived from the model above can be used to predict the frequency response of the gain or strength of the reflex, and phase or timing. For very low frequency rotations (below 0.1 Hz), the rotational stimulus must overcome the elastic restoring force of the cupula. Gain is directly related to acceleration (which is proportional to frequency) and phase is less than zero—eye velocity "leads" head velocity. For rotations between approximately 0.1 and 5 Hz, the restoring forces are easily overcome. Gain is near 1 (perfectly compensatory) and phase is nearly 0. Over this range, the canals act as velocity integrators so that eye velocity is directly compensatory to head velocity. However, at frequencies above 5 Hz, the effects of the short time constant begin to dominate as the brevity of acceleration for each half cycle fails to maximally deflect the cupula before the onset of the counterrotational acceleration of the next half cycle. At these higher frequencies, gain declines and phase becomes greater than zero—eye velocity "lags" head velocity.

Primary Canal Afferents

All vestibular afferent neurons have a resting discharge rate of approximately 90 spikes per second (range: 10 to 200 spikes/s). This resting discharge is required for bidirectional sensitivity. Excitatory canal rotation produces depolarization of hair cells, which leads to an increase in the neuronal firing rate. Rotation in the opposite direction causes hair cell hyperpolarization and

leads to a decrease in the firing rate. For low acceleration rotational stimuli, the modulation of firing rate around an individual neuron's mean is virtually symmetrical. At higher acceleration, however, the firing rate becomes increasingly asymmetrical because upward modulation is not limited, whereas downward modulation cannot go below zero.[5]

The transduction of head rotation in the yaw plane in the semicircular canals is graphically represented in **Fig. 3–4**. Leftward head rotation (indicated by the bold arrow) induces relative endolymph flow to the right (thin arrows) due to inertial forces of the fluid. This in turn causes ampullopetal cupular displacement in the left horizontal canal and ampullofugal displacement in the right horizontal canal. Hair cells in the crista of the left canal are depolarized, and those in the right canal are hyperpolarized. This causes an increase in the neuronal firing rate in the left vestibular nerve and a decrease in the neuronal firing rate in the right. Although the strongest input is provided by the ipsilateral canal (i.e., the canal on the side toward which the end is turned), this "push–pull" mechanism amplifies the asymmetric neural input to the vestibular nuclei.

Otolith Organs

Sensory Transduction

Otolith hair cell cilia are embedded in the gelatin layer of the otolithic membrane of the utricle and saccule that underlies the layer of otoconia (composed primarily of calcium carbonate crystals). Because the otoconia have a higher specific gravity than endolymph, their greater inertia causes them to be displaced upon the hair cell layer by applied linear acceleration (including gravity) in the plane of the otolithic membrane. As with all hair cells, maximal activation occurs along a vector deflecting the stereocilia toward the kinocilium. Compressive forces have no effect. Acceleration due to gravity exerts a constant shearing force on all portions of the macula except those perfectly aligned to the earth-horizontal plane. Hair cell activation can be changed by a static head tilt, which alters the

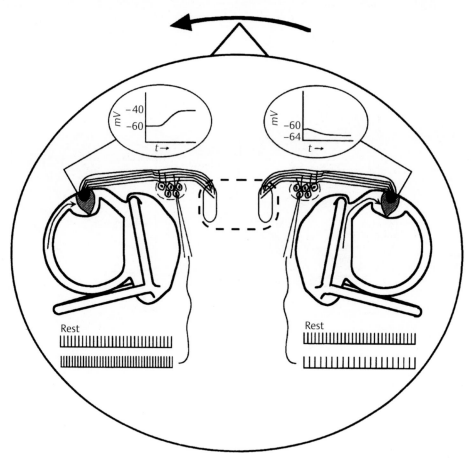

Figure 3–4 Binaural response of the horizontal canals to leftward head rotation in the yaw plane. The left canal hair cells depolarize, thus increasing the neural firing rate over the baseline activity. Conversely, hyperpolarization of the right canal hair cells causes a decrease in neural activity. Taken together, these two changes enhance the difference in signals to the brainstem that code rotation to the left.

orientation of the maculae with respect to the gravitational vector, or by translational movements of the head without change in head orientation, or a combination of both.[6]

The organ of sensory transduction in the otoliths consists of the maculae of the utricle and the saccule. The hair cells of both otolith organs are oriented at right angles to a central curvilinear axis called the striola. Oppositely oriented hair cells are separated by the striola, giving the maculae bidirectional sensitivity. The utricular macula is oriented roughly perpendicular to the earth-vertical plane in normal head position (i.e., roughly in the same plane as the horizontal semicircular canal), and the saccular macula roughly parallel to the earth-vertical plane. There are minimum and maximum stimuli to which the otoliths may respond. Threshold forces are approximately 1/20 of the acceleration of gravity (0.05g). Otolith responses are linear up to approximately 1g and saturate above this point (**Fig. 3–5**).[7]

Primary Otolith Afferents

Like semicircular canal afferents, otolith afferent neurons have a resting firing rate that is modulated up or down depending on hair cell activation by linear acceleration or gravity. Baseline neuronal activity is measured when hair cells are oriented parallel to the gravitational vector (and the otolithic membrane is oriented perpendicular to it) when no shear forces are present. This is also the orientation in which the hair cells have the greatest sensitivity to linear acceleration. Otolith afferent activity is modulated upward or downward depending on the combination of orientation by static head tilt, which alters the orientation of the maculae with respect to the gravitational vector, and translational movements of the head, which create transient linear forces. The firing rate of a particular neuron may not directly correlate with individual hair cell activation as in the canal afferents because otolith afferents collateralize to receive input from several hair cells, which may not be coplanar.[8]

Vestibular Efferents

Efferent neurons also are present in the semicircular canals and otoliths. Evidence exists that vestibular efferents modulate afferent neuron sensitivity or firing rates, but their exact function is far from clear. Further information on the hypothesized substrate and function of this system can be found elsewhere.[2,9]

◆ Vestibulo-Ocular Reflex

The purpose of the VOR is to stabilize images on the retina particularly during rapid impulsive head movements. These movements can be highly variable in frequency and velocity, such as voluntary changes in head position, subtle perturbations

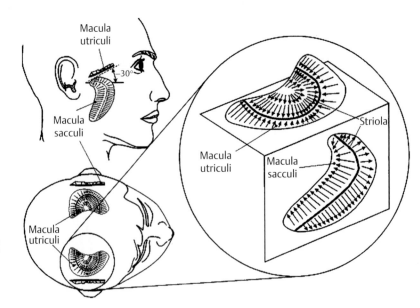

Figure 3–5 Orientation of the otolith organs. The utricle is oriented roughly perpendicular to gravity and the saccule lies parallel to gravity when the subject is upright. Arrows indicate orientation of hair cells and direction of maximal stimulation relative to the striola. (Courtesy of Kamran Barin, Ph.D.)

due to footfalls during locomotion, or transmitted effects of the cardiac pulse. The VOR is perhaps the best studied of all central reflexes because its stimulus transduction and central connections are relatively well understood, and its output is relatively easily measured. It is also an important diagnostic tool because by analyzing the reflex we can indirectly assess vestibular function.

Strictly speaking, the VOR encompasses all compensatory ocular responses to head movement. It may involve stimulation of any combination of the semicircular canals and otoliths, as head movements rarely occur in one plane. It also may involve observed effects of any combination of the extraocular muscles on the orbit, few of which have neatly oriented planes of activation.

Central Connections

Horizontal Canal Vestibulo-Ocular Reflex

The horizontal rotational component of the VOR is easiest to assess. Head rotation in the earth-horizontal plane primarily involves activation of the horizontal semicircular canals and minimal activation of other canals. Hair cells in the crista of the canal toward which the nose rotates are depolarized, whereas those in the contralateral side are hyperpolarized. Ipsilateral afferent firing rates are modulated upward from their resting rate, whereas contralateral afferent firing rates are modulated downward (**Fig. 3–4**).

Consider first the effects in the ipsilateral vestibular nucleus. Because the paired extraocular muscles operate in a push-pull fashion, central connections for the horizontal canal VOR consist of both excitatory and inhibitory pathways. The excitatory pathway consists primarily of a three-neuron arc comprising the vestibular afferent (cranial nerve VIII), an excitatory interneuron in the ipsilateral medial vestibular nucleus, and finally a motoneuron in the ipsilateral oculomotor and contralateral abducens nucleus. Activation causes deviation of the eyes in a direction counter to the rotational stimulus (**Fig. 3–6**).[2] There are two different inhibitory pathways. For

the ipsilateral lateral rectus, vestibular afferents contact an inhibitory interneuron in the ipsilateral medial vestibular nucleus that directly inhibits the lateral rectus motoneuron. For the contralateral medial rectus, vestibular afferents first contact an excitatory interneuron in the ipsilateral medial vestibular nucleus. This in turn contacts an inhibitory interneuron within the ipsilateral superior vestibular nucleus that inhibits the medial rectus motoneuron, permitting eye deviation as above. Both halves of the excitatory and inhibitory pathways are kept strictly separate from each other to allow for vergence effects while fixating targets at various distances.

In the contralateral vestibular nucleus, the downward modulation of afferent activity leads to concomitant modulation of the neuronal firing rates in the contralateral excitatory and inhibitory pathways, ultimately leading to activation of the same extraocular muscles in a complementary fashion by ipsilateral activity.

The pathways described account for conjugate vestibular-induced eye movements seen during head rotation. For rotations through small angles of movement, the eyes move smoothly in one direction opposite the head movement. When the angular displacement of the stimulus causes the globe to approach the limit of normal oculomotor range, the eyes are re-centered in the orbit by the saccadic system, resulting in nystagmus, which is traditionally named for the direction of the fast (saccadic) eye movement.

Anterior and Posterior Canal Reflexes

The anterior (superior) and posterior canals participate primarily in the vertical VOR in response to rotation in the pitch plane (around the interaural axis). Bilateral anterior canal stimulation causes upward eye deviation. Bilateral posterior canal stimulation causes downward eye deviation. Unilateral stimulation of any of these canals results in an unopposed torsional component in addition to those mentioned. This torsional component is always such that the upper poles of the globes deviate away from any individual canal. This results in torsional nystagmus with quick phases directed toward the

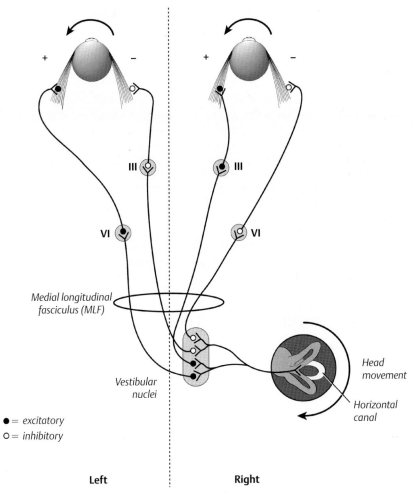

+   III   –

+   III   –

VI

VI

Medial longitudinal fasciculus (MLF)

Head movement

Vestibular nuclei

Horizontal canal

● = *excitatory*
○ = *inhibitory*

Left   **Right**

Figure 3–6 Right horizontal semicircular canal vestibulo-ocular reflex connections. Left vestibular nuclei and inhibitory pathways are not shown.

ipsilateral ear, with upbeat quick phases for posterior canal stimulation and downbeat quick phases for anterior canal activation.

Vestibulo-Ocular Cerebellar Connections

In addition to their principal projection to the vestibular nuclei, some primary canal afferents directly project to the cerebellar flocculus and paraflocculus. These connections permit functional adaptation of the VOR based on visual feedback through the accessory optic tract to cells in the cerebellar cortex. Various animal studies have shown that cerebellar lesions in these areas prevent gain adaptation of the VOR to minimizing or magnifying spectacles. Additional work has shown that specific brainstem and cerebellar neuron populations participate in adaptive modification of the VOR.[10]

◆ Otolith-Ocular Reflexes

Interaction between canal and otolith functions is important for compensating head movements while viewing near targets. When viewing targets at visual infinity (only a few meters in actual practice), the amount of eye movement required to refoveate an image following a linear head movement is negligible. For near targets, however, the compensatory eye movement required is a function of the vergence angle of the eyes and the relative position of the target with respect to the individual visual axis of each eye. This eye movement can be measured and the parameters of the linear VOR determined.[11,12] Another otolith-ocular reaction is ocular counterrolling, which may be seen as a torsional rotation of both eyes in response to a sustained lateral head tilt in the opposite direction.

Comparatively little is know about the central pathways of the otolith-ocular reflex, owing to the complex innervation pattern of the maculae. Each macular afferent carries information from several differentially oriented hair cells. Stimulation of small groups of hair cells can result in discrete eye movements, but the functional significance of this has not yet been determined.

◆ Visual-Vestibular Interaction

In addition to vestibular cues, visual tracking reflexes are important for stabilizing gaze during slow natural head movements. When a subject is rotated slowly at low frequencies in darkness, the VOR is unable to perfectly compensate for head movements. However, when a subject is rotated while viewing a visual target, the resultant eye movements are nearly perfectly compensatory. Two different visual systems—the optokinetic and smooth pursuit systems—combine with the VOR to augment the eye movements for a moving subject.

The optokinetic system augments vestibular input at lower accelerations and frequencies of rotation. This system involves peripheral retinal information transmitted via the accessory optic tract through the cerebellum via Purkinjes cells. The tracts ultimately terminate on secondary vestibular neurons in the vestibular nuclei, finally sharing a common pathway with the neurons of the VOR. If a stationary subject is presented with a full-field, high-contrast image that rotates around the subject, the eyes will reflexively follow. Nystagmus with quick phases directed counter to the direction of rotation and counter to the sensation of circumvection (self-rotation) will result.[5] The system relies on stimulation of the peripheral retina, and foveation of any specific part of the image is not required. The contribution of the optokinetic system enhances the VOR for earth-fixed or counterrotational visual stimuli, and inhibits the VOR for stimuli rotating in the same direction as the subject.

The smooth pursuit system is another mechanism of augmenting the VOR for rotational stimuli up to approximately 1 Hz. The purpose of smooth pursuit is to stabilize the image of a moving target on the fovea either when tracking a moving target with the head fixed or during combined eye-head tracking of a fixed or moving target. It is postulated that visual information is passed from cortical areas to the dorsolateral pontine nucleus through the cerebellum to the vestibular nuclei, from which signals traverse the same common pathways of the VOR. Visual tracking also is believed to be responsible for overriding the VOR when a subject is rotated while viewing a head-fixed target, known as fixation suppression. In addition, visual fixation of an earth-fixed target after sustained rotation largely nullifies the effect of the velocity storage mechanism, and nystagmus decays with a time constant similar to that of the cupula.[5]

There is also evidence for nonvisual parametric modulation of the VOR. Little is known about the anatomic substrate of this system, but it has been demonstrated to operate with a shorter latency and at higher frequencies than the above-mentioned visual tracking systems and is believed to combine with them in augmenting VOR gain in a context-specific manner.[13,14]

◆ Vestibulospinal Reflex

In addition to stabilizing gaze, the vestibular system plays an important role in maintaining posture via the vestibulospinal reflex (VSR). Vestibular information is integrated with visual and somatosensory modalities to supply input to the antigravity muscles of the neck, trunk, and extremities for the maintenance of posture during both standing and locomotion. The VSR is most important in setting antigravity muscle tone and participates with the somatosensory and visual systems and segmental reflexes to maintain posture when subjected to perturbations.

Central Connections

Somatosensory input to the vestibular nuclei has been demonstrated, including direct connections from (1) spinocerebellar tracts to the vestibular nuclei; (2) relays through

the inferior olive, posterior vermis, and anterior cortex of the cerebellum; and (3) the fastigial nuclei. Integration with visual systems is less understood. As smooth pursuit and optokinetic systems augment the VOR, pathways also are postulated for integration of these systems for the control of posture.

Quantification of the VSR is more difficult because the effector pathways are more complex than their VOR counterparts. First, motoneuron output acts on numerous muscles and joints that can require differing amounts of force depending on their specific orientation and the external forces acting upon them. Second, otolith function depends in large part on head orientation (as distinguished from body orientation). Third, the VSR depends on information provided by the neck stretch receptors reflex to account for head-on-body position changes. For these reasons, posture testing often is limited to detailed assessment of function (i.e., computed dynamic posturography) rather than to the parameters of a single reflex loop.[15]

◆ Plasticity and Adaptation

Vestibulo-Ocular Reflex

The VOR is a context-related reflex for maintaining stability of images upon the retina during head movement. In humans, this task is fulfilled by merging visual information from smooth pursuit and optokinetic pathways with the intrinsic VOR signal across a wide frequency of head movements. Prior experience via feedback from the retina serves to "tune" the VOR gain and phase to limit retinal slip and enhance gaze stability. When changes occur within either the visual world or vestibular function, this capacity to adapt is crucial for avoiding oscillopsia ("visual bobbing") during head movement.

Numerous animal studies support the ability of the VOR to adapt following injury. Following unilateral labyrinthectomy, for instance, the disappearance of spontaneous nystagmus within 24 to 48 hours is due to central rebalancing of the asymmetry in tonic activity at rest at the level of the vestibular nuclei.[16,17] Unilateral canal plugging experiments in squirrel monkeys also have shown an immediate 46% reduction in VOR gain during head rotation, which tended to revert back toward normal within 2 weeks in unrestricted animals with normal visual input.[18] In certain cases of total unilateral loss, however, dynamic VOR parameters do not recover as expected despite adequate visual and proprioceptive input; in such cases, saccadic substitution and modification of behavior are the main strategies for gaze stabilization. This is also the case with total bilateral vestibular loss where the animal is forced to rely solely on visual cues to substitute for absent vestibular function for gaze stabilization. As would be expected, neural substitution of visual for vestibular input is most effective during lower frequency and acceleration head movements where smooth pursuit and optokinetic reflexes are most robust.

In humans, a similar pattern is observed, although with greater variability. Partial unilateral losses tend to recover full VOR function within weeks of injury with little or no permanent deficit except for asymmetry on caloric testing. Total unilateral loss, however, represents a greater challenge to the patient. Although low frequency (<0.5 Hz) gain recovery is variable, in most cases a permanent phase lead remains, which implies persistent shortening of the vestibular time constant within the brainstem. In the low-frequency range of head movements, optokinetic and smooth pursuit systems can make up for the deficit of the VOR. However, high-acceleration yaw head movements toward the damaged ear elicit refixation saccades due to deficient ipsilateral (ampullopetal) VOR function and saturation of contralateral VOR (ampullofugal) neural activity, leading to inadequate fixation. Finally, rapid head shaking (>2 Hz over 20 seconds) elicits a post–head shake nystagmus in some individuals with the fast component directed toward the intact ear. This nystagmus has been demonstrated using scleral search coil technique in some patients up to 1 year following unilateral vestibular ablation surgery and is thought to represent ongoing dynamic asymmetry between the damaged and intact sides[19] (**Fig. 3–7**).

With total bilateral loss in humans, substitution of pursuit and saccadic eye movements is the primary strategy for gaze fixation. With practice, pursuit efficiency has been shown to increase, and efficient use of "catch-up" saccades helps to stabilize retinal images during head rotation. As previously noted, however, as the frequency or acceleration of head movement increases (>1–2 Hz, >2000 degrees/s^2), the efficiency

of tracking and preprogrammed saccadic eye movements decreases and oscillopsia occurs.

As mentioned above, changes in visual cues also have impact on VOR function. For example, magnifying prisms worn continuously by human subjects for 5 to 7 days produce a gradual increase in VOR gain in the dark due to increased eye movement required with every head movement against a magnified backdrop; reversing prisms can even cause a 180-degree shift in VOR phase. Such visual context-related VOR adaptation rapidly reverts to the normal state upon removal of the optical challenge.[20] These experiments prove that visual inputs have a great impact upon VOR function with one goal in mind—to ensure retinal fixation and, hence, visual acuity during head motion.

Vestibulospinal Reflex

The VSR is difficult to study in isolation, and therefore most evidence of adaptation following vestibular injury is based on overall recovery of posture. In monkeys, recovery of postural stability following unilateral labyrinthectomy occurred more rapidly in

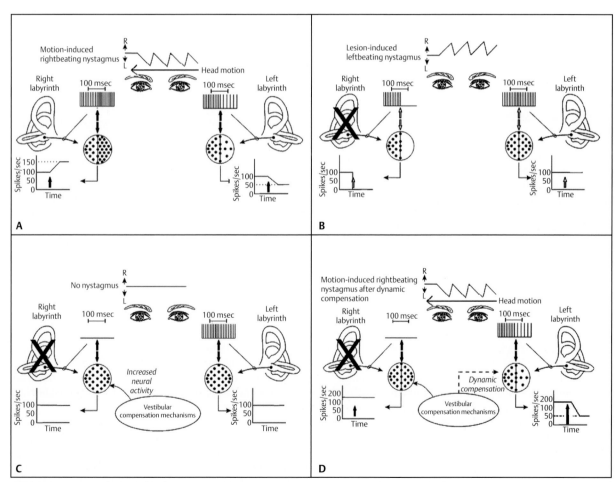

Figure 3–7 **(A)** Normal physiology. Head turns to the right lead to right beating nystagmus due to asymmetry in neural firing between the right and left labyrinths. **(B)** When the right labyrinth loses function, the imbalance between resting neural firing from the intact left labyrinth and ablated right side results in left beating nystagmus. **(C)** Within a matter of days, static compensation mechanisms equalize the firing rates between the two vestibular nuclei and there is no nystagmus at rest (static compensation). **(D)** Over a longer period of time, dynamic recalibration of the VOR occurs with head movements both ipsilateral and contralateral to the lesioned side resulting in less oscillopsia. This occurs by a combination of central factors including restoration of the contralesional VOR and augmentation of ipsilesional VOR movements perhaps due to increased contralesional resting firing rate allowing for better VOR modulation with movement toward the lesioned side. (Courtesy of Kamran Barin, Ph.D.)

unrestrained animals with normal visual input, although all animals recovered to the same level over time. In cases of bilateral vestibular ablation, both the speed and overall level of recovery of balance was affected.[21] In these cases, elimination or distortion of the visual world produced greater instability compared with normal animals. In humans, recovery of balance occurs rapidly following unilateral vestibular injury as measured by dynamic platform posturography. In patients with acquired bilateral loss, postural stability is heavily dependent on adequate proprioceptive input and, to a lesser extent, visual input; simultaneous perturbations to the support surface and visual surround produce a "free fall" response due to absence of any reliable sensory cue for orientation. In these patients, postural adaptation consists of maximal utilization of somatosensory and visual cues and avoidance of sensory conflict or deprivation.

In some instances, prolonged postural instability following vestibular injury or loss is attributed to poor resolution of conflict between the remaining sensory cues. These patients have difficulty whenever visual and somatosensory cues do not match and instability occurs when choosing the "orientationally incorrect" input. This problem may be viewed as a form of maladaptation following vestibular injury.

◆ Case Examples of Vestibular Pathophysiology

For a discussion of clinical and laboratory testing in the following cases, the reader is referred to Chapters 10 and 14.

Case 1: Unilateral Vestibular Loss

A 46-year-old woman experiences acute onset of vertigo, nausea, and vomiting upon arising one morning. No hearing loss, tinnitus, or other neurologic symptom was noted. Symptoms slowly faded after 24 hours. Physical findings included brisk left-beating spontaneous nystagmus (increased on left gaze), postural instability to the right, and a positive tandem Romberg sign. Three months after the onset of vertigo, the patient still complained of mid-dysequilibrium with rapid head motions (especially to the right) and a worsening of her balance when she was tired.

Comments

1. Acute loss of unilateral peripheral function creates a large imbalance in tonic vestibular input from the labyrinth to the brainstem, resulting in spontaneous nystagmus beating toward the intact side. Peripheral nystagmus is unidirectional and increases with gaze in the direction of the fast phase. Central rebalancing of tonic activity causes the spontaneous nystagmus to rapidly abate.

2. Patients with acute unilateral loss tend to feel that they are falling toward the lesioned side due to an ipsilateral reduction in extensor tone. Tandem Romberg testing sharpens the ability to detect this finding by narrowing the base of support.

3. Over weeks to months, the central nervous system adapts to the unilateral loss of function, and the severe symptoms of vertigo disappear. With high acceleration head movements toward the lesioned side, dynamic asymmetry between the two sides is brought out and the patient experiences

momentary dysequilibrium; during periods of exhaustion, prolonged bed rest or stress, symptoms of imbalance and even vertigo frequently reappear. Furthermore, in cases of poorly compensated unilateral loss, even movements toward the intact ear result in symptoms due to poor central calibration of the VOR after injury.

Case 2: Vestibulo-Ocular Bilateral Vestibular Loss

A 67-year-old man with diabetes, hypertension, and mild peripheral neuropathy presented with slowly progressive postural instability in the dark and decreased visual acuity while driving a car. Physical examination revealed decreased dynamic visual acuity with head shaking and refixation saccades with impulsive head movements in either direction. Romberg testing was abnormal in tandem stance or on 3-inch foam with or without eyes closed. Video-oculography (VOG) with caloric stimulation revealed absent caloric responses even to ice water. Rotational chair testing showed abnormal gain and phase of the VOR up to 1.0 Hz with normal visual-vestibular interaction. Dynamic platform posturography revealed instability on conditions 2 (platform still, eyes closed) and 3 (platform still, screen moving) and falls on conditions 5 (platform moving, eyes closed) and 6 (screen moving). The patient was referred for vestibular rehabilitation.

Comments

1. Acquired bilateral loss can be slow or rapid in onset depending on the etiology. In this case, progressive loss of function presumably was due to diabetic and hypertensive microangiopathy of the vestibular labyrinth. With symmetric loss of function, large tonic imbalances of peripheral input do not occur, and hence there rarely is nystagmus or severe vertigo.

2. Evidence for bilateral loss of VOR input includes reduced dynamic visual acuity and the presence of refixation saccades. In effect, when the speed of head movement exceeds the capacity of visual tracking, retinal slippage occurs and vision degrades. Refixation saccades directed back toward the target imply unwanted movement of the eyes with the head during head rotation and a compensatory ocular movement to realign the target on the retina.

3. Postural stability in patients with bilateral loss of vestibular function is heavily dependent on vision and proprioception. In this case with concomitant peripheral neuropathy, balance is easily degraded on tandem Romberg testing with or without visual input. When this patient walks in the dark, all three primary inputs (visual, vestibular, and proprioceptive) for balance are affected and his stability is severely impaired.

4. Video-oculography confirms bilateral dysfunction as noted in absent caloric responses. This, however, does not document the extent of VOR injury across the entire operative frequencies of the reflex. Rotary chair examination confirms broad-frequency damage through 1.0 Hz. Finally, even though visual tracking mechanisms are intact up to 1.0 Hz, head movements that exceed this frequency lead to oscillopsia.

5. Dynamic platform posturography documents vestibular loss of posture control mechanisms on conditions 5 and 6. The patient's poor proprioception due to neuropathy also

hampers his balance on conditions 2 and 3 where vision is impaired as well.

6. This type of patient can be helped by exercises designed to enhance remaining vestibular function and maximize utilization of alternative sensory inputs, along with instructions for modification of daily activities to avoid movements that exceed the capabilities of any remaining inputs (see Chapter 30).

Case 3:   Mixed Peripheral-Central Disease

A 75-year-old man with hypercholesterolemia and diabetes suffered acute vertigo and profound hearing loss in the left ear 6 months ago. Recovery of balance was slow due to inactivity and fear of falling. Over the next 6 months, the patient had three episodes of severe vertigo and diplopia and dysarthria lasting 15 minutes; one episode was accompanied by syncope for 5 minutes. Physical examination showed refixation saccades with rapid leftward head turns and impaired smooth pursuit in both directions despite normal visual acuity. Saccades were inaccurate with repeated overshoots. Romberg testing was abnormal with eyes closed and feet together or in the tandem stance. There was significant decrease in vibratory sense and joint proprioception in the lower extremities.

Comments

1. Acute loss of hearing and balance are due to infarction of the labyrinthine arterial supply off of the anterior inferior cerebellar artery. Subsequent spells of vertigo with diplopia, slurred speech, and syncope constituted transient ischemic attacks because labyrinthine malfunction alone could not account for all these central nervous system symptoms.

2. Abnormal smooth pursuit can be a central finding once alternative explanations (acuity, drugs, inattention, normal aging decline) are ruled out. Localization of the lesion on this finding alone is difficult. Unidirectional pursuit deficits, however, can be localized to the ipsilateral parietal cortex.

3. Saccadic dysmetria (hypermetric saccades) is an indicator of cerebellar dysfunction in the absence of drug effects. On the other hand, hypometric saccades may or may not be indicative of midline cerebellar disease.

4. Compensation for the peripheral (inner ear) injury in this patient is slow due to inactivity and damage within the compensatory mechanisms of the brain. Both visual tracking and postural somatosensation systems are affected by vascular degenerative processes.

5. In addition to appropriate treatment of his medical diseases, therapy for this patient consists of rehabilitative exercises to increase activity, and avoidance of rapid position changes, which cause brief loss of posture control. Due to complete loss of labyrinthine input from the left ear, rapid leftward head turns always will cause symptoms of visual blurring.

6. The loss of vibratory and joint sensation in the lower extremities complicates posture control in this patient because vestibular cues also are distorted and central compensatory mechanisms are impaired. It is especially important in this case to maximize visual input because it is the only remaining "intact" sensory input.

Case 4:   Motion Sensitivity Syndrome

A 47-year-old woman suffered from "car sickness" since childhood. She always had great difficulty reading in a car, riding in the backseat, going on carnival rides, and boat trips. Six months ago, after an extended trip around the world by air, boat, and train, the patient developed prolonged dysequilibrium and a sense of ground movement. Physical examination was entirely normal. A variety of medications was tried for this sensation to no avail. The patient severely limited her activities due to this sensation.

Comments

1. Motion sensitivity syndromes (motion intolerance, motion "sickness") are caused by sensory conflict among visual, vestibular, and somatosensory inputs in certain susceptible individuals. Symptoms often appear in childhood and may weaken or intensify in adulthood.

2. The physical examination in patients with motion sensitivity syndrome almost is always normal due to the fact that the problem does not lie in sensory inputs themselves but rather in how the brain coordinates these senses.

3. A severe form of motion sensitivity, termed maldebarquement syndrome, is seen after protracted travel with significant visual and vestibular stimulation. Following such a trip, patients can complain of disturbing sensations of motion for up to a year. Vestibular suppressive medications are employed with disappointing results; vigorous exercise, however, has been helpful to break this cycle.

4. Some motion-sensitive patients suffer from migraine headaches and associated dizziness and are treated successfully with diet modification and migraine prophylactic medications.

5. Treatment of motion sensitivity syndrome consists of avoidance of sensory conflict, vestibular suppressive medication, and general conditioning exercises.

References

1. Hudspeth AJ. Mechanoelectrical transduction by hair cells in the acousticolateralis sensory system. Annu Rev Neurosci 1983;6:187–215

2. Jackler RK, Brackmann DE, eds. Textbook of Neurotology. St. Louis: Mosby, 1993

3. Wilson VJ, Melvill-Jones G, eds. Mammalian Vestibular Physiology. New York: Plenum Press, 1979

4. Raphan T, Cohen B. Velocity storage and the ocular response to multidimensional vestibular stimuli. Rev Oculomot Res 1985;1:123–143

5. Baloh RW, Honrubia V, eds. Clinical Neurophysiology of the Vestibular System, 2nd ed. Philadelphia: FA Davis, 1990

6. Gresty MA, Bronstein AM, Brandt T, Dieterich M. Neurology of otolith function: peripheral and central disorders. Brain 1992;115:647–673

7. DeVris H. The mechanisms of the labyrinth otoliths. Acta Otolaryngol 1950;38:262–273

8. Bush GA, Perachio AA, Angelaki DE. Encoding of head acceleration in vestibular neurons: I. Spatiotemporal response properties to linear acceleration. J Neurophysiol 1993;69:2039–2055

9. Highstein SM. The central nervous system efferent control of the organs of balance and equilibrium. Neurosci Res 1991;12:13–30

10. Lisberger SG. Neural basis for motor learning in the vestibulo-ocular reflex of primates: III. Computational and behavioral analyses of sites of learning. J Neurophysiol 1994;72:928–953

11. Busettini C, Miles FA, Schwarz U, Carl JR. Human ocular responses to translation of the observer and of the scene: dependence on viewing distance. Exp Brain Res 1994;100:484–494

12. Furman JM. Role of posturography in the management of vestibular patients. Otolaryngol Head Neck Surg 1995;112:8–15

13. Cullen KE, Belton T, McCrea RA. A non-visual mechanisms for voluntary cancellation of the vestibulo-ocular reflex. Exp Brain Res 1991; 83: 237–252

14. Moller C, White V, Odkvist LM. Plasticity of compensatory eye movements in rotary tests. II: The effect of voluntary, visual, imaginary, auditory, and proprioceptive mechanisms. Acta Otolaryngol 1990;109: 168–178

15. Furman JM, Baloh RW. Otolith-ocular testing in human subjects. Ann N Y Acad Sci 1992;656:431–451

16. Cass SP, Kartush JM, Graham MD. Patterns of vestibular function following vestibular nerve section. Laryngoscope 1992;102:388–394

17. Curthoys IS, Halmagyi GM. Vestibular compensation: a review of the oculomotor, neural, and clinical consequences of unilateral vestibular loss. J Vestib Res 1995;5:67–107

18. Paige GD. Vestibuloocular reflex and its interactions with visual following mechanisms in the squirrel monkey. II: Inactivation of horizontal canal. J Neurophysiol 1983;49:152–168

19. Hain TC, Fetter M, Zee DS. Headshaking nystagmus in patients with unilateral peripheral vestibular lesions. Am J Otolaryngol 1987;8: 36–47

20. Proceedings: Changes in human vestibulo-ocular response induced by vision reversal during head rotation. J Physiol (London) 1973;234: 102–103

21. Igarashi M, Kato Y. Effect of different vestibular lesions upon body equilibrium function in squirrel monkeys. Acta Otolaryngol Suppl 1975; 330:91–99

4

Middle Ear Molecular Biology

Allen F. Ryan, Michelle Hernandez, and Stephen I. Wasserman

The process of hearing depends on specialized groups of cells working in concert to deliver acoustic information from the ear to the brain. The function of these specialized cells, in turn, requires the activation of specific sets of genes. In otologic disease states, the expression of genes in the cells of the ear may be altered. In addition, during infection, disease organisms bring their own genes into play. The gene sequences expressed in the ear therefore provide a potential wealth of information regarding normal otologic biology and disease. Methods to recover this information have been developed at a rapid rate, and are now being applied to clinical and basic science problems in otology. Such molecular information can be used for diagnostic purposes, and to increase our understanding of the etiologies of otologic diseases. Moreover, methods with which to manipulate gene expression directly are now under active development, and may in the future translate into gene therapy for use in otology. Molecular biology is also helping to elucidate the basic cellular processes that govern hearing. These processes include the expression of genes involved in middle and inner ear homeostasis, production of proteins unique to the ear, cochlear and vestibular transduction, neurotransmission, responses to inner ear damage, and hair cell regeneration.

This chapter briefly describes the basic methods of molecular biology. The molecular biology of the middle ear (ME) is also explored. We concentrate on immediate and future clinical applications of the basic molecular research being performed today. More specifically, the focus is on molecular diagnostics, pathogen genomes, and vaccine development as well as aspects of host biology that underlie inflammatory responses, tissue hyperplasia, and bacterial resistance in otitis media (OM). Factors that predispose patients to ME infections are also considered. We also describe current work on growth factors that contribute to the healing of tympanic membrane perforations.

◆ Basic Methods in Molecular Biology

A short review of the basic molecular processes that take place within a cell will facilitate an understanding of the information contained in this chapter. One of the most fundamental events that occur within a cell is transcription of a gene, encoded in the genomic DNA of the cell nucleus, into messenger RNA (mRNA). During transcription, a faithful RNA copy of the gene sequence is produced within the nucleus. This copy is then edited to remove segments, called introns, which are not required for the production of protein. The remaining RNA segments, called exons, are spliced together to form the mature mRNA, which is then exported to the cytoplasm for translation. The mRNA is translated into protein by ribosomes, which assemble amino acids sequentially according to the mRNA blueprint. Once the protein is produced, there can be substantial modifications to its structure via posttranslational processing. This can involve cleavage, phosphorylation, the addition of carbohydrate moieties, and other changes that alter the behavior of the protein.

A basic technique of molecular biology is DNA cloning. Segments of DNA can be isolated by digestion with enzymes that cleave the DNA at specific sites (restriction enzymes) and cloned into a variety of self-replicating DNA structures, called vectors, which have been derived by genetic engineering primarily from naturally occurring bacteriophages. When the vectors replicate within bacteria in the laboratory, millions of copies of the inserted DNA sequence are produced, and can then be analyzed.

A second basic method is reverse transcription. Viral enzymes known as reverse transcriptases are capable of producing complementary DNA (cDNA) copies of RNA. When this is applied to mRNA, it allows the rapid and efficient cloning of the mRNA sequences. Because RNA is a relatively ephemeral molecule, cDNAs provide a stable record of the mRNA. Together, reverse transcription and DNA cloning have revolutionized the study of genetics and protein chemistry.

A third method with wide application is the polymerase chain reaction (PCR), which relies on the repeated replication of double-stranded DNA. Through heating, double-stranded DNA separates to form single strands, whose specific sequences can then be replicated. With appropriate primers to recognize the sequence, two identical double-stranded DNA segments are then formed. This process is repeated many times, resulting in exponential amplification of the original DNA sequence. The use of DNA components that fluoresce when integrated into such copies allows the original amount of target DNA to be quantified in a process known as real-time or quantitative PCR (Q-PCR).

Tremendous strides have been made in DNA sequencing technology, which has led to the recent sequencing of not just the human, mouse, and chimp genomes, but also the genomes of many disease organisms. This includes pathogens that contribute to otologic diseases. It has been estimated that the cost of sequencing a human genome will decrease to around $1000 within 10 years, which could make patients' genome sequence part of their medical record. Rapid sequencing of cDNAs has also allowed us to profile thousands of cDNA sequences expressed by individual tissues and organs, including the inner ear.[1] The availability of genome sequences has allowed the development of gene arrays, or chips, which include essentially all genes, permitting rapid and comprehensive profiling of gene expression in tissue samples. Gene expression can be localized at the cellular level using in situ hybridization of mRNA, in which complementary probes are used to label mRNA in tissue sections.

The increase in sequence information has had a tremendous impact on genetics, allowing the identification of an increasing array of unique molecular markers for linkage analysis, a process by which inherited disorders are linked to a particular chromosomal location. The precision of linkage and the complete map of genes in the region have made the identification of disease-causing mutations significantly easier and faster.

In the experimental realm, techniques for engineering the DNA of animals have become commonplace, resulting in the generation of numerous gene deletion (knockout) mice for many genes. Methods to limit gene deletion to specific tissues (conditional knockouts) have allowed the analysis of deletions that may be embryonically lethal. Deletions that can be activated at a given time (inducible knockouts) allow developmental functions to be separated from the role of a gene in the adult. Gene substitution (knock-in) techniques allow animal models of specific human mutations to be created.

Although there have as yet been few applications to patients, gene therapy methods have advanced greatly with the development of improved viral vectors for induced gene expression. They have been used successfully in the ear, most spectacularly in hair cell regeneration.[2] In addition, gene silencing through such techniques as short, interference RNA (siRNA) promises to improve the treatment of dominant genetic disorders.

This review of molecular biology is necessarily limited, and is intended only as a brief introduction. For more detailed information on the methods outlined above, and on many other aspects of gene structure and function, many excellent reviews are available.[3–5]

◆ Molecular Biology of the Middle Ear

Host Responses During Otitis Media

From a molecular perspective, the normal tympanic cavity is a relatively quiescent tissue environment. With the exception of the ME muscles, the activities of the acoustic transmission apparatus are largely passive, and that of the remaining ME tissues are related primarily to homeostasis. Thus, the ME mucosa and eustachian tube maintain the gaseous environment of the ME and maintain a first line of defense against potential infection. However, in disease the ME becomes highly active and exhibits substantial levels of molecular activity. This activity determines the response of the ME to infection, and recent research has generated a substantial amount of new information regarding molecular events during OM. Also, variation in the molecular response to infection is thought to be a major component of differential sensitivity to this disease.

Mucosal Hyperplasia and Recovery

The mucosa that lines the ME cavity can undergo extensive modification during OM, involving changes in the expression of a large number of genes. In response to inflammation, the mucosa changes from a simple, squamous epithelial monolayer to a pseudostratified, respiratory epithelium with many cell layers. This respiratory epithelium has goblet and ciliated cells, and a greatly expanded stroma and vasculature. The hyperplasia of the mucosa is rapid, occurring in a few days, and involves extensive cell proliferation and differentiation. Recovery from OM is characterized by rapid loss of these additional cells, and return to a relatively simple epithelial morphology.

ME mucosal hyperplasia is almost certainly controlled in part by growth factors (GFs) through their interaction with specific transmembrane receptors. The role of GFs in the regulation of cellular growth and differentiation in other tissues is undisputed, and we have obtained substantial evidence that GFs play a similar role in the ME during OM.[6,7] GFs produce their effects on cells by interacting with specific transmembrane receptors. Although there are several classes of GF receptors, many are tyrosine kinase (TK) receptors, including those for the fibroblast GF (FGF), vascular endothelial GF (VEGF), and epidermal GF (EGF) families. GF binding leads to receptor dimerization and autophosphorylation of the intracellular TK domains. Once phosphorylated, the TK domains interact with cytoplasmic adaptor proteins to activate intracellular signaling cascades.[8,9] Many of the adaptor proteins that interact directly with GF receptors bind via src homology 2 (SH2) domains, and link to additional proteins via SH3 domains.[10] A wealth of signaling cascades can be activated. However, the mitogen-activated protein kinase (MAPK) pathways are perhaps the most closely associated with tissue proliferation. MAPK activation stimulates gene expression via transcription factors, including AP-1, Elk1, ATF-2, and CREB, that are often involved in the proliferative responses.[11]

Other transmembrane receptors are also likely to be involved in mucosal responses during OM. Several mammalian cell surface receptors directly recognize pathogens. These pathogen-associated receptor proteins (PARPs) include the Toll-like receptors (TLRs) and transforming GF-β receptors,[12] which recognize a variety of pathogen-associated molecular patterns (PAMPs). The best-studied PARPs are the TLRs. Recognized by their homology to the *Drosophila* Toll receptor, the 10 human (and 13 mouse) TLRs have been shown to be important mediators of responses to pathogenic organisms.[14] Because each receptor senses a distinct repertoire of conserved microbial molecules, collectively they can detect most if not all microbes.[15] Several elegant studies using epithelial cell lines derived from the human ME mucosa have linked TLR signaling to the production of mucin and cytokines in these cells.[16–19] Of particular importance for OM are the TLRs that respond to bacterial products. These include TLR4, which responds to the lipopolysaccharide (LPS) of gram-negative bacteria.[20] TLR1 and TLR2 respond to bacterial lipoproteins, lipopeptides, and other molecules, whereas TLR9 responds to CpG-containing DNA, from both gram-negative and gram-positive bacteria.[5] Given their distributions in other tissues[21,22] and ME epithelial cell lines,[16–19] TLRs should be present on a variety of cell types in the ME. Downstream signaling from these TLRs occurs via a family of adaptor molecules, especially MyD88 and MAL, which via a series of intermediates can activate the MAPKs as well as NF-κB. These events influence the expression of many genes involved in inflammation, tissue proliferation, apoptosis, and other processes.[5,15,23] MyD88-independent pathway for TLR4, involving TRAM and TRIF, is activated later and can activate NF-κB and produce interferon-β (IFN-β), leading to gene activation.[5,15,23] Thus there are multiple means by which TLRs might influence mucosal proliferation. MyD88 is also used as an adaptor for interleukin-1 (IL-1) signaling, activating many of the same downstream signaling cascades.[23] Other receptors that can mediate host cell responses to the bacterium nontypeable *Haemophilus influenzae* (NTHi) include the PAF receptor,[24] ganglioside receptors,[25] and β-glucan receptor.[26] Bacteria may also signal via direct mechanical action by the motile type IV pilus,[27] a pilus form recently demonstrated on NTHi.[28]

Although many groups have evaluated the proliferative response of ME tissue in cholesteatoma, fewer groups have studied the ME mucosa itself. However, several laboratories have evaluated GFs in the ME mucosa during OM. For example, Palacios et al[29] surveyed mRNAs encoding epithelial GFs in the ME mucosa of rats during experimental bacterial otitis. They observed rapidly increased expression of several EGF family members, including EGF itself, human GF (HGF), and neuregulin-α, but reported a downregulation of β-cellulin. Both EGF and HGF receptors were also upregulated. Yetiser et al[30] evaluated EGF levels in granulation tissue recovered from patients with OM, and found EGF levels comparable to those in skin but lower than those in cholesteatoma. These results suggest that several GFs have the potential to be involved in epithelial proliferation during OM.

Similarly, Jung et al[31] assessed mRNAs encoding isoforms of VEGF during OM. Expression of several VEGF isoforms increased within 1 hour of endotoxin instillation in the rat ME, and remained elevated for several days. VEGF expression was also elevated in chronic human ME effusions. Their data suggest that VEGF may be involved in neovascularization of the ME subepithelial tissue during otitis.

In vitro model systems have been developed for the evaluation of GF effects on the ME mucosa. For example, Palacios et al[32] exposed cultured explants of normal rat ME epithelium to several epithelial GFs. Significant enhancement of epithelial growth from the explants was observed with keratinocyte growth factor (KGF), β-cellulin, and EGF, whereas suppression of growth was observed with HGF and heregulin. Evidence of increased epithelial differentiation was observed with KGF, HGF, amphiregulin, and heregulin (**Fig. 4–1**).

Binding of GFs to their cognate receptors is linked to the cell nucleus, and then to cellular responses including proliferation and differentiation, by intracellular signaling pathways. To explore these pathways during OM, Palacios et al[33] developed an in vitro model of bacterially induced mucosal proliferation. They found that ME mucosa harvested 48 hours after instillation of NTHi into the ME exhibited greatly enhanced proliferation in culture. They evaluated the signaling events involved in this response using assays for activation of signal transduction molecules, as well as specific inhibitors of different pathways. They observed phosphorylation of the Erk MAPK immediately after instillation of bacteria in the ME, and then later during the resolution phase. Inhibitors of both the small G protein Ras and the Erk MAPK blocked bacterially induced proliferation in ME cultures. The results suggest that Ras-Erk signaling plays a critical role in ME proliferation during OM, and may also mediate aspects of recovery from OM. Palacios et al[34] used a similar strategy to evaluate signaling via p38 MAPK. This MAPK is activated early in OM, and as with Ras-Erk, inhibition reduced mucosal proliferation.

OM involves not only mucosal proliferation but also in many cases osteoneogenesis. Melhus and Ryan[35] assayed the expression of genes involved in bone formation during bacterial otitis in the rat, using quantitative PCR. They found that after a brief period of inhibition of genes associated with osteoclast activity, a prolonged period of expression of bone formation genes occurs. The regulation of mucosal proliferation and differentiation during OM offers opportunities for novel treatments designed to return the mucosa to its resting state.

Mucus Production

Mucins are an important structural component of the mucociliary transport system of the ME mucosa, especially of the eustachian tube, and as such contribute to ME defense again infection. With the exception of the region near the eustachian tube orifice, the normal ME mucosa has few goblet cells and produces mucus at low levels. However, during OM the population of goblet cells and the production of mucus can increase dramatically. Mucus can become an important component of ME effusions, contributing to their viscosity and persistence, and thence to the negative sequelae of OM.

Mucins are large, glycosylated proteins produced by mucosal epithelial cells, and are the major component of mucus. They protect epithelial surfaces by trapping infectious particles, including bacteria and viruses, for mucociliary clearance. Thus the expression of mucin genes in infectious diseases, including OM, is an important component of the host response to microbes. Of the 18 mucins identified, there is currently evidence that 11 are expressed in the ME of patients during OM.[36–40] Recently, substantial evidence has been obtained regarding how the genes encoding these mucins are regulated in the ME mucosa.

Lin et al[41] performed a gene array analysis of altered gene expression in the rat ME during pneumococcal infection. They observed upregulation of the *Muc2* and *Muc5* genes 6 weeks after inoculation. In addition, their morphology studies demonstrated a thickened mucosa and submucosa with increased expression of glycoproteins. Jono et al[38] reported that NTHi utilizes the TGF-β-Smad and TLR2-MyD88-TAK1-NIK-IKKβ/γ-IκBα pathways to upregulate *Muc2* mucin gene transcription. In contrast, Wang et al[39] and Jono et al[42] found that *Muc5Ac* transcription was upregulated by a TLR2-MyD88–dependent p38 MAPK pathway and downregulated by a phosphatidylinositol (PI$_3$)-kinase-Akt pathway. Also in contrast to *Muc2*, TGF-β-Smad signaling downregulates p38 by inducing MAPK phosphatase-1, thereby negatively

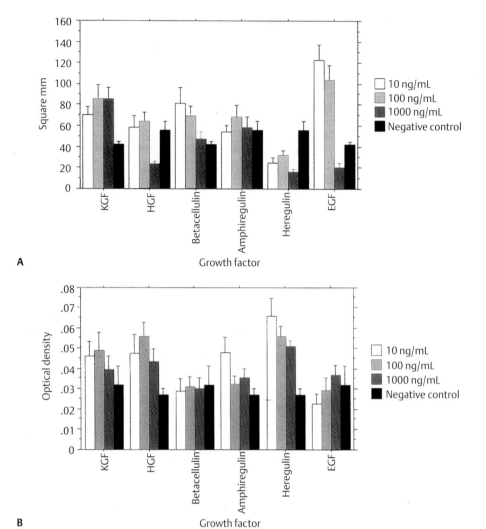

A

Growth factor

B

Growth factor

Figure 4–1 **(A)** Surface area (in millimeters squared) of epithelial growth of middle ear mucosa explants treated with different concentrations of specific growth factors (in nanograms per milliliter). Compared with the negative control (untreated) mucosa, treatment with epidermal growth factor (EGF), keratinocyte growth factor (KGF), and β-cellulin resulted in significant ($p < .05$) growth. Vertical lines represent 1 standard error (SE). **(B)** Optical density of middle ear mucosa epithelium treated with different concentrations of specific growth factors (in nanograms per milliliter) and stained with anticytokeratin antibody to evaluate the degree of differentiation of the cells. Compared with the negative control mucosa, treatment with heregulin, amphiregulin, human growth factor (HGF), and KGF resulted in significant differentiation. Vertical lines represent 1 SE.

regulating *Muc5Ac*. In addition to the studies performed using bacteria, Kim et al[43] found that bacterial LPS upregulates MUC5AC mRNA in the rat ME mucosa, with maximal expression 1 to 3 days after inoculation.

Because proinflammatory cytokines play a role in the pathogenesis of OM, Lin et al[44] assessed the effect of tumor necrosis factor-α (TNF-α) on rat ME mucin gene expression and found that TNF-α increased *Muc2* expression. Similarly, Smirnova et al[45,46] observed that TNF-α, IL-6, and IL-8 stimulated MUC5AC and MUC5B mucin secretion.

Chung et al[47] showed that MUC5AC was expressed in only a small portion of the goblet cells of ME mucosa from patients with mucoid OM. They concluded that both serous secretions and mucin might make the ME effusion more viscous and that mucins other than MUC5AC might have a major role in the viscosity of ME effusion.

As with mucosal proliferation, as our understanding of the regulation of mucin production increases, it may be possible

to design pharmacologic interventions that could reduce their production and enhance recovery from OM.

Innate Immunity

The concept of innate immunity has expanded significantly in the past decade, driven by the discovery of new families of natural antibiotic substances, and transmembrane receptors that respond to a wide variety of molecules produced by pathogens, such as the TLRs. These discoveries have revolutionized our concepts regarding the first line of defense in the ME.

Lim et al[48] demonstrated the importance of innate immune molecules in protecting the tubotympanum against OM pathogens. Their results show that β-defensin-1 (BD-1) and BD-2, surfactant proteins A and D, lysozyme, and lactoferrin are expressed in the ME and eustachian tube. They also found that the defensins and lysozyme have distinct and potent antimicrobial activity against NTHi, *Streptococcus pneumoniae,* and *Moraxella catarrhalis.* Moon et al[49] found BD-2 is expressed in the ME mucosa of humans and rats, and that its expression is upregulated by proinflammatory stimuli such as IL-1α, TNF-α, and LPS. Moreover, they demonstrated that transcriptional activation of the BD-2 gene is mediated through an Src-dependent Ras-Raf-MEK1/2-ERK pathway.

Stenfors et al[50] evaluated the coating of the bacteria with antibacterial substances, including lysozyme, lactoferrin, and immunoglobulins IgG, secretory IgA, and IgM. They also tested the microbes' ability to penetrate epithelial cells during infectious mononucleosis (IM) caused by Epstein-Barr virus. The samples studied were collected from the oropharynx of patients with current IM. Their results demonstrated a significant reduction in bacterial coating with IgG and S-IgA, whereas a significant increase in coating was observed with lactoferrin and IgM. No significant change in coating of the bacteria by lysozyme was seen. The authors concluded that reduced bacterial coating with IgG and S-IgA immunoglobulins, combined with bacterial penetration into epithelial cells, may exacerbate the bacterial colonization of oropharyngeal mucosal membranes observed during IM. This enhanced colonization may result in a greater frequency of infections such as OM and sinusitis.

The initiation of inflammatory responses to pathogens in acute OM is important for understanding innate immunity and the first line of defense against OM, and may lead to innovative strategies that harness these responses to enhance resistance to OM. However, it should be noted that a dysregulated innate immune response, with sustained production of proinflammatory mediators, could contribute to chronic ME disease.

Genetic Components of Otitis Media Susceptibility

The molecular response that occurs in the ME during OM is complex. It provides many opportunities for differences in OM phenotypes among individuals who may express different forms of critical proteins or may have mutations in critical genes. It has long been suspected that OM susceptibility can be an inherited trait because the susceptibility of siblings is correlated and because different racial groups often have different frequencies of OM. It is therefore reasonable to expect that genetic factors play a role in OM. Several genetic defects in immunity and other host response mechanisms have been reported to be associated with OM susceptibility. For example, studies of human leukocyte antigen (HLA) factors in otitis-prone versus normal children have revealed that HLA-2A is more prevalent in the otitis-prone population.[51] Similarly, a common mutation in the gene encoding mannan-binding protein, involved in complement activation, may also be more prevalent in otitis-prone children.[52] In addition, several genetic defects influence the morphology of the ME and eustachian tube,[53–57] which could influence OM susceptibility. However, it has been difficult to completely separate genetic from environmental factors.[58]

The strongest evidence supporting a genetic basis for otitis susceptibility has come from twin studies. Two recent investigations comparing OM in monozygotic and dizygotic twin pairs suggest that 60 to 70% of the variation in OM susceptibility is due to genetic factors.[59,60]

Identifying the genes involved will be challenging. Molecular genetic methodology should help to address this issue. Positional cloning techniques have been found to be extremely useful in identifying single genes causal in specific diseases, including Huntington's disease, cystic fibrosis, and Crouzon syndrome. It is unlikely that OM susceptibility is influenced only by a single gene. Analysis of OM patients with a statistical method known as quantitative trait locus may permit the identification of multiple genes relating to immunity, structure, and physiology that increase the susceptibility of individuals to the development of the disease. This technology has been recently used to identify multiple genes associated with insulin-dependent diabetes mellitus, and could be used to identify the molecular genetic underpinnings of OM.

Otitis Media in Mutant Mouse Strains

Genetic variation in humans can also be modeled in animals. In fact, some of the most useful molecular tools for research are natural and induced mutations. Mouse models of gene deletions and specific mutations can provide powerful insights into the role of individual genes, as they operate within the context of the intact organism, in OM. Recent developments in the use of mouse models for OM[35,61] have laid the foundation for the use of mutant mice to probe molecular mechanisms in this disease.

Ebmeyer et al[62] evaluated OM in mice with mutations in the gene encoding the mast cell stem cell factor Kit1. These mice completely lack mast cells, which are by far the most common leukocyte in the normal ME mucosa. They found that mast cell–deficient mice exhibited a significantly reduced ME response to bacterial infection, when compared with wild-type controls. Moreover, this deficit could be corrected by transplanting mast cells derived from the bone marrow of wild-type animals, which populated the ME mucosa (**Fig. 4–2**). This study suggests that mast cells are an important component of the innate immune response of the ME cavity during the initial stages of OM.

Rivkin et al[63] evaluated endotoxin-induced OM in *lpr/lpr* mice, which have a deficit in the apoptosis receptor Fas. They found that mucosal hyperplasia during OM was enhanced in *lpr/lpr* mice, when compared with wild-type controls. In addition, the recovery of the mucosa was significantly delayed in Fas-deficient mice. The results suggest that Fas-mediated apoptosis plays a role in the remodeling of the ME mucosa during OM-induced mucosal growth, and that the recovery of the mucosa during OM resolution involves apoptosis mediated by death ligands and receptors.

Several large mutagenesis projects have used tagged, single-base mutations to identify the genes associated with various phenotypes. The European ethylnitrosourea (ENU) mutagenesis project for dominant mutations has recently identified mice with mutations that increase the incidence of OM.[64] Identification of the proteins altered in these mutations will provide new information on mechanisms of OM susceptibility.

Gene Arrays

Another advantage of the mouse as a model is the availability of sequence data for this species. Complete sequencing of the mouse genome and years of transcription profiling in a variety of tissues have generated rich resources for probing

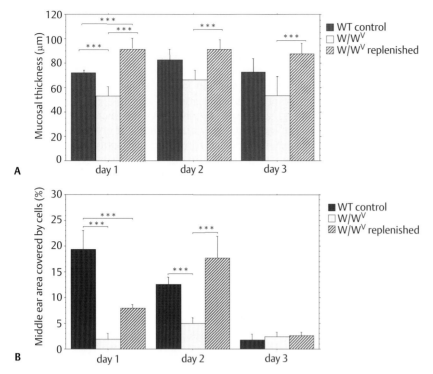

Figure 4–2 **(A)** Thickness of the middle ear (ME) mucosa in micrometers (μm) after challenge with nontypeable *Haemophilus influenzae* (NTHi). Mast cell–deficient animals (W/Wv) exhibited significantly less mucosal growth than wild-type (WT control) mice at 24 hours. The ME mucosal response to NTHi was restored when bone-marrow–derived mast cells were transplanted into mast cell–deficient mice (W/Wv replenished). Values are means ± SE; asterisks indicate statistical significance ($p \leq .05$); $n = 6–8$ for each group. **(B)** Percentage of the ME lumen that was filled with inflammatory cells after challenge with NTHi. Very few leukocytes infiltrated the MEs of mast cell–deficient mice. However, mast cell–replenished mice showed significant restoration of leukocyte infiltration. Values are means ± SE; asterisks indicate statistical significance ($p \leq .05$); $n = 6–8$ for each group.

murine gene expression. One application of these resources is the gene array or chip. Current arrays contain representative probes for virtually all of the genes in the mouse genome, such as the Affymetrix 2.0 array, which has more than 55,000 transcripts represented. Chung et al[65] used this array to assess gene expression in the mouse ME in the first 24 hours following exposure to NTHi. They observed 513 transcripts that were significantly upregulated 3 hours after inoculation, whereas only two transcripts were downregulated. At 6 hours, 658 upregulated transcripts were noted, as compared with 188 downregulated genes. By 24 hours after bacterial exposure, 1350 transcripts showed increased expression, whereas 1632 exhibited reduced expression. The results indicate that the initial response to infection involves the upregulation of a relatively small number of genes. This included, as expected, genes encoding inflammatory mediators or receptors. Genes encoding components of innate immune response, such as TLRs, were also affected. However, many of the genes identified were unexpected, and their roles must be explored. This technology shows great promise for identifying genes that are involved in the pathogenesis or resolution of OM, and for which we currently have no evidence to suggest a role.

Molecular Responses of Bacteria and Molecular Vaccine Strategies

Advances in genomics have by no means been confined to mammals. Complete genomes were produced for bacteria long before the human genome was sequenced, and the genomes of many additional microbial species and strains have since been generated. This includes organisms that are frequently involved in OM. These and other genetic developments have contributed to significant advances in our understanding of otitis pathogens. Genomics, molecular biology, and proteomics have been used to study the properties of bacterial genes and proteins, with the goal of understanding the basic process of infection and contributions of bacterial molecules to pathogenesis in infectious diseases including OM. This information is also being used translationally, to develop innovative approaches to the diagnosis, treatment, and prevention of OM, including vaccine development.

Streptococcus pneumoniae

S. pneumoniae is the most common species of bacterium isolated from the ME in OM. The genomes of a variety of *S. pneumoniae* strains have been published.[66–68] Wizemann et al[69] used the whole genome sequence of *S. pneumoniae* to identify novel microbial targets for vaccine development. They predicted virulence factors based on protein structure consistent with surface localization, and the presence of protein motifs related to secretion or surface binding. They identified 130 genes encoding such proteins. Immunization with 108 of these proteins revealed six that conferred protection against pneumococcal infection. Moreover, these six protective antigens showed broad distribution across several strains, and immunogenicity during human infection. This study demonstrates the power of genome-based methods to identify important bacterial proteins.

A powerful molecular technique known as signature-tagged mutagenesis was used by Lau and colleagues,[70] in concert with analysis of the *S. pneumoniae* type 3 genomic sequence, to identify and characterize genes required for pathogenesis. Nearly 2000 tagged mutations were created and screened for the inability to survive and replicate in mouse models of pneumonia and bacteremia; 186 of these mutants proved to be so attenuated, and 42 novel virulence genes were identified. Five mutations, in genes involved in gene regulation, cation transport, or stress tolerance, were shown to be highly attenuated when tested individually in a murine respiratory tract infection model.

Another powerful molecular tool, differential fluorescence induction (DFI) was used by Marra and colleagues[71] to screen for *S. pneumoniae* genes that vary their expression during infection, suggesting a functional role. Sequence encoding green fluorescent protein (GFP) was randomly inserted into the *S. pneumoniae* genome, and in many cases GFP expression was influenced by the promoter of an adjacent bacterial gene. GFP expression was then assessed under in vitro conditions chosen to mimic various aspects of the host in vivo environment, including changes in temperature, osmolarity, oxygen and iron concentration, as well as the presence or absence of blood in the media. A total of 25 genes whose promoters were induced twofold or greater under conditions that mimic infection were identified. They were then mutated to assess their role in virulence using at least two different infection models. More than 50% of these mutants were attenuated in at least one model system. Thus, the authors concluded that DFI is a useful tool for identifying bacterial virulence factors as well as identifying conditions that control their expression.

Nontypeable Haemophilus influenzae *(NTHi)*

Similar genomic and proteomic approaches are being used to understand pathogenesis of NTHi-induced OM, and to identify novel targets for therapeutics or vaccine development. van Schilfgaarde and colleagues[72] cloned NTHi genes involved in penetration between human lung epithelial cells. A chromosomal library of NTHi strain A960053 DNA was constructed in *Escherichia coli* DH5 to identify bacterial genes involved in paracytosis, the passage between cells. Two *E. coli* clones contained open reading frames (ORFs, protein coding sequences) homologous to genes in the published genomic sequence of *H. influenzae* strain Rd, encoding two small proteins of unknown function. Clones containing these ORFs showed significant increase in penetration of NCI-H292, a human bronchial epithelial cell line. Disruption of one of these genes (HI0636) by kanamycin cassette insertion had no effect on penetration, whereas disruption of the other (HI0638) resulted in loss of paracytosis. The authors concluded that the protein encoded by ORF HI0638 may function as a paracytin, whereas that encoded by HI0636 may have an auxiliary function.

van Ulsen et al[73] used a promoter trap library to identify NTHi genes expressed during interaction with epithelial cells of the lower airway (NCI-H292). A promoter trap vector was used to construct a genetic library of NTHi strain (A95006) (recovered from a patient with chronic obstructive pulmonary disease). Eight thousand chromosomal fragments were cloned upstream of a promoterless *cat* gene in *H. influenzae* strain Rd. Exposure of this library to NCI-H292 cells in the presence of chloramphenicol (Cam) resulted in 52 clones that were resistant to Cam, including genes belonging to the following functional classes: metabolic processes, stress response, gene expression, cell envelope biosynthesis, DNA-related processes and cell division, and ORFs containing genes of unknown function.

Mason and colleagues[74] recently used a similar promoter trap strategy for an OM isolate of NTHi. Their library was screened in a chinchilla model of acute OM to identify genes required for survival in the microenvironment of the ME. Genomic DNA fragments from NTHi strain 86–028NP were cloned upstream of the promoterless *gfpmut3* gene, and bacterial gene expression was monitored by differential fluorescence induction. Clones containing promoter elements that were induced in vivo and thus produced GFP were isolated by two-color fluorescence-activated cell sorter (FACS). Insert DNA was sequenced and compared with both the complete genomic sequence of strain Rd as well as the genome of strain 86–028NP, which has recently been sequenced.[75] A screen of 16,000 clones identified 52 clones with putative promoters that were regulated in vivo. Forty-four clones contained gene fragments encoding biosynthetic enzymes, metabolic and regulatory proteins, and hypothetical proteins of unknown function. An additional eight clones contained gene fragments unique to the OM isolate used as the host for the promoter trap library. Real-time RT-PCR was used to confirm the induction of putative promoter candidates in vivo in 26 of the 44 candidates with homology to ORFs in *H. influenzae* strain Rd. The authors concluded that these data provide insight into the response of NTHi as these bacteria sense and respond to the ME microenvironment during early events in OM.

Hou and Gu[76] have investigated the possibility of using detoxified LPS as a vaccine candidate for NTHi-induced OM. By screening a phage-display peptide library with a rabbit antibody specific for NTHi LPS, they identified peptides that mimic LPS and thus convert it into a nontoxic T-cell–dependent antigen. Using this strategy, they identified 56 phage clones found to share LPS mimicry molecules. Among these 56, 22 clones were sequenced resulting in four consensus sequences identified as NMMRFTSQPPNN, NMMNYIMDPRTH, NMMKYISPPIFL, and NMMRFTELSTPS. Three of the four synthetic peptides showed strong binding reactivity to the rabbit anti-LPS antibody and also to a mouse monoclonal antibody to NTHi LPS that had bactericidal activity in vitro. After conjugation to KLH, these peptides induced a 27- to 81-fold increase in serum anti-LPS in rabbits. Passive immunization of mice with these rabbit sera enhanced pulmonary clearance in a mouse model, an effect that was eliminated if the sera were preabsorbed with NTHi LPS. The authors concluded that mimotopes of LPS might be potential components of a peptide vaccine against NTHi.

Thoren et al[77] conducted a proteomic study of NTHi using sequential extraction and both analytical two-dimensional (2D) polyacrylamide gel electrophoresis (PAGE) and 2D semipreparative electrophoresis (PE) to study protein expression in NTHi strain A4. A total of 15 protein identities were obtained using these techniques including OMPs P2, P4, and 26, HtrA (a putative adhesin precursor), and elongation factor Tu. Although putative vaccine candidates were identified with both techniques, 11 of 15 proteins identified using the 2D PE approach were not identified by 2D PAGE, demonstrating the complementarity of the two systems.

Moraxella catarrhalis

Hays et al[78] used pulse field gel electrophoresis (PFGE) and polymerase chain reaction–restriction fragment length polymorphism (PCR-RFLP) analysis to study intragenomic variation in the *uspA1* and *uspA2* genes of *M. catarrhalis*. They found 19 pairs of PFGE-identical isolates among a set of 91 strains. Five pairs came from non–otitis-prone children, 11 pairs originated from otitis-prone children, and for three pairs, one originated from an otitis-prone and the other two from a non-prone child. No particular *M. catarrhalis* isolate was associated with either prone or non-prone children. One of the 19 pairs demonstrated both *uspA1* and *uspA2* intragenomic variation, whereas another exhibited *uspA2* intragenomic variation only. PCR-RFLP–obtained sequence data showed that these pattern differences reflected changes in predicted amino acid composition including changes in a 23 base pair NINNIY repeat region, a conserved binding site in UspA1 and UspA2 for the neutralizing antibody mAb17C7. The results may be useful for future design of UspA1 or UspA2 vaccine candidates.

To date, the genomes of several *M. catarrhalis* isolates have been sequenced; however, these sequences have been generated by private industry and are thus proprietary.

Bacterial Proteins as Sources of Defensive Strategies

Nell et al[79] investigated the capacity of rBPI21, a recombinant amino-terminal analog derived from bacterial permeability-increasing protein, to inhibit the effects of LPS on cultured human ME epithelium. The cultures were inspected after 4 weeks for the number of ciliated and secretory cells, thickness of the mucosal layer, and cell size. Endotoxin treatment resulted in an increase in the thickness of the mucosal layer and in the number of secretory cells. These changes were significantly diminished when endotoxin was added with rBPI21 to the culture medium, suggesting that this molecule may be useful in diminishing the effects of endotoxin.

Bacterial Phase and Strain Variation

Host efforts to eliminate bacteria and to develop defenses via cognate immunity can be complicated by the potential for phase variation that involves PAMPs. To evade both innate and cognate host defenses, pathogens have evolved effective strategies by which to vary their phenotypes. This is accomplished, in part, by generating genetic variation at contingency loci, hypermutable regions within their genomes that facilitate rapid changes in expression of genes likely to be the targets of host defenses.[80] Many of these genes, which are characterized by simple sequence tetranucleotide (e.g., AGTC, GCAA, CAAT) DNA repeats that rapidly accumulate reversible mutations, encode virulence factors. They allow the pathogens to generate a large number of phenotypes rapidly, which can be selected for survival by local conditions and host responses. For example, in NTHi strain Hd, a strain for which extensive genomic sequence is available, about 20 simple contingency loci have been identified in genes encoding LPS biosynthetic enzymes (*lic1–3, lgtC, lex2*), adhesins (*hmw1, hmw2, yadA* homolog, *hifA, hifB*),[81] iron acquisition proteins (*hgpA-C*, HI0635, 0661, 0712, 1565), and host restriction/modification proteins (*mod, hsd*). An additional six contingency loci have been identified in other strains. Contingency loci can move sequences in and out of frame to serve as on/off switches, or less commonly alter promoter regions to control the level of expression, as with the *hmw* genes.[81] Other means of genetic recombination may also contribute to phase variation in NTHi (e.g., gene conversion, transposition, and flip-flop[82]). Of course, environmental conditions can lead to changes in phenotype independent of phase variation, through the normal process of gene regulation. For example, although the gene responsible for ChoP decoration of LPS is phase-variable, its promoter is also sensitive to decreased oxygen tension.[83]

Strain differences are equally problematic for host defenses. Many different isotypes of pathogens important in OM have been identified, each with a different complement of genes. Collectively, the various strains of a disease organism can be thought of as having a collective genome, or "metagenome." Different strains can express different subsets of molecules from this metagenome. Ehrlich's group[84,85] recently estimated the number of genes that vary between strains of NTHi and *S. pneumoniae*. They found that, of a random sample of 771 genes from 10 NTHi OM isolates, approximately 10% were absent from the sequenced Rd genome. These genes varied widely in expression across strains, from 17% found in all 10 strains to a few genes occurring only in one strain.[85] Interestingly, they found a similar level of genetic variation across strains of *S. pneumoniae*.[84] These observations suggest that host signaling will vary across different bacterial strains. Allelic variation is another source of potential strain differences. Although there are marked similarities between the glycoforms produced by different NTHi isolates,[86] NTHi adhesins are known to vary between strains.[87] Thus strain variation must be taken into consideration in any study of bacterial OM.

Molecular Diagnostics

The identification of microorganisms in OM historically depended upon culture of viable bacteria. Because of the many antimicrobial substances that can be present in OM effusions, culture was often unsuccessful. More recently, molecular strategies for identification of ME pathogens have been developed.[88] Advances in microbial genomics now permit the detection of an increasing number of bacterial strains and viruses by PCR.[89]

◆ Tympanic Membrane Perforation

Chronic tympanic membrane (TM) perforations display resistance to healing due to a reduced or absent ability of cells to migrate inward from the periphery of the TM. Perforations in the TM that do not heal independently can be approached with surgical techniques such as myringoplasty or tympanoplasty using paper, fat, or fascial patches. Alternative approaches, however, have been explored using growth factors to promote cellular migration and membrane healing. Early reports on the efficacy in vivo of basic fibroblast growth factor (bFGF), epidermal growth factor, and eye-derived growth factor to promote healing in injured tissue have been encouraging.[90-96] Multiple studies have since been performed with bFGF, an 18-kD polypeptide that is a potent mitogen for a variety of cells including endothelial cells, smooth muscle cells, chondrocytes, keratinocytes, fibroblasts, and numerous mesenchymal cells.[97–99] The TM is considered to be well suited for bFGF application given that it is composed primarily of connective and epithelial tissue.

To understand how bFGF enhances TM healing, it is important to first understand the natural history of TM healing. Johnson and Hawke[99] demonstrated in 1987 that the first layer to close TM perforations is the stratum corneum. The stratum corneum has the ability to migrate and then generate a connective tissue scaffold upon which a fibrous layer may grow.[100] If the stratum corneum grows faster than the connective tissue scaffold, then inward epidermal invagination may occur and TM closure may be obstructed. bFGF has the ability to initiate early formation of the connective tissue scaffold, thereby preventing the early inward epidermal invagination and promoting cell growth, migration, and TM healing.[101] This hypertrophic subepithelial connective tissue reaction is characterized by intense fibroblast proliferation, neovascularization, and matrix deposition in a linear fashion that maintains the inward growth of the epithelial layer. The submucosal layer medial to the connective tissue scaffold shows a more modest hyperplastic response, and the mucosal layer maintains its monolayer structure. It remains to be answered whether bFGF directly affects the growth of the epidermal layer. However, EGF has been shown to endure TM healing.[102] Combined GF therapy is therefore an option. It also remains to be answered whether using a paper scaffold or cellulose membrane in addition to bFGF will enhance TM healing even further.

◆ Conclusion

The field of molecular biology remains a vibrant and rapidly developing area with research, and increasingly clinical, applications to otology. New techniques are constantly evolving. Moreover, genetic information in the form of genome sequences, expression profiles, and gene array data expands at an exponential pace as the cost of DNA sequencing decreases. Molecular advances are occurring in the ME on two broad fronts. Our understanding of the biology and genetics of ME tissues and responses to infection/inflammation has benefited greatly from the availability of gene sequences and from induced mutations. In addition, bacterial genetics has provided substantial new information on pathogenic mechanisms and has identified many new vaccine candidates. We can look forward to continuing advances in the future.

◆ Acknowledgment

This work is supported by the National Institutes of Health/(NIH)/National Institute on Deafness and Other Communication Disorders (NIDCD) grants DC000129 and DC006279, and by the Research Service of the Veterans Administration.

References

1. Morton CC. Gene discovery in the auditory system using a tissue specific approach. Am J Med Genet A 2004;130:26–28
2. Izumikawa M, Minoda R, Kawamoto K, et al. Auditory hair cell replacement and hearing improvement by Atoh1 gene therapy in deaf mammals. Nat Med 2005;11:271–276
3. Alberts B, Johnson A, Lewis J, Raff M, Roberts K, Walter P. Molecular Biology of the Cell, 4th ed. New York and London: Garland, 2002
4. Lewin B. Genes VIII. New York and Cambridge: Oxford University Press and Cell Press, 2004
5. Miklos D, Freyer GA, Crotty DA. DNA Science: A First Course, 2nd ed. Burlington, NC: Cold Spring Harbor Lab Press and Carolina Biological Supply Co., 2002
6. Ryan A, Baird A. Growth factors during proliferation of the middle ear mucosa. Acta Otolaryngol 1993;113:68–74
7. Ryan AF, Luo L, Baird A. Implantation of cells transfected with the FGF-1 gene induces middle ear mucosal proliferation. In: Lim D, ed. Recent Advances in Otitis Media with Effusion. Amsterdam: Kugler, 1997:248–325
8. Li H, Doyle W, Swarts J, Lo C, Hebda PA. Mucosal expression of genes encoding possible upstream regulators of Na+ transport during pneumococcal otitis media. Acta Otolaryngol 2003;123:575–582
9. Ortega N, Hutchings H, Plouët J. Signal relays in the VEGF system. Front Biosci 1999;4:D141–152
10. Vidal M, Gigoux V, Garbay C. SH2 and SH3 domains as targets for antiproliferative agents. Crit Rev Oncol Hematol 2001;40:175–186
11. Hancock JT. Cell Signaling. London: Longman, 1997
12. Abreu MT, Arditi M. Innate immunity and toll-like receptors: clinical implications of basic science research. J Pediatr 2004;144:421–429
13. Rao V, Krasan G, Hendrixson D, Dawid S, St Geme J. Molecular determinants of the pathogenesis of disease due to non-typeable Haemophilus influenzae. FEMS Microbiol Rev 1999;23:99–129
14. Palsson-McDermott EM, O'Neill LA. Signal transduction by the lipopolysaccharide receptor, Toll-like receptor-4. Immunology 2004; 113:153–162
15. Beutler B. Inferences, questions and possibilities in TLR signaling. Nature 2004;430:257–263
16. Imasato A, Desbois-Mouthon C, Han J, et al. Inhibition of p38 MAPK by glucocorticoids via induction of MAPK phosphatase-1 enhances nontypeable Haemophilus influenzae-induced expression of toll-like receptor 2. J Biol Chem 2002;277:47444–47450
17. Jones MK, Tomikawa M, Mohajer B, Tarnawski AS. Gastrointestinal mucosal regeneration: role of growth factors. Front Biosci 1999;4:D303–309
18. Li J. Exploitation of host epithelial signaling networks by respiratory bacterial pathogens. J Pharmacol Sci 2003;91:1–7
19. Shuto T, Xu H, Wang B, et al. Activation of NF-κB by nontypeable Haemophilus influenzae is mediated by toll-like receptor 2–TAK1-dependent NIK-IKK alpha/beta-I kappa B alpha and MKK3/6-p38 MAP kinase signaling pathways in epithelial cells. Proc Natl Acad Sci USA 2001;98:8774–8779
20. Poltorak A, He X, Smirnova I, et al. Defective LPS signaling in C3H/HeJ and C57BL/10ScCr mice: mutations in tlr4 gene. Science 1998;282:2085–2088
21. McGettrick AF, O'Neill LA. The expanding family of MyD88-like adaptors in Toll-like receptor signal transduction. Mol Immunol 2004;41:577–582
22. Strober W. Epithelial cells pay a Toll for protection. Nat Med 2004;10: 898–900
23. Akira S, Takeda K. Toll-like receptor signaling. Nat Rev Immunol 2004; 4:499–511
24. Swords WE, Moore ML, Godzicki L, Bukofzer G, Mitten MJ, VonCannon J. Nontypeable Haemophilus influenzae adhere to and invade human bronchial epithelial cells via in interaction of lipooligosaccharide with the PAF receptor. Mol Microbiol 2000;37:13–27
25. Kawakami K, Ahmed K, Utsunomiya Y, et al. Attachment of nontypable Haemophilus influenzae to human pharyngeal epithelial cells mediated by a ganglioside receptor. Microbiol Immunol 1998;42:697–702
26. Ahren I, Eriksson E, Egesten A, Riesbeck K. Nontypeable Haemophilus influenzae activates human eosinophils through beta-glucan receptors. Am J Respir Cell Mol Biol 2003;29:598–605
27. Howie HL, Glogauer M, So M. The N. gonorrhoeae type IV pilus stimulates mechanosensitive pathways and cytoprotection through a pilT-dependent mechanism. PLoS Biol 2005;3:e100 Epub 2005 Mar 22
28. Bakaletz L, Baker B, Jurisek J, et al. Demonstration of Type IV pilus expression and a twitching phenotype by Haemophilus influenzae. Infect Immun 2005;73:1635–1643
29. Palacios SD, Pak K, Kayali AG, et al. Participation of Ras and extracellular regulated kinase in the hyperplastic response of middle-ear mucosa during bacterial otitis media. J Infect Dis 2002;186:1761–1769
30. Yetiser S, Satar B, Aydin N. Expression of epidermal growth factor, tumor necrosis factor-alpha, and interleukin-1alpha in chronic otitis media with or without cholesteatoma. Otol Neurotol 2002;23:647–652
31. Jung HH, Kim MW, Lee JH, et al. Expression of vascular endothelial growth factor in otitis media. Acta Otolaryngol 1999;119:801–808
32. Palacios SD, Oehl HJ, Rivkin AZ, Aletsee C, Pak K, Ryan AF. Growth factors influence growth and differentiation of the middle ear mucosa. Laryngoscope 2001;111:874–880

33. Palacios SD, Pak D, Rivkin AZ, Bennett T, Ryan AF. Growth factors and their receptors in the middle ear mucosa during otitis media. Laryngoscope 2002;112:420–423

34. Palacios SD, Pak K, Rivkin AZ, et al. Role of p38 mitogen-activated protein kinase in middle ear mucosa hyperplasia during bacterial otitis media. Infect Immun 2004;72:4662–4667

35. Melhus A, Ryan AF. Expression of molecular markers for bone formation increases during experimental acute otitis media. Microb Pathog 2001;30:111–120

36. Hutton DA, Fogg FJ, Kubba H, Birchall JP, Pearson JP. Heterogeneity in the protein cores of mucins isolated from human middle ear effusions: evidence for expression of different mucin gene products. Glycoconj J 1998;15:283–291

37. Lin J, Tsuprun V, Kawano H, et al. Characterization of mucins in human middle ear and eustachian tube. Am J Physiol Lung Cell Mol Physiol 2001;280:L1157–L1167

38. Jono H, Shuto T, Xu H, et al. Transforming growth factor-b-Smad signaling pathway cooperates with NF-kB to mediate nontypeable Haemophilus influenzae-induced MUC2 mucin transcription. J Biol Chem 2002;277:45547–45557

39. Wang B, Lim DJ, Han J, Kim YS, Basbaum CB, Li JD. Novel cytoplasmic proteins of nontypeable Haemophilus influenza up-regulate human MUC5AC mucin transcription via a positive p38 MAP kinase pathway and a negative PI 3-kinase-Akt pathway. J Biol Chem 2002;277:949–957

40. Takeuchi K, Yagawa M, Ishinaga H, Kishioka C, Harada T, Majima Y. Mucin gene expression in the effusions of otitis media with effusion. Int J Pediatr Otorhinolaryngol 2003;67:53–58

41. Lin J, Tsuboi Y, Pan W, Giebink GS, Adams GL, Kim Y. Analysis by cDNA microarrays of altered gene expression in middle ears of rats following pneumococcal infection. Int J Pediatr Otorhinolaryngol 2002;65:203–211

42. Jono H, Xu H, Kai H, et al. TGF-β-Smad signaling pathway negatively regulates nontypeable Haemophilus influenzae-induced MUC5AC mucin transcription via MAPK phosphatase-1-dependent inhibition of p38 MAPK. J Biol Chem 2003;278:27811–27819

43. Kim YT, Jung HH, Ko TO, Kim SJ. Up-regulation of MUC5AC mRNA expression in endotoxin-induced otitis media. Acta Otolaryngol 2001;121:364–370

44. Lin J, Haruta A, Kawano H, et al. Induction of mucin gene expression in middle ear of rats by tumor necrosis factor-alpha: potential cause for mucoid otitis media. J Infect Dis 2000;182:882–887

45. Smirnova MG, Birchall JP, Pearson JP. In vitro study of IL-8 and goblet cells: possible role of IL-8 in the aetiology of otitis media with effusion. Acta Otolaryngol 2002;122:146–152

46. Smirnova MG, Birchall JP, Pearson JP. TNF-alpha in the regulation of MUC5AC secretion: some aspects of cytokine-induced mucin hypersecretion on the in vitro model. Cytokine 2000;12:1732–1736

47. Chung MH, Choi JY, Lee WS, Kim HN, Yoon JH. Compositional difference in middle ear effusion: mucous versus serous. Laryngoscope 2002;112:152–155

48. Lim DJ, Chun YM, Lee HY, et al. Cell biology of tubotympanum in relation to pathogenesis of otitis media – a review. Vaccine 2000;19 (suppl 1):S17–S25

49. Moon SK, Lee HY, Li JD, et al. Activation of a Src-dependent Raf-MEK1/2-ERK signaling pathway is required for IL-1alpha-induced upregulation of beta-defensin 2 in human middle ear epithelial cells. Biochim Biophys Acta 2002;1590:41–51

50. Stenfors LE, Bye HM, Raisanen S. Causes for massive bacterial colonization on mucosal membranes during infectious mononucleosis: implications for acute otitis media. Int J Pediatr Otorhinolaryngol 2002;65:233–240

51. Kalm O, Johnson U, Preliner K. Hereditary factors, including HLA, in otitis media. In: Mogi G, Honjo I, Ishii T, Takasaka T, eds. Recent Advances in Otitis Media. Amsterdam: Kugler, 1994:113–116

52. Garred P, Brygge K, Sorensen CH, Madsen HO, Thiel S, Svejgaard A. Mannan-binding protein-levels in plasma and upper-airways secretions and frequency of genotypes in children with recurrence of otitis media. Clin Exp Immunol 1993;94:99–104

53. Adams D, Gormley PK, Kerr AG, Smyth GD, Osterber P, Sloan J. Otological manifestations of a new familial polyostotic bone disorder. J Laryngol Otol 1991;105:80–84

54. Butler M. Allen GA, Haynes JL, Singh DN, Watson MS, Breg WR. Anthropometric comparison of mentally retarded males with and without the fragile X syndrome. Am J Med Genet 1991;38:260–268

55. Cole W, Hall RK, Rogers JG. The clinical features of spondyloepiphyseal dysplasia congenital resulting form the substitution of glycine 997 by serine in the alpha I(II) chain type II collagen. J Med Genet 1993;30:27–35

56. Granstrom G, Tjellstrom A. Ear deformities in mandibulofacial dysostosis. Acta Otolaryngol Suppl 1992;493:113–117

57. Hultcrantz M, Sylven L, Borg E. Ear and hearing problems in 44 middle-aged women with Turner's syndrome. Hear Res 1994;76:127–132

58. Jahrsdoerfer R, Jacobson JT. Treacher Collins syndrome: otologic and auditory management. J Am Acad Audiol 1995;6:93–102

59. Rasmussen F. Protracted secretory otitis media. The impact of familial factors and day-care center attendance. Int J Pediatr Otorhinolaryngol 1993;26:29–37

60. Casselbrant ML, Mandel EM, Rockette HE, et al. The genetic component of middle ear disease in the first 5 years of life. Arch Otolaryngol Head Neck Surg 2004;130:273–278

61. Kvestad E, Kvaerner KJ, Roysamb E, Tambs K, Harris JR, Magnus P. Otitis media: genetic factors and sex differences. Twin Res 2004;7:239–244

62. Ebmeyer J, Furukawa M, Pak K, et al. Role of mast cells in otitis media. J Allergy Clin Immunol 2005;116:1129–1135

63. Rivkin AZ, Palacios SD, Pak K, Bennett T, Ryan AF. The role of Fas-mediated apoptosis in otitis media: observations in the lpr/lpr mouse. Hear Res 2005;207:110–116

64. Hardisty RE, Erven A, Logan K, et al. The deaf mouse mutant Jeff (Jf) is a single gene model of otitis media. J Assoc Res Otolaryngol 2003;4:130–138

65. Chung WH, Furukawa M, Ebmeyer J, et al. Whole genome assessment of the initial response to bacterial infection in the middle ear, a gene array study. Submitted, 2006

66. Dopazo J, Mendoza A, Herrero J, et al. Annotated draft genomic sequence from a Streptococcus pneumoniae type 19F clinical isolate. Microb Drug Resist 2001;7:99–125

67. Tettelin H, Nelson KE, Paulsen IT, et al. Complete genome sequence of a virulent isolate of Streptococcus pneumoniae. Science 2001;293:498–506

68. Hoskins J, Alborn WE Jr, Arnold J, et al. Genome of the bacterium Streptococcus pneumoniae strain R6. J Bacteriol 2001;183:5709–5717

69. Wizemann TM, Heinrichs JH, Adamou JE, et al. Use of a whole genome approach to identify vaccine molecules affording protection against Streptococcus pneumoniae infection. Infect Immun 2001;69:1593–1598

70. Lau GW, Haataja S, Lonetto M, et al. A functional genomic analysis of type 3 Streptococcus pneumoniae virulence. Mol Microbiol 2001;40:555–571

71. Marra A, Asundi J, Bartilson M, et al. Differential fluorescence induction analysis of Streptococcus pneumoniae identifies genes involved in pathogenesis. Infect Immun 2002;70:1422–1433

72. van Schilfgaarde M, van Ulsen P, van Der Steeg W, et al. Cloning of genes of nontypeable Haemophilus influenzae involved in penetration between human lung epithelial cells. Infect Immun 2000;68:4616–4623

73. van Ulsen P, van Schilfgaarde M, Dankert J, et al. Genes of non-typeable Haemophilus influenzae expressed during interaction with human epithelial cell lines. Mol Microbiol 2002;45:485–500

74. Mason KM, Munson RS Jr, Bakaletz LO. Nontypeable Haemophilus influenzae gene expression induced in vivo in a chinchilla model of otitis media. Infect Immun 2003;71:3454–3462

75. Harrison A, Dwyer DW, Gillaspy A, et al. Genomic sequence of an otitis media isolate of nontypeable Haemophilus influenzae: comparative study with H. influenzae serotype d, strain KW20. J Bacteriol 2005;187:4627–4636

76. Hou Y, Gu XX. Development of peptide mimotopes of lipooligosaccharide from nontypeable Haemophilus influenzae as vaccine candidates. J Immunol 2003;170:4373–4379

77. Thoren K, Gustafsson E, Clevnert A, et al. Proteomic study of non-typable Haemophilus influenzae. J Chromatogr B Analyt Technol Biomed Life Sci 2002;782:219–226

78. Hays JP, van der Schee C, Loogman A, et al. Total genome polymorphism and low frequency of intra-genomic variation in the uspA1 and uspA2 genes of Moraxella catarrhalis in otitis prone and non-prone children up to 2 years of age. Consequences for vaccine design? Vaccine 2003;21:1118–1124

79. Nell MJ, Albers-Op 't Hof BM, Koerten HK, Grote JJ. Inhibition of endotoxin effects on cultured human middle ear epithelium by bactericidal permeability-increasing protein. Am J Otol 2000;21:625–630

80. Bayliss C, Field D, Moxon E. The simple sequence contingency loci of Haemophilus influenzae and Neisseria meningitides. J Clin Invest 2001;107:657–662

81. Dawid S, Barenkamp S, St Geme J. Variation in expression of the Haemophilus influenzae HMW adhesins: a prokaryotic system reminiscent of eukaryotes. Proc Natl Acad Sci U S A 1999;96:1077–1082

82. Cody A, Field D, Feil E, et al. High rates of recombination in otitis media isolates of non-typeable Haemophilus influenzae. Infect Genet Evol 2003;3:57–66

83. Wong S, Akerley B. Environmental and genetic regulation of the phosphorylcholine epitope of Haemophilus influenzae lipooligosaccharide. Mol Microbiol 2005;55:724–738

84. Ehrlich G. The distributed genome hypothesis: towards an understanding of bacterial persistence. Abstr Extraord Intl Symp on Recent Advances in OM 2005;5:47 (Amsterdam)

85. Shen K, Antalis P, Gladitz J, et al. Identification, distribution, and expression of novel genes in 10 clinical isolates of nontypeable Haemophilus influenzae. Infect Immun 2005;73:3479–3491

I Basic Science

86. Schweda E, Landerholm M, Li J, Richard Moxon E, Richards JC. Structural profiling of LPS glycoforms expressed by non-typeable Haemophilus influenzae: phenotypic similarities between NTHi strain 162 and the genome strain Rd. Carbohydr Res 2003;338:2731–2744

87. Ecevit I, McCrea K, Pettigrew M, Sen A, Marrs C, Gilsdorf J. Prevalence of the hifBC, hmw1A, hmw2A, hmwC, and hia genes in *Haemophilus influenzae* isolates. J Clin Microbiol 2004;42:3065–3072

88. Post JC, Ehrlich GD. The impact of the polymerase chain reaction in clinical medicine. JAMA 2000;283:1544–1546

89. Poxton IR. Molecular techniques in the diagnosis and management of infectious diseases: do they have a role in bacteriology? Med Princ Pract 2005;14(suppl 1):20–26

90. Klingbeil C, Cesar LB, Fiddes JC. Basic fibroblast growth factor accelerates tissue repair in models of impaired wound healing. Prog Clin Biol Res 1991;365:443–458

91. Gospodarowicz D, Greenburg G. The effects of epidermal and fibroblast growth factors on the repair of corneal endothelial wounds in bovine corneas maintained in organ culture. Exp Eye Res 1979;28:147–157

92. Davidson J, Klagsbrun M, Hill KE, et al. Accelerated wound repair, cell proliferation, and collagen accumulation are produced by a cartilage-derived growth factor. J Cell Biol 1985;100:1219–1227

93. Davidson J, Buckley A, Woodward S, Nichols W, McGee G, Demetriou A. Mechanisms of accelerated wound repair using epidermal growth factor and basic fibroblast growth factor. Prog Clin Biol Res 1988;266:63–75

94. Greenhalgh D, Sprugel KH, Murray MJ, Ross R. PDGF and FGF stimulate wound healing in the genetically diabetic mouse. Am J Pathol 1990;136:1235–1246

95. Lynch S. Interactions of growth factors in tissue repair. Prog Clin Biol Res 1991;365:341–357

96. Burgess W, Maciag T. The heparin-binding (fibroblast) growth factor family of proteins. Annu Rev Biochem 1989;58:575–606

97. Baird A, Bohlen P. Fibroblast growth factors. In: Sporn M, Roberts A, eds. Handbook of Experimental Pharmacology: Peptide Growth Factors. Berlin: Springer-Verlag, 1990:369–417

98. Gospodarowicz D. Fibroblast growth factor: Chemical structure and biologic function. Clin Orthop Relat Res 1990;257:231–248

99. Johnson A, Hawke M. The function of migratory epidermis in the healing of tympanic membrane perforations in guinea pigs. Acta Otolaryngol 1987;103:81–86

100. Fina M, Bresnik S, Baird A, Ryan AF. Improved healing of tympanic membrane perforations with basic fibroblast growth factor. Growth Factors 1991;5:265–272

101. Guneri EA, Tekin S, Yilmaz O, et al. The effects of hyaluronic acid, epidermal growth factor, and mitomycin in an experimental model of acute traumatic tympanic membrane perforation. Otol Neurotol 2003;24:371–376

102. Ma Y, Zhao H, Zhou X. Topical treatment with growth factors for tympanic membrane perforations: progress towards clinical application. Acta Otolaryngol 2002;122:586–599

5

Inner Ear Molecular Disorders

Joni K. Doherty, David J. Lim, and Rick A. Friedman

Much of what we know about the workings of the inner ear at the molecular level has been attained through analysis of mutations that result in hearing and balance dysfunction. Dissection of a particular mutation to determine its genomic location and gene product, including structure, subcellular location, and function, can provide vast information in terms of inner ear molecular mechanisms. Genetic mutations affecting the inner ear are being intensely studied in both humans and animal models, resulting in a dramatic increase in our understanding of the molecular biology of the inner ear. This chapter reviews the current state of our understanding based on such studies.

◆ Identification of Deafness Genes in Human Studies

Hearing loss (HL) is the most common sensory impairment in humans. At least one out of every 750 babies born in the United States has sensorineural HL (SNHL). Demographic studies estimate that approximately 50% of all congenital deafness can be traced to inheritable factors—most due to single gene mutations—and at least 90% are inherited as autosomal recessive (AR) traits. Of these, approximately 30% are syndromic and 70% are nonsyndromic. Considerable progress has been made in identifying and characterizing these deafness genes.

During the 1980s, advances in molecular genetic technology led to a rapidly progressive increase in the number of molecular markers that facilitate linkage analysis. These markers, or polymorphisms, define genetic locations and have enabled scientists to identify the approximate location of inherited mutations. Thus, gene mapping began to be applied to familial deafness in the late 1980s, resulting in the first definitive information regarding the physical site and nature of the mutations affecting the inner ear. The recent development of thousands of molecular tags for specific locations in the genome has dramatically enhanced the ability to link inherited disorders to their specific chromosomal location via recombination frequency analysis. When combined with information from prior localization studies of candidate genes or related animal mutations in the homologous chromosomal region, such linkage analysis has enabled the characterization of an increasing number of mutations that cause disorders of hearing. Approximately 200 deafness loci have been identified, including syndromic and nonsyndromic forms. Our knowledge of the identity and function of these genes has grown almost exponentially over the last decade. Today, more than 10 genetic mutations leading to congenital hearing loss can be identified with genetic testing (go to www.genetests.com for testing laboratory information). This has improved our ability to provide genetic counseling, and, in the future, may lead to gene therapy for otologic diseases. Gene identification also allows for determination of function via animal studies of homologous gene mutations that can be genetically engineered.

Syndromic Deafness

Genetic mutations causing congenital deafness in association with other morphologic or clinical features are referred to as syndromic deafness genes. Syndromic deafness accounts for 30% of inherited congenital hearing loss.[1] Linkage analysis has been facilitated by the fact that affected individuals are more easily distinguishable from unaffected members within a given population or family with respect to a specific syndrome. The specific mutations causing Alport syndrome, Waardenburg syndrome, Usher syndrome, branchio-oto-renal (BOR) syndrome, Pendred syndrome, X-linked deafness with perilymph gusher, neurofibromatosis type 2 (NF2), and many other forms of syndromic deafness, as well as nonsyndromic deafness, have been determined (**Fig. 5–1**), and many have been characterized, in terms of the molecular defect (**Table 5–1**). The mitochondrial DNA mutation leading to inherited susceptibility to aminoglycoside-induced hearing loss has also been identified.[2] Here, we will discuss the molecular genetics of inherited deafness. Chapter 22 discusses the clinical aspects of these syndromes in more detail.

Alport Syndrome

The first human mutation affecting the inner ear to be identified was that causing Alport syndrome, an X-linked disease associated with renal abnormalities and progressive HL.

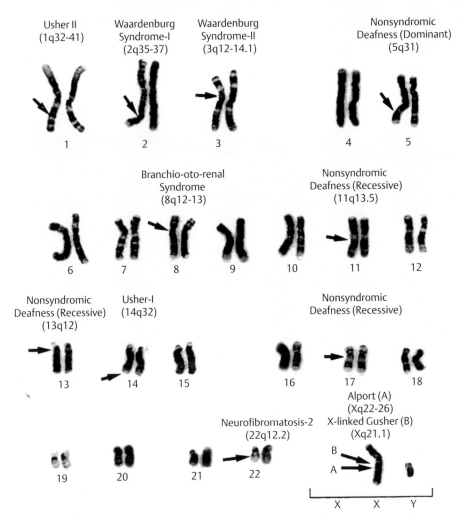

Figure 5–1 Human male karyotype with chromosomal locations of a few of the known deafness genes, including syndromic and one nonsyndromic loci. Arrows indicate the approximate location of each of the genes on each particular chromosome.

The mutated gene was initially linked to Xq22–26 and was subsequently identified as that encoding the α5 chain of type IV collagen, which plays a critical role in the formation of basement membranes.[3] Six subtypes of Alport syndrome have since been identified: types II, III, and IV are X-linked, whereas types I, V, and VI are inherited in an autosomal dominant (AD) fashion.[1]

Waardenburg Syndrome

Waardenburg syndrome (WS) can be inherited as an AD, AR, or sporadic mutation. WS type I (WS-I) is characterized by hearing loss and pigmentary abnormalities such as white forelock and heterochromia irides. Waardenburg syndrome type II (WS-II) is distinguished from WS-I by the presence of dystopia canthorum, which presents as lateral displacement of the medial canthi. The AD WS-I defect was initially localized to the long arm of chromosome 2 (2q35–37) because of a de novo chromosomal malformation,[4] and then further linked to a gene near 2q37.[5] This locus is homologous to the *Pax3* gene in *Splotch* mice, which had been proposed as a murine equivalent of WS-I (**Fig. 5–2**). Mutations in the *PAX3* gene of WS-I patients were subsequently shown to be responsible for WS-I and WS type III (WS-III).[6] *PAX3* encodes a transcription factor

(TF) that regulates expression of other genes. The PAX3 protein product plays a regulatory role in melanocyte differentiation during embryogenesis when they migrate from neural crest to various tissues, including the intermediate cells of the stria vascularis in the cochlea and the melanocytes apposing the dark cells of the vestibular labyrinth, where they are necessary for production of endolymph and the endolymphatic potential. In *VGA-9* mice, harboring a transgenic mutation of *Pax3* similar to that in *Splotch* mice (the murine equivalent of WS-I), the stria vascularis shows a lack of intermediate cells and disorganization of the basal layer (**Fig. 5–2**). WS-II has not shown linkage to the region of chromosome 2 that includes *PAX3*, and WS-II appears to be caused by mutation of either the microphthalmia-associated TF, MITF, which maps to 3p12.3–14.1, or *SNA12*, which is located at 8q11 and encodes the SLUG transcription factor.[1] Type IV Waardenburg (WS-IV) maps to still other sites: (1) 20q13.2–3, where the *EDN3* gene is located, encoding endothelin-3[7]; (2) 13q22, where *ENDRB* encodes the endothelin receptor, type B; and (3) 22q13, encoding the transcription factor SOX10. Endothelin signaling is involved in neuronal survival, and patients with WS-IV develop Hirschsprung disease (lack of autonomic innervation to the distal large colon) in addition to signs and symptoms of WS-II.[8]

Table 5–1 Summary of Genes Involved in Syndromic Hearing Loss

Syndrome	Inherit.	Gene (Locus)	Location	Gene Product	Function
Alport	XLD	COL4A5	Xq22	Collagen α5(IV)	Basement membrane
Apert	S, AD	FGFR2	10q26	FGF receptor 2	FGF receptor
Branchio-oto-renal	AD	EYA1	8q13.3	Eyes absent 1	Transcription factor
Charcot-Marie tooth peroneal muscular atrophy	XLD	GJB1	Xq13.1	Connexin 32	Gap junction protein
Chondrodystrophy with sensorineural deafness	AR	COL11A2	6p21.3	Collagen α2(XI)	Fibrillar cartilage collagen
Cockayne (classic form)	AR	CKN1	5q12.1	CKN1	RNA polymerase II transcription
Crouzon	AD	FGFR2	10q26	FGF receptor 2	FGF receptor
DiGeorge syndrome	AD, AR, S	(DGCR)	22q11	Contiguous del.	Gene deletion
Fanconi anemia A	AR	FANCA	16q24.3	FANCA	Nuclear prot. complex
Friedrich ataxia, type I	AR	FRDA1	9q13	Frataxin	Iron homeostasis, mit.
Gaucher type III	AR	GBA	1q21	Glucocerebroside	Lysosomal enzyme
Hunter	XLR	IDS	Xq28	Iduronate 2-sulfatase	Lysosomal enzyme
Hurler	AR	IDUA	4p16.3	α-L-iduronidase	Lysosomal enzyme
Jervell and Lange-Nielsen	AR	KCNQ1	11p15.5	Potassium channel	Delayed rectifier K⁺ ch.
Marfan syndrome	AD	FBN1	15q21.1	Fibrillin-1	Formation of microfibrils
Neurofibromatosis 2	AD, S	NF2	22q12.2	Merlin	Tumor suppressor
Noonan	AD	PTPN11	12q24.1	Tyrosine phosphatase	Protein dephosphorylation
Norrie	XLR	NDP	Xp11.4	Norrie disease protein	Neuroectodermal cell int.
Ocular albinism, SN deafness	A, digenic	MITF	3p13	Microphthalmia-assoc.TF	Transcription factor
Orofacial digital	XLD	(OFD1)	Xp22.2	Unknown	Unknown
Osteogenesis imperfecta	AD (AR)	COL1A2	7q22.1	Collagen α2	Fibrillar collagen
Osteopetrosis (Albers-Schönberg)	AR (AD)	CLCN7	16p13.3	Chloride channel 7	Chloride channel
Otopalatodigital	XL	(OPD1)	Xq28	Unknown	Unknown
Paget's disease of bone	AD	TNFRSF11	18q22.1	TNF receptor 11A	Activator of NF-κB
	AD	SQSTM1	5q35	Sequestosome 1	Ubiquitin-binding protein
Pendred	AR	SLC26A4	7q31	Pendrin	Anion transporter
Pfeiffer	AD	FGR1,2,3	8p,10q,4p	FGF receptor	FGF receptor
Refsum	AR	PHYH	10p12–15	Phytanoy-coenzyme A hydroxylase	Peroxisomal enzyme
Refsum, infantile form	AR	PEX1	7q21–22	Peroxisome bio. factor 1	Peroxisomal matrix prot.
Spondyloepiphyseal dysplasia	AD	COL2A1	12q13	Collagen α1(II)	Fibrillar collagen-cartilage
Stickler type I	AD	COL2A1	12q13	Collagen α1(II)	Fibrillar collagen-cartilage
Tay-Sachs	AR	HEXA	15q23–24	Hexosaminidase A	Degrades GM2 ganglioside
Townes-Brocks	AD	SALL1	16q12.1	C2H2 zinc finger TF	Homology to Drosoph. sal
Treacher Collins	AD	TCOF1	5q31–33	Nucleolar phosphoprot.	Nuc. Protein trafficking
Turner	Nondysjxn.	(X)	(X)	(single X chromosome)	(Chromosomal deletion)
Usher, type Ia	AR	(USH1A)	14q32		
Usher, type Ib	AR	MYO7A	11q13.5	Type 7 myosin	Myosin motor protein
Usher, type Ic	AR	USH1C	11p14–15	Harmonin	PDZ-domain protein
Usher, type Id	AR	CDH23	10q21–22	Cadherin 23	PDZ-dom., cell. adhesion
Usher, type Ie	AR	(USH1E)	21q21		
Usher, type If	AR	PCDH15	10q21–22	Protocadherin 15	Cellular adhesion
Usher, type Ig	AR	USH1G	17q24–25	SANS	PDZ-binding motif
Usher, type IIa	AR	USH2A	1q41	Usherin	?Extracellular matrix
Usher, type IIb	AR	(USH2B)	3p23–24		
Usher, type IIc	AR	(USH2C)	5q14–23		
Usher, type IIIa	AR	USH3A	3q21–25	Clarin 1	Transmembrane protein
Usher, type IIIb	AR	(USH3B)			
Velocardial facial	AD	(VCFS)	22q11	Frequent cont. gene del.	(Gene deletion)
Waardenburg, type I	AD	PAX3	2q35–37	Paired-box gene 3	Transcription factor
Waardenburg, type IIa	AD	MITF	3p12–14	Microphthalmia-assoc. TF	Transcription factor
Waardenburg, type IIb	AD	SNAI2	8q11	SLUG	Transcription factor
Klein-Waardenburg (type III)	AD, AR	PAX3	2q35–37	Paired-box gene 3	Transcription factor
Shah-Waardenburg (type IV)	AR	EDN3,	20q13	Endothelin-3	Ligand
	AD	EDNRB	13q22	Endothelin receptor B	Endothelin receptor
		SOX10	22q13	SOX10	Transcription factor
Wolfram	AR	WFS1			
Xeroderma pigmentosum	AR	XPA			

AD, autosomal dominant; AR, autosomal recessive; XLD, X-linked dominant; XLR, X-linked recessive; S, sporadic; FGF, fibroblast growth factor; mit., mitochondrial protein; TF, transcription factor; Nondysjxn., nondysjunction.

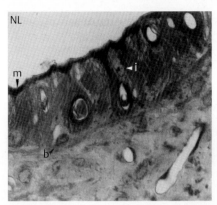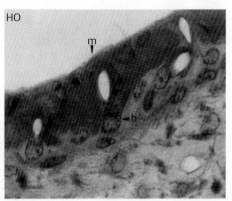

NL

HO

A

B

Figure 5–2 Loss of intermediate cells in the stria vascularis of transgenic VGA-9 mice, a murine equivalent of Waardenburg syndrome type I (WS-I) and very similar to *Splotch* mice. **(A)** There are three cell layers in the normal (NL) stria: basal (b), intermediate (i), and marginal (m). **(B)** Note the absence of the intermediate cells and the disorganization of the basal layer in the homozygous (HO) mouse. The marginal cells do not interdigitate with the basal cells and appear somewhat abnormal with larger, more cuboidal nuclei. Original magnification ×63.

Usher Syndrome

Usher syndrome (US) is inherited in an AR fashion and is characterized by deafness and retinitis pigmentosa. Usher syndrome type I (US-I) is characterized by severe HL and impaired vestibular function, whereas Usher syndrome type II (US-II) has less severe involvement of both. Additional subtypes based on severity and character of progression have been proposed: US-III and US-IV. Both US-I and US-II are genetically heterogeneous, with some US-I families linking to chromosome 14q32 and others linking to chromosome 11, and the *Shaker-1* mouse mutation, which maps to a region homologous to human 14q32, was shown to involve a gene encoding Myosin VII.[1] Based on this observation, Myosin VIIA was subsequently identified as the gene responsible for Usher syndrome Ib.[10] Although incompletely understood, the role of Myosin VIIA in the inner ear appears to involve inner hair cell (IHC) integrity. Myosin VIIA localizes to the cross-links between adjacent stereocilia and at the cuticular plate of IHCs (**Fig. 5–3**). It has been postulated to play a role in adaptation, which is the process of maintenance of lateral tip link tension and restoration of hair cell sensitivity after depolarization.[11–13] Myosin VIIA can move upward on the actin core within stereocilia, and may connect with cadherin-catenin complexes via the PDZ domain-containing protein harmonin in an adaptation motor to maintain stereocilia tension as well as lateral link tension within hair cells (HCs) (**Fig. 5–3**). Mutations in harmonin cause Usher syndrome Ic.[14] US-IIa links to chromosome 1q41, where the gene product, named Usherin, is encoded. Usherin contains laminin–epidermal growth factor (EGF) and fibronectin domains, and thus likely functions in extracellular matrix interactions.[1,15–18] Overall, at least nine distinct chromosomal locations have been linked to the various forms of US.[1,9]

Pendred Syndrome

Pendred syndrome is an AR disorder characterized by deafness and euthyroid goiter that results from mutation of the *PDS* gene, also called *SLC26A4*, which encodes the pendrin protein. Pendrin is a putative ion transport molecule that appears to function as an iodide (in the thyroid), chloride, bicarbonate, formate, and nitrate transporter.[19] Pendrin is discretely expressed in (1) the apical membrane of endolymphatic sac cells; (2) the transitional cells of the cristae ampullaris, utriculi, and sacculi; (3) on the apical surface of basal and intermediate cells within the stria vascularis in the cochlea of the embryonic mouse; and (4) in the apical membrane of cells in the spiral prominence and along the root processes of outer sulcus cells in the cochlea.[20] Based on studies of *PDS* knockout mice, pendrin appears to play a vital role in endolymph fluid homeostasis in the inner ear as well as maintenance of the endolymphatic potential.[20] The spectrum of inner ear abnormalities associated with *PDS* mutations ranges from isolated enlarged vestibular aqueduct (EVA) to classic Mondini malformation, or incomplete partition type II, with cystic apical and middle turns of the cochlea, lacking the interscalar septum, a mildly dilated vestibule, and EVA. Hearing is similarly variable, ranging from normal in early childhood to mild low-frequency conductive loss to profound SNHL. Stepwise progression of hearing loss is the typical pattern, and there have been no reported cases with normal hearing beyond early childhood. In association with Pendred syndrome, euthyroid goiter and a positive perchlorate discharge test are present.

Neurofibromatosis Type 2

Affecting 1 in 40,000 individuals, neurofibromatosis type 2 (NF2) is caused by a mutation at 22q12.2.[21] Individuals affected with NF2 characteristically develop bilateral vestibular nerve schwannomas, inevitably leading to HL and balance dysfunction. NF2 mutation is also associated with schwannomas of other cranial nerves, meningiomas, and spinal tumors. NF2 is inherited in an AD fashion, but approximately 50% of cases are sporadic. Mosaicism of *NF2* gene mutation also occurs in up to 25% of cases. The *NF2* gene encodes merlin, or schwannomin, an intracellular tumor suppressor protein expressed in Schwann cells. Merlin shares extensive homology with the erzin/radixin/moesin family, is negatively regulated by phosphorylation–mediated by p21-activated kinase 1 (PAK1) or focal adhesion kinase (FAK), and translocates to the cytoplasmic cell membrane in a paxillin-dependent manner, where it binds to ErbB2.[22] ErbB2 is a growth factor receptor tyrosine kinase that couples with ErbB3 when stimulated by neuregulin binding and activates intracellular signaling cascades, such as

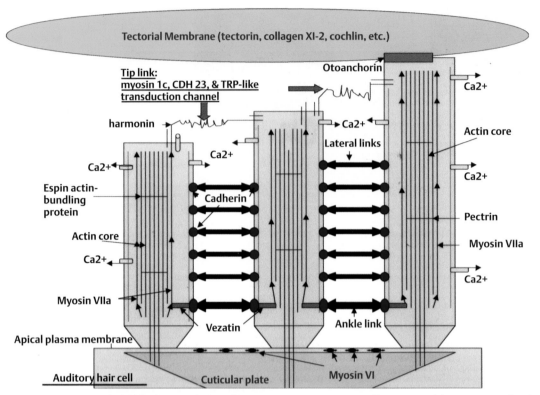

Figure 5–3 Auditory hair cell schematic diagram illustrating molecules involved in mechanosensory transduction of sound. The stereocilia are anchored into the cuticular plate at the apical aspect of the hair cell. The apical plasma membrane is anchored to the cuticular plate by myosin VI, acting in opposition to myosin VIIa, which is involved in elongation of stereocilia via association with the actin core. The tallest stereocilium is attached to the tectorial membrane via otoanchorin, and is connected by cross-links to the shorter stereocilia. The stereocilia contain a circumferential actin core linked by longitudinal pectrin filaments, and they are tapered at the base, which facilitates pivoting rather than bending motion. Movement results in opening of the transduction channels located at either end of the tip links (composed of myosin 1c, cadherin 23, and TRP-like channels) and linked to the myosin VIIa–actin core via harmonin, which is involved in maintenance of lateral link tension. Vezatin facilitates ankle link tension. (Adapted from Hone SW, Smith RJ. Understanding inner ear physiology at the molecular level. Adv Otorhinolaryngol 2002;61:1–10. Reprinted with permission.)

mitogen-activated protein kinase (MAPK) and pAkt/PI3-K, thus mediating Schwann cell proliferation and survival. Merlin also has been shown to translocate to the nucleus where it may affect gene expression in Schwann cells.[22] However, the role of merlin as a tumor suppressor gene is still poorly understood.

Other Deafness Syndromes

Apert syndrome is AD or, more commonly, sporadic, and results from mutation of the fibroblast growth factor receptor 2 (FGFR2) gene at 10q26. Congenital stapedial footplate fixation results in conductive HL and other craniofacial deformities as well as developmental delay, which are secondary to craniosynostosis in Apert syndrome.[1]

Branchio-oto-renal syndrome is AD in inheritance and is characterized by several branchial arch deformities, deafness, and renal anomalies. The mutation has been localized to a gene at 8q13.3, termed *EYA1* for the "eyes absent" phenotype associated with the orthologous mutation in *Drosophila*.[23,24]

X-linked deafness with a perilymph gusher is an X-linked progressive mixed deafness associated with a perilymph (cerebrospinal fluid) "gusher" during stapes surgery, as the name implies. It was linked to Xq21.1 by examination of cytogenetically visible deletion.[25–27] The gene mutation causing X-linked mixed deafness with stapes fixation, or *DFN3*, has recently been identified as *POU3F4*, which encodes the TF Brn-4, a member of the POU-domain family that is extensively expressed during cochlear development.[28] Although the phenotype associated with this disorder only involves the inner ear abnormality, it has historically been classified as a syndromic form of HL, because there is occasionally a radiographic finding of a bulbous distal internal auditory canal associated with the characteristic stapes gusher.

Other AD syndromic forms of HL include Crouzon, DiGeorge, Goldenhar (oculoauricular vertebral dysplasia), osteogenesis imperfecta, Paget, Noonan, Pfeiffer, Stickler, Townes-Brocks, Treacher Collins, and velocardial facial syndromes. Other AR syndromic HL syndromes include Cockayne, Fanconi anemia A, Friedrich ataxia, Hurler, Jervell and Lange-Nielsen, osteopetrosis (Albers-Schönberg), Refsum, Tay-Sachs, and xeroderma pigmentosum. X-linked syndromic deafness disorders include Charcot-Marie Tooth, Hunter, Norrie, otofacial digital, and otopalatodigital syndromes. **Table 5–2** lists the genetic defects associated with these disorders, and Chapter 22 discusses their clinical features in detail. Mitochondrial deafness syndromes are discussed in a separate section of this chapter. For a more complete and current review of syndromic deafness genes, go to the Online Mendelian Inheritance in Man Web site at http://www.ncbi.nlm.nih.gov/Omim/.

Table 5–2 Factors Affecting Inner Ear Development

Factor	Source	Target Cells	Action
Retinoic acid (RA)	Inner ear sensory epithelia	Supporting cells	Differentiation of supporting cells into hair cells
Nerve growth factor (NGF)	Cochlear and vestibular hair cells	Cochlear and vestibular neurons	Neurite extension
Brain derived neurotrophic factor (BDNF)	Cochlear and vestibular hair cells	Type II cochlear neurons, OHC afferents, vestibular neurons	Neurite extension
Neurotrophin-3 (NT-3)	Cochlear and vestibular hair cells	Type I cochlear neurons, IHC afferent neurons	Neurite extension
Basic fibroblast growth factor (bFGF)	OHC, IHC, spiral limbus, spiral ganglion neurons, stria vascularis	Cochlear and vestibular neurons	Neuronal development
Transforming growth factor-β (TGF-β)	Ubiquitous throughout cochlear epithelium	Cochlear and vestibular neurons	Neuronal development via ↑bFGF receptors (FGFR)

OHC, outer hair cell; IHC, inner hair cell.

Nonsyndromic Deafness

Although 30% of prelingual deafness is syndromic, 70% is nonsyndromic HL (NHL).[29] NHL is a diagnosis that applies to patients who suffer genetic HL without associated phenotypic abnormalities, and it results from mutations in an estimated 100 genes. Linkage analysis is very difficult in this group of patients due to the genetic heterogeneity. However, using relatively isolated populations and large families, linkage analysis has facilitated the identification of over 70 loci and cloning of more than 21 genes responsible for NHL. Identification of genetic mutations associated with deafness enables genetic testing, precise diagnosis, and genetic counseling. Human temporal bone studies have allowed observations of morphologic defects resulting from such mutations, providing speculative information of gene function. Animal studies utilizing homologous targeted mutations facilitate experimental studies of gene function, and have been the major tool in expanding our knowledge of inner ear protein functions. Because the number of DNA polymorphic markers for genetic NHL is increasing exponentially, up-to-date information can be found on the Hereditary Hearing Loss Homepage at http://dnalab-www.uia.ac.be/dnalab/hhh.

Molecules Involved in Ion Homeostasis

Maintaining the endolymphatic potential within the cochlear duct is essential for normal HC function, and it is postulated that the potassium content in endolymph is highly regulated via a bimodal recycling pathway. According to the predominant theory, potassium is recycled both medially and laterally within the cochlea. The medial pathway involves the spiral limbus interdental cells medial to the organ of Corti, which recycle potassium ions (K^+) back into the scala media after auditory HC depolarization (**Fig. 5–4**); see Chapter 1 for a description of cellular subtypes. The lateral pathway involves the supporting cells adjacent to HCs within the organ of Corti, that recycle K^+ through the spiral ligament and stria vascularis back into the scala media (**Fig. 5–4**). Potassium recycling requires a network of ion channels and transporters, including gap junctions assembled by connexins, the anion transporter pendrin, and potassium channels KCNQ and KCNE.[29]

Connexins

Currently, *GJB2*, which encodes connexin 26, is recognized as the most frequent gene mutation associated with congenital deafness in Caucasians. DFNA3, the dominantly inherited form, and DFNB1, the AR mutation, account for up to 50% of cases of congenital deafness. Although relatively small, with the entire coding sequence contained in one exon, more than 50 mutations within the *GJB2* gene account for HL. The most common is the 35delG mutation in European countries and the United States.[30] In contrast, the 235delC mutation accounts for 73% of *GJB2* mutations in the Japanese population.[31] The small coding region has facilitated genetic screening methods for *GJB2* mutations, which can now be done more rapidly and easily using microarray.[32] The role of connexin 26 in the inner ear is related to its function as a subunit of connexon gap junctions. Connexons are composed of hexameric connexin molecules forming a hemipore. The connexon hemipore of two adjacent cells will join to form a complete gap junction and allow intercellular diffusion of K^+. Other connexin proteins associated with NHL include connexin 30 (encoded by *GJB6*, associated with *DFNA3* and *DFNB1* loci), 31 (*DFNA2* locus, *GJB3* gene), and 43 (*GJA1*). Connexins form mostly homomeric connexons, but the heteromeric connexon of connexin 26 and connexin 32 is also expressed in the inner ear. Connexons appear to be essential for generation and maintenance of the endocochlear potential due to their role in K^+ recycling (**Fig. 5–4**).[33] There are two independent networks of intercellular connexons that seem to play an important role in recycling of K^+ ions: (1) the epithelial network within the basilar membrane adjacent to the organ of Corti both medially and laterally; and (2) the fibrocyte network, which is present within the spiral limbus (medially) and spiral ligament (laterally) and includes the basal, intermediate, and endothelial cells of the stria vascularis. The major pathway for K^+ recycling appears to involve the stria vascularis (**Fig. 5–4**), and connexons have been implicated as part of the structure required for this process, via transcellular circulation of K^+ through the spiral ligament and basal cells of the stria vascularis.[33]

Other Ion Transport Molecules

Another junctional protein important for fluid homeostasis in the inner ear is Claudin 14, a *CLDN14* gene product. Claudin 14 forms tight junctions within sensory epithelia of the cochlea

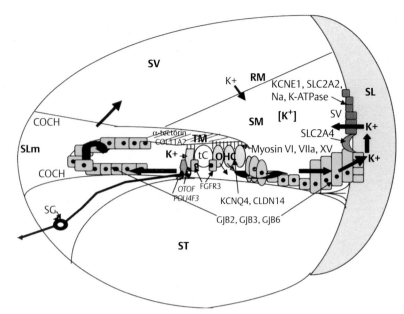

Figure 5–4 Schematic drawing of a cross section through a single turn of the cochlea illustrating potassium recycling pathways medially and laterally (arrows). (See text for description of genes and their role in ion homeostasis; see Chapter 1 for a more detailed description of cochlear anatomy, including cellular subtypes.) SG, spiral ganglia; SLm, spiral limbus; SV, stria vascularis; SL, spiral ligament; SV, scala vestibule; ST, scala tympani; SM, scala media; RM, Reissner's membrane; K⁺, potassium ion; TM, tectorial membrane; tC, Corti's tunnel; OHC, outer hair cell.

I Basic Science

and vestibular organs, and NHL results from mutation at the *DFNB29* locus (**Fig. 5–4**).[34]

PDS (SLC26A4) gene mutations that lead to EVA in isolation (i.e., in absence of goiter or a positive perchlorate discharge test) are a form of nonsyndromic deafness, *DFNB4*, and are thought to be part of a continuum of diseases caused by the same gene, where Pendred syndrome in association with Mondini malformation (as discussed earlier; see Syndromic Deafness) is at the opposite end of the spectrum.[35] Expression studies in *Xenopus* oocytes as well as mammalian cells, including knockout studies in mice, indicate that pendrin function can support chloride/formate, chloride/hydroxide, chloride/bicarbonate, chloride/nitrate, and chloride/iodide ion exchange.[19] Notably, *PDS* knockout mice develop severe hydrops, suggesting a role for pendrin in endolymphatic fluid homeostasis.

Potassium channels in the inner ear are encoded by the *KCNQ1–4* and *KCNE1–4* genes. Splice variants from these genes are expressed as subunits of the various isoforms of potassium channels present throughout the mammalian inner ear.[36] Together, the KCNE and KCNQ subunits form a functional potassium channel. The KCNE1 (minK) subunit IsK regulates the pore-forming KvLQT1 α-subunit encoded by KCNQ1, which is expressed at the apical surface of marginal cells in the stria vascularis (**Fig. 5–4**). Mutation in any of these genes can result in deafness, presumably secondary to lack of endocochlear potential generation. These potassium channels are expressed in cardiac tissue as well; Jervell and Lange-Nielsen syndrome results from mutations in either KCNE1 or KCNQ1.[36,37] KCNQ4 is expressed by cochlear outer hair cells (OHCs) and vestibular type I HCs. Several lines of evidence suggest that KCNQ4 channels are responsible for the resting K⁺ current described in OHCs and type I HCs, which likely influence their electrical properties. Furthermore, KCNQ4 is expressed in central auditory pathway nuclei, suggesting that defects in *KCNQ4*, which lead to *DFNA2*, contribute to both peripheral and central deafness.[38]

Transcription Factors

The POU-domain family of transcription factors contains the genes *POU4F3* and *POU3F4*, both of which have been identified in association with late-onset progressive NHL. These TFs are expressed in the late stages of inner ear development, and are important for neuronal differentiation and survival. *POU3F4* is expressed in the otic capsule in mesenchyme of the cochlear and the vestibular primordial.[39] Mutations in *POU3F4* are associated with X-linked progressive mixed HL due to stapes fixation with a progressive SNHL, termed *DFN3*.[25] It is associated with increased perilymphatic (cerebrospinal fluid) pressure and a gusher at stapedectomy, as discussed earlier (see Syndromic Deafness). Conversely, *POU4F3* is expressed in developing cochlear and vestibular hair cells.[40] A family with a dominantly inherited mutation in the *POU4F3* gene encoding a truncated Brn-3.1 resulting in late-onset nonsyndromic sensorineural deafness has been identified, and the deafness gene termed *DFNA15*.[41]

Proteins with Unknown Function

A common form of AD low-frequency nonsyndromic SNHL is caused by mutation of the *WFS1* gene designated DFNA6/14. *WFS1* encodes wolframin, a protein that localizes to the endoplasmic reticulum and is thought to play a role in protein sorting and trafficking, although the function is unknown.[42]

Cytoskeletal Proteins

Structural components of the cochlea and vestibular organs are highly organized, and their maintenance is essential for the function of hearing and balance, especially with respect to sensory HCs. Mutation in many of the genes that encode cytoskeletal proteins within hair cells leads to NHL. These include (1) a conventional myosin, *MYH9*; (2) four unconventional myosins, *MYO3A*, *MYO6*, *MYO7A*, and

MYO15; (3) stereocilin, a novel stereocilia-associated protein; (4) harmonin, a PDZ-domain protein; (5) a putative actin-polymerization protein, HDIA1; and (6) a cadherin, CDH23.[29]

Stereocilia are the main structures responsible for mechanosensory transduction in auditory and vestibular HCs. Stereocilia are cellular organelles that are organized into rows of increasing height to create the characteristic staircase pattern seen by electron microscopy. Unlike vestibular HCs, mature auditory hair cells do not contain a kinocilium. Stereocilia are exquisitely sensitive to mechanical vibration, and can easily be damaged by overstimulation, but undergo continuous renewal from tip to base to continue to function an entire lifetime.[43] Each stereocilium is composed of a rigid central structure containing several hundred parallel, polarized, and cross-linked actin filaments. Different members of the myosin family are present with these actin filaments in specific locations within stereocilia: myosin XVa (*MYO15A* gene product) is located at the tips, whereas myosin VIIa (encoded by *MYO7A*) is located alongside actin at cross-links of adjacent stereocilia, and myosin VI (gene product of *MYO6*) is present at the cuticular plate (**Fig. 5–3**). Myosins bind actin, forming the molecular motor units that generate movement via adenosine triphosphate (ATP) hydrolysis. The *MYO7A* gene, also the causative gene mutation associated with Usher Ib, is associated with two forms of nonsyndromic deafness: DFNB2, an AR disorder; and DFNA11, an AD disorder.[10,44]

Harmonin, encoded by *USH1C* at 11p14–15.2, is associated with NHL via mutations linking to the *DFNB18* locus. Harmonin contains a PDZ domain, which suggests that it may function as an assembling protein. PDZ (an acronym designated after three proteins that contain this domain—*PSD-95*, *d*iscs large, and *z*ona occludens—were identified) proteins organize protein complexes into their specific subcellular location, they anchor transmembrane proteins, and recruit cytosolic signaling molecules, and may bind directly to the actin cytoskeleton.[14]

A putative actin-polymerizing protein is expressed as the gene product of *HDIA1*, the human homologue of the *Drosophila* diaphanous gene.[45] *HDIA1* is a formin gene family member, of which most are involved in cytokinesis and establishing cell polarity.

A novel cadherin-like protein is encoded by *CDH23*, which is also linked to Usher type 1d, and mutation at the *DFNB12* locus results in NHL. Cadherins form adherin junctions, which are critically important during embryogenesis and organogenesis. Stereocilia organization is disrupted early during hair cell differentiation in mouse mutants.[46]

Synaptic Vesicle Trafficking

OTOF mutation, associated with *DFNB9*, is reported to be a frequent cause of recessive prelingual NHL in Spanish patients, and accounts for 4.4% of recessive prelingual NHL not due to *GJB2* (connexin 26) mutations.[47] *OTOF* encodes otoferlin, which has been identified as a calcium-triggered synaptic vesicle trafficking protein that interacts with syntaxin1 and SNAP25 of the SNARE complex for Ca^{2+}-dependent presynaptic vesicle exocytosis within IHCs. Otoferlin, therefore, appears to be important for afferent neural signaling, and mutations have also been found to be associated with auditory neuropathy.[48]

Extracellular Matrix Components

Overlying the auditory HCs within the organ of Corti is the tectorial membrane, which generates the shearing force that bends the stereocilia, opening transduction channels and initiating depolarization. This composes the mechanosensory transduction process that is necessary for hearing. Additionally, the tectorial membrane matrix acts as a second resonator and ensures that the OHC bundles are displacement coupled to the sound stimulus. Thus, it facilitates optimal electromechanical feedback to the basilar membrane from OHCs.[49] The tectorial membrane consists of collagen fibers and a noncollagenous matrix containing mostly α- and β-tectorin.[29] Otoancorin mediates the attachment of the tectorial membrane to the apical surface of the HCs (**Fig. 5–3**). *TECTA* encodes α-tectorin, *OTOA* encodes otoancorin, and *COL11A2* encodes the type XI collagen subunit 2. Mutation in any of these three genes results in SNHL, which can be dominant, recessive, NHL, or syndromic HL.[29]

COCH encodes cochlin, an extracellular matrix protein that is abundantly expressed throughout the inner ear, except sensory hair cells.[50] Mutations in *COCH* at the DFNA9 locus lead to late-onset, progressive NHL, which is characterized by acidophilic mucopolysaccharide deposits in the cochlea and vestibular organs,[51] SNHL, and vestibular symptoms similar to Meniere's disease.[52] Interestingly, only missense mutations of the COCH gene have been identified in association with DFNA9 NSHL.[53]

Mitochondrial Deafness

Mitochondrial mutations have recently been identified in association with some maternally inherited HLs. These can result from heteroplasmic or homoplasmic states with respect to the mitochondrial DNA pool. Heteroplasmy refers to a mixture (usually two, but "multiplasmy" has been reported) of mitochondrial genotypes, whereas homoplasmy refers to a single mitochondrial genotype present in all of the cells of the body.[54] Mitochondrial mutations are associated with some forms of syndromic as well as NHL.

The systemic neuromuscular syndromes MELAS (mitochondrial encephalopathy, lactic acidosis, and stroke-like episodes), MERRF (mitochondrial encephalomyopathy with ragged red fibers), and Kearns-Sayre syndrome frequently present with hearing loss, among other symptoms.[55] They are caused by heteroplasmic mitochondrial DNA mutations that manifest in nerves and muscle tissue, where energy requirements are highest, and, therefore, mitochondria are more abundant and active. HL results from generalized neuronal dysfunction.[56]

A form of inherited SNHL associated with diabetes mellitus results from several distinct heteroplasmic mutations in the mitochondrial transfer RNA (tRNA) genes. In these patients, HL develops after diabetes, but is of early onset with a severe phenotype. Interestingly, these include the A3243G mutation within the mitochondrial gene encoding $tRNA_{leu}(UUR)$, which is the same mutation that results in MELAS syndrome.[56]

A mitochondrial genome 1555A→G mutation within the gene encoding 12S ribosomal RNA is associated with aminoglycoside susceptibility to HL. Additionally, a progressive high-frequency SNHL and permanent tinnitus, even in the absence of exposure to aminoglycosides, may occur in individuals harboring this mutation, which is, thus, a form of

NHL.[57] HL presumably results from increased susceptibility to cochlear injury in response to various environmental factors.

Presbycusis is thought to be inherited as a mitochondrial mutation, but the specific mutation(s) have yet to be identified. It is thought to involve at least one of the genes for the oxidative phosphorylation pathway, and the mitochondrial cytochrome oxidase II gene is a likely candidate.[54,58]

Besides the particular mutation in a single gene, other factors may modify the observed clinical phenotype. Such factors may include the genetic background, modifying genes, and environmental factors, such as noise exposure and ototoxicity. Modifying genes can influence the phenotype resulting from a given mutation at another locus. An extreme example is DFNM1, which acts as a dominant suppressor of DFNB26.[59] Modifier genes may explain why the level of HL can range from mild to profound with identical NHL mutations, as well as the phenotypic variance of identical syndromic and mitochondrial mutations.[54]

Semicircular Canal Dysplasias

Another class of disorders resulting in SNHL, conductive HL, or mixed HL is semicircular canal dysplasia.[60] Although traditional hypotheses have held that semicircular canal dysplasias result from arrest in development during the sixth week of gestation, several cases of semicircular canal dysplasia or aplasia have been reported with normal cochlear development.[61,62] The majority are nonsyndromic, although 12.5% were associated with known syndromes in a series of 16 cases.[62] The genetic mutations leading to isolated semicircular canal abnormalities have yet to be identified.

◆ Identification of Deafness Genes Utilizing Transgenic Animal Studies

The study of mouse genetics has been indispensable in terms of the knowledge we have been able to glean about human development and disorders utilizing mice. Creating homologous mutations in experimental mouse models enables us to determine the function of genes mutated in human disorders. Techniques for developing animal models include creating transgenic animals, insertional mutagenesis, and site-directed mutagenesis.

Transgenic Animals

The insertion of a man-made gene into the genome of a normal mouse embryo can result in the production of a transgenic mouse. The artificial gene is composed of a tissue-specific promoter sequence linked to the sequence coding for the protein of interest. This construct is then inserted into the fertilized mouse embryo through various means, including physical injection or retroviral transfection. If the transgene inserts into the genomic DNA and if the embryo survives, the adult mouse will pass the gene on to future generations. In any transgenic animal, if there are cells that express a TF that interacts with the promoter, the gene product will be expressed in these cells and may affect their function. Thus, Rauch[63] showed that several lines of transgenic mice in which the *mos* proto-oncogene is driven by a constitutive retroviral promoter develop deafness and a shaker-waltzing phenotype (**Fig. 5–5**).

Insertional Mutagenesis

In a small percentage of the offspring of transgenic animals, the transgene is randomly inserted into another gene in the genome, resulting in a mutation and a phenotype change in the animal. This process is termed insertional mutagenesis. The position of the mutated gene is now marked by the transgene, which can facilitate its localization and identification. For example, Crenshaw et al[64] reported that one out of 14 transgenic mice with a v-*src* transgene developed an inner ear defect, including collapse of the pars superior and a shaker-waltzing phenotype. The collapse was concomitant with abnormal otoconia in the macula of the saccule and degenerated spiral ganglion cells, and was preceded by a period of neonatal endolymphatic hydrops. The mutation is autosomal dominant with complete penetrance and has been mapped to chromosome 1 near the interleukin-1 receptor.[65]

Site-Directed Mutagenesis

Site-directed mutagenesis or gene targeting is an ingenious technique that relies on the process of insertional mutagenesis. Basically, a mutant gene that confers antibiotic resistance and disrupts expression of a normal protein is flanked by sequences of a gene to be disrupted, and then it is inserted into an embryonic stem cell. The cultured cell then divides, and through homologous recombination, targeted insertional

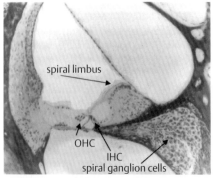
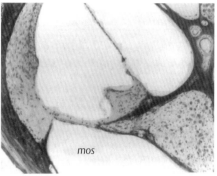

Figure 5–5 Twenty-micrometer sections of the organ of Corti of a transgenic animal overexpressing *mos*. Compared with normal **(A)**, note the total loss of hair cells, supporting cells, and pillar cells in the *mos* organ of Corti **(B)**. The tectorial membrane appears somewhat contracted and the normally convex surface of the spiral limbus is scooped out in a deep trough in the *mos* cochlea. There is also a marked loss of spiral ganglion cells in Rosenthal's canal. (Original magnification ×100.) (From Rauch S. Malformation and degeneration in the inner ear of *mos* transgenic mice. Ann Otol Rhinol Laryngol 1992;101:430–436. Reprinted with permission.)

mutagenesis occurs and simultaneously results in both gene deletion and antibiotic resistance in the progeny cells. The progeny cells are then selected for antibiotic resistance and inserted into a blastocyst, which is then implanted into the uterus of a mouse. The resulting offspring mice are chimeric, and subsequent breeding of the mice in which the germline is affected will eventually generate some homozygous mutants, if the mutation is not lethal. This method was used by Mansour et al[66] to generate mice with a mutation in the *int-2* gene, which encodes fibroblast growth factor 3 (FGF-3). Prior to production of this mutant mouse, Represa et al[67] had shown that disruption of *int-2* expression in vitro prevented inner ear development. The mutant mice created by Mansour et al, however, had normal induction of the inner ear despite having decreased FGF-3 production, suggesting the existence of a redundant pathway of induction. Interestingly, these mice did have hearing and vestibular defects that correlated with multiple inner ear abnormalities, indicating that such an alternative pathway still results in aberrant development.

Alternatively, the analysis of mutant mice with hearing and balance defects has facilitated our current understanding of inner ear development. The process of inner ear development is governed by complex gene interactions, which regulate a series of ontogenetic events. Generally, mutations in genes that play a role early in otocyst induction and patterning result in gross malformations, whereas mutations in genes expressed later tend to result in subtle inner ear structural abnormalities, often limited to discrete elements of the sensory neuroepithelium or dysregulation of inner ear homeostasis. Thus, phenotypic abnormalities can be used to predict the stage of development at which a particular gene is expressed. Some genes, however, display overlap in their developmental roles, such as those encoding Delta and Jagged—the Notch receptor ligands[68]—as discussed below.

Additionally, subtractive hybridization techniques using chicken embryos have led to the rapid identification of several inner ear genes that are expressed during development as unique inner ear proteins. Among them are otoancorin, β-tectorin, calbindin, type II collagen, and connexins.[69] Such genes are potential candidates for deafness genes based on their temporal expression, and several have subsequently been identified in humans in association with hereditary deafness.

◆ Inner Ear Development

The inner ear is a highly complex yet ordered structure in which induction and differentiation initiate and maturation completes the process of development. Studying gene expression during development and in animal models has enabled identification of factors that play essential roles in each stage of inner ear development. Although some of these observations have potential clinical implications, a complete review of developmental factors is beyond the scope of this chapter; only clinically relevant factors are covered. For a more comprehensive categorization of mouse models, go to www.ihr.mrc.ac.uk/hereditary/Mutants/Table.shtml.

Transcription Factors Involved in Inner Ear Development

The otic placode, which develops as an ectodermal thickening of either side of the neural plate in the hindbrain of mice at embryonic day 8.5 (E8.5), gives rise to all of the inner ear structures and cell types, except melanocytes and Schwann cells.[70] TF gene expression is thought to specify the patterning of inner ear development at this crucial stage.[71] Essential genes at this early stage that have been described include *Pax2*, *Hmx3*, *Hoxa1*, retinoic acid receptor (*RAR*), and *NeuroD1*.

Otx1 and Prx1/Prx2

The horizontal semicircular canal is absent in *Otx1* mutants and in double mutants of *Prx1* and *Prx2*.[72] Targeted deletion of *Otx1* results in normal development of the cochlea and all other vestibular structures, whereas in double mutants of *Prx1/2*, the other semicircular canals are delayed in development.

Pax

Disruption of either *Pax* gene in mice results in cochlear agenesis with absence of the spiral ganglion, while the vestibular apparatus is unaffected.[73,74] *Pax3*, or *p*aired bo*x* DNA-binding protein 3, encodes a TF essential for proper migration of melanocytes and organization of the stria vascularis (**Fig. 5–2**), and, thus, appears to play an essential role in endolymph production. *PAX3*, the human homolog, is mutated in WS-I, as described earlier in the chapter.

Hmx3

Hmx3 is expressed in the inner ear as well as in the second branchial arch. Targeted deletion of *Hmx3* results in vestibular dysgenesis.[71] *Hmx3* appears to play a role in separation of the utricular and saccular maculae and development of the semicircular canals. The sensory organ within the horizontal semicircular canal is absent in *Hmx3* mutants.

RAR

Three genes encode RAR subtypes α, β, and γ that are expressed in the mouse embryonic inner ear and are important in otocyst development.[75,76] These RARs bind all-*trans* retinoic acid, the major biologically active metabolite of vitamin A, as ligand and are activated to then bind retinoic acid response elements of target genes.

One such gene, which encodes bone morphogenic protein 4 (BMP4), plays a role in patterning of the semicircular canals (SCCs). BMP4 downregulation by retinoic acid, mediated by RAR action at a promoter site of the second intron of the *BMP4* gene, affects SCC formation.[77]

Other genes involved in the retinoic acid signaling pathways are also essential, such as the mouse gene *Hoxa1*, a homeobox gene that is a putative downstream target of RAR.[78] Mutations in RARα and RARγ, together, result in severe vestibular and cochlear malformations that are similar to *Hoxa1*-deficient mice. *Hoxa1* mutants display inner ear dysmorphogenesis with variable defects in the vestibular and cochlear components. Although RARs are widely expressed in the mouse inner ear, phenotypic defects are not displayed unless two or more receptors are absent, as in compound null mutants.[79] This fact underscores the redundancy of such receptor isoforms.

Furthermore, messenger RNA (mRNA) encoding RARβ has been found in the inner ear of embryonic mice.[80] In addition, when exposed to retinoic acid in vitro, embryonic supporting cells show premature differentiation into hair cells.[67] Retinoic acid or similar growth factors could thus eventually play a role in HC regeneration.

BETA2/NeuroD1

Another basic helix-loop-helix (bHLH) TF that is expressed in many cell types during development of the mammalian central nervous system is *BETA2/NeuroD1*. Its role in the inner ear is essential in that knockouts are deaf and have balance disorders, displayed by head tilting and circling.[81] Null mutations result in severely reduced numbers of cochlear and vestibular ganglion (CVG) cells in mice due to apoptosis after differentiation; therefore, the role of *BETA2/NeuroD1* appears to be in CVG cell survival. Additionally, mutants have defects in cochlear duct differentiation and patterning, sensory epithelium, and dorsal cochlear nucleus cells.

Math1

Determination of auditory and vestibular HC fate is an early event in embryogenesis and has not been completely elucidated. In mice, the bHLH TF *Math1* (also known as *Atoh1*, due to its homology with the *Drosophila* proneural gene *Atonal*) is expressed early in HC differentiation and *Math1* knockouts fail to develop HCs.[82] Moreover, inoculation of adenovirus with the *Math1* gene insert (Adv-Math1 vector) into the scala media of the mature guinea pig cochlea in vivo results in *Math1* overexpression in nonsensory cochlear cells and leads to the development of new HCs.[83] Furthermore, regenerated HCs in the adult guinea pig via inoculation with Adv-Math1 vectors following complete HC destruction restored hearing.[83] Axons extend from the auditory nerve toward some of the new HCs, suggesting that the new cells attract auditory neurons. Therefore, nonsensory cells in the mature cochlea retain the competence to generate new HCs after overexpression of Math1 in vivo and these investigators concluded that Math1 is necessary and sufficient to direct HC differentiation in these mature nonsensory cells.[83] However, the fact that Math1 is expressed in several mammalian cell lineages suggests that its role is contributory and essential but that it does not act alone in determining HC fate. It is likely that combinatorial coding in TF regulation of gene expression occurs as a unique process in specifying cell type and initiating differentiation. Math1 may also have a role in vestibular HC differentiation.

POU-Domain

At least two of the three members of the *Brn-3* subfamily of POU-domain *RF* genes also play a key role in auditory and vestibular sensory neuron development. The Brn-3.0 (or Brn-3a) and Brn-3.2 (or Brn-3b) proteins are expressed in some spiral ganglion and Scarpa's ganglion cells. The Brn-3.1 (or Brn-3c) protein is essential for auditory and vestibular HC development, and appears to function downstream of *Math1*. Brn-3.1 knockout mice are deaf and have impaired balance function due to absence of sensory HCs.[84,85] Localization studies in mice embryos have shown that Brn-3.1 is expressed early in HC lineage after fate is determined, but before HC morphology is distinguishable, and high-level expression continues throughout HC life. Brn-3.1 knockouts display normal migration of HC precursors, but HCs degenerate and undergo apoptosis by E18 in mice.[86] The human homologues are POU4F3 and POU3F4, mutations of which lead to late-onset progressive nonsyndromic SNHL, as discussed earlier in the chapter.

Growth Factors in Inner Ear Development

Growth factors have been implicated in the development and survival of inner ear neurons. Nerve growth factor (NGF), brain-derived growth factor (BDGF), neurotrophin-3 (NT-3), basic fibroblast growth factor (bFGF), and transforming growth factor-β (TGF-β) have all been shown to be important in early and late cochlear and vestibular neuronal development[87–90] (**Table 5–2**).

Both vestibular and cochlear HCs produce mRNA encoding neurotrophic factors, especially BDNF and NT-3. Cochlear and vestibular neurite extension in vitro is inhibited with antisense oligonucleotides to BDNF and NT-3, but it is enhanced when NGF, BDNF, or NT-3 is added to the media.[91,92] In addition, mice have been bred with gene knockouts of the *BDNF* gene, the *NT-3* gene, and with both genes.[91,92] BDNF knockout mice lose most vestibular as well as type II cochlear ganglion cells and OHC afferents. NT-3 knockouts lose type I cochlear ganglion cells in addition to IHC afferent neurons (**Fig. 5–6**). The mice without both genes lack vestibular and cochlear ganglion cells.[93] The importance of these neurotrophic factors for the survival of inner ear neurons suggests that they have the potential to protect these cells from degenerating. Therefore, they might have a role in preserving spiral ganglion neurons for stimulation by the cochlear implant. Other growth factors that have been identified as key players in inner ear development via animal models are discussed later.

Jagged/Delta

Exit from the cell cycle is crucial for induction of differentiation and maturation. Cell cycle exit in the cochlea seems to depend on expression of Notch1 and its ligands, Jagged1/2

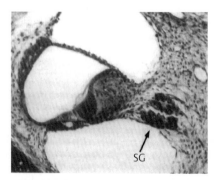

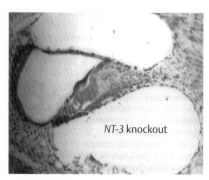

Figure 5–6 Loss of spiral ganglion (SG) neurons due to targeted mutation of the *NT-3* gene. **(A)** Hematoxylin and eosin (H&E)-stained section displays the organ of Corti from a wild-type mouse. **(B)** Absent spiral ganglions in an *NT-3* negative transgenic mouse. (Courtesy of T. Van De Water.)

and Delta, which may define boundaries and patterning of sensory cell development.[94] Mutants in Jagged1 and Notch display abnormal patterning of the cochlea.[68,95] Notch-Delta signaling plays a crucial role in primary cell fate determination through lateral inhibition. Early in development of the organ of Corti in chicks, Delta and Jagged expression by developing IHCs appears to result in lateral inhibition of HC differentiation, committing adjacent progenitor cells to the fate of supporting cells, and, possibly induces OHC development as well. Later in development, expression of Delta and Jagged appears to inhibit both IHC and OHC differentiation.[96,97]

Fgf3

Although the fibroblast growth factor-3 (FGF-3) is expressed widely in both brain and ear tissues, the role it appears to play in inner ear morphogenesis involves the endolymphatic duct (ELD) and sac. FGF-3 knockout mice display malformation of both the ELD and sac, among other abnormalities.[66,98]

Neurogenin1

Auditory and vestibular ganglion neurons fail to develop in mice with targeted deletion of *neurogenin1*.[99]

Shh

Mesenchymal–epithelial interactions appear to play an essential role in inner ear development, based on observations in mice. The protein product of Sonic hedgehog (*Shh*) is secreted by notochord in early development and is essential for ventral otic derivatives, such as the cochlear duct and cochleovestibular ganglion.[100] *Shh* interacts with both *Pax2* and BMPs during otocyst development, where it may induce mesenchymal condensation to form the bony otic capsule. *Shh* knockouts display a poorly mineralized otic capsule that occasionally lacks semicircular canals.[100]

Sensory Cell Differentiation and Development

The organ of Corti displays a distinct planar cell polarity (PCP) parallel to the sensory epithelium with uniformly oriented stereocilia on the apical HC surfaces. Development of this ordered structure involves convergent extension, but the process that dictates it is incompletely understood. Evidence for a PCP pathway exists, and it has been suggested that the mammalian homologue of the *Drosophila* gene *Dishevelled2* may play a role in polarizing HCs.[93]

Differentiation and development of the organ of Corti in mice arises from the zone of nonproliferating cells (ZNPCs), induced by a synchronous exit from the cell cycle promoted by the cyclin-dependent kinase inhibitor p27 kip1.[94] As discussed earlier, cell cycle exit also seems to depend on expression of Notch1 and its ligand, Jagged1, which may define boundaries and patterning of sensory cell development in the cochlea,[94] because Jagged1 and Notch mutants display abnormal patterning of the cochlea.[68,95]

Sensory cell fate determination is orchestrated by Notch-Delta signaling via lateral inhibition, which results in precise patterning of sensory neuroepithelia of the cochlea and vestibular apparatus. The Web site at www.ihr.mrc.ac.uk/Hereditary/genetable/index.shtml provides a table of genes expressed in mice and humans during inner ear development.

Myosins in Inner Ear Development

The mouse mutant Shaker-2 carries a *Myosin XV* mutation, for which the homologous human deafness gene is *DFNB3*, which results in shortened stereocilia.[11] Myosin XVa localizes to the tips of stereocilia of the cochlear and vestibular HCs, overlaps with the barbed ends of actin filaments, and extends into the apical plasma membrane. Myosin XVa is essential for the graded elongation of stereocilia in formation of the characteristic staircase pattern of the hair bundle[101] (**Figs. 5–3** and **5–4**).

A Myosin VI null mutation causes the mouse mutant Snell's waltzer, which displays fusion of the stereocilia at birth and subsequent HC degeneration. This finding, combined with immunofluorescence and electron microscopy studies, revealed the function of myosin VI as an anchor between the cuticular plate of stereocilia and the apical membrane of HCs (**Fig. 5–3**).[102]

POU4F3

This transcription factor may play a dual role. Although the mouse homologue *Pou4f3* determines late HC differentiation and mutations lead to HC death prior to complete differentiation, the human *POU4F3* is a dominant deafness gene (*DFNA15*), inducing adult-onset hearing loss. Thus, *POU4F3* may play a role in long-term HC survival in the human, but its role is clearly distinct from that in mice.[103]

◆ Basic Science Applications of Molecular Biology to Hearing

Molecular biology has been used to address many basic science questions in otology. In many cases, the potential exists for such studies to influence clinical care in the future. A discussion of some promising areas of research follows.

Unique Inner Ear Proteins

Genes that are expressed uniquely in the inner ear are potentially important for its function and might be involved in diseases limited to hearing or balance. The molecular methods used to identify unique inner ear proteins are based on the laboratory production of complementary DNA (cDNA) copies of mRNA, which is expressed in the inner ear. The cDNA copies are made by reverse transcription of mRNA from inner ear tissues. Once created, these inner ear–specific cDNAs can be inserted into bacteriophage vectors for replication and screening as a cDNA library.[104–106] Several inner ear cDNA libraries have been produced and are commercially available, including those from rat and mouse inner ear, rat OHCs, guinea pig organ of Corti, and human fetal cochlea.[105–108] These libraries have enabled researchers to identify several unique proteins, including two organ of Corti–specific proteins (OCP I and II) and tectorial membrane proteins (tectorins), that have little homology to other known protein.[109–112] Also, the gene coding for a unique inner ear collagen has been identified, which has 56% homology with collagen VIII and X.[113] Localization studies within the sunfish saccule showed a predominance of the collagen at the edge of the saccule, indicating that the collagen may be secreted into the otolithic membrane by supporting cells in that area.[113] Go to http://oto.wustl.edu/thc/history.htm for a comprehensive inner ear protein inventory.

Inner Ear Homeostasis

Numerous studies have investigated genes involved in cochlear homeostasis, and, in particular, the molecular basis of production and maintenance of ion gradients between cochlear fluids and cells. Such studies have particular relevance for disorders of fluid balance in the inner ear, including Meniere's disease. Expression of genes encoding isoforms of the sodium- and potassium-activated adenosine triphosphatase (Na,K-ATPase) has been studied by Ryan and Watts[114] and Fina et al,[115] who found that all three known α-isoforms and both known β-isoforms were expressed in different combinations in different rat cochlear tissues (**Fig. 5–7**). Moreover, only the α1- and β2-isoforms were expressed in the stria vascularis, a combination not found in isolation in any other bodily tissue. This is likely related to the uniquely high electrochemical gradient against which the stria vascularis must transport sodium and potassium (**Fig. 5–4**). Similarly, Furuta et al[116] found that different isoforms of the plasma membrane calcium ATPase (PMCA) were expressed by different cochlear cells. In particular, IHCs express high levels of PMCA1 mRNA, whereas OHCs express high levels of PMCA2, suggesting that the calcium regulation requirements of the two cell types are distinct.

Furthermore, as discussed earlier, the pendrin protein is involved in endolymph homeostasis through its role as an anion transporter in the inner ear. Targeted disruption of the *Pds* gene in mice leads to severe vestibular defects, endolymphatic hydrops with dilation of associated inner ear structures, reduced macular otoconia, and cochlear HC degeneration.[117] The finding of excess endolymph in such mice has led to the assumption that pendrin plays an essential role in endolymph resorption.

In contrast, two other ion transporters of the inner ear have been identified in mice as having an essential role in endolymph production: the Na-K-Cl cotransporter encoded by *Slc12a2*, which is expressed at the basolateral membrane of stria vascularis marginal cells, and the K+ channel Kcne1 or Isk, which is expressed at the apical surface of strial marginal cells (**Fig. 5–4**). In mice with targeted disruption of either gene, there is failure of endolymph production, resulting in endolymph compartment collapse, smaller than normal SCCs, and severe vestibular defects similar to those of *Pds* mutants.[118,119] Characterization of human homologs will likely expand our knowledge of related human audiovestibular disorders.

Connexins also play a crucial role in ion homeostasis in the inner ear via recycling of K+ to the endolymphatic compartment (**Fig. 5–4**), as discussed earlier (see Nonsyndromic Deafness). For an overview of current connexin-related research, go to www.crg.es/deafness/.

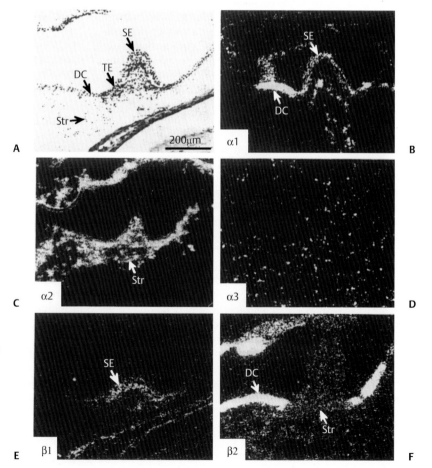

Figure 5–7 H&E-stained section **(A)** and dark-field autoradiographs **(B–F)** of Na,K-ATPase hybridization in rat ampullae of the semicircular canals. Intense expression of α1 **(B)** and β2 **(F)** was observed in the dark cell epithelium (DC), coupled with weak expression of β1 **(E).** Moderate expression of α1 **(B)** and β1 **(E)** was observed in the sensory epithelium (SE). The stroma (Str) underlying the supporting cells expressed strong levels of α2 **(C)** coupled with weak expression of the β2 isoform **(F).** However, some stromal cells (Str) located just beneath the sensory epithelium showed moderate α1 expression (arrow). An edge effect, caused by pooling of emulsion against the border of dense tissue, is visible along the bottom of the β1 panel, adjacent to the bone of the inner ear capsule. TE, transitional epithelium.

Also of importance in inner ear homeostasis is the Aquaporin family of water channels. Aquaporins (AQPs) are integral membrane proteins that are expressed in many isoforms in the inner ear, including AQP2, AQP5, and AQP6. Their function in water transport and location in the inner ear suggests a role in maintaining endolymphatic fluid balance, and they may play a role in Meniere's disease.[120,121] AQP activity may be regulated by antidiuretic hormone (ADH) or vasopressin, which is elevated in some patients with Meniere's disease.[122] Furthermore, the AQP4 knockout is deaf, underscoring the importance of AQPs in inner ear function.

Outer Hair Cell Electromotility

The discovery of otoacoustic emissions has led to their use as a tool in infant deafness screening, and audiologists already use them widely as part of their battery of diagnostic testing.[123] The basis for otoacoustic emissions is the electromotile activity of OHCs, first discovered in 1985, and thought to be responsible for both sharp tuning of the basilar membrane frequency response and for increased auditory sensitivity. Deflection of the HC stereocilia leads to a change in membrane voltage. For the OHC, unlike IHCs, this voltage response induces changes in cell length that affect the motion of the basilar membrane (discussed in Chapter 2). Several candidates for the OHC motor have under investigation, including AP-1–like proteins[124] and molecules containing a motif related to the S4 segment of voltage-gated ion channels, both of which change shape in response to changes in membrane voltage. Recently, however, prestin has been identified as the molecular motor protein of OHCs. Prestin was recently cloned from mammalian cochlear OHCs using subtractive hybridization.[125] Prestin localization and gene expression profile studies coincide with the pattern of OHC development of electromotility. Overexpression of prestin in normally nonmotile kidney cells results in nonlinear capacitance and motility that are normally only recordable in OHCs.[125] Furthermore, these properties can be reduced by salicylate, a well-known inhibitor of electromotility. Analysis of gene structure and amino acid sequence indicate that prestin is structurally homologous with the anion transporter family (SLC26) that includes PDS, DRA, and DTDST, which are chloride-iodide transporters, Cl^-/HCO_3^- exchangers, or sulfate transporters. Moreover, intracellular anions (chloride or bicarbonate) are essential for OHC electromotility and prestin's function.[125]

Mechanoelectric Transduction

The hearing and balance sensory systems require mechano-electrical transduction of sound and head movements. In the hearing process, a sound wave—a vibrational mechanical force—is transformed into an electrochemical signal that is transmitted as a nerve impulse to the brain. Investigation continues into the process of mechanoelectrical transduction, which is thought to occur as follows: When an acoustic stimulus is received, the stereociliary bundle on the apical surface of HCs is defected. The stereocilia are connected by filamentous structures at their tips, called tip links (**Fig. 5–3**). These are at least partially composed of cadherin 23 (CDH23) and myosin 1c (MYO1C), as well as a calcium channel.[11,13,126,127] If the stereocilia are deflected toward the kinocilium, tension on these tip links activates a mechanically sensitive channel, and a transduction current is induced.[128,129] If the deflection is

away from the kinocilium, the channel closes, and no current is produced. Evidence places the transduction channel, which is responsible for inducing the transduction current, on the stereocilia close to the tip links[129-131] (**Fig. 5–3**). If the stereocilia deflection is sustained, as frequently occurs in vestibular HCs, then the cells appear to actively adapt, by readjusting the attachment site of the tip links.[132] This adaptation maintains an appropriate level of tension at the tip links, and enables the HCs to maintain sensitivity over a wide range of stereociliary positions. The molecule that serves as a transduction channel has been identified as TRPN1 in zebrafish,[133] but the human homologue has not yet been identified. Molecular studies have identified prestin[134] as a candidate molecule for regulating the tensioning process, which appears to be controlled by 120-kD myosin motors that attach to the tip links and slide along the actin filaments that form the core of stereocilia.[130,135-138]

Neurotransmission

By understanding the patterns of neurotransmission within the inner ear, a pharmacologic approach to some forms of tinnitus might be developed. The afferent neurotransmitter from the HCs to the spiral ganglion neurons has not yet been identified. However, spiral ganglion and vestibular ganglion neurons strongly express genes encoding glutamate receptors of the α-amino-3-hydroxy-5-methyl-4- (AMPA), N-methyl-D-aspartate (NMDA), and kainate families,[138-143] implicating a glutamate-like neurotransmitter. The olivocochlear efferent neurotransmitter that operates from the brainstem to the inner ear is primarily acetylcholine,[144] acting at nicotinic acetylcholine receptors[145] that are strongly expressed in HCs.[146,147] Other receptors found in the cochlea include muscarinic acetylcholine, γ-aminobutyric acid (GABA), and ATP receptors,[148-151] whereas olivocochlear efferent neurons express enkephalin mRNA.[141]

Molecular Mechanisms of Inner Ear Damage

Ototoxicity

Inner ear damage commonly occurs as a result of acoustic overstimulation or through exposure to ototoxins. The list of ototoxins is impressive and includes aminoglycosides, macrolides, glycopeptide antibiotics such as vancomycin, loop diuretics, salicylates, nonsteroidal antiinflammatory drugs (NSAIDs), antimalarials such as quinine, and antineoplastic agents such as cisplatin, to name a few. Chapter 23 discusses this topic in more detail. Although the molecular mechanisms for ototoxicity of many of these agents are still incompletely elucidated, a great deal of investigation has taken place, especially with respect to aminoglycoside antibiotics. It is well established that the antimicrobial action of aminoglycosides occurs at the ribosomal level by arresting the synthesis of bacterial cell proteins. This results in an efflux of electrolytes and bacterial constituents, in turn resulting in bacterial cell death.[152] However, the ototoxic reaction, which results in OHC apoptosis, is still incompletely understood.

Aminoglycosides interfere with cell membrane lipids in two stages.[153-155] First, once a cell is exposed to the antibiotic, reversible binding of the aminoglycoside to the plasma membrane occurs. Second, energy-dependent uptake of the antibiotic occurs. Once inside the cell, the aminoglycoside interferes with basic cellular processes and ultimately disrupts the cellular membrane. The molecular mechanism of this latter process includes inhibition of the phosphoinositide pathway, which in turn affects calcium influx, activity of adenosine 3',5'-cyclic monophosphate (cAMP), cell membrane homeostasis, as well as many other basic cellular functions.[156] Histologically, HC stereocilia become edematous after aminoglycoside exposure. Together with the knowledge of the mitochondrially inherited susceptibility to aminoglycoside ototoxicity via a missense mutation in the 12S ribosomal RNA gene (discussed earlier), and with the understanding of HC stereocilia sensitivity (also discussed earlier), we might speculate that aminoglycoside antibiotics induce reversible damage to the stereocilia in most patients. In patients who harbor the mitochondrial 12S ribosomal RNA A1555G mutation, perhaps protein reproduction and turnover (i.e., recycling) cannot keep up with the rate of damage incurred within the stereocilia at certain antibiotic concentrations.

Cisplatin has been shown to induce apoptosis in a cochlear cell line, in a dose- and duration-dependent manner. Cisplatin was found to initiate the apoptosis pathway via activation of caspases. Specifically, caspase 8 activation induced mitochondrial translocation and activation of Bax, induction of mitochondrial permeability transition, release of cytochrome c into the cytosol, activation of caspase 9, and entry into the execution phase of apoptosis.[157]

Chemoprotection

In families with a genetic predisposition as well as in renal patients being treated with intravenous aminoglycosides, there is an increased likelihood of ototoxicity. The use of chemoprotectants to prevent the inner ear damage from occurring is being investigated. Of note, FGF-2 has been shown to protect neonatal HCs in vitro from neomycin ototoxicity, a fact consistent with the expression of FGF receptors on neonatal cochlear HCs.[158] Also, in vitro, glutathione has been shown to decrease gentamicin metabolite toxicity to outer HCs, and in vivo guinea pigs that were fed glutathione had less HL when exposed to gentamicin than did controls.[159] Many other candidates for aminoglycoside chemoprotection exist, and an excellent review is provided by Schacht.[160] Investigation also continues into substances that provide chemoprotection against other ototoxins, as in the case of sodium thiosulfate, fosfomycin, and lazaroids, which might provide protection against the chemotherapeutic cisplatinum.[161]

Cisplatin-induced HC death involves intracellular Ca^{2+} mobilization. The effect of calcium channel blocker, flunarizine (Sibelium), on cisplatin-induced HC apoptosis was recently investigated in a cochlear organ of Corti–derived cell line, HEI-OC1, and a neonatal (P2) rat organ of Corti explant.[162] Flunarizine significantly inhibited cisplatin-induced apoptosis. Surprisingly, flunarizine increased the intracellular calcium levels in vitro. The protective effect of flunarizine against cisplatin was not mediated by modulation of intracellular calcium level. Treatment of cisplatin resulted in ROS generation and lipid peroxidation in the HEI-OC1 cell line. Flunarizine inhibited lipid peroxidation and mitochondrial permeability transition in cisplatin-treated cells but did not attenuate ROS production. This study suggested that the protective mechanism of flunarizine on cisplatin-induced cytotoxicity is associated with direct inhibition of lipid peroxidation and mitochondrial permeability transition.[162]

Regeneration

Two separate but simultaneous experiments led to the discovery that birds are able to restore their HCs after injury from exposure to ototoxic drugs or noise. In 1987, Cruz et al[163] counted cochlear HCs in chickens that had been treated with gentamicin for 10 days and then allowed to survive from 1 to 21 days. Initially, the cochlear HC populations were depleted, but as time elapsed from the gentamicin exposure, the HC populations began to increase and approach those of normal controls. Also in 1987, Cotanche[164] observed through electron microscopy that the sensory epithelia of the chick cochlea could be repaired over the course of 10 days after exposure to excessive noise. The inevitable conclusion from both these experiments as well as from subsequent reports was that damage to avian HCs induces precursor cells, likely supporting cells within the basilar papilla, to reenter the mitotic cycle and differentiate into functioning HCs.[165]

The identities of cellular or molecular signals that can induce or regulate regenerative activity remain illusive, although evidence of diffusible factors regulating avian HC regeneration in paracrine fashion has been reported.[166] In 1994, Tsue et al[166] showed that normal inner ear epithelium displayed increased proliferation of supporting cells when exposed to damaged inner ear epithelium. Their model proposed that mitogen release in response to HC damage induces progenitor cells to differentiate into HCs and supporting cells. The mitogen release signal could be from HCs themselves, from scavenging phagocytes, or in response to decreased neuronal activity. This study implies the presence of factors that can upregulate supporting cells and promote regeneration, at least in the avian model. Although much investigation is being performed on mammalian systems, so far only vestibular HCs in mammals display a limited regenerative potential.[167] Perhaps with further research, factors that can promote regeneration of the sensory elements in the mammalian inner ear will be discovered.

◆ Future Considerations

In the last decade, the dramatic increase in our knowledge of molecular biology of the inner ear has translated into a remarkable increase in diagnostic and treatment capabilities for inner ear disorders. One such possibility is the detection of gene mutations involved in hereditary deafness, and additional genes are being identified at an almost exponential pace. Of great interest is the potential for development of gene therapy and of the delivery systems that will enable clinicians to bypass the blood–perilymph barrier and directly administer various pharmacologic therapies to the inner ear. Gene therapy has been applied experimentally in the *shiverer* mouse, which shows deficits in the amplitude and latency of auditory evoked potential (AEP) responses secondary to a mutation in the myelin basic protein gene. Yoo et al[168] demonstrated improved AEP responses in a *shiverer* mouse in which a transgene coding for normal myelin basic protein was integrated into its genome. Gene therapy of this nature might one day be applied to humans with genetic hearing loss, with the use of in vitro fertilization.

Research efforts at gene therapy are concentrating on the delivery of gene products or genes to the adult system. The development of such delivery systems for the inner ear is

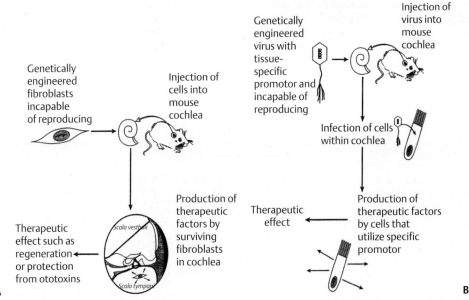

Figure 5–8 Schematics of proposed gene delivery systems utilizing genetically engineered fibroblasts **(A)** and viruses **(B)**. The fibroblasts and viruses are incapable of reproducing, but the viruses are additionally constructed with tissue-specific promoters. These modifications will minimize complications associated with the delivery systems.

being approached in several ways. The first approach is to infuse drugs directly into the inner ear with a microcatheter placed through the tympanic membrane, either against or through the round window membrane to gain entry into the scala tympani. This method has been used successfully in delivering neurotrophins to the scala tympani of guinea pigs to improve survival of neurons after ototoxin-induced damage.[169] An alternative approach is to embed the drug of choice into a polymer that, once placed in the inner ear, would protect the drug from degradation and help to sustain its release at a specific rate.[170] This approach, however, requires a second surgery to terminate the therapy. A third technique is to utilize carrier proteins that would link the drug of choice to endothelial cells lining the inner ear capillaries. These carrier proteins could then facilitate the transportation of the drug across the endothelial cell barrier and then release the drug into the endolymph or perilymph where the targeted cell population awaits. Early success with this technique has been achieved in brain when nerve growth factor was delivered across the blood–brain barrier utilizing an antitransferrin antibody as the carrier protein.[171]

Other approaches of gene therapy utilize the techniques of molecular biology (**Fig. 5–8**). Viral vectors that carry and express genes that encode therapeutic proteins or factors can be used to infect cochlear cells. The advantage of this approach is that the delivery of the inactivated viral vector requires only one procedure, and once transfection has occurred within the target site, the therapeutic factor can be continually produced. These viruses can be driven by specifically designed promoters but do not retain the ability to replicate. The viruses being investigated for this purpose include retroviruses, herpes viruses, adenoviruses, and adeno-associated viruses, with each virus having different cell type specificity. An in vivo report in 1992 documented that a herpes simplex viral vector, carrying a nerve growth factor gene, protected neurons of the dorsal root ganglion from the consequences of a traumatic injury.[172] Several laboratories are using herpes viruses and adenoviruses to induce gene expression in inner ear cells.[173–175] Expression of Math1, for example, delivered via viral vector with targeted gene expression in the organ of Corti may one day facilitate mammalian HC regeneration.

Another approach is transplantation of cells that have been genetically modified to produce therapeutic factors. This method involves injecting genetically engineered cells into the inner ear where they can release the therapeutic factors in large quantities. These cells, however, must be incapable of reproducing, as uncontrolled proliferation and neoplastic processes might potentially be induced otherwise. Two studies have shown that genetically engineered fibroblasts could be used to deliver growth factors to the cochlear duct.[169,176] The tools of molecular biology will enable us to further develop these and other delivery systems. For an up-to-date overview of progress in this area, go to www.nlm.nih.gov/medlineplus/genesandgenetherapy.html.

References

1. Friedman TB, Schultz JM, Ben-Yosef T, et al. Recent advances in the understanding of syndromic forms of hearing loss. Ear Hear 2003;24:289–302
2. Hu D, Qui WQ, Wu BT, et al. Genetic aspects of antibiotic induced deafness: mitochondrial inheritance. J Med Genet 1991;28:79–83
3. Barker D, Hostikka SL, Zhou J, et al. Identification of mutations in the COL4A5 collagen gene in Alport syndrome. Science 1990;248:1224–1227
4. Ishikiriyama S, Tonoki H, Shibuya Y, et al. Waardenburg syndrome type I in a child with de novo inversion (2q35-q37.3). Am J Med Genet 1989;33:505–507
5. Foy C, Newton V, Wellesley D, Harris R, Read AP. Assignment of the locus for Waardenburg syndrome type I to human chromosome 2q37 and possible homology to Splotch mouse. Am J Hum Genet 1990;46: 1017–1023
6. Hoth C, Milunsky A, Lipsky N, et al. Mutations in the paired domain of the human PAX3 gene caused Klein-Waardenburg syndrome (WS-III) as well as Waardenburg syndrome type I (WS-I). Am J Hum Genet 1993;52:455–462
7. Edery P, Attie T, Amiel J, et al. Mutation in the endothelin-3 gene in the Waardenburg-Hirschsprung disease (Shah-Waardenburg syndrome). Nat Genet 1996;12:442–444

8. Hofstra RM, Osinga J, Tan-Sindhunata G, et al. A homozygous mutation in the endothelin-3 gene associated with a combined Waardenburg type 2 and Hirschsprung phenotype (Shah-Waardenburg syndrome). Nat Genet 1996;12:445–447

9. Gibson F, Walsh J, Mburu P, et al. A type VII myosin encoded by the mouse deafness gene shaker-1. Nature 1995;374:62–64

10. Weil D, Blanchard S, Kaplan J, et al. Defective myosin VIIA gene responsible for Usher syndrome type 1B. Nature 1995;374:60–61

11. Friedman TB, Sellers JR, Avraham KB. Unconventional myosins and the genetics of hearing loss. Am J Med Genet 1999;89:147–157

12. Steel KP, Kros CJ. A genetic approach to understanding auditory function. Nat Genet 2001;27:143–149

13. Hasson T, Gillespie PG, Garcia JA, et al. Unconventional myosins in inner-ear sensory epithelia. J Cell Biol 1997;137:1287–1307

14. Verpy E, Leibovici M, Zwaenepoel I, et al. A defect in harmonin, a PDZ domain-containing protein expressed in the inner ear sensory hair cells, underlies Usher syndrome type 1C. Nat Genet 2000;26:51–55

15. Kimberling W, Weston MD, Moller C, et al. Localization of Usher syndrome type II to chromosome 1q. Genomics 1990;7:245–249

16. Lewis R, Otterud B, Stauffer D, Lalouel JM, Leppert M. Mapping recessive ophthalmic diseases: linkage of the locus for Usher syndrome type II to a DNA marker on chromosome 1q. Genomics 1990;7:250–256

17. Kaplan J, Gerber S, Bonneau D, et al. A gene for Usher syndrome type I (USH1A) maps to chromosome 14q. Genomics 1992;14:979–987

18. Kimberling W, Moller CG, Davenport S, et al. Linkage of Usher syndrome type gene (USH1B) to the long arm of chromosome 11. Genomics 1992;14:988–994

19. Scott DA, Karniski LP. Human pendrin expressed in Xenopus laevis oocytes mediates chloride/formate exchange. Am J Physiol Cell Physiol 2000;278:C207–C211

20. Royaux IE, Belyantseva IA, Wu T, et al. Localization and functional studies of pendrin in the mouse inner ear provide insight about the etiology of deafness in Pendred syndrome. J Assoc Res Otolaryngol 2003;4:394–404

21. Trofatter J, MacCollin MM, Rutter JL, et al. A novel moesin-radixin-like gene is a candidate for the neurofibromatosis 2 tumor suppressor. Cell 1993;72:791–800

22. Fernandez-Valle C, Tang Y, Richard J, et al. Paxillin binds schwannomin and regulates its density-dependent localization and effect on cell morphology. Nat Genet 2002;31:354–362

23. Abdelhak S, Kalatzis V, Heilig R, et al. A human homolog of the Drosophila eyes absent gene underlies branchio-oto-renal (BOR) syndrome and identifies a novel gene family. Nat Genet 1997;15:157–164

24. Smith R, Coppage KB, Ankerstjerne JKB, et al. Localization of the gene for branchiootorenal syndrome to chromosome 8q. Genomics 1992;14:841–844

25. Merry D, Lesko JG, Sosnoski DM, et al. Choroideremia and deafness with stapes fixation: a contiguous gene deletion syndrome in Xq21. Am J Hum Genet 1989;45:530–540

26. Cremers F, Van De Pol TJ, Diergaarde PJ, et al. Physical fine mapping of the choroideremi a locus using Xq21 deletions associated with complex syndromes. Genomics 1989;4:41–46

27. Bach I, Brunner HG, Beighton P, et al. Microdeletions in patients with gusher-associated, X-linked mixed deafness (DFN3). Am J Hum Genet 1992;51:38–44

28. de Kok YJ, van der Maarel SM, Bitner-Glindzicz M, et al. Association between X-linked mixed deafness and mutations in the POU domain gene POU3F4. Science 1995;267:685–688

29. Van Laer L, Cryns K, Smith RJ, Van Camp G. Nonsyndromic hearing loss. Ear Hear 2003;24:275–288

30. Kelsell DP, Di WI, Houseman MJ. Connexin mutations in skin disease and hearing loss. Am J Hum Genet 2001;68:559–568

31. Abe S, Usami S, Shinkawa H, Kelley PM, Kimberling WJ. Prevalent connexin 26 gene (GJB2) mutations in Japanese. J Med Genet 2000;37:41–43

32. Usami S, Koda E, Tsukamoto K, et al. Molecular diagnosis of deafness: impact of gene identification. Audiol Neurootol 2002;7:185–190

33. Chang EH, Van Camp G, Smith RJ. The role of connexins in human disease. Ear Hear 2003;24:314–323

34. Wilcox ER, Burton QL, Naz S, et al. Mutations in the gene encoding tight junction claudin-14 cause autosomal recessive deafness DFNB29. Cell 2001;104:165–172

35. Usami S, Abe S, Weston MD, Shinkawa H, Van Camp G, Kimberling WJ. Non-syndromic hearing loss associated with enlarged vestibular aqueducts is caused by PDS mutations. Hum Genet 1999;104:188–192

36. Schmitt N, Schwarz M, Peretz A, Abitbol I, Attali B, Pongs O. A recessive C-terminal Jervell and Lange-Nielsen mutation of the KCNQ1 channel impairs subunit assembly. EMBO J 2000;19:332–340

37. Schulze-Bahr E, Wang Q, Wedekind H, et al. KCNE1 mutations cause Jervell and Lange-Nielsen syndrome. Nat Genet 1997;17:267–268

38. Kharkovets T, Hardelin JP, Safieddine S, et al. KCNQ4, a K+-channel mutated in a form of dominant deafness, is expressed in the inner ear and the central auditory pathway. Proc Natl Acad Sci USA 2000;97:4333–4338

39. Phippard D, Heydemann A, Lechner M, et al. Changes in the subcellular location of the Brn4 gene product precede mesenchymal remodeling of the otic capsule. Hear Res 1998;120:77–85

40. Erkman L, McEvilly RJ, Luo L, et al. Role of transcription factors Brn-3.1 and Brn-3.2 in auditory and visual system development. Nature 1996;381:603–606

41. Vahava O, Morell R, Lynch E, et al. Mutation in transcription factor POU4F3 associated with inherited progressive hearing loss in humans. Science 1998;279:1950–1954

42. Bespalova IN, Van Camp G, Bom S, et al. Mutations in the Wolfram syndrome 1 gene (WFS1) are a common cause of low frequency sensorineural hearing loss. Hum Mol Genet 2001;10:2501–2508

43. Schneider ME, Belyantseva IA, Azevedo RB, Kachar B. Rapid renewal of auditory hair bundles. Nature 2002;418:837–838

44. Liu XZ, Walsh J, Tamagawa Y, et al. Autosomal dominant non-syndromic deafness caused by a mutation in the myosin VIIA gene. Nat Genet 1997;17:268–269

45. Lynch ED, Lee MK, Morrow JE, et al. Nonsyndromic deafness DFNA1 associated with mutation of a human homolog of the Drosophila gene diaphanous. Science 1997;278:1315–1318

46. Di Palma F, Holme RH, Bryda EC, et al. Mutations in Cdh23, encoding a new type of cadherin, cause stereocilia disorganization in walzer, the mouse model for Usher syndrome type 1D. Nat Genet 2001;27:103–107

47. Migliosi V, Modamio-Hoybjor S, Moreno-Pelayo MA, et al. Q829X, a novel mutation in the gene encoding otoferlin (OTOF), is frequently found in Spanish patients with prelingual nonsyndromic hearing loss. J Med Genet 2002;39:502–506

48. Varga R, Kelley PM, Keats BJ, et al. Non-syndromic recessive auditory neuropathy is the result of mutations in the otoferlin (OTOF) gene. J Med Genet 2003;40:45–50

49. Richardson RT, Wise A, O'Leary S, et al. Tracing neurotrophin-3 diffusion and uptake in the guinea pig cochlea. Hear Res 2004;198:25–35

50. Ikezono T, Omori A, Ichinose S, et al. Identification of the protein product of the Coch gene (hereditary deafness gene) as the major component of bovine inner ear protein. Biochim Biophys Acta 2001;1535:258–265

51. Robertson NG, Lu L, Heller S, et al. Mutations in a novel cochlear gene cause DFNA9, a human nonsyndromic deafness with vestibular dysfunction. Nat Genet 1998;20:299–303

52. Fransen E, Verstreken M, Verhagen WI, et al. High prevalence of symptoms of Meniere's disease in three families with a mutation in the COCH gene. Hum Mol Genet 1999;8:1425–1429

53. Robertson CP, Braun MM, Roelink H. Sonic hedgehog patterning in chick neural plate is antagonized by a Wnt3-like signal. Dev Dyn 2004;229:510–519

54. Fischel-Ghodsian N. Mitochondrial deafness. Ear Hear 2003;24:303–313

55. Sue CM, Lipsett LJ, Crimmins DS, et al. Cochlear origin of hearing loss in MELAS syndrome. Ann Neurol 1998;43:350–359

56. Reardon W, Ross RJM, Sweeney MG, et al. Diabetes mellitus associated with a pathogenic point mutation in mitochondrial DNA. Lancet 1992;340:1376–1379

57. Usami S, Abe S, Kasai M, et al. Genetic and clinical features of sensorineural hearing loss associated with the 1555 mitochondrial mutation. Laryngoscope 1997;107:483–490

58. Fischel-Ghodsian N, Bykhovskaya Y, Taylor K, et al. Temporal bone analysis of patients with presbycusis reveals high frequency of mitochondrial mutations. Hear Res 1997;110:147–154

59. Riazuddin S, Castelein CM, Ahmed ZM, et al. Dominant modifier DFNM1 suppresses recessive deafness FNB26. Nat Genet 2000;26:431–434

60. Lalwani AK. Evaluation of childhood sensorineural hearing loss in the post-genome world. Arch Otolaryngol Head Neck Surg 2002;128:88–89

61. Parnes LS, Chernoff WG. Bilateral semicircular canal aplasia with near-normal cochlear development. Ann Otol Rhinol Laryngol 1990;99:957–959

62. Yu KK, Mukherji S, Carrasco V, Pillsbury HC, Shores CG. Molecular genetic advances in semicircular canal abnormalities and sensorineural hearing loss: a report of 16 cases. Otolaryngol Head Neck Surg 2003;129:637–646

63. Rauch S. Malformation and degeneration in the inner ear of mos transgenic mice. Ann Otol Rhinol Laryngol 1992;101:430–436

64. Crenshaw EB 3rd, Ryan AF, Dillon SR, et al. Wocko: a neurological mutant generated in a transgenic mouse pedigree. J Neurosci 1991;11:1524–1530

65. Friedman RA. Wocko: A Transgenic Insertional Inner Ear Mutation. San Diego: University of California at San Diego Department of Molecular Pathology, 1994

66. Mansour SL, Goddard JM, Capecchi MR. Mice homozygous for a targeted disruption of the proto-oncogene INT-2 have developmental defects in the tail and ear. Development 1993;117:13–28

67. Represa J, Leon Y, Miner C, Giraldez F. The Int-2 proto-oncogene is responsible for induction of the inner ear. Nature 1991;353:561–563

68. Kiernan AE, Ahituv N, Fuchs H, et al. The Notch ligand Jagged1 is required for inner ear sensory development. Proc Natl Acad Sci U S A 2001; 98:3873–3878

69. Heller S, Sheane CA, Javed Z, Hudspeth AJ. Molecular markers for cell types of the inner ear and candidate genes for hearing disorders. Proc Natl Acad Sci U S A 1998;95:11400–11405

70. Carney PR, Silver J. Studies on cell migration and axon guidance in the developing distal auditory system of the mouse. J Comp Neurol 1983;215:359–369

71. Fekete DM, Wu DK. Revisiting cell fate specification in the inner ear. Curr Opin Neurobiol 2002;12:35–42

72. Acampora D, Mazan S, Avantaggiato V, et al. Epilepsy and brain abnormalities in mice lacking the Otx1 gene. Nat Genet 1996;14:218–222

73. Favor J, Sandulache R, Neuhauser-Klaus A, et al. The mouse Pax2(1Neu) mutation is identical to a human PAX2 mutation in a family with renal-coloboma syndrome and results in developmental defects of the brain, ear, eye, and kidney. Proc Natl Acad Sci USA 1996;93:13870–13875

74. Torres M, Gomez-Pardo E, Gruss P. Pax2 contributes to inner ear patterning and optic nerve trajectory. Development 1996;122:3381–3391

75. Glass CK, Direnzo J, Kurokawa R, Han Z. Regulation of gene expression by retinoic acid receptors. DNA Cell Biol 1991;10:623–638

76. Romand R, Sapin V, Dolle P. Spatial distributions of retinoic acid receptor gene transcripts in the prenatal mouse inner ear. J Comp Neurol 1998;393:298–308

77. Thompson DL, Gerlach-Bank LM, Barald KF, Koenig RJ. Retinoic acid repression of bone morphogenetic protein 4 in inner ear development. Mol Cell Biol 2003;23:2277–2286

78. Romand R, Hashino E, Dolle P, et al. The retinoic acid receptors RARalpha and RARgamma are required for inner ear development. Mech Dev 2002;119:213–223

79. Lohnes D, Mark M, Mendelsohn C, et al. Function of the retinoic acid receptors (RARs) during development (I). Craniofacial and skeletal abnormalities in RAR double mutants. Development 1994; 120: 2723–2748

80. Kelley MW, Xu XM, Wagner MA, et al. The developing organ of Corti contains retinoic acid and forms supernumerary hair cells in response to exogenous retinoic acid in culture. Development 1993;119:1041–1055

81. Liu M, Pereira FA, Price SD, et al. Essential role of BETA2/NeuroD1 in development of the vestibular and auditory systems. Genes Dev 2000;14:2839–2854

82. Bermingham N, Hassan B, Price S, et al. Math1: an essential gene for the generation of inner ear hair cells. Science 1999;284:1837–1841

83. Izumikawa M, Minoda R, Kawamoto K, et al. Auditory hair cell replacement and hearing improvement by Atoh1 gene therapy in deaf animals. Nat Med 2005;11:271–276

84. Erkman L, McEvilly RJ, Luo L, et al. Role of transcription factors Brn-3.1 and 3.2 in auditory and visual system development. Nature 1996; 381:603–606

85. Xiang M, Gan L, Li D, et al. Essential role of POU-domain factor Brn-3c in auditory and vestibular hair cell development. Proc Natl Acad Sci U S A 1997;94:9445–9450

86. Xiang M, Gao WQ, Hasson T, Shin JJ. Requirement for Brn-3c in maturation and survival, but not in fate determination of inner ear hair cells. Development 1998;125:3935–3946

87. Lefebvre P, Staecker H, Weber T, et al. TGFB1 modulates bFGF receptor message expression in cultured adult auditory neurons. Neuroreport 1991;2:305–308

88. Lefebvre P, Van de Water TR, Represa J, et al. Temporal pattern of nerve growth factor (NGF) binding in vivo and the in vitro effects of NGF on cultures of developing auditory and vestibular neurons. Acta Otolaryngol 1991;111:304–311

89. Lefebvre P, Van de Water TR, Weber T, et al. Growth factor interactions in cultures of dissociated adult acoustic ganglia: neuronotrophic effects. Brain Res 1991;567:306–312

90. Lefebvre P, Van de Water TR, Staecker H, et al. Nerve growth factor stimulates neurite regeneration but not survival of adult auditory nerves in vitro. Acta Otolaryngol 1992;112:288–293

91. Staecker H, Van de Water TR, Lefebvre PP, et al. NGF, BDNF and NT-3 play unique roles in the in vitro development and patterning of innervation of the mammalian inner ear. Brain Res Dev Brain Res 1996;92:49–60

92. Ernfors P, Lee KF, Jaenisch R. Mice lacking brain-derived neurotrophic factor develop with sensory deficits. Nature 1994;368:147–150

93. Wang J, Mark S, Zhang X, et al. Regulation of polarized extension and planar cell polarity in the cochlea by the vertebrate PCP pathway. Nat Genet 2005;37:980–985

94. Chen P, Johnson JE, Zoghbi HY, Segil N. The role of Math1 in inner ear development: uncoupling the establishment of the sensory primordium from hair cell fate determination. Development 2002; 129:2495–2505

95. Tsai H, Hardisty RE, Rhodes C, et al. The mouse slalom mutant demonstrates a role for Jagged1 in neuroepithelial patterning in the organ of Corti. Hum Mol Genet 2001;10:507–512

96. Daudet N, Lewis J. Two contrasting roles for Notch activity in chick inner ear development: specification of prosensory patches and lateral inhibition of hair-cell differentiation. Development 2005;132:541–551

97. Eddison M, Le Roux I, Lewis J. Notch signaling in the development of the inner ear: lessons from Drosophila. Proc Natl Acad Sci U S A 2000; 97:11692–11699

98. McKay IJ, Lewis J, Lumsden A. The role of FGF-3 in early inner ear development: an analysis in normal and Kreisler mutant mice. Dev Biol 1996;174:370–378

99. Ma Q, Chen Z, del Barco Barrantes I, et al. Neurogenin 1 is essential for the determination of neuronal precursors for proximal cranial sensory ganglia. Neuron 1998;20:469–482

100. Liu W, Li G, Chien JS, et al. Sonic hedgehog regulates otic capsule chondrogenesis and inner ear development in the mouse embryo. Dev Biol 2002;248:240–250

101. Belyantseva IA, Boger ET, Friedman TB. Myosin XVa localizes to the tips of inner ear sensory cell stereocilia and is essential for staircase formation of the hair bundle. Proc Natl Acad Sci U S A 2003;100:13958–13963

102. Avraham KB, Hasson T, Steel KP, et al. The mouse Snell's waltzer deafness gene encodes an unconventional myosin required for structural integrity of inner ear hair cells. Nat Genet 1995;11:369–375

103. Fekete DM. Development of the vertebrate ear: insights from knockouts and mutants. Trends Neurosci 1999;22:263–269

104. Davis J, Oberholtzer JC, Burns FR, et al. Use of the teleost saccule to identify genes involved in inner ear function. DNA Cell Biol 1995; 14:833–839

105. Ryan AF, Batcher S, Brumm D, O'Driscoll K, Harris JP. Cloning genes from an inner ear cDNA library. Arch Otolaryngol Head Neck Surg 1993;119:1217–1220. PMID: 8217081

106. Wilcox E, Fex J. Construction of a guinea pig organ of Corti cDNA library. Hear Res 1992;62:124–126

107. Robertson N, Khetarpal U, Gutierrez-Espeleta GA, et al. Isolation of novel and known genes from a fetal cochlear cDNA library using subtractive hybridization and differential screening. Genomics 1994;23:42–50

108. Beisel K, Kennedy JE, Morley BJ. Construction and assessment of a rat outer hair cell unidirectional cDNA library. Abstr Assoc Res Otolaryngol 1995;18:81

109. Chen H, Thalmann I, Adams JC, et al. cDNA cloning, tissue distribution, and chromosomal localization of Ocp2; a gene encoding a putative transcription-associated factor predominantly expressed in the auditory organs. Genomics 1995;10:389–398

110. Killick R, Legan PK, Malenczak C, Richardson GP. Molecular cloning of chick beta-tectorin, an extracellular matrix molecule of the inner ear. J Cell Biol 1995;129:535-547

111. Thalmann I, Suzuki H, McCourt DW, et al. Partial amino acid sequences of organ of Corti proteins OCP1 and OCP2: a progress report. Hear Res 1993;64:191–198

112. Killick R, Legan PK, Malenczak C, Richardson GP. Molecular cloning of chick beta-tectorin, an extracellular matrix molecule of the inner ear. J Cell Biol 1995;129:535–547

113. Davis J, Oberholtzer JC, Burns FR, Greene MI. Molecular cloning and characterization of an inner ear-specific structural protein. Science 1995;267:1031–1034

114. Ryan A, Watts AG. Expression of genes coding for α and β isoforms of Na/K-ATPase in the cochlea of the rat. Cell Mol Neurosci 1991;2:179–187

115. Fina M, Bresnik S, Baird A, Ryan AF. Improved healing of tympanic membrane perforations with basic fibroblast growth factor. Growth Factors 1991;5:265–272

116. Furuta H, Luo L, Helper K, Ryan AF. Evidence for differential regulation of calcium by outer versus inner hair cells: plasma membrane Ca-ATPase gene expression. Hear Res 1998;123:10-26

117. Everett LA, Belyantseva IA, Noben-Trauth K, et al. Targeted disruption of mouse Pds provides insight about the inner-ear defects encountered in Pendred syndrome. Hum Mol Genet 2001;10:153–161

118. Delpire E, Lu J, England R, Dull C, Thorn T. Deafness and imbalance associated with inactivation of the secretory Na-K-Cl co-transporter. Nat Genet 1999;22:192–195

119. Letts VA, Valenzuela A, Dunbar C, Zheng QY, Johnson KR, Frankel WN. A new spontaneous mouse mutation in the Kene1 gene. Mamm Genome 2000;11:831–835

120. Couloigner V, Berrebi D, Teixeira M, et al. Aquaporin-2 in the human endolymphatic sac. Acta Otolaryngol 2004;124:449–453

121. Fukushima M, Kitahara T, Fuse Y, et al. Changes in aquaporin expression in the inner ear of the rat after i.p. injection of steroids. Acta Otolaryngol Suppl 2004;553:13–18

122. Ferrary E, Sterkers O, Couloigne V. Hormonal regulation of endolymph homeostasis. Abst Meniere's Symp 2005;MS-2:39

123. Kemp D. Stimulated acoustic emissions from within the human auditory system. J Acoust Soc Am 1978;64:1386–1391

124. Kalinec F, Kachar B. Inhibition of outer hair cell electromotility by sulfhydryl specific agents. Neurosci Lett 1993;157:231–234

125. Zheng J, Madison LD, Oliver D. Prestin, the motor protein of outer hair cells. Audiol Neurootol 2002;7:9–12

126. Holt JR, Gillespie SK, Provance DW, et al. A chemical-genetic strategy implicates myosin-1c in adaptation by hair cells. Cell 2002; 108: 371–381

127. Siemens J, Lillo C, Dumont RA, et al. Cadherin 23 is a component of the tip link in hair-cell stereocilia. Nature 2004;428:950–955

128. Pickles J, Comis SD, Osborne MP. Cross-links between stereocilia in the guinea pig organ of Corti and their possible relation to sensory transduction. Hear Res 1984;15:103–112

129. Assad J, Shepherd GM, Corey DP. Tip-link integrity and mechanical transduction in vertebrate hair cells. Neuron 1991;7:985–994

130. Gillespie P, Wagner MC, Hudspeth AJ. Identification of a 120 kDa hair-bundle myosin located near stereociliary tips. Neuron 1993;11: 581–594

131. Hackney CM, Furness DN, Benos DJ, et al. Putative immunolocalization of the mechanoelectric transduction channels in mammalian cochlear hair cells. Proc Biol Sci 1992;248:215–221

132. Howard J, Hudspeth AJ. Mechanical relation of the hair bundle mediated adaptation in mechanoelectrical transduction by the bullfrog's saccular hair cells. Proc Natl Acad Sci U S A 1987;84:3064–3068

133. Sidi S, Friedrich R, Nicolson T. NomC TRP channel required for vertebrate sensory hair cell mechanotransduction. Science 2003;301: 96–99

134. Zheng J, Shen W, He DZ, et al. Prestin is the motor protein of cochlear outer hair cells. Nature 2000;405:149–155

135. Hudspeth A, Gillespie PG. Pulling springs to tune transduction: adaptation by hair cells. Neuron 1994;12:1–9

136. Metcalf A, Chelliah Y, Hudspeth AJ. Molecular cloning of a myosin 1 beta isozyme that may mediate adaptation by hair cells of the bullfrog's internal ear. Proc Natl Acad Sci U S A 1994;91:11821–11825

137. Soc C, Derfler BH, Buyks GM, Corey DP. Molecular Cloning of myosins from the bullfrog saccular macula: a candidate for the hair cell adaptation motor. Auditory Neurol 1994;1:63–75

138. Kuriyama H, Albin RL, Altschuler RA. Expression of NMDA-receptor mRNA in the rat cochlea. Hear Res 1993;69:215–220

139. Hunter C, Petralia RS, Vu T, Wenthold RJ. Expression of AMPA-selective glutamate receptor in morphologically-defined neurons of the mammalian cochlear nucleus. J Neurosci 1993;13:1932–1946

140. Niedzielski A, Wenthold RJ. Expression of AMPA, kainite and NMDA receptor subunits in cochlear and vestibular ganglia. J Neurosci 1995;15:2338–2353

141. Ryan AF, Brumm D, Kraft M. Occurrence and distribution of non-NMDA glutamate receptor mRNAs in the cochlea. Neuroreport 1991; 2: 643–646

142. Wenthold R, Martin MR. Neurotransmitters of the auditory nerve and central auditory system. In: Berlin C, ed. Hearing Science: Recent Advances. San Diego: College-Hill Press, 1984:342–369

143. Li HS, Niedzielski AS, Beisel KW, et al. Identification of a glutamate/aspartate transporter in the rat cochlea. Hear Res 1994;78:235–242

144. Housley GD, Ashmore JF. Direct measurement of the action of acetylcholine on isolated outer hair cells of the guinea pig cochlea. Proc Biol Sci 1991;244:161–167

145. Wackym P, Popper P, Lopez I, et al. Expression of alpha 4 and beta 2 nicotinic acetylcholine receptor subunit mRNA and localization of alpha-bungarotoxin binding proteins in the rat vestibular periphery. Cell Biol Int 1995;19:291–300

146. Elgoyhen A, Johnson DS, Boulter J, et al. Alpha 9: acetylcholine receptor with novel pharmacological properties expressed in rat cochlear hair cells. Cell 1994;79:705–715

147. Luo L, Bennett T, Jung HH, Ryan AF. Developmental expression of alpha 9 acetylcholine receptor mRNA in the rat cochlea and vestibular inner ear. J Comp Neurol 1998;393:320–331

148. Mockett BG, Housley GD, Thorne PR. Fluorescence imaging of extracellular purinergic receptor sites and putative ecto-ATPase sites on isolated cochlear hair cells. J Neurosci 1994;14:6992–7007

149. Drescher D, Upadhyay S, Wilcox, Fex J. Analysis of muscarinic receptor subtypes in the mouse cochlea by means of PCR. J Neurochem 1992;59:765–767

150. Drescher D, Green GE, Khan KM, et al. Analysis of GABA-A receptor subunits in the mouse cochlea by means of PCR. J Neurochem 1993;61:1167–1170

151. Housley GD, Greenwood D, Bennett T, Ryan AF. Identification of a short form of the P2xR1-purinoceptor subunit produced by alternative splicing in the pituitary and cochlea. Biochem Biophys Res Commun 1995;212:501–508

152. Edson R, Terrell CL. The aminoglycosides: streptomycin, kanamycin, gentamicin, tobramycin, amikacin, netilmicin, and sisomicin. Mayo Clin Proc 1987;62:916–920

153. Henley C, Schacht J. Pharmacokinetics of aminoglycoside antibiotics in blood, inner ear fluids and tissues and their relationship to ototoxicity. Audiology 1988;27:137–146

154. Schacht J. Molecular mechanisms of drug-induced hearing loss. Hear Res 1986;22:297–304

155. Williams SE, Zenner HP, Schacht J. Three molecular steps of aminoglycoside ototoxicity demonstrated in outer hair cells. Hear Res 1987; 30:11–18

156. Bartolami S, Planche M, Pujol R. Inhibition of the carbachol-evoked synthesis of inositol phosphates by ototoxic drugs in the rat cochlea. Hear Res 1993;67:203–210

157. Devarajan P, Savoca M, Castaneda MP, et al. Cisplatin-induced apoptosis in auditory cells: role of death receptor and mitochondrial pathways. Hear Res 2002;174:45–54

158. Low W, Dazert S, Baird A, Ryan AF. Fibroblast growth factor (FGF-2) protects rat cochlear hair cells in organotypical culture from aminoglycoside injury. J Cell Physiol 1996;167:443–450

159. Garetz SL, Rhee DJ, Schacht J. Attenuation of gentamicin ototoxicity by glutathione in the guinea pig in vivo. Hear Res 1994;77:81–87

160. Schacht J. Biochemical basis of aminoglycoside ototoxicity. Otolaryngol Clin North Am 1993;26:845–857

161. Chiodo A, Alberti PW. Experimental, clinical, and preventive aspects of ototoxicity. Eur Arch Otorhinolaryngol 1994;251:375–392

162. So HS, Park C, Kim HJ, et al. Protective effect of T-type calcium channel blocker flunarizine on cisplatin-induced death of auditory cells. Hear Res 2005;204:127–139

163. Cruz RM, Lambert PR, Rubel EW. Light microscopic evidence of hair cell regeneration after gentamicin toxicity in chick cochlea. Arch Otolaryngol Head Neck Surg 1987;113:1058–1062

164. Cotanche D. Regeneration of hair cell stereociliary bundles in the chick cochlea following severe acoustic trauma. Hear Res 1987;30:181–194

165. Rubel EW. Regeneration of hair cells. In: Dancer A, Henderson D, Salvi R, Hammernik R, eds. Noise-Induced Hearing Loss. St. Louis: Mosby, 1992:204–227

166. Tsue T, Oesterle EC, Rubel EW. Diffusible factors regulate hair cell regeneration in the avian inner ear. Proc Natl Acad Sci U S A 1994;91: 1584–1588

167. Warchol M, Lambert PR, Goldstein BJ, et al. Regenerative proliferation in inner ear sensory epithelia from adult guinea pigs and humans. Science 1993;259:1619–1622

168. Yoo T, Fujiyoshi T, Readhead C, Hood L. Restoration of auditory evoked potential by myelin basic protein (MBP) gene therapy in shiverer mice. Abstr Assoc Res Otolaryngol 1993;16:147

169. Staecker H, Galinovic-Schwartz V, Liu W, et al. The role of the neurotrophins in maturation and maintenance of postnatal auditory innervation. Am J Otol 1996;17:486–492

170. Leong K, D'Amore P, Marletta M, Langer R. Biodegradable polyanhydrides as drug-carrier matrices II. Biocompatibility and chemical reactivity. J Biomed Mater Res 1986;20:51–64

171. Pardridge W. Receptor mediated peptide transport through the blood brain barrier. Endocr Rev 1986;7:314–330

172. Federoff H, Geschwind MD, Geller AI, Kessler JA. Expression of NGF in vivo from a defective HSV-I vector prevents effects of axotomy on sympathetic ganglia. Proc Natl Acad Sci U S A 1992;89:1636–1640

173. Qun LX, Pirvola U, Saarma M, Ylikoski J. Neurotrophic factors in the auditory periphery. Ann N Y Acad Sci 1999;884:292–304

174. Weiss MA, Frisancho JC, Roessler BJ, Raphael Y. Viral-mediated gene transfer in the cochlea. Int J Dev Neurosci 1997;15:577–583

175. Dazert S, Battaglia A, Ryan AF. Transfection of neonatal rat cochlear cells in vitro with an adenovirus vector. Int J Dev Neurosci 1997;15: 595–600

176. Ryan A, Luo L. Delivery of a recombinant growth factor into the mouse inner ear by implantation of a transfected cell line. Abstr Assoc Res Otolaryngol 1995;18:47

6

Pharmacology of Otologic Drugs

Leonard P. Rybak

There has been a proliferation of publications dealing with the use of new and established drugs for the therapy of inner ear diseases. Novel ways of delivery of drugs to the inner ear have been tested in the last decade. This chapter discusses the pharmacology of several agents used to treat sensorineural hearing loss and vertigo and offers perspectives for the future for drug delivery to the inner ear.

◆ Corticosteroids

Indications

Naturally occurring corticosteroids are used to replace deficient hormone levels in patients with adrenocortical insufficiency. Various synthetic corticosteroids are used for pharmacologic effects because of their greater potency, longer duration of action, and superior efficacy in the treatment of disease states. Corticosteroids are used to treat a variety of nonotologic diseases, including disorders of the upper and lower respiratory tract, endocrine diseases, collagen diseases, skin disorders, neoplasms, allergic problems, and diseases of the eye and blood-forming organs.[1]

Corticosteroids are employed to treat a variety of otologic diseases, ranging from illnesses affecting the pinna and external auditory canal, such as contact dermatitis and eczema, and as an adjunct in combination with topical antibiotic solutions or powders to treat external otitis. These drugs may also be used in combination with antibiotics topically to treat otitis media in patients with an opening into the middle ear, whether it is a ventilation tube or a spontaneous perforation of the tympanic membrane. They are also frequently used to treat several inner ear disorders, including sudden sensorineural hearing loss, whether idiopathic or of suspected vascular, traumatic, or viral etiology; Meniere's disease; autoimmune inner ear disease; and certain vestibular disorders.

Mechanisms of Action

The glucocorticoids are the corticosteroids that are most commonly utilized to treat ear disease. These drugs are derivatives of the naturally occurring hormones in the adrenal cortex. These compounds affect carbohydrate, lipid, and protein metabolism by combining with their receptors in the tissues affected. Interaction with the receptors causes a change in gene expression within the cells. The resulting effects include immune suppression, membrane stabilization, antiinflammatory effects with a reduction in tissue edema, sodium transport regulation, and increased perfusion of target tissues.[2] Steroids have been shown to prevent hearing loss in patients with bacterial meningitis by inhibiting the actions of cell adhesion molecules, thereby reducing the inflammatory response to molecules released in response to the bacterial injury, such as the arachidonic acid metabolites.[3,4] Nevertheless, the exact molecular mechanisms by which steroids reverse or prevent hearing loss are not yet known.[2]

New mechanisms for the actions of glucocorticoids have been elucidated recently. These drugs clearly act on diverse targets through multiple mechanisms to control inflammation. The glucocorticoid receptor in humans is located on chromosome 5q31–32. The details of its regulation are detailed in a recent review article.[1] Glucocorticoids interacting with their receptor initiate a complex regulatory network that blocks several inflammatory pathways. The glucocorticoids can block the production of prostaglandins through three independent mechanisms: the induction and activation of annexin I, the induction of mitogen-activated protein kinase (MAPK) phosphatase 1, and the repression of transcription of cyclooxygenase 2. The latter step is accomplished by blocking the transcriptional activity of nuclear factor (NF)-κB. Glucocorticoids and their receptor also modulate the activity of other transcription factors.

By a nongenomic mechanism, glucocorticoids activate endothelial nitric oxide synthase, thus protecting against ischemia-reperfusion injury. Glucocorticoids can also decrease inflammation by decreasing the stability of messenger RNA (mRNA) for inflammatory proteins, such as vascular endothelial growth factor and cyclooxygenase 2.[1]

Pharmacokinetics

Corticosteroids, such as dexamethasone, are primarily metabolized in the liver and excreted by the kidneys. The most commonly used systemic glucocorticoids are hydrocortisone, prednisolone, methylprednisolone, prednisone, and dexamethasone. These drugs have good oral bioavailability. Plasma concentrations follow a biexponential pattern. Two-compartment models are used after intravenous administration, but one-compartment models are sufficient to describe pharmacokinetics after oral administration. Pharmacokinetic parameters such as the elimination half-life, and pharmacodynamic parameters such as the concentration producing the half-maximal effect, determine the duration and intensity of the effects of the glucocorticoids.[5] Measurable concentrations of steroids are reached in inner ear fluids, but the concentrations are much lower than those achieved following intratympanic administration (see below).

Adverse Reactions

A host of adverse reactions has been reported following systemic administration of corticosteroids. These tend to be more frequent and more severe following chronic administration. Adverse events include increased susceptibility to infection; disturbances in fluid and electrolyte balance (hypokalemia, retention of sodium and water); congestive heart failure and myocardial rupture after recent acute myocardial infarction; muscle weakness and wasting; disturbances in bone metabolism (osteoporosis, aseptic necrosis of the heads of the femur or humerus, compression fractures of the vertebrae); and tendon ruptures.

Endocrine problems found with corticosteroid therapy include suppression of growth in children; secondary lack of responsiveness to stress, such as trauma, illnesses, or surgery by the adrenal cortex and pituitary gland; carbohydrate intolerance especially in latent or insulin-dependent diabetics, making them relatively resistant to insulin; hirsutism; cushingoid changes in body habitus, including "buffalo hump" and cushingoid facies; as well as hypertension.

Gastrointestinal complications may include nausea, perforation of the bowel, peptic ulcers (especially when combined with oral non-steroidal anti-inflammatory drugs) with hemorrhage and possible perforation, pancreatitis, and ulcers of the esophagus.

Ophthalmologic complications include posterior subcapsular cataracts, increased intraocular pressure or glaucoma, and exophthalmos.

Neurologic side effects include seizures, increased intracranial pressure, headache, and psychological changes, including severe depression.

Skin changes include petechiae, increased fragility of the skin and capillaries with petechiae and ecchymosis, impairment of wound healing, diaphoresis, and acne.

Additional side effects such as thromboembolism, weight gain, increased appetite, and malaise may occur.[1,6] Dormant tuberculosis can become active.

Drug Interactions

Corticosteroids have a hyperglycemic effect and may increase the requirement for insulin or oral hypoglycemic drugs. A patient who requires insulin while taking corticosteroids may not be able to resume oral hypoglycemic drugs when steroids are stopped. The potassium balance needs to be monitored in patients receiving corticosteroids, especially when these patients are receiving concomitant diuretics, such as thiazides or loop diuretics, or when they are being treated concurrently with amphotericin B. Such combinations

can cause potassium depletion.[1] The hypokalemia induced by glucocorticoids may enhance the blockade of nondepolarizing neuromuscular blocking agents, which may lead to increased or prolonged respiratory depression or paralysis, resulting in apnea. Prolonged paralysis with cisatracurium for mechanical ventilation in combination with methylprednisolone resulted in acute motor axonal polyneuropathy manifested as flaccid quadriplegia with absent deep tendon reflexes.[7] Patients receiving digitalis glycosides may be more likely to experience arrhythmias or digitalis toxicity associated with hypokalemia.[8] The natriuretic and diuretic effects of diuretics may be decreased by the sodium- and fluid-retaining effects of corticosteroids.[8]

Corticosteroids given in combination with salicylates can result in increased clearance of salicylates. The efficacy of anticoagulants can be diminished by steroid therapy, and the dosage of the former may need to be adjusted when steroid therapy is initiated or discontinued. The risk of gastrointestinal ulceration or hemorrhage may be increased during concurrent use. The induction of hepatic enzymes by corticosteroids may increase the formation of a hepatotoxic acetaminophen metabolite, thereby increasing the risk of hepatotoxicity when they are used concurrently with high-dose or chronic acetaminophen therapy.[8]

The metabolism of corticosteroids is increased by drugs that induce drug metabolizing enzymes in the liver. Such drugs include phenobarbital, phenytoin, and rifampin. If one or more of these drugs is administered concurrently with corticosteroids, the maintenance dose of the latter may need to be increased to maintain the desired effect.

The simultaneous use of certain antibiotics, such as troleandomycin or erythromycin may reduce the clearance of corticosteroids, resulting in an exaggerated steroid activity or cushingoid side effects, and the dose of steroid may need to be reduced.[9]

Large doses of intravenous methylprednisolone can increase the plasma concentrations of cyclosporine in renal transplant patients. This may require that the physician reduce the dose of cyclosporine in the face of glucocorticoid therapy.[10]

Estrogens have a dual effect on the pharmacokinetics of corticosteroids. The former hormones increase the levels of corticosteroid-binding globulin, thus increasing the fraction of bound steroid and rendering it less active. On the other hand, the metabolism of corticosteroids is decreased, thus prolonging their half-life. Therefore, when estrogen therapy is begun, a reduction in the dose of glucocorticoids may be in order, and when estrogen therapy is discontinued in patients on concomitant corticosteroid therapy, the dose of the latter may need to be increased.[8]

Tricyclic antidepressants do not relieve, but rather may exacerbate, corticosteroid-induced mental disturbances, and they should not be used to treat these adverse effects (United States Pharmacopeia, 1999).

◆ Aminoglycoside Antibiotics

Indications

Aminoglycosides are polyanionic amino sugars that have been derived from soil bacteria. They were first developed in 1944 to treat gram-negative bacterial infections, such as those occurring in necrotizing otitis externa and chronic otitis media. The members of this family of drugs are streptomycin, kanamycin, neomycin, gentamicin, amikacin, tobramycin, and netilmicin. Intramuscular streptomycin has been used for vestibular ablation in patients with bilateral Meniere's disease, Meniere's disease in an only hearing ear, or in the second ear that is symptomatic after contralateral ablation.[11] Intratympanic gentamicin (see below) now has replaced intramuscular streptomycin.

Mechanisms of Action

The aminoglycosides are bactericidal. They are actively transported across the bacterial cell membrane, irreversibly bind to one or more specific receptor proteins on the 30S subunit of bacterial ribosomes, and interfere with an initiation complex between mRNA and the 30S subunit. DNA may be incorrectly read, and this can lead to the formation of nonfunctional proteins. Polyribosomes are split apart, resulting in inability to synthesize new proteins. This then accelerates uptake of the antibiotic molecules, disrupting the cytoplasmic membrane of the bacteria, leading to leakage of ions and other substances out of the bacterial cell, and then to cell death.[12]

The mechanisms of action of aminoglycosides in the treatment of Meniere's disease are not entirely clear. These are thought to include ablation of type I hair cells of the crista ampullaris of the semicircular canals and damage to the dark cells of the ampulla.[13]

Pharmacokinetics

Aminoglycosides are poorly absorbed after oral administration. They are well absorbed from intramuscular injection sites. These drugs may be absorbed in significant amounts from certain body surfaces, such as from the peritoneal or pleural cavity, following local irrigation of these body cavities.[12] They are absorbed through the round window membrane to a significant degree (see below).

Aminoglycosides are not significantly metabolized following systemic administration. They are not bound to serum proteins to any great extent (usually less than 10%). They are distributed to all body tissues and accumulate within cells. These drugs achieve high concentrations in highly perfused organs, like liver, lungs, and kidneys. Lower concentrations are found in muscle, fat, and bone. They are excreted by the kidney and a high concentration is found in the urine. Distribution half-life after systemic administration is quite short, 5 to 15 minutes. Elimination half-life is 2 to 4 hours in adults with normal renal function, but is significantly longer in neonates and in patients with renal insufficiency. The terminal half-life is greater than 100 hours and this is because of slow release from binding to intracellular sites.[12] Animal studies have shown that aminoglycosides may be detected in inner ear tissues up to a year after systemic administration.[14] To avoid systemic toxicity and to achieve selective vestibular ablation, especially in one ear only, aminoglycosides have been applied intratympanically for Meniere's disease (see below).

Adverse Reactions

Hypersensitivity reactions to aminoglycosides occasionally occur, and, when they are documented, cross-sensitivity to other members of this class of drugs must be considered. Hearing loss and nephrotoxicity are risks with any of the aminoglycosides. All aminoglycosides cross the placenta and cause nephrotoxicity or total, irreversible congenital deafness in children born to mothers treated with these drugs during pregnancy. All aminoglycosides have the potential to cause neuromuscular blockade. Very young infants have been reported to experience central nervous system depression, with stupor, flaccidity, coma, or deep respiratory depression. Caution needs to be exercised in the treatment of elderly patients because of age-related decrease in renal function and perhaps increased susceptibility to toxicity.[12] Systemic aminoglycosides can cause unintended severe bilateral vestibular loss, resulting in clumsiness, ataxia, and oscillopsia. Toxicity to peripheral nerves can also occur. Optic neuritis has been reported only following streptomycin.

Drug Interactions

Aminoglycoside antibiotics may interact with other nephrotoxic or ototoxic medications to produce a higher incidence or a greater severity of kidney damage or ototoxic injury, particularly loop diuretics.

Neuromuscular blocking agents used in patients receiving aminoglycosides may result in respiratory depression or skeletal muscle weakness after surgery.

◆ Methotrexate

Indications

Several reports have suggested that methotrexate may be useful for the treatment of immune-mediated and autoimmune inner ear disease (AIED). Hearing and balance were improved in patients with AIED and Meniere's disease treated with oral methotrexate.[15] Open-label studies demonstrate that this drug may be beneficial in some patients with mild AIED; controlled randomized trials do not support its use, however.[16,17] This drug is widely used to treat rheumatoid arthritis. It may be beneficial in systemic immune disease which secondarily affects the inner ear, e.g. Cogan's syndrome.

Mechanism of Action

Methotrexate is an antimetabolite that is an analogue of folic acid. In the treatment of cancer, it is specific for the S phase of cell division. Methotrexate inhibits the synthesis of DNA, RNA, thymidylate, and protein synthesis by binding irreversibility to the enzyme, dihydrofolate reductase. Rapidly dividing cells, including tumor cells and normal cells in the bone marrow, buccal and intestinal mucosa, cells in the urinary bladder, spermatogonia, and cells in the fetus have their growth inhibited by this drug. In nonmalignant conditions, such as AIED, methotrexate has a mild immunosuppressive action.[18]

Pharmacokinetics

Methotrexate is absorbed by the oral route, but the absorption is highly variable. It is moderately (approximately 50%) bound to serum proteins. It has only limited penetration of the blood–brain barrier. It is metabolized by the liver where metabolites are retained in the hepatocytes. The half-life for low doses is variable—from 3 to 10 hours. The clearance rates vary a great deal for individuals. Peak concentration after oral administration is 1 to 2 hours. Eighty to 90% of a dose is excreted primarily by the kidney as the unchanged molecule within 24 hours. Biliary excretion occurs to a slight extent—only 10% or less of methotrexate administered is eliminated in the bile.

Adverse Reactions

Methotrexate crosses the placenta and is teratogenic. It is also a potent abortifacient. It is potentially carcinogenic. Methotrexate can cause ulcerative stomatitis, gingivitis, and pharyngitis. It is also hepatotoxic. Gastrointestinal ulceration, bleeding, or perforation may occur with methotrexate. Bone marrow suppression from methotrexate may result in thrombocytopenia, with easy bruising and bleeding. Leukopenia may also occur, resulting in bacterial infections or septicemia.[18]

Drug Interactions

Methotrexate may increase the risk of hepatotoxicity when used in combination with alcohol or hepatotoxic medications, such as the sulfonamides. Methotrexate may cause an additive effect on the bone marrow when used in combination with bone marrow suppressant medications.

Oral neomycin may increase the absorption of methotrexate. Probenecid and weak organic acids such as salicylates may inhibit the renal tubular secretion of methotrexate, resulting in higher blood concentrations. Drugs that are highly protein bound, such as sulfonamides and salicylates may displace bound methotrexate in the blood, resulting in toxic concentrations of unbound methotrexate.[18]

◆ Etanercept

Indications

Etanercept is a dimeric fusion protein "decoy receptor" consisting of the extracellular ligand-binding protein of the human 75-kD tumor necrosis factor (TNF) receptor linked to the Fc portion of the human immunoglobulin (Ig) G1, the drug that has been approved for the treatment of rheumatic arthritis in adults and juveniles, psoriatic arthritis, ankylosing spondylitis, and psoriasis.[19,20] Animal studies suggested that prompt intervention with etanercept reduces inflammation and immune-mediated hearing loss in treated ears.[21] Recently, it has been used to treat immune-mediated cochleovestibular disorders.[22] It is administered twice weekly by subcutaneous injection of 25 mg per dose. Recent clinical studies suggest that etanercept therapy does not improve hearing loss in AIED compared with placebo,[23] but may stabilize hearing in a group of patients with pretreatment intractable progressive hearing loss.[22] Vertigo and tinnitus may be improved, however.[22]

Mechanism of Action

Etanercept binds to TNF, acting as a "decoy receptor," thereby blocking the interaction of TNF with cell surface receptors and preventing the proinflammatory effects of this cytokine. TNF has a pivotal role in inflammation, and its crucial role has been demonstrated in several autoimmune diseases.[20]

Pharmacokinetics

A single 25-mg dose of etanercept given subcutaneously (SC) to healthy adults is slowly absorbed from injection sites, reaching a peak concentration at 51 hours. Mean bioavailability was 58% following a single SC dose of 10 mg etanercept. It is assumed that the complex of etanercept with TNF is metabolized through peptide and amino acid pathways, with either recycling of amino acids or elimination in bile and urine. Age, body size, gender, and ethnic origin can have an effect on pharmacokinetics of etanercept.[20]

Adverse Reactions

Etanercept is generally safe and well tolerated. However, because TNF-α may play a role in host defense against tuberculosis and other infections, there is a risk of infection with the use of drugs like etanercept. Cases reports of tuberculosis in patients treated with etanercept have been reported to the Food and Drug Administration.[24] Fulminant pneumonia with adult respiratory distress syndrome can occur, especially in patients receiving both systemic corticosteroids and etanercept.[25]

Drug Interactions

Drug interactions of etanercept with warfarin, digoxin, and methotrexate were examined. To date no clinically relevant drug–drug interactions between etanercept and other commonly prescribed drugs have been detected.[20]

◆ Intratympanic Therapy

Over the past one to two decades, intratympanic drug therapy has become an increasingly utilized method to deliver drugs to the inner ear in higher concentrations than can be achieved by systemic administration, and to circumvent systemic toxicity of these agents. The inner ear is isolated from the rest of the body by the blood–labyrinth barrier.[26] This route of drug treatment has been utilized primarily to deliver corticosteroids or aminoglycosides to the inner ear. Other less frequently used medications applied by this route include antioxidants, growth factors, antiviral agents, diuretics, and volume expanders.[2] The drug selected for treatment may be injected through an intact tympanic membrane, through a ventilation tube, or through a myringotomy incision. For endoscopic guidance, various wicks and catheters have been devised to deliver the drug directly to the round window membrane of the patient to be treated.

Anatomy of the Round Window

The round window membrane is located in the medial wall of the middle ear within the round window niche. This membrane is partially obscured by the bony promontory. The latter may frequently have mucoperiosteal folds that may tend to obstruct access to the round window membrane. Such folds may be known as "false round window membranes."[27] Studies of adult human temporal bones have revealed that 21% had false round window membranes and 11% had a plug of fat or fibrous tissue obstructing the round window niche. Only 56% had no obstruction, whereas 22% had bilateral obstruction.[28]

In 41 living patients undergoing middle ear endoscopy prior to intratympanic therapy, 29 round windows appeared to be unobstructed, seven were partially obstructed, and five were completely obstructed by adhesions.[29]

The round window membrane is thicker around the edges and thinner in the center. The average thickness of the human round window membrane is approximately 70 μm, but it is much thinner in rodents, ranging from 10 to 14 μm in thickness, and in cats it varies from 20 to 40 μm in average thickness.[30] It consists of three layers: an epithelial layer facing the middle ear, a core of connective tissue, and an inner epithelial layer facing the inner ear.[27] Animal experiments have shown that the round window membrane acts as a semipermeable membrane, allowing the passage of cationic ferritin, horseradish peroxidase, 1-μm latex spheres, and neomycin-gold spheres.[27]

Principles of Pharmacokinetics of Intratympanic Drug Therapy

The inner ear is a geometrically complex organ containing spaces (scalae) filled with fluid, and each scala has multiple interfaces with other scalae and with other compartments, including the middle ear space and the systemic blood circulation. The scala tympani and scala vestibuli contain perilymph, which has characteristics of extracellular fluid, namely low potassium and high sodium concentrations. The scala media contains endolymph, a fluid high in potassium and a relatively high positive charge. Recent studies have revealed that inner ear fluids do not circulate to any significant degree and are not actively stirred. Therefore, drugs applied locally to the round window membrane enter the ear slowly, mainly by passive diffusion. The rate at which drugs spread depends on the physical properties of the diffusing molecules. Their molecular weight appears to have the greatest influence on their diffusion. Animal experiments suggest that the round window acts as a semipermeable membrane. A major process that determines drug concentration in the inner ear is clearance, which expresses the rate of removal of drugs from the inner ear fluids into the circulation. Large gradients of drug concentration can occur with intratympanic application, resulting in higher levels of drug near the round window, with diminishing concentrations at more apical locations in the inner ear.[31] Fluid sampling to determine the kinetics of locally applied drugs from animal cochleae has specific challenges, as discussed in a recent review.[31] A variety of drug application systems has been employed, varying from intratympanic injections of fluids to the use of wicks, catheters, implantable pumps, polymers, and gels in animal and human studies. Based on animal studies, it appears that the application protocol is a major factor that determines the drug level achieved in the inner ear. The time that the drug is present in the middle ear plays a primary role.[31] The differences in anatomy between animals and humans make it difficult to extrapolate the results from animal studies to clinical intratympanic therapy.[30]

Intratympanic Corticosteroid Therapy

Indications

Intratympanic administration of corticosteroids has been used to provide high concentrations of these antiinflammatory drugs to the inner ear tissues. Clinical otologic conditions that have been treated with this technique include sudden sensorineural hearing loss, Meniere's disease, tinnitus, and AIED.

Adverse Effects

Intratympanic steroid therapy has been associated with tympanic membrane perforation, chronic otitis media, disequilibrium and dysgeusia[32] (**Table 6–1**).

Pharmacokinetics

Intratympanic dexamethasone administration in animals resulted in greater concentrations in perilymph than those resulting from intravenous injection.[33] The perilymph kinetics of methylprednisolone, dexamethasone, and hydrocortisone were compared in the guinea pig after intratympanic administration. Methylprednisolone reached the highest concentration in both perilymph and endolymph. Concentrations in endolymph were greater than in perilymph. The peak perilymph concentrations were attained within the first hour, and then diminished rapidly. Peak endolymph levels occurred at 1 to 2 hours, followed by a rapid decline. Plontke and Salt[34] used computer simulation to determine the pharmacokinetics of steroids in the inner ear using the data published by Parnes et al[35] and Bachmann et al.[36] From these data, Plontke and Salt determined that the clearance half-time of these corticosteroids was 130 minutes. They calculated that continuous delivery resulted in the highest maximum concentration. On the other hand, a brief single application gave the lowest maximum concentration. Because of the rapid clearance half-time, it was ascertained that although the method of drug delivery and its concentration determined the absolute concentration at any given place in the scala tympani, it did not alter the relative concentration. A steady state is achieved within hours, and this is not significantly affected by additional drug application.[30,34]

Table 6–1 Adverse Effects of Intratympanic Corticosteroids

Event	Reference
Tympanic membrane perforation	
Temporary	Parnes et al, 1999[35]
Slow healing	Silverstein et al, 1996[42]
Chronic	Shulman and Goldstein, 2000[43]
	Doyle et al, 2004[6]
Ear blockage	Shulman and Goldstein, 2000[43]
Increased tinnitus intensity	Shulman and Goldstein, 2000[43]
Otitis media	
Acute	Doyle et al, 2004[6]
Chronic	Herr and Marzo, 2005[32]
Increased insulin requirement	Doyle et al, 2004[6]
Pain	
Methylprednisolone	Parnes et al, 1999[35]
Dexamethasone	Barrs et al, 2001[44]
Vertigo (temporary)	Doyle et al, 2004[6]
Dysequilibrium	Herr and Marzo, 2005[32]
Dysgeusia	Herr and Marzo, 2005[32]

Intratympanic Therapy with Aminoglycosides

Indications

The intratympanic use of aminoglycoside antibiotics, primarily gentamicin, has been primarily focused on the treatment of peripheral vertigo associated with unilateral Meniere's disease.

Adverse Effects

A major concern with the intratympanic administration of the ototoxic antibiotic gentamicin is hearing loss. However, a recent meta-analysis of articles reported clinical trials of patients diagnosed as having definitive Meniere's disease according to the criteria described by the Committee on Hearing and Equilibrium of the American Academy of Otolaryngology–Head and Neck Surgery 1985 or 1995 and receiving gentamicin administered into the middle ear by transtympanic injection or using a specially designed catheter. Toxic effects of intratympanic gentamicin on hearing and word recognition were found to be neither statistically significant nor clinically important. However, it was reported that patients treated with a titration regimen experienced a lesser degree of worsening of hearing and word recognition than those receiving the drug on a fixed dose regimen (0.02 dB and 0.4% in the former group versus 5.4 dB and 6.5% for the latter group).[37] However, another recently published meta-analysis of intratympanic gentamicin for Meniere's disease reported an estimated hearing loss of 25.1% from all studies combined. The weekly method of gentamicin dosing was associated with less hearing loss (13.1%) than the multiple daily dosing method, which resulted in hearing loss in nearly 35% of patients treated in this manner. Other delivery methods, so-called low-dose, titration, or continuous administration, displayed similar rates of hearing loss to the group as a whole.[38] The discrepancies between these two meta-analyses published in the same year likely represent differences in inclusion criteria between the two studies.

Pharmacokinetics

Gentamicin kinetics in the chinchilla inner ear varied according to whether the drug was administered by bolus intratympanic injection or by round window microcatheter infusion.[39] After transtympanic injection, a peak concentration of gentamicin was found in perilymph at 24 hours, followed by a decline in concentration that followed first-order kinetics. On the other hand, when the drug was applied by round window microcatheter infusion, a small peak was reached at 4 hours, followed by a slight decline. A higher, sustained peak concentration was measured at 24 hours and persisted for 72 hours. This was followed by a gradual decline in spite of continued infusion of gentamicin.[39] Plontke and colleagues[40] combined the data from studies in the chinchilla to create a computer simulation of gentamicin in the chinchilla and human. By combining these data, they determined that the peak concentration of gentamicin after a single application of a 10 mg/mL solution would occur between 600 to 700 minutes after application, followed by a rapid decline. Using this computer simulation and comparing the relative size of the human and chinchilla inner ear, they calculated that the drug levels in the vestibule would be similar for the chinchilla and human. Because of the greater length of the human cochlea, the concentration of gentamicin at the apex would be two orders of magnitude lower than at the base in humans, as opposed to being 10-fold lower in the chinchilla.[30,40] Comparing different protocols of drug administration using computer simulation, Plontke and colleagues found that continuous delivery of gentamicin resulted in the highest maximum concentration. Middle ear volume stabilization with fibrin glue gave intermediate maximum concentrations, and a single application of gentamicin without volume stabilization in the middle ear resulted in the lowest concentrations in perilymph.[30,40]

From animal studies, it appears that there is great variation in the maximum concentration of gentamicin after single-dose intratympanic administration; however, peak concentrations appear to be achieved in 8 to 24 hours. Elimination from perilymph appears to follow first-order kinetics and may be energy dependent. Continuous administration appears to lead to more predictable and stable concentrations.[30]

The Future of Intratympanic Therapy

The use of the intratympanic route to administer drugs, such as corticosteroids, is a rational approach to the treatment of diseases that may involve the release of inflammatory cytokines into the inner ear to reduce the damage caused by the latter molecules. This approach needs further study to define the ideal pharmacologic parameters for steroid delivery.[41] The use of computer simulation of concentration-time courses can guide the design of preclinical animal experiments and can help to estimate inner ear drug concentrations prior to designing clinical protocols.[31] The use of carrier substances, such as biopolymers to prolong the time that a drug remains in the middle ear and other methods of inner ear delivery, such as nanotechnology and gene therapy may provide exciting prospects for improving the therapy of inner ear diseases with intratympanic drug administration.

◆ Acknowledgment

Dr. Rybak is supported by National Institutes of Health (NIH) grant R 01-DC 02396.

References

1. Rhen T, Cidlowski JA. Antiinflammatory actions of glucocorticoids—new mechanism for old drugs. N Engl J Med 2005;353:1711–1723
2. Seidman MD, Vivek P. Intratympanic treatment of hearing loss with novel and traditional agents. Otolaryngol Clin North Am 2004;37: 973–990
3. Kaplan SL. Prevention of hearing loss from meningitis. Lancet 1997;350: 158–159
4. Coyle PK. Glucocorticoids in central nervous system bacterial infection. Arch Neurol 1999;56:796–801
5. Czock D, Keller F, Rasche FM, Haussler U. Pharmacokinetics and pharmacodynamics of systemically administered glucocorticoids. Clin Pharmacokinet 2005;44:61–98
6. Doyle KJ, Bauch C, Battista R, et al. Intratympanic steroid treatment: a review. Otol Neurotol. 2004;25:1034–1039
7. Fodale V, Pratico C, Girlanda P, et al. Acute motor axonal polyneuropathy after a cisatracurium infusion and concomitant corticosteroid therapy. Br J Anaesth 2004;92:289–293
8. United States Pharmacopeia Drug Information. Drug Information for the Health Care Professional, vol I, 19th ed. Englewood, CO: Micromedix, 1999:1000–1001

9. Szefler SJ, Rose JQ, Ellis EF, Spector SL, Green AW, Jusko WJ. The effect of troleandomycin on methylprednisolone elimination. J Allergy Clin Immunol 1980;66:447–451

10. Klintmalm G, Sawe J, von Bahr C, et al. Optimal cyclosporine plasma levels decline with time of therapy. Transplant Proc 1984;16:1208–1211

11. Monsell EM, Cass SP, Rybak LP, Nedzelski JM. Chemical treatment of the labyrinth. In: Brackman DE, Shelton C, Arriaga MA, eds. Otologic Surgery, 2nd ed. Philadelphia: WB Saunders, 2001:413–421

12. United States Pharmacopeia Drug Information. Drug Information for the Health Care Professional, vol I, 19th ed. Englewood, CO: Micromedix, 1999:70–72

13. Monsell EM, Cass SP, Rybak LP. Therapeutic use of aminoglycosides in Meniere's disease. Otolaryngol Clin North Am 1993;26:737–746

14. Aran JM. Current perspectives on inner ear toxicity. Otolaryngol Head Neck Surg 1995;112:133–144

15. Matteson EL, Tirzaman O, Facer GW, et al. Use of methotrexate for autoimmune hearing loss. Ann Otol Rhinol Laryngol 2000;109:710–714

16. Matteson EL, Fabry DA, Facer GW, et al. Open trial of methotrexate for autoimmune hearing loss. Arthritis Rheum 2001;45:146–150

17. Harris JP, Weisman MH, Derebery JM, et al. Treatment of corticosteroid-responsive autoimmune inner ear disease with methotrexate. A randomized controlled trial. JAMA 2003;290:1875–1883

18. United States Pharmacopeia Drug Information. Drug Information for the Health Care Professional, vol I, 19th ed. Englewood, CO: Micromedix, 1999:1969–1973

19. Atzeni F, Turiel M, Capsoni F, Doria A, Meroni P, Sarzi-Puttini P. Autoimmunity and anti-TNF-alpha agents. Ann N Y Acad Sci 2005;1051:559–569

20. Zhou H. Clinical pharmacokinetics of etanercept: a fully humanized soluble recombinant tumor necrosis factor receptor fusion protein. J Clin Pharmacol 2005;45:490–497

21. Wang X, Truong T, Billings PB, Harris JP, Keithley EM. Blockage of immune-mediated inner ear damage by etanercept. Otol Neurotol 2003;24:52–57

22. Matteson EL, Choi HK, Poe DS, et al. Etanercept therapy for immune-mediated cochleovestibular disorders: a multi-center, open-label, pilot study. Arthritis Rheum 2005;53:337–342

23. Cohen S, Shoup A, Weisman MH, Harris J. Etanercept treatment for autoimmune inner ear disease: results of a pilot placebo-controlled study. Otol Neurotol 2005;26:903–907

24. Rychly DJ, DiPiro JT. Infections associated with tumor necrosis factor-alpha antagonists. Pharmacotherapy 2005;25:1181–1192

25. Zimmer C, Beiderlinden M, Peters J. Lethal acute respiratory distress syndrome during anti-TNF-alpha therapy for rheumatoid arthritis. Clin Rheumatol 2006;25:430–432 [epub 2005 Oct 1]

26. Juhn SK, Rybak LP, Prado S. Nature of blood labyrinth barrier in experimental conditions. Ann Otol Rhinol Laryngol 1981;90:135–141

27. Goycoolea MV, Lundman L. Round window membrane: structure function and permeability: a review. Microsc Res Tech 1997;36:201–211

28. Alzamil KS, Linthicum FH Jr. Extraneous round window membranes and plugs: possible effect on intratympanic therapy. Ann Otol Rhinol Laryngol 2000;109:30–32

29. Silverstein H, Rowan PT, Olds MJ, Rosenberg SI. Inner ear perfusion and the role of round window patency. Am J Otol 1997;18:586–589

30. Banerjee A, Parner LS. The biology of intratympanic drug administration and pharmacodynamics of round window drug absorption. Otolaryngol Clin North Am 2004;37:1035–1051

31. Salt AN, Plontke SKR. Local inner-ear drug delivery and pharmacokinetics. Drug Discov Today 2005;10:1299–1306

32. Herr BD, Marzo SJ. Intratympanic steroid perfusion for refractory sudden sensorineural hearing loss. Otolaryngol Head Neck Surg 2005;132:527–531

33. Chandrasekhar SS, Rubinstein RY, Kwartler JA, et al. Dexamethasone pharmacokinetics in the inner ear: comparison of route of administration and use of facilitating agents. Otolaryngol Head Neck Surg 2000;122:521–528

34. Plontke SK, Salt AN. Quantitative interpretation of corticosteroid pharmacokinetics in inner ear fluids using computer simulations. Hear Res 2003;182:34–42

35. Parnes LS, Sun AH, Freeman DJ. Corticosteroid pharmacokinetics in the inner ear fluids: an animal study followed-up by clinical application. Laryngoscope 1999;109(suppl 91):1–17

36. Bachmann G, Su J, Zumegen C, Wittekindt C, Michel O. Permeabilitat des runden Fenstermembranen fur prednisolon-21-hydrogensuccinat. HNO 2001;49:538–541

37. Cohen-Kerem R, Kisilevsky V, Einarson TR, Kozer E, Koren G, Rutka JA. Intratympanic gentamicin for Meniere's disease: a meta-analysis. Laryngoscope 2004;114:2085–2091

38. Chia SH, Gamst AC, Anderson JP, Harris JP. Intratympanic gentamicin therapy for Meniere's disease: a meta-analysis. Otol Neurotol 2004;25:544–552

39. Hoffer ME, Allen K, Kopke RD, Weisskopf P, Gottshall K. Transtympanic versus sustained release administration of gentamicin: kinetics, morphology and function. Laryngoscope 2001;111:1343–1357

40. Plontke SK, Wood AW, Salt AN. Analysis of gentamicin kinetics in fluids of the inner ear with round window administration. Otol Neurotol 2002;23:967–974

41. Staecker H. Broadening the spectrum of treatment options for SNHL. Arch Otolaryngol Head Neck Surg 2005;131:734

42. Silverstein H, Choo D, Rosenberg S, Kuhn J, Seidman M, Stein I. Intratympanic steroid treatment of inner ear disease and tinnitus (preliminary report). Ear Nose Throat J 1996;75:468–488

43. Shulman A, Goldstein B. Intratympanic drug therapy with steroids for tinnitus control: a preliminary report. Int Tinnitus J 2000;6:10–20

44. Barrs DM, Keyser JS, Stallworth C, McElveen JT. Intratympanic steroid injections for intractable Meniere's disease. Laryngoscope 2001;111:2100–2104

II

Evaluation

7

Temporal Bone Imaging

Rebecca S. Cornelius

Imaging of temporal bone pathology relies primarily on computed tomography (CT) and magnetic resonance imaging (MRI).[1,2] Other modalities, including angiography and nuclear medicine imaging, have a role limited to specific clinical situations.

Imaging procedures of choice in various clinical situations are discussed in the subsections of this chapter. In general, MRI offers advantages of multiplanar imaging capability without requiring the patient to lie in uncomfortable positions. MRI provides better detail of soft tissue abnormalities as well as more specific characteristics of mass lesions. However, imaging time is usually considerably longer than with CT and requires a higher level of patient cooperation to achieve high-quality images. Likewise, patients with claustrophobia usually experience greater difficulty with MRI than with CT. Newer-generation helical multislice CT technology now allows for rapid scan times and high-quality multiplanar reconstructions, often obviating the need for scanning directly in two planes. A high-detail temporal bone CT performed using these techniques requires less than 10 minutes of patient time in the CT scanner and actual scan time of under 30 seconds for a single plane study.

MRI is contraindicated in some patients with implanted metallic devices or foreign bodies: pacemakers, certain aneurysm clips, cardiac valves, cochlear and other metallic implants, and metallic foreign bodies in the globe or orbit. MRI centers keep extensive lists of implanted devices that are known to be MRI compatible or incompatible. Radiologists and technologists operating MRI scanners should be able to determine whether a particular device implanted in a patient can be exposed to the magnetic field without risk.

The cost of CT examination is usually 20% to 40% less than MRI; however, in most instances of temporal bone evaluation, one test is clearly the procedure of choice over the other as far as diagnostic value. Thus, the issue of cost differential does not realistically come into play in most situations.

As a general guideline for choosing imaging modalities, readers are referred to the introductory chapter of *Imaging of the Temporal Bone* by Swartz and Harnsberger.[3] This covers in detail an algorithmic approach to imaging based on the patient's clinical presentation.

◆ Imaging of Diseases of the External Auditory Canal

Disease processes that affect the external auditory canal (EAC) include congenital dysplasias (**Fig. 7–1**), benign and malignant neoplasms, and inflammatory disease. These entities are covered in detail in Chapters 16 and 26.

Imaging of EAC disease is best accomplished with CT scanning to ensure that the cortex of the osseous portion of the EAC is fully evaluated.[3,4]

In patients with aggressive malignant neoplasms additional evaluation with MRI with gadolinium contrast enhancement may be warranted if there is evidence of intracranial extension. Extension into adjacent extracranial tissue such as the parotid space usually can be evaluated with either contrast-enhanced CT or MRI.

Likewise, patients with necrotizing external otitis (NEO) with suspicion of intracranial spread may require additional imaging with MRI. Detection of meningeal involvement and complications such as abscess or sinus thrombosis will be better detected with MRI than CT.

Extracranial spread into the temporomandibular joint, parapharyngeal space, and masticator space usually is adequately evaluated with contrast-enhanced CT,[5] but also is well evaluated with MRI. MRI also detects bony signal changes in osteomyelitis.[6,7]

Some studies advocate the use of radionuclide imaging in the diagnosis and follow-up of NEO. Both technetium-99m (Tc-99m) and gallium-67 citrate have been used.[7–9] Tc-99m is a bone-scanning agent that demonstrates increased uptake in areas of increased osteoblastic activity. It is more sensitive than CT for early changes of osteomyelitis in the skull base,[10] but does not delineate soft tissue changes, which are clearly seen with CT scanning. The bone scan will

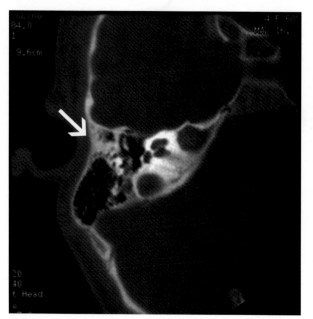

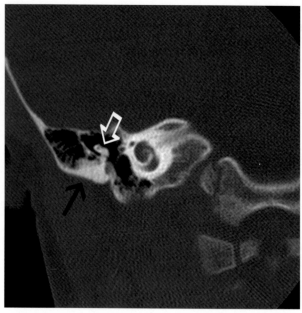

A

B

Figure 7–1 External auditory canal atresia. **(A)** Axial computed tomography (CT) image of external auditory canal (EAC) and middle ear shows absent EAC (solid arrow) as well as abnormal appearance of the ossicles. **(B)** Coronal CT image demonstrates absent EAC (solid arrow) as well as fusion of the ossicular mass to the lateral wall of the attic at the level of the atresia plate (open arrow). (Courtesy of Bernadette Koch, M.D.)

remain abnormal for months even if there is no active infection. Gallium-67 citrate scintigraphy is more specific for active infection, and serial scanning has been used to predict resolution of NEO.[11] However, there are documented cases of patients with recurrent or persistent NEO who have had normal gallium scans.[12]

Indium-111 white blood cell scan in combination with Tc-99m single photon emission computed tomography (SPECT) scan has also been shown to be useful in the diagnosis and follow-up of skull base osteomyelitis in patients with NEO.[13]

◆ Imaging of Diseases of the Mastoid and Middle Ear

Diseases of the mastoid and middle ear cavity include congenital anomalies (Chapter 1), inflammatory disease (Chapters 17 and 19), and neoplasms (Chapters 24 and 26).

The initial imaging evaluation of mastoid and middle ear pathology relies primarily on high-resolution noncontrast CT[14,15] (**Figs. 7–2** and **7–3**). MRI is extremely valuable in the assessment of patients with intracranial complications from otomastoiditis and cholesteatoma. Meningitis, subdural or epidural empyema, and intracranial abscess are much better demonstrated with MRI than CT. Sigmoid sinus thrombophlebitis is also better demonstrated on MRI. If findings of venous thrombosis are equivocal on routine spin-echo images, magnetic resonance venography can be utilized for confirmation. MRI is also superior in detecting encephaloceles, which may develop at sites of postsurgical or erosive defects in the tegmen.[16]

Paragangliomas including glomus tympanicum and jugulotympanicum involve the middle ear cavity. Their imaging evaluation is discussed later in this chapter.

◆ Imaging of Disease of the Inner Ear

Congenital malformations of the inner ear are covered in Chapters 1 and 22. Other processes that may lead to imaging evaluations include inflammatory disease, otodystrophies, and neoplasms.

Imaging of patients with suspected otodystrophy relies heavily on high-resolution CT scanning.[17–19] Otosclerosis is covered in detail in Chapter 20.[20–22] Other otodystrophies including fibrous dysplasia and Paget's disease demonstrate classic findings on CT.[3] Extensive areas of bony demineralization are evident with the cotton-wool appearance seen in calvarial bone in Paget's disease.[23,24] Patients with fibrous dysplasia demonstrate areas of enlarged dense bone with a ground-glass appearance to the matrix. Although patients with Paget's disease and those with fibrous dysplasia have visible abnormalities on MRI, the changes are frequently less diagnostic on MRI than on CT and do not warrant the added expense.

Imaging of patients with inner ear inflammatory disease is performed to exclude other causes of vertigo. Patients with acute labyrinthitis frequently show abnormal signal or enhancement within the membranous labyrinth on MRI. The findings are a nonspecific indication of inflammation.

Labyrinthitis ossificans can occur as a sequelae of labyrinthitis, most frequently following a bacterial infection. CT and MRI

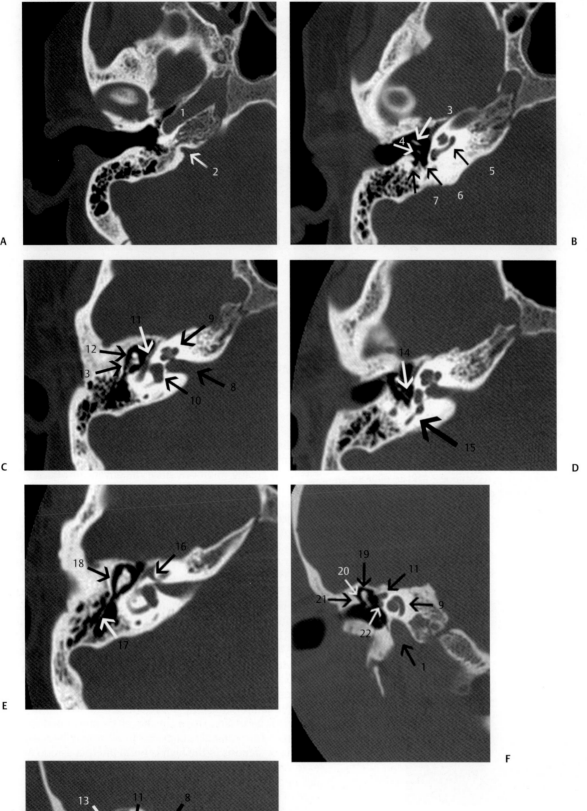

Figure 7–2 (A–E) Normal anatomy axial CT image. **(F,G)** Normal anatomy CT coronal image. 1, Carotid canal; 2, cochlear aqueduct; 3, malleus handle; 4, long process incus; 5, basal turn of cochlea; 6, sinus tympani; 7, facial recess; 8, internal auditory canal; 9, cochlea—2nd turn and apex; 10, vestibule; 11, tympanic segment facial nerve canal; 12, malleus head; 13, short process incus; 14, stapes crura; 15, posterior semicircular canal; 16, labyrinthine segment facial nerve canal; 17, Koerner's septum; 18, incus body; 19, tegmen; 20, Prussak's space; 21, scutum; 22, tensor tympani; 23, lenticular process of incus; 24, oval window.

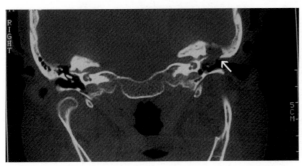
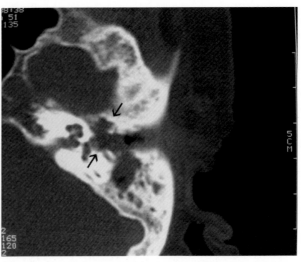

A   B

Figure 7–3 Cholesteatoma. **(A)** Coronal CT image shows soft tissue mass filling the attic with erosion of the ossicles and blunting of the scutum (arrow). **(B)** Axial CT image shows large soft tissue mass and absent ossicles as well as erosion of the medial and lateral walls of the attic (arrows).

are both useful in the detection of labyrinthitis ossificans (**Figs. 7–4** and **7–5**).[25,26] On MRI obliteration of the normal fluid signal within the membranous labyrinth on high-resolution T2-weighted sequences can be detected. In the early stages, MR findings may be more obvious than the CT findings of subtle labyrinthine sclerosis.[27]

Rare intralabyrinthine schwannomas are easily detected on gadolinium-enhanced MRI.[28]

With improved visualization of inner ear structures using 3D and high-resolution techniques, MRI is playing an increasing role in the detection and diagnosis of inner ear pathology.[29–45]

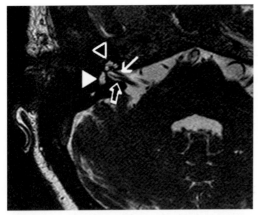

Figure 7–4 Normal anatomy axial three-dimensional Fourier transform–constructive interference in steady state (3DFT-CISS) magnetic resonance imaging (MRI). There is excellent visualization of the cochlear division (solid arrow) and vestibular division (open arrow) of cranial nerve VIII. Fluid signal intensity is seen within the vestibule (solid arrowhead) and cochlea (open arrowhead). Close examination of the cochlea demonstrates the modiolus and spiral lamina are visible as low signal intensity areas within the high signal fluid spaces of the cochlea.

◆ Imaging of Diseases of the Skull Base, Internal Auditory Canal, and Cerebellopontine Angle

The main categories of disease to be considered include neoplasms and cysts, inflammatory disease, and vascular lesions including normal vascular variants. Imaging of the skull base, internal auditory canal (IAC), and cerebellopontine angle (CPA) has been greatly improved since the advent of MRI.[46–49] This is the one area of temporal bone imaging where MRI clearly supplants CT as the initial imaging test of choice in most instances. MRI also plays a role in the evaluation of patients with pulsatile tinnitus. MRI/magnetic resonance angiography (MRA) can detect petrous carotid aneurysm, glomus tumor, atherosclerotic carotid stenosis, advanced fibromuscular dysplasia (FMD), and high-flow dural arteriovenous malformation/fistula.[50,51] However, many patients with objective pulsatile tinnitus require conventional angiography for more complete evaluation of lesions detected on MRI or for treatment purposes (**Fig. 7–6**). Low-flow dural fistulas may not be detected with MRI/MRA. Likewise, subtle FMD may be mistaken as an artifactual finding on MRA. Thus, it may be more cost-effective to proceed directly to conventional angiography in patients with objective pulsatile tinnitus. In patients with subjective pulsatile tinnitus, imaging to exclude several normal vascular variants is necessary. These are all well demonstrated with CT imaging.[51] Uncommonly subjective tinnitus may be related to kinking or stenosis in the high cervical internal carotid artery, or to venous sinus stenosis. MRA and MR venography can be of use in detecting such abnormalities. Pulsatile tinnitus is covered in more detail in Chapter 35.

MRI allows for excellent delineation of tumors and cysts of the skull base, IAC, and CPA.[52–54] Schwannomas of the fifth, seventh, and eighth cranial nerves typically demonstrate intermediate signal on T1-weighted images (T1WI), and high signal on T2-weighted images (T2WI).[55] They enhance intensely with gadolinium (**Figs. 7–7 and 7–8**). Even small intracanalicular acoustic schwannomas are easily detected with MRI with gadolinium and with high-resolution 3D technique (**Fig. 7–9**).[56–58]

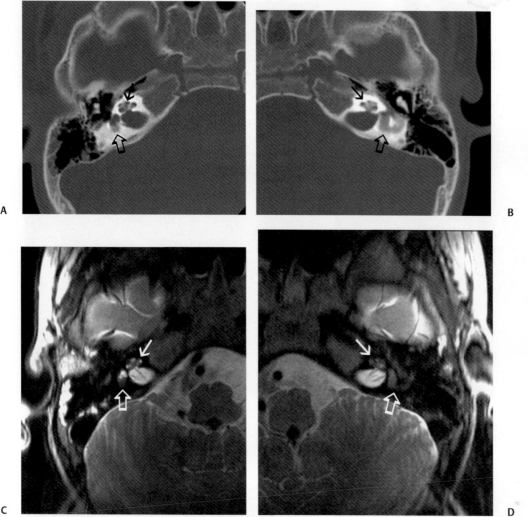

Figure 7–5 Labyrinthitis ossificans in a 3-year-old boy with a history of meningitis. **(A,B)** Axial CT images show subtle abnormal hazy sclerosis in the cochlea (solid arrows), vestibule, and semicircular canals (open arrows). **(C,D)** Axial high-resolution T2-weighted MRI demonstrates areas of obliteration of normal fluid signal within the cochlea (solid arrows), vestibule, and semicircular canals (open arrows). Compare with the normal appearance in **Fig. 7–4.** (Courtesy of Richard Wiggins, M.D.)

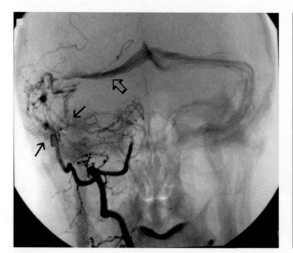
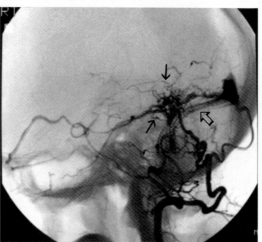

Figure 7–6 Dural fistula in a patient with pulsatile tinnitus. Vertebral angiogram anteroposterior (AP) **(A)** and lateral **(B)** projections shows multiple small arterial feeders from the vertebral artery (solid arrows) supplying a dural fistula along the lateral aspect of the transverse sinus. There is abnormal early filling of venous structures (open arrows) during the arterial phase due to the arteriovenous shunting. (Courtesy of Todd Abruzzo, M.D.)

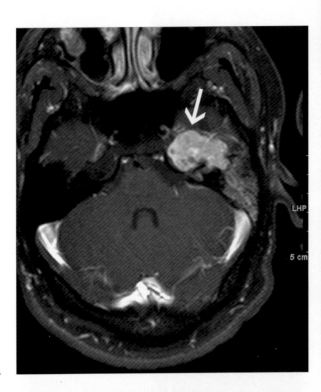

A

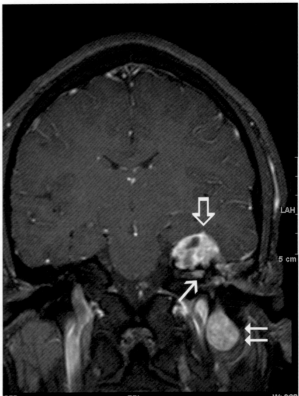

B

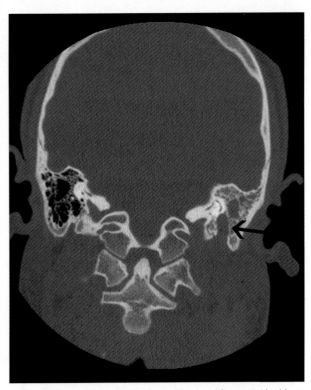

C

D

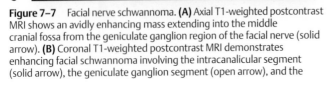

Figure 7–7 Facial nerve schwannoma. **(A)** Axial T1-weighted postcontrast MRI shows an avidly enhancing mass extending into the middle cranial fossa from the geniculate ganglion region of the facial nerve (solid arrow). **(B)** Coronal T1-weighted postcontrast MRI demonstrates enhancing facial schwannoma involving the intracanalicular segment (solid arrow), the geniculate ganglion segment (open arrow), and the descending segment as it exits the stylomastoid foramen (double arrow). **(C)** Coronal bone algorithm CT image shows soft tissue within the middle ear cavity from involvement of the tympanic segment as well as marked bony expansion and smooth erosion of the tegmen (arrows) from geniculate ganglion involvement. **(D)** Coronal bone algorithm CT image shows expansion of the mastoid segment of facial nerve canal (arrow).

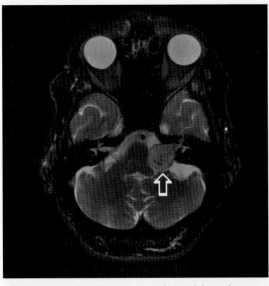

A

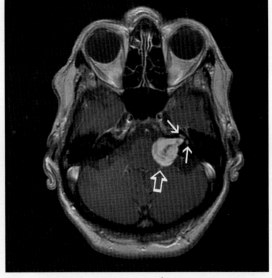

B

Figure 7–8 Vestibular schwannoma with translabyrinthine extension. **(A)** Axial T2-weighted MRI shows a large mass in the cerebellopontine angle (CPA) (open arrow) and internal auditory canal (IAC). **(B)** Axial

T1-weighted postcontrast MRI shows enhancing mass in the CPA (open arrow) and IAC. Enhancement extending into the vestibule and basal turn of the cochlea (solid arrows) usually is not extension of tumor.

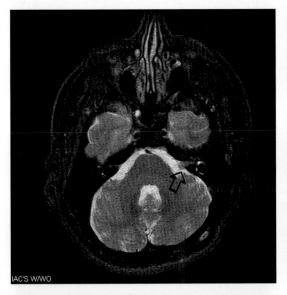

A   IAC'S W/WO

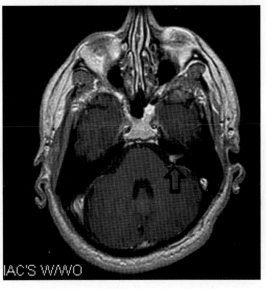

IAC'S W/WO   B

C   IAC'S W/WO

Figure 7–9 Intracanalicular vestibular schwannoma with slight extension to the CPA. **(A)** Axial T2-weighted MRI shows small mass within the IAC obliterating the normal cerebrospinal fluid (CSF) signal (open arrow). **(B,C)** Axial and coronal T1-weighted postcontrast MRI show small enhancing mass mostly within the IAC (arrows).

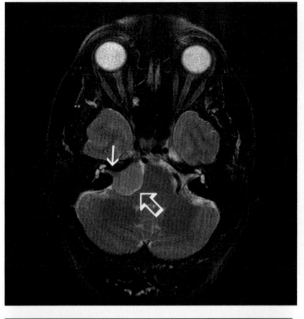

A

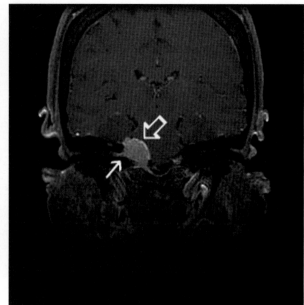

B

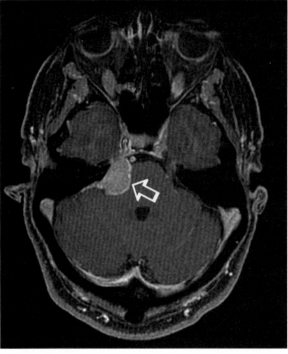

C

Figure 7–10   Cerebellopontine angle (CPA) meningioma. **(A)** Axial T2-weighted MRI shows an intermediate signal intensity mass in the CPA (open arrow) with minimal extension into the IAC (solid arrow). **(B,C)** Coronal and axial T1-weighted postcontrast MRIs show enhancing mass in CPA (open arrows) with small linear extension of enhancement into IAC (solid arrow). There is also an enhancing dural tail visible.

Meningiomas typically demonstrate intermediate signal on T1WI and T2WI, usually isointense to gray matter, with intense gadolinium enhancement. The multiplanar imaging capability of MRI allows for easier determination of the dural base of a meningioma (**Fig. 7–10**). Some meningiomas demonstrate increased signal on T2WI.

Epidermoid tumors, frequently seen in the CPA, have a characteristic appearance on MRI. Signal characteristics parallel cerebrospinal fluid (CSF), but are usually not identical. These lesions demonstrate low signal on T1WI and high signal on T2WI. They do not demonstrate enhancement. They usually have characteristic frond-like borders when occurring in the CPA. Differentiation from arachnoid cyst is sometimes difficult if the lesions have smooth borders. In these cases diffusion

weighted imaging is helpful, as epidermoid tumors demonstrate restricted diffusion.

Cholesterol granulomas of the petrous apex demonstrate characteristic findings on MRI, with high signal intensity seen on both T1- and T2WI.[59–62] This is in contrast to cholesteatoma, which has low T1 signal intensity.[62–66] CT findings are less specific, showing expansile smooth erosion of the petrous apex.[60,61,65,66,67] These are covered in detail in Chapter 25.

Dermoids and lipomas have characteristic fat signal on MRI. They demonstrate increased signal on T1WI and low signal on T2WI. T1WI with fat-suppression techniques is also useful, showing loss of high T1 signal with fat suppression.

Tumors of the skull base including chordoma, chondrosarcoma, and metastatic disease frequently require both MRI and

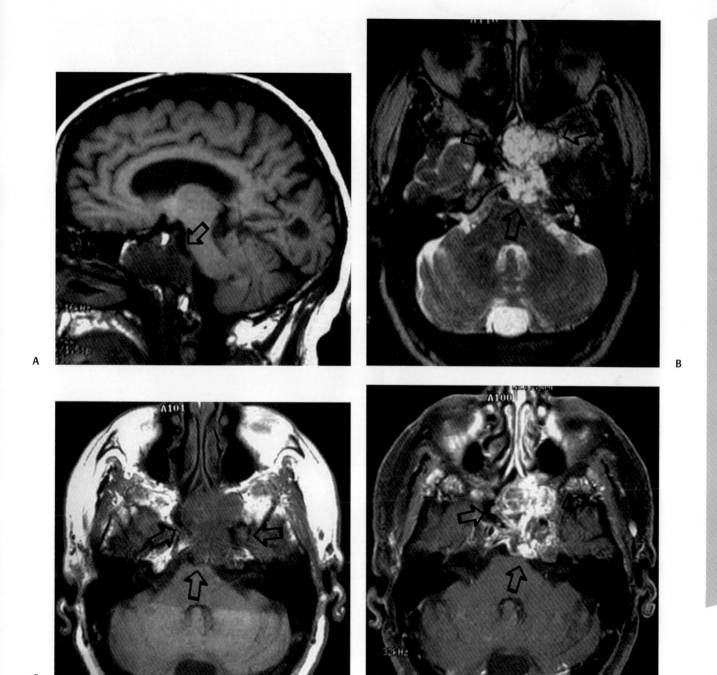

Figure 7–11 Skull base chondrosarcoma. **(A)** Sagittal T1-weighted MRI shows an intermediate signal intensity expansile mass replacing the normal high signal intensity marrow (open arrow). **(B)** Axial T2-weighted MRI shows mass with heterogeneous high signal intensity involving base of skull and petrous apex region (open arrows).

(C) Axial T1-weighted MRI shows replacement of normal fat signal in the skull base by the large soft tissue mass (open arrows). **(D)** Axial T1-weighted postcontrast MRI demonstrates heterogeneous enhancement within the mass (open arrows).

CT for complete evaluation.[68–72] CT is useful in evaluating subtle foraminal erosion[73–75] and for evaluating for chondroid matrix in chondrosarcoma or chordomas.[76–78] MRI provides elegant visualization of the skull base and intracranial and extracranial extent of tumor by virtue of its multiplanar imaging capabilities.[79–82] Intrinsic skull base tumors show replacement of normal fatty marrow signal on T1WI by abnormal intermediate signal intensity.[83] T2WI show abnormal increased signal (**Figs. 7–11** and **7–12**).[76] Chordomas tend to have extremely bright signal on T2-weighted images.[78,81,84–86]

Paragangliomas of the temporal bone may involve middle ear cavity (glomus tympanicum), jugular foramen (glomus jugulare), or both (glomus jugulotympanicum).[87] High-resolution CT with contrast should be used as the first step in the evaluation in patients with suspected temporal bone glomus tumor.[88,89] Glomus tympanicum can frequently be diagnosed and completely evaluated with CT only.[90,91] If the tumor is large enough to involve the eustachian tube, MRI may be necessary to differentiate fluid within the middle ear cavity from enhancing tumor mass.[92]

High-resolution CT is needed to assess for subtle bony erosion of the jugular foramen in small glomus jugulare tumors (**Fig. 7–13**).[93] Erosion of the bony plate between the jugular bulb and hypotympanum may be subtle, but can usually be

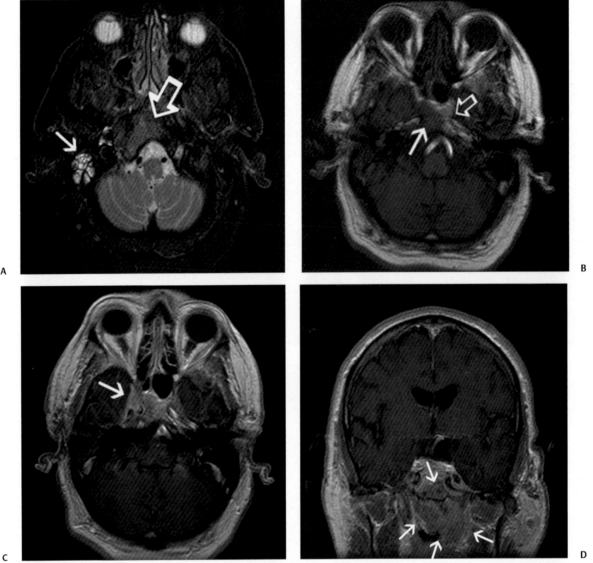

C

Figure 7–12 Nasopharyngeal carcinoma with skull base extension. **(A)** Axial T2-weighted MRI shows fluid signal within the left mastoid air cells due to eustachian tube obstruction (solid arrow). Abnormal increased signal is seen within the clivus (open arrow). **(B)** Axial T1-weighted MRI shows normal high signal intensity marrow signal in the clivus on the right (open arrow) and abnormal intermediate

signal infiltrating the left portion of the clivus (solid arrow). **(C)** Axial T1-weighted postcontrast MRI shows evidence of intracranial extension of enhancing tumor within the left cavernous sinus (solid arrow). **(D)** Coronal T1-weighted postcontrast MRI demonstrates the large left nasopharyngeal mass with skull base invasion (solid arrows).

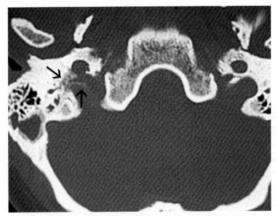

A

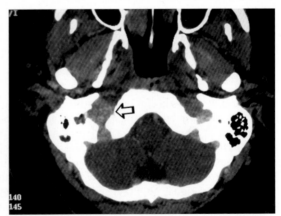

B

Figure 7–13 Glomus jugulare. **(A)** Axial bone algorithm CT image shows typical permeative pattern of bone erosion involving the margins of the jugular foramen and the jugular spine (arrows).

(B) Axial enhanced CT image at soft tissue algorithm demonstrates the enhancing mass within the jugular foramen (open arrow).

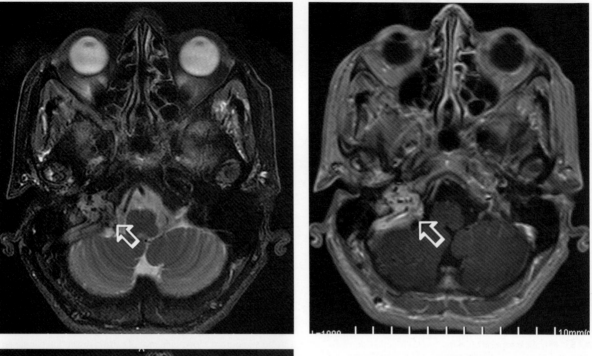

A

B

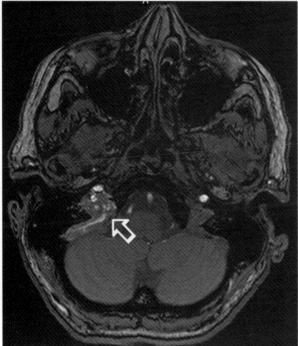

C

Figure 7–14 Glomus jugulare. **(A)** Axial T2-weighted MRI shows a mixed signal intensity mass in the right jugular foramen with a "salt-and-pepper" appearance (open arrow). Low signal intensity areas represent vascular flow voids. **(B)** Axial T1-weighted postcontrast MRI shows the mass enhances avidly and contains multiple low signal vascular flow voids (open arrow). **(C)** Axial source image from magnetic resonance angiography (MRA) sequence demonstrates multiple arterial vessels within the mass (open arrow).

detected with high-resolution CT in cases of glomus jugulotympanicum. In large glomus jugulare tumors MRI is useful for evaluation of intracranial extension, inferior extension in the neck, and evaluation for multicentric tumors. On MRI glomus tumors demonstrate intermediate signal on T1WI. Larger lesions demonstrate an inhomogeneous "salt-and-pepper" pattern with areas of foci of subacute hemorrhage and areas of low signal representing vascular flow voids. On T2WI the lesion usually has inhomogeneous bright signal with areas of low signal flow voids. The lesions demonstrate significant enhancement with gadolinium (**Fig. 7–14**).

A radionuclide imaging technique has been described that may be useful in evaluating for multicentric glomus tumors. Indium-111 octreotide, a somatostatin analogue, has been investigated in identifying tumors of neuroendocrine origin. Limitations of the technique include identification of small tumors. The smallest lesion detected in current studies was 2 to 3 cm.[94]

Petrous apicitis may be diagnosed earlier with MRI than with CT. T2WI demonstrate abnormal high signal intensity in the petrous apex. Gadolinium-enhanced images demonstrate abnormal enhancement within the petrous apex and adjacent

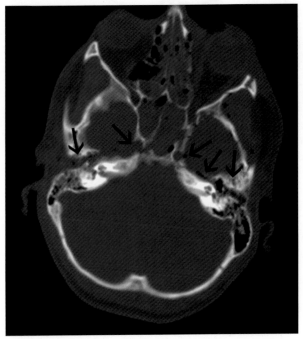

A

B

Figure 7–15 Petrous temporal bone fractures with extension into carotid canal and associated vascular injuries. **(A)** Axial CT image shows complex bilateral petrous temporal bone fractures with medial extension into both carotid canals (arrows). **(B)** Lateral view from carotid angiogram shows evidence of carotid dissection (single arrow), pseudoaneurysm (open arrow), and carotid-cavernous fistula (double arrow). Note the anterior venous drainage of the carotid cavernous fistula into the superior and inferior ophthalmic veins (open arrowheads).

leptomeninges.[3] CT imaging may show fluid-filled pneumatized petrous apex cells or in severe cases bone erosion.

◆ Imaging of Injuries Due to Trauma

This subject is covered in detail in Chapter 21. Evaluation of temporal bone fractures is best achieved with high-resolution CT scanning in axial projection with coronal reconstructions.[95–98]

If fractures are seen to extend into the carotid canal, further imaging is indicated to assess for vascular injury (**Fig. 7–15**). Conventional angiography is still considered the gold standard for evaluation though CT angiography is being increasingly utilized to evaluate for dissections.[99,100]

MRA is less useful in evaluation of vascular injury at the skull base level due to frequently encountered artifacts in this region.

References

1. Swartz JD. Current imaging approach to the temporal bone. Radiology 1989;171:309–317
2. Swartz JD. The temporal bone: imaging considerations. Crit Rev Diagn Imaging 1990;30:341–417
3. Swartz JD, Harnsberger HR. Imaging of the Temporal Bone, 2nd ed. New York: Thieme, 1992:1–19, 20–47, 154–191, 221–226, 330
4. Gassner EM, Mallouhi A, Jaschke WR. Preoperative evaluation of external auditory canal atresia on high-resolution CT. Am J Roentgenol 2004; 182:1305–1312
5. Rubin J, Curtin HD, Yu VL, et al. Malignant external otitis: utility of CT in diagnosis and follow-up. Radiology 1990;174:391–394
6. Gherini SG, Brackmann DE, Bradley WG. Magnetic resonance imaging and computerized tomography in malignant external otitis. Laryngoscope 1986;96:542–548

7. Chang PC, Fischbein NJ, Holliday RA. Central skull base osteomyelitis in patients without otitis externa: imaging findings. Am J Neuroradiol 2003; 24:1310–1316
8. Uri N, Gips S, Front A, et al. Quantitative bone and 67Ga scintigraphy in the differentiation of necrotizing external otitis from severe external otitis. Arch Otolaryngol Head Neck Surg 1991;117:623–626
9. Parisier SC, Lucente FE, Hirschman SZ, et al. Nuclear scanning in necrotizing progressive malignant external otitis. Laryngoscope 1982;92: 1016–1020
10. Ostfeld E, Aviel A, Pelet D. Malignant external otitis: the diagnostic value of bone scintigraphy. Laryngoscope 1981;91:960–964
11. Mendelson DS, Som PM, Mendelson CH, et al. Malignant external otitis: the role of computed tomography and radionuclides in evaluation. Radiology 1983;149:745–749
12. Kraus DH, Rehm SJ, Kinney SE. The evolving treatment of necrotizing external otitis. Laryngoscope 1988;98:934–939
13. Seabold JE, Simonson TM, Weber PC, et al. Cranial osteomyelitis: diagnosis and follow-up with In-111 white blood cell and Tc-99m methylene diphosphonate bone SPECT, CT, and MR imaging. Radiology 1995;196:779–788
14. Silver AJ, Janecka I, Wazen J, et al. Complicated cholesteatomas: CT findings in inner ear complications of middle ear cholesteatomas. Radiology 1987;164:47–51
15. Torizuka T, Hayakawa K, Satoh Y, et al. High resolution CT of the temporal bone: a modified baseline. Radiology 1992;184:109–111
16. Martin N, Sterkers O, Nahum H. Chronic inflammatory disease of the middle ear cavities: Gd-DTPA-enhanced MR imaging. Radiology 1990; 176:399–405
17. Swartz JD. The otodystrophies: diagnosis and differential diagnosis. Semin Ultrasound CT MR 2004;25:305–318
18. Odrezin GT, Krasikov N. CT of the temporal bone in a patient with osteopathia striate and cranial sclerosis. Am J Neuroradiol 1993;14:72–75
19. d'Archambeau O, Parizel PM, Koekelkoren E, et al. CT diagnosis and differential diagnosis of otodystrophic lesions of the temporal bone. Eur J Radiol 1990;11:22–30
20. Ziyeh S, Berlis A, Ross UH, Reinhardt MJ, Schumacher M. MRI of active otosclerosis. Neuroradiology 1997;39:453–457
21. Saunders JE, Derebery MJ, Lo WWM. Imaging case study of the month: magnetic resonance imaging of cochlear otosclerosis. Ann Otol Rhinol Laryngol 1995;104:826–829
22. Goh JPN, Chan LL, Tan TY. MRI of cochlear otosclerosis. Br J Radiol 2002; 75:502–505

23. Crain MR, Dolan KD. Internal auditory canal enlargement in Paget's disease appearing as bilateral acoustic neuromas. Ann Otol Rhinol Laryngol 1990;99:833–834

24. Alkadhi H, Rissmann D, Kollias SS. Osteogenesis imperfecta of the temporal bone: CT and MR imaging in Van der Hoeve-de Kleyn syndrome. Am J Neuroradiol 2004;25:1106–1109

25. Ball JB Jr, Miller GW, Hepfner ST. Computed tomography of single-channel cochlear implants. Am J Neuroradiol 1986;7:41–47

26. Swartz JD, Mandell DM, Faerber EN. Labyrinthine ossification: etiologies and CT findings. Radiology 1985;157:395–398

27. Arriaga MA, Carrier D. MRI and clinical decisions in cochlear implantation. Am J Otol 1996;17:547–553

28. Mafee MF, Lachenauer CS, Kumar A, et al. CT and MR imaging of intralabyrinthine schwannoma: report of two cases and review of the literature. Radiology 1990;174:395–400

29. Mark AS, Fitzgerald D. Segmental enhancement of the cochlea on contrast enhanced MR: correlation with the frequency of hearing loss and possible sign of perilymphatic fistula and autoimmune labyrinthitis. Am J Neuroradiol 1993;14:991–996

30. Stillman AE, Remley K, Loes DJ, et al. Steady state free procession imaging of the inner ear. Am J Neuroradiol 1994;15:348–350

31. Casselman JW, Kuhweide R, Deimling M, et al. Constructive interference in steady state 3-DFT MR imaging of the inner ear and cerebellopontine angle. Am J Neuroradiol 1993;14:47–57

32. Casselman JW, Kuhweide R, Ampe W, et al. Pathology of the membranous labyrinth: comparison of T1 and T2 weighted and gadolinium enhanced spin echo and 3-DFT-CISS imaging. Am J Neuroradiol 1993; 14:56–69

33. Mark AS, Seltzer S, Harnsberger HR. Sensorineural hearing loss: more than meets the eye? Am J Neuroradiol 1993;14:37–45

34. Tien RD, Felsberg GJ, MacFall J. Fast spin-echo high-resolution MR imaging of the inner ear. Am J Roentgenol 1992;159:395–398

35. Seltzer S, Mark AS. Contrast enhancement on MR scans in patients with sudden hearing loss and vertigo: evidence of labyrinthine disease. Am J Neuroradiol 1991;12:13–16

36. Harnsberger HR, Dart DJ, Parkin JL, et al. Cochlear implant candidates: assessment with CT and MR imaging. Radiology 1987;164:53–57

37. Brogan M, Chakeres DW, Schmalbrock P. High-resolution 3-DFT MR imaging of the endolymphatic duct and soft tissues of the otic capsule. Am J Neuroradiol 1991;12:1–11

38. Kim HJ, Song JW, Chon KM, Goh EK. Common crus aplasia: diagnosis by 3D volume rendering imaging using 3DFT-CISS sequence. Clin Radiol 2004;59:830–834

39. Dahlen RT, Harnsberger HR, Gray SD, et al. Overlapping thin-section fast spin-echo MR of the large vestibular aqueduct syndrome. Am J Neuroradiol 1997;18:67–75

40. Fitzgerald DC, Mark AS. Sudden hearing loss: frequency of abnormal findings on contrast-enhanced MR studies. Am J Neuroradiol 1998;19: 1443–1446

41. Lemmerling M, Vanzieleghem B, Dhooge I, Van Cauwenberge P, Kunnen M. CT and MRI of the semicircular canals in the normal and diseased temporal bone. Eur Radiol 2001;11:1210–1219

42. Naganawa S, Koshikawa T, Nakamura T, Fukatsu H, Ishigaki T, Aoki I. High-resolution T1-weighted 3D real IR imaging of the temporal bone using triple-dose contrast material. Eur Radiol 2003;13:2650–2658

43. Guirado CR, Martinez P, Roig R, et al. Three-dimensional MR of the inner ear with steady-state free precession. Am J Neuroradiol 1995;16: 1909–1913

44. Held P, Fellner C, Fellner F, Seitz J, Strutz J. MRI of inner ear anatomy using 3D MP-RAGE and 3D CISS sequences. Br J Radiol 1997;70:465–472

45. Stone JA, Chakeres DW, Schmalbrock P. High-resolution MR imaging of the auditory pathway. Magn Reson Imaging Clin N Am 1998;6: 195–217

46. Sartoretti-Schefer S, Wichmann W, Valavanis A. Idiopathic herpetic and HIV-associated facial nerve palsies: abnormal MR enhancement pattern. Am J Neuroradiol 1994;15:479–485

47. Han MH, Jabour BA, Andrews JC, et al. Nonneoplastic enhancing lesions mimicking intracanalicular acoustic neuroma on gadolinium-enhanced MR images. Radiology 1991;179:795–796

48. Madden GJ, Sirimanna KS. Cavernous hemangioma of the internal auditory meatus. J Otolaryngol 1990;19:288–291

49. Atlas MD, Fagan PA, Turner J. Calcification of internal auditory canal tumors. Ann Otol Rhinol Laryngol 1992;101:620–622

50. Remley KB, Coit WE, Harnsberger HR, et al. Pulsatile tinnitus and the vascular tympanic membrane: CT, MR and angiographic findings. Radiology 1990;174:383–389

51. Lo WW, Solti-Bohman LG. High-resolution CT of the jugular foramen: anatomy and vascular variants and anomalies. Radiology 1984;150: 743–747

52. Press GA, Hesselink JR. MR imaging of cerebellopontine angle and internal auditory canal lesions at 1.5T. AJR Am J Neuroradiol 1988;150:1371–1381

53. Martin N, Sterkers O, Nahum H. Haemangioma of the petrous bone: MRI. Neuroradiology 1992;34:420–422

54. Salzman KL, Davidson HC, Harnsberger HR, et al. Dumbbell schwannomas of the internal auditory canal. Am J Neuroradiol 2001;22:1368–1376

55. Sanna M, Zini C, Garroletti R, et al. Primary infratemporal tumors of the facial nerve: diagnosis and treatment. J Laryngol Otol 1990;104:765–771

56. Linskey ME, Lunsford LD, Flickinger JC. Neuroimaging of acoustic nerve sheath tumors after stereotaxic radiosurgery. Am J Neuroradiol 1991;12: 1165–1175

57. Mueller DP, Gantz BJ, Dolan KD. Gadolinium-enhanced MR of the post-operative internal auditory canal following acoustic neuromaresection via the middle fossa approach. Am J Neuroradiol 1992;13:197–200

58. Litt AW, Kondo N, Bannon KR, et al. Role of slice thickness in MR imaging of the internal auditory canal. J Comput Assist Tomogr 1990;14:717–720

59. Greenberg JJ, Oot RF, Wismer GL, et al. Cholesterol granuloma of the petrous apex: MR and CT evaluation. Am J Neuroradiol 1988;9:1205–1214

60. Griffin C, De La Paz R, Enzmann D. Magnetic resonance and CT correlation of cholesterol cysts of the petrous bone. Am J Neuroradiol 1987;8: 825–829

61. Latack JT, Graham MD, Kemink JL, et al. Giant cholesterol cysts of the petrous apex: radiologic features. Am J Neuroradiol 1985;6:409–413

62. Goldofsky E, Holliday RA, Hoffman RA, et al. Cholesterol cysts of the temporal bone: diagnosis and treatment. Ann Otol Rhinol Laryngol 1991; 100:181–187

63. Rosenberg RA, Hammerschlag PE, Cohen NL, et al. Cholesteatoma vs cholesterol granuloma of the petrous apex. Otolaryngol Head Neck Surg 1986;94:322–327

64. Morrison GA, Dilkes MG. View from within: radiology in focus. Cholesterol cyst and cholesterol granuloma of the petrous bone. J Laryngol Otol 1992;106:465–467

65. Latack JT, Kartush JM, Kemink JL, et al. Epidermoidomas of the cerebellopontine angle and temporal bone: CT and MR aspects. Radiology 1985; 157:361–366

66. Clifton AG, Phelps PD, Brookes GB. Cholesterol granuloma of the petrous apex. Br J Radiol 1990;63:724–726

67. Larson TL, Wong ML. Primary mucocele of the petrous apex: MR appearance. Am J Neuroradiol 1992;13:203–204

68. Horowitz SW, Leonetti JP, Behrooz AK, et al. CT and MR of temporal bone malignancies primary and secondary to parotid carcinoma. Am J Neuroradiol 1994;15:755–762

69. Lo WW, Applegate LJ, Carberry JN, et al. Endolymphatic sac tumors: radiologic appearance. Radiology 1993;189:199–204

70. Birzgalis AR, Ramsden RT, Lye RH, et al. Haemangiopericytoma of the temporal bone. J Laryngol Otol 1990;104:908–1003

71. Han JS, Huss RG, Benson JE, et al. MR imaging of the skull base. J Comput Assist Tomogr 1984;8:944–952

72. Osborn AG, Harnsberger HR, Smoker WR. Base of the skull imaging. Semin Ultrasound CT MR 1986;7:91–106

73. Ginsberg LE, Pruett SW, Chen MY, et al. Skull base foramina of the middle cranial fossa: reassessment of normal variation with high-resolution CT. Am J Neuroradiol 1994;15:283–291

74. Daniels DL, Williams AL, Haughton VM. Jugular foramen: anatomic and computed tomography study. Am J Roentgenol 1984;142:153–158

75. Lanzieri CF, Duchesneau PM, Rosenbloom SA, et al. The significance of asymmetry of the foramen of Vesalius. Am J Neuroradiol 1988;9: 1201–1204

76. Ginsberg LE. Neoplastic diseases affecting the central skull base: CT and MR imaging. Am J Roentgenol 1992;159:581–589

77. Meyers SP, Hirsch WL, Curtin HD, et al. Chondrosarcomas of the skull base: MR imaging features. Radiology 1992;184:103–108

78. Brown RV, Sage MR, Brophy BP. CT and MR findings in patients with chordomas of the petrous apex. Am J Neuroradiol 1990;11:121–124

79. Daniels DL, Czervionke LF, Pech P, et al. Gradient recalled echo MR imaging of the jugular foramen. Am J Neuroradiol 1988;9:675–678

80. Laine FJ, Braun IF, Jensen ME, et al. Perineural tumor extension through the foramen ovale: evaluation with MR imaging. Radiology 1990;174: 65–71

81. Oot RF, Melville GF, New PF, et al. The role of MR and CT in evaluating clival chordomas and chondrosarcomas. Am J Neuroradiol 1988;9:715–723

82. Laine FJ, Nadel L, Braun IF. CT and MR imaging of the central skull base. Part 2: Pathologic spectrum. Radiographics 1990;10:591–602, 797–821

83. West MS, Russell EJ, Breit R, et al. Calvarial and skull base metastases: comparison of nonenhanced and Gd-DTPA-enhanced MR images. Radiology 1990;174:85–91

84. Myers SP, Hirsch WL, Curtin HD, et al. Chordomas of the skull base: MR features. Am J Neuroradiol 1992;13:1627–1636

85. Sze G, Uichanco LS, Brant-Zawadzki MN, et al. Chordomas: MR imaging. Radiology 1988;166:187–191

86. Lipper MH, Call WS. Chordoma of the petrous bone. South Med J 1991; 84:629–631

87. Duncan AW, Lack EE, Deck MF. Radiological evaluation of paragangliomas of the head and neck. Radiology 1979;132:99–105

88. Chakeres DW, LaMasters DL. Paragangliomas of the temporal bone: high resolution CT studies. Radiology 1984;150:749–753

89. Lo WW, Solti-Bohman LG, Lambert PR. High-resolution CT in the evaluation of glomus tumors of the temporal bone. Radiology 1984;150: 737–742

90. Curtin HD. Radiologic approach to paragangliomas of the temporal bone. Radiology 1984;150:837–838

91. Larson TC, Reese DF, Baker HL, et al. Glomus tympanicum chemodectomas: radiographic and clinical characteristics. Radiology 987;163:801–806

92. Phelps PD, Cheesman AD. Imaging jugulotympanic glomus tumors. Arch Otolaryngol Head Neck Surg 1990;116:940–945

93. Rubinstein D, Burton BS, Walker AL. The anatomy of the inferior petrosal sinus, glossopharyngeal nerve, vagus nerve and accessory nerve in the jugular foramen. Am J Neuroradiol 1995;16:185–194

94. Whiteman ML, Serafini AN, Falcone AN, et al. In-111 octreotide scintigraphy in the evaluation of suspected lesions of the head and neck. Presented at the 1995 Annual Meeting of American Society of Neuroradiology, Chicago, IL, and 1995 29th Annual Scientific Conference and Postgraduate Course in Head and Neck Imaging, Pittsburgh, PA

95. Avrahami E, Chen Z, Solomon A. Modern high resolution CT diagnosis of longitudinal fractures of the petrous bone. Neuroradiology 1988;30: 166–168

96. Zimmerman RA, Bilaniuk LT, Hackney DB, et al. Magnetic resonance imaging in temporal bone fracture. Neuroradiology 1987;29:246–251

97. Swartz JD, Zwillenberg S, Berger AS. Acquired disruptions of the incudostapedial articulation: diagnosis with CT. Radiology 1989;171:779–781

98. Betz BW, Wiener MD. Air in the temporomandibular joint fossa: CT sign of temporal bone fracture. Radiology 1991;180:463–466

99. Rogers FB, Baker EF, Osler TM, Shackford SR, Wald SL, Vieco P. Computed tomographic angiography as a screening modality for blunt cervical arterial injuries: preliminary results. J Trauma 1999;46:380–385

100. Munera F, Soto JA, Palacio D, Velez SM, Medina E. Diagnosis of arterial injuries caused by penetrating trauma to the neck: comparison of helical CT angiography and conventional angiography. Radiology 2000;216: 356–362

8

Diagnostic Audiology

Craig W. Newman and Sharon A. Sandridge

Coupled with the patient's case history and physical examination, audiologic testing assists the physician in developing a medical, surgical, or rehabilitative treatment plan for patients with auditory disorders. Further, audiologic procedures may be used to quantify outcome when administered in a pre- and posttreatment protocol.

The audiologic test battery is composed of two major categories of procedures. The first group of tests involves behavioral or psychophysical techniques requiring the patient to take an active role in the test session by responding to some form of an auditory stimulus. These tests include pure-tone and speech audiometry. The second group of tests capitalizes on physiologic responses to auditory signals and does not require active participation by the patient. The latter category of relatively objective test procedures includes immittance studies, otoacoustic emissions, and auditory evoked potentials.

It may be noted by the more seasoned professional, that a discussion of the traditional behavioral diagnostic tests (e.g., tone decay, Short Increment Sensitivity Index [SISI]; Alternate Binaural Loudness Balancing [ABLB]; Bekesy Audiometry) has been omitted in this chapter. Although these tests may have some interest from an historical perspective, they hold little clinical value in today's audiologic test battery. It is our intent to provide the otolaryngology practitioner or resident with the most essential concepts and terms underlying contemporary diagnostic audiology.

◆ Pure-Tone Audiometry

Pure-tone audiometry is the most fundamental component of the audiologic evaluation. Results from pure-tone testing are used to (1) determine the severity of hearing loss; (2) diagnose the type (i.e., conductive, sensorineural, or mixed) of hearing loss by comparing air- and bone-conduction thresholds; (3) describe the configuration of hearing loss (i.e., pattern of pure-tone thresholds from low frequencies to high frequencies); (4) determine the intensity levels at which other audiologic procedures will be performed; and (5) determine the need for rehabilitative treatment.

Pure-tone audiometry is based on obtaining a series of thresholds. According to the American National Standards Institute (ANSI S3.20), threshold is defined as the "minimum effective sound pressure level of the signal that is capable of evoking an auditory sensation in a specified fraction of trials."[1] Clinically, the term *threshold* is defined as the lowest intensity at which the patient is able to respond to the stimulus 50% of the time (e.g., two out of four trials using a bracketing approach). For air-conduction testing, thresholds for single frequencies are assessed between octave intervals ranging from 250 Hz to 8000 Hz. When differences in thresholds of 20 dB or greater are obtained between adjacent thresholds, responses to inter-octave frequencies (750, 1500, 3000, or 6000 Hz) are determined. For bone-conduction testing, thresholds are measured at octave intervals between 250 and 4000 Hz.

Air-conduction measurements, using standard supraaural headphones or insert earphones, assess the entire peripheral auditory system including both the conductive (outer ear and middle ear) and sensorineural portions (cochlea and eighth nerve). In contrast, bone-conduction measurements are made using a bone oscillator typically placed on the mastoid prominence, although forehead placement is an alternative. Pure-tone signals transmitted via the bone oscillator cause the skull to vibrate, thereby stimulating the cochlea. For clinical purposes, bone-conduction audiometry is used to bypass conductive mechanisms and provide a measure of sensorineural reserve. It should be noted that tactile responses occur when signal levels are too intense, especially at low frequencies. In the latter case, patients respond to the vibration of the oscillator rather than to an auditory percept, leading to possible erroneous test results.

Clinical Procedures

Pure-tone thresholds are obtained using an audiometer that is calibrated to current ANSI specifications (ANSI S3.6) to ensure both the validity and reliability of test results.[2] Regardless of the make and model, all diagnostic audiometers have the capability of presenting calibrated pure-tone stimuli for air-and bone-conduction testing and speech stimuli using monitored

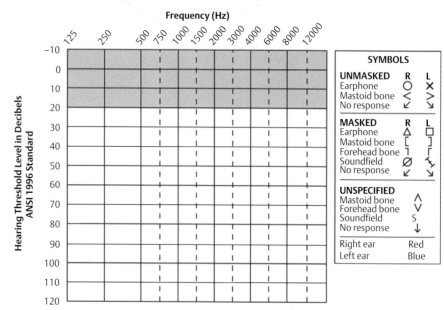

Figure 8–1 Example of an audiogram and a key of audiometric symbols.

live voice or recorded presentations. The results from pure-tone testing are recorded on a form called the *audiogram*, with frequency displayed on the abscissa and intensity in dB HL (hearing level) on the ordinate. **Fig. 8–1** shows a typical version of an audiogram and associated set of symbols used to document responses.

Obtaining valid and reliable pure-tone thresholds requires a skilled examiner. Without proper control of the following variables, results may be influenced by such factors as collapsed ear canals, false-positive/negative responses, equipment calibration, ambient noise in the test environment, earphone/bone-oscillator placement, visual cues given by examiner, ear selection, frequency sequencing, instructional set, response mode (use of handheld switch versus hand/finger raise), threshold procedure, and patient rapport.[3,4]

Audiogram Interpretation

Magnitude of Hearing Impairment

Several schemes have been developed to classify the degree of hearing impairment based on the pure-tone average (PTA) of 500, 1000, and 2000 Hz.[5] The two-frequency PTA (Fletcher average, which is the best two thresholds at 500, 1000, and 2000 Hz) is often a better predictor of hearing for speech than the three-frequency PTA. **Table 8–1** shows a classification scheme that is appropriate for adults; however, it is noteworthy that losses as minimal as 15 to 25 dB HL can have negative effects on the academic performance of children.[6] Calculating the PTA provides an overall estimate, albeit a loose one, of the impact a given hearing loss has on communication function.

Type of Hearing Loss

Three types of hearing loss, namely, conductive, sensorineural, and mixed, can be determined by comparing air-conduction thresholds to bone-conduction thresholds for each ear independently.

- *Conductive hearing loss* involves disorders of the outer ear, middle ear, or both. A conductive hearing loss is characterized by bone-conduction threshold responses obtained at 20 dB or better (reflecting normal cochlear or neural function) with air-conduction thresholds falling outside the normal limits. For illustrative purposes, the audiometric pattern for a bilateral conductive hearing loss is displayed in **Fig. 8–2A.** As shown, thresholds for air conduction are elevated (poorer hearing) for both ears. In contrast, masked bone-conduction thresholds fall within normal limits across the frequency range showing normal sensorineural function.
- *Sensorineural hearing loss* involves the cochlea, eighth cranial nerve, or both. A sensorineural hearing loss is characterized by a relatively equal (i.e., within 10 dB) elevation (i.e., poorer thresholds) of both air- and bone-conduction

Table 8–1 Hearing Loss Classification Scheme Based on Pure-Tone Average (PTA; 500, 1000, 2000 Hz) and Associated Communication Difficulty

PTA (in dB HL)	Category	Communication Difficulty
0–25	Normal	No significant difficulty
26–40	Mild	Difficulty understanding soft-spoken speech
41–55	Moderate	An understanding of speech at 3 to 5 feet
56–70	Moderately severe	Speech must be loud for auditory reception; significant difficulty in group settings
71–90	Severe	Loud speech may be understood at 1 foot from the ear; may distinguish vowel but not consonant sounds
90+	Profound	Does not rely on audition as primary mode of communication

Source: Adapted from Roeser RJ, Buckley KA, Stickney GS. Pure tone tests. In: Roeser RJ, Valente, M, Hosford-Dunn, H, eds. Audiology Diagnosis. New York: Thieme, 2000;239. Reprinted by permission.

HL, hearing level referring to the ANSI-1996 scale.

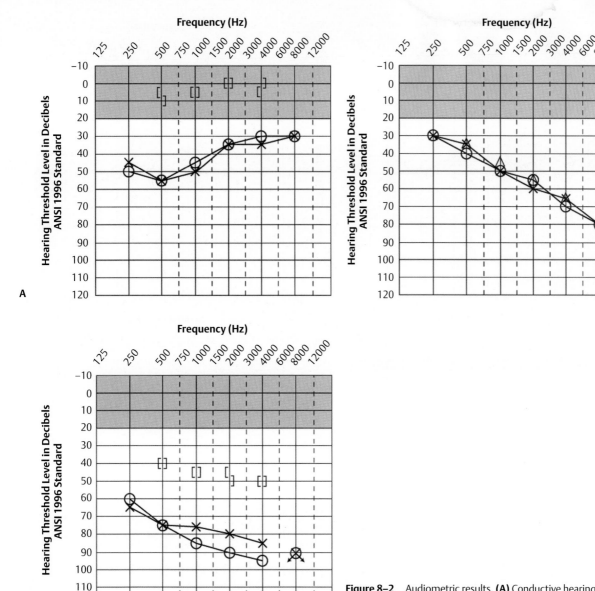

Figure 8–2 Audiometric results. **(A)** Conductive hearing loss. **(B)** Sensorineural hearing loss. **(C)** Mixed hearing loss.

thresholds that fall outside the normal limits. For example, audiometric findings for a bilateral sensorineural hearing loss are displayed in **Fig. 8–2B**. As can be seen, both air- and bone-conduction thresholds are elevated and interweaving.

- *Mixed hearing loss* is a combination of a conductive and sensorineural hearing loss. Mixed hearing losses are characterized by an elevation of both the air- and bone-conduction thresholds beyond the normal limits. Yet, as illustrated in **Fig. 8–2C**, air-conduction thresholds are even poorer (responses present at higher intensity levels) than bone-conduction responses. The difference between the air- and bone-conduction thresholds, known as the *air–bone gap*, reflects the degree of the conductive component contributing to the overall hearing loss.

Audiometric Configuration

A variety of audiometric configurations is used to describe patterns of pure-tone findings (**Fig. 8–3**). Often certain configurations are considered pathognomonic of specific otologic conditions. For example, a 4000-Hz notch is consistent with

noise exposure. A rising conductive loss reflects a stiffness tilt associated with middle ear effusion. In contrast, a sloping conductive loss reflects a mass tilt associated with such disorders as ossicular discontinuity, middle ear tumor, and thickened tympanic membrane. For patients with otosclerosis, the bone-conduction threshold often is reduced at 2000 Hz. The latter finding is referred to as the Carhart notch.

◆ Speech Audiometry

Results from speech audiometry are useful for (1) cross-checking the validity of pure-tone thresholds; (2) quantifying suprathreshold speech recognition, which assists the clinician in determining site of lesion; and (3) estimating communication function so that appropriate rehabilitative interventions can be recommended and outcome monitored. Although several speech tests are available, the following sections focus on the two major components of speech audiometry used routinely in diagnostic audiology, namely, the speech reception threshold (SRT) and suprathreshold word recognition testing.

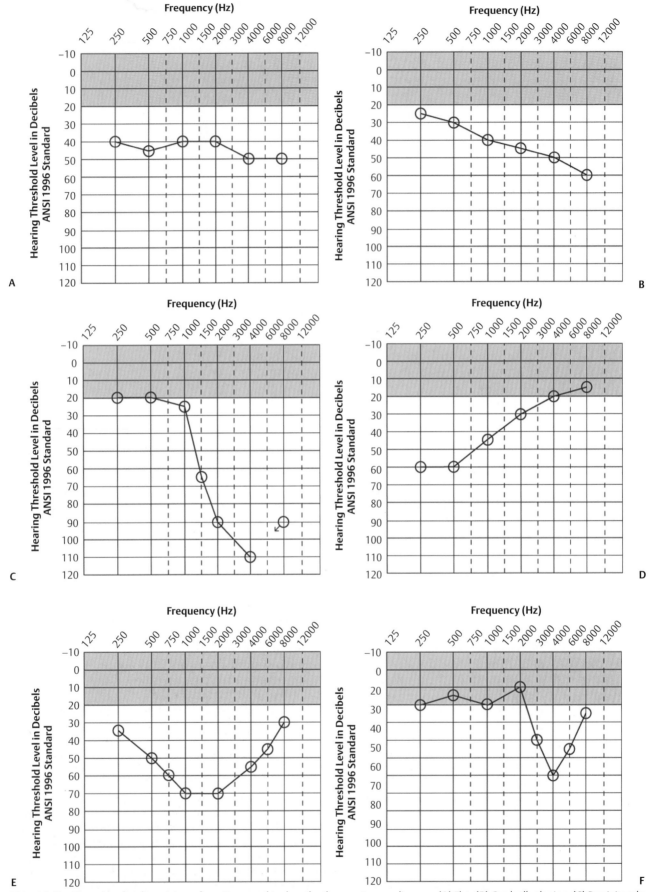

Figure 8–3 Examples of audiometric configurations used to describe the pure-tone audiogram. **(A)** Flat. **(B)** Gradually sloping. **(C)** Precipitously sloping. **(D)** Rising. **(E)** Trough. **(F)** Notch.

Speech Recognition Threshold

Similar to pure-tone thresholds, the SRT is the lowest hearing level at which the patient correctly recognizes speech stimuli 50% of the time for each ear independently. The most commonly used and recommended speech stimuli for obtaining SRTs are spondaic words.[5] A spondee is a bisyllabic word with equal stress on both syllables (e.g., baseball, hotdog, airplane). Because the PTA reflects hearing thresholds in the speech-frequency region and the SRT is measured using speech stimuli, close agreement between the latter two measures is expected. Accordingly, functional hearing loss (i.e., pseudohypoacusis) should be considered whenever there is an SRT-PTA discrepancy of more than 12 dB, especially when the SRT is better than would be predicted from the PTA.[7] In addition to functional hearing loss, a variety of other reasons must be considered when an SRT-PTA discrepancy exists, including (1) audiometer malfunction; (2) eighth cranial nerve disorders; (3) significant hearing loss with an island of normal hearing; and (4) cognitive or language disorders.

Word Recognition Testing

Materials and Procedures

Word recognition testing (WRT) is evaluated using monosyllabic phonetically balanced (PB) words. PB word lists contain all of the phonetic elements of connected discourse representative of everyday English speech. The most popular 50-item PB-word lists used today are the Central Institute for the Deaf (CID) Auditory Test W-22 and the Northwestern University Test No. 6.[8] These word lists are presented in an "open response" format wherein the set of possible responses to a test item is open and limited only by the patient's vocabulary. Because patients with severe hearing impairments often perform poorly on open response tests, alternative "closed response" multiple choice tests such as the California Consonant Test (CCT) have been developed.[9] In addition to monosyllabic word lists, several sentence-length materials such as the Everyday Speech Sentences[10] and Speech Perception in Noise (SPIN) test[11] have been developed to approximate a patient's speech understanding using contextual materials or hearing in the presence of a competing background noise.

Typically, WRT is performed at a 30- to 40-dB sensation level (i.e., above the SRT) or at the patient's most comfortable listening level (MCL) for each ear independently. Higher presentation levels, however, may be necessary to determine the patient's maximum word recognition score (i.e., PB Max). The evaluation of word recognition at multiple intensity levels is referred to as the performance-intensity (PI) function. For standardization purposes, it is preferable that PB word lists are presented using commercially available recordings rather than "live voice" presentations.

Scoring and Interpretation

Word recognition scores are expressed as the percentage of words correctly repeated from the 50 (full) or 25 (one-half) word lists. The obtained percent correct scores then are used in a classification scheme to estimate speech understanding ability. For example, word recognition scores of 90 to 100% are classified as excellent, 80 to 88% good, 70 to 78% fair, and below 70% is poor. It should be noted, however, that considerable variability on test-retest occurs especially as the number of test items is reduced from 50 words to 25 words, known as the "list size/measurement error trade-off."[12]

There are characteristic word recognition score patterns for different types of hearing loss. For patients with normal hearing sensitivity, PB Max occurs at or near 100% when the words are presented 35 to 40 dB above the SRT. Patients with conductive hearing loss perform similarly to normal individuals once the intensity level of the signal is increased to overcome the reduction in audibility caused by the conductive component. For patients with cochlear disorders, PB Max is generally reduced and is consistent with the severity of hearing loss. Further, no significant decline is expected in the word recognition score as intensity levels are increased. In contrast, patients with eighth nerve disorders may show word recognition scores disproportionately poorer in relationship to the severity of hearing loss. In addition, *rollover*, which is a decline in word recognition performance, occurs at higher intensity levels.

◆ Clinical Masking

Masking often is necessary during pure-tone and speech audiometry. In essence, clinical masking is used to eliminate the participation of the nontest ear when evaluating the test ear. To accomplish this, a noise is presented through an earphone to the nontest ear to prevent it from responding to the signal (air- or bone-conduction) presented to the test ear. Narrowband noise masking is used for pure-tone testing, whereas a wideband speech-frequency weighted noise is used for speech audiometry. *Crossover* of the signal is the actual transmission of sound arriving at the nontest cochlea. The amount of sound intensity needed before crossover occurs is a reflection of *interaural attenuation*. Accordingly, interaural attenuation is the loss of sound as the signal crosses over from the test ear to the nontest ear. The loss of sound is caused by the insulation properties of the head. To prevent crossover, the nontest ear must be masked.

For clinical purposes, minimum interaural attenuation for air-conduction testing is approximately 40 to 50 dB for supraaural earphones and 70 dB for insert phones. Thus, masking is required less frequently when insert phones are used compared with supraaural headphones. On the other hand, the minimum interaural attenuation for bone conduction is approximately 0 dB across test frequencies. Therefore, it is assumed that both cochleae are stimulated equally and simultaneously regardless of bone oscillator placement. Thus, the better cochlea theoretically always "hears" the signal, creating the need to mask for bone conduction when thresholds between ears are asymmetric. Moreover, too little or too much masking may be problematic. That is, *undermasking* refers to an insufficient amount of masking to produce the needed threshold shift, whereas *overmasking* occurs when the masking noise is so intense in the masked nontest ear that it crosses over to mask the test cochlea, yielding a false shift in threshold.

Unless the examiner uses appropriate masking levels and procedures, serious errors in diagnosing the type and severity of hearing loss may occur. That is, a hearing loss that is actually a sensorineural loss may be shown as a conductive hearing loss or a profound hearing loss may be viewed as a moderate loss. Recall that when a signal is presented to the poorer test ear at a sufficiently loud intensity level it may cross over to the opposite ear and be perceived by that ear. In fact, when testing a "dead ear"—an ear with no measurable hearing—the sound is expected to cross over and create what is referred to as a *shadow curve*. In this case, air-conducted signals have crossed over from the poorer ear and "mimic" thresholds of the better ear. Masking is needed to eliminate the shadow curve and obtain valid thresholds. Without masking to obtain valid thresholds, errors in the interpretation of the audiogram could result in unnecessary medical or surgical intervention or inappropriate rehabilitative recommendations.

◆ Immittance Measurement

Acoustic immittance measurements are considered a routine component of the audiologic test battery, serving at least two primary functions: (1) detecting middle ear disorders; and (2) differentiating cochlear from retrocochlear disorders. Acoustic immittance is a general term referring to *acoustic impedance* (Z_a) or *acoustic admittance* (Y_a). Whereas Z_a refers to opposition to the transfer of acoustic energy, Y_a refers to ease of sound flow through an acoustic system. Z_a and Y_a are direct reciprocals. Most commercially available immittance instrumentation available today actually measures Y_a (i.e., ease of energy flow). **Fig. 8–4** shows a schematic diagram of the major components and functions of an electroacoustic immittance meter.

Tympanometry

Tympanometry is a dynamic measure of immittance in the ear canal as a function of changes in pressure in the ear canal above and below atmospheric pressure. Ear canal pressure is expressed in units called decaPascals (daPa). The unit of immittance is the millimho (mmho). The graphic display of these measures, called the tympanogram, has been described using the following qualitative and quantitative analysis schemes.

Tympanometric Shape

As shown in **Fig. 8–5**, tympanograms have been classified qualitatively according to the height and location of the tympanometric peak[13]: (1) *type A*—single peak of normal height at or near atmospheric pressure, consistent with a normal middle ear; (2) *type A_s*—"shallow" tympanogram with a reduced peak height present at normal pressure, consistent with moderate middle ear fluid, otosclerosis or ossicular fixation; (3) *type A_d*—"deep" tympanogram with an increased peak height present at normal pressure, consistent with a hypermobile middle ear system such as disruption of the ossicular chain or tympanic membrane abnormality; (4) *type B*—flat tympanogram, associated with severe middle ear effusion or cerumen occlusion; and (5) *type C*—normal height occurring at negative pressure, associated with negative middle ear pressure.

Tympanometric Width

Tympanometric width (TW) is the width of the tympanogram (in daPa) measured at half of the height from the peak to the tail. Abnormally wide TW is considered an indication of middle ear dysfunction.[13] TWs should be considered abnormal when they exceed 235 daPa in infants, 200 daPa in older children, 300 daPa in children with high prevalence of middle ear disorders, and 110 daPa in adults.[14,15]

Equivalent Ear Canal Volume

Equivalent ear canal volume (V_{ea}) is an estimate of the volume of air trapped between the probe tip and the tympanic membrane. In the presence of a flat tympanogram, a large V_{ea} is useful for detecting tympanic membrane perforations or patency of tympanostomy tubes. A normal volume, however, may occur when active middle ear disease is present. An abnormal criterion for children is >1.0 cc, whereas a value of >2.0 cc for adults appears to effectively distinguish ears with intact tympanic membranes from those with perforations but without active disease.[13]

Acoustic Reflex Testing

Measuring acoustic reflexes for differential diagnosis purposes is especially helpful in (1) confirming middle ear disease; (2) distinguishing between sensory (cochlear) and neural (eighth nerve) disease; (3) identifying lower brainstem pathology; and (4) identifying the site of a facial nerve lesion. The *acoustic reflex threshold* is defined as the lowest intensity level at which a middle ear immittance change can

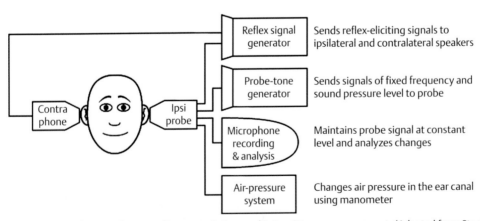

Figure 8–4 Schematic diagram of instrumentation used in immittance measurement. (Adapted from Stach BA. Clinical Audiology—An Introduction. San Diego, CA: Singular Publishing Group, 1998. Reprinted with permission.)

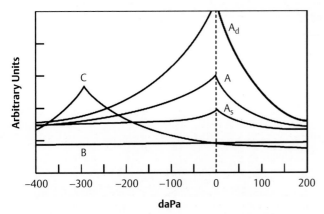

Figure 8–5 A group of five types of tympanograms based on tympanometric shape. Type A shows normal peak pressure and height. Type A_s shows a shallow peak. Type A_d shows a high or deep peak. Type B shows a flat tympanogram. Type C shows a negative pressure peak.

be detected in response to sound. Acoustic reflex thresholds in patients with normal hearing and normal middle ear function will occur between 70 and 100 dB HL. Comparison of acoustic reflex threshold levels for tones versus other broadband stimuli permits estimation of the degree of cochlear hearing loss. Suprathreshold analysis of the acoustic reflex includes reflex *adaptation* or *decay*. The clinical usefulness of measuring acoustic reflex thresholds and decay is described below along with some general rules for interpretation. First, however, a brief overview of the acoustic-stapedius reflex arc is presented.

Acoustic reflexes are measured by assessing changes in acoustic admittance of the ear caused by a contraction of the stapedius muscle. The acoustic reflex is a bilateral phenomenon. That is, when a high-intensity stimulus (i.e., usually

80 dB HL or greater) is presented to either ear of a patient with normal hearing to moderate cochlear hearing loss, the stapedius muscle reflexively contracts bilaterally. **Fig. 8–6** shows a block diagram of the ipsilateral (uncrossed) and contralateral (crossed) acoustic reflex pathway. The afferent portion of the reflex arc is the eighth nerve. Complex brainstem pathways lead from the cochlear nucleus on the stimulated side to the motor nucleus of the seventh nerve on both sides (ipsilateral and contralateral to the stimulus) of the brainstem. The efferent portion of the arc is the seventh nerve, which innervates the stapedius muscle.[16]

Principles of Interpretation

The following patterns are meant as general principles and should be interpreted only within the context of the entire audiologic evaluation.[17]

- *Middle ear disorders:* For bilateral middle ear disorders, acoustic reflexes typically are absent when both ipsilateral and contralateral ears are stimulated with the acoustic signal. In cases of a unilateral conductive disorder, stimulation of the unaffected ear will elicit an ipsilateral reflex, whereas the occurrence of a reflex caused by stimulating the contralateral affected ear will be determined by the severity of the conductive hearing loss in that abnormal ear.

- *Cochlear disorders:* Acoustic reflex thresholds in ears with cochlear disorders are determined by the degree of sensory hearing loss. Mild cochlear hearing loss has little effect on acoustic reflex thresholds. In contrast, reflexes probably will be absent when audiometric thresholds exceed 80 dB HL. When the cochlear hearing loss is <80 dB HL, acoustic reflex thresholds may be present but at reduced sensation levels. For example, a 55-dB cochlear hearing loss may show a reflex at 95 dB HL (expected HL for a patient with normal hearing), which is a 40-dB sensation level. Reduced reflex

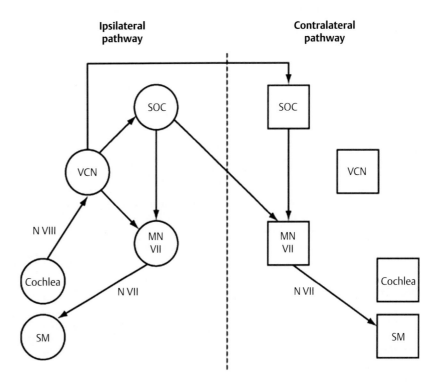

Figure 8–6 Schematic of the ipsilateral and contralateral acoustic stapedial reflex pathways. SM, stapedius muscle; N VIII, auditory nerve; VCN, ventral cochlear nucleus; SOC, superior olivary complex; MN VII, motor nucleus of the facial nerve; N VII, facial nerve.

sensation levels should be considered a strong diagnostic indicator of cochlear hearing loss.

- *Eighth nerve disorders:* Acoustic reflexes are absent with stimulation to the affected ear. It is noteworthy that the reflex is absent regardless of the degree of hearing loss. When reflexes are present, rapid decay may be observed. The most commonly used technique to measure reflex decay is half-life (i.e., time required for reflex magnitude to decrease to one-half of it maximum value) of a 500 or 1000 Hz tone presented at 10 dB SL re: acoustic reflex threshold. A half-life of ≤5 seconds over a 10-second stimulus period is clinically significant for an eighth nerve disorder.

- *Facial nerve disorders:* Acoustic reflexes are abnormal or absent when the probe is placed in the ear with facial nerve paralysis. Acoustic reflex responses are affected only if the site of lesion is central to the innervation of the stapedius muscle.

- *Brainstem disorders:* Patients with brainstem disorders may demonstrate normal ipsilateral reflexes with abnormalities in contralateral reflex measures. The exact site and size of the brainstem disorder will influence the crossed and uncrossed reflex patterns.

◆ Otoacoustic Emissions

Otoacoustic emissions (OAEs) are low-intensity sounds generated by the cochlea that emanate into the middle ear and are detected in the external auditory canal by a microphone. OAEs are considered by-products of outer hair cell motility, thereby providing an objective noninvasive technique for assessing preneural cochlear function. Applications of OAE include (1) screening for hearing loss in newborn and pediatric populations; (2) cross-checks for behavioral testing in difficult-to-test patients (including functional hearing loss); (3) differential assessment of sensory and neural hearing losses; and (4) ototoxicity monitoring. Although *spontaneous* OAEs can be recorded, *evoked* OAEs (EOAE), specifically transient-evoked (TEOAE) and distortion-product OAEs (DPOAE) provide the most clinically useful information.

Transient-Evoked Otoacoustic Emissions

Using time-synchronous averaging techniques, TEOAEs are accomplished using an 80 to 85 dB sound pressure level (SPL) transient (i.e., click or tone burst) signal that stimulates a wide range of frequencies in the cochlea. Although a broadband signal is used, cochlear response can be analyzed to provide frequency-specific information. **Fig. 8–7** is an example of a normal TEOAE response obtained from an adult ear. In general, the TEOAE will be absent when cochlear hearing loss exceeds approximately 30 dB HL. It is noteworthy that a conductive hearing loss may prevent a TEOAE even with normal cochlear function; responses may be present with patent tympanostomy tubes.

Distortion-Product Otoacoustic Emissions

DPOAEs reflect nonlinear processes of the cochlea and represent distortions of the test stimuli. That is, DPOAEs are recorded in response to presentation of a pair of primary

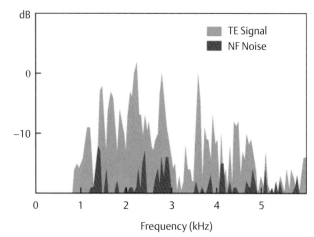

Figure 8–7 Example of a transient-evoked otoacoustic emission (TEOAE) obtained from an adult with normal hearing. The dark response shows the noise floor (NF), and the gray response is the transient evoked (TE) emission.

tones (i.e., F_1 and F_2). In response to F_1 and F_2, the outer hair cells generate a different frequency called the distortion product. The most robust distortion product typically is depicted at a frequency equal to $2F_1 - F_2$. **Fig. 8–8** is an example of a normal DPOAE in an adult ear. When emissions are present, it is likely that outer hair cells are functioning in the frequency region of the F_2 tone or approximately at the midpoint between F_1 and F_2. Although the presence of DPOAEs documents normal to near-normal cochlear function, the absence of the response does not indicate the magnitude of the hearing loss.

Differential Assessment

Recall that EOAEs provide an objective measure of preneural cochlear function, thereby assisting in the differentiation between sensory and neural dysfunction. Retrocochlear pathology is supported in patients having EOAEs with moderate to

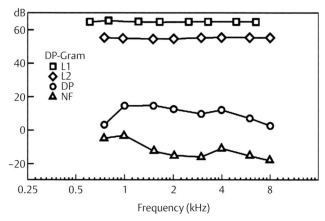

Figure 8–8 Example of a distortion-product otoacoustic emission (DPOAE) obtained from an adult with normal hearing. L1 and L2 represent the stimulus levels (in dB) for the primary tones. The lower line (Δ) is the noise floor (NF) and the line above it (o) is the distortion-product (DP) response.

profound hearing loss.[18] It should be noted, however, that sensory pathologies caused by inner hair cell damage will not produce EOAEs.

EOAEs have been especially helpful in the diagnosis of auditory neuropathy, which reflects the lack of synchronous activity in the auditory nerve. The audiologic picture for individuals with auditory neuropathy includes (1) mild to profound behavioral pure-tone thresholds; (2) normal OAEs; (3) the presence of cochlear microphonic; (4) elevated or absent acoustic reflexes; and (5) absent or abnormal auditory brainstem response recordings.

◆ Auditory Evoked Potential Measurement

Auditory evoked potentials (AEPs) are a series of bioelectric responses recorded using surface (for most clinical applications) electrodes and computer averaging techniques. AEP recordings reflect neural synchrony and transmission in the auditory system. The obtained waveforms consist of a series of peaks and troughs (i.e., wave components) that can be quantified by amplitude and latency measures. The following discussion focuses on those AEPs primarily used in clinical practice.

Electrocochleography

The electrocochleography (ECochG) response arises in the first 2 or 3 ms following an abrupt signal onset. **Fig. 8–9A** shows a normal ECochG waveform that consists of two cochlear potentials, the summating potential (SP) and compound action potential (AP) of the eighth nerve. Although the exact source of the SP is unknown, it is attributed to distortion products associated with basilar membrane and hair cell displacement. The AP arises from the distal portion of the eighth nerve.

Currently, the primary clinical application of ECochG is for the diagnosis and monitoring of Meniere's disease/endolymphatic hydrops. This is accomplished by comparing the amplitude relationships between the SP and AP, forming the SP/AP ratio.

In most clinical practices, noninvasive extratympanic or tympanic membrane electrodes are used for recording purposes. **Fig. 8–9B** illustrates an abnormal ECochG reflected by an abnormally large SP in comparison to the AP (SP/AP ratio). An SP/AP ratio of 0.45 or greater is considered abnormal, suggesting increased labyrinth pressure.[19] In addition, ECochG is used as an enhancement technique for wave I of the ABR when the patient has significant hearing loss or when recording conditions are less than optimal. Moreover, ECochG recordings intraoperatively have been helpful for monitoring cochlear and auditory nerve function during surgical procedures involving the auditory periphery.[20]

Auditory Brainstem Response

The auditory brainstem response (ABR) occurs during the first 10 ms following an appropriate signal. As shown in **Fig. 8–10**, the response is composed of a series of vertex-positive waves. In general, waves I and II are generated by the distal and proximal portions of the eighth nerve, respectively. Although the precise generator sites for later waves are less well defined, it is currently held that wave III represents the cochlear nucleus, wave IV the superior olivary complex with input from the cochlear nucleus and lateral lemniscus, and wave V is associated with the termination of fibers from the lateral lemniscus into the inferior colliculus.[16,21] Accordingly, it is best to assume that with the exceptions of waves I and II, the latter responses have multiple generator sites.

ABR commonly is used to estimate peripheral hearing sensitivity of patients who cannot (e.g., infants and young children, developmentally delayed children and/or adults) or will not (e.g., because of malingering) cooperate with behavioral testing. It is important to note that ABR testing is *not* a true test of hearing, but evaluates neural synchrony and

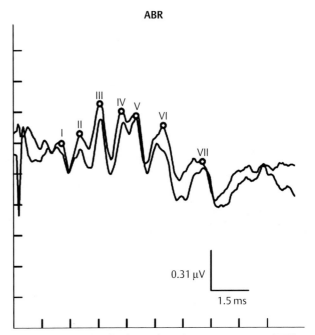

Figure 8–10　Example of an auditory brainstem response (ABR) recording obtained from a normal ear. The individual waves of the ABR are labeled with roman numerals I to VII.

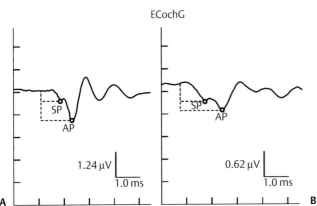

Figure 8–9　Example of electrocochleography (ECochG) recordings (SP, summating potential; AP, whole-nerve action potential) from **(A)** a normal ear and **(B)** patient with Meniere's disease showing an enlarged SP/AP ratio.

helps to estimate hearing thresholds. The process of hearing sensitivity prediction is a determination of the lowest level at which wave V of the ABR can be identified (**Fig. 8–11**). ABR thresholds may be determined using clicks (estimate of sensitivity from 1000 to 4000 Hz) or more frequency-specific tone pips.

ABR is also useful in otoneurologic assessment. ABR interpretation is typically based on latencies for waves I, III, and V wherein absolute latency values, interaural differences, interwave differences, and absent waves serve as diagnostic indices. It is noteworthy that there is not any one ABR pattern that is diagnostic for a particular disease process. Standard ABR latency measures are valuable in detecting extracanalicular and intracanalicular tumors larger than 1.0 cm; however, smaller tumors often go undetected using standard clinical techniques. Because gadolinium-enhanced magnetic resonance imaging (MRI) provides reliable identification, size, and location of tumors as small as 3.0 mm in the internal auditory canal, MRI is considered the gold standard for detecting vestibular schwannoma.[22] A new ABR measure, however, namely the stacked ABR, has been successful in detecting smaller tumors. Stacked ABR is obtained by using a derived-band procedure followed by a summation of wave V amplitudes.[23] The stacked ABR holds promise as a cost-effective method for detecting small tumors.

Finally, ABR is useful for neurophysiologic monitoring of surgical procedures that place hearing at risk during cerebellopontine angle surgery. During the surgical procedure, ABR responses are compared against baseline recordings. For example, wave V latency shifts of 1 ms or greater and amplitude reduction for wave V of greater than 50% have been considered clinically significant changes from baseline. According to Hall,[16] hearing preservation is best for patients with small tumors (less than 1.5 cm) and intact hearing (PTA of 30 dB or better and word recognition scores better that 70%).

Auditory Steady-State Response

The auditory steady-state response (ASSR) is a new tool that is gaining popularity with clinicians because of its good correlation with behavioral thresholds. The ASSR uses a continuous frequency-specific stimulus that is either frequency or amplitude modulated. The recorded response is generated in the EEG response rather than specifically in the auditory brainstem pathway as with the ABR. Whereas the ABR response is determined through the identification of peaks and troughs in the time domain, the presence or absence of the ASSR is determined through a series of statistical algorithms in the frequency domain. The ASSR can be recorded within 10 dB of the behavioral threshold. At the conclusion of testing, an ASSR audiogram can be generated, yielding ear-specific, frequency-specific, and threshold information.

Middle Latency Response

The middle latency response (MLR) is a series of waveforms occurring within the 10- to 50-ms time epoch. As shown in **Fig. 8–12A**, major peaks are denoted as Na, Pa, Nb, and Pb or P1. It has been suggested that primary and nonprimary components of the auditory thalamocortical pathway contribute to the MLR.[24] The major clinical applications of the MLR have included estimation of low-frequency hearing thresholds,[25] assessment of patients with cochlear implants,[26] and neurodiagnostic assessment of auditory pathway disease and central auditory processing disorders.[27]

Auditory Late Response

As seen in **Fig. 8–12B**, the auditory late response (ALR) is a response with latencies ranging from 50 to 250 ms (P1, N1, P2, N2) and amplitudes ranging from 3 to 10 μV. ALR is a cortical response that depends on the patient's state of arousal. Therefore, the patient cannot be sedated during the test session and must remain awake and attentive to the stimulus. The ALR has had limited use in threshold estimation and evaluation of central auditory processing and cortical function.[16]

P3/P300

The P3 or P300 is an endogenous response requiring active cognitive participation with multiple neural generator sites involving the frontal cortex, centroparietal cortex, and hippocampus.[28] It is elicited by what is referred to as the "oddball" paradigm. That is, a series of infrequently occurring target (deviant) stimuli are presented within a series of nontarget homogeneous (standard) stimuli. The patient's task is to attend to the deviant stimuli. As shown in **Fig. 8–12C**, the P3 response accompanies the occurrence of the rare, unexpected stimulus or the absence of the expected stimulus. P3 has been used to evaluate such psychological events as attention, alerting, arousal, and memory.

Figure 8–11 Example of an ABR latency-intensity function obtained from a child with normal hearing. Note the increase in wave V latency and decrease in amplitude as stimulus intensity decreases.

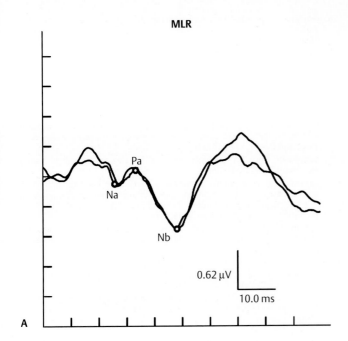

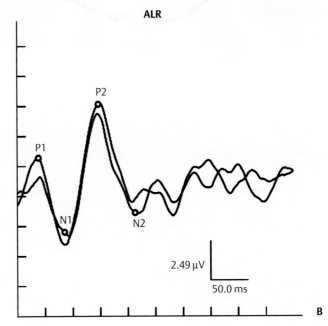

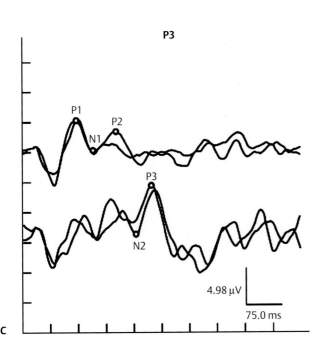

Figure 8–12 Examples of auditory evoked potential recordings from normal ears showing **(A)** middle latency responses (P, positive polarity; N, negative polarity), **(B)** auditory late responses, and **(C)** P3 response. The top P3 recordings are the averages of a standard (frequent) 500 Hz stimulus. The bottom P3 recordings are the average of a deviant (infrequent) 2000 Hz stimulus.

◆ Conclusion

Diagnostic audiology is dependent on examining the relationships among the behavioral and physiologic measures employed during the test session. Each procedure adds a piece of information to the audiologic picture of the patient. Several new techniques, such as wideband energy reflectance, laser-Doppler vibrometry, and the Cochlear Hydrops Analysis Masking Procedure (CHAMP™), hold promise as new tools in the clinician's armamentarium. Diagnostic procedures, especially those capitalizing on physiologic responses to auditory signals, continue to be refined and evolve as new technology and related clinical applications emerge.

References

1. American National Standards Institute. American National Standard Psychoacoustical Terminology. ANSI S3.2. New York: American Standards Institute, 1973

2. American National Standards Institute. American National Standard Specification for Audiometers. ANSI S3.6. New York: American Standards Institute, 1996

3. Silman S, Silverman CA. Auditory Diagnosis-Principles and Applications. San Diego, CA: Academic Press, 1991

4. Roeser RJ, Valente M, Hosford-Dunn H. Diagnostic procedures in the profession of audiology. In: Roeser RJ, Valente M, Hossford-Dunn, H, eds. Audiology Diagnosis. New York: Thieme, 2000:1–18

5. Martin FN, Greer Clark J. Introduction to Audiology. Boston: Allyn and Bacon, 2003

6. Bess FH, Humes LE. Audiology—The Fundamentals, 2nd ed. Baltimore: Williams & Wilkins, 1995

7. Ventry IM, Chaiklin JB. Evaluation configurations used in identifying adults with functional hearing loss. J Aud Res 1965;5;212–218

8. Martin FN, Champlin CA, Chambers J. Seventh survey of audiometric practices in the United States. J Am Acad Audiol 1998;9: 95–104

9. Owens E, Schubert ED. Development of the California Consonant Test. J Speech Hear Res 1977;20:463–474

10. Davis H, Silverman SR. Hearing and Deafness, 4th ed. New York: Holt, Rinehart and Winston, 1978

11. Kalikow DN, Stevens KN, Elliott LL. Development of a test of speech intelligibility in noise using sentence materials with controlled predictability. J Acoust Soc Am 1977;61:1337–1351

12. Thornton AR, Raffin MJM. Speech discrimination scores modified as a binomial variable. J Speech Hear Res 1978;21:507–518

13. Margolis RH, Hunter LL. Acoustic immittance measurements. In: Roeser RJ, Valente M, Hossford-Dunn H., eds. Audiology Diagnosis. New York: Thieme, 2000:381–424

14. Working Group on Acoustic Immittance Measurements and the Committee on Audiologic Evaluation, American Speech-Language-Hearing Association. Guidelines for screening for hearing impairment and middle-ear disorders. ASHA Suppl 1990;2:17–24

15. American Speech–Language Hearing Association. Guidelines for Audiologic Screening. Rockville, MD: American Speech–Language Hearing Association, 1997

16. Hall JW. Handbook of Auditory Evoked Responses. Boston: Allyn and Bacon, 1992

17. Wiley TL, Fowler CG. Acoustic Immittance Measures in Clinical Audiology: A Primer. San Diego, CA: Singular Publishing Group, 1997

18. Robinette MS, Glattke TJ. In: Roeser RJ, Valente M, Hossford-Dunn H, eds. Audiology Diagnosis. New York: Thieme, 2000:503–527

19. Ferraro JA, Ruth RA. Electrocochleography. In: Jacobson JT, ed. Principles and Applications in Auditory Evoked Potentials. Needham Heights, MA: Allyn and Bacon, 1994:101–122

20. Ferraro JA, Ruth RA. Cochlear potentials in clinical audiology. Audiol Neurootol 1997;2:241–256

21. Jacobson GP, Jacobson JT, Ramadan N, Hyde ML. Auditory brainstem response measures in acoustic nerve and brainstem disease. In: Jacobson JT, ed. Principles and Applications in Auditory Evoked Potentials. Needham Heights, MA: Allyn and Bacon, 1994:387–426

22. National Institutes of Health. Consensus Development Conference Statement. Acoustic Neuroma. December 11–13, 1991. Consensus statement. 9(4):1–24

23. Don M, Kwong B. Auditory brainstem response: differential diagnosis. In: Katz J, ed. Handbook of Clinical Audiology. Philadelphia: Lippincott Williams & Wilkins, 2002:274–297

24. Kraus N, Smith DI, McGee T. Midline and temporal lobe MLRs in the guinea pig originate from different generator systems: a conceptual framework for new and existing data. Electroencephalogr Clin Neurophysiol 1988;70:541–558

25. Scherg M, Volk SA. Frequency specificity of simultaneously recorded early and middle latency auditory evoked potentials. Electroencephalogr Clin Neurophysiol 1983;56:443–452

26. Kileny PR, Kemink JL. Electrically evoked middle-latency auditory potentials in cochlear implant candidates. Arch Otolaryngol Head Neck Surg 1987;113:1072–1077

27. Cacace AT, McFarland DJ. Middle-latency auditory evoked potentials: basic issues and potential applications. In: Katz J, ed. Handbook of Clinical Audiology. Philadelphia: Lippincott Williams & Wilkins, 2002:349–377

28. McPherson DL. Late Potentials of the Auditory System. San Diego, CA: Singular Publisher Group, 1996

9

Assessment of Auditory Processing Disorders

Robert W. Keith

Many practicing otolaryngologists, even Fellowship-trained otologists, are unfamiliar with central auditory processing and dysfunction. This chapter provides information on central auditory testing including the rationale for such tests. The chapter includes suggestions for ordering central auditory testing and a test battery approach is proposed. Finally, case histories showing results of central auditory testing are given.

◆ History of Central Auditory Disorders in Otoneurologic Diagnosis

Although many physicians are not familiar with the subject of central auditory disorders, otolaryngologists conducted some of the earliest systematic clinical research on this subject. Specifically, the classic works of Bocca, Calearo, and Antonelli published in the mid-1950s provided a basis for subsequent development of central auditory testing. Their early research, summarized by Calearo and Antonelli in the first edition of *Otolaryngology*[1] is informative reading even today.

Calearo and Antonelli noted that sensorineural hearing loss can be classified as cochlear and retrocochlear. Because retrocochlear disorders may include eighth cranial nerve and central pathways lesions, they defined central auditory lesions as involving the pathway between the cochlear nucleus and the temporal lobe cortex. This classification remains today, with the added notion of interhemispheric transmission of auditory information through the corpus callosum.

The single difference between testing conducted earlier and now is the *focus* or purpose of central auditory testing. In the 1950s and 1960s, the emphasis was on the identification of auditory pathway lesions. With the development of sophisticated diagnostic imaging techniques (e.g., magnetic resonance imaging), there is presently little need for auditory diagnosis of central lesions. Therefore, the current primary focus of central auditory testing is to describe functional disorders of communication.[2,3] Terms used to describe these disorders of listening and understanding include *auditory perceptual disorders, central auditory processing disorders,* and more recently *auditory processing disorders* (APDs).[4]

A secondary purpose, also discussed by Calearo and Antonelli,[1] continues to be experimental research into communication disorders related to various language and learning problems and central auditory pathway lesions.

The last few years have seen a remarkably increase of interest in APDs by professionals and the lay public. This interest is a result of the large body of research on APD that became available during previous decades in conferences, through increased communication through the Internet, and through commercialization of remediation programs. One negative factor is the lack of consensus on a precise definition of the term APD and how this disorder is unique. Two conferences held in 1993 and 2000 addressed issues of definitions of APD.

◆ Definition of Auditory Processing Disorder

APDs can be defined as dysfunctions of one or more of the basic processes involved in understanding spoken language, which may manifest themselves in an imperfect ability to listen.[5] An American Speech–Language Hearing Association (ASHA) ad hoc committee on central auditory processing[6] defined auditory processing disorders as "deficits in information processing of audible signals not attributed to impaired hearing sensitivity or intellectual impairment." Specifically, the committee stated that "APD" refers to limitations in the ongoing transmission, analysis, organization, transformation, elaboration, storage, retrieval, and use of information contained in audible signals. More simply stated, the auditory system is responsible for the following:

- Sound localization and lateralization
- Auditory discrimination
- Auditory pattern recognition
- Temporal aspects of audition including resolution, masking, and ordering
- Performance with competing signals
- Performance with degraded signals

Deficits in processing of those signals can be considered an APD.

More recently the Consensus Conference on the diagnosis of APD in school-aged children suggested, "An APD may be broadly defined as a deficit in the processing of information that is specific to the auditory modality."[4] The panel concluded that the problem may be exacerbated in unfavorable acoustic environments. It may be associated with difficulties in listening, speech understanding, language development, and learning. "In its pure form, however, it is conceptualized as a deficit in the processing of auditory input." These discussions about terminology suggest that APD contributes to developmental language disorders and interferes with academic achievement in the classroom.

The prevalence of APD is unknown as there is no gold standard for the disorder. Learning disabilities in children have a prevalence of 4 to 5%.[7,8] Many of these children have APD also, but the occurrence is unknown and estimates reported in the literature are speculative.

◆ Principles of Central Auditory Dysfunction

Calearo and Antonelli[1] summarized several principles attributed to Carhart that explain how the normal central nervous system (CNS) handles auditory messages:

1. *Channel separation:* A signal delivered to one ear is kept distinct from a different signal in the other ear.
2. *Binaural fusion:* If a single auditory message is divided into two bands by filtering or by switching, and these bands are delivered binaurally and simultaneously, fusion will take place (at the brainstem level) and the subject will experience one message only.
3. *Contralateral pathways:* Auditory messages from one ear cross at the brainstem level, and reach the temporal lobe of the opposite side.
4. *Hemispheric dominance for language:* Although one cerebral hemisphere (usually the left) is verbally dominant, the other hemisphere appears to possess limited verbal abilities. Adding to Bocca and Calearo, we now understand that linguistic information reaching the nondominant hemisphere (the right hemisphere from information presented to the left ear) crosses to the dominant language hemisphere through the densely myelinated fibers in the splenium of the corpus callosum.

Related to the above principles, the following additional principles apply to central auditory assessment:

1. Most diseases affecting central hearing pathways produce no loss in threshold sensitivity. Therefore, pure-tone tests do not generally identify APD.
2. Undistorted speech audiometry is not sufficiently challenging to the central auditory nervous system to identify the presence of a central auditory lesion/disorder.
3. Only tests of reduced acoustic redundancy (distorted speech materials called sensitized speech tests by Teatini[9]) are sufficiently challenging to the auditory nervous system to identify a central auditory lesion/disorder.

The rationale for use of sensitized speech testing was further described by Jerger[10] as the *subtlety principle,* in which the subtlety of the auditory manifestation increases as the site of lesion progresses from peripheral to central. More recently, Phillips[11] described these processes in a somewhat different way as "patterns of convergence and divergence in the ascending auditory pathway."

◆ Neurophysiologic Basis of Central Auditory Disorders

The auditory nervous system presents a complex interaction of neural signals that integrates acoustic information from both ears at nearly all levels of the central auditory nervous system from the cochlear nucleus to the auditory cortex. These neural pathways are not simply passive conductors of an electrical signal; auditory analysis takes place at all levels of the auditory system from cochlea to cortex.

The final common pathway is the auditory area of the cerebral cortex that lies in Heschl's gyrus. Anatomically the brain contains regions that are typically different in size on the two sides. The best-defined asymmetry is in the primary auditory reception area in centers known to be associated with language comprehension. This asymmetry is present in newborns.

What we know about auditory processing and the brain is as follows:

1. Language centers are usually situated in the left hemisphere. Ninety-five percent of persons are left-hemisphere dominant for language. Although production of speech is controlled from one hemisphere, there is a continuum of lateralization for speech perception. The right hemisphere is probably capable of processing paralinguistic aspects of language such as emotional tone, context, inference, and connotation. Therefore, motor speech production is a single hemisphere function, whereas speech perception is a dual hemisphere function that has implication for interpretation of auditory perceptual test results.
2. Maturation of neural structures, especially association fibers, takes place over many years. Sensory deprivation results in failure of certain neural centers to develop at least in the brainstem and probably cortically.[11]
3. Dominance for language is present in the left cerebral hemisphere at early ages, but the brain is sufficiently plastic to allow language to be controlled by other areas if early damage occurs.[12] Linguistic processing is more completely centered in dominant hemispheres in older persons who are less able to recover from damage to language centers.
4. Failure to establish cerebral dominance is associated with problems associated with language development, learning to read, and integration of information from the several senses. Causes of brain dysfunction include:
   a. Congenital abnormalities
   b. Anoxia
   c. Maternal virus
   d. Other birth injury or illness
   e. Head trauma
   f. Seizures
   g. Genetic factors
   h. Unknown factors

According to Ferry,[13] delay or deviation in language development is due to disordered brain functioning. Normal speech and language development is a reflection of an intact functioning brain. A speech or language delay, or auditory processing disorder, may be the only symptom or sign of neurologic impairment.

◆ Sensitized Speech Tests

Sensitized speech tests utilize various means of distortion of the speech stimuli to reduce the intelligibility of the message. Distortion can be accomplished by reducing the range of frequencies in the speech signal through filtering (filtered speech testing), by reducing the intensity level of speech above a simultaneously presented background noise (auditory figure ground testing), by interrupting the speech at different rates, and by increasing the rate of presentation (time-compressed speech). The basic principle of sensitized speech testing is that persons with normal hearing and a normal central auditory system can understand the distorted message. When a central auditory disorder is present, however, speech intelligibility is poor. The construct of sensitized speech testing is extremely powerful and forms the basis of all behavioral speech tests of central auditory function.

◆ Dichotic Testing

Other techniques for assessing the central auditory system are accomplished with simultaneous (dichotic) presentation of sentences, words, digits, or syllables to opposite ears. Dichotic test results describe maturation of the auditory nervous system in children and adolescents, specify the dominant hemisphere for language, access short-term auditory memory storage and retrieval, and identify breakdowns in cortical auditory function.

Different categories of diagnostic central auditory tests have been proposed. For example, the ASHA Committee on Disorders of Central Auditory Processing[6] used the following taxonomy:

1. Monotic (signals presented to one ear)
   a. Filtered speech (e.g., low-pass-filtered)
   b. Time-altered speech (e.g., time-compressed speech)
   c. Pattern recognition (e.g., frequency and duration patterns)
   d. Ipsilateral competing signals (e.g., auditory figure ground)
2. Dichotic (signals presented simultaneously to two ears called binaural separation tasks)
   a. Digits
   b. Syllables
   c. Words
   d. Sentences
3. Binaural (signals presented simultaneously to two ears called binaural integration tasks)
   a. Binaural fusion (low- and high-filtered speech bands presented simultaneously to opposite ears)
   b. Rapidly alternating speech
   c. Masking-level differences

Pattern recognition tests are used to assess nondominant hemisphere function and interhemispheric transfer of information. Two examples are the frequency-patterns and duration-patterns tests.[14–16]

◆ Auditory Processing Disorders in Clinical Populations

Adults

Research has been conducted in various adult patient populations including persons who are aging[17,18] and those with Parkinson's disease,[19] chronic alcoholism,[20] Alzheimer's disease,[21–23] multiple sclerosis, head trauma,[24–26] stroke,[2,27] learning disabilities and reading disorders,[28–30] and AIDS.[31] In all of these patient groups, results of central auditory tests were poorer than predicted on the basis of peripheral hearing levels. There are several purposes for administration of a central auditory test battery to adults[32]:

1. In chronic CNS disease, to assess progression and to describe functional impairment
2. In head injury and stroke, to monitor recovery and provide a framework for counseling families
3. In pre- and postoperative brain surgery patients, to determine functional disorders of communication
4. In learning-disabled adults, to describe auditory processing abilities
5. In persons with neurologic disease, to monitor degenerative cognitive function, and to assess the effectiveness of medical treatment
6. In patients with normal hearing who have histories of decreased ability to understand speech, to identify the presence of an APD
7. In aging patients, to study and describe auditory processing abilities related to changes that occur among healthy elderly persons and those with chronic disease.

Identification of central auditory disorders among these patient populations will assist when counseling affected individuals and their families about their communication abilities, identifying necessary changes in the patient's listening environment (both physical and psychological changes), and determining specific recommendations for rehabilitation.

Children

The literature is full of examples of APDs in children that are related to language, learning, reading, and other developmental disorders. Auditory processing test results provide the following information about children:

1. The test results describe the maturation level of the central auditory pathways, and through longitudinal studies on the same child demonstrate the development of auditory processing abilities.
2. The test results provide data to document the neurologic origin presumed to exist in children with specific learning disabilities.
3. The test results can aid in ruling out abnormalities of the central auditory pathways as contributing to a language-learning problem.

4. The test results describe whether language is appropriately located in the left hemisphere, or whether there is mixed or right hemisphere cerebral dominance for language.

5. The test results describe whether the auditory channel is weak or strong, and whether the classroom environment should be modified, tutoring or remedial material initiated, or assistive listening devices recommended to help the child in a learning environment.

6. The test results can be used to assess the effect of medication (for example, Ritalin) on central auditory abilities.

In summary, results of the auditory processing test battery are used to develop remedial strategies for auditory processing/language-learning disordered children.

◆ Factors Affecting Central Auditory Test Results

Many variables can affect central auditory test results. Speech intelligibility of distorted speech is reduced by both peripheral and central factors, so that hearing thresholds must always be known before interpreting auditory processing test results. Peripheral hearing loss, both conductive and sensorineural, can result in hearing asymmetry and cochlear distortion. Patients with peripheral hearing loss cannot be tested with most central auditory measures. Even a mild conductive hearing loss results in diminished performance on auditory processing tests. Subjects with low intellectual abilities perform at a level that is commensurate with their mental age, and allowance for that factor must be made when interpreting results of central auditory tests. Normal children and adults who are non–native speakers of English have difficulty performing on sensitized speech tasks presented in English, even years after being immersed in the language.[33,34] Marriage et al[35] found that even children who speak British-accented English have difficulty understanding American-accented speech on an auditory processing test battery. Examiners should be cautious when administering any test of auditory processing that uses American-accented speech to children who are not native speakers of English.

Regarding conductive hearing loss, in the past there was little available information on the long-term effects of early and prolonged otitis media with static or fluctuating hearing loss on auditory processing abilities. There is some evidence that otitis media can cause auditory learning problems.[36–44] The residual effects can be central auditory processing problems that may cause language and learning delays long after the middle ear disease has been resolved. The relationship between histories of otitis media and auditory processing disorders does not have a perfect correlation and controversy on that topic exists. Nevertheless, it is important to watch children with histories of frequent colds or chronic middle ear disease for signs of auditory language-learning problems.

As with most learning disabilities, APD can exist in combination with or because of other disorders. For example, auditory perceptual problems may stem from neurologic problems or brain injury resulting from head trauma, meningitis or other viral infections, seizure disorders, congenital anomalies such as agenesis of the corpus callosum, low birth weight, or other factors. Maternal drug and alcohol abuse may also result in APD in offspring. Additionally, there are undoubtedly genetic factors involved because many family members have similar educational histories of auditory learning problems. Some children with attention deficit hyperactive disorder (ADHD) have comorbidity with APD, and a diagnostic assessment is sometimes necessary to identify the primary problem. In fact, recent research has focused on attempts to differentiate between APD and ADHD, which have similar behavioral patterns. In general, the literature indicates that the presence of ADHD results in a general reduction of performance on tests of auditory processing. When questioned carefully, there are behavioral differences between the two entities and it is possible to separate them.[45,46] When possible, it is important to differentiate between ADHD and APD because they receive different treatments. Specifically, one does not treat children who have APD with medication.

◆ Behaviors of Individuals with Central Auditory Processing Disorders

The following observations are characteristic of children with auditory processing problems:

1. Most are male.
2. They have normal pure-tone hearing thresholds.
3. They generally respond inconsistently to auditory stimuli. They often respond appropriately, but at other times they seem unable to follow auditory instructions.
4. They have short attention spans and fatigue easily when confronted with long or complex activities.
5. They are distracted by both auditory and visual stimulation. These children are described as being at the mercy of their environment. Unable to block out irrelevant stimuli, they must respond immediately and totally to everything they see, feel, or hear, no matter how trivial.
6. They may have difficulty with auditory localization skills. This may include an inability to discern the source and distance of sound and an inability to differentiate soft and loud sounds.
7. They may listen attentively, but have difficulty following long or complicated verbal commands or instructions.
8. They frequently request that information be repeated.
9. They are often unable to remember information presented verbally for both short-term and long-term memory.
10. They sometimes have a significant history of chronic otitis media.

Other behavioral characteristics of children with central auditory processing disorder (CAPD) include having poor listening skills, taking a substantial amount of time to answer questions, having difficulty relating what is heard to the words seen on paper, and being unable to appreciate jokes, puns, or other humorous twists of language.

In addition to specific auditory behaviors, many of these children have significant reading problems, are poor spellers, and have poor handwriting. They may have articulation or language disorders. In the classroom they may act out frustrations that result from their perceptual deficits, or they may be shy and withdrawn because of the poor self-concept that results from multiple failures. Therefore, appropriate referrals for central auditory testing should be made for patients of any age who exhibit the symptoms listed above.

◆ Test Battery Approach

Examiners can arrive at a diagnosis of APD using a variety of indices. The ASHA Consensus Statement on Central Auditory Processing[47] recommends the following approach to assessment:

1. History of the patient's social, birth, health, developmental status, and auditory behavior
2. Systematic observation of auditory behavior including information obtained from available questionnaires and checklists.[21–24,48–51] For example, the Children's Auditory Performance Scale (CHAPS)[51] is a scaled questionnaire consisting of 25 items used to rate listening behavior in a variety of conditions. Responses from parents and teachers are quantified and the child's listening behaviors profiled. The scale can be used to identify children who should be tested for auditory processing abilities and to prescribe and measure the effects of intervention.
3. Tests of peripheral function, including pure-tone thresholds, speech recognition, acoustic immittance measures, and (when possible) otoacoustic emissions.
4. Central auditory tests including measures of the following:
   a. Temporal processes (gap detection tests)
   b. Localization and lateralization
   c. Low-redundancy monaural speech (time-compressed, filtered, interrupted, competing, etc.)
   d. Dichotic stimuli (competing nonsense syllables, digits, words, and sentences)
   e. Binaural interaction (e.g., masking-level differences)

When organized according to the ASHA categories, measures of auditory processing abilities include the following:

1. Temporal processes
   a. Random-gap detection test[52]
2. Low-redundancy monaural speech tests
   a. Time-compressed sentence test[53]
   b. Filtered words tests of SCAN-C[54] and SCAN-A[55]
   c. Auditory figure–ground tests: hearing-in-noise test, SPIN, QuickSIN, BKB SIN, competing words test of SCAN-C[54] and SCAN-A[55]
3. Dichotic stimuli (tests of binaural separation including competing nonsense syllables, digits, words, and sentences)
   a. Dichotic CV test[56]
   b. Dichotic digits test[57]
   c. Competing words tests
      i. Staggered Spondee Word test[58]
      ii. Competing words test of SCAN-C[54] and SCAN-A[55]
   d. Competing sentences test of SCAN-C[54] and SCAN-A[55]
   e. Dichotic sentence identification test[59]
4. Binaural integration
   a. Masking-level differences
   b. Binaural fusion test
5. Pattern recognition tests
   a. Frequency pattern test[14,15,60]
   b. Duration pattern test[16]

Interpretation

Tests of low redundancy monaural speech identify how a particular child performs under poor acoustic conditions such as listening under degraded conditions and competing conditions. For example, auditory figure-ground tests enable the examiner to assess a child's ability to understand speech in the presence of competing background noise. Difficulty understanding speech in the presence of background noise is a frequent complaint of individuals with auditory processing difficulties. Many children have poor ability to understand speech under noisy situations, in reverberant rooms, and in other unfavorable listening conditions. These children require management of the acoustic environment and occasionally use of an assistive listening device in the classroom.

Tests of dichotic listening ability are used to determine levels of auditory maturation and hemispheric dominance for language, and to identify disordered or damaged central auditory pathways. The advantage of testing binaural separation with signals at simple and more complex linguistic levels (e.g., digits, words, and sentences) is that it serves the purposes of test reliability, and it examines how performance, including ear advantage, changes with a different hierarchy of signal. Poor overall performance may indicate a developmental delay in maturation or underlying neurologic disorganization or damage to auditory pathways. Ear advantage is a powerful indicator of hemispheric organization. Normal-achieving children typically have a strong right ear advantage at younger ages with equal performance between ears as the child's auditory system matures. Left-ear advantages for all test conditions indicate the possibility of damage to the auditory reception areas of the left hemisphere, or failure to develop left hemisphere dominance for language. Abnormalities shown by dichotic test results correlate with a wide range of specific disabilities, including APD, language disabilities, learning disabilities, and reading disorders.

Tests of temporal processing identify perceptual disorders that lead to phonologic problems of reading and spelling. Tests of binaural integration identify brainstem dysfunction. Finally, tests of pattern recognition access nondominant hemisphere function and, if a verbal report is required, transfer of information from the nondominant to the dominant hemisphere.

Preferably, auditory tests are normed on large populations of typically performing children or adults. The use of normative scores with composite standard scores, percentile ranks, and a normative classification system enables the examiner to compare results with any other speech-language, educational, or psychological test that is standardized. Use of standard scores allows the examiner to identify performance profiles that lead to a better understanding of the child's language learning problem, which leads to appropriate intervention.[61–64]

◆ Electrophysiologic Tests of Auditory Processing Abilities

Both the ASHA Consensus Statement on Central Auditory Processing[47] and the Consensus Conference on the Diagnosis of APD in School-Aged Children[4] stated that electrophysiologic measures of auditory function is useful in the diagnosis of APDs. In fact one focus of the later conference was the increased use of electrophysiology in identifying auditory-specific

APD. The several types of auditory evoked measures available for these purposes include the auditory brainstem response (ABR), the middle latency response (MLR), late vertex auditory evoked response (LVAER), brain mapping, the P-300, and Mismatch Negativity (MMN). Early responses from the auditory brainstem can be obtained under medication. Unfortunately, middle latency and cortical evoked potentials are affected by sleep states and attention, and sedation will affect the result and interpretation. All of these techniques are well described in the literature and their use is increasing, especially in recent years in the investigation of APD. Nevertheless, their specific application to the routine clinical assessment of central auditory processing, language, and learning disabilities has yet to be determined. For example, at one time the MMN was considered to provide a promising avenue of studying auditory processing disorders in children. Kraus et al[65] described the MMN as "robust and consistently obtained in school-age children and adults … and may become a tool for clinical as well as research applications." Recent data, however, indicate that MMN in normal, healthy subjects may not be quite as robust as described. For example, Kurtzberg et al,[66] Dalebout and Stack,[67] Cunningham,[68] and Uwer and von Suchodoletz[69] all found MMN to be absent in 25 to 35% of normal children and adults. In addition, the results had poor repeatability on retest of the same child. Therefore, although MMN continues to be a promising research tool in groups of children, the use of this technique in the assessment of individual subjects should be approached with caution.

◆ Electrophysiologic Tests in Auditory Neuropathy

One reason to conduct electrophysiologic tests is to rule out auditory neuropathy. Although not considered a pure auditory processing disorder, this diagnostic entity is characterized by normal otoacoustic emissions, absent or abnormal ABR, and absent acoustic reflexes. These findings indicate that the affected person has auditory neuropathy with normal cochlear outer hair cell function with abnormal eighth cranial nerve neural synchrony or abnormal cochlear inner hair cell function. The identification of auditory neuropathy has significantly different remediation efforts than APD, including possible cochlear implantation.

In summary, advances in electrophysiologic measurements in the study of APD increased dramatically in the past two decades. In spite of problems in the application and interpretation of electrophysiologic responses, they add one more dimension to our understanding of auditory processing disorders. They currently provide invaluable information to the understanding of auditory processing disorders but it is premature to recommend their routine use in clinical diagnosis of APD. When they are better understood they will add substantial new information to the behavioral test battery.

◆ Remediation

The emphasis of this chapter so far has been on the diagnosis of APDs. In fact, diagnostic testing has greater value when remediation plans result. Many strategies exist for assisting children and adults found to have APD. The following is a brief overview of strategies for management and remediation of auditory processing disorders.[70]

In general, remediation for children with central auditory disorders falls into three categories including management of the environment, remediation of auditory perceptual skills, and use of cognitive strategies.

Management of the Environment

Management of the environment includes such strategies as preferential seating, use of FM and sound field systems, and attention to classroom acoustics. For example, when an auditory figure-ground deficit is identified, recommendations for remediation are directed toward management of the environment to enhance listening opportunities and to improve signal quality.[47] One way to improve speech understanding is to reduce competing acoustic signals in the listening environment by reducing background noise and reverberation time. Other methods are to increase the intensity of the signal through preferential seating, and the use of assistive listening devices such as FM systems or classroom amplification.[71-74] Trials with FM systems should be carefully monitored to be sure that the child, teachers, and parents understand the device, to ensure optimal fitting, and to minimize possible detrimental effects.[75] Classroom amplification has the additional benefit of helping all children including those with APD, mild or fluctuating hearing loss from otitis media, and children with ADHD. Direct intervention to help achieve better listening skills in noise through cognitive training and focusing of auditory attention may be beneficial. However, there is no evidence to support the improvement of auditory figure-ground perceptual deficits through such training. Specific recommendations for remediation of central auditory disorders can be found in several sources. [48,76-80]

Remediation of Auditory Perceptual Skills

Perceptual training is used to strengthen basic perceptual processes and teach specific academic skills. For example, auditory perceptual processes can be improved through direct techniques applied during individual therapy. The following list includes some of the auditory perceptual skills that can be strengthened:

- Speech sound discrimination (auditory discrimination)
- Auditory analysis
- Phonemic synthesis (auditory synthesis)
- Auditory memory
- Auditory figure-ground ability
- Prosody recognition
- Temporal processing deficit

Cognitive Strategies

Compensatory strategies are designed to teach the individual how to overcome residual dysfunction and maximize use of auditory information. These techniques are focused on improving learning and listening skills. For example, cognitive training involves teaching children to actively monitor and self-regulate their message comprehension skills and develop new problem-solving skills. Cognitive therapy may include language training, vocabulary development, and the teaching of organizational skills. Some organizational skills include teaching the child the following:

- How to follow directions
- How to use written notes
- Self-monitoring strategies
- To recognize what they know
- To learn to listen and anticipate
- To ask relevant questions
- To know how to answer questions

The past several years have experienced increased interest in computer-based remediation programs such as FastForward™ and Earobics™. In addition, several "sound therapy" techniques are being actively promoted by various groups. Little hard evidence exists to demonstrate the effectiveness of these techniques, which are largely unproven. They stand in contrast to such techniques as the Lindamood Bell Learning Processes© (www.lblp.com) and its various remediation programs. This program has been available for many years and appears to help children with APDs.

Finally, learning-disabled adolescents can benefit from vocational planning or college planning. Many colleges have special programs to provide individual assistance for learning-disabled students. For example, students with APDs may have difficulty learning a foreign language. Some colleges will substitute another course in place of a foreign language requirement when an APD is identified.

Diagnosis of an APD and recommendations for remediation/rehabilitation must be made as part of a multidisciplinary team decision. The purpose is to ensure that different aspects of the individual's speech, language, auditory, psychological, emotional, and physical function have been evaluated. Only after all these aspects have been examined can an APD be diagnosed and appropriate recommendations for treatment made. This is especially true when evaluating children and adolescents with language and learning problems.

Remediation of Adults with Auditory Processing Disorders

For adult patients much of the remediation process is in the form of counseling. All patients experiencing APDs and their families benefit from understanding patients' auditory capabilities and from learning day-to-day compensatory activities that can be used to ameliorate APD effects. Patients with head injury and stroke or those who have undergone brain surgery can be tested to determine their auditory processing abilities, monitor their recovery, and provide a framework for counseling families. Patients with chronic brain disease can be assessed to determine progression and to describe functional impairment. Finally, many of the environmental management suggestions made for children are helpful for adults including use of assistive listening devices and FM systems. Enactment of the Americans with Disabilities Act[81] provides accessibility of assistive listening devices in public places.

◆ Case Examples of Auditory Processing Disorders

The following two cases exemplify some of the principles discussed in this chapter. The first case is a child with evidence of neurophysiologic basis for an auditory processing and language-learning disorder. The second case demonstrates a child with a functional disorder of communication and possible delay in the development of auditory pathways that will improve over time.

Case 1: Child with Abnormal Ear Advantage and Neurologic Basis for Auditory Processing Disorder

This 7-year-old boy was referred to our center with a complex history of language, learning, auditory, and attention problems. He was the product of a normal pregnancy and delivery. He had normal physical development with no significant medical problems. He experienced slow language development with a significant language delay. At 3 years of age he used only an estimated 100 words.

Physical Examination

The physical examination was normal in all respects. It should be noted that his mother described him as always being strongly left-hand oriented from his earliest days.

Psychological Evaluation

A significant discrepancy was noted between his verbal and performance scores, with verbal IQ at 60 and performance IQ at 122. This child was noted to be eager to participate and cooperative but tired easily and became fidgety. All his performance was affected by his lack of impulse control.

Speech and Language Evaluation

Results of the Clinical Evaluation of Language Function (CELF)-R indicated a receptive language score in the 1st percentile and expressive language score in the 3rd percentile. His language scores were similarly depressed on the Test of Auditory Comprehension of Language (TACL)-3, Preschool Language Scale (PLS)-3, and Expressive One-Word Picture Vocabulary Test, 3rd edition.

Peripheral hearing testing found normal pure-tone thresholds with normal tympanometry.

Central auditory test results were as follows:

- SCAN-C composite performance was in the 8th percentile with no performance discrepancy among subtests. Another remarkable finding was a clear left ear advantage for all tests including filtered words, auditory figure ground, competing words, and competing sentences. That is, for all tests, he scored more correct responses in the left ear than in the right. For example, the competing words test found a right ear total raw score of 5 and a left ear total of 14, placing him in the 5th percentile.
- The Staggered Spondee Word test found a significant left ear advantage with 90% error on the right-competing and 35% error on the left-competing conditions.

Random-gap detection testing was not completed because he was unable to perform the test.

Electrophysiologic measures found normal ABRs bilaterally, a normal P-100 and P-200 with abnormal P-300.

Findings and Comments

There were several significant findings including the poor language performance and central auditory processing scores. The most significant finding was the strong left ear advantage found on all subtests. This finding is extremely unusual in the average 7-year-old where a strong right ear advantage is typical. These findings raised the concern of possible left hemisphere lesion, so the pediatrician ordered an MRI. The MRI results were normal with no evidence of any lesion and with normal symmetry of cerebral hemispheres.

The finding of strong left ear advantage is contrary to the normal auditory development of children. In the average child the right ear scores are substantially better than the left because of the left hemisphere dominance for language, and the direct right-ear-to-left-hemisphere anatomic connection. When a strong left ear advantage is found in a young child, several possibilities exist including the presence of a lesion of the left hemisphere, lack of a strong left dominant hemisphere for language, and mixed dominance for language or right hemisphere dominance. In the absence of a lesion of the brain, the findings indicate a neurophysiologic basis for the language disorder experienced by this child. The findings also help to explain the neurologic basis for the significant verbal-performance discrepancy found on psychological testing.

These test findings are unusual because of the extreme left ear advantage. Our clinical experience indicates that such children have greater language problems, require more intensive remediation, and have a long course of habilitation as a consequence of the neurologic basis for their disorder. The findings indicate the need for intensive language remediation to deal with all aspects of language development. His attention problems are a related issue that needs to be managed. Because of the plasticity of the brain, this child is likely to improve substantially over time. However the need for intensive language intervention cannot be overemphasized.

In summary, the central auditory test findings obtained on this language-delayed child indicate an underlying neurologic basis for the language disorder and indicate directions for intervention.

Case 2: Child with Delay in Auditory Maturation with Standard Score Discrepancies Among Intelligence, Language, and Auditory Processing Results

This pleasant, handsome 10-year-old boy interacts and communicates well with adults. His birth and developmental history are normal. He loves music and has perfect pitch. In conversation he is reported to do better if he is engaged visually while he is spoken to. His parents report that since kindergarten he has had difficulty in school, with problems following directions or "listening to instructions." He is beginning to have trouble following multistep instructions, and sometimes has difficulty completing tasks as instructed. His parents report that he is in the fifth grade and is "trying very hard to listen." Results of intelligence testing found no substantial discrepancy between verbal and performance IQs with a full-scale IQ in the 90th percentile with a standard score of approximately 120. He performs in the 90+ percentile on standardized psychoeducational tests; however, his parents report that this has led to his relaxed attitude toward study, as a lot of the material comes naturally to him. In spite of his intelligence, this child's grades are slipping and he recently received some F's. There is some question by the speech–language pathologist (SLP) about whether the child has attention deficit disorder, though the parents feel he does not. But he is one of the younger children in his class. Finally, he has no obvious problems with coordination or fine motor control, but he dislikes group sports because most of the other children are better coordinated, and he dislikes physical contact. His parents describe his handwriting as "atrocious."

Speech–Language Evaluation

Results of language testing found a total language standard score of 128. Both his receptive language and his expressive language were advanced. On a test of phonologic processing he was normal for awareness and memory but low average for rapid naming. Specifically he has difficulty whenever he is required to retrieve specific information or to name something. That is, given freedom to talk freely about the world he appears to be very intelligent. However, when he is required to give specific convergent knowledge his performance is low. He was in the 9th stanine for math and the 7th stanine for reading.

Test Results

Pure-tone threshold testing found thresholds at 5 dB for all frequencies with normal tympanometry. Speech reception thresholds were 5 dB HL with 100% word discrimination in quiet.

Results of the SCAN-C Test for Auditory Processing Disorders in Children–Revised were as shown in **Tables 9–1** and **9–2**.

Results of Filtered Words and Auditory Figure Ground subtests are in the normal range. The Competing Words subtest is normal in absolute terms, but the 16th percentile is low for normal processing. The Competing Sentence subtest results

Table 9–1 Scoring Summary

	Raw Score	Standard Score	% Rank	Confidence Level
Filtered words	34	10	50	7 to 13
Auditory figure ground	35	10	50	6 to 13
Competing words	36	7	16	4 to 10
Competing sentences	13	6	9	3 to 9
Scan composite	33	88	21	78 to 98

Table 9–2 Competing Words Ear Advantage

Right Ear First Task		Left Ear First Task	
RE correct	14	RE correct	8
LE correct	5	LE correct	9
Ear advantage	9	Ear advantage	–1
Right ear advantage	Yes	Right ear advantage	No
Left ear advantage	No	Left ear advantage	Yes
Prevalence	2%	Prevalence	15%

were in the 9th percentile. Moreover, the ear advantage scores found an atypical strong right ear advantage. The same finding was obtained on the Competing Words subtest, the Competing Sentences subtest, and the Staggered Spondee Word test. Ear advantage scores are powerful indicators of hemispheric dominance for language and maturational based language/learning disorders. The right ear advantage indicates that language is appropriately established in the left cerebral hemisphere but the atypical large right ear advantage in a child approaching 11 years of age indicates the presence of a developmental delay of the auditory system.

- *Random Gap Detection Test (RGDT):* The RGDT is a test of temporal processing (auditory timing) ability. Disorders of auditory timing are related to disorders of auditory discrimination, reading, and language. This child's gap detection thresholds of less than 5 ms are normal.
- *Duration pattern test (DPT):* The DPT is a measure of pattern recognition in the time domain, a cortical function reflecting hemispheric interaction between recognition of sound patterns of different duration, and providing a linguistic label of what was heard. This child's responses were completely normal.
- *Frequency pattern test (FPT):* The FPT is a measure of pattern recognition in the frequency (pitch) domain, a cortical function reflecting hemispheric interaction between recognition of sound patterns of different pitch, and providing a linguistic label of what was heard. This child's responses were 100%.
- *Staggered Spondee Word test (SSW):* The SSW is a dichotic test of binaural separation. The SSW stimuli represent both competing and noncompeting words presented to each ear simultaneously (**Table 9–3**).

The SSW results are abnormal, with the number of errors in the left-ear competing condition more than twice the typical finding for a child this age. When the SSW results are converted to Z scores and percentiles, the left competing condition result has a Z score of –4, which is below the 1st percentile. The right competing score Z score equals –1.3, which is approximately the 10th percentile.

- *Behavioral auditory testing:* This child's responses to auditory stimuli were characterized by slow responses that occurred at the end of nearly every response time interval allowed during the standardized tests. This delayed latency of response indicated that he was always at the "threshold" of understanding. The need for additional time to process auditory information indicates that listening under complex acoustic conditions to rapid or distorted speech is a difficult task that is frustrating and tiring.
- *Electrophysiologic testing:* A battery of electrophysiologic tests included the following:

- Auditory brainstem evoked potentials
- Middle latency auditory evoked potentials
- P-100
- P-300

Results of all tests were normal. The P-300 assesses auditory attention at the physiologic level. The P-300 response was present with a normal latency and large amplitude, indicating that attention processes as measured by this technique are completely normal.

Summary

This child was referred for CAPD testing because of a history of difficulty with listening, missing directions, and doing poorly in school. These difficulties occur even though the child is extremely bright, has good language skills, and is reading above grade level. He is a self-admitted "dawdler." Results on routine hearing testing found normal hearing thresholds. Tests of auditory processing abilities found normal duration and frequency processing, normal processing in the time domain, and normal auditory processing of minimally distorted speech and speech in noise. Tests of auditory maturation found delays in the development of his central auditory pathways. There are large discrepancies between the standard scores found on intelligence and language testing compared with auditory processing. These findings confirm that learning through the auditory modality may be difficult because this child's listening skills are those of a child who is chronologically younger. In addition, he was slow in responding during behavioral testing. That is, his responses always came at the end of time intervals allowed for response. His responses indicated a need for additional time to process auditory information. His high level of intelligence compensates somewhat for these deficiencies, but may cause him problems because the language closure he utilizes sometimes leads him down the wrong path, causing him to miss basic specific information, assignments, directions, etc. He was completely attentive throughout testing done on this date, with no evidence of attention deficit.

Electrophysiologic tests of auditory nervous system function confirm that there is no fundamental physiologic CNS disorder, that he is simply delayed in auditory maturation. The implication is that his auditory system will continue to mature and he will catch up with his peers at some time. Finally, the P-300 auditory evoked potential was normal, providing electrophysiologic confirmation of behavioral observations that this child does not have attention deficit disorder.

Recommendations

Results of this testing indicate normal peripheral hearing, with normal auditory processing for some fundamental perceptual tasks. The delay in auditory maturation found on several tests indicates that this child's listening ability is his weakest academic ability. Because his auditory processing is not strong, this child may hear some information inaccurately. For example, his auditory analysis and synthesis skills may be harmed by his cognitive ability. Specifically, this child has excellent top-down processing. His world knowledge, his knowledge of events, and his linguistic knowledge are at a high level. His processing is at a low level, however, so that

Table 9–3 Results of Staggered Spondee Word Test from Case 2

Staggered Spondee Conditions	Results (number of errors)	Normative Data (number of errors)
Right ear noncompeting	0	1
Right ear competing	1	3
Left ear competing	12	5
Left ear noncompeting	0	1

auditory subskills processing, short-term memory, and phonologic processing skills are comparatively weak. He guesses when he misses auditory information, but he sometimes guesses wrong, misses information, and does not get complete or accurate directions. This situation is exacerbated by his self-admitted dawdling.

The following basic classroom management techniques may help this child in classroom activities:

- Provide his teachers with information contained in this report.
- Provide the child with preferential seating, close to the teacher.
- Identify noise sources, reduce them, and move the child away from them.
- Alert the child to changes in topic, and supplement group instructions with individual checks of comprehension.
- Increase one-on-one instruction.
- Monitor his auditory comprehension, to be sure he has understood directions, correctly understands the assignments, and understands the material covered.
- Break new information into shorter segments.
- Assist him in developing organizational strategies.

This child can also help himself by taking responsibility for making the following changes:

- Increase his visual vigilance, and watch speakers for information to supplement what is heard.
- Increase his vigilance to the task at hand, and reduce the time wasted by dawdling.
- Begin moving toward an internal locus of control, and ask for clarification of auditory information when unsure or misses instructional material.

Finally, it was recommend that this child's auditory processing be rechecked in a year to document the rate of change in maturation.

References

1. Calearo C, Antonelli AR. Disorders of the central auditory nervous system. In: Paparella M, Shumrick D, eds. Otolaryngology, vol 2. Philadelphia: WB Saunders, 1973:407–425
2. Bergman M, Hirsch S, Solzi P, Mankowitz Z. The threshold-of-interference test: a new test of interhemispheric suppression in brain injury. Ear Hear 1987;8:147–150
3. Keith RW. Special issue: dichotic listening tests. Ear Hear 1983;4:6
4. Jerger J, Musiek F. Report of the consensus conference on the diagnosis of auditory processing disorders in school-aged children. J Am Acad Audiol 2000;11:467–474
5. ACLD Newsbriefs. ACLD Description: Specific Learning Disabilities, No. 166 (Sept-Oct 1986)
6. ASHA. Central auditory processing: current status of research and implications for clinical practice. Am J Audiol 1996;5:41–54
7. Roush W. Arguing over why Johnny can't read. Science 1995;267:1896–1898
8. Macmillan DL, ed. Development of Operational Definitions in Mental Retardations: Similarities and Differences with the Field of Learning Disabilities. Baltimore: Paul H. Brookes, 1993
9. Teatini GP. Speech audiometry. In: Rojskjaer C, ed. Second Danavox Symposium. Danavox Hearing Aid Company: Odense, Denmark: 1970
10. Jerger J. Audiological manifestations of lesions in the auditory nervous system. Laryngoscope 1960;70:417–425
11. Phillips DP. Central auditory processing: a view from auditory neuroscience. Am J Otol 1995;16:338–352
12. Gelfand SA. Long-term recovery and no recovery from the auditory deprivation effect with binaural amplification: six cases. J Am Acad Audiol 1995;6:141–149
13. Ferry PC. Neurological considerations in children with learning disabilities. In: Keith RW, ed. Central Auditory and Language Disorders in Children. Houston: College Hill Press, 1981:1–12
14. Pinheiro M. Tests of central auditory function in children with learning disabilities. In: Keith R, ed. Central Auditory Dysfunction. New York: Grune and Stratton, 1977:223–256
15. Musiek FE, Pinheiro ML. Frequency patterns in cochlear, brainstem and cerebral lesions. Audiology 1987;26:79–88
16. Musiek FE, Baran JA, Pinheiro M. Duration pattern recognition in normal subjects and patients with cerebral and cochlear lesions. Audiology 1990;29:304–313
17. Golding M, Carter N, Mitchell P, Hood LJ. Prevalence of central auditory Processing (CAP) abnormality in an older Australian population: the Blue Mountains Hearing Study. J Am Acad Audiol 2004;15:633–642
18. Jerger J, Chmiel R, Allen J, Wilson A. Effects of age and gender on dichotic sentence identification. Ear Hear 1994;15:274–286
19. Jerger J. Observations on auditory behavior in lesions of the central auditory pathway. Arch Otolaryngol 1960;71:797–806
20. Spitzer J, Ventry I. Central auditory dysfunction among chronic alcoholics. Arch Otolaryngol 1980;106:224–229
21. Grimes AM, Grady CL, Pikus A. Auditory evoked potentials in patients with dementia of the Alzheimer type. Ear Hear 1987;8:157–161
22. Keith RW, Stein L. Central auditory processing in patients with dementia of the Alzheimer's type. Unpublished research, 1987
23. Strouse AL, Hall JW III, Burger MC. Central auditory processing in Alzheimer's disease. Ear Hear 1995;16:230–238
24. Mueller H, Sedge R, Salazar A. Auditory assessment of neural trauma. In: Miner M, Wagner K, eds. Neurotrauma: Treatment, Rehabilitation and Related Issues. Boston: Butterworths, 1986
25. Musiek FE, Baran J, Shinn J. Assessment and remediation of an auditory processing disorder associated with head trauma. J Am Acad Audiol 2004;15:117–132
26. Bergemalm PO, Lyxell B. Appearances are deceptive? Long term cognitive and central auditory sequelae from closed head injury. Int J Audiol 2005;44:39–49
27. Baran JA, Bothfeldt RW, Musiek FE. Central auditory deficits associated with compromise of the primary auditory cortex. J Am Acad Audiol 2004;15:106–116
28. Hasbrouck J. Diagnosis of auditory perceptual disorders in previously undiagnosed adults. J Learn Disabil 1983;16:206–208
29. Walker MM, Shinn JB, Cranford JL, Givens GD, Holbert D. Auditory temporal processing performance of young adults with reading disorders. J Speech Lang Hear Res 2002;45:568–605
30. Crandell C, Leonard C. Comorbid auditory processing disorder in developmental dyslexia. Ear Hear 2003;24:448–456
31. Bankaitis AE, Keith RW. Audiological changes associated with HIV infection. Ear Nose Throat J 1995;74:353–359
32. Keith RW, Pensak ML. Central auditory function. Otolaryngol Clin North Am 1991;24:371–379
33. Gat IB, Keith RW. An effect of linguistic experience: auditory word discrimination by native and non-native speakers of English. Audiology 1978;17:339–345
34. Keith RW, Katbamna B, Tawfik S, et al. The effect of linguistic background on staggered spondiac word and dichotic consonant vowel scores. Br J Audiol 1987;21:21–26
35. Marriage J, King J, Lutman M. The reliability of the SCAN test: results from a primary school in the UK. Br J Audiol 2001;35:199–208
36. Holm VA, Kunze LH. Effect of chronic otitis media on language and speech development. Pediatrics 1969;43:833–839
37. Schlieper A, Kisilevsky H, Mattingly S, Yorke L. Mild conductive hearing loss and language development. A one year follow up study. Dev Behav Pediatr 1985;6:65–68
38. Brandes PJ, Ehinger DM. The effects of early middle ear pathology on auditory perception and academic achievement. J Speech Hear Disord 1981;46:301–307
39. Welsh L, Welsh J, Healy M. Effect of sound deprivation on central hearing. Laryngoscope 1983;93:1569–1575
40. Sak RJ, Ruben RJ. Recurrent middle ear effusion in childhood: implications of temporary auditory deprivation for language and learning. Ann Otol Rhinol Laryngol 1981;90:546–551
41. Hanson DG, Ulvested RF. Summary of discussion and recommendations made during the workshop on otitis media and development. Ann Otol Rhinol Laryngol 1979;88(5 pt 2 suppl 60):107–111
42. Lehmann MD, Charron K, Kummer A, et al. The effects of chronic middle ear effusion on speech and language development. A descriptive study. Int J Pediatr Otorhinolaryngol 1979;1:137–144

43. Menyuk P. Relationship of otitis media to speech processing and language development. In: Katz J, Stecker N, Henderson D, eds. Central Auditory Processing: A Transdisciplinary View. St. Louis: Mosby Year Book, 1992

44. Keogh T, Kei J, Driscoll C, et al. Measuring the ability of school children with a history of otitis media to understand everyday speech. J Am Acad Audiol 2005;16:301–311

45. Chermak GD, Tucker E. Behavioral characteristics of auditory processing disorder and attention-deficit hyperactivity disorder: predominantly inattentive type. J Am Acad Audiol 2002;13:332–338

46. Somers EK, Seikel JA. Behavioral signs of central auditory processing disorder and attention deficit hyperactivity disorder. J Am Acad Audiol 1998;9:78–84

47. Task Force on Central Auditory Processing Consensus Development. ASHA Consensus Statement on Central Auditory Processing. Washington, DC: American Speech-Language-Hearing Association, 1995

48. Willeford J, Burleigh J. Handbook of Central Auditory Processing Disorders in Children. Orlando, FL: Grune and Stratton, 1985

49. Fisher LI. Auditory Problems Checklist. Bemidji, MN: Life Products, 1976

50. Sanger DD, Freed JM, Decker TN. Behavioral profile of preschool children suspected of auditory language processing problems. Hearing J 1985;38:17–20

51. Smoski WJ, Brunt MA, Tannahill JC. Listening characteristics of children with central auditory processing disorders. Stanford University Libraries: Language Speech and Hearing Services in School 1992;23: 145–152

52. Keith RW. Random Gap Detection Test (RGDT). St. Louis: Auditec, 2000

53. Keith RW. Time Compressed Sentence Test. St. Louis: Auditec, 2002.

54. Keith RW. Development and standardization of SCAN-C: test for auditory processing disorders in children-revised. J Am Acad Audiol 2000; 11:438–445

55. Keith RW. SCAN-A: A Test for Auditory Processing Disorders in Adolescents and Adults. San Antonio: Psychological Corporation, 1994

56. Berlin CI, Porter RJ Jr, Lowe-Bell SS. Dichotic signs of the recognition of speech elements in normals, temporal lobectomies, and hemispherectomies. IEEE Trans. Audio Electroacoust AU 1973;21:189–195

57. Musiek FM, Baran JA, Pinheiro ML. Neuroaudiology: Case Studies. San Diego: Singular Publishing Group, 1994

58. Katz J. The Staggered Spondaic Word Test. In: Keith R, ed. Central Auditory Dysfunction. New York: Grune & Stratton, 1977

59. Fifer R, Jerger JF, Berlin CI, et al. Development of a dichotic sentence identification test for hearing impaired adults. Ear Hear 1983;4:300–305

60. Musiek FE, Pinheiro ML. Frequency patterns in cochlear, brainstem and cerebral lesions. Audiology 1987;26:79–88

61. Marlowe J, Engels TL, Keith RW. Screening for auditory disorders in psychiatric hospitals. In: Bess F, ed. Proceedings of the International Symposium on Screening Children for Auditory Function. Nashville: Bill Wilkerson Center Press, 1992

62. Katbamna B, Keith RW, Johnson JL. Auditory processing abilities in children with learning disabilities: A pilot study. J Ohio Speech Hear Assoc 1990;fall/winter:80–87

63. Keith RW, Rudy J, Donahue P, Katbamna B. Comparison of SCAN results with other auditory and language measures in a clinical population. Ear Hear 1989;10:382–386

64. Dietrich KN, Succop PA, Berger OG, Keith RW. Lead exposure and the central auditory processing abilities and cognitive development of urban children: the Cincinnati Lead Study cohort at age 5 years. Neurotoxicol Teratol 1992;14:51–56

65. Kraus N, Koch DB, McGee TJ, et al. Speech-sound discrimination in school-age children: psychophysical and neurophysiologic measures. J Speech Lang Hear Res 1999;42:1042–1060

66. Kurtzberg D, Vaughan HG Jr, Kreuzer JA, et al. Developmental studies and clinical applications of mismatch negativity: problems and prospects. Ear Hear 1995;16:105–117

67. Dalebout SD, Stack JW. Mismatch negativity to acoustic differences not differentiated behaviorally. J Am Acad Audiol 1999;10:388–399

68. Cunningham RF. Mismatch negativity in normally developing children. Unpublished Ph.D. dissertation, University of Cincinnati, 2000

69. Uwer R, von Suchodoletz W. Stability of mismatch negativites in children. Clin Neurophysiol 2000;111:45–52

70. Keith RW, Fallis RL. How Behavioral Tests of Central Auditory Processing Influence Management. Nashville: Vanderbilt Bill Wilkerson Center Press, 1998;137–143.

71. Flexer C, Millin JP, Brown L. Children with developmental disabilities: the effect of sound field amplification on word identification. Lang Speech Hear Serv Sch 1990;21:177–182

72. Committee on Amplification for the Hearing Impaired, ASHA. Amplification as a remediation technique for children with normal peripheral hearing. ASHA 1991;33(suppl 3):22–24

73. Chermak GD, Museik F. Managing central auditory processing disorders in children and youth. Am J Audiol 1992;1:61–65

74. Schneider D. Audiologic management of children with central auditory processing disorders. In: Katz J, Stecker N, Henderson D, eds. Central Auditory Process: A Transdisciplinary View. St. Louis: Mosby Year Book, 1992

75. American Speech-Language-Hearing Association. Guidelines for fitting and monitoring FM systems. ASHA 1994;36(suppl 12):1–9

76. Kahn MS. Learning problems of the secondary and junior college learning disabled student: suggested remedies. J Learn Disabil 1980;13: 445–449

77. Keith RW. Central Auditory and Language Disorders in Children. San Diego: College-Hill Press, 1981

78. Katz J, Stecker N, Henderson D. Central Auditory Process: A Transdisciplinary View. St. Louis: Mosby Year Book, 1992

79. Levinson P, Sloan C. Auditory Processing and Language. New York: Grune and Stratton, 1980

80. Willeford J, Burleigh J. Handbook of Central Auditory Processing Disorders in Children. Orlando: Grune and Stratton, 1985

81. Americans with Disabilities Act in Brief. Federal Register, Parts I, II, III 1991;IV:V

Suggested Readings

Bamiou DE, Liasis A, Boyd S, Cohen M, Raglan E. Central auditory processing disorder as the presenting manifestation of subtle brain pathology. Audiology 2000;39:168–172

Bankaitis AU. The effects of HIV on the ABR, AMLR, and SCAN-A in Adults. Unpublished Ph.D. Thesis, University of Cincinnati, 1995

Beasley D, Freeman B. Time altered speech as a measure of central auditory processing. In: Keith RW, ed. Central Auditory Dysfunction. New York: Grune and Stratton, 1977

Cherry R. The Selective Auditory Attention Test (SAAT). St Louis: Auditec of St Louis, 1980

Keith RW. SCAN: A Screening Test for Auditory Processing Disorders. New York: Psychological Corporation, Harcourt Brace Jovanovich, 1986

Keith RW, Engineer P. Effects of methylphenidate on the auditory processing abilities of children with attention deficit-hyperactivity disorder. J Learn Disabil 1991;24:630–636

Keller WD. Effects of methylphenidate (Ritalin) on auditory performance in children with attention and auditory processing disorders. J Speech Lang Hear Res 2000;43:893–901

Kraus N, McGee T. Testimony presented to the American Speech–Language Hearing Association Task Force on Central Auditory Processing; March 1993; Rockville, MD: American Speech–Language Hearing Association

Olsen W, Noffsinger PD, Kurdziel SA. Speech discrimination in quiet and in white noise by patients with peripheral and central lesions. Acta Otolaryngol 1975;80:375–382

Pinheiro ML. Tests of central auditory function in children with learning disabilities. In: Keith RW, ed. Central Auditory Dysfunction. New York: Grune and Stratton, 1977

Tillery K, Katz J, Keller WD. Effects of methylphenidate (Ritalin) on auditory performance in children with attention and auditory processing disorders. J Speech Lang Hear Res 2000;43:893–901

10

Laboratory Tests of Vestibular and Balance Functioning

Judith A. White

Laboratory vestibular testing includes a battery of quantitative tests that can be selected to provide assessment of the oculomotor system, caloric responses, positional and positioning nystagmus, vestibulo-ocular reflex (VOR) gain, phase and symmetry, vestibular-visual interaction, and postural control. Each test in the appropriately chosen test battery will add independent information to the assessment.

◆ Clinical Utility of Vestibular Testing

First it is important to consider which clinical questions laboratory vestibular testing can answer. Vestibular testing can identify a vestibular deficit and provide information to localize the lesion. This is appropriate when the diagnosis remains uncertain after the history and office physical examination of the dizzy patient (see Chapter 14) are completed. Laboratory vestibular testing is not a substitute for an accurate, thorough history. It should not replace the basic office physical examination of the dizzy patient, including spontaneous, gaze, positional, and positioning testing; head thrust and head shake testing; and office oculomotor assessment, including pursuit and saccade. For example, it would not be necessary to obtain laboratory vestibular testing when simple posterior semicircular canal benign paroxysmal positional vertigo is noted on office Dix-Hallpike testing.

Vestibular assessment can also be used to follow vestibular deficits over time. This is because the testing not only identifies a vestibular deficit, such as a caloric weakness in one ear, but also provides valuable information regarding the degree of compensation present to that deficit. Compensation is a central process that recalibrates the vestibular system after an acute unilateral vestibular loss. During the initial period following an acute unilateral vestibular loss, there may be spontaneous nystagmus beating away from the affected ear, positional and positioning nystagmus similarly beating away from the affected side, and a weakness of VOR gain when the patient rotates to the side of loss. Postural control may be abnormal when visual and proprioceptive cues are minimized.

After vestibular compensation to an acute unilateral vestibular loss, the vestibular assessment pattern changes. The caloric loss may remain, but spontaneous, positional, and gaze-evoked nystagmus disappear. Rotary chair VOR gain normalizes, and VOR asymmetry resolves. Postural control normalizes. The only persistent signs of a long-standing compensated vestibular loss may be VOR phase elevations and the caloric asymmetry. This information is useful in assessing response to vestibular rehabilitation. Following successful vestibular rehabilitation, the resolution of VOR asymmetry can be followed objectively using rotary chair testing (see Chapter 32). Similarly, the significance of an isolated caloric asymmetry identified during caloric testing can be determined by looking for associated indicators of an uncompensated versus compensated unilateral loss.

Vestibular testing is an important consideration prior to ablative vestibular procedures or surgery. Ensuring normal function on the unaffected side avoids inadvertently ablating the only functioning vestibular system. Preoperative vestibular testing may also help predict the course of recovery after procedures such as vestibular nerve section, intratympanic gentamicin, or acoustic neuroma resection. A robust response in the affected ear would predict significant vertigo after surgical ablation, similar to a bout of vestibular neuritis. A weak response suggests that some degree of chronic loss and compensation may have previously occurred, and predicts a more rapid recovery.

In summary, vestibular testing can identify and help localize vestibular lesions, and assess the degree of compensation present to these lesions. It is appropriate after a history and office physical examination leave the diagnosis in question, when initial treatment does not result in expected benefit, and prior to vestibular ablative surgical procedures.

◆ Limitations of Vestibular Testing

Vestibular testing has several limitations. It does not measure disability from vestibular deficits. Patients with similar test results may have widely varying functional capacity. Factors such as the demands of the workplace and environment, response to illness, concurrent medical problems, and psychosocial resources affect the degree of disability a patient may experience from a vestibular deficit.

An additional limitation of standard vestibular testing is that it does not assess the vertical canals or otolith function. Head-shake testing, the Halmagyi-Curthoys head thrust, caloric testing, and rotary-chair testing all assess the lateral (horizontal) canal and by extension the superior division of the vestibular nerve. Head-thrust testing in vertical canal planes can be performed, but may be uncomfortable for the patient because twisting of the neck is required at a high velocity and should only be performed by someone familiar with the technique. Most clinical vestibular laboratories limit assessment of the vertical canals to Dix-Hallpike positioning.

◆ Indications and Patient Preparation for Vestibular Testing

Vestibular testing begins with patient preparation. Typically, patients referred for testing have suffered from some type of dizziness or vertigo, and the prospect that testing will reproduce this symptom is daunting. Patient cooperation with test instructions, including concentration, is vital in obtaining accurate data. Psychological factors strongly affect test performance, and patients who are too anxious, preoccupied, or fatigued cannot perform the required tasks. Patients are prepared for the test with simple, clear instructions, and advised to get a good night's rest before the test. Reassurance, encouragement, and support during testing are very helpful. Patients are required to refrain from antihistamines, alcohol, sedatives, and benzodiazepines 24 to 48 hours prior to testing (exceptions for benzodiazepines are sometimes made for chronic low-dose use when discontinuation presents significant problems, but this compromises test accuracy). Other medications may also affect test sensitivity (notably antiepileptics, which should not be discontinued), and interpretation should note all medications taken and include their possible effects on the test results.

Vestibular test data quality is human operator dependent. The patient's frequent eye blinks, eye closure, poor concentration, and less than optimal performance may make vestibular test data useless, or inaccurately suggest oculomotor deficits, failure of fixation suppression, or other "central" findings. Computerized interpretation systems cannot replace the role of the experienced human operator in obtaining optimal, cooperative performance from patients, which yields valid and reliable data.

As computerized interpretation systems become faster, more accurate, and more sensitive, our tendency may be to only examine the computer screen graphics, or the printed results. However, each of the clinical interpretation systems in common usage analyzes eye movements in the x-y (horizontal and vertical) plane. These systems are sensitive to horizontal and vertical eye movements, whether sensed by skin electrodes or infrared video image analysis. Torsional eye movements are not accurately analyzed by commonly used computerized systems because torsion of the pupil is not accurately sensed in either a horizontal or vertical plane. We find it very useful to record the nystagmus seen during positional and positioning testing and replay and review it during interpretation. Various recording methods seem to work well,

including VCR, DVD, and hard drive digital recording. The most important teaching point in our vestibular laboratory is to look at the eye movement during positional and positioning testing, not the computer graphics.

The order of testing is planned to allow the patient to perform easier tests first. Computerized dynamic posturography may be performed first. Oculomotor and rotary chair testing is usually performed prior to positional and positioning testing. Caloric testing, usually the most unpleasant of the tests because it provokes brief vertigo, is performed last.

◆ Types of Vestibular Testing

Oculomotor Testing

Oculomotor testing consists of pursuit, saccade, spontaneous, gaze-evoked, and optokinetic nystagmus. The reader is directed to Leigh and Zee[1] for an excellent reference on the neurology of eye movements. Eye movements are assessed first in the vestibular test battery, to identify abnormalities and also to ensure that nystagmus can be recorded accurately during later vestibular stimulation. The presence of strabismus and poor vision should be noted and considered in test interpretation.

Calibration is performed by having the patient look at fixed points 1 m away, including center, left (27 cm), and right (27 cm). These lateral points correspond to approximately 15 degrees of eccentric gaze. Calibration is important for computerized interpretation systems because inaccurate calibration will affect measurement of the amplitude and direction of nystagmus throughout testing. Calibration errors are the most common reason caloric responses appear "reversed."

Nystagmus refers to rhythmic repetitive eye movements. The term is derived from the Greek expression used to describe the involuntary head nodding seen during napping while sitting up. Nystagmus may be visual or central in origin, and is commonly seen in individuals with congenital blindness. Vestibular nystagmus is specifically characterized by a slow and fast phase. The eyes deviate slowly to one direction and jerk rapidly back (fast phase). By convention, the direction of the nystagmus is named for the direction of the fast phase. The strength of the nystagmus is calculated by measuring the degrees that the eye moves in 1 second during the slow phase.

Vestibular test interpretation is greatly facilitated for beginners by recognizing the conventions used in strip recording. A line tracing of nystagmus will usually have time along the horizontal axis and eye deviation along the vertical axis. Looking at the strip recording from left to right shows the eye movement as time progressed in the testing (similar to electrocardiogram strips). An upward deflection of the line on the horizontal recording strip corresponds to a rightward eye movement (UP-RIGHT), and a downward deflection corresponds to a leftward eye movement. The vertical strip (if used) is easier to interpret because upward eye movement is also an upward deflection of the line, and a downward eye movement is a downward deflection of the line.

Nystagmus can be recorded by several methods. Visual inspection in room light is the least sensitive. Patients who can see objects visually fixate on them, and this reduces vestibular nystagmus by at least 50%. Electro-oculography (EOG) uses surface skin electrodes around the eye to

Spontaneous nystagmus

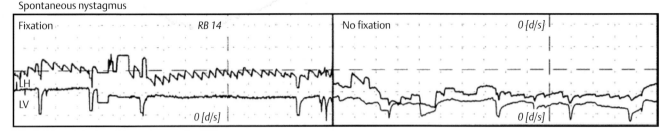

Scale = 10 degrees x 1 second

Figure 10–1 Rightward nystagmus (seen during fixation testing only)—a central finding.

record changes in the strength of the field generated by the corneo-retinal potential, and nystagmus is recorded in the dark or with eyes closed. EOG resolution is 1 degree and recording bandwidth is narrow (35 Hz), but electrical and muscle interference decreases sensitivity. Infrared video-oculography (IR-VOG) uses infrared recording cameras placed in goggles in front of the eyes, which must be kept open for the examination. Most clinical vestibular image analysis systems use the differing infrared reflectance of the sclera versus the iris to analyze eye movement. Resolution is high (0.1 degree) but bandwidth is limited by present recording speed technology and currently exceeds 100 Hz. This limitation does not usually affect the accuracy of clinical vestibular testing, but more advanced infrared systems are available at a considerably higher cost for research applications. The most complex technique, using magnetic search coils placed on the sclera, has very high resolution (0.02 degrees), high recording speed, and the advantage of torsional nystagmus recording. However, magnetic search coils are expensive and uncomfortable, with recording times limited to 30 minutes.

Spontaneous nystagmus is recorded with the patient sitting comfortably, and is recorded with and without visual fixation. Usually a small light located inside the infrared goggle is illuminated for fixation testing. The most common pattern of vestibular nystagmus is a persistent horizontal unidirectional nystagmus that diminishes at least 50% with fixation. It may be stronger when patients direct their gaze in the direction of

the fast phase (Alexander's law). It is usually seen in the acute period following a unilateral vestibular loss, and the fast phase beats away from the affected ear.

Spontaneous nystagmus that does not have these important characteristics (unidirectional, horizontal, diminishes with fixation, and worsens with gaze in the direction of the fast phase) should be considered potentially central. This includes vertical nystagmus (upbeat or downbeat), direction-changing nystagmus, irregular or disconjugate nystagmus, or nystagmus that worsens with fixation. Alcohol and anticonvulsants may cause atypical nystagmus.

A rightward spontaneous nystagmus is seen in **Fig. 10–1**. The fast phase of the nystagmus beats rightward (upward on a horizontal channel strip recording). The nystagmus is recorded only during fixation and disappears without fixation. This is a central finding because the nystagmus is worse with fixation. Another central spontaneous nystagmus is shown in **Fig. 10–2**. It beats leftward with fixation and rightward without fixation. This nystagmus is direction-changing.

Nystagmus is tested next in eccentric gaze. Fifteen to 30 degrees of eccentric gaze is sufficient; more may provoke a physiologic end-gaze nystagmus seen in many normal patients. Rightward, leftward, upward, and downward gaze are assessed. Unidirectional horizontal nystagmus may sometimes be seen when gazing away from the side of an acute vestibular loss, and other features of acute uncompensated

Spontaneous gaze test

Center gaze - fix

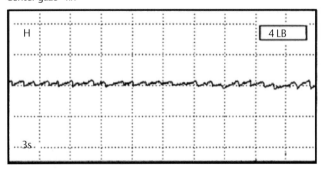

Center gaze - no fix

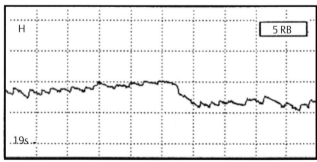

Scale = 10 degrees x 1 second

Figure 10–2 Direction-changing nystagmus that beats leftward in center gaze with fixation and rightward in center gaze without fixation—a central finding.

Spontaneous gaze test

Center gaze

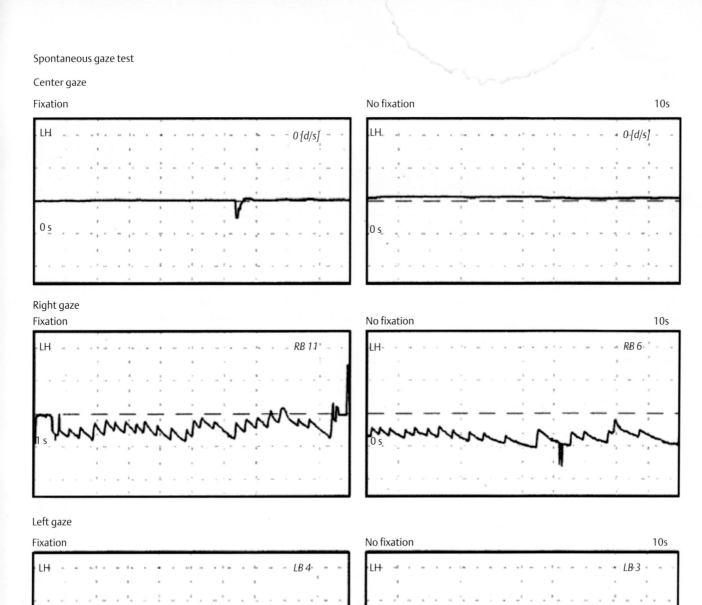

Scale = 10 degrees x 1 second

Figure 10–3   Gaze-evoked nystagmus.

vestibular loss are evident when this occurs (such as caloric weakness and VOR asymmetry). However, most other types of gaze-evoked nystagmus, such as direction-changing nystagmus, are considered a sign of central pathology. Anticonvulsants and alcohol may cause gaze-evoked nystagmus. **Fig. 10–3** shows a central gaze-evoked rightward nystagmus in right gaze (worse with fixation in this example, which is another central sign). Gaze-evoked nystagmus may be so severe that it interferes with the patient's ability to visually follow a moving object. **Fig. 10–4** shows right gaze-evoked nystagmus interfering with smooth pursuit tracking.

Saccades are extremely high acceleration (30,000 deg/sec^2) eye movements with a 200-ms latency and a 50- to 100-ms duration. They are used to volitionally redirect sight, or reflexively gaze toward a startling stimulus. Saccades are so fast that vision is obscured during the eye movement. Three features of saccades are usually assessed in vestibular testing: latency (delay between the presentation of the stimulus and beginning of the saccade, usually approximately 200 ms); accuracy; and peak velocity (norms vary with ocular displacement and are displayed on a special graph, ranging from 50 to 700 degrees/s). Saccades that are hypometric undershoot and

10 Laboratory Tests of Vestibular and Balance Functioning

135

Pursuit horizontal

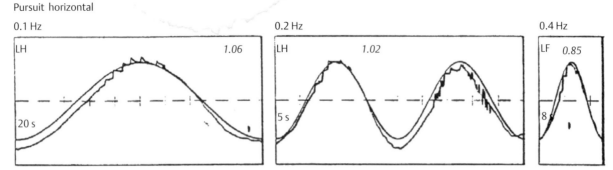

Figure 10–4 Gaze-evoked nystagmus affecting right smooth pursuit.

fail to reach the target. Hypometria must be severe and reproducible to be considered abnormal. Hypermetric saccades overshoot the target, and are more significant even if slightly abnormal.

Saccades are frequently noted to have bilateral mildly prolonged latency and mild hypometria in older, less alert, or poorly compliant patients. Drugs may affect saccades symmetrically (both leftward and rightward). Care should be taken not to attribute a central pathology in those situations. However, any asymmetric saccade abnormality is considered significant. Internuclear ophthalmoplegia (INO) is a central disorder that causes slowed or absent adduction (inward movement toward the nose) of the affected eye during conjugate eye movements, such as saccades or pursuit. It may be seen in both eyes in bilateral INO. It is seen in lesions of the median longitudinal fasciculus such as multiple sclerosis.

Pursuit eye movements allow clear viewing of objects moving slowly in the visual environment by allowing the eye to focus the image on the fovea. The match of eye speed to target speed is termed "gain." Pursuit performance is highly affected by age, alertness, attention, and cooperation.

Asymmetric pursuit is considered significant for a central or visual disorder, as is gain that is markedly decreased, with a substitution of saccades for normal smooth pursuit. This gives the appearance of "stair steps" on the eye movement tracing (**Fig. 10–5**) rather than normal smooth pursuit tracings (**Fig. 10–6**).

Optokinetic nystagmus is a combination of pursuit (foveal vision) and optokinetic (extrafovial) systems. It is best seen when the moving stimulus surrounds the patient in an environment without visual referents, such as traveling through a featureless tunnel with moving objects presented on the walls. This is used in amusement rides to trigger sensations of motion. In the vestibular laboratory visual stimuli are presented in the rotary chair booth surrounding the seated patient, and the ability of the eye movements to follow the visual stimuli is recorded as gain. Typically, optokinetic nystagmus abnormalities will be associated with other oculomotor system abnormalities, and as in all oculomotor test abnormalities, asymmetric responses are more likely to represent localized central pathology such as acute unilateral parieto-occipital lesions.

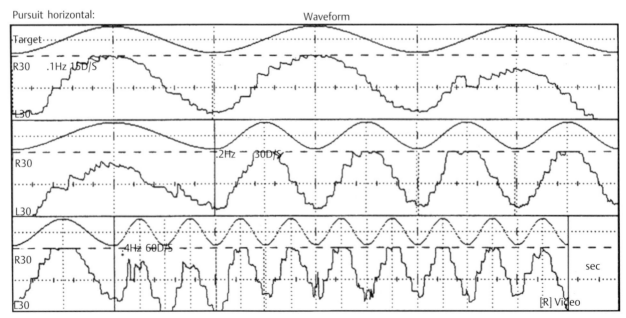

Figure 10–5 Saccadic pursuit, note stair-step pattern. (Courtesy of Micromedical Technologies, with permission.)

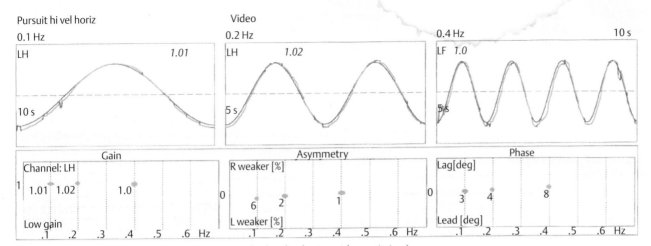

Figure 10–6 Normal pursuit. (Courtesy of Micromedical Technologies, with permission.)

In summary, oculomotor tests are affected by age, vision, medication, alertness, and cooperation. Central pathologic patterns are usually evident on several of the tests. Although base rates differ, the finding of oculomotor pathology is relatively rare in the outpatient clinical vestibular laboratory. Interpret oculomotor abnormalities cautiously, considering the effects of age, alertness, medication, and cooperation as well as vision. Bilateral findings are less often central in origin than are unilateral asymmetric findings. The demonstration of an intact oculomotor system during oculomotor testing allows valid interpretation of the vestibular responses obtained during the next steps: vestibulo-ocular testing and caloric testing. A sample normal oculomotor computer-generated report is shown in **Fig. 10–7**.

Vestibulo-Ocular Reflex Testing

The VOR is designed to stabilize vision during head movements. We can readily appreciate the effect of a normally functioning VOR by holding up a finger approximately 12 inches in front of our nose and staring at it while shaking our head quickly. The finger remains in clear focus because the vestibular system is stimulated by the head movements and generates corrective eye movements to allow the gaze to remain centered on the target. Moving the finger quickly back and forth in front of the eyes while keeping the head still results in visual blurring. The eyes cannot accurately follow high-velocity targets without help from the vestibular system.

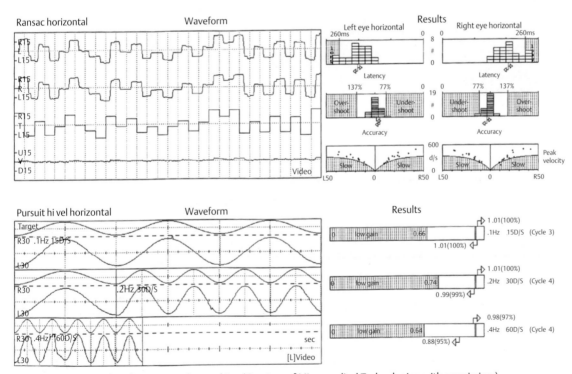

Figure 10–7 Normal oculomotor results graphics. (Courtesy of Micromedical Technologies, with permission.)

VOR gain refers to eye movements occurring in response to head movement. When the head is rotated to the left, the eyes turn to the right to allow vision to remain centered on the target. Similarly, right head rotation results in a leftward movement of the eyes to remain centered on the target. *Gain* is a measure of how closely the eye movements match the head movements. A perfect match would result in a gain of 1. VOR gain is usually assessed at several frequencies. The reader is referred to the excellent discussion of the VOR in Baloh and Halmagyi.[2]

Two related measurements of the VOR are related to gain. *Phase* refers to how quickly the eye movements begin, compared with the head movements. The timing of the eye and head movements is compared when phase is measured. Lastly, *symmetry* refers to how the eye movements during rightward head rotation compare with those during leftward head rotation. Normally the movements in both directions are symmetric.

Rotary chair testing is a method used to assess the gain, phase, and symmetry of the VOR under controlled conditions. Standard computer-generated frequencies are used (usually 0.05–0.50 Hz), which are frequencies commonly encountered during many normal physiologic head movements. The frequencies are commonly presented as sinusoids, with the chair rotating first to one side and then back to the other. The formula for the frequency is related to the inverse of the time it takes to complete one cycle of back and forth movement (Hz =1/cycle in seconds). Thus, a frequency of 0.2 Hz would take 50 seconds to complete, and 0.1 Hz would take 100 seconds to complete. The maximum chair speed is usually 60 degrees/s,

but chair speed varies depending on where in the sinusoid the measurement is taken, and is maximal halfway through each rotation. The chair slows as the end of one direction is reached, then briefly stops and begins rotation in the other direction. The movements of the chair are presented in a time strip and appear as a sinusoid moving left and right. The slow phase of the eye movements can be recorded on the same strip, but the eyes move rightward with left rotation of the chair and leftward with right rotation. The two recording lines appear as mirror images (**Fig. 10–8**). Standard computerized VOR summary analysis is shown in **Fig. 10–9**.

An alternate approach is to spin the patient in one direction at a given speed (120, 240, and sometimes 300 degrees/s are commonly chosen). This can be used to assess VOR gain during the "impulse" acceleration of starting and stopping. Once the patient reaches a constant speed the VOR declines. The "time constant" is used to measure the strength and duration of the VOR during these accelerations/decelerations.

Rotary chair testing is performed with the patient seated in a computer-controlled rotating chair inside a booth. Standardized stimulus frequencies make testing comparable across individuals and test sessions. The body is passively rotated en bloc (the head is fixed in a headholder to match the vestibular system's stimulus to the chair stimulus, and patients are not allowed to move their head about).

Neck turning to induce head rotation has been used to test VOR when rotary chair testing is unavailable, and is termed "autorotation." The patient shakes his or her head to produce VOR gain. Evidence suggests that autorotation results differ from gold standard rotary chair testing (American Academy of

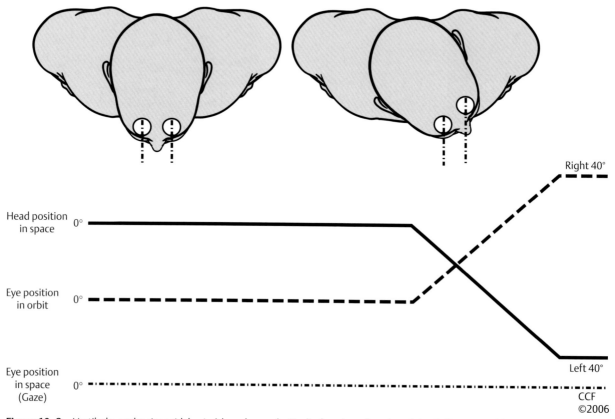

Figure 10–8 Vestibulo-ocular sinusoidal gain (slow phase velocity displayed as a function of time). (Courtesy of Micromedical Technologies, with permission.)

Rotational chair summary

VOR Summary

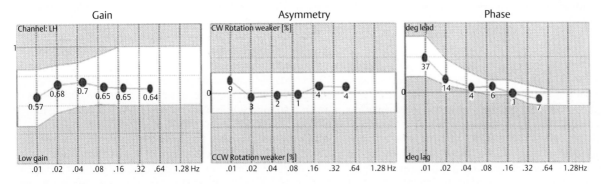

VFX Summary

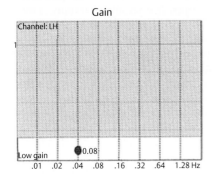

Asymmetry and Phase results are not calculated for Gains less than .2

VVOR Summary

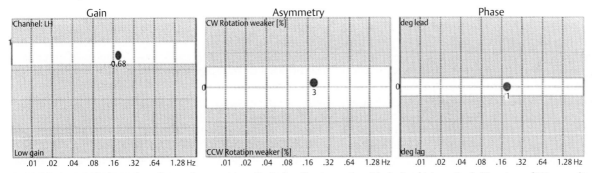

Figure 10–9 Vestibulo-ocular reflex testing summary (including fixation and vestibulovisual interaction). (Courtesy of Micromedical Technologies, with permission.)

Neurology, 2000). This may be due to the subject's anticipating the head rotation and learning to use saccadic compensatory movements, or to the effect of the cervical muscles on stabilizing the vestibulo-ocular gain. Although cervico-ocular gain is negligible in normal subjects (<0.05 degrees/s), it may play a far greater role in patients with bilateral vestibular loss.

Rotary chair testing of the VOR is performed in the dark to eliminate visual fixation. Visual stimuli are included in two additional portions of the test: fixation and visual-vestibular interaction testing. During vestibulo-ocular fixation (VFIX) a steady light rotating with the subject is used to test for the expected (>50%) decrease in vestibulo-ocular gain during visual fixation. During visual-vestibular interaction, visual stimuli are used to increase the perceived motion of the subject by projecting the visual images on the surround of the rotary chair, and the visual-vestibular ocular reflex (VVOR)

is usually greater than VOR. Central pathology can affect the integration of visual and vestibular inputs, resulting in abnormal VFIX and VVOR.

VOR testing is the only standardized test method that assesses the vestibular-ocular system at physiologic frequencies. The VOR is generated by both vestibular systems working together, and thus is an excellent measurement of compensation to acute unilateral vestibular loss. Complete compensation to a total unilateral vestibular loss will result in normal VOR gain and symmetry. (Phase may or may not remain elevated at low frequencies.)

The limitations of VOR testing include the high cost and space requirements of the rotary chair systems, the increased sophistication of analysis and interpretation required, and the limitation that only the lateral semicircular canals are tested during rotation around the fixed earth vertical axis. In addition, no lateralizing information is provided. As noted, in the context of a completely compensated total unilateral vestibular loss, VOR testing will be normal (except for possible low-frequency phase elevation).

Caloric Testing

Caloric testing has been the mainstay of vestibular assessment since Barany[3] described it in 1906 (and was subsequently awarded the Nobel Prize in 1915 for this work). It is the only vestibular test that provides lateralizing information because it compares responses of the left lateral semicircular canal with the right lateral semicircular canal. However, it is also the most inaccurate test in the vestibular armamentarium. It depends on the transmission of temperature stimuli through the external ear and mastoid to the lateral canal, and is affected by anatomic variability and conductivity (i.e., sclerotic mastoid bone secondary to infection, stenotic external canals, cerumen, or prior surgery) as well as patient cooperation. Most patients can suppress caloric nystagmus with concentration. Tasks to divert attention are used to try to circumvent this problem, such as naming foods, names, or states alphabetically.

The patient is placed in the dark in "caloric position," supine with the head elevated 30 degrees. This brings the lateral semicircular canals into earth vertical position. Standardized warm and cool stimuli are applied to the external canal. Water is the most dependable stimulus, but air has gained some popularity due to ease of use. Water can be also be used in a "closed loop" balloon system (Brookler-Grams irrigator, Grams Medical Products, Costa Mesa, CA) when prior surgery, infection, or perforation contraindicates open water irrigation.

The warm caloric irrigation (44°C) transmits heat to the lateral semicircular canal and stimulates ampullopetal flow of the endolymph (heat rises). This is stimulatory to the lateral canal, and nystagmus is generated with the fast phase beating toward the affected ear. The cool caloric stimulus (30°C) causes ampullofugal endolymph flow (cool endolymph is more dense and falls), inhibitory to the lateral canal. This generates nystagmus away from the affected ear. The simple mnemonic "COWS" can be memorized to remember the association: cold–opposite, warm–same. (The actual movement of the endolymph is probably more complex, demonstrated by the persistence of caloric responses in zero gravity, but for the purposes of everyday clinical use this model is valuable.)

Caloric stimuli are presented for 30 seconds, and nystagmus is calculated for the maximum slow phase velocity over 10 seconds. The operator or computer system may select the most representative tracing for this calculation. Order effects may be seen, and if a first irrigation is especially pronounced, it may be repeated later and the second value used. Stimuli are presented to each ear in an alternating bithermic manner [i.e., left warm (LW), right warm (RW), left cold (LC), right cold (RC)]. A 25 to 30% difference in caloric nystagmus between ears is considered significant (our laboratory uses a 28% cutoff). This is calculated using Jongkees's[4] formula: % caloric paresis = 100 × [(LC + LW) − (RC + RW)/(LC + LW + RC + RW)]. The strength of leftward nystagmus to rightward nystagmus can also be calculated: % directional preponderance (DP) = 100 × [(LC + RW) − (RC + LW)/(LC + LW + RC + RW)]. Greater than 30% directional

preponderance of nystagmus is considered abnormal, although this is a rather nonspecific finding in isolation. DP may be seen if spontaneous unidirectional nystagmus is present throughout caloric testing. An example of graphic caloric results is shown in **Fig. 10–10**.

Fixation is tested during peak caloric nystagmus. The patient is asked to stare at a strong fixed light. Usually the intensity of nystagmus diminishes by at least 50% after 2 seconds. After 10 seconds of fixation, the patient is returned to darkness and nystagmus should increase. Assuming normal vision, failure of fixation suppression is a strong central sign suggesting failure of visual-vestibular suppression. It is seen throughout caloric (and VOR) testing when there is central pathology, so isolated failure of fixation suppression is generally disregarded.

If caloric responses are low or absent, ice-water irrigation can be used. This is a much stronger stimulus and may be performed with the patient in the prone or supine position. In the prone position it is the strongest vestibular stimulus known because it causes ampullopetal endolymph flow and generated nystagmus toward the affected ear. Note that the direction of caloric nystagmus in the prone position is opposite that in the supine position because the canals are inverted. This alteration in ice-water–generated nystagmus direction may be a helpful sign when an overlying spontaneous nystagmus makes interpretation of low-amplitude ice-water–induced nystagmus problematic, and the patient can be tested in both the prone and supine positions to determine if there is a measurable vestibular response.

Observation of nystagmus that beats in the wrong direction during caloric testing (i.e., rightward nystagmus after left warm irrigation) is one of the most common problems prompting requests for assistance in vestibular laboratories. Several causes are likely. A moist ear will experience cooling even with warm air irrigation. Postsurgical ears may have configurations that prompt pressure-induced nystagmus due to pressure on ossicles or fenestra. Incorrect calibration is often responsible, and calibration before each caloric test may be helpful. True reversal of caloric nystagmus is very rare (less than 5 in 10,000) and is due to brainstem abnormalities. Perversion of nystagmus (vertical nystagmus without a horizontal component) after caloric stimulation is a central finding.

Caloric testing assesses very low frequency responses (0.003 Hz), far below physiologic frequencies encountered during active head or body movement. Caloric responses are subject to anatomic variability, medication effects (sedatives, benzodiazepines, antihistamines, alcohol, anticonvulsants), patient arousal, and compliance. For this reason, caloric testing is limited, and cannot confirm bilateral vestibular hypofunction. Total eye speeds for all four caloric irrigations of less than 22 degrees/s should be interpreted with caution. Rotary chair VOR testing is the gold standard to confirm bilateral vestibular hypofunction (American Academy of Neurology, 2000). Rotary chair responses may frequently be normal in patients with reduced caloric responses, especially in older patients. Jongkees's formula for the calculation of unilateral loss and directional preponderance is not accurate at low eye speeds less that 22 degrees/s total, and should not be calculated in that circumstance.

Isolated caloric weakness should also be interpreted with caution. If no other abnormalities are noted on vestibular testing, interpretation should note the weakness, but also suggests the possibility of anatomic variability or full vestibular

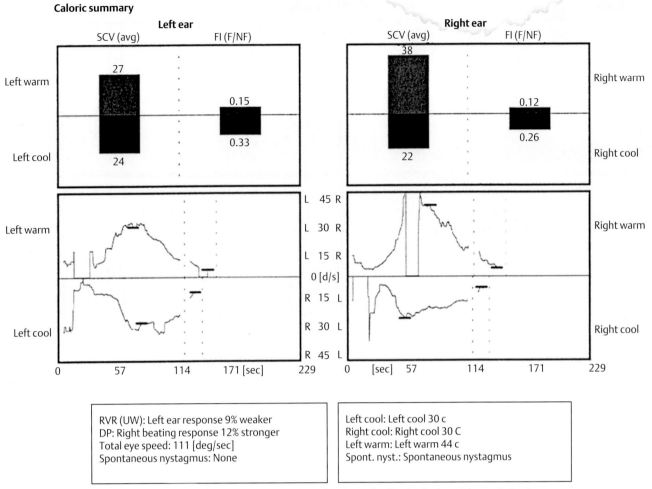

Caloric summary

RVR (UW): Left ear response 9% weaker
DP: Right beating response 12% stronger
Total eye speed: 111 [deg/sec]
Spontaneous nystagmus: None

Left cool: Left cool 30 c
Right cool: Right cool 30 C
Left warm: Left warm 44 c
Spont. nyst.: Spontaneous nystagmus

Figure 10–10　Graphic summary of caloric testing results. (Courtesy of Micromedical Technologies, with permission.)

compensation if a loss is actually present. The finding of isolated caloric asymmetry in the face of normal VOR testing and no positional or positioning nystagmus is unlikely to explain any recent symptoms the patient is experiencing.

Positional and Positioning Testing

Positional and positioning testing is usually performed prior to caloric testing. Any nystagmus is observed, and testing with IR-VOG has allowed recording and playback of the recorded video. This enables the interpreter to review the nystagmus during interpretation and substantially increases sensitivity to torsional nystagmus, which is not well recorded by standard image analysis or electro-oculography systems.

The patient is initially placed in a supine position with eyes open. The head is then rotated to the right lateral position for 10 seconds, brought back to midline for 10 seconds, and rotated to the left lateral position for 10 seconds before being returned to midline. The patient then returns to the sitting position. This maneuver detects horizontal nystagmus that may be related to lateral canal benign paroxysmal positional vertigo (BPPV). Lateral canal BPPV affects approximately 15% of patients with BPPV, and is usually not detected in Dix-Hallpike positioning due to stimulation of the posterior rather than lateral canal[5]

(**Fig. 10–11**). The paroxysmal positional nystagmus in lateral canal BPPV usually has less latency and a longer duration than that typically seen in posterior canal BPPV. It changes direction depending on the portion of the canal involved and the direction of the head. Geotropic (beating toward the ground; i.e., leftward in left ear down and rightward in right ear down positions, **Fig. 10–12**) nystagmus suggests canalithiasis in the distal lateral canal, with the worst nystagmus in the affected ear-down position (**Fig. 10–13**). Apogeotropic nystagmus beats toward the uppermost ear in lateral supine positions (**Fig. 10–14**), and suggests material proximal to or adherent to the cupula of the lateral canal (**Fig. 10–15**).

Positional nystagmus is best interpreted in the overall context of the vestibular battery. The nystagmus of lateral semicircular canal BPPV is seen in both right and left lateral positions, reverses direction during lateral supine head turns, and is usually pronounced (greater than 10 degrees/s). Other forms of horizontal nystagmus may be observed during positional testing (referred to as positional because the patient remains in a static position during recording). Unidirectional horizontal nystagmus beating away from an ear affected by acute unilateral vestibular loss, and seen in several positions, suggests a lack of vestibular compensation. In contrast, scattered positional nystagmus less than

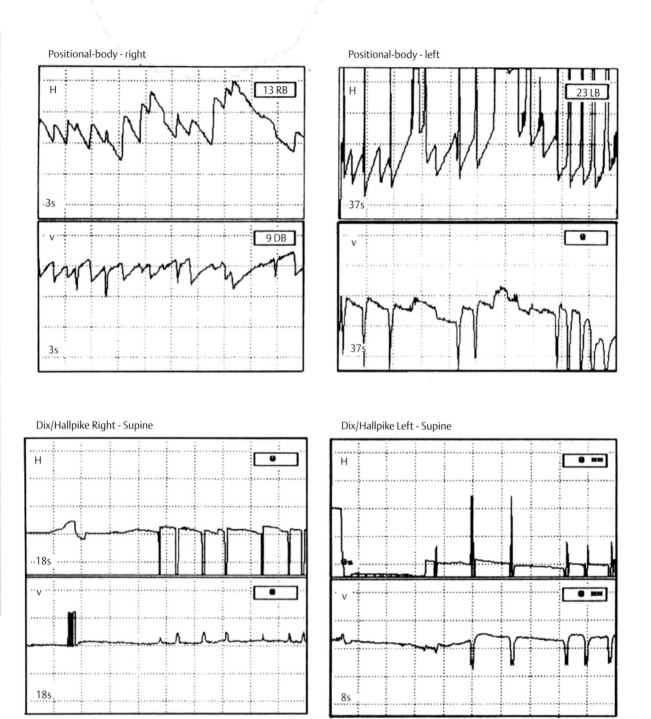

Figure 10–11 Positioning nystagmus demonstrating low sensitivity of Dix-Hallpike positioning compared with supine head turns in detecting horizontal nystagmus associated with lateral semicircular canal benign paroxysmal positional vertigo.

6 degrees/s and following no overall pattern is usually considered to be insignificant by many. Horizontal positional nystagmus greater than 6 degrees/s is usually noted, but it is a nonspecific, nonlocalizing finding that may be seen in central or peripheral vestibular disorders.

Dix-Hallpike positioning testing is performed next. In 1952, Dix and Hallpike[5] described the characteristic ipsidirectional torsional nystagmus provoked by the head maneuver they developed to identify posterior canal BPPV (**Fig. 10–16**). During this maneuver, the patient's head is turned 45 degrees to one side while he or she is seated. The patient is then moved quickly to a supine position with the neck slightly extended and the head remaining turned. When the undermost ear is affected, nystagmus is seen. The patient is then brought back up to a sitting position, and the nystagmus is noted to reverse direction. The maneuver is then performed on the other side. The characteristic nystagmus occurs after a delay of several seconds, declines after 10 to 30 seconds, and diminishes with repeated positional testing in the same sitting position.

Positional body   Video

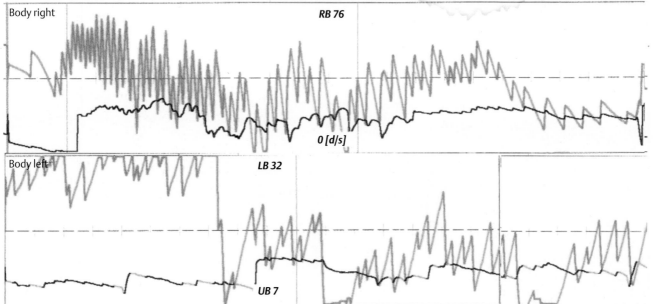

Body right   ***RB 76***

0 [d/s]

Body left   *LB 32*

UB 7

Figure 10–12   Geotropic horizontal nystagmus (nystagmus beats rightward when the head is turned right in the supine position and nystagmus beats leftward when the head is turned left in the supine position).

Computerized Dynamic Posturography

Postural control involves a complex interplay of visual, proprioceptive, and vestibular input. Computerized dynamic posturography (CDP) tests static postural control in a series of conditions designed to emphasize or minimize each of these inputs. The somatosensory system detects contact force and motion between the feet and contact surface, and utilizes tactile, deep pressure, joint receptor, and muscle proprioceptive input. Under normal conditions, the somatosensory system dominates balance control. Firm, fixed surfaces favor the somatosensory system, and classic Romberg testing utilizes these features by testing postural control on a stable surface with eyes closed.

The visual system relies on visual cues from the environment to assist in maintaining upright posture. It may be affected by decreased vision, or inappropriate dependence on visual stimuli (i.e., standing next to a moving bus and perceiving sway).

The vestibular system usually functions to allow head and eye movements that are independent in usual situations. In situations of decreased proprioceptive and visual input the vestibular system is crucial for maintaining upright postural control. Patients with bilateral vestibular hypofunction have great difficulty maintaining postural control on compliant surfaces in the dark, such as deep carpeting or uneven landscape.

CDP presents six different conditions to maximize or minimize input from the somatosensory, visual and vestibular

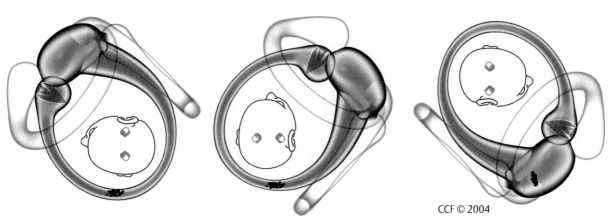

CCF © 2004

Figure 10–13   Illustration of supine positional testing in geotropic lateral semicircular canal benign paroxysmal positional vertigo. (Courtesy of the Cleveland Clinic Foundation, with permission.)

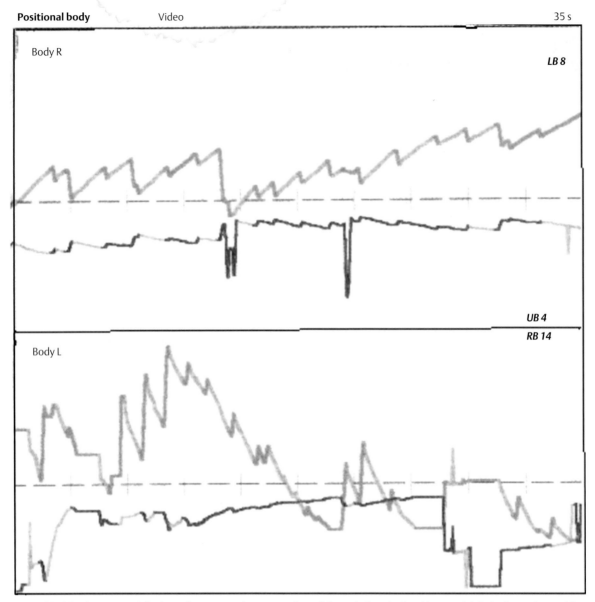

Body R

LB 8

UB 4
RB 14

Body L

Figure 10–14 Apogeotropic horizontal nystagmus (nystagmus beats leftward when the head is turned right in the supine position, and nystagmus beats rightward when the head is turned leftward in the supine position).

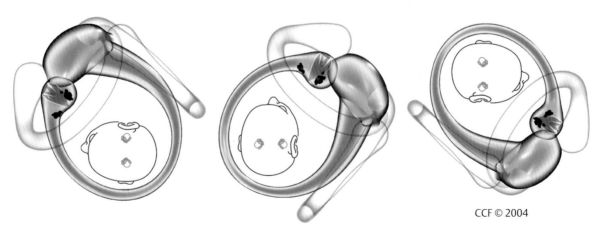

CCF © 2004

Figure 10–15 Illustration of supine positional testing in apogeotropic lateral semicircular canal benign paroxysmal positional vertigo. (Courtesy of the Cleveland Clinic Foundation, with permission.)

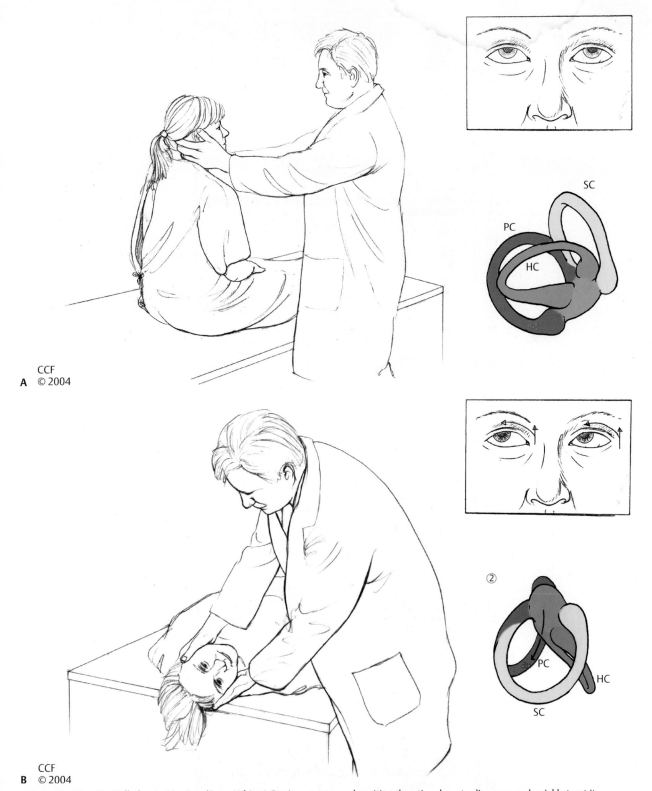

CCF
A © 2004

CCF
B © 2004

Figure 10–16 Dix-Hallpike positioning. (From White J. Benign paroxysmal positional vertigo: how to diagnose and quickly treat it. Cleve Clin J Med 2004;71:722–728, reprinted with permission. Copyright © 2004. The Cleveland Clinic Foundation. All rights reserved.) HC, horizontal canal; PC, posterior canal; SC, superior canal.

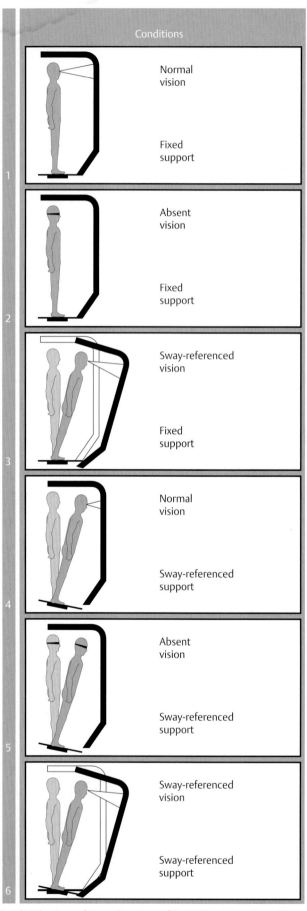

Conditions

1 — Normal vision / Fixed support

2 — Absent vision / Fixed support

3 — Sway-referenced vision / Fixed support

4 — Normal vision / Sway-referenced support

5 — Absent vision / Sway-referenced support

6 — Sway-referenced vision / Sway-referenced support

146   **Figure 10–17**   Sensory Organization Test (SOT)—six conditions. (Courtesy of NeuroCom International.)

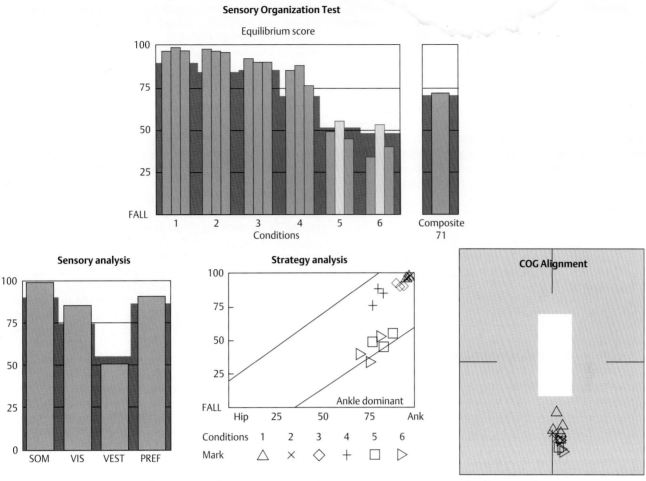

Figure 10–18   Graphic display of Computerized Dynamic Posturography Sensory Organization Test results. (Courtesy of NeuroCom International.)

systems (**Fig. 10–17**). Postural sway is assessed using force plate technology in six different conditions (sensory organization testing). Initially using a fixed platform the patient is tested with eyes open, eyes closed, or with a swaying visual surround. Next, the platform is allowed to sway and the tests are repeated with eyes open, eyes closed, and swaying surround. Normal subjects center their balance (center of gravity). When movement of the feet is not allowed, subjects fall if swaying more than 12.5 degrees from that base (termed the limits of stability). Patients are compared with age-matched norms and the degree of peak sway is reported, with 100% indicating no sway and 0% indicating sway approaching the limits of stability.

Interpretation of posturography begins with noting overall postural control. Subscale scores on somatosensory, visual and visual preference, and vestibular subscales are noted. The position of the center of gravity, the use of hip and ankle strategies to maintain postural control, and the pattern of falls are assessed. Posturography demonstrates which sensory systems the patient uses to maintain balance, but it does not directly assess deficits in those systems. Thus, a low score on the vestibular subscale suggests either that the patient is not using vestibular input when appropriate to maintain posture or that vestibular input may be deficient (as in bilateral

hypofunction) (**Fig. 10–18**). Posturography uniquely assesses the functional use of the vestibular system to achieve postural control. Thus, posturography is best included in a comprehensive vestibular test battery. An additional use of posturography is to identify patients with "aphysiologic" performance on various test conditions. Patients who fail easier conditions and pass harder conditions are demonstrating performance that is not consistent with known physiologic patterns, and may be identified by this pattern of test performance.

◆ Vestibular Test Battery Interpretation

Vestibular test battery interpretation is a complex process that involves a search for patterns of deficit. Understanding these patterns will allow stepwise interpretation, and assist with the prioritization of inconsistent results.

Interpretation begins with a review of oculomotor testing performance. Central oculomotor abnormalities are usually obvious and recurrent (see Oculomotor Testing, above). Computerized interpretation systems commonly over-read central pathology, such as symmetric prolonged saccade latency. The base rates of central pathology in the test population should be considered, as well as performance and medication effects. Demonstration of normal oculomotor function allows assessment to progress to the next level.

Next we check for spontaneous nystagmus. Spontaneous nystagmus may affect results on oculomotor, caloric, VOR symmetry, and directional preponderance. Any spontaneous nystagmus is noted, and its effect on the aforementioned tests is considered.

Caloric asymmetry is assessed next. Caloric asymmetry in our laboratory is defined by a greater than 28% difference between ears as calculated by Jongkees's formula (see Caloric Testing, above, for discussion of possible order effect). The next task of the interpreter once a caloric asymmetry is noted is to determine if this is an acute uncompensated unilateral loss versus a compensated loss.

The following pattern suggests acute uncompensated peripheral vestibular loss:

1. Spontaneous horizontal nystagmus away from the affected ear that decreases at least 50% with fixation
2. Positional or positioning nystagmus away from the affected ear, especially if seen in several positions
3. Gaze-evoked unidirectional horizontal nystagmus worse in the direction of gaze away from the affected ear
4. Asymmetric VOR gain, decreased with rotation toward the affected side
5. Low-frequency VOR phase elevation may be present (variable).
6. VOR gain may be normal or reduced.
7. Postur.ography may show a vestibular pattern of deficit.

In contrast, a unilateral caloric loss may be fully compensated. Features of this pattern include the following:

1. No spontaneous nystagmus
2. No gaze-evoked nystagmus
3. Minimal positional and positioning nystagmus (less than 6 degrees/s and not present in several positions)
4. Symmetric VOR gain
5. Low-frequency VOR phase elevation may be present (variable).
6. Normal VOR gain
7. Normal posturography
8. Asymmetric caloric responses

Patterns that are a mixture of acute uncompensated and compensated features are described as partially compensated. Therefore, when a caloric asymmetry greater than 28% is noted, the next step is to check for features that indicate whether this is a compensated or uncompensated loss.

Bilateral vestibular hypofunction is suggested by caloric responses less than 22 degrees/s total eye speed, and confirmed by rotary chair VOR that is two or more standard deviations below normal.[7] The time constant on impulse testing is less than 5 seconds, and sinusoidal VOR testing results indicate reduced VOR gain (at 0.05 Hz <0.20; at 0.2 Hz <0.21; at 1.0 Hz <0.62). Medication effects must be excluded.

One common question is how to prioritize vestibular test findings when results do not agree. Caloric stimuli are very low frequency (0.003 Hz), much lower than those assessed by rotary chair. Caloric responses are affected by anatomic variability and patient cooperation to a greater extent than other vestibular testing. Caloric weakness does not reflect the degree of compensation that may be present to a unilateral vestibular weakness. Caloric testing continues to be included in vestibular test batteries because it is the only test that provides lateralizing information.

Some of the most puzzling vestibular tests results are obtained in patients with Meniere's syndrome. As a rule, vestibular testing should not be used to lateralize the affected side in Meniere's syndrome. Audiograms are far more specific and reliable. Vestibular testing may show hyperfunction of the involved side, or nystagmus beating toward the involved ear as well as more classic patterns of unilateral loss. Variable portions of the test battery may be abnormal in atypical patterns. Perhaps the most useful application of vestibular testing in Meniere's patients is to document normal caloric function in the unaffected side prior to performing ablative procedures in the affected ear.

Migraine-associated dizziness may also show variable vestibular test findings, and both classic peripheral loss patterns and central patterns can be seen.[8] An additional feature of vestibular test results in migraineurs is the variability of results when retested, likely related to the fluctuating nature of the disorder.

◆ Additional Vestibular Tests

The standard vestibular test battery described above provides information about the lateral semicircular canals and by extension the superior division of the vestibular nerve. Newer test methods allow assessment of the saccular response (inferior vestibular nerve) and offer the promise of assessing otolith function.

Vestibular evoked myogenic potentials (VEMPs) measure changes in the static contraction of the ipsilateral sternocleidomastoid muscle in response to loud acoustic stimuli. The saccule has been shown to mediate this response, and VEMP testing is the first evoked response method available to assess saccular responses.[9] VEMP testing is also helpful in identifying dehiscence of the superior semicircular canal, where responses are abnormally elevated in affected ears.

The otolith organs (utricle and saccule) detect linear acceleration, in contrast to the semicircular canals, which detect angular acceleration. Linear vectors of force can be applied to each utricle by rotating a subject around a vertical axis while the subject is eccentrically displaced 4 cm. This centers one utricle on the axis of rotation and subjects the other side to a linear force vector. While rotating, patients feel as if they are being pushed outward toward the side of displacement (similar to standing on the edge of a merry-go-round). The response of each utricle can be contrasted when the subject is rotated with the right ear displaced laterally versus the left ear displaced laterally.

One response mediated by the utricles is the assessment of visual vertical. In the dark, a subject is asked to move a light bar until it appears vertical. The accuracy of the subject's placement is recorded. This technique can be affixed to the rotary chair to provide subjective visual vertical assessment during eccentric rotation. This protocol allows for comparison of right and left utricular function.[10]

Research applications use off-vertical axis rotation (OVAR) to tilt the entire rotary chair unit and allow for analysis of gravitational forces on utricular function in rotating subjects.[11] This method can be visualized as a spinning holiday tree tilting from side to side in its base. OVAR testing requires complex chair construction and interpretation and is mainly utilized by research laboratories.

References

1. Leigh RJ, Zee D. The Neurology of Eye Movements, 4th ed. Contemporary Neurology Series. New York: Oxford University Press, 2006

2. Baloh RW, Halmagyi GM. Disorders of the Vestibular System. New York: Oxford University Press, 1996

3. Barany R. Weitere untersuchungen uber den von vestibular-apparat des ohres reflektorisch aus gelosten rhythmischen nystagmus und seine begleiterscheinungen. Monatsschr Ohrenheik 1907;41: 477–541

4. Jongkees LBW. On the otoliths: their function and how to test them. In: Third symposium on the Role of the Vestibular Organs in Space Exploration. NASA Publication No. SP-152. Washington, DC: Government Printing Office, pp. 307–330

5. Dix MR, Hallpike CS. The pathology symptomatology and diagnosis of certain common disorders of the vestibular system. Proc R Soc Med 1952;45:341–354

6. Baloh RW, Hess K, Honrubia V, Yee RD. Low and high frequency sinusoidal rotation testing in patients with vestibular lesions. Acta Otolaryngol Suppl 1984;406:189–193

7. Halmagyi GM, Curthoys IS, Aw ST, Todd MJ. The human vestibulo-ocular reflex after unilateral vestibular deafferentation: the results of high-acceleration impulsive testing. In: Sharpe JA, Barber HO, eds. The Vestibulo-Ocular Reflex and Vertigo. New York: Raven Press, 1993:45–54

8. Furman JM, Schor RH, Schumann TL. Off-vertical axis rotation: a test of the otolith-ocular reflex. Ann Otol Rhinol Laryngol 1992;101:643–650

9. Kingma H. Function tests of the otolith or statolith system. Curr Opin Neurol 2006;19:21–25

10. Furman JM, Marcus DA, Balaban CD. Migrainous vertigo. Development of a pathogenetic model and structured diagnostic interview. Curr Opin Neurol 2003;16:5–13

11. White J, Coale K, Catalano P, Oas J. Diagnosis and management of lateral semicircular canal benign positional vertigo. Otolaryngol Head Neck Surg 2005;133:278–284

11

Clinical Evaluation of the Cranial Nerves

Abraham Jacob and D. Bradley Welling

Diagnostic evaluation of the cranial nerves (CNs) begins with understanding their anatomy, requires obtaining a detailed patient history, and calls for a thorough bedside evaluation. Cranial base imaging (Chapter 7) and the use of neuro-diagnostic electrical tests are becoming common clinical adjuncts for evaluating neural integrity. In modern otology and neurotology, the preoperative and intraoperative assessment of CN integrity may help optimize each patient's post-operative outcome.

◆ Anatomy and Bedside Evaluation of Cranial Nerves

The first step in assessing the CNs is understanding the anatomy and performing a basic bedside evaluation. **Fig. 11–1** illustrates the topographic anatomy of the brainstem. CNs I and II are direct extensions of the central nervous system (CNS), CNs III and IV arise from the midbrain, CNs V to VIII originate in the pons, and CNs IX to XII arise from the medulla.

Cranial Nerve I: Olfactory Nerve

The olfactory system is made up of specialized olfactory epithelium, olfactory bulbs, olfactory tracts, and their central projections. This epithelium, present along the superior concha, superior nasal septum, and nasal vault, is made up of bipolar sensory receptors that also serve as first-order neurons. Approximately 20 filaments traverse the cribriform plate and enter the anterior cranial fossa on each side of the crista galli. These first-order axons synapse with mitral and tufted cells (second-order neurons) in the olfactory bulbs. Central projections from the olfactory bulbs then travel primarily to the limbic system. These projections, termed olfactory tracts, arise from the posterior aspect of each olfactory bulb and project to the lateral (primary), intermediate, and medial olfactory areas. Periamygdaloid and prepiriform areas are thought to make up the primary olfactory cortex, whereas the entorhinal area functions as a secondary olfactory cortex.[1] The bedside evaluation of olfaction begins with a complete (including endoscopic) nasal, sinus, and nasopharyngeal examination. The patient is then asked to identify familiar aromatic odors delivered separately to each nostril. A variety of odorant delivery devices are commercially available.

Cranial Nerve II: Optic Nerve

Visual inputs, transformed into electrical signals by the retina, are transmitted centrally via the optic nerve (**Fig. 11–2**). This nerve enters the middle cranial fossa through the optic canal, an opening in the lesser wing of the sphenoid bone. It unites with the contralateral optic nerve at the optic chiasm where fibers from the medial (nasal) half of each retina cross into the contralateral optic tract. Each optic tract, central to the chiasm, travels to the lateral geniculate nucleus of the thalamus. Optic radiations then leave the thalamus, pass through the internal capsule, and terminate in each occipital lobe's primary visual cortex. The bedside evaluation of CN II includes testing basic visual acuity (Snellen chart), performing an ophthalmoscopic examination, testing pupillary response to light (afferent limb of a neural arc involving the second CN), and testing the patient's visual fields. Visual field defects can help localize the "site of lesion" along the visual pathway. A more detailed evaluation generally requires consultation with the ophthalmology service.

Cranial Nerves III, IV, and VI: Oculomotor Complex and Abducens Nerves

The oculomotor complex (oculomotor and Edinger-Westphal nuclei) is located in the midbrain ventral to the cerebral aqueduct (**Fig. 11–3**). The oculomotor nerve itself emerges ventrally from the caudal midbrain, passes between the posterior cerebral and superior cerebellar arteries, and enters the lateral aspect of the cavernous sinus. It then enters the orbit through the superior orbital fissure. Just inside the orbit, CN III splits into superior and inferior divisions. The superior division supplies motor input to the superior rectus and levator palpebrae muscles, whereas the inferior division innervates the medial rectus, inferior rectus, and inferior oblique. This inferior division also carries preganglionic parasympathetic fibers from the Edinger-Westphal nucleus to the ciliary ganglion. Postganglionic fibers travel to the ciliary body and constrictor pupillae muscles.

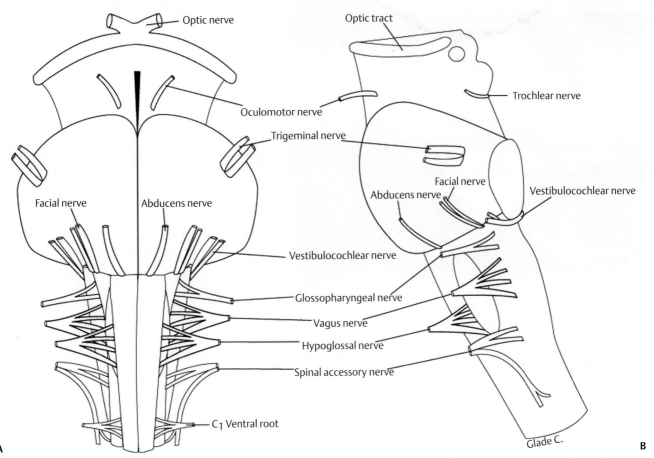

Figure 11–1 Topographic anatomy of the cranial nerves (CNs) at the brainstem in frontal **(A)** and lateral **(B)** views. Note that CNs I and II are direct extensions of the central nervous system, CN III and IV arise from the midbrain, CN V to VIII originate in the pons, and CN IX to XII arise from the medulla. (See Figure 11–3 for CN I)

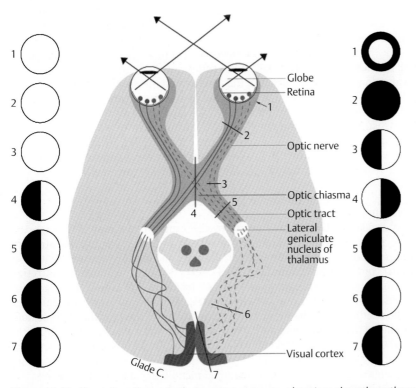

Figure 11–2 The optic pathway. As shown, injuries at various locations along the pathway result in characteristic visual field defects, noted by the darkened areas.

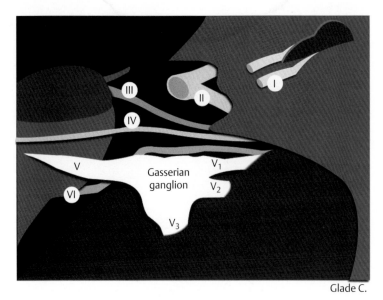

Figure 11–3   Diagram of the anterior and middle cranial fossae depicting the first (olfactory), second (optic), third (oculomotor), fourth (trochlear), fifth (trigeminal), and sixth (abducens) CNs. Note the dorsal origin of the trochlear nerve as well as the ascent of the abducens nerve along the clivus.

Glade C.

The trochlear nerve innervates the superior oblique muscle. Its fibers originate in the midbrain caudal to the oculomotor complex. Interestingly, this nerve decussates within the brainstem before exiting on its dorsal surface. The trochlear nerve travels along the lateral wall of the cavernous sinus just inferior to the oculomotor nerve prior to entering the orbit through the superior orbital fissure. This nerve has the longest intracranial course of any CN.

The abducens nerve provides motor input to the lateral rectus muscle. Its nucleus is located in the pons anterior to the fourth ventricle and adjacent to the facial motor nucleus. Axons from the ipsilateral seventh CN loop around the abducens nucleus prior to leaving the brainstem. CN VI exits the ventral pontomedullary junction, travels rostrally along the clivus, passes through Dorello's canal, and emerges within the cavernous sinus. It enters the orbit through the superior orbital fissure.

CNs III, IV, and VI move the globe, regulate pupil diameter, and help retract the upper eyelid. The bedside evaluation of these nerves requires inspection of the upper eyelids for ptosis, assessment of each upper lid for adequate lid retraction during eye opening, testing extraocular motion, measuring pupil size and symmetry, and testing both the direct and consensual pupillary response to light.

Cranial Nerve V: Trigeminal Nerve

The principal brainstem nuclei of CN V are the motor (masticator) nucleus and the pontine (sensory) trigeminal nucleus (**Figs. 11–3** and **11–4**). A rostral extension of the pontine nucleus makes up the mesencephalic nucleus, whereas its caudal extension into the dorsal gray matter of the spinal cord is called the nucleus of the spinal trigeminal tract. The trigeminal nerve emerges from the mid-lateral pons as a large sensory and smaller motor root. Its principal sensory ganglion, the semilunar or Gasserian ganglion, is situated in Meckel's cave along the anterior-medial floor of the middle cranial fossa. From the ganglion, three divisions of the nerve (ophthalmic V_1, maxillary V_2, and mandibular V_3) exit the intracranial space through the superior orbital fissure, foramen rotundum, and foramen ovale, respectively. The ophthalmic division divides into its four terminal branches (the frontal nerve, nasociliary nerve, lacrimal

nerve, and a meningeal branch) within the orbit. The maxillary division splits into a meningeal branch, the zygomatic nerve, infraorbital nerve, and the superior alveolar nerve within the pterygopalatine fossa. The peripheral ganglion of the maxillary nerve, the pterygopalatine ganglion, is located within the pterygopalatine fossa. The mandibular nerve traverses the foramen ovale and enters the infratemporal fossa. Here it divides into its terminal branches, the auriculotemporal nerve, the buccal nerve, the lingual nerve, and the inferior alveolar nerve. The peripheral ganglion of the trigeminal nerve, the otic ganglion, is situated in the infratemporal fossa. The trigeminal nerve provides motor innervation to the muscles of mastication, the mylohyoid, the anterior belly of the digastric muscle, the tensor tympani, and the tensor veli palatini muscles. It also receives general sensory information from the face and scalp (up to the vertex of the head) ocular conjunctiva, paranasal sinuses and nasal cavity, oral cavity (including tongue and dentition) anterior ear canal, lateral surface of the tympanic membrane, and the meninges of the anterior and middle cranial fossa.

Primary bedside evaluation of the trigeminal nerve assesses cutaneous sensation of the face and scalp, intraoral sensation along the tongue, buccal mucosa, floor of mouth, and alveolar ridges, and evaluates the corneal reflex (afferent limb mediated by CN V_1). The muscles of mastication can be tested for symmetry by having patients clench their teeth.

Cranial Nerve VII: Facial Nerve

CN VII emerges from the caudal pons, passes through the cerebellopontine angle (CPA), and enters the internal auditory canal (IAC), where it assumes an anterior-superior position at the fundus (**Fig. 11–5**). Several named segments characterize its intratemporal course, including the labyrinthine, geniculate, tympanic (horizontal), and mastoid (vertical) segments. The nerve exits the temporal bone through the stylomastoid foramen and divides at the pes anserinus into temporozygomatic and cervicofacial trunks. These primary branches then split into five terminal branches: the frontal (temporal), orbital, buccal, marginal mandibular, and cervical nerves.

The facial nerve contains parasympathetic fibers from the superior salivatory nucleus, motor fibers from the facial motor nucleus, taste afferents to the nucleus solitarius, and general

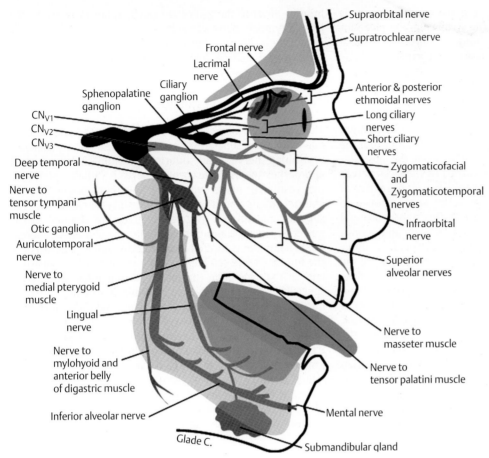

Figure 11–4 Diagrammatic representation of the V₁, V₂, and V₃ divisions of the trigeminal nerve.

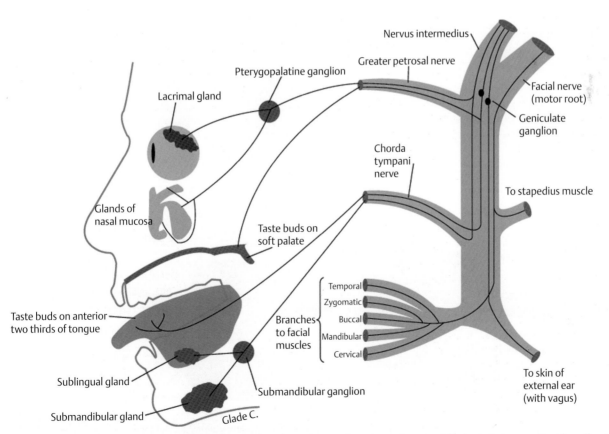

Figure 11–5 Facial nerve innervation. This nerve stimulates lacrimation and nasal secretions, contributes to taste sensation along the soft palate and anterior tongue, is motor to the mimetic facial musculature, and sensory to the skin of external auditory meatus.

sensory afferents to the spinal trigeminal tract. The nerve is motor to the stapedius muscle, the stylohyoid, the posterior belly of digastric, the auricular muscles, muscles of facial expression, the buccinator, and the platysma. Parasympathetic innervation of the lacrimal gland occurs via the greater superficial petrosal nerve. The chorda tympani nerve stimulates salivation from the submandibular and sublingual glands. Special sensory fibers within the chorda tympani also transmit taste afferents from the anterior two-thirds of the tongue, whereas the greater superficial petrosal nerve mediates taste from the posterior soft palate. General sensation from the posterior meatal skin of the ear canal is also carried by the facial nerve.

The initial patient examination should classify the extent of facial weakness (House-Brackmann scale) and approximate the location of nerve injury. The upper face enjoys bilateral central motor innervation. As a result, brainstem and peripheral facial nerve injuries cause a complete, unilateral paralysis, whereas injuries rostral to the facial motor nucleus spare the upper face. Because the facial and abducens nuclei are in close proximity within the pons, concomitant facial paralysis and lateral rectus palsy suggest a brainstem lesion. Involvement of the facial nerve in the CPA usually occurs late in CPA diseases. Other CNs, especially CN VIII, are typically involved prior to the onset of facial weakness. The physical examination may help localize the site of intratemporal facial nerve injury. Disruption of the nerve at the stylomastoid foramen causes facial paralysis without changes in taste, lacrimation, or salivation. Lesions near the geniculate ganglion result in facial paralysis, altered lacrimation, decreased salivation, and taste dysfunction. Injuries distal to the geniculate ganglion but proximal to the chorda tympani nerve cause facial paralysis, loss of taste, and diminished salivation but do not affect lacrimation. Injuries distal to the stylomastoid foramen affect specific peripheral branches of the nerve.

Cranial Nerve VIII: Vestibulocochlear Nerve

The vestibulocochlear nerve (**Fig. 11–6**) exits the brainstem as one nerve but separates into the cochlear nerve, superior vestibular nerve, and inferior vestibular nerve as it approaches the IAC. The cochlear nerve is initially inferior to the vestibular nerve within the CPA but rotates into an anterior-inferior position by the time it reaches the IAC. The superior and inferior vestibular nerves are situated in the posterior-superior and posterior-inferior quadrants, whereas the facial nerve is located in an anterior-superior position at the fundus. Nerve cell bodies in the spiral ganglion (hearing) and Scarpa's ganglion (balance) transmit information from specialized sensory end-organs within the cochlea (organ of Corti), the utricle and saccule (maculae), and the semicircular canals (cristae).

The auditory pathway begins with cochlear hair cells that transduce mechanical energy into electrical impulses. These impulses are transmitted along the auditory nerve to the ipsilateral cochlear nucleus by the neurons of the spiral ganglion. From the cochlear nucleus, ipsilateral and contralateral auditory pathways are generated. The majority of fibers cross the brainstem and synapse in the contralateral superior olivary

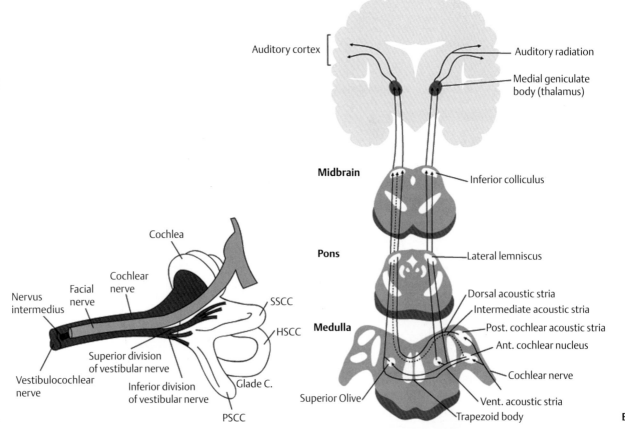

Figure 11–6 **(A)** Anatomy of the seventh (facial) and eighth (vestibulocochlear) CNs. At the fundus of internal auditory canal, the facial nerve is in the anterior-superior quadrant, the cochlear nerve is in the anterior-inferior quadrant, and the superior and inferior vestibular nerves are in the posterior-superior and posterior-inferior quadrants. **(B)** The central auditory pathways. Note the bilateral representation of auditory inputs at multiple levels within the brainstem. SSCC, HSCC, PSCC; superior, horizontal, and posterior semicircular canals.

complex or pass through the lateral lemniscus to the inferior colliculus. Information is then relayed to the medial geniculate body of the thalamus from which it is transmitted to the primary auditory complex of the temporal lobe.

The bedside evaluation for hearing includes the whisper test and a tuning fork examination. A 512-Hz tuning fork lateralizes toward the ear with a conductive hearing loss and away from the ear with a sensorineural hearing deficit. The Rinne is positive if air conduction (tuning fork next to the pinna) is greater than bone conduction (tuning fork placed on the antrum or mastoid tip). Bone conduction greater than air conduction typically reflects a 25-dB conductive hearing loss (negative Rinne). Bedside balance testing includes evaluating the patient's gait and performing the Rhomberg or tandem Rhomberg tests. Spontaneous, gaze, positional, and positioning nystagmus should also be sought. A post–head-shake nystagmus will beat away from an ear with unilateral vestibular loss. The presence of a post–head-thrust refixation saccade reflects a vestibular weakness in the ear toward which the head is thrust. Detailed descriptions regarding these and other tests are covered in other chapters.

Cranial Nerve IX: Glossopharyngeal Nerve

The ninth CN provides motor innervation to the stylopharyngeus muscle (nucleus ambiguus), supplies parasympathetic input to the parotid gland (inferior salivatory nucleus), innervates the carotid body and carotid sinus (nucleus solitarius), provides general sensation (trigeminal tract) and taste (nucleus solitarius) to the posterior third of the tongue, and is sensory to a portion of the ear canal and internal surface of the tympanic membrane (trigeminal tract). It exits the medulla as rootlets, which enter the jugular foramen. Superior and inferior glossopharyngeal ganglia are present within the foramen. As the nerve enters the jugular foramen, the tympanic branch (Jacobson's nerve) separates and enters the middle ear through the inferior (hypotympanic) canaliculus. A plexus is formed on the promontory of the cochlea after which the nerve reconstitutes as the lesser petrosal nerve. This petrosal nerve enters the middle cranial fossa, descends through the foramen ovale, and synapses with the otic ganglion in the infratemporal fossa. Parasympathetic fibers from CN IX eventually join the auriculotemporal nerve (V_3) within the otic ganglion.

Bedside examination of CN IX involves testing the afferent limb of the oropharyngeal gag reflex and evaluating supraglottic sensation during flexible fiberoptic laryngoscopy. Xerostomia, particularly during mastication, may reflect parotid dysfunction secondary to CN IX palsy.

Cranial Nerve X: Vagus Nerve

A complete description of CN X (**Fig. 11–7**) anatomy is beyond the scope of this text. In brief, vagal rootlets emerge from the medulla and join as they enter the jugular foramen. The superior

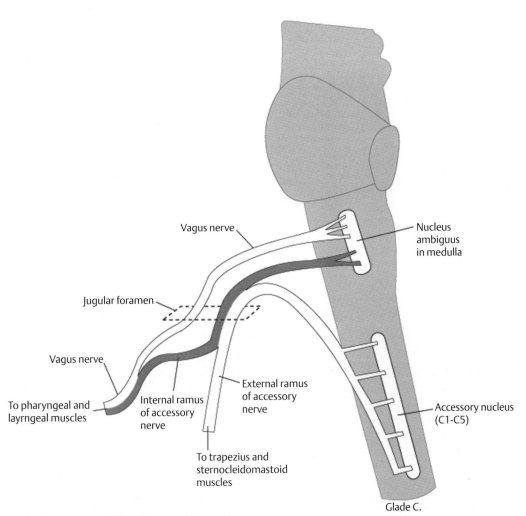

Vagus nerve

Nucleus ambiguus in medulla

Jugular foramen

Vagus nerve

Internal ramus of accessory nerve

External ramus of accessory nerve

To pharyngeal and layrngeal muscles

To trapezius and sternocleidomastoid muscles

Accessory nucleus (C1-C5)

Glade C.

Figure 11–7 The tenth (vagus) and eleventh (spinal accessory) CNs. Note that some fibers initially traveling with the eleventh nerve join the vagus nerve distal to the jugular foramen.

(jugular) and inferior (nodose) ganglia of CN X are located within this foramen. Some fibers from the caudal aspect of the nucleus ambiguus exit the brainstem within the spinal accessory nerve (CN XI) but later join CN X after it exits the skull base. Motor branches from the vagus nerve (nucleus ambiguus) include the pharyngeal branch, the superior laryngeal nerve, and the recurrent laryngeal nerve. Parasympathetic fibers (dorsal vagal nucleus) innervate glands within the pharyngeal, laryngeal, gastric, and intestinal mucosa. Visceral sensation from the gut is transmitted to the nucleus solitarius. General sensory afferents from the pharynx, larynx, skin of the external auditory canal (auricular branch), external surface of the tympanic membrane (auricular branch), and meninges of the posterior fossa travel with CN X to the trigeminal tract and nucleus.

Bedside otolaryngologic testing of the vagus nerve includes inspection of the palate during swallowing or phonation; a bedside swallow evaluation to rule out aspiration; appraisal of voice quality for hypernasality, hoarseness, or breathiness; and fiberoptic laryngoscopy to examine vocal cord motion.

Cranial Nerve XI: Spinal Accessory Nerve

The accessory nucleus is located within the spinal cord. Axons from lower motor neurons emerge as rootlets that ascend through the foramen magnum into the posterior cranial fossa.

These are joined by fibers of the nucleus ambiguus to form CN XI (**Fig. 11–7**). The spinal accessory nerve exits the posterior fossa through the jugular foramen and provides motor innervation to the sternocleidomastoid (SCM) and trapezius muscles. Dysfunction of this nerve is manifest by a winged scapula, shoulder weakness, an inability to abduct the arm past 100 degrees, and weakness when turning the head toward the contralateral side.

Cranial Nerve XII: Hypoglossal Nerve

The hypoglossal nerve provides motor input to the ipsilateral tongue by innervating all intrinsic and extrinsic tongue musculature except the palatoglossus muscle (vagus nerve). The hypoglossal nucleus is located within the medulla. Nerve rootlets exit between the pyramids and olive to form a common trunk, which then traverses the hypoglossal (anterior condylar) canal. Hypoglossal nerve weakness is manifest by deviation of the tongue toward the weaker side during protrusion.

◆ Nerve Injury

Seddon's[2] 1943 three-tier classification of neural injury was later expanded in 1951 by Sunderland[3] into a five-tier system (**Fig. 11–8**). Sunderland used the terms *first-* and *second-degree*

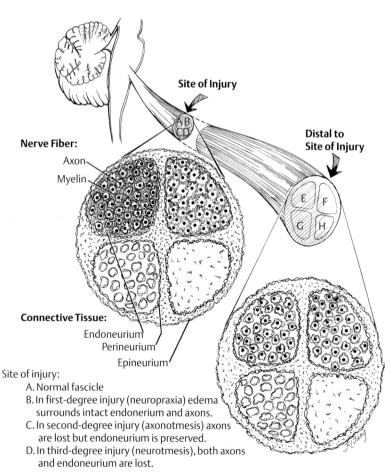

Site of injury:
  A. Normal fascicle
  B. In first-degree injury (neuropraxia) edema surrounds intact endonerium and axons.
  C. In second-degree injury (axonotmesis) axons are lost but endoneurium is preserved.
  D. In third-degree injury (neurotmesis), both axons and endoneurium are lost.

Distal to site of injury, several days later:
  E. Normal fascicle
  F. After first-degree injury, fascicles are normal distally.
  G. After second-degree injury, Wallerian degeneration has occurred and axons are lost distally.
  H. After third-degree injury, loss of endoneurium at the site of injury prevents guidance of regenerating fibers into distal nerve segment.

Figure 11–8 Cross-sectional model of microanatomic changes in mild to moderate CN injury. The effects of neural injury dictate the potential for successful, appropriate patterns of fiber regeneration across the site of nerve injury, (Courtesy of John K. Niparko, MD).

injury in place of Seddon's *neurapraxia* and *axonotmesis*, while subclassifying Seddon's *neurotmesis* into third-, fourth-, and fifth-degree injuries. A first-degree injury (neurapraxia) is a conduction block resulting from edema and compression at the site of injury. Once remyelination occurs, complete recovery usually occurs within days or weeks, or up to 3 months if demyelination has occurred. Second-degree injury (axonotmesis) results in Wallerian degeneration distal to the injured site. Electromyographic (EMG) testing confirms the denervation, but reinnervation is expected as axons grow toward their target musculature roughly 1 mm/day. A second-degree injury is more severe than a first-degree conduction block, but endoneurial tubules remain intact to guide regenerating axons. Complete recovery is expected. Seddon used the term *neurotmesis* to mean complete disruption of the nerve. Sunderland's subclassification divided neurotmesis into third-degree injury (endoneurial disruption without loss of perineurium or epineurium), fourth-degree injury (disruption of endoneurium and perineurium), and fifth-degree injury (transection of endoneurium, perineurium, and epineurium). Third-degree injuries usually recover some function but with varying degrees of synkinesis. Fourth- and fifth-degree injuries do not recover. Unfortunately, electrical tests are unable to differentiate between axonotmesis and neurotmesis because both undergo Wallerian degeneration. One should recognize that each nerve trunk (within its epineurial sheath) contains numerous perineurial fascicles, which in turn ensheath large numbers of axon-containing endoneurial tubules. A compound nerve action potential and the resulting muscle twitch it engenders reflect the net effect of the electrical activity within the entire nerve trunk.

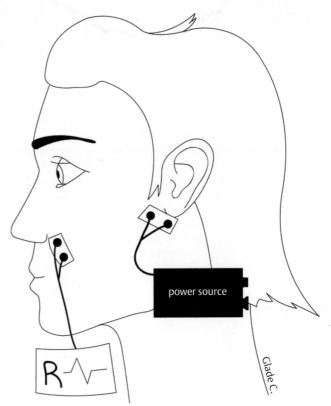

Figure 11–9 Electroneurography (ENoG) uses suprathreshold electrical stimuli applied bilaterally at the stylomastoid foramina to elicit a maximal contraction on each side. Bipolar pads placed along the nasolabial folds record the compound action potential from the underlying mimetic musculature.

◆ Preoperative Electrophysiologic Testing of the Seventh Cranial Nerve

The preoperative status of CNs VII and VIII are of particular interest to the otologist and are covered elsewhere in this text. The following section describes electrophysiologic testing of the facial nerve using the nerve excitability test, maximal stimulation test, electroneurography, and EMG.

The nerve excitability test (NET) uses an electrical current to stimulate the facial nerve at the stylomastoid foramen. A minimum threshold stimulus for initiating perceptible facial motion on the uninjured side is established first. This threshold is then compared with the threshold obtained from the injured side. A 3.5-mA or greater difference in thresholds between the two sides represents a significant difference. Assessing the mimetic response is qualitative and subject to interobserver variability.

The maximal stimulation test (MST) delivers suprathreshold stimuli at the stylomastoid foramen bilaterally while an observer grades the maximal mimetic response obtained from each side. This test is qualitative and subject to interobserver variability.

Electroneurography (ENoG) is a quantitative electrical test of facial nerve function. As with MST, suprathreshold electrical stimuli are applied bilaterally at the stylomastoid foramina to elicit a maximal contraction on each side. In its original description, bipolar pads placed along the nasolabial folds recorded the compound action potential from the underlying mimetic musculature (**Fig. 11–9**). Direct measurement of these potentials using EMG electrodes is now referred to as evoked electromyography (EEMG). Both techniques provide similar information. The amplitude of these potentials is proportional to the number of functional motor axons present within the facial nerve.[4] Peak-to-peak amplitude differences between the normal and involved sides of the face are expressed mathematically as percent-degeneration of axons within the injured nerve. ENoG is a time-limited study and should be performed between 3 and 21 days after neural injury. Wallerian degeneration distal to the site of an intracranial or intratemporal facial nerve injury takes place within 72 hours, and a proximally injured nerve continues to stimulate at the stylomastoid foramen until that time. Therefore, ENoG is unreliable for the first 3 days after the onset of facial paralysis. This test also becomes unreliable after 3 weeks. By this time, axons in varying stages of degeneration and regeneration create desynchronous neural activity. Clinically, ENoG has been used to determine when surgical intervention might be appropriate for patients with facial paralysis.[5,6]

Either spontaneous or voluntary EMG activity can be recorded from mimetic muscles innervated by all five terminal branches of the facial nerve. Spontaneous EMG activity is classified as normal (di- or triphasic), polyphasic potentials, or fibrillation potentials. The presence of fibrillation potentials reflects relatively recent denervation at the motor end plate, whereas long-standing denervation results in electrical silence.[7,8] Testing spontaneous EMG is most useful during nerve regeneration. The presence of polyphasic EMG potentials in a patient with complete clinical facial paralysis reflects active neuronal reinnervation. In fact, these polyphasic potentials can precede functional recovery by several weeks.

Fisch[5] suggested that greater than 90% degeneration on ENoG within 3 weeks of facial nerve injury justifies surgical decompression. More recently, Gantz and associates,[6] in a multicenter clinical trial of Bell's palsy, demonstrated that patients with greater than 90% degeneration on ENoG testing and no evidence of voluntary potentials on EMG within 14 days of facial paralysis had improved outcomes with surgical decompression. Outcomes in patients electing middle fossa decompression medial to the geniculate ganglion were compared with those patients who refused surgery. Those undergoing surgical decompression exhibited a House-Brackmann (HB) grade I or II in 91% of cases, whereas the control group had a 58% chance of an unfavorable HB grade III or IV recovery at 7 months. In 1999, Chang and Cass[9] extensively reviewed the literature on facial nerve injury in temporal bone trauma. They suggested that patients with greater than 95% degeneration within 2 weeks of injury may benefit from decompression. Note that in both studies antiviral medications were not used.

◆ Intraoperative Cranial Nerve Monitoring

Cranial base surgery risks mechanical, ischemic, and thermal damage to CNs. Improved anesthetic techniques, better surgical instruments, control of perioperative infections, and better postoperative care have reduced mortality rates significantly. Attention is now also focused on preserving CN function. Intraoperative nerve monitoring has been increasingly utilized during cranial base surgery to achieve this goal.

Background

During the late nineteenth and early twentieth centuries, Krause[10] and Frazier[11] described using monopolar electrical current for stimulating the facial nerve. Surgeons were limited to assessing the neuromuscular mimetic response by physical examination until 1979, when Delgado and associates[12] introduced intraoperative, recordable facial EMG. Sugita and Kobayashi[13] then coupled the EMG to a loudspeaker, making muscle activity audible to the surgeon. Innovations in monitoring have since continued. In 1991, Schmid and colleagues[14] reported central magnetic stimulation of the facial nerve. Neurophysiologic monitoring has become a profession in itself with various societies and certifying bodies including the American Board of Registered Electrodiagnostics Technologists (ABRET), the Certification in Neurophysiological Intraoperative Monitoring (CNIM), and the American Board of Neurophysiologic Monitoring (ABNM).

Modern vestibular schwannoma (VS) surgery successfully preserves the anatomic integrity of the facial nerve in more than 90% of cases.[15,16] Attention is also now turned to hearing preservation during VS procedures. Since the initial description of the human auditory brainstem response in 1971,[17] intraoperative auditory brainstem response (ABR), electrocochleography, otoacoustic emissions, and direct eighth nerve monitoring have emerged as potentially useful techniques designed to save hearing.

Equipment

A complete inventory of monitoring equipment is beyond the scope of this text. However, a brief overview is warranted. CNs III to VII and IX to XII are typically monitored using spontaneous or evoked EMG. Multichannel EMG devices are capable of recording electrical activity in several muscle groups simultaneously. Because the operating room is an electrically and acoustically hostile environment, these systems must mute their audible responses upon detecting interference from other equipment. High- and low-pass acoustic filters can help reduce signal artifacts.[18]

Several electrode designs are available. These include monopolar or bipolar surface and needle electrodes. Bipolar needle electrodes inserted directly into the muscles being monitored provide the best signal-to-noise ratio. Insulated needle electrodes or hook-wire electrodes allow for deeper insertions when necessary. When placing bipolar recording electrodes, the operator must take care not to allow contact between the EMG needles to prevent short circuits. Stimulator probes also come in monopolar and bipolar varieties. Insulated monopolar probes are less bulky and provide 1-mm spatial resolution.[19] Equipment manufacturers now make surgical dissection instruments coupled directly to monopolar stimulating probes.

Intraoperative ABR, electrocochleography (ECochG), otoacoustic emissions (OAEs), and direct eighth nerve monitoring are techniques used to monitor the vestibulocochlear nerve. Intraoperative ABR requires a sound source, surface electroencephalogram (EEG) electrodes and amplifiers, a computer for averaging ABR sweeps, and a monitor for displaying the tracing. ECochG also requires a sound source but can utilize a variety of different recording electrodes. Transtympanic electrodes provide the best ECochG tracing but risk tympanic membrane perforation and subsequent cerebrospinal fluid (CSF) leakage. Tympanic membrane electrodes placed in contact with the eardrum generate the next-best signal-to-noise ratio without the risk of perforation. Direct eighth nerve monitoring techniques use wire electrodes, wick electrodes, or the recently available Cueva electrode. The Cueva electrode (Ad-Tech, Racine, WI) is a C-shaped monopolar electrode that can be attached directly to the cochlear nerve (**Fig. 11–10**). Recording otoacoustic emissions requires a sound source and microphones placed within the ear canal.

Laryngeal EMG recordings (tenth nerve monitoring) from each vocal fold can now be obtained using the Medtronic-Xomed (Jacksonville, FL) endotracheal tube with built-in EMG electrodes (**Fig. 11–11**).

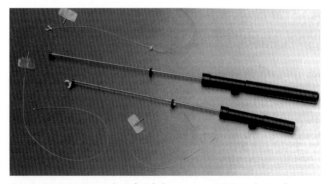

Figure 11–10 Examples of eighth nerve monitoring electrodes include the flat electrode used during middle fossa procedures and the Cueva C-shaped electrode. (From Yingling CD, Ashram YA. Intraoperative monitoring of cranial nerves in skull base surgery. In: Jackler RK, Brackmann DE, eds. Neurotology, 2nd ed. Philadelphia: Elsevier Mosby, 2005:958–994. Reprinted with permission.)

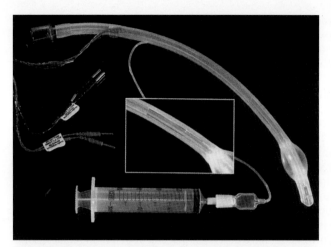

Figure 11–11 The laryngeal electromyographic endotracheal tube (Medtronic Xomed, Jacksonville, FL). Central stimulation of the vagus nerve results in recurrent laryngeal nerve activation and monitored EMG activity within the vocalis muscle. (From Yingling CD, Ashram YA. Intraoperative monitoring of cranial nerves in skull base surgery. In: Jackler RK, Brackmann DE, eds. Neurotology, 2nd ed. Philadelphia: Elsevier Mosby, 2005:958–994. Reprinted with permission.)

Stimuli

There is some debate regarding the optimal type, intensity, and duration of the stimulus applied during intraoperative evoked EMG. Constant-voltage stimulation adjusts the current applied through the stimulator probe to account for changes in tissue resistance over time. Constant-current stimulation adjusts voltage to keep current flow stable.[18] Surgeon preference usually dictates the type of stimulus used. Hughes and colleagues[20] have suggested that applying short-duration stimuli may lower the potential for neural damage. Some earlier animal studies by the same group call this conclusion into question.[21] Most surgeons use electrical stimuli of between a 50- and 200-μs duration. Some guidelines for facial nerve stimulus intensity during surgery are 0.05 to 0.2 mA for intracranial stimulation, 0.1 to 0.3 mA for intratemporal stimulation, and 0.1 to 0.5 mA for extracranial stimulation.[18]

Facial Nerve Monitoring

Acoustically coupled EMG remains the gold standard for intraoperative facial nerve monitoring.[22,23] Spontaneous EMG

recordings detect direct mechanical stimulation of the nerve, whereas stimulus-evoked EMG helps surgeons identify the nerve during difficult dissections. Prass and Leuders[24] described two patterns of EMG activity (**Fig. 11–12**). "Burst" activity refers to short, synchronized motor unit potentials resulting from direct stimulation, whereas "train" activity reflects asynchronous, often prolonged motor unit responses secondary to nerve irritation or traction. Trains are more frequently observed from nerves that have sustained preoperative compression, stretch, or ischemic injury.[18] Irrigation with warm saline usually quells a train response.

Large solid CPA tumors or smaller cystic tumors may splay the facial nerve, making it difficult to identify it anatomically even with high-power magnification. In such situations, electrophysiologic monitoring may be useful in "finding" the nerve. After establishing threshold intensity for stimulation using an easily identified segment of nerve, suprathreshold stimuli are used to "search" for the nerve. Although a positive response does help the operator, a negative response can mean anything from the nerve not being present in that location to a monitor malfunction, temporary nerve dysfunction, effects from anesthesia, electrical interference, or probe failure. Therefore, the monitor is not a substitute for a thorough knowledge of the anatomy, surgical experience, and good judgment.

Intraoperative facial nerve monitoring can help predict postoperative facial function. Several studies have found a higher rate of HB grade I or II outcomes and fewer HB V or VI in monitored patients.[25–30] In a series of 67 patients, Fenton and coworkers[31] reported that all patients with an EMG response after tumor removal recovered facial function to at least an HB grade III. Electrical silence portends a bad outcome.[32] Beck and associates[33] found that a nerve stimulated to 500 μV with a 0.05-mA current correlates with a postoperative HB grade I or II. Neff and colleagues[16] found that if the facial nerve stimulated to 240 μV with a 0.05-mA stimulus, this predicted an HB grade I or II outcome in 85% of patients. Mandpe and coworkers[34] reported that only 41% of patients stimulating to less than 200 μV achieved an HB grade I or II recovery.

The 1991 National Institutes of Health (NIH) consensus conference on vestibular schwannoma advocated routine facial nerve monitoring during neurotologic resection.[35] The decision to monitor other otologic cases, however, should be left to the surgeon's discretion. In a survey by Roland and Meyerhoff,[36] 95% of otologists and neurotologists believed that facial monitoring should be used only in high-risk ear

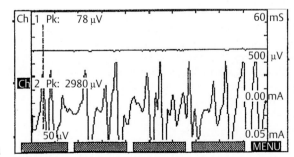

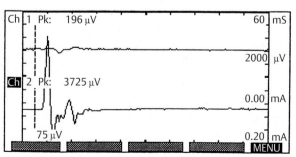

Figure 11–12 Intraoperative, two-channel monitoring of the facial EMG. **(A)** Traction applied to a motor nerve may evoke prolonged trains of motor unit activity that are temporally unrelated to the duration of the traction. These potentials reflect asynchronous, autoregenerative neural discharges. **(B)** During posterior fossa and middle ear surgery the facial nerve may be activated electrically. Effective stimulation yields a single compound MAP, synchronized to the delivered stimulus. MAP, muscle action potential.

procedures. The monitor should not be considered the standard of care for all otologic cases and certainly does not excuse poor operative technique.

Monitoring Other Cranial Nerves

CNs III, IV, and VI may be monitored directly by inserting long, insulated needle electrodes into the extraocular muscles. Although this is technically feasible, the potential for globe injury limits its utility. Instead, shorter bipolar electrodes can be placed in proximity to the extraocular muscles to obtain electrical signals by volume conduction. Electrodes may be placed along the medial infraorbital rim (inferior rectus or inferior oblique muscles, CN III), the lateral orbital rim (lateral rectus muscle, CN VI), and along the superior orbital rim just lateral to the supratrochlear foramen (superior oblique muscle, CN IV).[37]

The motor division of the mandibular nerve (V_3) can be monitored using EMG electrodes placed in either the temporalis or masseter muscles. Because of interference from overlying mimetic muscles, recording from the masseter requires deep electrode insertion. Monitoring the temporalis muscle is ideal but may be limited during neurotologic cases by the sterile surgical field.

The stylopharyngeus muscle (CN IX) can be monitored by placing electrodes into the ipsilateral posterior soft palate. As mentioned earlier, Medtronic-Xomed now offers a commercially available endotracheal tube with integrated EMG electrodes for monitoring CN X (**Fig. 11–11**). EMG monitoring of the SCM or trapezius muscle provides information about CN XI, and the hypoglossal nerve can be monitored with electrodes placed directly into the tongue.

◆ Intraoperative Monitoring of Auditory Function

Auditory function may be monitored using the ABR, the eighth nerve compound action potential (CNAP; also called direct eighth nerve monitoring, DENM), OAE, and ECochG. Multiple modalities can be used simultaneously.

Intraoperative Auditory Brainstem Response

The ABR is a set of seven peaks named by consecutive roman numerals. Only patients with a discernible wave I on ABR preoperatively can be monitored with intraoperative ABR, and normalized latency values for ABR are not useful in these patients. Each patient must have a baseline ABR established just prior to the start of the operation. Click stimuli >70 dB sound level (SL) are typically delivered at 20 to 30 clicks per second.[37] Each ABR sweep is filtered and averaged by a computer, which then engenders interpretable waveforms. The delay from stimulus to readable waveform may be up to several minutes. Acoustic interference from instruments such as electrocautery or the drill is a significant limitation of intraoperative ABR. Cerebellar retraction, dissection, acoustic trauma, temperature changes, and interruptions to cochlear blood flow can also affect the ABR.[37]

Matthies and Samii[38] reported the utility of intraoperative bilateral ABR in more than 200 VS resections. Temporary or permanent losses of waves V, I, and III occurred in 21%, 27%, and 29% of patients, respectively. Wave III disappearance reflecting loss of activity in the first brainstem nucleus was the earliest and most sensitive sign of trauma to the auditory nerve. Other clinicians prefer to monitor wave V. Much of the more recent literature on intraoperative ABR monitoring compares this modality to other, newer monitoring techniques.

Direct VIII Nerve Potentials

The eighth CNAP (or DENM) is measured directly using specifically designed electrodes (**Fig. 11–10**). These high amplitude responses require minimal signal averaging and permit nearly real-time data acquisition.[18] In general, monopolar electrodes are used more frequently than bipolar electrodes. Rosenberg and colleagues,[39] however, reported a specially designed flush-tipped, bipolar electrode to help define the cochlear-vestibular cleavage plane during vestibular nerve section. Moller and coworkers[40] have described placement of a monopolar recording electrode in the lateral recess of the fourth ventricle. Using this technique, potentials were recorded directly from the cochlear nucleus (rather than the eighth nerve trunk). They purport that the electrode is not in the way during tumor dissection, and CNAPs were recorded 20 to 50 times faster than ABR tracings. The Cueva electrode (Ad-Tech), with its unique C-shape can be attached directly to the cochlear nerve (**Fig. 11–10**). Unfortunately, most electrode designs are limited because the electrode must be placed on a clear segment of normal cochlear nerve. The cochlear nerve is not readily visible, however, early in middle fossa cases. Therefore, during these procedures, Roberson et al.[41] has described using a plate electrode placed along the floor of the IAC.

Stretching the nerve increases response latency first before affecting the response amplitude.[42] CNAP amplitudes then decline progressively with greater amounts of auditory nerve damage.[42] Yamakami and coworkers[43] found DENM to be more useful than ABR in 10 patients undergoing CPA tumor surgery. Hearing was preserved in eight of the 10 patients postoperatively. ABR was useless in six of the 10 patients due to severe artifacts. This group found that DENM more accurately predicted postoperative hearing outcome.

Electrocochleography

Electrocochleography records the cochlear microphonic (CM), summating potential (SP), and the eighth nerve action potential (AP) in response to sound stimuli. Therefore, ECochG reflects only the status of the cochlea and distal auditory nerve. It has found limited utility during acoustic neuroma or jugular foramen surgery. Bojrab and colleagues[44] found ECochG to be useful in localizing the endolymphatic sac during shunt surgery for Meniere's disease. However, it did not predict either postoperative hearing status or improvement in vertigo. Krueger and Storper[45] found that the SP/AP ratio decreased by more than 25% in 93% of the Meniere's patients after sectioning the vestibular nerve. Mullatti and colleagues[46] noted that the CNAP of the ECochG was 2.5 times greater in amplitude than the wave I of the ABR and required minimal signal averaging.

Otoacoustic Emissions

Otoacoustic emissions (OAEs) reflect intact outer hair cell function within the organ of Corti. Filipo and coworkers[47] found that transient-evoked otoacoustic emissions (TEOAEs) were markedly affected by ambient operating room noise and were unreliable for intraoperative monitoring. Telischi and colleagues[48] reported that changes in distortion-product otoacoustic emissions (DPOAEs) were exquisitely sensitive to interruptions in cochlear blood flow. Recordings could be obtained as frequently as every 2 seconds and provided nearly real-time data. Morawski and associates[49] used DPOAEs monitoring in 20 patients undergoing resection of acoustic tumors using a retrosigmoid approach. They found that DPOAEs from the basal regions (high frequency) of the cochlea were more readily affected by surgical manipulation than those from middle and apical segments (middle and low frequencies). Microcoagulation of small vessels, tumor debulking, and compression or stretch of IAC contents resulted in altered DPOAEs. This group felt that the DPOAEs did not assist the surgeon during tumor dissection, but the presence of DPOAEs at the end of the procedure correlated with postoperative hearing outcomes.

Hearing Outcomes

Numerous variables confound interpretation of clinical outcomes for hearing preservation. The technical skill of the surgeon, the surgical approach used, different types of monitoring equipment, and various criteria for meaningful postoperative hearing affect the interpretation of available data.

Several studies have compared ABR, ECochG, and DENM. Yamakami and colleagues[43] found ABR recordings to be unsatisfactory in six of 10 patients undergoing hearing-preservation approaches for CPA tumors, whereas CNAPs were obtained in all 10 patients intraoperatively. The authors felt that CNAP amplitude more consistently predicted postoperative hearing results. Defining hearing preservation as any measurable hearing, Tucker and coworkers[50] also compared ABR with CNAPs. The presence of both ABR and CNAP at the end of resection was associated with successful hearing preservation, whereas their absence was associated with loss of hearing in 75.5% of cases. Unfortunately, no association was found between ABR, CNAP, and hearing preservation in nearly 25% of cases. Using postoperative pure-tone thresholds and word recognition scores as outcome measures, Battista and colleagues[51] compared ABR, ECochG, and DENM retrospectively in 66 patients. Overall, 24% of patients retained useful hearing. Forty-percent of DENM patients retained their hearing, whereas only 18% of ABR and 17% of ECochG patients retained theirs. Jackson and Roberson[52] compared CNAP with ABR in 25 patients undergoing hearing preservation acoustic tumor surgery. Pure-tone average <50 dB and word recognition >50% was used to define successful hearing preservation. CNAPs were obtained in 92% of patients, whereas ABR was recordable in only 48%. For tumors less than or equal to 2 cm, hearing was preserved in 67% of those monitored with CNAPs. ABR monitoring did not significantly alter hearing preservation rates. Danner and associates[53] retrospectively compared use of DENM using the Cueva electrode in one group of patients with intraoperative ABR in another cohort. A total of 77 patients undergoing retrosigmoid resection of vestibular schwannomas were included in the study. In the DENM group, hearing was preserved in 71% of patients with tumors 1 cm or less and 32% with tumors between 1 and 2.5 cm. Hearing preservation using ABR was 41% and 10%, respectively. These authors concluded that DENM was superior to ABR in preserving hearing. In comparing ABR, CNAP, and ECochG, Colletti and associates[54] found that CNAPs were most predictive of hearing preservation. In fact, irreversible loss of

CNAPs was 100% predictive of poor postoperative hearing. Comparing ABR monitoring alone to ABR with simultaneous DENM, Colletti and Fiorino[55] found that the ABR-only group had significantly poorer pure tone outcomes (82 dB) than the dual-monitored group (54 dB). They felt that multimodality monitoring might provide additional clinical benefit.

◆ Conclusion

Accurately assessing CN function begins at the initial physician–patient encounter and continues throughout the evaluation and treatment period. Electrical testing is now part of the surgeon's technologic armamentarium, helping the operator preserve function while removing the disease. With improvements in anesthesia, perioperative care, and microsurgical techniques, complete tumor removal and patient survival are expected outcomes. Minimizing patient morbidity with respect to CN function has now become the next challenge in the practice of otology and neurotology.

References

1. Snell RS. Clinical Neuroanatomy: A Review with Questions and Explanations, 3rd ed. Philadelphia: Lippincott Williams Wilkins, 2001
2. Seddon HJ. Three types of nerve injury. Brain 1943;66:237–288
3. Sunderland S. Nerve and Nerve Injuries, 2nd ed. New York: Churchill Livingstone, 1978
4. Esslen E. The Acute Facial Palsies. Berlin: Springer-Verlag, 1977
5. Fisch U. Prognostic value of electrical tests in acute facial paralysis. Am J Otol 1984;5:494–498
6. Gantz BJ, Rubinstein JT, Gidley P, et al. Surgical management of Bell's palsy. Laryngoscope 1999;109:1177–1188
7. Dumitru D, Walsh NE, Porter LD. Electrophysiologic evaluation of the facial nerve in Bell's palsy. A review. Am J Phys Med Rehabil 1988;67:137–144
8. Barwick DD, Fawcett PRW. The clinical physiology of neuromuscular disease. In: Walton J, ed. Disorders of Voluntary Muscle. Edinburgh, England: Churchill Livingstone, 1988:1015–1080
9. Chang CY, Cass SP. Management of facial injury due to temporal bone trauma. Am J Otol 1999;20:96–114
10. Krause F. Surgery of the Brain and Spinal Cord, vol 2. New York: Rebman, 1912
11. Frazier CH. Intracranial division of the auditory nerve for persistent aural vertigo. Surg Gynecol Obstet 1912;15:524–529
12. Delgado TE, Bucheit WA, Rosenholtz HR, Chrissian S. Intraoperative monitoring of facial muscle evoked responses obtained by intracranial stimulation of the facial nerve: a more accurate technique for facial nerve dissection. Neurosurgery 1979;4:418–421
13. Sugita K, Kobayashi S. Technical and instrumental improvements in the surgical treatment of acoustic neurinomas. J Neurosurg 1982;57:747–752
14. Schmid UD, Moller AR, Schmid J. Transcranial magnetic stimulation excites the labyrinthine segment of the facial nerve: an intraoperative electrophysiological study in man. Neurosci Lett 1991;124:273–276
15. Kartush J, Lundy L. Facial nerve outcome in acoustic neuroma surgery. Otolaryngol Clin North Am 1992;25:623–647
16. Neff BA, Ting J, Dickinson SL, Welling DB. Facial nerve monitoring parameters as a predictor of postoperative facial nerve outcomes after vestibular schwannoma resection. Otol Neurotol 2005;26:728–732
17. Jewett DL, Williston JS. Auditory evoked far fields averaged from the scalp of humans. Brain 1971;94:681–696
18. Martin WH, Mishler ET. Intraoperative monitoring of auditory evoked potentials and facial nerve electromyography. In: Katz ed. Handbook of Clinical Audiology, 5th ed. Philadelphia: Lippincott Williams & Wilkins, 2002:323–348
19. Kartush JM, Niparko JK, Bledsoe SC, Graham MD, Kemink JL. Intraoperative facial nerve monitoring: a comparison of stimulating electrodes. Laryngoscope 1985;95:1536–1540
20. Hughes G, Chase S, Dudley A, et al. Safety of electrical stimulation of peripheral nerves. Potentials. In: Portmann M, ed. The Facial Nerve. Paris: Masson, 1985:381–384

21. Hughes GB, Bottomy MB, Dickins JR, et al. A comparative study of neuropathologic changes following pulsed and direct current stimulation of the mouse sciatic nerve. Am J Otolaryngol 1980;1:378–384

22. Nadol JB Jr, Chiong CM, Ojemann RG, et al. Preservation of hearing and facial nerve function in resection of acoustic neuromas. Laryngoscope 1992;102:1153–1158

23. Beck DL, Benecke JE Jr. Intraoperative facial nerve monitoring. Technical aspects. Otolaryngol Head Neck Surg 1990;102:270–272

24. Prass RL, Leuders H. Acoustic (loudspeaker) facial electromyographic monitoring: Part 1. Evoked electromyographic activity during acoustic neuroma resection. Neurosurgery 1986;19:392–400

25. Kwartler JA, Luxford WM, Atkins J, Shelton C. Facial nerve monitoring in acoustic tumor surgery. Otolaryngol Head Neck Surg 1991;104:814–817

26. Hammerschlag P, Cohen N. Intraoperative monitoring of facial nerve function in cerebellopontine angle surgery. Otolaryngol Head Neck Surg 1990;103:681–684

27. Harner SG, Daube JR, Beatty CW, Ebersold MJ. Intraoperative monitoring of the facial nerve. Laryngoscope 1988;98:209–212

28. Kartush JM. Electroneurography and intraoperative facial nerve monitoring in contemporary neurotology. Otolaryngol Head Neck Surg 1989;101:496–503

29. Benecke JE Jr, Calder HB, Chadwick G. Facial nerve monitoring during acoustic neuroma removal. Laryngoscope 1987;97:697–700

30. Leonetti JP, Matz GJ, Smith PG, Beck DL. Facial nerve monitoring in otologic surgery: clinical indications and intraoperative technique. Ann Otol Rhinol Laryngol 1990;99:911–918

31. Fenton JE, Chin RY, Shirazi A, Fagan PA. Prediction of postoperative facial nerve function in acoustic neuroma surgery. Clin Otolaryngol Allied Sci 1999;24:483–486

32. Nakao Y, Piccirillo E, Falcioni M, et al. Prediction of facial nerve outcome using electromyographic responses in acoustic neuroma surgery. Otol Neurotol 2002;23:93–95

33. Beck DL, Atkins JS Jr, Benecke JE Jr, Brackmann DE. Intraoperative facial nerve monitoring: prognostic aspects during acoustic tumor removal. Otolaryngol Head Neck Surg 1991;104:780–782

34. Mandpe AH, Mikulec A, Jackler RK, et al. Comparison of response amplitude versus stimulation threshold in predicting early postoperative facial nerve function after acoustic neuroma resection. Am J Otol 1998;19:112–117

35. National Institutes of Health Consensus Statement. Acoustic neuromas. NIH Consensus Development Conference, Bethesda MD, December 11–13, 1991

36. Roland PS, Meyerhoff WL. Intraoperative electrophysiological monitoring of the facial nerve: is it standard of practice? Am J Otolaryngol 1994;15:267–270

37. Yingling CD, Ashram YA. Intraoperative monitoring of cranial nerves in skull base surgery. In: Jackler RK, Brackmann DE eds. Neurotology, 2nd ed. Philadelphia: Elsevier Mosby, 2005:958–994

38. Matthies C, Samii M. Management of vestibular schwannomas (acoustic neuromas): the value of neurophysiology for intraoperative monitoring of auditory function in 200 cases. Neurosurgery 1997;40:459–466 discussion 466–8

39. Rosenberg SI, Martin WH, Pratt H, et al. Bipolar cochlear nerve recording technique: a preliminary report. Am J Otol 1993;14:362–368

40. Moller AR, Jho HD, Jannetta PJ. Preservation of hearing in operations on acoustic tumors: an alternative to recording brain stem auditory evoked potentials. Neurosurgery 1994;34:688–692 discussion 692–3

41. Roberson J, Senne A, Brackmann D, et al. Direct cochlear nerve action potentials as an aid to hearing preservation in middle fossa acoustic neuroma resections. Am J Otol 1996;17:653–657

42. Moller AR. Evoked Potentials in Intraoperative Monitoring. Baltimore: Williams & Wilkins, 1988

43. Yamakami I, Oka N, Yamaura A. Intraoperative monitoring of cochlear nerve compound action potential in cerebellopontine angle tumour removal. J Clin Neurosci 2003;10:567–570

44. Bojrab DI, Bhansali SA, Andreozzi MP. Intraoperative electrocochleography during endolymphatic sac surgery: clinical results. Otolaryngol Head Neck Surg 1994;111:478–484

45. Krueger WW, Storper IS. Electrocochleography in retrosigmoid vestibular nerve section for intractable vertigo caused by Meniere's disease. Otolaryngol Head Neck Surg 1997;116:593–596

46. Mullatti N, Coakham HB, Maw AR, et al. Intraoperative monitoring during surgery for acoustic neuroma: benefits of an extratympanic intrameatal electrode. J Neurol Neurosurg Psychiatry 1999;66:591–599

47. Filipo R, Delfini R, Fabiani M, et al. Role of transient-evoked otoacoustic emissions for hearing preservation in acoustic neuroma surgery. Am J Otol 1997;18:746–749

48. Telischi FF, Widick MP, Lonsbury-Martin BL, et al. Monitoring cochlear function intraoperatively using distortion product otoacoustic emissions. Am J Otol 1995;16:597–608

49. Morawski K, Namyslowski G, Lisowska G, et al. Intraoperative monitoring of cochlear function using distortion product otoacoustic emissions (DPOAEs) in patients with cerebellopontine angle tumors. Otol Neurotol 2004;25:818–825

50. Tucker A, Slattery WH, Solcyk L, et al. Intraoperative auditory assessments as predictors of hearing preservation after vestibular schwannoma surgery. J Am Acad Audiol 2001;12:471–477

51. Battista RA, Wiet RJ, Paauwe L. Evaluation of three intraoperative auditory monitoring techniques in acoustic neuroma surgery. Am J Otol 2000;21:244–248

52. Jackson LE, Roberson JB Jr. Acoustic neuroma surgery: use of cochlear nerve action potential monitoring for hearing preservation. Am J Otol 2000;21:249–259

53. Danner C, Mastrodimos B, Cueva RA. A comparison of direct eighth nerve monitoring and auditory brain stem response in hearing preservation surgery for vestibular schwannoma. Otol Neurotol 2004;25:826–832

54. Colletti V, Fiorino FG, Mocella S, Policante Z. ECochG, CNAP and ABR monitoring during vestibular schwannoma surgery. Audiology 1998;37:27–37

55. Colletti V, Fiorino FG. Advances in monitoring of seventh and eighth cranial nerve function during posterior fossa surgery. Am J Otol 1998;19:503–512

12

Otologic Photography and Videography

Eiji Yanagisawa and Ken Yanagisawa

The first American photographic documentation of the tympanic membrane[1] occurred in 1887 when Randall and Morse[2] published a series of normal and pathologic images of the tympanic membrane. Since that time, many different methods of tympanic membrane photography have evolved.[3–16] Open tube photography was popularized using a variety of different cameras including the Cameron, Brubaker-Holinger, and Kowa.[3–6] Buckingham[3] first adapted the Brubaker-Holinger camera to ear photography in the mid-1950s, and produced beautiful, high-quality images of the tympanic membrane and middle ear. Smith et al[6] described an inexpensive method of producing high-resolution images of the tympanic membrane using a Kowa Fundus camera. Both of these methods produced small images that required editing and enlargement to be appreciated when projected. The introduction of the Carl Zeiss operating microscope in the late 1950s made it feasible to obtain enlarged images of the tympanic membrane. A variety of attachments was subsequently created that permitted 35 mm and video cameras to document images via photo adapters.[8,9] An alternative, less expensive method of photographing the tympanic membrane through the eyepiece of the microscope with a 35 mm single lens reflex (SLR) camera was described by Hughes et al[7] and Yanagisawa et al.[8]

The development of the Hopkins telescope was a significant advancement in endoscopic technology.[8–15] Rather than air-containing spaces between conventional lenses, glass rods with polished ends separated by small air lenses were used, greatly improving image quality, brightness, and magnification. Many clinicians including Konrad et al,[10] Chen et al,[11] Chole,[12] Nomura,[13] Yanagisawa,[8] and Hawke[14] have refined the techniques for improving the quality of images captured with the telescope. Several excellent textbooks of telescopic tympanic membrane photography have been published.[17–21] Selkin[16] has recommended fiberscopic photography as an alternative means to capture images of the tympanic membrane. Transtympanic endoscopy of the middle ear was pioneered by Nomura[13] in 1982 and advocated by Poe et al[22] as an office procedure to precede middle ear exploration using a 2-mm or smaller telescope by which they could take acceptable pictures of the middle ear structure.

With the advent of video cameras, Yanagisawa extensively used videography[23–26] as an ideal method for endoscopic documentation because it provides a real-time record of anatomic structures and their movements, and allows instantaneous review, confirming adequate image capture. He advocated the wider use of videography and video printers in otolaryngology.[23–27] Excellent still images could be produced from videotapes using an analog video printer.[23–28]

We are now in the era of digital imaging.[29,30] There are currently several newer digital image capture systems. One of us (E.Y.) had the opportunity to use one of these systems, the Stryker Digital Capture System (SDCS; Kalamazoo, MI) and found it to be very effective and promising. It is a device that quickly transports surgical images to a high-density computer disk. Image capture time is very fast, taking approximately 1 second. Stored images can be viewed, selected, and easily retrieved. It costs approximately $11,000.[30]

With the widespread use of still digital cameras, their use in otorhinolaryngologic endoscopy has been recommended.[30–34] Melder and Mair[31] compared an off-the-shelf digital camera with a standard single lens reflex 35 mm endoscopic camera and introduced a simple, inexpensive, and easily available endoscopic digital photography system. They stated that digital photography offers numerous advantages over analog photography. They predicted digital imaging would soon replace 35 mm camera photography.

Haynes et al[34] described the microscopic photographic technique with the handheld digital camera placed in contact with one of the microscope ocular lenses. Using this practical and inexpensive technique, it was possible to take beautiful pictures of a variety of microsurgical procedures through the eyepiece of the microscope.

This chapter discusses traditional (film) photography, digital (filmless) photography, and videography of the ear.

◆ Traditional (Film) Photography

Telescopic Film Photography

A majority of the tympanic membrane pictures shown in this book were taken with a Hopkins 4.0 mm telescope (Karl Storz 1215A, Culver City, CA) attached to an Olympus OM2 SLR camera with a 100-mm Zuiko lens (**Fig. 12–1A**). The 1–9

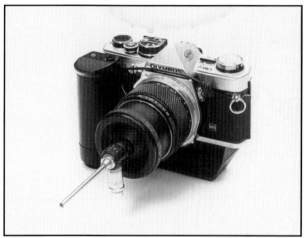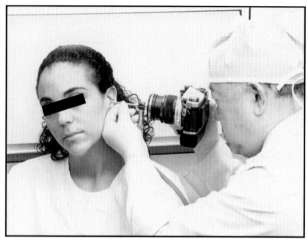

A B

Figure 12–1 Telescopic film photography of the ear. **(A)** Equipment recommended for telescopic film photography includes the Olympus OM2 SLR 35 mm camera with autowinder, the 100-mm macrolens, the Karl Storz quick-connect adapter, and the Hopkins 4 mm 0-degree 1215A ototelescope. **(B)** The technique of telescopic film photography.

An Olympus OM-2 SLR camera with a Hopkins 4 mm 0-degree 1215A ototelescope is held in one hand while the tip of the telescope and the head of the patient is supported by the other hand to prevent injury to the ear canal.

focusing camera screen and the autowinder were used. For the light source, Karl Storz flash generator (No. 558) was used. The distance of the lens of the camera was set at infinity and the shutter speed at 1/30 second. The intensity dial of the flash generator was set at 1. Best results were obtained with the aperture set at f/5.6 when Ektachrome Daylight film ASA 200 was used.

In this technique, the 4 mm telescope attached to the Olympus OM2 SLR camera is carefully inserted into the ear canal while the camera is held in one hand and the tip of the telescope and the head of the patient are supported by the other hand to prevent injury to the ear canal and the tympanic membrane (**Fig. 12–1B**).

The authors have also used a nonflash technique with a Nikon N8008 camera with the 55-mm Nikkor lens and 2X teleconverter. The camera was set at the automatic mode and f-stop at 5.6. The Karl Storz light source 610 was used.

The advantages of the telescopic technique include the following: (1) The entire tympanic membrane can be visualized, because the tip of the telescope can be passed through the narrow isthmus of the ear canal (**Fig. 12–2**). This is not the case in the microscopic techniques. (2) The wide-angle view of the telescope allows an almost infinite depth of field, so that all areas of the tympanic membrane are in focus. (3) No cropping or enlargement is required when the finished slides return from the processing laboratory. Using the 100-mm lens, the diameter of the image measures 21 mm on the finished slide.

The disadvantages of the telescopic technique include the following: (1) Lens fogging can be annoying, and frequent dips into warm water or anti-fog solution are needed. (2) Care must be taken not to touch the ear canal or the tympanic membrane. We recommend holding the camera in the right hand and grasping the telescope several centimeters from

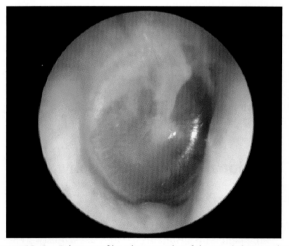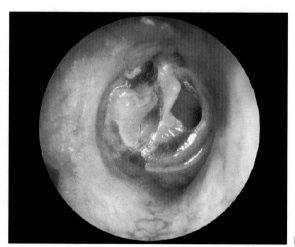

A B

Figure 12–2 Telescopic film photography of the ear. **(A)** Normal right tympanic membrane. **(B)** Right postoperative tympanoplasty with incus repositioning.

the tip in the left hand to stabilize the scope as well as to prevent excessive length from sliding into the ear canal (**Fig. 12–1B**). A pediatric patient is placed in the supine position with the head held steady by an assistant.

Microscopic Film Photography

Using the Zeiss operating microscope with a 250-mm lens, 35 mm still photographs can be taken with a SLR camera with or without a photoadapter.

Microscopic Film Photography Through the Eyepiece of the Microscope (Without a Photoadapter)

Microscopic photography through the eyepiece of the microscope using a 35 mm SLR camera without a photoadapter[8,9] requires the following equipment: (1) 35 mm SLR camera such as Olympus OM2 or Nikon 8008, with a 50-mm macrolens ("aperture-preferred" mode); (2) Ektachrome tungsten film ASA 320 (**Fig. 12–3A**).

With the eyepiece of the microscope set at 0, the tympanic membrane image is viewed through the microscope, centered, and focused. The focus on the camera is set at infinity with the aperture open maximally (typically f-3.5). The macrolens of the camera is placed gently but snugly against the eyepiece (**Fig. 12–3A**). The tympanic membrane is centered and photographs are taken.

The advantages of this technique include the following: (1) The technique is easy and simple to perform. (2) If you own a SLR camera and a macrolens, the technique is inexpensive. (3) Magnification changes can be made through the microscope. Surprisingly good pictures can be taken using this inexpensive technique (**Fig. 12–4A,B**).

The disadvantages of this technique include the following: (1) It may be difficult to hold the camera perfectly still on the microscope eyepiece. (2) Medical procedures must be interrupted to take the photograph. (3) Bright illumination is required or a film with high speed/high ASA rating (ASA 160 pushed to 320 or ASA 320 film).

Microscopic Film Photography with a Photoadapter

Microscopic photography using an SLR camera with a photoadapter requires the following equipment: (1) a Zeiss operating microscope; (2) a Zeiss beam splitter; (3) a photoadapter, such as Zeiss TV photoadapter, Zeiss-Urban dual adapter, or Design for Vision adapter (Storz Instruments, St. Louis, MO) (**Fig. 12–3B**); (4) an adapter ring for the SLR camera; (5) an automatic 35 mm SLR camera such as an Olympus OM2 or Nikon 8008; and (6) Ektachrome film ASA 400. The image is identified, centered, and focused through the operating microscope. Magnification is selected to best demonstrate the otologic findings. The camera is attached to a side arm via the beam splitter and photoadapter (**Fig. 12–3B**). It is set on automatic mode, and selected photographs are taken by depressing the shutter release button. Bracketing of exposures both under and over is recommended.

The advantages of this technique include the following: (1) The camera is steady. (2) The procedure is not interrupted. (3) Different magnifications of the microscope are readily available. (4) Simultaneous video and still photography can be performed if appropriate television still photoadapters are used. This is a more dependable technique of photography because the camera is fixed (**Fig. 12–4C,D**).

The disadvantages of this technique include the following: (1) The photoadapter and beam splitter are expensive. (2) An adapter ring for SLR camera is needed.

◆ Digital Photography (Filmless Photography)

Digital imaging is the newest technology for permanently recording images without film or videotape. An image obtained via a video camera is converted to an electronic signal that a computer can read, record, and store in a digital fashion.[30]

There are three primary approaches to creating digital images. The first is to convert a photograph or slide into a still digital image using an image scanner connected to

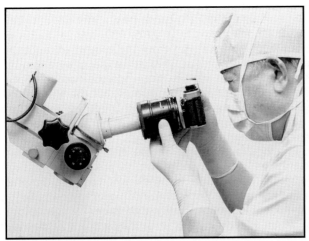
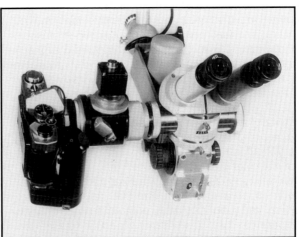

A   B

Figure 12–3 Microscopic still photography of the ear. **(A)** Technique of microscopic film photography through the eyepiece of the microscope without photoadapter. Recessed housing of the macrolens of an SLR camera is held against the eyepiece of the microscope. Make sure the optical line of the microscope and the camera is straight. The tympanic membrane is focused through the camera viewfinder and photographs are taken. **(B)** The technique of microscopic film photography with a photoadapter. The SLR camera is attached to the operating microscope using the photoadapter and the beam splitter. The subject is focused through the camera viewfinder and photographs are taken.

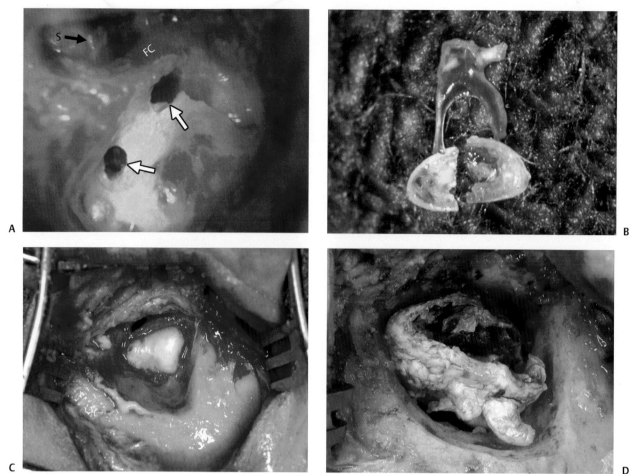

Figure 12–4 Microscopic film photography through the eyepiece of the microscope without a photoadapter. **(A)** Left mastoid cavity with opened horizontal semicircular canal (arrows) during labyrinthectomy. S, stapes; FC, facial canal. **(B)** Otosclerotic stapes removed during total stapedectomy. Microscopic film photography with a photoadapter. **(C)** Cholesteatoma filling the medial portion of the left mastoid cavity. **(D)** Large cholesteatoma filling the left mastoid cavity.

a computer. The second is to convert an analog signal from a video camera or videotape into streaming digital video with an image capture board installed in a computer. Such hardware is universally compatible with either a Macintosh- or a PC-based system. Using this method, the senior author has produced excellent images for his publications.[23-27] He uses ¾-inch prerecorded videotapes, a Macintosh computer, Avid Media Suite Pro video editing software, Adobe Photoshop, and a Sony digital dye-sublimation printer. Several easy and useful video editing applications are commercially available such as that by Pinnacle studio (Mountain View, CA). The third is to capture the image directly with a charge-coupled device (CCD) digital camera. This method bypasses conversion and starts with a digital image at the time of capture. Components of a digital imaging system include a digital camera, computer, removable memory storage, digital video recorder, and color digital printer.

Digital still cameras, like conventional film-based cameras, come in point-and-shoot and SLR models. Utilizing fixed lenses and a built-in flash, point-and-shoot cameras are inexpensive, easy to use, and generally smaller and lighter than SLR cameras. The disadvantages of point-and-shoot models include less flexibility in controlling the features of the camera and lower resolution. In contrast, SLR cameras have modified the typical film-based 35 mm camera by replacing the film advanced system with the CCD and processing hardware and liquid crystal diode (LCD) screen. SLR-derived digital cameras are usually larger than point-and-shoot digital cameras and more expensive, but produce superior quality images.

There are many digital still cameras available that can be used for endoscopy including the (1) Nikon CoolPix 5000[32]; (2) Olympus C-4040; (3) Canon Power Shot G6[31]; (4) Canon EOS 20D[33]; (5) Nikon D70, D70S, D50; and (6) Kodak Easy Share DX7630 Zoom. Selecting the camera for endoscopic photography depends on whether the user needs a step-up or step-down ring in addition to an endoscopic adapter. Specific digital camera adapters are available for the Nikon CoolPix 5000 and Olympus C4040. Rapid technologic advances have led to constant improvements in features and size of the camera, thus often lowering the price.

For medical use, one should choose a 3.1 or greater megapixel digital camera, which produces high-quality images.[32] It should also be lightweight, compact, convenient, affordable, and easy to handle. Additional advantages of digital imaging include the ability, at the time of image capture, to highlight selected areas of interest by scrolling or magnifying within the LCD display. Furthermore, digital images are easily annotated or edited utilizing commercially available applications such as Adobe Photoshop. Digital imaging is an effective and convenient method for storing, delivering, and archiving multiple images within a compact medium.

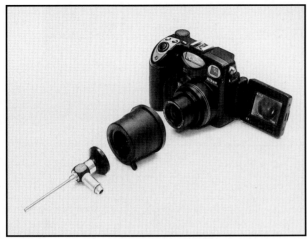
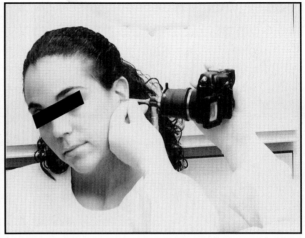

A   B

Figure 12–5 Telescopic digital photography of the ear. **(A)** Equipment recommended for telescopic digital photography of the ear includes a digital camera (e.g., Nikon CoolPix 5000), an endoscopic digital camera mounting adapter, and a Hopkins 4 mm ototelescope. The Nikon CoolPix 5000 has a LCD monitor that flips and twists. **(B)** Technique of telescopic digital photography. A Hopkins telescope attached to a Nikon CoolPix 5000 is carefully inserted into the ear canal. When the desired image is visualized, gently press the shutter release button on the camera halfway. When the image becomes focused, press the shutter release button all the way.

We chose the Nikon CoolPix 5000 (**Fig. 12–5A**), which is a 5.0-megapixel CCD camera with a 3X zoom lens, with a focal range of 7.1 to 21.4 mm (equivalent to 28 to 85 mm in the 35 mm format) producing high-resolution images (2560×1920 pixels).[32] Its small size and compact design is an advantage. The Nikon CoolPix 5000 has an LCD that allows for better visualization before image capture as well as immediate review. The flip-out and twist LCD monitor has proved to be extremely useful. It is an adjustable monitor that folds out and swivels to allow photographs to be framed with the camera held at arm's length, or folds back onto the camera body to make a more compact unit. The camera can also be connected to an external monitor or television through the audiovisual output cable. The Nikon CoolPix 5000 allows image transfer to a computer hard drive via a universal serial bus (USB) cable.

The Nikon CoolPix 5000 camera costs approximately $700 or less and the digital camera mounting adapter is about $275, totaling $975.[32] The adapter is manufactured by Precision Optics Corporation Inc. of Gardner, Massachusetts.

Telescopic Digital Photography

Telescopic digital photography requires (1) a Hopkins 4 mm 0-degree telescope (**Fig. 12–5A**), (2) a light source (Karl Storz 615, 610, 481C, Xenon Nova) and light cable, (3) a digital camera (e.g., Nikon CoolPix 5000), (4) an endoscopic digital camera mounting adapter, and (5) a computer. No step-up/-down ring is necessary. We use the Nikon CoolPix 5000 because (1) it is compact and easy to use, (2) it is affordable (in the middle range), and (3) it has a good macrofocus ability.

With the patient in a sitting position, the telescope is carefully advanced into the ear canal (**Fig. 12–5B**). Select the size of the images by controlling the zoom button. When the desired image is visualized, gently press the shutter release button on the camera halfway. The green light on the viewfinder will light up and flash. Wait until this flashing light becomes a steady light, indicating it is focused. Press the release button all the way down to take a picture.

An advantage of digital imaging is that you can immediately observe the image you have taken in the LCD monitor. If it is unsatisfactory, you can repeat it. You do not have to wait for an hour or longer, as in the case of film photography. The system we use usually takes very good pictures (**Fig. 12–6A,B**).

A disadvantage of digital imaging is that it may take some time for the camera to focus the image. The images on the LCD monitor may become too dark or too bright and it may be difficult to see and focus. This may depend on the angle at which you view the LCD. But these cases are rare. You have to get accustomed to each digital camera.

Microscopic Digital Photography

Microscopic Digital Photography Through the Eyepiece of the Microscope (Without a Photoadapter)[34]

This is a "digital" version of microscopic film photography through the eyepiece of the microscope without a photoadapter. In this technique, instead of a standard 35 mm automatic SLR camera, a digital still camera is used. The technique is practically the same as the microscopic film photography through the eyepiece.

To take a picture, make sure that the microscope is stable and fixed. The subject is centered and focused through the microscope first. The front end of the digital camera is placed gently but snugly against the eyepiece of the microscope (**Fig. 12–7A**) or the assistant's observation tube (**Fig. 12–7B**). The size of the image is adjusted using the digital zoom. The microscope and the digital camera are held still, making sure that the optical line of the long axis of the microscope eyepiece is aligned with the digital camera. When the images are chosen, depress the shutter release button halfway. The flashing green light in the viewfinder box changes to a steady green when images are focused. Depress the shutter release button all the way. The picture is immediately reviewed in the LCD monitor of the digital camera (**Fig. 12–8**). If the captured image is unsatisfactory, repeat this procedure until the desired image is obtained.

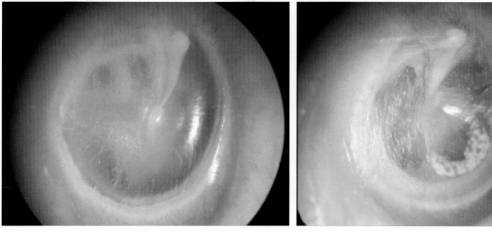

A

B

Figure 12–6 Telescopic digital photography of the ear. **(A)** Right normal tympanic membrane. **(B)** Right atrophic tympanic membrane with healed perforation.

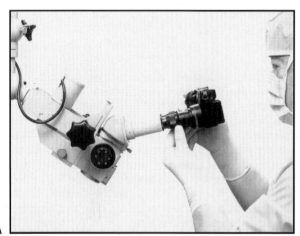

A

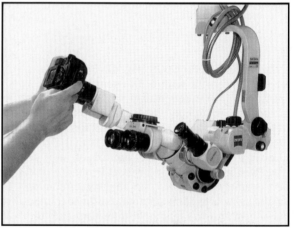

B

Figure 12–7 Microscopic digital photography of the ear.
(A) Microscopic digital photography through the eyepiece of the microscope. The camera is handheld and the tip of the camera is held against the eyepiece of the microscope. The ear is centered and

focused. When the subject is in focus, depress the shutter release button all the way. **(B)** Microscopic digital photography through the eyepiece using the assistant observation tube. When the pictures are taken in this way, the operation is not interrupted.

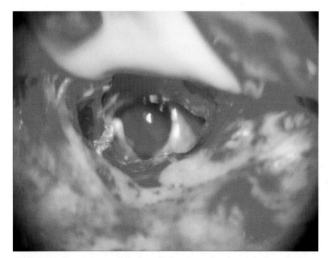

Figure 12–8 Microscopic digital photography through the eyepiece of the microscope. Intraoperative image during repair of a subtotal perforation of the right tympanic membrane. The image may not be ideal but may improve with experience.

The largest disadvantage of this technique is the potentially cumbersome orientation between the long axis of the microscope eyepiece and the digital camera. Optional accessories available from the manufacturer may facilitate this process with compatible hardware. The endoscopic digital camera mounting adapter can be used to stabilize the digital camera. The other disadvantage is that, in the operating room, sterile operative procedures are interrupted because the assistant has to take the picture or the surgeon has to change gloves to take the picture.

Assuming that the microscope is available in the operating room, this is the least expensive way to photograph the middle ear in the operating room. This technique provides acceptable images although not ideal (**Fig. 12–8**).

Microscopic Digital Photography with a Photoadapter

This is a more expensive but more desirable method of digital photography because the digital camera is fixed. This technique requires (1) a digital camera (e.g., Nikon CoolPix 5000), (2) a digital camera mounting adapter (the connections between the digital camera and the photoadapter are so variable, readers are advised to check with the company), (3) a photoadapter for the Zeiss microscope, and (4) an optical beam splitter (50/50). The authors have not had the opportunity to try this technique.

◆ Videography

With the technical improvements in video documentation devices including video cameras, video recorders, high-intensity lighting, high-quality endoscopes, and video printers, video imaging has become our recommended procedure of choice for otologic documentation.

Unlike film still photography where there is a delay in seeing the final image, as well as concern whether the image was captured on film successfully, video documentation permits instantaneous imaging. The previously described digital photography techniques now permit immediate image verification. With the use of video printers, nearly instantaneous video printouts of outstanding quality can be obtained, even at the time of the otologic examination.

Equipment required for videography includes a video camera, a light source, a video recorder, a video monitor, and a video printer.

- *Video cameras:* The best resolution and brightness of images are obtained with compact three-chip CCD video cameras such as the Karl Storz Tricam, Stryker 782, or Karl Storz Image 1 (primarily made for endoscopic videography). These cameras are expensive ($16,000 to $20,000 or more), but produce superior images with outstanding color and clarity. A less expensive single lens chip camera, such as the Karl Storz Telecam, provides adequate images.

- *Light sources:* Xenon light sources such as the Karl Storz 487C, 610, or 615C Xenon Nova are recommended. Standard illuminators such as the Pilling (Fort Washington, PA) 2X Luminator and Karl Storz miniature light source 481C also give satisfactory results.

- *Video recorders:* Many video recorders have been used, including the ¾-inch or ½-inch VHS, S-VHS, and DVD. We favor the ¾-inch format (Sony VO 5600, VO 5700), but for those beginning with new systems, we recommend DVD, S-VHS, or VHS. However, users should check with the video technician in their facility. For a digital DV or DVCAM recorder, the Sony DSR20, DVCAM recorder and the Sony DSR V10 video Walkman minirecorder are available, $3500 and $2300, respectively.

- *Video monitors:* Any Sony or Panasonic monitor is adequate. Innovations in display design (e.g., high-definition televisions, plasma screen displays, or LCD monitors) may take full advantage of the superior image quality afforded by newer digital capture devices.

- *Video printers:* We use the Sony UP5000, UP5100, or UP5600, which produces the best images but is costly—approximately $7000. The Sony CVP M3 is more affordable and produces acceptable images.

The videoprints can be used directly in publications. The videoprints or pictures of the video monitor image can alternatively be copied with a digital camera for digital presentation.

The advantages of video imaging are the following: (1) reliable images of high color and resolution quality; (2) immediate images that can be easily recorded and played back at a later time for more careful analysis; and (3) nearly instantaneous video printouts for patient charts, teaching, publication, and effective communication with referring physicians.

The disadvantages of video imaging are the following: (1) the equipment is costly; (2) the equipment becomes outdated quickly; (3) the multiple tape formats make for potential compatibility problems when playing back tapes at other locations; and (4) the video images will fade with time. We recommend that hardcopy prints or preferably digitized images on computer format be made because the image quality from videotape degrades after 10 to 20 years.

Telescopic Videography

Telescopic Video-Otoscopy in the Office

Video-otoscopy may be performed with the 4 mm 0-degree (adult and older children) or 2.7 mm 0-degree (younger children) rigid telescopes. A light-sensitive and lightweight CCD video camera (single chip or three chip CCD camera) is used for video recording (**Fig. 12–9A**).

With the patient in the sitting position, the telescope, which is attached to the video camera, is dipped into warm water to prevent fogging and passed into the ear canal. The video camera should be held in one hand while the other hand holds the distal tip of the telescope to protect it from injuring the ear canal or the tympanic membrane (**Fig. 12–9A**). When the desired image is seen on the video monitor screen, focus is confirmed, and video recording is begun. Hard copies of the selected video image can be easily obtained using a color video printer (**Fig. 12–9B**). These can be used for medical records, teaching, patient education, and physician referrals. Mastoidectomy cavities can be thoroughly examined by angling the tip of the telescope. A retrograde telescope (30, 70, or 120 degrees) may be helpful to visualize hidden areas of the mastoidectomy cavity in some cases.

The advantages of this technique include the following: (1) It is a simple and safe technique that permits excellent visualization of the entire ear canal and tympanic membrane (**Fig. 12–10A,B**). (2) It is a fast technique, with the entire procedure taking less than 3 minutes to perform. (3) Video image recording can be immediately confirmed, and video prints can be nearly instantaneously made using a color video printer. (4) The video camera can be connected to one of the digital capture systems, resulting in almost simultaneous digital images. It is the authors' opinion that this is the most useful technique of imaging of the tympanic membrane (**Fig. 12–10A,B**).

The disadvantages of this technique include the following: (1) The equipment is expensive. (2) Lens fogging can be annoying. Frequent dips into warm water or anti-fog solution are needed. (3) Some image distortion occurs due to the wide-angle effect of the telescope lens. (4) Care must be taken not to touch the ear canal skin or the tympanic membrane.

Telescopic Pneumatic Video-Otoscopy

The mobility of the tympanic membrane can best be documented by pneumatic video-otoscopy. Although there are several excellent commercially available video-pneumatic

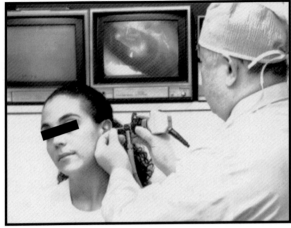
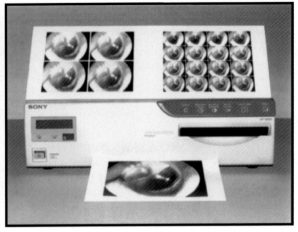

Figure 12–9   Telescopic video-otoscopy. **(A)** Technique of telescopic video-otoscopy. A Hopkins 4 mm 0-degree ototelescope is attached to the Stryker 3-chip CCD camera and used to examine the left ear canal. **(B)** Color video printers. Color video images obtained from the video camera can be printed almost simultaneously with a Sony UP5000 Mavigraph color video printer. Note that single or multiple image printouts can be produced.

otoscopes, video-pneumatic otoscopy can be simply accomplished by the Welch-Allen (Skaneateles Falls, NY) otoscope technique.

A simple and effective method of documenting pneumatic otoscopy has been described using an adapted Welch-Allen otoscope head.[23] The open end of the otoscope head with the pneumatic bulb attached is filled with Mack's ear plug molds, and a 4-mm central opening through the ear plug mold is made with a hemostat. The telescope is then passed through the hole so that the telescope tip extends just beyond the tip of the speculum. To produce a better seal within the ear canal, a rubber tourniquet may be wrapped around the tip of the speculum. Video adapters are then attached to the eyepiece of the telescope and video recordings with pneumatic insufflation documented.

The normal tympanic membrane moves readily with pneumatic otoscopy. Decreased mobility may be observed in patients with serous otitis media and tympanosclerosis. Excessive mobility may be noted with an atrophic tympanic membrane or ossicular discontinuity.

Telescopic Transtympanic Middle Ear Videography

Transtympanic middle ear endoscopy has been described as an office procedure using a small diameter telescope such as the 1.9 mm 0- or 30-degree telescope attached to a video camera.[22,27] Structures that can be well visualized and documented include the promontory, round window, oval window, stapes suprastructure, long process of the incus, and with the 30-degree telescope, the sinus tympani, facial nerve, pyramidal eminence, cochleariform process, and eustachian tube orifice. Poe et al[22] described the diagnosis of a labyrinthine fistula using this technique.

Telescopic Videography of the Ear in the Operating Room

The main advantage of performing telescopic videography of the ear in the operating room is that the patient remains immobile during the procedure while under general anesthesia. We sometimes reexamine the patient with this technique

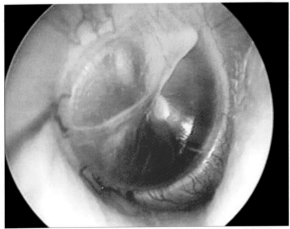
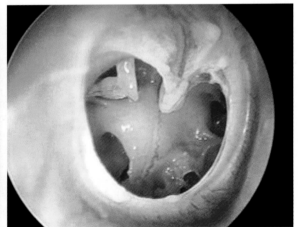

Figure 12–10   Telescopic video-otoscopy. **(A)** Glomus jugulare tumor of the right ear. **(B)** Subtotal tympanic membrane perforation of the right ear.

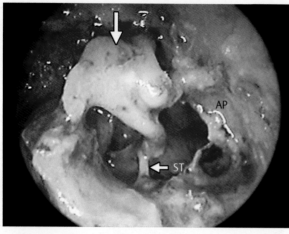 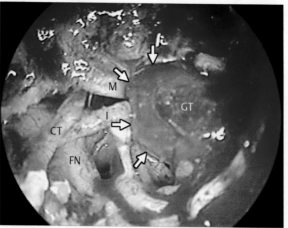

Figure 12–11 Telescopic videography of the ear in the operating room. **(A)** Fused malleus and incus (arrow) found in a patient with right congenital atresia of the ear canal. AP, atresia plate; ST, stapedial tendon.

(B) Intraoperative view of right middle ear showing glomus tumor (GT), malleus (M), incus (I), chorda tympani (CT), and facial nerve (FN).

to obtain better, clearer images for permanent records and teaching (**Fig. 12–11A,B**). Also, intraoperative documentation during middle ear surgery can be performed with the telescope, allowing excellent depth of field, color reproduction, and clear images. Nearly instantaneous video printouts can be produced using the color video printer.

Microscopic Videography

Microscopic videography of the ear is the most convenient and useful method of documenting and teaching of otologic surgery (**Figs. 12–12** and **12–13A,B**).

Videomicroscopic documentation requires (1) a Zeiss operating microscope, (2) a Zeiss beam splitter, (3) a photoadapter (Design for Vision, Ronkonkoma, NY; Zeiss; or Zeiss-Urban dual adapter), and (4) a video camera such as the single-chip CCD cameras with a C-mount coupler including Telecam (Chatham, MA) microscopic camera head (20210136U) or three-chip cameras such as the Sony DXC-970 MD, Tricam camera, Stryker camera, or Karl Storz Image 1 camera. An endoscopic camera can also be attached to the C-mount of a photoadapter of the Zeiss microscope utilizing a special endocamera adapter (Karl Storz). With their small size and weight, the miniature CCD cameras interfere minimally with the operative procedure.

With the patient lying supine, an ear speculum is used to expose the tympanic membrane or ear canal lesion. The microscope is positioned to visualize the lesion, and appropriate magnification is selected. The video camera is whitebalanced. The image is centered and focused on the video monitor and video recording is begun.

The advantages of this technique include the following: (1) It is an easy and effective technique that requires no interruption of surgery. (2) Different magnifications are readily available using the magnification dial of the microscope. (**Figs 12–13A,B**) (3) Digital images can be obtained in real time if the video camera is connected to the digital capture system, thus obviating the need for analog-to-digital conversion later.

The disadvantages of this technique include the following: (1) The photoadapter and beam splitter are expensive. (2) The depth of field is shallow. (3) It is difficult to photograph the entire tympanic membrane through the transcanal approach.

We believe microscopic videography of the ear is the single best method of documenting and teaching otologic surgery. Live images of the procedure can be observed on video monitors placed in the operating room, permitting ear, nose, and throat (ENT) residents and all operating room personnel to learn and understand the fundamentals of otologic surgery. The images obtained with a single-chip CCD (Telecam DX camera) are usually adequate. Images of the highest quality can be obtained with a three-chip CCD video camera such as the Tricam, Stryker, or Karl Storz Image 1. Nearly instantaneous video printouts of surgical anatomy and pathology can be made using the color video printers, which can be placed in the patient's chart or sent to the referring physician. If the video camera is attached to a digital capture system, almost simultaneous digital images are possible.

Figure 12–12 The technique of microscopic videography of the ear. Stryker 782 3-chip CCD video camera (other cameras such as the Tricam 3-chip CCD, Sony DXC-C33 3-chip CCD, Image-1 3-chip CCD, and Telecam 1-chip CCD can be used) attached to the Zeiss TV adapter and beam splitter of the microscope with an appropriate adapter. Make sure that the proper connection between the video camera and the photoadapter is chosen.

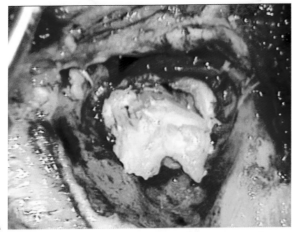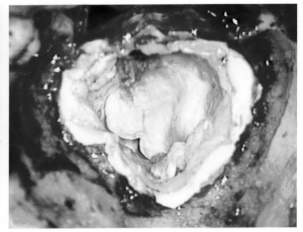

A   **B**

Figure 12–13   Microscopic videography of the ear. **(A)** Cholesteatoma filling the right mastoid cavity. **(B)** Closer view of cholesteatoma contents.

◆ Conclusion

During the past four decades, photographic techniques for the tympanic membrane have changed dramatically from the open tube (speculum) photography of Buckingham to microscopic photography with a photoadapter and through the eyepiece of the microscope, to telescopic film photography, and to digital filmless telescopic and microscopic photography.

Today, telescopic video otoscopy with a video camera in the office is the most useful procedure. This technique permits immediate exact diagnosis, patient counseling, and adequate treatment. The quality of the images is outstanding, and high-resolution images can be obtained nearly instantaneously using the video printer. The image from the videoprint can be digitized.

Microscopic videography in the operating room is the most useful and convenient method of otologic teaching and documentation. Telescopic digital photography of the ear in the office is a very economical advanced way of tympanic membrane photography. There is no question that filmless digital photography will continue to replace single-lens 35 mm film photography, but it is not always easy to perform.

Microscopic digital photography through the eyepiece of the microscope is a practical and inexpensive method for documenting the surgical procedures of the ear. Microscopic digital photography using a photoadapter is costly but may be the ideal method for capturing digital images.

With the continued advances in computer technology and the ability to digitize video images into computer memory, image storage will continue primarily in digitized formats. Digital images should last nearly indefinitely compared with other formats such as 35 mm slides and videotape where image distortion or degradation occurs. Digital imaging remains the ideal modality for otologic photography in the future.

◆ Acknowledgments

The authors acknowledge the assistance of the late John K. Joe, M.D., and Ronald Hirokawa, M.D., both of the Yale University School of Medicine.

References

1. Pensak ML, Yanagisawa E. Tympanic membrane photography: historical perspective. Am J Otol 1984;5:324–332
2. Randall BA, Morse HL. Photographic Illustrations of the Anatomy of the Human Ear, Together with Pathological Conditions of the Drum Membrane. Philadelphia: P Blakiston's, 1887
3. Buckingham RA. Endoscopic otophotography. Laryngoscope 1963;73:71–84
4. Brubaker JD, Holinger PH. Recent progress in open tube endoscopic and cavity still and motion picture photography. J Biol Photogr Assoc 1957;24:104–113
5. Holinger PH, Tardy ME Jr. Photography in otorhinolaryngology and bronchoesophagology. In: English GM, ed. Otolaryngology. rev. ed. Vol. 5. ch 22 Philadelphia: Lippincott, 1988, pp 1–21
6. Smith HW, Rosnagle RS, Yanagisawa E. Tympanic membrane photography. Arch Otolaryngol 1974;99:125–127
7. Hughes GB, Yanagisawa E, Dickins JRE, et al. Microscopic otologic photography using a standard 35 mm camera. Am J Otol 1981;2:243–247
8. Yanagisawa E. Effective photography in otolaryngology-head and neck surgery: tympanic membrane photography. Otolaryngol Head Neck Surg 1982;90:399–407
9. Yanagisawa E. Documentation of otologic surgery. In: Yanagisawa E, Gardner G, eds. The Surgical Atlas of Otology and Neuro-Otology. New York: Grune & Stratton, 1983
10. Konrad HR, Berci G, Ward P. Pediatric otoscopy and photography of the tympanic membrane. Arch Otolaryngol 1979;105:431–433
11. Chen B, Fry TL, Fischer ND. Otoscopy and photography–a new method. Ann Otol Rhinol Laryngol 1979;88:771–773
12. Chole RA. Photography of the tympanic membrane: a new method. Arch Otolaryngol 1980;106:230–231
13. Nomura Y. Effective photography in otolaryngology-head and neck surgery: endoscopic photography of the middle ear. Otolaryngol Head Neck Surg 1982;90:395–398
14. Hawke M. Telescopic otoscopy and photography of the tympanic membrane. J Otolaryngol 1982;11:35–39
15. Gonzalez C, Bluestone CD. Visualization of a retraction pocket/cholesteatoma: indications for use of the middle ear telescope in children. "How I Do It." Laryngoscope 1986;96:109–110
16. Selkin SG. Endoscopic photography of the ear, nose, and throat. Laryngoscope 1984;94:336–339
17. Chole RA. Color Atlas of Ear Disease. New York: Appleton-Century-Crofts, 1982
18. Hawke M, Keene M, Alberti PW. Clinical Otoscopy—A Text and Colour Atlas. Edinburgh: Churchill Livingstone, 1984
19. Hawke M. Clinical Pocket Guide to Ear Disease. Philadelphia: Lea & Febiger, 1987
20. Owens TW. Ear Disease—A School Nurse Manual of Common Ear Problems. Houston: Peanut, 1992
21. Wormald PJ, Browning GG. Otoscopy—A Structural Approach. San Diego: Singular, 1996
22. Poe DS, Rebeiz EE, Pankratov MM, Shapshay SM. Transtympanic endoscopy of the middle ear. Laryngoscope 1992;102:993–996

II Evaluation

23. Yanagisawa E, Carlson RD. Telescopic video-otoscopy using a compact home video color camera. Laryngoscope 1987;97:1350–1355

24. Yanagisawa E. The use of video in ENT endoscopy: its value in teaching. Ear Nose Throat J 1994;73:754–763

25. Mambrino L, Yanagisawa E, Yanagisawa K, Gallo O. Endoscopic ENT photography: a comparison of pictures by standard color films and newer color video printers. Laryngoscope 1991;101:1229–1232

26. Yanagisawa K, Shi JM, Yanagisawa E. Color photography of video images of otolaryngological structures using a 35 mm SLR camera. Laryngoscope 1987;97:992–993

27. Yanagisawa E. Color Atlas of Diagnostic Endoscopy in Otorhinolaryngology. New York: Igaku Shoin, 1997

28. Silverstein H, Seidman M, Rosenberg S. Documentation is a snap. Laryngoscope 1992;102:1395–1398

29. Spiegel JH, Singer MI. Practical approach to digital photography and its applications. Otolaryngol Head Neck Surg 2000;123:152–156

30. Yanagisawa E, Joe JK, Yanagisawa R. Digital imaging in otolaryngology-head and neck surgery. In: Citardi MJ, ed. Computer-Aided Otorhinolaryngology—Head and Neck Surgery. New York: Marcel Dekker, 2002, 117–134

31. Melder PC, Mair EA. Endoscopic photography—digital or 35 mm? Arch Otolaryngol Head Neck Surg 2003;129:570–575

32. Manarey CRA, Anand VK. Office-based digital photography in rhinology. Laryngoscope 2004;114:593–595

33. Benjamin B. Digital photography of the larynx. Ann Otol Rhinol Laryngol 2002;111:603–608

34. Haynes DS, Moore BA, Roland P, Olson GT. Digital microphotography: a simple solution. Laryngoscope 2003;113:915–919

13

Clinical Evaluation of Hearing Loss

Alyssa R. Terk and John F. Kveton

The number of people with a severe-to-profound hearing impairment in the United States in 2001 ranged from 464,000 to 738,000, with 54% of them over the age of 65.[1] The incidence of significant hearing loss in infants ranged from 1:1000 to 1:2000. The average lifetime cost for one person with hearing loss is estimated to be $417,000 (in 2003 dollars) (includes productivity loss in the workplace and household). This represents costs over and above those experienced by a person who does not have a disability.[2]

Given the prevalence of hearing loss, a cost-effective and accurate diagnostic approach is essential to assess the degree and nature of hearing loss and to arrive at the underlying cause. Patients may undergo assessment for hearing loss (**Fig. 13–1**) because of their subjective complaints or because they belong to groups that have been shown to be at risk for hearing loss, such as low birth weight infants, or those receiving ototoxic chemotherapy. In either case, an understanding-of the differential diagnosis of hearing loss is helpful in guiding clinical evaluation.

◆ Differential Diagnosis of Hearing Loss

A critical step in establishing a differential diagnosis is to determine whether the hearing loss is conductive, sensorineural, mixed, or central.

A sensorineural hearing loss (SNHL) may be caused by a lesion of the cochlea or the auditory nerve. A conductive hearing loss is caused by a lesion affecting the mechanism that transmits sound energy from the external environment to the cochlea and may involve the external ear, the tympanic membrane, or the contents of the middle ear. Some patients may have both sensorineural and conductive hearing loss simultaneously, in which the hearing loss is categorized as mixed. Conditions that may be associated with mixed hearing loss include chronic otitis media, acquired cholesteatoma, temporal bone trauma, certain hereditary syndromes, and otosclerosis. Central hearing loss is caused by a lesion along the neural pathway either from the inner ear to the auditory region of the brain or in the brain itself.

History and physical examination findings are extremely important in narrowing the list of clinical possibilities. To refine the differential diagnosis, information from the audiogram as well as data obtained from impedance testing and speech audiometry are used. Further examinations can be performed such as laboratory testing and diagnostic imaging to further narrow the diagnosis.

The differential diagnosis for a patient with unilateral SNHL varies considerably from that for a patient with bilateral slowly progressive SNHL. However, for the purposes of giving a broad overview, differential diagnoses for sensorineural and conductive hearing loss are discussed in this chapter (**Tables 13–1** and **13–2**).

Sensorineural Hearing Loss

Sensorineural hearing loss can be categorized in different ways. One scheme uses age of onset. Congenital hearing loss is that which is present from birth, whether due to hereditary factors, prenatal exposure or infection, or perinatal events. In contrast, hereditary hearing loss may not be present at birth. More than 50% of congenital hearing loss is due to genetic factors, 25% is acquired, and 25% is of unknown etiology. Causes of congenital SNHL include a variety of genetic disorders, intrauterine infections, exposure to teratogenic agents, prematurity, perinatal anoxia, and hyperbilirubinemia. Some of these factors may result in inner ear aplasia; however, such deformities may also exist without identifiable cause. Although the mechanism is not understood, low-birth-weight infants (<2500 g) are also at increased risk for SNHL as well as problems with figure/ground differentiation and auditory memory.[3] Congenital infections that can cause hearing loss include toxoplasmosis, rubella, cytomegalovirus (CMV), herpes simplex virus (HSV), and syphilis.

Delayed-onset hearing loss can be caused by a variety of factors, including infection, trauma, and ototoxic medications. Genetic factors can also cause delayed-onset hearing loss. Hereditary hearing loss may be dominant, recessive, X-linked, or mitochondrially inherited, and may exist with or without abnormalities in other organ systems (i.e., syndromic versus nonsyndromic).

Of the 50 to 60% of congenital hearing loss that is hereditary, approximately 70% is nonsyndromic, of which 80% is

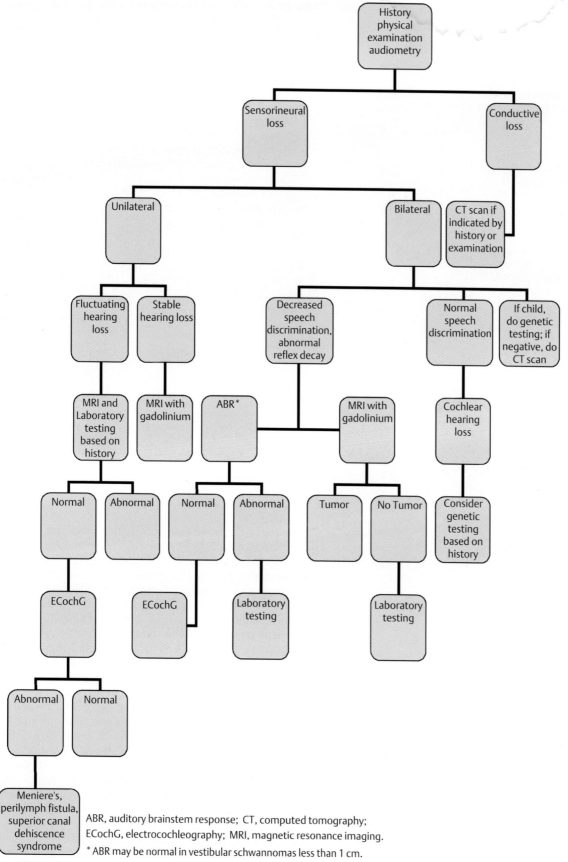

ABR, auditory brainstem response; CT, computed tomography;
ECochG, electrocochleography; MRI, magnetic resonance imaging.
* ABR may be normal in vestibular schwannomas less than 1 cm.

Figure 13–1 Algorithm for clinical assessment of hearing loss.

Table 13–1 Differential Diagnosis of Sensorineural Hearing Loss

Congenital
    Genetic disorders
        Usher's syndrome, Jervell and Lange-Nielsen syndrome
        Pendred syndrome
    Intrauterine infection (TORCH syndrome: toxoplasmosis, rubella, cytomegalovirus, and herpes simplex)
    Teratogens
    Perinatal anoxia—hypoxia
    Prematurity
    Low birth weight
    Hyperbilirubinemia
    Inner ear dysplasia
Hereditary—delayed onset
    Dominant (e.g., Paget's disease, dominant progressive hearing loss)
    Recessive (e.g., DFNB1, connexin 26 mutations—35delG, 167delT, connexin 30 mutations)
    X-linked (e.g., Alport's syndrome)
    Mitochondrial (e.g., MIDD)
Infectious
    Postmeningitis
    Chronic otitis media
    Syphilis
    Viral (CMV, HSV, HIV)
    Lyme disease
    Tuberculosis
Inflammatory
    Systemic immune and autoimmune disease
    Primary autoimmune ear disease
Neoplastic
    Primary tumors arising within the temporal bone
    Metastatic tumors
Metabolic
    Diabetes
    Hypothyroidism
    Hyperlipidemia
Traumatic
    Temporal bone fracture
    Perilymph fistula
    Barotrauma
    Noise exposure
    Auditory concussion
    Traumatic brain injury
    Postsurgical
Vascular-hematologic
    Hypertension
    Vascular occlusion/emboli
    Inner ear hemorrhage
Miscellaneous
    Meniere's disease
    Presbycusis
    Cochlear otosclerosis
    Multiple sclerosis
    Ototoxicity
    Radiation injury

Table 13–2 Differential Diagnosis of Conductive Hearing Loss

Congenital
    Ossicular fusion/malformation
    Ossicular fixation
    Atresia of the external auditory canal
    Congenital cholesteatoma
Hereditary
    Otosclerosis
    Osteogenesis imperfecta
    Paget's disease (osteitis deformans)
    Osteopetrosis (Albers-Schönberg disease)
    Crouzon's syndrome
    Marfan's syndrome
Infectious-inflammatory
    Otitis media with effusion
    Acquired cholesteatoma
    Otitis externa
Neoplastic
    Ear canal tumor
    Glomus tumor
    Histiocytosis
    Fibrous dysplasia
Traumatic
    Tympanic membrane perforation
    Ossicular discontinuity
    Hemotympanum
Mechanical
    Cerumen impaction
    Foreign body of the ear canal
    Exostoses
    Superior canal dehiscence syndrome

13q12. The connexin gene codes a protein called gap junction protein β2 (GJB2). Connexin 26 and connexin 30 as well as other connexins fit together to compose gap junctions. These are expressed in the cochlea where they are thought to aid in returning potassium ions to the endolymph following hair cell stimulation. The most common mutation in connexin 26 is the 35delG mutation with a carrier rate estimated at 2.5% in the general population. Other mutations have been found in specific ethnic groups, such as 167delT in Ashkenazi Jews and 235delC in Korean and Japanese populations. Genetic mutations in the connexin 30 gene have also been implicated in some nonsyndromic hearing loss.

Infectious agents and inflammatory processes can lead to SNHL. The infectious agents include both bacteria and viruses. Some individuals with otitis media may develop SNHL through round window membrane permeability to bacterial toxins.[5] Tuberculosis may be associated with otitis media as well as SNHL.[6,7] The spirochetes causing both syphilis and Lyme disease can involve the perilymph, resulting in sudden or fluctuating SNHL. In one study, Lyme titers were positive in 20% of patients with sudden SNHL.[8]

Cytomegalovirus, HSV, and human immunodeficiency virus (HIV) can lead to SNHL. In HIV, the hearing loss may result from the opportunistic infections characteristic of the acquired immunodeficiency syndrome, ototoxic medications used to treat infections, or possibly direct effects of the virus upon the cochlea.[7] Specifically, nucleoside analog reverse

inherited in an autosomal recessive manner.[4] Many loci have been mapped, including autosomal recessive, autosomal dominant, and X-linked loci. The gene coding for connexin 26 (Cx26) is located at locus *DFNB1* on human chromosome transcriptase inhibitors reduce mitochondrial DNA content, which may contribute to auditory dysfunction in older patients with HIV-1 infection.[9]

Approximately 5 to 35% of patients are left with SNHL following bacterial meningitis.[10] Since the introduction of the *Haemophilus influenzae* type B vaccine, most cases of bacterial meningitis are caused by *Streptococcus pneumoniae*. Bacterial meningitis is the most common cause of acquired SNHL in children (85%).[11,12] Inflammatory processes can be associated with SNHL. These include systemic diseases such as Cogan's syndrome, relapsing polychondritis, Wegener's granulomatosis, lupus erythematosus, Takayasu's disease, and giant cell arteritis. In addition, primary autoimmune hearing loss may present without systemic manifestations.[13]

SNHL may result from primary tumors arising within the temporal bone as well as from metastatic lesions. The most common neoplasm causing SNHL is vestibular schwannoma. Squamous cell cancer and paragangliomas arising within the temporal bone may also cause SNHL, though they are more commonly associated with conductive hearing loss.[14] Metastatic lesions to the temporal bone include those with a proclivity for bony metastases such as carcinoma of the breast, lung, and prostate.[15]

Associations have been suggested but not conclusively proven between several metabolic disorders and SNHL. These include diabetes mellitus, in which microangiopathy has been postulated to lead to auditory damage; hypothyroidism; and hyperlipoproteinemia. Hypertension as well as vascular and hematologic problems are also thought to cause hearing loss. Decreased blood flow to the inner ear may result from narrowed blood vessels, as in atherosclerosis or diabetes mellitus (DM), or from abnormal flow or coagulability, as in sickle cell and hypercoagulable disorders. Platelet dysfunction, thrombocytopenia, and hypocoagulable states can also lead to hemorrhage within the inner ear, thus causing hearing loss.[16,17] A rare maternally inherited form of deafness and diabetes (MIDD) has also recently been discovered, in which a mitochondrial gene defect results in type 2 diabetes and bilateral SNHL presenting at an average age of 35 years.[18]

Trauma can cause SNHL in several ways. Both longitudinal and transverse fractures of the temporal bone can disrupt the labyrinth, although this is more likely to occur with the latter. Perilymphatic fistula can result from both blunt injuries to the head and barotrauma. Head trauma may also cause concussive injury to the inner ear or traumatic brain injury with central hearing loss. Surgical trauma may result in SNHL. Excessive noise exposure damages the outer hair cells of the cochlea, causing hearing loss with a specific pattern on audiogram. Other conditions known to lead to SNHL include Meniere's disease, cochlear otosclerosis, multiple sclerosis, ototoxic drugs, radiation injury, and aging (presbycusis).

Conductive Hearing Loss

Congenital causes of conductive hearing loss include ossicular fixation and ossicular malformations, as well as atresia or stenosis of the external auditory canal. These anomalies may exist in conjunction with other craniofacial abnormalities and possibly with SNHL.

Hereditary delayed-onset conductive hearing loss can be caused by otosclerosis, which is thought to be an autosomal dominant disease with incomplete penetrance.[19–21] Osteogenesis imperfecta tarda, another autosomal dominant

disorder, leads to delayed-onset conductive hearing loss by causing stapes fixation or ossicular fracture. Other hereditary causes of conductive hearing loss include osteopetrosis, Marfan's disease, Paget's disease, and Crouzon's syndrome. The presence of congenital cholesteatoma in the middle ear can also cause conductive hearing loss.

The most common cause of conductive hearing loss is otitis media with effusion, which can be either acute or chronic. Cholesteatoma or granulation tissue caused by chronic otitis media can interfere with the transmission of sound to the oval window, sometimes even causing ossicular erosion. Other sequelae of infection that may cause conductive hearing loss include tympanosclerosis and atelectasis of the middle ear. Another infectious cause of conductive hearing loss is severe otitis externa, in which edema of the ear canal interferes with hearing. Trauma may also lead to conductive hearing loss, caused by tympanic membrane (TM) perforation, hemotympanum, or ossicular discontinuity.

Rarer causes of conductive hearing loss include neoplasms involving the external auditory canal or middle ear. These may be benign or malignant. A more recent discovery is the superior canal dehiscence syndrome causing a conductive hearing loss in the face of intact middle ear function and normal stapes reflexes.[22] Lastly, mechanical occlusion of the external auditory canal from cerumen, foreign bodies, or large exostoses can also cause conductive hearing loss.

◆ History

The history is the first and most important step in the clinical evaluation of hearing loss. The history may identify individuals with hearing loss and can direct the clinician to the appropriate testing.

History in Infants and Children

Family history, pregnancy history, and birth history are particularly important in the clinical evaluation of infants and children because they can identify factors that may increase the risk of hearing loss. Given that only approximately 10% of newborns fall into the high-risk category and 50% of infants with significant hearing loss do not have any high-risk features, screening patients only through a high-risk register will miss half the diagnoses of SNHL.

Universal newborn hearing screening measures have thus been mandated by the federal government. This involves testing of all babies with either auditory brainstem response (ABR), otoacoustic emissions (OAEs), or both. The Joint Committee on Infant Hearing released a statement in 2000 stating that in "all infants' hearing should be screened using objective, physiologic measures to identify those with congenital or neonatal onset hearing loss. Audiologic evaluation and medical evaluations should be in progress before 3 months of age."[23]

Further questions important in the history of the child with hearing loss include history of bacterial meningitis or other infections associated with hearing loss, history of head trauma associated with loss of consciousness or skull fracture, use of ototoxic medications including intravenous (IV) antibiotics, recurrent or persistent otitis media with effusion for more than 3 months, and parental concern about hearing, speech, language, or development.

Parental concerns have often been found to be correct. Appropriate speech development can be assessed based on age-appropriate milestones as published by Matkin's group[24,25]:

1. Absence of differentiated babbling or vocal imitation by 12 months
2. Failure to use single words by 18 months
3. A single-word vocabulary of 10 words or less by 24 months
4. A vocabulary of less than 100 words, failure to use two-word combinations, and unintelligible speech at 30 months
5. A vocabulary of less than 200 words, no use of telegraphic sentences, and clarity less than 50% at 36 months
6. A vocabulary of less than 600 words, no use of simple sentences, and clarity of less than 80% at 48 months.

Developmental milestones also exist for receptive abilities. From birth to 4 months, infants should startle to loud sounds, quiet to their mother's voice, and cease activity when sound is presented at a conversational level. From 5 to 6 months, infants should be able to localize to sound in the horizontal plane, imitate sounds in their own speech repertoire, and vocalize reciprocally with an adult. Between 7 and 12 months, infants should localize to sound in any plane and respond to their name. By 13 to 15 months, children should be able to point in the direction of an unexpected sound as well as to familiar objects or people when asked. Between 16 and 18 months, children should begin to follow simple directions without cues and should be able to be trained to reach toward a midline toy when a sound is presented. Finally by 19 to 24 months, children should be able to point to parts of the body when named.[14]

Additionally, the Joint Committee recommends monitoring hearing in children at risk every 6 months between the ages of 29 days and 3 years, even if they passed the initial hearing screening test. These include children at risk for delayed-onset SNHL or conductive hearing loss.[26]

History in General

The history should include the patient's age, duration, and progression of symptoms. It is important to establish whether the hearing loss is unilateral or bilateral, sudden in onset or gradual, stable or fluctuating. Associated otologic symptoms such as tinnitus, otalgia, aural fullness, and otorrhea should be inquired about, as well as any vertigo or instability suggestive of vestibular dysfunction.

After the otologic history has been taken, further questioning should establish the existence of other systemic illnesses, symptoms of those illnesses, history of infections, and history of head trauma. Particular attention should be paid to both current and prior medications for ototoxic potential, taking care to include over-the-counter and homeopathic drugs[27,28] (**Table 13–3**). Any allergies should be noted. A complete review of systems should be performed. Family history of hearing loss or anomalies associated with syndromic hearing loss (such as the pigmentation abnormalities in Waardenburg's syndrome) should be reviewed. The occupational history should be obtained with careful questioning of noise exposure, not only in the workplace but also at so-called leisure activities of firing ranges and concerts. History of prior otologic and neurologic surgery should be reviewed as well.

Table 13–3 Ototoxic Drugs

| Aminoglycoside antibiotics |
| Streptomycin |
| Dihydrostreptomycin |
| Kanamycin |
| Gentamicin |
| Neomycin |
| Amikacin |
| Tobramycin |
| Netilmicin |
| Vancomycin |
| Erythromycin |
| Chemotherapeutic agents |
| Cisplatin (stria) |
| Nitrogen mustard |
| Loop diuretics (stria vascularis) |
| Furosemide |
| Ethacrynic acid |
| Salicylates |
| Quinine |

◆ Physical Examination

The physical examination begins with examination of the external ear. The size, shape, and position of the pinna should be noted. In cases of microtia, the degree of external malformation can be used to assess the development of the middle ear because a more deformed auricle is more likely to be associated with a greater degree of middle ear atresia.[29] The preauricular area should be examined carefully for pits or skin tags, whereas postauricular inspection should make note of tenderness, erythema, swelling, or evidence of prior surgery. Even before the external auditory canal is inspected visually, pain may be elicited by traction on the pinna, suggesting otitis externa.

Visual inspection of the external auditory canal and TM can be performed with the handheld otoscope or the microscope. Both afford the opportunity for pneumatic otoscopy; the latter may provide improved visualization and capacity to use instruments. In either case, the examination should include thorough inspection of the bony and cartilaginous ear canal. Cerumen, foreign bodies, pus, fungal infection, keratinaceous debris, and granulation tissue may be noted. The canal itself may be erythematous and edematous or dry and flaky. Sagging of the posterosuperior canal wall suggests mastoid disease. Step-offs of the superior canal may be evidence of temporal bone fracture.

For optimal visualization, the canal should be carefully but thoroughly cleaned, and if indicated, material from the canal may be sent for culture. Polyps, osteomas, or exostoses may partially or completely occlude the ear canal, making visualization of the TM difficult. However, under optimal circumstances, the entire TM should be inspected, making note of perforations, sclerotic areas, and retraction pockets.

The color of the TM provides additional clinical information. The normal TM is pearly gray. However, serous fluid may make it appear amber, whereas hemotympanum appears bluish. Masses may appear behind the TM and may be white (cholesteatoma), blue (dehiscent jugular bulb), or red (glomus tumor or more rarely aberrant carotid artery). Pneumatic otoscopy can be performed to assess drum movement. Poor mobility suggests fluid in the middle ear space, whereas a healed perforation may be flaccid and hypermobile. Pneumatic otoscopy can also be used to perform the fistula test by applying positive and negative pressure and observing the patient for nystagmus.

A thorough head and neck examination can provide important clues. Initial examination may reveal physical findings suggestive of syndromic hearing loss, such as white forelock or facial asymmetry. Examination of the eyes should include assessment of pupillary function, evaluation of extraocular movements, and inspection for spontaneous or gaze nystagmus. Eye examination may also reveal abnormalities such as blue sclerae and heterochromia iridis that can be associated with hearing loss. In addition to the nasal examination, either mirror or fiberoptic examination of the nasopharynx may be performed, especially if presence of a unilateral serous effusion in an adult is noted.[30,31]

The oral cavity should be examined for abnormalities such as the stigmata of submucous cleft or more overt palatal malformations. Information can also be obtained from neck examination, such as the presence or absence of bruits in patients with pulsatile tinnitus or the presence of a neck mass in a patient with a suspected temporal bone neoplasm. In the patient with SNHL, further valuable data can be obtained by performing a thorough examination of the cranial nerves. In a patient who presents with vestibular complaints in addition to hearing loss, assessment should also include observation of the patient's gait, Romberg test, and tests of position sense such as the finger-nose and heel-shin tests.

Tuning fork examination can also be performed as part of the initial physical examination. Although tuning fork tests do not provide the objectivity of formal audiometric testing, they are inexpensive and easy to administer and can be administered in situations where formal audiometric testing would be cumbersome, such as at the bedside. The Rinne and Weber tests as performed with a 512-Hz tuning fork continue to play a role in the initial physical examination and assessment of the patient with suspected hearing loss.

Lastly, the physician may acquire additional information that may be pertinent by performing a more generalized physical examination where appropriate. For example, pigmentation abnormalities such as café-au-lait spots and vitiligo may suggest congenital disorders associated with hearing loss. Similarly, limb, stature, or phalangeal abnormalities may be associated with syndromic hearing loss. Cardiovascular examination may reveal bruits or murmurs that point to the possibility of vascular or embolic disease. Stigmata such as rheumatoid nodules, skin rashes, or neuromuscular abnormalities may identify systemic diseases with otologic manifestations.

◆ Audiologic Testing (also see Chapter 8)

All patients suspected of having hearing loss should undergo audiologic examination, including pure-tone threshold testing for air and bone as well as assessment of speech threshold and discrimination. Subjective assessment tests rely on the participation of the patient, whereas physiologic tests do not rely on the patient's interaction with the audiologist.

Subjective Hearing Assessment

For children under 3 years or those with developmental delay, visual reinforcement audiometry (VRA) or conditioned play audiometry (CPA) replaces conventional audiologic examination.[32,33] VRA is commonly used in children between the ages of 6 and 24 months. A signal is presented in the sound field, and the child is conditioned to turn toward the sound by the activity of a toy that is located close to the sound source. A normal-hearing 6-month-old responds to sound stimuli of 20 dB or higher.[34]

For older children (2 to 6 years), CPA can be used. In this technique, the child is taught to perform a simple task, such as dropping a toy into a bucket or stacking a ring on a pole, in response to auditory signals. In CPA the child wears headphones, and pure-tone thresholds for both air and bone can be obtained. In small children, speech reception testing can be performed by allowing the child to point to a picture, rather than repeating the word.

For children younger than 6 months, physiologic tests of the auditory system provide greater accuracy than behavioral observation audiometry techniques.

For children older than 6 years and for adults, a pure-tone audiogram is used to assess hearing in cooperative patients. Both air conduction and bone conduction thresholds are obtained across the frequency range of 250 to 8000 Hz.[35] The span between 500 and 3000 Hz is the most significant, as this range includes the majority of human speech sounds. In pure-tone testing, normal hearing is defined as less than 25 dB. Mild includes 25 to 40 dB; moderate hearing loss 40 to 60 dB, severe 60 to 90 dB, and profound greater than 90 dB.

Immittance Measures

In addition to basic audiometry, tests that may aid in identifying the cause of hearing loss include tympanometry and acoustic reflex testing. Tympanometry provides information about the compliance of the tympanic membrane and can be used to assess middle ear pathology as a cause of hearing loss. Tympanometry in infants younger than 4 months old should be obtained by using a probe frequency of 600 to 1000 Hz because when tested with a standard probe tone frequency of 226 Hz infants with otitis media with effusion can reveal a normal-appearing tympanogram due to extensibility of skin in the ear canal.

Acoustic reflex testing assesses a reflex arc that involves the eighth nerve, the brainstem, the facial nerve, and the stapedius muscle. An acoustic signal presented to one ear can produce bilateral reflex contraction of the stapedius muscle, producing a change in impedance. The threshold of the acoustic reflex can be measured as well as the duration of the response to a sustained signal. Although both middle ear and retrocochlear pathology may result in absent or abnormal reflexes, they are usually present in mild to moderate cochlear disorders. Abnormal decay of acoustic reflexes is suggestive of retrocochlear pathology. Kumar et al,[22] in their review of 200 cases of unilateral SNHL, have suggested that acoustic reflex testing be included in the battery of tests designed to identify the site of the lesion.

In otosclerosis, the tympanogram can be normal but reflexes are absent. In superior canal dehiscence, the tympanogram is normal and reflexes are present.

Lastly, in cases where pseudohypoacusis is suspected, either because of the clinical scenario or because of inconsistent responses on basic audiologic testing, additional tests can be used. The presence of normal acoustic reflexes with responses characteristic of a profound SNHL on pure-tone testing suggests a functional problem. The Stenger test can be used to test asymmetrical hearing loss, whereas the Doerfler-Stewart test is used to test cases of bilateral hearing loss that are thought to be nonorganic. Other tests monitor the patient's spoken responses in the presence of masking noise or with delayed auditory feedback of his or her own voice.

Physiologic Hearing Assessment

Physiologic tests of the auditory system that may provide clinical information in cases of hearing loss include ABR, OAEs, and electrocochleography (ECochG). These tests may provide information about auditory thresholds in infants or in patients who are unwilling or unable to cooperate with basic audiologic testing. In addition, these tests may identify the site of the lesion in cases of SNHL.

Auditory Brainstem Response

The ABR tests the auditory pathway from the eighth nerve to the midbrain. Surface electrodes are used to measure evoked electrical responses to an acoustic signal, commonly a wideband click. The ABR is a noninvasive test that does not depend on the patient's level of consciousness or cooperation, and it has been widely used as a screening test for hearing loss in newborn infants.[23] Identification of threshold hearing levels is thought to be most accurate in cases of flat hearing loss because the wideband click includes a range of frequencies that stimulate the entire cochlea. To elicit more frequency-specific threshold sensitivity, a stimulus with a narrower frequency band can be used, such as a tone pip. In frequency-specific testing, masking may be necessary with high-intensity signals.[24] In addition, in cases of asymmetric hearing loss, it has been used to detect acoustic neuromas because of the delay in response latency produced by these tumors. Because the ABR can be normal in small (<1 cm) vestibular schwannomas, MRI with gadolinium contrast enhancement remains the gold standard for diagnosis of suspected tumor. Extremely large tumors may also produce abnormalities in the ABR of the contralateral ear.[25] This may be useful in cases where hearing loss is too profound to permit ABR testing on the ipsilateral side. The ABR can also identify demyelinating diseases such as multiple sclerosis that result in changes in wave morphology and deterioration wave V morphology with increased stimulation. In infants, the auditory nerve and brainstem structures continue to develop for 18 to 24 months of age as reflected in decreasing interpeak latencies in the ABR.[36]

Otoacoustic Emissions

OAEs, discovered by Kemp[26] in 1978, are produced by the cochlea. These signals may be spontaneous (SOAEs) or may be produced in response to external stimulation. Different patterns of OAEs are produced by different stimuli. The most commonly used in clinical practice are transient-evoked OAEs (TEOAEs) and distortion-product OAEs (DPOAEs). The former are produced by a tone pip or broadband tone click like that used for the ABR. The latter are produced by using two tones of different frequency simultaneously. Less commonly used are stimulus-frequency OAEs (SFOAEs), which are evoked by pure-tone stimuli and provide frequency-specific responses. For all types, testing is noninvasive; a probe in the ear canal is used to produce the stimulus and record the response.

The presence of OAEs generally indicates that hearing is present because positive OAEs indicate functioning outer hair cells. OAEs are affected by outer and middle ear pathology, so that the absence of OAEs does not necessarily indicate hearing loss. The presence of OAEs with absent ABR waveforms has been recognized by Berlin et al[38] as an unusual type of hearing loss known as auditory dyssynchrony (auditory neuropathy). Approximately 7 to 10% of these patients have no observable symptoms other than an absent ABR. Most others show minimal benefit from hearing aid trials based on behavioral audiograms, and some respond extremely well to cochlear implants even when the audiogram is not consistent with severe-to-profound hearing loss. In auditory dyssynchrony, the pure-tone audiogram is not felt to predict hearing abilities. Cochlear implants bypass the site of neuropathy, which is thought to be at or near the spiral ganglion, and thus can produce good results.

Electrocochleography

ECochG measures evoked potentials arising from the cochlea and the auditory nerve, usually using a broadband click stimulus. The responses that provide the most clinical information are the summating potential and the compound action potential of the eighth nerve. ECochG can provide information about auditory thresholds. In addition, Meniere's disease and vestibular schwannomas can produce characteristic changes in the summating potential and the action potential, respectively.[39,40] However, because the most accurate data are produced by a transtympanic needle electrode, ECochG has not found widespread clinical use. With the development of electrodes that do not require TM penetration, this test may find greater clinical application in the future.

◆ Vestibular Testing

The need for formal vestibular testing is determined primarily by the patient's history and physical examination. In children, vestibular screening tests should be performed in children with SNHL using a commonsense approach, such as when the hearing impairment is caused by a factor that also causes vestibular systems as in Pendred and Usher syndrome, aminoglycoside toxicity, bacterial meningitis, perilymphatic fistula, inner ear dysplasia, CHARGE syndrome (coloboma, heart disease, atresia choanae, retarded growth and retarded development or central nervous system anomalies, genital hyperplasia, and ear anomalies or deafness), and when there is a balance or motor delay.[41]

◆ Laboratory Testing

Testing is usually directed at uncovering underlying systemic diseases that may result in hearing loss, and the need for a specific test can be determined by the history and physical examination. Basic hematologic evaluation should include a complete blood count, platelet count, and sedimentation rate. Coagulation studies may include prothrombin and partial thromboplastin time. Blood chemistries include serum electrolytes, BUN, creatinine, and urinalysis. Metabolic abnormalities may be revealed by thyroid function tests, fasting blood sugar or glucose tolerance, adrenocorticotrophic hormone (ACTH)-cortisol stimulation tests, and determination of serum cholesterol and triglycerides.

When the differential diagnosis includes immune-mediated hearing loss, the laboratory evaluation may include both nonspecific and specific tests. The Otoblot test (OTOblot™ anti-68kd [hsp-70] Antibody Western Blot Assay, IMMCO, Buffalo, NY) is an available Western blot assay to measure antibodies against the bovine heat shock protein (bHSP) 70. If the test is positive the patient is more likely to respond well to steroids. Conversely, a negative Otoblot test does not rule out autoimmune inner ear disease.[42,43] If a systemic collagen vascular disorder is suspected, general tests such as rheumatoid factor (RF) and antinuclear antibodies (ANAs) may be performed.

When indicated, laboratory tests for infectious diseases should be performed. Testing for syphilis should be performed by the fluorescent treponemal antibody absorption (FTA-abs) test. In suspected cases of neurosyphilis a lumbar puncture should be done. Cerebrospinal fluid studies should include opening pressure, cell count with differential, protein, glucose, Venereal Disease Research Laboratory (VDRL) test, culture, and Gram stain. Other serum tests include Lyme titers and tests for viral illnesses such as CMV. Specific immunoglobulin M (IgM) antibody assays should be performed if intrauterine infection is suspected, as IgM does not cross the placenta.

Because Jervell and Lange-Nielsen syndrome with prolonged Q-T interval on electriocardiography (EKG) may be the only hereditary ear disorder which can lead to sudden death, some clinicians routinely obtain EKG in children with congenital profound hearing loss, especially if there is a history of syncopal episodes.

◆ Genetic Testing

In 1997 the discovery was made that mutations in *GJB2,* the gene that encodes connexin 26 (Cx26), were responsible for up to half of cases of autosomal recessive nonsyndromic hearing loss.[44] Connexin 26 mutation screening is becoming more popular, though traditionally it has been performed by geneticists and genetic counselors to provide families appropriate counseling. Autosomal recessive nonsyndromic hearing loss caused by mutations in connexin 26 is known as DFNB1, which is characterized by a prelingual, nonprogressive bilateral loss. No abnormal computed tomography (CT) findings or laboratory findings have been associated with DFNB1; therefore, testing positive for a Cx26 mutation may eliminate the need for further laboratory or CT studies.[45]

◆ Radiologic Evaluation

In the evaluation of temporal bone pathology, high-definition CT with fine cuts of the temporal bone and magnetic resonance imaging (MRI) provide excellent information. High-definition CT with fine cuts in both the axial and coronal planes provides information about the bony anatomy of the

temporal bone. This study should be performed in all children and considered in older patients with progressive hearing loss and craniofacial anomalies. The reported incidence of CT anomalies is 6.8 to 31%, with the most common abnormality being the dilated vestibular aqueduct (DVA).[46,47] Other abnormalities diagnosed include Mondini dysplasia, common cavity deformity of the cochlea, and abnormalities of semicircular canals. For imaging pathology of the CPA and central nervous system, MRI with gadolinium contrast is preferable.

Additional imaging outside the head and neck may be indicated in patients who are suspected of having syndromic hearing loss with pathology involving other systems. For example, cardiac echo may be necessary in chromosome dysjunction (e.g., trisomy 13), and a renal ultrasound is recommended in Alport's syndrome and branchio-oto-renal syndrome.

◆ Involvement of Specialists

Complete evaluation of the child with hearing loss may involve a team of specialists, including pediatricians, geneticists, and ophthalmologists. Ophthalmologists are extremely helpful as half of severely to profoundly deaf children have ocular abnormalities.[48] Similarly, in adults, hearing disorders may require consultation with specialists such as allergists, rheumatologists, neurologists, or endocrinologists to assess associated problems.

◆ Conclusion

Clinical evaluation of the patient with hearing loss requires an understanding of the differential diagnosis of conductive and SNHL. Patients may require evaluation because of their subjective complaints or because of identifiable risk factors for hearing loss, particularly in children. A complete history and physical examination provides important information narrowing the differential diagnosis for the individual patient. Basic audiologic testing provides information about the nature, degree, and symmetry of hearing loss. Additional testing to identify the site of lesion and underlying pathologic process may include more extensive audiologic testing, physiologic assessment of the auditory system, vestibular testing, laboratory tests, and radiologic studies. On the basis of this evaluation, the physician can choose appropriate treatment or rehabilitation for the individual patient.

References

1. Blanchfield BB, Feldman JJ, Dunbar JL, Gardner EN. The severely to profoundly hearing-impaired population in the United States: prevalence estimates and demographics. J Am Acad Audiol 2001;12: 183–189

2. Centers for Disease Control and Prevention. Economic costs associated with mental retardation, cerebral palsy, hearing loss, and vision impairment–United States, 2003. MMWR Morb Mortal Wkly Rep 2004;53: 57–59

3. Van Naarden K, Decouflè P. Relative and attributable risks for moderate to profound bilateral sensorineural hearing impairment associated with lower birth weight in children 3 to 10 years old. Pediatrics 1999; 104:905–910

4. Erbe CB, Harris KC, Runge-Samuelson CL, Flanary VA, Wackym PA. Connexin 26 and connexin 30 mutations in children with non-syndromic hearing loss. Laryngoscope 2004;114:607–611

5. Engel F, Blatz R, Schliebs R, Palmer M, Bhakdi S. Bacterial cytolysin perturbs round window membrane permeability barrier in vivo: possible cause of sensorineural hearing loss in acute otitis media. Infect Immun 1998;66:343–346

6. Bhalla RK, Jones TM, Rothburn MM, Swift AC. Tuberculous otitis media—a diagnostic dilemma. Auris Nasus Larynx 2001;28:241–243

7. Kotnis R, Simo R. Tuberculous meningitis presenting as sensorineural hearing loss. J Laryngol Otol 2001;115:491–492

8. Lorenzi MC, Bittar RS, Pedalini ME, Zerati F, Yoshinari NH, Bento RF. Sudden deafness and Lyme disease. Laryngoscope 2003;113:312–315

9. Simdon J, Watters D, Bartlett S, Connick E. Ototoxicity associated with use of nucleoside analog reverse transcriptase inhibitors: a report of 3 possible cases and review of the literature. Clin Infect Dis 2001;32:1623–1627

10. Wellman MB, Sommer DD, McKenna J. Sensorineural hearing loss in postmeningitic children. Otol Neurotol 2003;24:907–912

11. Kulahli I, Ozturk M, Bilen C, et al. Evaluation of hearing loss with auditory brainstem responses in the early and late period of bacterial meningitis in children. J Laryngol Otol 1997;111:223–227

12. Richardson M, Williamson T, Reid A, et al. Otoacoustic emissions as a screening test for hearing impairment in children recovering from acute bacterial meningitis. Pediatrics 1998;102:1364–1368

13. Ruckenstein MJ. Autoimmune inner ear disease. Curr Opin Otolaryngol Head Neck Surg 2004;12:426–430

14. Swartz JD. Lesions of the cerebellopontine angle and internal auditory canal: diagnosis and differential diagnosis. Semin Ultrasound CT MR 2004;25:332–352

15. Gloria-Cruz TI, Schachern PA, Paparella MM, Adams GL, Fulton SE. Metastases to temporal bones from primary nonsystemic malignant neoplasms. Arch Otolaryngol Head Neck Surg 2000;126:209–214

16. Kazmierczak H, Doroszewska G. Metabolic disorders in vertigo, tinnitus, and hearing loss. Int Tinnitus J 2001;7:54–58

17. Hirano K, Ikeda K, Kawase T, et al. Prognosis of sudden deafness with special reference to risk factors of microvascular pathology. Auris Nasus Larynx 1999;26:111–115

18. Guillausseau PJ, Massin P, Dubois-LaForgue D, et al. Maternally inherited diabetes and deafness: a multicenter study. Ann Intern Med 2001;134 (9 pt 1):721–728

19. Menger DJ, Tange RA. The aetiology of otosclerosis: a review of the literature. Clin Otolaryngol 2003;28:112–120

20. Niedermeyer HP, Arnold W. Etiopathogenesis of otosclerosis. ORL J Otorhinolaryngol Relat Spec 2002;64:114–119

21. Chole RA, McKenna M. Pathophysiology of otosclerosis. Otol Neurotol 2001;22:249–257

22. Minor LB, Carey JP, Cremer PD, Lustig LR, Streubel S. Dehiscence of bone overlying the superior canal as a cause of apparent conductive hearing loss. Otol Neurotol 2003;24:270–278

23. American Academy of Pediatrics. Year 2000 position statement: principles and guidelines for early hearing detection. Pediatrics 2000;106:798–817

24. Roush J, Matkin ND. Infants and Toddlers with Hearing Loss. Baltimore: York Press, 1994

25. Matkin ND, Wilcox AM. Considerations in the education of children with hearing loss. Pediatr Clin North Am 1999;46:143–152

26. Chole RA, McKenna M. Pathophysiology of otosclerosis. Otol Neurotol 2001;22:249–257

27. Tange RA. Ototoxicity. Adverse Drug React Toxicol Rev 1998;17:75–89

28. Humes HD. Insights into ototoxicity. Analogies to nephrotoxicity. Ann N Y Acad Sci 1999;884:15–18

29. Kountakis SE, Helidonis E, Jahrsdoerfer RA. Microtia grade as an indicator of middle ear development in aural atresia. Arch Otolaryngol Head Neck Surg 1995;121:885–886

30. Low WK, Lim TA, Fan YF, Balakrishnan A. Pathogenesis of middle-ear effusion in nasopharyngeal carcinoma: a new perspective. J Laryngol Otol 1997;111:431–434

31. Low WK, Goh YH. Uncommon otological manifestations of nasopharyngeal carcinoma. J Laryngol Otol 1999;113:558–560

32. Sininger YS. Audiologic assessment in infants. Curr Opin Otolaryngol Head Neck Surg 2003;11:378–382

33. Johnson KC. Audiologic assessment of children with suspected hearing loss. Otolaryngol Clin North Am 2002;35:711–732

34. Kumar A, Maudelonde C, Mafee M. Unilateral sensorineural hearing loss: analysis of 200 consecutive cases. Laryngoscope 1986;96:14–18

35. Schulman-Galambos C, Galambos R. Brain stem evoked response audiometry in newborn hearing screening. Arch Otolaryngol 1976; 105:86–90

36. Jackler RK. A 73-year-old man with hearing loss. JAMA 2003;289: 1557–1565

37. Kemp DT. Stimulated acoustic emissions from within the human auditory system. J Acoust Soc Am 1978;64:1386–1391

38. Berlin CI, Morlet T, Hood LJ. Auditory neuropathy/dyssynchrony: its diagnosis and management. Pediatr Clin North Am 2003;50: 331–340

39. Ruth RA, Lambert PR, Ferraro JA. Electrocochleography: methods and clinical applications. Am J Otol 1988;9(suppl):1–11

40. Orchik DJ, Shea JJ Jr, Ge X. Transtympanic electrocochleography in Meniere's disease using clicks and tone-bursts. Am J Otol 1993;14: 290–294

41. Angeli S. Value of vestibular testing in young children with sensorineural hearing loss. Arch Otolaryngol Head Neck Surg 2003; 129:478–482

42. Mathews J, Rao S, Kumar BN. Autoimmune sensorineural hearing loss: is it still a clinical diagnosis? J Laryngol Otol 2003;117:212–214

43. Mathews J, Kumar BN. Autoimmune sensorineural hearing loss. Clin Otolaryngol 2003;28:479–488

44. Kelsell DP, Dunlop J, Stevens HP, et al. Connexin 26 mutations in hereditary non-syndromic sensorineural deafness. Nature 1997; 387:80–83

45. Greinwald JH Jr, Hartnick CJ. The evaluation of children with sensorineural hearing loss. Arch Otolaryngol Head Neck Surg 2002;128: 84–87

46. Hone SW, Smith RJ. Medical evaluation of pediatric hearing loss. Laboratory, radiographic, and genetic testing. Otolaryngol Clin North Am 2002;35:751–764

47. Mafong DD, Shin EJ, Lalwani AK. Use of laboratory evaluation and radiologic imaging in the diagnostic evaluation of children with sensorineural hearing loss. Laryngoscope 2002;112:1–7

14

Clinical Evaluation of the Dizzy Patient

Judith A. White

◆ History

The history is the cornerstone of all medical evaluation. For the dizzy patient, it is the most valuable portion of the evaluation. Symptoms of dizziness may not be active at the time the patient is seen in the office, and the historical account may be all that is available to the clinician. An accurate and detailed history leads to the correct diagnosis in 70% of dizzy patients, when compared with final diagnostic conclusions after all evaluation is completed by a vestibular specialist.[1]

Obtaining a complete, accurate, and detailed history may be challenging in the dizzy patient. Even the most conscientious, motivated patient may have difficulty describing symptoms. One reason is that equilibrium is largely an unconscious sensation. We have few words to describe its absence. The catchall term *dizziness* is commonly used to describe vertigo, syncope or near-syncope, imbalance or ataxia, disequilibrium, light-headedness, and poor concentration. We explain to patients that although they are being seen to evaluate their dizziness, we need to find a more exact description of their symptoms. Initial open-ended questioning can be rapidly focused onto key symptoms such as vertigo.

Vertigo is an illusion of rotatory movement. The nearly universal childhood experience of turning around rapidly and repeatedly in one location and then stopping suddenly and experiencing the illusion of the room spinning in front of your eyes can be used to describe vertigo to patients. Asking specifically "Do things move in front of your eyes when you are dizzy?" can also be helpful.

Syncope, fainting, and loss of consciousness are never vestibular in origin, and suggest the need for cardiac consultation. Even the severe drop attacks experienced by Meniere's syndrome patients are not associated with loss of consciousness (unless patients knock themselves out inadvertently from a head injury while dropping from loss of extensor tone).

Imbalance only while walking, difficulty walking, stumbling, ataxia, and other movement disorders suggest neurologic and/or musculoskeletal diagnoses, particularly when active head movements are well tolerated in a sitting position. In contrast, vestibular disorders (including bilateral vestibular loss) cause symptoms of visual blurring (oscillopsia) during rapid head movements, occurring both while sitting and upright/ambulating.

Light-headedness, disequilibrium, and "things moving around inside my head" are nonspecific complaints, and further diagnostic evaluation may be necessary to determine if there is an underlying vestibular component to these complaints.

After the patient and clinician have agreed on as specific a description of the symptom as possible, the duration of the specific symptom is reviewed next, which is particularly important in vestibular evaluation. Vertigo may last only seconds in benign paroxysmal positional vertigo, but the ensuing nausea or mild disequilibrium may persist for hours. Many patients may not initially differentiate between the character and the intensity of symptoms and inaccurately report "I have been dizzy for 3 weeks" when further questioning elicits a history of sudden brief vertigo with certain position changes accompanied by mild nonspecific disequilibrium. Similarly, the severe vertigo of Meniere's syndrome may last for hours but the patient may feel "off" for days thereafter.

Patients are asked to describe in detail the first episode of dizziness, as well as the most recent episode, and to give an estimate of how many episodes in total have occurred. Details include exactly what they were doing when symptoms occurred (e.g., looking up on a high shelf, or sitting quietly at a desk) and how long each symptom lasted. Any associated symptoms, such as hearing change or loss, or tinnitus, are noted. Focal neurologic symptoms such as diplopia, visual loss, headache, numbness, and weakness are inquired about specifically. Provoking factors such as position change, pressure changes (sneezing, lifting) or loud noises are specifically reviewed.

The patient's medical history also establishes risk factors and has impact on the likelihood of some diagnoses. Cerebrovascular pathology is more likely in patients with advanced age, valvular heart disease, smoking, hypertension, diabetes, and cardiac arrhythmias. Prior history of ear surgery, pain, and drainage makes an otologic source more likely. A history of prior transient focal neurologic deficits (such as a numb hand or visual loss) increases the possibility that imbalance or dizziness may be due to multiple sclerosis. Prior exposure to ototoxic or vestibulotoxic medications such as chemotherapeutic agents (especially cis-platinum) or aminoglycosides are important historic points suggesting bilateral vestibular hypofunction. Oncologic disease may give rise to paraneoplastic neurologic disorders such as cerebellar ataxia. Renal disease, cardiac arrhythmias, and some ophthalmologic conditions suggest syndromic vestibular disorders with or without hearing loss.

Migraine is increasingly recognized as an etiology for many episodic vestibular symptoms. Approximately 25% of patients meeting defined criteria for migraine experience otherwise unexplained episodic dizziness.[2] Familiarity with migraine classification criteria may be helpful in making the diagnosis of migraine-associated dizziness, and they are outlined below. Note that migraine headaches may occur with or without classic aura such as visual loss, scintillating scotomata, and peri-oral numbness (**Table 14–1**).[3]

The International Classification of Headache Disorders (ICHD-II) has included vertigo as part of aura only in basilar-type migraine, which also requires other symptoms from the posterior circulation, such as posterior headache, bilateral visual auras, or diplopia. However, the association of the vestibular symptoms and headache may be inconsistent in migraine-associated dizziness (MAD). Vestibular symptoms may precede headache, occur variably (most commonly), or be totally unrelated to headache.[4] The duration of vestibular symptoms may also be variable, ranging from minutes to days, and the nystagmus seen can have peripheral, central, or mixed features.[4] Regardless of duration and association with headache, however, most investigators require discrete episodes of vestibular symptoms.

Because neither of these ICHD-II definitions includes the type of vertigo most commonly associated with migraine, additional criteria for "migrainous vertigo" or "migraine-associated dizziness" have been proposed by Neuhauser et al[5] (**Table 14–2**) and have been generally accepted; these criteria form the basis of a structured diagnostic interview, the Structured Interview for Migrainous Vertigo (SIM-V).[6]

Questionnaires are often recommended for clinical evaluations of dizzy patients. We find that a one- or two-page questionnaire mailed to the patient prior to the appointment, along with a request to bring outside audiologic, vestibular, and neurologic evaluations, medication lists, and previous brain imaging studies can be time-saving and allow the patient to organize the history prior to the appointment.

Prior diagnoses that patients may have received may not be necessarily accurate. One recent review[7] found that only 31% of consulted neurologists, 16% of otolaryngologists, and 2% of primary care providers performed positional testing in patients complaining of positional vertigo. They suggest this leads to inaccurate diagnosis and contributes to the average North American testing costs of $2000 per patient.[8]

◆ Differential Diagnosis of Common Vestibular Disorders

The four most common vestibular syndromes have classic distinguishing historic features. A review of the pathophysiology of these disorders can be found in Chapter 27.

Benign paroxysmal positional vertigo (BPPV) is the most commonly recognized vestibular disorder. The incidence of BPPV ranges from 10.7[9] to 64[10] per 100,000, and increases by 38% with each decade of life.[10] However, recent data suggest that this disorder may be more common than current

Table 14–1 International Classification of Headache Disorders—II

Criteria for migraine without aura (1.1)
A. At least five attacks fulfilling criteria B to D
B. Headache attacks lasting 4 to 72 hours (untreated or unsuccessfully treated)
C. Headache has at least two of the following characteristics:
 1. Unilateral location
 2. Pulsating quality
 3. Moderate or intense intensity
 4. Aggravation by or causing avoidance of routine physical activity (e.g., walking or climbing stairs)
D. During headache at least one of the following:
 1. Nausea or vomiting
 2. Photophobia and phonophobia
E. Not attributed to another disorder

Criteria for basilar-type migraine (1.2.6)
A. At least two attacks fulfilling criteria B to D
B. Aura consisting of at least two of the following fully reversible symptoms, but no motor weakness:
 1. Dysarthria (slurred speech)
 2. Vertigo (dizziness)
 3. Tinnitus (illusory noise)
 4. Hypacusia (reduced hearing)
 5. Diplopia (double vision)
 6. Simultaneous bilateral visual aura in both temporal and nasal fields
 7. Ataxia (imbalance)
 8. Decreased level of consciousness
 9. Simultaneous bilateral paresthesias
C. At least one of the following
 1. At least one aura symptom develops gradually over 5 or more minutes or different aura symptoms occur in succession for 5 or more minutes
 2. Each aura symptom lasts for at least 5 minutes but not greater than 60 minutes
D. Headache fulfilling criteria for ICHD-II migraine without aura begins during the aura or follows aura within 60 minutes
E. Not attributed to another disorder

Source: International Classification of Headache Disorders, 2nd ed. Cephalalgia 2004;24:1–160. Reprinted by permission.

Table 14–2 Neuhauser Criteria for Migrainous Vertigo

1. Recurrent episodic vestibular symptoms (attacks)
2. Migraine headache meeting International Headache Society (IHS) 1988 criteria
3. At least one of the following migrainous symptoms during at least two of these attacks:
 a. Migraine-type headache
 b. Visual or other auras
 c. Photophobia
 d. Phonophobia
4. Other causes ruled out by appropriate investigations

Source: Neuhauser H, Leopold M, von Brevern M, et al. The interrelations of migraine, vertigo and migrainous vertigo. Neurology 2001;56:436–441. Reprinted by permission.

population estimates indicate. In one study, Oghalai et al[11] noted that 9% of randomly selected geriatric patients in an urban clinic who had undergone positional testing had positive results and undiagnosed BPPV.

Characteristically, patients complain of brief vertigo lasting seconds to minutes provoked by position change such as lying back, rolling over, bending over, or arising quickly, or by looking up. The position of the head during hairdresser or dentist appointments may provoke vertigo. Patients may learn to avoid positions provoking vertigo, and unexpected falls in the elderly have been attributed to unrecognized BPPV. There is no associated hearing change or tinnitus. Although the majority of episodes last less than 2 months, some persist for over a year. Recurrence is common (15% per year).

The second most common vestibular disorder is vestibular neuritis. It is characterized by the sudden onset of prolonged severe incapacitating vertigo. Antiemetic and vestibular-suppressive medication may be needed in the acute period, which typically lasts approximately 3 days. This is commonly followed by weeks of gradually resolving disequilibrium and intolerance of rapid head movement. When hearing loss accompanies vestibular neuritis, the more generalized involvement of the labyrinth (including the cochlear and vestibular nerves) is termed labyrinthitis. Prompt identification of neuritis facilitates appropriate treatment (including steroids and vestibular rehabilitation techniques, see Chapter 32), which can improve outcome. Magnetic resonance imaging (MRI) with contrast of the brain is helpful in excluding an acoustic neuroma or other structural pathology.

The third most common vestibular disorder is Meniere's syndrome. Historic features include episodic spontaneous vertigo lasting at least 20 minutes (but typically less than 24 hours) with associated hearing loss, aural fullness, and tinnitus. In 1995 the Committee on Hearing and Equilibrium of the American Academy of Otolaryngology released guidelines for the diagnosis and evaluation of therapy in Meniere's disease.[12] "Certain" Meniere's disease is based on histopathologic confirmation, which is limited to postmortem examination. "Definite" Meniere's disease requires two or more definite spontaneous episodes of vertigo 20 minutes or longer, audiometrically documented hearing loss on at least one occasion, tinnitus or aural fullness in the treated ear, and other possible causes have been excluded. The hearing loss may take several forms: The arithmetic mean of hearing thresholds at 0.25, 0.5, and 1 kHz is 15 dB or more higher than the average of 1, 2, and 3 kHz; or the average threshold at 1, 2, and 3 kHz is 20 dB or more poorer than the other ear. "Probable" Meniere's disease is similar, with the exception that only one definite episode of vertigo is required. "Possible" Meniere's disease includes episodic vertigo without hearing loss or sensorineural hearing loss (fluctuating or fixed) with disequilibrium but without definitive vertigo episodes.

Occasionally episodic vertigo occurs without any identified hearing loss or lateralizing otologic symptoms. In patients with a history of migraine (ICHD-II criterion 3), this may represent migraine-associated dizziness. However, both migraine-associated dizziness and Meniere's syndrome are diagnoses of exclusion, and they have been noted to coexist in a greater-than-expected percentage of the population.[13] Neural imaging studies are appropriate in these patients. Repeated examination, especially when symptoms are active, may clarify cases with confusing historic features. Repeated audiologic evaluation may be particularly helpful. An empiric therapeutic trial may be undertaken with low-sodium diet (1500 to 2000 mg/day) and diuretic such at triamterene/hydrochlorothiazide 37.5 mg/25 mg once daily. Response to this empiric trial supports a diagnosis of Meniere's syndrome. Alternately, an empiric trial of a migraine preventive such as topiramate suggests a non-vestibular cause, such as migraine-associated dizziness.[14]

Less common vestibular disorders may also be identified because of their characteristic history. Patients complaining of vertigo, instability, and blurred vision when exposed to loud noises or pressure changes such as sneezing or straining may have dehiscence of the superior semicircular canal. This leads to unusual pressure and sound sensitivity in the affected ear, and possible low-frequency conductive hearing loss with suprathreshold bone curve and abnormal vestibular evoked myogenic potential testing. Computed tomography (CT) scan of the temporal bones with fine cuts reconstructed in the plane of the superior semicircular canal show a dehiscence in the bone overlying the superior semicircular canal.[15]

◆ Physical Examination

Physical examination of the dizzy patient begins with the standard otologic exam, including thorough visualization of the tympanic membrane to exclude structural ear disease such as cholesteatoma or chronic suppurative otitis media.

Vital signs including systolic and diastolic blood pressure and pulse are taken with the patient in the sitting, lying, and standing positions to elicit possible postural orthostatic cardiovascular instability. Auscultation of the heart and carotid arteries augments the cardiovascular portion of the examination. Level of alertness, speech intelligibility, and affect are noted.

Cranial nerves are briefly surveyed with attention to gross visual acuity, ocular motion in the nine cardinal directions of gaze (neutral, up, down, left, right, up and left, down and left, up and right, down and right), ocular alignment, facial sensation to light touch, facial movement symmetry, palate elevation symmetry, shoulder shrug and head turn strength and symmetry, and lateral tongue motion.

The oculomotor exam is important to detect central and visual abnormalities. Oculomotor abnormalities will also affect the sensitivity of the vestibular exam that will follow. Smooth pursuit is assessed by slowly moving a finger or pen in both the lateral and vertical planes at a distance of about 8 inches in front of the patient using the best corrected vision (i.e., eyeglasses on, if possible). Finger movement that is too rapid will elicit rapid catch-up saccades and is the most frequent error in performing this exam. Testing should be restricted to the central 30 degrees of vision (15 degrees to the left and 15 degrees to the right or up and down) to avoid provoking end-gaze physiologic nystagmus. Breakup of pursuit is significant, and can suggest visual problems (especially in the elderly), attentional problems, or central pathology. Nystagmus that is provoked by eccentric gaze should be noted (this may indicate peripheral vestibular pathology if seen in one direction of lateral gaze only, and suggest central pathology if seen bilaterally or in the vertical plane). Abnormal findings in pursuit are noted and then corroborated in saccade testing.

Saccades are tested in vertical and horizontal planes by asking the patient to rapidly look from the examiner's nose to a finger placed approximately 15 degrees lateral or vertical to neutral eye position. Several repetitions are optimal in each direction (right, left, up and down). Particular attention is paid

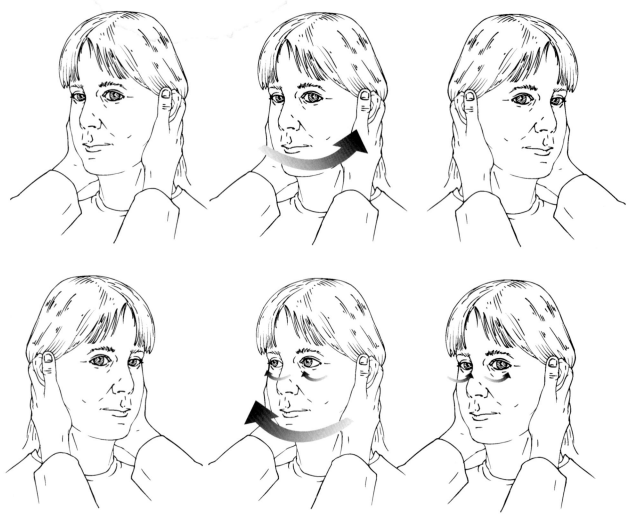

Figure 14–1 Halmagyi-Curthoys head-thrust test, illustrating normal gaze stability with head thrust left, and impaired gaze stability with head thrust right. The subjects must make a compensatory saccade to bring gaze back to center after head thrust right. (From Cleveland Clinic Foundation. Reprinted by permission.)

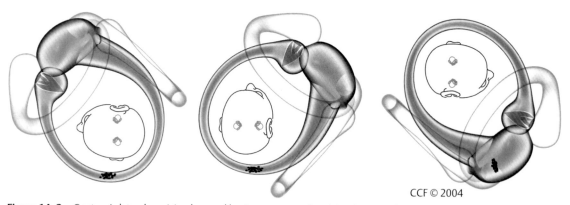

CCF © 2004

Figure 14–2 Geotropic lateral semicircular canal benign paroxysmal positional vertigo (LSC-BPPV). The left ear is viewed from above as the patient lies supine. Head position is indicated. In the central figure, the patient is supine and canalith material is in the distal lateral semicircular canal. On the left side of the figure, the patient has rolled onto the left ear and the canalith material moves towards the left LSC cupula, causing an ampullopetal endolymph current that is excitatory. On the right of the figure, the patient has rolled onto the right ear and the canalith material moves away from the cupula, causing an ampullofugal endolymph flow that is inhibitory. Nystagmus beats towards the undermost ear. (From Cleveland Clinic Foundation. Reprinted by permission.)

to the accurate movement of the eyes to the target (without undershoot or overshoot) and to conjugate movement of both eyes. If one or both eyes fail to move in conjugate gaze, or move more slowly, a possible internuclear ophthalmoplegia is noted and further evaluation of possible central pathology is warranted. Care is taken to note long-standing strabismus prior to interpreting saccade and pursuit abnormalities as central indicators.

Spontaneous nystagmus is examined both with and without visual fixation. Frenzel lenses are very useful for this purpose, and are available in optical and infrared versions for office use. Infrared video systems project to video monitors and can be interfaced with computerized image analysis systems. Nystagmus is named for the fast phase (relative to the patient's perspective). Thus, nystagmus with a fast phase (beat) toward the patient's right ear is termed rightward nystagmus. Nystagmus due to a peripheral vestibular abnormality should decrease with visual fixation (fixation suppression). Nystagmus that does not decrease by 50% with fixation or that becomes worse with fixation is a strong predictor of central pathology. We also repeat eccentric gaze testing using Frenzel lenses to eliminate visual fixation because this may bring out nystagmus that was not previously observed during pursuit and saccade testing in room light.

Office testing of vestibulo-ocular reflex gain by rotating the exam chair while wearing Frenzel lenses to eliminate visual fixation can give a screening estimate of vestibular function, but the stimulus is not standardized and computer analysis is not possible. Vestibular autorotation testing has been developed using motion-detecting sensors on the head to assess the stimulus frequency while the patient shakes the head wearing Frenzel infrared recording goggles. However, this method may allow for vestibulo-colic (neck) reflexes and anticipatory saccades to affect gain, and the gold standard remains computerized rotary chair testing with standardized stimulus frequencies and analysis.[16] This vestibular laboratory method was discussed in Chapter 10.

Head-thrust testing (developed by Halmagyi and Curthoys[17]) facilitates evaluation of the high-frequency vestibulo-ocular reflex to each side. The patient is placed facing the examiner with the head tilted down approximately 30 degrees to place the lateral semicircular canals in earth horizontal position. The examiner grasps the patient's head in both hands and asks the patient to keep his or her gaze on the examiner's nose. The head is then slowly rotated back and forth laterally until an unexpected high-velocity low-amplitude thrust is made to bring the head from lateral to midline. The normal patient keeps the eyes on the examiner's nose without difficulty. The patient with a weak peripheral vestibular system cannot stabilize vision in this situation and the eyes slide past the target and are redirected to the examiner's nose with a compensatory saccade immediately after the thrust. This abnormality is seen when the thrust is in the direction of the weak ear (**Fig. 14–1**).

The final, and most important, vestibulo-ocular office test is positional and positioning testing. With Frenzel lenses in place, the patient is initially placed in a supine position with the eyes open. Any nystagmus is observed. The head is then rotated to the right lateral position for 10 seconds, brought

back to midline for 10 seconds, and rotated to the left lateral position for 10 seconds before being returned to midline. The patient then returns to the sitting position. This maneuver detects horizontal nystagmus that may be related to lateral canal BPPV. Lateral canal BPPV[18] affects approximately 15% of patients with BPPV, and is usually not detected in Dix-Hallpike positioning because that positioning stimulates the posterior rather than the lateral canal. The paroxysmal positional nystagmus in lateral canal BPPV usually has less latency and a longer duration than that typically seen in posterior canal BPPV. It changes direction depending on the portion of the canal involved and the direction of the head. Geotropic (beating toward the ground, i.e., leftward in the left-ear-down position and rightward in the right-ear-down position) nystagmus suggests canalithiasis in the distal lateral canal, with the worst nystagmus in the affected-ear-down position (**Fig. 14–2**). Apogeotropic nystagmus beats toward the uppermost ear in the lateral supine position, and suggests material proximal to or adherent to the cupula (**Fig. 14–3**). If lateral canal testing is negative in supine lateral turns, Dix-Hallpike positioning testing is performed next.

In 1952, Dix and Hallpike[19] described the characteristic ipsidirectional torsional nystagmus provoked by the head maneuver they developed to identify posterior canal BPPV. During this maneuver, the patient's head is turned 45 degrees to one side while he or she is seated. The patient is then moved quickly to a supine position with the neck slightly extended and the head remaining turned. When the undermost ear is affected, nystagmus is seen. The patient is then brought back up to a sitting position, and the nystagmus is noted to reverse direction. The maneuver is then performed on the other side. The characteristic nystagmus occurs after a delay of several seconds, declines after 10 to 30 seconds, and diminishes with repeated positional testing in the same sitting (**Fig. 14–4**). Posterior semicircular canal BPPV responds to Semont, Epley, or canalith repositioning maneuvers[20] (**Fig. 14–5**). See Chapter 32 for a review of these techniques.

The neurotologic office exam is completed with assessment of postural stability, gait, and cerebellar function. Finger-to-nose and heel-to-shin testing and rapid alternating movements are assessed. Postural control is assessed by observing gait, with attention to broad-based, shuffling, or ataxic gait. In appropriate patients (older patients, diabetics, and those complaining of leg numbness or ataxia) vibration sense is tested at the ankle and compared with the wrist. A Rydel Seiffer (Barthelmes Zella-Mefilis, Thuringan, Germany) or other 128 Hz tuning fork can be used. Decreased lower extremity vibration sense suggests neurologic processes, such as peripheral neuropathy. Proprioception is assessed with toes-up or toes-down positioning. A survey of reflexes and motor strength can be included as needed if deficits are suspected.

An audiogram remains one of the most helpful tests in the clinical evaluation of the dizzy patient. Asymmetric hearing loss and low-frequency hearing loss (sensorineural or conductive) are suggestive of an otologic source for dizziness and provide valuable diagnostic information.

At the completion of the clinical evaluation of the dizzy patient, the clinician usually has obtained characteristic historical and examination findings that correctly suggest the

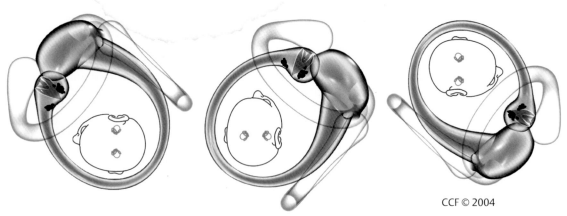

CCF © 2004

Figure 14–3 Apogeotropic lateral semicircular canal benign paroxysmal positional vertigo (LSC-BPPV). The left ear is viewed from above, as the patient lies supine. Head position is indicated. In the central figure, the patient is supine and canalith material is in the proximal lateral semicircular canal, possibly adherent to the cupula. On the left side of the figure, the patient has rolled onto the left ear, causing an ampullofugal endolymph current that is inhibitory. On the right of the figure, the patient has rolled onto the right ear, causing an ampullopetal endolymph flow that is excitatiry. Nystagmus beats away from the undermost ear. (From Cleveland Clinic Foundation. Reprinted by permission.)

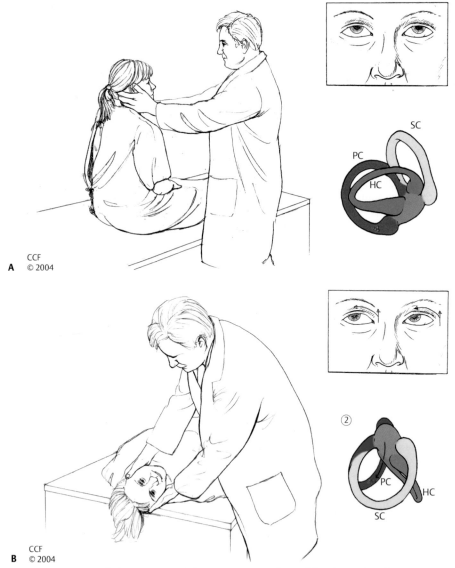

A CCF © 2004

B CCF © 2004

Figure 14–4 Dix-Hallpike positioning. **(A)**. Starting position (seated, head turned 45 degrees to the right). Position of the eyes is shown on the right. **(B)**. Lying position (head turned 45 degrees to the right). Characteristic upbeat and right torsional nystagmus is illustrated; canalith material can travel down the long arm of the posterior semicircular canal, causing ampullofugal endolymph flow and stimulation of the cupula. White J. Benign paroxysmal positional vertigo: How to diagnose and quickly treat it. (Cleve Clin J Med 2004;[71]9:722-728. From Cleveland Clinic Foundation. Copyright © 2004. All rights reserved. Reprinted by permission.)

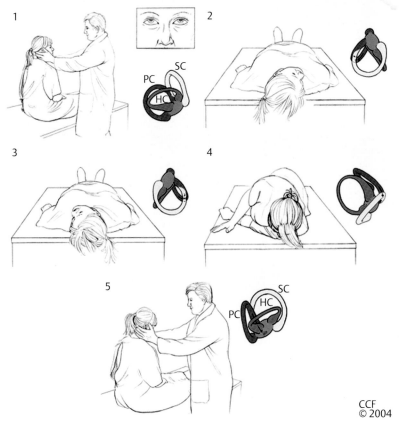

Figure 14–5 Canalith repositioning procedure for right posterior semicircular canal benign paroxysmal positional vertigo. The patient begins in the seated position with the head turned 45 degrees towards the examiner (rightwards, see Box 1). The patient is placed in the right Dix-Hallpike position and the characteristic nystagmus may be observed (Box 2). The patient remains supine and the head is slowly rotated towards the opposite ear (Box 3). The patient rolls onto the opposite shoulder and directs the head into a nose-down position (Box 4). After any nystagmus subsides, the patient is assisted in returning to the original position (Box 5). White J. Benign paroxysmal positional vertigo: How to diagnose and quickly treat it. (Cleve Clin J Med 2004;[71]9:722–728. From Cleveland Clinic Foundation. Copyright © 2004. All rights reserved. Reprinted with permission.)

diagnosis. In cases such as BPPV vertigo, treatment may begin immediately and no further assessment is needed. In other cases, additional information is needed. Neural imaging studies and vestibular testing may be appropriate.

See Chapter 10 for a discussion of vestibular testing.

References

1. Gufoni M, Guidetti G, Nutti D, et al. The role of clinical history in the evaluation of balance and spatial orientation disorders in the elderly. Acta Otorhinolaryngol Ital 2005;25(suppl 79)5–10

2. Baloh RW. Neurotology of migraine. Headache 1997;37:615–620

3. International Classification of Headache Disorders, 2nd ed. Cephalalgia 2004;24:1–160

4. von Brevern M, Zeise D, Neuhauser H, et al. Acute migrainous vertigo: Clinical and oculographic findings. Brain 2005;128:365–374

5. Neuhauser H, Leopold M, von Brevern M, et al. The interrelations of migraine, vertigo and migrainous vertigo. Neurology 2001;56: 436–441

6. Furman JM, Marcus DA, Balaban CD. Migrainous vertigo: development of a pathogenetic model and structured diagnostic interview. Curr Opin Neurol 2003;16:5–13

7. von Brevern M, Lezius F, Tiel-Wilck K, Radtke A, Lempert T. Benign paroxysmal positional vertigo: current status of medical management. Otolaryngol Head Neck Surg 2004;130:381–382

8. Li JC, Li CJ, Epley J, et al. Cost-effective management of benign positional vertigo using canalith repositioning. Otolaryngol Head Neck Surg 2000;122:334–339

9. Mizukoshi K, Watanabe Y, Shojaku H, et al. Epidemiological study on benign paroxysmal positional vertigo. Acta Otolaryngol Suppl 1988;447:67–72

10. Froehling D, Silverstein MD, Mohr DN, et al. BPPV: incidence and prognosis in a population-based study in Olmsted County Minnesota. Mayo Clin Proc 1991;66:596–601

11. Oghalai JS, Manolidis S, Barth JL, et al. Unrecognized benign paroxysmal positional vertigo in elderly patients. Otolaryngol Head Neck Surg 2000;122:630–634

12. Committee on Hearing and Equilibrium guidelines for the diagnosis and evaluation of therapy in Meniere's disease. Otolaryngol Head Neck Surg 1995;113:181–185

13. Radtke A, Lempert T, Gretsky MA, et al. Migraine and Meniere's disease-is there a link? Neurology 2002;59:1700–1704

14. Fife T, White J. Treating migraine-associated vertigo with topiramate. Presented at the 2006 Annual meeting of the American Neurotology Society, Chicago

15. Minor LB, Solomon D, Zinreich JS, Zee DS. Sound– and/or pressure-induced vertigo due to bone dehiscence of the superior semicircular canal. Arch Otolaryngol Head Neck Surg 1998;124:249–258

16. Fife TD, Tusa RJ, Furman JM, et al. Assessment: Vestibular testing in adults and children Report of the Therapeutic and Technology Subcommittee of the American Academy of Neurology. Neurology 2000;55:1431–1441

17. Halmagyi GM, Curthoys IS. A clinical sign of canal paresis. Arch Neurol 1988;45:737–739

18. White J, Coale K, Catalano P, Oas J. Diagnosis and management of lateral semicircular canal benign positional vertigo. Otolaryngol Head Neck Surg 2005;133:278–284

19. Dix MR, Hallpike CS. Pathology, symptoms and diagnosis of certain disorders of the vestibular system. Proc R Soc Med 1952;45:341–354

20. White J, Savvides P, Cherian N, Oas J. Canalith repositioning for benign paroxysmal positional vertigo. Otol Neurotol 2005;26:704–710

III

Management

15

Disorders of the Auricle

Benjamin D. Liess and William C. Kinney

The external ear is a unique part of the human sensory system. Its structure, prominent position, and complex function predispose the auricle to disorders not seen in other parts of the human body. Congenital defects of the auricle result from disruption of complex developmental events and may lead to many combinations of both external and middle ear disorders. The prominent position of the ear makes it more susceptible to both mechanical and thermal trauma and also affects how the auricle heals from the trauma. A unique set of local infectious and systemic diseases manifests in the ear and may represent a primary process or an associated finding. Multiple dermatologic conditions involve the auricle and should be treated as part of the general dermatologic illness. In addition to systemic infectious etiologies, both immunologic and metabolic disease states may develop auricular manifestations. The auricle is also subject to various neoplastic processes. This chapter assists the otolaryngologist in recognizing and understanding the various disease entities that can involve the auricle.

◆ Congenital Disorders of the Auricle

Congenital disorders of the auricle involve a wide range of deformities, each requiring a different surgical approach for correction. Rogers[1] classified these defects in descending order of severity in terms of deformity: microtia,[2] lop ear,[3] constricted ear, and prominent or protruding ear.[4] Weerda[2] combined the classification systems of Rogers and Tanzer and expanded on this classification by correlating the defect with degree of developmental dysplasia (**Table 15–1**). Other findings not seen in these classification systems include preauricular pits and sinuses as well as preauricular appendages.

Heredity is a factor in specific defects. Preauricular pits and sinuses appear to be dominant characteristics in some families.[3] Deafness and auricular deformities have been reported as characteristics of both dominant and recessive genetic disorders. For example, ear deformities occur in families of patients with mandibulofacial deformities such as Treacher-Collins syndrome.[4] Additionally, the incidence of microtia may vary among ethnic groups. In one series by

Table 15–1 Classification of Auricular Defects

Constricted ear (cup or lop), cryptotia
Prominent ear (first-degree dysplasia)
Hypoplasia of superior third of auricle (first-degree dysplasia)
Hypoplasia of middle third of auricle (second-degree dysplasia)
Anotia (third-degree dysplasia)
Complete hypoplasia (third-degree dysplasia) with atresia of external auditory canal
Complete hypoplasia (third-degree dysplasia) without atresia of external auditory canal
Hypoplasia of entire superior third

Source: Adapted from Weerda H. Classification of congenital deformities of the auricle. Facial Plast Surg 1988;5:385–388. Reprinted by permission.

Harris et al,[5] the incidence was estimated to be 1 to 3 per 10,000 live births. In contrast, the incidence of microtia is estimated to be 1 in every 4000 live births among the Japanese and 1 in every 900 to 1200 among Navajo Native Americans.[6]

The embryologic relationship of the auricle to the middle ear produces a range of concurrent defects in the middle ear and surrounding structures that must be evaluated when an auricular deformity is present. Middle ear deformities can vary from a narrow external auditory canal with minimal ossicular defects to fused ossicles with an absence of mastoid pneumatization. Specific abnormalities of the ossicles include a shortened long process of the malleus that may be attached to the anterior canal wall or complete absence; the malleus and incus may be underdeveloped or a single mass of bone; and stapes abnormalities including defects in the superstructure or even complete absence of the footplate. Facial nerve disorders can include loss of the bony fallopian canal covering, bulging of the nerve over the oval window, or running of the nerve inferior to the oval window. Changes in the tympanic bone, temporomandibular joint, mastoid, and location of dura also have been associated with deformities of the auricle.[7] Additionally, children with external ear abnormalities have a mildly increased risk of concurrent renal abnormalities[8] and may need to undergo a clinical genetics evaluation to screen for additional anomalies.

Congenital Deformities

Microtia represents a range of findings from complete agenesis to a somewhat small ear with an atretic canal. The most common finding is a vertically oriented sausage-like or "peanut" ear (**Fig. 15–1**). Twice as many males are affected, with the right side being involved more often. Bilateral microtia is relatively rare but is seen frequently in patients with Treacher-Collins syndrome or bilateral craniofacial microsomia.

Constricted ear is a term coined by Tanzer[9] to represent deformities in which the encircling helix is tight. This term includes the "cup ear," which refers to an increase in the conchal bowl size (**Fig. 15–2**), and "lop ear," with inferior bending of the superior helix (**Fig. 15–3**). Repair may involve reshaping existing tissue or require supplemental skin and supporting structures. Stahl's ear (**Fig. 15–4**) represents a variant of constricted ear. It is characterized by a third crus with a flattened scaphoid fossa and deficient antihelix.

Auricular atresia results from abnormal development of the first branchial cleft (ear canal) and arch (auricle) (also see Chapter 1). Lack of recanalization of the canal occurs during the same embryologic period as ossicular formation. As expected, ossicular abnormalities are commonly associated. Children with this anomaly may develop otitis media and cholesteatoma[10] with ear pain and fever. If clinical suspicion exists, computed tomography (CT) studies may delineate a pathologic process.

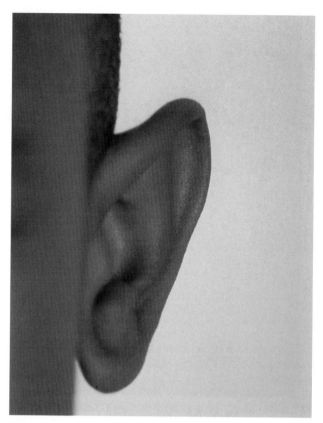

Figure 15–2   Cup ear.

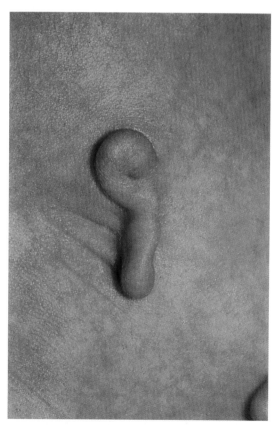

Figure 15–1   Peanut ear

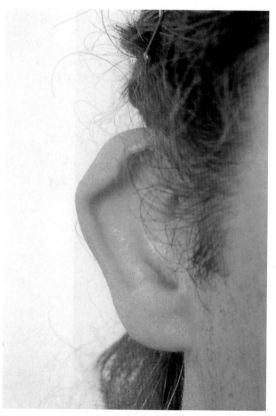

Figure 15–3   Lop ear.

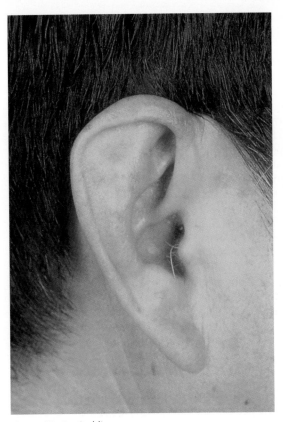

Figure 15–4 Stahl's ear.

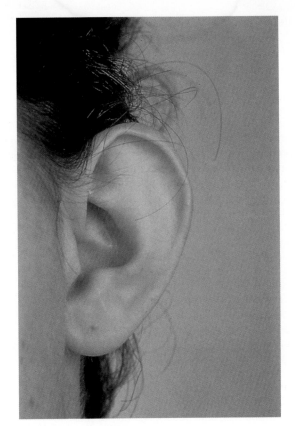

Figure 15–5 Prominent ear.

Cryptotia is the failure of the superior auriculocephalic sulcus to form, with the underlying cartilage buried beneath the scalp. The deformity occurs commonly in Japan, with an incidence as high as 1 in 400 births.[11]

Protrusion of the auricle with subsequent folding of the helix and antihelix occurs between the third and sixth month of gestation. Any interference with this process may result in a prominent ear (**Fig. 15–5**). Of known defects, the most common finding is failure of the antihelix to fold. Widening of the concha may also be seen. These findings are usually bilateral with a heredity influence, as they are seen in first-degree relatives.

Auricular appendages are common and result from the presence of accessory auricular hillocks. They usually appear anterior to the auricle and most often are unilateral. Skin alone or skin with underlying cartilage may be present. Children with preauricular appendages may have an associated unilateral hearing loss; therefore, complete audiologic testing may be necessary.[12] These appendages may appear as part of Goldenhar syndrome. Auricular sinuses are pit-like depressions occurring in a triangular area just anterior to the auricle (**Fig. 15–6**). The embryologic basis for these sinuses is unclear, but is thought to be caused by failed closure of the dorsal part of the first branchial groove. Some sinuses appear to be a portion of ectoderm sequestered during formation of the auricle.[13]

Congenital Syndromes

Treacher-Collins syndrome (mandibulofacial dysostosis) is an autosomal dominant hereditary malformation caused by abnormal development of the first branchial arch. Deformities

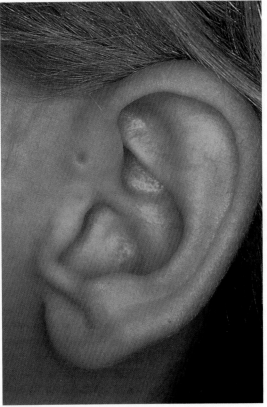

Figure 15–6 Preauricular sinus.

of the auricle are common and usually are bilateral but may be unilateral. Associated findings include auricular deformities, atresia or stenosis of the external auditory canal, middle ear anomalies resulting in a conductive hearing loss, lower eyelid notching, diminished nasofrontal angle, cheek flattening, mandibular hypoplasia, palatal defects, and dental anomalies.[14,15]

Branchio-oto-renal syndrome (Melnick Fraser syndrome) is an autosomal dominant disorder with both branchial arch and renal anomalies. Auricular findings include preauricular sinuses or auricular appendages. Additionally, an associated sensorineural, conductive, or mixed hearing loss may exist. Although it is unclear why the association among multiple organ systems exists, it remains important for any child with branchial arch anomalies to be evaluated for concurrent otologic and renal deformities.[16]

Goldenhar syndrome (oculoauriculovertebral dysplasia) has been described as autosomal dominant, but other factors in addition to heredity may have a role. Ear findings include microtia, preauricular sinuses or appendages, and external auditory canal atresia.[17]

Townes-Brocks syndrome (anus-hand-ear syndrome or renal ear and radical [REAR] syndrome) is an autosomal dominant disorder with multiple abnormalities including malformations of the external and middle ear with sensorineural hearing loss, hand deformities, renal anomalies (mainly hypoplastic kidney), and anorectal malformations. Auricular findings include microtia, "satyr" or "lop" ear, and preauricular tags or pits.[18]

Nager syndrome (preaxial acrofacial dysostosis) is an autosomal dominant condition resulting from abnormal development of the first and second branchial arches. Characteristics of this condition include the absence of radius, radioulnar synostosis, and hypoplasia or absence of the thumbs. Acrofacial dysostosis is characterized mainly by lower lid ptosis, cleft palate, severe micrognathia, and malar hypoplasia. Auricular findings include atresia, aplasia, and dysplasia of the auricle, along with multiple deformities of the external, middle, and internal ear with related hearing loss.[19]

Miller syndrome (postaxial acrofacial dysostosis) is an inherited disorder characterized by distinctive craniofacial malformations that occur in association with abnormalities of the outer aspects of the forearms and lower legs. Craniofacial malformations may include malar hypoplasia, micrognathia, cleft lip and palate, "cup-shaped" ears, and ectropion.[20]

Surgical Correction

The need for surgical correction of a congenitally malformed auricle is based on multiple variables including, but not limited to, the severity of deformity, associated middle ear anomalies, unilateral versus bilateral involvement, and the degree of inner ear function. The immediate role of the otologist is to assess hearing and select an appropriate hearing aid. In the newborn, auditory brainstem response testing is performed. In the older child, a combination of auditory brainstem response testing and behavioral audiometry is employed. Jahrsdoerfer and Hall[21] recommend a CT scan after age 3 years to evaluate the middle ear structures. Glasscock and colleagues[22] obtain plain films in the infant to assess bony atresia of the external auditory canal, portions of the labyrinth and cochlea, and internal auditory canal. They reserve CT scan for the older child. In the case of auricular atresia,

intraoperative facial nerve monitoring to identify the commonly aberrant nerve is recommended to help prevent iatrogenic facial paralysis.[23,24]

Disagreement exists whether the malformed auricle or atretic external auditory canal should be repaired first. The reconstructive surgeon believes that repairing the auricle after the atresia decreases cartilage viability because of changes in blood supply and scarring resulting from previous surgery. The otologist would first correct the atresia, believing that proper positioning of the new auricle is dependent on appropriate placement of the new external auditory canal. Investigation has shown that a reconstructed auricle can be repositioned successfully with careful soft tissue elevation,[4] but this additional procedure is avoidable if the atresia is addressed first. Timing for surgical correction of the deformity also is controversial. In patients with unilateral microtia and a normal opposite ear, Glasscock and colleagues[22] prefer to wait until the patient is age 18 and able to make a decision based on the risks and benefits involved. Jahrsdoerfer and Hall[21] perform most of the repairs on patients between the ages of 4 and 6 years. Brent[4] suggests that optimal timing for unilateral repair is when the patient is 6 to 7 years old, after the rib cartilage has matured and the child can perform postoperative care. Exceptions for postponement of auricular repair in unilateral cases include cases of a chronically draining fistula involving the ear or extensive cholesteatoma. For bilateral microtia, Jahrsdoerfer and Hall suggest repair of at least one side before the child starts school.

◆ Auricular Trauma

Auricular trauma can result from blunt, penetrating, or thermal injury. The auricle is susceptible to such trauma because of its prominent and unprotected position. Unlike the eyes, the auricle has no reflex to protect against impending injury. In addition to immediate damage from the traumatic event, complications of auricular trauma such as chondritis with loss of cartilage support can be cosmetically deforming.

Often, auricular trauma will require surgical reconstruction. In most cases, prophylactic antibiotics and tetanus prophylaxis are warranted. Photographs or drawings may be helpful for planning a repair and documenting the extent of injury. In a multitrauma patient, stabilization and treatment of other injuries take precedence over auricular trauma.

Blunt Trauma

Shearing forces occurring with blunt trauma may produce an auricular hematoma (**Fig. 15–7**). Commonly seen in wrestlers and boxers, this hematoma forms when blood vessels of the perichondrium are traumatically separated from their underlying cartilage. Additional accumulation of blood further separates the perichondrium from the cartilage. Because cartilage receives oxygen and nutrients solely from the perichondrium, this separation may result in cartilage necrosis. Early treatment is necessary to prevent growth of ectopic fibrinocartilage from the perichondrium, resulting in a thickened external ear or "cauliflower ear" (**Fig. 15–8**). The pathogenesis of auricular hematoma has been studied and confirmed in an animal model.[25]

Auricular hematoma originally was treated with repeated aspirations and bandaging, but unfortunately such treatment

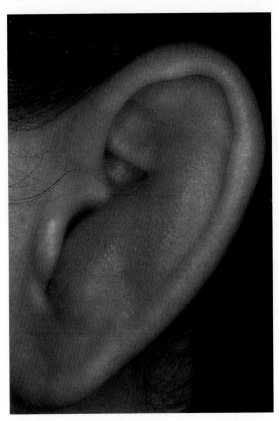

Figure 15–7 Auricular hematoma.

often resulted in a thickened auricle. Current methods for treatment include aspiration followed by pressure dressing involving a plaster mold[26] or reinforced collodion dressing,[27] anterior auricular incision with cartilage fenestration and hematoma evacuation,[28] postauricular incision with resection of cartilage and hematoma evacuation followed by cotton bolster dressings[29] or through-suturing,[30] and continuous portable suction drainage.[31,32] Schuller and associates[33] describe a technique of incising the hematoma, removing the clot, debriding any compromised cartilage, and then suturing dental rolls in place to bolster and reshape the auricle. This technique is technically simple and highly reliable. Antibiotic ointment and oral antistaphylococcal antibiotics commonly are prescribed. Bolsters are removed in 7 to 14 days. The advantage of this technique is that the patient may return to work or to sports activities with protective headgear the next day.

In the event of late treatment where fibrinocartilage has formed, the old clot and growth of new cartilage can be excised along with auricular skin until a normal contour is achieved as compared with the other ear. The ear can be repaired successfully with minimal distortion of normal tissue.[28] Fortunately, such extensive deformity has become a rarity. Generally these procedures are without risk; however, hematoma may reaccumulate or infection may be introduced prompting initiation of antibiotics.

Lacerations and Abrasions

Lacerations of the auricle may range from a simple laceration requiring primary closure to complete avulsion. The auricle, like the face, has excellent blood supply and heals remarkably well. Proper surgical technique with atraumatic handling of tissue, minimal debridement, realignment of known anatomic landmarks, and meticulous approximation of tissue edges will provide the best results. If cartilage exposure occurs, the risk of infection increases and antibiotic prophylaxis may be required.

Simple Lacerations

Approximation of the cartilage, perichondrium, and skin edges is required for a good result. Some prefer to avoid direct suturing of cartilage and believe that only approximation of the skin is required, citing concerns of weakening of the structural integrity.[34] Appropriate sutures include a through-and-through nonabsorbable stitch to approximate all three layers or a figure-of-eight closure of perichondrium and cartilage using an absorbable suture and simple skin closure. Advantages of the latter approach include better stabilization of the cartilage with no overriding of repaired edges and better approximation of auricular skin. If perichondrium-to-perichondrium suturing is employed, some cartilage may have to be removed.

Complex Lacerations

The same principles of repair apply to complex lacerations. However, because the laceration is complex, correct alignment of the fragments may be difficult. Temporary sutures may be helpful in realigning auricular landmarks. Debridement may be necessary to create adequate margins for reapproximation but should be kept to a minimum.

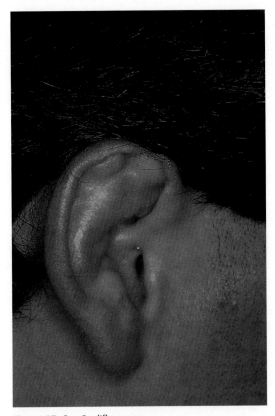

Figure 15–8 Cauliflower ear.

Abrasions

Abrasions of the auricle can result from a motorcycle or bicycle accident or another event resulting in a dragging injury across the ground. These wounds are contaminated and may have embedded debris. Persistent, gentle scrubbing can be used to clean the ear and remove dirt and particulate matter. The auricle should be covered with an antibiotic-impregnated gauze and a pressure dressing applied for 24 hours. Local wound care is employed after the dressing is removed to allow for reepithelialization.

Partial Tissue Loss

Partial tissue loss includes avulsions of the skin alone or full-thickness loss of the auricle. If the avulsion results in skin loss only with preservation of the perichondrium, then a split- or full-thickness skin graft may be applied directly. Potential donor sites include the upper eyelid or the cranial surface of the auricle. When trauma to skin and perichondrium involves the concha or antihelix, cartilage may be removed and a skin graft placed directly on the posterior perichondrium. This cartilage removal will not result in loss of support. When skin and perichondrium loss involves other parts of the auricle, pedicled flaps of postauricular skin may be used. For larger defects, a temporoparietal fascia flap may be used with a split-thickness skin graft.[35]

Full-thickness loss of the helix of less than 2 cm can be converted to a wedge repair with primary closure. Cupping of the auricle may result, but this can be corrected at closure with the excision of side triangles at the apex of the wedge. Larger defects of the marginal rim can be repaired with a chondrocutaneous advancement flap as described by Antia and Buch[36] or with a modified Antia-Buch repair.[37] Skin and cartilage are incised laterally with undermining of skin medially to allow for advancement of the helical rim. Some defects may require bringing additional material into the defect to minimize the decrease in ear size. Options include advancement flaps from adjacent areas with cartilage grafting and staged procedures with implanting of the exposed cartilage in the postauricular skin. Further reconstruction with a cartilage graft occurs during a second procedure.

Auricular Avulsions

Near-total or total avulsion of the auricle may be seen with animal or human bites, knife injuries, or motor vehicle accidents. Careful debridement of devitalized tissue along with wound cleaning and irrigation should occur with each case. Successful reattachment usually is more cosmetic than reconstruction. If the avulsed segment remains partially attached, an attempt should be made to regain position. In these situations, the blood supply may be adequate for partial or complete repair.

Reattaching the avulsed segment as a composite graft often results in various degrees of venous congestion and requires blood thinning agents to decrease clotting and improve blood flow.[38] Multiple stab wounds or medicinal leeches[38] also may improve tissue survival. Mladick et al[39] described a "pocket principle" for the treatment of auricular avulsions where the skin of the avulsed segment is dermabraded and reattached in its correct anatomic position. The auricle then is buried beneath a postauricular incision or "pocket." After 10 to 14 days, the auricle is removed from the pocket and allowed to reepithelialize.

Microvascular replantation of near total or total auricular avulsion is an effective surgical option. Anastomosis to the superficial temporal vessels either directly or via vein graft was first described by Pennington et al.[40] Although a technically challenging procedure, successful operation with excellent aesthetic outcome has been reported, even in unfavorable cases.[41–45] These authors describe the necessity of meticulous dissection and careful handling of tissue during direct vessel anastomosis and venous graft repair to avoid complications. As with the composite graft technique, blood thinners and medicinal leeches may assist with ear perfusion and subsequent neovascularization and healing.

In the event of complete avulsion, the avulsed segment should be transported in a cold, sterile container, and reattached as soon as possible. If the ear cannot be saved, then an auricular prosthesis held in place by osseointegrated implants or total auricular reconstruction may be needed.

Animal bites require special consideration not seen with other forms of trauma. Documentation of what type of animal, when the injury occurred, status of tetanus immunization, and rabies status of the animal should be completed as part of the initial evaluation. Photo documentation of animal bites may be needed in the event that legal action is taken by the injured party.

All animal bites to the auricle require debridement, irrigation, and prophylactic antibiotics along with a 24-hour checkup. Common organisms seen with both human and non-human bites are listed in **Table 15–2**. A majority of wounds contain both aerobic and anaerobic organisms. Careful cleaning and wound irrigation is required. Surgical repair follows the principles outlined above. Stucker and colleagues[46] recommend delayed repair of severe or older human bites to allow for initial antibiotic treatment to decrease the degree of bacterial presence from the traumatic inoculation. For the uncomplicated injury less than 5 hours old, they recommend primary repair. If delayed repair is chosen, local wound care should be employed until the wound is clean and shows signs of granulation tissue formation.

Thermal Injuries

Frostbite

Frostbite is a localized injury resulting from exposure of tissue to subfreezing temperatures (**Fig. 15–9**). Frostbite injury may be divided into four degrees. First degree presents with edema and erythema and in approximately 1 week the superficial skin layers slough. Second degree begins with the development of blisters and may progress to bulla formation. Upon

Table 15–2 Bacteriology of Human and Nonhuman Bites

Human Bites	Nonhuman Bites
Streptococcus species	*Streptococcus* species
Aerobic *Streptococcus* species	Aerobic *Streptococcus* species
Aerobic *Staphylococcus aureus*	Anaerobic *Staphylococcus aureus*
Haemophilus species	*Pasteurella multocida*
Bacteroides species	*Bacteroides* species
Eikenella corrodens	*Fusobacterium* species

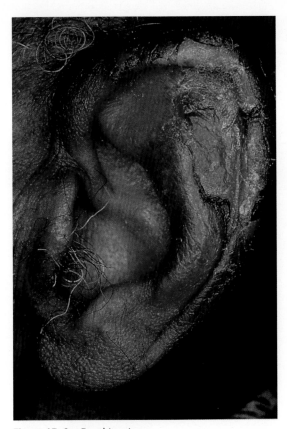

Figure 15–9 Frostbite pinna.

desiccation of the blisters an eschar will form; when the eschar sloughs, healthy tissue will appear. Third degree consists of dermal and possible subcutaneous tissue damage resulting in an eschar that may take months to heal. Fourth degree presents with damage to the deeper tissues and underlying bone, which often leads to tissue necrosis, gangrene, and autoamputation. The extent of injury depends on the duration of exposure, temperature, and whether contact with metal, moisture, or protective ointment occurs.[47]

Tissue loss is caused by direct cellular and vascular injury. At a cellular level, chondrocytes show a greater degree of devastation compared with epidermal cells. Vascular injury results from separation of the vascular endothelium from the underlying lamina, thought to be caused by ice crystal formation.[48] Resultant tissue necrosis then is caused by erythrocyte extravasation, interstitial edema, and decreased blood flow. Endothelial cells at the injury site release chemical mediators, including arachidonic acid metabolites, which directly stimulate contraction of vascular and nonvascular smooth muscle, modulate platelet aggregation, and influence histamine release.[49]

Treatment of auricular frostbite first requires rapid rewarming of the affected tissue. Wet cloths at 38° to 42°C are applied to the ear and changed as needed until the ear is thawed.[50] The auricle should be kept clean and both physical pressure upon the ear and vasoconstrictors should be avoided. Prophylactic antibiotics are recommended and early debridement generally is discouraged because several months may be required to assess the extent of self-healing. Heggers and colleagues[51] recommend debridement of blisters because they contain arachidonic acid metabolites that may further damage the auricle.

Burns

The auricle is at risk of extensive injury from a burn because of its prominent position and tissue composition. Lack of subcutaneous tissue leaves the perichondrium and cartilage with little protection. Exposed cartilage is at increased risk of chondritis (**Fig. 15–10**). Dowling et al[52] estimated that infection occurred in up to 25% of auricular burns.

Burn injury is classified as first, second, and third degree. First-degree (superficial) burns involve only the epidermis and present with erythema, warmth, and no blisters, and are painful to touch. Minimal treatment is needed. Second-degree (partial-thickness) burns involve the epidermis and part of the dermis and appear red, blistered, and may be swollen and painful to touch. They can be further classified as superficial or deep, depending on the amount of dermis involved. Third-degree (full thickness) burns involve the epidermis and dermis and appear erythematous, mottled, white, brown, or charred, and lack all but deep sensation. Local tissue loss may result from both direct heat injury and tissue ischemia. Ischemia is due to both increased vascular permeability to fluid from platelet microthrombi damage to small vessels, and release of chemical mediators similar to those seen in frostbite injury.

Treatment of auricular burns is similar to treatment of burns in other locations. This treatment may be remembered with the six C's of care: (1) remove clothing, (2) cool the burn, (3) clean the burn site, (4) chemoprophylaxis with tetanus immunization, (5) cover the burn site with appropriate dressings, and (6) comfort the patient with analgesics. Topical mafenide acetate (Sulfamylon) cream is recommended due to excellent eschar and cartilage penetration along with clinical

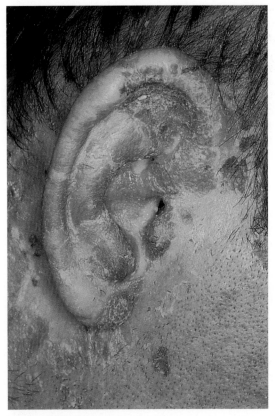

Figure 15–10 Burn pinna.

efficacy in reducing the incidence of chondritis. Exposed cartilage must be covered with vascularized tissue. A complication of cartilaginous involvement in burn injury is suppurative chondritis, commonly caused by *Pseudomonas aeruginosa*. In chondritis, appropriate antibiotics may be given intravenously or by direct injection into the ear multiple times each day, in addition to topical application of Sulfamylon cream. Principles of reconstruction described for avulsion may be used to correct any resulting defect.

◆ Infections of the Auricle

Infections of the external ear include primary infections of the auricle and infections of the external auditory canal. This discussion focuses on infections of the auricle but includes those processes that may overlap with the external auditory canal. Infections of the external ear may be primary or secondary to underlying disease or injury.

Bacterial Infections

Impetigo

Impetigo is a highly contagious superficial spreading infection involving the superficial layers of the epidermis. Impetigo of the auricle commonly occurs when an infection of the lateral external auditory canal and concha extends to the auricle. The clinical presentation may be bullous or nonbullous. Bullous impetigo presents with rapidly appearing superficial clusters of fragile blisters or large bullae. Rupture of the blisters produces a raw area surrounded by a ragged fringe of epidermis called a "collarette of scale."[53] Lymph nodes are not frequently involved. Bullous impetigo is commonly caused by *Staphylococcus aureus,* which has been cultured from blisters. Nonbullous impetigo (impetigo contagiosa) presents a single erythematous macule that becomes vesicular and easily ruptures, leaving a "honey-colored" crust over the erosion. This commonly expands into surrounding areas and may have associated local lymphadenopathy.[54] Some disagreement exists concerning the causative agent, but most concur that staphylococcal organisms are responsible for cases in temperate climates and streptococcal organisms for those in tropical environments.[53] The ear may be autoinoculated when children scratch the external meatus after touching another affected area of the body.

Before initiating antibiotic treatment, wound cultures should be obtained. Local wound care is appropriate in addition to topical antistaphylococcal agents, including mupirocin, which have been proven equally effective as oral agents.[55,56] Treatment of nonbullous impetigo should begin promptly to decrease the likelihood of poststreptococcal glomerulonephritis. Due to penicillin resistance among organisms, β-lactamase–resistant antimicrobials are recommended first, followed by macrolides, when oral agents are necessary for extensive involvement.[54]

Erysipelas

Erysipelas is a superficial subcutaneous infection of the skin typically caused by group A β-hemolytic streptococci involving the dermis and local lymphatics. Infection may spread across anatomic boundaries (**Fig. 15–11**). Auricular involvement

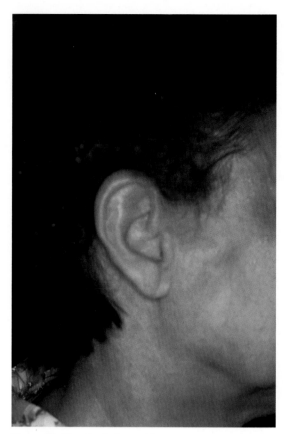

Figure 15–11 Erysipelas auricle.

commonly is due to autoinoculation during ear cleaning or scratching. The affected area is warm, erythematous, and painful with an expanding zone of involvement that is irregular, sharply elevated, and clearly demarcated from uninvolved skin.[57] Systemic symptoms commonly include fever, chills, and malaise. Treatment begins with analgesics and oral antibiotics, commonly penicillin, to cover streptococcal organisms. Patients without improvement in 48 hours may require intravenous antibiotics.

Perichondritis and Chondritis

Perichondritis is an infection of the external ear caused by trauma, burns, ear piercing, and insect bites. If untreated, perichondritis will progress to chondritis with necrosis of cartilage and auricular deformity. Clinically, perichondritis presents with diffuse swelling, erythema, and extreme tenderness of the auricle (**Fig. 15–12**). Fever and chills may be present. This is usually caused by *S. aureus* or *P. aeruginosa*.[58] Chondritis indicates the infection has progressed, and areas of fluctuance suggest abscess formation. Treatment consists of surgical drainage and debridement of devitalized tissue followed by administration of systemic antibiotics, commonly a fluoroquinolone due to antipseudomonal and antistaphylococcal activity and excellent cartilage penetration. However, in patients under 18 years of age, another antibiotic with adequate coverage may be chosen due to possible adverse effects on developing cartilage. Treatment with drainage and indwelling catheter irrigation with antibiotic solution has been reported.[59,60]

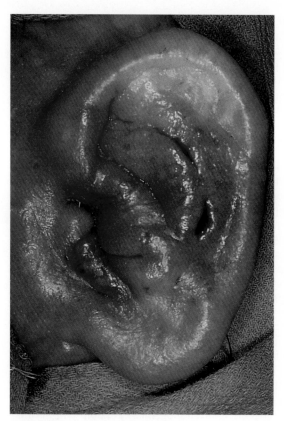

Figure 15–12 Perichondritis auricle.

Viral Infections

Herpes Zoster Oticus

Herpes zoster oticus, or Ramsay Hunt syndrome, is the most common viral infection of the auricle, caused by reactivation of latent varicella zoster virus in the seventh cranial nerve in the geniculate ganglion. This syndrome is characterized by an acute facial nerve palsy along with an erythematous rash on the ear or in the mouth. Ramsay Hunt syndrome differs from Bell's palsy, which does not present with cutaneous involvement. Unlike Bell's palsy, recovery of full facial mobility with Ramsay Hunt syndrome is less than 50%.

Clinically, herpes zoster oticus begins with a dull ache in the retro- or infra-auricular area that progresses to deep, severe pain. Soon, auricular erythema and swelling develop followed by vesicle eruption involving the lateral external auditory canal and concha (**Fig. 15–13**) 3 to 7 days after the onset of pain.[61] Culture of vesicle beds reveal varicella zoster virus. This syndrome is estimated to cause 3 to 12% of all cases of facial nerve paralysis.[62] Other cranial nerves also may be involved, including the cochleovestibular nerve, which results in hearing loss and vertigo. Less commonly involved nerves are cranial nerves V, IX, X, XI, and XII. Clinical symptoms begin to resolve in 10 to 14 days.

Treatment includes warm compresses, analgesics prednisone, and antivirals. Scratching should be discouraged to avoid secondary infection. During facial paralysis, routine eye care and protection of the cornea is required. In one study, patients who began prednisone and acyclovir within 3 days of onset of symptoms demonstrated significant improvement in overall recovery.[63] One currently used regimen consists of prednisone 60 mg

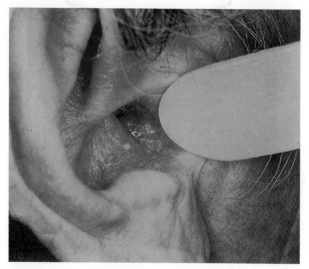

Figure 15–13 Herpes zoster.

daily for 14-21 days (longer than in Bell's palsy) and valacyclovir 1.5 grams twice daily for 14 days. Vestibular suppressives and analgesics may help associated symptoms.

◆ Dermatologic Conditions of the Auricle

Allergic contact dermatitis and seborrheic dermatitis are two important conditions that the otologist should recognize. Seborrheic dermatitis is a common cause of external otitis. Allergic contact dermatitis, although less common, can confound pathologic conditions and limit the available treatment options for many external ear disorders.

Allergic Contact Dermatitis

Allergic contact dermatitis is an inflammatory condition of the skin presenting with erythema, edema, and scaling that develops hours to weeks after exposure to the pathogen. A strong immunogenic reaction against a harmless agent creates a hypersensitivity reaction caused by a specific antigen or irritant. The auricle is a common site because of its exposure to many products, both medicinal and cosmetic, that contain antigenic or irritant substances. The physician should maintain a high index of suspicion for contact dermatitis in any patient who appears to worsen after treatment has been initiated. Once suspected, a careful history and patch testing may be used to delineate sensitivity to a substance.

Allergic contact dermatitis is a classic example of delayed hypersensitivity reaction. On a cellular level, a hapten (a small chemical molecule) binds skin Langerhans cells, also known as antigen-presenting cells (APCs) or dendritic cells, and stimulates an inflammatory response. The APCs travel to local lymph nodes for induction of hapten sensitization and activation of antigen-dependent T cells. T lymphocytes migrate back to the affected area and release cytokines and chemokines, which further amplify the inflammatory response. Local dendritic cells again are stimulated, releasing additional inflammatory mediators, perpetuating the cycle of inflammation. Although the precise mechanism of irritant contact dermatitis remains under investigation, it is well known that an irritant substance stimulates cytokine presentation to skin cells. This attracts additional cells involved in the immune-mediated process, perpetuating the cycle.[64] Greater understanding of this intricate process may allow for development of immunomodulators and new therapies to alleviate this troublesome condition.

Topical antibiotics, steroids, pharmaceutical solvents, preservatives, and jewelry containing nickel are the most common causes of allergic contact dermatitis involving the auricle. Many physicians use topical neomycin in combination with bacitracin and polymyxin B for treatment of external otitis. Unfortunately, sensitivity to neomycin is common,[65] and neomycin can cross-react with other antimicrobial drugs administered systematically (**Fig. 15–14**). Of greatest concern is the potential for cross-reaction with gentamicin. A study of 100 neomycin-sensitive patients with no prior exposure to gentamicin demonstrated 40 patients who developed an adverse cross-reaction to gentamicin.[66] Consequently, in critically ill patients, gentamicin treatment may not be possible. Contact allergy to topical corticosteroids, including hydrocortisone, also is well recognized. The possibility of an allergic reaction to a preparation solvent also should be kept in mind. Propylene glycol is a commonly used vehicle for topical corticosteroid, antibiotic, and antifungal preparations. The concentration of propylene glycol in each preparation varies depending on desired drug penetration and release. Cutaneous reaction to propylene glycol is either an allergic or irritant response, depending on the preparation concentration. Many topical preparations contain preservatives to extend the shelf life, which may cause an allergic contact dermatitis. These include parabens, imidazolidinyl urea, quaternium 15, butylated hydroxyanisole (BHA), formaldehyde, DMDM hydantoin, methylisothiazolinone/methylchloroisothiazolinone (Kathon

CG), bronopol, and diazolidinyl urea.[67] Both propyl and methyl paraben are commonly used in topical antibiotic and fungal preparations. Because they are weak antigens, many otherwise sensitive patients can tolerate their application. Finally, nickel is one of the most common contact allergens and is frequently a composite metal in jewelry. Fortunately, its use is decreasing as a result of this well-documented allergy.

Seborrheic Dermatitis

Seborrheic dermatitis is a scaly, superficial, eczematous dermatitis that can affect the auricle and is a common cause of otitis externa. The disease primarily affects sebaceous skin and may present in a variety of ways, ranging from an unnoticed dermatitis to an erythematous, pruritic, scaling, oozing dermatitis evolving into a secondary bacterial infection.[68] The cause of seborrheic dermatitis is uncertain but believed to be related to the yeast-like organism *Malassezia furfur* (formerly *Pityrosporum ovale*). Studies linking *Malassezia* to seborrheic dermatitis are based on cutaneous resolution of the condition after treatment with specific antifungal preparations; however, not all patients achieve a complete response. As a result, some authors discount infection with *Malassezia* as the sole cause of this disease. Webster[69] proposed that an immune hypersensitivity to *Malassezia* caused local skin changes. Because *Malassezia* is a part of the normal human skin flora, an unknown event may occur to cause it to become either pathogenic or immunogenic.[70] Possible triggers may include a change in local sebum production, an increase in skin alkalinity, or, in the case of the auricle, occlusion of the external canal leading to a local environmental change.

Conservative treatment for seborrheic dermatitis aims to decrease yeast colonization and inflammation (**Table 15–3**). Each has in common an element of activity against *Malassezia*. For more extensive involvement, oral ketaconazole is the most effective antimycotic drug against *Malassezia*. The use of a combination of ketaconazole and topical steroid cream is also effective.[70] The book editor (G.B.H.) prefers Locoid (cortisone butyrate) 0.1% topical solution, four drops in the ear canal for 5 minutes, which then drain out, repeated three times daily

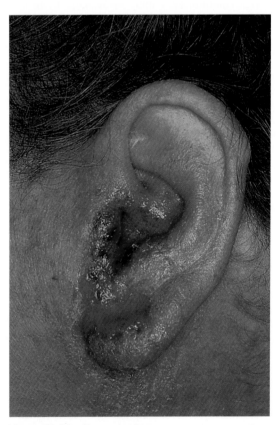

Figure 15–14 Neomycin allergy.

Table 15–3 Topical Preparations for the Treatment of Seborrheic Dermatitis with Activity Against *Malassezia furfur*

Selenium sulfide (2.5%)
Zinc pyrithione (1%)
Corticosteroids
Sulfur (2% aqueous cream)
Tar (coal tar solution USP 0.1%)
Salicylic acid (2% aqueous cream)
Ultraviolet B radiation
Propylene glycol (5% to 40%)
Imidazoles (ketoconazole, itraconazole, metronidazole, fluconazole)
Pimecrolimus cream (1%)
Terbinafine
Butenafine
Tacrolimus
Ciclopiroxolamine (1%)
Lithium gluconate

Source: Adapted from Gupta AK, Madzia SE, Batra R. Etiology and management of seborrheic dermatitis. Dermatology 2004;208:89–93. Reprinted by permission.

for the first week and then in decreasing amounts until maintenance therapy prevents itching and other symptoms. Water should be kept out of the canal.

◆ Systemic Diseases of the Auricle

Many systemic diseases can involve the auricle, and auricular manifestations can be the initial presentation. Otologists must be familiar with the presenting signs and symptoms of these diseases so that an accurate diagnosis can be made. Systemic diseases with auricular manifestations can be divided into infectious, immunologic, and metabolic disorders. Our discussion focuses on those diseases that affect the auricle or the external auditory canal.

Infectious Disorders

Herpes Simplex

Herpes simplex virus (HSV) is ubiquitous, but humans are the only known reservoir.[61] This disease affects mainly the orolabial and genital regions and is transmitted through direct contact with an infected individual. Infection involves ectodermally derived tissue with subsequent retrograde axonal transport to neuronal cell bodies of sensory ganglia. HSV infection presents as groups of vesicles on an erythematous base, and symptoms of pain, pruritus, or paresthesia may precede or coincide with onset of the rash. Vesicle eruption may involve the auricle or external canal. HSV also may cause ocular infection, facial paralysis (Bell's palsy), and neonatal encephalitis. Once infected, a person may experience recurrent clinical outbreaks. The disease is self-limited, requiring only local care with compresses, analgesia, and topical antibiotics if bacterial superinfection arises. Antiviral therapy with acyclovir, pencyclovir, famcyclovir, valacyclovir, foscarnet, and docosanol cream (10%) have variable benefit in hastening healing and preventing transmission of the virus.[71] Antivirals combined with prednisone (in immunocompetent patients) may speed recovery.

Human Immunodeficiency Virus

Human immunodeficiency virus (HIV) is a growing global epidemic affecting people of all ages. Both adults and children with HIV may have their first manifestation of the disease as an ear, nose, or throat disorder or present with a protracted history of head and neck disease, including serial or unusual ear infections with or without mastoid involvement, sensorineural hearing loss, vestibular dysfunction, sinonasal disease, ocular or periorbital cellulitis, oral candidiasis, bilateral parotid swelling (especially in children), or severe infections with common organisms. Physicians should be alert for other systemic findings including generalized lymphadenopathy, hepatosplenomegaly, and growth retardation in children. Uncommon pathogens affecting this set of patients include pseudomonas, aspergillus, rhizopus, mycobacterium, candida, and other opportunistic organisms.[72,73]

HIV does not involve the auricle directly but rather predisposes the patient to a range of infectious diseases that can involve the auricle. Complicated bacterial and fungal infections of the external auditory canal can lead to perichondritis. Treatment consists of local cleaning; topical, oral, or intravenous antibiotics; antifungals or antivirals; and debridement when appropriate. *Pneumocystis carinii* infection of unilateral or bilateral external auditory canals is a well-known extrapulmonary manifestation that may evolve into mastoiditis. Pentamidine prophylaxis has reduced the incidence of otic involvement.[74,75] Acute invasive external otitis may occur in an immunosuppressed individual and manifest with severe life-threatening infection.[76] Kaposi's sarcoma, a spindle cell tumor, may occur with advanced AIDS and involve the auricle, external auditory canal, eardrum, and middle ear.[77] AIDS patients also have been documented to develop non-Hodgkin's lymphoma of the ear lobe.[78,79]

Leprosy

Mycobacterium leprae is responsible for leprosy, also known as Hansen's disease. Although endemic in many parts of the world,[80] few cases are reported today in the United States. Auricle lesions can occur in up to 70% of cases.[81] Characteristic lesions of the auricle include infiltrating nodules, loss of cartilage, and ulceration. Current therapy involves multidrug therapy consisting of dapsone, clofazimine, and monthly rifampin.[80]

Immunologic Disorders

Wegener's Granulomatosis

Wegener's granulomatosis is an autoimmune vasculitis that primarily affects the upper and lower respiratory tract and kidneys with variable expression at each anatomic site. The frequent demonstration of cytoplasmic antineutrophil cytoplasm antibodies (c-ANCAs) in sera of patients with Wegener's has facilitated an earlier diagnosis of the disease when it may involve only the ear, nose, or throat. Otolaryngologists should be aware of this disease and associated symptomatology to assist with early detection and treatment, possibly preventing renal or pulmonary involvement.[82,83] With disease progression, otolaryngologists should be part of a multidisciplinary team. Head and neck manifestations most commonly present in the nasal passages and paranasal sinuses. Primary involvement of the auricle is rare, but the disease can present in a manner similar to relapsing polychondritis. Findings include a red, tender, brawny, diffuse swelling of the pinna that is exacerbated during active disease.[84] Other otologic manifestations include ear lobe deformities, external otitis, serous or purulent otitis media, hearing loss, vertigo, and facial nerve palsy.[85]

Diagnosis requires a clinical history with findings of nasal, pulmonary, or renal involvement and serum measurement of c-ANCA. A diagnostic tissue specimen of an involved structure is necessary for accurate diagnosis. Therefore, in the case of auricular involvement, concurrent nasal disease is usually extensive enough to provide tissue for diagnosis, without the need for auricular biopsy. Early treatment includes trimethoprim-sulfamethoxazole. More extensive disease may be treated with immunosuppressives or cytotoxic drugs, including corticosteroids, methotrexate, or cyclophosphamide.[82,86]

Relapsing Polychondritis

Relapsing polychondritis is a rare idiopathic disease presenting as recurrent episodes of inflammation and destruction of articular and nonarticular cartilage. Auricular chondritis is the most common initial manifestation, which is heralded by the sudden onset of swelling, warmth, pain, and erythema of the cartilaginous portion of both external ears (**Fig. 15–15**).[87] Additional structures may include the eye, cochleovestibular organ, nose, trachea, larynx, and both pulmonary and cardiovascular systems. Multiple theories account for disease manifestations including (1) a hypersensitivity reaction with release of proteolytic enzymes and dissolution of cartilage, (2) antibody formation to type II collagen, (3) deposition of immune complexes, and (4) abnormalities of cell-mediated immunity.[88] Treatment options are guided by the degree of involvement and include nonsteroidal antiinflammatory drugs (NSAIDs), oral corticosteroids, colchicine, methotrexate, azathioprine, cyclosporine, and cyclophosphamide.[89]

Lupus Erythematosus

Lupus erythematosus is an autoimmune disease with both systemic manifestations and cutaneous involvement usually of the scalp, ears, or neck. Discoid lupus erythematosus is a subset that presents with cutaneous lesions. The discoid lesion is a well-demarcated, erythematous, infiltrated plaque with epidermal atrophy, telangiectasia, and scaling.[90] Lesions occur primarily in photosensitive areas and may involve the auricle in up to 44% of patients.[91] With time, cutaneous lupus progresses to scarring, skin atrophy, and areas of central hypopigmentation with a surrounding hyperpigmented border. Treatment includes sunscreen application, avoiding excessive sun exposure, topical steroids, retinoids, and hydrochloroquine.[92] The natural progression of lesions consists of hypo- or hyperpigmentation followed by scarring.[93] Approximately 5% of patients with

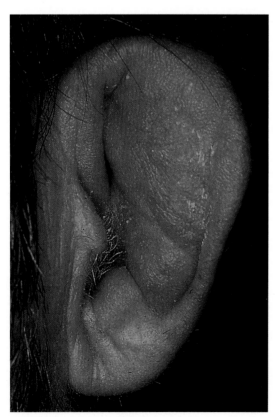

Figure 15–15 Relapsing polychondritis.

discoid lupus erythematosus eventually develop systemic lupus erythematosus.[81]

Rheumatoid Arthritis

Auricular involvement of rheumatoid arthritis is manifested by the formation of cutaneous and subcutaneous rheumatoid nodules on the external ear. Nodules may become necrotic and painful. Treatment is the same as that for systemic manifestations of the disease.

Metabolic Disorders

Gout

Gout develops from errors in purine metabolism resulting in hyperuricemia with deposition of urate in nonarticular tissue. Subcutaneous urate deposits, called tophi, are commonly found on the rim of the external ear, knee, and metatarsophalangeal joint. Clinically, patients present with painful subcutaneous nodules that may express a chalky white material containing sodium biurate.[84] Monosodium urate crystals can be seen on histopathologic examination. A defect in hypoxanthine guanine phosphoribosyl-transferase has been identified in familial clusters that results in excess uric acid production. First-line therapy should include NSAIDs and supplemental opiates for acute attacks, along with dietary changes, alcohol abstinence, and initiation of long-term medication. Current therapeutic recommendations include long-term probenecid or sulfapyrazone, colchicine for a short period in the acute setting for decreased renal excretion, allopurinol for overproduction of uric acid, systemic corticosteroids, and corticotropin.[94]

Ochronosis

Ochronosis is a form of alkaptonuria, an autosomal recessive disorder in which the metabolism of homogentisic acid to fumaric and acidoacetic acid is blocked owing to a lack of renal and hepatic homogentisic acid oxidase. Clinically, this enzyme deficiency causes homogentisic acid excretion in the urine along with its deposition in connective tissue. This results in ochronosis, a brown-black pigmentation in and deterioration of cartilage, bone, and cardiac valves, along with production of renal and prostate stones. Patients usually present in the third decade of life with the following signs: pigmentation of sclera (Osler's sign), pigmentation of auricular cartilage, and bluish nodules on the ears, nose, oral mucosa, and fingers. Ochronotic arthropathy involving the major joints also can develop. Treatment consists of a low-protein diet to decrease homogentisic acid accumulation, and oral ascorbic acid, which may counteract the homogentisic acid inhibition of lysyl hydroxylase activity. Investigation into nitarsone therapy, which inhibits the production of homogentisic acid, may demonstrate an additional safe and effective treatment modality.[95]

Auricular Ossification

Auricular ossification is a form of ectopic ossification resulting in replacement of elastic cartilage by bone. Auricular involvement may be unilateral, bilateral, or partial and most often occurs after frostbite injury. Concurrent involvement of the external auditory canal results in otalgia during ear manipulation or when the patient lies upon the affected auricle. Although seen more commonly after local trauma, it also can be seen after radiation therapy and in various endocrinopathies including hypopituitarism, Addison's disease, or thyroid or parathyroid disorders. Patients with von Meyenburg's syndrome (systemic chondromalacia) and familial cold hypersensitivity also may develop auricular calcification.[96,97] In cases of trauma, two cell types are postulated to be involved in new bone formation: an immediately reacting cell type present in periosteal connective tissue, and a slowly reacting cell type in the mesenchymal endomysium. The latter group can differentiate into osteoblasts and produce osseous matrix.[98]

Chondrodermatitis Nodularis Chronica Helicus

Chondrodermatitis nodularis chronica helicus is a perforating dermatosis in which dermal elements are exuded through the epidermis. This event occurs almost exclusively in white men over 40 years of age and is rarely seen in women or African Americans. Clinically, it presents as a solitary nodule on the superior rim of the helix, more often on the right ear (**Fig. 15–16**), though multiple lesions can occur. The nodule is tender and flesh-colored with an erythematous rim and a central crust overlying an ulcer. Various theories account for the pathogenesis: (1) an inciting event damages the cartilage, producing an inflammatory response creating a nodule[99]; (2) the lesion itself represents a perforating necrobiotic granuloma that is actinically induced[100]; (3) hyperkeratosis leads to superficial skin perforation[101]; (4) hypothermia or circulatory insufficiency creates an environment conducive to nodule formation; and (5) nodule formation is an idiopathic event.[102] Histopathology shows epidermal hyperplasia with

central ulceration capped by hyperkeratotic and parakeratotic scale. Edema, fibrinoid necrosis of dermal collagen, and granulation tissue surround the dermal necrobiosis. An inflammatory lymphohistiocytic infiltrate and perichondritis are present.[100] Although spontaneous resolution of the chondrodermatitis nodularis chronica helicus does not occur, some patients report spontaneous relief of associated pain. Treatment options include conservative management, intralesional steroids, carbon dioxide laser ablation, cryosurgery, and primary excision.[103]

◆ Neoplasms of the Auricle

The prominent position of the auricle gives it greater exposure to environmental factors, such as cold temperature and sunlight, that may play a role in the development of malignant neoplasms. The types of tumors that arise from the auricle are limited because of its composition of skin and cartilage. Neoplasms arising from the skin and skin appendages occur with greater frequency than from cartilage. Primary neoplasms of the auricular cartilage are rare.

Clinically, neoplasms of the auricle can be benign or malignant. Typically, benign lesions present with a painless slow-growing mass noted during personal grooming or incidentally by a relative or friend. Malignant neoplasms also may present as a painless mass but can progress to a painful, pruritic mass with intermittent bleeding. Advanced lesions with bone involvement can cause severe pain. A mass anterior to the auricle in the neck may indicate auricular carcinoma metastasis to a regional lymph node.

Benign Neoplasms

Sebaceous Cyst

A sebaceous cyst is a keratinous occlusion of a follicular ostium with accumulation of sebaceous material from the sebaceous gland. With time, the gland becomes atrophic while the cyst continues to grow secondary to continued keratin production. The cyst tends to occur in the postauricular area or on the earlobe. Differential diagnosis includes an epidermal inclusion cyst and a dermoid cyst. Epidermal inclusion cysts result from inoculation of epidermis into the dermis by trauma, such as ear piercing, infection, or penetration by a foreign body. The dermoid cyst is epidermal tissue trapped along the lines of fusion of embryonic skin flaps.[104] Treatment for the sebaceous cyst involves surgical excision with care taken to ensure removal of the overlying skin. If the cyst is infected, excision should be delayed until the infection has resolved.

Keloids

Keloids are benign overgrowths of dermal scar tissue in response to local trauma and are found commonly on the ear as a result of ear piercing, insect bites, or acne. Keloids should not be confused with hypertrophic scars. Hypertrophic scars are seen in wounds closed under tension and are confined to the boundaries of the initial scar, whereas keloids grow outward, spreading into adjacent tissue beyond its original borders (**Fig. 15–17**). Patients may report associated pain, pruritus, and physical deformity in the affected area. Histologically, keloids are composed of abundant hyalinized

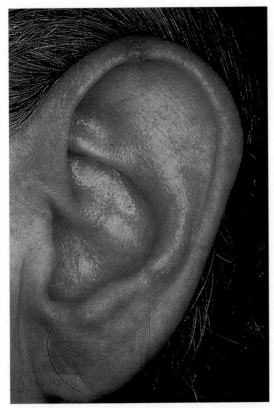

Figure 15–16 Chondrodermatitis.

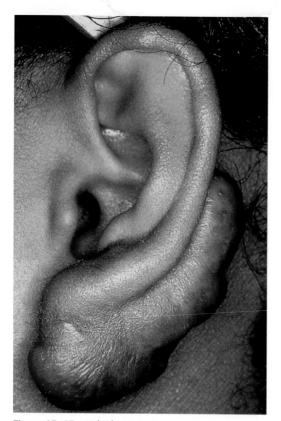

Figure 15–17 Keloid.

collagen bundles, extracellular matrix, and fibronectin, whereas hypertrophic scars lack these components.[105] Treatment of keloids includes surgical excision, laser therapy, intradermal steroid injection, cryotherapy, occlusive Silastic sheeting, pressure earrings, or even radiation therapy (reserved for severe, refractory cases).[106] The need for clinical follow-up and likelihood of recurrence should be discussed with each patient.

Pseudocyst of the Auricle

Pseudocyst of the auricle is an asymptomatic, unilateral swelling of the auricle most frequently seen in middle-aged men. Common nomenclature for this manifestation includes intracartilaginous cyst, endochondral pseudocyst, and cystic chondromalacia of the auricle. It often presents in the upper portion of the antihelix within the scaphoid or triangular fossa. Histologically, the inner surface of the cyst has no epithelial lining and therefore is considered a pseudocyst. Cystic fluid is straw colored, and cultures are typically sterile. Although the pathogenesis of this lesion remains uncertain, several mechanisms have been proposed: (1) repetitive minor trauma results in cartilaginous disruption and formation of cystic spaces; (2) embryologic malformation of the auricle creates areas of altered structural resistance, potentially leading to the creation of spaces in which fluid can collect; and (3) chondrocyte lysosomal enzymes are released, resulting in the dissolution of cartilage and creation of a pseudocyst.[107] The latter mechanism, although possible, has been discounted because increased levels of lysosomal enzyme have not been found in the cystic fluid, and an increase in the number of lysosomes in the chondrocytes has not been shown. Treatment

may involve simple aspiration, compression suturing, use of sclerosing agents, and surgical removal of the anterior wall of the cyst.[107] Success is determined by resolution of the cyst with preservation of the anatomic structure and appearance of the auricle.

Malignant Neoplasms

Squamous Cell Carcinoma

Squamous cell carcinoma (SCC) is a neoplasm of keratinocytes originating from the surface epithelium. It represents one half to two thirds of all skin cancers that involve the auricle.[108,109] SCC of the ear commonly presents in areas of severe actinic change as an indurated plaque or nodule that may ulcerate and bleed (**Fig. 15–18**). Differential diagnosis includes keratoacanthoma and actinic keratosis. In situ SCC presents as a scaly red patch that may clinically resemble seborrheic dermatitis.

When SCC involves the auricle, it is difficult to control. Local spread can involve the external auditory canal, temporomandibular joint, temporal bone, parotid or mandible, and metastasis is reported in 12 to 18% of patients.[110,111] Bailin and colleagues[112] showed local tumor extension along perichondral, periosteal, and neurovascular planes, thus demonstrating occult malignancy can spread beyond clinically visible lines. This subclinical spread may explain the difficulty controlling these lesions. Therapeutic approaches include Mohs' micrographic surgery in the absence of regional disease, primary excision, and primary excision with postoperative radiation therapy. When the lesion is confined to the auricle, prognosis is good. For lesions smaller than 1 cm in

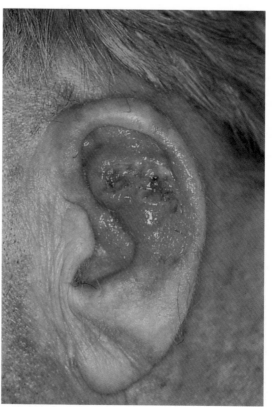

Figure 15–18 Squamous carcinoma.

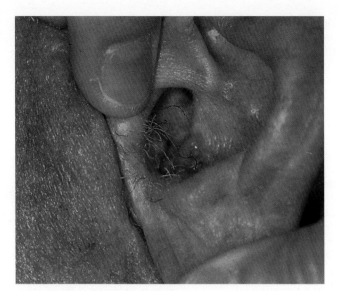

Figure 15–19 Basal cell carcinoma.

diameter, Shockley and Strucker[108] have shown a cure rate as great as 95% for initial and salvage surgery combined.

Basal Cell Carcinoma

Basal cell carcinoma (BCC) is the most common skin cancer and consists of five main subtypes. Nodular BCC is a pearly, ulcerative telangiectatic papule with rolled borders, commonly referred to a "rat bite ulcer" (**Fig. 15–19**). Superficial BCC is waxy, scaly, indurated, and irregular in appearance, often mimicking eczema. Morpheaform (sclerosing or fibrosing) BCC is a flat or depressed, yellow, indurated lesion with indistinct borders that is very aggressive with a high rate of recurrence and associated poor prognosis. Pigmented BCC appears similar to nodular except that it has a greater amount of pigmentation and resembles a melanoma. Fibroepithelioma is an elevated, firm, sessile or pedunculated, erythematous lesion. The occurrence of BCC on the auricle is relatively uncommon, representing only 1.5% of all BCC of the head and neck.[113] BCC is commonly found in areas of severe actinic damage marked by actinic keratoses. The tumor is believed to arise from pluripotential cells in the basal layer of the epidermis and consists of cords, strands, and sheets of small, uniform cells invading the dermis.[109] Treatment with electrodesiccation and curettage, cryotherapy, or laser resection have all been successful[114]; however, the mainstay of treatment for small, nonaggressive tumors remains primary surgical excision. Mohs' micrographic surgery is effective for resecting tumors with ill-defined margins, large tumors, tumors with aggressive histology, recurrent tumors, tumors with a high recurrence risk located in the "H zone" (lateral aspects of the face and midface) or tumors in areas where cosmetic reconstruction is challenging (ears, eyes, nose, nasolabial folds, lips). Reconstruction requires techniques similar to those described for repair of traumatic injury or congenital deformity. Primary BCCs have reported recurrence rates of 5% after surgical excision and 19% after curettage and electrodesiccation.[115] Recurrence of BCC is reported to be 10% after radiation therapy and 40% after curettage and electrodesiccation.[116] Regional metastases tend to occur in areas with multiple recurrences.[117]

Once diagnosed with BCC, a patient has a 44% likelihood of developing a second BCC. Therefore, 5 years of follow-up are recommended for a primary BCC and 10 years for a recurrent BCC.[116,118]

Melanoma

Malignant melanoma is the third most common cutaneous carcinoma. Byers and colleagues[119] reported that malignant melanoma of the external ear accounts for 7% of all melanomas of the head and neck. Three main morphologic subtypes of melanoma exist and each can occur in the head and neck area. Superficial spreading melanoma presents as an irregularly shaped, brown-to-black patch that may include tan, pink, gray, blue, red, or white areas. An ulcerative appearance often indicates vertical phase growth. Nodular melanoma is a very aggressive lesion with a poor prognosis commonly presenting as a blue-to-black nodule or plaque with a smooth or ulcerated surface. Lentigo maligna melanoma is an irregular tan, brown, or black macular lesion that usually extends radially and has a good prognosis. Byers et al found lesion thickness to be the most important prognostic factor in melanoma involving the ear.[119] Lesions less than 3 mm in depth had a nodal metastasis incidence of 21%, whereas for lesions with depth greater than 3 mm the incidence was 61%. The authors found a 5-year survival rate of 12% in patients with positive nodes and a 75% rate for those with negative nodes. Primary treatment of malignant melanoma remains wide surgical excision, but some success has been reported with Mohs' micrographic surgery. Using the fixed tissue technique, Mohs[120] reported a 5-year cure rate of 75%. The role of elective neck dissection when the neck is clinically negative remains controversial. Therapy also can involve sentinel lymph node biopsy, which provides the most accurate prognostic information.[121] Current adjuvant treatments include dacarbazine and interleukin-2; however, many treatment protocols are under investigation.[122–125]

Rhabdomyosarcoma

Rhabdomyosarcoma is the most common childhood tumor to involve the auricle, and the auricle is the third most common site of presentation after the orbit and nasopharynx. Clinically, the lesion is painful and may cause otorrhea. Bleeding and bone destruction occur as the lesion progresses. If the lesion is confined to the auricle, primary excision may be attempted. Recurrent disease usually presents with medial extension to involve the meninges. For unresectable lesions the preferred treatment consists of vincristine, dactinomycin, and cyclophosphamide; or vincristine, dactinomycin, and ifosfamide; or vincristine, ifosfamide, and etoposide. Each protocol is combined with surgery and may include radiation therapy. This extensive treatment regimen is reported of equal effectiveness for patients with local or regional rhabdomyosarcoma and is superior treatment for embryonal tumors compared with previous therapies.[126]

Mohs' Micrographic Surgery

Mohs' micrographic surgery, or microscopically controlled surgery, is a technique of skin cancer removal in which the cancer is excised layer by layer, with careful mapping and microscopic examination of frozen sections to ensure complete tumor removal.[127–129] The complete excision of tumor and associated microscopic tumor cells is of utmost importance. Microscopic residuum from incompletely excised tumor has an associated greater rate of recurrence, resulting in lower long-term cure rates and significantly poorer prognosis. Thus, preservation of natural function and cosmesis are of lesser concern than complete tumor excision. Because small margins of 2 to 3 mm are taken with each layer, the maximum amount of normal skin can be preserved. Larger initial margins may be taken based on the expected biologic behavior of certain tumors, such as multiply recurrent BCC, SCC, or dermatofibrosarcoma protuberans. Using horizontally oriented sections of tissue allows both lateral and deep margins to be examined and provides histologically controlled, staged tissue removal. In contrast, routine frozen section margin evaluations may assess as little as 1% of the excised specimen margins.[130,131] Systemic mapping and microscopic analysis with Mohs' micrographic surgery allow removal of micrographic extensions of skin cancer that may not yet be clinically visible or palpable.

Mohs developed a fixed-tissue technique, called chemosurgery, in the 1930s that involved application of a zinc chloride fixative paste to the tumor before excision. This method prevented dissemination of tumor cells if the excision was performed through tumor-laden skin and also created a bloodless field. Disadvantages included pain secondary to application of the fixative paste, and the necessity of a delayed repair after demarcation and sloughing of the final layer of fixed tissue. In addition, a delay of up to 24 hours was necessary between the fixative paste application, removal, and the excision. Currently, the method most commonly used is the fresh-tissue technique, which does not use fixative paste. Most fresh-tissue Mohs' surgery procedures are performed on an outpatient basis using local anesthesia. Extensive cases may necessitate general anesthesia and an interdisciplinary team approach. Turner and colleagues[132] described a "slow Mohs" approach using permanent instead of frozen sections, citing the technical superiority of their method. However, because their results were nearly the same and their treatment required extended periods of excision and reconstruction ranging from 2 to 28 days, additional study is necessary before this method becomes standard. Perhaps a combination of approaches will guide future treatment.

BCC and SCC are the most common tumor types treated with Mohs' micrographic surgery. However, any tumor that grows in continuity with a low metastatic potential and has an increased tendency to recur after routine surgical excision may be a candidate. Mohs' surgery is indicated for very large skin cancers, recurrent tumors, tumors likely to recur (in the H zone), tumors with ill-defined margins, tumors with aggressive histology, and tumors where restoring function or cosmetic reconstruction proves challenging (ears, eyes, nose, nasolabial folds, lips). Fixed-tissue Mohs' surgery may still be used for very large or deeply invasive tumors, vascular tumors, tumors in vascular sites, tumors involving bone, and melanoma.

Treatment options for nonmelanoma skin cancer include surgical excision, liquid nitrogen cryotherapy, electrodesiccation and curettage, and radiation therapy. Cure rates of 90% or higher may be achieved with these modalities in properly selected tumors. Mohs' micrographic surgery provides cure rates of 97% to 99% for primary skin cancers and 90% or higher for recurrent tumors.[128,129,133,134] Because nonmelanoma skin cancers of the ear can have significant subclinical extensions along the perichondrium and embryonic fusion planes, the tendency to recur after standard surgical excision as well as Mohs' surgery may be greater than for comparably sized tumors in other anatomic locations. In treating 338 BCCs and SCCs of the ear and periauricular skin with Mohs' surgery, Robins[135] reported a 6.8% recurrence rate. The highest recurrence rate was in the postauricular region. Mohs[136] reported cure rates of 98.4% and 91.7% in treating 375 BCCs and 337 SCCs of the ear, respectively.

Reconstructive options after Mohs' surgery for tumors of the auricle include secondary-intention healing, primary closure, and flap or graft repair. An auricular prosthesis may be indicated after extensive tumor removal in patients who do not desire or are not good candidates for reconstruction. Patients with multiply recurrent tumors who require close surveillance of wounds healed by secondary intention may also benefit from a prosthesis. Delayed reconstruction then may be considered after a tumor-free follow-up interval of at least 1 year.

◆ Conclusion

The external ear plays an important role in the human sensory system and it is not spared from involvement in disease. The otolaryngologist plays an essential role in the identification and treatment of diseases of the auricle. Management is dependent on proper recognition and treatment. Treatment of congenital auricular deformities requires identification of associated congenital anomalies so that a proper repair can be planned. Successful auricular repair after trauma is dependent on recognizing the extent of injury, using proper surgical technique, and preventing sequelae. Primary auricular infections must be identified and treated to prevent deformity. Systemic disease involvement and dermatologic conditions of the auricle are best managed by identifying and treating the underlying cause. Finally, early recognition of neoplasms of the auricle is essential for proper treatment and successful outcome.

References

1. Rogers B. Microtia, lop, cup and protruding ears: four directly inherited deformities? Plast Reconstr Surg 1968;41:208–231
2. Weerda H. Classification of congenital deformities of the auricle. Facial Plast Surg 1988;5:385–388
3. Wildervanck LS. Hereditary malformations of the ear in three generations: marginal pits, preauricular appendages, malformations of the auricle and conductive deafness. Acta Otolaryngol 1962;54:553–560
4. Brent B. Reconstruction of the auricle. In: McCarthy JG, ed. Plastic Surgery. Philadelphia: WB Saunders, 1990:2094–2152
5. Harris J, Kallen B, Robert E. The epidemiology of anotia and microtia. J Med Genet 1996;33:809–813
6. Aase JM, Tegtmeier RE. Microtia in New Mexico: evidence for multifactorial causation. Birth Defects Orig Artic Ser 1977;13:113–116
7. Crabtree JA, Harker LA. Developmental abnormalities of the ear. In: Cummings CW, Fredrickson JM, Harker LA, et al, eds. Otolaryngology-Head and Neck Surgery. St. Louis: Mosby Year Book, 1993:2746–2755
8. Queisser-Luft A, Stolz G, Wiesel A, et al. Associations between renal malformations and abnormally formed ears: analysis of 32,589 newborns and newborn fetuses of the Mainz Congenital Birth Defect Monitoring System. In: XXI David W. Smith Workshop on Malformation and Morphogenesis. San Diego, CA: 2000:60
9. Tanzer RC. The constricted (cup and lop) ear. Plast Reconstr Surg 1975;55:406–415

10. Miyamoto RT, Fairchild TH, Daugherty HS. Primary cholesteatoma in the congenitally atretic ear. Am J Otol 1984;5:283–285

11. Crabtree JA, Harker LA. Developmental abnormalities of the ear. In: Cummings CW, Fredrickson JM, Harker LA, et al, eds. Otolaryngology-Head and Neck Surgery. St. Louis: Mosby Year Book, 1993:2746–2755

12. Jansen T, Romiti R, Altmeyer P. Accessory tragus: report of two cases and review of the literature. Pediatr Dermatol 2000;17:391–394

13. Moore KL. The Developing Human. 4th ed. Philadelphia: WB Saunders, 1988:412–419

14. Argenta LC, Iacobucci JJ. Treacher Collins syndrome: present concepts of the disorder and their surgical correction. World J Surg 1989;13:401–409

15. Hunt JA, Hobar PC. Common craniofacial anomalies: the facial dysostoses. Plast Reconstr Surg 2002;110:1714–1728

16. Pierides AM, Athanasiou Y, Demetriou K, et al. A family with branchio-oto-renal syndrome: clinical and genetic correlations. Nephrol Dial Transplant 2002;17:1014–1018

17. Rollnick BR, Kaye CI, Nagatoshi K, et al. Oculoauriculovertebral dysplasia and variants: phenotypic characteristics of 294 patients. Am J Med Genet 1987;26:361–375

18. Powell CM, Michaelis RC. Townes-Brocks syndrome. J Med Genet 1999;36:89–93

19. Danziger I, Brodsky L, Perry R, et al. Nager's acrofacial dysostosis. Case report and review of the literature. Int J Pediatr Otorhinolaryngol 1990;20:225–240

20. Vigneron J, Stricker M, Vert P, et al. Postaxial acrofacial dysostosis (Miller) syndrome: a new case. J Med Genet 1991;28:636–638

21. Jahrsdoerfer RA, Hall JW III. Congenital malformations of the ear. Am J Otol 1986;7:267–269

22. Glasscock ME, Schwaber MK, Nissen AJ, et al. Management of congenital ear malformations. Ann Otol Rhinol Laryngol 1983;92:504–509

23. Linstrom CJ, Meiteles LZ. Facial nerve monitoring in surgery for congenital auricular atresia. Laryngoscope 1993;103:406–415

24. McKinnon BJ, Jahrsdoerfer RA. Congenital auricular atresia: update on options for intervention and timing of repair. Otolaryngol Clin North Am 2002;35:877–890

25. Ohlsen L, Skoog T, Sohn S. Pathogenesis of cauliflower ear: and experimental study in rabbits. Scand J Plast Reconstr Surg 1975;9:34–39

26. Escat M. Simplified treatment of hematoma of the ear. Otorhinolaryngol Int 1946;30:181–182

27. Kelleher JC, Sullivan K, Baibak G, et al. The wrestler's ear. Plast Reconstr Surg 1967;40:540–546

28. O'Donnell BP, Eliezri YD. The surgical treatment of traumatic hematoma of the auricle. Dermatol Surg 1999;25:803–805

29. Davis PK. An operation for hematoma auris. Br J Plast Surg 1971;24:277–279

30. Vuyk HD, Bakkers EJ. Absorbable mattress sutures in the management of auricular hematoma. Laryngoscope 1991;101:1124–1126

31. Eliachar I, Golz A, Joachims HZ, et al. Continuous portable vacuum drainage of the auricular hematomas. Am J Otolaryngol 1983;4:141–143

32. Martin RJ, Carey VM, Philbert RF, et al. Prevention of haematomas after auricular injuries. Br J Oral Maxillofac Surg 2000;38:238–240

33. Schuller DE, Damkle SD, Strauss RH. A technique to treat wrestler's auricular hematoma without interrupting training or competition. Arch Otolaryngol Head Neck Surg 1989;115:202–205

34. Walike J, Larrabee WF Jr. Repair of the cleft earlobe. Laryngoscope 1985;95:876–877

35. Brent B, Byrd HS. Secondary ear reconstruction with cartilage grafts covered by axial, random, and free flaps of temporoparietal fascia. Plast Reconstr Surg 1983;72:141–152

36. Antia NH, Buch VI. Chondrocutaneous advancement flap for the marginal defect of the ear. Plast Reconstr Surg 1967;39:472–477

37. Bialostocki A, Tan ST. Modified Antia-Buch repair for full-thickness upper pole auricular defects. Plast Reconstr Surg 1999;103:1476–1479

38. Cho BH, Ahn HB. Microsurgical replantation of a partial ear, with leech therapy. Ann Plast Surg 1999;43:427–429

39. Mladick RA, Horton CE, Adamson JE, Cohen BI. The pocket principle: a new technique for the reattachment of a severed ear part. Plast Reconstr Surg 1971;48:219–223

40. Pennington DG, Lai MF, Pelly AD. Successful replantation of a completely avulsed ear by microvascular anastomosis. Plast Reconstr Surg 1980;65:820–823

41. Schonauer F, Blair JW, Moloney DM, et al. Three cases of successful microvascular ear replantation after bite avulsion injury. Scand J Plast Reconstr Surg Hand Surg 2004;38:177–182

42. Nath RK, Kraemer BA, Azizzadeh A. Complete ear replantation without venous anastomosis. Microsurgery 1998;18:282–285

43. Concannon MJ, Puckett CL. Microsurgical replantation of an ear in a child without venous repair. Plast Reconstr Surg 1998;102:2088–2096

44. Kind GM, Buncke GM, Placik OJ, et al. Total ear replantation. Plast Reconstr Surg 1997;99:1858–1867

45. Juri J, Irigaray A, Juri C, et al. Ear replantation. Plast Reconstr Surg 1987;80:431–435

46. Stucker FJ, Shaw GY, Boyd S, Shockley WW. Management of animal and human bites in the head and neck. Arch Otolaryngol Head Neck Surg 1990;116:789–793

47. Lehmuskallio E, Lindholm H, Koskenvuo K, et al. Frostbite of the face and ears: epidemiological study of risk factors in Finnish conscripts. BMJ 1995;311:1661–1663

48. Gilmer PA. Trauma of the auricle. In: Bailey BJ, Johnson JT, Kohut RI, et al, eds. Head and Neck Surgery–Otolaryngology. Philadelphia: JB Lippincott, 1993:1557–1563

49. Marzella L, Jesudass RR, Manson PN, et al. Morphologic characterization of acute injury to vascular endothelium of skin after frostbite. Plast Reconstr Surg 1989;83:67–75

50. Sessions DG, Stallings JO, Mills WJ Jr, et al. Frostbite of the ear. Laryngoscope 1971;81:1223–1232

51. Heggers JP, Robson MC, Manavalen K, et al. Experimental and clinical observations on frostbite. Ann Emerg Med 1987;16:1056–1062

52. Dowling JA, Foley FD, Moncrief JA. Chondritis in the burned ear. Plast Reconstr Surg 1968;42:115–122

53. Williams RE, MacKie RM. The staphylococci. Dermatol Clin 1993;11:201–206

54. Brown J, Shriner DL, Schwartz RA, et al. Impetigo: an update. Int J Dermatol 2003;42:251–255

55. Dagan R. Impetigo in childhood: changing epidemiology and new treatments. Pediatr Ann 1993;22:235–240

56. Gisby J, Bryant J. Efficacy of a new cream formulation of mupirocin: comparison with oral and topical agents in experimental skin infections. Antimicrob Agents Chemother 2000;44:255–260

57. Bisno AL, Stevens DL. Streptococcal infections of skin and soft tissues. N Engl J Med 1996;334:240–245

58. Simplot TC, Hoffman HT. Comparison between cartilage and soft tissue ear piercing complications. Am J Otolaryngol 1998;19:305–310

59. Bassiouny A. Perichondritis of the auricle. Laryngoscope 1981;91:422–431

60. Linstrom CJ, Lucente FE. Infections of the external ear. In: Bailey BJ, Johnson JT, Kohut RI, et al, eds. Head and Neck Surgery–Otolaryngology. Philadelphia: JB Lippincott, 1993:1542–1555

61. Mofid M, Dover JS, Skerlev M, et al. Herpes simplex. Semin Neurol 1992;12:312–321

62. Uri N, Greenberg E, Meyer W, et al. Herpes zoster oticus: treatment with acyclovir. Ann Otol Rhinol Laryngol 1992;101:161–162

63. Murakami S, Hato N, Horiuchi J, et al. Treatment of Ramsay Hunt syndrome with acyclovir-prednisone: significance of early diagnosis and treatment. Ann Neurol 1997;41:353–357

64. Sebastiani S, Albanesi C, De PO, et al. The role of chemokines in allergic contact dermatitis. Arch Dermatol Res 2002;293:552–559

65. Prystowsky SD, Nonomura JH, Smith RW, et al. Allergic hypersensitivity to neomycin: relationship between patch reactions and 'use' tests. Arch Dermatol 1979;115:713–715

66. Pirila V, Hirvonen ML, Rouhunkoski S. The pattern of cross-sensitivity to neomycin. Secondary sensitization to gentamicin. Dermatologica 1968;136:321–324

67. Fransway AF. The problem of preservation in the 1990s: I. Statement of the problem, solution(s) of the industry, and current use of formaldehyde and formaldehyde-releasing biocides. Am J Contact Dermatitis 1991;2:6–23

68. Clark RAF, Hopkins TT. The other eczemas. In: Moschella SJ, Hurley HJ, eds. Dermatology. Philadelphia: WB Saunders, 1992:465–503

69. Webster G. Seborrheic dermatitis. Int J Dermatol 1991;30:843–844

70. Gupta AK, Madzia SE, Batra R. Etiology and management of seborrheic dermatitis. Dermatology 2004;208:89–93

71. Simmons A. Clinical manifestations and treatment considerations of herpes simplex virus infection. J Infect Dis 2002;186(suppl 1):S71–S77

72. Hoare S. HIV infection in children–impact upon ENT doctors. Int J Pediatr Otorhinolaryngol 2003;67(suppl 1):S85–S90

73. Rinaldo A, Brandwein MS, Devaney KO, et al. AIDS-related otological lesions. Acta Otolaryngol 2003;123:672–674

74. Gherman CR, Ward RR, Bassis ML. Pneumocystis carinii otitis media and mastoiditis as the initial manifestation of the acquired immunodeficiency syndrome. Am J Med 1988;85:250–252

75. Menger DJ, v d Berg RG. Pneumocystis carinii infection of the middle ear and external auditory canal. Report of a case and review of the literature. ORL J Otorhinolaryngol Relat Spec 2003;65:49–51

76. Lasisi OA, Bakare RA, Usman MA. Human immunodeficiency virus and invasive external otitis—a case report. West Afr J Med 2003;22:103–105

77. Lalwani AK, Sooy CD. Otologic and neurotologic manifestations of acquired immunodeficiency syndrome. Otolaryngol Clin North Am 1992;25:1183–1197

78. Ziegler JL, Beckstead JA, Volberding PA, et al. Non-Hodgkin's lymphoma in 90 homosexual men. Relation to generalized lymphadenopathy and the acquired immunodeficiency syndrome. N Engl J Med 1984;311:565–570

79. Kieserman SP, Finn DG. Non-Hodgkin's lymphoma of the external auditory canal in an HIV-positive patient. J Laryngol Otol 1995;109:751–754

80. Ustianowski AP, Lockwood DN. Leprosy: current diagnostic and treatment approaches. Curr Opin Infect Dis 2003;16:421–427

81. Schleuning AJ, Andersen PE. Otologic manifestations of systemic disease. In: Bailey BJ, Johnson JT, Kohut RI, et al, eds. Head and Neck Surgery–Otolaryngology. Philadelphia: JB Lippincott, 1993:1747–1753

82. Rasmussen N. Management of the ear, nose, and throat manifestations of Wegener granulomatosis: an otorhinolaryngologist's perspective. Curr Opin Rheumatol 2001;13:3–11

83. Jennings CR, Jones NS, Dugar J, et al. Wegener's granulomatosis–a review of diagnosis and treatment in 53 subjects. Rhinology 1998;36:188–191

84. McDonald TJ. Manifestations of systemic disease in the external ear. In: Cummings CW, Fredrickson JM, Harker LA, et al, eds. Otolaryngology–Head and Neck Surgery. St. Louis: Mosby Year Book, 1993:2901–2905

85. Murty GE. Wegener's granulomatosis: otorhinolaryngological manifestations. Clin Otolaryngol Allied Sci 1990;15:385–393

86. McDonald TJ, DeRemee RA. Head and neck involvement of Wegener's granulomatosis. In: Gross WL, ed. ANCA-Associated Vaculitides: Immunological and Clinical Aspects. New York: Plenum Press, 1993:309–313

87. White JW. Miscellaneous inflammatory disorders. In: Moschella SJ, Hurley HJ, eds. Dermatology. Philadelphia: WB Saunders, 1992:594–604

88. Foidart JM, Abe S, Martin GR, et al. Antibodies to type II collagen in relapsing polychondritis. N Engl J Med 1978;299:1203–1207

89. Kent PD, Michet CJ Jr, Luthra HS. Relapsing polychondritis. Curr Opin Rheumatol 2004;16:56–61

90. Laman SD, Provost TT. Cutaneous manifestations of lupus erythematosus. Rheum Dis Clin North Am 1994;20:195–212

91. Prystowsky SD, Herndon JH Jr, Gilliam JN. Chronic cutaneous lupus erythematosus (DLE): a clinical and laboratory investigation of 80 patients. Medicine (Baltimore) 1976;55:183–191

92. Ruzicka T, Sommerburg C, Goerz G, et al. Treatment of cutaneous lupus erythematosus with acitretin and hydroxychloroquine. Br J Dermatol 1992;127:513–518

93. Tuffanelli DL. Discoid lupus erythematous. Clin Rheum Dis 1982;8:327–341

94. Terkeltaub RA. Clinical practice. Gout. N Engl J Med 2003;349:1647–1655

95. Phornphutkul C, Introne WJ, Perry MB, et al. Natural history of alkaptonuria. N Engl J Med 2002;347:2111–2121

96. McKusick VA, Goodman RM. Pinnal calcification. JAMA 1962;179:230–232

97. Barkan A, Glantz I. Calcification of auricular cartilages in patients with hypopituitarism. J Clin Endocrinol Metab 1982;55:354–357

98. DiBartolomeo JR. The petrified auricle: comments on ossification, calcification and exostoses of the external ear. Laryngoscope 1985;95:566–575

99. Goette DK. Chondrodermatitis nodularis chronica helicis: a perforating necrobiotic granuloma. J Am Acad Dermatol 1980;2:148–154

100. Moschella SL, Cropley TG. Diseases of the mononuclear phagocytic system (the so-called reticuloendothelial system). In: Moschella SJ, Hurley HJ, eds. Dermatology. Philadelphia: WB Saunders, 1992:1031–1141

101. Yoshinaga E, Enomoto U, Fujimoto N, et al. A case of chondrodermatitis nodularis chronica helicis with an autoantibody to denatured type II collagen. Acta Derm Venereol 2001;81:137–138

102. Santa Cruz DJ. Chondrodermatitis nodularis chronica helicis: a transepidermal perforating disorder. J Cutan Pathol 1980;7:70–76

103. Moncrieff M, Sassoon EM. Effective treatment of chondrodermatitis nodularis chronica helicis using a conservative approach. Br J Dermatol 2004;150:892–894

104. Paletta FX. Premalignant and malignant lesions of the skin- general considerations. In: Stark RB, ed. Plastic Surgery of the Head and Neck. New York: Churchill Livingstone, 1987:222–224

105. Muir IFK. Premalignant and malignant lesions of the skin- keloid and hypertrophic scar. In: Stark RB, ed. Plastic Surgery of the Head and Neck. New York: Churchill Livingstone, 1987:260–265

106. Hom DB. Treating the elusive keloid. Arch Otolaryngol Head Neck Surg 2001;127:1140–1143

107. Christian MM, Mink KR, Wagner RF Jr. Asymptomatic swelling of a man's ear. Auricular pseudocyst. Arch Dermatol 1998;134:1627–1630

108. Shockley WW, Stucker FJ Jr. Squamous cell carcinoma of the external ear: a review of 75 cases. Otolaryngol Head Neck Surg 1987;97:308–312

109. Silerman AR, Neiland ML. Pathology of selected skin lesions. In: Bames L, ed. Surgical Pathology of the Head and Neck. New York: Marcel Dekker, 1985:1571–1580

110. Afzelius LE, Gunnarsson M, Nordgren H. Guidelines for prophylactic radical lymph node dissection in cases of carcinoma of the external ear. Head Neck Surg 1980;2:361–365

111. Cassisi NJ, Dickerson DR, Million RR. Squamous cell carcinoma of the skin metastatic to parotid nodes. Arch Otolaryngol 1978;104:336–339

112. Bailin P, Levine HL, Wood BG, Tucker HM. Cutaneous carcinoma of the auricular and periauricular region. Arch Otolaryngol 1980;106:692–696

113. Batsakis JG. Tumors of the Head and Neck, 2nd ed. Baltimore: Williams & Wilkins, 1979

114. Estrem SA, Renner GJ. Special problems associated with cutaneous carcinoma of the ear. Otolaryngol Clin North Am 1993;26:231–245

115. Thissen MR, Neumann MH, Schouten LJ. A systematic review of treatment modalities for primary basal cell carcinomas. Arch Dermatol 1999;135:1177–1183

116. Rowe DE, Carroll RJ, Day CL Jr. Long-term recurrence rates in previously untreated (primary) basal cell carcinoma: implications for patient follow-up. J Dermatol Surg Oncol 1989;15:315–328

117. Cassisi NJ. Neoplasms of the auricle. In: Cummings CW, Fredrickson JM, Harker LA, et al., eds. Otolaryngology–Head and Neck Surgery. St. Louis: Mosby Year Book, 1993:2965–2970

118. Marcil I, Stern RS. Risk of developing a subsequent nonmelanoma skin cancer in patients with a history of nonmelanoma skin cancer: a critical review of the literature and meta-analysis. Arch Dermatol 2000;136:1524–1530

119. Byers RM, Smith JL, Russell N, et al. Malignant melanoma of the external ear. Review of 102 cases. Am J Surg 1980;140:518–521

120. Mohs FE. Fixed-tissue micrographic surgery for melanoma of the ear. Arch Otolaryngol Head Neck Surg 1988;114:625–631

121. Gershenwald JE, Mansfield PF, Lee JE, et al. Role for lymphatic mapping and sentinel lymph node biopsy in patients with thick (> or =4 mm) primary melanoma. Ann Surg Oncol 2000;7:160–165

122. Rigel DS, Carucci JA. Malignant melanoma: prevention, early detection, and treatment in the 21st century. CA Cancer J Clin 2000;50:215–240

123. Moschos SJ, Kirkwood JM, Konstantinopoulos PA. Present status and future prospects for adjuvant therapy of melanoma: time to build upon the foundation of high-dose interferon alfa-2b. J Clin Oncol 2004;22:11–14

124. Slingluff CL Jr, Petroni GR, Yamshchikov GV, et al. Immunologic and clinical outcomes of vaccination with a multiepitope melanoma peptide vaccine plus low-dose interleukin-2 administered either concurrently or on a delayed schedule. J Clin Oncol 2004;22:4474–4485

125. Panelli MC, Wang E, Monsurro VV, et al. Overview of melanoma vaccines and promising approaches. Curr Oncol Rep 2004;6:414–420

126. Crist WM, Anderson JR, Meza JL, et al. Intergroup Rhabdomyosarcoma Study-IV: results for patients with nonmetastatic disease. J Clin Oncol 2001;19:3091–3102

127. Mohs FE. Premalignant and malignant lesions of the skin—microscopically controlled surgery for skin cancer. In: Stark RB, ed. Plastic Surgery of the Head and Neck. New York: Churchill Livingstone, 1987:253–259

128. Mohs FE. Chemosurgery: Microscopically Controlled Surgery for Skin Cancer. Springfield, IL: Charles C. Thomas, 1978:3–29

129. Swanson NA. Mohs surgery: technique, indications, applications, and the future. Arch Dermatol 1983;119:761–773

130. Bennett RG. The meaning and significance of tissue margins. Adv Dermatol 1989;4:343–355

131. Davidson TM, Haghighi P, Astarita RW, et al. Mohs for head and neck mucosal cancer. Report on 111 patients. Laryngoscope 1988;98:1078–1083

132. Turner RJ, Leonard N, Malcolm AJ, et al. A retrospective study of outcome of Mohs' micrographic surgery for cutaneous squamous cell carcinoma using formalin fixed sections. Br J Dermatol 2000;142:752–757

133. Rowe DE, Carroll RJ, Day CL Jr. Mohs surgery is the treatment of choice for recurrent (previously treated) basal cell carcinoma. J Dermatol Surg Oncol 1989;15:424–431

134. Rowe DE, Carroll RJ, Day CL Jr. Prognostic factors for local recurrence, metastasis, and survival rates in squamous cell carcinoma of the skin, ear, and lip. Implications for treatment modality selection. J Am Acad Dermatol 1992;26:976–990

135. Robins P. Chemosurgery: my 15 years of experience. J Dermatol Surg Oncol 1981;7:779–789

136. Mohs FE. Chemosurgery: Microscopically Controlled Surgery for Skin Cancer. Springfield, IL: Charles C. Thomas, 1978:85–105

16

Diseases of the External Auditory Canal

Chad A. Zender, Sam J. Marzo, and John P. Leonetti

The external auditory canal (EAC) is a bony and cartilaginous tube lined by a thin layer of stratified squamous epithelium. The main function of the EAC is to transmit sound from the pinna to the middle ear. The EAC also has a self-cleaning mechanism. Namely, desquamated skin from the tympanic membrane (TM) migrates down the canal shaft toward the canal orifice. Secretions from ear canal glands lubricate the canal, repel water, and are bacteriostatic. The proper function of the ear canal is necessary for optimal hearing. The various tissues in the EAC can be involved in multiple pathologic processes including viral and bacterial infections, inflammatory disorders, traumatic conditions, developmental anomalies, and benign and malignant lesions. This chapter provides an overview of EAC diseases and their management.

◆ Embryology

An understanding of the developmental anatomy of the external auditory canal is important for physicians treating diseases in this area. The external canal develops primarily from the first branchial cleft. This cleft eventually develops into the fibrocartilaginous EAC. Several medial ossification centers later develop into the bony external auditory canal. Between the eighth and 20th gestational week a solid core of epithelium grows toward the middle ear. By the 21st week, this core begins to resorb, and the innermost layer of ectoderm remains, forming the lining of the bony external canal and the lateral aspect of the TM.[1] Embryologic malformations, such as congenital aural canal atresia, can occur if the reabsorption process does not occur or is incomplete. This process is generally completed by 28 weeks. Development of the middle ear and inner ear occurs earlier in fetal life, with formation of the cochlea, membranous labyrinth, and ossicular chain by 16 weeks. These distinctions are important because patients with congenital aural atresias might have well-developed middle and inner ears, thus allowing the potential for favorable surgical intervention.

◆ Anatomy

The lateral third of the EAC is fibrocartilaginous, and is composed of an epithelial lining, subcutaneous soft tissue, and cartilage. The cartilaginous portion frequently has several gaps known as the fissures of Santorini, which may allow for the anterior spread of malignant neoplasms of the EAC into the parotid gland, which lies just anterior to this portion of the canal. The medial two thirds of the canal is bony and has a thin layer of periosteum and a thin epithelial lining, but lacks substantial subcutaneous soft tissue. This latter characteristic makes it very sensitive to manipulation and prone to trauma. The loss of hair in the ear canal signifies the transition from the cartilaginous portion of the canal to the bony portion, which lacks hair follicles. The ear specialist must be extremely gentle when cleaning, examining, and working in this portion of the ear canal. The epithelial lining of the ear has both apocrine and sebaceous glands that are responsible for producing cerumen. Cerumen is thought to have protective properties, acidifying the ear and creating an environment that is less conducive to infectious overgrowth.[2] The cerumen along with the desquamated epithelial lining has a lateral migratory pattern that allows the ear to self-clean.

The innervation of the EAC is via the fifth, seventh, and tenth cranial nerves and the greater auricular nerve. The tenth nerve contribution, known as Arnold's nerve, is responsible for the cough reflex that can be elicited by touching or irritating the inferior portion of the EAC. The blood supply to the EAC is via the superficial temporal artery and the posterior auricular artery.[3]

◆ Physiology

Cerumen is a naturally occurring substance of the EAC. It is composed of a combination of sebaceous and apocrine gland secretions in addition to desquamated squamous epithelium.[3] Cerumen is thought to be a bacteriostatic/fungostatic substance whose function is to waterproof the canal. Its components make it extremely hydrophobic and it has an acidic pH, both of which are important in preventing infection.

Constant epithelial proliferation occurs in the EAC and on the lateral surface of the TM. These epithelial proliferation centers have varying locations throughout the TM and EAC.[4] The EAC has an inherent ability for the lateral migration of cerumen and desquamated epithelium. Some cytokeratins are seen specifically in hyperproliferative cells. Studies looking at the cytokeratin content of keratinocytes of the EAC have found some areas to be populated with both normal and hyperproliferative cells. The hyperproliferative subtypes are believed to be important for the lateral epithelial migratory pattern, which is necessary for the EAC to remain free of desquamated epithelium.[5]

◆ Pathology

Obstructive Masses

Cerumen Impaction

Impaction of cerumen is one of the most common causes of conductive hearing loss (**Fig. 16–1**). It classically presents with muffled or decreased hearing, but it may be accompanied by other symptoms like fullness, pruritus, or even pain. This is a frequent problem in the elderly, especially in the face of contributing factors such as increased ear canal hair, hearing aids, medications, or use of Q-tips. Primary care doctors frequently see these patients before an otolaryngologist, and are sometimes unable to adequately cleanse the canal. Repeated unsuccessful attempts can result in trauma to the canal with swelling and inflammation. Treatment with a topical antibiotic-steroid mixture can decrease ear canal edema. Topical softening agents such as carbamide peroxide or mineral oil for several days may also make debridement of cerumen impactions easier.

There are several methods available to the physician for cerumen removal. Irrigation with a white vinegar (acetic acid) and water mixture often is utilized. The mixture should be kept near body temperature (98°F) to prevent vertigo from horizontal semicircular canal stimulation. This method has its limitations, and may induce damage to the canal, TM, or even the middle/inner ear.[6] It can be useful as first-line treatment of impacted cerumen by primary care personnel. Softening agents like carbamide peroxide (Debrox™), hydrogen peroxide, and mineral oil may also be utilized. They can be used alone or as an adjunct to office debridement. Some agents (e.g., triethanolamine polypeptide oleate), if used for long periods of time, can cause inflammation of the EAC, and cause a chemically induced otitis externa.

Perhaps the safest way to remove cerumen is by using binocular microscopic otoscopy. This method allows direct binocular visualization with depth perception and the use of two hands. Small loops, right-angle hooks, suction aspirators, and forceps can safely be used to remove cerumen, hairs, and other debris. If a severe impaction precludes complete removal of the cerumen, the patient may be prescribed softening drops and told to return in several days for completion of the procedure. If the canal has been traumatized, especially in the diabetic patient, the use of antibiotic drops for several days is advisable to prevent infection.

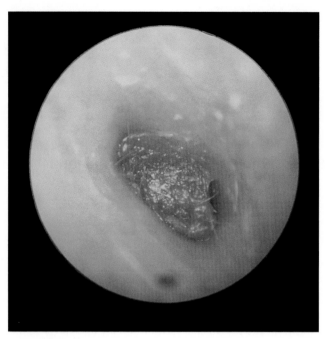

Figure 16–1   Cerumen.

Foreign Bodies

Foreign bodies in the EAC are another frequently encountered problem (**Figs. 16–2** through **16–4**). Common objects include beads, crayons, rocks, food matter, and insects. Small alkali batteries can cause chemical burns, and removal should be performed as soon as possible, followed by topical treatment with antibiotic/steroid drops.[7] Other small objects such are rocks can frequently be removed in the office under binocular vision. A right-angle hook can often be positioned medial to the object and used to pull it laterally, facilitating removal.

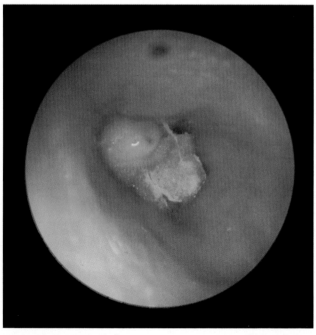

Figure 16–2   Cotton ball.

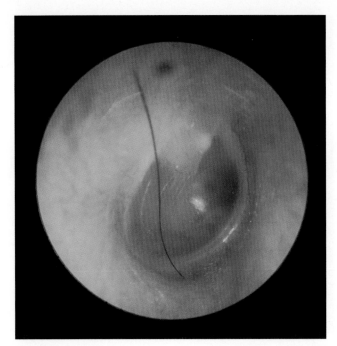

Figure 16–3 Hair.

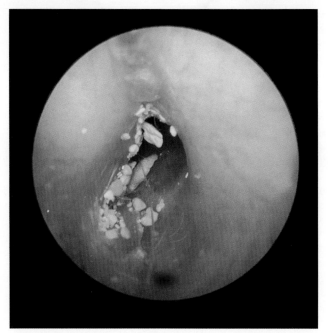

Figure 16–4 Pebble.

Small beads and other spherical objects can sometimes be removed with suction. Local ear canal injection with lidocaine can allow office removal of impacted objects.

Young children with foreign bodies in their ears can sometimes be restrained. However, in the uncooperative child, a general anesthetic might be necessary. Food matter like popcorn or beans may also be encountered, and irrigation should be avoided because of the propensity for these foods to swell. Insects (**Fig. 16–5**) enter the ear canal at night while the patient is sleeping, but because of their inability for retrograde mobility, and not enough room to turn around, they cannot exit the canal. Patients will often complain of an itching or tickling sensation in the ear and "hear" something in the affected ear if the insect is still alive. In such cases, an

insecticidal liquid (alcohol or lidocaine) can be placed in the ear canal for several minutes.[8] Once the insect has died, it can then be removed safely. Except for batteries, which require prompt removal, foreign bodies in the ear canal can usually be removed safely within several days of onset.

Exostosis and Osteomas

Exostoses are bony outgrowths of the EAC (**Fig. 16–6**). They are frequently multiple and bilateral, and are associated with

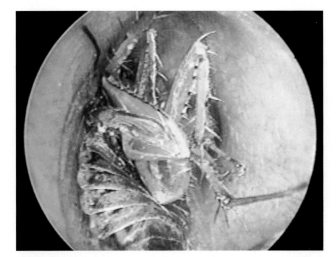

Figure 16–5 Insect.

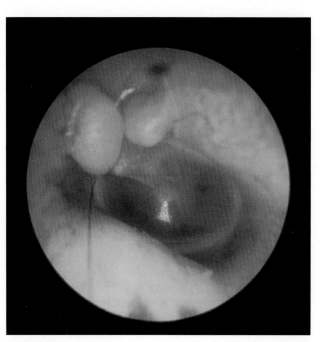

Figure 16–6 Exostosis.

swimming and water sports. However, their exact pathophysiology is not completely understood.[9,10] Van Gilse[11] proposed that exposure to cold water for long periods of time produces erythema of the canal and a periosteal reaction that induces exostosis formation. More recent research shows that these lesions are not unique to humans, and are found in other mammals that spend considerable amounts of time in the water.[12] These benign growths usually do not involve the suture lines and consist of broad-based lamellar bone.[13] Usually these lesions are asymptomatic, but with excessive growth they can impair water and cerumen drainage from the EAC, resulting in otitis externa and hearing loss. The vast majority of these lesions are asymptomatic and require no treatment. Patients with recurring cerumen impactions medial to the exostoses might require frequent office debridement or use of softening agents such as mineral oil. Patients with obstructing exostoses and conductive hearing losses might benefit from surgical correction via canalplasty. This is generally performed through an endaural or postauricular approach. It is important to preserve as much canal skin as possible to prevent potential EAC stenosis. As these lesions are broad-based, removal is best performed using high-speed cutting and diamond burs. Small canal skin defects can be covered with a fascia graft and allowed to heal, in which case the graft acts as a scaffold and the epithelium migrates across during the healing process. Larger defects might require a small skin graft, which can usually be obtained from the postauricular area. Recurrent disease is not uncommon.[14]

Osteomas are bony lesions that are usually unilateral, and almost always found attached to the tympanosquamous or tympanomastoid suture (**Fig. 16–7**). These lesions differ from exostosis in that they are less common and solitary.[13] The typical location also differs in that these lesions are usually more laterally based. These neoplasms are less likely to be symptomatic, but when they obstruct the canal or impede cerumen migration, they should be removed, usually through an endaural or postauricular approach.

Keratosis Obturans and Canal Cholesteatoma

These two diseases initially were considered to be the same entity, but insight generated by Piepergerdes et al[15] helped to elucidate key differences. Keratosis obturans usually is circumferential in its bony destruction, affects a younger age group, and usually is bilateral. It also has an affiliation for younger patients with bronchiectasis and chronic sinusitis. Its exact etiology is unknown, but it is thought to result from abnormal epithelial kinetics and loss of the lateral migration pattern of the squamous epithelium. Canal cholesteatoma is different in that it usually affects an older age group, is unilateral, and frequently is associated with a dull-aching, chronically draining ear.[16] These lesions are not circumferential in their destruction pattern. They typically result from trauma to the EAC, either postsurgical or self-inflicted. Nontraumatic EAC cholesteatomas are a much rarer entity.

The treatment of keratosis obturans is conservative. These patients generally require serial office debridements under the microscope. Topical therapy with antibiotic or steroid drops is reserved for disease that has a corresponding inflammatory or infectious component. Surgical therapy is generally not indicated.

Canal cholesteatomas usually can initially be managed conservatively, especially in the elderly or debilitated patient.[17]

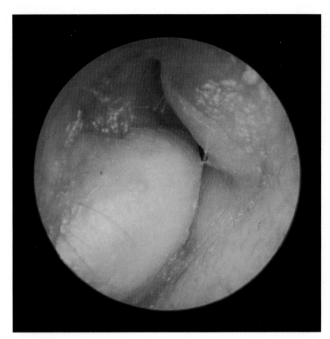

Figure 16–7 Osteomas.

Such patients are typically seen on a regular basis for office debridement. A softening agent, such as mineral oil can be used by the patient several days prior to the visit to facilitate cleaning under the microscope. In younger patients or in those with progressive, symptomatic disease, surgical intervention may be necessary. This usually requires an endaural or postauricular approach. Normal-appearing ear canal skin should be preserved. The TM and ossicular chain are usually not involved with EAC cholesteatomas, and should be preserved. Next a canalplasty is performed, with removal of disease until healthy appearing bone is identified. Small canal skin defects can be covered with a fascia graft, whereas larger defects might require a small skin graft from the postauricular area.

Inflammatory Polyp

Inflammatory polyps of the middle ear can present as masses in the EAC (**Fig. 16–8**). These lesions typically are seen with chronic otitis media with or without cholesteatoma. Other causes include foreign bodies in the EAC or TM, such as retained pressure-equalizing tubes; canal cholesteatoma; osteoradionecrosis; necrotizing otitis externa; benign tumors such as ceruminomas, cystadenomas, pleomorphic adenomas; and malignant tumors, such as squamous cell carcinoma. Most benign inflammatory polyps are not painful, and will respond to office debridement and topical therapy with steroid-antibiotic drops. Polyps that persist despite conservative treatment for several weeks indicate an underlying disease process. The most common causes are chronic otitis media and cholesteatoma. Perforations and retractions of the tympanic membrane are usually seen. Temporal bone computed tomography (CT) can help determine the extent of disease. Pain is always worrisome, and is common with necrotizing otitis externa and squamous cell carcinoma. Suspicious lesions should be biopsied. A negative biopsy may indicate no cancer or a nonrepresentative sample. It may be necessary to perform deeper biopsies under local or even

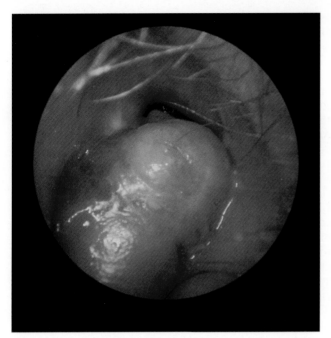

Figure 16–8 Large obstructing polyp.

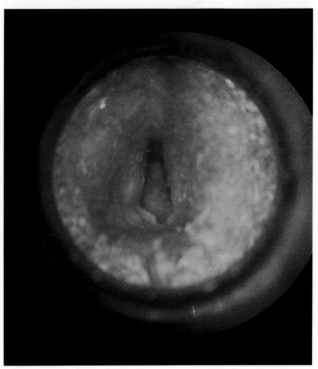

Figure 16–9 External otitis.

general anesthesia to make sure they are representative of the disease process. All polyps should be treated until resolved.

Ear Canal Infections

Otitis Externa

Bacterial otitis externa is a common problem for the otologist as well as the general practitioner (**Fig. 16–9**). Infections can range from a brief problem in an immunocompetent individual to a devastating life-threatening infection in the immunocompromised individual. Individuals who are at risk for necrotizing otitis externa are discussed below.

Acute otitis externa is a common problem in swimmers. Swimming in contaminated water (lakes and rivers) increases the risk of pseudomonas otitis externa.[18] The increase in moisture in the EAC causes edema and a more favorable environment for bacterial overgrowth. Cerumen has an acidic pH, and helps prevent bacterial growth in the EAC. A lack of cerumen and exposure to moisture predisposes to infection. Cleaning with cotton applicators can traumatize the thin epithelial lining of the bony EAC, which then predisposes to infection. Patients who wear hearing aids also are at increased risk of otitis externa because of the moist environment that is created in the ear canal and because of occasional EAC trauma. All of the above factors can create an environment that is optimal for bacterial growth, particularly pseudomonas and to a lesser degree staphylococcal species.[19]

Patients with acute otitis externa typically present with unilateral pain and tenderness of the external ear. The pain often is quite severe, and significantly increases with manipulation of the pinna. There is usually some edema of the EAC, and less often some erythema and tenderness in the preauricular soft tissue. Patients may complain of drainage, but typically not as much as patients with chronic otitis media.

Binocular microscopy shows an edematous canal, occasionally so severe that the speculum cannot be inserted. It is extremely important to remove as much EAC discharge and debris as can be performed safely. Properly cleaning the ear canal helps topical medications to resolve edematous and inflamed tissue. Occasionally the infection swells the external canal to the point that it is completely closed, and in these cases it is necessary to place a small wick for 4 or 5 days to allow the antibiotic drops to penetrate the EAC. Forceps are used to place a 1.5-cm piece of absorbable sponge or longer gauze strip, which is able to "wick" the topical antibiotic drops into the inflamed canal. In patients with disease involving the preauricular soft tissue and in recalcitrant cases that have failed a course of topical antibiotics, systemic antibiotic therapy may be necessary. Because ciprofloxacin has the greatest pseudomonas coverage of the quinolones, it is frequently the oral antibiotic of choice for severe acute otitis externa. Oral quinolones should be reserved for adult patients because of possible effects on cartilage growth plates in the pediatric population. Because of increased antibiotic use, bacterial sensitivities have changed, as have recommendations for the treatment of acute otitis externa.[19] Aminoglycosides (gentamicin/tobramycin) along with neomycin and polymixin are available as otic solutions and have proven efficacy against external otitis. However, concerns about ototoxicity have limited their use to ears in which the TM is intact.[20]

Newer antibiotics like Floxin™ (floxacin) and Ciprodex™ (ciprofloxacin/dexamethasone) have a safer therapeutic profile and are preferred for external otitis with tympanostomy tubes, or in association with otitis media. Treatment duration varies, but will typically last 7 to 10 days. A recent pediatric study investigated a regimen of ofloxacin once daily for 7 days and found that it was effective in eradicating 96% of the organisms.[21]

Necrotizing External Otitis

In the immunocompromised patient otitis externa can be a much more aggressive infection, seen most frequently in the poorly controlled diabetic patients (**Fig. 16–10**). It is also more frequent in patients with HIV and AIDS. AIDS patients are typically younger and may not have EAC granulation tissue, which is common in patients with diabetes.[22,23] Necrotizing external otitis (NEO) is a progression of acute otitis externa in the immunocompromised host. Historically termed "malignant otitis externa," the disease can involve the temporal bone and skull base, and is essentially osteomyelitis. It usually begins as an episode of acute otitis externa, but because of the host's compromised immune status, the infection is able to spread beyond the epithelium and soft tissue of the ear canal, and penetrate the periosteum, involving the underlying temporal bone. A chronic infection then occurs, manifesting with granulation tissue formation in the EAC. Granulation and reactive inflammatory tissue replace a significant portion of the bony EAC and can mimic malignant disease. A high index of suspicion should exist in immunocompromised patients with otitis externa. Biopsies should be performed to rule out malignant disease and to obtain tissue necessary for bacterial and fungal cultures. It may be necessary to anesthetize the EAC with injected lidocaine or even perform deep biopsies under general anesthesia to obtain representative tissues samples. The disease can be fatal if not aggressively treated. The infectious organism is typically pseudomonas, but other organisms have been implicated.[24,25]

Disease extension can produce intratemporal and intracranial complications through involvement of neurovascular pathways. Inferior extension into the mastoid portion of the temporal bone can produce facial paresis and paralysis. Medial extension into the petrous apex can produce fifth and sixth nerve signs. Inferomedial extension can involve the jugular foramen, with resulting paralysis of the lower cranial nerves (IX, X, and XI), resulting in hoarseness, dysphonia, and

aspiration. Extension of disease to the dura lining the medial and superior surface of the temporal bone can result in vascular (sigmoid sinus thrombosis), and intracranial complications (otitic hydrocephalus, meningitis).

These patients typically present to the otolaryngologist and otologist because they have failed topical therapy provided by their primary care physician or internist. Success in treating this disease is dependent on its early diagnosis and treatment. Any immunocompromised individual with ear pain needs to be evaluated in a timely manner, and NEO should always be suspected in this patient population. Usually the otalgia is severe, despite analgesics, and may prevent the patient from sleeping. Some patients may be febrile and can appear toxic. Frequently the diabetic patient has difficulty with glycemic control, likely secondary to the inflammatory process. Binocular examination usually shows edema and drainage in the EAC, and the pathognomonic finding is granulation tissue at the bony-cartilaginous junction. The granulation tissue should be biopsied as discussed above. The ear should be cleaned to allow topical antibiotic medications to reach the diseased tissues. Laboratory studies including a complete blood count (CBC), metabolic profile, and erythrocyte sedimentation rate (ESR) should be obtained. The patient should be started empirically on oral ciprofloxacin 750 mg p.o. b.i.d. and topical Ciprodex. A CT scan of the temporal bones, bone scan, and gallium scan should be ordered. The CT scan shows the extent of bony erosion and the extension of the disease. Both the bone scan and gallium scan show areas of increased uptake in the affected temporal bone and skull base. However, the bone scan remains positive indefinitely, and the gallium scan no longer enhances this area once the disease process has resolved.[26]

Infectious disease consultation can be helpful to titrate antibiotics once the culture results are known and to decide the length of therapy. Because infections may be polymicrobial, an antipseudomonal cephalosporin or penicillin might be necessary in addition to oral ciprofloxacin.[27] It is also important to optimize the immune status in the immunocompromised individual, and the patient's internist or family practitioner can be helpful in this regard. Diabetic patients require tight control of blood glucose levels. Neutropenic patients also need to have their immune status optimized. These patients should be seen on a regular basis, and emergently if intratemporal or intracranial complications are suspected. Magnetic resonance imaging can be helpful in the diagnosis of suspected intracranial extension.

Hyperbaric oxygen (HBO) therapy may have a role in treating patients with NEO, although there is generally no consensus. HBO increases the wound levels of oxygen, enhancing the abilities of phagocytes, promotes wound healing, and increases vascularization.[28] Treatment consists of 20 dives, administered once a day, 5 days a week, for 4 weeks.[29] HBO may be helpful in patients with disease not responding to conventional antibiotic therapy, patients with recurrent disease, or in patients with intratemporal or intracranial complications.

The role of surgical therapy in NEO is also not well defined. Surgery in not indicated in patients with disease that is responding to parenteral and topical antibiotics. Aside from biopsy, patients with persistent granulation tissue, necrotic cartilage, bony sequestra, and abscesses can benefit from surgical debridement.[30] Most cranial nerve palsies that occur in NEO are not from compression, but from extension of

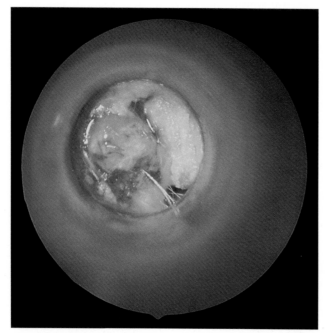

Figure 16–10 Necrotizing otitis.

the disease process, so it is unclear if nerve decompression is helpful.

With appropriate antimicrobial therapy, approximately 80 to 100% of patients can be cured.[31] Patients should be treated until the granulation tissue and pain resolve, and this may require 6 months of treatment. The ESR and gallium scan can be helpful in that therapy should generally be continued until these studies have normalized. Patients should be followed closely for recurrent disease, which can manifest with a recurrence of otalgia.

Furuncle

A furuncle is an abscess that typically arises from a hair follicle in the EAC (**Fig. 16–11**). It usually presents with a localized swelling in the lateral hair-bearing portion of the ear canal. The infection usually begins as a phlegmon and can proceed to an abscess. It is usually caused by *Staphylococcus aureus.* Treatment of the phlegmon consists of topical antibiotic drops or ointment, warm compresses, and oral antibiotics. Incision and drainage under local anesthesia is performed when the phlegmon progresses to an abscess.

Otomycosis

External otitis due to fungal overgrowth is a common problem especially in patients with hearing aids (**Figs. 16–12** and **16–13**), which create a moist environment. *Aspergillus* is the most common fungus isolated from patients with otomycosis, but other fungi have also been implicated.[32] The patient frequently presents with pruritus, drainage, and decreased hearing. Pain also can be a symptom, but it is usually not as severe as in bacterial otitis externa. Binocular microscopy typically reveals an edematous ear canal, sometimes with granulation, and frequently the fungal hyphae can be visualized. Usually black granular debris or soft tan discharge appearing like "wet newspaper" will be seen.

This diagnosis is best made by the physical examination, and it should also be suspected in patients treated for bacterial otitis externa that is persistent or not responding to treatment. Several options are available for treatment. Meticulous cleaning is critically important. Empiric treatment with acetic acid mixtures can begin soon after diagnosis and often are

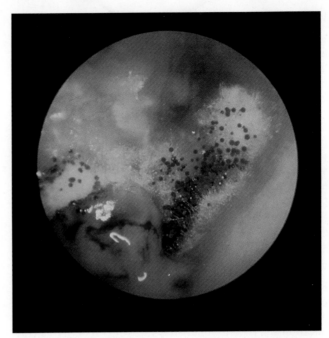

Figure 16–12 Otomycosis.

indicated for 10 to 14 days. Patients should follow water precautions during treatment. Some refractory cases require specific antifungals, but these often are off-label. Clotrimazole is an effective antifungal with activity against *Aspergillus*, but must be used with caution in patients with perforations of the TM, due to potential ototoxicity. In difficult cases with extensive disease that do not respond to topical antifungals, cultures may be helpful. Rarely are intravenous antifungals indicated in immunocompetent patients. Infectious disease consultation may be beneficial in such cases.

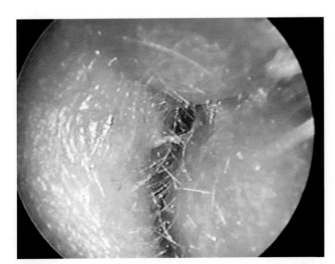

Figure 16–11 Furuncle.

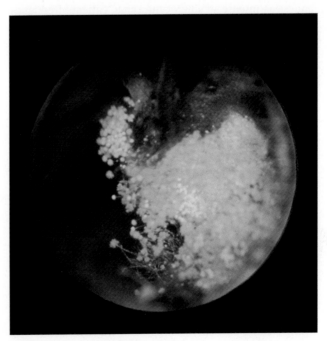

Figure 16–13 Otomycosis.

Viral Infections

Viral infections involving the EAC are much less common than bacterial or fungal infections, but can be quite severe. Varicella-Zoster virus can manifest as Ramsay Hunt syndrome, characterized by severe ear pain usually preceding vesicular eruptions on the pinna and EAC. Varicella zoster results from reactivation of latent virus usually in the geniculate ganglion, less often in the spiral or vestibular ganglion.[33] It may cause seventh nerve paralysis, hearing loss, and vertigo. This infection is quite painful, and should be treated aggressively with acyclovir or one of the other viral DNA polymerase inhibitors. If a seventh nerve paralysis is found in a patient with a normal immune system, systemic steroids may be prescribed to speed recovery. The role of facial nerve decompression in these cases is unclear.

Bullous Myringitis

Bullous myringitis is believed secondary to viral or mycoplasmal infection of the tympanic membrane and medial portion of the ear canal. It can be associated with upper respiratory infection and is more common in the winter months. Patients typically present with severe otalgia, serosanguinous otorrhea, and hearing loss. Approximately one third of patients also have serous otitis media.[34] The hearing loss can be conductive, mixed, or sensorineural, with the sensorineural component completely recovering in approximately 60% of patients.[35] Treatment consists of topical antibiotic/steroid drops, analgesics, oral quinolone, or macrolide antibiotics for 7 to 10 days (for mycoplasma involvement), and occasional myringotomy.

Dermatologic Disease

Dermatitis

Dermatitis of the EAC (also know as chronic external otitis and seborrheic external otitis) may be the result of several irritants. Chemical irritants and allergens affecting the EAC may manifest as intense itching of the canal. Patients frequently complain of itching and dry flaky skin. There may be a history of eczema involving other sites, but it may only be limited to the EAC. Patients frequently report using cotton swabs or other instruments such as toothpicks or bobby pins to scratch the canal in an attempt to relieve itching. These instruments can cause lacerations of the canal, leading to a secondary bacterial infection.

Allergic dermatitis is best treated by avoidance. Hairsprays, perfumes, cosmetics, and hearing aid mold material can all be EAC irritants. Careful elimination helps resolve symptoms. Once resolution has occurred, the patient may start to reuse such items one at a time, watching for a return of symptoms to identify the offending agent. If the agent can be identified, a more hypoallergenic material should be used if the device is necessary (such as hearing aids). In patients whose symptoms persist or are severe, a topical steroid cream or even systemic steroids may be used for a short period of time to expedite resolution of symptoms.

Patients with chronic otitis media may develop dermatitis as a result of chronic drainage from a chronically infected middle ear. The infectious drainage irritates the canal causing itching and edema. Treatment involves cleaning of the ear and removing any drainage or crusts to allow topical medications to reach the middle ear and thus treat the source of the infection. Topical antibiotic drops containing a quinolone antibiotic along with steroid are effective in treating the infection, and also help decrease any secondary inflammation of the EAC.

Most patients with chronic external otitis/dermatitis have no topical allergy, no microbial infection, and no chronic otitis media. They may or may not have a more generalized dermatologic condition. Treatment has both an acute phase and a maintenance phase to prevent recurrence. If the canal is swollen shut, a steroid-impregnated gauze wick is inserted for 2 or 3 days. The patient returns, the wick is removed, and the ear canal is carefully cleaned. If the dermatitis produces copious canal debris, the patient should irrigate the canal with 2 to 3 ounces (or more) of dilute white vinegar (50% white vinegar and 50% water boiled 5 minutes then cooled to body/room temperature) prior to instilling drops. Then four drops of otic solution are placed in the canal for 5 minutes. One particularly effective solution is Locoid™ (hydrocortisone butyrate) 0.1% topical solution, which also contains alcohol, mineral oil, and other soothing ingredients. After 5 minutes the drops are removed from the canal. This flush and drop treatment is repeated at least 3 times daily for the first week. The patient can return to the physician for cleaning and a progress report if necessary. In the second week, this flush/drop combination is continued twice a day, in the third week once a day, then every other day until the patient titrates the treatment to prevent itching and other symptoms. As water aggravates the condition, the patient should remain on dry ear precautions indefinitely.

Canal Atresia

As discussed in the beginning of the chapter, failure of the canalization of EAC can result in various degrees of canal (and auricular) atresia (see Chapter 1, Fig. 1–28). This occurs more commonly unilaterally, but may also occur bilaterally. The incidence of canal atresia is 1 in 10,000 to 1 in 20,000 births.[36] Canal atresia can be isolated, or associated with various syndromes. It may be accompanied by microtia or several middle ear anomalies. All of these factors play a role in selecting patients who are amenable to surgical correction. In patients with canal atresia in association with microtia, it is preferable to repair the microtia first, and this is generally performed when the patient is 6 to 8 years old. The reasons for this are several. At age 8, the pinna is almost adult size. Also, most microtia reconstructions are staged and utilize the skin in the pre- and postauricular area. If the canal atresia is repaired first (usually through a postauricular approach), then this skin can no longer be used.

Preoperative Evaluation

Proper patient selection is important when considering congenital canal atresia repair. The surgical procedure can be difficult secondary to the lack of normal landmarks and the potential for an aberrant facial nerve. The facial nerve may also have a more lateral course. Absence of a tympanic membrane and an abnormal ossicular chain may make location of the horizontal semicircular canal difficult. Grading systems have been developed to help decide which candidates may best benefit from surgical repair. Jahrsdoerfer et al[37] developed a preoperative grading system that utilized temporal bone CT scanning and clinical evaluation of the external ear (**Table 16–1**). Based on their system, a patient with at least a 60% chance (6 out of 10 possible points) of having a 15- to 25-dB speech reception threshold (SRT) postoperatively would be a good surgical candidate. A CT scan is pivotal in the preoperative evaluation of these patients. CT scanning is useful in identifying potential anomalies in the cochlea, vestibule, semicircular canals, endolymphatic duct, internal auditory canal, and course of the facial nerve. Finally, it is important to obtain a preoperative audiogram to document a functioning cochlea. The vast majority of these patients have a 50- to 60-dB conductive hearing loss from loss of function of the EAC and middle ear structures.

Nonsurgical modalities of treatment should also be discussed with the patient and family members. Hearing aids can be beneficial. Patients with unilateral atresia may not desire or want to wear hearing devices even though the benefits of binaural hearing are significant. Patients with bilateral atresia should be aided early to optimize speech development. Previously if the atresia was severe and bilateral, it was not possible for patients to use even small traditional hearing devices. Now with development of bone-anchored hearing aids (BAHAs), even patients with severe microtia and atresia can be aided early without the bulky external devices that were required in the past. Some studies support the use of bilateral BAHAs to improve localization of sound and speech perception.[38] This allows the patient to have excellent hearing during their lengthy staged surgical correction. These devices utilize a titanium implant placed directly into the bone just above the postauricular area. The implant becomes osseointegrated several months after implantation. The patient is then fitted with a sound processor that snaps onto the titanium abutment, which vibrates the temporal bone and cochlea, bypassing the EAC and middle ear structures.

Surgical Treatment

Surgical correction of the atretic ear canal most commonly is performed in a single stage. Occasionally a second stage is required. The first stage addresses the external ear with

Table 16–1 Jahrsdoerfer Grading System of Candidacy for Atresia Repair

Parameter	Points
Stapes present	2
Oval window open	1
Normal facial nerve	1
Malleus-incus complex present	1
Appearance of external ear	1
Middle ear space	1
Normal round window	1
Well-pneumatized mastoid	1
Incus-stapes connection	1
Total Points	**Type of Candidate**
10	Excellent
9	Very good
8	Good
7	Fair
6	Marginal
5 or less	Poor

canaloplasty, tympanoplasty, and meatoplasty. Two surgical approaches are possible: a direct approach using the root of the zygoma and the glenoid fossa as primary landmarks, or a posterior approach utilizing a mastoidectomy and early identification of the facial nerve. In either approach one must be very cognizant of the facial nerve, and in all cases facial nerve monitoring is used. The middle ear structures are identified, the stapes is checked for mobility, and a decision is made about the malleus/incus complex. It may be necessary to remove the malleus/incus complex, especially if it is fixed. An ossiculoplasty can be performed if necessary. Another option is to use a laser to mobilize the malleus/incus complex. If the stapes is fixed, a stapedectomy should be performed at a second stage. A canaloplasty and meatoplasty are performed. A bony trough for the location of the tympanic annulus is created. A fascia graft is used to construct a new TM. This graft is placed over the malleus/incus complex, or on top of the ossiculoplasty. A split-thickness skin graft is harvested from the ipsilateral thigh and used to line the new ear canal. Laterally, this graft is sutured to the meatoplasty. The meatoplasty should be large enough to allow for routine examination and good visualization of the TM and middle ear. Because the skin graft does not have the same migration kinetics as a normal ear, regular visits are necessary and frequent cleaning is required. Current advances in atresia repair utilizing lasers, thinner split-thickness skin grafts, Silastic sheets, and wicks in the EAC have improved outcomes.[39]

Neoplasms

Benign Neoplasms

Benign neoplasms of the EAC are rare, and usually arise from ceruminous glands. These tumors usually present as a painless mass in the cartilaginous portion of the ear canal. As the tumors enlarge, patients can develop pain, aural fullness, hearing loss, and otorrhea. The two most common types of benign EAC neoplasms are ceruminous adenoma and pleomorphic adenoma. Biopsies should be obtained with a margin of normal tissue to rule out invasion and to help distinguish these benign tumors from adenoid cystic carcinoma and ceruminous adenocarcinoma. The treatment of benign tumors of the EAC is wide local excision with negative margins.[40]

Malignant Neoplasms

Malignancies of the temporal bone are fortunately rare, with an estimated incidence of 1 to 6 per 1,000,000, and malignancies of the EAC comprise approximately 25% of those cases[41] (**Figs. 16–14** through **16–16**). Squamous cell carcinoma is the most common malignancy of the EAC in adults. In children sarcomas are the most frequent malignancy of the temporal bone. Other malignancies seen in the EAC include adenoid cystic carcinoma and acinic cell carcinoma.[42] The presentation of these lesions varies significantly. They may present with pain, drainage, and hearing loss mimicking benign disease, or they may be completely asymptomatic. Because symptoms can imitate benign diseases like chronic otitis externa, the diagnosis can be delayed, and therefore all patients with nonresolving "granulation tissue" should be biopsied to confirm the diagnosis. A negative biopsy may not be diagnostic. Multiple biopsies may be necessary, sometimes even under general anesthesia if necessary.

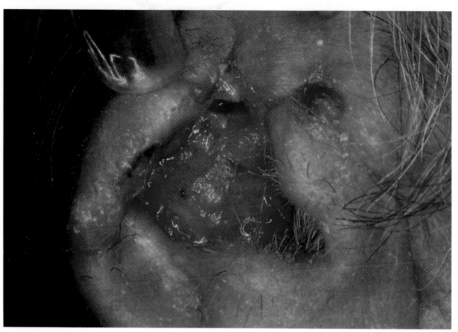

Figure 16–14   Invasive squamous cell carcinoma.

Preoperative imaging should include a CT scan of the temporal bone to assess bony destruction. MRI gives superior detail in assessing local soft tissue invasion. Staging is based on clinical and radiographic findings (see Chapter 26). Most centers treating malignant disease of the temporal bone utilize a multidisciplinary team including an otologist, head and neck surgical oncologist, reconstructive surgeon, medical oncologist, and radiation therapist. Many patients present with advanced disease, and a combination of surgery and radiation is often required. The surgical procedure required is usually a form of lateral temporal bone resection, with the extent of surgery based on staging. Chapter 26 further discusses this disorder.

Osteoradionecrosis

Osteoradionecrosis (ORN) of the temporal bone is a complication occurring from radiation treatment of skull base malignancies (**Fig. 16–17**), but idiopathic variants do exist.[43] Patient presentation varies, and symptoms include ear fullness, hearing loss, pain, discharge, tinnitus, and bloody otorrhea. On binocular microscopy there is often debris in the canal,

Figure 16–15   Basal cell carcinoma.

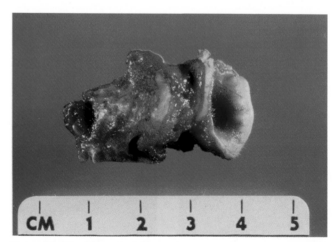

Figure 16–16   External canal resection specimen.

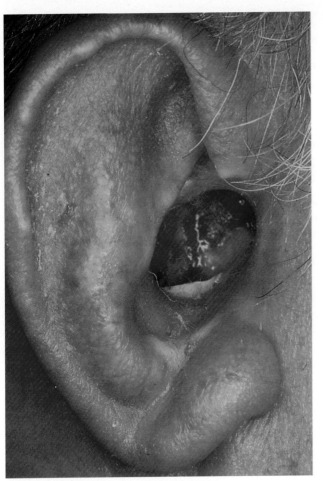

Figure 16–17 Postoperative osteoradionecrosis.

with occasional granulation tissue. There may be single or multiple areas of exposed EAC bone. The devascularized bone is often yellowish in color, spiculated, and soft. Neighboring granulation tissue should be biopsied if persistent. ORN may be localized or diffuse,[44] with localized disease occurring because the EAC is in the radiation portal (as in nasopharyngeal carcinoma) and diffuse disease occurring from direct high-dose radiation therapy to the temporal bone. Localized ORN usually is a less aggressive form of disease and often responds to serial office debridements and topical antibiotic therapy. Diffuse ORN is more lethal, and the necrotic temporal bone is at risk for intratemporal and intracranial neurovascular complications. In such cases, the management is very like the treatment of NEO. Surgical debridement, intravenous antibiotics, and HBO therapy may all be required.

References

1. Gulya AJ. Developmental anatomy of the temporal bone and skull base. In: Glasscock ME III, Gulya AJ, eds. Surgery of the Ear, 5th ed. Lewiston, NY: BC Decker, 2002:3–8

2. Okuda I, Bingham B, Stoney P, Hawke M. The organic composition of ear wax. J Otolaryngol 1991;20:212–215

3. Gray H. Anatomy of the Human Body. Philadelphia: Lea & Febiger, 1918; www.bartleby.com/107/, 2000

4. Kakoi H, Anniko M, Kinnefors A, Rask-Andersen H. Auditory. Epidermal cell migration. VII. Antigen expression of proliferating cell nuclear antigens, PCNA and Ki-67 in human tympanic membrane and external auditory canal. Acta Otolaryngol 1997;117:100–108

5. Vennix PP, Kuijpers W, Peters TA, Tonnaer EL, Ramaekers FC. Epidermal differentiation in the human external auditory meatus. Laryngoscope 1996;106:470–475

6. Bapat U, Nia J, Bance M. Severe audiovestibular loss following ear syringing for wax removal. J Laryngol Otol 2001;115:410–411

7. Capo JM, Lucente FE. Alkaline battery foreign bodies of the ear and nose. Arch Otolaryngol Head Neck Surg 1986;112:562–563

8. Antonelli PJ, Ahmadi A, Prevatt A. Insecticidal activity of common reagents for insect foreign bodies of the ear. Laryngoscope 2001;111:15–20

9. Hurst W, Bailey M, Hurst B. Prevalence of external auditory canal exostoses in Australian surfboard riders. J Laryngol Otol 2004;118:348–351

10. Kroon DF, Lawson ML, Derkay CS, Hoffmann K, McCook J. Surfer's ear: external auditory exostoses are more prevalent in cold water surfers. Otolaryngol Head Neck Surg 2002;126:499–504

11. van Gilse PHG. Des observations ulterieures sur la genes des exostoses du conduit externe par l'irriations d'eau froide. Acta Otolaryngol (Stockh) 1938;26:343

12. Stenfors LE, Sade J, Hellstrom S, Anniko M, Folkow L. Exostoses and cavernous venous formation in the external auditory canal of the hooded seal as a functional physiological organ. Acta Otolaryngol 2000;120:940–943

13. Graham MD. Osteoma and exostosis of the external auditory canal. A clinical histopathologic and scanning microscopic study. Ann Otol Rhinol Laryngol 1979;88:566–572

14. Timofeev I, Notkina N, Smith IM. Exostoses of the external auditory canal: a long-term follow-up study of surgical treatment. Clin Otolaryngol Allied Sci. 2004;29:588–594

15. Piepergerdes MC, Kramer BM, Behnke EE. Keratosis obturans and external auditory canal cholesteatoma. Laryngoscope 1980;90:383–891

16. Persaud RA, Hajioff D, Thevasagayam MS, Wareing MJ, Wright A. Keratosis obturans and external ear canal cholesteatoma: how and why we should distinguish between these conditions. Clin Otolaryngol 2004;29:577–581

17. Garin P, Degols JC, Delos M. External auditory canal cholesteatoma. Arch Otolaryngol Head Neck Surg 1997;123:62–65

18. Hajjartabar M. Poor-quality water in swimming pools associated with a substantial risk of otitis externa due to Pseudomonas aeruginosa. Water Sci Technol 2004;50:63–67

19. Roland PS, Stroman DW. Microbiology of acute otitis externa. Laryngoscope 2002;112(7 pt 1):1166–1177

20. Bath AP, Walsh RM, Bance ML, Rutka JA. Ototoxicity of topical gentamicin preparations. Laryngoscope 1999;109(7 pt 1):1088–1093

21. Torum B, Block SL, Avila H, et al. Efficacy of ofloxacin otic solution once daily for 7 days in the treatment of otitis externa: a multicenter, open-label, phase III trial. Clin Ther 2004;26:1046–1054

22. Weinroth SE, Schessel D, Tuazon CU. Malignant otitis externa in AIDS patients: case report and review of the literature. Ear Nose Throat J 1994;73:772–778

23. Ress BD, Luntz M, Telischi FF, Balkany TJ, Whiteman ML. Necrotizing external otitis in patients with AIDS. Laryngoscope 1997;107:456–460

24. Munoz A, Martinez-Chamorro E. Necrotizing external otitis caused by Aspergillus fumigatus: computed tomography and high resolution magnetic resonance imaging in an AIDS patient. J Laryngol Otol 1998;112: 98–102

25. Soldati D, Mudry A, Monnier P. Necrotizing otitis externa caused by Staphylococcus epidermidis. Eur Arch Otorhinolaryngol 1999;256: 439–441

26. Parisier SC, Lucente FE, Som PM, Hirschman SZ, Arnold LM, Roffman JD. Nuclear scanning in necrotizing progressive "malignant" external otitis. Laryngoscope 1982;92(9 pt 1):1016–1019

27. Gehanno P. Ciprofloxacin in the treatment of malignant external otitis. Chemotherapy 1994;40(suppl 1):35–40

28. Davis JC, Gates GA, Lerner C, et al. Adjuvant hyperbaric oxygen therapy in malignant external otitis. Arch Otolaryngol Head Neck Surg 1992; 118:89–93

29. Mader JT, Love JT. Malignant external otitis: Cure with adjunctive hyperbaric oxygen therapy. Arch Otolaryngol 1982;108:38–40

30. Babiatzki A, Sade J. Malignant external otitis. J Laryngol Otol 1987;101: 205–210

31. Johnson MP, Ramphal R. Malignant external otitis: Report on therapy with ceftazidime and review of therapy and prognosis. Rev Infect Dis. 1990;12:173–180

32. Kaur R, Mittal N, Kakkar M, Aggarwal AK, Mathur MD. Otomycosis: a clinicomycologic study. Ear Nose Throat J 2000;79:606–609

33. Kuhweide R, Van de Steene V, Vlaminck S, Casselman JW. Ramsay Hunt syndrome: pathophysiology of cochleovestibular symptoms. J Laryngol Otol 2002;116:844–848 Review.

34. Marais J, Dale BA. Bullous myringitis: a review. Clin Otolaryngol Allied Sci 1997;22:497–499

35. Hariri MA. Sensorineural hearing loss in bullous myringitis. A prospective study of eighteen patients. Clin Otolaryngol Allied Sci 1990;15:351–353

36. De La Cruz A, Chandrasekhar SS. Congenital malformation of the temporal bone. In: Brackmann DE, Shelton C, Arriaga M, eds. Otologic Surgery. Philadelphia: WB Saunders, 2001:54–67

37. Jahrsdoerfer RA, Yeakley JW, Aguilar EA, Cole RR, Gray LC. Grading system for the selection of patients with congenital aural atresia. Am J Otol 1992;13:6–12

38. Van der Pouw KT, Snik AF, Cremers CW. Audiometric results of bilateral bone-anchored hearing aid application in patients with bilateral congenital aural atresia. Laryngoscope 1998;108(4 pt 1):548–553

39. Teufert KB, De la Cruz A. Advances in congenital aural atresia surgery: effects on outcome. Otolaryngol Head Neck Surg 2004;131:263–270

40. Hicks GW. Tumors arising from the glandular structure of the external auditory canal. Laryngoscope 1983;93:326–340

41. Morton RP, Stell PM, Derrick PPO. Epidemiology of cancer of the middle ear cleft. Cancer 1984;53:1612–1617

42. Kinney SE, Wood BG. Malignancies of the external ear canal and temporal bone. Laryngoscope 1987;97:158–164

43. Goufas G. Diagnosis and pathogenesis of benign necrotic osteitis of the external ear canal. Ann Otolaryngol Chir Cervicofac 1954;71:390–396

44. Ramsden RT, Bulman CH, Lorigan BP. Osteoradionecrosis of the temporal bone. J Laryngol Otol 1975;89:941–956

17

Otitis Media

Nathan Sautter and Keiko Hirose

Treatment of children and adults with otitis media (OM) is a substantial component of the practice of otolaryngology–head and neck surgery. OM is second only to viral upper respiratory tract infection as the most common reason for visits to pediatricians. In a prospective study of children in the greater Boston area, 93% of children had one or more episode of acute otitis media (AOM) and 74% had at least three episodes of AOM during the first 7 years of life.[1] Epidemiologic studies at the University of Pittsburgh revealed a 90% incidence of OM in urban children within the first 2 years of life.[2] The vast majority of OM occur in children, and although the greater part of these cases resolves by adolescence, the disease may also occur in adults. Tympanostomy with tube placement is the primary surgical treatment for OM and remains the most common surgical procedure performed under general anesthesia in the United States.

In spite of substantial research, controversy exists regarding optimal therapy and treatment guidelines, which vary widely across the United States and in other nations. The large annual health care expenditure in the United States for treatment of OM, estimated at more than $5 billion, has caused health care providers and payers to adopt several tactics aimed at reducing costs.

The first attempt at development of an evidence-based and cost-effective clinical treatment guideline for OM was introduced by the Agency for Health Care Policy and Research (AHCPR)[3] in 1994. These recommendations were updated in 2004 by the Subcommittee on Otitis Media with Effusion, composed of experts selected by the American Academy of Otolaryngology–Head and Neck Surgery in conjunction with the American Academy of Pediatrics and the American Academy of Family Physicians.[4] These recommendations apply to children aged 2 months to 12 years without developmental disabilities or an underlying medical condition causing predisposition to OM. The evidence-based guidelines proposed by the Subcommittee are intended to maximize efficiency of health care expenditures while maintaining the highest standard of care. They are intended as a guide, not a substitute, for clinical judgment.

◆ Terminology

OM is an infectious, inflammatory condition of the middle ear associated with an effusion behind an intact tympanic membrane. It also may be associated with several inciting factors, most commonly upper respiratory tract infection and eustachian tube dysfunction. OM may be classified according to the composition of the effusion: serous (SOM), mucoid (MOM), and purulent (POM). Each classification is not in itself a distinct entity; that is, a specific etiology may not be inferred by the composition of the effusion. Rather, OM is a dynamic process encompassing a somewhat broad spectrum of disease. For example, SOM may progress to MOM, and POM typically progresses to SOM during the course of resolution.

Acute otitis media usually is characterized by rapid onset of otalgia and erythema of the tympanic membrane in the presence of middle ear effusion. Otalgia and fever are more evident in younger children and may be absent in older children. Erythema of the tympanic membrane without middle ear effusion is called acute myringitis and may be mistaken for AOM. Erythema of the tympanic membrane also is seen in a small proportion of chronic middle ear effusions. *Recurrent acute otitis media* (RAOM) is a term commonly assigned to patients with multiple self-limited episodes of AOM punctuated by periods of time in which the patient is symptom-free, either with or without a persistent middle ear effusion. Current practice guidelines define RAOM as three or more episodes of AOM within 6 months, or four or more episodes within a year.

Chronic otitis media with effusion (COME) refers to an accumulation of inflammatory liquid in the middle ear cleft without other signs of inflammation (e.g., fever, otalgia). Alternative names assigned to COME in the literature include glue ear, chronic secretory otitis media, serous otitis media, persistent otitis media, and silent otitis media. Effusions resulting from barotrauma, skull fracture, or leakage of cerebrospinal fluid are not included in this category. Many, if not most, chronic effusions result from resolving AOM. It is appropriate to think of AOM and COME as two points along a continuum of the same disease process. An antecedent history of AOM, however, is not necessary for diagnosis of COME. Chronic effusions of unknown duration as well as all cases of OM persisting more than 30 days are classified as COME. Chronic otorrhea through a perforated tympanic membrane is termed chronic suppurative otitis media and may be associated with cholesteatoma.

◆ Risk Factors

Known risk factors for OM include recent upper respiratory infection (URI), male gender, a greater number of siblings in the home, attending day care, family history, bottle (rather than breast) feeding, and smoking in the home.[5] Familial susceptibility to OM may result from defects in the immune system or in the biologic structure of the middle ear, palate, and eustachian tube. Inherited disorders of mucociliary clearance such as Kartagener's syndrome or cystic fibrosis may predispose to OM. Socioeconomic factors within a family that may contribute to the development of OM include overcrowding, poor diet, and lack of access to health care. Certain ethnic groups, notably Native Americans, have a high prevalence of OM presumably due to differences in the anatomy of the eustachian tube and skull base.[6] Children in day care have a greater incidence of OM than those reared at home because of endemic URI in groups. Similarly, children in early grade school have an increased incidence of OM. Some authors have also suggested that environmental allergy, food allergy, and gastroesophageal reflux disease contribute to the development of OM, although a definite link between any of these conditions and OM has yet to be established.[7,8]

◆ Pathophysiology

Acute Otitis Media

AOM is an inflammatory disorder induced by microorganisms in the middle ear (**Figs. 17–1** through **17–6**) characterized by the presence of an effusion (often purulent), and frequently associated with otalgia and fevers, particularly in younger children. The most likely route of bacterial entry into the middle ear is from reflux of infected secretions from the nasopharynx through the eustachian tube, which is known to occur in otitis-prone children. Three factors appear to facilitate bacterial reflux into the middle ear: bacterial colonization of the nasopharynx, incompetence of the protective function of the eustachian tube, and a negative pressure in the middle ear in relation to the nasopharynx.

AOM is principally a sequel of viral URI.[9,10] Viral rhinitis breaks down mucosal barriers and mechanisms of muciliary clearance that prevent bacterial adherence and growth in both the nose and nasopharynx. In addition, swelling of the nasal mucosa alters the aerodynamics of the upper airway.

The bacteriology of AOM has been studied extensively. In a large study at the University of Pittsburgh, the most predominant bacteria cultured from acute middle ear effusions were *Streptococcus pneumoniae* (35%), *Haemophilus influenzae* (23%) and *Moraxella catarrhalis* (14%).[11] These same three pathogenic bacteria appear in the nasopharynx following an URI.[12,13] Pillsbury et al[14] demonstrated higher bacterial colony

counts in the adenoids of children with recurrent OM than in those undergoing adenoidectomy for adenoid hypertrophy without OM. Bernstein et al[15] have identified the alterations in the microecology of the nasopharynx in children with RAOM. It would appear that loss of the immunologic function of the adenoid and colonization of the nasopharynx with pathogenic bacteria are important factors in the pathophysiology of OM. Normalization of the nasopharyngeal flora in conjunction with a marked decrease in the colonization of pathogenic bacteria has been demonstrated following adenoidectomy in otitis-prone children.[13]

Eustachian tube dysfunction is generally held to be an underlying cause of OM. However, controversy remains about

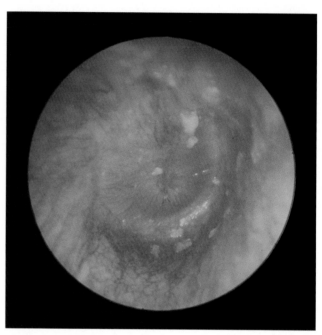

Figure 17–1   Acute otitis media.

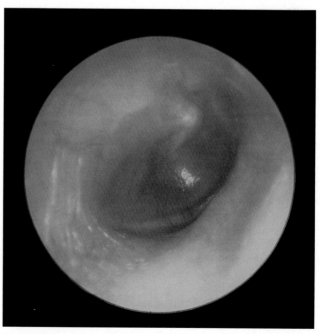

Figure 17–2   Acute otitis media with effusion.

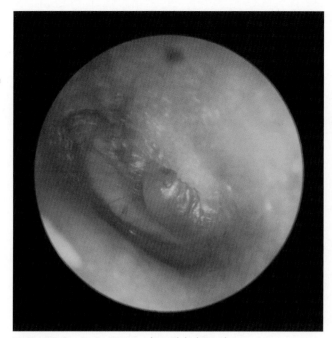

Figure 17–3 Acute otitis media with bulging drum.

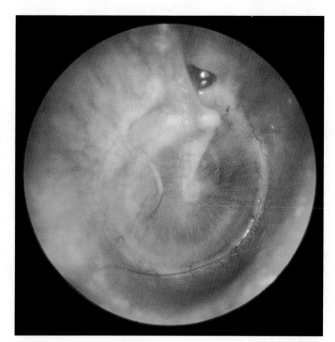

Figure 17–4 Acute otitis media, exudative stage.

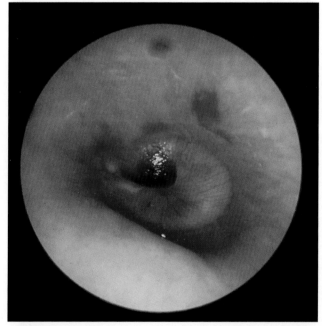

Figure 17–5 Acute otitis media with bleb.

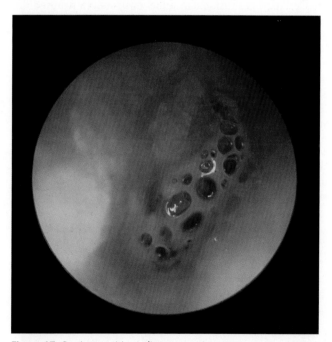

Figure 17–6 Acute otitis media, suppurative stage.

whether eustachian tube dysfunction causes or is a result of OM. The eustachian tube has three functions: protection of the middle ear, clearance of middle ear secretions, and equalization of pressure between the nose and middle ear. The child's eustachian tube is short, horizontal, and composed of relatively flaccid cartilage. The protective function of the tube is less effective, and retrograde reflux of nasopharyngeal secretions may occur more readily than in the mature eustachian tube.[16]

Clearance of secretions results mainly from ciliary action. Viral upper respiratory infection is known to cause transient ciliary dysfunction; it is presumed that ciliary function of the middle ear and eustachian tube mucosa is also impaired during AOM. Fluid accumulates as a consequence of ciliary paralysis, and clearance of fluid follows recovery of ciliary function. However, thick viscous fluid may occlude the tube secondarily because of its rheologic properties. Pressure equalization is normally mediated by tubal opening from contraction of the tensor veli palatini muscle in response to stimuli mediated by the tympanic plexus.[17] Normal function of the tensor veli palatini muscle is impaired in patients with submucous or complete cleft palate and is thought to be the main reason for the resultant eustachian tube dysfunction.

The third factor in the genesis of AOM may result from either excessive negative pressure in the middle ear or positive pressure in the nasopharynx. Obstruction of the nose secondary to viral rhinitis may result in the equivalent of the Toynbee maneuver, that is, holding the nostrils closed during swallowing. Because most URIs result in nasal obstruction, swallowing during an URI may increase the nasopharyngeal pressure, which will open the tube and tend to push secretions into the middle ear space. Nose blowing also increases nasopharyngeal pressures. Sniffing is a common symptom of URI and it is known to produce negative middle ear pressure, which may facilitate the reflux process by creating a negative pressure differential that would pull on any material entering the eustachian tube.[18]

Chronic Otitis Media with Effusion

COME was virtually unknown before antimicrobial therapy began in the 1940s (**Figs. 17–7** through **17–10**). Whether this is the result of widespread use of antibiotics or better diagnostic methods is unclear. However, perforations of the tympanic membrane are less prevalent after antimicrobial therapy than in the preantibiotic era. Such perforations permitted adequate drainage of the ear and prevented COME.

Early researchers postulated that COME was a primary disorder of multiple causes resulting from the hydrops ex vacuo theory; that is, eustachian tube obstruction resulted in, sequentially, under-aeration of the middle ear, negative middle ear pressure, and fluid transudation.[19] When the drop in pressure is acute, these observations adequately explain the development of effusion as in barotrauma.[20] However, applying this concept to the pathogenesis of COME does not fully explain more recent observations about the disorder. The Greater Boston Collaborative Otitis Media Study found persistent effusion following AOM for 1 month in 40%, for 2 months in 20%, and for 3 months or longer in 10% of cases.[21] More recently, Rosenfeld and Kay[22] performed a literature search and meta-analysis of the literature to estimate the natural history of untreated OM. In patients with middle ear effusion following an untreated episode of AOM, 59% resolved

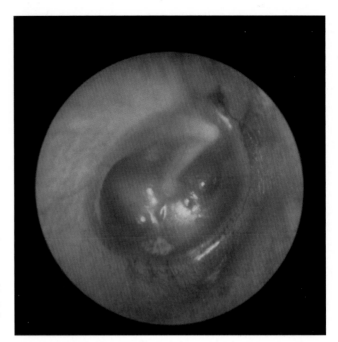

Figure 17–8 Serous otitis media with retracted drum.

within 1 month and 74% resolved within 3 months. Patients with chronic middle ear effusions (observed to be present for longer than 3 months) exhibited 26% resolution within 6 months and 33% resolution by 1 year. Many investigators have demonstrated pathogenic bacteria in the fluid obtained from the middle ears of children with COME.[23] The Pittsburgh Otitis Media Research Center study confirmed similar bacteriology in cultured effusions from children with AOM and COME. Children with chronic effusion had a positive culture 70% of the time.[2] In one study, reverse-transcriptase polymerase chain reaction (RT-PCR) analysis of culture-negative chronic effusions in children revealed the presence of bacterial messenger RNA (mRNA) (hence, viable and metabolically active

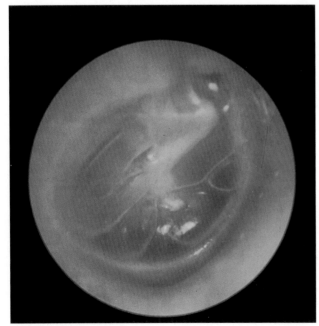

Figure 17–7 Serous otitis media.

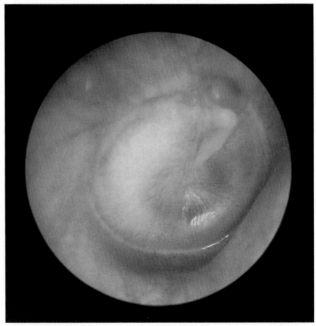

Figure 17–9 Serous otitis media, advanced.

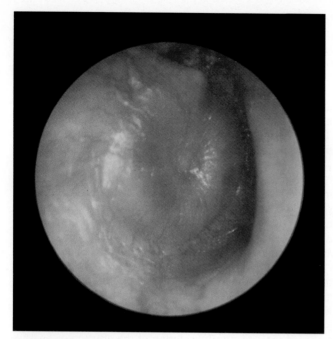

Figure 17–10 Mucoid otitis media.

bacteria) in a significant proportion of effusions.[24] It is possible that, in many chronic effusions, bacteria may be present in an attenuated form, existing as biofilms on the mucosal surface. This was demonstrated by Ehrlich et al[25] in a chinchilla model of OM using *H. influenzae.* Studies in experimental OM[26] have demonstrated that eustachian tube obstruction does not result in mucoid effusion in the absence of bacterial infection. Normal middle ear gas is now known to be hypoxic and hypercapneic in relation to inspired air,[27] and chronic eustachian tube obstruction per se does not result in severe negative middle ear pressure.[28]

Thus, the preponderance of available evidence supports the theory that (1) secretory changes in the middle ear in COME are histologic sequelae of chronic infection, rather than a separate pathologic disorder; (2) the majority of cases of COME begin as acute infection of the middle ear; (3) postinflammatory alterations in the middle ear mucosa and eustachian tube (e.g., goblet cell metaplasia and hypersecretion) lead to persistence of effusion; and (4) dysfunction of the eustachian tube is an important part of the process.

◆ Diagnosis

The diagnosis of OM is made primarily on a clinical basis. Symptoms such as fever, otalgia, otorrhea, irritability, and decreased hearing should raise suspicion for the presence of OM. In patients with a previous history of OM or with a given history of a preceding URI, the likelihood of middle ear effusion is even greater. COME may be asymptomatic and often is detected incidentally during well-child visits to the pediatrician. Direct visualization of the tympanic membrane with an otoscope is necessary for confirmation of the diagnosis. An erythematous, opaque, and bulging tympanic membrane is consistent with AOM. Clear or amber-colored fluid may be seen with COME; bubbles or an air-fluid level may also be visible behind the tympanic membrane. Pneumatic otoscopy

is useful if the diagnosis is in doubt; decreased TM mobility with pneumotoscopy may indicate the presence of fluid in the middle ear. Tympanometry, acoustic reflectometry, and ultrasonography may be useful adjuncts in the diagnosis of OM.[29,30] Tympanometry combined with otoscopy has been demonstrated to raise the sensitivity and specificity of the diagnosis of OM to greater than 90%,[31] whereas pneumatic otoscopy alone has been shown to have 85% sensitivity and 75% specificity in the diagnosis of OM, although this may vary based on the individual clinician's training and experience.[32] Accordingly, the official recommendation of the Subcommittee on Otitis Media with Effusion is the use of pneumatic otoscopy as the primary diagnostic method for OM with tympanometry reserved as a confirmatory test when the diagnosis is in doubt.[4] In the absence of other otologic abnormalities, audiometry may demonstrate a mild or moderate (20–40 dB) conductive hearing loss but is not useful for the initial diagnosis of OM. It is important to document the laterality and duration of the effusion.

The history should also include questions regarding the risk factors for learning and speech disabilities, duration of symptoms, quality of life issues, and the presence of the aforementioned environmental risk factors.

The incidence of OM in adults is much less common than in children. In the absence of an obvious inciting factor (e.g., viral URI, barotrauma) a careful search for the underlying etiology should be undertaken. An adult with unilateral middle ear effusion should undergo evaluation for a nasopharyngeal mass, including nasopharyngoscopy.

◆ Medical Management

Acute Otitis Media

Clearance of an acute episode of OM usually follows control of the infecting organism through immunologic defense. Most clinicians, however, agree that antimicrobial therapy hastens clearance. The majority of cases are due to aerobic organisms with *S. pneumoniae, H. influenzae,* and *M. catarrhalis*—the three most commonly isolated organisms in acute middle ear effusions. Routine culture of the middle ear contents is not done in practice. Tympanocentesis may provide some information regarding the composition and cause of the effusion, but it is not routinely performed and is not considered a therapeutic procedure for any form of OM. It should be reserved for cases in which the clinician suspects a rare or resistant bacterial etiology, or in newborns or immunocompromised patients with OM. In cases of AOM with negative cultures, either the causative agent (virus, anaerobes) is uncertain or the diagnosis is wrong.

Traditional therapy in the United States is amoxicillin 40 mg/kg/day for 7 to 10 days.[33] Although shorter courses probably are adequate, the evidence is incomplete. The principal reasons for use of an antimicrobial are to lower the risk of meningitis in babies and shorten the duration of symptoms in a minority of patients. In a meta-analysis of 5400 children with AOM, Rosenfeld et al[33] observed clinical resolution within 7 to 14 days in 81% of untreated children and in 94% of children treated with antibiotics. These findings are similar to those in a later meta-analysis.[34] Current practice conventions suggest that treatment with another agent, such as amoxicillin clavulanate, is indicated when symptoms fail to resolve after 3 days of treatment. These conventions should be studied in more detail because in some cases the fever is due to a systemic viral infection, and the redness of the tympanic membrane in a crying infant is mistakenly used as evidence of AOM. In such cases, lack of effusion in the middle ear should be considered as clinical evidence against a diagnosis of AOM, and a second antimicrobial agent, therefore, would not be indicated. Further, presence of effusion even up to 3 months after an episode of AOM is not unusual and is not, in itself, an indication for a second or later round of antimicrobial therapy. If the clinician is concerned about lack of response to the agent used, cultures of the middle ear via tympanocentesis is a time-honored method for clarifying the pathogenesis of the signs and symptoms. The role of antimicrobial treatment for AOM is being studied closely, but there is certainly no consensus regarding optimal treatment.

Alternative agents are higher-dose amoxicillin (80–90 mg/kg/day); the second- and third-generation cephalosporins such as cefaclor, cefuroxime, and cefpodoxime; macrolide antibiotics; the combination of sulfisoxazole and erythromycin (Pediazole); or trimethoprim/sulfamethoxazole. Doses are based on body weight.

In an alternative strategy used in many European countries antimicrobial agents are withheld pending spontaneous resolution, which occurs in a majority of cases.[22,35] Children are given analgesics and antipyretics; antimicrobials are started if the infection persists after several days or if the tympanic membrane ruptures. Another treatment strategy that is gaining in popularity is "safety net" antibiotic prescriptions.[36] Parents of children with AOM are given a prescription for antibiotics and are instructed to fill it only if symptoms persist for 48 hours.

There are no proven preventive measures for AOM other than avoidance of risk factors. A Finnish study of the efficacy of pneumococcal conjugate vaccine (Prevnar) in prevention of AOM in children showed only a modest benefit of 6% reduction in the total number of episodes.[37] Although this same vaccine is very effective in preventing invasive pneumococcal infections, its efficacy in prevention of mucosal disease (such as OM) appears to be slight.

Recurrent Acute Otitis Media

The first step in treatment of patients with recurrent or chronic OM should be manipulation of any existing environmental risk factors whenever possible. When this fails, other medical or surgical therapies are considered. Prophylactic medical therapy for RAOM has fallen out of favor. A common practice in the past has been long-term administration of antibiotics for prophylactic purposes. This practice, however, is no longer recommended in the face of rising indices of antibiotic resistance.[38] It was estimated in 1995 that approximately 25% of pneumococci were penicillin-resistant, and approximately 25% of *H. influenzae* isolates and 90% of *M. catarrhalis* isolates produced β-lactamase.[39] Due to these alarming statistics, some authors have advocated earlier surgical intervention in place of repeated courses of antibiotics as primary treatment of RAOM.[40]

Chronic Otitis Media with Effusion

Although Mandel et al[41] demonstrated a small effect of antimicrobial therapy in COME, clinical experience indicates that the effectiveness is further reduced as the number of treatments increases. It is not uncommon to see children with persistent COME who have received four or more courses of antimicrobials in a 3-month period. For these children, additional antimicrobial therapy is futile. Rosenfeld and Post[42] found in a meta-analysis of existing studies that the benefit of antimicrobial therapy in COME is slight. Treatment with prolonged courses of antibiotics when the efficacy is doubtful is not prudent in the face of rising microbial resistance to antibiotics. Because most effusions resolve spontaneously after treating AOM, withholding additional treatment in favor of watchful waiting for 3 months is recommended. Updated AHCPR guidelines recommend observation of nonacute OM for 3 months in children who are not otherwise at risk for speech, language, or hearing problems. At-risk children may undergo expedited treatment at the discretion of the clinician. A single course of antibiotics over 10 to 14 days may be used as an alternative treatment in children who are poor surgical candidates or whose parents request additional therapy prior to surgery. If there is no resolution after 3 months, an audiogram is indicated. Surgery is indicated if there is a conductive hearing loss of 20 dB above normal threshold. If no hearing loss is detected, the child should be reexamined at 3- to 6-month intervals until resolution of the effusion or hearing loss is identified. If tympanic membrane or middle ear pathology (e.g., retraction of the tympanic membrane) is noted, surgery is indicated at that time.[4]

Certain nonantimicrobial medical therapies have been used as alternatives or adjuncts to antibiotics. Studies of short-term corticosteroid therapy have had conflicting results. Schwartz et al[43] found otoscopic improvement in the treated subjects, whereas Lambert[44] found no difference in outcomes between the corticosteroid group and the control group. Rosenfeld et al[45] performed a meta-analysis of the published studies and found that the odds ratio for clearance was 3.6 in steroid-treated children. A later meta-analysis failed to show any benefit of oral steroids over placebo as treatment for OM.[46] It has not been shown that the long-term benefits of corticosteroid therapy outweigh the risks when used as treatment for OM. Accordingly, the AHCPR does not recommend the use of corticosteroids as treatment of OM, citing lack of proof of long-term efficacy.[4] A preliminary randomized placebo-controlled trial evaluating the effectiveness of homeopathic remedies in the treatment of AOM could not rule out a positive treatment effect over placebo, but further study is necessary prior to any conclusions.[47] Antihistamines and decongestants are ineffective treatments for OM.

◆ Surgical Management

Otitis media is the most common indication for a surgical procedure in children. Surgical therapy is recommended only when initial medical therapy fails. Thus, medical and surgical therapy are sequential, not alternative. Over the past two decades, several prospective randomized clinical trials have validated the efficacy of surgical therapy of OM. The goal of surgical therapy is correction of the underlying pathophysiologic condition, if possible, to prevent recurrent OM and remediation of symptoms, primarily conductive hearing loss, especially during the key periods for development of speech and language. Where inadequate ventilation of the middle ear is the principal problem, insertion of tympanostomy tubes

(TTs), also known as PE (pressure equalization) tubes, is the treatment of choice. Where infection of the middle ear from reflux of nasopharyngeal organisms is the chief problem, adenoidectomy is the treatment of choice. In most cases of COME, both conditions exist concurrently and, thus, the combined operation may be indicated.

Therapy for OM differs by the age of the patient and whether the process is acute or chronic. Because antimicrobial therapy is the standard of treatment for AOM in the United States (this is a controversial issue in Europe[35]), patients with occasional, isolated episodes of AOM do not generally come to the attention of the otolaryngologist.[48] Therefore, only recurrent or chronic cases are considered here.

Tympanostomy Tubes

Tympanostomy tubes were popularized by Armstrong[49] and insertion of TTs is the most common operation performed in children (**Figs. 17–11** through **17–14**). The TT serves as an artificial eustachian tube to ventilate the middle ear and equalize the middle ear pressure to atmospheric. The TT also serves as a portal for topical delivery of medications to the middle ear space. Middle ear clearance also is aided because negative pressure cannot occur from the piston effect as a bolus of thick fluid is moved into the eustachian tube by ciliary action. The greater efficacy of TT in OM as opposed to simple drainage by myringotomy has been established.[50]

The finding that the time to recurrence of OM after myringotomy is the same as after extrusion of TTs[51] suggests that ventilation of the middle ear provides palliation of the symptoms of OM rather than correcting the underlying problem. Permanent cure of OM is accomplished only with time, allowing for maturation of the immune system and eustachian tube. Therefore, using TTs that remain in place and ventilate the ear for a longer duration compared with myringotomy alone is a logical choice.

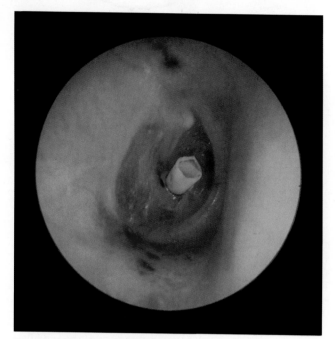

Figure 17–12   Long shaft tympanostomy tube.

The major differences among the multitude of available tubes relate to lumen size, length, and retention time. In general, the short grommet tubes extrude sooner than the long, T-shaped tubes. The larger the bore of the tube and the longer it stays in place, the more likely is a persistent perforation of the tympanic membrane. A similar rate of perforations is seen after TT insertion using short-term grommets as compared with myringotomy alone.[51] Long-term tubes have a greater perforation rate but greater freedom from OM during their sojourn. Closure of such persistent perforations is easily accomplished with a fat graft myringoplasty as an outpatient procedure.[52]

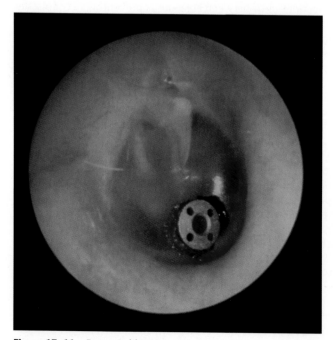

Figure 17–11   Reuter Bobbin tympanostomy tube.

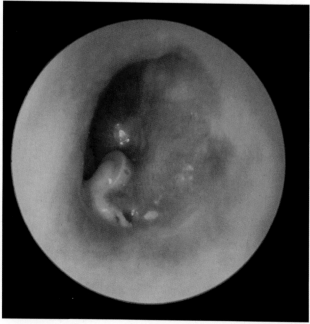

Figure 17–13   Purulent otitis following tympanostomy tube.

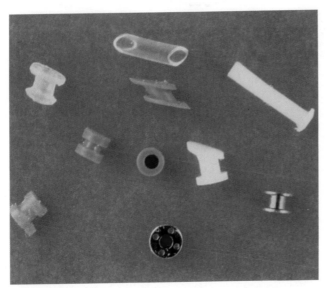

Figure 17–14 Various tympanostomy tubes.

Patients with TTs need periodic monitoring. The modified T tubes, which are slightly shorter than the original Goode T tubes,[53] will remain in situ for 2 to 5 years. Patients are examined at 6-month intervals to ensure tubal patency, freedom from infection, and proper position of the tube. These tubes are generally well tolerated, but occasionally granulation tissue will form around the base of the tube, and this usually responds well to topical steroid/antibiotic preparations.

Adenoidectomy

Adenoidectomy was once the primary surgical treatment offered to children with OM. During the 1960s and 1970s, adenoidectomy was used less often because of the popularity of TTs and because several studies, which would be considered flawed by today's standards, failed to show a significant effect of adenoidectomy on outcome. Three separate, prospective, randomized clinical trials have shown that adenoidectomy significantly reduces morbidity from COME.[51,54,55] These studies have demonstrated that (1) adenoidectomy is an effective treatment for patients with OM, and (2) the effect is independent of the size of the adenoid.

Given that (1) children in the San Antonio study[51] receiving adenoidectomy had a significant reduction in morbidity as compared with those who did not have their adenoid removed, (2) if adenoidectomy was done the outcome in hearing and time with effusion was similar whether a TT was used or not, and (3) the complication rate from adenoidectomy was very low, an argument can be made to perform adenoidectomy and myringotomy with or without TT insertion as the primary procedure for COME in children 4 years of age and older.[56] Paradise and Bluestone[56] have argued that adenoidectomy, being slightly riskier and more expensive than TT insertion, should be reserved for recurrent cases.

The study of Paradise et al[55] showed that the adenoidectomy effect did not differ by age (about one third of the children were under 4 years of age). Common knowledge indicates that there is little physiologic difference between a 3-year-old and a 4-year-old child. The effect of adenoidectomy was greater for the younger children in the San Antonio study.[51] Therefore, one could make the case that high-risk children should have adenoidectomy at a younger age to accrue the greatest benefit. Adenoidectomy in children over 18 months has been shown to be a safe procedure.[58] When recurrence rate is factored into the initial cost of adenoidectomy versus TT, the cost per quality-adjusted life-year is essentially the same.[48]

Certainly, the preceding arguments are logical but not validated; therefore, clinicians have to decide this matter in their own practice according to local costs and practice guidelines. Two important, parallel misconceptions by some physicians still influence clinical decisions about adenoidectomy: first, adenoidectomy is indicated for OM if the adenoid is enlarged; and second, the small adenoid is normal. The three clinical trials on adenoidectomy[51,54,55] have all shown that the size of the adenoid is irrelevant to outcome. Adenoid hyperplasia is a reaction of the healthy adenoid to antigenic stimulation, whereas the chronically infected adenoid, which is associated with OM,[58] is small because it is unable to mount an immune response. The decision for adenoidectomy, therefore, should be based on the severity and persistence of the middle ear disease, not on the size of the adenoid. Until direct methods for evaluating adenoid pathology are found, it is well to remember that the status of the middle ear may indirectly indicate the status of the adenoid in children with histories of OM.

Children being considered for adenoidectomy should be free of defects of the soft palate. The most insidious problem is submucous cleft of the soft palate, which can be suspected by a bifid uvula, a bluish-white band (zona pellucida) in the midline of the palate (where the muscles are absent), absence of a spine on the posterior edge of the hard palate, and a groove in the posterior surface of the soft palate seen on fiberoptic nasopharyngoscopy.

Surgical Treatment of Recurrent Acute Otitis Media

Many children with RAOM have normal otoscopy between episodes but some retain effusion, and therefore could be categorized also as having COME. The chief goal for those whose infections clear between episodes is preventing new episodes of infection. Although antimicrobial prophylaxis was commonly used in the past,[59] overreliance on long-term treatment with low-dose antimicrobial therapy appears to be a contributing factor to the emergence of resistant strains of S. pneumoniae. Therefore, surgical prophylaxis is being considered more frequently.[60] Depending on the child's age, TTs, adenoidectomy, or both should be considered.

Gebhart[61] was the first to demonstrate a reduction in the number of new episodes of AOM following the insertion of TTs. Subsequently, TT placement has become the primary surgical prophylaxis against RAOM. The current recommendation of the Academy of Otolaryngology–Head and Neck Surgery is placement of TTs in otherwise healthy children with three or more episodes of AOM in 6 months, or four or more episodes within a year.[62] TT insertion is recommended for infants and children under the age of 18 months who fail medical therapy whether there is residual fluid in the middle ear or not. In otitis-prone children 18 months and older adenoidectomy with TT placement is the preferred second procedure if the child fails initial TT placement. If the child is in the older range of the AOM group (i.e., 3 years or older) and the middle ears are well aerated, adenoidectomy and myringotomy without TT is preferred in selected cases. This cannot be recommended for all children with RAOM because the efficacy of adenoidectomy for prevention of AOM has not been studied rigorously.

Paradise et al,[55] in studying children with recurrent OM despite TT placement, found a significant reduction in the incidence of AOM in the first year following adenoidectomy but not in the second year. A study of adenoidectomy in the management of RAOM has demonstrated that although adenoidectomy and adenotonsillectomy may be effective in treating COME, the results when compared with tympanostomy tubes alone were not favorable for RAOM.[63] The efficacy of controlling RAOM with ear tubes alone did not warrant the added risk of the additional procedures of adenoidectomy or adenotonsillectomy as first-line therapy. A study of the Ontario, Canada, hospital database demonstrated a decreased need for subsequent surgery when TT placement in conjunction with adenoidectomy was performed as the initial surgical intervention in children (age 19 and younger) as opposed to TT placement alone. A small added benefit was seen with adenotonsillectomy plus TT versus adenoidectomy alone with TT placement.[64]

Nonetheless, adenoidectomy is a logical method for surgical prophylaxis against RAOM, both in patients with refractory disease and in patients with failure to resolve infections after ear tubes alone. Adenoidectomy has been shown to be a safe procedure for children over 18 months.[58] The AHCPR currently recommends TT placement as the preferred initial procedure for surgical treatment of OM. In recurrent or refractory cases, adenoidectomy plus myringotomy (with or without TT placement) is recommended as the second surgical procedure.[4]

Surgical Treatment of Chronic Otitis Media with Effusion

The indication for surgery for COME is failure of medical therapy to clear the middle ear effusion and restore hearing to normal levels within a reasonable time. Updated AHCPR guidelines recommend surgical treatment (consisting of TT, adenoidectomy, or both) for bilateral effusions that have not cleared in 3 months, or a unilateral effusion that persists for 6 months. Documentation of hearing loss (20 dB HL or more in the better ear) is the current treatment guideline.[4]

In children with documented learning difficulties and bilateral conductive hearing loss, a case can be made to proceed with surgery after 60 days. It is helpful to note that the time criterion is used as an index of the likelihood of spontaneous resolution; many effusions clear within 30 to 60 days, and surgery should not be performed in such self-limited cases. Once an effusion has persisted for 90 days it is possible that it may persist for months or even years. Maw[65] noted an average duration of effusion in the untreated ear of 7.8 years. In such a circumstance there is little doubt that correction of the hearing loss should be done to avoid speech delays. Although the evidence that mild to moderate conductive hearing loss causes speech delay is inconsistent, it is clear that these occur in many cases and it seems prudent, therefore, to prevent the problem rather than to seek remedial education after the fact.

Early treatment principles for COME were based on the theory that secretory OM was primarily due to eustachian tube obstruction and that ventilation of the middle ear was both necessary and sufficient treatment. It now appears that ventilation of the middle ear via TT bypasses the problem but does not correct the underlying disorder, whereas adenoidectomy appears to modify the underlying pathophysiology. Gates et al[51] compared adenoidectomy (and myringotomy) with TT and found no significant differences in the outcome variables, including hearing. Further, it was demonstrated that outcome after adenoidectomy did not vary with the size of the adenoid. Although adenoidectomy and myringotomy with or without TT insertion is a more expensive and slightly riskier procedure than TT insertion, it has fewer relapses and is equally cost-effective.

Selecting patients for adenoidectomy should be done on the basis of the severity of their middle ear disease. The presence of infection of the adenoid as seen with a transnasal fiberoptic scope would support a consideration of adenoidectomy; however, in many cases the infectious nature of the process is not obvious to clinical inspection and is evident on histologic examination. Parents should be made aware of the risks and benefits of adenoidectomy. If adenoidectomy is chosen, bilateral myringotomy (with or without TT placement) and suction evacuation of the middle ear is always done.

Benefits and Limitations of Surgical Treatment

Recurrent AOM often is associated with considerable morbidity from fever, malaise, pain, anorexia, and inadequate sleep. These associated symptoms may produce behavioral changes in children, such as poor attention span and irritability, and lead to social isolation. These symptoms may result in impaired learning and poor socialization. In addition to the disruptive effects upon the child's behavior, OM produces a mild to moderate conductive hearing loss due to the middle ear effusion. Because the hearing level fluctuates, the child has difficulty in developing a consistent hearing strategy. Such hearing losses may impair communication and create additional difficulties in interpersonal relations, affect the development of speech and language skills, and, perhaps, retard intellectual achievement.[66,67] A further problem is the impact of sickness upon family dynamics. Time lost from work or social activities due to illness of a child may impose additional hardships upon family relationships. In addition, otitis-prone children are often perceived as being unhealthy, which affects their relations within the family. These considerations contribute substantially to the quality of life in families with frequent episodes of OM.

Patients and parents are advised that surgical therapy for OM is generally not curative, but it does correct the hearing loss and generally reduces the number and severity of subsequent episodes. TTs correct the conductive hearing loss as long as they remain open and in place. However, when the tube extrudes, many patients experience recurrent OM. Adenoidectomy removes a source of infection from the nasopharynx and is associated with a reduction in the number of new episodes. Removal of the adenoid often improves sleep and decreases mouth breathing. The cost-effectiveness of surgical therapy for COME has been shown to be high.[48]

Technical Considerations

Myringotomy and Tympanostomy Tube Insertion

Sterilization of the external auditory canal is not routinely performed because of the low rate of infection and the lack of efficacy. Thorough cleaning of the canal is important for seeing the tympanic membrane and for postoperative care. In most cases, the incision is made parallel to the annulus fibrosis in the anteroinferior quadrant of the tympanic membrane. Care is taken to avoid separating the epithelium from the fibrous layer as this predisposes to tympanosclerosis. The fluid is removed with a 5-French cannula, or if very mucoid, a 7F cannula. It is important to position the tube so that the lumen is directly in the line of sight so that it may be inspected postoperatively and suctioned as needed.

Postoperative use of topical antimicrobial drops is often used now that non-ototoxic otic formulations are widely available. They are useful in younger children and in cases of purulent or mucoid effusion. The ototoxicity of some of these preparations precludes their use in situations where absorption through the round window membrane is possible, such as in ears with normal middle ear mucosa. In cases of thickened mucosa the risk of absorption appears to be low, but there have been few documented episodes of sensorineural loss and vestibular loss in humans from this use. Quinolone antibiotics, which are noncochleotoxic, are now available in a topical otic solution and an ophthalmic solution. Topical quinolone solutions are approved and used quite commonly for both routine postoperative prophylaxis and treatment of ears draining from AOM.[68–70]

The choice of tympanostomy tube is dictated by the surgeon's experience and the treatment goals. The choice of tubes available is staggering in number and variety. However, direct comparison of tubes using a prospective randomized study design with stratification by important risk factors has not been done. Three considerations influence the choice of tube: duration of intubation, risk of water contamination, and ease of removal. For short-term intubation (as with placement for a severe AOM), a short grommet is a logical choice. For long-term intubation (e.g., for an 11-month-old boy in day care with eight documented episodes of AOM, persistent effusion, a strong family history of OM, and smoking in the family) a long-stemmed TT may be a better choice. The short, wide-bore tubes offer little resistance to water entry into the middle ear, compared with the long-shafted TTs. Finally, the long tubes can be easily removed in the office, whereas removal of the short grommet tubes with rigid flanges may require a general anesthetic. The risk of otorrhea and permanent perforation increases with the duration of the intubation. However, the risk of recurrent effusion appears to lessen as the duration of intubation increases. Thus, there is a trade-off between effectiveness and complications. It is necessary to discuss with the parents the possibility of a permanent perforation rate of 15% that might be expected with a long-stemmed tube staying for 5 years, in light of 5 years freedom from effusion, and the 90% closure rates of such perforations with an outpatient fat-graft myringoplasty. It may be argued that the 15% perforation rate, which is lower than the 34% reoperation rate with grommets, is acceptable. However, it is important to involve the parents in such discussions so that they understand the implications of the choices available to them.

Adenoidectomy

General anesthesia is used for children and most adults, and the airway is assured by endotracheal intubation. The middle ears are aspirated through a myringotomy incision (see above). The patient is placed in the Rose position with the neck extended over a roll. A mouth gag is inserted and the soft palate is retracted with a catheter. The adenoid is excised with curved

curettes of various sizes and shapes using a large mirror and either a headlight or the operating microscope to inspect the nasopharynx to assure completeness of removal. Adenoid curettes are available in several sizes and configurations. Those with an angulated handle are easier to use than those with a straight handle. A 10F catheter is used to retract the soft palate. A malleable suction cautery may be used to control bleeding.

Careful instrumentation minimizes injury to the prevertebral fascia and muscles, which might otherwise result in excessive bleeding. Curved biting forceps are useful to remove tissue not accessible by the curette. The basket adenotome is seldom used because its curved shape may promote incomplete removal. Adenoidectomy is being done with cautery or the microdebrider in some hospitals. The effectiveness and cost-effectiveness of such approaches have not been evaluated.

Bleeding usually stops promptly; pressure applied for a few minutes via sponges in the nasopharynx appears to assist the process, as does irrigation with saline at room temperature. Suction electrocautery permits precise coagulation of bleeding vessels and avoids the risk of stenosis from indiscriminate field cauterization.

The goal of the surgery is complete removal of the midline adenoid pad to achieve smooth reepithelialization of the nasopharynx. Curettage of the tissue in the fossa of Rosenmuller is not done for fear of scar tissue formation and contracture that might contribute to eustachian tube reflux. Care must be taken to avoid direct injury to the eustachian tube that might result in stenosis. Inadequate removal of adenoid tissue may be avoided by careful inspection of the nasopharynx with a mirror.

Following adenoidectomy, mild ear pain is common. Acetaminophen is prescribed for pain control. The child is able to eat normally as soon as nausea from the anesthetic has subsided. Transient hypernasal speech may occur in a small percentage of cases, but frank regurgitation of liquids through the nose is rare. These transient sequelae may occur after removal of a large adenoid mass. Palatal and pharyngeal wall compensation occurs quickly, and permanent voice change is highly unusual in patients with normal palate anatomy.

◆ Documentation

Current cost-containment strategies by third-party payers have led to increasing scrutiny of the indications for surgical treatment of OM. A variety of schemes has been developed to verify the history, physical findings, and prior treatment. Criteria for precertification vary among the payers in spite of widely circulated indications used by otolaryngologists. As a result, an increasing burden is placed upon the staff of the surgeon's office to collect the additional information over and above that needed for patient care. A written summary from the referring pediatrician should fulfill the documentation requirements of most payers.

Demonstration of an enlarged adenoid classically has been required to justify adenoidectomy. Now that it is known that the size of the adenoid is not related to outcome, basing the decision on adenoid size is no longer justified. However, some insurer's precertification programs have not understood this concept and require a separate diagnosis code for adenoidectomy. Rather than use the International Classification of Diseases (ICD-9) code for adenoid hypertrophy (474.12) wrongly, the ICD-9 code (474.2) for the archaic term *adenoid vegetations,* which Meyer[71] used to indicate the chronically infected adenoid, may be more appropriate.

◆ Complications and Sequelae

The complications of untreated AOM are well known, despite being relatively rare (see Chapter 19). OM may progress to mastoiditis, which if also untreated, may lead to such infectious intracranial complications as meningitis and brain abscess. Untreated mastoiditis may also result in Bezold's abscess, subperiosteal abscess, and permanent hearing loss.

A well-studied and long-debated topic is the effect of OM-associated conductive hearing loss on speech and language development in children. Over 100 clinical studies have sought to determine if speech and language development is delayed or impaired in children with OM, but most are flawed due to intrinsic study design difficulties. Paradise et al[72] reported the results of a prospective, randomized clinical trial evaluating the difference between time-appropriate and delayed (after 9 months) TT insertion on speech and language development in children 3 years of age. Various indicators of developmental outcomes then were measured, which did not differ significantly between early and late treatment groups. Roberts et al[73] performed a meta-analysis of similar prospective trials evaluating speech and language development in children with OM between 1 and 5 years of age. A very small negative association was seen with OM early in life and later speech and language development. The general consensus among many clinicians is that any impairment suffered as a result of OM early in life is temporary, and speech and language skills return to normal with time.[66]

Intraoperative complications following TT placement are few and rarely severe. Accidental displacement of the tube into the middle ear may require elevation of a tympanomeatal flap for recovery. Persistent perforation of the TM following TT removal or extrusion occurs in 1 to 15% of cases depending on the size of the tube, the number of intercurrent infections, and the duration of intubation. If the child is older, it may be possible to close the perforation with cautery to the edges with trichloroacetic acid and application of a paper patch. More often, however, the standard treatment, after it is seen that the ear is dry, is to perform a fat-graft myringoplasty. This offers an effective remedy that can be performed on an outpatient basis. Recurrence of effusion is not uncommon after extrusion or removal of TTs.

The most prevalent sequela of TT placement is purulent otorrhea. In young children the organisms recovered are often the same as with AOM. In older children *Pseudomonas* sp. usually are grown. Some cases are due to water contamination of the ear; others are the result of AOM. In the past, water precautions (keeping the ears dry) were universally recommended for patients with tubes, and many clinicians continue to recommend such precautions. In our experience, however, only a small percentage of patients develop purulent otorrhea following submersion in water. These patients must follow strict water precautions to prevent future episodes. Most children are able to continue normal activities such as swimming without any problems following TT placement. Initial treatment should consist of topical antibiotic drops. The topical quinolone preparations (ciprofloxacin, ofloxacin) have been shown to be as effective as oral antibiotics, better tolerated,

and without risk of ototoxicity.[68,74] An oral antibiotic agent effective against β-lactamase may be used if the discharge continues for more than 48 hours despite topical treatment. Fortunately, most episodes clear promptly.

If the discharge fails to resolve promptly with this regimen, office cleaning of the canal, softening any debris in the tube (if necessary) with hydrogen peroxide and opening by gentle suctioning, and culture for identification and antimicrobial sensitivity are performed. Repeated office cleaning and continued use of topical drops usually suffice. If not, the tube is removed and the middle ear inspected and cultured. If the middle ear looks healthy, the tube is replaced; if there is significant inflammation the tube is removed and medical treatment is continued. Rarely, a resistant organism may require intravenous antimicrobial therapy, either at home (with visiting nurse support) or in the hospital. The choice of agent depends on the sensitivity of the organism. In most cases a resistant *Pseudomonas* sp. is found. With home intravenous therapy becoming available in many cities, prolonged use of intravenous antipseudomonal agents may be practical. If the otorrhea continues, imaging studies to look for cholesteatoma or other structural abnormalities is considered, and mastoidectomy with tympanoplasty may be performed. Fortunately, this is seldom necessary.

Recently, biofilms have been implicated as a potential cause of chronic TT otorrhea. With the aid of electron microscopy, biofilms were visualized on the surface of TTs removed from children with refractory posttympanotomy otorrhea.[75] New strategies such as the use of phosphorylcholine-coated tubes[76] may help eliminate biofilms as a potential cause of chronic TT otorrhea.

The most common complication of adenoidectomy is postoperative bleeding. However, the incidence is low: of 250 cases done by 13 surgeons, only one child required operative treatment for bleeding and none needed blood transfusion.[51] Helmus et al[77] noted that only four patients in 1000 (0.4%) bled after outpatient adenoidectomy and that all instances occurred in the first 6 postoperative hours and were managed without transfusion.[77] Other less common complications include nasopharyngeal stenosis and velopharyngeal incompetence (VPI). Stenosis results from excessive tissue destruction such as might occur from excessive use of the electrocautery, excessive curettage of the fossa of Rosenmuller, and removal of the lateral pharyngeal bands. Transient VPI may occur after removal of a large adenoid but resolves spontaneously in the majority of cases. Persistent VPI is a significant concern to both surgeons and parents as impaired speech can be devastating. The majority of such cases are due to an undetected submucous cleft palate. Preoperative evaluation with fiberoptic nasopharyngoscopy is useful in detecting an occult posterior submucous cleft. In patients with a known history of cleft palate or submucous cleft palate, adenoidectomy is contraindicated. In cases of severe nasal airway obstruction, an inferior adenoidectomy may be performed with great caution.

References

1. Teele DW, Klein JO, Rosner B. Epidemiology of otitis media during the first seven years of life in children in greater Boston: a prospective, cohort study. J Infect Dis 1989;160:83–94
2. Bluestone CD. Studies in otitis media: Children's Hospital of Pittsburgh-University of Pittsburgh progress report–2004. Laryngoscope 2004;114 (11 pt 3 suppl 105):1–26

3. Stool SE, and Otitis Media Guideline Panel. Otitis media with effusion in young children. Clinical practice guideline no. 12. Rockville, MD: Department of Health and Human Services, Public Health Service, Agency for Health Care Policy and Research, 1994

4. Rosenfeld RM, Culpepper L, Doyle KJ, et al. Clinical practice guideline: Otitis media with effusion. Otolaryngol Head Neck Surg 2004;130 (5 suppl):S95–118

5. Bluestone CD, Klein JO. Otitis Media in Infants and Children, 2nd ed. Philadelphia: WB Saunders, 1995

6. Doyle WJ. A functiono-anatomic description of eustachian tube vector relations in four ethnic populations: an osteology study. Pittsburgh: University of Pittsburgh, 1977

7. Aydogan B, Kiroglu M, Altintas D, et al. The role of food allergy in otitis media with effusion. Otolaryngol Head Neck Surg 2004;130:747–750

8. White DR, Heavner SB, Hardy SM, Prazma J. Gastroesophageal reflux and eustachian tube dysfunction in an animal model. Laryngoscope 2002; 112:955–961

9. Henderson FW, Collier AM, Sanyal MA, et al. A longitudinal study of respiratory viruses and bacteria in the etiology of acute otitis media with effusion. N Engl J Med 1982;306:1377–1383

10. Giebink GS, Payne EE, Mills EL, Juhn SK, Quie PG. Experimental otitis media due to Streptococcus pneumoniae: immunopathogenic response in the chinchilla. J Infect Dis 1976;134:595–604

11. Bluestone CD, Stephenson JS, Martin LM. Ten-year review of otitis media pathogens. Pediatr Infect Dis J 1992;11(8 suppl):S7–11

12. Howie VM, Ploussard JH. Simultaneous nasopharyngeal and middle ear exudates in otitis media. Pediatrics Digest 1971;13:31–35

13. Dhooge I, Van Damme D, Vaneechouette M, et al. Role of nasopharyngeal bacterial flora in the evaluation of recurrent middle ear infections in children. Clin Microbiol Infect 1999;5:530–534

14. Pillsbury HC III, Kveton JF, Sasaki CT, Frazier W. Quantitative bacteriology in adenoid tissue. Otolaryngol Head Neck Surg 1981;89(3 pt 1):355–363

15. Bernstein JM, Faden HF, Dryja DM, et al. Micro-ecology of the nasopharyngeal bacterial flora in otitis-prone and non-otitis-prone children. Acta Otolaryngol 1993;113:88–92

16. Bluestone CD, Paradise JL, Beery QC. Physiology of the eustachian tube in the pathogenesis and management of middle ear effusions. Laryngoscope 1972;82:1654–1670

17. Eden AR, Laitman JT, Gannon PJ. Mechanisms of middle ear aeration: anatomic and physiologic evidence in primates. Laryngoscope 1990; 100:67–75

18. Aschan G, Ekvall L, Magnusson B. Reverse aspiratory middle ear disease: a neglected pathogenic principle. In: Munker G, Arnold W, eds. Physiology and Pathophysiology of the Eustachian Tube and Middle Ear. New York: Thieme-Stratton, 1980:90–96

19. Politzer A. A Textbook of Diseases of the Ear. Philadelphia: Henry C. Lea's Son, 1883:107

20. Swarts JD, Alper CM, Seroky JT, et al. In vivo observation with magnetic resonance imaging of middle ear effusion in response to experimental underpressures. Ann Otol Rhinol Laryngol 1995;104:522–528

21. Teele DW, Klein JO, Rosner BA. Epidemiology of otitis media in children. Ann Otol Rhinol Laryngol 1980;89(3 pt 2):5–6

22. Rosenfeld RM, Kay D. Natural history of untreated otitis media. Laryngoscope 2003;113:1645–1657

23. Giebink GS, Mills EL, Huff JS, et al. The microbiology of serous and mucoid otitis media. Pediatrics 1979;63:915–919

24. Rayner MG, Zhang Y, Gorry MC, et al. Evidence of bacterial metabolic activity in culture-negative otitis media with effusion. JAMA 1998;279: 296–299

25. Ehrlich GD, Veeh R, Wang X, et al. Mucosal biofilm formation on middle-ear mucosa in the chinchilla model of otitis media. JAMA 2002;287: 1710–1715

26. Goldie P, Hellstrom S, Johansson U. Vascular events in experimental otitis media models: a comparative study. ORL J Otorhinolaryngol Relat Spec 1990;52:104–112

27. Segal J, et al. Mass spectometric analysis of composition in the guinea pig middle ear-mastoid system. In: Lim DJ, Bluestone CD, eds. Recent Advances in Otitis Media with Effusion, Philadelphia: BC Decker, 1983:68–70

28. Cantekin EI, Doyle WJ, Phillips DC, Bluestone CD. Gas absorption in the middle ear. Ann Otol Rhinol Laryngol Suppl 1980;89(3 pt 2):71–75

29. Discolo CM, Byrd MC, Bates T, et al. Ultrasonic detection of middle ear effusion: a preliminary study. Arch Otolaryngol Head Neck Surg 2004; 130:1407–1410

30. Babb MJ, Hilsinger RL Jr, Korol HW, et al. Modern acoustic reflectometry: accuracy in diagnosing otitis media with effusion. Ear Nose Throat J 2004;83:622–624

31. Finitzo T, Friel-Patti S, Chinn K, Brown O. Tympanometry and otoscopy prior to myringotomy: issues in diagnosis of otitis media. Int J Pediatr Otorhinolaryngol 1992;24:101–110

32. Kaleida PH, Stool SE. Assessment of otoscopists' accuracy regarding middle-ear effusion. Otoscopic validation. Am J Dis Child 1992;146:433–435

33. Rosenfeld RM, Vertrees JE, Carr J, et al. Clinical efficacy of antimicrobial drugs for acute otitis media: metaanalysis of 5400 children from thirty-three randomized trials. J Pediatr 1994;124:355–367

34. Glasziou PP, Del Mar CB, Sanders SL, Hayem M. Antibiotics for acute otitis media in children. Cochrane Database Syst Rev 2000;1:CD000219

35. van Buchem FL, Peeters MF, van 't Hof MA. Acute otitis media: a new treatment strategy. Br Med J (Clin Res Ed) 1985;290:1033–1037

36. Siegel RM, Kiely M, Bien JP, et al. Treatment of otitis media with observation and a safety-net antibiotic prescription. Pediatrics 2003;112 (3 pt 1):527–531

37. Eskola J, Kilpi T, Palmu A, et al. Efficacy of a pneumococcal conjugate vaccine against acute otitis media. N Engl J Med 2001;344:403–409

38. Paradise JL. Managing otitis media: a time for change. Pediatrics 1995; 96(4 pt 1):712–715

39. Barnett ED, Klein JO. The problem of resistant bacteria for the management of acute otitis media. Pediatr Clin North Am 1995;42:509–517

40. Bluestone CD. Role of surgery for otitis media in the era of resistant bacteria. Pediatr Infect Dis J 1998;17:1090–1098 discussion 1099–100

41. Mandel EM, Rockette HE, Bluestone CD, Paradise JL, Nozza RJ. Efficacy of amoxicillin with and without decongestant-antihistamine for otitis media with effusion in children. Results of a double-blind, randomized trial. N Engl J Med 1987;316:432–437

42. Rosenfeld RM, Post JC. Meta-analysis of antibiotics for the treatment of otitis media with effusion. Otolaryngol Head Neck Surg 1992;106:378–386

43. Schwartz RH, Puglese J, Schwartz DM. Use of a short course of prednisone for treating middle ear effusion. A double-blind crossover study. Ann Otol Rhinol Laryngol Suppl 1980;89(3 pt 2):296–300

44. Lambert PR. Oral steroid therapy for chronic middle ear perfusion: a double-blind crossover study. Otolaryngol Head Neck Surg 1986;95:193–199

45. Rosenfeld RM, Mandel EM, Bluestone CD. Systemic steroids for otitis media with effusion in children. Arch Otolaryngol Head Neck Surg 1991; 117:984–989

46. Butler CC, Van Der Voort JH. Oral or topical nasal steroids for hearing loss associated with otitis media with effusion in children. Cochrane Database Syst Rev 2002;4:CD001935

47. Jacobs J, Springer DA, Crothers D. Homeopathic treatment of acute otitis media in children: a preliminary randomized placebo-controlled trial. Pediatr Infect Dis J 2001;20:177–183

48. Gates GA. Cost-effectiveness considerations in otitis media treatment. Otolaryngol Head Neck Surg 1996;114:525–530

49. Armstrong BW. A new treatment for chronic secretory otitis media. AMA Arch Otolaryngol 1954;59:653–654

50. Mandel EM, Rockette HE, Bluestone CD, Paradise JL, Nozza RJ. Myringotomy with and without tympanostomy tubes for chronic otitis media with effusion. Arch Otolaryngol Head Neck Surg 1989;115: 1217–1224

51. Gates GA, Avery CA, Prihoda TJ, Cooper JC Jr. Effectiveness of adenoidectomy and tympanostomy tubes in the treatment of chronic otitis media with effusion. N Engl J Med 1987;317:1444–1451

52. Gross CW, Bassila M, Lazar RH, et al. Adipose plug myringoplasty: an alternative to formal myringoplasty techniques in children. Otolaryngol Head Neck Surg 1989;101:617–620

53. Goode RL. T-tube for middle ear ventilation. Arch Otolaryngol 1973;97: 402–403

54. Maw AR. Chronic otitis media with effusion (glue ear) and adenotonsillectomy: prospective randomised controlled study. Br Med J (Clin Res Ed) 1983;287:1586–1588

55. Paradise JL, Bluestone CD, Rogers KD, et al. Efficacy of adenoidectomy for recurrent otitis media in children previously treated with tympanostomy-tube placement. Results of parallel randomized and nonrandomized trials. JAMA 1990;263:2066–2073

56. Paradise JL, Bluestone CD. Adenoidectomy and chronic otitis media (letter). N Engl J Med 1988;318:1470

57. Gates GA, Muntz HR, Gaylis B. Adenoidectomy and otitis media. Ann Otol Rhinol Laryngol Suppl 1992;155:24–32

58. Brodsky L, Koch RJ. Bacteriology and immunology of normal and diseased adenoids in children. Arch Otolaryngol Head Neck Surg 1993; 119:821–829

59. Maynard JE, Fleshman JK, Tschopp CF. Otitis media in Alaskan Eskimo children. Prospective evaluation of chemoprophylaxis. JAMA 1972;219: 597–599

60. Bluestone CD, Klein JO. Clinical practice guideline on otitis media with effusion in young children: strengths and weaknesses. Otolaryngol Head Neck Surg 1995;112:507–511

61. Gebhart DE. Tympanostomy tubes in the otitis media prone child. Laryngoscope 1981;91:849–866

62. AAO-HNS. 2000 Clinical Indicators Compendium. Alexandria, VA: American Academy of Otolaryngology-Head and Neck Surgery, 2000

63. Paradise JL, Bluestone CD, Colborn DK, et al. Adenoidectomy and adeno-tonsillectomy for recurrent acute otitis media: parallel randomized clinical trials in children not previously treated with tympanostomy tubes. JAMA 1999;282:945–953

64. Coyte PC, Croxford R, McIsaac W, et al. The role of adjuvant adenoidectomy and tonsillectomy in the outcome of the insertion of tympanostomy tubes. N Engl J Med 2001;344:1188–1195

65. Maw R. Glue Ear in Childhood. Cambridge, England: Cambridge University Press, 1995

66. Klein JO, et al. Otitis media with effusion during the first three years of life and development of speech and language. In: Lim DJ, Bluestone CD, eds. Recent Advances in Otitis Media with Effusion. Philadelphia: BC Decker, 1984:332–335

67. Hubbard TW, Paradise JL, McWilliams BJ, et al. Consequences of unremitting middle-ear disease in early life. Otologic, audiologic, and developmental findings in children with cleft palate. N Engl J Med 1985; 312:1529–1534

68. Barlow DW, Duckert LG, Kreig CS, et al. Ototoxicity of topical otomicrobial agents. Acta Otolaryngol 1995;115:231–235

69. Dohar JE, Garner ET, Nielsen RW, Biel MA, Seidlin M. Topical ofloxacin treatment of otorrhea in children with tympanostomy tubes. Arch Otolaryngol Head Neck Surg 1999;125:537–545

70. Goldblatt EL. Efficacy of ofloxacin and other otic preparations for acute otitis media in patients with tympanostomy tubes. Pediatr Infect Dis J 2001;20:116–119 discussion 120–122

71. Meyer W. Adenoid vegetations in the nasopharyngeal cavity: their pathology, diagnosis and treatment. Med Surg Trans 1870;53: 191–215

72. Paradise JL, Feldman HM, Campbell TF, et al. Effect of early or delayed insertion of tympanostomy tubes for persistent otitis media on developmental outcomes at the age of three years. N Engl J Med 2001;344: 1179–1187

73. Roberts JE, Rosenfeld RM, Zeisel SA. Otitis media and speech and language: a meta-analysis of prospective studies. Pediatrics 2004;113(3 pt 1):e238–e248

74. Goldblatt EL, Dohar J, Nozza RJ, et al. Topical ofloxacin versus systemic amoxicillin/clavulanate in purulent otorrhea in children with tympanostomy tubes. Int J Pediatr Otorhinolaryngol 1998;46: 91–101

75. Post JC. Direct evidence of bacterial biofilms in otitis media. Laryngoscope 2001;111:2083–2094

76. Berry JA, Biedlingmaier JF, Whelan PJ. In vitro resistance to bacterial biofilm formation on coated fluoroplastic tympanostomy tubes. Otolaryngol Head Neck Surg 2000;123:246–251

77. Helmus C, Grin M, Westfall R. Same-day-stay adenotonsillectomy. Laryngoscope 1990;100:593–596

18

Chronic Otitis Media

Peter C. Weber

This chapter discusses medical and surgical management of chronic otitis media (COM), including dry perforation, mucosal disease, cholesteatoma, surgical techniques, and surgical complications. Acute otitis media and meningeal complications of disease are covered in Chapters 17 and 19.

◆ Office Management

Chronic Otitis Media Without Cholesteatoma

Tubotympanic disease as described in 1965 by Thorburn[1] consists of two types.[2] Type I is a chronic perforation that may occasionally drain due to colds, weather changes, or water in the ear but rarely presents significant problems to the patient. When the ear is dry the middle ear mucosa is pink, healthy, and normal (**Fig. 18–1**). Type II is a persistent mucosal infection. Typically the patient presents with a 3- to 6-month history of chronic discharge from the ear, which may or may not have been associated with a respiratory infection, and hearing loss (**Fig. 18–2**).

More than likely, the type II patient has already been treated for several months with multiple courses of systemic and topical antibiotics, and cultures have been obtained. Cultures can be helpful; however, sensitivities do not reflect that topical therapy results in concentrations much greater than those achieved by systemic antibiotics,[3] and bacteria are usually known from published studies. *Pseudomonas aeruginosa* and *Staphylococcus aureus* are most common,[4–7] and *Escherichia coli* and *Streptococcus pneumoniae* are less so. Foul-smelling drainage also suggests anaerobic *Streptococcus* or *Bacteroides*.[8,9] *Bacteroides* often responds to chloramphenicol in drop or powder form, but *Pseudomonas* does not. Persistent drainage despite antibiotics may indicate *Mycobacterium* or even cerebrospinal fluid (CSF) leak.[10,11] Cultures and β_2-transferrin testing are helpful in those cases.

Physical examination of the ear may demonstrate a perforation with significant granulation tissue and purulent discharge (**Fig. 18–3**). A high-resolution computed tomography (CT) scan usually shows middle ear soft tissue extending into the attic and often fluid within the mastoid air cells.[12] I typically do not obtain a CT scan unless surgery is required (see below).

COM without cholesteatoma is distinctly different from persistent middle ear effusion requiring myringotomy and tube insertion and from a chronic draining tube requiring tube removal and antibiotics. Such treatment almost always results in a dry ear, although persistent perforation may sometimes occur. Instead, COM describes somebody who drains fluid time and again after a tube is placed then removed. The patient may have chronic eustachian tube dysfunction, chronic mucosal disease with attic block, or chronic serous mastoiditis. Many cases of COM can be traced back to an underperforming eustachian tube with effusion and drum retraction (**Fig. 18–4**).

Many patients with COM without cholesteatoma will need surgery; however, medical therapy should be tried first. The ear should be cleaned so that drops can reach the middle ear. Cleaning begins in the office and continues at home with irrigations of 50–50 alcohol and vinegar (essentially acetic acid). The patient repeats the washings several times daily with the ear turned up as described by Sheehy[7] or turned down as preferred by others. The dropper and rubber bulb are filled with solution, the tip of the dropper is placed in the ear opening, and the bulb is compressed and decompressed gently, swishing the solution back and forth to clear the canal. The solution should be near body temperature to avoid dizziness. If acetic acid solution causes pain, Sheehy also has described using one-half strength Betadine (providine–iodine). Washings are continued for about 1 week. Steroid antibiotic drops are then added or can be started immediately after each washing.

The preferred medicated drop is a fluoroquinolone with steroid[13] because it is not ototoxic and because corticosteroids can help reduce granulation tissue and edema in the middle ear as well as scaling and itching of the external canal (dexamethasone may be even better than hydrocortisone in this regard[14]). Rarely, a fungal infection can occur with fluoroquinolone drops. Potentially ototoxic drops (tobramycin, Cortisporin, Colimycin) have been used quite safely for decades, probably because a barrier over the round window membrane is formed by chronic disease. However, if middle ear mucosa heals with treatment but the patient continues to use ototoxic drops, they could then penetrate the inner ear and cause vestibulopathy or hearing loss. Thus, the clinician should inform the patient if a potentially ototoxic drop is

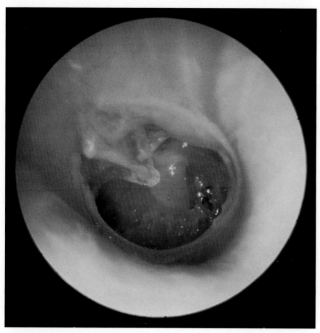

Figure 18–1 Near total perforation caused by "necrotizing otitis media" from ß-hemolytic streptococcus.

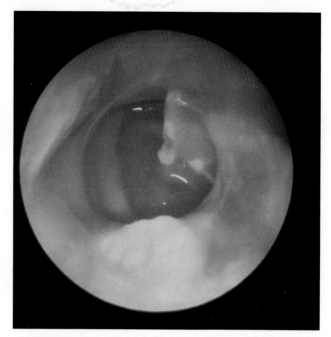

Figure 18–2 Chronic suppurative otitis media.

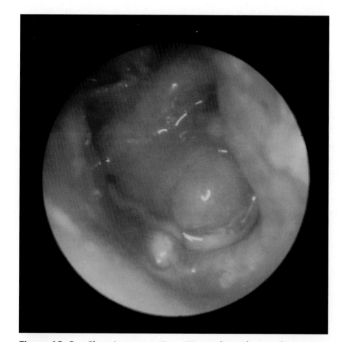

Figure 18–3 Chronic suppurative otitis media with granuloma.

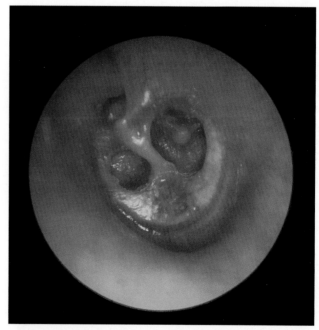

Figure 18–4 Serous otitis media with retraction.

to be used. However, risks are rare and if fluoroquinolones fail, it may be necessary to use these types of drops. Also, the author generally avoids Cortisporin (neomycin/polymixin/hydrocortisone) in chronically draining ears because topical allergy to neomycin can occur and be difficult to recognize.

After washing, antibiotic powder may be useful. A mixture of chloramphenicol, amphotericin, and boric acid powder can be quite effective as it creates an environment that is very resistant to bacterial and fungal growth. If the patient has not had any oral antibiotic treatment prior to the first visit, I usually treat with one course. However, the topical drop is more important.

Intravenous antibiotics are almost never needed unless there are complications such as petrositis, labyrinthitis, or meningitis. Surgery for COM without cholesteatoma usually is withheld until the ear is dry or maximum improvement is reached.

Cholesteatoma

Cholesteatomas grow by forming a keratinizing stratified epithelial layer and fibrous subepithelial layer called the *matrix*. The matrix is constantly desquamating sheets of keratin into the cholesteatoma sac. This keratin or dead skin accumulates in concentric layers. As the sac expands it erodes surrounding bone, even the hard bone of the labyrinth.

Cholesteatoma can be congenital or acquired. Congenital cholesteatomas almost always are seen in children, although adults may present with petrous apex or intracranial epidermoids. By definition, congenital cholesteatomas have no history of perforation, myringotomy, or otorrhea and have a normal tympanic membrane.[15–19] The vast majority are found in the anterior-superior quadrant, although at times they may be found in the posterior-superior quadrant, within the tympanic membrane (TM) itself, or in the petrous apex. The pathogenesis of congenital cholesteatoma is controversial, although most theories have some merit: fetal epithelial cells are trapped in the middle ear; inflamed tympanic membrane cells invaginate into the middle ear; squamous metaplasia transforms middle ear mucosa into keratinizing epithelium.[17]

Acquired cholesteatoma is far more common than congenital, and usually results from retraction of the TM in the pars flaccida or posterior-superior quadrant (**Figs. 18–5** through **18–7**). This slowly occurs and may not be detected until the patient complains of drainage or hearing loss. Previous ear surgery or drum perforation may also be a site for acquired cholesteatoma as keratin can invaginate and proliferate on the undersurface of the perforation. Usually, however, epithelium from the lateral tympanic membrane, which goes around the edge of a perforation, stops growing 1–2 mm on the medial surface, where it abuts the mucosal layer.

Diagnosis of cholesteatoma is usually not difficult, as both congenital and acquired types usually can be seen on microscopic examination in the office. Patients with acquired disease usually complain of foul-smelling discharge and often bleeding. Normally, hearing is down and this can be verified with audiometric studies. Patients may have slight otalgia or headache and occasionally mild dizziness. Diseased mucosa, granulation tissue, and keratin debris may be confined to the epitympanum. Occasionally, drainage and granulation tissue can make it difficult to see the keratin sac (**Fig. 18–3**; also see Chapter 16, **Fig. 16–8**).

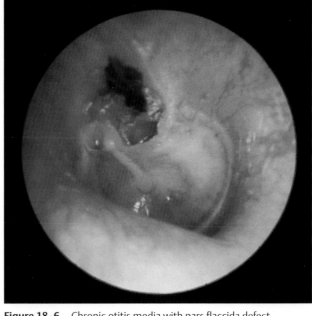

Figure 18–6   Chronic otitis media with pars flaccida defect.

Cholesteatoma is a surgical disease, but again antibiotic-steroid drops should be started to decrease the inflammation and granulation tissue prior to surgery. Although medical treatment will not cure cholesteatoma, it can decrease bleeding during surgery. Cholesteatoma still must be removed to obtain a safe, dry ear.

Although one could obtain culture and sensitivity studies, the most likely organisms are pseudomonas or a bacillus, and culture results do not alter the treatment. Culture and sensitivities often are obtained if a complication is suspected (see Chapter 19). Many otologists do not obtain CT scans of the temporal bones for cholesteatoma surgery, but I usually do to

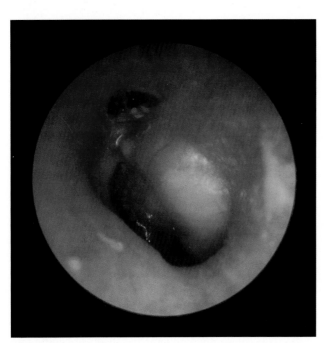

Figure 18–5   Cholesteatoma behind posterior drum.

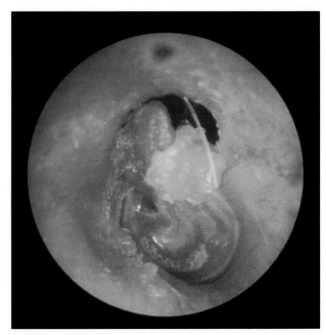

Figure 18–7   Attic erosion.

identify possible erosion of the tegmen, facial nerve dehiscence, and labyrinth fistula so that the patient may be better informed about the potential risks of surgery. The patient should know that cholesteatoma can cause not only hearing loss but also facial paralysis, dizziness, meningitis, and other intracranial complications.

◆ Surgical Management

Whether treating chronic mucosal disease, cholesteatoma, or benign perforation, the surgeon's primary goal is to obtain a safe, dry ear. The approach and technique vary depending on training and experience. However, basic principles apply to all procedures to achieve a good result. These principles and the author's preferences are presented.

Preoperative Counseling

Patients should understand that a safe, dry ear is the primary goal of surgery so they do not have unrealistic expectations such as perfect hearing. Indeed, the treatment plan often requires two staged procedures and hearing will temporarily be worse because ossicular reconstruction often is delayed until the second step. Even without cholesteatoma, attic mucosal disease often requires incus removal; failure to do so may not completely eradicate disease or restore ventilation. Free flow of irrigant from the mastoid into the middle ear is a good indication that disease has been removed and aeration is adequate. The author performs second-look surgery with ossicular reconstruction 6 to 12 months after the first stage (see below). The patient should realize that hearing in the operated ear will not be perfect despite reconstruction, but optimally it will be better. The patient may wish to use amplification after repair.

Indications, risks, benefits, alternatives, and personnel are discussed. The success rate for a safe, dry ear is roughly 90%.[20] Risks include but are not limited to partial or total hearing loss (which can occur 1–2% of the time), vertigo, disequilibrium, facial nerve paralysis, CSF leak, tinnitus, infection, bleeding, meningitis, perilymph fistula, otorrhea, stenosis/fistulization of the external auditory canal, pain, headaches, cosmetic deformities, loss of taste, and visual changes, all of which occur very infrequently.

Underlying sinonasal disease should be treated prior to ear surgery to improve postoperative eustachian tube function. Even if the eustachian tube is not blocked by sinonasal disease, its function is improved anyway by removing disease from the protympanum.

Terminology

Glasscock's group[20–23] well described the history of ear surgery. In chronic ear surgery, *residual* cholesteatoma refers to disease that is intentionally or unintentionally left behind after surgery, and *recurrent* cholesteatoma refers to that which forms in a postoperative retraction pocket.

Although many clinicians define *tympanoplasty* as closure of a TM perforation, it is really an operation that removes middle ear disease and reconstructs hearing with or without TM grafting. Tympanoplasty may be performed with or without mastoidectomy. Medial (underlay) grafting with temporalis fascia (or areolar tissue) was first performed by Storrs[24] in 1961 in the United States and remains one of the most common techniques. Prior to this, early techniques employed a small rubber disk attached to a silver wire by Toynbee[25] in 1853, skin grafts by Berthhold[26] in 1878, and paper patch 10 years later.[27] In the 1950s Wullstein[28] and Zollner[29] used split- and full-thickness skin grafts to repair chronically diseased ears, not just drum perforations, for better healing and hearing, and in 1967 Goodhill[30] first described using tragal cartilage for attic reconstruction to minimize recurrent cholesteatoma. Approaches for repair include transcanal, Lempert incision, and postauricular[31] procedures.

Atticotomy is appropriate for disease lateral to the incus body and malleus head, which does not extend anterior to the head of the malleus, posterior to the short process of the incus, or medial to either. It involves removal of the scutum to expose the attic tympanum. By removing this medial portion of the lateral epitympanic wall, the posterior external auditory canal wall is preserved, allowing removal of cholesteatoma confined to the epitympanum, repair of an attic retraction pocket, or gaining exposure for stapedectomy or lateral chain fixation procedures. Once disease is removed, reconstruction of the scutal wall is important to prevent recurrence of disease[32] (see Tympanoplasty, later in chapter). Cartilage obtained from the tragus or cymba can be used to reconstruct the scutum (**Fig. 18–8**).

Cortical (simple) mastoidectomy removes the lateral aspect of mastoid bone with exposure of the middle fossa tegmen, sigmoid sinus, and antrum. Opening the facial recess can be performed if desired. This procedure is the workhorse for many ear surgeries in that it provides ventilation from the middle ear to the mastoid, eradicates disease, and provides exposure for many procedures including endolymphatic sac surgery, labyrinthectomy, and cochlear implantation. *Intact canal wall* tympanoplasty with mastoidectomy was first described by Jansen[33] in the 1950s, a dramatic improvement over techniques and instrumentation[34–37] since the first recorded mastoidectomy by Jean Louis Petit in 1774[38] in Paris.

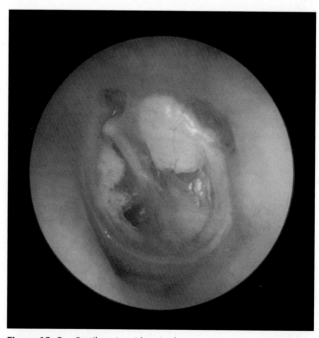

Figure 18–8 Cartilage is evident in the posterior-superior quadrant after tympanoplasty.

Modified radical mastoidectomy differs from intact canal wall mastoidectomy in that the posterior external auditory canal wall is removed. A meatoplasty is also routinely performed to better ventilate the mastoid and facilitate postoperative care. *Modified* radical mastoidectomy by definition includes grafting the TM to cover the mesotympanum or protympanum. The operation is also commonly referred to as *canal-wall-down* (CWD) surgery and *open* technique.

Although surgeons prefer to keep the posterior canal wall up, indications to take it down include extensive disease, residual epithelium over a labyrinthine fistula, recurrent attic cholesteatoma, and patient inability to come for follow-up or unwillingness to undergo two-staged procedures. Removing the lateral attic wall minimizes the chance of recurrent attic disease.[39] Recently, Gantz et al[40] described a procedure of removing the canal wall, eradicating disease, and then replacing the canal wall.

The Bondy[41] *modified radical mastoidectomy*, first performed in 1910, is rarely used today for attic cholesteatoma. The medial wall of the cholesteatoma sac is preserved over the intact TM and ossicular chain. Most otologists instead completely remove disease using an intact canal wall technique with second-stage ossicular reconstruction.

Radical mastoidectomy differs from modified radical mastoidectomy in that the TM is not grafted, that is, the middle ear space is not reconstructed and the eustachian tube is obliterated. The posterior canal wall is removed and meatoplasty performed. A radical mastoidectomy usually is performed in revision cases when disease (usually cholesteatoma) is so extensive that it cannot be completely removed.

Preoperative Preparation, Anesthesia, and Incisions

The operating theater is set up with the anesthesiologist at the foot of the patient and the scrub nurse directly opposite the surgeon so that instruments can be easily passed back and forth while working under the microscope. I prefer using general anesthesia for all patients, although transcanal surgery can easily be done under local anesthesia or monitored anesthesia care (MAC). The postauricular incision site is injected with 1% lidocaine–1/100,000 epinephrine, although other concentrations can be used. I do not shave any of the patient's hair whatsoever on any otologic surgery, including chronic ear, skull base, and craniotomy surgery. Studies have indicated that the rate of infection is certainly no worse and may indeed be less than if one does shave the patient.[42] The ear canal is injected with 1% lidocaine–1/40,000 epinephrine. The actual concentration of epinephrine for vasoconstriction may not matter significantly. Lidocaine does decrease some of the pain, and the patient does not have to be quite as deep in anesthesia. To monitor the facial nerve, I do not allow patients to be paralyzed for the procedure. However, a short-acting paralytic agent can be used for endotracheal intubation. Also, if a medial graft tympanoplasty is performed and the middle ear is packed with Gelfoam, nitrous oxide can be used because any lateral pressure will better adhere the graft to the undersurface of the tympanic membrane. However, for lateral graft tympanoplasty even with packing the middle ear, nitrous oxide should not be used because it may increase graft lateralization or blunting. I recommend extubation at the end of the procedure while the patient is "deep" to avoid an increase in middle ear pressure. Postoperatively, an anti-nauseant can be used to minimize straining.

After prepping with iodinated solution (Betadine), the microscope is used to make vascular strip and tympanomeatal incisions (**Fig. 18–9**). For transcanal work, a tympanomeatal flap incision is used (**Fig. 18–10**). Under direct vision the postauricular incision is then made (**Fig. 18–11**) a few millimeters behind the crease, which makes closure more cosmetic. A temporalis areolar tissue graft is harvested, saving fascia for revision should it be needed. A Palva flap is then raised (**Fig. 18–12**) by making cuts along the tegmen tympani line and mastoid tip, then connected posteriorly to create a rectangle of tissue. Many surgeons instead use a T incision; however, the Palva flap helps fill in a mastoid defect, especially in CWD surgery, and decreases caving in or cosmetic deformity

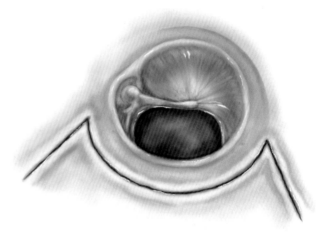

Figure 18–9 Figure demonstrates the use of the tympanomeatal and vascular strip incisions for postauricular approach. The horizontal incision parallels and is close to the annulus in this particular incision. The incision at the 6 o'clock position actually starts at 6 o'clock but comes out more at the 7 to 8 o'clock position, as this makes it easier to identify the incision on a postauricular approach. The incision at the 12 o'clock position is angled upward into the incisura of the avascular plane between the helical and antihelical cartilage. Other canal incisions can be used, as the surgeon prefers.

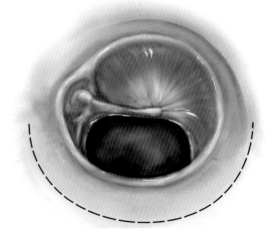

Figure 18–10 The tympanomeatal incision for transcanal work demonstrates a slightly larger distance between the annulus (about 8 mm) and the horizontal cut. The reason for this is that if the scutum needs to be curetted it will facilitate closer much easier. If the flap does not lay forward easily, the superior radial incision should be extended beyond 12 o'clock.

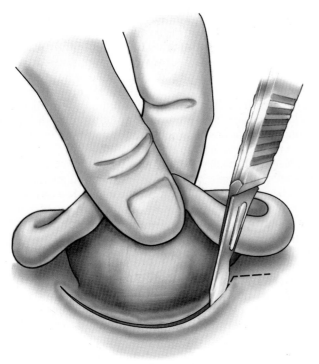

Figure 18–11 The postauricular incision.

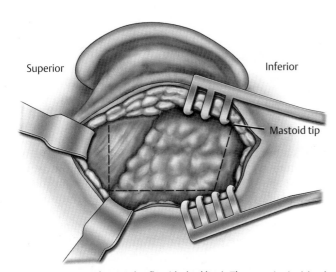

Superior

Inferior

Mastoid tip

Figure 18–12 A large Palva flap (dashed line). The superior incision is usually made several millimeters above the actual temporal line, and the inferior incision angles slightly toward the mastoid tip. A T-incision also can be used.

postauricularly. Alternatively, if one is doing a lateral graft tympanoplasty without mastoidectomy, then a small curved linear incision just posterior to the external auditory canal may be made because no drilling will occur in the mastoid area.

Surgical Technique

Tympanoplasty

Tympanoplasty itself can be divided into two techniques: medial/underlay and lateral/overlay. In the *medial* graft technique the perforation edges are freshened. I use a small cup

forceps to gently pull a rim of tissue off the edge of the perforation, which also removes any underlying skin. The tympanomeatal flap is elevated and reflected anteriorly. A small piece of Gelfilm placed onto the floor of the middle ear helps prevent adhesions and allows the mesotympanum to be filled with Gelfoam quite easily, as the Gelfoam readily slides across the Gelfilm. The graft is placed medial to the TM and, after ensuring it is in the exact place, the middle ear is filled with Gelfoam (**Fig. 18–13**). This graft-then-Gelfoam order makes for easier placement of the graft. For anterior-superior perforations that are not marginal, an anterior wall tympanomeatal flap can be created in much the same fashion. If the anterior bony overhang prevents adequate visualization, it can be drilled away after back-elevating the skin over this hump, just like pulling up a window shade.

The *lateral* graft technique is quite useful for total or near-total perforations, marginal perforations, and revision cases after medial graft failure. The lateral graft technique differs in that the entire epithelial layer over the TM must be removed to prevent intratympanic cholesteatoma formation (**Fig. 18–14**). The posterior canal incision is extended circumferentially around the ear canal. This skin is elevated 360 degrees down to the level of the annulus. Starting inferiorly, the squamous portion of the TM is removed in continuity with canal skin. I routinely elevate the skin both anterior and posterior to the short process of the malleus, and then gently pull it down to the malleus with a small cup forceps to remove the skin all in one piece. This skin is then saved and moistened for later use. If there is no concern about middle ear pathology, the annulus is left intact. If there is concern about ossicular erosion or other types of disease, then the annulus is dissected out of the annular ring and the middle ear is explored.

A 1-mm trough is drilled just lateral to the annulus anteriorly, and the anterior-superior and anterior-inferior regions are enlarged and squared off slightly to provide a better area for the lateral graft to sit. Care is taken not to expose the temporomandibular joint. The fascia graft is then fashioned. A good rule for sizing the fascia for a lateral graft is to use the

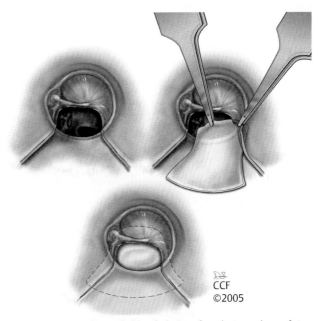

DS
CCF
©2005

Figure 18–13 In the medial (underlay) graft technique, the graft is placed medial to the malleus and drum remnant.

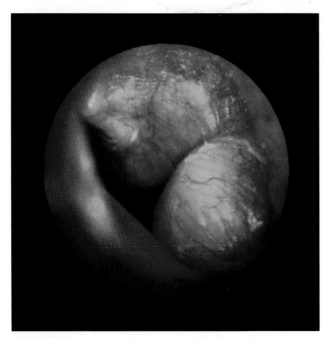

Figure 18–14 Intratympanic and canal cholestoma after a lateral graft technique.

fingernail of the index finger. A small slit is cut in the superior portion of the graft. The graft is slipped under the malleus and the slit gives two pieces to wrap around the malleus handle to prevent lateralization. The anterior portion of the graft is placed into the trough/ledge drilled on top of the annulus (**Fig. 18–15**). The posterior portion then comes up the posterior canal wall. Next the harvested skin is used as a graft. Drilling the anterior wall makes it difficult to put the skin back in one piece because it will not perfectly fit. Therefore, the skin can be cut into strips or pieces and placed back creating a sulcus anteriorly and also placing some posteriorly on the drum. A small rolled piece of Gelfoam is then placed into the sulcus anteriorly to prevent blunting. The vascular strip is replaced and the remainder of the canal filled with Gelfoam. The patient is started on antibiotic drops to help dissolve the packing and prevent infection. After 2 weeks one half to two thirds of the packing are removed, and the patient returns about 6 weeks later.

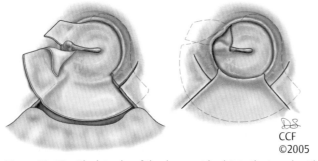

DS
CCF
©2005

Figure 18–15 The lateral graft has been put back into the trough with the skin graft then placed back over the anterior-inferior-superior region to help keep the graft from blunting anteriorly. The graft also shows the slit in the middle, which is then wrapped around the malleus to help keep it from lateralizing. The tympanomeatal flap and further skin grafts are being put back down over the fascia graft.

Another option to pack the canal is to use a Rosebud pack. Parachute silk is used to line the medial ear canal and new TM. Small cotton pledgets dipped in antibiotic ointment are placed on the silk-lined drum and into the sulcus to create pressure on the drum. A second Rosebud packing is placed into the external auditory canal on top of the first. This is left in place for 10 to 14 days. With a closed or repaired eardrum it is possible to use a less expensive medication such as Cortisporin otic suspension; just be aware of recognizing neomycin reactions. Of course a fluoroquinolone can be used.

Cartilage tympanoplasty is indicated when the scutum has been eroded by disease or drilled to facilitate full removal of disease. Reconstruction in this area should include a cartilage graft to prevent a future retraction pocket. Cartilage may be taken from either the tragus or the cymba region of the auricle (**Fig. 18–16**). Perichondrium is left on both sides of the cartilage, and then raised on one side to create a cartilage flap with perichondrial extension. In most cases the ossicular chain is preserved or reconstructed (sometimes at a second stage); therefore, a mobile TM is necessary. A large piece of cartilage to block off the epitympanum is appropriate but not so large that it adheres to the external canal and becomes non-mobile. Thus, cartilage can be scored and placed in an L-shaped fashion where one piece supports the scutal wall and the other grafts the TM (**Fig. 18–17**). A fascia graft then can be placed over the cartilage and the eardrum repaired as previously discussed. These patients need to be followed long-term because recurrence rates over 20 years may be as high as 60%.

Second-Look Surgery and Ossicular Reconstruction

Occasionally the cholesteatoma will be small and easily removed in one piece. The surgeon should be confident that no residual disease remains. In these cases, ossicular reconstruction can take place immediately. Second-look surgery is needed when disease is more extensive, and ossicular reconstruction is performed at that time, usually 6 to 12 months after initial surgery. Because many prostheses are covered by cartilage to prevent extrusion, reconstruction can be combined with cartilage tympanoplasty as described above.

The published rate of residual cholesteatoma is as high as 30%[20]; 85% of residual disease is in the epitympanum, 10% in the mesotympanum, and 5% in the mastoid. Usually, at the second look, residual cholesteatoma is quite small, just a pearl that is easily removed. Ossicular reconstruction then employs a total ossicular reconstruction prosthesis (TORP) if the stapes is absent or a partial ossicular reconstruction prosthesis (PORP) if the stapes is present. Most prostheses are made of titanium, hydroxyapatite or porous polyethylene. Which brand or type used is really a matter of personal choice as they all seem to give good results when placed by competent surgeons. Results usually are better with PORPs than TORPs.

Mastoidectomy

Prior to performing a mastoidectomy, disease in the mesotympanum is first removed to help identify landmarks so that one can ascertain how deep one is in a mastoid, especially if it is sclerotic, and to improve hemostasis with adrenalin-soaked Gelfoam prior to grafting. Several basic rules for mastoidectomy then are followed: (1) "As you go deep go wide," that is, the mastoid bowl should be saucerized to improve exposure and

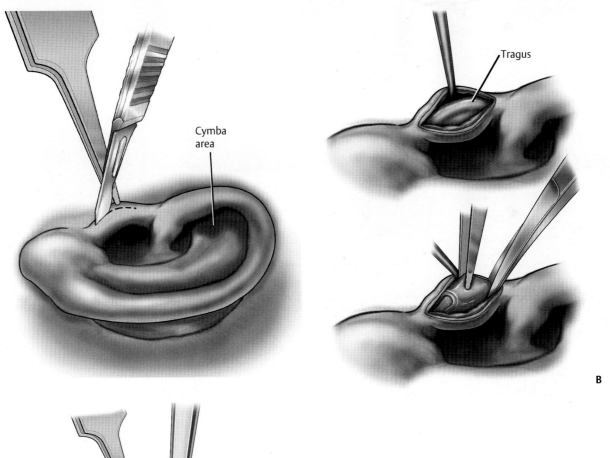

Cymba
area

Tragus

A

B

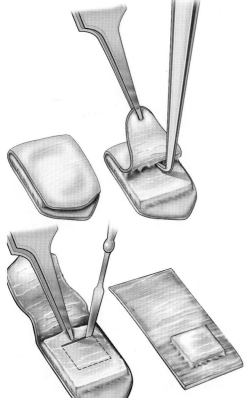

C

Figure 18–16 The stripping of the perichondrium off of one side of the tragal cartilage graft and then removing enough cartilage as needed to fit into the defect. The location for the cymbal of cartilage can be obtained underneath the antihelix and the tragus where cartilage is routinely harvested as well.

18 Chronic Otitis Media

243

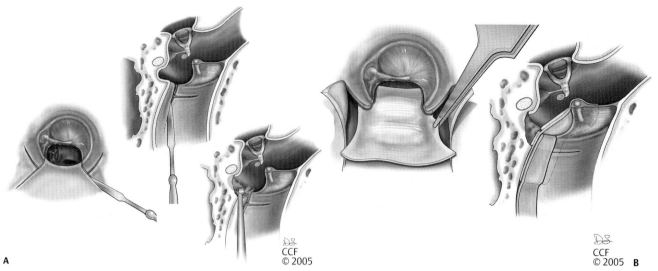

Figure 18–17 **(A)** The placement of a medial graft to repair a TM perforation; this can be used with cartilage especially if a total ossicular reconstruction prosthesis (TORP) or a partial ossicular reconstruction prosthesis (PORP) will be needed. **(B)** This figure demonstrates that piece of cartilage sliding medially. Graft placement is illustrated in the normal surgical position; the other figures are viewed superiorly for clarity.

III Management

minimize risk from drilling in a confined space (**Fig. 18–18**). (2) "The tegmen is your friend," that is, drilling high along the tegmen minimizes risk to the lateral canal and facial nerve as you approach the antrum. This is especially important for sclerotic mastoids, which are not well aerated and may have bone, not air, overlying the lateral semicircular canal.[3]

If possible some bone should be left over the tegmen and sigmoid sinus to protect dura and minimize risk of CSF leak and bleeding.[43] The posterior wall of the external canal should be thinned to avoid drilling under a ledge. Drilling proceeds from one safe area to the next. All disease from affected air cells should be removed or infection often recurs.

Some clinicians always identify the facial nerve because they believe the nerve then is less likely to be injured. Others do so only if the nerve is involved with disease. I identify the nerve if disease is in this area; otherwise I leave it alone. However, facial nerve landmarks must always be kept in mind. In the mesotympanum the tensor tympani, lateral semicircular canal, and stapedial tendon are good landmarks to identify the tympanic segment and geniculate ganglion. The facial nerve lies superior to the cochleariform process and oval window. In many normal patients the distal tympanic segment may be dehiscent along its inferior border just above the oval window niche. The second genu is just anterior/inferior and slightly medial to the lateral semicircular canal as the nerve enters the vertical segment. From there to the stylomastoid foramen the nerve courses slightly from medial to lateral. The digastric ridge is the best landmark for the stylomastoid foramen.

The pyramidal process separates the facial recess laterally from the sinus tympani medially. The incus should be removed and facial recess opened if significant disease fills the posterior epitympanum or posterior-superior mesotympanum. The facial recess is bounded medially by the facial nerve, laterally by the chorda tympani, and superiorly by the incus buttress (**Fig. 18–19**). Disease in the sinus tympani medial to the facial nerve may defy removal. It has been suggested that the sinus tympani may be reached by a retrofacial air cell tract if there is adequate aeration between the facial nerve and the posterior semicircular canal.[43] The author has suggested that the distance (mastoid to middle ear) be less than 2½ mm and the width or height distance between the canal and the facial nerve be greater than 2 mm.

If possible, a small cholesteatoma sac should be removed in one piece; a larger sac usually is removed piecemeal.

Figure 18–18 The saucerization of a mastoid bowl identifying the tegmen.

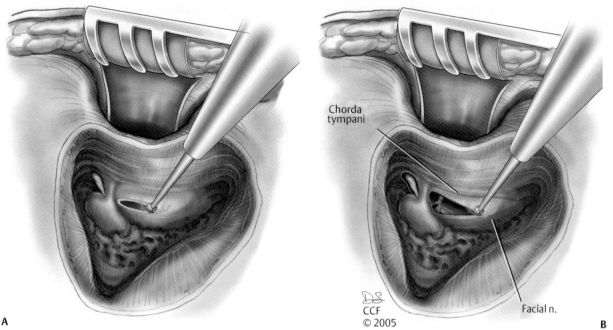

A

B

Chorda tympani

Facial n.

CCF © 2005

Figure 18–19   A facial recess is bounded by the chorda tympani, facial nerve, and incus buttress.

Canal-Wall-Down Mastoidectomy

The reasons for performing a CWD mastoidectomy already have been discussed, but the surgeon must consider the disadvantages of this procedure as well. Hearing results generally are worse because the eardrum is located at a lower level and vibrates less well; cartilage reconstruction of the drum may prevent this. The cavity tends to collect wax and other debris and must be cleaned periodically as an outpatient procedure, usually every 6 months. Larger cavities do not tolerate water, and a custom-fitted earmold often is needed during swimming. Most of all, the technical aspects of the operation must be performed carefully to maintain a safe, dry ear that is easily cleaned in the office. A high facial ridge, dependent mastoid tip, and small meatus must be avoided.

The incus and malleus are removed. The facial nerve is identified and posterior canal bone lowered down to it and the lateral canal, dividing the chorda tympani. The external canal wall remnants (buttresses) are drilled superiorly to the tegmen, anteriorly to the root of the zygoma, and inferiorly to the floor of the hypotympanum and mastoid tip. The small bony overhang separating the anterior epitympanum and eustachian tube is removed. All infected mucosa must be removed; none should remain especially in undrilled tip cells. Drilling away the mastoid may allow some obliteration in this area, resulting in a smaller cavity with less chance of drainage.

The tympanoplasty technique is relatively the same, although a larger piece of fascia is used and is draped up over the facial ridge and semicircular canals into the mastoid bowl. A prosthesis can easily be placed by raising up the fascia or can be delayed until a second stage. If desired, cartilage can be placed to reconstruct the drum.

Meatoplasty

Meatoplasty often is performed before drilling a CWD mastoid so that soft tissue hemostasis is obtained before delicate middle ear work is begun. A large meatoplasty facilitates office examination and cleaning and provides good aeration to the mastoid bowl, thus preventing chronic drainage. Many surgeons advocate removal of 1 cm or 40% of conchal cartilage to create a rather large opening and prevent cupping of the ear from tension during closure. Such a large piece is removed because the meatus will contract by approximately 25% over time. However, a large meatus can be cosmetically undesirable, and I prefer a more limited procedure called *incisural* meatoplasty. An incision at 12 o'clock between the tragal and conchal cartilages is made similar to an endaural incision; however, it stops just at the top of the meatus. This opening is large enough to place the surgeon's thumb or forefinger in the ear canal opening. To protect against constriction a suture is placed posteriorly from the vascular strip area to the temporalis fascia posteriorly to keep the meatus opened. The ear canal/meatus is then packed open. I use Gelfoam for a couple of layers, then ¼-inch gauze soaked in bacitracin (actually two pieces of gauze so if the top piece is accidentally pulled out, the other remains).

Postoperative Care

I remove the gauze packing in 7 to 10 days because otherwise it tends to become odorous with purulent discharge. Antibiotic drops then are used to promote healing and dissolve the Gelfoam. Six to 8 weeks are needed for the mastoid to epithelialize. During this time patients may have areas that develop granulation tissue, which can be treated locally with drops, powder, or silver nitrate if necessary.

◆ Complications

Complications from chronic ear surgery are many and varied but fortunately are less than 1% risk.[44–46] In contrast, complications can be relatively frequent if disease is left untreated.[46] This section discusses facial nerve injuries, tegmen dehiscence

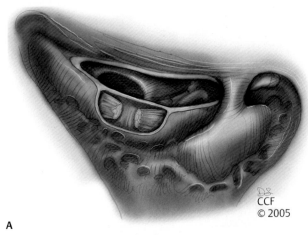 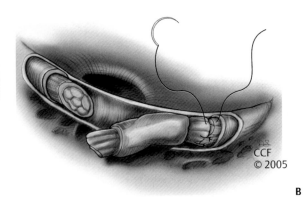

A

B

Figure 18–20 Repair of the facial nerve.

with or without CSF leak, hemorrhage from sigmoid sinus or carotid artery, semicircular canal fistula, and stapes dislocation. Some of these are further discussed in Chapter 19. I believe that infectious complications are minimized by administering prophylactic antibiotics, which are on call to the operating room, and by not shaving the patient's hair.[47]

Facial Paralysis

One of the most dreaded complications is facial paralysis. The best way to avoid facial nerve injury is to thoroughly understand its anatomy.[48–50] Although the risk of facial nerve injury is quite low, less than 1% for primary cases, it can be as high as 4 to 10% in revision cases.[51]

I routinely order a preoperative CT scan to see if disease directly involves the facial nerve; however, many surgeons do not do this. Use of intraoperative facial nerve monitoring also is helpful but not required.[52,53] The surgeon should bear in mind that 50% of normal nerves have a small 0.4-mm dehiscence in the tympanic segment.[54] Other areas of dehiscence can involve the geniculate ganglion, facial recess, and the mastoid area (most commonly when the mucosa of an air cell covers the facial nerve).[55] In these cases, the stimulator and monitor can identify the nerve.

If the nerve is injured, one hopes that the surgeon will recognize this in the operating room rather than in the recovery room when the patient awakens. The surgeon first determines the degree of injury. Minimal erythema and contusion do not require treatment. The nerve actually is quite hardy and can be manipulated without significant effect.[56,57] However, if bruising or contusion is more extensive, the nerve should be decompressed locally by removing 5 to 10 mm of bone from both sides of injury.[58] Opening the nerve sheath probably causes more harm than good.[59,60] High-dose steroids (prednisone 60–80 mg daily) also are recommended for 7 to 10 days. The patient should be taught how to use ophthalmic drops and ointment and a moisture chamber at bedtime.

Occasionally, the injury is more extensive: partial or total transection. This type of injury is particularly emotional not only for the patient but also for the surgeon, who often underestimates the degree of injury because he or she wants to believe the nerve is not injured so much. Moreover, injury usually is more extensive than it appears, even to an objective observer. If less than one third of the nerve is cut, the surgeon

should decompress on either side of the injury.[61] If greater than one third of the nerve is cut, then repair is needed to provide a better chance for recovery to House-Brackmann grade 3.[62,63]

Primary repair is preferred because only one anastomosis is required. However, if anastomosis cannot be performed without tension, a graft is needed. Some extra length can be obtained by drilling out the stylomastoid foramen; however, this also disrupts some of the blood supply. Indeed, the final outcome of one anastomosis versus two may not be clinically significant.[59,64]

All bone spicules are removed from the nerve. Nerve repair uses 9-0 or 10-0 monofilament suture (**Fig. 18–20**), which can be difficult but helped by using the immobile bed of the fallopian canal. If the nerve ends are stable they can be held together by fibrin glue, Gelfoam, or Cargile[59,60,65] without suture. The ends should be cut obliquely to increase the surface area for axon regeneration.[62,66] If a graft is required, either the greater auricular or sural nerve can be used. The greater auricular nerve usually provides adequate length and already is in the operative field.[59] A line is drawn from the mastoid tip to the angle of the jaw; a second line bisects the first and extends perpendicularly toward the neck. Two-thirds down this second line an incision is made onto the sternocleidomastoid muscle where the greater auricular nerve can be found[62] (**Fig. 18–21**).

The patient and family must be counseled about realistic expectations. If the nerve was grafted, 6 to 9 months are required before any voluntary movement is seen and final recovery will not be known for 1 year. At best, the final outcome in grafting is approximately 75% of normal[64] (House-Brackmann grade 3 or 4 is common). Synkinesis is expected.[67]

When facial nerve injury is discovered in the recovery room rather than in the operating room, the surgeon should consider whether tight packing in a mastoid cavity or local anesthetic block at the nerve trunk may be responsible. Packing should be loosened or removed. In both cases function usually returns within 2 hours. If not, the surgeon should determine first if facial muscles are weak or paralyzed. Voluntary movement indicates that the nerve is not transected and the prognosis is excellent. High-dose steroids are given and the patient is observed closely for a day or so. If palsy progresses to paralysis, injury is more severe than believed at first and electroneurography (ENoG) is used if 72 hours have elapsed since surgery. If the compound action potential is reduced by 95%, the nerve is explored within 1 to 3 days if possible.[68,69] Neural

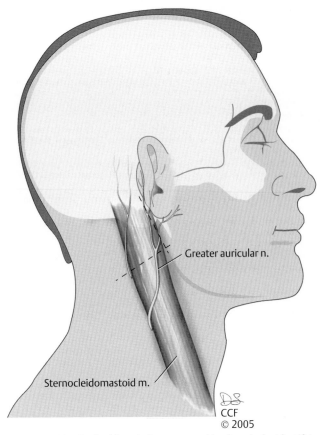

Figure 18–21 Dashed lines indicate external land marks for identifying the greater auricular nerve (see text for details).

Greater auricular n.

Sternocleidomastoid m.

DS
CCF
© 2005

If bleeding occurs when raising a tympanomeatal flap, then Surgicel and Gelfoam are used to pack the middle ear onto the bulb. The tympanomeatal flap is replaced and the ear canal is packed for at least 1 week.[58,72] Injury during myringotomy usually can be controlled with external canal packing.

Injury to the *carotid artery* is exceedingly rare because a congenitally dehiscent exposed carotid artery itself is very rare, less than 1%.[73] The artery is normally covered by thick bone and lies medial to the eustachian tube orifice, anterior-medial to the cochlea, and anterior-inferior to the cochleari-form process. Imaging studies preoperatively again can help identify a suspected anomaly. Vigilance when dissecting in this area is essential because the petrous carotid may not pulsate normally, making it more difficult to identify.[48]

Bleeding from the artery wall is simply controlled with Surgicel because it arises from minor vessels along the wall. However, major bleeding must be controlled immediately by packing and pressure. Once hemorrhage is controlled, then definitive management can be decided: temporary balloon occlusion with secondary repair or grafting, permanent balloon occlusion, or surgical ligation.[58,74] There is risk of stroke with balloon occlusion even in normal people.[75]

Dural Injury and Cerebrospinal Fluid Leak

During mastoid surgery the tegmen/dura is commonly exposed because its identification is used in performing safe mastoid surgery.[59] Exposure of tegmen dura requires no further corrective action.[60] However, large defects may result in a meningoencephalocele over a long period of time. Even so, I would not treat exposed dura immediately because the incidence of meningoencephalocele is so low, but would rather wait until a problem actually develops. Dural violation, on the other hand, whether by drill, instruments, or cautery, does require some corrective action. The site of the injury dictates the repair. Middle fossa tegmen dura is normally thick and associated with a significant amount of arachnoid tissue. Arachnoid tissue actually helps form fibrous scar to seal a CSF leak. With small (1 cm) areas of injury. Some bone is removed all around the site to allow placement of a fascia or muscle plug/graft.[58] A piece of Gelfoam can be used to help hold this graft in place after it is tucked under the bony edges. For large defects middle cranial fossa craniotomy with a fascia-bone-fascia graft sandwich is required to repair the dural defect.[48] Antibiotic coverage in all CSF leaks is recommended.

A CSF leak in the posterior fossa dura is more challenging because there is little arachnoid tissue in this area. Thus, even though fascia grafts are tucked in and around the bone circumferentially and Gelfoam is placed, the patient also may require lumbar-subarachnoid drainage and bed rest for 2 to 3 days.[60] Occasionally, a posterior fossa leak requires sealing with connective tissue, bone wax, and abdominal fat graft. Consultation with neurosurgery is recommended if either a middle or posterior fossa leak does not quickly resolve.

Semicircular Canal Fistula

It is actually more common to injure the membranous labyrinth when dissecting cholesteatoma off a dehiscent canal than it is to inadvertently drill into a semicircular canal. A drilling accident probably occurs less than 0.1% of the time.[76] Opening a bony canal itself does not necessarily lead to hearing loss. Significant damage more often occurs with suction into the vestibular system. If the bony labyrinth is entered, the

growth (axon budding) may be maximal 3 to 4 weeks postinjury, but exploration should proceed without undue delay anyway.[59,70]

Vascular Injuries

Occasionally the *sigmoid sinus* may be injured. Mild bleeding usually comes from small, torn dural vessels that lie on the sinus and are easily cauterized with bipolar cautery. If a small laceration of the sinus occurs, Gelfoam covered temporarily by a small cottonoid will suffice. The area is left alone and cottonoid removed at closure. More substantial laceration requires packing with Surgicel, either extraluminally[71] or intraluminally. Intraluminal packing has the risk of embolization, which is minimized by leaving a long tail of Surgicel posteriorly over the mastoid edge until closure. Anesthesia should be notified when a tear occurs so that the patient can be monitored and treated quickly if an air embolus develops.

The injured *jugular bulb* also can bleed profusely. The bulb may be high (above the inferior annulus of the eardrum) in up to 7% of people.[72] Occasionally high jugular bulbs may be dehiscent, making them especially prone to injury. Again, bleeding usually is easily controlled with pressure from Gelfoam or by packing with Surgicel. In the rare event that this treatment fails and bleeding is profuse, control may require internal jugular vein ligation in the neck and extraluminal or intraluminal packing of the sigmoid/jugular bulb in the mastoid. Bleeding still can persist via backflow from the inferior petrosal vein out the jugular dehiscence so pressure on the bulb must be maintained.

surgeon should not suction but rather should seal the fistula with bone wax, fascia, or muscle.[77–79]

More commonly, cholesteatoma causes a fistula. Preoperative CT scanning can usually identify this pathology. If a labyrinthine fistula is suspected, cholesteatoma sac contents should first be removed and the matrix carefully inspected for deformity or blue coloration, indicating the membranous labyrinth is exposed. If the fistula is small, slow, gentle removal of the sac over it sometimes can be accomplished; if larger, the matrix should be left over the fistula to avoid inner ear trauma. Either the canal wall is taken down and the matrix exteriorized, or the wall is left intact and the fistula is reassessed at a second stage. Some fistulas can heal; some residual epithelium can simply disappear.[58] Definitive management is decided at the second stage. Profound sensorineural hearing loss occurs in 3 to 22% of patients with disease-induced canal fistula.[44] The surgeon also should note that if a lateral canal fistula is present, almost always the tympanic facial nerve is dehiscent.

Oval window fistulization is more often iatrogenic from dissection of disease off the footplate and stapes, or the stapes can be dislocated when raising a tympanomeatal flap or manipulating the ossicular chain. In cholesteatoma surgery, it is better to leave a little cholesteatoma and disease on the stapes and return in 6 to 9 months when it should be easier to remove (it should form a small pearl), than to pursue total removal and risk stapes injury.[58] If the footplate can be put back into position, it should be covered with connective tissue. One must make sure that it will not sink into the vestibule. If the footplate cannot be returned to its position, then it should be removed and the oval window sealed with fascia. If there is fistulization of the footplate but the footplate is still in place and intact, then the fistula is sealed with fascia or muscle. Hearing loss and dizziness may occur short-term but symptoms often improve over time.

Certainly, iatrogenic injuries do occur. The key to avoidance is attention to detail. When injury does occur, the surgeon must know in advance how to handle it.

References

1. Thorburn IA. Chronic disease of the middle ear. In: Scott-Brown WG, Balantyne JC, Groves J, eds. Diseases of the Ear, Nose, and Throat, 2nd ed. London: Butterworth, 1965

2. Procter B. Chronic otitis media and mastoiditis. In: Paparella M, Shumrick D, Gluckman J, Meyerhoff W, eds. Otolaryngology, vol 2, 3rd ed. Philadelphia: WB Saunders, 1991:1349–1376

3. Weber PC, Roland PS, Hannlay M, et al. The developments of antibiotic resistant organisms with use of oto-topical medications. Otolaryngol Head Neck Surg 2004;130:S89–S94

4. Harker LA, Koontz FB. Bacteriology of cholesteatoma: clinical significance. Otolaryngol Head Neck Surg 1977;84:683–686

5. Brook I. Aerobic and anaerobic bacteriology of cholesteatoma. Laryngoscope 1981;91:250–253

6. Brook I. Bacteriology and treatment of chronic otitis media. Laryngoscope 1979;89:1129–1134

7. Sheehy JL. Chronic tympanomastoiditis. In: Gates G, ed. Current Therapy in Otolaryngology Head and Neck Surgery, 4th ed. Toronto: BC Decker 1990:19–22

8. Fairbanks DNF. Otic topical agents. Otolaryngol Head Neck Surg 1980;88: 327–331

9. Fairbanks DNF. Topical therapeutics for otitis media. Otolaryngol Head Neck Surg 1981;89:381–385

10. Anderson CW, Stevens MH. Synchronous tuberculous involvement of both ears and the larynx in a patient with active pulmonary disease. Laryngoscope 1981;91:906–909

11. Windle-Taylor PC, Bailey CM. Tuberculous otitis media: a series of 22 patients. Laryngoscope 1980;90:1039–1044

12. Mafee MF. MRI and CT in the evaluation of acquired and congenital cholesteatoma of the temporal bone. J Otolaryngol 1993;22: 239–248

13. Roland PS, Stewart MG, Hannley M, et al. Consensus Panel on Role of Potentially Ototoxic Antibiotics for Topical Middle Ear Use: introduction, methodology, and recommendations. Otolaryngol Head Neck Surg 2004;130:S51–S56

14. Alcon paper.

15. Levenson MJ, Parisier SC, Chute P, et al. A review of twenty congenital cholesteatomas of the middle ear in children. Otolaryngol Head Neck Surg 1986;94:560–567

16. Nelson M, Roger G, Koltai PJ, et al. Congenital cholesteatomas: classification, management and outcome. Arch Otolaryngol Head Neck Surg 2002;128: 810–814

17. Weber PC, Adkins WY. Congenital cholesteatomas in the tympanic membrane. Laryngoscope 1997;107:1181–1184

18. Potsic WP, Samadi DS, Marsh RR, Wetmore RF. A staging system for congenital cholesteatoma. Arch Otolaryngol Head Neck Surg 2002;128: 1009–1012

19. Karmody CS, Byanattis V, Blevins N, et al. The origin of congenital cholesteatoma. Am J Otol 1998;19:292–297

20. Glasscock ME, Haynes DS, Storper, et al. Surgery for chronic ear disease. In: Hughes GB, Pensak ML, eds. Clinical Otology, 2nd ed. New York: Thieme, 1997:215–232

21. Jackson CG. Cholesteatoma: the method of. In: Gates GA, ed. Current Therapy in Otolaryngology Head and Neck Surgery-4. Toronto: BC Decker 1990:23–28

22. Jackson CG, Glasscock ME, Nissen AJ, et al. Open mastoid procedures: contemporary indications and surgical technique. Laryngoscope 1985; 95:1037–1040

23. Glasscock ME, Jackson CG, Nissen AJ, Schwaber MK. Post-auricular under-surface tympanic membrane grafting: a follow-up report. Laryngoscope 1982;92:718–727

24. Storrs LA. Myringoplasty with the use of facial grafts. Arch Otolaryngol 1961;74:65

25. Toynbee J. On the Use of an Artificial Membrane Tympanic in Cases of Deafness Dependent upon Perforations in Destruction of the Natural Organ. London: J. Churchill, 1853

26. Berthold E. Ueber myringoplastick. Wier Med Bull 1878;1:627

27. Blake CJ. Transactions of the First Congress of the International Otological Society. New York: D. Appelton, 1887

28. Wullstein H. Funktionelle Operationen im mittelohr mit Hilfe des freien Spaltlappen-Transplantates. Arch Ohrenheilkd 1952;161:422

29. Zollner F. The principles of plastic surgery of the sound conduction apparatus. J Laryngol Otol 1955;69:637–652

30. Goodhill V. Tragal perichondrium and cartilage in tympanoplasty. Arch Otolaryngol 1967;85:480–491

31. Glasscock ME 3rd. Tympanic membrane grafting with fascia: overlay vs. undersurface technique. Laryngoscope 1973;83:754–770

32. Weber PC, Gantz BJ. Cartilage reconstruction of scutal defects in canal wall-up mastoidectomies. Am J Otolaryngol 1998;19:178–183

33. Jansen C. Ulur Radikaoperationen Und Tympanoplastik. Sitz Ber. Fontbild, Arztekamm. Ob., vol 18, 1958

34. Kessel J. Uber das Ausschneiden des Tromelfells, Hammers ad Ambosses bei Undurchgangigkeit det Tube. Arch Ohr Nas Kehlkophfheilk 1885; 22:196

35. Zaufal E. Technik der Trepanation des Prc. Mastoid. Nach Kuster'schen Grundsatzen. Ohrenheilkd 1890;30:291

36. Stacke L. Stacke's Operationsmethode. Arch Ohrenheilkd 1893;35:145

37. Schwartze HH, Eysell CG. Uber die Kunstliche Eroffnung des Warzenfortsatzes. Arch Ohrenheilkd 1873;7:157

38. Petit JL. Traite des Maladies Chirurgicales. Paris: 1774.

39. Hirsch BE, Kamerer DB, Doshi S. Single stage management of cholesteatoma. Otolaryngol Head Neck Surg 1992;106:351–354

40. Gantz BJ, Wilkinson EP, Hansen MR. Canal wall reconstruction tympanomastoidectomy with mastoid obliteration. Laryngoscope 2005;115: 1734–1740

41. Bondy G. Totalaufmeisselung mit Erhaltung von Tromelfell und Gehorknochelchen. Monatsschr Ohrenheilk 1910;44:15

42. Miller JJ, Weber PC, Patel S, Ramey J. Intracranial surgery: to shave or not to shave? Otol Neurotol 2001;22:908–911

43. Sheehy JL. Surgery of chronic otitis media. In: English G, ed. Otolaryngology, vol 1. Philadelphia: JB Lippincott, 1984

44. Dawes FR. Early complications of surgery for chronic otitis media. J Otolaryngol Otol 1999;133:803–810

45. Kempf HG, Johann K, Lenarz T. Complications in pediatric cochlear implant surgery. Eur Arch Otorhinolaryngol 1999;256:128–132

46. Greenberg MD, Jayson S, Manolidis S. High incidence of complications encountered in chronic otitis media surgery in a U.S. metropolitan public hospital. American Academy of Otolaryngology–Head and Neck Surgery 2001;125:623–627

47. Miller J, Weber P, Patel S. Intracranial surgery to shave or not to shave? Otol Neurotol 2001;22:908–911

48. Bellucci R. Iatrogenic surgical trauma in otolaryngology. J Laryngol Otol Suppl 1983;8:13–17

49. May M, Wiet RJ. Iatrogenic injury-prevention and management. In: May M, ed. The Facial Nerve. New York: Thieme, 1986:549–560

50. Wiet RJ. Iatrogenic facial paralysis. Otolaryngol Clin North Am 1982;15: 773–788

51. Wiet RJ, Herzon GD. Surgery of the mastoid. In: Wiert RJ, Causse JB, eds. Complications in Otolaryngology-Head and Neck Surgery, vol 1. Philadelphia: BC Decker, 1986:25–31

52. Roland PS, Meyerhoff WL. Intraoperative electrophysiological monitoring of the facial nerve: is it standard of practice? Am J Otolaryngol 1994; 15:267–270

53. Green JD, Shelton C, Brackmann DE. Iatrogenic facial nerve injury (letter). Laryngoscope 1995;105:444–445

54. Baxter A. Dehiscence of the fallopian canal. J Otolaryngol Otol 1971;85:587–594

55. Schuknecht HF, Guyle AJ. Anatomy of the Temporal Bone with Surgical Implications. Philadelphia: Lea & Febiger, 1986

56. Sheehy JL. Facial nerve in surgery of chronic otitis media. Otolaryngol Clin North Am 1974;7:493–503

57. Neely JG. Surgery of acute infections and their complications. In: Brackmann DE, Shelton C, Arriaga MA, eds. Otologic Surgery. Philadelphia: WB Saunders, 1994:201–210

58. Wiet RJ, Harvet SA, Bauer GP. (1994) Management of complications of chronic otitis media. In: Brackmann DE, Shelton C, Arriaga MA, eds. Otologic Surgery. Philadelphia: WB Saunders, 1994:257–276

59. Smyth, Gordon GDL, Toner JG. Mastoidectomy: canal wall down techniques. In: Brackmann DE, Shelton C, Arriaga MA, eds. Otologic Surgery. Philadelphia: WB Saunders, 1994:225–239

60. Paparella MM, Meyerghoff WL, Morris MS, Dacosta SS. Mastoidectomy and tympanoplasty. In: Paparella MM, Shumrick D, Gluckman JL, Meyerhoff WL, eds. Otolaryngology, vol 2, 3rd ed. Philadelphia: WB Saunders, 1991:1405–1439

61. May M, et al. Trauma to the facial nerve: external, surgical, iatrogenic. In: May M, Schaitkin BM, eds. The Facial Nerve, 2nd ed. New York: Thieme, 2000:367–382

62. Adkins WY, Osguthorpe JD. Management of trauma of the facial nerve. Otolaryngol Clin North Am 1991;24:587–611

63. Brackmann D. Otoneurosurgical procedures. In: May M, ed. The Facial Nerve. New York: Thieme, 1986:589–618

64. Fisch U, Rouleau M. Facial nerve reconstruction. J Otolaryngol 1980;9: 487–492

65. Fisch U, Lanser MJ. Facial nerve grafting. Otolaryngol Clin North Am 1991;24:691–708

66. Yamamoto E, Fisch U. Experiments on facial nerves suturing. ORL J Otorhinolaryngol Relat Spec 1974;36:193–204

67. Fisch U. Facial nerve grafting. Otolaryngol Clin North Am 1974;7:517–529

68. Barrs DM. Facial nerve trauma: Optimal timing for repair. Laryngoscope 1991;101:835–848

69. May M. Facial reanimation after skull base trauma. In: May M, ed. The Facial Nerve. New York: Thieme, 1986:421–440

70. McQuarrie IG, Grafstein B. Axon outgrowth enhanced by previous nerve injury. Arch Neurol 1973;29:53–55

71. Moloy PJ, Brackmann DE. "How I do it." Control of venous bleeding in otologic surgery. Laryngoscope 1986;96:580–582

72. Graham MD. The jugular bulb: its anatomic and clinical considerations in contemporary otology. Laryngoscope 1977;87:105–125

73. Goldman NC, Singleton GT, Holly EH. Aberrant internal carotid artery presenting as a mass in the middle ear. Arch Otolaryngol 1971;94: 269–273

74. Andrews JC, Valavanis A, Fisch U. Management of the internal carotid artery of the skull base. Laryngoscope 1989;99:1224–1229

75. de Vries EJ, Sekhar LN, Janecka IP, et al. Elective resection of the internal carotid artery without reconstruction. Laryngoscope 1988;98:960–966

76. Palva T, Karja J, Palva A. Immediate and short-term complications of chronic ear surgery. Arch Otolaryngol Head Neck Surg 1976;102:137–139

77. Jahrsdoerfer RA, Johns ME, Cantrell RW. Labyrinthine trauma during ear surgery. Laryngoscope 1978;88:1589–1595

78. Canalis RF, Gussen R, Abemayor E, Andrews J. Surgical trauma to the lateral semicircular canal with preservation of hearing. Laryngoscope 1987;97:575–581

79. Cullen JR, Kerr AG. "How I do it." Iatrogenic fenestration of a semicircular canal: a method of closure. Laryngoscope 1986;96:1168–1169

19

Complications of Otitis Media

Jerry W. Lin, Mukesh Prasad, and Samuel H. Selesnick

Acute otitis media (AOM) is one of the most prevalent illnesses in children in the United States. A 1989 prospective study by Teele et al[1] demonstrated that 83% of children suffered at least one episode of AOM during their lifetime, whereas 46% of children had at least three episodes of AOM by age 3. More recent evidence by Block et al[2] in 2001 suggested that the incidence and frequency of episodes of AOM are trending even higher. The use of antibiotic therapy in the treatment of AOM continues to be an active area of clinical investigation, resulting in continual modifications of the guidelines for treatment of AOM. Recent revisions in the management guidelines of AOM have focused on decreasing the use of antibiotics for initial therapy[3] (see Chapter 17).

The use of antibiotics for AOM has reduced the incidence of acute suppurative mastoiditis. Conversely, Hoppe et al[4] have shown that withholding initial antibiotic therapy for AOM is associated with a rising incidence of mastoiditis. A comparison of the rates of mastoiditis in children from countries with different philosophies for initial antibiotic therapy for AOM has shown that those children in countries with prescription rates of 76% or less have approximately twice the rate of mastoiditis as those in countries with prescription rates of 96% or greater.[5] Although the rates of mastoiditis are quite low (4 per 100,000 children) even in those countries with lower prescription rates, the trend toward withholding initial antibiotic therapy requires the clinician to maintain an increasingly high clinical awareness of the signs and symptoms of complications of AOM.

This chapter reviews complications of both acute and chronic otitis media. Complications from otitis media can be organized into extracranial and intracranial areas of involvement, although one does not necessarily preclude the other. Extracranial complications can remain within the temporal bone or can extend beyond its confines (**Table 19–1**).

◆ Extracranial Complications

Intratemporal Extension

Acute Mastoiditis

Acute mastoiditis is an inflammatory process of the mastoid air cells of the temporal bone. It is characterized by hyperemia

of the mucosal lining of the mastoid air cells with development of fluid and pus within the air cells. Prolonged infection can lead to osteitis and subsequent destruction of the bony trabeculae that delineate the mastoid air cells. Loss of these bony trabeculae results in coalescence of the air cells, which become filled with pus. Once acute mastoiditis has progressed to the point of "coalescence," surgical management is required.[6] In the event that coalescent mastoiditis continues untreated, the process of bony erosion and abscess formation can extend to adjacent structures, resulting in myriad complications, many of which are discussed in this chapter.

As mastoid air cells are contiguous with the middle ear space via the aditus ad antrum, so must mastoiditis be considered an extension of otitis media. Patients with mastoiditis typically present with the symptoms of AOM such as fever, ear pain, and conductive hearing loss. Purulent otorrhea arises in cases of tympanic membrane perforation. Physical examination can reveal edema and erythema of the postauricular soft tissue with pain and tenderness over the mastoid process. Anterior and inferior displacement of the pinna often results in proptosis of the ear. Otoscopic examination may reveal fullness or "sagging" of the posterior-superior external canal wall, secondary to periosteal thickening near the antrum. In addition, the tympanic membrane may show evidence of AOM; if the tympanic membrane is perforated, inflamed middle ear mucosa may be seen through the perforation.

Bacterial cultures obtained from the middle ear in patients with acute mastoiditis most commonly reveal those pathogens involved in uncomplicated AOM: *Streptococcus pneumoniae*, *Haemophilus influenzae*, and *Moraxella catarrhalis*. *Streptococcus pyogenes* and *Staphylococcus aureus* are frequently found in persistent acute mastoiditis. Less common organisms include *Pseudomonas aeruginosa* and gram-negative organisms such as *Escherichia coli* and *Klebsiella pneumonia*.[7–9]

The discovery of antibiotics and their application to infectious diseases in the middle of the twentieth century greatly reduced the frequency of progression of AOM to acute mastoiditis. Prior to the use of antibiotics, one quarter to one half of patients with AOM could be expected to develop acute mastoiditis.[10] In a review in 2001, the incidence of acute mastoiditis in patients with AOM was 0.04 to 0.07%.[11]

Table 19–1   Complications of Otitis Media

Extracranial
  Intratemporal
    Mastoiditis
    Ossicular erosion
    Sensorineural hearing loss
    Facial nerve paralysis
    Otic capsule fistula
    Suppurative labyrinthitis
    Petrous apicitis
  Extratemporal
    Subperiosteal abscess
    Zygomatic abscess
    Bezold's abscess
    Cervical/postauricular fistula
    Extramastoid cholesteatoma
Intracranial
  Meningitis
  Brain abscess
  Subdural empyema
  Epidural abscess
  Lateral sinus thrombosis
  Otitic hydrocephalus
  Meningoencephalocele

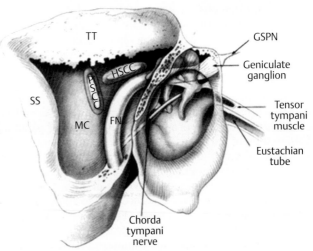

Figure 19–1   Surgical anatomy of the middle ear and mastoid after a cortical mastoidectomy includes the mastoid cavity (MC), the facial nerve (FN), the horizontal semicircular canal (HSCC), the posterior semicircular canal (PSCC), the sigmoid sinus (SS), the tegmen tympani (TT), and the greater superficial petrosal nerve (GSPN). (From Selesnick SH, Jackler RK. Facial paralysis in suppurative ear disease. Operative techniques in Otolaryngology. Head Neck Surg 1992;3:61–68. Reprinted by permission.)

A computed tomography (CT) scan of the temporal bone is the optimal imaging modality for the diagnosis of acute mastoiditis. Opacification of the mastoid air cells and the middle ear space can be observed due to mucosal edema as well as fluid or pus collection. Careful attention must be paid to the bony trabeculae defining the mastoid air cells. Haziness of these structures suggests demineralization and loss of integrity of the bony septa. This disease process may progress to complete destruction of the bone, resulting in coalescent mastoiditis and necessitating surgical intervention.

If acute mastoiditis is diagnosed prior to radiographic observation of coalescence, it may be successfully treated conservatively with myringotomy and intravenous antibiotics.[12] With earlier intervention, mucosal edema in the antrum may be reduced to allow for adequate clearance of fluid or pus from the mastoid air cells into the middle ear and out the eustachian tube as well as the myringotomy site. Acute mastoiditis that persists despite conservative management requires direct drainage of the infected contents of the mastoid air cells via a cortical mastoidectomy (**Fig. 19–1**).[12,13] Despite the powerful antibiotics available today, acute mastoiditis remains a serious otologic infection. In a recent retrospective review in 1996 of 124 patients with acute mastoiditis, Gliklich et al[14] reported that 62% required surgical intervention.

Extension of the infectious process within the temporal bone can manifest as myriad functional disabilities. Spread of infection from the middle ear to the inner ear typically occurs via direct extension either through areas of bony destruction or through preformed openings in the bone, such as the round window, the oval window, or preexisting dehiscences of the temporal bone.

Ossicular Erosion

Chronic suppurative otitis media commonly results in a conductive hearing loss. Conduction of sound through the middle ear is compromised by the presence of pus in the middle ear space; however, damage to the ossicular chain may also contribute to the hearing loss. Typically, bony erosion occurs at the stapes suprastructure and the incus, whereas the malleus is less often involved. Treatment entails prosthetic reconstruction of the ossicular chain once the suppurative otitis media has been controlled.

Sensorineural Hearing Loss

Occasionally, sensorineural hearing loss may be found in patients with chronic otitis media. In fact, sensorineural hearing loss has been positively correlated with the duration and severity of otitis media.[15] The mechanism of hearing loss is not completely understood. The most commonly proposed theory is that pathologic changes in the round window membrane can render it more permeable to bacterial toxins. Thus passage of chemical toxins from the middle ear into the inner ear via the round window may damage the cochlear apparatus.[16,17] A study in 2004 has shown that introduction of fluorescence-labeled endotoxin into the middle ear can lead to accumulation of intense fluorescence in the basal turn of the cochlea.[18] Consistent with this observation, another study detailing cochlear morphology in the setting of chronic otitis media described loss of outer and inner hair cells in the basal turn of the cochlea.[19] Nevertheless, studies that found no cochlear pathology and described improvement of hearing following treatment of otitis have led to postulation of otitic change in middle ear resonance or change in mechanics of sound transmission as the etiology of the sensorineural hearing loss.[20] Clarification of the mechanism of hearing loss remains an active area of investigation.

Facial Nerve Paralysis

Facial nerve paralysis is a rare complication of otitis media. Of all cases of peripheral facial paralysis, those secondary to otitis media comprise 6 to 8%.[21] The timing of the development of facial paralysis after onset of otitis media is important to consider as it suggests the pathophysiology of the symptoms and, more importantly, has implications for the treatment of the disease. Facial palsy that occurs in the acute setting, that is, within 2 weeks of onset of otitis, likely represents injury to a dehiscent, exposed facial nerve by bacterial toxins with resultant neural edema. Inflammatory edema, as it extends to portions of the nerve that are contained within a bony canal, leads to compression of the nerve and neuropraxia secondary to ischemia.[22] Treatment of acute onset of facial nerve paralysis in the setting of otitis media includes intravenous antibiotics and wide myringotomy to decompress the middle ear. Typically, complete resolution of nerve palsy is expected.[23]

If facial paralysis occurs after 2 weeks of otitis media, it is more likely that bony erosion has occurred to allow access of bacterial toxins to the facial nerve (**Fig. 19–2**). Bony erosion also can occur in the setting of cholesteatoma that has eroded through the fallopian canal and compresses the facial nerve directly. In these cases, mastoidectomy with facial nerve decompression is indicated.[24] The nerve should be identified, any granulation tissue should be exenterated, and the facial nerve should be decompressed several millimeters distal and proximal to the area of involvement. In cases of cholesteatoma invasion of the fallopian canal, all cholesteatoma must be removed to relieve pressure on the facial nerve. Intraoperative facial nerve monitoring may supply meaningful information.

Otic Capsule Fistula

The endosteal bone that forms the otic capsule is subject to damage from an inflammatory process that is engendered by infection or more typically, by cholesteatoma. A fistula arises when the endosteal bone layer has been eroded, leaving only the endosteal membrane to separate the perilymphatic space from the infectious or cholesteatomatous process in the middle ear

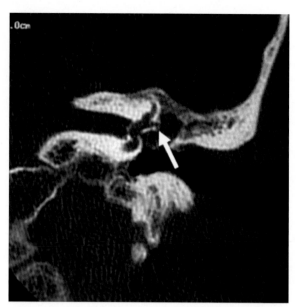

Figure 19–3 Lateral semicircular canal erosion. In this coronal CT scan of the temporal bone, the endosteal bone covering the lateralmost aspect of the lateral semicircular canal (white arrow) has been eroded by an epitympanic cholesteatoma.

(**Fig. 19–3**).[25] The lateral semicircular canal is more frequently involved than the superior or posterior semicircular canals; the cochlea is rarely involved. The incidence of otic capsule fistula in the setting of chronic otitis media is 3.6 to 12.9%.[26–28]

Patients who develop otic capsule fistulas typically present with dizziness and a chronically draining ear. Interestingly, the severity of symptoms depends on the rate of change in the size of the fistula rather than the absolute size of the fistula.[29] A fistula test can be performed, although studies have suggested that this test is not highly sensitive or reliable. In a positive fistula test, positive pressure applied to the middle ear with a pneumatic otoscope results in nystagmus toward the ipsilateral ear. When the pressure is reversed, the nystagmus also reverses, and its fast component is directed toward the contralateral ear. Positive and negative pressures applied to the middle ear induce ampullopetal and ampullofugal movement of the endolymph, respectively (in the lateral semicircular canal), resulting in perception of rotation and resultant nystagmus. Otic capsule fistulas involving the superior or posterior semicircular canals respond to fistula tests with pure vertical or complex nystagmus. The fistula test can be falsely positive with an abnormally mobile stapes. If the labyrinth is not functional, the fistula test can be falsely negative.

A patient in whom an otic capsule fistula is suspected should undergo a CT scan of the temporal bone. The scan, in addition to suggesting the presence of cholesteatoma, is often useful in identifying an otic capsule fistula. Surgical treatment of an otic capsule fistula focuses on leaving the cholesteatoma matrix intact over the site of the fistula until the entire middle ear has been explored and cleared of cholesteatoma. Once attention is directed back to the fistula, its size should be assessed. For fistulas less than 2 mm in diameter, the cholesteatoma often can be removed without violating the membranous labyrinth. Once the fistula has been exposed, it is quickly repaired with a tissue seal such as a fascia or vein graft. Fistulas greater than 2 mm typically are left with the protective cholesteatoma matrix intact.[23] This is best

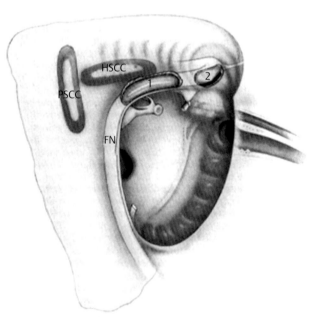

Figure 19–2 Typical sites of facial nerve (FN) erosion by cholesteatoma and otitis media. The posterior portion of the tympanic segment and the second genu (1) and the anterior portion of the tympanic segment near the first genu (2) are most commonly affected. HSCC, horizontal semicircular canal; PSCC, posterior semicircular canal. (From Selesnick SH, Jackler RK. Facial paralysis in suppurative ear disease operative techniques. Otolaryngol Head Neck Surg 1992;3:61–68. Reprinted by permission.)

performed with a canal-wall-down mastoidectomy procedure. Cochlear fistulas are not explored to avoid complete sensorineural hearing loss, vertigo, and development of a dead ear. Even with care, sensorineural hearing loss after removal of cholesteatoma matrix from large fistulas can occur as frequently as 56% of the time.[26]

Suppurative Labyrinthitis

Suppurative labyrinthitis is an uncommon complication of chronic otitis media or mastoiditis that results from bacterial invasion of the inner ear via either the round or oval window or through a labyrinthine fistula created by cholesteatoma.[30] Initially, as bacterial toxins enter the inner ear, the labyrinth becomes irritated and hyperactive with ensuing nystagmus toward the infected ear. As bacteria enter the middle ear and frank purulence develops, the neuroepithelium of the inner ear becomes irreversibly damaged and inner ear function is lost. At this point, spontaneous nystagmus shifts away from the infected ear toward the opposite side. The onset of suppurative labyrinthitis is characterized by sudden profound sensorineural hearing loss and severe vertigo. Additionally, patients with suppurative labyrinthitis suffer from severe nausea and vomiting, falling away from the affected ear, and past-pointing. Because perilymph is directly continuous with the cerebrospinal fluid (CSF), meningitis often ensues via the cochlear aqueduct.

Treatment consists of intravenous antibiotics and surgical drainage of purulence from the middle ear as well as debridement of granulomatous tissue or cholesteatoma. Restoration of labyrinthine and cochlear function is not a concern as the inner ear damage is permanent. Rather, control and eradication of the infectious process is paramount to avert meningitis, which often presents with the classic signs of headache, fever, photophobia, and obtundation.

Petrous Apicitis

Petrous apex air cells exist in approximately 30% of normal temporal bones.[13] Pneumatization of petrous apex air cells typically occurs by two routes: anterior and posterior (**Fig. 19–4**). The anterior or apical air cells lie in three general areas corresponding to three pneumatization tracts: (1) the hypotympanic tract, (2) the peritubal tract, and (3) the perilabyrinthine tract (see Chapter 1). The posterior or perilabyrinthine air cells are divided into two areas of pneumatization: the supralabyrinthine and infralabyrinthine tracts.[31,32] In cases of chronic otitis media or mastoiditis, the air cells of the petrous apex—like those of the mastoid—are subject to extension of inflammation and infection from the middle ear. As in mastoiditis, advancement of the disease process occurs by local extension through areas of bony erosion or by thrombophlebitic spread.

Petrositis presents with a triad of symptoms first described by Gradenigo[33] in 1904: retro-orbital pain, purulent otorrhea, and diplopia secondary to lateral rectus palsy. Irritation of the fifth cranial nerve within Meckel's cave can cause retro-orbital pain as well as a more generalized trigeminal neuralgia. Lateral rectus dysfunction is a result of inflammation of the sixth cranial nerve as it passes through Dorello's canal between the petrous bone and the petroclinoid ligament. Other symptoms associated with petrositis include fever, vertigo, hearing loss, and facial nerve dysfunction. Meningismus suggests intracranial extension of the infectious process.

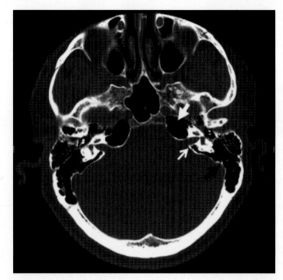

Figure 19–4 Pneumatization of the petrous apex air cells. In this axial CT scan through the petrous apex of the temporal bones, anterior (thick white arrow) and posterior (thin white arrow) petrous apex air cells are well pneumatized and easily visualized. Perisinus mastoid air cells are also well pneumatized (black arrow).

Petrous apicitis is treated with intravenous antibiotics and surgical decompression and drainage of the petrous apex. A low threshold for surgical intervention must be maintained, as infection in the petrous apex has no natural route of drainage and thus has a greater likelihood of eroding through the confines of the petrous bone to involve the middle cranial fossa, the posterior cranial fossa, or the cavernous sinus. Surgical approaches to the petrous apex are as varied as the pneumatization tracts of the petrous apex air cells. Posterior approaches for the hearing ear include decompression through the (1) subarcuate tracts (through the superior semicircular canal),[34] (2) tracts along the sinodural angle (posterior to the superior semicircular canal and superior to the lateral semicircular canal), and (3) the infralabyrinthine tracts.[35] Anterior approaches can be made along (4) infracochlear tracts[34] as well as (5) tracts anterior to the cochlea between the carotid artery and the middle fossa dura.[36] Surgical management of petrous apicitis includes a complete mastoidectomy, skeletonization of the semicircular canals, and exploration of all suspicious petrous air cell tracts. If the patient is deaf, a translabyrinthine approach offers the widest decompression.

Extratemporal Extension

The mucosal inflammation, fluid and pus collection, and bony destruction of mastoiditis can extend within and even out of the temporal bone via several routes. Most commonly, necrosis and demineralization of the mastoid bone allow for direct extension of the infectious process. Disease also can spread through healthy intact bone by thrombophlebitic or hematogenous dissemination. In cases of extratemporal extension, the surgeon also should be suspicious of concurrent intracranial complications.

Subperiosteal Abscess

First described by Bezold[37] in 1908, the subperiosteal abscess represents lateral extension of acute mastoiditis through the thin bone of the lateral mastoid cortex typically superior to the insertion of the sternocleidomastoid muscle. The pinna is displaced anteriorly, inferiorly, and laterally, resulting in proptosis of the ear. Examination of the postauricular soft tissue reveals edema, erythema, and a deep fluctuance. Treatment of the subperiosteal abscess is surgical drainage via a postauricular incision and a simple mastoidectomy. In this case, pus is encountered upon incising the periosteum superficial to the mastoid bone. A myringotomy also is performed, and the patient is treated with intravenous antibiotics.

Zygomatic Abscess

Rarely, extension of acute mastoiditis anteriorly via anterior air cells can lead to infectious involvement of the root of the zygoma. Perforation can occur anteriorly under the lower edge of the temporalis muscle, resulting in soft tissue edema and erythema of the cheek anterior to the ear. Surgical management of a zygomatic abscess involves a cortical mastoidectomy to access and remove the anterior mastoid air cells and drainage of the facial abscess, if possible, via the postauricular incision.

Bezold's Abscess

Also described by Bezold[37] at the beginning of the twentieth century was extension of acute mastoiditis inferiorly to the mastoid tip. Perforation of the mastoid tip medial to the insertion of the sternocleidomastoid muscle results in the infectious process extending into the digastric groove and into deep neck spaces including the parapharyngeal space, the carotid sheath, and the retropharyngeal space. Unabated infection can extend into the mediastinum via the so-called danger space. Patients with Bezold's abscesses usually present with diffuse edema of the lower mastoid area as well as a fluctuant neck mass. Surgical management includes drainage of the neck collection as well as cortical mastoidectomy with exenteration of air cells inferiorly to the mastoid tip. Careful identification and preservation of the facial nerve must be performed as the mastoid tip is approached. The neck must then be explored, and all involved deep neck spaces drained.

Cervical/Postauricular Fistula

Once the suppurative process of acute mastoiditis has eroded through its bony confines, it may extend through the soft tissue to the surface of the skin, forming a fistulous tract. A mastoid periosteal abscess may evolve into a postauricular fistula. Rarely, the deep neck space infection of Bezold's abscess can migrate to the skin surface and present as a cervical fistula. During surgical treatment of a postauricular or cervical fistula, the bony involvement is addressed with a simple mastoidectomy, any neck collection is drained, and the fistula is excised completely.

Extramastoid Cholesteatoma

Cholesteatoma represents cystic growth of keratinizing epithelium accompanied by an inflammatory process that is not necessarily infectious in nature but can demineralize and erode through the bony septa of the mastoid air cells as well as the lateral mastoid cortex. Therefore, extramastoid extension of a cholesteatoma should be considered an extramastoid complication of otitis media.[38] The cholesteatoma must be exenterated from all involved areas. As with the mastoidectomy for Bezold's abscess, the facial nerve must be identified and preserved as cholesteatoma is removed from areas near the mastoid tip.

◆ Intracranial Complications

In the antibiotic era, intracranial complications of otitis media are quite rare. A 1995 review of 24,321 patients reported an intracranial complication rate of 0.36%.[39] Nevertheless, intracranial involvement, when it does occur, can be quite devastating; the same review reported a mortality rate of 18.4% in those patients who developed intracranial complications. Therefore, signs of meningismus or symptoms suggestive of intracranial pathology must be carefully noted particularly after antibiotic therapy has already begun.

Meningitis

Meningitis is the most common intracranial complication of otitis media. Middle ear infections can progress to the brain by several routes: direct extension through bone eroded by inflammatory processes, through preformed pathways via the round window and the cochlear aqueduct, or by thrombophlebitic spread. Because these routes involve infection of intermediate areas between the inner ear and the meninges (i.e., mastoid air cells), meningitis rarely occurs in the absence of another preexisting complication of otitis media.

Early meningitis presents as fever and persistent headache. As the disease progresses, patients may develop photophobia, lethargy, irritability, and neck stiffness. Patients with fully established disease become obtunded and develop seizure activity. Physical examination is often marked by a positive Kernig's or Brudzinski's sign. Kernig's sign is the inability to extend the leg when the thigh is flexed against the abdomen. Brudzinski's sign is the involuntary flexion of the hips and knees when the neck is flexed.

A magnetic resonance image (MRI) of the brain with gadolinium contrast is the optimal imaging tool to confirm the diagnosis by meningeal enhancement. MRI scans also can identify the suppurative focus from which the meningitis arose as well as other intracranial complications of otitis media such as abscess formation or lateral sinus thrombosis. A lumbar puncture (LP) must be performed to establish the diagnosis as well as to determine the offending organism(s). An LP is performed only after the MRI shows no abscess or hydrocephalus. Typically, an LP shows elevated opening pressure, elevated protein level, pleocytosis, and low glucose level. Bacterial cultures of the CSF most commonly yield *H. influenzae* type B and *S. pneumoniae*. *S. pyogenes*, *Staphylococcus epidermidis*, and *S. aureus* also can be found. Meningitis secondary to chronic otitis media may yield gram-negative or anaerobic bacteria.

Treatment of bacterial meningitis begins with stabilization of the patient and initiation of broad-spectrum intravenous antibiotics. Once the meningitic infection has been controlled, the suppurative focus must be surgically removed. Because otogenic meningitis rarely occurs in the absence of other complications of otitis media (e.g., mastoiditis, labyrinthitis, or petrous apicitis), concomitant complications need to be surgically addressed as well.

Brain Abscess

Brain abscesses typically arise from hematogenous or thrombophlebitic extension of extradural infections. The development of a brain abscess usually occurs over the course of several days to several weeks. Initially, inflammation and edema of the white matter surrounding the infected vasculature manifests as encephalitis. The clinical presentation is very similar to that of meningitis including persistent headache, moderate fever, chills, nausea, vomiting, neck stiffness, and altered mental status. An intermediate, quiescent phase ensues as the inflammatory process attempts to contain and encapsulate the focus of encephalitis by means of reactive gliosis. If successfully contained, the focus of infection may respond to antibiotics and be resorbed without need for surgical intervention. More frequently, infection progresses to an expanding granulomatous lesion with central necrosis and abscess formation. At this point, focal neurologic defects become apparent as the expanding abscess and its surrounding edema compress the brain. Although abscesses can occur anywhere in the brain, they are typically found in the ipsilateral temporal lobe or cerebellum.

Treatment of a brain abscess includes intravenous antibiotics and a combined otologic and neurologic surgical procedure. Neurosurgical drainage of the abscess is done concomitantly with otologic decompression and debridement of the suppurative focus within the temporal bone. Occasionally, in patients with severe symptoms, neurosurgical drainage and neurologic stabilization must be completed first, followed by the otologic procedure after the patient is stable.

Subdural Empyema

Subdural empyema is a collection of purulence between the dura mater and the arachnoid mater. Like brain abscesses, subdural empyemas can be seeded through thrombophlebitic spread; however, direct extension through bone also can occur. Subdural empyemas are rare complications of otitis media, occurring more commonly as complications of frontal or ethmoid sinusitis.[40] Because a subdural empyema collects in an already-existing space, the infection progresses more rapidly than a brain abscess, and can extend throughout the subdural space until limited by specific boundaries such as the falx cerebri, tentorium cerebelli, and base of the brain. Initial symptoms can be mild and nonspecific such as fever, headache, and general malaise. As the infection progresses, however, signs of meningitis become apparent. Eventually, expansion of the empyema can compress the brain, leading to focal neurologic signs such as aphasia, hemianopsia, hemiplegia, or cranial nerve palsies.

Diagnosis of subdural empyema can be made by either CT scan or MRI scan. Treatment entails intravenous antibiotics, neurosurgical drainage of the empyema, and otologic surgical management of the middle ear and mastoid disease.

Epidural Abscess

Epidural abscess results from direct superior, posterior, or medial extension of coalescent mastoiditis through eroded bone into the middle or posterior fossa. In the middle fossa, purulence collects between the dura mater and the thin bony plate of the tegmen. Posterior fossa collections occur in the posterior petrous pyramid or just superior to the sigmoid

sinus. Perisinus abscesses can predispose the patient to lateral sinus thrombosis.[41]

Many epidural abscesses can be asymptomatic and are identified only during workup for a concomitant disease. Typically intracranial pressure is normal, and no focal neurologic deficits are observed until the abscess grows to a large size. An epidural abscess can readily be identified by MRI or CT (**Fig. 19–5**). Once identified, the abscess can be drained and debrided via a cortical mastoidectomy approach. Management of the disease also includes intravenous antibiotics.

Lateral Sinus Thrombosis

A perisinus abscess can induce a mural thrombus within the lateral (a.k.a. sigmoid) sinus. The mural thrombus then can organize and expand to completely occlude the lateral sinus. Formation of an obliterating thrombus can lead to a multitude of sequelae. The thrombus can extend anterograde to occlude the jugular or subclavian veins. More dangerous, retrograde extension can lead to cavernous sinus thrombosis. In addition, retrograde extension can occlude the torcula herophili, thereby compromising the superior and inferior sagittal sinus drainage pathways and leading ultimately to a thrombotic cerebrovascular accident. Infected thrombus can break off into the systemic circulation resulting in septic embolization. Obliterating thrombus also can predispose the affected vessels to perforation and subsequent hemorrhage.

Lateral sinus thrombosis typically presents with low-grade, intermittent fever that can progress to a spiking, picket-fence pattern secondary to the dissemination of septic emboli into the systemic circulation.[42] Torticollis and neck tenderness also are common particularly along the course of the internal jugular vein; occasionally a cord can be palpated within the internal jugular vein. *Griesinger's sign*, or edema of the lateral mastoid soft tissue, may be observed secondary to thrombosis

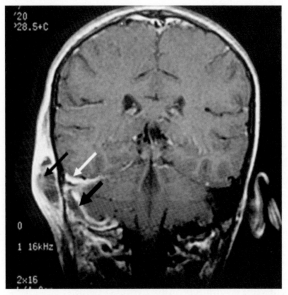

Figure 19–5 Perisinus epidural abscess. This contrast-enhanced coronal T1-weighted magnetic resonance image demonstrates multiple intracranial complications of mastoiditis including focal meningitis (white arrow), lateral sinus thrombosis (thick black arrow), and perisinus epidural abscess (thin black arrow).

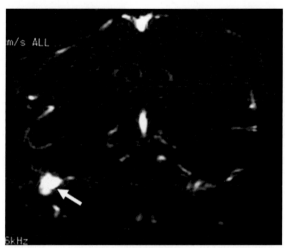

Figure 19–6 Lateral sinus thrombosis. This magnetic resonance venogram demonstrates left-sided lateral sinus thrombosis. Note the enhancement consistent with flow in the right lateral sinus (white arrow) but absence of enhancement in the left lateral sinus.

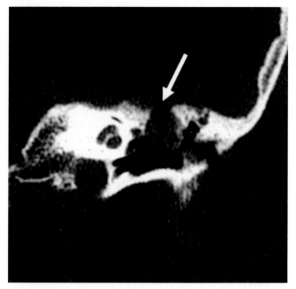

Figure 19–7 Erosion of the tegmen tympani. This coronal CT scan of the temporal bone demonstrates erosion of the tegmen tympani by an epitympanic cholesteatoma.

of a mastoid emissary vein. Less commonly, extension of the thrombus to the jugular bulb may cause palsies of cranial nerves IX, X, and XI.

Diagnosis of lateral sinus thrombosis can be made by CT scan or MRI scan.[43] A magnetic resonance venogram (MRV) can be particularly helpful in showing the degree of thrombus extension within the venous system (**Fig. 19–6**). Additionally, diagnosis can be suggested by characteristic CSF pressure findings. Normally, CSF pressure, as measured by spinal needle in the subarachnoid space, increases when the internal jugular vein is compressed. The lack of increase in CSF pressure during compression of the internal jugular vein ipsilateral to a thrombosed lateral sinus is termed a positive *Queckenstedt test.*

Lateral sinus thrombosis is treated with intravenous antibiotics and surgical decompression and evacuation of the sinus. A complete mastoidectomy is performed with exposure of the lateral sinus as well as the diseased dura. All granulation tissue and infectious debris must be removed. The sinus is then aspirated with a large-bore needle. If frank pus is obtained, the sinus is then opened and as much thrombus as possible is evacuated. Ligation of the internal jugular vein is controversial and is reserved for cases where septic emboli persist despite surgical management.[41] The role of anticoagulation also is controversial; though theoretically indicated, the efficacy remains to be determined.

Otitic Hydrocephalus

Otitic hydrocephalus is a rare complication of otitis media that is often associated with lateral sinus thrombosis. Its pathophysiology is poorly understood. One hypothesis suggests that a meningitic process may interfere with arachnoid granulations and reabsorption of CSF into the subarachnoid space, resulting in elevation of intracranial pressure (ICP) in a manner consistent with a communicating hydrocephalus.[44]

Symptoms and signs include headache, vomiting, papilledema, visual disturbance, cranial nerve VI palsy due to stretch, and mental status changes. MRI of the brain typically shows a normal ventricular size, but LP reveals increased ICP.

Treatment of otitic hydrocephalus includes management of the middle ear and mastoid disease that is the source of the hydrocephalus—with intravenous antibiotics and possible surgical debridement. Treatment is also directed toward relief of the elevated ICP: steroid therapy, diuretics, hyperosmolar agents, and, as a last resort, decompression of CSF by serial LP or ventriculostomy.

Meningoencephalocele

Herniation of the brain inferiorly into the mastoid cavity can occur when the integrity of the tegmen has been compromised. Tegmen compromise can occur by multiple mechanisms including congenital dehiscence, erosion by a chronically infected middle ear mucosa or cholesteatoma (**Fig. 19–7**), or injury from a previous mastoidectomy. A meningoencephalocele can be asymptomatic, although it more commonly is associated with CSF otorrhea or rhinorrhea. Herniated brain tissue is nonfunctional. CT scan of the temporal bone best identifies the bony defect of the tegmen and the herniating tissue. Treatment consists of surgical exploration of the mastoid cavity, removal of herniated tissue, and repair of the tegmen.[45,46] If the bony deficit is <1.0 cm and localized to the tegmen mastoideum, it can sometimes be approached via a mastoidectomy and reinforced with tissue grafts such as abdominal fat. If the bony deficit is >1.0 cm or localized to the epitympanic tegmen, a combined mastoidectomy and middle fossa approach is used to repair the tegmen.

◆ Conclusion

The advent of antibiotic therapy has significantly decreased the incidence of complications of otitis media. Delays in initial diagnosis of otitis media, current trends toward decreasing the use of antibiotics for initial therapy of otitis media, and the development of antibiotic-resistant bacteria all may contribute to recent observations of slight increases in complication rates of otitis media. Thus, the otolaryngologist must be increasingly vigilant and prepared for the diagnosis and management of these complications.

References

1. Teele DW, Klein JO, Rosner BA. Epidemiology of otitis media during the first seven years of life in children in Greater Boston: a prospective, cohort study. J Infect Dis 1989;160:83–94

2. Block SL, Harrison CJ, Hedrick J, Tyler R, Smith A, Hedrick R. Restricted use of antibiotic prophylaxis for recurrent acute otitis media in the era of penicillin non-susceptible *Streptococcus pneumoniae*. Int J Pediatr Otorhinolaryngol 2001;61:47–60

3. Subcommittee on Management of Acute Otitis Media. Diagnosis and management of acute otitis media. Pediatrics 2004;113:1451–1465

4. Hoppe JE, Koster S, Bootz F, Niethammer D. Acute mastoiditis—relevant once again. Infection 1994;22:178–182

5. Van Zuijlen DA, Schilder AG, Van Balen FA, Hoes AW. National differences in incidence of acute mastoiditis: relationship to prescribing patterns of antibiotics for acute otitis media. Pediatr Infect Dis J 2001;20:140–144

6. Shambaugh GE, Glasscock ME. Surgery of the Ear. Philadelphia: WB Saunders, 1980:195–199

7. Hawkins DB, Dru D, House JW, Clark RW. Acute mastoiditis in chidren: a review of 54 cases. Laryngoscope 1983;93:568–572

8. Zapalac JS, Billings KR, Schwade ND, Roland PS. Suppurative complications of acute otitis media in the era of antibiotic resistance. Arch Otolaryngol Head Neck Surg 2002;128:660–663

9. Nussinovitch M, Yoeli R, Elishkevitz K, Varsano I. Acute mastoiditis in children: epidemiologic, clinical, microbiologic, and therapeutic aspects over past years. Clin Pediatr (Phila) 2004;43:261–267

10. Mygind H. Subperiosteal abscess of the mastoid region. Ann Otol Rhinol Laryngol 1910;19:259

11. Ghaffar FA, Wordemann M, McCracken GH Jr. Acute mastoiditis in children: a seventeen-year experience in Dallas, Texas. Pediatr Infect Dis J 2001;20:376–380

12. House HP, Crabtree JA. Mastoiditis. In: Maloney WH, ed. Otolaryngology. Hagerstown, MD: Harper & Row, 1967

13. Gulya AJ, Glasscock ME III, eds. Surgery of the Ear. Philadelphia: BC Decker, 2002

14. Gliklich RE, Eavey RD, Iannuzzi RA, Camacho AE. A contemporary analysis of acute mastoiditis. Arch Otolaryngol Head Neck Surg 1996;122:135–139

15. English GM, Northern JL, Fria TJ. Chronic otitis media as a cause of sensorineural hearing loss. Arch Otolaryngol 1973;98:18–22

16. Goycoolea MV, Paparella MM, Juhn SK, Carmpenter AM. Oval and round window changes in otitis media. Potential pathways between middle and inner ear. Laryngoscope 1980;90:1387–1391

17. Paparella MM, Oda M, Hiraide F, Brady D. Pathology of sensorineural hearing loss in otitis media. Ann Otol Rhinol Laryngol 1972;81:632–647

18. Takumida M, Anniko M. Localization of endotoxin in the inner ear following inoculation into the middle ear. Acta Otolaryngol 2004;124:772–777

19. Cureoglu S, Schachern PA, Paparella MM, Lindgren BR. Cochlear changes in chronic otitis media. Laryngoscope 2004;114:622–626

20. Walby AP, Berrera A, Schuknecht HF. Cochlear pathology in chronic suppurative otitis media. Ann Otol Rhinol Laryngol Suppl 1983;103:1–19

21. Fisch U. Current surgical treatment of intratemporal facial palsy. Clin Plast Surg 1979;6:377–388

22. Antoli-Candela F Jr, Stewart TJ. The pathophysiology of otologic facial paralysis. Otolaryngol Clin North Am 1974;7:309–330

23. Popovtzer A, Raveh E, Bahar G, Oestreicher-Kedem Y, Feinmesser R, Nageris BI. Facial palsy associated with acute otitis media. Otolaryngol Head Neck Surg 2005;132:327–329

24. Selesnick SH, Jackler RK. Facial paralysis in suppurative ear disease. Operative techniques. Otolaryngol Head Neck Surg 1992;3:61–68

25. Gacek RR. The surgical management of labyrinthine fistulae in chronic otitis media with cholesteatoma. Ann Otol Rhinol Laryngol 1974;83:1–19

26. Palva T, Kårjå J, Palva A. Opening of the labyrinth during chronic ear surgery. Arch Otolaryngol Head Neck Surg 1971;93:75–78

27. Sanna M, Zini C, Gamoletti R, Taibah AK, Russo A, Scandellari R. Closed versus open technique in the management of labyrinthine fistula. Am J Otol 1988;9:470–475

28. Sheehy JL, Brackmann DE. Cholesteatoma surgery: management of the labyrinthine fistula—a report of 97 cases. Laryngoscope 1979;89:78–87

29. Dawes JDK, Watson RT. Labyrinthine fistulae. J Laryngol Otol 1978;92:83–98

30. Schuknecht HF. Pathology of the Ear. Philadelphia: Lea & Febiger, 1993

31. Allam AF, Schuknecht HF. Pathology of petrositis. Laryngoscope 1968;78:1813–1832

32. Allam AF. Pneumatization of the temporal bone. Ann Otol Rhinol Laryngol 1969;78:49–64

33. Gradenigo G. Ueber circumscripte leptomeningitis mit spinalen symptomen. Arch Ohrenheilk 1904;51:60–62

34. Freckner P. Some remarks on the treatment of apicitis (petrositis) with or without Gradenigo's syndrome. Acta Otolaryngol (Stockh) 1932;17:97

35. Farrior JB. Anterior hypotympanic approach for glomus tumor of the infratemporal fossa. Laryngoscope 1984;94:1016–1021

36. Lempert J. Complete apicectomy (mastoidotympanoapicectomy). Arch Otolaryngol Head Neck Surg 1937;25:144

37. Bezold F, Siebenmann F. Textbook of Otology (Holinger J, trans.). Chicago: EH Cosgrove, 1908:208

38. Luetje CM. Extramastoid cholesteatoma in chronic ear disease: a report of two cases. Laryngoscope 1979;89:1755–1759

39. Kangsanarak J, Navacharoen N, Fooanant S, Ruchphaopunt K. Intracranial complications of suppurative otitis media: 13 years' experience. Am J Otol 1995;16:104–109

40. Bernardini GL. Diagnosis and management of brain abscess and subdural empyema. Curr Neurol Neurosci Rep 2004;4:448–456

41. Cummings CW, Frederickson JM, Harker LA, Krause CJ, Shuller DE, Richardson MA. Otolaryngology Head and Neck Surgery. St. Louis: Mosby, 1998

42. Teichgraeber JF, Per-Lee JH, Turner JS. Lateral sinus thrombosis: modern perspective. Laryngoscope 1982;92:744–751

43. Hulcelle PJ, Dooms GC, Mathurin P, Cornelis G. MRI assessment of unsuspected dural sinus thrombosis. Neuroradiology 1989;31:217–221

44. Hughes GB. Complications of otitis media. In: Hughes GB, Pensak ML, eds. Clinical Otology. New York & Stuttgart: Thieme, 1997

45. Glasscock ME, Dickens JRE, Jackson CG, Wiet RJ, Feenstra L. Surgical management of brain tissue herniation into the middle ear and mastoid. Laryngoscope 1979;89:1743–1754

46. Graham MD. Surgical management of dural and termporal bone herniation into the radical mastoid cavity. Laryngoscope 1982;92:329–331

20

Otosclerosis

Michael J. McKenna and Ronald K. de Venecia

Otosclerosis is a bone disease that is unique to the human temporal bone.[1] One of the most common causes of acquired hearing loss, otosclerosis has a well-established hereditary predisposition, with about 50% of affected individuals having other known affected family members.[2] Otosclerosis occurs within the endochondral layer of the temporal bone, usually in certain sites of predilection that are associated with globuli interossei or so-called embryonic rests. The most common site of occurrence of otosclerosis is the fissula ante fenestram just anterior to the stapes footplate.[3,4] As the lesion enlarges and spreads, it encroaches on the stapes footplate and produces a conductive hearing loss (clinical otosclerosis). In some cases, the lesion may spread to involve the cochlea and result in an irreversible sensorineural hearing loss (SNHL).[5,6] However, the majority of lesions do not encroach on the footplate or cochlea; such lesions remain small and asymptomatic (histologic otosclerosis).[7] The small histologic foci are 10-fold more common than the larger lesions that result in clinical manifestations.[8] Despite intensive investigation, the etiology of otosclerosis remains unknown.

◆ Pathology

Histopathologically, the otosclerotic process is characterized by a wave of abnormal bone remodeling, resulting in the replacement of otic capsule bone with a hypercellular woven bone, which may undergo further remodeling, resulting in a mosaic sclerotic appearance. The initial remodeling process consists predominantly of mononuclear cells, including histiocytes and bone cells, many of which show degeneration with cellular lysis and release of cytoplastic contents.[9] There is a distinct absence of acute inflammatory cells.[10] Although the most common site of predilection is the fissula ante fenestram that lies in close proximity to the anterior portion of the stapes footplate, otosclerosis also may occur in other sites including the round window, sometimes resulting in round window obliteration. The degree of stapes footplate involvement from otosclerosis is highly variable. In the majority of cases, otosclerosis results in anterior stapes fixation without involvement of the posterior footplate or the posterior annular ligament. In

many cases, as the otosclerotic process begins to develop anterior to the footplate, the footplate becomes posteriorly displaced. This results in a jamming of the posterior footplate within the oval window and the development of a low-frequency conductive hearing loss[11,12] (**Fig. 20–1**). With bony fixation of the footplate, there is conductive hearing loss across all frequencies. This has long been recognized by stapes surgeons, who often were reluctant to operate on patients without a negative Rinne at 512- and 1024-Hz (bone conduction louder than air conduction) prior to the advent of the laser. These patients had a higher risk for footplate mobilization or a floating footplate upon down-fracture of the stapes superstructure. In some cases, the otosclerotic lesion may overgrow the footplate, resulting in obliterative otosclerosis. It is not possible to differentiate between obliterative otosclerosis and bony ankylosis of the footplate without oval window obliteration on audiometric testing alone.

Large active otosclerotic lesions that involve the cochlear capsule and penetrate the cochlear endosteum can result in a progressive SNHL.[7,13] Until recently, there was no clear explanation for the cause of the SNHL in these patients. Temporal bone studies have failed to demonstrate a loss of sensory cells, both hair cells and spiral ganglion cells, in proportion to the degree of SNHL.[14,15] The only pathologic correlation between SNHL and otosclerosis has been the penetration of the cochlear endosteum with hyalinization of the spiral ligament.[16] Recent investigations have revealed that the spiral ligament is a dynamic organ that plays an important role in maintaining normal cochlear physiology. It plays a critical role in the recirculation of potassium ions within the cochlea.[17,18] Disturbance of this function is one plausible explanation that can account for the degree of SNHL that occurs in these patients.

When a careful history is taken, between 10% and 20% of patients relate symptoms of dizziness or vertigo.[19] The symptoms are highly variable, ranging from benign paroxysmal positional vertigo, to waxing and waning disequilibrium, to vertigo of Meniere's type. In some cases, although uncommon, otosclerosis may involve the endolymphatic duct, resulting in hydrops and symptoms of Meniere's disease. This is important to recognize, as this is an absolute contraindication for stapedectomy, as hydrops may result in saccular dilatation, predisposing the

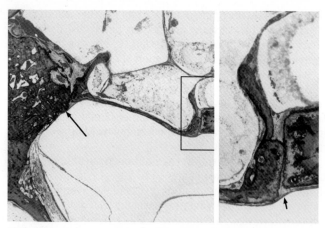

Figure 20–1 Fixation of the footplate by an anterior focus of otosclerosis (large arrow). The otosclerotic process also has resulted in posterior displacement of the footplate. Inset: Higher magnification view of the posterior footplate, which has become jammed against the bony annulus (small arrow).

membranous labyrinth to injury upon fenestration of the footplate. For reasons that are unclear, some patients who have a history of giddiness or waxing and waning disequilibrium without true vertigo experience an improvement in their vestibular symptoms following stapedectomy.[20]

◆ Etiology

Although the precise etiology of otosclerosis has yet to be elucidated, significant progress has been made over the past 20 years. Fundamentally, otosclerosis is an active remodeling process of bone that occurs within the endochondral layer of the temporal bone that under normal circumstances undergoes virtually no remodeling following development.[21,22] In this respect, the otic capsule is unique and different from all other bones in the body. To understand why this abnormal remodeling process occurs in the first place, it is important to first understand why the otic capsule is devoid of postdevelopmental remodeling. Sorensen et al[23,24] have studied otic capsule remodeling in several species and have shown that remodeling in the otic capsule is markedly inhibited compared with other bones and that this inhibition is most prevalent in direct proximity to the inner ear. These studies have led to the hypothesis that the inner ear itself may play a direct role in the inhibition of otic capsule remodeling by producing substances that diffuse into the surrounding bone and prevent remodeling. We have recently discovered that the spiral ligament produces a compound called osteoprotegerin (OPG), which is secreted into the perilymph and diffuses into the surrounding otic capsule bone.[25] OPG is a potent inhibitor of bone remodeling. It acts by inhibiting the recruitment, formation, and activity of osteoclasts, which resorb bone. Knockout mice that lack OPG have active otic capsule remodeling that closely resembles otosclerosis.[26] We suspect that there are other factors involved in the inhibition of otic capsule remodeling other than OPG, although as of yet they have not been clearly defined.

One hypothesis that has gained considerable support over the past 15 years is that otosclerosis may be related to a persistent measles virus infection within the otic capsule.[27]

The evidence to support this hypothesis includes the demonstration of (1) viral-like particles within osteoblasts and preosteoblasts in active otosclerotic lesions by electron microscopy, (2) measles antigens within active lesions using immunohistochemical techniques, and (3) measles virus gene products in active otosclerotic lesions using reverse transcription/polymerase chain reaction techniques.[28–35] This hypothesis would account for the fact that otosclerosis appears to involve only the human otic capsule, as measles virus affects only humans and closely related primates. It would also account for the significant decline in incidence of new cases of otosclerosis, which is well correlated with the measles virus vaccination.[36,37]

Otosclerosis is most common among whites, uncommon among Asians, and extremely rare in blacks. Otosclerosis is estimated to occur histologically in 10% of the white population and results in hearing loss in 0.5%.[6] The clinical prevalence of otosclerosis is estimated to be twice as common in females as in males.[38]

Familial aggregation of individuals affected by otosclerosis has been recognized for many years.[39,40] Most studies support a pattern of autosomal dominant transmission with incomplete penetrance in the range of 20 to 40%.[41] The most compelling evidence for an underlying genetic cause for otosclerosis comes from studies on monozygotic twins with clinical otosclerosis, in which concordance has been found in nearly all cases.[42] However, information does not exist on the genetic transmission of histologic otosclerosis. It is not known whether the genetic basis of inheritance is related to the formation of an otosclerosis focus within the temporal bone or the tendency for a lesion to progress once it has begun, or both. Most studies on families with otosclerosis support a pattern of autosomal dominant transmission with incomplete penetrance. A study of 65 pedigrees with otosclerosis in Tunisia suggests that otosclerosis is primarily heterogenetic, and in 13% of clinical cases studied, affected individuals who carry a dominant gene with nearly complete penetrance.[43] Linkage analyses of large and unrelated families have revealed linkage to distinctly different loci, indicating that otosclerosis is heterogenetic.[44–48] The otosclerosis phenotype may result from several different gene defects. Each of the families that have been studied thus far is atypical in that the penetrance is nearly complete, with approximately half of all individuals in each family being affected. Although a strong familial component exists, several studies have reported that sporadic otosclerosis represents 40 to 50% of all clinical cases.

There is evidence to suggest that some cases of otosclerosis may be related to defects in expression of the *COL1A1* gene. Association analysis using multiple polymorphic markers has revealed a significant association between both familial and sporadic cases of clinical otosclerosis and the *COL1A1* gene.[49,50] The association has been found to increase from the 3' to the 5' region of the gene. Studies of the allelic expression of the *COL1A1* gene in patients with clinical otosclerosis have revealed reduced expression of one *COL1A1* allele in some cases, similar to that which has been described in many cases of type I osteogenesis imperfecta.[51,52] Type I osteogenesis imperfecta shares both clinical and histologic similarities with otosclerosis. Approximately half of all patients with type I osteogenesis imperfecta develop hearing loss that is clinically indistinguishable from otosclerosis. It is also well known that some patients with clinical otosclerosis have blue sclera, a feature that is found in virtually all patients with type I osteogenesis imperfecta.[53] The histopathology of temporal bones from patients with type I osteogenesis imperfecta is identical to that observed in patients with otosclerosis.[54,55]

Although the etiology of otosclerosis is not clearly understood at present, the above studies have brought us much closer to understanding the basic nature of the disease. Otosclerosis is clearly a heterogenetic and possibly a multifactorial disease process. It is fundamentally a disturbance in the physiologic pathways or factors that normally serve to inhibit otic capsule remodeling. As we develop a better understanding of otic capsule physiology and factors that account for its unique absence of remodeling, we will gain a better understanding of the processes that result in abnormal remodeling including otosclerosis.

◆ History of Otosclerosis Surgery

The history of otosclerosis surgery is among the most interesting and colorful chapters in all of otolaryngology. Students of otology are strongly encouraged to read the biography of Howard House, *For the World to Hear,*[56] as it not only chronicles the history of otosclerosis surgery during the last century but also provides insight into the personalities of some of the great leaders in our field. Stapedectomy was first introduced as a treatment for otosclerosis in the late 1800s by Blake and Jack in Boston and shortly thereafter by DeRossi in Italy. Although initial results were encouraging, there were cases of infection that resulted in meningitis and death and led to a condemnation of all stapes surgery by prominent leaders in the field. It was John Shea Jr. in 1956 who, with the benefit of improved instrumentation and employing the operating microscope, reintroduced stapedectomy using a polyethylene strut and vein graft. Although most otologists were skeptical at the time, within 10 years it became widely apparent that stapedectomy was the most reliable and safest technique for the restoration of hearing in patients with otosclerosis and stapes fixation. What followed was one of the most exciting periods in modern otology and occupied much of the agenda of the American Otological Society, including papers and discussions. There has been an evolution in the two fundamental steps of the operation: fenestration of the oval window and introduction of a prosthesis. The fenestration of the oval window evolved from a technique of total stapedectomy with removal of the stapes footplate with micropicks; to partial stapedectomy; to the small fenestra technique, initially using microdrills; and ultimately to the introduction of otologic lasers. Similarly there has been an evolution in the development of prostheses from polyethylene tubes to fat- and gel-wires and ultimately to the piston prostheses of varying sizes and materials. Throughout this period, there have been significant improvements in the operating microscope, including superior optics and brighter illumination. Although it is not clear what the future holds in terms of further technologic innovations, with the advancements in robotic and computer technology, the evolution of stapes surgery will certainly continue.

◆ Diagnosis

History

Most often, otosclerosis results in a gradually progressive, conductive, or mixed hearing loss. In approximately 70% of cases, both ears are affected over time. Typically, onset occurs between the ages of 20 and 40. Juvenile onset is known to occur but is relatively uncommon and warrants further investigation of other possible causes. A progressive, purely SNHL may also occur as a result of cochlear otosclerosis, but this too is relatively rare and warrants investigation of other possible causes. In patients with a past history of infection, other possible causes of the conductive hearing loss need to be considered. A family history of hearing loss can be elicited in many cases. A family history of otosclerosis or another family member who has undergone a successful stapedectomy makes the diagnosis of otosclerosis far more likely.

A history of dizziness or vertigo, although uncommon, is certainly not rare. Approximately 10 to 20% of patients, if questioned, give some past history of vestibular symptoms. The range of vestibular symptoms is highly variable, including positional vertigo, waxing and waning disequilibrium, and severe vertigo of the Meniere's type. Although rare, Meniere's disease may occur in patients with otosclerosis, and it is essential to establish this prior to considering stapedectomy. As mentioned above, stapedectomy in a patient with otosclerosis and Meniere's disease is contraindicated. Some patients with superior canal dehiscence syndrome present with both conductive hearing loss and vestibular symptoms. The conductive hearing loss may closely mimic that seen in otosclerosis.[57] Often these patients complain of severe autophony. A diagnosis of superior canal dehiscence syndrome should be suspected in a patient with a low-frequency conductive hearing loss with bone conduction thresholds that rise above 0 dB. Acoustic reflex testing also is helpful in differentiating otosclerosis from superior semicircular canal dehiscence (SSCD) syndrome as it should be present in SSCD and abnormal in otosclerosis.

Physical Examination

Otoscopic examination usually reveals normal-appearing tympanic membranes. Pneumo-otoscopy with magnification is helpful in both ruling out the presence of a middle ear effusion and assessing malleus mobility. The presence of tympanosclerosis or a retraction pocket should lead to the consideration of conductive hearing loss of other cause. Occasionally, a vascular hue can be seen near the stapes, known as *Schwartze's sign* (**Fig. 20–2**), which is the result of hyperemic middle ear mucosa over an area of active otosclerosis.

Tuning fork tests, both Weber and Rinne at 512 Hz and 1024 Hz, should be performed. The results should be correlated with a complete audiogram.

Audiologic Testing

All patients undergo standard audiometry including pure-tone audiometry with air and bone testing and speech discrimination testing. It is important that true bone conduction thresholds be determined as this may be helpful in differentiating the conductive hearing loss in otosclerosis from that seen in SSCD. Patients with SSCD often demonstrate bone conduction thresholds above 0 dB. If the audiologist stops testing at 0 dB, this will not be appreciated. Until recently we had abandoned stapedial reflex testing as part of the standard audiometric evaluation in patients with conductive hearing loss. However, with the recognition of SSCD as a potential cause for conductive hearing loss and the fact that patients with SSCD have normal acoustic reflex testing, we have begun testing the stapedial reflex in these patients.

Early in the development of conductive hearing loss from otosclerosis, patients typically demonstrate a low-frequency

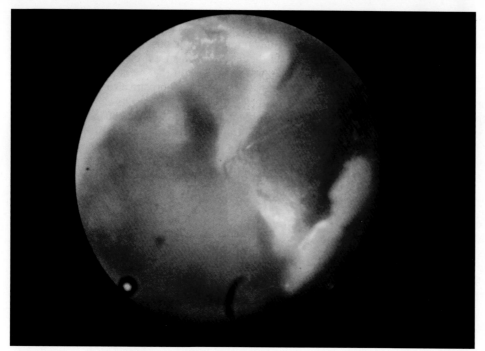

Figure 20–2 Schwartze's sign.

conductive loss that narrows in the high frequencies. This low-frequency conductive loss is related to the posterior displacement of the footplate as a result of an encroaching anterior otosclerotic lesion. The jammed footplate with impaired mobility maintains the capacity for transmission in the higher frequencies. With bony ankylosis of the footplate, the conductive hearing loss flattens across all frequencies.

It is not unusual for patients with otosclerosis and conductive hearing loss to have a depression in the bone conduction thresholds that is most significant at 2000 Hz, termed a *Carhart notch*, which is thought to represent an audiologic artifact, possibly from an affect of stapes fixation on middle ear resonance. It often resolves following a successful stapedectomy. For this reason, it is important that all patients who are tested postoperatively also have both air and bone thresholds tested.

Word recognition scores or speech discrimination is usually normal unless there is a significant sensorineural component to the hearing loss.

◆ Surgical Management by Stapedectomy

Indications

In general there should be a conductive hearing loss of at least 25 dB in frequencies 250 to 1 kHz or higher as determined by both audiometry and the presence of a negative Rinne at 512 Hz (bone > air conduction). The presence of a concomitant SNHL in the affected ear is not necessarily a contraindication for stapes surgery. It does, however, require some thoughtful consideration. If a hearing aid will still be required after successful stapedectomy, the procedure may be considered if it would result in improved performance with amplification. If both ears are involved, generally the poorer hearing ear is operated first. If the operation is a success, the patient may be a candidate for a contralateral stapedectomy after a year has gone by and the hearing in the operated ear has remained stable.

In some cases of advanced otosclerosis it may be difficult on the basis of audiometry to determine whether or not a patient might benefit from a stapedectomy. Often the tuning fork tests are more helpful than the audiogram under such circumstances. Often these patients have very poor speech discrimination scores preoperatively because of an inadequate presentation level, which is at the limit of the audiometer. These patients may demonstrate a dramatic improvement in their speech discrimination following stapedectomy.

Contraindications

Stapedectomy on an only-hearing ear is almost always contraindicated. One exception may be a case of a profound mixed loss, which is beyond the level of benefit of a conventional hearing aid. Such a patient would otherwise be considered a cochlear implant candidate, and a stapedectomy may be considered as the first option prior to proceeding with implantation. Stapedectomy is contraindicated in cases of active infection of the middle ear or external auditory canal. It is also contraindicated in patients with tympanic membrane perforations. Patients in whom vestibular function is absolutely critical for their employment should be given special consideration. Stapedectomy is contraindicated in ears with Meniere's disease and relatively contraindicated in patients with a contralateral otologic problem, which may threaten the hearing in their contralateral ear over time.

Informed Consent

All patients being considered for stapedectomy should be counseled regarding the potential benefits of amplification as a nonsurgical option to help improve their hearing. Patients should be made aware that there is no window of opportunity and that any delay in deciding to proceed with surgery does not impact the eventual result. After describing the details of the surgical procedure in a manner that the patient can easily understand, all of the potential risks should be discussed, including failure of the surgery to improve hearing by virtue of residual conductive hearing loss; creation of a SNHL, either partial or complete; vestibular dysfunction; perforation of the tympanic membrane; facial nerve dysfunction; disturbance in taste; development of a perilymph fistula; and late failure of the procedure. It is prudent to inform all patients to expect some disturbance in taste related to manipulation of the chorda tympani nerve, as this occurs in most cases. Thus the patient will be reassured that this was expected and does not constitute a complication. Nevertheless, this issue deserves further discussion and is included below under Early Postoperative Complications.

Anesthesia

Primary stapedectomy can be performed with either local or general anesthesia. The primary advantage of local anesthesia is the time saved in putting patients to sleep and waking them up. There may be some advantage in monitoring vestibular symptoms, but this is certainly not borne out by differences in results with local and general anesthesia. General anesthesia provides assurance of absolute control of head motion and prevention of pain. In recent times, over half of our patients have selected general anesthesia.

Positioning

The patient is placed in a supine head-hanging position with the head turned to the opposite shoulder. A downward tilt of the head of about 10 to 15 degrees helps bring the ear canal into a straight upright position and places the tympanic membrane in an approximate horizontal plane. A head rest that is separable from the remainder of the operating table is preferred to facilitate appropriate positioning. The headrest is fitted with a fastening mechanism for a self-retaining speculum holder with sufficient degrees of freedom to allow manipulation of the speculum during surgery. The external auditory meatus is injected in four quadrants with 1% Xylocaine with 1:100,000 epinephrine. The bony canal is then injected at 12 o'clock and 6 o'clock with 2% Xylocaine with 1:50,000 epinephrine.

Surgical Technique

Exposure

A posterior tympanomeatal flap is developed such that there is some redundancy in the posterior-superior aspect to cover the area of bone that may be curetted to provide optimal visualization of the oval window (**Fig. 20–3**). Bone is curetted from the posterosuperior portion of the tympanic annulus until both the pyramidal process and the tympanic segment of the facial nerve are easily visualized. Every effort should be made to preserve the chorda tympani nerve unless it severely obstructs access to the oval window niche. The round window is inspected and its patency should be noted in the operative note. The ossicular chain is palpated and the mobility of the malleus, incus, and stapes is established. The incudostapedial joint is separated with a joint knife (**Fig. 20–4**). The stapedial tendon is sectioned with the laser (**Fig. 20–5A**). Any mucosal folds or adhesions are taken down with the laser until the crural arches and footplate are clearly visualized. Using a laser, a posterior crurotomy is accomplished at the junction of the posterior crus and the footplate (**Fig. 20–5B**). If the anterior crus is visualized, this too is divided with the laser

(**Fig. 20–5C**). The superstructure is then down-fractured onto the promontory and removed from the middle ear. It is helpful to remove any remnant of the posterior crus extending above the level of the footplate because it often obstructs introduction of the prosthesis later in the operation. A thick mucous membrane that obscures the footplate also can be coagulated with the laser (**Fig. 20–5D**) to improve its exposure.

Prior to proceeding with fenestration of the footplate, it is important to control all mucosal bleeding that may occur as a result of removal of the superstructure. Usually such bleeding stops spontaneously over a period of a few minutes. If it does

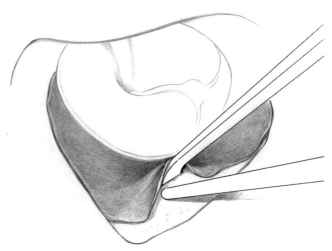

Figure 20–3 Development of a posterior tympanomeatal flap. A triangular segment of meatal skin is incised with a roller knife then elevated to the tympanic annulus. (From Nadol JB Jr, McKenna MJ, eds. Surgery of the Ear and Temporal Bone, 2nd ed. Philadelphia: Lippincott Williams & Wilkins, 2005:276. Reprinted by permission.)

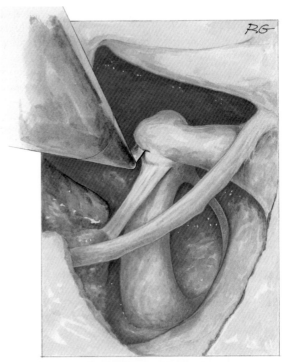

Figure 20–4 Separation of the incudostapedial joint using a joint knife. (From Nadol JB Jr, McKenna MJ, eds. Surgery of the Ear and Temporal Bone, 2nd ed. Philadelphia: Lippincott Williams & Wilkins, 2005:277. Reprinted by permission.)

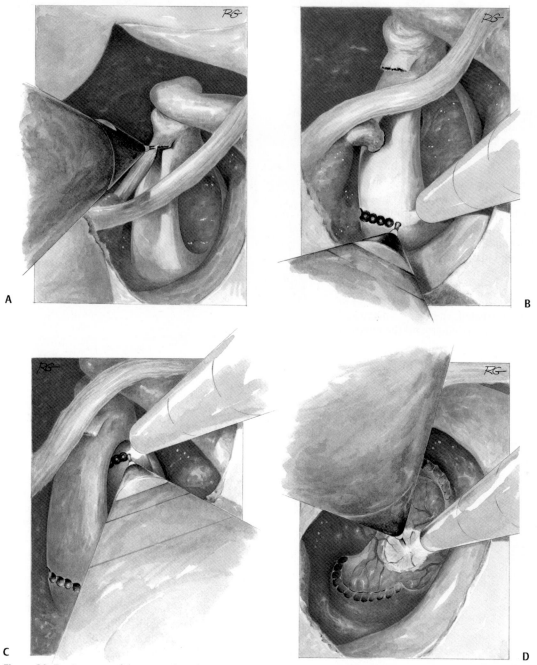

A

B

C

D

Figure 20–5 Exposure of the stapes footplate using the handheld laser. **(A)** The stapedius tendon is separated. **(B)** A posterior crurotomy is performed. **(C)** If visible, the anterior crus is divided. **(D)** The laser beam is withdrawn approximately 2 mm from the footplate to coagulate thick mucosa overlying the lateral surface of the footplate. (From Nadol JB Jr, McKenna MJ, eds. Surgery of the Ear and Temporal Bone, 2nd ed. Philadelphia: Lippincott Williams & Wilkins, 2005:277–279. Reprinted by permission.)

not, a small cotton ball soaked in epinephrine solution can be placed within the oval window niche until the bleeding ceases. Any bleeding during the process of fenestration will impair the surgeon's view and necessitate suctioning in proximity to an open vestibule, which can result in inner ear injury.

Fenestration

Fenestration is usually accomplished with the laser. Our experience has been with the argon and potassium titanyl phosphate (KTP) lasers, both of which are in the visible range and can be passed through a fiberoptic cable and delivered with a handheld instrument. Others have had success with the CO_2 laser, which must be attached to the operating microscope and has a separate co-axial aiming beam. Advantages of the laser include: (1) hemostatic properties; (2) precision that far exceeds other handheld instruments; (3) the ability to vaporize the posterior crus, therefore reducing the chance of a floating footplate; (4) the ability to create a precise fenestra in the footplate without excessive footplate or perilymph motion thus minimizing the risk of acoustic trauma; and (5) the ability to fenestrate a floating footplate without the risk of depressing the footplate into the vestibule, which is an inherent risk of other fenestration techniques. It has been our experience that neither the argon nor the KTP laser is effective in fenestrating thick footplates. If it is apparent that the footplate is thick and that the laser beam is not penetrating through the footplate as evidenced by a small amount of perilymph emanating through the central char, then fenestration is accomplished using the Skeeter drill and a 0.7-mm diamond bur. Because the argon and KTP lasers are delivered through a fiberoptic bundle, it becomes defocused at a very short distance beyond the tip of the probe. Therefore, to use the laser as a cutting tool, the tip of the probe needs to be in nearly direct contact with the bone. To use the laser as a coagulating instrument, the tip is withdrawn 2 to 3 mm, allowing the beam to defocus. The fiberoptic bundle delivers a spot size of approximately 200 μm. A rosette of laser spots is created in the thinnest portion of the footplate. The rosette should measure about 5 spot sizes in diameter in each dimension (**Fig. 20–6**). It is better to err on the side of a slightly large fenestra than one that is too small to admit a 0.6 mm piston and requires additional enlargement once the fenestra has been opened. To avoid thermal injury to the inner ear, 2 to 3 seconds should elapse between pulses to allow for the heat to dissipate. Once the rosette is created, the char is dispersed with a straight pick that is gently passed around the edges of

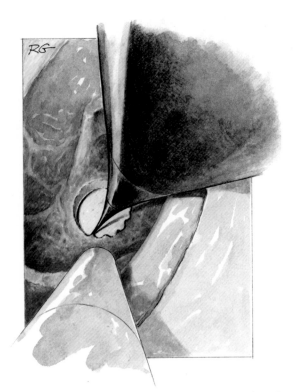

Figure 20–7 The fenestra is completed using a straight pick to disperse the char. A 24-French-guage suction is held near but never over the fenestra. (From Nadol JB Jr, McKenna MJ, eds. Surgery of the Ear and Temporal Bone, 2nd ed. Philadelphia: Lippincott Williams & Wilkins, 2005:281. Reprinted by permission.)

the fenestra (**Fig. 20–7**). On occasion, a portion of the footplate may be relatively thicker and will remain intact, despite having been treated with the laser. Under such circumstances, the Skeeter drill with a 0.7-mm diamond bur is gently used to enlarge the fenestra. The diameter of the hole can be measured with either a measuring stick or a 0.6-mm footplate rasp, which should pass easily through the fenestra.

Measuring the Length of the Prosthesis

A measuring stick with a diameter of 0.6 mm and calibrated for length can be used to determine simultaneously the adequacy of the size of the fenestra and the required length of the piston prosthesis to be used. We utilize a 4-mm standard measuring stick and measure from the medial aspect of the long process of the incus to the fenestra (**Fig. 20–8**).

Placement and Attachment of the Prosthesis

The prostheses are available from several instrument suppliers in 3.25- to 4.75-mm lengths at increments of 0.25 mm. The combined length of the piston head and rod (exclusive of the loop) is used to identify the length of the prosthesis (**Fig. 20–9**). The length of the prosthesis should be 0.25 mm longer than the measurement between the fenestra and the medial edge of the long process of the incus. In cases where it is anticipated that the prosthesis will require bending to accomplish a perpendicular entry into the fenestra, an additional 0.25 mm should be added.

Several stapes prostheses are commercially available and in current use. We are currently utilizing a Teflon piston with platinum wire and ribbon prosthesis. It is fashioned after the Schuknecht stainless steel wire Teflon piston and has the

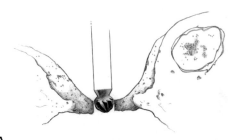

A

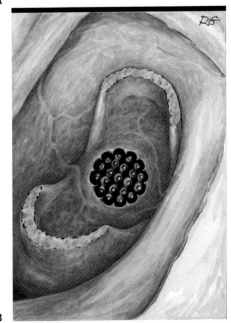

B

Figure 20–6 Two methods of fenestration. **(A)** A microdrill with a 0.7-mm cutting bur and then a diamond bur is used to fenestrate the footplate. **(B)** The laser is used to create a rosette of burn spots that should measure 5 spot-sizes in diameter to create a 0.7-mm fenestra. Each burn spot has a black periphery representing charred bone, a more central halo of white representing vaporized bone, and a central pinhole representing complete fenestration, through which a small amount of perilymph can be seen to emanate. (From Nadol JB Jr, McKenna MJ, eds. Surgery of the Ear and Temporal Bone, 2nd ed. Philadelphia: Lippincott Williams & Wilkins, 2005:280. Reprinted by permission.)

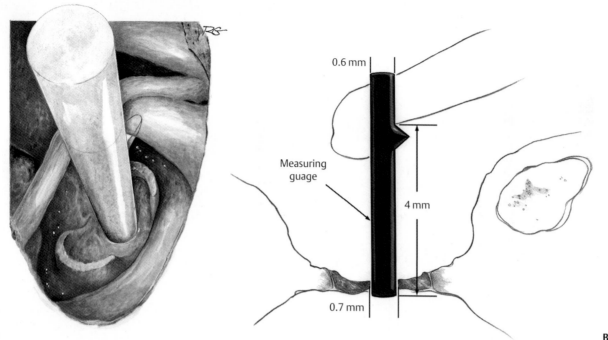

A

B

Figure 20–8 Measuring the length of the prosthesis. **(A)** A measuring stick with a diameter of 0.6 mm and calibrated for length is placed just through the fenestra to determine its diameter and the required length of the piston prosthesis to be used. **(B)** We measure from the medial aspect of the long process of the incus to the fenestra. The 0.6-mm diameter measuring stick should easily pass through a 0.7-mm-wide fenestra. A 4-mm standard measuring stick is shown. An additional 0.25 mm is added to allow for adequate penetration into the vestibule. Thus in this example a 4.25 mm × 0.6 mm prosthesis would be needed. (From Nadol JB Jr, McKenna MJ, eds. Surgery of the Ear and Temporal Bone, 2nd ed. Philadelphia: Lippincott Williams & Wilkins, 2005:281. Reprinted by permission.)

advantage of a platinum wire shaft and a platinum ribbon hook (**Fig. 20–10**). The wire allows easy alteration of the angulation once the prosthesis is in place, and the platinum ribbon hook provides a wider purchase on the incus. In addition, the platinum is also somewhat easier to crimp because it does not have the metallic "memory" of stainless steel. At the time of this writing, a recently developed prosthesis with a Teflon piston and nitinol wire has been introduced and seems to be gaining widespread acceptance. This so-called "smart" prosthesis makes use of a metal, nitonol, that can be crimped by heat activation of the open loop.[58] It has the advantage of not requiring mechanical crimping, and a very secure crimp can be accomplished either by heating the wire with a laser burst or by small bipolar forceps. There has been some concern, however, that one component of this metal alloy is nickel, which may not be highly biocompatible.

The prosthesis is introduced by first grasping the open loop with a smooth alligator forceps and adjusting the angle of the prosthesis with respect to the alligator forceps in accordance to what the surgeon views when looking through the operating microscope. Slightly loosening the grip on the prosthesis and gently tapping the prosthesis posteriorly against the annulus or anteriorly against the incus can further adjust this angle. Ideally, the prosthesis is gently introduced into the fenestra and then around the long process of the incus. In some cases it is difficult to accomplish this with a single move, and it is best to gently place the prosthesis upright within the oval window niche. The loop can then be manipulated with either a straight pick or a small hook such that it is properly positioned around the long process of the incus. The prosthesis should extend into the vestibule for 0.25 mm. Some consider crimping the prosthesis to be the most difficult part of the stapedectomy procedure, hence the rising popularity of the nitinol or "smart"

prosthesis. A variety of crimping forceps are commercially available. Adjust the microscope and the angle of introduction of the crimping forceps so that both blades of the forceps are easily visualized as it engages the loop to facilitate crimping. The loop is gently engaged with both blades of the forceps and then crimped to the incus with sufficient firmness to create a stable linkage. After the prosthesis is crimped, adjustments may be made in the angle of the prosthesis by bending the wire portion of the shaft with a right-angled hook to achieve optimal functional orientation within the fenestra. Usually this would entail a direct perpendicular drop into the fenestra. However, in cases of an overhanging facial nerve, the prosthesis can be bent inferiorly to avoid excessive contact with the nerve, which will impede its mobility. The prosthesis must move freely within the fenestra. This can be assessed by gently elevating the long process of the malleus while watching the motion of the prosthesis. If there is differential motion between the wire loop and incus, friction between the Teflon shaft and margins of the fenestra should be assumed and a modification of the angle made. Despite this, if the prosthesis does not have absolute freedom of movement at the level of the fenestra, the source of impedance must be identified or a good hearing result will not be achieved. Possibilities include a fenestra that is too small or a fleck of bone at the margin of the fenestra that is contacting the piston. The prosthesis should be removed, the fenestra examined and enlarged if necessary with a small rasp. Once the prosthesis has been secured and the freedom of mobility confirmed, a small pledget of Gelfoam soaked in normal saline is placed around the base of the piston. In cases where the fenestra is significantly larger than the piston, a tissue graft is preferred. Subcutaneous fat from the postauricular area on the ear lobe can be harvested, cut into small pieces, and placed around the base of the piston with a

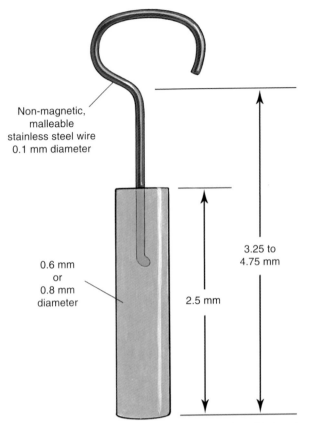

Non-magnetic, malleable stainless steel wire 0.1 mm diameter

0.6 mm or 0.8 mm diameter

3.25 to 4.75 mm

2.5 mm

Figure 20–9 The Teflon stainless steel wire prosthesis (designed in 1960 by H. F. Schuknecht and H. Treace) is commercially available in lengths from 3.25 to 4.75 mm and diameters of 0.6 or 0.8 mm. The non-magnetic wire is MRI-compatible. (From Nadol JB Jr, McKenna MJ, eds. Surgery of the Ear and Temporal Bone, 2nd ed. Philadelphia: Lippincott Williams & Wilkins, 2005:282. Reprinted with permission.)

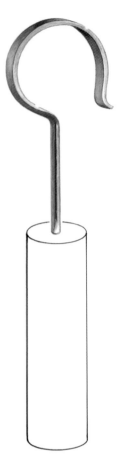

Figure 20–10 The MEEI prosthesis is a modification of the Schuknecht piston prosthesis. The platinum ribbon hook affords a wider and more secure grasp onto the incus, whereas the cylindrical platinum wire shaft can be easily bent to any angle necessary for a perpendicular entry of the Teflon piston into the fenestra. Additionally, the platinum is relatively easy to crimp. (From Nadol JB Jr, McKenna MJ, eds. Surgery of the Ear and Temporal Bone, 2nd ed. Philadelphia: Lippincott Williams & Wilkins, 2005:282. Reprinted by permission.)

straight pick. The tympanomeatal flap is then returned to its anatomic position and stabilized either with Gelfoam or silk packing. Antibiotic prophylaxis begun intraoperatively is generally continued for 1 week postoperatively while the packing is in place. Most patients are discharged from the hospital on the same day as their surgery. They are instructed to avoid any vigorous activity, keep water away from the ear, and refrain from blowing their nose.

◆ Results

Expert results usually are defined as closure of the air-bone gap to 10 dB or less in 90% or more patients, with 1% or less incidence of profound sensorineural hearing loss (anacusis).

◆ Complications During and After Stapedectomy

Intraoperative Problems and Complications

Exostoses of the External Auditory Canal

Small exostoses that do not impair the surgeon's ability to elevate a tympanomeatal flap and access the oval niche do not pose a problem and may be left intact. However, moderate or severe exostoses may severely limit exposure and should be managed as a separate procedure prior to performing a stapedectomy. In such cases, a stapedectomy can be performed at a later date once the healing of the external canal is complete.

Tears in the Tympanomeatal Flap

Tears in the tympanomeatal flap or tympanic membrane that occur during elevation of the flap and drum should be repaired at the completion of the procedure. When this occurs, it has been our practice to harvest a piece of tragal perichondrium and use it as an underlay graft overlapping the defect by several millimeters. Although many of these tears may heal without grafting, the extra few minutes involved in harvesting the perichondrium and placing the graft will serve to prevent the need for another operation in most patients.

High Jugular Bulb

A superiorly located jugular bulb may come into juxtaposition with the tympanic annulus and is vulnerable to injury during elevation of the tympanomeatal flap. Thus, it is important that the flap be elevated with direct visualization especially when working inferiorly. Tears of the jugular bulb result in profuse bleeding and constitute an alarming, although not serious, complication. The bleeding can be controlled by elevating the head of the operating table and with the use of hemostatic packing such as Surgicel or Gelfoam. Modest pressure over the packing for a few minutes generally results in cessation of the bleeding. If the bleeding is readily controlled, the operation may be continued. If, however, the tear is large and the bleeding is difficult to control, the procedure should be terminated.

Disarticulation of the Incus

Disarticulation or partial subluxation of the incus can occur during curetting or while separating the incudostapedial joint. If partial subluxation occurs, the operation may be completed, although the incus will be hypermobile and crimping will be more difficult. In most cases of partial subluxation, the incudomalleal joint will heal and the end result will be satisfactory. If, however, complete dislocation of the incus occurs as is evidenced by complete freedom on movement in both the medial to lateral and anterior to posterior dimensions, it is best to remove the incus and use a malleus attachment prosthesis.

Overhanging Facial Nerve

In rare cases, the facial nerve may be dehiscent and may completely fill the oval window niche. If the nerve is noted to be contacting the promontory inferior to the footplate with complete visual obstruction of the oval window, it is best to abort the procedure and replace the tympanomeatal flap. However, in the majority of cases of dehiscent overhanging facial nerves, the operation can be completed by using a microdrill and small diamond bur to create a fenestra that passes through the inferior aspect of the annular ligament. A small amount of bone can be removed over the promontory to facilitate exposure and free passage of the prosthesis. This technique of creating a marginal bur hole is similar to that used for removal of a floating footplate when the laser is not available. Unlike the case of a marginal bur hole for a floating footplate, the fenestration may incorporate the inferior aspect of the fixed footplate. Often in cases of overhanging facial nerve, the wire of the prosthesis needs to be bent inferiorly to allow for perpendicular decent of the prosthesis into the bur hole and avoid contact with the facial nerve. Because of this requirement, a longer prosthesis is necessary.

Obliterative Otosclerosis of the Oval Window

Otosclerosis that obliterates the oval window niche cannot be easily managed or removed with the laser. However, the laser is helpful in cauterizing the surrounding mucosa to prevent any bleeding. Obliteration of the oval window niche with otosclerosis requires removal of the obliterating bone first by saucerization followed by fenestration (**Fig. 20–11**). This is performed in incremental stages by first using a 1-mm diamond or cutting bur with gradual repeated drilling and saucerization until the bone has been thinned and the blue hue of the vestibule visualized. Final fenestration is then accomplished with the 0.7-mm diamond bur, which should be epicentered in the saucerized cavity. In these cases it is best to measure the distance between the incus and vestibule prior to fenestration, as it is often difficult to assess the depth of penetration of the measuring stick once the fenestra has been created.

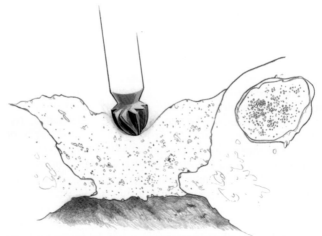

Figure 20–11 Saucerization of obliterative otosclerosis of the oval window is incrementally performed starting with a 1-mm diamond or cutting bur to remove bone until the blue hue of the vestibule is seen. Final fenestration is then performed with either a 0.7-mm diamond bur or the laser. (From Nadol JB Jr, McKenna MJ, eds. Surgery of the Ear and Temporal Bone, 2nd ed. Philadelphia: Lippincott Williams & Wilkins, 2005:292. Reprinted by Permission.)

Round Window Otosclerosis

Complete obliteration of the round window with otosclerosis can result in residual conductive hearing loss following stapedectomy. However, experience has shown that it is impossible to determine at surgery whether or not the round window niche is completely obliterated or partially obliterated. For this reason, it is advisable to complete the stapedectomy even in the presence of round window obliteration. Often, the hearing will be significantly improved despite the appearance of complete obliteration at surgery. However, if the hearing fails to improve postoperatively, revision surgery is not indicated. It is important that the surgeon examines the patency of the round window and notes this in the operative report. Past efforts to remove otosclerosis from the obliterated round window niche have universally resulted in SNHL and should never be attempted.

Persistent Stapedial Artery

During early development, the stapedial artery traverses the obturator foramen of the stapes and then regresses prior to birth. The remnant of this artery is often encountered at surgery as a small vessel that crosses the footplate and can be easily coagulated with the laser. This does not constitute a persistent stapedial artery. A true persistent stapedial artery may be found in 1 in 5000 cases and in some cases may be of a caliber where it nearly fills the obturator foramen of the stapes. It cannot be safely coagulated with either bipolar forceps or the laser. In most cases the persistent stapedial artery occupies the anterior half of the obturator foramen, leaving a potential space in the posterior half of the footplate where fenestration can be safely accomplished. If such is the case, stapedectomy may be performed using the technique described above. If there is a concern regarding the adequacy of available footplate area to perform a stapedectomy, the procedure should be aborted.

Malleus Ankylosis

Fixation of the malleus may be encountered at the time of primary stapedectomy, but in some cases it is clearly overlooked. When the malleus is rigidly fixed as a result of bony fixation in the epitympanum, the findings at surgery are not subtle and can be easily established by gentle palpation of the malleus. The incidence of malleus fixation is somewhat controversial. Studies of the temporal bone collection at the Massachusetts Eye and Ear Infirmary reveal an incidence of 0.5%.[59] The condition does not appear to be related to otosclerosis.[60] Others have reported a higher incidence of malleus fixation and have attributed it to the underlying otosclerotic process, although the exact relationship is unclear.[61,62] When malleus fixation is encountered, the condition must be rectified if a satisfactory hearing result is to be obtained from stapedectomy. This is best accomplished by removal of the incus and the head of the malleus and reconstruction with a malleus attachment prosthesis.

Perilymph Gushers and Oozers

Occasionally, fenestration of the footplate results in the free flow of fluid from the vestibule into the middle ear. When the flow is torrential, it is often referred to as a "perilymph" gusher but is actually cerebrospinal fluid (CSF). A constant but persistent trickle of fluid that wells up through the fenestra is often called a "perilymph" oozer. Perilymph gushers occur as a result of a defect in the cribrose area of the internal auditory canal and are most often found in congenital anomalies of the inner ear. In many cases, the stapes fixation is likely of congenital origin as well. Perilymph oozers, on the other hand, are most often the result of a persistent cochlear aqueduct.[63] In most cases the occurrence of either a gusher or oozer is unanticipated. In the case of a perilymph gusher, it is nearly impossible to perform a stapedectomy until the flow of fluid has been curtailed. This very rapid flow of fluid through the vestibule is deleterious to the health of the inner ear and should be initially controlled by packing the fenestra with either a tissue graft, if immediately available, or a cotton pledget.

The pressure head can then be lowered by placing a lumbar drain and removing spinal fluid. Stapedectomy should be accomplished using a tissue graft, either perichondrium or vein to prevent problems with persistent postoperative leakage. In the case of a perilymph oozer, lumbar drainage is usually not necessary. However, a tissue seal of perichondrium or vein should be utilized. If a perilymph gusher is anticipated, a lumbar drain can be placed prior to the fenestration to avoid the problems associated with turbulent flow through the vestibule; however, a hearing aid is a better option.

Floating or Depressed Footplate

A floating footplate may occur in an ear with minimal stapes fixation and result from down-fracture of the stapes superstructure. It is a relatively rare occurrence with the use of the operating laser, as the laser precludes the need for mechanical force. If, during stapedectomy, the footplate is either mobilized or becomes free-floating, the footplate may be fenestrated safely with the laser as long as the footplate is thin. If the laser is not available or the footplate is thick, the best option is to remove the footplate by first creating a marginal bur hole inferior to the annular ligament. Once the bur hole has been completed, a small hook can be passed through it and under the inferior lip of the footplate. The footplate is then gently elevated and removed (**Fig. 20–12**). The stapedectomy is then completed using a tissue seal consisting of perichondrium, vein, or small pieces of ear lobe fat packed around the base of the piston. An alternative technique is to onlay a tissue graft over the footplate and complete the reconstruction with a bucket-handle or wire prosthesis.

There is no good solution for the depressed footplate, one that has settled down into the vestibule. It is a near certainty that the patient will suffer immediate and protracted vertigo. A footplate that is depressed in a trapdoor or tilted configuration may sometimes be removed by engaging the nondepressed margin with a small hook at the crural remnant. If the footplate is totally depressed, no attempt should be made to

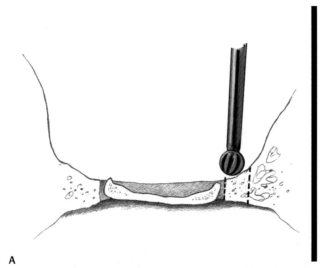
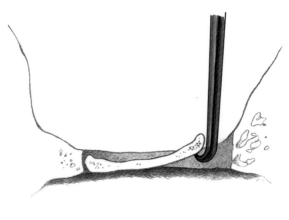

A

B

Figure 20–12 Management of a floating or subluxed footplate with a marginal bur hole technique. **(A)** A marginal bur hole of 0.7-mm diameter or less is completed inferior to the annular ligament to allow for entry of a 0.3-mm angulated hook. **(B)** The hook is used to gently elevate and remove the footplate. (From Nadol JB Jr, McKenna MJ, eds. Surgery of the Ear and Temporal Bone, 2nd ed. Philadelphia: Lippincott Williams & Wilkins, 2005:296. Reprinted by permission.)

remove it. A tissue graft and prosthesis should be introduced, although the results are highly variable.

Early Postoperative Complications

Chorda Tympani Nerve

The main issues are: (1) what range of postoperative symptoms is possible; (2) what final outcome is likely; (3) how does loss of the nerve on one sie affect informed consent/counseling for the contralateral side? In a minority of cases, the nerve is tucked well up under the scutum; the exposure is excellent; no bone curetting is needed; surgery is simple and fast; and no postoperative change of taste or numbness is perceived postoperatively. In a minority of cases, the nerve cannot be preserved because it interferes with exposure; it is intentionally removed; the patient experiences temporary decreased taste and sensation on the ipsilateral tongue, and gradual improvement occurs spontaneously over 3–6 months as the opposite nerve and other taste/smell mechanisms compensate for the loss. In a majority of cases, some curetting of bone, exposure and manipulation of the nerve are required, and at least the nerve probably dries out some and at the worst is stretched. Dryness creates temporary symptoms which resolve quickly. Stretching creates the most severe and permanent symptoms of all: metallic taste, unpleasant taste, inability to taste some things while others are greatly accentuated. Unless these symptoms resolve in 3–6 months, the nerve probably should be resected totally. If the surgeon identifies significant stretching during surgery, the nerve can be resected then.

The management dilemma and relative risks increase significantly if the first nerve has been resected and the second, contralateral stapes surgery is planned. The surgeon should make every effort to obtain the first operative note to determine the status of the first chorda nerve. If present, routine counseling for the second ear can proceed. If absent, the patient must accept the possible risk of a significant permanent drop in taste if the second nerve cannot be preserved. Other taste and smell pathways compensate some for this loss, but usually it remains abnormal in some way.

So critically important are the issues to potential patients who require normal taste for their profession—chefs, wine stewards etc.—that they indeed may opt for a hearing aid instead of surgery even on the first ear, let alone the second.

Facial Palsy

Facial paralysis following stapedectomy is alarming to both the patient and surgeon. There are two possible causes. The first is related to the use of local anesthetics at the time of surgery. If, after 3 hours, the facial paralysis persists, it is unlikely related to local anesthesia and almost certainly related to nerve trauma incurred at the time of surgery. If the operating surgeon is aware of the nerve having been manipulated or mildly traumatized at the time of surgery but is confident that the nerve is anatomically intact, then no intervention is necessary other than those necessary to prevent corneal exposure and perhaps a course of corticosteroids. If, however, the operating surgeon does not recall manipulating or traumatizing the nerve during the surgery, the patient should be returned to the operating room for facial nerve exploration and examination. In rare cases the facial nerve

may pass inferior to the oval window and fan out over the promontory in a flattened configuration that is not easily recognized. If the continuity of the nerve is confirmed, then observation is in order. If the nerve has been severely traumatized or transected, then repair with a short cable graft may be required. Fortunately, this is rarely ever necessary.

Otitis Media

Acute otitis media in the early postoperative period is a rare but worrisome complication. The patients are at high risk for developing suppurative labyrinthitis and meningitis. Patients should be admitted to the hospital and the packing removed. If there is suppuration in the ear canal, cultures should be taken and the patient started on broad-spectrum intravenous antibiotic coverage. Steroids may also be helpful in minimizing inner ear damage. Acute otitis media that occurs months following stapedectomy can be treated in the usual fashion with oral antibiotics.

Vertigo

The occurrence of vertigo either during surgery or immediately thereafter is indicative of a labyrinthine insult. This may be the result of air entering the vestibule during the procedure, blood within the vestibule, or mechanical trauma to the utricle, which lies in close proximity to the oval window. These patients should remain in the hospital and be managed with vestibular suppressives and steroids. Air within the vestibule usually resolves within 24 to 48 hours. Vertigo that is protracted beyond 48 hours is suggestive of a more serious insult and is often associated with SNHL. Even if these patients recover with a good hearing result, vestibular testing should be performed prior to considering a contralateral stapedectomy. Thoughtful consideration should be given to any patient in whom a stapedectomy is being considered when the contralateral ear has significantly reduced vestibular function.

Reparative Granuloma

Exuberant reactive granulation tissue in response to surgery or the placement of a foreign body (prosthesis) is now a rare complication following stapedectomy.[64,65] Decades ago the complication was common when contaminated gelatin sponge (Gelfoam) was used to seal the oval window, after faulty sterilization with ethylene oxide. The typical history is one of an uncomplicated procedure after which the patient does well for the first several days following surgery. Patients then develop symptoms of labyrinthitis with vertigo, spontaneous nystagmus toward the unoperated ear, and tinnitus. Usually the onset is between 5 days and 2 weeks. Examination of the ear upon removal of the packing often reveals an inflamed middle ear space without frank purulence. These patients are best served by returning them to the operating room for exploration of the ear under general anesthesia with the removal of the prosthesis and granulation tissue prior to sealing the fenestra with a tissue graft. In most cases there is a permanent SNHL. Vestibular symptoms usually resolve within a period of weeks. Steroids may also be helpful in reducing the degree of injury.

Delayed Facial Paralysis

Delayed facial paralysis following stapedectomy is an uncommon occurrence that may result either from minor trauma to the facial nerve during surgery with a delayed neuropraxia or possibly activation of a viral neuritis as is seen in Bell's palsy.

Sensorineural Hearing Loss

SNHL following stapedectomy can occur immediately or in a delayed manner anywhere from weeks to months following the procedure. SNHL that occurs in the early postoperative period can be attributed to surgical trauma. The overall incidence in the hands of experienced surgeons is under 1%.[66] High-tone hearing loss above 4000 Hz is likely related to acoustic trauma caused by excessive manipulation of either the footplate or the prosthesis.

Conductive Hearing Loss

Unexpected conductive hearing loss that occurs immediately following stapedectomy can be attributed to one or more of the following conditions: (1) malfunction of the prosthesis, (2) failure to recognize malleus fixation, (3) failure to recognize round window obliteration, (4) middle ear effusion or hemotympanum, or (5) the presence of an unrecognized superior canal dehiscence. In these cases, a high-resolution noncontrast CT scan may be helpful in ruling out superior canal dehiscence and round window obliteration. Ultimately, reexploration may be necessary to establish the cause. Occasionally the cause remains unknown ("inner ear conductive hearing loss") and reexploration is not helpful.

At a recent meeting of the Otosclerosis Study Group, the question was asked, "Should the ear be re-explored for significant/identical conductive loss which persists after surgery? The group concensus, consisting of experts world-wide, was that the ear should not be explored if there was never any gain and if the surgery was performed by a recognized expert. If the hearing improved, then dropped, or if the surgeon's skill was questionable, the ear should be explored. Often, however, no obvious abnormality is found and no benefit achieved.

Late Postoperative Complications

Perilymph Fistula

The development of a perilymph fistula can occur in either the early or late postoperative period. The classic symptoms are fluctuating SNHL and mild to moderate episodic unsteadiness. The diagnosis should be suspected in patients who have a positive fistula test or in whom Hallpike positional testing results in vertigo and nystagmus with the affected ear in a down position. Exploratory tympanotomy is indicated when a perilymph fistula is suspected, and the oval window is sealed with connective tissue.

Delayed-Onset Conductive Hearing Loss

The development of a delayed conductive hearing loss following a successful stapedectomy is relatively common. The exact incidence is unknown. We suspect that it is in the range of 5% of patients who have a successful stapedectomy. The most common cause is erosion of the long process of the incus at the prosthesis attachment site, which results in displacement of the prosthesis.[67] Other less common causes are new bone formation within the oval window niche, which restricts the movement of the prosthesis and delayed round window obliteration.

◆ Cochlear Otosclerosis

It is well established that some patients with advanced otosclerosis develop a progressive irreversible SNHL. The diagnosis should be suspected in patients with known otosclerosis who develop a progressive SNHL, and in patients who have a family history of otosclerosis. The loss is usually gradual and worse for the high frequencies. In some cases the diagnosis can be confirmed with a high-resolution noncontrast CT scan, which may demonstrate areas of lucency within the otic capsule. Many clinicians have used sodium fluoride with calcium (Florical™) in an effort to slow or stabilize the SNHL caused by otosclerosis, yet the efficacy of this treatment has not been well established. The only controlled prospective study demonstrates a weak effect at best.[68] Some of the new biphosphate compounds that have been developed to treat other bone disorders including osteoporosis may prove to be of greater efficacy in preventing SNHL from otosclerosis.[69,70] Although difficult to conduct, these studies are essential to further progress in this area.

◆ Editor's Note

This chapter beautifully represents the state of the art. Less experienced stapes surgeons may wish to read the only publication in the history of otolaryngology-head and neck surgery publications that lists consecutive case results beginning with case #1, which suggests that 50 cases as a primary surgeon are needed to achieve "expert" results (Hughes GB: The learning curve in stapes surgery. Laryngoscope 101: 1280-1284,1991).

References

1. Wang P-C, Merchant SN, McKenna MJ, Glynn RJ, Nadol JB Jr. Does otosclerosis occur only in the temporal bone? Am J Otol 1999;20: 162–165
2. Morrison AW. Genetic factors in otosclerosis. Ann R Coll Surg Engl 1967; 41:202–237
3. Nager T. Histopathology of otosclerosis. Arch Otolaryngol 1969;89: 341–363
4. Lindsay JR. Histopathology of otosclerosis. Arch Otolaryngol 1973;97: 24–29
5. Ghorayeb BY, Linthicum FH. Otosclerotic inner ear syndrome. Ann Otol Rhinol Laryngol 1978;87:85–90
6. Hueb MM, Goycoolea MV, Paparella MM, Oliviera JA. Otosclerosis: the University of Minnesota Temporal Bone Collection. Otolaryngol Head Neck Surg 1991;105:396–405
7. Schuknecht HF. Myths in Neurotology. Am J Otol 1992;13:124–126
8. Schuknecht HF, Kirchner JC. Cochlear otosclerosis: fact or fantasy. Laryngoscope 1974;84:766–782
9. Guild SR. Histologic otosclerosis. Ann Otol Rhinol Laryngol 1944;53: 246–266
10. McKenna MJ, Gadre AK, Rask-Andersen H. Ultrastructural characterization of otospongiotic lesions in celloidin sections. Acta Otolaryngol (Stockh) 1990;109:397–405
11. Altermatt HJ, Gerber HA, Gaeng D, Muller C, Arnold W. Immunohistochemical findings in otosclerotiic lesions. HNO 1992;40:476–479

12. Cherukupally SR, Merchant SN, Rosowski JJ. Correlations between pathologic changes in the stapes and conductive hearing loss in otosclerosis. Ann Otol Rhinol Laryngol 1998;107:319–326

13. Schuknecht HF, Barber W. Histologic variants in otosclerosis. Laryngoscope 1985;95:1307–1317

14. Kwok OT, Nadol JB Jr. Correlation of otosclerotic foci and degenerative changes in the Organ of Corti and spiral ganglion. Am J Otolaryngol 1989;10:1–12

15. Nelson EG, Hinojosa R. Questioning the relationship between cochlear otosclerosis and sensorineural hearing loss: a quantitative evaluation of cochlear structures in cases of otosclerosis and review of the literature. Laryngoscope 2004;114:1214–1230

16. Doherty JK, Linthicum FH Jr. Spiral ligament and stria vascularis changes in cochlear otosclerosis: effect on hearing level. Otol Neurotol 2004; 25:457–464

17. Weber PC, Cunningham CD, Schulte BA. Potassium recycling pathways in the human cochlea. Laryngoscope 2001;111:1156–1165

18. Salt AN, Melichar J, Thalman R. Mechanisms of endocochlear potential generation by stria vascularis. Laryngoscope 1987;97:985–991

19. Cody DT, Baker HL Jr. Otosclerosis: vestibular symptoms and sensory neural hearing loss. Ann Otol Rhinol Laryngol 1978;87:778–796

20. Birch L, Elbrond O. Stapedectomy and vertigo. Clin Otolaryngol 1985;10: 217–223

21. Frisch T, Sorensen MS, Overgaard S, et al. Volume-referent bone turnover estimated from the interlabel area fraction after sequential labeling. Bone 1998;22:677–682

22. Nadol JB Jr. Pathoembryology of the middle ear. Birth Defects Orig Artic Ser 1980;16:181–209

23. Sorensen MS, Bretlau P, Jorgensen MB. Human perilabyrinthine bone dynamics. A functional approach to temporal bone histology. Acta Otolaryngol Suppl 1992;496:1–27

24. Sorensen MS, Jorgensen MB, Bretlau P. Remodeling patterns in the bony otic capsule of the dog. Ann Otol Rhinol Laryngol 1991;100:751–758

25. Zehnder AF, Kristiansen AG, Adams JC, Merchant SN, McKenna MJ. Osteoprotegrin in the inner ear may inhibit bone remodeling in the otic capsule. Laryngoscope 2005;115:172–177

26. Zehnder AF, Kujawa SG, Kristiansen AG, Adams JC, McKenna MJ. Osteoprotegrin (OPG) knockout mice have abnormal otic capsule remodeling and progressive hearing loss. Assoc Res Otolaryngol Abs 2005;28:650

27. Ferlito A, Arnold W, Rinaldo A, et al. Viruses and otosclerosis: chance association or true causal link? Acta Otolaryngol 2003;123: 741–746

28. McKenna MJ, Mills BG, Galey FR, Linthicum FH Jr. Filamentous structures morphologically similar to viral nucleocapsids in otosclerotic lesions in two patients. Am J Otol 1986;7:25–28

29. McKenna MJ, Mills BG. Immunohistochemical evidence of measles virus antigens in active otosclerosis. Otolaryngol Head Neck Surg 1989;101: 415–421

30. McKenna MJ, Mills BG. Ultrastructural and immunohistochemical evidence of measles virus in active otosclerosis. Acta Otolaryngol Suppl 1990;470:130–139

31. McKenna MJ, Kristiansen AG, Haines J. Polymerase chain reaction amplification of a measles virus sequence from human temporal bone sections with active otosclerosis. Am J Otol 1996;17:827–830

32. Niedermeyer HP, Arnold W. Otosclerosis: a measles virus associated inflammatory disease. Acta Otolaryngol 1995;115:300–303

33. Arnold W, Niedermeyer HP, Lehn N, Neubert W, Hofler H. Measles virus in otosclerosis and the specific immune response of the inner ear. Acta Otolaryngol 1996;116:705–709

34. Niedermeyer HP, Arnold W, Schuster M, et al. Persistent measles virus infection and otosclerosis. Ann Otol Rhinol Laryngol 2001;110: 897–903

35. Karosi T, Konya J, Szabo LZ, Sziklai I. Measles virus prevalence in otosclerotic stapes footplate samples. Otol Neurotol 2004;25:451–456

36. Niedermeyer HP, Arnold W, Schwub D, Busch R, Wiest I, Sedlmeier R. Shift of the distribution of age in patients with otosclerosis. Acta Otolaryngol 2001;121:197–199

37. Vrabec JT, Coker NJ. Stapes surgery in the United States. Otol Neurotol 2004;25:465–469

38. Browning GG, Gatehouse S. The prevalence of middle ear disease in the adult British population. Clin Otolaryngol 1992;17:317–321

39. Hammerschlag V. Zur frage der vererbbarkeit der otosklerose. Wien Klin Rdsch. 1905;19:5–7

40. Albrecht W. Über die vererbung der konstitutionell sporadischen taubstummheit der hereditären labyrithschwerhörigkeit und der otosklerose. Arch Ohr Nas Kehlkopfheilk 1923;110:15–48

41. Sabitha R, Ramalingam R, Ramalingam KK, Sivakumaran TA, Ramesh A. Genetics of otosclerosis. J Laryngol Otol 1997;111:109–112

42. Fowler EP. Otosclerosis in identical twins: a study of 40 pairs. Arch Otolaryngol 1966;83:324–328

43. Ben Arab S, Bonaïti-Pellié C, Belkahia A. A genetic study of otosclerosis in a population living in the north of Tunisia. Ann Genet 1993;36:111–116

44. Tomek MS, Brown MR, Mani SR, et al. Localization of a gene for otosclerosis to chromosome 15q25-q26. Hum Mol Genet 1998;7:285–290

45. Van Den Bogaert K, Govaerts PJ, Schatteman I, et al. A second gene for otosclerosis, OTSC2, maps to chromosome 7q34–36. Am J Hum Genet 2001;68:495–500

46. Chen W, Campbell CA, Green GE, et al. Linkage of otosclerosis to a third locus (OTSC3) on human chromosome 6p21.3–22.3. J Med Genet 2002; 39:473–477

47. Van Den Bogaert K, Govaerts PJ, De Leenheer EM, et al. Otosclerosis: A genetically heterogeneous disease involving at least three different genes. Bone 2002;30:624–630

48. Van Den Bogaert K, De Leenheer EM, Chen W, et al. A fifth locus for otosclerosis, OTSC5, maps to chromosome 3q22–24. J Med Genet 2004; 41:450–453

49. McKenna MJ, Kristiansen AG, Körkkö J. Sequence analysis of COC1A1 and COL1A2 genes in clinical otosclerosis: no evidence for mutations in the coding regions of the genes. Otorhinolaryng Nova 2001;11:267–270

50. McKenna MJ, Nguyen-Huynh AT, Kristiansen AG. Association of Otosclerosis with Sp1 binding site polymorphism in COL1A1 gene: evidence for a shared genetic etiology with osteoporosis. Otol Neurotol 2004;25:447–450

51. McKenna MJ, Kristiansen AG, Bartley ML, Rogus JJ, Haines JL. Association of COL1A1 and otosclerosis. Evidence for a shared genetic etiology with mild osteogenesis imperfecta. Am J Otol 1998;19:604–610

52. McKenna MJ, Kristiansen AG, Tropitzsch AS. Similar COL1Al expression in fibroblasts from some patients with clinical otosclerosis and those with type 1 osteogenesis imperfecta. Ann Otol Rhinol Laryngol 2002; 111:184–189

53. Fowler EP. The incidence (and degrees) of blue sclerae in otosclerosis and other ear disorders. Laryngoscope 1949;59:406–416

54. Schuknecht HF. Pathology of the Ear. Cambridge, MA: Harvard University Press, 1974

55. Nager GT. Osteogenesis imperfecta of the temporal bone and its relation to otosclerosis. Ann Otol Rhinol Laryngol 1988;97:585–593

56. Hyman S. For the World to Hear: A Biography of Howard P. House, M.D. Pasadena, CA: Hope Publishing House, 1990

57. Mikulec AA, McKenna MJ, Ramsey MJ, et al. Superior semicircular canal dehiscence presenting as conductive hearing loss without vertigo. Otol Neurotol 2004;25:121–129

58. Rajan GP, Atlas MD, Subramaniam K, Eikelboom RH. Eliminating the limitations of manual crimping in stapes surgery? A preliminary trial with the shape memory Nitinol stapes piston. Laryngoscope 2005;115:366–369

59. Nadol JB Jr, Schuknecht HF. Surgery for otosclerosis and fixation of the stapes. In: Nadol JB Jr, Mckenna MJ, eds. Surgery of the Ear and Temporal Bone, 2nd ed. Philadelphia: Lippincott Williams & Wilkins, 2005:273–303

60. Harris JP, Mehta RP, Nadol JB. Malleus fixation: clinical and histopathologic findings. Ann Otol Rhinol Laryngol 2002;111:246–254

61. Guilford FR, Anson BJ. Ossification of the malleus. Trans Am Acad Ophthalmol Otolaryngol 1967;71:398–407

62. Katzke D, Plester D. Idiopathic malleus head fixation a cause of a combined conductive and sensorineural hearing loss. Clin Otolaryngol 1981; 6:39–44

63. Schuknecht HF, Reisser C. The morphologic basis for perilymphatic gushers and oozers. Adv Otorhinolaryngol 1988;39:1–12

64. Kaufman RS, Schuknecht HF. Reparative granuloma following stapedectomy: a clinical entity. Ann Otol Rhinol Laryngol 1967;76:1008–1017

65. Seicshnaydre MA, Sismanis A, Hughes GB. Update on reparative granuloma: Survey of the American Otological Society and the American Neurology Society. Am J Otol 1994;15:155–160

66. Glasscock ME III, Storper IS, Haynes DS, Bohrer PS. Twenty-five years of experience with stapedectomy. Laryngoscope 1995;105:899–904

67. Han WW, Incesulu A, McKenna MJ, Rauch SD, Nadol JB Jr, Glynn RJ. Revision stapedectomy: intraoperative findings, results, and review of the literature. Laryngoscope 1997;107:1185–1192

68. Bretlau P, Salomon G, Johnsen NJ. Otospongiosis and sodium fluoride. A clinical double-blind, placebo-controlled study on sodium fluoride treatment in otospongiosis. Am J Otol 1989;10:20–22

69. Kennedy DW, Hoffer ME, Holliday M. The effects of etifronate disodium on progressive hearing loss from otosclerosis. Otolaryngol Head Neck Surg 1993;109:461–467

70. Brookler KH, Tanyeri H. Etidronate for the neurotologic symptoms of otosclerosis: preliminary study. Ear Nose Throat J 1997;76:371–376

21

Temporal Bone Trauma

May Y. Huang and Paul R. Lambert

Temporal bone trauma occurs in 30 to 75% of head injuries.[1–7] Compared with the face and skull, the temporal bone is very dense and requires a tremendous amount of force to sustain fracture. The majority of temporal bone injuries are associated with other multiple traumas following motor vehicle accidents. Temporal bone trauma also may be associated with industrial accidents, recreational injuries, falls, assaults, or self-inflicted injuries. Types of temporal bone trauma include blunt trauma without fracture, blunt trauma with fracture, penetrating trauma, compressive injuries, and thermal injuries. Trauma may cause injury to specific parts of the external, middle, or inner ear in addition to other structures within the temporal bone. Frequently, the history of the type of temporal bone injury facilitates evaluation of the spectrum of potential sequelae.

◆ Anatomic Considerations

The temporal bone is a wedge-shaped bone in the lateral skull base that is bordered by the middle fossa tegmen superiorly, the posterior fossa tegmen posteriorly, the temporomandibular joint anteriorly, the clivus and foramen magnum medially, and the infratemporal fossa inferiorly. The temporal bone is divided into four regions: squamous, petrous, mastoid, and tympanic. Its posterosuperior border is called the petrous ridge, which lies along the long axis of the temporal bone at about a 45-degree angle posterior to the midcoronal plane. The squamous portion articulates with the sphenoid bone anteriorly and the parietal bone posteriorly, thus forming the roof of the infratemporal fossa and the medial wall of the temporal fossa. At the base of the skull, the petrous and mastoid portions of the temporal bone lie lateral to the occipital bone at the foramen magnum. The petrous apex is separated from the clivus (the fusion of the occipital and sphenoid bones anterior to the foramen magnum) by the foramen lacerum. At the inferior aspect of the base of the skull medial to the styloid process lie the jugular and carotid foramina.

Vital structures that reside within the anatomic confines of the temporal bone include audiovestibular mechanoreceptors; cranial nerves V, VI, VII, and VIII; the sigmoid sinus; and the jugular bulb. Injury to these vital structures needs to be considered in evaluation of temporal bone trauma.

The seventh and eighth cranial nerves arise from the pons, enter the posterior aspect of the temporal bone at the porus acusticus, and then course laterally in the internal auditory canal toward the vestibule. The cochlea and semicircular canals lie anteroinferiorly and posterosuperiorly, respectively, with respect to the internal auditory canal.

The course of the facial or seventh nerve within the temporal bone can be described in segments: the meatal segment within the internal auditory canal, the labyrinthine segment within the internal auditory canal, the labyrinthine segment and geniculate ganglion, the tympanic segment in the middle ear, and the mastoid segment. From the internal auditory canal the facial nerve passes through the facial hiatus into the labyrinthine segment of the fallopian canal. At the geniculate ganglion it gives off the greater superficial petrosal nerve (preganglionic parasympathetic innervation for lacrimation) and then turns posteroinferiorly (first genu) along the medial wall of the tympanic cavity. It passes superior to the cochleariform process and the oval window. Inferior to the horizontal semicircular canal it turns (second genu) into the mastoid segment. It gives off the stapedial branch and the chorda tympani branch (special visceral afferent innervation for taste and preganglionic parasympathetic innervation for submandibular and sublingual glands) before exiting the temporal bone through the stylomastoid foramen.

The trigeminal of fifth cranial nerve exits the pons and travels anterolaterally from the posterior fossa to the trigeminal ganglion by passing over the petrous apex just deep to the attachment of the tentorium cerebelli. Its branches exit the middle fossa via the superior orbital fissure, foramen rotundum, and foramen ovale.

The abducens or sixth cranial nerve travels forward from the pons through the dura over the clivus, passing through Dorello's canal at the petrous apex. The internal carotid artery enters the carotid canal at the inferior aspect of the petrous temporal bone (anterior to the jugular fossa), courses superiorly, and then turns anteromedially just medial to the cochlea and the eustachian tube. The internal carotid artery exits the petrous apex just above the foramen lacerum, ascends in the carotid siphon just lateral to the sella turcica, traverses the cavernous sinus, and enters the dura just medial to the anterior clinoid process.

The middle meningeal artery arises from the maxillary artery in the infratemporal fossa. It enters the temporal bone via the foramen spinosum, runs laterally in the dura over the middle fossa tegmen, and then branches into frontal and parietal branches. It gives rise to the superficial petrosal branch that enters the canal of the greater superficial petrosal nerve.

The sigmoid sinus extends from the transverse sinus to the jugular bulb, coursing from superior to inferior in the dura along the posterolateral aspect of the temporal bone. It receives the greater and lesser petrosal sinuses from the cavernous sinus, as well as the mastoid emissary vein. The jugular bulb lies medial to the vertical segment of the facial nerve and posterior to the ascending portion of the internal carotid artery.

◆ Classifications of Types of Temporal Bone Trauma

Trauma with Fracture

Temporal bone fractures most commonly arise from blunt trauma. They have been traditionally classified as longitudinal or transverse, with respect to the long axis of the temporal bone as viewed from the middle fossa (**Fig. 21–1**).

Longitudinal fractures are the most common fractures of the temporal bone, constituting approximately 70 to 90% of temporal bone fractures.[1–7] This fracture typically results from a direct blow to the temporal or parietal aspects of the head. Symptoms at presentation include conductive hearing loss, bloody otorrhea, and loss of consciousness. Longitudinal fractures are bilateral in 8 to 29% of cases. The facial nerve is injured in approximately 15%. Due to the higher incidence of this type of fracture, however, facial nerve injury is most commonly caused by longitudinal fractures.

The longitudinal fracture line roughly parallels the long axis of the temporal bone in the coronal plane. Classically this fracture extends from the squamous portion of the temporal bone to the anterior portion of the petrous apex in the area of the foramen lacerum and foramen ovale. The fracture thus passes through the posterosuperior aspect of the external auditory canal, the tympanic membrane, and the roof of the middle ear

(**Figs. 21–2** and **21–3**). These fractures commonly disrupt the ossicles or lacerate the skin of the ear canal, but usually spare the otic capsule. Fractures extending through the mastoid rather than the ear canal can result in hemotympanum without laceration of the tympanic membrane.

Transverse fractures are far less common, accounting for 20 to 30% of temporal bone fractures. Transverse fractures usually are associated with a blow to the occiput. Symptoms include profound sensorineural hearing loss (SNHL), vertigo, and severe head injury. In approximately 50% of these fractures, a facial paralysis occurs.[5,7–9]

The transverse fracture extends from the posterior fossa across the petrous pyramid to the foramen spinosum in a more sagittal plane. Transverse fractures extend through the internal auditory canal or the otic capsule. Fractures that arise near the porus acusticus can alternatively end at the oval or round window and produce hemotympanum without laceration of the tympanic membrane (**Figs. 21–4** and **21–5**).

Few temporal bone fractures are purely longitudinal or transverse. From 50 to 75% of both pediatric and adult temporal bones, fractures could be classified as mixed in their axis of orientation.[4,7] In addition, there are not only two axes of orientation but also three planes of orientation by which to

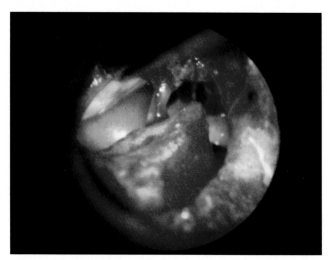

Figure 21–2 Temporal bone fracture.

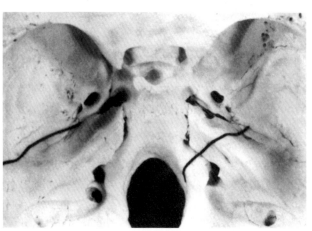

Figure 21–1 Diagram of a longitudinal fracture (left) and a transverse temporal bone fracture (right) as viewed from the middle fossa.

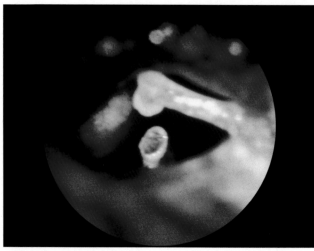

Figure 21–3 Traumatic separation incus-stapes.

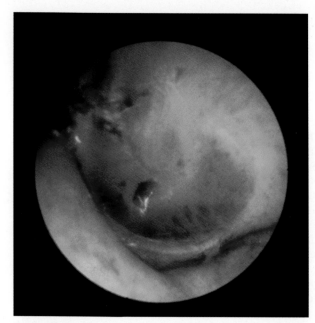

Figure 21–4 Traumatic hemotympanum.

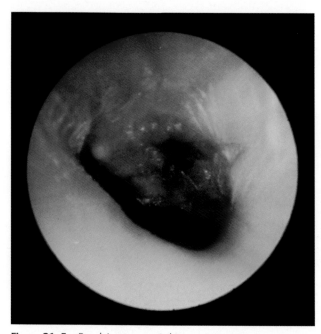

Figure 21–5 Resolving traumatic hemotympanum.

describe fractures. Fractures in the oblique plane of orientation are the most common.[10–12] As seen from the middle fossa, oblique fractures extend roughly between the coronal and axial planes, across the mastoid cortex, external auditory canal, petrotympanic fissure, and glenoid fossa.

As in adults, pediatric temporal bone fractures are commonly longitudinal or oblique.[13,14] The etiology of pediatric temporal bone fractures includes a higher incidence of falling from heights and automobile-pedestrian accidents. Facial nerve injury and cerebrospinal fluid (CSF) leak may be less common than in adults. The sites of temporal bone injury and their management are similar.

Penetrating Temporal Bone Trauma

The most common type of penetrating trauma affecting the temporal bone is a low-velocity gunshot wound.[15] Temporal bone injuries from the typical 0.22-mm to 0.38-mm caliber handgun are most commonly associated with a facial entrance wound rather than one on the side of the head. Mixed or comminuted fractures are most likely; there is no typical pattern of injury. Gunshot wounds of the temporal bone can create a wide variety of specific injuries including trauma to the major vessels, laceration of the dura, and destruction of the middle ear, inner ear, cranial nerves, and central nervous system. The facial nerve is injured in approximately 50% of cases. Usually the associated paralysis is immediate in onset and results from direct nerve injury.

Trauma Without Fracture

Injury to structures of the temporal bone can occur without temporal bone fracture. Such trauma is best enumerated by etiology. Barotrauma, thermal, foreign body, and compressive injuries frequently involve the external and middle ear. Concussive injuries or barotraumas more commonly involve the inner ear.

Blunt head trauma without fracture of the temporal bone may result in SNHL[2,16,17] from direct hair cell damage, disruption of inner ear membranes, or fracture of the oval window. A conductive hearing loss can result from ossicular damage or disruption of the tympanic membrane.

Foreign bodies used to remove cerumen, such as hair pins, cotton-tip applicators, pens, pencils, and toothpicks, can traumatize the external auditory canal or the tympanic membrane and result in localized laceration, hematoma, or infection. Injuries from foreign bodies can extend through the tympanic membrane to the middle and inner ear, causing hearing loss with or without vertigo.[18,19]

Compressive injuries to the ear can result from being slapped or struck on the side of the head or from falling on the water surface during water sports (e.g., waterskiing or diving). These may result in laceration of the tympanic membrane. More significant compressive injuries result from blast injuries. Bomb explosions can cause disruption and implosion of the tympanic membrane as well as high-frequency SNHL due to disruption of the inner ear.[20,21]

Otitic barotrauma or aerotitis occurs when sudden and severe negative middle ear pressure results in trauma to the ear.[22–31] It can be precipitated by concurrent sinonasal inflammation. Symptoms typically include excruciating otalgia during descent flying or ascent from underwater diving. Failure of the eustachian tube to open and adequately equilibrate middle ear pressure with atmospheric pressure causes hyperemia, edema, and ecchymosis of the middle ear mucosa with possible rupture of the tympanic membrane. Perilymph fistulas have also been reported after barotraumas, characterized by fluctuating SNHL and vertigo.[32–42]

Thermal injuries involve the temporal bone as well. Hot slag injuries sustained during welding can cause a perforation of the tympanic membrane that is difficult to repair (**Fig. 21–6**) as well as inner ear injury. Also, lightning bolt injuries to the temporal bone can occur from lightning conducted through a telephone to the ear. SNHL, vertigo, tinnitus, and facial paralysis potentially result from devitalized bone and soft tissue.[43–47]

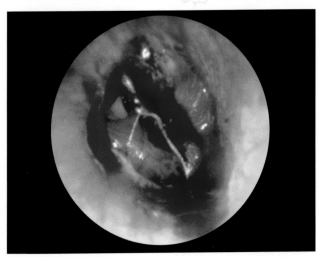

Figure 21–6 Large traumatic perforation.

◆ Mechanisms of Injury

Auditory

Conductive hearing loss can arise from injury to the external auditory canal, tympanic membrane, or middle ear. Conductive hearing loss can become evident in the acute setting or on a delayed basis. Acutely, the ear canal often is filled with clotted blood, debris, or hematoma. The tympanic membrane may be lacerated, perforated, or completely disrupted. The middle ear may be filled with blood or cerebrospinal fluid. The ossicular chain may be interrupted (**Fig. 21–7**). Incudostapedial joint separation is the most common ossicular injury, secondary to longitudinal temporal bone fracture.[4,48–55] Dislocation of the incus is the second most common finding, followed by fracture of the stapes superstructure. Fracture of the malleus is the least common. Delayed conductive hearing loss can be due to stenosis of the external auditory canal, or ossicular fixation. Ossicular fixation due to fibrous adhesion or bony ankylosis most commonly involves the head of the malleus and the body of the incus.

Severe head trauma of any type is associated with a high incidence of SNHL.[2,56,57] Approximately one third of patients

Audiogram

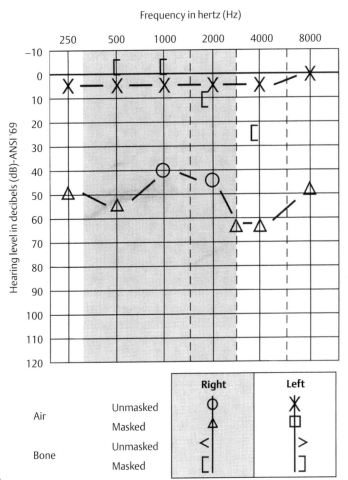

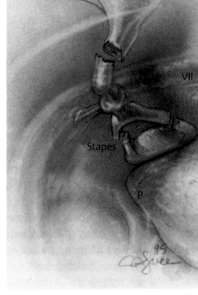

Figure 21–7 **(A)** Audiogram showing persistent maximal conductive hearing loss many years after a fall. CT scan showed no temporal bone fracture. **(B)** Diagram of ossicular findings in same patient. Findings during middle ear exploration included fractures of the lenticular process of the incus and both crura of the stapes, as well as incudostapedial joint separation. A stapes prosthesis was successfully placed.

with significant closed head injury experience hearing loss, and up to one half of them also have loss of consciousness. SNHL may result from injury to the inner ear, the eighth nerve, or the central auditory system. The inner ear and internal auditory canal may be directly involved, as in a transverse fracture. As many as one third of longitudinal fractures produce high-frequency SNHL, thought to arise from cochlear concussion.[58-65] Degeneration of the hair cells in the basal turn of the cochlea may be due either to production of a pressure wave being transmitted through bone to the cochlea or to sudden acceleration-deceleration of the head with sudden movement of the stapes footplate. Disruption of the basilar membrane or tear of the oval window membrane with perilymph fistula may occur with excessive stapes footplate excursion. Traction on the eighth cranial nerve and brainstem contusion are more central etiologies for SNHL.

Vestibular

Benign paroxysmal positional vertigo is the most common form of disequilibrium after head injury.[16,17,63,64] It occurs in nearly half of patients with longitudinal temporal bone fractures and in one fifth of patients who suffer blunt head trauma without fracture. Typically the onset of symptoms immediately follows the injury. This clinical entity is thought to be due to disruption of the utricular macula. Detached otoconia enter the posterior semicircular canal and render the ampulla sensitive to gravity and thus changes in head position.[57,65-70]

Traumatic perilymph fistulas may result from fracture or subluxation of the stapes, penetrating trauma, and barotrauma.[22-42] Transverse fractures may directly involve the vestibule or semicircular canals and cause a leak of inner ear fluids.[71] A perilymph fistula (PLF) is a persistent, abnormal communication between the inner ear and middle ear or the mastoid. Trauma is the third most common cause of PLF, after iatrogenic injuries and idiopathic causes,[41] although the traumatic event can involve a relatively minor head injury. The defect is found in the oval window or the round window. Symptoms can include tinnitus, disequilibrium with or without vertigo, aural fullness, and SNHL that may be fluctuating. Patients often describe a popping sensation in the affected ear at the time the fistula occurs. Symptoms cannot reliably predict the site of the fistula. The duration of symptoms is variable but can persist for months. Bilateral PLF is not uncommon.[38] The mechanisms of PLF formation are described as implosive or explosive. Implosive PLF such as barotrauma results in inward motion of the oval widow or round window. Explosive PLF results from increased intracranial pressure (e.g., the Valsalva maneuver) transmitted to the labyrinth, possibly by way of an abnormally patent cochlear aqueduct or internal auditory canal. Patients with congenital anomalies such as enlarged vestibular aqueduct are predisposed to PLF from minor head trauma.[39] Because the symptom complex caused by PLF is varied, the diagnosis of this entity can be difficult. A specific history of barotrauma or straining coincident with the onset of the symptoms provides some confidence in the diagnosis.

Injury to the labyrinth is more frequently caused by concussion of the labyrinth than fracture. Concussive injury produces shock waves through the inner ear fluids that disrupt labyrinthine membranes.[58-62] Traction on the eighth nerve also may result in vestibular symptoms. Brainstem contusion or hemorrhage can involve vestibular nuclei, although trauma

to the brainstem usually arises in conjunction with diffuse brain injury.[57,65-70,72] Isolated brainstem contusion is unusual. Typical presentation includes multiple cranial nerve palsies, elevated intracranial pressure, and focal neurologic signs.

Facial Nerve

In 80 to 90% of longitudinal fractures, the site of facial nerve trauma is located in the perigeniculate region or just distal to it in the tympanic segment[5,8,9,73-75] (**Fig. 21–8**). Impingement from bone spicules is the most common mechanism of early-onset paralysis, followed by neural contusion. Transverse fractures usually injure the facial nerve in the labyrinthine portion, at or proximal to the geniculate ganglion. The geniculate region may be particularly sensitive to shearing forces in blunt head trauma; its bony covering is frequently dehiscent in this area compared with the surrounding labyrinthine and tympanic segments. In addition, the ganglion is tethered by the takeoff of the greater superficial petrosal nerve. Other mechanisms of injury to the intratemporal facial nerve include transection by fracture, hematoma within the nerve sheath, and edema with constriction in the fallopian canal.

Histopathologically, the extent of facial nerve injury can be classified as neuropraxia, axonotmesis, or neurotmesis (see Chapter 9).[76] Neuropraxia is defined as cessation of axoplasmic flow without degeneration of the axon. Axonotmesis describes degeneration of axons with maintenance of the endoneurial sheaths. In neurotmesis, the axons and their endoneurium degenerate. A more detailed classification of neural injuries has been presented by Sunderland,[77] who described five levels of injury based on the status of the

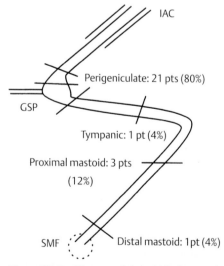

Site of lesion

n = 26 patients

IAC

Perigeniculate: 21 pts (80%)

GSP

Tympanic: 1 pt (4%)

Proximal mastoid: 3 pts (12%)

SMF

Distal mastoid: 1pt (4%)

Figure 21–8 Diagram of the middle fossa and mastoid exposure of the intratemporal facial nerve. Arrows indicate the frequency of facial nerve injury at each site in 26 patients following longitudinal temporal bone fracture. IAC, internal auditory canal; GSP, greater superficial petrosal (nerve); SMP, stylomastoid foramen. (Adapted from Lambert PR, Brackmann DE. Facial paralysis in longitudinal temporal bone fracture: a review of 26 cases. Laryngoscope 1984;94:1022–1026. Reprinted with permission.)

endoneurium, perineurium, and epineurium. During the first 2 to 3 days of a complete paralysis, or before significant Wallerian degeneration has occurred, electrical tests are not reliable in distinguishing between different levels of injury. Once axonal degeneration has occurred, electrical testing can differentiate neuropraxia from the other injury types. Electrical testing cannot distinguish between axonotmesis and neurotmesis, although the rapidity with which electrical excitability is lost can provide some indirect measure.[9,75,77–84] Any type of trauma to the facial nerve will cause a spectrum of neural injuries. If most of the nerve fibers are neuropraxic only, recovery will be excellent and occur rapidly. Recovery will also be excellent if the injury does not progress beyond the level of axonotmesis, although it will be delayed compared with the neuropraxic state, as regrowth of the axons to the motor end-plates occurs. Because the endoneurial tubules are lost in neurotmesis, regenerating axons will become misdirected, resulting in synkinesis, or encounter fibrosis, producing a residual weakness.

Intracranial

Intracranial injuries include trauma to the dura, brain parenchyma, and other neural or vascular structures. Fractures with dural tears or fractures through the otic capsule or internal auditory canal can result in leakage of CSF. Leaks can present as otorrhea, rhinorrhea (via the eustachian tube), or fluid behind an intact tympanic membrane. Multiple cranial nerves can be injured including V, VI, IX, X, XI, and XII. Introduction of air through the fracture into the cranial vault results in pneumocephalus. Mechanisms of brain injury include hemorrhage, contusion, infarct, and edema with increased intracerebral pressure. Herniation of brain through fractures results in encephalocele or meningoencephalocele. Bony fragments also can impinge directly on the brain and cause devitalization of the central nervous system.

Vascular

The location of hematomas can be extradural or subdural. In the region of the temporal bone, hematomas typically arise from injury to the middle meningeal artery. Direct vascular injury can be arterial or venous. Mechanisms of direct injury to the internal carotid arterial system include transaction, laceration, thrombosis, aneurysm, and pseudoaneurysm formation. Fracture or penetrating injury in the mastoid area can lacerate or thrombose the sigmoid dural venous sinus. Associated venous injury includes avulsion of the superior or inferior petrosal sinuses, injury to the jugular bulb, or injury to the cavernous sinus.

◆ Evaluation

Overall stabilization of the multiple-trauma patient precedes evaluation of specific temporal bone injuries. The history of the traumatic events and any loss of consciousness should be ascertained. Initial assessment is performed with emergency department personnel and includes level of consciousness, adequacy of the upper and lower airway, hemodynamic stability, and central neurologic deficits. The otolaryngologist may need to perform intubation, tracheotomy, or cricothyroidotomy emergently. Life-threatening injuries, such as shock, hemorrhage, expanding hematoma, tension pneumothorax, or cardiac arrhythmia, are the physician's first priority. In addition, the cervical spine must not be manipulated until instability has been ruled out by lateral neck plain films, preferably in flexion and extension. A pertinent medical history should be elicited from the patient or family members.

Examination of the head and neck can proceed once the patient has been stabilized. This examination must be performed deftly and thoroughly because many people may converge on the patient in the emergency room. Development of a methodical examination prevents the omission or repetition of part of the examination. It is suggested that one proceed from cranial to caudal, including the temporal bones. Examination of cranial nerves can be included with each region. Starting with the scalp and upper third of the face, rule out open skull or sinus fractures. Examine the reactivity and symmetry of the pupils and visual acuity. Check for restriction of extraocular motion, proptosis, enophthalmos, diplopia, and traumatic telecanthus. In the midface, rule out a nasal fracture, septal hematoma, CSF rhinorrhea, hypesthesia, asymmetry, malocclusion, and trismus. When evaluating the lower third and mandible, examine intraorally for fractures, edema, missing teeth, and hypesthesia. For each third of the face, take note of fractures (point tenderness, crepitus, and bony step-off), laceration, and facial motion. Examine lower cranial nerve function if possible, including the larynx and hypopharynx. Palpate the neck for trauma to the airway, hematoma, crepitus, and midline shift.

If there are no life-threatening emergencies, a focused history is taken and an examination of the temporal bone is performed. Pertinent history includes vertigo, hearing loss, otalgia, otorrhea, rhinorrhea, pulsatile tinnitus, and facial paralysis. Try to ascertain from other observers whether there was immediate or delayed onset of any facial paralysis. Vertigo may be episodic or intermittent, positional or spontaneous. On physical examination, look for postauricular ecchymosis or *Battle's sign*, which is consistent with temporal bone fracture. Periorbital ecchymosis or raccoon eyes are also indicative of a base of skull fracture. The auricle should be examined for external trauma, especially avulsion or denuded cartilage. The external auditory canal should be cleaned under an otomicroscope to facilitate examination. Signs of trauma in the external auditory canal include lacerations, ecchymoses, hematomas, and the presence of CSF. At the level of the tympanic membrane and the middle ear, document hemotympanum or other middle ear fluid (e.g., CSF), perforation, and any visible ossicular landmarks. If CSF otorrhea is seen, cleaning should stop and the ear should be packed to create a biologic dressing.

Tuning forks can be useful for evaluation of hearing at the bedside. Lateralization of the tone to the afflicted ear is consistent with a conductive hearing loss and preservation of sensorineural function. Formal audiograms are usually obtained after the patient is otherwise stable and alert. Many conductive hearing losses will improve in the first few months, as middle ear fluid resolves or as loose ossicular connections restabilize. The conductive loss from persistent ossicular discontinuity will commonly exceed 30 to 45 dB. Ossicular discontinuity can result in type A_D (abnormally high peak admittance) tympanogram and the loss of stapedial reflexes in the affected ear.

The presence and directionality of any spontaneous nystagmus should be documented. Vertigo associated with spontaneous nystagmus or with decrease or absence of ipsilateral caloric response on electronystagmography (ENG) is indicative of injury to the peripheral vestibular system. The patient with positional or intermittent vertigo should be evaluated by positioning the head with the affected ear in the dependent position (Hallpike maneuver). Severe rotatory nystagmus lasting less than a minute with latency of onset and fatiguability is consistent with benign paroxysmal positional vertigo. Symptoms of traumatic perilymph fistula include SNHL that may fluctuate, tinnitus, and vertigo. Delayed onset of symptoms can be difficult to distinguish from Meniere's disease or delayed endolymphatic hydrops. A positive fistula test (using pneumatic otoscopy or ENG with an immittance device) can help confirm a suspected fistula, and the ENG may show ipsilateral caloric weakness.

The leak of clear watery fluid from the ear or from the nose, or clear fluid behind an intact tympanic membrane, indicates CSF leak. Flow will increase with the head hanging forward in the dependent position or with the Valsalva maneuver. Because otorrhea or rhinorrhea after trauma is typically mixed with bloody secretions, demonstration of the *ring sign* at the bedside adds support to the diagnosis. To demonstrate the ring sign, drop the fluid onto tissue paper and look for the CSF to spread and create a clear halo around the centrally located bloody secretion. Other methods of confirming a CSF leak include detection of leakage of fluorescin or radionuclides after placement of these substances into the subarachnoid space. The definitive test for identification of CSF is to analyze the fluid for the presence of β_2-transferrin.[85–99] Methods for the localization of persistent leaks have evolved over time. Iohexol high-resolution computed tomography (CT) scans have been successfully used to demonstrate site of leak. The CT or magnetic resonance imaging (MRI) may also show an encephalocele related to the fracture line, which may underlie the leak of CSF.

Most importantly, the function of all branches of the facial nerve should be evaluated for later comparison.[100] In case of diminished or absent facial motion, symptoms of eye pain, diminished visual acuity, and epiphora should be noted. Corneal sensation and Bell's phenomenon should be documented. Central facial paralysis should not affect the forehead motion due to contralateral innervation. Extratemporal facial nerve injury should be suspected when there is sparing of some branches of the facial nerve or there is soft tissue injury medial to the lateral canthus of the eye.

If there is only facial paresis, no electrophysiologic testing is warranted. Complete facial paralysis suggests an intratemporal injury and warrants electrophysiologic testing. Commonly used tests include the maximal stimulation test (MST), electromyography (EMG), and electroneurography (ENoG). The Hilger stimulator can be used to deliver a suprathreshold nerve stimulus at the bedside; persistent normal facial motion after 48 to 72 hours postinjury helps to quantitate the degree and progression of Wallerian degeneration. Following denervation, EMG will demonstrate fibrillation potentials. Recovery of facial movement will be preceded by the appearance of polyphasic reinnervation potentials on EMG.

Topognostic testing has been used to help determine the site of facial nerve injury, but it has not been consistently reliable. Topognostic testing and imaging may influence the surgical approach if exploration is indicated; however, most fractures require exploration of the perigeniculate area. An abnormal Schirmer's lacrimation test may indicate facial nerve injury at or proximal to the greater superficial petrosal nerve (normal is 15 mm in 5 minutes). Stapedial reflexes should be obtained during the audiogram. An intact acoustic reflex with acute facial paralysis indicates a lesion in the mastoid or extratemporal segment of the facial nerve.

Temporal lobe injury may manifest as hemiplegia, expressive aphasia, seizures, or auditory, olfactory, or visual hallucinations. Central nervous system injuries include contusion of the brain parenchyma, edema, microvascular hemorrhage or infarct, and encephalopathy. These can be heralded by changes in level of consciousness, headache, seizures, loss of cognitive function, personality/behavioral changes, incoordination, spasticity/paralysis, or cranial nerve deficits. A funduscopic examination is important to rule out increased intracranial pressure manifested by papilledema.

High-resolution CT scan (1.5-mm-thick axial and coronal cuts) is the image technique of choice for radiographic evaluation of a temporal bone fracture[12,101–103] (**Fig. 21–9**). This can usually be performed electively once the patient is stable, and it facilitates the diagnosis and prognosis of the structures injured in and around the temporal bone. The site of fracture, the site(s) of facial nerve injury, dislocation of ossicles, and the site of a CSF leak can often be determined. Penetrating trauma in this region may require an angiogram. The CT scan also is important in ruling out adjacent skull fractures, intracranial hematoma or hemorrhage, and parenchymal injury of the brain. Indications for immediate radiographic evaluation include open skull fractures, intracranial hemorrhage, blindness due to arterial occlusion, evidence of cavernous sinus injury, and any evidence of increased intracranial pressure.

Surgical intervention specific to the temporal bone typically is based more on clinical findings and other diagnostic and prognostic tests (e.g., electrophysiologic tests, audiometry) than on CT results.

◆ Treatment

Auditory

Hemotympanum can result in up to a 30- to 45-dB conductive hearing loss initially. Usually, the hemotympanum is self-limited and clears by the fourth to sixth week. Myringotomy for drainage of the hemotympanum is not generally recommended due to the potential for infection.

Small traumatic perforations of the tympanic membrane often heal with conservative management over several weeks. Careful examination is needed to ensure that none of the perforation edges has become infolded, creating the risk for development of a cholesteatoma. A cigarette paper patch can be applied to a small perforation once the edges have been freshened. Unless there is gross contamination of the middle ear, antibiotic ear drops are not necessary. Keeping the ears free from water exposure is advised. For uncomplicated perforations that persist longer than several months, a variety of procedures can be offered to the patient. Similarly, fat myringoplasties have been employed with success. A type I tympanoplasty via a transcanal or postauricular approach traditionally has been recommended, especially if the perforation is large, difficult to visualize, or complicated by ossicular discontinuity or chronic infection.

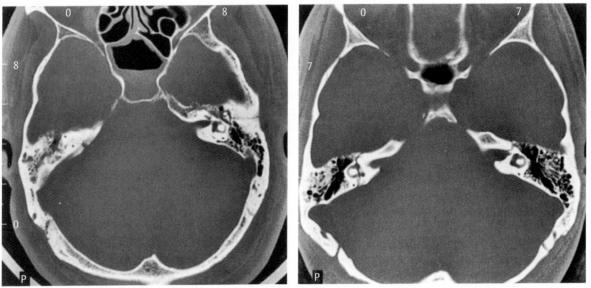

Figure 21–9 **(A)** Axial CT scan image (bone window) of a left longitudinal temporal bone fracture due to a fall with loss of consciousness. **(B)** Axial scan image (bone window) of a right transverse temporal bone fracture sustained in a motor vehicle accident. The fracture traverses the labyrinth.

Patients with persistent conductive hearing losses greater than 25 dB may be eligible for middle ear exploration with ossicular reconstruction. Hearing aids or conservative management are alternatives, depending on the patient's overall hearing status. Timing of the surgery is elective after hearing has stabilized; wait at least 3 months for any spontaneous healing to occur (suspected stapes fracture with PLF requires urgent surgery). Surgical options for a dislocated incus include incus interposition or transposition, or the use of an ossicular reconstruction prosthesis. Injuries involving the stapes footplate may necessitate repair by tissue graft or partial or total stapedectomy. Ossicular reconstruction can be accomplished by autograft (e.g., ossicle, bone, cartilage) or alloplastic material (e.g., stapes prosthesis, total or partial ossicular reconstruction prostheses). Fractured fragments dislocated into the vestibule are not removed due to the risk of SNHL.

Most patients with transverse fractures have a profound, irreversible SNHL. The majority of patients who have mild closed head injuries and have only low-frequency SNHL may recover hearing thresholds in the first couple of days; high-frequency losses are much less likely to recover. The vast majority of patients with temporal bone fractures and SNHL do not improve significantly with time. Moderate to severe losses may benefit from a hearing aid. Persistent nonpulsatile tinnitus after temporal bone trauma is usually associated with hearing loss and can be difficult to ameliorate. In patients who might otherwise benefit from a hearing aid, the aid may also mask tinnitus in the daytime. Background noise such as white noise or music from a radio can be used at night, or a more formal tinnitus masker can be fitted if there is sufficient residual inhibition.

Vestibular

The course of benign paroxysmal positional vertigo (BPPV) is usually self-limited with resolution of symptoms in 3 months.[57,65–70] Therapeutic maneuvers such as that of Epley may be efficacious and provide immediate resolution. Surgical interventions such as singular neurectomy or vestibular nerve section are rarely required.

Most of the symptoms of vestibular injury are self-limited and gradually resolve in 6 months. During that time the patient should be as active as possible and use the minimal amount of vestibular sedative needed, to facilitate central vestibular compensation. For severe continuous or prolonged episodes of vertigo, short courses of meclizine or diazepam may be helpful. Persistent vertigo or unsteadiness following head trauma suggests a possible central cause or failure of central compensation. In cases of failure of compensation, vestibular dysfunction would include vestibular nerve section (useful hearing) and a labyrinthectomy (no useful hearing)[104–109] (see Chapter 27).

Urgent middle ear exploration is recommended to repair an obvious traumatic perilymph leak, to attempt hearing preservation, and to resolve disequilibrium.[32–42] Some otologists avoid urgent surgery for fear of doing more harm than good. There are no uniform criteria for selecting patients for middle ear exploration. A history of antecedent trauma, vertigo, and SNHL favor the diagnosis of PLF. Symptoms include tinnitus, vertigo with or without disequilibrium, aural fullness, and SNHL that may be fluctuating. The sensitivity of the fistula test may be as low as 60%,[38] so the diagnosis is based primarily on symptoms, a high index of clinical suspicion, and middle ear exploration. ENG may show abnormalities. The most common ENG finding is spontaneous nystagmus, which can be directed either away from or toward the affected ear. Positional nystagmus and ipsilateral vestibular hypofunction have been seen as well. Surgical repair of PLF will most likely improve vertigo; hearing and tinnitus can improve, according to some reports. The patient should be cautioned against the Valsalva maneuver, heavy lifting or straining, or flying for at least several weeks postrepair; scuba diving or other activities that can produce severe pressure changes within the ear may be contraindicated in the long term.

Facial Paralysis

Initial management of facial nerve dysfunction should include corneal protection. For significant lagophthalmos with incomplete eye closure, liberal use of eyedrops during the daytime is prescribed. Nightly application of ophthalmic ointment and eye protection (bubble protector, moisture chamber) are enforced to prevent exposure keratitis.

More definitive treatment is based on prognosis. Overall, facial nerve paresis (incomplete loss of facial nerve function)

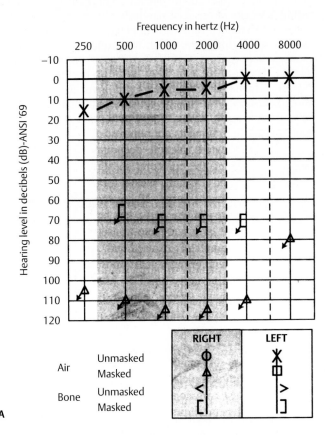

		RIGHT	LEFT
Air	Unmasked	O	X
	Masked	△	☐
Bone	Unmasked	<	>
	Masked	[	]

A

↙ or ↘ attached to symbol indicates "no response" at maximum output of the audiometer.

Figure 21–10 **(A)** Audiogram demonstrating profound right sensorineural hearing loss due to a transverse temporal bone fracture. Associated findings included horizontal spontaneous nystagmus and complete facial paralysis. **(B)** Electroneurography of the right facial nerve in the same patient after a transverse temporal bone fracture. The amplitude of the compound action potential was 36% of the response from the contralateral facial nerve 8 days postinjury. **(C)** Serial electroneurography of the facial nerve showed a decrease in the amplitude of the compound muscle action potential to 18% within 3 weeks of injury. This patient did not undergo facial nerve exploration and began to show clinical return of function 1 month postinjury.

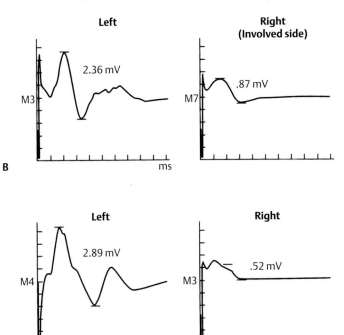

carries an excellent prognosis, and conservative management is recommended.[5,110–115] Electrical testing is not necessary in this setting.

After paralysis, spontaneous nerve regeneration can be detectable by EMG as early as 3 weeks after injury. Reinnervation potentials usually precede the clinical return of motor function, which is usually apparent by 1 to 2 months. The role of steroids is unclear.

Clinical management of complete paralysis is based on electrophysiologic testing.[9,75,77–84] Delay in the onset of the facial paralysis or the ability to stimulate the nerve more than 48 to 72 hours postinjury confirms that the nerve has not been transected. In either situation, however, the nerve still may be severely injured and require surgical intervention to maximize recovery potential. ENoG should be used to follow progression of neural degeneration for 2 to 3 weeks posttrauma

(**Fig. 21–10**). After 3 weeks, a false-negative response to ENoG may be due to asynchronous firing from regenerating axons. An EMG should be performed to rule out the presence of any voluntary potentials.

For complete facial nerve paralysis, early facial nerve exploration for decompression or repair is recommended if there is greater than 90% degeneration of the ENoG response within 2 weeks of onset of paralysis.[11,73,75,116–124] Studies have suggested that such rapid loss of electrical excitability indicates a severe injury in which a significant proportion of axons will progress from axonotmesis to neurotmesis (**Fig. 21–11**). EMG can be used to identify fibrillation potentials or polyphasic reinnervation potentials. Exploration for immediate-onset paralysis is indicated if there is obvious nerve transection, which is very likely in penetrating temporal bone trauma.

III Management

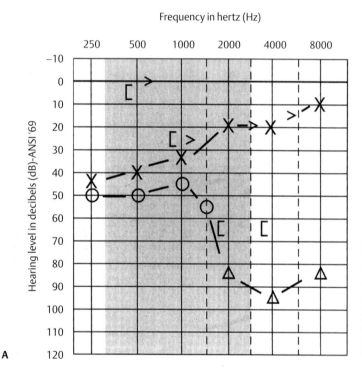

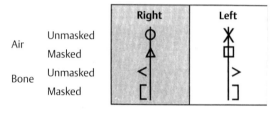

Figure 21–11 **(A)** Audiogram after a mixed right temporal bone fracture showing right mixed hearing loss. **(B)** Electroneurography of the right facial nerve in same patient showed no response 19 days postinjury, and there was no response to Hilger facial nerve stimulation. The patient underwent right facial nerve exploration and decompression via a middle fossa approach. The fracture had partially transected the labyrinthine segment of the facial nerve. Recovery of facial function 6 months later was poor, and this patient underwent a hypoglossal-to-facial nerve anastomosis.

Although it is the authors' bias to consider strongly surgical exploration for patients meeting the criteria noted above, it is acknowledged that conclusive studies demonstrating the efficacy of facial nerve decompression are lacking. Brodie and Thompson[125] as well as other authors[126] have reported small series of patients who met the surgical criteria but were treated only with observation. Good recovery was reported in approximately 50 to 60% of these patients.

Patients with a complete paralysis who are initially seen several months after injury present a diagnostic dilemma, although decompression still may be indicated.[9,77,127,128] A history of sudden onset of facial paralysis suggests a more severe injury. An EMG is obtained to detect evidence of reinnervation potentials or voluntary motor potentials. In this setting, failure to regenerate can be due to a transection injury or severe intraneural fibrosis. Exploration of the nerve at this time may optimize any chance for recovery. Nerve graft results seem better if performed within the first 12 months. In some instances, excision of a fibrotic segment with primary anastomosis or interposition graft as long as 12 to 18 months postinjury has resulted in recovery of facial tone and some mimetic movement. Viability of facial muscles should be confirmed by EMG fibrillation potentials. If more than 12 to 18 months have elapsed without clinical evidence of facial motion, substitution procedures (e.g., hypoglossal-to-facial anastomosis), muscle transpositions, or static sling procedures may be required.

The surgical approach to exploration and decompression of the facial nerve is based on the status of the hearing and the anticipated sites of injury.[11,73,75,116–124] In most cases, exploration of the nerve needs to include the perigeniculate region. For most longitudinal temporal bone fractures, both middle cranial fossa and transmastoid explorations of the facial nerve are required (**Fig. 21–12**). The nerve is exposed by a translabyrinthine approach in cases of a transverse fracture with severe to profound SNHL (**Fig. 21–13**). Impinging bone fragments are removed and any intraneural hematoma evacuated. Nerve decompression usually extends from the meatal foramen to the vertical segment of the facial nerve. If greater than 50% of the cross-sectional area of the nerve has been lost, the injury should be treated as a complete transection. The traumatized region is completely excised and, if possible, rerouting of the nerve with primary anastomoses is accomplished. A greater auricular nerve graft is interposed if primary anastomosis without tension cannot be achieved.[129–133] Temporizing measures for eye protection include tarsorrhaphy or implantation of gold eyelid weight. These procedures are reversible if facial motion should return.

Exceptions to this management plan arise in the case of the neonate with complete facial paralysis. Neonatal facial paralysis is most commonly caused by birth trauma or by developmental neuromuscular anomalies. Facial paralysis following birth trauma has been associated with forceps delivery and with decompression of the head and face during prolonged or difficult spontaneous delivery. The temporal bone is softer in the neonate, and the facial nerve is more superficially located. Birth trauma results in compression or crushing of the facial nerve within the fallopian canal but transection of the nerve has not been reported. Neonatal traumatic facial paralysis is usually unilateral and accompanied by facial ecchymosis, Battle's sign, or hemotympanum. In contrast, developmental anomalies presenting with facial paralysis are usually associated with maldevelopment of the face or ear and multiple or bilateral cranial nerve deficits, including abnormal eighth nerve findings.

In contrast to adults, electrophysiologic testing for neonatal facial paralysis should be done soon after birth. The primary clinical concern is documentation of the presence of neuromuscular integrity, to distinguish traumatic from developmental paralysis. Spontaneous and complete recovery occurs in greater than 90% of neonatal facial paralysis. Usually recovery is detectable within the first 4 weeks of life due to the excellent prognosis and the unlikelihood of nerve transection.[134–139] Observation and conservative management are recommended for 5 weeks before considering surgical exploration.

Intracranial

Treatment of parenchymal brain injury and intracranial complications depends on the site and the type of injury. Consultation with a neurologist or neurosurgeon should be obtained. Management of a confirmed CSF leak depends on duration, site, and presence of complications.[86–99] Conservative management is acceptable initially. Most leaks resolve spontaneously within the first 3 to 5 days after injury. Coverage with antibiotics is controversial and often not recommended, to prevent masking the early symptoms of meningitis or selecting for resistant organisms. Patients are initially treated with strict bed rest and head elevation; a lumbar drain may be necessary if this early conservative approach is unsuccessful. Leaks that persist beyond 10 to 14 days require surgical intervention due to the risk of meningitis. Surgical approaches to close a CSF leak depend on the site of leak and the hearing status. A transmastoid and middle fossa approach used alone or in combination allows both repair of the leak and reduction or resection of any encephalocele in cases of intact hearing. The transmastoid approach and repair with abdominal fat graft can be used if hearing has been lost, and obliteration of the eustachian tube and middle ear with soft tissue may be employed to isolate any dural dehiscence from the external environment.

Vascular

Intracranial vascular complications require neurosurgical consultation.[140–144] Hemorrhage from the sigmoid or petrosal sinuses can usually be managed by transmastoid exposure followed by extraluminal packing at the site of injury. Occasionally ligation of the internal jugular vein distally is also required. Arterial hemorrhage is most quickly managed by balloon occlusion or embolization.

◆ Other Considerations

Recurrent Conductive Hearing Loss

Adhesions to the ossicles in the epitympanum and posterior mesotympanum as well as displacement of an ossicular prosthesis or repositioned incus may cause a conductive hearing loss during follow-up. Scarring in the external auditory canal leads to canal stenosis and secondary infection or cholesteatoma of the canal. Treatment of these conditions is primarily surgical, involving middle ear exploration and canaloplasty.

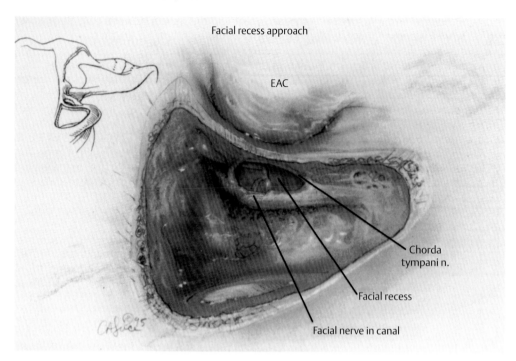

Facial recess approach

EAC

Chorda
tympani n.

Facial recess

Facial nerve in canal

A

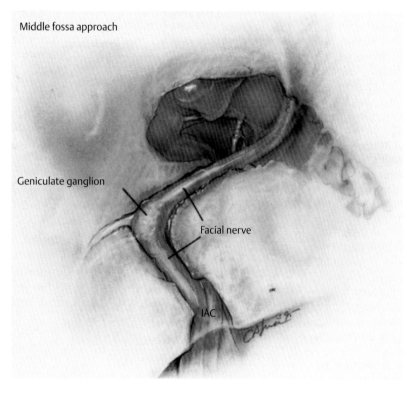

Middle fossa approach

Geniculate ganglion

Facial nerve

IAC

B

Figure 21–12 **(A)** Diagram of the transmastoid-facial recess approach to the facial nerve. This approach should be combined with the middle fossa approach **(B)** because of the high likelihood of coexisting injury to the mastoid segment of the nerve. EAC, external auditory canal; IAC, internal auditory canal.

Cholesteatoma

Cholesteatoma may involve the pneumatized spaces of the temporal bone as a delayed complication of penetrating or blunt trauma, particularly after a longitudinal fracture.[145,146] The cholesteatoma primarily results from trapped or ingrown squamous epithelium of the external auditory canal. Treatment is surgical removal of the cholesteatoma from the canal, middle ear, or mastoid by transcanal or transmastoid approaches.

Delayed Endolymphatic Hydrops

Delayed endolymphatic hydrops with SNHL, episodic vertigo, aural fulness, and tinnitus can arise many years after transverse temporal bone and other fractures of the skull base.[71,147] Trauma or obstruction to the vestibular aqueduct is thought to be the mechanism responsible for hydrops, which has also been associated with these symptoms.

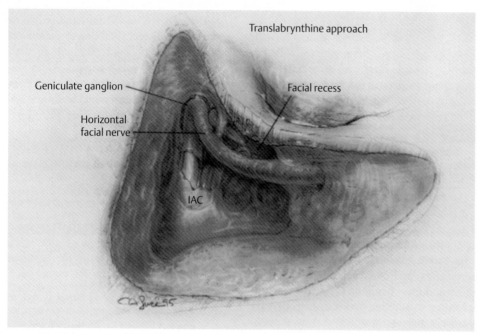

Figure 21–13 Diagram of translabyrinthine exposure of the facial nerve from the tympanic segment to the internal auditory canal (IAC) can be used for transverse temporal bone fractures without residual hearing.

Encephalocele

Temporal bone fractures heal primarily by fibrous union. The middle cranial fossa is usually sealed off from the ear within 3 to 4 weeks by a combination of mucosa, bone, and fibrous tissue from the endosteal and periosteal layers of the osseous labyrinth. An encephalocele or meningoencephalocele results from failure to adequately heal the fracture site and associated dural injury. If the dura is uninjured and the intracranial pressure remains within normal limits, then sizable middle fossa tegmen defects can be tolerated without formation of an encephalocele. In fact, spontaneous asymptomatic tegmen dehiscences frequently are found at surgery and at autopsy. Traumatic encephaloceles may be asymptomatic or may present in various ways: a pulsatile soft mass in the external auditory canal that increases in size with Valsalva, recurrent meningitis, or herniation into the middle ear resulting in conductive hearing loss.[148–150]

Diagnosis of the tegmen defect is best accomplished by high-resolution axial and coronal CT scans, but the presence of central nervous system tissue and CSF in the herniated tissue is best identified on an MRI scan. Treatment is surgical reduction with excision of the herniated brain and repair of the tegmen defect. Surgical approach is transmastoid for small defects; this can be combined with a middle fossa approach for larger defects.

Otitic Meningitis

Meningitis can complicate a traumatic encephalocele or CSF leak.[86–89] Meningitis can also occur as a delayed consequence of a temporal bone fracture months or years later, even without a CSF leak. In such cases, incomplete healing of the fracture line provides a pathway for pathogens to access the CSF space. Recurrent meningitis is not unusual, and is usually associated with otitis media. One should look for a middle ear effusion that could represent an acute or resolving otitis media or CSF. Signs and symptoms of meningitis include fever, headache, meningismus, positive Kernig's or Brudzinski's sign, and changes in level of consciousness or mental status. Diagnosis is based on lumbar puncture with examination of the CSF for protein, glucose, Gram stain, cell count, and culture, after CT scan to rule out obstructive hydrocephalus. Intravenous antibiotics that provide central nervous system penetration and broad coverage of middle ear and upper respiratory organisms should be initiated immediately. Continued antibiotic treatment is based on culture results and sensitivities of the organisms, as well as the clinical response. Pneumococcus is the most frequent organism.

Pneumocephalus and Pneumolabyrinth

Pneumocephalus is a rare complication that denotes the entry of air into the cranial vault through a traumatic breach in the continuity of the dura and the bone.[151–154] Presenting symptoms can be vague. Headache, meningismus, aphasia, vomiting, visual alteration, decreased level of consciousness, hemiplegia, seizures, and other neurologic signs can occur. The diagnosis is readily made on CT scan. Uncomplicated pneumocephalus usually resolves spontaneously by resorption of the air. Persistent pneumocephalus or pneumocephalus associated with a persistent CSF leak is an indication for surgical repair of the defect. Tension pneumocephalus requires urgent surgical intervention. Entry of air into the labyrinth is also rare, but when seen on CT scan it indicates a fracture of the otic capsule or dislocation of the stapes.[155]

Temporomandibular Joint Trauma

The tympanic, petrous, and squamous portions of the temporal bone are situated about the posterior aspect of the glenoid fossa. Trauma to the mandible in cases of multiple trauma can result in posterior displacement of the mandibular condyle and thus results in a fracture of the external auditory canal. Uncommonly, there can be traumatic displacement of the condyle into the middle fossa with pneumocephalus, which must be emergently reduced and repaired. Fractures of the temporal bone can conversely extend into the glenoid fossa resulting in air in the temporomandibular joint and joint dysfunction.[152–154,156–158]

Carotid-Cavernous Fistula

Carotid-cavernous fistula (CCF) may present immediately or years following a penetrating skull base trauma.[159] CCF can be classified as direct or indirect. Direct communication between the intracavernous internal carotid artery and the cavernous sinus is the most common type, and is most frequently caused by trauma. Indirect fistulas usually arise spontaneously and involve an abnormal connection between the cavernous sinus and the dural branches of either the internal or external carotid artery (middle meningeal artery, accessory meningeal artery, or the artery of the foramen rotundum). Symptoms usually result from shunting of blood into the superior ophthalmic vein, but can also present with a steal syndrome. Orbital findings include pulsatile proptosis or tinnitus, chemosis, lid edema, orbital bruit, ophthalmoplegia, glaucoma, decreased visual acuity, and severe epistaxis.

Diagnosis is based on angiography and imaging of the skull base. Direct CCF due to trauma requires intervention; progressive monocular blindness occurs in 50% of untreated cases. If facial nerve exploration is also needed, CCF repair should proceed first to avoid severe hemorrhage if fragments in the cavernous sinus are inadvertently manipulated. CCF can be surgically repaired by ligating the carotid proximally in the neck and distally at the supraclinoid carotid segment. Alternatively, the carotid artery can be preserved with selective embolization of the CCF.

References

1. Murphy AG. The ear and cranial trauma. Arch Otolaryngol 1935; 21:686–693
2. Podoshin L, Fradis M. Hearing loss after head injury. Arch Otolaryngol 1975;101:15–18
3. Singh SP, Adeloye A. Hearing loss in missile head injuries. J Laryngol Otol 1971;85:1183–1187
4. Tos M. Prognosis of hearing loss in temporal bone fractures. J Laryngol Otol 1971;85:1147–1159
5. Grove WE. Skull fractures involving the ear. A clinical study of 211 cases. Laryngoscope 1939;49:678–706, 833–867
6. Griffin JE, Altenase MM, Schaefer SD. Bilateral longitudinal temporal bone fractures: a retrospective review of seventeen cases. Laryngoscope 1979;89:1432–1435
7. Proctor B, Gurdjian ES, Webster JE. The ear in head trauma. Laryngoscope 1956;66:16–59
8. Fisch U. Facial paralysis in fractures of the petrous bone. Laryngoscope 1974;84:2141–2154
9. Harker L, McCabe BF. Temporal bone fractures and facial nerve injury. Otolaryngol Clin North Am 1974;7:425–431
10. Ghorayeb BY, Yeakley JW. Temporal bone fractures: longitudinal or oblique? The case for oblique temporal bone fractures. Laryngoscope 1992;102:129–134
11. McHugh HE. The surgical treatment of facial paralysis and traumatic conductive deafness on fractures of the temporal bone. Ann Otol Rhinol Laryngol 1959;68:855–889
12. Aguillar EA 3rd, Yeakley JW, Ghorayeb BY, et al. High resolution CT scans of temporal bone fractures: association of facial paralysis with temporal bone fractures. Head Neck Surg 1987;9:162–166
13. McGuirt WF Jr, Stool S. Temporal bone fractures in children: a review with emphasis on long-term sequelae. Clin Pediatr (Phila) 1992;31:12–18
14. Williams WT, Ghorayeb BY, Yeakley JW. Pediatric temporal bone fractures. Laryngoscope 1992;102:600–603
15. Duncan NO III, Coker NJ, Jenkins HA, Canalis RF. Gunshot injuries of the temporal bone. Otolaryngol Head Neck Surg 1986;94:47–55
16. Griffith MV. The incidence of auditory and vestibular concussion following minor head injury. J Laryngol Otol 1979;9:253–265
17. Barber HO. Head injury, audiological and vestibular findings. Ann Otol Rhinol Laryngol 1969;78:239–252
18. Silverstein H, Fabian RL, Stoll SE, Hong SW. Penetrating wounds of the tympanic membrane and ossicular chain. Trans Am Acad Ophthalmol Otolaryngol 1973;77:ORL125–135
19. Arragg FG, Paparella MM. Traumatic fracture of the stapes. Laryngoscope 1964;74:1329–1332
20. Kerr AG, Byrne JET. Concussive effects of bomb blast on the ear. J Laryngol Otol 1975;89:131–143
21. Roberto M, Hamernik RP, Turrentine GA. Damage of the auditory system associated with acute blast trauma. Ann Otol Rhinol Laryngol Suppl 1989;140:23–34
22. Armstrong HG, Heim JW. The effects of flight on the middle ear. JAMA 1937;109:417–421
23. King PF. Otitic barotrauma. Proc R Soc Med 1966;59:543–554
24. Bayliss GJ. Aural barotoma in naval divers. Arch Otolaryngol 1968; 88:141–147
25. Soss SL. Sensorineural hearing loss with diving. Arch Otolaryngol 1971;93:501–504
26. Freeman P, Edmonds C. Inner ear barotrauma. Arch Otolaryngol 1972;95:556–563
27. Pullen FW II, Rosenberg GJ, Cabeza CH. Sudden hearing loss in divers and fliers. Laryngoscope 1979;89:1373–1377
28. Farmer JC, Thomas WG, Youngblood DG, Bennett PB. Inner ear decompression sickness. Laryngoscope 1976;86:1315–1326
29. Gray RF, Barton RPE. Clinical records. Round window rupture. J Laryngol Otol 1981;95:165–177
30. Fraser JG, Harborow PC. Labyrinthine window rupture. J Laryngol Otol 1975;89:1–7
31. Althaus SR. Perilymph fistulas. Laryngoscope 1981;91:538–562
32. Goodhill V. Leaking labyrinth lesions, deafness, tinnitus and dizziness. Ann Otol Rhinol Laryngol 1981;90:99–106
33. Feldmann H. Sudden hearing loss with delayed onset following head trauma. Acta Otolaryngol 1987;103:379–383
34. Fee GA. Traumatic perilymphatic fistulas. Arch Otolaryngol 1968; 88:477–480
35. Tonkin JP, Fagan P. Rupture of the round window membrane. J Laryngol Otol 1975;89:733–756
36. Kohut RI, Waldorf RA, Haenel JL, Thompson JN. Minute perilymph fistulas: vertigo and Hennbert's sign without hearing loss. Ann Otol Rhinol Laryngol 1979;88:153–159
37. Thompson JN, Kohut RI. Perilymph fistula: variability of symptoms and results of surgery. Otolaryngol Head Neck Surg 1979;87: 898–903
38. Goodhill V. Traumatic fistulae. J Laryngol Otol 1980;94:123–128
39. Grimm RJ, Hemenway WG, LeBray PR, Black FO. The perilymph fistula syndrome defined in mild head trauma. Acta Otolaryngol Suppl 1989;464:1–40
40. Paparella MM. Interactive inner-ear/middle-ear disease, including perilymph fistula. Acta Otolaryngol Suppl 1991;485:36–45
41. Glasscock ME III, Hart MJ, Rosdeutscher JD, Bhansali SA. Traumatic perilymphatic fistula: how long can symptoms persist? A follow-up report. Am J Otol 1992;13:333–338
42. Seltzer S, McCabe BF. Perilymph fistula: the Iowa experience. Laryngoscope 1986;96:37–49
43. Glasscock ME, McKennan KX, Levine SC. Persistent traumatic perilymph fistulas. Laryngoscope 1987;97:860–864
44. Wright JW, Silk KL. Acoustic and vestibular defects in lightning survivors. Laryngoscope 1974;84:1378–1387
45. Weiss KS. Otologic lightning bolts. Am J Otolaryngol 1980;1:334–337
46. Jones DT, Ogren FP, Roh LH, Moore GF. Lightning and its effect on the auditory system. Laryngoscope 1991;101:830–834
47. Bergstrom L, Neblett LW, Sando I, Hemenway WG, Harrison GD. The lightning-damaged ear. Arch Otolaryngol 1974;100:117–121
48. Youngs R, Deck J, Kwok P, Hawke M. Severe sensorineural hearing loss caused by lightning. A temporal bone case report. Arch Otolaryngol Head Neck Surg 1988;114:1184–1187
49. Hough JV. Restoration of hearing loss after head trauma. Ann Otol Rhinol Laryngol 1969;78:210–226
50. Does IE, Bottema T. Post-traumatic conductive hearing loss. Arch Otolaryngol 1965;82:331–339

51. Wright JW, Taylor CG, Bizal JA. Tomography and the vulnerable incus. Ann Otol Rhinol Laryngol 1969;78:263–279

52. Cannon CR, Jahresdoerfer RA. Temporal bone fractures. Arch Otolaryngol 1983;109:285–288

53. Spector G, Pratt LL, Randall G. A clinical study of delayed reconstruction in ossicular fractures. Laryngoscope 1973;83:837–851

54. Hough J, Stuart W. Middle ear injuries in skull trauma. Laryngoscope 1968;78:899–937

55. Bellucci RJ. Traumatic injuries of the middle ear. Otolaryngol Clin North Am 1983;16:633–650

56. Strohm M. Trauma of the middle ear. Clinical findings, postmortem observation and results of experimental studies. Adv Otorhinolaryngol 1986;35:1–254

57. Schuknecht HF, Davison RC. Deafness and vertigo from head injury. Arch Otolaryngol 1956;63:513–528

58. Schuknecht HF. A clinical study of auditory damage following blows to the head. Ann Otol Rhinol Laryngol 1950;59:331–358

59. Makishima K, Snow JB. Pathogenesis of hearing loss in head injury: studies in man and experimental animals. Arch Otolaryngol 1975;101:426–432

60. Makishima K, Sobel SF, Snow JB. Histopathologic correlates of otoneurologic manifestations following head trauma. Laryngoscope 1976; 86:1303–1314

61. Lindsay JR, Zajtchuk J. Concussion of the inner ear. Ann Otol Rhinol Laryngol 1970;79:699–709

62. Schuknecht HF. Mechanism of inner ear injury from blows to the head. Ann Otol Rhinol Laryngol 1969;78:253–262

63. Kirikae I, Eguchi K, Okamoto M, Nakamura K. Histopathological changes in the auditory pathway in case of fatal head injury. Acta Otolaryngol 1969;67:341–349

64. Rantanen T, Aantaa E, Salmivalli A, et al. Audiometric and electronystagmographic studies of patients with traumatic skull injuries. Acta Otolaryngol 1966;224(suppl):256–259

65. Pearson BW, Barber HO. Head injury: some otoneurologic sequelae. Arch Otolaryngol 1973;97:81–84

66. Dix MR, Hallpike CS. The pathology, symptomatology and diagnosis of certain common disorders of the vestibular system. Ann Otol Rhinol Laryngol 1952;61:987–1016

67. Schuknecht HF. Cupololithiasis. Arch Otolaryngol 1969;90:765–778

68. Parker DE, Covell WP, von Gierke HE. Exploration of vestibular damage in guinea pigs following mechanical stimulation. Acta Otolaryngol 1968;239:7–59

69. Cawthorne T. Positional nystagmus. Ann Otol Rhinol Laryngol 1954;63:481–490

70. Cawthorne TE, Hallpike CS. A study of the clinical features and pathological changes within the temporal bones, brain stem and cerebellum of an early case of positional nystagmus of the so-called benign paroxysmal type. Acta Otolaryngol 1957;48:89–103

71. Gordon N. Post-traumatic vertigo with special reference to positional nystagmus. Lancet 1954;266:1216–1218

72. Rizvi SS, Gibbin KP. Effect of transverse temporal bone fracture on the fluid compartment of the inner ear. Ann Otol Rhinol Laryngol 1979;88:741–748

73. Windle WF, Groat RA, Fox CA. Experimental structural alterations in the brain during and after concussion. Surg Gynecol Obstet 1944; 79:561–572

74. Lambert PR, Brackmann DE. Facial paralysis in longitudinal temporal bone fracture: a review of 26 cases. Laryngoscope 1984;94:1022–1026

75. Travis LW, Stalnaker RL, Melvin JW. Impact trauma of the human temporal bone. J Trauma 1977;17:761–766

76. Coker NJ, Kendall KA, Jenkins HA, Alford BR. Traumatic intratemporal facial nerve injury: management rationale for preservation of function. Otolaryngol Head Neck Surg 1987;97:262–269

77. Sunderland S. Nerve and Nerve Injuries, 2nd ed. New York: Churchill-Livingstone, 1978

78. Esslen E. Electrodiagnosis of facial palsy. In: Miehlke A, ed. Surgery of the Facial Nerve, 2nd ed. Philadelphia: WB Saunders, 1973:45–51

79. May M, Harvey JE, Marovits WF. The prognostic accuracy of the maximal stimulation test compared with that of the nerve excitability test in Bell's palsy. Laryngoscope 1971;81:931–938

80. Fisch U. Prognostic value of electrical tests in acute facial paralysis. Am J Otol 1984;5:494–498

81. Hughes GB. Electroneurography: objective prognostic assessment of facial paralysis. Am J Otol 1982;4:73–76

82. Kamerer DB. Intratemproal facial nerve injuries. Otolaryngol Head Neck Surg 1982;90:612–615

83. Coker NJ, Fordice JO, Moore S. Correlation of the nerve excitability test and electroneurography in acute facial paralysis. Am J Otol 1992;13:127–133

84. Coker NJ. Facial electroneurography: analysis of techniques and correlation with degenerating motor neurons. Laryngoscope 1992;102:747–759

85. Lewis BI, Adour KK, Kahn JM, Lewis AJ. Hilger facial nerve stimulator: a 25-year update. Laryngoscope 1991;101:71–74

86. McGuirt WF Jr, Stool SE. Cerebrospinal fluid fistula: the identification and management in pediatric temporal bone fractures. Laryngoscope 1995;105:359–365

87. Dula DJ, Fales W. The "ring sign": is it a reliable indicator for cerebral spinal fluid? Ann Emerg Med 1993;22:718–720

88. Ryall RG, Peacock MK, Simpson DA. Usefulness of beta2-transferrin assay in the detection of cerebrospinal fluid leaks following head injury. J Neurosurg 1992;77:737–739

89. Fransen P, Sindic CJ, Thauvoy C, Laterre C, Stroobandt G. Highly sensitive detection of beta-2 transferrin in rhinorrhea and otorrhea as a marker for cerebrospinal fluid (C.S.F.) leakage. Acta Neurochir (Wien) 1991;109:98–101

90. Irjala K, Suonpaa J, Laurent B. Identification of CSF leakage by immunofixation. Arch Otolaryngol 1979;105:447–448

91. Miller RH. Cerebrospinal fluid rhinorrhea and otorrhea. Clin Neurosurg 1972;19:263–270

92. Hicks GW, Wright JW Jr, Wright JW III. Cerebrospinal fluid otorrhea. Laryngoscope 1980;90(suppl 25):1–25

93. Dandy WE. Treatment of rhinorrhea and otorrhea. Arch Surg 1944;49:75–85

94. Calcaterra TC, Rand RW. Tympanic cavity obliteration for cerebrospinal fluid otorhinorrhea. Arch Otolaryngol 1973;97:388–390

95. MacGee EE, Gauthen JC, Brackett CE. Meningitis following acute traumatic cerebrospinal fluid fistula. J Neurosurg 1970;33:312–316

96. Klastersky J, Sadeghi M, Brihaye J. Antimicrobial prophylaxis in patients with rhinorrhea or othorrhea: a double-blind study. Surg Neurol 1976;6:111–114

97. Pollak AM, Pauw BK, Marion MS. Temporal bone histopathology: resident's quiz. Otogenic pneumococci meningitis after transverse temporal bone fracture during childhood. Am J Otolaryngol 1991;12:56–58

98. Oberascher G. Cerebrospinal fluid otorrhea – new trends in diagnosis. Am J Otol 1988;9:102–108

99. Westmore GA, Whittam DE. Cerebrospinal fluid rhinorrhea and its management. Br J Surg 1982;69:489–492

100. Leech PJ, Paterson A. Conservative and operative management for cerebrospinal fluid leakage after closed head injury. Lancet 1973; 1:1013–1016

101. House JW. Facial nerve grading systems. Laryngoscope 1983; 93:1056–1069

102. Schubiger O, Valvanis A, Stuckamnn G, Antonucci F. Temporal bone fractures and their complications: examination with high resolution CT. Neuroradiology 1986;28:93–99

103. Kahn JB, Syewart MG, Diaz Marchan PJ. Acute temporal bone trauma: Utility of high resolution computed tomography. Am J Otol 2000;21:743–752

104. Haberkamp TJ, Harvey SA, Daniels DL. The use of gadolinium-enhanced magnetic resonance imaging to determine lesion site in traumatic facial paralysis. Laryngoscope 1990;100:1294–1300

105. Gotten N. Survey of one hundred cases of whiplash injury after settlement of litigation. JAMA 1956;162:865–867

106. Toglia JU, Rosenberg PE, Ronis ML. Posttraumatic dizziness. Vestibular, audiologic, and mediological aspects. Arch Otolaryngol 1970;92:485–492

107. Tuohimaa P. Vestibular disturbances after acute mild head injury. Acta Otolaryngol Suppl 1978;359:3–67

108. Ylikoski J, Palva T, Sanna M. Dizziness after head trauma: clinical and morphologic findings. Am J Otol 1982;3:343–352

109. Gacek RR. Transection of the posterior ampullary nerve for the relief of benign paroxysmal positional vertigo. Ann Otol Rhinol Laryngol 1974;83:596–605

110. Garcia-Ibanez E, Garcia-Ibanez JL. Middle fossa vestibular neurectomy: a report of 373 cases. Otolaryngol Head Neck Surg 1980;88:486–490

111. Turner JWA. Facial palsy in closed head injuries. Lancet 1944;246:756–757

112. Potter J. Facial palsy following head injury. J Laryngol Otol 1964;78:654–657

113. Curtin JM. Fractures of the skull and intratemporal lesions affecting the facial nerve. Adv Otorhinolaryngol 1977;22:202–206

114. Kettel K. Peripheral facial paralysis in fractures of the temporal bone. Arch Otolaryngol 1950;51:25–41

115. McKennan KX, Chole RA. Facial paralysis in temporal bone trauma. Am J Otol 1992;13:167–172

116. Adegbite AB, Khan MI, Tan L. Predicting recovery of facial nerve function following injury from a basilar skull fracture. J Neurosurg 1991;75:759–762

117. Adour K, Boyajean J, Kahn Z, Schneider GS. Surgical and nonsurgical management of facial paralysis following closed head injury. Laryngoscope 1977;87:380–390

118. Alford BR, Sessions RB, Weber SC. Indications for surgical decompression of the facial nerve. Laryngoscope 1971;81:620–635

119. Fisch U. Total facial nerve decompression and electroneurography. In: Silverstein H, Norrell H, eds. Neurologic Surgery of the Ear. Birmingham, AL: Aesculapis, 1977:chapter 4

120. Sillman JS, Niparko JK, Lee SS, Kileny PR. Prognostic valve of evoked and standard electromyography in acute facial paralysis. Otolaryngol Head Neck Surg 1992;107:377–381

121. Yanagihara N. Transmastoid decompression of the facial nerve in temporal bone fracture. Otolaryngol Head Neck Surg 1982;90:616–621

122. May M, Klein SR. Facial nerve decompression complications. Laryngoscope 1983;93:299–305

123. Fisch U, Esslen E. Total intratemporal exposure of the facial nerve. Arch Otolaryngol 1972;95:335–341

124. House WF, Crabtree JA. Surgical exposure of petrous portion of seventh nerve. Arch Otolaryngol 1965;81:506–507

125. Brodie HA, Thompson TC. Management of complications from 820 temporal bone fractures. Am J Otol 1997;18:188–197

126. Chang CY, Cass SP. Management of facial nerve injury due to temporal bone trauma. Am J Otol 1999;20:96–114

127. May M. Total facial nerve exploration: transmastoid, extra-labyrinthine, and subtemporal. Results. Laryngoscope 1979;89:906–916

128. Brodsky L, Eviatar A, Daniller A. Post-traumatic facial nerve paralysis. Three cases of delayed temporal bone exploration with recovery. Laryngoscope 1983;93:1560–1565

129. Felix H, Eby TL, Fisch U. New aspects of facial nerve pathology in temporal bone fractures. Acta Otolaryngol 1991;111:332–336

130. Coker NJ. Management of traumatic injuries to the facial nerve. Otolaryngol Clin North Am 1991;24:215–227

131. Fisch U. Facial nerve grafting. Otolaryngol Clin North Am 1974;7:517–529

132. Fisch U, Lanser MJ. Facial nerve grafting. Otolaryngol Clin North Am 1991;24:691–708

133. Barrs DM. Facial nerve trauma: optional timing for repair. Laryngoscope 1991;101:835–848

134. Fisch U, Dobie RA, Gmur A, Felix H. Intracranial facial nerve anastomosis. Am J Otol 1987;8:23–29

135. McHugh HE. Facial paralysis in birth injury and skull fractures. Arch Otolaryngol 1963;78:443–455

136. Grundfast KM, Guarisco JL, Thomsen JR, Koch B. Diverse etiologies of facial paralysis in children. Int J Pediatr Otorhinolaryngol 1990;19:223–239

137. Orobello P. Congenital and acquired facial nerve paralysis in children. Otolaryngol Clin North Am 1991;24:647–652

138. Bergman I, May M, Stool S, Wessel HB. Neonatal traumatic facial palsy. Laryngoscope 1986;96:381–384

139. Kumari S, Bhargava SK, Choudhury P, Ghosh S. Facial palsy in the newborn: clinical profile and long term follow-up. Indian Pediatr 1980;17:917–922

140. Smith JD, Cromby RC, Harker LA. Facial paralysis in the newborn. Otolaryngol Head Neck Surg 1981;89:1021–1024

141. Du Trevou M, Bullock R, Teasdale E, Quin RO. False aneurysms of the carotid tree due to unsuspected penetrating injury of the head and neck. Injury 1991;22:237–239

142. Meder JF, Gaston A, Merienne L, Goden-Hardy S, Fredy D. Traumatic aneurysms of the internal and external arteries. One case and a review of the literature. J Neuroradiol 1992;19:248–255

143. Chandrasekaran S, Zainal J. Delayed traumatic extradural hematomas. Aust N Z J Surg 1993;63:780–783

144. Goodwin JR, Johnson MH. Carotid injury secondary to blunt head trauma; case report. J Trauma 1944;37:119–122

145. Pollanen MS, Dreck JHN, Blenkinsop B, Farkas EM. Fracture of the temporal bone with exsanguinations: pathology and mechanisms. Can J Neurol Sci 1992;19:196–200

146. Freeman J. Temporal bone fractures and cholesteatoma. Ann Otol Rhinol Laryngol 1983;92:558–560

147. Bottrill ID. Post-traumatic cholesteatoma. J Laryngol Otol 1991;105:367–369

148. Clark SK, Rees TS. Posttraumatic endolymphatic hydrops. Arch Otolaryngol 1977;103:725–726

149. Golding-Wood DG, Williams HO, Brookes GB. Tegmental dehiscence and brain herniation into the middle ear cleft. J Laryngol Otol 1991;105:477–480

150. Ramsden RT, Latif A, Lye RN, Dutton JEM. Endaural cerebral hernia. J Laryngol Otol 1985;99:643–651

151. Kamerer DB, Caparosa RJ. Temporal bone encephalocele—diagnosis and treatment. Laryngoscope 1982;92:878–882

152. Andrews JC, Canalis RF. Otogenic pneumocephalus. Laryngoscope 1986;96:521–528

153. Tarlov IM, Mule J. Traumatic pneumocephalus associated with cerebrospinal fluid otorrhea. Am J Roentgenol Radiol Ther 1956;56:179–184

154. Lunsford LD, Maroon JC, Sheptak PE, Albin MS. Subdural tension pneumocephalus: report of two cases. J Neurosurg 1979;50:525–527

155. Weissman JL, Curtin HD. Pneumolabyrinth: a computed tomographic sign of temporal bone fracture. Am J Otolaryngol 1992;13:113–114

156. Betz BW, Wiener MD. Air in the temporomandibular joint fossa: CT sign of temporal bone fracture. Radiology 1991;180:463–466

157. Engevall S, Fischer K. Dislocation of the mandibular condyle into the middle cranial fossa: review of the literature and report of a case. J Oral Maxillofac Surg 1992;50:524–527

158. Avrahami E. CT of intact but nonfunctioning temporomandibular joints following temporal bone fracture. Neuroradiology 1994;36:142–143

159. Roland JT Jr, Hammerschlag PE, Lewis WS, Choi I, Berenstein A. Management of traumatic facial nerve paralysis with carotid artery cavernous sinus fistula. Eur Arch Otorhinolaryngol 1994;251:57–60

22

Hereditary Hearing Impairment

Daniel I. Choo and John H. Greinwald Jr.

Although many areas of medicine have benefited from the exponentially expanding knowledge base of molecular genetics and the underlying molecular biology of human diseases, few branches of medicine have been as dramatically affected as clinical otology and the diagnosis and management of patients with hereditary hearing impairment (HHI). Over the course of just one decade, genes responsible for some of the most common forms of HHI have been identified, and "routine" laboratory assays to identify mutations of these genes have become almost uniformly available in most major medical centers across the United States. These advances in the molecular genetics of hearing loss have translated into a markedly improved ability of clinicians to precisely diagnose the cause of hearing loss in a large population of patients in whom all traditional diagnostic testing would previously have been uninformative.

Given the fact that hearing impairment is the most common sensory deficit in the United States (affecting 2 to 3 per 1000 live births) and affects about 28 million Americans, this improved diagnostic ability has tremendous clinical relevance. Furthermore, as many as 5% of children have a demonstrable hearing loss by 18 years of age, with that incidence reaching 40 to 50% by age 75. Taking into account the aging demographic of the United States population, it becomes apparent that more accurate, efficient, and cost-effective diagnosis and management of patients with hearing loss are requisite. This chapter illustrates how the emerging era of molecular medicine translates into the field of clinical otology, particularly the care of patients with HHI (see also Chapter 5).

◆ Basic Principles and Nomenclature in Human Genetics

To meaningfully discuss the genetic mechanisms of HHI, a grasp of some basic terminology is required. The core material composing the human genome is linear strands of deoxyribonucleic acid (DNA) whose precise sequence of base pairs creates *genes* that are organized into 23 pairs of *chromosomes*: 22 autosomes and 1 pair of sex chromosomes (in total, 46 chromosomes). An X and a Y chromosome for males and 2 X chromosomes for females determine sex.

Genes have been further dissected to identify regions within their DNA sequence that have specific functions. In general, each gene contains (1) DNA that has the actual coding sequence(s) (called *exons*) that contain the information for synthesizing proteins; (2) interspersed (noncoding) DNA between these exons (called *introns*); and (3) regulatory regions of DNA before and after the exons that are referred to as *upstream* or *downstream* regions, respectively. Particularly relevant for most genes are upstream regions termed *promoters* that bind regulatory proteins and determine when genes will be actively read or *transcribed* and made into messenger RNA (mRNA). mRNA is then *translated* or made into protein by cells to carry out the actual function of that gene.

Mutations are abnormal alterations of the DNA sequence in genes that then impact their ability to guide cellular processes. *Nonsense* mutations, for example, result in an early "stop" in the transcription or reading of the DNA. No mRNA or protein is synthesized. In contrast, *missense* mutations result in an abnormal transcript or protein that is synthesized but abnormal because of the mutation. In this case, the abnormal protein may not function normally and contribute to the phenotype.

The other relevant terminology can best be explained by discussing a specific example of genetic hearing impairment: gap junction β2 (*GJB2*)-related HHI. (*GJB2*-related hearing loss is discussed in greater detail later in this chapter.) *GJB2* refers to the specific gene located on chromosome 13 at a *locus* (or position on the chromosome) designated 13q11; "13" refers to the chromosome number, with "q11" further specifying a position along the long arm of chromosome 13. Every person carries two copies of the *GJB2* gene in every cell of the body. One copy (or *allele*) of the *GJB2* gene is inherited from the biologic mother whereas the other allele is inherited from the biologic father. Several variants or forms of the *GJB2* gene (and most other genes) exist. If both alleles of the *GJB2* gene are identical, then the individual is *homozygous* at the *GJB2* locus. If the alleles are different, then the individual is *heterozygous* for *GJB2*. This description of an individual's genetic composition is termed the *genotype* for any given trait. In distinction, the physical trait(s) that a person displays (in this case, hearing impairment) is termed the *phenotype*. In the case of HHI, the onset and nature of the hearing impairment (i.e., the phenotype) can be largely determined by the patient's genotype (i.e., which alleles of the *GJB2* gene a person carries).

Alleles also can function in a *dominant* or *recessive* manner depending on whether the presence of a single allele can determine/produce a phenotype (dominant) or whether two copies of an allele are required to produce a phenotype (recessive). In most cases of *GJB2*-related hearing impairment, both copies of a person's *GJB2* gene need to be abnormal to cause a hearing impairment (i.e., autosomal recessive). In other autosomal dominant processes, one abnormal copy of the gene (even in the presence of one normal allele) is sufficient to produce a phenotype (e.g., some forms of Waardenburg's syndrome caused by *MITF* mutations). Dominant traits typically do not skip generations, and there is a 50% chance that a heterozygous parent will transmit the abnormal allele to offspring. In contrast, recessive traits do not typically appear in each generation, and there is a 25% chance that two heterozygous parents would produce an affected child.

One feature that can affect this simple inheritance concept is the phenomenon of *penetrance* (or ability of the gene to manifest the phenotypic traits). In some autosomal dominant disorders, a patient may carry an abnormal gene but not display any physical abnormalities (i.e., incomplete penetrance). Furthermore, dominant disorders also can show *variable expressivity*, whereby different family members who carry the same abnormal gene can present with different manifestations of the abnormality. In the case of HHI, this might present as varying degrees of hearing impairment in family members all carrying the same genetic abnormality.

Sex-linked or X-linked traits demonstrate a different inheritance pattern due to males carrying only one X chromosome. For example, an X-linked recessive trait can lack phenotypic expression if carried in a female who is heterozygous. However, male offspring of this female would have a 50% chance of inheriting the gene, and expression of the gene would occur in a male child because of the lack of a second X chromosome. The female offspring of an X-linked female carrier have a 50% risk of carrying such a trait. But because males inherit their father's Y chromosome (i.e., not the X-linked recessive allele), they are unaffected and do not become carriers. In contrast, females inherit their father's X-linked allele and necessarily become carriers of the allele.

There are circumstances in which diseases or phenotypes are caused by abnormalities that involve all or portions of chromosomes (as opposed to individual genes as described above). Most of these chromosomal abnormalities result in clinical conditions with developmental delays and a spectrum of congenital anomalies, the exception being instances in which sex chromosomes are affected. As an example, trisomy 21 (Down syndrome) is caused by the presence of a third copy of an entire chromosome (chromosome 21). Individuals with extra X or Y chromosomes tend to have milder phenotypes such as Klinefelter syndrome (47, XXY or XYY) or Turner syndrome (45 X).

Remarkable advances in the knowledge base of molecular biology and human genetics of normal and impaired hearing have been made over the past several years. However, greater detail into these topics is beyond the scope of this chapter. For further reading and more in-depth review of these areas, the reader is referred to resources such as the Hereditary Hearing Loss Homepage (www.webhost.ua.ac.be/hhh).

◆ Autosomal Recessive Disorders of Hearing

Overall, most genetic hearing disorders are transmitted in an autosomal recessive mode of inheritance. Furthermore, for those hearing impairments presenting in childhood, roughly 80% are inherited recessively. In the vast majority of patients (80–90%), the HHI is nonsyndromic (i.e., with no other abnormalities/phenotypes that can be identified). From a clinical perspective, this poses significant challenges in the workup and evaluation of an otherwise healthy-appearing child presenting with sensorineural hearing impairment (SNHI). Although most children do not have any other anomalies, a thorough evaluation is necessary to identify the 10 to 20% of patients who have other features that would point toward a syndromic etiology and potentially a different evaluation and management pathway. A very common scenario is to identify an isolated child with SNHI in a family with no known history of HHI. The medical evaluation of such a patient requires methodical history taking and physical examination (in addition to ancillary testing, such as genetic testing) to differentiate nongenetic causes of hearing impairment from those that are inherited in an autosomal recessive fashion. The sections below cover the different categories of autosomal recessive, autosomal dominant, sex-linked, mitochondrially related and gross chromosomal abnormality–related HHI. To further structure the discussion, each category is then subdivided into syndromic and nonsyndromic forms of HHI where appropriate.

Autosomal Recessive Nonsyndromic Hearing Impairment (ARNSHI)

The rapidly advancing field of auditory molecular genetics has shown that ARNSHI is a genetically heterogeneous disorder, meaning that many genetic causes have been identified that can cause HHI. As an illustration, 41 loci for ARNSHI have already been reported. The nomenclature for these genetic loci uses the prefix DFNB, with DFN indicating deafness and B indicating an autosomal recessive mode of inheritance. (In contrast, the prefix DFNA would be used for deafness transmitted in an autosomal dominant fashion A, discussed below). To date, 22 genes have been identified as being involved in ARNSHI (**Table 22–1**) with DFNB1 (the first autosomal recessive disorder) responsible for 30 to 40% of all cases of ARNSHI.

DFNB1

The gene identified at the DFNB1 locus is *GJB2*, which encodes for a protein called connexin 26.[1–4] Connexin 26 represents one of a family of gap junction proteins that form intercellular channels that allow low molecular weight molecules to travel from cell to cell. In the inner ear, connexin 26 is one of several gap junction proteins expressed in the epithelia lining the cochlea and has been reported to be involved in potassium recycling that is critical to hair cell transduction of sound stimuli into electrical signals.

Table 22–1 Genetic Defects Associated with Hearing Impairment

Gene (protein)	Locus	Mode of Inheritance/Syndrome	Phenotype
CDH23 (cadherin 23)	DFNB12	ARNSHL	Sensorineural hearing loss
	Usher 1C	AR syndromic	Congenital hearing loss, retinitis pigmentosa, and variable vestibular areflexia
COCH (cochlin)	DFNA9	ADNSHL	Onset of hearing loss occurs between ages 20 to 30; profound at high frequencies, and displays variable progression to anacusis by ages 40 to 50; vestibular dysfunction is variable
COL2A1 (collagen 2A1) COL11A2 (collagen11A2) COL11A1 (collagen 11A1)	Stickler	AR syndromic	Ocular, Pierre Robin sequence, SNHL
COL4A3 (collagen 4A3) COL4A4 (collagen 4A3) COL4A5 (collagen 4A5)	Alport	X-linked AR syndromic AD syndromic	Progressive, high-frequency, sensorineural deafness, nephritis
DDP (deafness/dystonia peptide)	DDP (previously called DFN1)	XL syndromic	Early-onset deafness with mental retardation in adulthood
DIAPH1 (diaphanous)	DFNA1	ADNSHL	Fully penetrant, nonsyndromic sensorineural progressive low-frequency hearing loss
EDNRB (endothelin receptor)	Waardenburg type 4	AD syndromic	Combined with Hirschsprung disease
EYA1 (eyes absent 1)	Branchio-oto-renal	AD syndromic	Hearing loss is usually stable; may be conductive, sensorineural, or mixed; 2% of children with profound deafness have BOR syndrome
GJB2 (connexin 26)	DFNA3	ADNSHL	Severe to profound SNHL
	DFNB1	ARNSHL	Stable mild to profound SNHL
GJB6 (connexin 30)	DFNA4	ARNSHL	Severe to profound SNHL
ICERE-1 (inversely correlated with estrogen receptor expression)	DFNA5	ADNSHL	Progressive hearing loss starting in the high frequencies
KVLQT1 (potassium gated voltage channels) KCNE1 (potassium channel, voltage-gated, isk-related subfamily, member 1)	Jervell and Lange-Nielsen	AR syndromic	Severe to profound hearing loss, prolonged QT interval, syncope
MITF (microphthalmia associated transcription factor)	Waardenburg type 2	AD syndromic	Same as type I but without dystopia canthorum
MYO1A (myosin 1A)	DFNA48	ADNSHL	Bilateral moderate to severe hearing loss
MYO7A (myosin 7A)	DFNB2 DFNA11 Usher 1B	ARNSHL ADNSHL AR syndromic	Profound congenital deafness, vestibular areflexia, and progressive retinitis pigmentosa Flat audiogram at young ages and some progression at the high frequencies
MYO15 (myosin 15)	DFNB3	ARNSHL	Profound deafness
NDP (Norrin)	Norrie	X-linked syndromic	Ocular symptoms (pseudotumor of the retina, retinal hyperplasia, hypoplasia, necrosis of the inner layer of the retina, cataracts), phthisis bulbi, progressive sensorineural hearing loss, and mental retardation
OTOF (Otoferlin)	DFNB9	ARNSHL	Severe to profound SNHL
PAX3 (paired box gene 3)	Waardenburg type 1	AD syndromic	Pigmentary abnormalities of hair, iris, and skin (often white forelock and heterochromia iridis); sensorineural deafness, dystopia canthorum (lateral displacement of the inner canthus of each eye)
	Waardenburg type 3		Type 1 and upper limb abnormalities

Continued

Table 22–1   *(Continued)*

Gene (protein)	Locus	Mode of Inheritance/Syndrome	Phenotype
POU3F4 (POU domain 3, transcription factor 4)	DFN 3	X-linked	Fixed stapes
POU4F3 (POU domain 4, transcription factor 3)	DFNA15	ADNSHL	Progressive hearing loss
SLC26A4 (Pendrin)	DFNB4	ARNSHL	EVAS, Mondini, goiter, SNHL
	Pendred	AR syndromic	
TCOF1 (Treacle)	Treacher Collins	AD syndromic	Coloboma of the lower eyelid, micrognathia, microtia, hypoplasia of the zygomatic arches, macrostomia, hearing loss
TECTA (α-tectorin)	DFNA8/12	ADNSHL	Prelingual severe to profound sensorineural deafness
	DFNB21	ARNSHL	
USH1C (USH1C)	DFNB21	ARNSHL	Profound congenital deafness, vestibular areflexia, and progressive retinitis pigmentosa
	Usher 1C	AR syndromic	
USH2A (USH2A) *SNAI2* (snail, homologue of *Drosophila*)	Usher 2A	AR syndromic	
tRNA$^{ser(UCN)}$	tRNA$^{ser(UCN)}$	Mitochondrial	Mild to severe, can be progressive
12rRNA	12rRNA	Mitochondrial	Mild to severe, usually associated with aminoglycoside exposure

ARSNHL, autosomal recessive sensorineural hearing loss; ADSNHL, autosomal dominant sensorineural hearing loss; AR syndromic, autosomal recessive syndromic; AD syndromic, autosomal dominant syndromic.

Source: Adapted from Van Camp G, Smith RJH. Hereditary Hearing Loss Homepage. http://webhost.ua.ac.be/hhh. Reprinted with permission. For a more comprehensive and current list of genes related to nonsyndromic and common syndromic hearing impairment, refer to this Web site. Additional information about these genes can be obtained from the Online Mendelian Inheritance in Man Web site (http://www.ncbi.nlm.nih.gov/entrez/query.fcgi?db=OMIM).

Although *GJB2*-related HHI has been identified in almost all regions of the world, certain ethnic backgrounds and populations display different rates of specific *GJB2* mutations. For example, deletion of a guanine residue at nucleotide position 35 (35delG) is one of the most common mutations found in patients with ARNSHI and is particularly common in those of European descent. In contrast, a deletion of a thymine at position 167 (167delT) is much more common in Ashkenazi Jewish populations, whereas a 235delC mutation is more frequently identified in Asian patients.

Overall, DFNB1 is believed to cause 20% of all childhood HHI and among those children with more severe degrees of hearing impairment (e.g., thresholds >70 dB), almost 40% are due to DFNB1. Examining those pediatric patients with milder forms of hearing impairment, the rate of *GJB2* mutations drops to a smaller but nonetheless significant rate of 10 to 15%. Further illustrating the clinical relevance of DFNB1 is the estimated frequency of heterozygous carriers of deafness-causing *GJB2* mutations in the Caucasian U.S. population of 1 in 40. Taking together the high frequency of mutations in *GJB2* and the relatively small size of this gene, these factors make genetic screening and molecular diagnosis of *GJB2*-related hearing loss extremely feasible and attractive.

Related to *GJB2* HHI, mutations of *GJB6* also have been found in association with *GJB2* mutation, termed a double heterozygous state that may be another deafness-causing genotype. A large deletion of the *GJB6* upstream region has been found by itself to produce a severe hearing impairment phenotype.[5] However, the greater significance of *GJB6* mutations may lie in the fact that as many as 10% of patients with ARNSHI and *GJB2* mutation also carry a large deletion of *GJB6*.

Also, the colocalization of *GJB2* and *GJB6* to the same region of chromosome 13 may indicate these genes share a common regulatory region (i.e., a locus control region). Accordingly, gap junction gene mutations have an obvious importance in HHI, and although the basic molecular and cellular mechanisms of gap junction–related hearing impairment remain somewhat nebulous, this initial ability to molecularly diagnose patients with specific genetic mutations responsible for their HHI presents a clinically useful and necessary first step in translating molecular genetics to the patient care arena.

Recently published data demonstrate how these molecular data can be incorporated into clinical practice to improve efficient diagnosis and cost-effectiveness.[6] For pediatric patients with ARNSHI and moderately severe or worse hearing thresholds (e.g., >60 dB), *GJB2* testing is recommended as the first line of evaluation. If hearing thresholds are better than 60 dB, *GJB2* testing should be considered after temporal bone computed tomography (CT) has been performed. For these patients with normal temporal bone CT scans, *GJB2* testing is then appropriate. If the CT scan is abnormal, then genetic testing for *SLC26A4* (Pendred gene) mutations should be obtained.

Interestingly, *GJB2* mutation data have now been analyzed to correlate specific mutations with degrees of hearing impairment.[7] As an example, patients with two nonsense mutations (biallelic nonsense mutations, e.g., 35delG/35delG) have an extremely high likelihood of ultimately demonstrating a bilateral severe to profound hearing impairment. In contrast, patients with two missense mutations (e.g., M34T/M34T) are much more likely to demonstrate mild to moderate hearing impairments. Such prognostic factors have gained tremendous relevance since the implementation of universal newborn hearing screening programs across the United States. As infants are identified at birth after not passing their newborn hearing screening, clinicians will be challenged with determining management strategies as early as possible to maximize the infant's hearing and language skill development and to take advantage of early windows of opportunity, including cochlear implantation at 12 months of age for those infants with more severe degrees of hearing impairment. By obtaining GJB2 genotyping shortly after confirming a hearing impairment, clinicians can assimilate these molecular genetic data and more accurately identify those infants who are likely to demonstrate severe-to-profound hearing impairments and may require different and earlier interventions to let them reach their full communicational potential. For example, if auditory neuropathy-dyssynchrony occurs at the level of the spinal ganglion, cochlear implantation results still may be surprisingly good.

Otoferlin

One other noteworthy form of ARNSHI is HHI due to mutations of the Otoferlin (OTOF) gene.[8,9] OTOF mutations have been associated with a specific form of hearing impairment known as auditory neuropathy or auditory dyssynchrony (AD). AD is audiometrically characterized by an abnormal auditory brainstem response (ABR) with limited waveforms other than the cochlear microphonic. Additionally, patients with AD often demonstrate present otoacoustic emissions (OAEs), suggesting intact cochlear outer hair cell function. In these patients with AD, behavioral hearing thresholds can range from mild to profound hearing loss. Estimates indicate that 5 to 10% of patients with SNHI have AD. The optimal management of these patients is challenging, as some do not benefit from traditional amplification or other assistive listening devices. Through an improved understanding of the molecular genetics and biology of AD, improved therapies may become apparent.

Autosomal Recessive Syndromic Hearing Impairment

Jervell and Lange-Nielsen Syndrome

Jervell and Lange-Nielsen (JLN) syndrome represents a rare but very significant form of syndromic HHI. In JLN, infants are typically identified with a severe-to-profound congenital hearing impairment. The critical comorbidity is a prolongation of the QT interval on electrocardiography that can cause episodes of syncope or sudden cardiac death. If properly identified after presentation with a congenital hearing impairment, these infants can be managed with beta-blockers (e.g., propranolol), which are effective in controlling the cardiac condition. Accordingly, an astute clinician can detect a potentially life-threatening cardiac condition in infants by obtaining an electrocardiogram on infants with severe-to-profound SNHI. Other patients with SNHI and unexplained seizures or a family history of syncope or sudden death should similarly be sent for an electrocardiogram if not a full cardiologic evaluation.

Genetically, some cases of JLN can be attributed to mutations of a potassium channel gene, KVLQT1.[10] Other mutations of this gene have been identified but are associated with isolated cardiac conduction defects and not SNHI. Mutations of KCNE1 have also been identified in some families with JLN,[11] indicating again that the causes of ARNSHI can be heterogeneous.

Pendred Syndrome and Enlarged Vestibular Aqueduct Syndrome

Although the association of goiter and SNHI has been known since the late 1800s, the molecular basis for Pendred syndrome (euthyroid goiter and SNHI)[12,13] was not elucidated until much more recently.[14-16] The Pendred syndrome gene (PDS) is also referred to as SLC26A4 (solute carrier family 26, member 4) and encodes for the Pendrin protein that functions as an anion transporter. The hearing impairment in Pendred syndrome varies in terms of severity as well as age of onset. Some patients display a profound loss from birth, whereas others show later onset SNHI of lesser severity. Diagnostic imaging studies routinely show cochlear hypoplasias (Mondini-type deformities) in concert with enlarged vestibular aqueducts. However, mutations of the PDS gene have been identified in some patients with isolated enlarged vestibular aqueducts on CT imaging (see later in chapter).

Previously, the diagnostic test for Pendred syndrome was an abnormal perchlorate discharge test that identified defects in the organification of iodine that was typical of patients with Pendred syndrome. However, this assay is not specific for Pendred syndrome, and its sensitivity has not been definitively determined. Thyroid function testing for patients with suspected Pendred syndrome is still routinely recommended. It is noteworthy to mention that goiter typically does not manifest until 8 years of age or later, and exogenous thyroid hormone therapy is often the most appropriate therapy. Genetic testing for PDS mutations provides another manner for identifying these patients who often present at a young age with SNHI and CT abnormalities of the inner ear. For families with the full Pendred phenotype (i.e., hearing impairment and euthyroid goiter), there is little evidence of genetic heterogeneity. About 1 to 2% of patients with severe-to-profound hearing impairment can be attributed to PDS mutations.

In comparison with classic Pendred syndrome, enlarged vestibular aqueduct syndrome (EVAS) can also present with varying degrees of SNHI but without any goiter. The typical hearing loss patterns are flat or downsloping with either SNHI or mixed hearing impairment noted on audiometric testing. The cause of a common low-frequency conductive hearing loss component is not known. Progressive hearing impairment is seen in roughly 25% of patients with EVAS, and associations of hearing changes with head trauma have been commonly described. Because of this phenomenon, patients should be counseled regarding the avoidance of specific activities or sports in which head trauma could be routinely anticipated. Vestibular symptomatology is reported in 5 to 10% of patients. CT findings show either isolated enlargement of the vestibular aqueducts or incomplete partitioning of the cochlea, or both. PDS mutations in patients with EVAS have been reported to be identified in as many as 50% of some Asian EVAS populations.[17] In the United States, PDS mutations are found in about 5 to 10% of patients with EVAS.

Usher Syndrome

Usher syndrome is characterized by retinitis pigmentosa and hearing impairment and accounts for roughly half of the deaf and blind persons in the United States. As with some other hereditary syndromes, Usher syndrome has been clinically recognized for over a century, but only recently have the molecular genetic underpinnings for this disorder been identified. Linkage studies have shown this disorder to be genetically heterogeneous with different genetic loci responsible for at least three clinically discrete subtypes of Usher syndrome. The severity and progression of the hearing impairment and the extent of vestibular system dysfunction determine the different Usher subtypes.[18–21] Type 1 Usher's patients (USH1) display congenital profound SNHI and absent vestibular function. Usher type 2 (USH2) patients show moderate SNHI and normal vestibular function, whereas Usher type 3 patients (USH3) have progressive hearing loss and variable degrees of vestibular dysfunction. Notably, USH3 has primarily been reported in Norwegian cohorts.

As reflected in **Table 22–1**, several different causative genes have been identified for USH1, and at least three have been confirmed for USH2. USH1 is most commonly the result of mutations in the myosin VII gene (*MYO7A*), an unconventional myosin whose gene product is necessary for normal stereocilia formation and function in hair cells. Quite differently, USH2 is frequently caused by mutations of USH2A that encodes for an extracellular matrix protein (usherin).[22] The exact function of USH2A remains to be elucidated.

In the clinical evaluation of Usher syndrome patients an ophthalmologic consultation is requisite. Electroretinographic studies can reveal abnormalities in patients as early as the second or third year of life before funduscopic exams can reveal any lesions. Early diagnosis can dramatically impact the planning and management for an affected child, not only in terms of medical management but also for educational programs.

◆ Autosomal Dominant Disorders of Hearing

At least 20 genes have already been identified that can produce an autosomal dominant HHI when mutated. In addition, another 18 loci associated with autosomal dominant HHI have been mapped to specific chromosomal locations. As such, advances in molecular genetics have greatly enhanced our understanding of the causes and mechanisms involved in this form of HHI.

Diagnosing an autosomal dominant HHI in a patient is fairly straightforward when classic dominant inheritance pattern and a distinct phenotype (e.g., distinct pattern of hearing loss) are apparent. However, variable expressivity (as described above) may lead to different affected members of the same family displaying different degrees and patterns of hearing impairment, making it more difficult to discern the classic autosomal dominant pattern of HHI. As mentioned above, autosomal dominant nonsyndromic hearing impairment loci are designated DFNA with a following number indicating the order of discovery of the genetic locus (e.g., DFNA1).

Autosomal Dominant Nonsyndromic Hearing Impairment

In reviewing the reported forms of ADNSHI, the vast majority (except for DFNA3 and DFN8/12) show progressive hearing impairment with onset around 20 to 30 years of age. However, certain forms of ADNSHI may not manifest until significantly older ages, for example, DFNA10 and DFNA13.[23,24] Further variability in the nature of ADNSHI is seen with respect to the degree of progression and audiometric pattern of hearing impairment. For example, almost all DFNA-associated hearing impairments are typically progressive but incomplete, with patients usually performing well with hearing aids/amplification. The exceptions are DFNA3 and DFNA8/12, which can be congenital in onset and stable. Rarely, ADNSHI progresses to profound deafness (i.e., DFNA1) with patients potentially requiring cochlear implantation if auditory rehabilitation is desired.

Table 22–1 presents summary data on ADNSHI and the genes and loci that have been associated with each form of hearing impairment. The genes involved in autosomally transmitted HHI are significantly heterogeneous as noted in autosomal recessive hearing impairments, encoding for voltage-gated potassium channels (*KCNQ4*, DNFA2), various connexins (including connexin 26, 30, and 31, which map to the DFNA2, DFNA11, and DFNB1 loci), *Tecta* (a tectorial membrane component), *COL11A2* (a collagen gene responsible for DFNA13), transcription factors (for example, *POU4F3*, DFNA15), developmentally important genes (*HDIA1*, causing DFNA1), unconventional myosins (*MYO7A*, causing DFNA11, in addition to DFNB2 and USH1B), and structural binding proteins (e.g., *COCH*, DFNA9). Several DFNA loci represent novel genes whose functions have yet to be determined (e.g., DFNA5).[25–30]

It is noteworthy to point out that certain genes such as *GJB2* or *MYO7A*, when mutated, can cause different diseases or forms of hearing impairment. For example, *GJB2* mutations have been linked with both an autosomal dominant and recessive form of HHI as discussed above. Similarly, *MYO7A* mutations have been reported in Usher syndrome as well as DFNA11 and DFNB2. The molecular biology and mechanisms responsible for these genotype-phenotype correlations remain unclear.

Studies of DFNA9 and the *COCH* gene also provide one of the first genes that have been linked to vestibular disorders that appear to be relevant to Meniere's disease (a symptom complex of fluctuating SNHI, tinnitus, aural fullness, and episodic vertigo). By examining the functions of *COCH*, investigators may be able to gain insight into the molecular processes causing disorders such as Meniere's and autoimmune SNHI.

Autosomal Dominant Syndromic Hearing Impairment

Melnick-Fraser or Branchio-Oto-Renal Syndrome

Characterized by anomalies of the branchial-derived structures, renal anomalies and hearing impairment, branchio-oto-renal (BOR) syndrome has been reported to affect as many as 2% of children in schools for the deaf.[31] Phenotypically, the hearing impairment in BOR syndrome can be conductive in nature due to abnormalities of the auricle, external auditory canal, or middle ear ossicles. However, SNHI or mixed hearing impairment is also seen and can be due to a spectrum of cochlear hypoplasias or dysplasias. As many as 40% of BOR patients demonstrate cochlear abnormalities on high-resolution CT scanning. External ear defects can include ear pits, periauricular skin tags, and appendages as well as varying degrees of microtia. Cervical cysts and sinuses due to branchial cleft anomalies similarly present in a highly variable fashion. The renal anomalies can be mild and asymptomatic or severe with agenesis and renal failure. Such severe manifestations provide the indications for obtaining some type of renal evaluation (urinalysis, renal ultrasound, intravenous pyelogram, etc.) to rule out morbid renal anomalies in children who present with hearing impairment, ear anomalies, and branchial cleft lesions.

Genotypically, BOR syndrome has been linked to mutations of the *EYA1* gene on chromosome 8q13.[32] The *EYA1* gene is an evolutionarily conserved gene first identified in *Drosophila* as the *eyeless* gene. This transcription factor regulates gene expression during embryogenesis and appears to be specifically involved in morphogenesis of the ear, branchial structures, and kidney.[33,34] Some genetic heterogeneity of BOR syndrome is suggested by the fact that only 15% of affected individuals show *EYA1* mutations. It is noteworthy to mention, however, that more precise and rigorous criteria for clinically diagnosing BOR syndrome would greatly improve the accuracy of diagnosis. Using more stringent criteria for BOR syndrome, as many as 40% of this more narrowly defined population can be found to carry mutations of the *EYA1* gene. The criteria for BOR syndrome can be broken down into major and minor criteria with diagnosis based on three major criteria, two major and two minor criteria, or one major criterion and an affected first-degree relative.[35]

Neurofibromatosis

Two distinct forms of neurofibromatosis have been clinically and genetically defined: neurofibromatosis 1 (NF1, or classic neurofibromatosis) and neurofibromatosis 2 (NF2, or central neurofibromatosis). Although both forms of neurofibromatosis are associated with skin lesions (café-au-lait spots) and multiple neurofibromas, NF2 is distinguished by bilateral acoustic neuromas (vestibular schwannomas). The molecular genetics of NF1 and NF2 highlight how seemingly similar clinical diseases that share multiple features in common can be caused by very distinct genetic defects. The gene responsible for NF1 is caused by a neural growth factor, neurofibromin, that maps to chromosome 17q11.[36] In contrast, NF2 is caused by mutations of *schwannomin,* a classic tumor-suppressor gene, located on chromosome 22q12.[37] Such genetic data also highlight the critical importance of precise clinical diagnosis, as subtle phenotypic differences may help distinguish diseases that clinically appear similar but are in fact genetically diverse. Searching for common genetic etiologies among disparate clinical entities can lead investigators down erroneous pathways.

NF1 (also referred to as von Recklinghausen disease) is a relatively common disease affecting roughly 1 in 3000 persons per year. Diagnostic criteria for NF1 include multiple café-au-lait spots of certain size and number, cutaneous and plexiform neurofibromas, pseudarthrosis, Lisch nodules of the iris, and optic gliomas. Although not as common as skin lesions, central and peripheral nervous system neurofibromas do occur in NF1, producing problems such as blindness, hearing impairment, and mental retardation. Approximately 5% of NF1 patients develop vestibular schwannomas. For this and other potential neurologic reasons, hearing needs to be routinely monitored in patients with NF1. Any changes in hearing warrant diagnostic imaging (i.e., gadolinium-enhanced magnetic resonance imaging) to rule out retrocochlear pathology.

The hallmark feature in NF2 is bilateral acoustic neuromas. Although typically slow growing lesions, these vestibular schwannomas can be detected as early as the second decade of life. Lesions can remain asymptomatic for years, but clinicians are challenged with optimally timing intervention to maintain hearing and facial nerve function. Tinnitus and vestibular symptoms can be identified in many young adults with NF2, and other central nervous system lesions need to be ruled out in patients with any neurologic symptoms or deficits.

For both NF1 and NF2, early diagnosis and counseling can greatly improve the overall management of patients and family. The availability of genetic tests for neurofibromin and schwannomin now provides clinicians with objective data regarding the diagnosis and prognosis for presymptomatic family members who are at risk for NF1 or NF2.

Otosclerosis

Typically presenting as a gradually progressive conductive hearing loss, otosclerosis appears to be inherited in an autosomal dominant manner with decreased penetrance. Penetrance is estimated to be between 25% and 40%. Mean age of onset for hearing impairment is in the third decade of life, with women being more frequently affected than men. Exacerbation of hearing loss during pregnancy is a commonly reported phenomenon. Such observations suggest that additional factors (e.g., hormonal regulation) may also be involved in modifying the phenotypic manifestation of this HHI. Additional research has also identified measles virus particles in affected otosclerotic bone, suggesting a potential role for the viral genome in the pathogenesis of otosclerosis or perhaps in modifying the phenotypic expression of otosclerosis.[38]

The pathologic abnormality in otosclerosis is the replacement of normal bone in the middle and inner ear by otosclerotic bone. Fixation of the stapes footplate results in the progressive conductive hearing loss component. If the otosclerotic process progressively involves the cochlea, an SNHI can also develop.

As with many of the other HHI disorders discussed in this chapter, otosclerosis is a genetically heterogeneous disease with at least four different loci having been mapped from studies of large kindreds affected by otosclerosis: OTSC1 (chromosome 15q26), OTSC2 (7q34–36), OTSC3 (6p21–22) and OTSC4 (3q22–24).[38–42]

Stickler Syndrome

In addition to SNHI or a mixed sensorineural and conductive hearing impairment, individuals affected by Stickler syndrome also demonstrate hypermobility and enlargement of joints that is associated with early-onset arthritis, severe nearsightedness that can result in retinal detachment, cataracts, Robin sequence–like facial dysmorphology, and occasionally spondyloepiphyseal dysplasia. Hearing is impaired in about 80% of individuals, and 15% overall show a progressive hearing impairment over time. Three different types of Stickler syndrome have been identified and are believed to be due to genetic heterogeneity with variable expressivity.

Stickler syndrome type 1 (STL1) is the classically described syndrome associated with mutations of the collagen 2A1 (*COL2A1*) gene. The STL1 phenotype includes cleft palate, midface hypoplasia, progressive myopia, vitreoretinal degeneration, variable degrees of hearing loss, joint degeneration, abnormal epiphyseal development, and irregularities of the vertebral bodies. Different mutations of COL2A1 can result in more severe disease (e.g., Kniest syndrome and spondyloepiphyseal dysplasia congenita), which are associated with progressive SNHI.[43] Stickler syndrome type 2 (STL2) is caused by mutations of a different collagen gene (COL11A1) but manifests with the same craniofacial and hearing abnormalities as those seen in STL1. Stickler syndrome type 3 (STL3) is caused by mutations in the COL11A2 gene and results in a slightly milder form of the syndrome that largely lacks the ophthalmologic abnormalities. Palatal and joint abnormalities are present, but nearsightedness and vitreoretinal degeneration are typically not observed. From a molecular mechanistic perspective, these differences between STL3 and STL1 and -2 can potentially be explained by the fact that the two collagen genes (COL2A1 and COL11A1) associated with STL1 and STL2 are expressed in all the organs that are affected in those syndromes. In contrast, STL3 is caused by mutations of COL11A2, which is not expressed in the vitreous,[43] and therefore mutations of this gene would be not be expected to directly cause abnormalities in the vitreous.

Treacher Collins Syndrome (Mandibulofacial Dysostosis)

Treacher Collins syndrome involves abnormalities of the jaw, face, and ears, with significant variability in the phenotype. Bilateral microtia and aural atresia are common with individuals showing either pure conductive hearing loss or mixed hearing loss due to inner ear malformations in association with the external ear deformities. Approximately 30% of children with Treacher Collins demonstrate ossicular abnormalities that contribute to the conductive hearing loss. SNHI varies from mild to severe and is largely dependent on the degree of inner ear dysplasia. Although defects of vestibular apparatus can also be noted on CT scanning, clinically significant vestibular disorders are rare.

Hypoplastic zygomas result in downward slanting palpebral fissures that are characteristic of Treacher Collins syndrome. Bilateral colobomas of the upper eyelid and a symmetric but hypoplastic mandible are also commonly observed.

Many individuals affected by Treacher Collins syndrome demonstrate mutations of the TCOF1 gene, which is normally expressed during early craniofacial development. Although inheritance is typically autosomal dominant, new mutations of TCOF1 are identified in as many as 60% of affected individuals.

Waardenburg Syndrome

Waardenburg syndrome is classically described as hearing impairment, a white forelock, heterochromic iridis, dystopia canthorum, and synophrys. However, the study of Waardenburg syndrome highlights the phenomenon of variable expressivity in hereditary disorders. For example, pigmentary abnormalities traditionally associated with Waardenburg's syndrome include the white forelock, heterochromic iridis, premature graying, and vitiligo. Yet only 20 to 30% of individuals affected by Waardenburg syndrome demonstrate a white forelock and the age at initial appearance of a white forelock is quite variable. Similar variability in the craniofacial features (such as the dystopia canthorum, broad nasal root, and synophrys) is also commonly observed. Such variability makes clinical phenotyping challenging, but careful study has established at least four different types of Waardenburg syndrome.

Waardenburg syndrome 1 (WS1) is distinguished from WS2 by the presence of dystopia canthorum (absent in WS2). Hearing loss also differentiates WS1 and WS2. SNHI is observed in 20% of WS1 patients, whereas more than half of WS2 patients audiologically demonstrate an SNHI. Interestingly, enlarged vestibular aqueducts have been reported in as many as 50% of Waardenburg patients.[44] WS3 and WS4 are far less common than WS1 and WS2. WS3 is also referred to as Klein-Waardenburg syndrome and is characterized by bony malformations of the hands and forearms in addition to the abnormalities seen in WS1. WS4 (also referred to as Waardenburg-Shah syndrome) can be distinguished by an apparent association with Hirschsprung disease and either an autosomal recessive or autosomal dominant manner of transmission.

Consistent with this phenotypic variability is genetic heterogeneity in the gene mutations that have been identified in individuals with Waardenburg syndrome. PAX3, MITF, EDNRB, and EDN3 mutations have all been reported in WS. However, the vast majority of cases of WS1 are associated with mutations of the PAX3 gene, which is located on 2q37. PAX3 has been extensively studied as a developmentally critical regulatory gene that controls morphogenesis of the face and inner ear. Mouse models carrying targeted mutation of the PAX3 gene result in a murine mutant named Splotch, which displays pigmentary and eye abnormalities in the heterozygotes that are reminiscent of the WS phenotype observed in humans.[45,46] Interestingly, hearing loss is not observed in Splotch mice unless homozygous for PAX3 mutations. In contrast, WS2 has been associated with mutation of the microphthalmia-associated transcription factor (MITF) mapped to 3p12–14.[47] MITF mutations are found in about 20% of WS2 individuals, whereas a novel mutation of SNAI2[44] has recently been identified. Studies have demonstrated that MITF can potentially activate the promotor of SNAI2 and therefore provides a tenable mechanism by which both genes may produce a similar phenotype. WS3 and WS4 have also been associated with specific mutations: PAX3 with WS3, and endothelin-B receptor (EDNRB) and endothelin 3 (EDN3) with WS4.[45,48,49]

◆ Sex-Linked Disorders of Hearing

Sex-linked HHI accounts for 1 to 2% of cases. However, due to the nature of X-linked disorders, up to 5% of nonsyndromic profound SNHI in males can be attributed to sex-linked disorders. To date, no genes on the Y chromosome have been implicated as causing hearing impairment when mutated. Accordingly, the following discussion focuses solely on X-linked conditions.

Sex-Linked Nonsyndromic Hearing Impairment

Of the four loci identified on the X chromosome, the best studied is the DFN3 locus that encodes for the POU3F4 gene (a transcription factor). Mutations of POU3F4 result in stapes fixation with a perilymphatic gusher (as might be identified at the time of stapes surgery). The HHI observed in this syndrome is typically mixed and progressive in nature.

The clinical significance of this genetic condition is obvious in that patients presenting with an HHI that follows an X-linked inheritance pattern should be considered at higher risk for stapes surgery. Preoperative CT scanning showing abnormal enlargement of the internal auditory canal or deficient bone at the base of the cochlea warrants conservative nonsurgical management of the conductive hearing loss and avoids a stapes "gusher" with profound hearing loss postoperatively.

Sex-Linked Syndromic Hearing Impairment

Norrie Syndrome

Norrie syndrome is a fairly rare neurodevelopmental disorder characterized by a rapidly progressive vision loss with exudative vitreoretinopathy and ocular degeneration that results in microphthalmia. Progressive SNHL also begins in the 20- to 30-year age range and affects almost one third of patients. In some families, progressive mental deterioration is also observed. Linkage studies have identified NDP as the gene responsible for Norrie syndrome. The gene product, norrin, is very similar to developmentally important transforming growth factor-β, which is involved in vasculogenesis. Mutations of NDF alone can cause progressive mental retardation,[50,51] but in other cases, affected individuals have shown large deletions of the NDP region that include contiguous monoamine oxidase genes, which also plausibly explain the variable neurocognitive deterioration.

Otopalatodigital Syndrome

Hypertelorism, craniofacial defects of the supraorbital region, a flattened midface, small nose, and cleft palate compose the typical head and neck manifestations of otopalatodigital syndrome. In addition, affected persons are short in stature, have very broad fingers and toes of variable length and have an extremely wide space between the first and second toes. The hearing impairment in otopalatodigital syndrome is a conductive hearing loss due to ossicular abnormalities and is typically amenable to surgical reconstruction or amplification. Linkage studies have mapped the genetic locus to Xq28.

Wildervanck Syndrome

Wildervanck syndrome has been described as including the Klippel-Feil malformation of fused cervical vertebrae, SNHI, or a mixed hearing impairment, and abducens nerve palsy. Lack of lateral rectus function results in retraction of the eye on lateral gaze (Duane retraction syndrome). Hearing loss in Wildervanck syndrome is almost always seen in women and suggests that the trait is possibly X-linked dominant or perhaps lethal in males. Isolated Duane retraction syndrome also carries a small risk of SNHI (about 10%).[52]

Alport Syndrome

The classic ear-kidney disorder is Alport syndrome, which consists of progressive glomerulonephritis and progressive SNHI. Renal disease typically progresses on to end-stage renal failure and can present as early as infancy with micro-hematuria. Males are affected much more severely than females, with death occurring by the third decade due to

uremia if not managed early and effectively. Loss of hearing may not begin until the mid-20s with a somewhat variable rate of progression. Alport syndrome is yet another genetically heterogeneous disorder and has been associated with mutations of the COL4A5[53] in 85% of cases. However, mutation of an autosomal type 4 collagen gene can also produce a recessive form of Alport syndrome that also is more severe in males.

Deafness Dystonia Syndrome

This extremely rare disorder is a neurodegenerative syndrome originally described as a nonsyndromic disorder (DFN1). However, refined clinical evaluation of these individuals reveals myopia, cortical blindness, dystonia, fractures, and cognitive deterioration along with the progressive SNHI that more accurately compose the overall syndrome. Mutations of the DDP gene have been identified in individuals affected by deafness dystonia syndrome. At the cellular level, DDP is hypothesized to be important in the process of mitochondrial protein transport.

◆ Mitochondrial DNA Disorders of Hearing

In discussing mitochondrial genetic disorders, it is important to highlight the significant differences between the nuclear chromosomes and the mitochondrial DNA. Mitochondria are intracellular organelles that are largely responsible for generating energy (in the form of adenosine triphosphate, ATP) used by the cell. Uniquely, mitochondria contain their own relatively small circular loops of DNA that are about 16 kilobases (kb) in length. This small mitochondrial genome contains the genes for mitochondrial proteins that are required for oxidative phosphorylation and ATP generation. Each mitochondrion contains anywhere from two to 10 copies of this small genome, and spontaneous mutation of this DNA is more common in mitochondrial genomes compared with nuclear genomes. This is hypothesized as being due to less efficient DNA repair mechanisms in the mitochondria.

Mitochondrial genetics is also significantly different from nuclear genetics because sperm typically do not contain and hence do not transmit a significant number of mitochondria to the ovum. As a result, almost the entire mitochondrial gene transfer occurs from mother to offspring. Furthermore, it is relevant to note that each cell may contain as many as several hundred mitochondria. If the mother is *homoplasmic* for a mitochondrial mutation, all of the offspring are affected, and it is likely that all/most of the mitochondria carry DNA with a specific mutation. In contrast, if only a small percentage of the mitochondria carry abnormal genomes (*heteroplasmy*), the phenotype may be modified and different tissues within the same person can carry differing fractions of mutated mitochondria within their cells.

Mitochondrial Nonsyndromic Hearing Impairment

Several mitochondrial genetic mutations have recently been identified that result in a nonsyndromic SNHI. Many of these mutations occur in genes encoding for a ribosomal RNA 12s component or for transfer RNA genes. Persons carrying these mutations typically show mild and occasionally progressive hearing impairment. Perhaps of greater significance, however, are data that reveal that patients carrying certain mitochondrial DNA mutations are predisposed to SNHI induced by exposure to aminoglycoside antibiotics. Given the fact that specific mitochondrial mutations such as A1555G are found in about 2% of the hearing impaired population and 0.5% of the general population in the U.S., this has huge potential clinical relevance. In addition to the A1555G mutation, the 961 and 1494 mitochondrial loci have also been linked to aminoglycoside-induced hearing loss. To further highlight the clinical significance of mitochondrial genetic predisposition to aminoglycoside-induced hearing loss, it is worthwhile to examine the use of gentamicin in the neonatal populations. Among all low-birth-weight infants, approximately half are exposed to gentamicin at least once during their neonatal period. For those extremely low-birth-weight infants, almost all children receive one or more courses of gentamicin. In these populations, the prevalence of predisposing mitochondrial DNA mutations may be in the 1 to 2% range. Accordingly, screening high-risk infants for 12S rRNA mutations could potentially identify those infants likely to develop an irreversible SNHI.

The mechanism by which aminoglycosides and mitochondrial DNA mutations produce hearing loss has recently been elucidated to a greater extent. The bactericidal effect of gentamicin, for example, is known to occur because of binding of the aminoglycoside to the 16s ribosomal RNA (rRNA) of bacteria. Mutations of the human 12s rRNA result in an rRNA that is remarkably similar to the bacterial 16s rRNA, thereby making it amenable to binding with aminoglycoside antibiotics and subsequently generating the ototoxicity.[54,55]

Mitochondrial Syndromic Hearing Impairment

Common features in mitochondrial syndromic diseases are a progressive neuromuscular degeneration with ataxia that is likely related to the deficient energy production by mitochondria with mutated genomes in the affected muscles and neural tissues that typically have significant energy requirements. In addition, ophthalmoplegia and SNHI are routinely seen in these syndromic mitochondrial disorders:

- MELAS refers to mitochondrial syndromic encephalopathy, lactic acidosis, and stroke. Clinical variability in this syndrome is common. SNHI occurs in roughly one-third of patients with other symptoms including intermittent vomiting, limb weakness, partial visual loss, seizures, headaches, diabetes, short stature, heart problems, and renal insufficiency. Mutations of a lysine-transfer RNA (tRNA[lys]) have been associated with this syndrome.

- MIDD refers to maternally inherited diabetes and deafness. As in MELAS, mutations of the tRNA[lys] have been identified in patients with MIDD. Other large genetic deletions, insertions, and point mutations in a tRNA[glu] have also been reported.[56,57]

- Kearns-Sayre syndrome (KSS) is characterized by ataxia, short stature, ophthalmoplegia, retinopathy, delayed puberty, and SNHI.

- MERRF (myoclonic epilepsy with ragged red fibers) is typified by epilepsy, ataxia, and SNHI. Some individuals develop optic atrophy as well.

References

1. Rabionet R, Gasparini P, Estivill X. Molecular genetics of hearing impairment due to mutations in gap junction genes encoding beta connexins. Hum Mutat 2000;16:190–202

2. Wilcox SA, et al. High frequency hearing loss correlated with mutations in the GJB2 gene. Hum Genet 2000;106:399–405

3. Kelsell DP, et al. Connexin 26 mutations in hereditary non-syndromic sensorineural deafness. Nature 1997;387:80–83

4. Kelley PM, et al. Novel mutations in the connexin 26 gene (GJB2) that cause autosomal recessive (DFNB1) hearing loss. Am J Hum Genet 1998;62:792–799

5. Del Castillo I, Moreno-Pelayo MA, Del Castillo FJ, et al. Prevalence and evolutionary origins of the del(GJB6-D13S1830) mutation in the DFNB1 locus in hearing-impaired subjects: a multicenter study. Am J Hum Genet 2003;73:1452–1458

6. Preciado D, Lim LH, Cohen A, et al. A diagnostic paradigm for childhood idiopathic sensorineural hearing loss. Otolaryngol Head Neck Surg 2004;131:804–809

7. Lim LH, et al. Genotypic and phenotypic correlations of DFNB1-related hearing impairment in the Midwestern United States. Arch Otolaryngol Head Neck Surg 2003;129:836–840

8. Yasunaga S, et al. A mutation in OTOF, encoding otoferlin, a FER-1-like protein, causes DFNB9, a nonsyndromic form of deafness. Nat Genet 1999;21:363–369

9. Varga R, et al. Non-syndromic recessive auditory neuropathy is the result of mutations in the otoferlin (OTOF) gene. J Med Genet 2003;40:45–50

10. Neyroud N, et al. A novel mutation in the potassium channel gene KVLQT1 causes the Jervell and Lange-Nielsen cardioauditory syndrome. Nat Genet 1997;15:186–189

11. Schulze-Bahr E, et al. KCNE1 mutations cause Jervell and Lange-Nielsen syndrome. Nat Genet 1997;17:267–268

12. Reardon W, et al. Enlarged vestibular aqueduct: a radiological marker of Pendred syndrome, and mutation of the PDS gene. QJM 2000;93:99–104

13. Reardon W, et al. Pendred syndrome—100 years of underascertainment? QJM 1997;90:443–447

14. Everett LA, et al. Pendred syndrome is caused by mutations in a putative sulphate transporter gene (PDS). Nat Genet 1997;17:411–422

15. Sheffield VC, et al. Pendred syndrome maps to chromosome 7q21–34 and is caused by an intrinsic defect in thyroid iodine organification. Nat Genet 1996;12:424–426

16. Usami S, et al. Non-syndromic hearing loss associated with enlarged vestibular aqueduct is caused by PDS mutations. Hum Genet 1999;104:188–192

17. Wu CC, Chen PJ, Hsu CJ. Specificity of SLC26A4 mutations in the pathogenesis of inner ear malformations. Audiol Neurootol 2005;10:234–242

18. Weil D, et al. Defective myosin VIIA gene responsible for Usher syndrome type 1B. Nature 1995;374:60–61

19. Smith RJ, et al. Localization of two genes for Usher syndrome type I to chromosome 11. Genomics 1992;14:995–1002

20. Kimberling WJ, et al. Localization of Usher syndrome type II to chromosome 1q. Genomics 1990;7:245–249

21. Chaib H, et al. A newly identified locus for Usher syndrome type I, USH1E, maps to chromosome 21q21. Hum Mol Genet 1997;6:27–31

22. Eudy JD, et al. Mutation of a gene encoding a protein with extracellular matrix motifs in Usher syndrome type IIa. Science 1998;280:1753–1757

23. McGuirt WT, et al. Mutations in COL11A2 cause non-syndromic hearing loss (DFNB13). Nat Genet 1999;23:413–419

24. O'Neill ME, et al. A gene for autosomal dominant late-onset progressive non-syndromic hearing loss, DFNA10, maps to chromosome 6. Hum Mol Genet 1996;5:853–856

25. Kubisch C, et al. KCNQ4, a novel potassium channel expressed in sensory outer hair cells, is mutated in dominant deafness. Cell 1999;96: 437–446

26. Lynch ED, et al. Nonsyndromic deafness DFNA1 associated with mutation of a human homolog of the Drosophila gene diaphanous. Science 1997;278:1315–1318

27. Govaerts PJ, et al. Clinical presentation of DFNA8-DFNA12. Adv Otorhinolaryngol 2002;61:60–65

28. Verhoeven K, et al. A gene for autosomal dominant nonsyndromic hearing loss (DFNA12) maps to chromosome 11q22–24. Am J Hum Genet 1997;60:1168–1173

29. Vahava O, et al. Mutation in transcription factor POU4F3 associated with inherited progressive hearing loss in humans. Science 1998; 279:1950–1954

30. Brown MR, et al. A novel locus for autosomal dominant nonsyndromic hearing loss, DFNA13, maps to chromosome 6p. Am J Hum Genet 1997;61:924–927

31. Chen A, et al. Phenotypic manifestations of branchio-oto-renal syndrome. Am J Med Genet 1995;58:365–370

32. Abdelhak S, et al. A human homologue of the Drosophila eyes absent gene underlies branchio-oto-renal (BOR) syndrome and identifies a novel gene family. Nat Genet 1997;15:157–164

33. Zou D, et al. Eya1 and Six1 are essential for early steps of sensory neurogenesis in mammalian cranial placodes. Development 2004;131: 5561–5572

34. Kalatzis V, et al. Eya1 expression in the developing ear and kidney: towards the understanding of the pathogenesis of Branchio-Oto-Renal (BOR) syndrome. Dev Dyn 1998;213:486–499

35. Chang EH, et al. Branchio-oto-renal syndrome: the mutation spectrum in EYA1 and its phenotypic consequences. Hum Mutat 2004;23: 582–589

36. Skuse GR, Kosciolek BA, Rowley PT. Molecular genetic analysis of tumors in von Recklinghausen neurofibromatosis: loss of heterozygosity for chromosome 17. Genes Chromosomes Cancer 1989;1: 36–41

37. Wolff RK, et al. Analysis of chromosome 22 deletions in neurofibromatosis type 2-related tumors. Am J Hum Genet 1992;51:478–485

38. Niedermeyer HP, Arnold W. Otosclerosis: a measles virus associated inflammatory disease. Acta Otolaryngol 1995;115:300–303

39. Van Den Bogaert K, et al. A fifth locus for otosclerosis, OTSC5, maps to chromosome 3q22–24. J Med Genet 2004;41:450–453

40. Van Den Bogaert K, et al. Otosclerosis: a genetically heterogeneous disease involving at least three different genes. Bone 2002;30: 624–630

41. Van Den Bogaert K, et al. A second gene for otosclerosis, OTSC2, maps to chromosome 7q34–36. Am J Hum Genet 2001;68:495–500

42. Di Leva F, et al. Otosclerosis: exclusion of linkage to the OTSC1 and OTSC2 loci in four Italian families. Int J Audiol 2003;42:475–480

43. Snead MP, Yates JR. Clinical and molecular genetics of Stickler syndrome. J Med Genet 1999;36:353–359

44. Sanchez-Martin M, et al. SLUG (SNAI2) deletions in patients with Waardenburg disease. Hum Mol Genet 2002;11:3231–3236

45. Hoth CF, et al. Mutations in the paired domain of the human PAX3 gene cause Klein-Waardenburg syndrome (WS-III) as well as Waardenburg syndrome type I (WS-I). Am J Hum Genet 1993;52:455–462

46. Tassabehji M, et al. Waardenburg's syndrome patients have mutations in the human homologue of the Pax-3 paired box gene. Nature 1992;355:635–636

47. Hughes AE, et al. A gene for Waardenburg syndrome type 2 maps close to the human homologue of the microphthalmia gene at chromosome 3p12-p14.1. Nat Genet 1994;7:509–512

48. Edery P, et al. Mutation of the endothelin-3 gene in the Waardenburg-Hirschsprung disease (Shah-Waardenburg syndrome). Nat Genet 1996;12:442–444

49. Attie T, et al. Mutation of the endothelin-receptor B gene in Waardenburg-Hirschsprung disease. Hum Mol Genet 1995;4:2407–2409

50. Berger W, et al. Isolation of a candidate gene for Norrie disease by positional cloning. Nat Genet 1992;1:199–203

51. Chen ZY, et al. Isolation and characterization of a candidate gene for Norrie disease. Nat Genet 1992;1:204–208

52. Eisemann ML, Sharma GK. The Wildervanck syndrome: cervico-oculo-acoustic dysplasia. Otolaryngol Head Neck Surg 1979;87:892–897

53. Barker DF, et al. Identification of mutations in the COL4A5 collagen gene in Alport syndrome. Science 1990;248:1224–1227

54. Prezant TR, et al. Mitochondrial ribosomal RNA mutation associated with both antibiotic-induced and non-syndromic deafness. Nat Genet 1993;4:289–294

55. Zhao H, et al. Maternally inherited aminoglycoside-induced and nonsyndromic deafness is associated with the novel C1494T mutation in the mitochondrial 12S rRNA gene in a large Chinese family. Am J Hum Genet 2004;74:139–152

56. Jin H, et al. A novel X-linked gene, DDP, shows mutations in families with deafness (DFN-1), dystonia, mental deficiency and blindness. Nat Genet 1996;14:177–180

57. van den Ouweland JM, et al. Mutation in mitochondrial tRNA(Leu)(UUR) gene in a large pedigree with maternally transmitted type II diabetes mellitus and deafness. Nat Genet 1992;1:368–371

23

Nonhereditary Hearing Impairment

Edwin M. Monsell, Michael T. Teixido, Eric L. Slattery, Mark D. Wilson, Brian Kung, and Gordon B. Hughes

The most common causes of hearing loss in our society today are age and occupational noise exposure.

◆ Presbycusis

Presbycusis, the hearing of old age, encompasses the loss of peripheral auditory sensitivity, a decline in word recognition abilities, and associated psychological problems and communication issues. The auditory system is particularly prone to the effects of aging. The cells of the auditory system, being specialized neural structures, belong to the "fixed postmitotic" group of cells of the body and cannot reproduce.[1] Because of this, cells that can no longer function properly due to accumulated errors in DNA transcription,[1] inefficient protein syntheses,[2] or accumulation of insoluble pigments[3] cannot be replaced by new cells.

Many factors have been implicated in the pathogenesis of presbycusis, including genetic predispositions, occupational exposures, diet, cardiovascular disease, smoking, alcohol abuse, and head trauma.[4-6] Rosen et al[4] coined the term *socioacusis* to describe the socioeconomic factors that contribute to more severe presbycusis in industrialized societies than in rural Africa. They suggested that diet and noise exposure were more important than socioeconomic factors per se. Rosenhall et al[5] studied hearing levels at ages 70 to 85 years in a longitudinal study and found a weak correlation between hearing loss and smoking, alcohol abuse, and head trauma in men, and between hearing loss and intake of pharmaceutical agents (especially salicylates) in women. Gates et al[6] found a small but statistically significant association between cardiovascular disease and hearing status in the elderly that is greater for women than for men and more in the low than in the high frequencies. Pearlman[7] proposed a working clinical definition of "classic presbycusis" that required (1) bilaterally symmetric sensorineural hearing loss, (2) absent or partial recruitment, (3) a negative history for noise exposure, and (4) poorer speech discrimination than predicted by pure-tone sensitivity. Decline of word recognition out of proportion to pure-tone sensitivity has been termed *phonemic regression*.[8] It is thought to be due to a decline in central auditory function

and may be important in auditory rehabilitation. Not all cases of presbycusis show these classic features.

Epidemiologic cross-sectional surveys of elderly subjects have shown that hearing thresholds increase steadily with increased frequency and age, that women hear substantially better than men in higher frequencies, and that thresholds for the right and left ears tend to be similar for the majority of adults.[9-12]

Jerger et al[13] reviewed large-scale surveys of hearing published during the past 50 years and revealed a "gender reversal" phenomenon in the average audiograms of the elderly; above 1 kHz, men showed greater average loss than women, but below 1 kHz, women showed greater average loss than men. The effect increases with both age and degree of hearing loss and remains after persons with a history of noise exposure are excluded from the analysis.

Presbycusis usually reflects a gradual decline in hearing sensitivity but may be highly variable in its age of onset and rate of progression. Among the 1662 subjects in the Framingham cohort, pure-tone thresholds increased with age.[14] The rate of change with age did not differ by gender, although men had poorer threshold sensitivity. Word recognition ability declined with age more rapidly in men than in women and was poorer in men than in women at all ages.[14]

A subclassification of seven types of presbycusis has been suggested, based in part on studies that attempted to relate histopathologic findings and characteristic audiometric shapes. The seven types are sensory, neural, strial, cochlear conductive, indeterminate, central presbycusis, and middle ear aging.[1]

Sensory Presbycusis

Sensory presbycusis results in a steeply down-sloping audiometric configuration beginning just above the speech frequencies, with slow deterioration of hearing sensitivity beginning in middle age.[1,15] Steeply sloping changes in pure-tone thresholds are predominantly an expression of degeneration of the organ of Corti. The lesion is often restricted to the mid-first turn of the cochlea, has sharply defined boundaries, and may involve only the outer hair cells or both the outer and inner hair cells.[16] A sensory lesion restricted to the outer hair cells causes a 50-dB threshold elevation for those frequencies having their tonotopic locus within the area of the lesion.[16] Advanced lesions show loss of supporting cells, degeneration of the sensory cells, and replacement by epithelioid cells.[1,17,18] Typically, the sensory lesion occurs above the speech frequencies, and discrimination scores are well preserved.

Neural Presbycusis

In neural presbycusis, first-order neurons are lost, often with preservation of sensory cells.[1,17,18] Although a severe sensory lesion that involves the sustentacular elements of the organ of Corti may be associated with retrograde degeneration of cochlear neurons,[19] neuronal degeneration does not further aggravate a sensory hearing loss because the neural loss is obscured by the preexisting hair cell loss.[16] The typical audiometric pure-tone pattern in neural presbycusis is a downsloping high-frequency configuration, relatively more flat than that seen in sensory presbycusis. Speech frequencies are affected, and there exists a decline in speech discrimination scores that is disproportionate to the degree of pure-tone hearing loss. Thus, neural presbycusis may be a cause of phonemic regression. Pathologically, neurons are lost through the cochlea but more so in the basal turn.[1,20] In primary neuronal degeneration, the number of primary auditory neurons lost must exceed 50% of the neonatal normal level before word recognition scores are affected.[21]

Strial Presbycusis

Because the stria vascularis has no tonotopic organization, it cannot cause hearing losses with discrete frequency boundaries. A logical inference has been made that strial atrophy results in a degradation in the quality of endolymph, which results in a uniform elevation of threshold for all frequencies.[16] An effect on word discrimination scores would not be expected. A relatively flat pattern of pure-tone thresholds is seen. Speech discrimination scores are well preserved, often not declining until the pure-tone average exceeds 50 dB.[1] This type of hearing loss is the only condition in which strial atrophy occurs as an isolated acquired lesion.[22] The pattern of atrophy may be patchy or uniform, or may occur predominantly in the apical half of the cochlea. Large intracellular vacuoles, cystic structures, or basophilic deposits may be seen.[1,23] Similar patterns of strial damage are also seen in hearing loss due to other causes, such as ototoxicity. The volumetric loss of stria vascularis must exceed 30% before pure-tone thresholds are affected.[24]

Cochlear Conductive and Indeterminate Presbycusis

Cochlear conductive presbycusis refers to an age-related decrease in pure-tone sensitivity and word discrimination score with no histopathologic findings.[22] Hearing loss usually starts in mid-life with slow progression. It is proposed that this hearing loss results from excessive stiffness of the basilar membrane with impaired mechanical-electrical transduction of sound energy.[22] The greatest effect on hearing sensitivity would be expected to be at the basal end, where the basilar membrane is shortest. The resulting audiometric configuration would be a down-sloping linear pattern.

In Schuknecht et al's[23] original study, 11.9% of patients had sensory presbycusis, 30.7% had neural presbycusis, 34.6% had strial presbycusis, and 22.8% had conductive presbycusis. In a later study, Schuknecht[1] reported that 25% of all cases of presbycusis show no histopathologic correlates of hearing loss. He classified these as cases of indeterminate presbycusis. It has been postulated that the malfunction is caused by impaired cochlear mechanics, altered biochemistry, or histologic changes that cannot be resolved or demonstrated by light microscopy.[16,25]

Frequency selectivity, which is important in the understanding of human speech, refers to the ability of the ear to discriminate between two simultaneously occurring sounds of different spectral composition. Using psychoacoustic tuning curves, Matschke[26] found that frequency selectivity mainly concerns frequencies above 2 kHz and is significantly impaired by progressive loss of outer hair cells in the basal parts of the cochlea in old age. Although pure-tone audiograms show high-frequency hearing loss earlier in life, frequency selectivity is not significantly disturbed before age 60.[26] Another study did not demonstrate a statistically significant correlation between speech discrimination and frequency selectivity.[27] These studies illustrate the point that explanations of indeterminate presbycusis based on the limitations of light microscopy fail to acknowledge the contribution of central auditory factors to auditory disability. The scheme of sensory, neural, strial, and cochlear conductive or indeterminate presbycusis is conceptually useful, but of limited clinical applicability.

Central Presbycusis

Central presbycusis is the central integrative and synthesizing hearing disability that reflects a progressive deterioration of the central nervous system.[28] Although the existence of central presbycusis follows from the aging of the brain, studies of central auditory deficits in aging populations have been confounded by the effects of aging on the auditory periphery, which affects the measurement of central auditory function.[29] Nonetheless, several studies suggest a strong relationship between hearing ability and central auditory function.[29–31] Fire et al[32] found a significant correlation between self-perceived hearing handicap and central auditory nervous system status in 30 elderly adults. Substantial evidence for a biochemical basis for central presbycusis has been presented by Caspary et al,[33] who have demonstrated substantial, selective, and age-related loss of the inhibitory neurotransmitter γ-aminobutyric acid (GABA) in the central nucleus of the inferior colliculus of rats. Neurons in the central nucleus of the inferior colliculus are important in the localization of sound in space and are sensitive to differences in interaural time.[34,35] Nevertheless, the functional significance of these changes remains unclear. Thus, Kelly-Ballweber and Dobie[36] found equivalent performance on central auditory tests in elderly subjects and audiometrically matched young adults.

Middle Ear Aging

Degenerative changes in the middle ear can also influence hearing in the elderly population. Nixon et al[37] showed that a mean air–bone gap of 12 dB occurred in a group of elderly patients, typically at 2000 to 4000 Hz. They proposed that hearing loss resulted from loosening of the ligaments and articulations of the ossicles. Belal and Stewart[38] also demonstrated arthritis and ankylosis of the ossicles with aging in histopathologic preparations. Old ear canals lose some of their rigidity. The resulting collapse under the audiologist's headphones may result in a false air–bone gap. This phenomenon may be avoided by placing a short length of rigid plastic tubing in the external ear canal or by using insert earphones.

Hearing loss has been linked to depression and cognitive decline in the elderly,[39,40] but the reported relationship may be due to other factors associated with aging and hearing loss.[41]

It is the responsibility of the otolaryngologist to distinguish presbycusis from hearing loss that can occur from pathologic processes other than aging. Thus, a complete otologic history, physical examination, and audiometric testings are appropriate components of the evaluation. One important treatable cause of hearing loss that is more prevalent in the middle-aged and elderly is Paget's disease of bone.[42] A high-frequency sensory loss and a low-frequency air–bone gap are characteristic when the temporal bone is involved.[43,44] The hearing loss may progress at a more rapid rate than presbycusis.[45] Histopathologic correlates are lacking.[46] Treatment, which is associated with little or no morbidity, may stabilize the process,[47] although it is questionable that established Pagetic hearing loss can be reversed. Paget's disease may cause hearing loss even when its manifestations are not obvious on physical examination. Early detection is important. Patients may be screened for Paget's disease with a test for serum alkaline phosphatase; the disease may be confirmed by high-resolution computed tomograpy (CT) imaging of the temporal bones.[45] There is no known medical or surgical treatment for true presbycusis. When other pathologic processes, such as infection, Meniere's disease, otosclerosis, Paget's disease, and so on, have been ruled out or treated, auditory rehabilitation of presbycusis is appropriate (see Chapter 30).

◆ Noise-Induced Hearing Loss

Some important principles emerge from the physics of sound and a few well-established observations. We are more susceptible to noise-induced hearing loss (NIHL) from sound at frequencies within the audible spectrum than from sound outside that spectrum. Since the 1960s, sound level meters have incorporated a weighting standard, called the A-network, that has a relationship of frequency to sound pressure level similar to an inversion of the human audibility curve. Such measurements reflect the risk that measured sounds could damage human hearing and are expressed in dBA.

Damage to human hearing may begin when one is subjected to 8-hour daily exposures of continuous sound at 85 dBA.[48] As might be expected, higher sound intensities may be safe if the duration of exposure is shorter. Sound intensity is energy per unit area per unit of time. A 3-dBA increase measured by a sound pressure meter is equivalent to doubling of the sound intensity. Thus, for halving the time of daily exposure from 8 hours to 4 hours, it would be logical that the safe level of sound intensity could be increased by 3-dBA to 88-dBA. However, there is evidence that shorter daily durations of exposure are more likely to be intermittent in the workplace. Intermittent sound exposure may result in less NIHL even if the total intensity of exposure is the same. Thus, the Occupational Safety and Health Administration (OSHA) of

the U.S. Department of Labor has adopted a 5-dB trading rule. According to these regulations, for every halving of the duration of noise exposure, the intensity can be increased by 5 dB without increasing risk of NIHL.[49] Other groups have used a more conservative 3- or 4-dB trading rule, reflecting that there is no universal agreement that any one rule is best.[50,51]

A noise-induced temporary threshold shift (TTS) is defined as the reversible increase in the threshold of audibility for an ear at a given frequency following exposure to noise. A true TTS must be distinguished from physiologic phenomena of sensory adaptation, such as residual masking.[52] In experimental studies, a TTS is often measured 2 minutes after cessation of the noise.[53] OSHA requires hearing conservation programs to test hearing sensitivity at least 14 hours after exposure to noise to establish a worker's baseline hearing levels.[49] In 1930, when the average workday was 16 hours,[53] TTSs of 25 to 30 dB were common.[53] A daily exposure to sound levels that do not produce a TTS will not result in a permanent threshold shift (PTS) over a worker's lifetime.[54]

The NIHL is usually bilaterally symmetrical, but asymmetries of 15 dB or more are not uncommon.[55] In pure NIHL, profound hearing loss is rare. Low-frequency thresholds are rarely lower than 40 dB, and high-frequency thresholds are rarely lower than 75 dB. NIHL does not progress after cessation of noise exposure.[55] After 15 years of continuous exposure, NIHL may continue to progress, but at a much slower rate.[48,56]

There are at least several reasons why the 3- to 6-kHz region of the cochlea is most affected when the ear is exposed to high levels of broadband noise. The acoustic resonances of the ear canal and middle ear enhance the sensitivity to sounds from 1 to 4 kHz.[57] The acoustic reflex attenuates sound at frequencies below 2 kHz.[58] It is possible that mechanical forces may be stronger in the 3- to 6-kHz region due to the geometry of the cochlea, or that its blood supply may be more tenuous there.[17,59] The principle of special vulnerability of this region is supported by the fact that hearing loss in head trauma also affects this region preferentially.[48]

Permanent threshold shift was studied in detail by Passchier-Vermeer, who followed patients after 10 years of noise exposure.[60] When data were corrected for presbycusis, 0-dB PTS was seen for noise exposure of 80 dB or less in an 8-hour day. Noise of 85 dB produced 10 dB PTS at 4000 Hz; 90-dB noise produced a 20-dB shift at 4000 Hz but none in the speech range (500, 1000, and 2000 Hz). Noise intensity greater than 90 dB produced shifts greater than 20 dB, including the speech range.[60] Laboratory and field studies have resulted in the development of tables that predict levels of noise-induced PTS.[60]

Impulse noise is more difficult to measure than continuous noise. At a sufficient sound pressure level to produce a threshold shift, the amount of shift is proportional to the number of pulses given.[61]

There is much interest in factors that might potentiate or reduce the risk of NIHL. Animal experiments have demonstrated that magnesium may have a protective effect.[62] This protection is thought to be mediated at the level of the cell membrane by preventing excessive inflow of calcium, which is already great during periods of heavy noise stimulation.[63] Excessive intracellular calcium plays an important role in cell death.[64] The inverse relationship between NIHL and serum magnesium concentration has also been demonstrated in humans in the range of normal serum magnesium concentrations.[65] A placebo-controlled double-blind study involving 320 military recruits demonstrated that magnesium has a protective effect.[63] The total group received a drink containing either magnesium aspartate or placebo (sodium aspartate) every working day during a 2-month training period. In the placebo group, the percentages of ears with PTS greater than 25 dB after exposure to firearm noise were twice as high as those in the magnesium group. Long-term follow-up of the study group demonstrated that noise-induced PTS was significantly more frequent and more severe in the placebo group than in the magnesium group.[66] Long-term additional intake of a small dose of oral magnesium was not accompanied by any notable side effects in this study group.[66]

In 1987 the remarkable regenerative powers of hair cells in the chick cochlea following damage from intense sound exposure were demonstrated.[67–70] Hair cell regeneration, recovery of the cellular surface areas, and partial restoration of the tectorial membrane were noted to occur during a 12- to 15-day postexposure interval, with substantial recovery of auditory thresholds.[69–72] Details of initial structural damage, the associated consequences of hearing loss, and recovery from both noise damage[73] and ototoxic drug damage[74] have been documented. A study has demonstrated limited regeneration in rat vestibular hair cells in an intensely vitamin A–enriched environment.[75] Currently, there is no clinical application of cochlear hair cell regeneration, although this remains an area of intense investigation and development.

Lindgren and Axelsson[76] have demonstrated that noise with simultaneous exercise may increase the susceptibility to TTS. Aspirin in mild to moderate doses has not been shown to exacerbate TTS or PTS in chinchillas,[77] but neomycin or cisplatin may do so.[78] Iron deficiency has been shown to cause predisposition to TTS and PTS in rats.[79] Increased inner ear melanin and brown eye color have been demonstrated to decrease the susceptibility to TTS.[80,81] The function of melanin in the cochlea has not yet been established, although it may be associated with scavenging of oxygen free radicals. There is no statistically significant evidence that elderly persons or those with preexistent PTS are necessarily more susceptible to further PTS. As noted earlier, NIHL does not progress if there is no further exposure to hazardous noise.

Canlon et al[82] demonstrated that prior exposure to a moderate-level acoustic stimulus can reduce damage caused by later exposure to the same stimulus at high intensity. Guinea pigs were preexposed to a low-level acoustic stimulus before exposure to a stimulus known to yield a PTS. This pretreatment resulted in about 20 dB less TTS than in animals not preexposed and also resulted in complete recovery after 2 months.[82] The middle ear muscles do not play an important role in the mediation of this resistance to noise trauma provided by "acoustic conditioning."[83,84]

Clinicians have long been concerned about the risk of overamplification by hearing aids. To ensure that no NIHL occurs from a hearing aid, the output levels from the aid must be such that they would not cause injury to a person with normal hearing.[85] This constraint may be difficult to satisfy for users with severe to profound sensorineural hearing loss. In these patients, some risk of hearing damage must be accepted in exchange for the advantage gained from the use of a hearing aid.[56,85]

Pathology

A primary loss of sensory cochlear cells is evident in the corresponding area of maximal PTS. The earliest changes are usually seen in the outer hair cells and consist of loss of rigidity and fusion of stereocilia. Resolution of a TTS is associated with the regaining of stereociliary rigidity.[86] Initially (in guinea pigs) only the tips of the stereocilia are affected.[87,88] In the lesions of PTS in the guinea pig, Gao et al[87] observed that the base of the stereocilia was always damaged, the continuity of the cuticular plate was broken, and extracuticular cytoplasm was seen. The continuity of the cuticular plate may play an important role in determining the reversibility of threshold shifts. A proliferation of smooth endoplasmic reticulum with mitochondrial swelling can be seen in these early cases.[88,89] Further changes include vacuolization of the cells,[88] pyknosis of the nuclei,[90] depletion of respiratory enzymes,[91] and hair cell lysis.[88] Lim and Melnick proposed that these changes were caused by metabolic exhaustion. Changes in cochlear blood flow have also been implicated.[92]

Acoustic Trauma

Acoustic trauma is distinct from other forms of NIHL in that it refers to sudden mechanical disruption of cochlear and other auditory structures from bursts of intense acoustic energy (i.e., impulse noise). Sound intensity levels above 180 dB can rupture or produce hemorrhages within the human tympanic membrane or disrupt or fracture the ossicular chain.[93] Impact noise greater than 140-dB peak sound pressure level may result in a PTS from a single exposure. Such damage is termed *acoustic trauma.* Some early models of cordless telephones incorporated the ringer into the receiver, resulting in cases of acoustic trauma. Because the noise source was in the low-frequency region, a low-frequency NIHL was produced. These devices have been redesigned to eliminate this risk.[94–96] Because the rise time of impulse pressure waves is much more rapid than neural response in the auditory system, impulse sounds are seldom accurately perceived and middle ear protective reflexes are ineffective.

Management

Because there is no effective treatment for NIHL, the most effective management is prevention. If noise exposure is unavoidable, ear protectors may at least reduce the level of exposure.[97–99] If working properly, the most effective muffs and plugs may attenuate ambient sound by as much as 30 dB.

The Committee on Hearing and Equilibrium of the American Academy of Otolaryngology–Head and Neck Surgery established guidelines for initiating a hearing conservation program.[97] These recommendations included difficulty communicating by speech in the presence of noise, the presence of head noises or ringing in the ears after working in noise for several hours, or a temporary loss of hearing that lasts for several hours after exposure to noise. NIHL has prompted otologic referral criteria for workers exposed to industrial noise.[100–105] First, noise levels at work must be assessed. Noise should be characterized as steady (turbine), intermittent, or impulse. Eighty-five dBA is the limit for an 8-hour working day of continuous noise exposure.[50]

Counseling issues may include advice to avoid exposure to noise particularly after exposure to ototoxic drugs. This advice may need to be observed for months after treatment with aminoglycosides, as they may be retained in hair cells for many months. Nonoccupational noise exposure from power tools and recreational use of firearms should be avoided.

Environmental controls to minimize noise include reduction of noise at the source, reduction of noise transmitted through the building structure, and revision of work procedures to minimize duration of noise exposure.[97] If hearing loss continues to progress despite appropriate measures, it may be necessary for the physician to recommend job reassignment.

Audiologic and medical referral criteria for occupational hearing conservation programs were established by the Medical Aspects of Noise Committee of the American Council of Otolaryngology.[106] Workers should be referred according to the criteria listed below:

If the average hearing level at 500, 1,000, 2,000, and 3,000 Hz is greater than 30 dB; if there is more than 15-dB difference in average hearing between the ears at 500, 1,000, and 2,000 Hz or more than 30 dB at 3,000, 4,000, and 6,000 Hz; if there is a change from previous audiograms of more than 15 dB in the speech range, 20 dB at 3,000 Hz or 30 dB at 4,000-6,000 Hz; or if variable or inconsistent responses are measured.[107]

Medical criteria for referral include significant, persistent, or recurrent otologic symptoms.[106]

The percentage hearing handicap is a binaural assessment that may be calculated using guidelines of the Committee on Hearing and Equilibrium of the American Academy of Otolaryngology–Head and Neck Surgery:

The average of the hearing thresholds at 500, 1,000, 2,000, and 3,000 Hz should be calculated for each ear, and the percent impairment for each ear may be then calculated by multiplying by 1.5% the amount by which the above average hearing threshold level exceeds 25 dB (up to a maximum of 92 dB). The hearing handicap may then be calculated by multiplying the smaller percentage (better ear) by 5, adding this figure to the larger percentage, and dividing the total by 6.[107]

This percentage hearing handicap can then be applied to statutes and rules pertaining to occupational hearing loss.[108–110]

In evaluating claims for compensation for occupational hearing loss, it is necessary to confirm the presence of hearing loss, its magnitude, and possible etiologies, including functional hearing loss. It is essential to determine whether occupational noise exposure likely exceeded a time-weighted average of 85 dB. One must also allocate the proportion of hearing loss that may be attributed to NIHL.[48,111]

It is quite easy for use of portable headphone audio devices to exceed current OSHA recommendations. Similarly, sound levels measured at rock concerts often exceed 95 dB, and TTSs have been measured frequently in conjunction with both.[112–115] Nonetheless, guidelines for recreational sound exposure have not been established. Much needs to be done to communicate the risks of recreational noise exposure.

◆ Idiopathic Sudden Hearing Loss

Sudden hearing loss (SHL) has been defined as 30 dB or more sensorineural hearing loss occurring in at least three contiguous audiometric frequencies within 3 days or less.[116,117] Although this definition is useful for clinical research, in some patients sudden losses of less magnitude may be quite disruptive, especially if there is a preexisting loss or if the loss occurs in the better hearing ear. Slower loss over more than 3 days usually is described as "rapidly progressive" as opposed to "immediate."[118] Although conductive hearing loss also can be sudden, SHL refers only to sensorineural loss. Approximately 4000 new cases of SHL occur annually in the United States[119] and 15,000 annually worldwide,[120,121] accounting for about 1% of all cases of sensorineural hearing loss.[122] The incidence of SHL increases with age,[121] with no consistent sexual predominance[1] or geographic clustering.[123] The disorder may be cyclical or seasonal.[124] There is a 4 to 17% incidence of bilaterality during the patient's lifetime.[119]

Etiology

Histopathologic studies have demonstrated atrophy of the organ of Corti, stria vascularis, and tectorial membrane.[125,126] Changes were most often seen in the basal turn of the cochlea; however, in some specimens, all turns of the cochlea were involved. The degeneration of neural structures appeared significantly less than that in structures of the cochlea, with vascular channels appearing to be open in all specimens. These pathologic findings were not thought uniformly to represent vascular occlusion of the cochlea similar to that in experimental studies,[127,128] but rather more closely resembled those changes seen in viral hearing loss such as that occurring with measles, mumps, and rubella.[129–131]

There is a 5 to 65% prevalence of previous viral illness in patients with SHL,[119,132–135] but until recently investigators could not determine whether this finding was statistically significant.[136] In 1983 Wilson et al[134] found seroconversion to mumps, rubeola, varicella zoster, cytomegalovirus, and influenza B viruses in 63% of 122 patients with SHL and in 40% of controls. The many infectious agents that have been associated with sudden or progressive sensorineural hearing loss are discussed in a review.[137] Perhaps the strongest evidence for viral etiology comes from identification of viruses in the inner ear using indirect immunofluorescence. Cytomegalovirus, mumps, and rubeola have been identified in inner ears of patients suffering from SHL.[138]

Recoverable sensorineural hearing loss can be induced experimentally by temporary vascular occlusion.[139] Many well-documented cases of vascular disease have resulted in SHL, including leukemia, sickle cell disease, vasculitis, and embolization during coronary bypass surgery.

Immunologic causes of SHL include primary "autoimmune" inner ear disease,[140–143] temporal arteritis,[144] Wegener's granulomatosis,[145] Cogan's syndrome,[146] polyarteritis nodosa,[147] and delayed contralateral endolymphatic hydrops.[148] Immune-mediated SHL can be either primary and localized to the inner ear, or secondary due to generalized systemic immune disease.[149]

Up to 13% of patients with acoustic neuromas may present with SHL.[150] Of these patients, 23% may recover auditory function spontaneously[150] or with steroid therapy.[150,151] Although the prevalence is low, any patient with sensorineural hearing loss, including SHL, even with recovery, should be suspected of having an acoustic neuroma. The contralateral SHL associated with acoustic neuroma surgery averages 16.5 dB in high frequencies and 19.5 in low frequencies and typically returns to normal within 3 months.[152] This SHL may be caused by autoimmunity[149] or by postoperative hypotonia of the cerebrospinal fluid (CSF) or labyrinthine fluids.[152] The prevalence of acoustic neuroma in SHL is higher when associated with other cranial nerve involvement (ipsilateral facial numbness), papilledema, or ataxia. The diagnosis is confirmed by appropriate radiologic studies of the internal auditory canal.[153–156]

Other proposed causes of sudden sensorineural hearing loss include diabetes mellitus,[157] perilymphatic hypertension,[158] autonomic imbalance[159] cochlear hydrops, perilymphatic fistula, and operative complications of nonotologic surgery.[153] There is anecdotal evidence supporting an association between SHL and manipulation of the cervical spine. Injury to the vertebral artery is a proposed mechanism of injury.[160,161]

Evaluation

The evaluation and treatment of SHL should be considered a medical urgency, if not an emergency. The first priority is to discover those potential causes for which there is proven effective treatment, such as autoimmune disease. A thorough history may give clues leading to the discovery of a known cause. The circumstances and characteristics of the onset of hearing loss should be determined. Some patients may have preexistent hearing loss that was discovered accidentally. A history of trauma or noise exposure should be reviewed. Associated otologic symptoms should be identified, including vertigo or imbalance, tinnitus, and aural pressure.

Patients generally volunteer pertinent information; however, some patients may not readily speak about certain events. Examples include alcohol intoxication with secondary traumatic injury or childhood activities done without parental permission. Medical conditions that can be associated with SHL include diabetes, syphilis, and chronic renal and cardiovascular disease.

Usually the physical examination is otherwise normal. Baseline testing should include an otoscopic and complete neurotologic examination. Basic audiometry may-provide prognostic clues. A down-sloping or flat moderate to severe sensorineural hearing loss has a poor prognosis.[162] Mild low-frequency losses have the best prognosis. Spontaneous improvement is often followed by further recovery. The presence of vertigo is a poor prognostic finding, often corroborated by abnormal vestibular function testing.

Laboratory blood tests generally are not very helpful but can include fluorescent treponemal antibody-absorption (FTA-abs) test. Tests seeking confirmation of autoimmunity, such as sedimentation rate, C-reactive protein, rheumatoid factor, and antinuclear antibody, are nearly always noncontributory. Antigen-specific Western blot immunoassay is commercially available now at IMMCO Diagnostics, Buffalo, New York. CT or magnetic resonance imaging (MRI) studies of the head are important if trauma or tumor is suspected.

Natural History

The natural history of SHL is highly variable, probably because its pathogenesis is multifactorial. Many patients with SHL improve without treatment of any kind. Because most spontaneous improvement occurs in the first 2 weeks after onset, the prognosis is worse the longer the symptoms last. Studies are prone to selection bias, in that patients might not all be seen in the same stage of disease. In 15% of patients, the hearing loss progresses.[136]

Treatment

Although many treatment regimens have been proposed for idiopathic SHL,[163] at present independent studies have not consistently supported the use of any one treatment modality. The treatment that has been the most widely accepted is corticosteroids, such as prednisone, 1 mg/kg of lean body mass per day for 7 to 14 days.[164,165] If hearing levels improve, the course of treatment can be extended. Inhalations of carbogen (95% oxygen with 5% carbon dioxide) have been advocated by some because they may increase cochlear blood flow, at least temporarily.[166] A low-salt diet and diuretic therapy, as commonly used in classic Meniere's disease, has been advocated.[137]

There are few clinical trials in SHL. Wilson and coworkers[116] studied 33 patients treated with steroids. Some received dexamethasone, 4.5 mg twice daily for 4 days, followed by a short tapering dose; others received methylprednisolone, 16 mg for 3 days, which was tapered for the next 8 days. Although the study design contained several flaws, preliminary results suggested that steroids had statistically significant benefits on the recovery of hearing in patients with moderate hearing losses. Moskowitz et al[167] confirmed Wilson et al's results in 36 patients treated with dexamethasone, 0.75 mg four times daily for 3 days, followed by a tapering dose during a total of 12 days. Conversely, Byl,[168] found no treatment benefit in an 8-year prospective study of 225 patients with SHL.

The great majority of patients with SHL can be managed in the ambulatory setting with oral corticosteroids (e.g., 1 mg/kg of prednisone for 7 to 14 days), possibly with salt restriction and diuretics. Follow-up audiometry is scheduled along with hearing aid evaluation in selected patients. Appropriate tests are conducted to exclude acoustic tumors. Vestibular suppressives are used if needed. Histamine, peripheral vasodilators, and other less commonly proposed medical treatments have little evidential basis to be recommended at this time.[169] The intratympanic application of steroids in SHL has been suggested (see below).[170,171] A randomized clinical trial by Tucci et al[172] showed no benefit to adding the antiviral medication valacyclovir to standard systemic steroid treatment in SHL.

Because intratympanic (IT) steroids for idiopathic SHL can be given in high concentration without systemic side-effects and risks, this route of administration is becoming increasingly popular. At the time this chapter was written, two important studies were underway, one of them recently completed. Drs. Battaglia and Cueva at Kaiser San Diego (California) performed a multi-center, double-blinded, placebo-controlled randomized study to compare hearing results in idiopathic sudden sensorineural hearing loss (ISSNHL) patients who received either a high-dose prednisone taper (HDPT), IT-dexamethasone alone, or IT-dexamethasone and HDPT. Fifty-one patients with less than a 6-week history of ISSNHL were randomized to one of the three arms and followed prospectively. The ISSNHL patients treated with both IT-dexamethasone and HDPT experienced statistically significantly improved hearing recovery compared with treatment with HDPT or IT-dexamethasone alone (see final publication for details).[173]

While these results might suggest that every patient with ISSNHL should receive combined systemic and IT steroids, many patients cannot tolerate systemic steroids or cannot take them because of other medical problems. These patients would like to know if IT therapy is equally effective as systemic therapy. This question will be answered by another multi-center, randomized study headed by Steven D. Rauch, M.D. of the Massachusetts Eye and Ear Infirmary.[174] Hopefully preliminary results will be available in 2008-2009.

In SHL the treating physician's primary responsibilities include the following: (1) to diagnose and treat underlying causes, (2) to discuss the risks and potential benefits of treatment with the patient, (3) to treat aggressively or not at all, (4) to arrange rehabilitation for those patients whose hearing does not improve, (5) to exclude the diagnosis of retrocochlear tumor, and (6) to offer follow-up for possible delayed symptoms and contralateral ear disease.

◆ Ototoxicity

Ototoxicity is "the tendency of certain therapeutic agents and other chemical substances to cause functional impairment and cellular degeneration of the tissues of the inner ear, and especially of the end-organs and neurons of the cochlear and vestibular divisions of the eighth cranial nerve."[175] Ototoxicity must be distinguished from neurotoxicity, the process by which drugs and other substances may alter hearing or equilibrium by acting at the level of the brainstem or central connections of the cochlear and vestibular nuclei. Ototoxicity has been recognized since the late 1800s, when it was observed that quinine and acetylsalicylic acid (ASA) produced dizziness, tinnitus, and hearing loss. Since World War II, other drugs, often more toxic, have joined the list of ototoxic substances: aminoglycoside antibiotics, loop diuretics, macrolide antibiotics, and some antineoplastic agents.

Aminoglycosides

The aminoglycosides are highly polar, polycationic compounds, predominantly 4,6-diglycosylated 2-deostreptamines. The first aminoglycoside, streptomycin, was isolated from soil bacteria in 1943, followed by dihydrostreptomycin and neomycin (1949), kanamycin (1957), gentamicin, amikacin, tobramycin, netilmicin, dibekacin, and sisomicin. The bacterial activity of the aminoglycosides, largely against gram-negative and enterococcal infections, results from inhibition of protein synthesis at the level of the ribosome. Aminoglycoside ototoxicity has been reviewed by Forge and Schacht[176] and recently by Roland and Rutka.[177]

Dihydrostreptomycin was developed to treat tuberculosis; its use was quickly abandoned, however, because of the severe and unpredictable cochlear ototoxicity it produced. It differs from streptomycin only by the reduction of an aldehyde to an alcohol. Neomycin, which is also predominantly cochleotoxic, is used only topically or orally for bowel preparation before bowel surgery.[178]

It has been estimated that ototoxicity due to aminoglycoside use ranges in prevalence from 2 to 15% overall, with values of 2.4% for netilmicin, 6.1% for tobramycin, 8.6% for gentamicin, and 13.9% for amikacin in a survey of prospective studies by Kahlmeter and Dahlager.[179] A randomized, prospective study by Matz and Lerner[180] found a prevalence of ototoxicity of 5% for gentamicin and 7.5% for amikacin. Proposed risk factors for aminoglycoside-induced ototoxicity have included the type of aminoglycoside, concomitant exposure to other ototoxic drugs (loop diuretics, chemotherapeutic agents),

noise exposure, duration of therapy, total dose, plasma level, perilymph level, age, sex, liver dysfunction, renal dysfunction, bacteremia, dehydration, and hyperthermia. A prospective study found that of the latter 11 variables, only age increased risk significantly.[181]

The highly polar nature of the aminoglycosides accounts for their water solubility, renal excretion, and difficulty with traversing plasma membranes passively. They must be transported actively or engulfed by pinocytosis to reach the interior of cells. Only 1 to 3% of the oral dose is absorbed. Aminoglycosides have very strong tissue-binding properties and may be found in the urine of patients with normal renal function as long as 20 days after the cessation of therapy.[182] Animal experiments indicate that the serum half-life of aminoglycosides is about 80 minutes.[182] The concentration of aminoglycoside in the perilymph rises slowly, reaching its peak 2 to 5 hours after injection, at a level 3 to 5% of peak serum level.[183] The half-life of aminoglycoside in the perilymph has been reported to be from 3 to 15 hours[182,183]; however, ototoxicity does not correlate with drug concentration in inner ear tissue or fluids, and inner ear fluid concentrations at no time exceed serum levels.[184–187] Gentamicin can be found localized in hair cells for weeks to months, even without electrophysiologic signs of ototoxicity.[188] Ototoxicity does not correlate with nephrotoxicity; furthermore, damage to the auditory and vestibular systems occurs somewhat independently.

A mitochondrial mutation (A1555G) in the 12S rRNA gene was shown initially in Chinese families to predispose to ototoxicity from aminoglycosides. Only the cochlea is affected.[189]

Pathophysiology

In animals exposed to aminoglycosides the loss of hair cells of the organ of Corti is most severe in the basal turn of the cochlea and is progressively less toward the apex. The inner row of the outer hair cells is affected first, followed by the outer two rows. The inner hair cells and the rest of the organ of Corti are damaged only in cases of severe toxicity. Evidence of damage to other cochlear structures has also been noted, including the stria vascularis, spiral ligament, spiral prominence, outer sulcus, and Reissner's membrane.[190] Nerve fibers can be damaged after hair cell derangement, but this is thought to be secondary to the changes in the hair cells; ganglion cells do not seem to be affected directly.[191,192] Histologic and clinical cases of asymmetric and unilateral cochleotoxicity have been reported.[193]

Electrochemical studies of animal models of cochlear toxicity demonstrated that aminoglycosides produced a reduction in the endolymphatic potential and cationic content of endolymph.[194] Reduction of the levels of adenosine triphosphatase and succinic acid dehydrogenase has been found in the stria vascularis and may explain changes in endolymph composition.[195,196]

Animal studies of aminoglycoside toxicity suggest that the type I hair cells of the crista ampullaris are damaged earlier than the type II cells. The summit of the crista appears to be the area damaged first, followed by the sloping regions. The hair cells of the saccule appear to be less sensitive to aminoglycoside toxicity than those of the utricle.[182]

Human vestibulotoxicity has also shown good agreement with animal models. Loss of hair cells, type I more than type

II, and vacuolization of the remaining hair cells have been described in the cristae.[191,195] Hair cell loss and vacuolization have also been observed in the maculae of the utricle and saccule.[193,197]

Aminoglycosides cause both acute and chronic ototoxic effects. Acute effects manifest with neuromuscular and auditory blockage, is reversible, and is attributed to calcium antagonism and channel blockade.[198–201] Postsynaptic excitatory amino acid blockade has also been postulated.[202]

Aminoglycosides bond with extremely high affinity to polyphosphoinositides.[176] Polyphosphoinositides are membrane lipids involved in intracellular second messenger systems and are also sources of substrates for precursors in the synthesis of prostaglandins and leukotrienes.[203]

Several lines of evidence reviewed by Schacht[176,204] strongly suggest that oxygen and nitrogen free radical species are the primary mechanisms of permanent cellular injury in aminoglycoside ototoxicity. Priuska showed with nuclear magnetic resonance spectroscopy that gentamicin can act as an iron chelator. Priuska and Schacht proposed that a redox active gentamicin-Fe(II) complex activates molecular oxygen in a process that generates reactive oxygen species and damages the cell. Cell death occurs primarily by apoptosis.

A role for ornithine decarboxylase has also been proposed; neomycin and gentamicin are known to inhibit both the cochlear and renal enzymes. Induction of ornithine decarboxylase is important in cellular response to injury, and inhibition could lead to the accumulation of toxic moieties.[205]

It has been postulated that there exists an as yet unidentified metabolite of the aminoglycosides that is the true toxic agent. This hypothesis has been proposed to explain several observations, including the poor correlation between drug levels and ototoxicity and the delay seen before chronic toxicity occurs. This hypothesis also may account for the observation that gentamicin does not destroy isolated hair cells in vitro, but does so after incubation with liver cytosolic fraction or when injected systemically, applied locally, or in organ culture.[206–208] Distribution of such a transforming agent in different amounts in susceptible tissues may also account in part for the differential toxicity in the kidney, cochlea, and vestibular organs.

Some compounds have been proposed to confer partial protection from aminoglycoside ototoxicity, including sulfhydryl compounds and free radical scavengers, though other free radical scavengers have not been effective.[209–211] Clinical trials are needed to determine the clinical effectiveness and safety of chemoprotective strategies.

Streptomycin

Streptomycin was the first effective antibacterial agent employed against tuberculosis. As early as 1945, however, it was observed that 2 to 3 g/day of streptomycin would damage or destroy vestibular function in 2 to 4 weeks.[190] This effect was dose-dependent and cumulative. Adverse effects on hearing, although reported, were far less common.

McGee and Olszewski[212] gave cats 200 mg/kg/day of streptomycin and found that nystagmus developed after 12 days and a sloping sensorineural hearing loss developed after 28 days. Temporal bone sections revealed the previously noted changes in the cristae, with little, if any, damage to the maculae. Changes in the cochlea were confined to the basal turn

and varied from loss of outer hair cells to total destruction of the organ of Corti.

Dihydrostreptomycin

Unlike streptomycin, the ototoxic effects of dihydrostreptomycin can occur long after the drug has been withdrawn. Hearing loss has been reported as long as 5 months after discontinuation of the drug and after a patient has received as little as 4 g.[190] Animal experiments have demonstrated histopathologic changes similar to those caused by streptomycin. There seems, however, to be greater damage to the outer hair cells, involving both the basal and middle turns of the cochlea.[212] Dihydrostreptomycin has been discontinued for clinical use.

Gentamicin, Tobramycin, and Amikacin

Many clinical studies have investigated the ototoxicity of gentamicin, tobramycin, and amikacin. Results have been difficult to compare due to lack of control of confounding variables and variability in methods. Tests of cochlear function have been limited primarily to pure-tone audiometry, and assessment of vestibular ototoxicity usually has not included clinical tests of vestibular function.

In 1980 Fee[182] conducted a prospective study of 113 patients who received 138 courses of gentamicin or tobramycin. Dosages were modified to maintain blood levels within the recommended safe ranges, and patients were followed with pure-tone audiometry and electronystagmography. Toxicity was defined as sensorineural hearing loss of 20 dB or greater or reduction by 33% or more of slow-phase nystagmus velocity 90 seconds after irrigation. Cochlear toxicity developed in 16.4% of patients receiving gentamicin and in 15.3% of patients receiving tobramycin. Vestibular toxicity developed in 15.1% of patients receiving gentamicin and in 4.6% of patients receiving tobramycin. The only statistically significant difference between the two drugs was vestibular toxicity (which was less for tobramycin). Cochlear and vestibular toxicity progressed after discontinuation of treatment with either drug. The same type of hearing loss demonstrated in Fee's study has been observed with amikacin administration by the authors (**Fig. 23–1**).

Aminoglycoside cochlear toxicity has generally been thought to involve frequencies above 6 kHz. In Fee's[182] study, however, 27% of patients developed significant change only in the 1- to 4-kHz range. Decreased pure-tone sensitivity was unilateral in 91% of patients. Toxicity was first noted 3 to 35 days after the onset of therapy. Fifty-five percent of the patients recovered their loss of pure-tone sensitivity within 1 week to 6 months. Nonrecovery was associated with hearing losses greater than 25 dB, delayed onset, immediate onset that progressed despite discontinuation of the drug, and continuation of the drug after the onset of toxicity. In cases of vestibular toxicity, the mean depression of slow-phase velocity was 45%. The mean time of appearance of vestibular toxicity was 11.5 days after onset of treatment. Fifty-three percent of patients recovered within 10 days to 9 months.[182]

Most patients who developed cochlear or vestibular ototoxicity were asymptomatic. Less than 5% of patients reported any symptoms; these included decreased hearing, tinnitus, otalgia, and dizziness. Development of symptoms did not correlate well with measurable ototoxicity.[182]

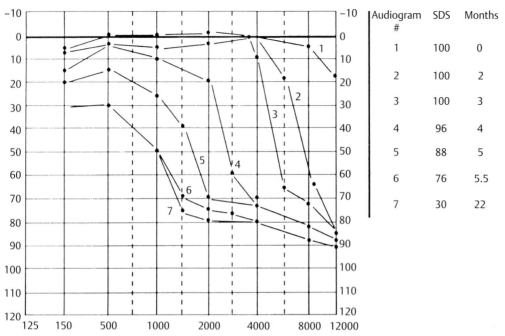

Audiogram #	SDS	Months
1	100	0
2	100	2
3	100	3
4	96	4
5	88	5
6	76	5.5
7	30	22

Figure 23–1 A family of audiometric curves showing progressive hearing loss in a 41-year-old woman treated with amikacin for a life-threatening, disseminated atypical mycobacterial infection that was sensitive only to that drug. Treatment was stopped after 4 months, but the hearing loss continued to progress, with an eventual loss of speech discrimination score (SDS) to 30% at 22 months after the beginning of treatment. (Courtesy of Edwin M. Monsell, M.D., Ph.D.)

Lerner and Matz[183] conducted a prospective study of comparative ototoxicity of gentamicin and amikacin using two groups of 54 patients each. Drug dosages were modified to keep plasma levels within the recommended range. Cochlear toxicity was defined as a 15-dB or greater loss of pure-tone sensitivity at two or more frequencies, in one or both ears. Vestibular toxicity was defined as a decrease of at least 50% in either maximum slow-phase velocity or frequency after aural irrigation. In the gentamicin-treated group, 7% of patients developed cochlear toxicity and 4% developed vestibular toxicity. Only half the patients in these categories were symptomatic at the time of testing. Unilateral toxicity, reversible losses, and onset of toxicity after discontinuation of the drug were all observed. In the amikacin-treated group, 9% of patients developed cochlear toxicity and 6% developed vestibular toxicity. Less than half of the patients in either category were symptomatic when losses were determined. As was observed with gentamicin, there were cases of unilateral involvement, delayed onset of toxicity, and reversibility.

Black et al[213] conducted a prospective study of amikacin ototoxicity in a group of 44 patients. Drug dosage was determined by weight (serum levels were not monitored). Patients were followed with pure-tone audiometric tests and were questioned for the development of tinnitus and vertigo; significant hearing loss was defined as at least 15-dB loss of pure-tone sensitivity. Significant hearing loss was detected in 24% of the patients, and among these, roughly half had unilateral hearing loss. Audiometric recovery was later documented in 23% of this group. Hearing losses were confined primarily to frequencies of 8 kHz or above, but in 25% of the patients frequencies as low as 2 kHz were involved. No patient complained of vertigo. Eighty-four percent of the patients who developed hearing loss were asymptomatic.

Although these three studies varied somewhat in the incidence of ototoxicity, they agreed on several points: (1) Aminoglycoside ototoxicity could be unilateral and reversible. (2) Aminoglycoside cochlear toxicity was not confined to the frequencies above 8 kHz. (3) Most patients who developed measurable ototoxicity were asymptomatic at the time of discovery. (4) Gentamicin, previously thought to be primarily vestibulotoxic, also caused cochlear toxicity. (5) Gentamicin, tobramycin, and amikacin could cause ototoxicity after they were withdrawn (**Fig. 23–1**).

The relatively high incidence of ototoxicity associated with aminoglycosides has led to efforts to identify factors that may predispose to ototoxicity. Previously implicated risk factors include preexisting hearing loss, prior noise exposure, previous ear infection, previous exposure to aminoglycosides, duration of therapy, total dosage, and previous or concomitant exposure to other ototoxic drugs.[214,215] Analysis of Fee's[182] series demonstrates three factors that were associated with increased risk of ototoxicity from gentamicin and tobramycin: duration of therapy greater than 10 days, decreased pure-tone sensitivity on the initial audiogram, and "severe illness." Black and associates'[213] prospective study of amikacin ototoxicity did not show any positive correlations with age, mean daily dose, or pretreatment audiogram. Risk factors included duration of therapy longer than 10 days, administration of greater than 15 g of amikacin, previous exposure to aminoglycosides, peak serum levels greater than 32 µg/mL, and trough levels greater than 10 µg/mL. Two large retrospective studies, which together included more than 5000 patients, support the potential risks of previous aminoglycoside exposure and high daily doses.[214,215]

Much recent work has been done concerning aminoglycoside dosing, challenging some prior assumptions. It is now accepted that efficacy, safety, and ototoxicity are not significantly different for once-daily versus thrice-daily dosing and may be improved with the former.[216–218] Furthermore, ototoxicity seems to be predicted most by the total dose rather than by serum peak and trough levels or any other factor.[219] The suggestions are to adjust the dose of aminoglycosides according to creatinine clearance rather than serum levels.[220] There may still be an important role for monitoring cochlear and vestibular function because only a small number of patients develop symptoms at the time they have measurable ototoxocity (see Recommendations for Management, later in chapter).

Loop Diuretics

Furosemide and ethacrynic acid are members of a family of drugs called "loop diuretics" because they produce diuresis by blocking reabsorption of sodium and chloride in the proximal renal tubule. Other members of this group include bumetanide, piretamide, azosemide, triflocin, and indapamide. These drugs are excreted almost entirely by the kidney. The serum half-like of furosemide is normally 47 to 53 minutes, but has been found to be significantly prolonged in neonates and in patients with renal failure.

Pathophysiology

Animal experiments demonstrated that furosemide and ethacrynic acid produced a dose-related, reversible reduction in endocochlear potential.[221,222] Intravenous furosemide increased endolymphatic sodium concentration and decreased potassium concentration.[222] Behavioral studies in guinea pigs confirmed that these changes correlated with temporary alterations in auditory sensitivity.[223]

Histologically, the major changes that have been observed in animal temporal bones involved the stria vascularis: intercellular edema, capillary narrowing, and degeneration of the intermediate cell layer.[221,223,224] Degenerative changes of the outer hair cells, primarily of the basal turn, have also been observed, but less commonly.[190,222] Electron microscopy has revealed mitochondrial deformation and pathologic intracellular vesicles.[224] Changes in the vestibular labyrinth have also been observed, with degeneration of both type I and type II hair cells in the ampullae and maculae.[224]

Matz and Hinojosa[225] and Arnold and colleagues[220] reported results of histologic examination of temporal bones of patients who had experienced ototoxicity from loop diuretics. Matz and Hinojosa found edema of the stria vascularis, loss of outer hair cells in the basal turn of the cochlea, and cystic degeneration of the hair cells in the ampulla of the posterior canal and in the macula of the saccule.[225] Arnold and associates identified endolymphatic hydrops present throughout the cochlea and alterations in the stria vascularis, with the most severe changes confined to the basal turn.[222] Stria vascularis pathology consisted of edema, thickening, and cystic degeneration. No reduction in the number of hair cells in the organ of Corti was found. It was noted, however, that these cells stained more darkly than normal, particularly in the region of the basal turn. Electron microscopic analysis of the hair cells demonstrated increased granularity of the ground substance and mitochondrial abnormalities. Similar cytoarchitectural changes were noted in type I and type II cells of the cristae and maculae.

Animal and human temporal bone studies indicate that the stria vascularis is the major site of loop diuretic ototoxicity. Furosemide has been demonstrated to inhibit oxidative phosphorylation in rat kidney mitochondria as well as succinic dehydrogenase activity in the hair cells of the guinea pig organ of Corti.[221] It seems likely that loop diuretics exert their ototoxic effect by some type of enzyme inhibition. Such an action in the stria vascularis could inhibit this structure's ability to maintain ionic homeostasis and thereby produce experimental reversible decrease in endocochlear potential and auditory sensitivity.

Clinical Studies

Clinical experience with ethacrynic acid and furosemide indicates that they may produce transient or permanent hearing loss following either oral or intravenous administration.[222,226] Reversible hearing loss appears to be more common, occurring in 26 of 29 patients in the review by Gallagher and Jones.[227] When reversible, hearing loss generally recovers within 30 minutes to 54 hours.[227] Reversible tinnitus and vertigo also have been reported after administration of loop diuretics.[222]

Clinical studies also have suggested that rapid intravenous infusion of furosemide increases the incidence of ototoxicity. In a study conducted with uremic patients, Bosher[224] found those who received furosemide at a rate of 25 mg/min developed ototoxicity, whereas those whose dosage rate was 5.6 mg/min or less developed no symptoms of ototoxicity.

Patients at greatest risk for loop diuretic ototoxicity are those with renal compromise, possibly those receiving aminoglycoside antibiotics, and premature infants.[224,227] Because loop diuretics are eliminated by glomerular filtration, renal impairment prolongs their serum half-life. This increase in serum half-life may permit elevation of perilymph concentration of these drugs, thereby increasing their ototoxicity. In their review of furosemide ototoxicity, Gallagher and Jones[227] found that 19 of 29 patients had renal impairment. Although suggested in many clinical reports, the apparent synergistic action of loop diuretics and aminoglycosides in the production of ototoxicity has yet to be established conclusively. These drugs have also been found to have a prolonged serum half-life in premature infants, although the reason for this is unclear.

Salicylates

The ototoxic potential of acetylsalicylic acid (ASA) has been recognized at least since 1899, when it was first used to treat rheumatic fever.[226] Before it was possible to measure serum drug levels, hearing loss, tinnitus, and vertigo were used to establish the dosage of ASA used in the treatment of gout and rheumatic fever.[228]

Pathophysiology

The mechanism of ASA ototoxicity appears to be multifactorial. Usually, no unequivocal histopathologic abnormalities are found.[228–231] Biochemical abnormalities are suspected.[232] Recent studies have pointed to the importance of subcisternal organelles in outer hair cells in the active cochlear amplifier and outer hair cell motility and have demonstrated the reversible disruption of this mechanism by ASA.

Quinine

Quinine is an alkaloid compound derived from the bark of the cinchona tree, native to certain parts of South America.[229] Its major use has been in the treatment of malaria, although it has largely been superseded by less toxic synthetic drugs. Quinine also is employed in the treatment of nocturnal leg cramping. Quinidine, its stereoisomer, sometimes is used in the treatment of cardiac arrhythmias.[226] The cinchona alkaloids primarily are degraded by the liver and then are eliminated by glomerular filtration. Plasma levels fall rapidly upon termination of therapy, and only negligible concentrations can be detected after 24 hours.

Pathophysiology

Animal experiments have demonstrated characteristic changes in the temporal bones of subjects in whom decreased hearing had been caused by quinine intoxication. Hawkins[175] found capillary vasoconstriction in the stria vascularis, suprastrial ligament, tympanic lip, and basilar membrane of guinea pigs. Ruedi et al[233] reported atrophy of the stria vascularis with decreased cellularity and vacuolization. In addition, they noted degenerative changes of the organ of Corti; these changes were most severe in the basal turn of the cochlea, ranging from loss of outer hair cells to destruction of the organ of Corti.

Clinical Studies

Patients receiving multiple full doses of quinine (approximately 2 g/day), or a single dose in cases of hypersensitivity, may develop a toxicity syndrome known as cinchonism: tinnitus, decreased hearing, vertigo, headache, nausea, and disturbed vision.[226] These symptoms generally resolve rapidly upon withdrawal of the drug; however, cases of irreversible hearing loss and tinnitus have been reported.[175]

Erythromycin

Erythromycin, a macrolide antibiotic discovered in 1952, is employed primarily in the treatment of infections caused by β-hemolytic streptococci, *Streptococus pneumoniae*, staphylococci, and *Legionella*, and in individuals with penicillin sensitivity. Erythromycin exerts its therapeutic effect by inhibiting bacterial protein synthesis at the level of the ribosome.[226] Several different esters of this drug have been developed for both oral and intravenous use, including stearate, estolate, lactobionate, ethylsuccinate, and gluceptate esters. Erythromycin is concentrated in the liver, and 95 to 97% is excreted in its active form in the bile. The remainder is excreted in the urine, also in its active form.[226] Some studies have suggested that its half-life may be prolonged in cases of severe renal failure.[234]

Clinical Studies

Ototoxicity has been reported following oral administration of the stearate ester and intravenous administration of the lactobionate and gluceptate esters.[235,236] Ototoxicity has been characterized by tinnitus, vertigo, subjective hearing loss, and a flat, sensorineural hearing loss, and has been reported with doses 500 mg twice daily.[237] The risk of toxicity is greater with decreased renal function.[234-236,238] Erythromycin ototoxicity is thought to be nearly always reversible. Recovery generally begins within 24 hours of discontinuation of the drug. The only common denominator in reports of erythromycin ototoxicity has been that these patients have received large doses of the drug, usually 4 g/day or more.[234]

Cisplatin

Cisplatin (*cis*-diamminedichloroplatinum II) is a potent cell cycle nonspecific agent used to treat a wide variety of solid tumors. Recognized side effects include ototoxicity, neurotoxicity, nephrotoxicity, gastrointestinal toxicity, and myelosuppression.[239] Most patients treated with cisplatin experience tinnitus, and many have symptomatic hearing loss or otalgia.[239-241] Carboplatin is less ototoxic than cisplatin.[243]

Pathophysiology

The mechanism of ototoxicity is unknown. Animal studies have demonstrated that cisplatin produced a loss of pure-tone auditory sensitivity initially greatest in the high frequencies.[244] In both guinea pigs and rhesus monkeys, this loss has been found to be reversible in its early stages.[244-246] Histopathologic examination of animal temporal bones after induction of cisplatin ototoxicity has shown primarily loss of outer hair cells in the cochlea. These changes have been most pronounced in the region of the basal turn. Ultrastructural changes in the stria vascularis, affecting mostly the marginal cells, have been reported.[247] In addition, collapse of Reissner's membrane in the basal turn also has been noted.[244] Vestibular ototoxicity by cisplatin has not been confirmed to date.[239] The phosphonic acid derivative fosfomycin blocks both ototoxicity and nephrotoxicity of cisplatin in animal models without reducing its antitumor effect.[184] Poly-L-aspartic acid, with known benefit for nephrotoxicity, has as yet undefined value for ototoxicity.[248]

Clinical Studies

Early clinical studies suggested that cisplatin produced an irreversible, dose-related sensorineural hearing loss in the 4 to 8 kHz range in 11% of patients.[240,241,249] At the time these studies were conducted, nephrotoxicity was the major limiting factor in total dosage that could be administered. More recently, techniques of aggressive hydration and diuresis have permitted considerably larger dosages of cisplatin to be employed. These techniques lessen renal toxicity, but not ototoxicity. Fosfomycin has been shown to be protective of ototoxicity and does not inhibit tumoricidal activity in vitro.[250,251] However, nausea from fosfomycin may limit its use in some patient populations.

In a prospective study of 32 patients receiving cisplatin, Reddel et al[242] found that 47% developed a sensorineural hearing loss of 15 dB or greater after receiving a mean cumulative dose of 203 mg/m². The incidence and degree of hearing loss increased with increasing cumulative dose of cisplatin. Although loss of pure-tone sensitivity initially was worse in the 6- to 8-kHz range, losses in the 3- to 4-kHz range became evident as cumulative doses increased. In other studies, patients followed 12 to 18 months after discovery of hearing loss have not shown any evidence of reversibility.[239] Bolus administration of cisplatin has been associated with significantly greater incidence of hearing loss than slow infusion over 2 hours.[240]

Instances of presumed vestibular toxicity, as evidenced by vertigo and disequilibrium, also have been reported in patients receiving cisplatin.[239,252] The incidence of reported vestibular toxicity has not been as great as that of cochlear toxicity; however, symptoms of vestibular toxicity may well be overlooked or minimized in debilitated cancer patients.

Other Potentially Ototoxic Agents

Detailed discussion of other *potentially* ototoxic agents is beyond the scope of this chapter. These agents can include propylene glycol,[253] methylmercury,[254] povidone-iodine,[255] potassium bromate,[256] industrial solvents (styrene and toluene),[257] vancomycin, chloramphenicol, bleomycin, nitrogen mustard, carbon monoxide, gold, lead, arsenic, alcohol, nicotine, caffeine, and nonsteroidal antiinflammatory drugs. Some of these compounds are more neurotoxic than ototoxic.

Recommendations for Management

The rapid administration of bolus doses of ototoxic drugs and their concomitant administration (especially loop diuretics and aminoglycosides) should be avoided. Once-daily dosing of aminoglycosides has shown promise to reduce toxicity.[216–218,258] A positive family history of hearing loss from aminoglycosides may help prevent deafness in other family members due to the A1555G mitrochondrial mutation.[189]

The use of topical otic drops containing neomycin continues to be widespread. Despite appropriate concern, hearing loss from the use of topical neomycin is remarkably rare, especially when it is used in the treatment of chronic suppurative otitis media. Reasonable caution in the use of ototopical neomycin is advisable, although difficult to define.

The early development of symptoms with erythromycin, ASA, and quinine provides a useful warning in alert patients. Excluding hypersensitivity, irreversible ototoxicity generally occurs with these agents only when high doses are continued after the development of symptoms. If symptoms appear, these agents should be withdrawn promptly, if possible. Total daily doses of erythromycin greater than 4 g, or 1.5 g in the presence of renal impairment, should be used with caution.[259]

Because a uniform method of monitoring for all drugs is not reasonable or practical, the authors suggest that monitoring for ototoxicity be individualized depending on the particular drug being employed. During monitoring of cochlear function, particular attention should be paid to pure-tone thresholds at 8 kHz and above, because a decrease in sensitivity to high-frequency sounds is the most sensitive auditory change for most ototoxic agents. Oto-acoustic emissions show promise as another method for monitoring.[260] Vestibular tests should be considered even after a patient has received aminoglycosides for several days, as the earliest reported incidence of ototoxicity was 5 days after beginning therapy.[182]

When a patient is referred for evaluation of possible ototoxicity, the audiologist-otolaryngologist team should identify possible ototoxicity and make appropriate recommendations based on clinical findings and test results. In many cases, there are no alternatives to the ototoxic medication. It may be appropriate for the physician prescribing the ototoxic medication to renew the discussion of informed consent if the medication is to be continued.

◆ Miscellaneous Causes of Sensorineural Hearing Loss

Hypoxemia

Many experimental studies have documented inner ear pathology following vascular occlusion. Kimura and Perlman[127] found rapid, progressive loss of hair cells after arterial occlusion of the labyrinthine artery. First inner hair cells, then outer, supporting, and strial cells degenerated. Eventually, the labyrinth ossified. Inner hair cells appear to be more sensitive than outer hair cells to mild hypoxia over an extended period time.[261] Venous occlusion also produced strial damage, hair cell loss, and hemorrhagic lesions.[128,262] Anoxia appears to potentiate noise-induced hearing loss.[263,264]

Many medical conditions can predispose to vascular occlusion, in which isolated hearing loss has been reported, including leukemia,[265–267] Buerger's disease,[268] macroglobulinemia,[268] fat embolism,[269] cardiac bypass,[270–273] sickle cell disease,[274,275] cryoglobulinemia,[276,277] nonotologic surgery,[155] Hand-Schüller-Christian disease,[278] and vasculitis.[279] Hypoxemia without vascular occlusion has been associated with a high risk of sensorineural hearing loss in infants.[280]

Hildesheimer et al[281] developed an animal model to study cochlear hypoxia. The vessels emerging from one side of the basilar artery were supplied exclusively by the homolateral vertebral artery. Because blood flow was laminar, mixing between the two sides did not normally occur. Changes in the cochlear action potentials on one side were induced by ipsilateral axillary artery retrograde perfusion of poorly oxygenated blood. Interestingly, Kitamura and Berreby[282] reported similar unilateral pathology in the inner ear of a patient who experienced occlusion of the ipsilateral vertebral artery 17 days before death.

Diabetes Mellitus

Whether diabetes mellitus results in hearing loss through vascular impairment, metabolic pathways, both, or not at all is a continuing and unresolved controversy. Hearing loss has been reported in diabetes mellitus,[283–290] though in some reports there was also significant generalized vascular disease.[291] Others have suggested that hearing loss may result from diabetic neuropathy.[292] Still, not all studies have correlated diabetes with hearing loss.[157,293–300] Although duration of diabetes has not been correlated with the degree of hearing loss,[284,285] severity of diabetes has.[284,289] Cullen and Cinnamond[285] found no correlation between insulin dosage and family history of diabetes and hearing thresholds.

Diabetic neuropathy has been suggested as the mechanism of sensorineural hearing loss.[292] In a retrospective study Duck et al[298] suggested that hypertensive end-organ disease of the cochlea may be amplified by coexisting diabetes, with increased hearing loss in the 4- to 8-kHz range.

Wackym and Linthicum[300] examined temporal bones of eight diabetics who had significantly more hearing loss than age- and sex-matched controls. Microangiopathy was found in the endolymphatic sac, stria vascularis, and basilar membrane in patients with diabetes. Sensorineural hearing loss was strongly correlated with involvement of endolymphatic sac and basilar membrane vessels. Earlier histologic studies showed vascular changes consistent with atherosclerosis in the stria vascularis and basement membrane, but no degeneration of the organ of Corti.[291,297]

Infection

Viral Infection

Viruses are believed to cause directly or indirectly many hearing disorders. Their presumed role in SHL has been discussed previously. Most evidence is inferential. Serum viral titers can establish the presence of viral infection but cannot prove viral infection was the direct cause of hearing loss. Cytomegalovirus (CMV), mumps, and rubeola have been identified in inner ears of patients suffering from SHL.[138] CMV[301–303] and mumps[304,305] have been cultured from inner ear fluids. Rubeola inclusion bodies have been identified in the inner ear.[306]

Rubella has been closely related epidemiologically with hearing loss.[131,307] Other viruses implicated in sensorineural hearing loss include herpes simplex, varicella zoster, Epstein-Barr virus, hepatitis virus, variola, adenovirus, influenza and parainfluenza, polio virus, encephalitis viruses, and infectious mononucleosis.[301,308] Severe sensorineural hearing loss with encephalitis following live measles virus vaccination has been reported.[309] There have been nine reports of sensorineural hearing loss after measles, mumps, and rubella (MMR) immunization.[310] Careful review revealed that in three cases the deafness was unrelated to MMR immunization and in six cases the cause was unknown and MMR remained a possible etiology.[310] Hall and Richards[311] considered the possibility of mumps in 33 children with profound acquired unilateral sensorineural hearing loss. Fifteen gave a history of mumps, 12 of whom contracted the infection between the last normal and first abnormal hearing tests.

CMV infection is currently reported as the most common cause of congenital viral-induced deafness.[312] Nonetheless, neonatal auditory screening based on the presence of risk criteria fails to identify the majority of cases of hearing loss caused by CMV infection.[313] A prospective study in which 1644 children were tested during a 9-year period has shown that the prevalence of CMV in the urine of children with sensorineural hearing loss but no immediate family history of deafness was nearly twice that (13%) found in other children with impaired hearing and those with normal hearing (7%).[314] A recent association has been shown between patients with congenital CMV infection who have CMV viremia detected by polymerase chain reaction (PCR) in early infancy and increased likelihood for hearing loss.[315] Ganciclovir treatment may improve outcome in symptomatic cases.[316]

Temporal bone pathology in viral-induced hearing loss generally consists of strial atrophy with hair cell loss. Labyrinthitis and auditory nerve inflammation also have been reported.[301,305,308,317,318] A large review of 52 pairs of infant and children temporal bones demonstrated no evidence of CMV endolabyrinthitis, even in a single case with extensive congenital CMV infection.[312] Reye's syndrome has also been reported to cause diffuse central nervous system pathology along with severe inner ear degeneration.[319,320]

Human Immunodeficiency Virus

Human immunodeficiency virus (HIV), the causative agent of acquired immunodeficiency disorder (AIDS), is associated with many otologic findings.[321,322] Hausler et al[322] reported that 57% of AIDS patients and 45% of non-AIDS HIV-infected individuals had abnormal results in various audiologic, vestibular, and electrophysiologic tests, with a seronegative control group registering only 12% abnormalities. Chandrasekhar et al[321] reported that up to 33% of HIV-infected individuals in various stages of the disease have ear disease. Aural fullness was present in 34%, dizziness in 32%, hearing loss in 29%, tinnitus in 26%, otalgia in 23%, and otorrhea in 5%. Hearing loss is reported in 21 to 49% of infected individuals, and has a varying degree of incidence, magnitude, and range of loss.[323–325]

Hearing loss has been attributed to direct infection by the HIV virus, opportunistic infection (bacterial, viral, parasitic, and fungal), central nervous system disease, malignancies (e.g., lymphoma and Kaposi's sarcoma), and ototoxic therapy.[323,326] Reactivation of varicella, CMV, and latent syphilis, along with cryptococcus, are more common infections that can affect the eighth cranial nerve.[323] Audiologic evaluation of individuals separated according to Centers for Disease Control and Prevention (CDC) guidelines of HIV progression, showed a worsening of hearing at all ranges tested in later stages of the disease with a significant correlation at 500, 2000, and 8000 Hz.[321] Soucek and Michaels reported hearing impairment >20 dB in 69% of HIV subjects. Almost all impaired patients displayed diminished otoacoustic emissions, suggesting impairment of outer hair cell function. Delayed and desynchronized latencies between intervals I-V of brainstem auditory-evoked responses have been reported in HIV patients as well, suggesting central dysfunction.[322,326–328] Furthermore, these central changes usually occur early in the progression of the disease, often during HIV's subclinical phase.[329–332]

Temporal bone pathology studies have shown multiple abnormalities in patients with HIV. Chandrasekhar et al[333] originally described many abnormalities with light and electron microscopy, including severe petrositis with marrow replacement, mastoiditis, ossicular destruction, precipitations in the perilymphatic and endolymphatic spaces of the vestibule and of the semicircular canals, and subepithelial elevation of the sensory epithelium of the saccule and utricle. Further studies have shown large aggregations of HIV-like particles around the tectorial membrane and in endolymphatic structures, suggesting these extracellular areas may be able to support HIV or opportunistic infection.[332] Ultrastructural investigation also has shown shortened and fused cilia of the hair cells. Pathologic changes consistent with viral infection occurred within hair cells and in connective/support cells of the cochlea.[334] Similar HIV-like particles, inclusion bodies, and other viral ultrastructural changes were observed in vestibular structures such as the labyrinthine wall, supporting cells, maculae, and cristae.[335] The inner ear has been shown to have changes suggestive of CMV infection, Kaposi's sarcoma in the eighth cranial nerve, and fungal infection by disseminated Cryptococcus.[336]

Otitis media, usually with effusion, chronic otitis media, acute otitis media, otitis externa, and progression of latent otosyphilis have been described at higher frequencies in HIV patients.[324,337–339] Histologic studies have also shown otitis media, which may have been a preterminal event in some cases.[338]

Ototoxicity due to antiretroviral therapy, including azidothymidine (AZT), dideoxyinosine (DDI), and dideoxycytidine (DDC), has been described. Hearing loss and tinnitus due to these agents can present with sudden or gradual onset.[323,340] Auditory dysfunction from these drugs may be caused by a reduction in mitochondrial DNA.[341-343] It has been suggested that drug effects may compound synergistically with age-related and, possibly, HIV-related mitochondrial DNA reduction to cause hearing loss.[340,344-346]

Otitic Syphilis

Syphilitic inner ear disease results from vasculitis and obliterative endarteritis.[347] Pathology of syphilitic labyrinthitis consists of diffuse osteitis, severe hydrops, and degeneration of the membranous labyrinth.[348] Electrocochleographic features of hydropic syphilitic lesions resemble those in Meniere's disease.[349]

The diagnosis of otitic syphilis may be straightforward when the patient presents with primary or secondary disease and acute ear symptoms; however, the majority of patients present with late disease, delayed otologic symptoms, and otherwise normal physical examinations.[350-352] Despite a sensitivity of 100% and a specificity of 98%, the predictive value of a positive FTA-abs (or microhemagglutination–*Treponema pallidum* [MHA-TP]) still is only 22% in an otologic population because the prevalence of disease is so low.[353] The FTA-abs assay does not distinguish between active and treated disease. A Western blot assay can eliminate the possibility of a false-positive result and can confirm whether the infection is active.[354] This assay can be used to refute the diagnosis by demonstrating that the FTA-abs result was falsely positive for syphilis or that the infection is inactive.[354] Because the predictive value of a positive test is so low and the sensitivity of the FTA-abs is twice as great as the sensitivity of the rapid plasma reagent (RPR),[353] the authors advise that the RPR assay is an inadequate screening test for suspect patients in otology.

Treatment of otologic syphilis combines penicillin and steroids.[352,355,356] Because most patients have latent disease in which the spirochete replicates more slowly (up to 90 days), prolonged penicillin treatment is necessary. The authors recommend benzathine penicillin, 2.4 million units intramuscularly for each of 3 consecutive weeks, followed by a similar dose every other week for a total of 3 months of treatment. Tetracycline or erythromycin, 500 mg by mouth four times daily for 3 months, is given to penicillin-allergic patients. Prednisone, 20 mg four times daily for at least 10 days, is given to reduce presumed vasculitis. Maintenance prednisone (10 mg every other day) is continued if hearing does not stabilize. In 75% of patients, improvement in pure-tone sensitivity or speech discrimination score can be obtained.[357] Otosyphilis can and does present at any stage of HIV infection and should be considered in seropositive patients presenting with otologic complaints.[358]

Bacterial Infection

The relationship between bacterial otitis media and sensorineural hearing loss[359-361] has been discussed in Chapter 17. Berlow and coworkers[362] prospectively studied 47 patients with bacterial meningitis to evaluate the onset and the degree of sensorineural hearing loss and to describe the audiometric pattern. The prevalence of sensorineural hearing loss in this population was 11%. Late-onset hearing loss was not

observed; however, one patient developed progressive hearing loss. Both bilateral and unilateral hearing loss were noted. The degree of hearing loss varied from mild to profound, with no consistent audiometric pattern. Statistical analysis revealed that patients in the hearing-impaired group and normal hearing group did not differ significantly in the types of therapy they received.

Fungal Infection

Although fungal involvement of the inner ear is not common, one case of temporal bone mucormycosis has been reported.[363]

Renal Disease

Sensorineural hearing loss is frequently found in patients with renal failure,[364] but the underlying mechanisms remain controversial. Many forms of congenital renal failure (e.g., Alport's syndrome[365,366]) combine hearing loss with renal failure.[367] Many drugs also produce both ototoxicity and renal toxicity. This is related in part to the demonstrated shared antigenicity between the kidney and labyrinth.[368] Ikeda et al[369] developed an animal model to investigate the relationship between renal failure and hearing loss and demonstrated significant decreases in the cochlear microphonic and cochlear nerve action potentials in the uremic state. No pathologic alterations were visible in the cochlea by light microscopy, suggesting that the etiology of the hearing loss was due mainly to metabolic disturbances such as uremic toxins, electrolyte imbalance, or endocrine abnormalities. These conclusions are corroborated by the experience of Antonelli et al[370] and Kustel et al,[371] who have found consistent and significant lengthening of the interpeak latencies in the auditory brainstem response in uremic patients. In one study high-frequency thresholds were significantly higher in patients with chronic renal disease.[372]

Hearing loss in patients undergoing dialysis and renal transplantation[373,374] may be caused by electrolyte imbalance, accumulated toxic factors, or osmotic shifts during dialysis.[375] Significant fluctuation in low-frequency thresholds immediately following dialysis is commonly observed.[375] An association between child and adolescent chronic renal disease with hemodialysis and high-frequency hearing loss also exists.[376,377] Hearing loss is not proportional to the blood urea nitrogen (BUN) or creatinine levels or to the number of dialyses,[373] and appears not to become manifest after a single episode of hemodialysis.[378] Even when such factors as ototoxicity are eliminated, the true prevalence of hearing loss related to renal failure is difficult to identify precisely. Both collapse of the endolymphatic space and deposits in the stria and vestibular apparatus have been observed histologically in patients with renal failure.[379]

Hypothyroidism

Hypothyroidism has been associated with hearing loss,[380] which although generally reported as a high-frequency sensorineural loss,[381] may also be conductive.[382] Anand et al[382] studied 20 patients with hypothyroidism who were then treated to the euthyroid state. Eighty percent demonstrated hearing loss when compared with randomly selected age- and sex-matched controls. Twelve had sensorineural hearing loss, whereas four had mixed hearing loss. Auditory brainstem responses showed prolonged absolute wave V latency, prolonged interpeak latencies, and decreased wave amplitudes. Following treatment with levothyroxine, a significant reversibility of sensorineural and conductive hearing loss was observed, although brainstem responses did not change. These results suggest a site of lesion at many levels in the auditory system from the middle ear to retrocochlear sites. Di Lorenzo et al[383] described similar changes in auditory brainstem potentials with hypothyroidism that was correctable with levothyroxine. A study with rats subjected to thyroidectomies suggests that a potential treatment window exists with complete recovery of auditory dysfunction before 5 months and incomplete recovery after 7 months.[384] Pathologic changes in hypothyroidism include sensory cell loss and thickening of the basilar membrane.[385]

Perilymph Fistula

Probably the only universally acceptable statement about perilymphatic fistula is that it is controversial.[386–388] Attempts have been made to relate a history of hearing loss to histologic evidence of patency of the fissula ante fenestram and microfissures of the temporal bone, with conflicting results.[389,390] Otic capsule anomalies on CT[391] positive fistula test,[386] increased summating potential-to-action potential ratio on electrocochleography,[392] clinical history,[386] and progressive or fluctuating sensorineural hearing loss[391] suggest perilymph fistula. Most clinicians have tended to rely more on a clinical history of recent head trauma or exacerbation of symptoms with lifting or straining than on tests.[386,387,393] A key impediment to progress has been the lack of a gold standard for the diagnosis. β_2-transferrin may be a sensitive and specific chemical marker of perilymph, CSF, and aqueous humor that can be detected in very small samples.[394–396] To date, no studies with more than a handful of patients have been presented. No study satisfies all critics on what the proper clinical signs and findings should be, what the natural history of the untreated disorder is, or what treatment response should be anticipated (see Chapter 19). Many cases attributed to perilymphatic fistulas may have been due to the superior semicircular canal dehiscence syndrome.[397,398]

◆ Other Causes

Other causes of hearing loss include head trauma,[399] multiple sclerosis,[400–402] hypercholesterolemia,[403] sarcoidosis,[404,405] and mucopolysaccharidosis.[406,407]

◆ Acknowledgments

Our thanks to Karen Mielke and Wendy Lynn, who helped with manuscript preparation.

References

1. Schuknecht H. Pathology of the Ear, 2nd ed. Philadelphia: Lea & Febiger, 1993
2. Andreasen E. Studies on endolymphatic system in normal rats at different ages, under normal conditions and during inanition and restitution after starving. Acta Pathol Microbiol Scand Suppl 1943;49:1
3. Ishii T, Murakami Y, Kimura RS, Balogh K Jr. Electron microscopic and histochemical identification of lipofuscin in the human inner ear. Acta Otolaryngol 1967;64:17–29
4. Rosen S, Burgman M, Plaster D, et al. Presbycusis study of a relatively noise free population in the Sudan. Ann Otol Rhinol Laryngol 1962;71:727–743
5. Rosenhall U, Sixt E, Sundh V, Svanborg A. Correlations between presbyacusis and extrinsic noxious factors. Audiology 1993;32:234–243
6. Gates G, Cobb J, D'Agostino R, Wolf P. The relation of hearing in the elderly to the presence of cardiovascular disease and cardiovascular risk factors. Arch Otolaryngol Head Neck Surg 1993;119:156–161
7. Pearlman R. Presbycusis: the need for a clinical definition. Am J Otol 1982;3:183–186
8. Gaeth J. A study of phonemic regression associated with hearing loss. Northwestern University, 1948
9. Rowland M. Basic data on hearing levels of adults 25 to 74 years: United States 1971–1975. Vital Health Stat 11 1980;(215):I–vi, 1–49
10. Beasely W. Characteristics and distribution of impaired hearing in the population of the United States. J Acoust Soc Am 1940;12:114–121
11. Glorig A, Wheeler D, et al. 1954 Wisconsin State Fair Hearing Survey, Amer Acad of Opthalmol and Otolaryngol 1957
12. Glorig A, Roberts J. Hearing levels of adults by age and sex: United States 1960–1962. Vital Health Statistics 1965
13. Jerger J, Chmiel R, Stach B, Spretnjak M. Gender affects audiometric shape in presbyacusis. J Am Acad Audiol 1933;4:42–49
14. Gates G, Cooper JJ, Kannel W, Miller N. Hearing in the elderly: the Framingham cohort, 1983–1985. Part I. Basic audiometric test results. Ear Hear 1990;11:247–256
15. Zunehmendern A. Ein nues gestez. Arch Ohr Waskehlkheilk 1899;32:53
16. Schuknecht H. Auditory and cytocochlear correlates of inner ear disorders. Otolaryngol Head Neck Surg 1994;110:530–538
17. Crowe S, Guild S, Polvogt LM. Observations on pathology of high tone deafness. Bull Johns Hopkins Hosp 1934;54:315–379
18. Saxen A. Pathologie und klinik der aterschinerhorigkeit nacht unter suchungen von fund aiero Saxen. Acta Otolaryngol Suppl (Stockh) 1937;23
19. Suzuka Y, Schuknecht HF. Retrograde cochlear neuronal degeneration in human subjects. Acta Otolaryngol Suppl 1988;450:1–20
20. Bredberg G. Cellular pattern and nerve supply of the human organ of Corti. Acta Otolaryngol 1968;236(suppl):1–135
21. Pauler M, Schuknecht H, Thornton A. Correlative studies of cochlear neuronal loss with speech discrimination and pure-tone thresholds. Arch Otorhinolaryngol 1986;243:200–206
22. Schuknecht H. Further observations on the pathology of presbycusis. Arch Otolaryngol 1964;80:369–382
23. Schuknecht H, Watanuki K, Takahashi T, et al. Atrophy of the stria vascularis, a common cause for hearing loss. Laryngoscope 1974;84:1777–1821
24. Pauler M, Schuknecht H, White J. Atrophy of the stria vascularis as a cause of sensorineural hearing loss. Laryngoscope 1988;98:754–759
25. Nadol JB Jr. Electron microscopic findings in presbycusic degeneration of the basal turn of the human cochlea. Otolaryngol Head Neck Surg 1979;87:818–836
26. Matschke R. Frequency selectivity and psychoacoustic tuning curves in old age. Acta Otolaryngol Suppl 1990;476:114–119
27. Bonding P. Frequency selectivity and speech discrimination in sensorineural hearing loss. Scand Audiol 1979;8:205–215
28. Welsh L, Welsh J, Healy M. Central presbycusis. Laryngoscope 1985;95:128–136
29. Gatehouse S. The contribution of central auditory factors to auditory disability. Acta Otolaryngol Suppl 1990;476:182–188
30. van Rooij JC, Plomp R. Auditive and cognitive factors in speech perception by elderly listeners. Acta Otolaryngol Suppl 1990;476:177–181
31. Rizzo SR Jr, Gutnick HN. Cochlear versus retrocochlear presbyacusis: clinical correlates. Ear Hear 1991;12:61–63
32. Fire K, Lesner S, Newman C. Hearing handicap as a function of central auditory abilities in the elderly. Am J Otol 1991;12:105–108
33. Caspary D, Raza A, Lawhorn Armour B, Pippin J, Arneric S. Immunocytochemical and neurochemical evidence for age-related loss of GABA in the inferior colliculus: implications for neural presbycusis. J Neurosci 1990;10:2363–2372
34. Aitkin L. The cytoarchitecture of the mammalian auditory midbrain. In: Aitkin L, ed. The Auditory Midbrain: Structure and Function in the Central Auditory Pathway. Clifton, NJ: Humana, 1986:31–46
35. Carney L, Yin T. Responses of low-frequency cells in the inferior colliculus to interaural time differences of clicks. J Neurophysiol 1989; 62:144–161
36. Kelly-Ballweber D, Dobie R. Binaural interaction measured behaviorally and electrophysiologically in young and old adults. Audiology 1984;23:181–194

37. Nixon JC, Glorig A, High WS. Changes in air and bone conduction thresholds as a function of age. J Laryngol Otol 1962;76:288–298

38. Belal A, Stewart T. Pathological changes in the middle ear joints. Ann Otol Rhinol Laryngol 1974;83:159–167

39. Herbst K, Humphrey C. Hearing impairment and mental state in the elderly living at home. BMJ 1956;281:903–905

40. Uhlmann R, Larson E, Rees T, Koepsell T, Duckert L. Relationship of hearing impairment to dementia and cognitive dysfunction in older adults. JAMA 1989;261:1916–1919

41. Thomas P, Hunt W, Garry P, et al. Hearing acuity in a healthy elderly population: effects on emotional, cognitive, and social status. J Gerontol 1983;38:321–325

42. Lutman M. Hearing disability in the elderly. Acta Otolaryngol Suppl 1990;476:239–248

43. Harner SG, Rose DE, Facer GW. Paget's disease and hearing loss. Otolaryngology 1978;86(6 pt 1):ORL 869–874

44. Monsell E, Cody D, Bone H, et al. Hearing loss in Paget's disease of bone: the relationship. Hear Res 1995;83:114–120

45. Baraka M. Rate of progression of hearing loss in Paget's disease. J Laryngol Otol 1984;98:573–575

46. Khetarpal U, Schuknecht H. In search of pathologic correlates for hearing loss and vertigo in Paget's disease. A clinical and histopathologic study of 26 temporal bones. Ann Otol Rhinol Laryngol Suppl 1990;145:1–16

47. El Sammaa M, Linthicum FJ, House H, House J. Calcitonin as treatment for hearing loss in Paget's disease. Am J Otol 1986;7:241–243

48. Dobie R. Medical-Legal Evaluation of Hearing Loss. New York: Van Nostrand Reinhold, 1993

49. U.S. Department of Labor, Occupational Safety and Health Administration. Occupational Noise Exposure: Hearing Conservation Amendment Final Rule. Report No. 48. Washington, DC: OSHA, 1983

50. National Institutes of Health. Noise and Hearing Loss. Report No. 8(1). Washington, DC: NIH, 1990

51. International Organization for Standardization. Standard 1999.2. Geneva:150:1989

52. Meister F. Der einfluss ein winkdauer bei der beschallung des ohers. Larmbekamfung 1973;10:89–91

53. Peyser A. Geshundheitswesen und krankenfursorge. Chthretishe und experimenulle grundlagen des person lichen schallscutzes. Dtsch Med Wochenschr 1930;56:150–157

54. Ward E, Cushiing E, Burns E. Effective quiet and moderate TTS: implications for noise exposure standards. J Acoust Soc Am 1976;59:160–165

55. American College of Occupational Medicine and Noise and Hearing Conservation Committee. Occupational noise-induced hearing loss. J Occup Med 1989;31:996

56. International Organization for Standardization. Acoustics-Determination of Occupational Noise Exposure and Estimation of Noise-Induced Hearing Impairment, 1999

57. Pierson L, Gerhardt K, Rodriguez G, Yanke R. Relationship between outer ear resonance and permanent noise-induced hearing loss. Am J Otolaryngol 1994;15:37–40

58. Borg E, Nilsson R. Acoustic reflex in industrial noise. In: Silman S, ed. The Acoustic Reflex: Basic Principles and Clinical Applications. Orlando, FL: Academic Press, 1984:413–440

59. Schuknecht H, Tonndorf J. Acoustic trauma of the cochlea from surgery. Laryngoscope 1960;70:479–505

60. Sataloff J. The otologist in industry. Ear Nose Throat J 1980;59:238–242

61. Ward W. General auditory effects of noise. Otolaryngol Clin North Am 1979;12:473–492

62. Gunther T, Ising H, Joachims Z. Biochemical mechanisms affecting susceptibility to noise-induced hearing loss. Am J Otol 1989;10:36–41

63. Joachims Z, Netzer A, Ising H, et al. Oral magnesium supplementation as prophylaxis for noise-induced hearing loss: results of a double blind field study. Schriftenr Ver Wasser Boden Lufthyg 1993;88:503–516

64. Farber JL, Chien KR, Mittnacht S Jr. Myocardial ischemia: the pathogenesis of irreversible cell injury in ischemia. Am J Pathol 1981;102:271–281

65. Joachims Z, Ising H, Gunther T. Noise-induced hearing loss in humans as a function of serum Mg concentration. Magnesium Bull 1987;9:130–131

66. Attias J, Wiesz G, Almog S, et al. Oral magnesium intake reduces permanent hearing loss induced by noise exposure. Am J Otolaryngol 1994;15:26–32

67. Corwin J, Cotanche D. Regeneration of sensory hair cells after acoustic trauma. Science 1988;240:1772–1774

68. Ryals B, Rubel E. Hair cell regeneration after acoustic trauma in adult Coturnix qual. Science 1988;240:1774–1776

69. Cotanche D. Regeneration of the tectorial membrane in the chick cochlea following severe acoustic trauma. Hear Res 1987;30:197–206

70. Cotanche D. Regeneration of hair cell stereociliary bundles in the chick cochlea following severe acoustic trauma. Hear Res 1987;30:181–195

71. Cotanche D, Dopyera CE. Hair cell and supporting cell response to acoustic trauma in the chick cochlear. Hear Res 1990;46:29–40

72. Adler H, Kenealy J, Dedio R, Saunders J. Threshold shift, hair cell loss, and hair bundle stiffness following exposure to 120 and 125 dB pure tones in the neonatal chick. Otolaryngol 1992;112:444–454

73. Saunders J, Adler H, Publiano F. The structural and functional aspects of hair cell regeneration in the chick as a result of exposure to intense sound. Exp Neurol 1992;115:13–17

74. Cotanche D, Lee K, Stone J, Picard D. Hair cell regeneration in the bird cochlea following noise damage or ototoxic drug damage. Anat Embryol (Berl) 1994;189:1–18

75. Warchol M, Lambert P, Goldstein B, Forge A, Corwin J. Regenerative proliferation in inner ear sensory epithelia from adult guinea pigs and humans. Science 1993;259:1619–1622

76. Lindgren F, Axelsson A. The influence of physical exercise on susceptibility to noise-induced temporary threshold shift. Scand Audiol 1988;17:11–17

77. Bancroft B, Boettcher F, Salvi R, Wu J. Effects of noise and salicylate on auditory evoked-response thresholds in the chinchilla. Hear Res 1991;54:20–28

78. Byrne C. Synergistic interactions of noise and other ototraumatic agents. Ear Hear 1987;8:192–212

79. Sun A, Wang Z, Xiao S, et al. Noise-induced hearing loss in iron-deficient rats. Acta Otolaryngol 1991;111:684–690

80. Barrenas M, Lindgren F. The influence of inner ear melanin on susceptibility to TTS in humans. Scand Audiol 1990;19:97–102

81. Canlon B, Borg E, Flock A. Protection against noise trauma by preexposure to a low level acoustic stimulus. Hear Res 1988;34:197–200

82. Canlon B, Borg E, Flock A. Protection against noise trauma by preexposure to a low level acoustic stimulus. Hear Res 1988;34:197–200

83. Ryan AF, Bennett TM, Woolf NK, Axelsson A. Protection from noise-induced hearing loss by prior exposure to a nontraumatic stimulus: role of the middle ear muscles. Hear Res 1994;72:23–28

84. Henderson D, Subramaniam M, Papazian M, Spongr V. The role of middle ear muscles in the development of resistance to noise induced hearing loss. Hear Res 1994;74:22–28

85. Macrae J. Prediction of deterioration in hearing due to hearing aid use. J Speech Hear Res 1991;34:661–670

86. Hunter-Duvar I. Morphology of the Normal Acoustically Damaged Cochlea. Chicago: Seminar of the International Telephone and Telegraph Research Institute;1977:421–428

87. Gao W, Ding D, Zheng X, Ruan F, Liu Y. A comparison of changes in the stereocilia between temporary and permanent hearing losses in acoustic trauma. Hear Res 1992;62:27–41

88. Lim D, Melnick W. A scanning and transmission electron microscopic observation. Arch Otolaryngol 1971;94:294–305

89. Lim D, Dunn D. Anatomic correlates of noise induced hearing loss. Otolaryngol Clin North Am 1979;12:493–513

90. Liberman M, Kiang N. Acoustic trauma in cats. Cochlear pathology and auditory-nerve activity. Acta Otolaryngol Suppl 1978;358:1–63

91. Vosteen K. Die erschoepfung der phonoreceptoren nach funtioneller vels duug. Arch Nas-Kehlk Heilk 1958;172:489

92. Quirk W, Seidman M. Cochlear vascular changes in response to loud noise. Am J Otol 1995;16:322–325

93. Von Gierke H. The effects of sonic boom on people: review and outlook. J Acoust Soc Am 1966;39(suppl):S43–S50

94. Singleton G. Cordless telephones. A threat to hearing. Ann Otol Rhinol Laryngol 1984;93:565–568

95. Orchik DJ, Schumaier DR, Shea J, Moretz WH Jr. Intensity and frequency of sound levels from cordless telephones. A pediatric alert. Clin Pediatr (Phila) 1985;24:688–690

96. Gerling I, Jerger J. Cordless telephones and acoustic trauma: a case study. Ear Hear 1985;6:203–205

97. Catlin FI, Doerfler LG, Linthicum FJ, et al. Guide for conservation of hearing and noise. Trans Am Acad Ophthalmol Otolaryngol Suppl 1973.

98. Berger E. The performance of hearing protectors in industrial noise environments. Sound Vibrat 1980;May:14–17

99. Dancer A, Grateau P, Cabanis A, et al. Effectiveness of earplugs in high-intensity impulse noise. J Acoust Soc Am 1992;91:1677–1689

100. Dobie R. Time for action in hearing conservation. Otolaryngol Head Neck Surg 1983;91:347–349

101. Alberti P, Blair R. Occupational hearing loss: an Ontario perspective. Laryngoscope 1982;92:535–539

102. Dobie R, Archer R. Results of otologic referrals in an industrial hearing conservation program. Otolaryngol Head Neck Surg 1981;89:294–301

103. Dobie R. Otologic referral criteria. Otolaryngol Head Neck Surg 1982;90:598–601

104. Fox M. Workmen's compensation hearing loss claims. Laryngoscope 1980;90:1077–1081

105. Dobie RA. Industrial audiometry and the otologist. Laryngoscope 1985;95:382–385

106. The otologic referral criteria for occupational hearing conservation programs. Medical Aspects of Noise Committee. American Council of Otolaryngology. Otolaryngol Clin North Am 1979;12:635–636

107. Catlin F, American Academy of Otolaryngology Committee on Hearing and Equilibrium. Guide for the evaluation of hearing handicap. Otolaryngol Clin North Am 1979;12:655–663

108. Fox M, Bunn JJ. Worker's compensation aspects of noise induced hearing loss. Otolaryngol Clin North Am 1979;12:705–724

109. Fox M. Hearing loss statutes in the United States and Canada. Natl Saf News 1972;105:55–56

110. Department of Defense. Instruction Bulletin 6055. Washington, DC: DOD, 1978

111. Osguthorpe J, Klein J. Hearing Compensation Evaluation, 1st ed. Alexandria, VA: American Academy of Otolaryngology–Head and Neck Surgery Foundation, 1989

112. Yassi A, Pollock N, Tran N, Cheang M. Risks to hearing from a rock concert. Can Fam Physician 1993;39:1045–1050

113. Drake-Lee A. Beyond music: auditory temporary threshold shift in rock musicians after a heavy metal concern. J R Soc Med 1992;85:617–619

114. Turunen-Rise I, Flottorp G, Tvete O. A study of the possibility of acquiring noise-induced hearing loss by the use of personal cassette players (Walkman). Scand Audiol Suppl 1991;34:133–144

115. Lee P, Senders C, Gantz B, Otto S. Transient sensorineural hearing loss after overuse of portable headphone cassette radios. Otolaryngol Head Neck Surg 1985;93:622–625

116. Wilson W, Byl F, Laird N. The efficacy of steroids in the treatment of idiopathic sudden hearing loss. A double-blind clinical study. Arch Otolaryngol 1980;106:772–776

117. Whitaker S. Idiopathic sudden hearing loss. Am J Otol 1980;1:180–183

118. Terayama Y, Ishibe Y, Matsushima J. Rapidly progressive sensorineural hearing loss (rapid deafness). Acta Otolaryngol Suppl 1988;456:43–48

119. Jaffe B. Clinical studies in sudden deafness. Adv Otorhinolaryngol 1973;20:221–228

120. Van Dishoeck H, Beirmna T. Sudden perceptive deafness and viral infection. Ann Otol Rhinol Laryngol 1957;66:163–180

121. Byl F. Seventy-six cases of presumed sudden hearing loss occurring in 1973: prognosis and incidence. Laryngoscope 1977;87:817–825

122. Danino J, et al. Idiopathic sudden deafness. Ear Nose Throat J 1982;61:54–60

123. Mattox D, Simmons F. Natural history of sudden sensorineural hearing loss. Ann Otol Rhinol Laryngol 1977;86:463–480

124. Megighian D, Bolzan M, Barion U, Nicolai P. Epidemiological considerations in sudden hearing loss: a study of 183 cases. Arch Otorhinolaryngol 1986;243:250–253

125. Schuknecht H, Kimura R, Naufal P. The pathology of sudden deafness. Acta Otolaryngol 1973;76:75–97

126. Beal D, Hemenway W, Lindsay J. Inner ear pathology of sudden deafness. Histopathology of acquired deafness in the adult coincident with viral infection. Arch Otolaryngol 1967;85:591–598

127. Kimura R, Perlman HB. Arterial obstruction of the labyrinth. I. Cochlear changes. Ann Otol Rhinol Laryngol 1958;67:5–24

128. Kimura R, Perlman HB. Extensive venous obstruction of the labyrinth. A. Cochlear changes. Ann Otol Rhinol Laryngol 1956;65:332–350

129. Lindsay JR, Davey PR, Ward PH. Inner ear pathology and deafness due to mumps. Ann Otol Rhinol Laryngol 1960;69:918–935

130. Lindsay JR, Hemenway WG. Inner ear pathology due to measles. Ann Otol Rhinol Laryngol 1954;63:754–741

131. Lindsay JR, Carruthers DG, Hemenway WG, et al. Inner ear pathology following maternal rubella. Ann Otol Rhinol Laryngol 1953;62:1201–1218

132. Rowson K, Hinchcliffe R. A virological and epidemiological study of patients with acute hearing loss. Lancet 1975;1:471–473

133. Massab H. The role of viruses in sudden deafness. Adv Otorhinolaryngol 1973;20:229–235

134. Wilson W, Veltri R, Laird N, Sprinkle P. Viral and epidemiologic studies of idiopathic sudden hearing loss. Otolaryngol Head Neck Surg 1983;91:653–658

135. Veltri R, Wilson W, Sprinkle P, Rodman S, Kavesh D. The implication of viruses in sudden hearing loss: primary infection or reactivation of latent viruses? Otolaryngol Head Neck Surg 1981;89:137–141

136. Simmons B. Sudden sensorineural hearing loss. In: English GM, ed. Otolaryngology. Hagerstown, MD: Harper and Row, 1976

137. Hughes GB, Freedman MA, Haberkamp TJ, Guay ME. Sudden sensorineural hearing loss. Otolaryngol Clin North Am 1996;29:393–405

138. Cole R, Jahrsdoerfer R. Sudden hearing loss: an update. Am J Otol 1988;9:211–215

139. Bailey C, Graham M, Lawrence M. Recovery from prolonged sensorineural hearing loss. Am J Otol 1982;4:1–8

140. Hughes G, Barna B, Kinney S, Calabrese L, Nalepa N. Clinical diagnosis of immune inner ear disease. Laryngoscope 1988;98:251–253

141. Brookes G. Immune complex-associated deafness: preliminary communication. J R Soc Med 1985;78:47–55

142. McCabe B. Autoimmune inner ear disease: results of therapy. Adv Otorhinolaryngol 1991;46:78–81

143. Harris J. Autoimmunity of the inner ear. Am J Otol 1989;10:193–195

144. Wolfovitz E, Levy Y, Brook J. Sudden deafness in a patient with temporal arteritis. J Rheumatol 1987;14:384–385

145. Kempf H. Ear involvement in Wegener's granulomatosis. Clin Otolaryngol 1989;14:451–456

146. Cote D, Molony T, Waxman J, Parsa D. Cogan's syndrome manifesting as sudden bilateral deafness: diagnosis and management. South Med J 1993;86:1056–1060

147. Rowe-Jones J, Macallan D, Sorooshian M. Polyarteritis nodosa presenting as bilateral sudden onset cochleovestibular failure in a young woman. J Laryngol Otol 1990;104:562–564

148. Gulya A. Infections of the labyrinth. In: Bailey B, ed. Head and Neck Surgery–Otolaryngology. Philadelphia: JB Lippincott, 1993

149. Harris J, Low N, House W. Contralateral hearing loss following inner ear injury: sympathetic cochleolabyrinthitis? Am J Otol 1985;6:371–377

150. Berg H, Cohen N, Hammerschlag P, Waltzman S. Acoustic neuroma presenting as sudden hearing loss with recovery. Otolaryngol Head Neck Surg 1986;94:15–22

151. Berenholz L, Eriksen C, Hirsh F. Recovery from repeated sudden hearing loss with corticosteroid use in the presence of an acoustic neuroma. Ann Otol Rhinol Laryngol 1992;101:827–831

152. Walsted A, Salomon G, Thomsen J, Tos M. Hearing decrease after loss of cerebrospinal fluid. A new hydrops model? Acta Otolaryngol 1991;111:468–476

153. Millen S, Toohill R, Lehman R. Sudden sensorineural hearing loss: operative complications in nonotologic surgery. Laryngoscope 1982;92:613–617

154. Shaan M, Vassalli L, Landolfi M, Taibah A, Russo A, Sanna M. Atypical presentation of acoustic neuroma. Otolaryngol Head Neck Surg 1993;109:865–870

155. Ogawa K, Kanzaki J, Ogawa S, Tsuchihashi N, Inoue Y. Acoustic neuromas presenting as sudden hearing loss. Acta Otolaryngol Suppl 1991;487:138–143

156. Curtin H, Hirsh WJ. Imaging of acoustic neuromas. Otolaryngol Clin North Am 1992;25:553–607

157. Wilson W, Laird N, Moo-Young G, et al. The relationship of idiopathic sudden hearing loss to diabetes mellitus. Laryngoscope 1982;92:155–160

158. Goode R. Perilymph hypertension and the indirect measurement of cochlear pressure. Laryngoscope 1981;91:1706–1713

159. Haug O, Draper W, Haug S. Stellate ganglion blocks for idiopathic sensorineural hearing loss. Arch Otolaryngol 1976;102:5–8

160. Brownson R, Zollinger W, Madeira T, Fell D. Sudden sensorineural hearing loss following manipulation of the cervical spine. Laryngoscope 1986;96:166–170

161. Miller M. Spinal manipulation therapy. A cause of sudden hearing loss and tinnitus? Hearing Instruments 1995;11:11–13

162. Mattox D. Medical management of sudden hearing loss. Otolaryngol Head Neck Surg 1980;88:111–113

163. Norris C. A review of their clinical efficacy, mechanisms of action, toxicity, and place in therapy. Drugs 1988;36:754–772

164. Veldman J, Hanada T, Meeuwsen F. Diagnostic and therapeutic dilemmas in rapidly progressive sensorineural hearing loss and sudden deafness. A reappraisal of immune reactivity in inner ear disorders. Acta Otolaryngol 1993;113:303–306

165. Moscicki R, San Martin J, Quintero C, Rauch S, Nadol JJ, Bloch K. Serum antibody to inner ear proteins in patients with progressive hearing loss. Correlation with disease activity and response to corticosteroid treatment. JAMA 1994;272:611–616

166. Fisch U. Management of sudden deafness. Otolaryngol Head Neck Surg 1983;91:3–8

167. Moskowitz D, Lee K, Smith H. Steroid use in idiopathic sudden sensorineural hearing loss. Laryngoscope 1984;94:664–666

168. Byl FM Jr. Sudden hearing loss: eight years' experience and suggested prognostic table. Laryngoscope 1984;94:647–661

169. Shea J. Vasodilator treatment. Huntsville, AL: Strode, 1981:279–283

170. Rauch SD. Intratympanic steroids for sensorineural hearing loss. Otolaryngol Clin North Am 2004;37:1061–1074

171. Banerjee A, Parnes L. Intratympanic corticosteroids for sudden idiopathic sensorineural hearing loss. Otol Neurotol 2005;26:878–881

172. Tucci DL, Farmer JC Jr, Kitch RD, Witsell DL. Treatment of sudden sensorineural hearing loss with systemic steroids and valacyclovir. Otol Neurotol 2002;23:301–308

173. Battaglia A, Cueva R: Treatment of idiopathic sudden sensorineural hearing loss (ISSNHL) with intratympanic dexamethasone and/or prednisone taper. Otol Neurotol 2007 (in press)

174. Rauch SD, Carey JP, Gantz BJ, Hammerschlag P, Harris JP, Hughes GB, Lee DJ, Reda DJ, Telian SA, et al: Sudden hearing loss multicenter treatment trial. NIH Grant U01 DC006296

175. Hawkins J. Drug ototoxicity. In: Keidel W, Neff W, eds. Handbook of Sensory Physiology, vol 3. New York: Springer, 1976:704–748

176. Forge A, Schacht J. Aminoglycoside antibiotics. Audiol Neurootol 2000;5:3–22

177. Roland P, Rutka J. Ototoxicity. Hamilton, Ontario: BC Decker, 2004

178. Matz G. Aminoglycoside cochlear ototoxity. Otolaryngol Clin North Am 1993;26:705–712

179. Kahlmeter G, Dahlager J. Aminoglycoside toxicity and review of medical studies published between 1975 and 1982. J Antimicrob Chemother 1984;13(suppl):9–22

180. Matz G, Lerner S. Prospective studies of aminoglycoside ototoxicity in adults. In: Lerner S, Matz G, Hawkins JJ, eds. Aminoglycoside Ototoxicity. Boston: Little, Brown, 1981:327–337

181. Gatell J, Ferran F, Araujo V, et al. Univariate and multivariate analyses of risk factors predisposing to auditory toxicity in patients receiving aminoglycosides. Antimicrob Agents Chemother 1987;31:1383–1387

182. Fee WE Jr. Aminoglycoside ototoxicity in the human. Laryngoscope 1980;90(suppl 24):1–19

183. Lerner S, Matz G. Aminoglycoside ototoxicity. Am J Otolaryngol 1980;1:169–179

184. Ohtani I, Ohtsuki K, Aikawa T, et al. Mechanism of protective effect of fosfomycin against aminoglycoside ototoxicity. Auris Nasus Larynx 1984;11:119–124

185. Ohtsuki K, Ohtani I, Aikawa T, et al. The ototoxicity and the accumulation in the inner ear of the various aminoglycoside antibiotics. Ear Res Jpn 1982;13:85–87

186. Tran Ba Huy P, Bernard P, Schacht J. Kinetics of gentamicin uptake and release in the rat: comparison of inner ear tissues. J Clin Invest 1986;77:1492–1500

187. Dulon D, Aran J, Zajic G, Schacht J. Comparative uptake of gentamicin, netilmicin, and amikacin in the guinea pig cochlea and the vestibule. Antimicrob Agents Chemother 1986;30:96–100

188. Hiel H, Bennani H, Erre JP, Aurousseau C, Aran J. Kinetics of gentamicin in cochlear hair cells after chronic treatment. Acta Otolaryngol 1992;112:272–277

189. Fischel-Ghodsian N. Genetic factors in aminoglycoside ototoxicity. In: Roland P, Rutka J, eds. Ototoxicity. Hamilton: BC Decker, 2004:144–152

190. Schuknecht H. Pathology of the Ear. Cambridge: Harvard University Press, 1974

191. Huizing E, de Groot J. Human cochlear pathology in aminoglycoside ototoxicity–a review. Acta Otolaryngol 1987;436:117–125

192. Hinojosa R, Lerner S. Cochlear neural degeneration without hair cell loss in two patients with aminoglycoside ototoxicity. J Infect Dis 1987;156:449–455

193. Johnsson L, Hawkins JJ, Kingsley T, Black F, Matz G. Aminoglycoside-induced cochlear pathology in man. Acta Otolaryngol Suppl 1981; 383:1–19

194. Mendelsohn M, Katzenberg I. The effect of kanamycin on the cation content of the endolymph. Laryngoscope 1972;82:397–403

195. Iinuma T, Mizukoshi O, Daly JF. Possible effects of various ototoxic drugs upon the ATP-hydrolyzing system in the stria vascularis and spiral ligament of the guinear pig. Laryngoscope 1967;77:159–170

196. Musebeck K, Schatzle W. Experimentelle studien zur ototoxicitate des dihydrostreptomycins. Arch Ohr-Nos-u Kehlk–Heilik 1962;181:41–48

197. Keene M, Hawke M, Barber H, Farkashidy J. Histopathological findings in clinical gentamicin ototoxicity. Arch Otolaryngol 1982;108:65–70

198. Corrado A, de Morais I, Prado W. Aminoglycoside antibiotics as a tool for the study of the biological role of calcium ions. Historical overview. Acta Physiol Pharmacol Latinoam 1989;39:419–430

199. Takada A, Schacht J. Calcium antagonism and reversibility of gentamicin-induced loss of cochlear microphonics in the guinea pig. Hear Res 1982;8:179–186

200. Dulon D, Zajic G, Aran J, Schacht J. Aminoglycoside antibiotics impair calcium entry but not viability and motility in isolated cochlear outer hair cells. J Neurosci Res 1989;24:338–346

201. Nakagawa T, Kakehata S, Akaike N, et al. Effects of Ca^{2+} antagonists and aminoglycoside antibiotics on Ca^{2+} current in isolated outer hair cells of guinea pig cochlea. Brain Res 1992;580:345–347

202. Perez M, Soto E, Vega R. Streptomycin blocks the postsynaptic effects of excitatory amino acids on the vestibular system primary afferents. Brain Res 1991;563:221–226

203. Schacht J. Molecular mechanisms of drug-induced hearing loss. Hear Res 1986;22:297–304

204. Schacht J. Mechanism for aminoglycoside ototoxicity: basic science research. In: Roland P, Rutka J, eds. Ototoxicity. Hamilton, Ontario: BC Decker, 2004:93–100

205. Henley CE, Mahran L, Schacht J. Inhibition of renal ornithine decarboxylase by aminoglycoside antibiotics in vitro. Biochem Pharmacol 1988;37:1679–1682

206. Darrouzet J. Essais de protection de l'organe de Corti contre l'ototoxicité des antibiotiques. Rev Laryngol 1967;3–4:187–203

207. Crann S, Huang M, McLaren J, Schacht J. Formation of a toxic metabolite from gentamicin by a hepatic cytosolic fraction. Biochem Pharmacol 1992;43:1835–1839

208. Huang M, Schacht J. Formation of a cytotoxic metabolite from gentamicin by liver. Biochem Pharmacol 1990;40:R11–R14

209. Schacht J. Biochemical basis of aminoglycoside ototoxicity. Otolaryngol Clin North Am 1993;26:845–856

210. Pierson M, Moller AR. Prophylaxis of kanamycin-induced ototoxicity by a radioprotectant. Hear Res 1981;4:79–87

211. Bock G, Yates G, Miller J, Moorjani P. Effects of N-acetylcysteine on kanamycin ototoxicity in the guinea pig. Hear Res 1983;9:255–262

212. McGee T, Olszewski J. Streptomycin sulfate and dihydrostreptomycin. Arch Otolaryngol 1962;75:295

213. Black R, Lau W, Weinstein R, Young L, Hewitt W. Ototoxicity of amikacin. Antimicrob Agents Chemother 1976;9:956–961

214. Jackson GG, Arcieri G. Ototoxicity of gentamicin in man: a survey and controlled analysis of clinical experience in the United States. J Infect Dis 1971;124(suppl):S130–137

215. Neu H, Bendush C. Ototoxicity of tobramycin: a clinical overview. J Infect Dis 1976;134(suppl):S206–S218

216. Galloe A, Graudal N, Christensen H, Kampmann J. Aminoglycosides: single or multiple daily dosing? A meta-analysis on efficacy and safety. Eur J Clin Pharmacol 1995;48:39–43

217. Barclay M, Begg E, Hickling K. What is the evidence for once-daily aminoglycoside therapy. Clin Pharmacokinet 1994;27:32–48

218. Tulkens P. Pharmacokinetic and toxicological evaluation of a once-daily regimen versus conventional schedules of netilmicin and amikacin. J Antimicrob Chemother 1991;27(suppl C):49–61

219. Beaubien A, Ormsby E, Bayne A, et al. Evidence that amikacin ototoxicity is related to total perilymph area under the concentration-time curve regardless of concentration. Antimicrob Agents Chemother 1991;35:1070–1074

220. Cronberg S. Simplified monitoring of aminoglycosides. J Antimicrob Chemother 1994;34:819–827

221. Rybak L. Pathophysiology of furosemide ototoxicity. J Otolaryngol 1982;11:127–133

222. Arnold W, Nadol JJ, Weidauer H. Ultrastructural histopathology in a case of human ototoxicity due to loop diuretics. Acta Otolaryngol 1981;91:399–414

223. Quick C, Hoppe W. Permanent deafness associated with furosemide administration. Ann Otol Rhinol Laryngol 1975;84:94–101

224. Bosher S. Ethacrynic acid ototoxicity as a general model in cochlear pathology. Adv Otorhinolaryngol 1977;22:81–89

225. Matz G, Hinojosa R. Histopathology following use of ethacrynic acid. Surg Forum 1973;24:488–489

226. Goodman L, Gillman A. The Pharmacological Basis of Therapeutics. New York: Macmillan, 1975

227. Gallagher K, Jones J. Furosemide-induced ototoxicity. Ann Intern Med 1979;91:744–745

228. Myers E, Bernstein J. Salicylate ototoxicity. Arch Otolaryngol 1965; 82:483–493

229. Hawkins J. Iatrogenic toxic deafness in children. In: McConnell F, Ward P, eds. Symposium on Deafness in Childhood. Nashville: Vanderbilt University Press, 1967

230. Perez de Moura LF, Hayden RC Jr. Salicylate ototoxicity. A human temporal bone report. Arch Otolaryngol 1968;87:368–372

231. Bernstein J, Weiss A. Further observations on salicylate ototoxicity. J Laryngol Otol 1967;81:915–925

232. Jung T, Rhee C, Lee C, Park Y, Choi D. Ototoxicity of salicylate, nonsteroidal antiinflammatory drugs, and quinine. Otolaryngol Clin North Am 1993;26:791–810

233. Ruedi L, Furrer W, Luthy F, et al. Further observations concerning the toxic effects of streptomycin and quinine on the auditory organ of guinea pigs. Laryngoscope 1967;62:333–351

234. Thompson P, Wood RP 2nd, Bergstrom L. Erythromycin ototoxicity. J Otolaryngol 1980;9:60–62

235. Miller S. Erythromycin ototoxicity. Med J Aust 1982;2:242–243

236. Beckner R, Gantz N, Hughes J, Farricy J. Ototoxicity of erythromycin gluceptate. Am J Obstet Gynecol 1981;139:738–739

237. van Marion WF, van der Meer JW, Kalff MW, Schicht SM. Ototoxicity of erythromycin. Lancet 1978;2:214–215

238. Karmody C, Weinstein L. Reversible sensorineural hearing loss with intravenous erythromycin lactobionate. Ann Otol Rhinol Laryngol 1977;86:9–11

239. Chapman P. Rapid onset hearing loss after cisplatinum therapy: case reports and literature revieew. J Laryngol Otol 1982;96:159–162

240. Lippman A, Helson C, Helson L, Krakoff I. Clinical trials of cis-diamminedichloroplatinum (NSC-119875). Cancer Chemother Rep 1973;57:191–200

241. Kovach J, Moertel C, Schutt A, Reitemeier R, Hahn R. Phase II study of cis-diamminedichloroplatinum (NSC-119875) in advanced carcinoma of the large bowel. Cancer Chemother Rep 1973;57:357–359

242. Reddel R, Kefford R, Grant J, et al. Ototoxicity in patients receiving cisplatin: importance of dose and method of drug administration. Cancer Treat Rep 1982;66:19–23

243. Gratton M, Smyth B. Ototoxicity of platinum compounds. In: Roland P, Rutka J, eds. Ototoxicity. Hamilton, Ontario: BC Decker, 2004:60–75

244. Komune S, Asakuma S, Snow JJ. Pathophysiology of the ototoxicity of cis-diamminedichloroplatinum. Otolaryngol Head Neck Surg 1981; 89:275–282

245. Fleischman R, Stadnicki S, Ethier M, Schaeppi U. Ototoxicity of cis-dichlorodiammine platinum (II) in the guinea pig. Toxicol Appl Pharmacol 1975;33:320–332

246. Stadnicki S, Fleischman R, Schaeppi U, Merriam P. Cis-dichlorodiamminoplatinum (II) (NSC-119875): hearing loss and other toxic effects in rhesus monkeys. Cancer Chemother Rep 1975;59:467–480

247. Kohn S, Fradis M, Pratt H, et al. Cisplatin ototoxicity in guinea pigs with special reference to toxic effects in the stria vascularis. Laryngoscope 1988;98:865–871

248. Kishore B, Ibrahim S, Lambricht P, Laurent G, Maldague P, Tulkens P. Comparative assessment of poly-L-aspartic and poly-L-glutamic acids as protectants against gentamicin-induced renal lysosomal phospholipidosis, phospholipiduria and cell proliferation in rats. J Pharmacol Exp Ther 1992;262:424–432

249. Piel I, Meyer D, Perlia C, Wolfe U. Effects of cis-diamminedichloroplatinum (NSC-119875) on hearing function in man. Cancer Chemother Rep 1974;58:871–875

250. Schweitzer V, Dolan D, Abrams G, Davidson T, Snyder R. Amelioration of cisplatin-induced, ototoxicity by fosfomycin. Laryngoscope 1986; 96:948–958

251. Olson J, Turelson J, Street N. In vitro interaction of cisplatin and fosfomycin on squamous cell carcinoma cultures. Arch Otolaryngol Head Neck Surg 1994;120:1253–1257

252. Schaefer S, Wright C, Post J, Frenkel E. Cis-platinum vestibular toxicity. Cancer 1981;47:857–859

253. Morizono T, Paparella M, Juhn S. Ototoxicity of propylene glycol in experimental animals. Am J Otolaryngol 1980;1:393–399

254. Wilpizeski C, Lowry L, Zook B. Horizontal nystagmus in methylmercury poisoned squirrel monkeys. Laryngoscope 1982;92:161–168

255. Morizono T, Sikora M. The ototoxicity of topically applied povidone-iodine preparations. Arch Otolaryngol 1982;108:210–213

256. Matsumoto I, Morizono T, Paparella M. Hearing loss following potassium bromate: two case reports. Otolaryngol Head Neck Surg 1980;88:625–629

257. Odkvist L, Larsby B, Tham R, Hyden D. Vestibulo-oculomotor disturbances caused by industrial solvents. Otolaryngol Head Neck Surg 1983;91:537–539

258. Nordstrom L, Lerner S. Single daily dose therapy with aminoglycosides. J Hosp Infect 1991;18(suppl A):117–129

259. Schweitzer V, Olson N. Ototoxic effect of erythromycin therapy. Arch Otolaryngol 1984;110:258–260

260. Campbell K, Durrant J. Audiologic monitoring for ototoxicity. Otolaryngol Clin North Am 1993;26:903–914

261. Sawada S, Mori N, Mount RJ, Harrison RV. Differential vulnerability of inner and outer hair cell systems to chronic mild hypoxia and glutamate ototoxicity: insights into the cause of auditory neuropathy. J Otolaryngol 2001;30:106–114

262. Belal A Jr. Pathology of vascular sensorineural hearing impairment. Laryngoscope 1980;90:1831–1839

263. Chen GD. Effect of hypoxia on noise-induced auditory impairment. Hear Res 2002;172:186–195

264. Chen GD, Liu Y. Mechanisms of noise-induced hearing loss potentiation by hypoxia. Hear Res 2005;200:1–9

265. Frazer J. Affections of the labyrinth and eighth nerve in leukemia. Ann Otol Rhinol Laryngol 1928;37:361

266. Druss J. Aural manifestations of leukemia. Arch Otolaryngol 1945; 42:267

267. Schuknecht H, Igarashi M, Chasin W. Inner ear hemorrhage in leukemia. Laryngoscope 1965;76:662

268. Kirikae I, Nomura Y, Shitara T, et al. Sudden deafness due to Buerger's disease. Arch Otolaryngol 1962;75:502–505

269. Jaffe B. Sudden deafness—a local manifestation of systemic disorders: fat emboli, hypercoagulation and infections. Laryngoscope 1970;80:788–801

270. Shapiro M, Purn J, Raskin C. A study of the effects of cardiopulmonary bypass surgery on auditory function. Laryngoscope 1981;91: 2046–2052

271. Plasse H, Mittleman M, Frost J. Unilateral sudden hearing loss after open heart surgery: a detailed study of seven cases. Laryngoscope 1981;91:101–109

272. Young I, Mehta G, Lowry L. Unilateral sudden hearing loss with complete recovery following cardiopulmonary bypass surgery. Yonsei Med J 1987;28:152–156

273. Ness J, Stankiewicz J, Kaniff T, Pifarre R, Allegretti J. Sensorineural hearing loss associated with aortocoronary bypass surgery: a prospective analysis. Laryngoscope 1993;103:589–593

274. Friedman E, Herer G, Luban N, Williams I. Sickle cell anemia and hearing. Ann Otol Rhinol Laryngol 1980;89:342–347

275. Orchik D, Dunn J. Sickle cell anemia and sudden deafness. Arch Otolaryngol 1977;103:369–370

276. Nomura Y, Tsuchida M, Mori S, Sakurai T. Deafness in cryoglobulinemia. Ann Otol Rhinol Laryngol 1982;91:250–255

277. Barr D, Reeder G, Wheeler C. Cryoglobulinemia. A report of two cases with discussion of clinical manifestations, incidence, and significance. Ann Intern Med 1950;32:6–29

278. Tos M. A survey of Hand-Schuller-Christian's disease in otolaryngology. Acta Otolaryngol 1966;62:217–218

279. Hughes G, Kinney S, Barna B, Calabrese L. Practical versus theoretical management of autoimmune inner ear disease. Laryngoscope 1984;94:758–767

280. Salamy A, Eldredge L, Tooley W. Neonatal status and hearing loss in high-risk infants. J Pediatr 1989;114:847–852

281. Hildesheimer M, Rubinstein M, Muchnik C, Sahartiv E. A model for research on cochlear hypoxia. Laryngoscope 1983;93:615–620

282. Kitamura K, Berreby M. Temporal bone histopathology associated with occlusion of vertebrobasilar arteries. Ann Otol Rhinol Laryngol 1983;92:33–38

283. Harner SG. Hearing in adult-onset diabetes mellitus. Otolaryngol Head Neck Surg 1981;89:322–327

284. Kurien M, Thomas K, Bhanu T. Hearing threshold in patients with diabetes mellitus. J Laryngol Otol 1989;103:164–168

285. Cullen J, Cinnamond M. Hearing loss in diabetics. J Laryngol Otol 1993;107:179–182

286. Celik O, Yalcin S, Celebi H, Ozturk A. Hearing loss in insulin-dependent diabetes mellitus. Auris Nasus Larynx 1996;23:127–132

287. Dalton DS, Cruickshanks KJ, Klein R, Klein BE, Wiley TL. Association of NIDDM and hearing loss. Diabetes Care 1998;21:1540–1544

288. de Espana R, Biurrun O, Lorente J, Traserra J. Hearing and diabetes. ORL J Otorhinolaryngol Relat Spec 1995;57:325–327

289. Kakarlapudi V, Sawyer R, Staecker H. The effect of diabetes on sensorineural hearing loss. Otol Neurotol 2003;24:382–386

290. Ma F, Gomez-Marin O, Lee DJ, Balkany T. Diabetes and hearing impairment in Mexican American adults: a population-based study. J Laryngol Otol 1998;112:835–839

291. Jorgensen MB, Buch NH. Studies on inner ear function and cranial nerves in diabetes. Acta Otolaryngol 1961;53:350–364

292. Friedman S, Schulman R, Weiss S. Hearing and diabetic neuropathy. Arch Intern Med 1975;135:573–576

293. Sieger A, White N, Skinner M, Spector G. Auditory function in children with diabetes mellitus. Ann Otol Rhinol Laryngol 1983;92:237–241

294. Miller J, Beck L, Davis A, Jones D, Thomas A. Hearing loss in patients with diabetic retinopathy. Am J Otolaryngol 1983;4:342–346

295. Harner S. Hearing in adult-onset diabetes mellitus. Otolaryngol Head Neck Surg 1981;89:322–327

296. Parving A, Eberling C, Balle V, Parbo J, Dejgaard A, Parving H. Hearing disorders in patients with insulin-dependent diabetes mellitus. Audiology 1990;29:113–121

297. Costa OA. Inner ear pathology in experimental diabetes. Laryngoscope 1967;77:68–75

298. Duck SW, Prazma J, Bennett PS, Pillsbury HC. Interaction between hypertension and diabetes mellitus in the pathogenesis of sensorineural hearing loss. Laryngoscope 1997;107(12 pt 1):1596–1605

299. Jorgensen MB. The inner ear in diabetes mellitus. Histological studies. Arch Otolaryngol 1961;74:373–381

300. Wackym P, Linthicum FJ. Diabetes mellitus and hearing loss: clinical and histopathologic relationships. Am J Otol 1986;7:176–182

301. Davis L, Johnsson L. Viral infections of the inner ear: clinical, virologic, and pathologic studies in humans and animals. Am J Otolaryngol 1983;4:347–362

302. Strauss M, Davis G. Viral disease of the labyrinth. I. Review of the literature and discussion of the role of cytomegalovirus in congenital deafness. Ann Otol Rhinol Laryngol 1973;82:577–583

303. Pappas D. Hearing impairments and vestibular abnormalities among children with subclinical cytomegalovirus. Ann Otol Rhinol Laryngol 1983;92:552–557

304. Westmore G, Pickard B, Stern H. Isolation of mumps virus from the inner ear after sudden deafness. BMJ 1979;1:14–15

305. Smith G, Gussen R. Inner ear pathologic features following mumps infection. Arch Otolaryngol 1976;102:108–111

306. Bordley J, Kapur Y. Histopathologic changes in the temporal bone resulting from measles infection. Arch Otolaryngol 1977;103:162–168

307. Wild N, Sheppard S, Smithells R, Holzel H, Jones G. Onset and severity of hearing loss due to congenital rubella infection. Arch Dis Child 1989;64:1280–1283

308. Beg J. Bilateral sensorineural hearing loss as a complication of infectious mononucleosis. Arch Otolaryngol 1981;107:620–622

309. Brodsky L, Stanievich J. Sensorineural hearing loss following live measles virus vaccination. Int J Pediatr Otorhinolaryngol 1985;10:159–163

310. Stewart B, Prabhu P. Reports of sensorineural deafness after measles, mumps, and rubella immunization. Arch Dis Child 1993;69:153–154

311. Hall R, Richards H. Hearing loss due to mumps. Arch Dis Child 1987;62:189–191

312. Strauss M. A clinical pathologic study of hearing loss in congenital cytomegalovirus infection. Laryngoscope 1985;95:951–962

313. Hicks T, Fowler K, Richardson M, Dahle A, Adams L, Pass R. Congenital cytomegalovirus infection and neonatal auditory screening. J Pediatr 1993;123:779–782

314. Peckham C, Stark O, Dudgeon J, Martin J, Hawkins G. Congenital cytomegalovirus infection: a cause of sensorineural hearing loss. Arch Dis Child 1987;62:1233–1237

315. Bradford RD, Cloud G, Lakeman AD, et al. Detection of cytomegalovirus (CMV) DNA by polymerase chain reaction is associated with hearing loss in newborns with symptomatic congenital CMV infection involving the central nervous system. J Infect Dis 2005;191:227–233

316. Lagasse N, Dhooge I, Govaert P. Congenital CMV-infection and hearing loss. Acta Otorhinolaryngol Belg 2000;54:431–436

317. Zajtchuk JT, Matz GJ, Lindsay JR. Temporal bone pathology in herpes oticus. Ann Otol Rhinol Laryngol 1972;81:331–338

318. Suboti R. Histopathological findings in the inner ear caused by measles. J Laryngol Otol 1976;90:173–181

319. Hinojosa R, Lindsay J. Inner ear degeneration in Reye's syndrome. Arch Otolaryngol 1977;103:634–640

320. Rarey K, Davis J, Deshmukh D, et al. Structural and functional alterations of the inner ear associated with Reye's syndrome. 1984

321. Chandrasekhar SS, Connelly PE, Brahmbhatt SS, Shah CS, Kloser PC, Baredes S. Otologic and audiologic evaluation of human immunodeficiency virus-infected patients. Am J Otolaryngol 2000;21:1–9

322. Hausler R, Vibert D, Koralnik IJ, Hirschel B. Neuro-otological manifestations in different stages of HIV infection. Acta Otolaryngol Suppl 1991;481:515–521

323. Gurney TA, Murr AH. Otolaryngologic manifestations of human immunodeficiency virus infection. Otolaryngol Clin North Am 2003;36:607–624

324. Kohan D, Rothstein SG, Cohen NL. Otologic disease in patients with acquired immunodeficiency syndrome. Ann Otol Rhinol Laryngol 1988;97(6 pt 1):636–640

325. Rarey KE. Otologic pathophysiology in patients with human immunodeficiency virus. Am J Otolaryngol 1990;11:366–369

326. Lalwani A, Sooy C. Otologic and neurotologic manifestations of acquired immunodeficiency syndrome. Otolaryngol Clin North Am 1992;25:1183–1197

327. Hart CW, Cokely CG, Schupbach J, Dal Canto MC, Coppleson LW. Neurotologic findings of a patient with acquired immune deficiency syndrome. Ear Hear 1989;10:68–76

328. Welkoborsky HJ, Lowitzsch K. Auditory brain stem responses in patients with human immunotropic virus infection of different stages. Ear Hear 1992;13:55–57

329. Bankaitis AE. The effects of click rate on the auditory brain stem response (ABR) in patients with varying degrees of HIV-infection: a pilot study. Ear Hear 1995;16:321–324

330. Castello E, Baroni N, Pallestrini E. Neurotological auditory brain stem response findings in human immunodeficiency virus-positive patients without neurologic manifestations. Ann Otol Rhinol Laryngol 1998;107:1054–1060

331. Pagano MA, Cahn PE, Garau ML, et al. Brain-stem auditory evoked potentials in human immunodeficiency virus-seropositive patients with and without acquired immunodeficiency syndrome. Arch Neurol 1992;49:166–169

332. Reyes-Contreras L, Silva-Rojas A, Ysunza-Rivera A, Jimenez-Ruiz G, Berruecos-Villalobos P, Romo-Gutierrez G. Brainstem auditory evoked response in HIV-infected patients with and without AIDS. Arch Med Res 2002;33:25–28

333. Chandrasekhar S, Siverls V, Sekhar H. Histopathologic and ultrastructural changes in the temporal bones of HIV-infected human adults. Am J Otol 1992;13:207–214

334. Pappas DG Jr, Chandra HK, Lim J, Hillman DE. Ultrastructural findings in the cochlea of AIDS cases. Am J Otol 1994;15:456–465

335. Pappas DG Jr, Roland JT Jr, Lim J, Lai A, Hillman DE. Ultrastructural findings in the vestibular end-organs of AIDS cases. Am J Otol 1995;16:140–145

336. Michaels L, Soucek S, Liang J. The ear in the acquired immunodeficiency syndrome: I. Temporal bone histopathologic study. Am J Otol 1994;15:515–522

337. Linstrom CJ, Pincus RL, Leavitt EB, Urbina MC. Otologic neurotologic manifestations of HIV-related disease. Otolaryngol Head Neck Surg 1993;108:680–687

338. Morris MS, Prasad S. Otologic disease in the acquired immunodeficiency syndrome. Ear Nose Throat J 1990;69:451–453

339. Soucek S, Michaels L. The ear in the acquired immunodeficiency syndrome: II. Clinical and audiologic investigation. Am J Otol 1996;17:35–39

340. Simdon J, Watters D, Bartlett S, Connick E. Ototoxicity associated with use of nucleoside analog reverse transcriptase inhibitors: a report of 3 possible cases and review of the literature. Clin Infect Dis 2001;32:1623–1627

341. Brinkman K, ter Hofstede HJ, Burger DM, Smeitink JA, Koopmans PP. Adverse effects of reverse transcriptase inhibitors: mitochondrial toxicity as common pathway. AIDS 1998;12:1735–1744

342. Brinkman K, Kakuda TN. Mitochondrial toxicity of nucleoside analogue reverse transcriptase inhibitors: a looming obstacle for long-term antiretroviral therapy? Curr Opin Infect Dis 2000;13:5–11

343. Lewis W, Dalakas MC. Mitochondrial toxicity of antiviral drugs. Nat Med 1995;1:417–422

344. Johns DR. Seminars in medicine of the Beth Israel Hospital, Boston. Mitochondrial DNA and disease. N Engl J Med 1995;333:638–644

345. Shigenaga MK, Hagen TM, Ames BN. Oxidative damage and mitochondrial decay in aging. Proc Natl Acad Sci U S A 1994;91:10771–10778

346. Simonetti S, Chen X, DiMauro S, Schon E. Accumulation of deletions in human mitochondrial DNA during normal aging: analysis by quantitative PCR. Biochim Biophys Acta 1992;1180:113–122

347. McNulty J, Fassett R. Syphilis: an otolaryngologic perspective. Laryngoscope 1981;91:889–905

348. Belal AJ, Linthicum FJ. Pathology of congenital syphilitic labyrinthitis. Am J Otolaryngol 1980;1:109–118

349. Nagasaki T, Watanabe Y, Aso S, Mizukoshi K. Electrocochleography in syphilitic hearing loss. Acta Otolaryngol Suppl 1993;504:68–73

350. Zoller M, Wilson W, Nadol JJ, Girard K. Detection of syphilitic hearing loss. Arch Otolaryngol 1978;104:63–65

351. Balkany T, Dans P. Reversible sudden deafness in early acquired syphilis. Arch Otolaryngol 1978;104:66–68

352. Hendershot E. Luetic deafness. Laryngoscope 1973;83:865–870

353. Hughes G, Rutherford I. Predictive value of serologic tests for syphilis in otology. Ann Otol Rhinol Laryngol 1986;95:250–259

354. Birdsall H, Baughn R, Jenkins H. The diagnostic dilemma of otosyphilis. A new Western blot assay. Arch Otolaryngol Head Neck Surg 1990;116:617–621

355. Pillsbury H, Shea J. Luetic hydrops–diagnosis and therapy. Laryngoscope 1979;89:1135–1144

356. Patterson M. Congenital luetic hearing impairment. Treatment with prednisone. Arch Otolaryngol 1968;87:378–382

357. Hughes G, Haberkamp T. Other auditory disorders. In: Hughes G, ed. Textbook of Clinical Otology. New York: Thieme Stratton, 1985:129

358. Smith M, Canalis R. Otologic manifestations of AIDS: the otosyphilis connection. Laryngoscope 1989;99:365–372

359. Aviel A, Ostfeld E. Acquired irreversible sensorineural hearing loss associated with otitis media with effusion. Am J Otolaryngol 1982;3:217–222

360. Paparella MM, Goycoolea MV, Meyerhoff WL. Inner ear pathology and otitis media. Ann Otol Rhinol Laryngol Suppl 1980;89:249–253

361. Paparella M, Morizono T, Le CT, et al. Sensorineural hearing loss in otitis media. Ann Otol Rhinol Laryngol 1984;93(6 pt 1):623–629

362. Berlow S, Caldarelli D, Matz G, Meyer D, Harsch G. Bacterial meningitis and sensorineural hearing loss: a prospective investigation. Laryngoscope 1980;90:1445–1452

363. Gussen R, Canalis R. Mucormycosis of the temporal bone. Ann Otol Rhinol Laryngol 1982;91:27–32

364. Kligerman A, Solangi K, Ventry I, Goodman A, Weseley S. Hearing impairment associated with chronic renal failure. Laryngoscope 1981;91:583–592

365. Alport A. Hereditary familial congenital hemorrhagic nephritis. BMJ 1927;1:504–506

366. Bubalo F, Davidson D. Recent developments in hereditary nephritis (Alport's syndrome). Indiana Med 1991;84:860–866

367. Rosenberg AL, Bergstrom L, Troost BT, Bartholomew BA. Hyperuricemia and neurologic deficits. N Engl J Med 1970;282:992–997

368. Quick C, Fish A, Brown C. The relationship between cochlea and kidney. Laryngoscope 1973;83:1469–1482

369. Ikeda K, Kusakari J, Arakawa E, et al. Cochlear potentials of guinea pigs with experimentally induced renal failure. Acta Otolaryngol Suppl 1987;435:40–45

370. Antonelli A, Bonfioli F, Garrubba V, et al. Audiological findings in elderly patients with chronic renal failure. Acta Otolaryngol Suppl 1990;476:54–68

371. Kustel M, Buki B, Gyimesi J, Mako J, Komora V, Ribari O. Auditory brain stem potentials in uraemia. ORL J Otorhinolaryngol Relat Spec 1993;55:89–92

372. Zeigelboim BS, Mangabeira-Albernaz PL, Fukuda Y. High frequency audiometry and chronic renal failure. Acta Otolaryngol 2001;121:245–248

373. Mitschke H, Schmidt P, Kopsa H, Zazgornik J. Reversible uremic deafness after successful renal transplantation. N Engl J Med 1975;292:1061–1063

374. Rizvi S, Holmes R. Hearing loss from hemodialysis. Arch Otolaryngol 1980;106:751–756

375. Hutchinson JC Jr, Klodd DA. Electrophysiologic analysis of auditory, vestibular and brain stem function in chronic renal failure. Laryngoscope 1982;92:833–843

376. Nikolopoulos TP, Kandiloros DC, Segas JV, et al. Auditory function in young patients with chronic renal failure. Clin Otolaryngol Allied Sci 1997;22:222–225

377. Stavroulaki P, Nikolopoulos TP, Psarommatis I, Apostolopoulos N. Hearing evaluation with distortion-product otoacoustic emissions in young patients undergoing haemodialysis. Clin Otolaryngol Allied Sci 2001;26:235–242

378. Serbetcioglu MB, Erdogan S, Sifil A. Effects of a single session of hemodialysis on hearing abilities. Acta Otolaryngol 2001;121:836–838

379. Bergstrom L, Thompson P, Sando I, Wood R. 2. Renal disease. Its pathology, treatment, and effects on the ear. Arch Otolaryngol 1980;106:567–572

380. Horvath A, Lloyd H. Perceptive deafness and hypothyroidism. BMJ 1956;1:431–433

381. Post J. Hypothyroid deafness: a clinical study of sensorineural deafness associated with hypothyroidism. Laryngoscope 1964;74:221–232

382. Anand V, Mann S, Dash R, Mehra Y. Auditory investigations in hypothyroidism. Acta Otolaryngol 1989;108:83–87

383. Di Lorenzo L, Foggia L, Panza N, et al. Auditory brainstem responses in thyroid diseases before and after therapy. Horm Res 1995;43:200–205

384. Lai CL, Lin RT, Tai CT, Liu CK, Howng SL. The recovery potential of central conduction disorder in hypothyroid rats. J Neurol Sci 2000;173:113–119

385. Anniko M, Rosenkvist U. Tectorial and basilar membranes in experimental hypothyroidism. Acta Otolaryngol 1982;108:218–220

386. Hughes G, Sismanis A, House J. Is there consensus in perilymph fistula management? Otolaryngol Head Neck Surg 1990;102:111–117

387. House J, Morris M, Kramer S, Shasky G, Coggan B, Putter J. Perilymphatic fistula: surgical experience in the United States. Otolaryngol Head Neck Surg 1991;105:51–61

388. Maitland CG. Perilymphatic fistula. Curr Neurol Neurosci Rep 2001;1:486–491

389. Kohut R, Hinojosa R, Ryu J. Perilymphatic fistulae: a single-blind clinical histopathologic study. Adv Otorhinolaryngol 1988;42:148–152

390. el Shazly M, Linthicum FJ. Microfissures of the temporal bone: do they have any clinical significance? Am J Otol 1991;12:169–171

391. Reilly J, Kenna M. Congenital perilymphatic fistula: an overlooked diagnosis? Am J Otol 1989;10:496–498

392. Meyerhoff W, Yellin M. Summating potential/action potential ratio in perilymph fistula. Otolaryngol Head Neck Surg 1990;102:678–682

393. Goto F, Ogawa K, Kunihiro T, Kurashima K, Kobayashi H, Kanzaki J. Perilymph fistula—45 case analysis. Auris Nasus Larynx 2001;28:29–33

394. Weber P, Kelly R, Bluestone C, Bassiouny M. Beta2-transferrin confirms perilymphatic fistula in children. Otolaryngol Head Neck Surg 1994;110:381–386

395. Thalmann I, Kohut R, Ryu J, Comegys T, Senarita M, Thallman R. Protein profile of human perilymph: in search of markers for the diagnosis of perilymph fistula and other inner ear disease. Otolaryngol Head Neck Surg 1994;111:273–280

396. Weber PC, Bluestone CD, Kenna MA, Kelley RH. Correlation of beta-2 transferrin and middle ear abnormalities in congenital perilymphatic fistula. Am J Otol 1995;16:277–282

397. Mikulec AA, McKenna MJ, Ramsey MJ, et al. Superior semicircular canal dehiscence presenting as conductive hearing loss without vertigo. Otol Neurotol 2004;25:121–129

398. Minor LB. Superior canal dehiscence syndrome. Am J Otol 2000;21:9–19

399. Browning GG, Swan IR, Gatehouse S. Hearing loss in minor head injury. Arch Otolaryngol 1982;108:474–477

400. Dix M. Observations upon the nerve fiber deafness of multiple sclerosis with particular reference to the phenomenon of loudness recruitment. J Laryngol Otol 1965;79:695–706

401. Rose R, Daly J. Reversible temporary threshold shift in multiple sclerosis. Laryngoscope 1964;74:424–432

402. Drulovic B, Ribaric-Jankes K, Kostic V, Sternic N. Multiple sclerosis as the cause of sudden "pontine" deafness. Audiology 1994;33:195–201

403. Morizono T, Sikora M. Experimental hypercholesterolemia and auditory dysfunction in the chinchilla. Otolaryngol Head Neck Surg 1982;90:814–818

404. Jahrsdoerfer R, Thompson E, Johns M, Cantrell R. Sarcoidosis and fluctuating hearing loss. Ann Otol Rhinol Laryngol 1981;90:161–163

405. Brihaye P, Halama A. Fluctuating hearing loss in sarcoidosis. Acta Otorhinolaryngol Belg 1993;47:23–26

406. Hayes E, Babin R, Platz C. The otologic manifestations of mucopolysaccharidoses. Am J Otol 1980;2:65–69

407. Friedmann I, Spellacy E, Crow J, Watts R. Histopathological studies of the temporal bone in Hurler's disease. J Laryngol Otol 1985;99:29–41

24

Benign Neoplasms of the Temporal Bone

Lawrence R. Lustig and Robert K. Jackler

The benign tumors of the temporal bone comprise a diverse spectrum of lesions that have largely been responsible for defining the specialty of neurotology and skull base surgery. In spite of their benign histopathologic characteristics, however, these lesions may be locally destructive. Prompt diagnosis and treatment is therefore necessary to prevent further worsening of audiologic, vestibular, facial, or lower cranial nerve dysfunction that are so common upon presentation (**Table 24–1**).

◆ Schwannoma

The most common tumor of the temporal bone and cerebellopontine angle is the schwannoma, accounting for 6% of *all* intracranial tumors, and 91% of all tumors in and around the temporal bone.[1,2] Schwannomas are benign tumors of the nerve sheath, which historically have also been referred to as neuromas, neurofibromas, neurinomas, and neurilemmomas.[3] Within the temporal bone, schwannomas arise in three anatomic loci: the internal auditory canal (IAC) from the eighth cranial nerve, the fallopian canal from the seventh cranial nerve, and the jugular foramen from cranial nerves IX to XI.

Vestibular Schwannoma/Acoustic Neuroma

Vestibular schwannomas, more commonly known as acoustic neuromas (ANs), are the most commonly occurring schwannoma of the temporal bone, and by inference, the most commonly encountered tumor in otology. An overwhelming majority of ANs arise de novo as a solitary lesion. Diagnosis typically occurs after the sixth decade, with a slightly higher incidence in females.[4] Neurofibromatosis type 2 (NF2), accounting for only 5% of tumors, is associated with bilateral ANs and tends to present earlier in life (**Fig. 24–1**). Recent studies suggest that undiagnosed ANs may be present in as much as 2/10,000 of the population.[5] Schwannomas, as their name implies, are derived from Schwann cells. Their point of origin is repeatedly described in the literature as arising at the transition zone between central and peripheral myelin, known as the Obersteiner-Redlich zone, though one small series indicates that most vestibular nerve schwannomas may in fact originate lateral to the glial-schwannian junction of the nerve.[6,7] The tumors arise with an equal frequency from the superior and inferior divisions of the vestibular nerve, and usually originate within the medial portion of the IAC, though a fraction arise extrameatally or in the lateral IAC.[8]

The elucidation of the underlying genetics of ANs is derived from the study of NF2 patients. The specific defect for NF2 leading to bilateral ANs has been genetically mapped to chromosome 22.[9] The gene product, termed *merlin*, is believed to be a tumor-suppressor gene, requiring both copies of the gene to be dysfunctional for tumorigenesis to occur. NF2 patients

Table 24–1 Primary Temporal Bone Neoplasms

Site	Benign	Malignant
Pinna	Hemangioma	Basal cell carcinoma
		Squamous cell carcinoma
		Melanoma
EAC	Osteoma	Squamous cell carcinoma
	Neurofibroma	Adenoidcystic carcinoma
Middle ear	Adenoma	Squamous cell carcinoma (rare)
	Glomus tympanicum	Rhabdomyosarcoma
	Schwannoma (CN VII)	
Mastoid	Adenoma	Squamous cell carcinoma (rare)
	Schwannoma (CN VII)	Papillary adenocarcinoma
IAC	Schwannoma (CN VIII>>VII)	
	Meningioma	
	Ossifying hemangioma	
Jugular foramen	Glomus jugulare	
	Meningioma	
	Schwannoma (CN IX-XII)	
Petrous apex	Chondroma	Chondrosarcoma
		Chordoma
		Metastases

EAC, external auditory canal; IAC, internal auditory canal.

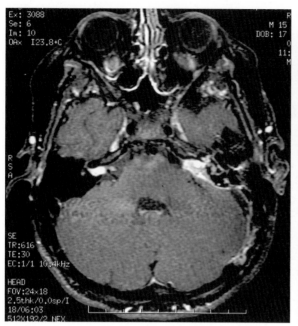

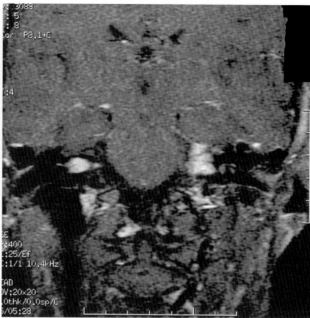

A

B

Figure 24–1 A patient with neurofibromatosis type 2 (NF2) and bilateral vestibular schwannomas. The T1-weighted MRI scan with gadolinium enhancement in the axial plane **(A)** shows a characteristic tumor of the right internal auditory canal with a small cerebellopontine angle component. The tumor on the left, which has the appearance of a meningioma with dural tail enhancement, was found to be a vestibular schwannoma at surgery. The coronal view **(B)** shows the tumors in this same patient.

are therefore born with one defective gene, leading to a lifelong propensity toward AN development. Patients with sporadically arising ANs, by contrast, have acquired defects of both gene copies, leading to the formation of tumor.[10,11] The precise role of the *merlin* gene product remains unclear, but has been shown to exert its activity by inhibiting phosphatidylinositol 3-kinase.[12,13]

Macroscopically, ANs are smooth-walled gray or yellowish masses. Though they have been traditionally described as being well encapsulated, studies indicate that they do not possess a true capsule.[14] Microscopically, two morphologic patterns can be discerned. The *Antoni A* pattern consists of densely packed spindle-shaped cells with darkly staining nuclei. When they appear in a whorled configuration, it is referred to as a Verocay body. The *Antoni B* pattern consists of a more diffusely arranged cell pattern with increased pleomorphism (**Fig. 24–2**). Any tumor may contain one or both patterns. The clinical significance of these two patterns is unclear, though the Antoni B type tends to predominate in larger tumors. The immunoperoxidase stain S-100 is positive and is used to confirm the diagnosis of schwannoma.[15–17]

The majority of ANs are benign and slow-growing tumors. Though the average growth rate for tumors has been estimated to be between 0.1 and 0.2 cm in diameter per year, the range is variable and 10 to 15% have a growth rate greater than 1 cm per year.[18,19] The growth rate has been shown to be

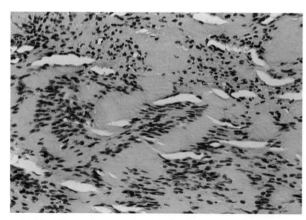

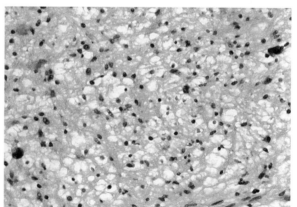

A

B

Figure 24–2 Histopathology of vestibular schwannomas. These hematoxylin and eosin (H&E) stains demonstrate the two common types of histopathology seen in vestibular schwannomas. The *Antoni A* pattern **(A)** consists of densely packed spindle-shaped cells with darkly staining nuclei. When they appear in a whorled configuration it is referred to as a Verocay body. The *Antoni B* pattern **(B)** consists of a more diffusely arranged cell pattern with increased pleomorphism. This pattern tends to predominate in larger tumors, though any tumor may contain one or both patterns. The clinical significance of these two patterns is unclear.

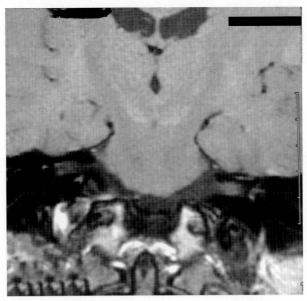
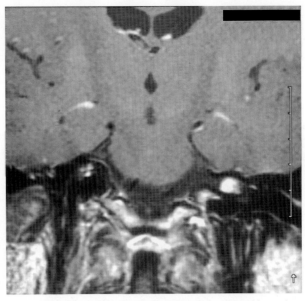

A   B

Figure 24–3 A coronal MRI of a small left intracanalicular vestibular schwannoma measuring about 8 mm. The tumor is barely visible on the T1-weighted images without gadolinium enhancement **(A)**, whereas with gadolinium **(B)** the tumor is markedly enhanced.

related to the concentration of vascular endothelial growth factor.[20] The tumors usually originate in the IAC. Growth then carries the tumor into the cerebellopontine angle cistern, where it commonly involves the seventh and eighth cranial nerves. Further enlargement causes brainstem compression and fifth nerve involvement, and eventually hydrocephalus.

The clinical presentation of patients with AN reflects the tumor growth pattern. Asymmetrical sensorineural hearing loss, occurring in 95% of patients, is believed to be secondary to direct compression of the tumor on cranial nerve VIII within the IAC, or due to compression of the nerve's vascular supply. The hearing loss is sudden in onset in about one fourth of cases.[4] Additional symptoms include high-pitched, continuous, asymmetrical tinnitus; vertigo; disequilibrium and ataxia (up to 70% incidence in larger tumors); facial sensory disturbances (50%); facial twitching (10%); headaches (40%); nystagmus; and decreased corneal reflexes.[4] Audiometric testing typically reveals asymmetrical sensorineural hearing loss predominating in the high frequencies, though this configuration is not strictly found. Speech discrimination scores often are out of proportion to the degree of pure-tone hearing thresholds. There is usually either an absent stapedial reflex or reflex decay, but this is not sufficiently reliable to be of much diagnostic value.[21] Auditory brainstem response (ABR) testing is also used to assist in identifying retrocochlear pathology. The presence of a wave I and absence of waves II to V is the most specific finding for AN, though one must be wary for both false-positive (>80%) and false-negative (12–18%) ABRs.[22,23]

Contrast-enhanced magnetic resonance imaging (MRI) provides the gold standard for the diagnosis of the AN, which is able to detect tumors as small as 1 mm. The well-demarcated lesions are isointense on T1-weighted images and demonstrate some signal increase on T2-weighted images with areas of heterogeneity[24] (**Fig. 24–3**). After gadolinium administration, enhancement is striking, more so than most other benign extraaxial tumors.[25] High-resolution computed tomography (CT), though not as sensitive as MRI for small tumors, reliably demonstrates a smoothly marginated, contrast-enhancing

mass within the cerebellopontine angle (CPA) in tumors over 1.5 cm in diameter[25] (**Fig. 24–4**).

Although the tumors are slow growing and benign, in most-cases treatment is recommended because growth may lead to multiple cranial neuropathies, brainstem compression, hydrocephalus, and death. In selected cases, a conservative "watch and wait" approach may be appropriate, such as in the

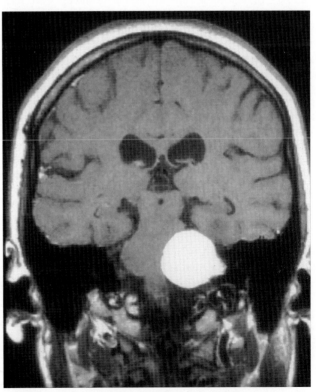

Figure 24–4 A 4-cm vestibular schwannoma with brainstem compression is shown in this coronal T1-weighted MRI scan with gadolinium enhancement.

elderly or medically infirm.[26,27] The first priority of surgery or radiation therapy is to alleviate the risk of progressive intracranial tumor growth, and it is secondarily concerned with preservation of facial nerve function and sparing of useful hearing. A variety of techniques have been employed to achieve these ends, including the translabyrinthine, retrosigmoid, and middle fossa approaches. The decision of which to use depends on the tumor size, its depth of penetration within the IAC, the degree of hearing loss, and the experience of the surgical team (**Table 24–2**).[28,29] A recent surgical trend also includes near-total tumor resection (remnant ≤2.5 mm in length and ≤2 mm thick) followed by expectant observation in an effort to improve facial nerve outcomes.[30] In such a scenario, recurrences have been shown to be about 3%. Intraoperative cranial nerve monitoring is routinely employed to assist with neural preservation during tumor resection. The results after surgery are dependent on the experience of the surgical team.[31] The expected mortality is less than 2% in most major centers, with tumor-related mortality limited to those with large tumors. Complications occur in about 20% of cases, and most commonly include cerebrospinal fluid (CSF) leakage, meningitis, and chronic headache.[32–34] Less common are traumatic parenchymal injury from intraoperative retraction, arterial or venous cerebral infarct, postoperative hemorrhage into the CPA, and air embolism.[35,36] Anatomically the facial nerve is preserved in 82 to 97% of cases, with an overwhelming majority having grade 1 or 2 facial nerve function 1 year after surgery. Whether anatomic preservation correlates with postoperative nerve function, however, is subject to debate.[37,38] Hearing preservation surgery may be attempted for tumors with less than a 1.5 cm intracranial component, and that meet the "50/50" rule, speech reception threshold less than 50 dB and a speech discrimination score of greater than 50%, though these rules are not strict and are even now being redefined and broadened.[39–42] Though results vary widely from center to center, useful hearing is commonly preserved in about one fourth of cases attempted, though in the most favorable tumors hearing preservation may be as high as 70% in experienced centers.[43,44]

Stereotactic radiosurgery ("gamma-knife") is being increasingly employed as an alternative to surgery in a growing number of centers with acceptable morbidity and a similar spectrum of functional deficits, though the long-term control rates have not yet been conclusively established. For those unable to tolerate the risk of surgery, radiation may represent a viable alternative.[45–49] There is also growing acceptance that for large tumors, a subtotal resection of tumor, leaving the tumor capsule behind to preserve existing cranial nerve function, followed by radiation or gamma knife treatment,

represents an alternative treatment option.[50] Several larger series with adequate (10 years or greater) follow-up have shown that following single dose radiotherapy, 20 to 25% of tumors remain stable, 50 to 75% of tumors shrink in size, and 2 to 13% show further growth.[51–54] However, these rates need to be tempered by the observation that in untreated tumors followed over a 3-year period, 50% of tumors remain stable, 14% shrink, and 37% enlarge.[55] Though older dosing regimens were associated with a 37% incidence of facial palsy, newer dosing algorithms are rarely associated with facial nerve weakness following stereotactic radiotherapy.[53] Preservation of useful hearing (>50% speech reception threshold and 50% word recognition scores) has been shown to occur in 47 to 79% of radiation tumors.[53,54,56,57] However, should a patient undergo stereotactic radiotherapy for a vestibular schwannoma and subsequently need surgical resection for a continually growing tumor, the facial nerve function preservation rates are not as good as compared with when there was no prior radiotherapy.[58–60] Further, because of the risk of a radiation-induced malignancy, radiotherapy for these lesions should only be cautiously used in younger individuals.[61]

The major dilemma in vestibular schwannoma management is a young healthy patient with good hearing and an intracanalicular tumor: to treat or wait and rescan in 6-12 months. First, the patient must understand that the least risk to hearing is to do nothing; however, even small tumors can suddenly cause hearing to drop. Also, in theory, facial nerve injury during surgery is greater if the tumor grows in the 6-12 month follow-up interval. Even the risk of partial but significant hearing loss with gamma knife (about 25% chance) outweighs most other considerations. Wait and re-scan has become the standard for initial management of intracanalicular schwannomas for many neurotologists. One major exception is significant dizzy attacks, which are best managed by tumor surgery which sections the vestibular nerve.

Jugular Foramen Schwannoma

Though schwannomas are the second most common lesion of the jugular foramen behind glomus tumors, overall they are relatively rare, representing about 3% of all intracranial schwannomas.[62,63] In fact, the largest series, that of Tan et al[62] in 1990, includes only 14 patients, with less than 100 cases in the world literature reported up to that time. Schwannomas presenting in this region arise from cranial nerves IX to XII. As with vestibular schwannomas, these tumors probably occur at the transition zone between the central and peripheral myelin. Histologically, the tumors resemble vestibular schwannomas.[64]

Table 24–2 Surgical Approaches for the Management of Acoustic Neuroma

Approach	Advantages	Disadvantages
Retrosigmoid	Excellent exposure	Increased incidence of postop headaches
	Hearing preservation possible	Higher incidence of CSF leak
		Need for more vigorous cerebellar retraction
Translabyrinthine/anterosigmoid	Lower surgical morbidity	Inability to preserve hearing
	More facial nerve reconstructive options	
Middle fossa	Superior hearing preservation results	Increased risk of transient facial neuropraxia
		Unsuitable for tumors with large CPA component

CPA, cerebellopontine angle; CSF, cerebrospinal fluid.

Three tumor growth patterns have been recognized for jugular foramen schwannomas.[65] Tumors arising in the distal portion of the foramen may expand inferiorly out of the skull base. More proximally arising tumors can expand into the posterior fossa. Others arise in the middle of the foramen and either expand primarily into bone or become bilobed, with an expansion both out of the skull base and into the posterior fossa.

The most common presenting symptoms are hoarseness, swallowing difficulties, and vertigo.[62–65] Other symptoms may include shoulder weakness, headache, nausea, vomiting, facial numbness or spasm, dysphagia, and visual disturbances. On exam, cranial nerve X is dysfunctional in 63% of cases presenting, and may be accompanied by deficits of cranial nerves IX (55%), XI (41%), and XII (36%).[66] Cranial nerve V and VII dysfunction is less common on examination, as are hemifacial spasm, nystagmus, ataxia, and papilledema.[62]

High-resolution CT typically demonstrates a well-demarcated, smoothly marginated expansion of the foramen walls (**Fig. 24–5**). MRI is superior for diagnosis, and demonstrates a lesion isointense to brain parenchyma on contrast-enhanced T1-weighted images, whereas T2-images usually reveal a high signal intensity. The addition of gadolinium causes a marked signal increase. Differentiation from paragangliomas is made possible by noting the morphologically smooth manner of bony erosion as compared with a more irregular pattern with glomus tumors and meningiomas. In contrast to glomus tumors, flow voids are notably absent.[63] Angiography is often undertaken under the presumption that the tumor is a paraganglioma, and has little use diagnostically for schwannomas unless one anticipates a possible surgical need to evaluate the carotid or jugulosigmoid venous systems.[63]

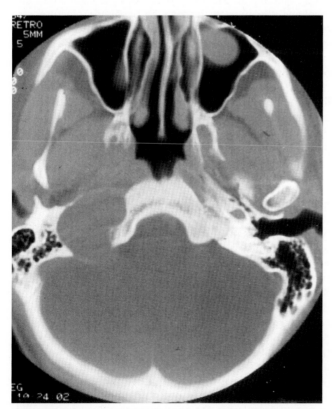

Figure 24–5 An axial CT scan of a right-sided jugular foramen schwannoma. Note the smooth enlargement of the jugular foramen. The patient presented with headaches, hoarseness, and dysphagia.

As with vestibular schwannomas, the treatment is primarily surgical.[67] Because of the variability of tumor presentation, the surgical approach must be individualized. Techniques for exposure of the jugular foramen have become increasingly routine in recent years.[68,69] Jugular foramen schwannomas, because they often possess an intracranial component, frequently require a transjugular posterior fossa craniotomy. Complete removal often causes paralysis of cranial nerves IX to XI, leading to postoperative hoarseness, dysphagia, and shoulder weakness in many cases.[66] Vocal cord medialization procedures can help compensate for paralytic laryngeal dysfunction.

Facial Nerve Schwannoma

Schwannomas of the facial nerve are uncommon lesions, accounting for only 1.2% of all temporal bone tumors.[1] Though its true incidence is not known, one study was able to identify only one case out of 1400 temporal bones analyzed.[70] Schwannomas have been identified along the entire course of the facial nerve, although intratemporal tumors appear to be much more common than the intracranial variety.[71,72] Within the temporal bone, the most common sites of involvement, in decreasing frequency, are geniculate ganglion, horizontal and vertical segments, IAC, and labyrinthine segment. A small percentage, however, display an unusual multicentricity evidenced by multiple discrete intraneural connections, sometimes described as a string of pearls.[73] The tendency for growth longitudinally along the lumen of the fallopian canal may lead to tumor prolapse into the middle ear, IAC, and CPA, and out of the stylomastoid foramen.

In contrast to ANs, facial nerve schwannomas tend to be slower growing and are often present for years before detection.[74] However, because of the facial nerve's intimate relationship with the sensory organs, otic capsule erosion is more common, occurring in up to 30% of cases.[72]

Facial nerve dysfunction (palsy or twitch) is the hallmark of the clinical presentation. It occurs due to compression of the nerve within the fallopian canal. The most common pattern is slowly progressive palsy, often accompanied by hyperfunction manifested as limited twitch or full hemifacial spasm. Recurrent acute paralytic episodes with partial or even complete recovery may also occur. Patients are commonly misdiagnosed with Bell's palsy with the first episode of paralysis. Successive bouts of palsy then ensue, with increasingly poorer facial nerve function. This presentation of recurrent, progressively more severe episodes of facial palsy is a classic characteristic of facial nerve schwannoma. The facial nerve is surprisingly resistant to compression. It has been estimated that 50% of facial nerve fibers must degenerate before clinical signs of a palsy are detected.[74,75] In one study of 48 patients with facial nerve neuromas, 26 presented with normal facial function.[72] Thus, patients without functional recovery from an idiopathic facial paralysis after 3 months or with a history of recurrent Bell's Palsy should have an enhanced MRI scan to search for tumor or facial nerve pathology.[74] Patients may also present with normal facial nerve function and a conductive hearing loss.[72] Additional presenting symptoms include vertigo from a labyrinthine fistula and sensorineural hearing loss from cochlear invasion.[56,76–78] Prolonged pain should also raise one's suspicion for a diagnosis other than idiopathic facial palsy.[72–74] Examination of the ear may demonstrate a mass behind the drum in up to 29% of cases.[74] Because biopsy of a facial nerve schwannoma in the middle ear usually results in a facial paralysis, appropriate imaging studies are recommended prior to biopsy of any middle ear tumor. Site of lesion tests, such as the Schirmer's test of lacrimation and stapedial reflex testing, while theoretically attractive, are not completely reliable and have been made largely obsolete by CT and MRI.

Radiographically, facial nerve schwannomas are similar to those arising in other portions of the temporal bone. They are hypointense on T1 images, hyperintense on T2 images, and show marked enhancement with gadolinium. An enhancing enlargement of varying thickness along a large segment of facial nerve is considered highly suggestive of schwannoma. Although high-resolution CT can identify these tumors due to their osseous erosion, MRI is a more sensitive diagnostic tool.[79]

The treatment for facial nerve schwannomas is primarily surgical.[51,76–78] The primary goal in management of an intratemporal facial nerve schwannoma is maintenance of facial function. With good facial function, it is usually best to leave the tumors alone as resection and grafting lead to at best a House-Brackmann grade of 3/6 (facial weakness at rest with good eye closure). For lesions limited to the transverse or descending portions of the nerve, a tympanomastoid approach may be used.[80] Lesions that involve the labyrinthine segment, IAC, or geniculate ganglion require the addition of an extradural middle cranial fossa approach. If cochlear function has been destroyed, then a translabyrinthine approach may be utilized.[74] At surgery, it is occasionally possible to remove a facial nerve schwannoma with preservation of its nerve of origin. More commonly, however, nerve repair with an interposition graft is needed. This may be accomplished with either a greater auricular or sural nerve graft. In general, those patients with long-standing facial nerve paralysis (>12 months) tend to have poorer postoperative facial nerve function. Because a common presentation for facial nerve schwannomas is a conductive hearing loss, it is not uncommon to first identify these tumors intraoperatively during an exploratory tympanotomy with the intent to perform a stapedectomy. In such a scenario, if a soft tissue mass is identified leaning on or eroding the stapes superstructure at tympanotomy, the surgeon should halt the procedure and perform imaging studies, and not biopsy the lesion.

◆ Paraganglioma (Glomus Tumor)

The most common tumor of the middle ear and second most common tumor found in the temporal bone is the paraganglioma, more commonly known as a glomus tumor but occasionally referred to as a chemodectoma.[81] Paraganglia, the origin of these tumors, exist throughout the temporal bone, including on the jugular dome, the promontory of the middle ear, and along Jacobson's and Arnold's nerves, and account for the predilection of glomus tumors toward these anatomic sites.[82] The term *glomus* was mistakenly attached to these tumors when it was believed that their origin was similar to true glomus (arteriovenous) complexes, and though now recognized as inaccurate, the nomenclature has persisted.[83]

Although most glomus tumors appear to arise sporadically, there are reports of families with several members affected by glomus tumors, with an unusual *genomic imprinting* mode of inheritance.[84,85] In this manner of transmission, tumors only occur in the offspring of an affected female when there is transmittance of the gene through a carrier male, accounting for the observed tumor occurrence in "skipped" generations.[86]

A genetic marker for familial paragangliomas has been localized to chromosome 11, though a precise genetic cause has not been identified as of yet.[85] There is a clear predilection for these tumors to arise in females, and patients usually present after the fifth decade of life.[81–84,86,87]

Glomus tumors are typically reddish-purple, vascular, and lobulated masses. Histologically they resemble normal paraganglia with clusters of chief cells, characteristically termed *zellballen* (literally translated as "cell balls") in a highly vascular stroma. This pattern is enhanced on silver staining, which is useful diagnostically. Sustentacular cells and nerve axons, seen in the normal paraganglion, are rarely seen in the tumor, however.[88,89]

Glomus tumors contain the neural crest cell–derived chief cells, which are included in the diffuse neuroendocrine system (DNES). As a result, they have the potential to produce catecholamines, producing a physiologic response similar to pheochromocytomas. Fortunately, this is extremely rare, occurring in only 1 to 3% of glomus tumors.[83,89,90] Nevertheless, it is reasonable to perform preoperative evaluation for the presence of catecholamine-producing tumors in all patients, because life-threatening intraoperative hypertension is possible. Elevation of urine catecholamine levels (three to five times normal) requires differentiation from pheochromocytomas, and occasionally may require selective renal vein sampling for adequate diagnosis.[91]

Glomus tumors involving the temporal bone are divided into two categories based on their anatomic location. Other classification schemes further subdivide these tumors according to size and extent of invasion (**Table 24–3**).[91] Those arising along the course of Jacobson's nerve and involving primarily the tympanic cavity are termed *glomus tympanicum*. Paragangliomas arising from the dome of the jugular bulb and involving the jugular foramen and related structures are termed *glomus jugulare*. Both types are marked by slow, progressive growth, spreading via the pathways of least resistance, such as the temporal bone air-cell tracts, neural foramina, vascular channels, bony haversian systems, and the eustachian tube.[91–94] Advanced lesions of either type have the ability to invade cranial nerves.[95] However, the clinical presentation and operative management of each may be markedly different, and thus each is discussed individually. *Glomus vagale* tumors arise beneath the cranial base in proximity to cranial nerve X. A small minority of vagale tumors involve the temporal bone via retrograde spread through the jugular foramen.

The appearance of a paraganglioma on MRI reflects its highly vascular nature. Glomus tumors are isointense on T1-weighted images and brightly enhance with gadolinium. They typically possess numerous signal voids due to the numerous vascular channels within them. On T2-weighted images, they demonstrate increased signal intensity in the solid portions of the tumor with persistent flow void in the vascular portions.[24] Because paragangliomas can be multiple, some advocate that the imaging study should be carried down to the level of the carotid bifurcation to determine if multiple tumors exist.[96] Angiography is an additional important aspect of the evaluation of glomus tumors, but should be deferred until the preoperative period when both diagnostic and therapeutic (embolization) measures can be accomplished in a single study. The study allows the determination of arterial supply, degree of vascularity, degree of arteriovenous shunting, evidence of major venous sinus occlusion, and confirmation of the diagnosis another advantage of angiography is that it can single-handedly evaluate both the internal and external

Table 24–3 Classification Schemes for Glomus Tumors

Glasscock/Jackson Classification of Glomus Tumors	
Tumor	**Description**
Glomus tympanicum	
Type I	Small mass limited to the promontory
Type II	Tumor completely filling the middle ear space
Type III	Tumor filling the middle ear and extending into the mastoid
Type IV	Tumor filling the middle ear, extending into the mastoid or through the tympanic membrane to fill the external auditory canal; +/–internal carotid artery involvement
Glomus jugulare	
Type I	Small tumors involving the jugular bulb, middle ear, and mastoid
Type II	Tumor extending under the internal auditory canal; might have intracranial extension
Type III	Tumor extending into petrous apex; might have intracranial extension
Type IV	Tumor extending beyond petrous apex into clivus or infratemporal fossa; might have intracranial extension
Fisch Classification of Glomus Tumors	
Type A	Tumors limited to the middle ear cleft (Glomus tympanicum)
Type B	Tumors limited to the tympanomastoid area with no bone destruction in the infralabyrinthine compartment of the temporal bone
Type C	Tumors involving the infralabyrinthine compartment with extension into the petrous apex
Type D1	Tumors with intracranial extension ≤2 cm in diameter
Type D2	Tumors with intracranial extension >2 cm in diameter

Sources: Jackson CG. Skull base surgery. Am J Otol 1981;3:161–171; Oldring D, Fisch U. Glomus tumors of the temporal region: Surgical therapy. Am J Otol 1979;1:7–18. Reprinted by permission.

carotid systems for evidence of multiple early lesions. Embolization is usually performed at the time of angiography as a preoperative maneuver to limit surgical blood loss.[97,98] Magnetic resonance angiography and venography are newer modalities that can also aid in the diagnosis of vascular lesions of the temporal bone including glomus tumors. The role of these newer radiographic modalities in the evaluation of glomus tumors is currently being defined.[99]

Glomus Tympanicum

Glomus tympanicum is a paraganglioma that arises from the promontory of the middle ear. Because of the vascularity of these tumors, pulsatile tinnitus is often the first presenting symptom.[92] Further growth causes conductive hearing loss as ossicular mobility is inhibited, which occurs in approximately half of all patients.[91] Continued expansion may cause the glomus tympanicum to erode laterally through the drum, mimicking a friable, bleeding polyp, or it may expand medially causing facial nerve dysfunction, sensorineural hearing loss, or vertigo.[81–84,86,88–93] Rarely, it may present as a eustachian tube mass or epistaxis.[100,101] In one large series of 71 patients, presenting symptoms, in order of decreasing frequency, were pulsatile tinnitus (76%), hearing loss (conductive 52%, mixed 17%, sensorineural 5%), aural pressure/fullness (18%), vertigo/dizziness (9%), external canal bleeding (7%), and headache (4%).[93] *Brown's sign*, which consists of a pulsatile, purple-red middle ear mass that blanches with positive pneumatic otoscopy, is a frequently mentioned distinguishing sign but is of little clinical value.[102]

The differentiation between tympanicum and jugulare tumors is not always possible by physical examination alone because both lesions typically involve the middle ear.[91] Furthermore, other vascular lesions of the middle ear, such as an aberrant carotid artery or a high-riding jugular bulb, may mimic a glomus tumor, and thus radiographic evaluation prior to biopsy or surgical intervention is important.

Temporal bone CT can identify an intact plate of bone at the lateral aspect of the jugular fossa, indicating that a tumor is limited to the middle ear and aiding its identification as a glomus tympanicum. CT is also useful for evaluating the degree of bony erosion and the tumor's relationship to surrounding temporal bone structures.[91–93,95,96] MRI, although not as good evaluating bony changes within the temporal bone as CT, is superior in identifying the extent of the tumor and defining the relationship of tumor to surrounding structures once it has extended beyond the confines of the middle ear.[103] Angiography, although useful for larger lesions, is not required for small glomus tympanicum tumors limited to the middle ear.

Surgery is the principal mode of therapy for glomus tympanicum tumors. Patients with small lesions limited to the promontory that can be completely visualized by otoscopy and are confined to the mesotympanum on CT scan can be approached via a transcanal incision and a tympanomeatal flap to expose the middle ear. Larger lesions are best exposed postauricularly via an extended facial recess approach.[104] Using these methods, complete tumor removal can be achieved in greater than 90% of cases.[93] Lasers are often used to assist with resection of these vascular tumors.[105] Closure of the air–bone gap can be expected in a majority of patients, whereas about 10% suffer some sensorineural worsening.

Glomus Jugulare

Glomus jugulare tumors arise from paragangliomas situated near the dome of the jugular bulb or the proximal portions of Arnold's or Jacobson's nerves. In contrast to the small confines of the middle ear where growth of a glomus tympanicum causes early symptoms, growth of a tumor in the jugular foramen region may remain clinically silent for years. Patients may not seek medical attention until the tumor has caused dysfunction of the lower cranial nerves or grown into the middle ear causing symptoms similar to a glomus tympanicum

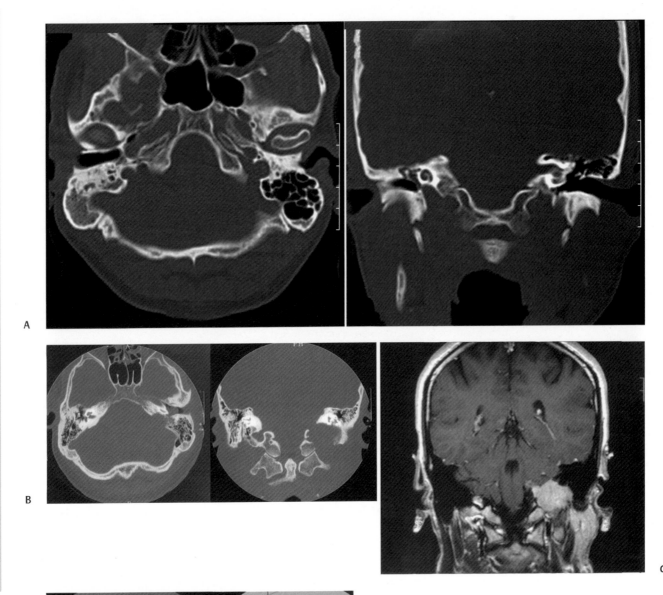

A

B

C

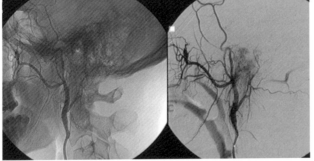

D

Figure 24–6 Glomus tumors. A glomus tympanicum **(A)** is limited to the middle ear space, typically arising on the promontory of the cochlea. The figure shows both the axial (left) and coronal (right) views, demonstrating opacification within the right middle ear space. A clear bony demarcation between the hypotympanum and jugular foramen/dome of the jugular bulb can be seen, which allows this tumor to be distinguished from a glomus jugulare. In contrast, a glomus jugulare **(B)** can erode through the hypotympanum, presenting in the middle ear in a similar fashion. However, in this case, the middle ear presentation is the "tip of the iceberg," as shown in axial (left) and coronal (right) CT images of this left glomus jugulare. A T1-weighted MRI scan from this patient is also shown **(C)**, demonstrating its intracranial extent. Preoperative angiography **(D)**, employed just prior to embolization to minimize blood loss in these highly vascular tumors, demonstrates the feeding vessels, often branches of the ascending pharyngeal artery.

(pulsatile tinnitus, hearing loss). Growth of the glomus jugulare may carry the tumor into the neck intraluminally within the jugular vein, into the lower reaches of the posterior cranial fossa, or proximally into the sigmoid or even transverse sinus[81,94] (**Fig. 24–6**). Middle fossa extension is rare, however.

Due to their proximity to the hearing apparatus, pulsatile tinnitus, hearing loss, otalgia, and aural fullness are the most frequent presenting symptoms.[93] Because cranial nerves IX to XI lie adjacent to the jugular bulb, they are frequently involved, as discovered upon the patient's clinical presentation, and lead to symptoms such as hoarseness and dysphagia.[87,90,91,93,106,107] Vertigo, facial weakness, and headache are additional presenting symptoms. The thin plate of bone separating the dome of the jugular bulb from the middle ear is frequently eroded by tumor, enabling access into the middle ear. This accounts for the finding of a middle ear mass or external auditory canal mass on exam in about 70% of patients, despite its origin within the jugular foramen.[93] Though a tenth cranial nerve deficit is the most commonly encountered cranial nerve deficit upon presentation (24% of cases), cranial nerves VII through XII are susceptible to injury depending on the size and location of the lesion.[66,87,90,91,93,106,107] Because cranial nerve XII is least likely to be involved with tumor, its dysfunction is usually indicative of more extensive disease.[66]

The radiographic appearance of a glomus jugulare is similar to the glomus tympanicum, yet there are a few important distinctions. As mentioned above, an intact plate of bone at the lateral aspect of the jugular fossa indicates that the tumor is limited to the middle ear and probably not a glomus jugulare. Further, the *carotid crest*, a vertically oriented triangular wedge of bone between the jugular bulb and the carotid artery, is often eroded with a glomus jugulare, a sign considered to be pathognomonic by many. Both of these findings can be demonstrated by high-resolution CT (**Fig. 24–6**). MRI is important to define the extent of tumor, particularly intracranially (posterior fossa) and extracranially (upper neck), and assists with surgical planning. The tumor appearance is similar to a glomus tympanicum, though generally much more extensive.

Angiography is also very important during the evaluation of glomus jugulare and its vascular supply (**Fig. 24–6**). Because an angiogram is needed immediately prior to surgical resection with embolization of the feeding vessels, the angiogram should be held off until just prior to surgery to avoid the need for a second angiogram. The tumor's primary arterial supply generally comes from the ascending pharyngeal artery. Lager tumors may also receive branches from the internal carotid system (caroticotympanic) or the vertebral-basilar system. These large vascular lesions also commonly involve the sigmoid sinus and inferior petrosal sinus. The intrapetrous carotid genu is usually eroded in larger lesions though it may also become occluded. Blood loss during tumor resection can be significant; thus preoperative embolization can help with intraoperative hemostasis. Angiography can also aid in determining the amount of contralateral blood flow to the brain, and provide an indication of whether the carotid artery can be sacrificed without the risk of inducing an infarct, though this topic is controversial and not without pitfalls.[91,107]

Treatment of the glomus jugulare can be complicated due to its origin in a surgically difficult location and its ability to involve a variety of critical neurovascular structures. Further, some argue that equal results can be obtained treating these lesions with either surgery or radiation therapy. Reports suggest, however, that with contemporary techniques there is an acceptably low disability rate following surgical resection, with a low probability of tumor recurrence and a good quality of life.[93,94,107–109] Depending on the size and location of the tumor, it may be approached either by a canal-wall-up or canal-wall-down mastoidectomy, an infratemporal fossa approach, a translabyrinthine approach, a transcochlear approach, or a combination of any of the above. The transjugular approach,

consisting of a lateral craniotomy conducted through a partial petrosectomy traversing the jugular fossa combined with resection of the sigmoid sinus and jugular bulb, which often have been occluded by disease, is another popular approach.[110] Because larger tumors tend to infiltrate cranial nerves, larger tumors are associated with a higher incidence of postoperative neural deficits.[106] One of the key surgical principles involves exposing the jugular fossa and gaining control of the vessels above and below the lesion. Facial nerve rerouting may be required for larger tumors with evidence of carotid erosion, though a majority of tumors can be resected with the facial nerve left in situ using the fallopian bridge technque.[68] Surgical complications most commonly include CSF leak (12%) and aspiration (5%).[93] New postoperative lower cranial deficits as a result of surgery occur in approximately one fourth to one half of cases.[68] In many of these cases, rehabilitation with speech therapy, vocal cord medialization procedures, and facial nerve reanimation techniques can offer adequate functional outcomes.

Radiation therapy is advocated in some centers as a first-line therapy for advanced glomus jugulare tumors or advanced patient age.[111–116] One review of 24 published series suggested that the difference in treatment failures between surgery and radiation was less than 10%.[117] However, lack of sufficient follow-up data as well as a bias toward the inclusion of inoperable tumors receiving radiation may bias these conclusions. Further, there does not exist an adequately controlled clinical trial comparing the two modalities, though limited studies comparing both modalities do exist.[113] The possibility of a rare but lethal radiation-induced tumor of the temporal bone must also be factored into the clinical decision to use this modality.[118] Thus, although most agree that radiation is indicated for incompletely resected tumors or those with positive surgical margins, the superiority of either modality still remains in question, and treatment must be individualized.

Having presented the advantages and disadvantages of surgery versus gamma knife/fractionated stereotactic radiotherapy for glomus jugulare, the issue can be more clearly stated: If you were 60+-years old with a 5 cm tumor eroding the base of skull, filling the middle ear, extending anteriorly toward the carotid artery and eustachian tube, but not (yet) affecting the VII, IX, or X cranial nerves, what would you do? A traditional surgical approach would be translabyrinthine-transcochlear with anterior re-routing of the facial nerve, intra/extraluminal packing of the lateral sinus, ligation of the internal jugular vein, and systematic removal of all tumor following primarily the course of the internal carotid artery. When the tumor in the jugular bulb is removed, packing the petrosal sinuses must be tight to insure hemostasis, which in turn can traumatize nerves IX-XI. For the sake of discussion, we will ignore issues of reconstructing the wound. In most cases, the patient is deaf (and temporarily dizzy), with a temporary facial paralysis which will never return completely to normal, often vocal palsy/paralysis and dysphagia with risk of possible aspiration pneumonia, and reduced mobility of the shoulder. Moreover, despite perioperative embolization, hemorrhage and multiple transfusions can be dramatic, and not infrequently some tumor is left behind.

One distinction which supports surgery is to operate on those patients who preoperatively already have lower cranial nerve deficits (Mario Sanna, M.D., personal communication. At the time of this writing he is doing more glomus jugulare surgery than anyone else worldwide). Another approach to

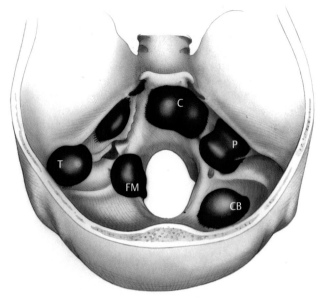

Figure 24–7 Meningioma of skull base. This illustration demonstrates common areas of meningioma occurrence within the skull base that may impinge on the temporal bone. These include the posterior petrous pyramid (P), tentorium (T), clivus (C), cerebellum (CB), or foramen magnum (FM).

contributing veins, at neural foramina, and from arachnoid cells anywhere along the arachnoid membrane[122] (**Fig. 24–7**). The etiology of meningiomas remains uncertain, though an association with progesterone levels and breast cancer has been demonstrated.[123] Genetically, cytogenetic losses on chromosomes 1, 7, 10, and 14 and telomerase activation have been observed in clinically aggressive meningiomas, whereas monosomy 22 has been shown to be a common early molecular event in tumor formation.[120] Several candidate growth regulatory genes have been identified, including the NF2 gene *merlin*, tumor suppressor in lung cancer-1 *(TSLC1)*, protein 4.1B, and *p53/MDM2* and *S6-kinase* genes.[120] Meningiomas have a clear association with NF2, and it has been estimated that one fifth of adolescents with a meningioma have NF2. There is also a four times higher incidence of meningiomas in patients who have received radiation therapy to the head.[124]

Meningiomas almost always involve the temporal bone secondarily due to spread from an adjacent region.[121,125–127] Most reports of primary middle ear meningiomas date from before the era of modern imaging when it was difficult to distinguish the point of origin.[119,122–127] It is thus likely that many of these older reports actually described intracranial meningiomas that secondarily invaded the structures of the temporal bone.[128] Today, the vast majority demonstrably have a dural origin, with several potential pathways to the middle ear. Those meningiomas that have been described as arising primarily from within the temporal bone were believed to arise from the internal auditory meatus and canal, the jugular foramen, the geniculate ganglion, and the sulcus of the greater and lesser superficial petrosal nerves.[119,122–127] Extratemporal meningiomas are far more common, and usually originate at the CPA attached to the posterior surface of the petrous pyramid. Tumors arising in this location account for up to 7 to 12% of all meningiomas.[121,129] In decreasing frequency, the other sites of origin of extratemporal meningiomas are the tentorium, clivus, cerebellar convexity, and foramen magnum. A majority of these extratemporal meningiomas of the posterior fossa arise from the porus acusticus or adjacent to the superior petrosal sinus.[122] Once an extratemporal meningioma has invaded the temporal bone, additional spread is common; about 40% will have spread extratemporally into the nasopharynx, retromaxillary space, retromandibular space, cervical space, parapharyngeal space, sphenoid sinus, pterygopalatine fossa, or the orbit.[122] Rarely, a meningioma will reside entirely within the IAC, mimicking an AN in both its clinical and radiographic presentation.[127,130]

Meningiomas tend to be lobulated, tough, white-gray masses that are well circumscribed and indent the adjacent

management is to debulk those portions of tumor which do not incur cranial nerve deficits to attain a size more easily treated by gamma knife. Finally, a reasonable option is to treat the entire tumor with gamma knife or fractionated stereotactic radiosurgery to hopefully prevent tumor growth and postpone deficits. In this latter option, the main issue is timing of radiation therapy, which remains controversial.

This management dilemma is hotly debated by many experienced neurotologists. Quality of life issues have swayed *many* former surgeons toward radiation therapy.

◆ Meningioma

Meningiomas, the second most common brain tumors in adults, accounting for up to one fifth of all intracranial neoplasms, are the second most common tumor of the central nervous system (CNS) after gliomas.[119,120] In spite of this prevalence, they account for only 10% of the tumors involving the CPA.[121] These slow-growing, benign tumors are growths of dural fibroblasts, pial cells, and arachnoid villi. They preferentially arise along the major venous sinuses and their

Table 24–4 World Health Organization (WHO) Classification of Meningiomas

Grade 1	Grade 2	Grade 3
Meningothelial meningioma	Chordoid meningioma	Papillary meningioma
Fibrous (fibroblastic) meningioma	Clear cell meningioma	Rhabdoid meningioma
Transitional (mixed) meningioma	Atypical meningioma	Anaplastic meningioma
Psammomatous meningioma		
Angiomatous meningioma		
Microcystic meningioma		
Secretory meningioma		
Lymphoplasmacyte-rich meningioma		
Metaplastic meningioma		

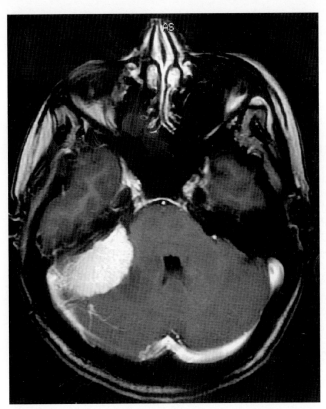

Figure 24–8 A large cerebellopontine angle meningioma, as demonstrated by this axial, T1-weighted MRI scan with gadolinium enhancement. The tumor shows characteristic features of a meningioma, including dural "tails."

nervous tissue, often growing "en-plaque" to cover a wide surface of the cranial base. Hyperostosis of the adjacent skull or penetration into adjacent bone is sometimes found. Histologically, four subcategories can be identified. *Syncytial* or *meningotheliomatous* lesions (55%) consist of an irregular arrangement of epithelial-like cells with abundant cytoplasm. *Fibroblastic* lesions (15%) demonstrate palisading spindle cells with interwoven reticulin collagen fibers and occasional psammoma bodies. *Transitional* tumors (30%) have features of both with prominent psammoma bodies, whereas *angioblastic* tumors (5%) are highly cellular with poorly defined cell cytoplasm.[129-131] The World Health Organization has recently come up with a grading scale that has become widely implemented (**Table 24–4**).

Meningiomas involving the temporal bone, in keeping with other meningiomas, affect women by a ratio of 2:1 and commonly are diagnosed in the middle and later decades of life.[122] The symptoms at presentation, in order of decreasing frequency, are progressive hearing loss, headaches, vertigo, tinnitus, otorrhea, otalgia, facial weakness or loss of taste, diplopia or visual disturbances, dysphagia, dysarthria, dysphonia, nausea and vomiting, facial pain or paresthesias, exophthalmos, lower limb hemiparesis or paraparesis, and periauricular swelling or neck mass.[122,127] Meningiomas may also gain access to the middle ear, mimicking an otitis media with a hyperemic tympanic membrane, granulation tissue, facial nerve involvement, and conductive hearing loss. In contrast to patients with an AN, who uniformly present with hearing loss, only 60% of patients with meningiomas involving the temporal bone present with hearing loss.[132] For meningiomas primarily involving the jugular foramen, the chief presenting symptoms and signs are pulsatile tinnitus, a middle ear mass, and dysfunction of the lower cranial nerves manifesting as hoarseness, dysphagia, and dysarthria.[133]

MRI with gadolinium is currently the most effective radiologic study for diagnosis, as it differentiates meningiomas from the more common ANs (**Fig. 24–8**). On T1-weighted images, meningiomas are isointense to slightly hypointense in relation to surrounding brain tissue. Their appearance on T2-weighted images is highly variable, though they tend to be less intense than ANs. There is moderate enhancement with gadolinium.[134] Whereas ANs tend to involve the entire IAC, forming an acute angle with the posterior surface of the petrous bone, meningiomas tend to be broad based, project asymmetrically into the IAC, and occasionally have calcifications or cystic changes and a dural "tail" sign.[135,136] If the MRI appearance is suspicious for a highly vascular tumor, then angiography with embolization is indicated, and also helps to differentiate a meningioma from a glomus tumor.[133] High-resolution CT may be of value in determining bony involvement.[137-139]

Although meningiomas are benign tumors, they are locally destructive and have the ability to invade cranial nerves. Surgical excision, therefore, is the treatment of choice. Conservative management may be selected in smaller lesions, in the elderly, or in those unable to tolerate surgical excision. The surgical approach is determined by several factors, including the size, the location relative to other critical neurovascular structures, and the status of hearing. The propensity of meningiomas to spread within the osseous haversian canals necessitates a surgical resection of adjacent bone to ensure tumor eradication. Surgical routes employed vary according to the anatomic peculiarities of each tumor, and include the middle fossa, suboccipital, translabyrinthine, transcochlear, and combined translabyrinthine-suboccipital approaches.[129] Hearing preservation is much more likely in CPA meningiomas as compared with ANs. Therefore, a labyrinth-sparing procedure is chosen for CPA meningiomas when the hearing is good, regardless of the tumor size. Hearing preservation is successful in about one third of meningiomas.[140] The role of radiotherapy is controversial.[141-143] Though there is an increasing trend to use radiotherapy as a primary treatment modality, it is more commonly used following a subtotal tumor resection.[143,144] Stereotaxic photon-beam radiosurgery, or "gamma-knife," is also being increasingly used as a viable treatment option for skull base meningiomas.[141,145,146]

Because meningiomas tend to invade cranial nerves and encircle other critical neurovascular structures, complete excision is often difficult. Even with gross total resection, recurrence rates approach 30% in some series.[147] Long-term follow-up is thus warranted after tumor extirpation with periodic radiologic evaluation.

◆ Adenomatous Tumors

Adenomatous tumors involving the temporal bone are rare lesions.[148] In the medical literature prior to the 1990s, all adenomatous tumors of the middle ear and temporal bone were grouped together, making historical comparisons difficult. Two distinct clinical and histopathologic subtypes have since been identified: a *mixed pleomorphic cell* pattern and a *papillary* pattern.[149] *Carcinoid* tumors are also recognized by some as a distinct clinical subtype of adenomatous tumors, though others group these tumors with the mixed pleomorphic cell type. Adenomatous tumors also include some lesions that have previously been reported as "ceruminomas," an ambiguous and misleading term used to describe a diverse group of glandular tumors of the middle ear and mastoid.[150]

Mixed Pleomorphic Cell Pattern (Mucosal Adenoma)

Mixed tumors are the more common and benign of the two major subtypes of adenomas and are always confined to the middle ear and mastoid. This pattern demonstrates acinar, solid, trabecular, and carcinoid-like histopathologic features. Some bone involvement is always seen and cholesteatoma or inflammation is nearly always present. Rarely, the otic capsule or facial nerve may be involved. These tumors are believed to arise from the poorly differentiated basement membrane cells within the normal mucosa of the middle ear, promontory, and eustachian tube.[149–151]

The majority of patients with mixed pleomorphic tumors of the middle ear are male, and typically present between the ages of 20 and 60. These tumors are commonly diagnosed preoperatively as chronic otitis media. Rarely, they have been reported to involve the adjacent posterior fossa.[152] Conductive hearing loss is often present as a result of tumor growth occluding the sound transducing mechanism, whereas otorrhea, facial nerve weakness, and tinnitus are variably present. Examination typically demonstrates a soft tissue middle ear mass. High-resolution CT scans conform to the clinical exam, and usually demonstrate a soft tissue middle ear and mastoid mass without associated bone destruction.

Because these lesions are commonly confused with chronic otitis media, the diagnosis is often made intraoperatively during a mastoidectomy and tympanoplasty. Despite the benign implication of their diagnosis, however, the mixed pleomorphic pattern tumors have a high likelihood of recurrence, with the ability to invade bone and soft tissue. Thus, complete surgical resection is necessary for cure, and long-term follow-up is mandatory to evaluate for recurrence.[151]

Papillary Pattern (Endolymphatic Sac Adenoma)

Adenomatous tumors with a papillary pattern are rarer and more aggressive lesions.[148] Historically, these lesions have also been called endolymphatic sac tumors, Heffner's tumors, low-grade papillary adenocarcinoma, and aggressive papillary middle ear tumors. In contrast to their more benign counterpart, these papillary neoplasms typically demonstrate adjacent bone invasion and extension into the petrous apex. Involvement of the facial nerve and middle or posterior cranial fossa dura is also commonly seen.[149,151,153–155] The tumors have been traditionally believed to arise in the endolymphatic sac, with subsequent extension into the posterior fossa and endolymphatic duct, providing access to the vestibule, mastoid process, and retrofacial air cells and facial nerve.[156,157] Histologically, these tumors are composed of a single- to double-layered epithelial lining with a variable cytoplasm and hyalinization. All papillary tumors invade adjacent bone and demonstrate glandular features that suggest the origin is from endolymphatic sac.[149,151,156–158]

Clinically, these tumors may behave aggressively and have a lethal potential. There is a female preponderance, and patients usually present at between 20 and 60 years of age. Symptoms at presentation include hearing loss and facial nerve paralysis, vertigo, and tinnitus.[89] On high-resolution CT scanning, the lesions are typically located near the vestibular aqueduct, centered between the sigmoid sinus and the IAC. Involvement of the IAC, jugular bulb, and mastoid is common, as is erosion of the bone toward the vestibule of the labyrinth (**Fig. 24–9**).[149,151,156]

Treatment is primarily surgical, with complete excision and adequate margins the surgical goal. This is usually accomplished via a translabyrinthine approach, which removes the dura, jugular bulb, and any involved cranial nerves.[159] Postoperative radiation is controversial because there is still debate about whether the tumor is malignant or benign and whether it displays clinical and pathologic features of both. With gross total surgical removal, a 90% cure rate has been reported. When radiation therapy is used after incomplete tumor extirpation, only 50% respond, though the numbers reported are very small and not statistically valid.[149,151,156,159]

Carcinoid Tumor

Although some believe that all carcinoid tumors of the middle ear should be classified as mixed pleomorphic adenomatous tumors, others consider them to be a unique histopathologic subtype of adenomatous tumors.[160–162] The first case was reported in 1980 by Murphy et al,[163] and less than 20 additional cases have been reported since then.[160,161,164–168] Carcinoid tumors are slow-growing but locally invasive lesions found in the middle ear. These rare lesions are believed to arise from the enterochromaffin cells of the endocrine system, and thus have the ability to secrete a variety of peptide hormones. Unlike similar lesions in other parts of the body, however, middle ear carcinoid tumors do not secrete large amounts of these hormones and thus are not associated with the systemic manifestations of carcinoid syndrome, such as flushing, wheezing, abdominal cramps, and diarrhea.[162]

Histologically, the tumors demonstrate ribbons and cords of trabecular, cuboidal cells. Argyrophil staining is positive in 80% of cases. Immunohistochemical stains are positive for cytokeratin AE-1, AE-3, serotonin, and neuron-specific enolase. Electron microscopy shows neurosecretory granules.[162]

Tumors present in both sexes between the second and sixth decades. Patients typically present with conductive hearing loss and the feeling of ear blockage. Tinnitus and transient facial paresis have also been described. Examination often demonstrates an intact but bulging drum. However, in less than half of all cases will a middle ear mass actually be seen. CT scan is useful for identifying the extent of middle ear involvement, as well as the status of the ossicles and facial nerve. Bony erosion or destruction is never seen.[160–162,164–168]

Definitive therapy involves complete tumor excision. Because the ossicles are frequently enveloped by tumor, which may extend into the mastoid, the surgeon should be prepared to perform a tympanomastoidectomy and ossicular reconstruction concurrently. With adequate excision, recurrence is unlikely. The role of radiotherapy is controversial, and currently is only considered after incomplete tumor excision or when the tumor has spread beyond the middle ear and mastoid.[162]

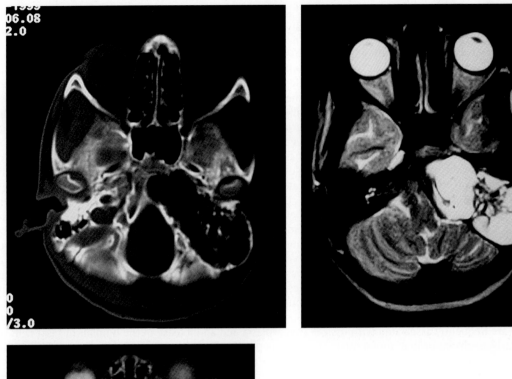

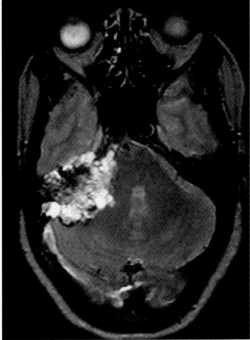

Figure 24–9 An endolymphatic sac adenoma, which has also been classified as a low-grade adenocarcinoma, can be locally destructive. A CT **(A)** and MRI **(B)** demonstrate a large endolymphatic sac tumor in the same patient that was locally destructive but not invasive. An MRI scan demonstrates a right-sided endolymphatic sac tumor from another patient **(C)**.

Glandular Tumors of the External Auditory Canal

The general term *ceruminoma* has been applied to a diverse spectrum of tumors originating from the glandular structures of the external auditory canal. The rarity of these lesions has contributed to this use of one term for different tumors. The most extensive review of the topic comprises only 32 cases over a 32-year period.[150] In fact, these tumors represent a variety of glandular tumors ranging from benign to malignant. The benign tumors include *ceruminomous adenomas,* similar to the mixed-pleomorphic pattern of the middle ear; *pleomorphic adenomas,* which are salivary gland choristomas (see below); and *cylindromas,* which are exceedingly rare tumors arising from the pilosebaceous units of the external canal.[150]

One study evaluating the ultrastructure of these tumors demonstrated apocrine caps, microvilli, cell junctions, secretory granules, vacuoles, lipid droplets, and siderosomes, which are the characteristic features of apocrine glands.[169] Presentation of the benign ceruminomous adenoma typically includes external auditory canal obstruction with hearing loss. Treatment for benign tumors includes conservative local excision with a skin graft to the operative site. Radiotherapy is not necessary.[150]

Choristomas

Choristoma is the pathologic term given to a benign cohesive mass of aberrant tissue or scattered cells in an inappropriate anatomic location. It is an extremely rare lesion in the temporal bone.[170] Although most reports are of salivary gland choristomas, neural and sebaceous choristomas have also been described.[171–174] It has been postulated that salivary gland tissue becomes trapped during fusion of the tympanic, mastoid, and squamous portions of the temporal bone, leading to the formation of salivary choristomas.[172,174] Neural rests of tissue are believed to gain access to the middle ear via Hyrtl's (tympanomeningeal) fissures during development, giving rise to the less common neural choristoma.[171–173]

Microscopically, choristomas of the middle ear are characterized by well-formed serous and mucous acini arranged randomly or in a lobular formation. Mucinous microcysts and fibroadipose tissue components have also been described.[170] Macroscopically, the tumors are lobulated and firm. Occasionally the tumor is attached to the middle ear by a fine stalk.

Choristomas have been reported in patients ranging in age from 5 to 52 years and there is no sex predilection. They are typically unilateral, although bilateral involvement has been reported. Choristomas typically arise in the posterosuperior tympanum, though they may vary in size and fill the entire tympanic cavity.[170] They are frequently associated with ossicular anomalies, particularly an absent or malformed incus or stapes, and facial nerve dehiscence or displacement is also common.[175] Because of this frequent association, a second branchial arch embryologic etiology has been proposed.[176]

Although tumors have been described in all ages, they typically present in the first two decades.[174] These benign tumors grow slowly and tend to produce few symptoms other than a conductive hearing loss in the affected ear, correlating with the degree of ossicular involvement. CT typically demonstrates a middle ear mass lesion without bony erosion. Angiography fails to demonstrate a tumor blush typically seen with vascular tumors of this region, further aiding in their differentiation.

Treatment is determined by the size and location of the tumor. Small tumors or those attached solely by a thin stalk may be readily excised. Larger or broad-based tumors, however, must be approached with a degree of caution. Because of its frequent association with the facial nerve, temporary or permanent palsy has been reported postoperatively in 25% of cases after tumor resection.[175] Attempts at ossiculoplasty to correct the conductive hearing loss have yielded success in approximately two thirds of cases. Because there is often little to no tumor growth over time and there is no reported evidence of malignant degeneration, conservative management with serial examinations is acceptable in those wishing to forgo surgery.

◆ Hemangiomas and Vascular Malformations

Historically, the literature on benign vascular tumors has lacked a rational or consistent nomenclature, and has contributed to widespread misunderstanding of these lesions.[177] The term hemangioma has historically been used to describe any vascular lesion, and is commonly preceded by descriptive but confusing and unhelpful terms such as strawberry, cavernous, and capillary. In 1982 a new system of classification of vascular tumors was developed based on the clinical behavior and growth characteristics of these lesions. The classification groups vascular tumors under two categories, hemangiomas and vascular malformations.[178] Hemangiomas usually present during the first month of life, and are characterized by a rapid growth period (proliferative phase) followed by a slow period of involution. Hemangiomas are further categorized on the basis of depth within the dermis, as cutaneous (entirely within papillary dermis), subcutaneous (into the reticular dermis or subcutaneous fat), or compound (containing elements of both).[178,179] In contrast, vascular malformations are always present at birth, and grow in proportion to body growth without regression. They can be arterial, capillary, venous, lymphatic, or any combination of these. Some authors have further divided these vascular malformations into low-flow lesions (venous malformations) and high-flow lesions (arteriovenous malformations).[177]

Unfortunately, the otologic literature does not differentiate between these two types of lesions, making clinical comparisons difficult.[180] To add a further element of confusion, some authors have reported that vascular lesions of the temporal bone frequently contain elements of both hemangiomas and vascular malformations.[181] However, a majority of the vascular lesions of the temporal bones are probably not hemangiomas but rather subcategories of vascular malformations. Histologically, hemangiomas are characterized by endothelial hyperplasia and an increase in the number of mast cells during the proliferative phase, followed by fibrosis, fatty infiltration, decreased cellularity, and normalization of the mast cell count during involution of the lesion. In contrast, vascular malformations are collections of abnormal vessels with normal endothelium and mast cell counts.[177] Using these histologic criteria, the term cavernous hemangioma, frequently used to describe lesions in the otologic literature, is more appropriately classified as a vascular malformation. Alternatively, the term capillary hemangioma probably describes a true hemangioma, but as Glasscock[182] has pointed out, this has not been reported in the temporal bone.[180,183]

Vascular malformations of the temporal bone are rare entities, composing less than 1% of all temporal bone tumors.[1,184] The overwhelming majority of these lesions present within the IAC or at the geniculate ganglion.[184–187] Rarely, they may arise within the middle ear or external auditory canal.[181–184,188–192] Tumor predilection for this region is believed to be due to the extensive blood supply surrounding Scarpa's ganglion and the geniculate ganglion. A majority of tumors are smaller than 1 cm at the time of presentation.[181–184,193]

Patients typically present after the third decade of life. When the geniculate ganglion is the site of origin, a seventh cranial nerve dysfunction (weakness and/or twitch) is nearly always present. Overall, facial nerve dysfunction is present in about 80% of temporal bone vascular malformations, and is usually the reason patients seek medical attention.[184] Other symptoms noted on clinical presentation include tinnitus, conductive hearing loss (more commonly with geniculate ganglion malformations), progressive sensorineural hearing loss (more commonly with IAC tumors), and vertigo.[184,185,194]

Radiographically, high-resolution CT and MRI define the lesion and provide complementary information. MRI demonstrates all tumors within the IAC and some tumors near the geniculate.[185] The lesions appear hyperintense on T2-weighted images, and tend to be more hyperintense than acoustic schwannomas.[184,194,195] Some geniculate ganglion lesions are difficult to visualize on MRI, but intratumoral calcium can be detected on high-resolution CT.[195] Venous malformations of the geniculate region may be differentiated from other temporal bone tumors based on radiographic appearances. A focal, enhancing lesion of the geniculate ganglion that is sessile on the middle fossa floor, erodes bone diffusely, has irregular margins, and contains flecks of calcification is most likely a meningioma. Facial nerve schwannomas typically cause smoothly marginated expansion and tend to be less focal, extending along the fallopian canal longitudinally.

The treatment of choice is surgical excision, with removal by drill of normal bony margins. The choice of surgical approach depends on the tumor location and size, but a middle fossa, transmastoid, or translabyrinthine approach is commonly employed. Because of the destructive nature of these benign tumors, intratemporal facial nerve grafting is frequently required. Facial nerve repairs are more often required for geniculate vascular malformations than for those originating within the IAC.[181,184,185,194,195] When facial paralysis is of recent origin, or partial function remains, the native facial nerve can often be preserved. In long-standing complete palsies, however, a graft is almost always required.

Surgery is generally successful at eradicating lesions, with a low likelihood of recurrence after complete excision. Results of facial nerve function following repair are good (House-Brackmann grade 2–4/6) except when nerve repair is delayed more than 1 year from the onset of the palsy.[181,184,194,195] For patients undergoing middle fossa or transmastoid procedures, approximately two thirds can expect postoperative hearing preservation to within 10 dB of preoperative speech thresholds.[181]

◆ Langerhans' Cell Histiocytosis (Eosinophilic Granuloma)

Langerhans' cell histiocytosis, previously referred to as histiocytosis X and reticuloendotheliosis, may occur in solitary or multiple forms. The diffuse disease spectrum comprises three clinical entities. *Eosinophilic granuloma* is the most mild form, and consists of multifocal bony erosions limited to the skull, long bones, ribs, vertebrae, pelvis, maxilla, and mandible.[196,197] *Hand-Schüller-Christian syndrome* and *Letterer-Siwe disease* are the more chronic and severe forms of Langerhans' cell histiocytosis, respectively, and are both marked by multiorgan involvement.[198] The underlying pathology in all three diseases is proliferating Langerhans' cells, a histiocyte involved in cell-mediated immunity, osteoclastic activity, and eosinophilic infiltration.[196] It is unknown what causes the abnormal proliferation or even whether the Langerhans' cells are normal or pathologic. Proposed theories for the genesis of the disease cite metabolic, genetic, infectious, neoplastic, and immunologic causes.[196–199]

The eosinophilic granuloma consists of a soft friable red mass containing histiocytes, eosinophils, lymphocytes, plasma cells, and multinucleated giant cells. The presence of histiocytes, with characteristic Birbeck granules (trilaminar rod-shapes organelles within the nuclear cytoplasm) seen under electron microscopy is considered diagnostic.[196]

Solitary eosinophilic granuloma most commonly appears in children over 5 years of age and in young adults, in contrast to the more severe systemic forms of Langerhans' cell histiocytosis, which tend to occur in infants and young children.[196] Temporal bone lesions have been described within the lateral mastoid and the petrous apex, and may also involve the entire temporal bone. Otologic involvement in Langerhans' cell histiocytosis has been estimated from 15 to 61% of patients, and may be the sole presenting symptom in 5 to 25% of

children.[200,201] The lesions typically present as a painful postauricular soft tissue swelling. Otorrhea, granulation tissue within the external auditory canal, and otitis externa are also common at presentation, making differentiation from routine chronic otitis media difficult.[197,202] Conductive hearing loss by either soft tissue obstruction or, less commonly, ossicular erosion may also be present. Sensorineural hearing loss from destruction of the bony labyrinth has also been described.[200] Facial palsy may be associated with the more severe forms of Langerhans' cell histiocytosis in about 3% of cases.[203]

Skull and plain radiographs demonstrate destructive, osteolytic lesions of the temporal bone, which is commonly mistaken for suppurative mastoiditis, cholesteatoma, or a metastatic osteolytic lesion.[200] A CT scan reveals a destructive lesion and is helpful in demarcating the areas of temporal bone involvement. On MRI, the lesion is usually hypointense on T1- and T2-weighted images, but highlights with gadolinium.[197]

Once the diagnosis is made, treatment consists of conservative curettage, followed by low-dose radiotherapy.[197,200] Intralesional steroid injections have also been successful in some reported cases.[204] When there is multisystem involvement, chemotherapy and intravenous steroids are advocated.[197]

When the disease is limited to the temporal bone, the eosinophilic granuloma typically resolves after local excision or radiation without recurrence.[201] Surgery usually consists of curetting the bony cavity created by the tumor. However, the disease may progress to a more disseminated form, and thus close follow-up observation is warranted.[197] With multisystem, nonosseous involvement, the prognosis is much poorer, with mortality reported at about 40%.[200]

References

1. Brackmann DE, Bartels LJ. Rare tumors of the cerebellopontine angle. Otolaryngol Head Neck Surg 1980;88:555–559
2. Mahaley MS Jr, Mettlin C, Natarajan N, Laws ER Jr, Peace BB. Analysis of patterns of care of brain tumor patients in the United States: a study of the Brain Tumor Section of the AANS and the CNS and the Commission on Cancer of the ACS. Clin Neurosurg 1990;36:347–352
3. Ahn MS, Jackler RK, Lustig LR. The early history of the neurofibromatosis. Evolution of the concept of neurofibromatosis type 2. Arch Otolaryngol Head Neck Surg 1996;122:1240–1249
4. Selesnick S, Jackler R, Pitts L. The changing clinical presentation of acoustic tumors in the MRI era. Laryngoscope 1993;103:431–436
5. Lin D, Hegarty JL, Fischbein NJ, Jackler RK. The prevalence of "incidental" acoustic neuroma. Arch Otolaryngol Head Neck Surg 2005;131:241–244
6. Sterkers J, Perre J, Viala P, Foncin J. The origin of acoustic neuromas. Acta Otolaryngol 1987;103:427–431
7. Xenellis JE, Linthicum FH Jr. On the myth of the glial/Schwann junction (Obersteiner-Redlich zone): origin of vestibular nerve schwannomas. Otol Neurotol 2003;24:1
8. Jackler R. Acoustic neuroma (vestibular schwannoma). In: Jackler R, Brackmann D, eds. Neurotology. St. Louis: Mosby, 1994:729–785
9. Seizinger BR, Martuza RL, Gusella JF. Loss of genes on chromosome 22 in tumorigenesis of human acoustic neuroma. Nature 1986;322: 644–647
10. Wolff R, Frazer K, Jackler R, Lanser M, Pitts L. Analysis of chromosome 22 deletions in neurofibromatosis type 2-related tumors. Am J Hum Genet 1992;51:478–485
11. Lanser M, Sussman S, Frazer K. Epidemiology, pathogenesis, and genetics of acoustic tumors. Otolaryngol Clin North Am 1992;25:499–520
12. Gronholm M, Teesalu T, Tyynela J, et al. Characterization of the NF2 protein merlin and the ERM protein ezrin in human, rat, and mouse central nervous system. Mol Cell Neurosci 2005;28:683–693
13. Rong R, Tang X, Gutmann DH, Ye K. Neurofibromatosis 2 (NF2) tumor suppressor merlin inhibits phosphatidylinositol 3-kinase through binding to PIKE-L. Proc Natl Acad Sci U S A 2004;101:18200–18205
14. Kuo T, Blevins N, Jackler R. Are acoustic neuromas encapsulated tumors? Otolaryngol Head Neck Surg 1997;117:606–609
15. Rutka JADG. Controversies in the histopathology of acoustic neuromas and their biological behavior. In: Tos M, Thomsen J, eds. Proceedings of

the first international conference on acoustic neuroma. Amsterdam: Kugler, 1992:199–202

16. Hebbar G, McKenna M, Linthicum F. Immunohistochemical localization of vimentin and s-100 antigen in small acoustic tumors and adjacent cochlear nerves. Am J Otol 1990;11:310–313

17. Nager G. Acoustic neuromas: Pathology and differential diagnosis. Arch Otolaryngol 1969;89:252–279

18. Nedzelski J, Schessel D, Pfleiderer A, Kassel E, Rowed D. Conservative management of acoustic neuroms. Otolaryngol Clin North Am 1992;25:691–705

19. Bederson J, von Ammon K, Wichmann W, Yasargil M. Conservative treatment of patients with acoustic tumors. Neurosurgery 1991;28:646–651

20. Caye-Thomasen P, Werther K, Nalla A, et al. VEGF and VEGF receptor-1 concentration in vestibular schwannoma homogenates correlates to tumor growth rate. Otol Neurotol 2005;26:98–101

21. Kanzaki J, Ogawa K, Ogawa S, et al. Audiological findings in acoustic neuroma. Acta Otolaryngol Suppl 1991;487:125–132

22. Wilson D, Hodgson R, Gustafson M, Hogue S, Mills L. The sensitivity of auditory brainstem response testing in small acoustic neuromas. Laryngoscope 1992;102:961–964

23. Weiss M, Kisiel D, Bhatia P. Predictive value of brainstem evoked response in the diagnosis of acoustic neuroma. Otolaryngol Head Neck Surg 1990;103:583–585

24. Hasso AN, Ledington JA. Imaging modalities for the study of the temporal bone. Otolaryngol Clin North Am 1988;21:219–244

25. Breger R, Papke R, Pojunas K, Haughton V, Williams A, Daniels D. Benign extraaxial tumors: contrast enhancement with Gd-DTPA. Radiology 1987;163:427–429

26. Shin YJ, Fraysse B, Cognard C, et al. Effectiveness of conservative management of acoustic neuromas. Am J Otol 2000;21:857–862

27. Raut VV, Walsh RM, Bath AP, et al. Conservative management of vestibular schwannomas—second review of a prospective longitudinal study. Clin Otolaryngol 2004;29:505–514

28. Jackler R, Pitts L. Selection of surgical approach to acoustic neuroma. Otolaryngol Clin North Am 1992;25:361–387

29. Colletti V, Fiorino F. Middle fossa versus retrosigmoid-transmeatal approach in vestibular schwannoma surgery: a prospective study. Otol Neurotol 2003;24:927–934

30. Bloch DC, Oghalai JS, Jackler RK, Osofsky M, Pitts LH. The fate of the tumor remnant after less-than-complete acoustic neuroma resection. Otolaryngol Head Neck Surg 2004;130:104–112

31. Thomsen J, Tos M, Harmsen A. Acoustic neuroma surgery: results of translabyrinthine tumour removal in 300 patients. Discussion of choice of approach in relation to overall results and possibility of hearing preservation. Br J Neurosurg 1989;3:349–360

32. Mosek AC, Dodick DW, Ebersold MJ, Swanson JW. Headache after resection of acoustic neuroma. Headache 1999;39:89–94

33. Sanna M, Falcioni M, Rohit. Cerebro-spinal fluid leak after acoustic neuroma surgery. Otol Neurotol 2003;24:524

34. Schaller B, Baumann A. Headache after removal of vestibular schwannoma via the retrosigmoid approach: a long-term follow-up-study. Otolaryngol Head Neck Surg 2003;128:387–395

35. Wiet R, Teixido M, Liang J. Complications in acoustic neuroma surgery. Otolaryngol Clin North Am 1992;25:389–412

36. Sanna M, Khrais T, Russo A, Piccirillo E, Augurio A. Hearing preservation surgery in vestibular schwannoma: the hidden truth. Ann Otol Rhinol Laryngol 2004;113:156–163

37. Lalwani A, Butt F, Jackler R, Pitts L, Yingling C. Facial nerve outcome after acoustic neuroma surgery: a study from the era of cranial nerve monitoring. Otolaryngol Head Neck Surg 1994;111:561–570

38. Kartush J, Lundy L. Facial nerve outcome in acoustic neuroma surgery. Otolaryngol Clin North Am 1992;25:623–647

39. Shelton C. Hearing preservation in acoustic tumor surgery. Otolaryngol Clin North Am 1992;25:609–621

40. Chee GH, Nedzelski JM, Rowed D. Acoustic neuroma surgery: the results of long-term hearing preservation. Otol Neurotol 2003;24:672–676

41. Friedman RA, Kesser B, Brackmann DE, Fisher LM, Slattery WH, Hitselberger WE. Long-term hearing preservation after middle fossa removal of vestibular schwannoma. Otolaryngol Head Neck Surg 2003;129:660–665

42. Yates PD, Jackler RK, Satar B, Pitts LH, Oghalai JS. Is it worthwhile to attempt hearing preservation in larger acoustic neuromas? Otol Neurotol 2003;24:460–464

43. Sanna M. Hearing preservation: a critical review of the literature. In: Tos M, Thomsen J, eds. Proceedings of the First International Conference on Acoustic Neuroma. Amsterdam: Kugler, 1992:631–638

44. Friedman WA, Foote KD. Linear accelerator-based radiosurgery for vestibular schwannoma. Neurosurg Focus 2003;14:e2

45. Wiet R, Zappia J, Hecht C, O'Connor CA. Conservative management of patients with small acoustic tumors. Laryngoscope 1995;105:795–800

46. Rowe JG, Radatz M, Walton L, Kemeny AA. Stereotactic radiosurgery for type 2 neurofibromatosis acoustic neuromas: patient selection and tumour size. Stereotact Funct Neurosurg 2002;79:107–116

47. Bolsi A, Fogliata A, Cozzi L. Radiotherapy of small intracranial tumours with different advanced techniques using photon and proton beams: a treatment planning study. Radiother Oncol 2003;68:1–14

48. Chakrabarti I, Apuzzo ML, Giannota SL. Acoustic tumors: operation versus radiation–making sense of opposing viewpoints. Part I. Acoustic neuroma: decision making with all the tools. Clin Neurosurg 2003;50:293–312

49. De Salles AA, Frighetto L, Selch M. Stereotactic and microsurgery for acoustic neuroma: the controversy continues. Int J Radiat Oncol Biol Phys 2003;56:1215–1217

50. Iwai Y, Yamanaka K, Ishiguro T. Surgery combined with radiosurgery of large acoustic neuromas. Surg Neurol 2003;59:283–289 discussion 289–91

51. Chung JW, Ahn JH, Kim JH, Nam SY, Kim CJ, Lee KS. Facial nerve schwannomas: different manifestations and outcomes. Surg Neurol 2004;62:245–252

52. Hasegawa T, Kida Y, Kobayashi T, Yoshimoto M, Mori Y, Yoshida J. Long-term outcomes in patients with vestibular schwannomas treated using gamma knife surgery: 10-year follow up. J Neurosurg 2005;102:10–16

53. Lunsford LD, Niranjan A, Flickinger JC, Maitz A, Kondziolka D. Radiosurgery of vestibular schwannomas: summary of experience in 829 cases. J Neurosurg 2005;102(suppl):195–199

54. Wowra B, Muacevic A, Jess-Hempen A, Hempel JM, Muller-Schunk S, Tonn JC. Outpatient gamma knife surgery for vestibular schwannoma: definition of the therapeutic profile based on a 10-year experience. J Neurosurg 2005;102(suppl):114–118

55. Walsh RM, Bath AP, Bance ML, Keller A, Tator CH, Rutka JA. The natural history of untreated vestibular schwannomas. Is there a role for conservative management? Rev Laryngol Otol Rhinol (Bord) 2000;121:21–26

56. Chung HT, Ma R, Toyota B, Clark B, Robar J, McKenzie M. Audiologic and treatment outcomes after linear accelerator-based stereotactic irradiation for acoustic neuroma. Int J Radiat Oncol Biol Phys 2004;59:1116–1121

57. Flickinger JC, Kondziolka D, Niranjan A, Lunsford LD. Results of acoustic neuroma radiosurgery: an analysis of 5 years' experience using current methods. J Neurosurg 2001;94:1–6

58. Limb CJ, Long DM, Niparko JK. Acoustic neuromas after failed radiation therapy: challenges of surgical salvage. Laryngoscope 2005;115:93–98

59. Roche PH, Regis J, Deveze A, Delsanti C, Thomassin JM, Pellet W. [Surgical removal of unilateral vestibular schwannomas after failed gamma knife radiosurgery] Neurochirurgie 2004;50:383–393. French

60. Slattery WH III, Brackmann DE. Results of surgery following stereotactic irradiation for acoustic neuromas. Am J Otol 1995;16:315–319 discussion 319–21

61. Lustig LR. Radiation-induced tumors of the temporal bone. In: Jackler RK, Driscoll CL, eds. Tumors of the Ear and Temporal Bone. Philadelphia: Lippincott Williams & Wilkins, 2000

62. Tan LC, Bordi L, Symon L, Cheesman AD. Jugular foramen neuromas: a review of 14 cases. Surg Neurol 1990;34:205–211

63. Horn K, Hankinson H. Tumors of the jugular foramen. In: Jackler R, Brackmann D, eds. Neurotology. St. Louis: Mosby, 1994:1059–1068

64. Gacek R. Pathology of jugular foramen neurofibroma. Ann Otol Rhinol Laryngol 1983;92:128–133

65. Kaye A, Hahn J, Kinney S, Hardy R, Bay J. Jugular foramen schwannomas. J Neurosurg 1984;60:1045–1053

66. Lustig L, Jackler R. The variable relation between the lower cranial nerves and jugular foramen tumors: Implications for neural preservation. Am J Otol 1996;17:658–668

67. Ramina R, Maniglia JJ, Fernandes YB, et al. Jugular foramen tumors: diagnosis and treatment. Neurosurg Focus 2004;17:E5

68. Pensak M, Jackler R. Removal of jugular foramen tumors without re-routing the facial nerve. The fallopian bridge technique. Otolaryngol Head Neck Surg 1997;117:586–591

69. Van Calenbergh F, Noens B, Delaere P, et al. Jugular foramen schwannoma: surgical experience in six cases. Acta Chir Belg 2004;104:435–439

70. Jung TT, Jun BH, Shea D, Paparella MM. Primary and secondary tumors of the facial nerve. A temporal bone study. Arch Otolaryngol Head Neck Surg 1986;112:1269–1273

71. Dort J, Fisch U. Facial nerve schwannomas. Skull Base Surg 1991;1:51–56

72. O'Donoghue GM, Brackmann DE, House JW, Jackler RK. Neuromas of the facial nerve. Am J Otol 1989;10:49–54

73. Janecka IP, Conley J. Primary neoplasms of the facial nerve. Plast Reconstr Surg 1987;79:177–185

74. O'Donoghue G. Tumors of the Facial Nerve. In: Jackler R, ed. Neurotology. St. Louis: Mosby, 1994

75. Saito H, Saito S, Sano T, Kagawa N, Hizawa K, Tatara K. Immunoreactive somatostatin in catecholamine-producing extra-adrenal paraganglioma. Cancer 1982;50:560–565

76. Peco MT, Palacios E. Intracranial and intratemporal facial nerve schwannoma. Ear Nose Throat J 2002;81:312

77. Sarma S, Sekhar LN, Schessel DA. Nonvestibular schwannomas of the brain: a 7-year experience. Neurosurgery 2002;50:437–448

78. Ulku CH, Uyar Y, Acar O, Yaman H, Avunduk MC. Facial nerve schwannomas: a report of four cases and a review of the literature. Am J Otolaryngol 2004;25:426–431

79. Parnes LS, Lee DH, Peerless SJ. Magnetic resonance imaging of facial nerve neuromas. Laryngoscope 1991;101:31–35

80. Liu R, Fagan P. Facial nerve schwannoma: surgical excision versus conservative management. Ann Otol Rhinol Laryngol 2001;110:1025–1029

81. Spector GJ, Maisel RH, Ogura JH. Glomus tumors in the middle ear. I. An analysis of 46 patients. Laryngoscope 1973;83:1652–1672

82. Guild S. The glomus jugulare, a nonchromaffin paraganglion, in man. Ann Otol Rhinol Laryngol 1953;62:1045–1071

83. Gulya AJ. The glomus tumor and its biology. Laryngoscope 1993;103:7–15

84. Heutink P, van der Mey AG, Sandkuijl LA, et al. A gene subject to genomic imprinting and responsible for hereditary paragangliomas maps to chromosome 11q23-qter. Hum Mol Genet 1992;1:7–10

85. Heth J. The basic science of glomus jugulare tumors. Neurosurg Focus 2004;17:E2

86. van der Mey AG, Maaswinkel-Mooy PD, Cornelisse CJ, Schmidt PH, van de Kamp JJ. Genomic imprinting in hereditary glomus tumours: evidence for new genetic theory. [see comments] Lancet 1989;2:1291–1294

87. Alford B, Guilford F. A comprehensive study of tumors of the glomus jugulare. Laryngoscope 1962;72:765–787

88. Batsakis J. Tumors of the Head and Neck: Clinical and Pathological Considerations, 2nd ed. Baltimore: Williams & Wilkins, 1979

89. Glenner G, Grimley P. Tumors of the extra-adrenal paraganglion system (including chemoreceptors). In: Atlas of Tumor Pathology, 2nd ed. Washington, DC: Armed Forces Institute of Pathology, 1974:1–90

90. Gulya A. Paraneoplastic disorders. In: Jackler R, ed. Neurotology. St. Louis: Mosby, 1994:535–542

91. Jackson CG. Neurotologic skull base surgery for glomus tumors. Diagnosis for treatment planning and treatment options. Laryngoscope 1993;103:17–22

92. House WF, Glasscock ME. Glomus tympanicum tumors. Arch Otolaryngol 1968;87:550–554

93. Woods CI, Strasnick B, Jackson CG. Surgery for glomus tumors: the Otology group experience. Laryngoscope 1993;103:65–70

94. Jackson CG, Kaylie DM, Coppit G, Gardner EK. Glomus jugulare tumors with intracranial extension. Neurosurg Focus 2004;17:E7

95. Makek M, Franklin DJ, Zhao JC, Fisch U. Neural infiltration of glomus temporale tumors. Am J Otol 1990;11:1–5

96. Arriaga MA, Lo WW, Brackmann DE. Magnetic resonance angiography of synchronous bilateral carotid body paragangliomas and bilateral vagal paragangliomas. Ann Otol Rhinol Laryngol 1992;101:955–957

97. Dowd C, Halback V, Higashida R, Heishima G. Diagnostic and therapeutic angiography. In: Jackler R, Brackmann D, eds. Neurotology. St. Louis: Mosby, 1994:399–436

98. Moret J, Picard L. Vascular architecture of tympanojugular glomus tumors. Sem Interventional Radiol 1987;4:291–308

99. Sismanis A, Smoker WR. Pulsatile tinnitus: recent advances in diagnosis. Laryngoscope 1994;104:681–688

100. Lum C, Keller AM, Kassel E, Blend R, Waldron J, Rutka J. Unusual eustachian tube mass: glomus tympanicum. AJNR Am J Neuroradiol 2001;22:508–509

101. Tatla T, Savy LE, Wareing MJ. Epistaxis as a rare presenting feature of glomus tympanicum. J Laryngol Otol 2003;117:577–579

102. Brown L. Glomus jugulare tumor of the middle ear: Clinical aspects. Laryngoscope 1953;63:281–292

103. Lo WW, Solti-Bohman LG, Lambert PR. High-resolution CT in the evaluation of glomus tumors of the temporal bone. Radiology 1984;150:737–742

104. Jackson CG. Basic surgical principles of neurotologic skull base surgery. Laryngoscope 1993;103:29–44

105. Durvasula VS, De R, Baguley DM, Moffat DA. Laser excision of glomus tympanicum tumours: long-term results. Eur Arch Otorhinolaryngol 2005;262:325–327

106. Jackson C, Cueva R, Thedinger B, Glasscock M. Cranial nerve preservation in lesions of the jugular fossa. Otolaryngol Head Neck Surg 1991;105:687–693

107. Jackson CG. Glomus tympanicum and glomus jugulare tumors. Otolaryngol Clin North Am 2001;34:941–970

108. Miman MC, Aktas D, Oncel S, Ozturan O, Kalcioglu MT. Glomus jugulare. Otolaryngol Head Neck Surg 2002;127:585–586

109. House JW, Fayad JN. Glomus jugulare. Ear Nose Throat J 2004;83:800

110. Oghalai JS, Leung MK, Jackler RK, McDermott MW. Transjugular craniotomy for the management of jugular foramen tumors with intracranial extension. Otol Neurotol 2004;25:570–579

111. Bari ME, Kemeny AA, Forster DM, Radatz MW. Radiosurgery for the control of glomus jugulare tumours. J Pak Med Assoc 2003;53:147–151

112. Foote RL, Pollock BE, Gorman DA, et al. Glomus jugulare tumor: tumor control and complications after stereotactic radiosurgery. Head Neck 2002;24:332–339

113. Gottfried ON, Liu JK, Couldwell WT. Comparison of radiosurgery and conventional surgery for the treatment of glomus jugulare tumors. Neurosurg Focus 2004;17:E4

114. Pollock BE. Stereotactic radiosurgery in patients with glomus jugulare tumors. Neurosurg Focus 2004;17:E10

115. Saringer W, Khayal H, Ertl A, Schoeggl A, Kitz K. Efficiency of gamma knife radiosurgery in the treatment of glomus jugulare tumors. Minim Invasive Neurosurg 2001;44:141–146

116. Sheehan J, Kondziolka D, Flickinger J, Lunsford LD. Gamma knife surgery for glomus jugulare tumors: an intermediate report on efficacy and safety. J Neurosurg 2005;102(suppl):241–246

117. Carrasco V, Rosenma J. Radiation therapy of glomus jugulare tumors. Laryngoscope 1993;103:23–27

118. Lustig LR, Jackler RK, Lanser MJ. Radiation-induced tumors of the temporal bone. Am J Otol 1997;18:230–235

119. Nager G, Masica D. Meningiomas of the cerebellopontine angle and their relation to the temporal bone. Laryngoscope 1970;80:863–895

120. Lusis E, Gutmann DH. Meningioma: an update. Curr Opin Neurol 2004;17:687–692

121. Ferlito A, Devaney KO, Rinaldo A. Primary extracranial meningioma in the vicinity of the temporal bone: a benign lesion which is rarely recognized clinically. Acta Otolaryngol 2004;124:5–7

122. Nager G, Heroy J, Hoeplinger M. Meningiomas invading the temporal bone with extension into the neck. Am J Otolaryngol 1983;4:297–324

123. Lesch K, Gross S. Estrogen receptor immunoreactivity in meningiomas. Comparison with the binding activity of estrogen, progesterone, and androgen receptors. J Neurosurg 1987;67:237–243

124. Modan B, Baidatz D, Mart H, Steinitz R, Levin S. Radiation-induced head and neck tumours. Lancet 1974;1:277–279

125. Roberti F, Sekhar LN, Kalavakonda C, Wright DC. Posterior fossa meningiomas: surgical experience in 161 cases. Surg Neurol 2001;56:8–20 discussion 20–21

126. Selesnick SH, Nguyen TD, Gutin PH, Lavyne MH. Posterior petrous face meningiomas. Otolaryngol Head Neck Surg 2001;124:408–413

127. Thompson LD, Bouffard JP, Sandberg GD, Mena H. Primary ear and temporal bone meningiomas: a clinicopathologic study of 36 cases with a review of the literature. Mod Pathol 2003;16:236–245

128. Chang CY, Cheung SW, Jackler RK. Meningiomas presenting in the temporal bone: the pathways of spread from an intracranial site of origin. Otolaryngol Head Neck Surg 1998;119:658–664

129. Singh AD, Selesnick SH. Meningiomas of the posterior fossa and skull base. In: Jackler RK, Brackmann DE, eds. Neurotology, 2nd ed. St. Louis: Mosby, 2005:792–840

130. Langman A, Jackler R, Althaus S. Meningioma of the internal auditory canal. Am J Otol 1990;11:201–204

131. Morris J, Schoen W. The nervous system. In: Robbins S, Cotran R, Kumar V, eds. Pathologic Basis of Disease, 5th ed. Philadelphia: WB Saunders, 1984:1370–1436

132. Laird F, Harner S, Laws E, Reese J. Meningiomas of the cerebellopontine angle. Otolaryngol Head Neck Surg 1985;93:163–167

133. Malony TB, Brackmann DE, Lo WW. Meningiomas of the jugular foramen. Otolaryngol Head Neck Surg 1992;106:128–136

134. Curati W, Grai M, Kingsley D, King T, Scholtz C, Steiner R. MRI in acoustic neuroma: a review of 35 patients. Neuroradiology 1986;28:208–214

135. Lalwani AK, Jackler RK. Preoperative differentiation between meningioma of the cerebellopontine angle and acoustic neuroma using MRI. Otolaryngol Head Neck Surg 1993;109:88–95

136. Wilms G, Plets C, Goossens L, Goffin J, Vanwambeke K. The radiological differentiation of acoustic neurinoma and meningioma occurring together in the cerebellopontine angle. Neurosurgery 1992;30:443–446

137. Itoh T, Harada M, Ichikawa T, Shimoyamada K, Katayama N, Tsukune Y. A case of jugular foramen chordoma with extension to the neck: CT and MR findings. Radiat Med 2000;18:63–65

138. Laudadio P, Canani FB, Cunsolo E. Meningioma of the internal auditory canal. Acta Otolaryngol 2004;124:1231–1234

139. Rinaldi A, Gazzeri G, Callovini GM, Masci P, Natali G. Acoustic intrameatal meningiomas. J Neurosurg Sci 2000;44:25–32

140. Glasscock M, Minor L, McMenomey S. Meningiomas of the cerebellopontine angle. In: Jackler R, Brackmann D, eds. Neurotology. St. Louis: Mosby, 1994:795–821

141. Chamberlain MC, Blumenthal DT. Intracranial meningiomas: diagnosis and treatment. Expert Rev Neurother 2004;4:641–648

142. Milker-Zabel S, Zabel A, Schulz-Ertner D, Schlegel W, Wannenmacher M, Debus J. Fractionated stereotactic radiotherapy in patients with benign or atypical intracranial meningioma: long-term experience and prognostic factors. Int J Radiat Oncol Biol Phys 2005;61:809–816

143. Tonn JC. Microneurosurgery and radiosurgery—an attractive combination. Acta Neurochir Suppl (Wien) 2004;91:103–108

144. Barbaro N, Gutin P, Wilson C, Sheline G, Boldrey E, Wara W. Radiation therapy in the treatment of partially resected meningiomas. Neurosurgery 1987;20:525–528

145. Kondziolka D, Lunsford L, Flickinger J. The role of radiosurgery in the management of chordoma and chondrosarcoma of the cranial base. Neurosurgery 1991;29:38–46

146. Liscak R, Kollova A, Vladyka V, Simonova G, Novotny J Jr. Gamma knife radiosurgery of skull base meningiomas. Acta Neurochir Suppl (Wien) 2004;91:65–74

147. Mirimanoff R, Dosoretz D, Linggood R, Ojemann R, Martuza R. Meningioma: analysis of recurrence and progression following neurosurgical resection. J Neurosurg 1985;62:18–24

148. Polinsky MN, Brunberg JA, McKeever PE, Sandler HM, Telian S, Ross D. Aggressive papillary middle ear tumors: a report of two cases with review of the literature. [see comments] Neurosurgery 1994; 35:493–497, discussion 497

149. Benecke JE Jr, Noel FL, Carberry JN, House JW, Patterson M. Adenomatous tumors of the middle ear and mastoid. Am J Otol 1990;11:20–26

150. Mills RG, Douglas-Jones T, Williams RG. "Ceruminoma"—a defunct diagnosis. J Laryngol Otol 1995;109:180–188

151. Batsakis JG. Adenomatous tumors of the middle ear. Ann Otol Rhinol Laryngol 1989;98:749–752

152. Peters BR, Maddox HE III, Batsakia JG. Pleomorphic adenoma of the middle ear and mastoid with posterior fossa extension. Arch Otolaryngol Head Neck Surg 1988;114:676–678

153. Batsakis JG, el-Naggar AK. Papillary neoplasms (Heffner's tumors) of the endolymphatic sac. Ann Otol Rhinol Laryngol 1993;102:648–651

154. Richards PS, Clifton AG. Endolymphatic sac tumours. J Laryngol Otol 2003;117:666–669

155. Stendel R, Suess O, Prosenc N, Funk T, Brock M. Neoplasm of endolymphatic sac origin: clinical, radiological and pathological features. Acta Neurochir (Wien) 1998;140:1083–1087

156. Heffner DK. Low-grade adenocarcinoma of probable endolymphatic sac origin: a clinicopathologic study of 20 cases. Cancer 1989;64:2292–2302

157. Poe DS, Tarlov EC, Thomas CB, Kveton JF. Aggressive papillary tumors of temporal bone. Otolaryngol Head Neck Surg 1993;108:80–86

158. Noel FL, Benecke JE Jr, Carberry JN, House JW, Patterson M. Adenomas of the mastoid and middle ear. Otolaryngol Head Neck Surg 1991;104: 133–134

159. Li JC, Brackmann DE, Lo WW, Carberry JN, House JW. Reclassification of aggressive adenomatous mastoid neoplasms as endolymphatic sac tumors. Laryngoscope 1993;103:1342–1348

160. Devaney KO, Ferlito A, Rinaldo A. Epithelial tumors of the middle ear—are middle ear carcinoids really distinct from middle ear adenomas? Acta Otolaryngol 2003;123:678–682

161. Torske KR, Thompson LD. Adenoma versus carcinoid tumor of the middle ear: a study of 48 cases and review of the literature. Mod Pathol 2002;15:543–555

162. Krouse JH, Nadol JB Jr, Goodman ML. Carcinoid tumors of the middle ear. Ann Otol Rhinol Laryngol 1990;99:547–552

163. Murphy GF, Pilch BZ, Dickersin GR, Goodman ML, Nadol JB Jr. Carcinoid tumor of the middle ear. Am J Clin Pathol 1980;73:816–823

164. Blaker H, Dyckhoff G, Weidauer H, Otto HF. Carcinoid tumor of the middle ear in a 28-year-old patient. Pathol Oncol Res 1998;4:40–43

165. Chan KC, Wu CM, Huang SF. Carcinoid tumor of the middle ear: a case report. Am J Otolaryngol 2005;26:57–59

166. Mooney EE, Dodd LG, Oury TD, Burchette JL, Layfield LJ, Scher RL. Middle ear carcinoid: an indolent tumor with metastatic potential. Head Neck 1999;21:72–77

167. Nikanne E, Kantola O, Parviainen T. Carcinoid tumor of the middle ear. Acta Otolaryngol 2004;124:754–757

168. Shibosawa E, Tsutsumi K, Ihara Y, Kinoshita H, Koizuka I. A case of carcinoid tumor of the middle ear. Auris Nasus Larynx 2003;30(Suppl): S99–102

169. Schenk P, Handisurya A, Steurer M. Ultrastructural morphology of a middle ear ceruminoma. ORL J Otorhinolaryngol Relat Spec 2002;64: 358–363

170. el-Naggar AK, Pflatz M, Ordonez NG, Batsakis JG. Tumors of the middle ear and endolymphatic sac. Pathol Annu 1994;29:199–231

171. Gulya AJ, Glasscock ME, Pensak ML. Neural choristoma of the middle ear. Otolaryngol Head Neck Surg 1987;97:52–56

172. Nelson EG, Kratz RC. Sebaceous choristoma of the middle ear. Otolaryngol Head Neck Surg 1993;108:372–373

173. Gyure KA, Thompson LD, Morrison AL. A clinicopathological study of 15 patients with neuroglial heterotopias and encephaloceles of the middle ear and mastoid region. Laryngoscope 2000;110:1731–1735

174. Rinaldo A, Ferlito A, Devaney KO. Salivary gland choristoma of the middle ear. A review. ORL J Otorhinolaryngol Relat Spec 2004;66: 141–147

175. Kartush JM, Graham MD. Salivary gland choristoma of the middle ear: a case report and review of the literature. Laryngoscope 1984;94:228–230

176. Abadir WF, Pease WS. Salivary gland choristoma of the middle ear. J Laryngol Otol 1978;92:247–252

177. Jackson IT, Carreno R, Potparic Z, Hussain K. Hemangiomas, vascular malformations, and lymphovenous malformations: classification and methods of treatment. Plast Reconstr Surg 1993;91:1216–1230

178. Mulliken JB, Glowacki J. Hemangiomas and vascular malformations in infants and children: a classification based on endothelial characteristics. Plast Reconstr Surg 1982;69:412–422

179. Waner M, Suen JY, Dinehart S. Treatment of hemangiomas of the head and neck. Laryngoscope 1992;102:1123–1132

180. Buchanan DS, Fagan PA, Turner J. Cavernous haemangioma of the temporal bone. J Laryngol Otol 1992;106:1086–1088

181. Shelton C, Brackmann DE, Lo WW, Carberry JN. Intratemporal facial nerve hemangiomas. Otolaryngol Head Neck Surg 1991;104:116–121

182. Glasscock ME, Smith PG, Schwaber MK, Nissen AJ. Clinical aspects of osseous hemangiomas of the skull base. Laryngoscope 1984;94:869–873

183. Mazzoni A, Pareschi R, Calabrese V. Intratemporal vascular tumours. J Laryngol Otol 1988;102:353–356

184. Dufour JJ, Michaud LA, Mohr G, Pouliot D, Picard C. Intratemporal vascular malformations (angiomas): particular clinical features. J Otolaryngol 1994;23:250–253

185. Barrera JE, Jenkins H, Said S. Cavernous hemangioma of the internal auditory canal: a case report and review of the literature. Am J Otolaryngol 2004;25:199–203

186. Aquilina K, Nanra JS, Brett F, Walsh RM, Rawluk D. Cavernous angioma of the internal auditory canal. J Laryngol Otol 2004;118:368–371

187. Gjuric M, Koester M, Paulus W. Cavernous hemangioma of the internal auditory canal arising from the inferior vestibular nerve: case report and review of the literature. Am J Otol 2000;21:110–114

188. Tokyol C, Yilmaz MD. Middle ear hemangioma: a case report. Am J Otolaryngol 2003;24:405–407

189. Reeck JB, Yen TL, Szmit A, Cheung SW. Cavernous hemangioma of the external ear canal. Laryngoscope 2002;112:1750–1752

190. Limb CJ, Mabrie DC, Carey JP, Minor LB. Hemangioma of the external auditory canal. Otolaryngol Head Neck Surg 2002;126:74–75

191. Hecht DA, Jackson CG, Grundfast KM. Management of middle ear hemangiomas. Am J Otolaryngol 2001;22:362–366

192. Bijelic L, Wei JL, McDonald TJ. Hemangioma of the tympanic membrane. Otolaryngol Head Neck Surg 2001;125:272–273

193. Fisch U, Ruttner J. Pathology of intratemporal tumors involving the facial nerve. In: Fisch U, ed. Facial Nerve Surgery. Birmingham: Aesculapius, 1977:448–456

194. Eby TL, Fisch U, Makek MS. Facial nerve management in temporal bone hemangiomas. Am J Otol 1992;13:223–232

195. Lo WW, Shelton C, Waluch V, et al. Intratemporal vascular tumors: detection with CT and MR imaging. Radiology 1989;171:445–448

196. Goldsmith AJ, Myssiorek D, Valderrama E, Patel M. Unifocal Langerhans' cell histiocytosis (eosinophilic granuloma) of the petrous apex. Arch Otolaryngol Head Neck Surg 1993;119:113–116

197. Cunningham MJ, Curtin HD, Jaffe R, Stool SE. Otologic manifestations of Langerhans' cell histiocytosis. Arch Otolaryngol Head Neck Surg 1989; 115:807–813

198. Nolph MB, Luikin GA. Histiocytosis X. Otolaryngol Clin North Am 1982;15:635–648

199. Arico M, Danesino C. Langerhans' cell histiocytosis: is there a role for genetics? Haematologica 2001;86:1009–1014

200. McCaffrey TV, McDonald TJ. Histiocytosis X of the ear and temporal bone: review of 22 cases. Laryngoscope 1979;89:1735–1742

201. Bayazit Y, Sirikci A, Bayaram M, Kanlikama M, Demir A, Bakir K. Eosinophilic granuloma of the temporal bone. Auris Nasus Larynx 2001;28:99–102

202. DeRowe A, Bernheim J, Ophir D. Eosinophilic granuloma presenting as chronic otitis media: pitfalls in the diagnosis of aural polyps in children. J Otolaryngol 1995;24:258–260

203. Tos M. Facial palsy in Hand-Schuller-Christian's disease. Arch Otolaryngol 1969;90:563–567

204. Fradis M, Podoshin L, Ben-David J, Grishkan A. Eosinophilic granuloma of the temporal bone. J Laryngol Otol 1985;99:475–479

25

Cystic Lesions of the Petrous Apex

Michael C. Byrd, Gordon B. Hughes, Paul M. Ruggieri, and Joung Lee

◆ Anatomy of the Petrous Apex

The petrous bone can be divided into two main compartments: anterior and posterior. The internal auditory canal acts as the partition. The anterior compartment (the petrous apex) is the larger of the two; it lies anteromedial to the cochlea and is more frequently involved in disease. Pneumatization can vary, and is indirectly proportional to the amount of bone marrow that comprises the compartment. The more bone marrow found within the petrous apex, the less air, and vice versa. Approximately one third of adults have pneumatization, and pneumatization is usually symmetric bilaterally.

Many authors describe the petrous apex as a three-sided pyramid with an anterior, posterior, and inferior surface. It is located between the clivus in the anteromedial position and the otic capsule in the posterolateral position. The anterior surface forms the floor of the middle cranial fossa. The internal carotid artery passes through this area to the cavernous sinus; the tensor tympani muscle and eustachian tube are located just lateral to the artery. The facial hiatus can be found along the anterior border with the greater superficial petrosal nerve carrying parasympathetics to the sphenopalatine ganglion. Near the anterior apex, the Gasserian ganglion of the trigeminal nerve rests in Meckel's cave. The posterior surface faces the posterior cranial fossa. Along the superior and inferior edges the superior and inferior petrosal sinuses can be found. The abducens nerve courses along with the superior petrosal sinus to enter the cavernous sinus through a tight fold of dura known as the petroclinoid ligament, or Dorello's canal. Posterior to the apex is the internal auditory meatus. The inferior surface lies along the horizontal plane and contains the carotid artery canal meatus.

◆ Pathology of Petrous Apex Lesions

Petrous apex lesions are rare. They can be categorized as primary or secondary. This chapter focuses on primary cystic lesions of the petrous apex, such as cholesterol granuloma, cholesteatoma, and mucocele, as well as petrous apicitis, retained fluid, and asymmetric petrous apex pneumatization.

Primary Cystic Lesions

Cholesterol granuloma is a foreign body giant cell reaction to cholesterol deposits, with chronic inflammation, fibrosis, and vascular proliferation all contained within a fibrous capsule. The first reported case of an otologic cholesterol granuloma was in the late nineteenth century.[1] Cholesterol granulomas are 10 times more common than petrous apex cholesteatomas and 40 times more common than mucoceles.

These lesions tend to remain clinically silent until expansile growth produces headache, or encroachment on adjacent cranial nerves causes hearing loss, imbalance, facial weakness, or diplopia. Two theories have been proposed concerning the development of cholesterol granulomas. The classic hypothesis is known as the obstruction-vacuum theory, which entails a series of events. First, mucosal swelling occludes petrous air cell outflow tracts, resulting in gas trapping, which leads to vacuum formation. In this vacuum, pressure causes transudation of blood into the mucosal surfaces. Anaerobes then begin to break down the red blood cells, liberating cholesterol granules. The cholesterol granules initiate the inflammatory cascade, resulting in bony erosion and foreign body reaction.[2–4]

A second theory on cholesterol granuloma formation has recently been proposed.[5] The new hypothesis is known as the exposed marrow theory. The theory states that during development there is aggressive pneumatization of the petrous apex resulting in the formation of a pathologic communication between mucosa-lined air cells and the marrow they gradually replace. The communication between the marrow and mucosa creates hemorrhage into the apical air cells. Once the blood becomes trapped in these cells, anaerobic bacteria digest the red cells, again releasing the cholesterol granules. The inflammatory cascade begins, resulting in a foreign body reaction and bony erosion.[2–4,6]

Primary cholesteatomas consist of stratified squamous epithelial lining surrounding desquamated keratin, and originate from epithelial rests within the petrous apex. Because these lesions expand into the area of least resistance, they have variable shapes. They can become quite large without producing symptoms; however, as they expand, compression and irritation of surrounding structures produce signs and symptoms similar to those of cholesterol granuloma.

Various theories on the development of petrous apex cholesteatomas have been proposed. Congenital onset is thought to be caused by the presence of epidermoid cells in the petrous apex during fetal development. A second hypothesis proposes migration of the external meatus ectoderm. In fetal development the internal and external meati are in close connection, which may result in trapping of epithelial remnants in the foramen lacerum.[7–10]

An exceedingly rare lesion of the petrous apex is the *primary mucocele*. The first reported case of petrous apex mucocele was in 1979.[11] The etiology of the mucocele is uncertain; however, several theories have been postulated. Mucosal thickening, bony overgrowth, or fibrosis may obliterate the outflow tract resulting in mucocele formation, or nests of seromucinous tissue may be responsible for the development of mucoceles through mucus retention.[10,12] It is logical to assume that, given the nature of ventilation and drainage of the petrous apex air cells, some individuals will develop a mucocele in these pneumatic spaces as a consequence of an upper respiratory tract infection. This situation is analogous to disease of the paranasal sinuses. As in the sinuses, the mucocele becomes expansile, resulting in bony erosion.

Other Lesions

Petrous apicitis can be classified as acute, subacute, or chronic. Acute apicitis usually involves an acute episode of otitis media or mastoiditis, potentially resulting in the formation of an apical abscess. More commonly, petrous apicitis results from chronic otitis media, with *Pseudomonas aeruginosa* being the predominant bacteria causing the infection. Long-standing infection can also potentially result in osteomyelitis. Prior to the era of antibiotics, suppurative disease of the petrous apex was often fatal. The classically described syndrome included a triad of signs and symptoms: (1) discharging ear, (2) deep retro-ocular pain, and (3) abducens paralysis.[3,12–15] This syndrome was known as Gradenigo's triad. Petrous apicitis should be suspected whenever a chronic suppurative ear is associated with deep pain. The pain is usually a result of either dural involvement over the apex or direct irritation of the Gasserian ganglion in Meckel's cave. Apicitis should also be suspected when cranial nerve palsies occur.

Retained fluid is a serous effusion trapped in apical air cells. By definition, retained fluid does not destroy bone; however, headache and pressure symptoms may prompt surgery if serial computed tomography (CT) scanning does not show resolution. The clinical entity of apical retained fluid is poorly understood, but may be analogous to chronic serous mastoiditis or may be an initial step toward cholesterol granuloma formation.

Asymmetric fatty marrow in the petrous apex is usually noted as an incidental finding on radiographic imaging (**Fig. 25–1**). It is the residual fatty marrow in the nonpneumatized or less pneumatized petrous apex that causes concern. Correct identification of this normal variant is essential to prevent misdiagnosis or unnecessary workup and treatment.[4,12] In a review of 500 CT scans, Roland et al[16] found 34 patients with some asymmetry of pneumatization of the petrous apex.

◆ Clinical Presentation and Assessment of Petrous Apex Lesions

Symptoms

Petrous apex lesions can be asymptomatic, and can be discovered only by coincidence on magnetic resonance imaging (MRI). Leonetti and colleagues[17] performed a retrospective chart review to categorize a group of petrous apex lesions that were noted incidentally on MRI in 88 patients. These incidental findings included asymmetric fatty bone marrow, inflammation, cholesterol granuloma, and cholesteatomas. Asymmetric fatty bone marrow was the predominant finding in this review. Therefore, the clinician should remember that a petrous apex lesion noted on MRI may or may not be related to the initial presenting symptoms. The physician should not overreact.

Most published reports of symptomatic petrous apex lesions include primary and secondary neoplasms and list hearing loss as the most common presenting symptom. Nonneoplastic, primary cystic lesions of the petrous apex more often present with headache, head pain, or aural pressure. Symptomatic petrous apex disease is usually a result of an expansile lesion, and can be correlated with anatomic structures: headache from tension on the dura of the middle cranial fossa; conductive hearing loss from serous effusion resulting from eustachian tube dysfunction or compression; facial pain due to impingement and compression on the trigeminal ganglion of Meckel's cave; syncope from carotid artery occlusion; and tinnitus, vertigo, facial paralysis, and sensorineural hearing loss due to involvement of the otic capsule or the internal auditory canal. Ophthalmoplegia from anterior extension into the cavernous sinus is rare. Syncope from carotid compression is also rare. Petrous apex lesions usually remain undetected for extended periods because patients complain of vague nonspecific symptoms that delay diagnosis.

Diagnosis

Although headache and head pain from cystic petrous apex lesions can be retro-ocular, they also can be temporoparietal and periauricular. Therefore, the differential diagnosis for referred otalgia should be considered: migraine, temporomandibular joint (TMJ) syndrome, cervical myalgia, fibromyalgia, odontogenic abscess, head and neck malignancy, temporal arteritis, inflammatory sinusitis, carotidynia, trigeminal neuralgia, glossopharyngeal neuralgia, and gastroesophageal reflux disease.

First a thorough history should be taken and physical examination performed. A neurotologic examination should focus on cranial nerve function. A careful head and neck examination is performed with focused attention on the ear and nasal cavity. Often audiologic testing including pure tone and speech audiometry is obtained. In some cases, electronystagmography and auditory brainstem response testing are employed. If no cause is identified at this point, radiologic evaluation is recommended.

Radiologic Findings

CT and MRI are most helpful in evaluating a possible petrous apex lesion. Petrous apex lesions vary in composition, and each has certain radiographic characteristics that distinguish it from other lesions (**Table 25–1**). CT is particularly helpful

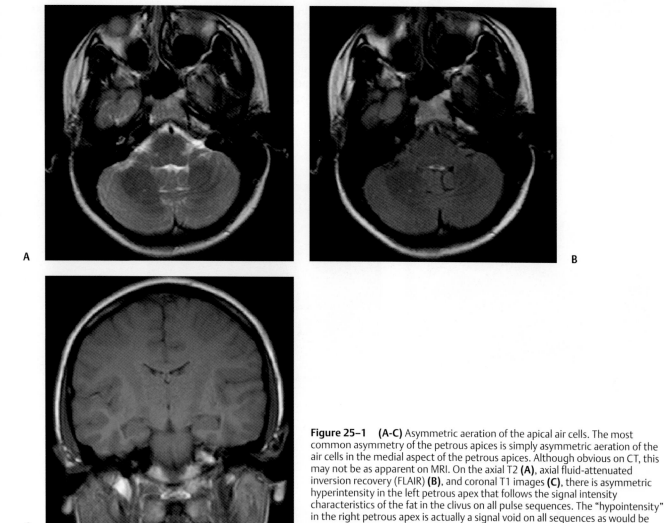

A

B

C

Figure 25–1 **(A-C)** Asymmetric aeration of the apical air cells. The most common asymmetry of the petrous apices is simply asymmetric aeration of the air cells in the medial aspect of the petrous apices. Although obvious on CT, this may not be as apparent on MRI. On the axial T2 **(A)**, axial fluid-attenuated inversion recovery (FLAIR) **(B)**, and coronal T1 images **(C)**, there is asymmetric hyperintensity in the left petrous apex that follows the signal intensity characteristics of the fat in the clivus on all pulse sequences. The "hypointensity" in the right petrous apex is actually a signal void on all sequences as would be expected with aerated air cells.

in identifying bone destruction. MRI is most useful in differentiating smoothly marginated lesions versus bone-eroding lesions. Additional MRI information is obtained with intravenous administration of the contrast agent gadolinium–diethylenetriamine pentaacetic acid (DTPA). As a rule, non-neoplastic lesions do not enhance or have only a rim of enhancement. Magnetic resonance angiography (MRA) is also helpful to evaluate the carotid and vertebrobasilar arterial systems. In addition to CT and MRI, arteriography helps evaluate possible vascular lesions. If surgical intervention is warranted, often the status of the carotid artery is important in determining the approach, anticipating complete or incomplete cyst resection, and judging the feasibility of artery resection and repair.

At times, bone scintigraphy may be the most sensitive means of early detection of petrous apex pathology. However, due to the intricate and complex anatomy of the skull base and face, routine planar bone scintigraphy may not be diagnostic. Several reports have demonstrated that single photon emission computed tomography (SPECT) improves the sensitivity for detecting abnormalities of the skull base and allows better localization of the pathology.[18]

Table 25–1 Imaging Features of Primary Petrous Apex Lesions

Lesion	MRI (T1)	MRI (T2)	Enhancing	Expansile
Cholesterol granuloma	High	High	No	Yes
Cholesteatoma	Low-medium	High	No	Yes
Mucocele	Low-variable	High	No	Yes
Petrous apicitis	Low	High	Yes	No

High, high attenuation and signal; low, low attenuation and signal.

On CT scan *cholesterol granuloma* appears as a smoothly marginated expansile mass typically located in the anteromedial petrous apex (**Fig. 25–2A**). The density is usually similar to brain density. There is no enhancement of these lesions with intravenous contrast material. They are distinguished from other smoothly marginated lesions of the apex by the presence of extensive pneumatization in the contralateral petrous apex.

On MRI scan, the appearance of cholesterol granuloma is so characteristic as to be diagnostic in the majority of cases.[12]

These lesions are hyperintense on both T1- and T2-weighted MRI images and do not enhance following administration of gadolinium contrast (**Fig. 25–2B-D**).

Cholesteatomas of the petrous apex have two origins: congenital and acquired. Congenital cholesteatomas were frequently overdiagnosed in the older literature; many of these were probably cholesterol granulomas, a much more common entity, but were not well appreciated until recently. On CT imaging cholesteatoma of the petrous apex appears as a smoothly marginated expansile lesion that does not

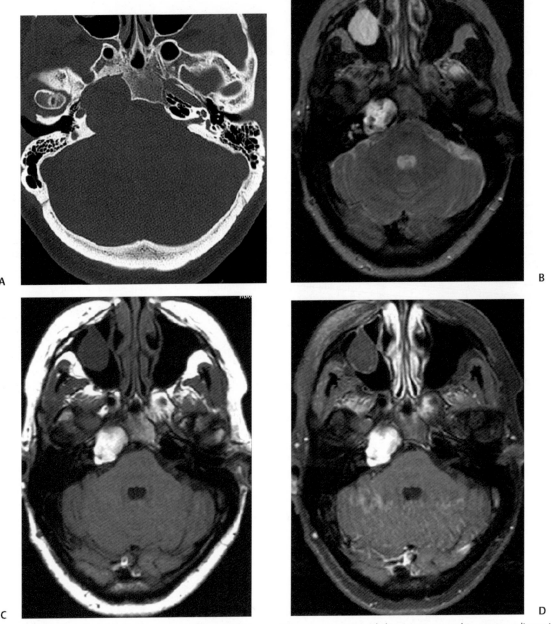

A

B

C

D

Figure 25–2   **(A)** Cholesterol granuloma. On the axial CT image, the mass is obviously expansile and protrudes into the cerebellopontine angle cistern. There is a thin rim of surrounding, reactive sclerosis as would be expected with a slowly growing process. The thin residual rim of bone protruding into the cistern is barely perceptible. **(B)** Axial T2-weighted fast spin echo MRI demonstrates a large, well-defined heterogeneously hyperintense mass in the right petrous apex that appears to be mildly expansile and impinges on the right carotid canal. **(C)** The mass is also prominently hyperintense on the corresponding axial T1-weighted spin echo image. The signal intensity characteristics on T1 and T2 are quite typical for a cholesterol granuloma, presumably due to prior hemorrhage. **(D)** Fat suppression eliminates the high signal intensity of the fat in the normal petrous apex to make the lesion more obvious but has no impact on the signal of the cholesterol granuloma itself. No enhancement can be appreciated along the periphery of the mass given the cystic nature of the process and the absence of a confluent soft tissue component.

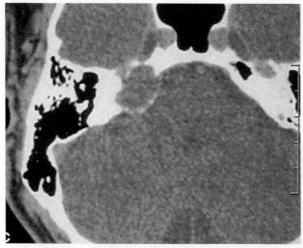

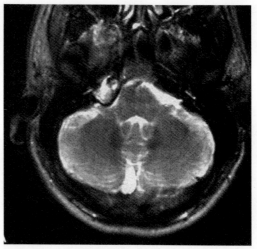

A

B

Figure 25–3 **(A)** Epidermoid/congenital cholesteatoma. High-resolution axial CT demonstrates a sharply delineated, expansile, cystic mass in the right petrous apex that extends into the right cerebellopontine angle cistern and is comparable in appearance to the cholesterol granuloma on CT. **(B)** These masses can be distinguished

from a cholesterol granuloma on MRI as the cholesteatomas are typically hyperintense on T2-weighted images, hypointense on T1-weighted images shown here, and do not enhance following gadolinium administration.

enhance with administration of intravenous contrast material. It may be hypodense to adjacent brain tissue, although this is variable (**Fig. 25–3A**). Cholesteatomas are generally not distinguishable from cholesterol granulomas on CT imaging. On MRI imaging, cholesteatomas have low signal intensity on T1-weighted images and high signal intensity on T2-weighted images (**Fig. 25–3B**). They do not enhance following administration of gadolinium contrast. The low signal intensity on T1-weighted imaging helps distinguish cholesteatomas from cholesterol granulomas. Cholesteatomas, however, can have intermediate signal intensity on T1-weighted imaging, making it sometimes difficult to differentiate them from cholesterol granulomas. It has been postulated that such lesions possess high lipid content.

On CT scan, a *mucocele* of the petrous apex appears as a soft tissue density filling the air cells with signs of bony destruction or bowing. The delicate septations that partition the air cells typically become destroyed and less delineated on CT scanning. By comparison the contralateral petrous air cells reveal similar pneumatization and are often aerated (**Fig. 25–4A**). On

MRI scan, petrous apex mucoceles have a similar appearance to that of cholesteatoma, with low signal intensity on T1-weighted images and high signal intensity on T2-weighted images (**Fig. 25–4B**). A rim of enhancement may be seen following administration of gadolinium contrast. The rim results from contrast accumulation in the hyperemic mucosal lining of the cyst. One must remember that with MRI alone it is almost impossible to distinguish a mucocele from a cholesteatoma. CT imaging must also be performed to assess the integrity of the bony architecture.

Petrous apicitis is an unusual infection of the petrous air cells occurring secondary to extension of a middle ear infection or mastoiditis. Since the advent of antibiotic therapy, petrous apicitis has become uncommon. On CT imaging, petrous apicitis appears as a nonexpansile lesion that may have irregular margins. There may also be some bony destruction similar to that seen with osteomyelitis of the skull base (**Fig. 25–5**). Apicitis does not enhance following administration of intravenous contrast, although if an abscess has formed, the lesion will have rim enhancement. On MRI,

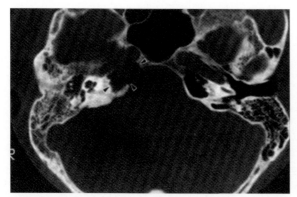

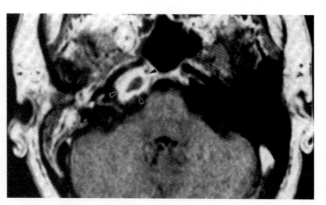

A

B

Figure 25–4 **(A)** Mucocele. CT imaging demonstrates irregular bony erosion of the posterior wall with good aeration of the contralateral petrous apex. Bony remodeling is clearly evident on imaging. Arrows that point to bony erosion and remodeling caused by the mucocele.

(B) T2-weighted MRI scan reveals medium- to high-signal intensity with rim enhancement (arrows) being a distinct possibility after gadolinium administration.

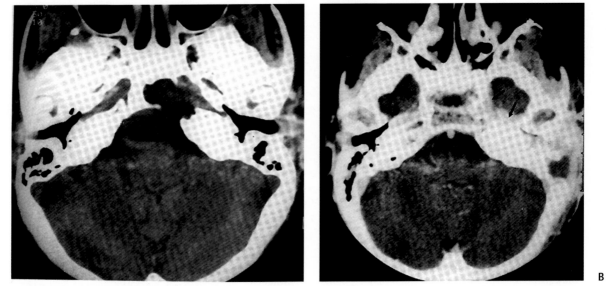

Figure 25–5 **(A,B)** Petrous apicitis. High-resolution axial unenhanced CT demonstrates an extensive, ill-defined lytic process involving the medial aspect of the left petrous apex (arrows).

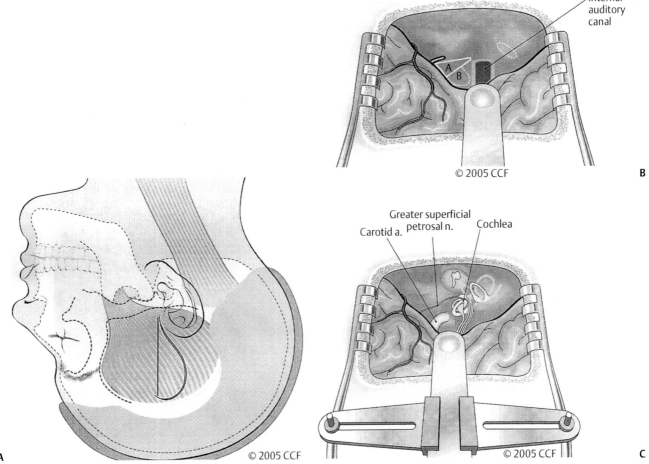

Figure 25–6 Middle cranial fossa approach. **(A)** A vertical or flap incision can be used. **(B)** Bone is removed from Kawase's triangle (solid line) and more medially to the superior petrosal sinus (dashed line). **(C)** The carotid artery and cochlea must be preserved. (From the Cleveland Clinic Foundation. Reprinted with permission.)

petrous apicitis demonstrates low signal intensity on T1-weighted images and high signal intensity on T2-weighted images. Rim enhancement following the administration of gadolinium contrast is dependent on whether a true abscess has formed. An abscess will have rim enhancement. Chronic apicitis demonstrates a heterogeneous appearance on T2-weighted imaging.

◆ Treatment

Surgical Approaches

Many surgical approaches to the petrous apex have been described for treatment of cystic lesions, depending on cyst type and location, patient hearing, and surgeon preference. Cholesterol granuloma can be removed or drained; cholesteatoma should be removed if possible. Some approaches preserve hearing; others do not. Some offer removal, and others use drainage. The one used most often for cyst removal with hearing preservation is the middle cranial fossa approach. The one used most often for cyst drainage with hearing preservation is the infracochlear-hypotympanic approach. Others include the infralabyrinthine, translabyrinthine, transcochlear, and transsphenoidal approaches. The retrosigmoid-suboccipital approach has been abandoned because of frequent chemical meningitis from cerebrospinal fluid (CSF) contamination.

The *middle cranial fossa approach* (**Fig. 25–6**) provides exposure for complete removal of the cyst unless it surrounds the carotid artery, and is preferred when the cyst lies adjacent to the cochlea. Bone is removed from Kawase's triangle, which has its base at the trigeminal nerve and apex at the geniculate ganglion (**Fig. 25–6B**). Additional bone is removed medially to the superior petrosal sinus. Care is taken to stay anterior to the basal turn of the cochlea (**Fig. 25–6C**). Below the cochlea, an additional 2 mm of posterior bone can be removed. The carotid artery lies deep to the greater superficial petrosal nerve, and is reddish and pulsatile. The cyst usually is more medial, bluish, and nonpulsatile. The cyst is exposed as much as possible, and then opened. Cholesterol granuloma contains thick, brown liquid. The fluid is suctioned out and the cyst wall is bluntly dissected from the bone and removed. Sometimes the posterior wall of the cyst is preserved to minimize risk to the cochlea and internal auditory canal. Usually a pressure equalizing tube is placed in the eardrum.

The *infracochlear (hypotympanic) approach* is usually a more conservative procedure to provide drainage, ventilation, or decompression of a cholesterol granuloma, mucocele, or effusion, and is best used when a large, expansile cyst lies near well-developed air cells in the hypotympanum. This approach is not designed for excision. Through a postauricular incision the ear is reflected anteriorly together with the transected lateral ear canal skin (**Fig. 25–7A,B**). The medial canal skin is elevated superiorly and left attached to the malleus umbo. The air cell tract below the cochlea is opened between the carotid artery and jugular bulb (**Fig. 25–7C,D**). These air cells connect the middle ear with the petrous apex, and can gently be curetted or drilled away to enhance drainage. The round window provides the superior line of dissection. Remaining below the round window prevents risk of injury to the internal auditory canal structures. Once the cyst is entered, a catheter may be placed to maintain drainage and aeration. A pressure equalizing tube can be placed in the drum.

The *transcochlear approach* to the petrous apex provides greater exposure and control of the carotid artery for larger lesions, but is less used for management of benign cysts because it destroys hearing and balance.

The *transsphenoidal approach* is useful only when a cyst forms a large surface area against the posterior wall of the sphenoid sinus. The lateral and superior walls of the sphenoid sinus are examined for indentations of the pituitary gland, optic nerve, maxillary nerve, and carotid artery. Once the wall of the cyst is identified, it is opened and drained.

Radiologic Confirmation of Petrous Apex Lesions

When the head, neck, and neurotologic examinations in the office are normal, a gadolinium contrasted MRI of the brain, base of skull, and infratemporal fossa is recommended. The clinician should bear in mind that an "abnormal" petrous apex finding on MRI may or may not be the cause of the symptoms. Both T1- and T2-weighted images should be compared. If MRI shows an apical cyst, a CT scan should also be obtained to further characterize the lesion.

Indications for Surgery

Surgery is indicated when the patient is symptomatic, when other causes are ruled out, and particularly when the CT scan shows the lesion to be expansile and eroding bone. Patients with expansile lesions usually present with headache or head pain and less often with other symptoms such as sensorineural hearing loss, vertigo, facial weakness, or dizziness. If the clinician is uncertain whether an apical cyst is the cause of symptoms, CT and MRI can be repeated in 6 months to check for cyst growth and bone destruction.

General Surgical Principles

General surgical principles are to (1) adequately drain or resect the lesion, (2) preserve hearing when possible, and (3) minimize the risk of cranial nerve and carotid artery injury and CSF leak. Treatment of cholesterol granuloma continues to be a constant debate among neurotologists. The infracochlear approach provides drainage of the cyst. Removal through the middle cranial fossa has more risk to hearing if the surgeon inadvertently enters the cochlea or internal auditory canal. Conservative near-total removal offers good long-term control with minimal morbidity from surgery. The infracochlear and middle cranial fossa approaches are recommended depending on the surgeon's experience and preference and cyst location.

Simple drainage of cholesteatoma is not curative. Total resection is possible when the lesion is small and separate from the carotid artery. Larger lesions tend to circumferentially involve the carotid artery. The risk to the carotid artery can be minimized by increasing exposure through the transcochlear and infratemporal fossa approaches, which allow for circumferential dissection of the carotid artery but sacrifice hearing. Generally, subtotal removal of cholesteatoma is recommended through the middle cranial fossa approach when the lesion is confined to the petrous apex and hearing is good. Serial MRI scans can then be used to follow any future progression of disease.

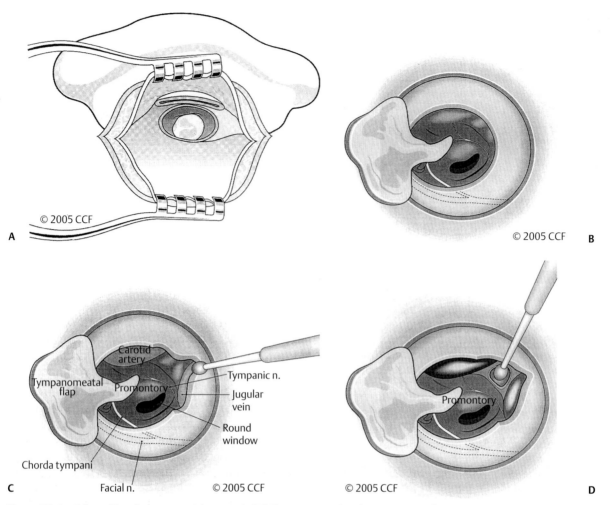

Figure 25–7 Infracochlear (hypotympanic) approach. **(A)** The ear canal skin is transected. Through a postauricular incision the lateral skin is retracted forward and medial skin is elevated. **(B)** The medial canal skin is elevated and left attached to the malleus umbo.

(C,D) Hypotympanic bone is removed between the carotid artery and jugular vein. (From the Cleveland Clinic Foundation. Reprinted with permission.)

References

1. Brackmann DE, Toh EH. Surgical management of petrous apex cholesterol granulomas. Otol Neurotol 2002;23:529–533
2. Jackler RK, Cho M. A new theory to explain the genesis of petrous apex cholesterol granuloma. Otol Neurotol 2003;24:96–106
3. Cristante L, Puchner MA. A keyhole middle fossa approach to large cholesterol granulomas of the petrous apex. Surg Neurol 2000;53:64–71
4. Muckle RP, De la Cruz A, Lo WM. Petrous apex lesions. Am J Otol 1998;19:219–225
5. Jackler RK, Cho M. A new theory to explain the genesis of petrous apex cholesterol granuloma. Otol Neurotol 2003;24:96–106
6. Brackmann DE, Toh EH. Surgical management of petrous cholesterol granuloma. Otol Neurotol 2002;23:529–533
7. Robert Y, Dubrulle F, Carcasset S, Hennequin C, Gaillandre L. Petrous bone extension of middle ear acquired cholesteatoma. Acta Radiol 1996;37:166–170
8. Profant M, Steno J. Petrous apex cholesteatoma. Acta Otolaryngol 2000;120:164–167
9. Atlas MD, Moffat DA, Hardy DG. Petrous apex cholesteatoma: diagnostic and treatment dilemmas. Laryngoscope 1992;102:1363–1368
10. Arriaga MA, Brackmann DE. Differential diagnosis of primary petrous apex lesions. Am J Otol 1991;12:470–474
11. Delozier HL, Perkins CW, Gacek RR. Mucocele of the petrous apex. J Laryngol Otol 1979;93:177–180
12. Chang P, Fagan PA, Atlas MD, Roche J. Imaging destructive lesions of the petrous apex. Laryngoscope 1998;108:599–604
13. Hentschel S, Durity F. Petrous apex granulomas: CT and MR imaging. Can J Neurol Sci 2002;29:169–170
14. Chole RA, Donald PJ. Petrous apicitis clinical indications. Ann Otol Rhinol Laryngol 1983;92:544–551
15. Peron DL, Schuknecht HF. Congenital cholesteatoma with other anomalies. Arch Otolaryngol 1975;101:498–505
16. Roland PS, Meyerhoff WL, Judge LO, Mickey BE. Asymmetric pneumatization of the petrous apex. Otolaryngol Head Neck Surg 1990;103:80–88
17. Leonetti JP, Shownkeen H, Marzo SJ. Incidental petrous apex findings on magnetic resonance imaging. Ear Nose Throat J 2001;80:200–206
18. Frates MC, Oates E. Petrous apicitis: evaluation by bone SPECT and magnetic resonance imaging. Clin Nucl Med 1990;15:293–294

26

Malignant Tumors of the Temporal Bone

Chandra M. Ivey and Myles L. Pensak

Malignant tumors of the temporal bone are often diagnosed at late stages of disease and portend a dismal prognosis. Symptoms are often analogous with those of chronic suppurative ear disease, and thus, in the absence of a high suspicion for malignancy, are treated as such. Electrophysiologic and neuroradiologic investigations may assist in the suggestion of malignant characteristics, and this heightened suspicion combined with contemporary skull base surgical techniques, adjuvant radiotherapy, and chemotherapy may improve survival rates over time. This chapter summarizes the pathobiology of temporal bone malignancies, the current literature on management options available at this time, and pain management options for palliative treatment for patients with these tumors.

◆ Anatomy of the Temporal Bone

The temporal bone is positioned between the middle and posterior cranial fossa and is constituted of four distinct segments: petrous, squamous, mastoid, and tympanic.[1] The petrous portion of the temporal bone contributes to the skull base of both the middle and posterior fossa, and is directed anteriorly and medially, juxtaposing the clivus and sphenoid. The squamous portion contributes to the lateral skull enclosing the temporal lobe of the brain. The mastoid portion contributes to the inferior-lateral skull base, and both enlarges and pneumatizes over the first few years of life to eventually overlie the stylomastoid foramen. The tympanic segment, although poorly developed at birth, forms the majority of the bony external auditory canal (EAC) and grows to maturity by age 3. The foramen of Huschke delineates the inadequate closure of the tympanic ring anteriorly.

Pneumatization of the petrous and mastoid portions of the temporal bone vary widely. The mesotympanum defines the largest pneumatized space and communicates directly with the eustachian tube anteriorly. This space communicates with the mastoid central air-cell tract via the aditus ad antrum, which then in turn may lead to perilabyrinthine, retrofacial, perisinus, apical, epitympanic, and sinodural air-cell tracts.[2]

Although there are many natural retardants to tumor spread within the temporal bone, some specific anatomic relationships within this region may assist in the extension of malignancy. The natural cleavage planes within the fibroelastic cartilage of the EAC, the fissures of Santorini, may allow delivery of tumor anteriorly to the parotid gland and posteriorly to the soft tissue lateral to the mastoid process. Incomplete closure of the foramen of Huschke also permits anterior spread into the parotid and glenoid fossa. If tumor invades the middle ear space, and thus the mesotympanum, there is potential for spread anteriorly through the eustachian tube to the infratemporal fossa and parapharyngeal space. This area also provides unimpeded access to all areas of the petrous bone through the central air-cell tract. Although the bony partitions of the temporal bone may retard direct tumor spread, as bony erosion occurs over time, access is allowed anteriorly toward the infratemporal fossa, inferiorly toward the jugular fossa, superiorly into the middle cranial vault, or posteriorly toward the posterior fossa.

Although there are recognized pathways of lymphatic drainage from the area around the temporal bone, metastatic spread from the area is not common.[3-6] When lymphadenopathy occurs, it is often associated with a secondary inflammatory process rather than with direct tumor involvement, but metastases have been reported in 10 to 15% of cases.[7,8]

Lymph nodes within the parotid and preauricular region receive drainage from the conchal bowl, cartilaginous canal, tragus, and fossa triangularis. Infraauricular lymph nodes receive drainage from the lobule and antitragus. Postauricular, or deep jugulodigastric lymphatics, along with spinal accessory lymphatics receive drainage from the helix and antihelix. The EAC lymphatics drain anteriorly into the preauricular and parotid lymph nodes, inferiorly into the upper cervical and deep internal jugular nodes, and posteriorly into the postauricular nodes. The middle ear has a reticular lymphatic network surrounding the eustachian tube and draining into the upper jugular and retropharyngeal lymph nodes. The inner ear has no known lymphatic drainage.

◆ Clinical Presentation and Assessment of Malignant Temporal Bone Tumors

Often indistinguishable from chronic suppurative otitis, patients with temporal bone malignancies commonly present with aural discharge, fullness, and hearing loss. Although bloody drainage may occur, it is more concerning in conjunction with pain. Symptoms more alarming for malignancy are cranial neuropathies, including facial paralysis and cochleovestibular deficits. Signs of meningeal involvement, including severe headache, may be late findings. **Table 26–1** lists the signs and symptoms found in the University of Cincinnati tumor registry recorded for patients with malignant temporal bone tumors from 1984 to 2005.

A complete history and neurotologic examination is essential in the evaluation of a temporal bone tumor. Audiometric, electrophysiologic, and neuroradiologic studies may also assist in defining the extent of tumor growth and the involvement of surrounding structures. Baseline studies can elaborate the etiology of hearing loss; audiometrics, including discrimination scores and acoustic reflexes, along with auditory brainstem response (ABR) may be used to assess retrocochlear pathology. Impedance assessments and tympanometry may help define middle ear involvement. Electronystagmography, rotation chair analysis, and platform posturography are of limited value, but will be abnormal if the integrity of the vestibular apparatus has been compromised.

Contemporary imaging techniques such as computed tomography (CT) and magnetic resonance imaging (MRI) have become gold standards for temporal bone assessment.[9–11] Adjuvant studies such as angiography, magnetic resonance angiography (MRA), and magnetic resonance venography (MRV) may also help in evaluation.[12]

CT performed at 1-mm intervals in a high-density bone window mode provides significant information regarding the status of the temporal bone and skull base. Bony erosion or disruption of the EAC, tegmen, or jugular foramen/carotid canal region may suggest the presence of a malignant process. The ossicles, semicanal of the tensor tympani muscle, and the eustachian tube are well defined on CT, and extratemporal involvement, including parotid, infratemporal fossa, and intracranial extension, can be easily appreciated[11,13] (**Fig. 26–1**).

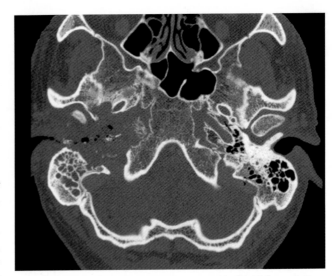

Figure 26–1 Extensive bone erosion is noted in this high-resolution axial computed tomography (CT) of the temporal bone.

Although MRI does not define bony erosion as well as CT does, it provides information about soft tissue involvement within the middle ear or other pneumatized spaces.[11,12] MRI may also show enhancement of the foramina, elucidating the spread of tumor along these pathways as well as extratemporal spread to surrounding structures. Dural violation as well as vascular involvement may be easily defined on MRI. MRA and MRV also display tumor vascularity, and may assist in further characterization of the tumor, as well as the patency of the surrounding vasculature due to analysis of flow voids (**Fig. 26–2B**).

Invasive vascular studies are performed less frequently for simple characterization of tumors since the increasing use of MRA and MRV. These studies may still assist in defining a patient's vascular arborization and thus the ability to tolerate internal artery compromise by means of xenon-131–assisted or balloon-occlusion studies. Carotid artery sacrifice may be indicated based on involvement of primary tumor or by the need for vascular control if heavy intraoperative bleeding is encountered. Embolization, although infrequently used, may be helpful in the perioperative setting to decrease bleeding from highly vascular tumors.

Although radionuclide studies are less helpful in initial evaluation of malignancy due to inflammation present in the area, they may be used to differentiate between recurrence and areas of osteoradionecrosis or infection.

Staging criteria for temporal bone malignancy have been published, but as of yet there is no universally accepted system. Although the American Joint Committee on Cancer uses the same staging system that has been applied to cutaneous malignancies at other sites, the unique anatomy of the temporal bone makes these criteria inadequate. Suggested staging systems have focused on tumor size and clinical appearance, as well as CT appearance of tumors.[12,14,15] **Tables 26–2** and **26–3** list the proposed staging systems from Arriaga et al and Pensak et al. Recently, Nakagawa et al[16] modified the Pittsburgh staging system to include tumors with infratemporal fossa involvement into the T3 category. Interestingly, research from this group has displayed an increased survival benefit for these tumors after radical surgery and preoperative radiation that has not been previously demonstrated.

Table 26–1 Signs and Symptoms of Malignant Temporal Bone Tumors

Signs	Percentage of Cases in Which Present	Symptoms	Percentage of Cases in Which Present
Canal mass or lesion	92%	Pain	72%
Aural drainage	84%	Hearing loss	66%
Periauricular swelling	29%	Pruritus	42%
Facial paralysis	20%	Bleeding	24%
Neck nodes	8%	Headache	20%
Temporal mass	6%	Tinnitus	20%
		Facial numbness	10%
		Vertigo	8%
		Hoarseness	4%

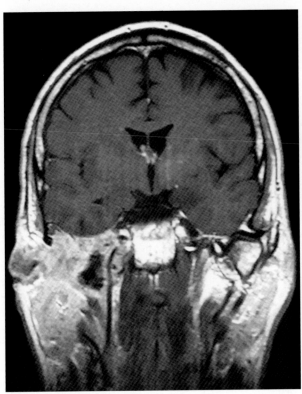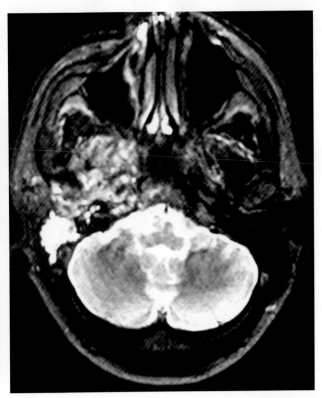

A
B

Figure 26–2 **(A,B)** Significant infratemporal fossa invasion is reflected by loss of soft tissue planes on magnetic resonance imaging (MRI) scan in both coronal and axial planes.

Table 26–2 Pittsburgh Staging System for Malignant External Auditory Canal Tumors

Stage	Description/Definition
T1	Tumor limited to external auditory canal without bony erosion or evidence of soft tissue extension
T2	Tumor with limited external auditory canal bony erosion (not full thickness) or radiographic finding consistent with limited (<0.5 cm) soft tissue involvement
T3	Tumor eroding the osseous external auditory canal (full thickness) with limited (<0.5 cm) soft tissue involvement or tumor involving the middle ear and/or mastoid or patients presenting with facial paralysis
T4	Tumor eroding cochlea, petrous apex, medial wall of the middle ear, carotid canal, jugular foramen, or dura, or with extensive (>0.5 cm) soft tissue involvement
N status	Involvement of lymph nodes is a poor prognostic finding and automatically places patient in an advanced stage [either stage III (T1N1) or stage IV (T2-T4N1)]
M status	Distant metastasis indicates a poor prognosis and immediately places patient in stage IV

Table 26–3 University of Cincinnati Grading System for Temporal Bone Tumors

Grade	Description/Definition
I	Tumor in a single site, 1 cm or smaller
II	Tumor in a single site, larger than 1 cm
III	Transannular tumor extension
IV	Mastoid or petrous air-cell invasion
V	Periauricular or contiguous extension (extratemporal/dural invasion)
VI	Neck adenopathy, distant anatomic site, or infratemporal fossa extension

◆ Pathology of Malignant Temporal Bone Tumors

Squamous cell carcinoma accounts for about 85% of malignancies of the EAC and petrous bone, although basal cell carcinoma (BCC) accounts for the majority of lesions on the pinna.[17–20] Other primary tumors of the temporal bone include glandular tumors, rhabdomyosarcoma, regionally invasive cancers, and metastatic disease, altogether accounting for the other 15% of tumors found in this region.[21–23] **Table 26–4** lists benign, aggressive benign, and malignant tumors of the temporal bone, and **Table 26–5** lists malignant tumors of metastatic origin found to invade the temporal bone.

Squamous Cell Carcinoma[24–30]

Squamous cell carcinoma most frequently appears within the cartilaginous portion of the EAC. Presenting patients are in the fifth to sixth decade and often have a history of chronic aural drainage, pain, and hearing loss. Misdiagnosis as suppurative otitis media or otitis externa accounts for these patients initially being treated with multiple courses of topical and systemic antibiotics without symptom resolution prior to biopsy being performed. As tumor extension occurs, chronic otalgia and cranial nerve damage (sensorineural hearing loss, facial weakness) become evident. Chewing and swallowing may become involved with tumor extension into the glenoid fossa and infratemporal fossa. Although significant local growth of these tumors may be evident at diagnosis, regional lymphatic metastasis is infrequent.

Although no etiologic factors have been found to explain squamous cell carcinoma of the EAC, predisposing conditions

Table 26–4 Benign, Aggressive Benign, and Malignant Temporal Bone Tumors

Benign	Aggressive Benign	Malignant
Meningioma, low grade	Chondroblastoma	Squamous cell
Schwannoma	Plasmacytoma	Basal cell
Paraganglioma	Hemangiopericytoma	Ceruminous gland tumor
Osteoma	Hemangioendothelioma	Rhabdomyosarcoma
Adenoma	Meningioma, high grade	Melanoma
Chordoma		Adenoidcystic
Lipoma		Chondrosarcoma
		Endolymphatic sac tumor
		Adenocarcinoma
		Chondrosarcoma
		Glioma
		Astrocytoma
		Medulloblastoma
		Neuroblastoma

Table 26–5 Metastatic Temporal Bone Tumors

Breast carcinoma
Renal carcinoma
Thyroid carcinoma
Lung carcinoma
GI/hepatocellular adenocarcinoma
Osteoblastoma
Non-Hodgkin's lymphoma
Leukemia
Melanoma

that have been examined include radiotherapy to the area, chronic otitis media, chronic otitis externa, cholesteatoma, and lymphoproliferative disorders. A select group of these patients have a common history of radium exposure. Squamous cell carcinoma is the second most common tumor of the auricle and is often related to sun exposure and local trauma.

On inspection, these tumors frequently appear granular and are quite friable with ill-defined borders. Manipulation may provoke bleeding, thus heightening suspicion and leading to biopsy.

Basal Cell Carcinoma[30–35]

BCC often presents on the helical rim, and can be found anywhere in the periauricular area. These tumors are associated with excessive sun exposure and are found with high prevalence in older Caucasian males. These tumors erode perichondrium and periosteum as they enlarge, and often set up conditions conducive to secondary infection at the site. Basal cell tumors often grow more slowly than squamous cell carcinomas, but are still able to deeply infiltrate surrounding tissues if left to progress. As these lesions do not illicit pain until deeply infiltrating, they are often neglected and late diagnosis ensues.

The most common variant of BCC is the nodular type; this variant, along with the superficial and ulcerative variants, is less aggressive than the morpheaform and basaloid variants. Because of their common location on the auricle, these tumors are often removed with the assistance of Mohs' micrographic surgery in an effort to minimize the removal of non-involved tissues. This method has been shown to be effective as long as there is no involvement of the EAC.

Glandular Tumors[15,22,36–39]

Despite the fact that the skin of the EAC contains ceruminous, modified apocrine, and sebaceous glands, glandular tumors of the EAC are very uncommon. More frequently, regionally invasive salivary gland tumors extending from the parotid gland are encountered. In most low-grade tumors of this region, including adenoidcystic carcinoma despite its propensity for neural invasion, surgery with preservation of the facial nerve has become the mainstay. Tumors such as high-grade adenocarcinoma, high-grade mucoepidermoid, and acinic cell carcinoma continue to be dealt with in an aggressive fashion with nerve sacrifice when involved.

Primary low-grade adenocarcinoma of the endolymphatic sac, or aggressive papillary cystadenoma, are found to invade the temporal bone. These are very rare tumors, but have been diagnosed in clinical connection with von Hippel–Lindau (VHL) disease. Certain mutations within the VHL gene locus have been shown to correlate with loss of a tumor-suppressor gene, both in familial and sporadic VHL. It is thought that further genetic research may be able to predict solely with genetic testing which VHL patients will develop endolymphatic sac tumors.

Rhabdomyosarcoma[40–42]

Rhabdomyosarcoma is the most common soft tissue sarcoma of childhood. The embryonal variant is the most likely to affect the head and neck, and 4 to 7% of these lesions involve the temporal bone. Unfortunately, 20% of children diagnosed with this lesion have metastatic spread at the time of presentation. These children often present with aural discharge and with friable polyps within the ear. Otalgia and facial nerve weakness may also be present. Disease presenting within the temporal bone portends poor prognosis, as patients often have incurable local disease.

Multimodal treatment for rhabdomyosarcoma has improved outcome significantly. Multidrug chemotherapy with radiation or surgery has come to be the mainstay of treatment. Surgical options are often used for biopsy and debulking of disease, as complete surgical excision within this area is extremely difficult, deforming, and unnecessary in light of recent chemotherapeutic options.

Metastatic Tumors[43–58]

A variety of metastatic tumors have been diagnosed within the temporal bone. Hematopoietic lesions including lymphoma and leukemia may invade the temporal bone. Plasmacytoma may also be found in this region. The lesions may manifest as a granular, friable mass in the middle ear or mastoid.

Malignant or highly aggressive benign intracranial tumors may occasionally invade the temporal bone, including seeding from meningeal carcinomatosis in rare cases. Primary brain tumors with invasion into the temporal bone may include medulloblastoma, neuroblastoma, malignant meningioma, and choroid plexus tumors. Likely hematogenous spread from the breast, kidney, thyroid, lung, liver, and gastrointestinal system has also been documented.

◆ Clinical Management

Once a malignancy involving the temporal bone has been recognized, it is important to determine the resectability of the tumor, along with the functional status of the patient. Limitations of both CT and MRI may prevent distinction between tumor and inflammatory process or cholesterol granuloma within the air-cell system and petrous apex, making it difficult to fully evaluate extent of tumor. Most protocols would exclude surgical intervention in patients with gross intraparenchymal brain invasion, extensive infratemporal fossa involvement, or extension along the internal carotid artery to the cavernous sinus.[59-62] Patients with severe intercurrent systemic disease, especially cardiopulmonary in origin, may not tolerate the extended surgical intervention necessary for tumor resection. Palliative radiation may be offered as a treatment option in these cases.[63-66]

Total en bloc resection of the temporal bone has been advocated for the treatment of temporal bone malignancies, but a piecemeal approach has also been developed due to studies displaying the improbability of not violating tumor margins during surgical excision.[67,68] Although debate continues as to which approach shows the best clinical outcome, some standard surgical options have been traditionally outlined for resection of disease.

Surgical Excision

Wedge Resection

If tumor is exclusively located on the auricle without extension into the temporal bone, a wedge resection is often adequate treatment.[69] Mohs' microsurgical techniques also offer an alternative that spares noninvolved tissue in these smaller tumors.[35] Briefly, the skin surrounding the lesion and the underlying auricular cartilage is removed. The defect may be closed primarily or with the application of a split-thickness skin graft.

Sleeve Resection

Lesions in the ear canal lateral to the bony cartilaginous junction may be amenable to a composite sleeve resection (see **Fig. 26–3**).[70,71] With this technique, a medial incision is completed initially to ensure that the bony cartilaginous region is not involved. Then a lateral cut is made to encompass the lesion, surrounding skin, and underlying cartilage. This is removed, and reconstruction may utilize split-thickness skin grafting.

Lateral Temporal Bone Resection

Lesions of the ear canal that lie juxtaposed to the bony cartilaginous junction or extend medially without gross violation of the tympanic annulus may be treated with a lateral temporal bone resection (see **Fig. 26–3**).[72-76] This may be performed in conjunction with a parotidectomy for completeness. A superiorly or postauricularly based flap is created to isolate

the noninvolved auricle centered around an "apple core" circumscribing the lesion. A cortical mastoidectomy and extended facial recess are drilled. The incudostapedial joint is separated and the roof of the middle ear is dissected from the tegmen plate. The zygomatic root is sectioned and the floor is separated just lateral to the facial nerve, jugular bulb, and internal carotid artery. The skin and cartilage of the auricle plus the EAC, tympanic ring and membrane, and malleus-incus complex are removed. A split-thickness skin graft with bolster packing is used for closure.

Subtotal Temporal Bone Resection

This resection removes the temporal bone lateral to the internal carotid artery, medially to the internal auditory canal (IAC), and inferiorly to the jugular foramen, leaving only the petrous apex.[77-79] A temporal craniotomy is performed to allow access to the IAC and demonstrate the absence of tumor along the floor of the middle fossa. Tumor may resected if it involves dura only, but if extension into the temporal lobe parenchyma is found, the tumor is considered inoperable. The temporal lobe is identified superiorly and the posterior fossa is uncovered posteriorly. The carotid and jugular veins are identified within the neck and followed superiorly to the skull base. The jugular bulb and sigmoid sinus are also completely unroofed with a mastoidectomy. Anteriorly, the facial nerve is identified within the parotid gland. The mandibular condyle is sectioned and the bone is severed cleanly from the middle fossa dura superiorly, internal carotid artery anteroinferiorly, and the IAC medially. Often, piecemeal removal of residual areas of tumor is necessary after this resection. A myocutaneous flap or regional flap may be used for closure. Recently, free vascular flaps have been employed successfully for closure.[80]

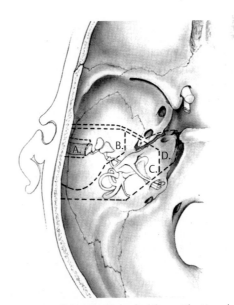

Figure 26–3 **(A)** Lesions lateral to the cartilaginous bony external auditory canal junction are amenable to sleeve resection. **(B)** Extension to the bony external auditory canal that does not violate the middle ear or mastoid is often managed with a lateral temporal bone resection. **(C)** The margins of a subtotal temporal bone resection are shown extending to the internal auditory canal medially. **(D)** In a total temporal bone resection the petrous apex is taken. Some authors have advocated sacrifice of the internal carotid artery.

Total Temporal Bone Resection

This resection includes the petrous apex with the removed specimen.[81–85] The petrous apex is isolated from the cavernous sinus at the anterior medial aspect of the bony carotid artery. The carotid is then mobilized anteriorly and medially during resection, or may be resected with the specimen. The 5-year survival rate after total temporal bone resection is no different from that after subtotal temporal bone resection, but it carries greater risk of bleeding, stroke, multiple craniopathies, and death.

Radiation Therapy

Radiation therapy is used in conjunction with surgical excision to treat temporal bone malignancies.[63–66] The radiation protocol is individualized to each patient, but often uses a wedged-pair photon radiation field with total dosage of 7000 rads, whereas brain exposure is held to 6000 rads. Preauricular, postauricular, and subdigastric nodes are usually encompassed within the radiation field setup.

More recently, intensity-modulated radiation therapy as an adjunct to external beam radiation has been trialed on selected tumors of the head and neck, including temporal bone carcinoma. Proper dosimetry and accurate target volume delineation have led to excellent reported local-freedom-from progression rates.[86] Stereotactically guided gamma knife surgery to date has been published only for treatment of benign temporal bone disease.[87]

Primary radiotherapy is indicated in palliation and eradication of pain from bony metastasis in head and neck cancer. Pain relief has been reported in 70 to 90% of patients treated for bony metastasis in this manner.[88] Others question the use of radiotherapy for pain and feel that the same results may be achieved with proper analgesics.[31]

Complications of radiotherapy are well recognized and can range from minor to severe. Radiation of the auricle may cause desquamation, irritation, dryness, and necrosis of the remaining cartilage. Within the EAC, thickening of the canal epithelium and tympanic membrane has been documented, along with loss of cerumen glands leading to severe dryness. Within the middle ear eustachian tube dysfunction may lead to effusion. Osteoradionecrosis may occur at the bony EAC, mastoid, or skull base due to devascularization of the bone. Radiation-induced tumors, parenchymal brain necrosis, and carotid artery pseudoaneurysm, although extremely rare, may occur following radiation to the temporal bone.[89–91]

Chemotherapy

Chemotherapeutic regimens are the mainstay of treatment for pediatric rhabdomyosarcoma with adjuvant radiation and surgery when indicated.[42] Single- and multidrug regimen chemotherapy is being evaluated for use in head and neck cancer with metastasis. Treatment under investigation include taxanes, cisplatin, and 5-fluorouracil.[92] Unfortunately, the use of chemotherapeutic agents has not yet been shown to significantly impact survival rates.

Pain Management and Quality of Life

Patients diagnosed with temporal bone malignancies may present with pain. Pain may be attributed to the primary tumor mass, bony erosion, or compromise of vascular and nervous structures as the tumor infiltrates areas around the temporal bone, such as the cerebellopontine angle, infratemporal fossa, temporomandibular joint, or upper cervical region. Unfortunately, cancer pain is often underestimated and undertreated.[93] Treatment options available, usually consisting of combination surgery and radiation therapy, have been found to cause significant increases in pain when evaluated using quality-of-life survey techniques.[94] Myofascial spasm may also contribute to discomfort after surgical disruption of normal functional muscle groups.

Pharmacologic management of pain in the head and neck region includes identification and control of both somatic and neuropathic pain. Somatic pain control guidelines have been adopted by the World Health Organization and outline treatment plans beginning with mild analgesics plus nonsteroidal antiinflammatory medication, progressing to mild opiates, and finally to opioid analgesics.[95] Effective treatment for neuropathic pain may begin with amitriptyline and carbamazepine. Nerve blocks, especially for malignancies involving the cranial nerves and sympathetic/parasympathetic chains, may be indicated for effective pain management.[96]

◆ Conclusion

Diagnosis and management of temporal bone malignancy continues to be a formidable challenge, despite advances in microsurgical techniques. Although tumors limited to the auricle or confined to the EAC portend relatively favorable prognosis, it is often not possible preoperatively to fully appreciate the tumor extent. Temporal bone resection is difficult, and may not allow for en bloc excision of malignancy. Establishment of clean margins is further encumbered by inadequate tumor volume in frozen section specimens, sampling error, and significant quantities of bone in the sample specimen. There is significant variability in survival data for temporal bone cancer, with data generally showing 5-year cure rates ranging from 25 to 50%.

In cases where complete resection is questioned, adjunctive radiation therapy may be employed. Although there has been agreement that radiation therapy alone has proven ineffective for complete treatment of temporal bone malignancy, its use in the postoperative period has been shown to increase survivorship in patients once gross tumor has been removed. Chemotherapy has been indicated in only a limited set of tumor types.

Surgical and adjuvant intervention for temporal bone malignancy represents a possibility for life-sustaining treatment in light of a rare and dire tumor, especially after frequent delay in diagnosis. High suspicion for these tumors, along with adequate assessment and treatment of pain accompanying both disease and treatment, may allow potentially favorable outcomes despite the often poor prognosis accompanying diagnosis.

References

1. Anson BJ, Donaldson JA, eds. Surgical Anatomy of the Temporal Bone. Philadelphia: WB Saunders, 1981
2. Schuknecht H. Pathology of the Ear, 2nd ed. Philadelphia: Lea & Febiger, 1993
3. Lewis JS. Surgical management of tumors of the middle ear and mastoid. J Laryngol Otol 1983;97:299–311

4. Goodwin WJ, Jess RH. Malignant neoplasms of the external auditory canal and temporal bone. Arch Otolaryngol 1980;106:675–679

5. Kinney SE, Wood BG. Malignancies of the external ear canal and temporal bone: surgical techniques and results. Laryngoscope 1987; 97:158–164

6. Chung SJ, Pensak ML. Tumors of the temporal bone. In: Jackler R, Brackmann D, eds. Neurotology, 2nd ed. Philadelphia: Elsevier Mosby, 2005

7. Pensak ML. Skull base surgery. In: Glasscock ME, Shambaugh GE, eds. Surgery of the Ear. Philadelphia: WB Saunders, 1990;503–533

8. Arena S, Keen M. Carcinoma of the middle ear and temporal bone. Am J Otol 1988;9:351–356

9. Phelps PD, Lloyd GAS. The radiology of carcinoma of the ear. Br J Radiol 1981;54:103–109

10. Arriaga M, Curtin H, Takahashi H, et al. Staging proposal for external auditory meatus carcinoma based on computer tomography findings. Ann Otol Rhinol Laryngol 1990;99:714–721

11. Friedman DP, Rao VM. MR and CT of squamous cell carcinoma of the middle ear and mastoid complex. AJNR Am J Neuroradiol 1991;12:872–874

12. Ball JB Jr, Pensak ML. Fundamentals of magnetic resonance imaging. Am J Otol 1987;8:81–85

13. Swartz JD, Russell KB, Wolfson RJ, et al. High resolution computed tomography in evaluation of the temporal bone. Head Neck Surg 1984; 6:921–931

14. Pensak ML, Gleich LL, Gluckman JL, et al. Temporal bone carcinoma: Contemporary perspectives in the skull base surgical era. Laryngoscope 1996;106:1234–1237

15. Stell PM, McCormick MS. Carcinoma of the external auditory meatus and middle ear: prognostic factors and a suggested staging system. J Laryngol Otol 1985;99:847–850

16. Nakagawa T, Natori Y, Kumamoto Y, et al. Squamous cell carcinoma of the external auditory canal and middle ear: proposal of modification of Pittsburgh TNM staging system. American Otological Society 138th annual meeting, Boca Raton, Florida, 2005

17. Batsakis JG, eds. Tumors of the Head and Neck, 2nd ed. Baltimore: Williams & Wilkins, 1979

18. Gacek R, Goodman M. Management of malignancy of the temporal bone. Laryngoscope 1977;87:1622–1634

19. Clairmont AA, Conley JJ. Primary carcinoma of the mastoid bone. Ann Otol Rhinol Laryngol 1977;86:306–309

20. Case records of the Massachusetts General Hospital. N Engl J Med 1989; 320:921–931

21. Wiatrak BJ, Pensak ML. Rhabdomyosarcoma of the ear and temporal bone. Laryngoscope 1989;99:1188–1192

22. Pulec JL. Glandular tumors of the external auditory canal. Laryngoscope 1977;87:1601–1612

23. Perzin KH, Gullane P, Conley J. Adenoid cystic carcinoma involving the external auditory canal: a clinicopathologic study of 16 cases. Cancer 1982;50:2873–2883

24. Lewis JS. Squamous carcinoma of the ear. Arch Otolaryngol 1973;97:41–42

25. Tucker WN. Cancer of the middle ear: a review of 89 cases. Cancer 1965;18:642–650

26. Lewis JS. A guide to cancer of the ear. CA Cancer J Clin 1977;27:42–46

27. Arena S, Keen M. Carcinoma of the middle ear and temporal bone. Am J Otol 1988;9:351–356

28. Conley J, Schuller DE. Malignancies of the ear. Laryngoscope 1976;86: 1147–1163

29. Crabtree JA, Britton BH, Pierce MK. Carcinoma of the external auditory canal. Laryngoscope 1976;86:405–415

30. Ahmad I, Das Gupta AR. Epidemiology of basal cell carcinoma and squamous cell carcinoma of the pinna. J Laryngol Otol 2001;115:85–86

31. Adams GL, Paparella MM, el Fiky FM. Primary and metastatic tumors of the temporal bone. Laryngoscope 1971;81:1273–1285

32. Parkin JL, Stevens MH. Basal cell carcinoma of the temporal bone. Otolaryngol Head Neck Surg 1979;87:645–647

33. Harwood AR, Keane TJ. Malignant tumors of the temporal bone and external ear: medical and radiation therapy. In: Alberti PW, Reuben RJ, eds. Otologic Medicine and Surgery, vol 2. London: Churchill Livingstone, 1988

34. Spector JG. Management of temporal bone carcinomas: a therapeutic analysis of two groups of patients and long term follow-up. Otolaryngol Head Neck Surg 1991;104:58–66

35. Glied M, Berg D, Witterick I. Basal cell carcinoma of the conchal bowl: Interdisciplinary approach to treatment. J Otolaryngol 1998; 27:322–326

36. Cannon CR, McLean WC. Adenoid cystic carcinoma of the middle ear and temporal bone. Otolaryngol Head Neck Surg 1983;91:96–99

37. Choo D, Shotland L, Mastroianni M, et al. Endolymphatic sac tumors in von Hippel-Lindau disease. J Neurosurg 2004;100:480–487

38. Irving RM. The molecular pathology of tumours of the ear and temporal bone. J Laryngol Otol 1998;112:1011–1018

39. Kawahara N, Kume H, Ueki K, et al. VHL gene inactivation in an endolymphatic sac tumor associated with von Hippel-Lindau disease. Neurology 1999;53:208–210

40. Feldman BA. Rhabdomyosarcomas of the head and neck. Laryngoscope 1982;92:424–440

41. Raney RB Jr, Lawrence W Jr, Maurer HM. Rhabdomyosarcoma of the ear in childhood. Report from the Intergroup Rhabdomyosarcoma Study-I. Cancer 1983;51:2356–2361

42. Durve DV, Kanegoankar RG, Albert D, Levitt G. Paediatric rhabdomyosarcoma of the ear and temporal bone. Clin Otolaryngol 2004;29:32–37

43. Zechner G, Altmann F. The temporal bone in leukemia: histological studies. Ann Otol Rhinol Laryngol 1969;78:375–387

44. Harbert F, Liu JC, Berry RG. Metastatic malignant melanoma to both VIIIth nerves. J Laryngol Otol 1969;83:889–898

45. Hoshino T, Hirade F, Normura Y. Metastatic tumor of the inner ear: a histopathological report. J Laryngol Otol 1972;86:697–707

46. Maddox HE 3rd. Metastatic tumors of the temporal bone. Ann Otol Rhinol Laryngol 1967;76:149–165

47. Stucker FJ, Holmes WF. Metastatic disease of the temporal bone. Laryngoscope 1976;86:1136–1140

48. Paparella MM, el Fiky FM. Ear involvement in malignant lymphoma. Ann Otol Rhinol Laryngol 1972;81:352–362

49. Takahara T, Sando I, Bluestone CD, et al. Lymphoma invading the anterior Eustachian tube: temporal bone histopathology of functional tubal obstruction. Ann Otol Rhinol Laryngol 1986;95:101–105

50. Thomas JR, David WE. Breast carcinoma metastatic to the temporal bone. Mo Med 1975;72:77–78

51. Brown NE, O'Brien DA, Megerian CA. Metastatic hepatocellular carcinoma to the temporal bone in a post-liver transplant patient. Otolaryngol Head Neck Surg 2004;130:370–371

52. Ruenes R, Palacios E. Plasmacytoma of the petrous temporal bone. Ear Nose Throat J 2003;82:672

53. Koral K, Curran JG, Thompson A. Primary non-Hodgkin's lymphoma of the temporal bone: CT findings. Clin Imaging 2003;27:386–388

54. Chang CY, O'Halloran EK, Fisher SR. Primary non-Hodgkin's lymphoma of the petrous bone: Case report. Otolaryngol Head Neck Surg 2004;130: 360–362

55. Musacchio M, Mont'Alverne F, Belzile F, et al. Posterior cervical haemangiopericytoma with intracranial and skull base extension. J Neuroradiol 2003;30:180–187

56. Ohba S, Kurokawa R, Yoshida K, Kawase T. Metastatic adenocarcinoma of the dura mimicking petroclival meningioma. Neurol Med Chir (Tokyo) 2004;44:317–320

57. Kim HL, Im SA, Lim GY, et al. High grade hemangioendothelioma of the temporal bone in a child. Korean J Radiol 2004;5:214–217

58. Gaudet EL Jr, Nuss DW, Johnson DH Jr, Miranne LS Jr. Chondroblastoma of the temporal bone involving the temporomandibular joint, mandibular condyle, and middle cranial fossa: case report and review of the literature. Cranio 2004;22:160–168

59. Arena S. Treatment of carcinoma of the temporal bone. Am J Otol 1983;5: 56–61

60. Conley J, Schuller DE. Malignancies of the ear. Laryngoscope 1976;86: 1147–1163

61. Ariyan S, Sasaki CT, Spenser D. Radical en bloc resection of the temporal bone. Am J Surg 1981;142:443–447

62. Graham MD, Sataloff RT, Kemink JL, et al. Total en bloc resection of the temporal bone and carotid artery for malignant tumors of the ear and temporal bone. Laryngoscope 1984;94:528–533

63. Million RR, Cassisi NJ. Temporal bone. In: Million RR, Cassisi NJ, eds. Management of Head and Neck Cancer: A Multidisciplinary Approach. Philadelphia: JB Lippincott, 1984

64. Wang CC. Radiation therapy in the management of carcinoma of the external auditory canal, middle ear, or mastoid. Radiology 1975;116:713–715

65. Gabriele P, Mannano M, Albera R, et al. Carcinoma of the auditory meatus and middle ear. Results of the treatment of 28 cases. Tumori 1994; 80:40–43

66. Korzeniowski S, Pszon J. The results of radiotherapy of cancer of the middle ear. Int J Radiat Oncol Biol Phys 1990;18:631–633

67. Lewis JS. Surgical management of tumors of the middle ear and mastoid. J Laryngol Otol 1983;97:299–311

68. Neely JG, Forrester M. Anatomic consideration of the medial cuts in subtotal temporal bone resection. Otolaryngol Head Neck Surg 1982;90: 641–645

69. Bailin PL, Levine HL, Wood BG, et al. Cutaneous carcinoma of the auricular and periauricular region. Arch Otolaryngol 1980;106:692–696

70. Kinney SE, Wood BG. Malignancies of the external ear canal and temporal bone: surgical techniques and results. Laryngoscope 1987;97:158–164

71. Krepsi YP, Levine TM. Management and therapy of tumors of the temporal bone. In: Alberti PW, Reuben RJ, eds. Otologic Medicine and Surgery. New York: Churchill-Livingstone, 1988

72. Schramm VL. Temporal bone resection. In: Sekhar LN, Schramm VL, eds. Tumors of the Cranial Base: Diagnosis and Treatment. Mount Kisco, NY: Futura, 1987

73. Arena S. Tumor surgery of the temporal bone. Laryngoscope 1974;84: 645–670

74. Conley J. Cancer of the middle ear. Trans Am Otol Soc 1965;53:189–207

75. Goodwin WJ, Jess RH. Malignant neoplasms of the external auditory canal and temporal bone. Arch Otolaryngol 1980;106: 675–679

76. Kinney SE, Wood BG. Surgical treatment of skull base malignancy. Otolaryngol Head Neck Surg 1984;92:94–99

77. Hilding DA, Selker R. Total resection of the temporal bone for carcinoma. Arch Otolaryngol 1969;89:636–645

78. Kinney SE. Clinical evaluation and treatment of ear tumors. In: Thawley E, Panje WR, eds. Comprehensive Management of Head and Neck Tumors. Philadelphia: WB Saunders, 1987

79. Lewis JS. Temporal bone resection: review of 100 cases. Arch Otolaryngol 1975;101:23–25

80. Wax MK, Burkey BB, Bascom D, Rosenthal EL. The role of free tissue transfer in the reconstruction of massive neglected skin cancers of the head and neck. Arch Facial Plast Surg 2003;5:479–482

81. Wu BT, Wang FT. Long term observation of total temporal bone resection in carcinoma of the middle ear and temporal bone. Chin Med J (Engl) 1984;97:205–210 [Engl]

82. Sekhar LN, Schramm VL Jr, et al. Operative management of large neoplasms of the lateral and posterior cranial base. In: Sekhar LN, Schramm VL, eds. Tumors of the Cranial Base: Diagnosis and Treatment. Mount Kisco, NY: Futura, 1987

83. Lesser RW, Spector GJ, Devineni VR. Malignant tumors of the middle ear and external auditory canal: a 20-year review. Otolaryngol Head Neck Surg 1987;96:43–47

84. Stucker FJ, Holmes WF. Metastatic disease of the temporal bone. Laryngoscope 1976;86:1136–1140

85. Tabb HG, Komet H, McLaurin JW. Cancer of the external auditory canal: treatment with radical mastoidectomy and irradiation. Laryngoscope 1964;74:634–654

86. Lee N, Xia P, Fischbein NH, et al. Intensity-modulated radiation therapy for head and neck cancer: the UCSF experience focusing on target volume delineation. Int J Radiat Oncol Biol Phys 2003;57:49–60

87. Linskey ME, Johnstone PAS, O'Leary M, Goetsch S. Radiation exposure of normal temporal bone structures during stereotactically guided gamma knife surgery for vestibular schwannomas. J Neurosurg 2003;98:800–806

88. Buckley JG, Ferlito A, Shaha AR, Rinaldo A. The treatment of distant metastases in head and neck cancer—present and future. ORL J Otorhinolaryngol Relat Spec 2001;63:259–264

89. Hsieh ST, Guo YC, Tsai TL, et al. Parosteal osteosarcoma of the mastoid bone following radiotherapy for nasopharyngeal carcinoma. J Chin Med Assoc 2004;67:314–316

90. Wang PC, Tu TY, Liu KD. Cystic brain necrosis and temporal bone osteoradionecrosis after radiotherapy and surgery in a patient of ear carcinoma. J Chin Med Assoc 2004;67:487–491

91. Auyeung KM, Lui WM, Chow LCK, Chan FL. Massive epistaxis related to petrous carotid artery pseudoaneurysm after radiation therapy: emergency treatment with covered stent in two cases. AJNR Am J Neuroradiol 2003;24:1449–1452

92. de Mulder PH. The chemotherapy of head and neck cancer. Anticancer Drugs 1999;10(suppl 1):S33–S37

93. Griepp ME. Undermedication for pain: an ethical model. ANS Adv Nurs Sci 1992;15:44–53

94. Whale Z, Lyne PA, Papanikolaou P. Pain experience following radical treatment for head and neck cancer. Eur J Oncol Nurs 2001;5:112–120

95. World Health Organization. Cancer Pain Relief and Palliative Care: Report of a WHO Expert Committee. Geneva: WHO, 1990

96. Vecht CJ, Hoff AM, Kansen PJ, de Boer MF, Bosch DA. Types and causes of pain in cancer of the head and neck. Cancer 1992;70:178–184

27

Vestibular Disorders

Mitchell K. Schwaber

Dizziness is the term used to describe a myriad of patient perceptions, including lightheadedness, syncope, disequilibrium, panic attacks, motion intolerance, visual disturbances, and true vertigo. It is the clinician's responsibility to determine which of these perceptions the patient is experiencing by obtaining a careful history, often using descriptions in laymen's terms. True vertigo is characterized by the perception that the external world is spinning, whirling, or swaying, and it is usually indicative of a vestibular disorder. Furthermore, true vertigo is usually accompanied by nystagmus. On the other hand, patients with nonvestibular dizziness more often perceive a sensation of movement or disorientation within their head, rather than the perception of the external world spinning. Also, nonvestibular dizziness is rarely accompanied by nystagmus. Chapter 14 discusses other features that can be helpful in differentiating vestibular and nonvestibular dizziness.

Once the clinician has established that the patient is experiencing vertigo, it is important next to determine if hearing loss is present or not. Depending on this determination, the most likely diagnosis can soon be reached.

◆ Episodic Vertigo with Hearing Loss

The differential diagnosis of episodic vertigo with hearing loss includes Meniere's syndrome and Meniere's disease, perilymph fistula, temporal bone fracture, syphilitic labyrinthitis, vascular occlusion of the labyrinthine artery, labyrinthine fistulas, labyrinthitis, and acoustic tumor. To rapidly differentiate these diagnoses, temporal bone fracture follows obvious head trauma; labyrinthine fistulas and labyrinthitis are associated with ear infections, pain, and drainage, or ear surgery; vascular occlusion is associated with a sudden single episode of vertigo with nearly total loss of hearing; Meniere's syndrome is associated with ear fullness, fluctuating hearing loss, and episodic vertigo without antecedent factors; perilymph fistula is associated with sensorineural loss, vertigo, and disequilibrium that occur after an event associated with straining, lifting, or a surgical procedure; syphilitic labyrinthitis can be indistinguishable from Meniere's syndrome and should be considered in any case that does not have a ready explanation,

particularly when bilateral; acoustic tumor is usually associated with progressive sensorineural hearing loss, tinnitus, and usually only disequilibrium; ototoxicity is associated with the development of hearing loss, loss of balance, and ataxia during or immediately following a course of intravenous antibiotic therapy. Further information concerning each follows.

Meniere's Syndrome and Meniere's Disease

Meniere's syndrome is defined as the clinical disorder associated with the histopathologic finding of endolymphatic hydrops. Clinically, Meniere's syndrome includes the following features: recurrent, spontaneous episodic vertigo; hearing loss; aural fullness; and tinnitus. Under the most recent guidelines of the American Academy of Otolaryngology–Head and Neck Surgery,[1] either tinnitus or fullness or both must be present on the affected side to establish the diagnosis. Recognized causes of Meniere's syndrome include (1) idiopathic, also known as Meniere's disease; (2) posttraumatic, following head injury or ear surgery; (3) postinfectious or delayed-onset Meniere's syndrome following a viral infection, usually mumps or measles; (4) late-stage syphilis; (5) classic Cogan's syndrome with episodic vertigo, hearing loss, interstitial keratitis, without syphilis; (6) variant Cogan's syndrome with episodic vertigo, hearing loss, uveitis, or other ocular inflammation and without syphilis and other immune-mediated inner ear diseases.

Although Meniere's disease is by far the most common cause of Meniere's syndrome and the terms are often used interchangeably, it should be remembered that a patient has an idiopathic etiology only when the known causes have been excluded.

Clinical Presentation

Meniere's disease is characterized by a history of increasing ear fullness with roaring tinnitus, followed by a sensation of blocked hearing. If the symptoms further worsen, a definitive vertigo spell may occur within a few minutes. Alternatively, patients may note the sudden onset of vertigo with little or no warning. Friberg et al[2] found that the disorder begins with hearing loss alone in 42%, vertigo alone in 11%, vertigo with hearing loss in 44%, and tinnitus alone in 3%.

The definitive vertigo spell is spontaneous rotational vertigo lasting 20 minutes or longer, with accompanying nausea, vomiting, and other autonomic symptoms. Most vertigo episodes last from 2 to 4 hours, although some can last for more than 6 hours. During the episode of vertigo, horizontal or horizontal-rotary nystagmus is *always* present. Following the vertigo episode, the patient may note that the hearing in the involved ear is markedly diminished. Disequilibrium may follow the definitive episode and may last for several days. Although the clinician might strongly suspect that the patient has Meniere's disease, definitive diagnosis depends on the occurrence of two or more definitive episodes lasting 20 minutes or longer.

The hearing loss that occurs with Meniere's disease typically begins with acoustic distortion that can be best described as a tinny quality to the signal. Another description is that only the higher-intensity peaks of certain frequencies are heard, whereas the rest of the frequencies are somewhat clipped or muffled. Loudness recruitment or loudness intolerance is also noted early in the illness, and is usually described by the patient as ordinary sounds being painfully loud in the affected ear. Early in the illness, many patients experience fluctuating hearing, with recovery beginning within a few hours of the episode. Hearing recovery may occur several days or months after a severe episode of vertigo. Either a shift of 10 dB or more in the average threshold of 0.5, 1, 2, and 3 kHz or a shift in speech discrimination of 15% is considered a significant change.

The hearing loss that accompanies Meniere's disease typically follows one of three forms[1]: (1) a low-frequency sensorineural loss that is greatest at 250 Hz, 500 Hz, and at 1 kHz, with a normal threshold at 2 kHz, and a sensorineural loss above 2 kHz (**Fig. 27–1**); (2) a flat, moderately severe sensorineural loss at 500 Hz, 1 kHz, 2 kHz, and 3 kHz; (3) in patients with bilateral hearing loss, an asymmetry of greater than 25 dB in one ear. Most patients with Meniere's disease, however, do experience a loss of hearing in the affected ear that slowly worsens over time, although it is extremely rare for a patient to lose all of the hearing in the ear. For most patients with Meniere's disease, the hearing threshold usually stabilizes at 50 to 60 dB levels, with a flat configuration ("burned out ear").

Aural pressure, positional vertigo, and roaring tinnitus are extremely common between definitive episodes of severe vertigo, as is instability with fast movements as well as a constant rocking sensation. Following the onset, there may be a period of remission that can confuse the clinical picture. Over time, however, Meniere's disease progresses from an early stage, through a middle stage, to a late or burn-out stage.

Meniere's disease also presents in several atypical clinical forms, including Lermoyez's variant, the otolithic crisis of Tumarkin or "drop attacks," cochlear Meniere's disease, vestibular Meniere's disease, and delayed-onset Meniere's syndrome. Lermoyez's variant is associated with hearing improvement before, during, or after the vertigo episode. The otolithic crisis or drop attack is characterized by a sudden falling that is often accompanied by sudden firing of the extensor muscles of the extremities. The otolithic crisis is thought to represent firing of primitive muscle reflexes in response to sudden decompression of the saccule or utricle.

Cochlear and vestibular Meniere's disease may represent early or possible Meniere's disease, although the Committee on Hearing and Equilibrium[1] has recommended that the use of these terms be discontinued. Cochlear Meniere's disease is

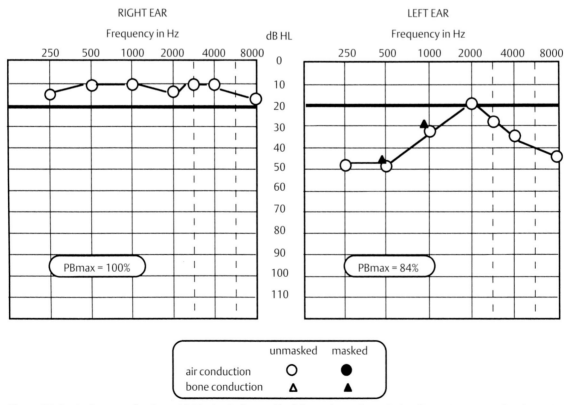

Figure 27–1 Audiogram of patient with Meniere's disease. The left ear shows the typical audiometric pattern of early Meniere's disease. PBmax, maximum-phonetic balance, or word-recognition, score.

characterized by the auditory symptoms of Meniere's disease, but none of the vestibular symptoms. Cochlear Meniere's disease is thought to represent endolymphatic hydrops (ELH) confined to the cochlear duct. Vestibular Meniere's disease is characterized by the vestibular symptoms of Meniere's disease without the auditory symptoms. Although many of these patients progress to the classic form, other clinical entities include migraine, recurrent vestibular neuritis, and cochleovestibular nerve compression syndrome.[3-5]

Delayed-onset Meniere's disease syndrome or postinfectious Meniere's syndrome represents a distinct clinical entity, in which a patient with a long-standing unilateral sensorineural hearing loss begins to experience episodic vertigo indistinguishable from classic Meniere's disease. There are two forms of the illness, ipsilateral and contralateral, indicating which ear is thought to be causing the problem. In the ipsilateral form, the deafened ear is usually found to have a caloric weakness on electronystagmography (ENG) testing. In the contralateral form, the better hearing ear begins to show fluctuating sensorineural levels, and on caloric testing shows a significant weakness. Schuknecht et al[6] identified features in the temporal bones of these patients that suggested that these findings are due to a subclinical viral infection in childhood, but many clinicians feel delayed contralateral endolymphatic hydrops is immune or autoimmune.

The incidence of Meniere's disease varies considerably in the various populations in which it has been studied.[7] In the United States the incidence has been reported as between 15 and 40 per 100,000 per year, whereas in the United Kingdom the incidence is reported as 157 per 100,000. The incidence in Sweden is reported as 50 per 100,000. The symptoms of Meniere's disease typically start at age 35 to 45, although later onset certainly occurs. There does seem to be a slight female-to-male preponderance, although the true incidence in males is probably underreported.

One third to one half of all patients have bilateral Meniere's disease, and the vast majority becomes symptomatic in the other ear within the first 3 years of onset. Several reports suggest that Meniere's disease, in particular bilateral Meniere's disease, might be an immunologically related disorder.[8,9] Hereditary, viral, noise, and allergic factors have also been identified, although their exact significance remains to be determined.[10-12]

Histopathology

Hallpike and Cairns[13] and Yamakawa[14] first reported the histopathologic finding of ELH in the temporal bones of patients with symptoms suggestive of Meniere's syndrome. Most of the distention is seen in the cochlear and saccular ducts (**Fig. 27–2**), although occasionally the walls of the utricle and the ampullae are distorted. In some cases, the Reissner's membrane is so distended that the space of the scala vestibulae is completely taken up by the scala media. Ruptures of the membranous labyrinth, fistulas between the endolymph and perilymph, collapse of the membranous labyrinth, and vestibular fibrosis further characterize the histopathologic picture in ELH.[15]

Altmann and Kornfield[16] noted that only minimal histopathologic changes are seen in the sensory epithelia of these cases. However, other investigators have identified a variety of ultrastructural abnormalities including loss of inner and outer hair cells, and spiral ligament fibrocytes,[17] as well as decreased strial vascularity.[18]

Endolymphatic hydrops has been documented at autopsy in a wide variety of disorders,[19] including acoustic trauma, autoimmune inner ear disease, chronic otitis media, Cogan's syndrome, congenital deafness, fenestration of the otic capsule, leukemia, Mondini dysplasia, otosclerosis, serous labyrinthitis, syphilis, temporal bone trauma, and viral labyrinthitis.

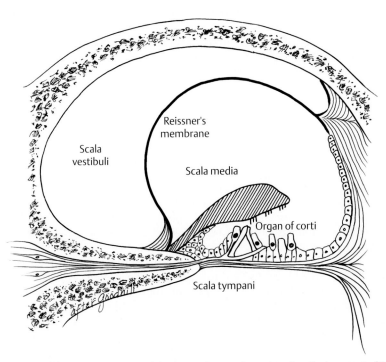

Figure 27–2 Histopathology of Meniere's disease, demonstrating displacement of Reissner's membrane and disruption of the organ of Corti by endolymphatic hydrops.

Pathophysiology

The exact mechanism by which idiopathic ELH occurs remains unproven, although it has become a central theory that ELH causes the symptoms of Meniere's syndrome. Specifically, this theory states that it is the increased pressure that causes the ear fullness, the hyperacusis and distorted hearing, and the unsteadiness and disequilibrium. Furthermore, the theory holds that, if the membranous labyrinth breaks, the patient then suffers a severe episode of vertigo, with a decline in hearing and resultant tinnitus.

On the other hand, Rauch et al,[20] in reviewing the temporal bone collection of the Massachusetts Eye and Ear Infirmary, have suggested that ELH does not cause the symptoms of Meniere's syndrome, but rather is an epiphenomenon. These investigators theorize that ELH is perhaps an indicator of inner ear membrane dysfunction or failure, and that some other factor or factors usually affect fluid management within the inner ear. Altered fluid management then produces both symptoms and ELH. Similar conclusions were reached by Swart and Schuknecht,[21] who reported the results of long-term destruction of the endolymphatic sac in monkeys.

Although the central role of ELH in Meniere's syndrome remains controversial, several pathophysiologic mechanisms have been proposed to explain its development. The most prevalent theory of pathophysiology of ELH is that the distention of the endolymphatic system occurs because of excessive accumulation of endolymph, primarily due to altered resorption by the endolymphatic duct and sac.[22] Altered resorption could be due to perisaccular and vestibular epithelial fibrosis,[23–26] altered glycoprotein metabolism,[27,28] viral infection of the inner ear,[6,29,30] or immune-mediated injury.[31,32] In addition, anatomic abnormalities in the bony structures surrounding the endolymphatic duct might also influence the development of ELH.[26,33] A bony abnormality might cause only a marginal obstruction of the duct, but when added to these other factors would result in a much more severe obstruction to endolymph flow.

As a corollary to the theory of excessive accumulation of endolymph, increased endolymphatic pressure is thought by many to cause the symptoms in these cases.[34,35] Furthermore, Zenner et al[36] have demonstrated experimentally that the hearing loss and tinnitus of ELH could be caused by ruptures of the membranes lining the endolymphatic space, so that potassium-rich endolymph intoxicates the sensory and neural structures. As a result of this potassium influx into the perilymph, the outer hair cells are depolarized, with shortening and loss of motility. Both fluctuating and chronic hearing loss in Meniere's syndrome can be explained by this model.

Other data tend to contradict the pressure hypothesis in EHL. For one thing, although various hearing abnormalities are commonly demonstrated[35] in experimental hydrops, vestibular dysfunction is rarely observed in these models. Also, Long and Morizono[37] measured the pressure gradients in experimental hydrops using microelectrode recording techniques, and found differences between endolymph and perilymph pressure that approximated 0.5 mm Hg. These investigators suggested that as pressure gradients increased, various corrective mechanisms such as an ion balance, endolymph secretion, and absorption are modulated to return the gradient to 0 mm Hg.

Kitahara et al,[38] in a series of elegant pressure studies using artificial endolymph, demonstrated that the auditory and vestibular abnormalities found in ELH most likely arise from biochemical rather than pressure alterations. Juhn et al[39] essentially concluded the same in their review of the subject. Following obliteration of the endolymphatic duct of guinea pigs, experimental findings, in addition to ELH, include a decrease in the endocochlear potential,[40] an increase in intracochlear calcium,[41] alterations in potassium permeability and in the inhibition of the electrogenic transport processes,[42] and increased endolymphatic fluid protein content.[43] Furthermore, Juhn et al found that infusion of epinephrine into the bloodstream results in increased osmolality of the serum and the perilymph, and postulated that this contributes to the development of episodic attacks in ELH.

In summary, evidence exists that the symptoms of Meniere's disease may be due to membranous ruptures or to some alteration in the biochemical gradients within the endolymphatic space. Undoubtedly, our theories of the pathophysiology of Meniere's disease will seem rather primitive and naive in the future. At this writing, however, most investigators believe that idiopathic ELH or Meniere's disease is a multifactorial illness, and that individuals might have more than one factor simultaneously contributing to the development of this problem. The proposed factors include autoimmune reactions, allergic responses, blocked venous drainage, excess endolymph production or decreased resorption, autonomic imbalances, viral infections, vascular irregularities, bony labyrinthine or mastoid air cell maldevelopment, migraine, noise, otosclerosis, and hereditary degeneration. In addition, it is well know among clinicians that patients with Meniere's disease often have relatives with similar symptoms and many also have a childhood history of car sickness or motion intolerance. Whether any of these factors are proven in the future remains to be seen.

Evaluation

The single most important step in the evaluation of the patient with recurrent vertigo and hearing loss is the medical history. An experienced clinician can often formulate the most likely diagnosis through history alone, and if Meniere's syndrome is suspected, the history should then focus on the exclusion of other conditions that can mimic this disorder. Specifically, the diagnoses of perilymph fistula, ototoxicity, chronic labyrinthitis, syphilis, autoimmune inner ear syndrome, and acoustic tumor should be excluded.

Perilymph fistula is usually associated with sudden, severe sensorineural loss with disequilibrium, and only occasional vertigo episodes. However, fluctuating hearing loss and ear fullness can also be seen with this disorder. Most cases of perilymph fistula are associated with straining, barometric pressure changes, or trauma, although definitive exclusion can only be accomplished through surgical exploration in some cases. Ototoxicity should be suspected if the patient has received intravenous therapy for an infection, more specifically receiving an aminoglycoside in the majority of cases. Ototoxicity should be further suspected if the patient complains of unsteadiness, staggering gait, movement of the visual field when walking, and a loss of balance rather than vertigo.

Chronic labyrinthitis should be suspected if the patient gives a history of ear drainage, ear pain, or prior ear surgery. Late-stage syphilitic labyrinthitis should be suspected in any patient with prior treatment for syphilis and with slowly progressive sensorineural hearing loss and progressive disequilibrium. Late-stage syphilitic labyrinthitis can also be clinically indistinguishable from Meniere's disease, with the only differentiating point being positive serology tests or interstitial keratitis on slit-lamp examination. Autoimmune inner ear syndrome should be suspected in patients with rapidly progressive or bilateral sensorineural hearing loss with episodic vertigo. These patients may have other autoimmune disorders such as systemic lupus erythematosa, rheumatoid arthritis, or vasculitis. Also there may have been a positive response to steroid therapy in the past in these cases. Acoustic tumor cases are characterized by progressive unilateral sensorineural hearing loss, decreased speech discrimination, tinnitus, and disequilibrium rather than episodic vertigo.

On completing the initial history, the details of the illness including onset, associated symptoms, and duration and frequency of vertigo episodes, and the provoking factors should be determined. The presence of roaring tinnitus, ear fullness, and fluctuating hearing loss, and their relationship to the episodic vertigo should also be noted. The past medical history, the response to any prior treatments, and the family history of illness should then be recorded. Any related medical illnesses, such as adult-onset diabetes mellitus, migraine, or vascular insufficiency, in addition to their treatments, are then noted.

The next step in the evaluation of the patient with suspected Meniere's syndrome is to perform the otolaryngologic and head and neck examination. Any external or middle ear disease is noted, as are any related findings. Attention is then turned to the neurotologic examination. Spontaneous nystagmus, usually with the fast component beating away from the affected ear, is often visible with Frenzel glasses. Head-shake nystagmus is then elicited by having the patient rapidly shake the head back and forth 15 to 20 times, and then observing spontaneous nystagmus beating away from the affected ear. The Romberg, Quix, and rapid turning tests often show a drift toward the affected side, particularly if the patient has recently experienced vertigo. *Hennebert's sign* should be sought or a fistula test should be performed with either a pneumatic otoscope or by compressing the tragus into the canal. A deviation of the eyes away from the ear being tested is considered to be an objective positive test and is noted in some Meniere's disease patients. A sensation of sway may be reported by the patient and is considered to be a subjectively positive symptom of dysfunction.

The audiometric evaluation of these patients includes a pure-tone audiogram with speech discrimination testing, tympanometry and imittance testing, and acoustic reflex decay testing. The pattern of results seen with Meniere's disease was described earlier (see Clinical Presentation). Acoustic reflex decay is an indicator of retrocochlear abnormality, and suggests the need for additional studies to exclude the possibility of a tumor in the cerebellopontine angle. If the initial evaluation suggests the possibility of Meniere's disease, additional studies to confirm the diagnosis may be obtained, including dehydration testing, electrocochleography (ECochG), and otoacoustic emissions.

Dehydration tests are performed using either furosemide 20 to 40 mg p.o., urea, or glycerol 75 to 100 cc p.o. These agents cause a rapid diuresis, and as a result improved hearing thresholds can be noted in patients with early Meniere's disease.[44] Although this information proves useful in some circumstances, most clinicians do not routinely use this study because of the unpleasant side effects of the test as well as the

availability of other diagnostic studies. Alternatively, many clinicians utilize ECochG in the evaluation of these patients.[45]

ECochG[45] uses computerized signal-averaging techniques to record the electrical signals from the cochlea and the auditory nerve in response to an auditory signal. Electrodes used for this study include transtympanic needles placed on the promontory of the cochlea, tympanic membrane electrodes, and ear canal electrodes. The major advantage of all three is an improved signal-to-noise ratio, so that the action potential or $N - 1$ is accentuated. With a variety of stimuli, including clicks and tone bursts with alternating polarity, the summating potential (SP) and action potential (AP) are further accentuated. Meniere's disease is characterized by an enhanced SP, and, relative to the amplitude of the AP, an increased SP/AP ratio (**Fig. 27–3**). An SP/AP ratio above 0.40 is thought by many clinicians to indicate ELH,[45] although the test-retest reliability and specificity of this value remain in question.[46] This information is helpful in cases where the diagnosis is not certain, such as differentiating nonhydropic sensorineural loss from early Meniere's disease, and in the evaluation of the opposite ear in suspected bilateral Meniere's disease.[47] Otoacoustic emissions may provide information concerning the status of the outer hair cells in ELH, but the clinical value of this test is not certain at present.

Vestibular testing provides limited though useful information in the evaluation of Meniere's disease patients. Vestibular studies commonly employed include ENG, rotational testing, and computerized dynamic platform posturography (CDP). Vestibular function in Meniere's disease patients fluctuates and is extremely variable, and as a result test data may be completely normal even in cases with active episodic vertigo. ENG enables separate evaluation of each labyrinth, and abnormalities including decreased caloric response and positional nystagmus are noted in 50% of Meniere's disease patients.[48] ENG can be helpful to confirm the presence of a vestibular disorder, either by documentation of a deficit or by reproducing the symptoms for the patient.

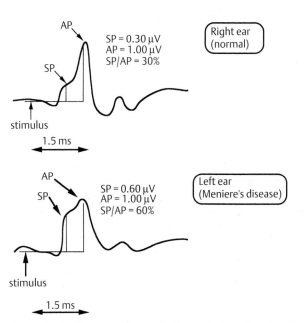

Figure 27–3 Electrocochleography demonstrates enhancing SP and SP/AP ratio in the left ear. SP, summating potential; AP, action potential.

Standard rotary chair testing has limited usefulness in the evaluation of patients with unilateral Meniere's disease, because is evaluates both labyrinths simultaneously. During an acute vertigo episode, rotational testing can show an altered vestibulo-ocular reflex (VOR), specifically phase shift, decreased gain, and an asymmetric response. However, between episodes, rotary chair testing is usually normal. However, O'Leary and Davis[49] have reported that with active head rotation or so-called vestibular autorotation in the vertical plane, Meniere's disease patients typically demonstrate markedly increased gain. Rotational testing can be extremely helpful in the evaluation of compensation following vestibular surgery, bilateral vestibular disorders, and gentamicin treatment. When compensation has occurred, the VOR symmetry and gain are usually within the normal range.

The vestibular evoked myogenic potential (VEMP) can be used to evaluate the status of the saccule and the inferior vestibular nerve. The VEMP actually measures the contractions of the sternocleidomastoid muscle in response to acoustic stimulation of the saccule, that is, the sacculocolic reflex. VEMPs are records using a 750-Hz tone burst, at 95 dB HL. The stimulus rate is 4.3/second, with masking in the contralateral ear. The response is recorded using electrodes placed on the sternocleidomastoid muscle, which is placed under stretch tension. Usually 200 responses are averaged, and the threshold response is sought by lowering the signal intensity in 10 dB steps.

The VEMP response is a biphasic wave recorded between 13 and 23 ms after the stimulus, and its peaks are labeled P_{13} and P_{23}, respectively. Alternatively, these two waves are labeled P1 and N1, as noted in **Figure 27–4**. The amplitude varies between 10 and 300 μV. The asymmetric ratio between sides utilizes a formula similar to that used for ENG. The peak-to-peak amplitude (A) is measured for both the left and right ears, A_L and A_R, respectively (**Fig. 27–4**):

$$\text{Asymmetric ratio (AR)} = \frac{A_L - A_R}{A_L + A_R} \times 100$$

A percent difference greater than 35% is considered significant.

In approximately half of patients with active Meniere's disease,[50] the VEMP is asymmetric on the side of the affected ear; this is thought to indicate saccular hydrops,[51] but no definitive data have yet proved this point. However, an asymmetric VEMP does indicate abnormal vestibular function, and therefore may confirm a history of Meniere's syndrome or early ELH.

The CDP is useful in determining if a patient in fact has vestibular dysfunction,[48] in measuring compensation after vestibular surgery, and in providing objective data to confirm the presence of a vestibular handicap. It is also useful in determining the proper physical therapy regimen for patients with stabilized vestibular deficits. However, it does not lateralize the side in Meniere's disease nor does it provide pathognomonic findings to confirm Meniere's disease.

Laboratory evaluation of patients with Meniere's syndrome is aimed at excluding several readily identifiable disorders that can affect the patient with Meniere's syndrome. These laboratory studies include fluorescent tregonemal antibody absorption (FTA-abs) or microhemagglutination–*Treponema pallidum* (MHA-TP) to exclude syphilis, fasting blood glucose

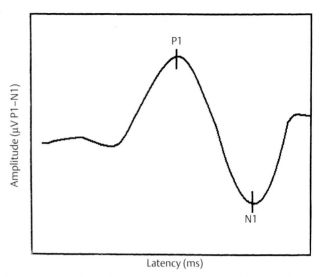

Figure 27–4 Vestibular evoked myogenic potential. P1 and N1 denote the peaks of biphasic waveforms.

to exclude adult-onset diabetes mellitus, cholesterol and triglyceride studies, and thyroid function tests. In addition, a large number of clinicians routinely obtain laboratory studies to exclude immune-related illnesses, particularly in bilateral Meniere's syndrome. These studies include the sedimentation rate, antinuclear antibody, rheumatoid factor, serum immunoglobulins, and, in some cases of atopy, the radioallergosorbent test (RAST).[19] If there is a strong suspicion of autoimmune inner ear syndrome, Cogan's syndrome, or variant Cogan's syndrome, specific testing with humerol heat shock protein-70 (HSP-70) or cellular COCH-protein testing may be obtained. Many clinicians use a positive response to a corticosteroid trial to denote a positive test for these disorders.

Finally, on rare occasions acoustic tumors can present with episodic vertigo. If during the course of evaluating patients with suspected Meniere's syndrome, the clinical features or audiometric or vestibular findings suggest the possibility of an acoustic tumor or another mass lesion, additional imaging studies should be performed. These studies should also be performed prior to any definitive surgical procedure. Diagnostic imaging usually includes magnetic resonance imaging (MRI) scans—either a focused internal auditory canal study (fast spin echo) or a contrasted study with gadolinium agents such as Magnevist. In some cases, auditory brainstem responses or high-resolution computed tomography (CT) scans of the temporal bone might provide additional information.

Classification and Staging

The Committee on Hearing and Equilibrium[1] of the American Academy of Otolaryngology–Head and Neck Surgery has recently updated the diagnosis and classification of Meniere's disease, as noted in **Table 27–1**. The diagnosis takes into account the certainty of the clinical diagnosis and includes possible, probable, definite, and certain Meniere's disease. A single definitive episode of vertigo with documented hearing loss is considered probable Meniere's disease, whereas multiple episodes with hearing loss are definite Meniere's disease. In staging

Meniere's disease, the Committee recommends that the stage be related to the hearing level only, as noted in **Table 27–2**. This staging system is in contrast to prior staging systems that were based on the frequency of vertigo episodes. The hearing level is based on a four-tone average of 0.5, 1, 2, and 3 kHz, obtained from the worst audiogram in the prior 6 months. The Committee noted that not all patients would progress through these stages in sequence. To quantify the episodic vertigo, the Committee recommended that the results be reported by comparing the number of episodes per month between 18 and 24 months postsurgery to the 6 months prior to the treatment. A ratio of the number of episodes between these two time intervals is multiplied by 100, to create a numerical value and related lettered classification, as noted in **Table 27–3**.

Medical Management

The medical management of Meniere's disease is directed at decreasing the fluid volume of the endolymph, increasing the circulation of the inner ear, or altering the immune reactivity or blockage of the endolymphatic duct.[19] None of these proposed regimens has ever been shown in a double-blind controlled study to be effective.[52] Despite that fact, most

Table 27–1 Diagnosis of Meniere's Disease

Certain Meniere's disease
Definite Meniere's disease, plus histopathologic confirmation
Definite Meniere's disease
Two or more definitive spontaneous episodes of vertigo 20 minutes or longer
Audiometrically documented hearing loss on at least one occasion
Tinnitus or aural fullness in the treated ear
Other causes excluded
Probable Meniere's disease
One definitive episode of vertigo
Audiometrically documented hearing loss on at least one occasion
Tinnitus or aural fullness in the treated ear
Other causes excluded
Possible Meniere's disease
Episodic vertigo of the Meniere type without documented hearing loss, or
Sensorineural hearing loss, fluctuating or fixed, with disequilibrium but without definitive episodes
Other causes excluded

Table 27–2 Staging of Definite and Certain Meniere's Disease*

Stage	Four-Tone Average (dB)
1	≤25
2	26–40
3	41–70
4	>70

*Staging is based on the four-tone average (arithmetic mean rounded to the nearest whole number) of the pure-tone thresholds at 0.5, 1, 2, and 3 kHz of the worst audiogram during the interval 6 months before treatment. This is the same audiogram that is used as the baseline evaluation to determine hearing outcome from treatment. Staging should be applied only to cases of definite or certain Meniere's disease.

Table 27–3 Summary of Reporting Guidelines

Numerical Value*	Class
0	A (complete control of definitive spells)
1 to 40	B
41 to 80	C
81 to 120	D
>120	E
Secondary treatment initiated due to disability from vertigo	F

*Numerical value = $(X/Y) \times 100$, rounded to the nearest whole number, where X is the average number of definitive spells per month for the 18 to 24 months after therapy and Y is the average number of definitive spells per month for the 6 months before therapy.

clinicians utilize one or more of these management strategies in an effort to alter the natural history of the disorder.

The most common management strategy is the use of a low-sodium diet and diuretic to decrease endolymph volume.[19] It is possible that this treatment strategy actually affects the inner ear through an unrecognized indirect mechanism, such as altering the ionic balance in some way. For most clinicians, a low-sodium diet is targeted at 1500 to 2000 mg of salt per day. This can be achieved by avoiding table salt and using a salt substitute, and avoiding obviously salty foods such as pickles, salty snacks, salty meats, and pizzas. To this diet is added a diuretic, usually a combination of hydrochlorothiazide 25 mg and triamterene 37.5 mg, taken daily with orange juice or fruit to restore potassium. Occasionally, furosemide 20 to 40 mg per day is recommended, although potassium supplementation is required with this drug. The vast majority of patients tolerate this regimen quite well, although muscle cramps, itching, and weakness do occur. In cases where significant side effects occur, the dose can be decreased to one half. Alternatively, a carbonic anhydrase diuretic such as astemizole can be prescribed. Vertigo control varies between 50 and 70% with this regimen.[52]

Vasodilator therapy is based on the belief by many clinicians that Meniere's disease is related to decreased inner ear blood flow. In this treatment strategy, the patient is instructed to avoid caffeine and nicotine completely. A vasodilating drug such as niacin, papaverine, or β-histamine is prescribed to improve the blood flow.[19] Lastly, the patient is told to avoid stressful situations and to begin a walking program for aerobic conditioning and for stress control. Although the effectiveness of this regimen in controlling Meniere's disease can be questioned, it is extremely beneficial to the patient both physically and psychologically and has few side effects.

A third treatment strategy is to alter the immune response, using either corticosteroids or allergic desensitization. These agents act by decreasing inflammation, and theoretically they alter the fluid mechanics of the inner ear. Whether the endolymphatic sac function or the autoimmune response to inner ear membranes is actually changed is a matter of conjecture.

A course of corticosteroids is often recommended[19] for patients with (1) active unilateral Meniere's disease with episodic vertigo unresponsive to vestibular suppressives and low-salt diet with diuretics; (2) Meniere's disease with a sudden decrease in hearing threshold; or (3) bilateral Meniere's disease, Cogan's syndrome, or suspected autoimmune inner ear syndrome. This treatment strategy typically takes one of two forms. The first is to use a dose pack of methylprednisolone, dexamethasone, or another corticosteroid. Although this regimen is convenient, questions have arisen as to whether the duration and dose are sufficient to suppress the immune response. The second regiment is to use prednisone 60 to 80 mg per day for 7 days, with a tapered dose over the next 7 days. Response to either regimen would indicate steroid responsiveness, in which case future prolonged use can be discussed with the patient. The side effects of short-term steroid use include appetite stimulation, irritability, heartburn and digestive disorder, and insomnia. The indigestion can be readily controlled using an antacid or an H2 blocker.

If steroid responsiveness is confirmed, longer-term steroid therapy may be useful. This consists of either low-dose or high-dose regimens. In many patients, prednisone 10 to 20 mg per day or dexamethasone 4 mg every other day seems to decrease the frequency and severity of episodic vertigo as well as stabilize a fluctuating sensorineural hearing loss. The dose of prednisone can be increased as necessary, as in autoimmune inner ear syndrome or in syphilitic labyrinthitis. As expected, higher doses of prednisone result in far greater side effects, including Cushing's syndrome, cataracts, avascular necrosis of the hip joint, pulmonary effusions, and worsened control of diabetes mellitus. To avoid many of these side effects, methotrexate 10 to 15 mg per week can sometimes help, enabling the prednisone dosage to be decreased or discontinued. Alternatively, plasmapheresis can be used to remove white blood cells and serum in these cases, enabling the dosage of prednisone to be decreased. If the symptoms can be stabilized for 1 year, the immune-suppressing drugs can usually be tapered and discontinued. Other medical treatments that are occasionally indicated for patients with Meniere's syndrome are (1) antibiotic therapy for syphilitic labyrinthitis, (2) allergic desensitization for inhalant or food allergies, and (3) calcium channel blockers with amitriptyline in patients with either vestibular Meniere's disease associated with headache or vestibular migraine. Furthermore, in patients with abnormalities discovered during the course of the laboratory evaluation, appropriate therapy can often improve many of the symptoms.

Vestibular suppressives and antiemetics also play a significant role in the management of patients with Meniere's syndrome. Vestibular suppressives are drugs with variable anticholinergic, sedative, and antiemetic effects that can be used to lessen the severity of the vertigo as well as the associated autonomic effects.[19] Some of the most useful are meclizine 12.5 to 25 mg p.o. three times per day, dimenhydrinate 25 mg p.o. or p.r. every 6 to 8 hours, diazepam 2.5 to 5 mg p.o twice or three times per day, and alprazolam 0.5 mg p.o. twice or three times per day. The major side effect of these drugs is drowsiness, and the patient should avoid the use of alcohol or other nervous system depressants when taking them. Patients should also avoid driving while taking vestibular suppressives. Glycopyrrolate (Robinul) 1 to 2 mg p.o twice daily or metoclopramide (Reglan) 10 mg p.o. twice daily are effective antinauseants with few side effects. Antinauseants

can be used on a continuous basis, whereas most vestibular suppressives should be used only as indicated.

Gates et al[53] have described a new medical treatment for Meniere's disease using a device to deliver transtympanic micropressure to the inner ear (Meniett, Medtronix Corp.). The treatment theoretically lowers fluid pressure in the inner ear, and is self-administered by the patient two or three times per day. The physician places a tympanostomy tube, and instructs the patient as to how to place the ear plug that delivers the micropressure pulses. The Meniett device reportedly does have short-term efficacy, and appears to be safe. It is primarily used for patients who wish to avoid surgery, such as deafferentation procedures, and is helpful in the management of patients with bilateral Meniere's disease. Some control of tinnitus and vertigo occurs in 50 to 60% of cases, and in our experience usually lasts for up to 18 months.

Some Meniere's disease patients continue to have severe debilitating vertigo despite oral or suppository medication. In these cases, hospitalization is often indicated for rehydration and for intravenous therapy to lessen the symptoms. Droperidol 1.25 to 2.5 g can be given intravenously, very slowly over 60 minutes. Although the drug is effective in stopping acute vertigo, it does cause drowsiness, and failure to administer it slowly can result in Parkinsonian-like anticholinergic side effects. Alternatively, diazepam 5 to 10 mg intravenously is also effective in controlling the episode of vertigo in these cases.

Most patients with bilateral Meniere's disease or with Meniere's disease in an only-hearing ear respond to the medical management described above. In some patients, however, uncontrollable episodic vertigo continues, and surgery should be considered.

Surgical Management

If a patient continues to have episodic vertigo in spite of an adequate trial or medical therapy (usually for 3 months), surgical management should be considered. Episodic vertigo occurring once a month or more often is considered life altering, and these patients are usually prepared to have a procedure to stop the vertigo if the clinician recommends it. The type of procedure recommended depends on the duration and stage of the Meniere's disease, the status of hearing in the involved and contralateral ear, as well as the desires of the patient. The clinician should identify the various options for the patient, and should contrast the relative advantages and disadvantages of each, as listed in **Table 27–4**.

Transtympanic Gentamicin Perfusion

Transtympanic gentamicin perfusion (TGP) is the easiest, least invasive surgical treatment available for Meniere's disease. It is performed in the outpatient clinic setting and is very cost-effective relative to the other procedures. In this procedure, the gentamicin penetrates the round window, mixes in the perilymph of the scala tympani, and travels through the cochlea, ultimately reaching the sensory neuroepithelia of the vestibule and the semicircular canals. Because gentamicin is relatively more vestibulotoxic than it is cochleotoxic, this usually results in a vestibular deficit without a hearing loss. A vestibular deficit occurs in 80% of cases, whereas sensorineural hearing loss occurs in just 10%. When the gentamicin causes a vestibular deficit, the episodic vertigo is significantly modified, and the episodes are then described as

Table 27–4 Surgical Management of Meniere's Disease

Procedure	Special Indications	Control of Vertigo	Hearing Loss	Cost	Risk of Procedure
Transtympanic gentamicin perfusion	Hearing loss <50 dB, 50% PBs Medically infirm Bilateral Meniere's disease	80–85%	5–10%	Low	Low
Transmastoid endolymphatic sac procedure	Early Meniere's Fluctuating SNHL; possibly with middle ear exploration	60–65%	<5%	Moderate	Low
Transmastoid labyrinthectomy	Hearing loss >50–60 dB <50% PBs	95%	Total	Moderate	Low-moderate
Retrosigmoid vestibular nerve section	Meniere's for >1–2 years usually <50 dB >50% PBs Good health	90%	<5%	High	Moderate

PBs, speech discrimination score using phonetically balanced words; SNHL, sensorineural hearing loss.

being mostly a sense of unsteadiness. The need for vestibular suppressives markedly diminishes in these cases. This improvement often lasts for months to years, but because regeneration of sensory epithelia does occur, some patients begin to have episodic vertigo once again. These patients can be either re-treated with TGP or can then undergo another procedure.

TGP can be used for patients with either fluctuating or fixed sensorineural hearing loss, and either unilateral or bilateral Meniere's disease. It is ideal for patients who might otherwise be considered a candidate for a retrosigmoid vestibular nerve section, which can then be performed should TGP fail. TGP is also an alternative to transmastoid labyrinthectomy, particularly in medically infirm patients.

TGP is performed through the tympanic membrane under microscopic vision. After anesthetizing the tympanic membrane, small incisions are made over the anterior and posterior portion of the tympanic membrane (**Fig. 27–5**). Five to 10 mL of gentamicin solution, buffered to a pH of 6.4, is drawn into a tuberculin syringe. The desired concentration is about 30 mg %. Using a 25-gauge spinal needle, the solution is slowly infused into the middle ear through the anterior incision.

After the middle ear is filled, the patient is told to remain in the supine position with the head partly turned to allow the drug to make contact with the round window membrane. Patients may feel a slight vertigo sensation during the perfusion because of the caloric effect of the solution, and may also feel a slight burning sensation.

TGP is performed once a week until an effect is noted. The gentamicin effect can be seen with a single perfusion, and this effect is typically noted within 5 days. When the gentamicin effect occurs, patients typically note a pulling or swaying sensation or a sense of disequilibrium. Spontaneous nystagmus away from the treated ear can also be seen with Frenzel glasses at this point. If the gentamicin effect is noted or if a hearing loss occurs, TGP is discontinued. Most patients demonstrate the gentamicin effect with one to three perfusions. Some clinicians give a single perfusion and wait a full month to guide the effect.

Endolymphatic Sac Surgery

Few procedures in otologic surgery have been as controversial as endolymphatic sac surgery. Opinions regarding the efficacy of this procedure vary from those who conclude that the procedure is effective in over 80% of cases to those who believe that the procedure is no better than a placebo or sham procedure.[55–60] Despite this controversy, most clinicians recommend endolymphatic surgery because it is a nondestructive procedure that can be performed on an outpatient basis. Endolymphatic sac surgery offers the possibility of vertigo control with little risk of morbidity. Theoretically, endolymphatic sac surgery improves the function of a scarified endolymphatic sac or opens a blocked endolymphatic duct. As a consequence, the pressure in the endolymphatic space is thought to decrease. Alternatively, endolymphatic sac surgery might cause a temporary subclinical labyrinthitis that perhaps alters the pattern of Meniere's disease.

Most clinicians recommend endolymphatic sac surgery for Meniere's disease cases in which the hearing continues to fluctuate and for early Meniere's disease within the first 2 to 3 years of onset. Endolymphatic sac surgery is also recommended in cases in which the possibility of perilymph fistula has not been excluded, because middle ear exploration can be easily performed at the same setting. Some clinicians recommend endolymphatic sac surgery only in cases where an enlarged summating potential or an increased SP/AP ratio is observed on ECochG.

Figure 27–5 Transtympanic gentamicin perfusion, right ear, surgical position.

In this procedure, the endolymphatic sac is exposed after performing a simple mastoidectomy through a postauricular incision. The endolymphatic sac is found embedded in the dura posteroinferior to the posterior semicircular canal (**Fig. 27–6A**). It extends down inferiorly, under the vertical segment of the facial nerve and toward the top of the jugular bulb. The superior margin of the endolymphatic sac is defined by a line that extends the plane of the lateral semicircular canal and runs perpendicular to the posterior semicircular canal, the so-called *Donaldson's line*. In most Meniere's disease cases, the endolymphatic sac is placed a little more inferior than in normals. Once identified, the sac can be decompressed by removing the overlying bone, or it can be opened (**Fig. 27–6B**) and its lumen probed. The sac can be shunted into the mastoid, using a variety of tubing or sheeting materials. The incision is closed with buried absorbable sutures and the wound dressed.

The patient is followed at increasing intervals over the next 6 months. In cases where the procedure is effective, vertigo episodes are absent or occur significantly less often. Ear fullness and tinnitus are usually improved in the majority of patients also. In some patients, the hearing threshold markedly improves or stabilizes, although this occurs less often than vertigo improvement.

Transmastoid Labyrinthectomy

A traditional procedure for Meniere's disease, transmastoid labyrinthectomy (TML) cures a high percentage of patients with episodic vertigo without entailing an intracranial procedure. By removing the vestibular neuroepithelium, the vestibular function in the operated ear is completely ablated. This results in control of vertigo in more than 90% of cases. Unfortunately, the hearing is also lost with this procedure. It is possible that patient selection plays a significant role in the outcome of TML, as the clinician is much more likely to recommend this procedure only to those patients with unequivocal unilateral vestibular dysfunction. Generally, a preoperative ENG must show normal caloric function in the opposite ear. TML usually requires postoperative hospitalization until the patient can tolerate oral intake and can ambulate with assistance. Transcanal labyrinthectomy is an

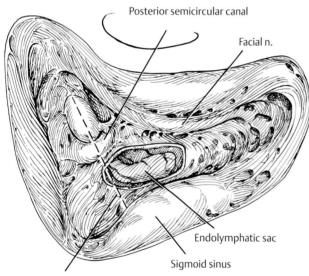

Posterior semicircular canal

Facial n.

Endolymphatic sac

Sigmoid sinus

A Donaldson's line

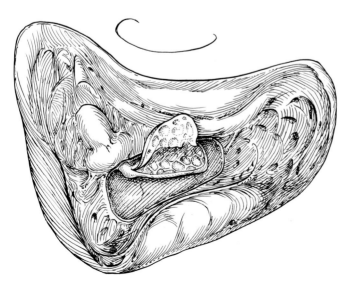

B

364

Figure 27–6 Endolymphatic sac surgery, right ear surgical position. **(A)** Relationship of endolymphatic sac with Donaldson's line (dotted line). **(B)** The sac is opened.

III Management

alternative procedure to TML, and although it can be performed with less exposure, it is difficult to be certain that all of the sensory neuroepithelium has been removed with this procedure. Translabyrinthine vestibular nerve section is an alternative to TML, which adds the section of the vestibular nerve to the removal of the sensory neuroepithelium. Translabyrinthine vestibular nerve section, as compared with TML, is associated with greater complications, including headache and cerebrospinal fluid (CSF) leak, without any noticeable improvement in results.

TML is the procedure indicated in patients with unilateral Meniere's disease and severe sensorineural hearing loss. Most clinicians use a hearing criteria of a pure-tone average greater than 70 dB and speech discrimination worse than 30%. These criteria are flexible, however, and under certain circumstances, a clinician might use a pure-tone average of 50 dB and speech discrimination of 50%. Factors that might influence these criteria are hearing loss in the contralateral ear, age, and prior otologic procedures.

TML is performed through a postauricular incision (**Fig. 27–7**). After completing a simple mastoidectomy, the semicircular canals are carefully identified by removing the surrounding air cells. The location of the vertical segment of the facial nerve is also verified. The lateral, superior, and upper half of the posterior semicircular canals are opened, with care taken to avoid injury to the tympanic segment and second genu of the facial nerve. On opening the ampullated ends of the lateral and superior canals, the sensory neuroepithelium is removed. The bridge of bone between the crus of the lateral canal is then opened, allowing removal of the utricle and the saccule. The inferior portion of the posterior semicircular canal, under the vertical segment of the facial nerve, is carefully opened and the posterior canal ampulla is removed. After careful inspection to be certain of the complete removal, the postauricular incision is closed with buried absorbable sutures.

Retrosigmoid Vestibular Nerve Section

Retrosigmoid vestibular nerve section (RVNS) is an effective procedure for the control of episodic vertigo with preservation of hearing (**Fig. 27–8**). Following Silverstein's and Norrell's[61] introduction of the retrolabyrinthine approach to vestibular nerve section, the procedure has undergone a slow evolution to the current approach.[62] RVNS offers superior,

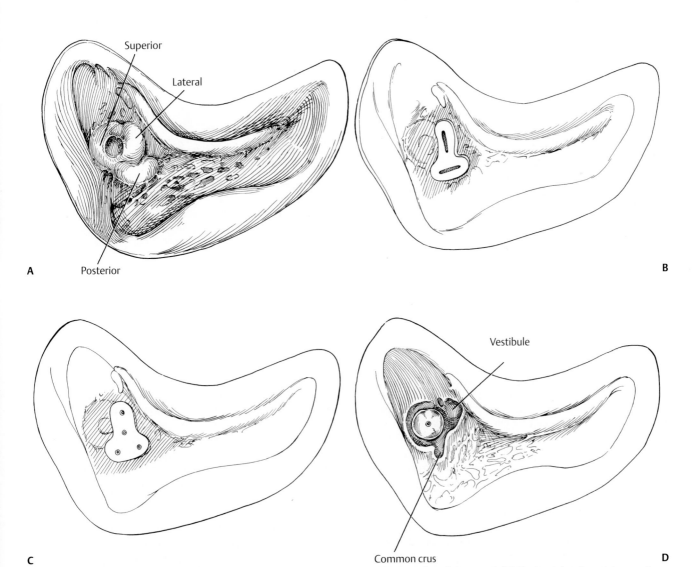

A Superior
Lateral
Posterior

B

C

D Vestibule
Common crus

Figure 27–7 Transmastoid labyrinthectomy. Right ear, surgical position. **(A)** The labyrinth is skeletonized. **(B)** The lateral and posterior canals are fenestrated. **(C)** Deeper bone removal reveals two pairs of "snake eyes." **(D)** The superior canal is opened and followed to the vestibule.

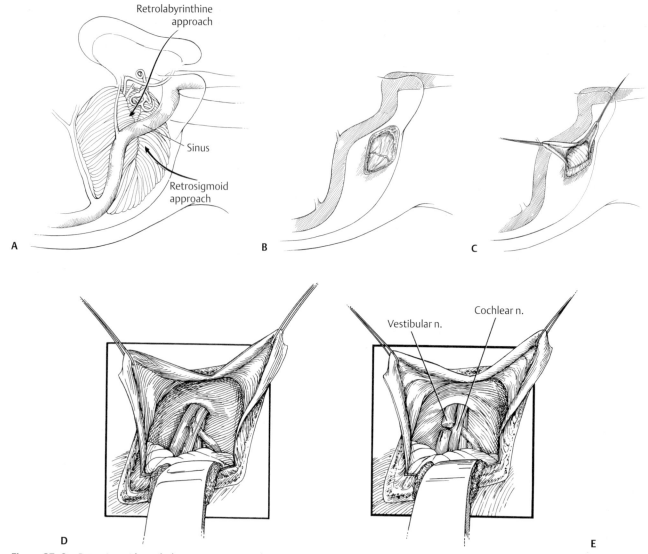

Figure 27–8 Retrosigmoid vestibular nerve section, right ear, surgical position. **(A)** Retrolabyrinthine and retrosigmoid approaches are compared. **(B)** Bone removal. **(C)** Dural opening. **(D)** Cochleovestibular nerve demonstrating cleavage plane between divisions. **(E)** Vestibular nerve (superior portion of eighth nerve complex) is sectioned.

readily obtained exposure of the cochleovestibular nerve with a low incidence of complications. The ease and rapidity of the exposure makes RVNS the preferred approach over the middle fossa vestibular nerve section for the vast majority of clinicians. The vestibular nerve can be selectively sectioned through the retrosigmoid approach, and, if necessary, the internal auditory canal can be drilled for additional exposure of the branches. However, a complete or near-complete vestibular nerve section can be performed in virtually every case with this exposure. RVNS requires hospitalization for several days after surgery, in addition to an overnight stay in the intensive care unit for monitoring. As a consequence, RVNS is also a more costly procedure for the control of episodic vertigo.

RVNS is indicated in patients with unilateral Meniere's disease and with a fixed or stable sensorineural loss in the serviceable range. It is much more effective for the episodic vertigo of Meniere's disease than other vestibular disorders, perhaps as a result of better patient selection in this group of patients.[62] RVNS can also be employed if other procedures such as TGP or

endolymphatic sac surgery have failed. Successful elimination of episodic vertigo occurs in nearly 90% of cases. Neither the hearing nor the ELH appears to be altered by the procedure.

The procedure is performed with the patient in the supine position with the head turned away and secured in Mayfield pins. At the inception of the procedure, the patient is given mannitol 100 g intravenously, furosemide 40 mg intravenously, and Solu-Cortef 125 mg intravenously. These drugs, coupled with hyperventilation of the patient, result in decreased CSF volume and pressure. A C-shaped incision (or standard suboccipital incision) is made behind the ear and the skin and the musculoperiosteum are elevated to the level of the mastoid. Several mastoid emissary veins must be controlled during this process. The posterior portion of the mastoid is opened with the drill to identify the location of the sigmoid sinus. The bony plate immediately behind the sigmoid sinus is outlined with the drill, removed, and set aside for replacement at closure. This exposes dura for about 5 cm in length and width, behind the sigmoid sinus and below the transverse sinus. The dura is opened in the cruciate, and the dural leaves are retracted with sutures. The blade of the self-retaining retractor is used to gently retract the cerebellum from inferior. After draining the CSF from the basal cistern, the cerebellum can usually be retracted to provide adequate exposure of the cochleovestibular nerve. The arachnoid surrounding the nerve is gently dissected to further expose the cochleovestibular and facial nerves.

The cleavage plane between the vestibular and cochlear portions of the nerve is then identified (**Fig. 27–7D**), and usually a small blood vessel runs in the plane. The superior half of the nerve or the vestibular portion is sectioned using a 90-degree back-cutting knife and microscissors. In most cases, the bundles within the nerve clearly differentiate the vestibular portion. Care is taken to avoid injuring the facial nerve. On completing the nerve section, the subarachnoid space is inspected for bleeding, and if none is seen, the dura is closed. The bone plate is then replaced (a titanium plate can also be used), and the incision closed in multiple layers.

Middle Fossa Vestibular Nerve Section

This procedure has advantages over the RVNS. The middle fossa approach is primarily extradural and offers the opportunity to visualize the separate nerve bundles discretely (**Fig. 27–9**). As a result, some clinicians are of the opinion that the middle fossa approach enables a more complete and thorough nerve section. However, the middle fossa exposure is somewhat more difficult as compared with RVNS, including the orientation of the procedure as well as the greater difficulty sectioning the inferior vestibular nerve, and probably slightly higher risk of hearing loss and facial palsy.

Other procedures are no longer performed by most clinicians, including streptomycin perfusion of the lateral semicircular canal and streptomycin perfusion of the middle ear.[63] Cochleosacculotomy is performed infrequently in elderly patients with Meniere's disease who would otherwise be candidates for TML. In each of these procedures, the incidence of sensorineural hearing loss is extremely high. In addition, critical review of data regarding the use of microvascular decompression of the cochleovestibular nerve has led to the conclusion by most clinicians that this procedure is not effective for episodic vertigo of Meniere's disease.[64]

Cochleosacculotomy

Cochleosacculotomy was designed to create a permanent fistula in the saccale, thus in theory decompressing an acute attack of endolymphatic hydrops. The theory is compelling but the fistula does not persist. Instead, many clinicians think cochleosacculotomy creates a mini-labyrinthectomy, which may indeed explain its benefits. As mentioned, the typical candidate is an elderly patient with disabling vertigo attacks and hearing so poor that he normally would be a candidate for transmastoid labyrinthectomy. As noted, however, a transmastoid labyrinthectomy (and gentamicin) causes postoperative imbalance, often for weeks. Prolonged postoperative imbalance in an elderly patient invites disaster from falls: broken hips, fractured skulls etc. Unlike these more traditional treatments, cochleosacculotomy does *not* produce postoperative dizziness and imbalance. The patient can walk out of the hospital the same day and resume routine activities. Add to this distinct advantage the simplicity of surgery: a 30-minute transcanal procedure under local anesthesia with mild sedation. A tympanomeatal flap is raised and a 4 mm right-angled pick is inserted through the round window membrane superiorly into the vestibule. At least 80% of patients achieve complete control of vertigo attacks and also drop attacks. You may argue that the risk of profound hearing loss is about one in three. That is very true, but these patients would have been candidates for labyrinthectomy anyway. You may argue that symptoms may return after several years, and that also is very true. However, these are *elderly* patients who may or may not live long enough to recur symptoms.

If vestibular surgery results in stable vestibular function, the patient may benefit from vestibular rehabilitation.

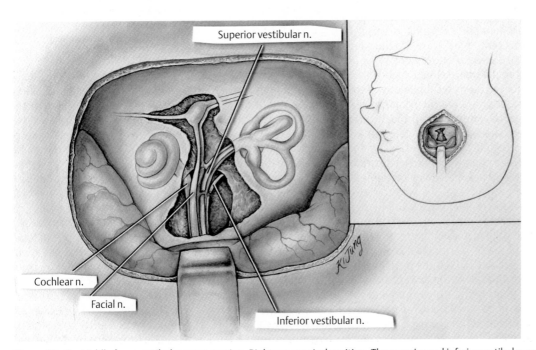

Figure 27–9 Middle fossa vestibular nerve section. Right ear, surgical position. The superior and inferior vestibular nerves are cut.

Vestibular exercises can help in the early stages of vestibular compensation after TML and after RVNS. Specific vestibular rehabilitation therapy can also aid in vestibular compensation, and particularly in cases with persistent disequilibrium.

Perilymph Fistula

A patient with a perilymph fistula (PLF) can present with symptoms virtually indistinguishable from those of Meniere's syndrome. There are four recognized patterns of this disorder[65]: (1) vertigo episodes without hearing loss, (2) hearing loss without vertigo, (3) a Meniere's syndrome pattern, and (4) a miscellaneous pattern with disequilibrium but not episodic vertigo. Unlike Meniere's syndrome, PLF is usually associated with either an implosive or an explosive event, such as straining or causing the ear to pop. PLF also occurs after stapedectomy. It should be noted, however, that spontaneous PLFs have been discovered at the time of endolymphatic sac surgery for classic Meniere's disease.

Middle ear exploration is recommended to repair an obvious traumatic perilymph leak, to attempt hearing preservation, and to resolve the disequilibrium. There are no uniform criteria for selecting patients for middle ear exploration, but a history of antecedent trauma, vertigo, and sensorineural hearing loss favors the diagnosis of PLF. The diagnosis is based primarily on the presentation of the symptom complex and a high index of clinical suspicion. Middle ear exploration is performed through a transcanal approach. Either perichondrium or temporalis fascia is used to seal the round (or oval) window. Surgical repair of PLF will most likely improve vertigo; hearing and tinnitus can improve according to some reports. After surgery the patient should be cautioned against heavy lifting or straining for several weeks.

Superior Semicircular Canal Dehiscence (Fig. 27–10)

Superior semicircular canal dehiscence (SSCD) is a syndrome characterized by vertigo and oscillopsia induced by loud sounds or by stimuli that change middle ear or intracranial pressure.[66] Specifically, the Tullio phenomenon (visual distortion caused by loud sounds), Hennebert's sign, and Valsalva maneuvers all elicit vestibular symptoms. These findings are thought to be caused by the excessive movement of perilymph, as a result of a defect in the bony semicircular canal.

Approximately 70% of patients have an air–bone gap on the affected side, and the tuning fork tests typically confirm this finding. Some of these patients have undergone exploration of the middle ear for possible stapedectomy, at which time a mobile stapes footplate was found. The explanation for the air–bone gap is an increased sensitivity to bone conduction, again caused by increased perilymph movement with skull vibration. Stapes reflexes are present.

The VEMP is very useful in the evaluation of patients suspected to have SSCD. As described earlier, the VEMP records the sacculocolic reflex, specifically recording the contractions of the sternocleidomastoid muscle. The response is typically recorded at 95 dB levels, but in cases of SSCD the response can be recorded at 75 or 80 dB HL levels in the affected ear. In addition, patients with an air–bone gap would not be expected to have a response at such lower thresholds. Theoretically, acoustic stimulation of the saccule is increased by excessive perilymph movement, resulting in increased response of the sternocleidomastoid muscle.

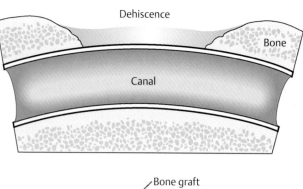

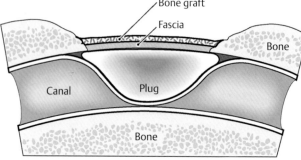

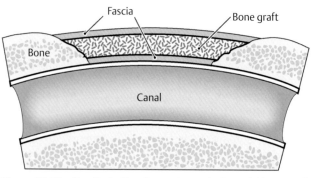

Figure 27–10 Top illustration demonstrates the bony dehiscence of the superior semicircular canal. Middle illustration demonstrates plugging of the canal with soft tissue and covering the defect with fascia and bone graft. Bottom illustration demonstrates resurfacing of canal.

High-resolution temporal bone CT scans are used to document the presence of SSCD. Using coronal views in the plane of the superior canal, the bony labyrinth is specifically visualized and inspected for thinning or dehiscence. The affected ear is also compared with the contralateral side, using 0.5-mm cuts. Minor[66] has reported that CT scans of the temporal bone have 100% sensitivity, 99% specificity, and a positive predictive rate of 93%. However, Vrabek (personal communication) has presented findings that suggest 9% of all normals have thin bone over the superior semicircular canal.

Most patients with SSCD have mild to moderate symptoms, which can be managed with an ear plug or avoidance of loud sounds. However, some patients are debilitated by their symptoms, and in these cases surgical repair should be considered. Two approaches have been reported: (1) resurfacing of the dehiscence with bone or bone cement, and (2) soft tissue plugging of the canal to diminish the excessive perilymph movement. Minor[66] recommends superior canal occlusion or plugging through either a middle fossa or transmastoid approach. Although this approach does carry a small risk of hearing loss, nearly 90% of patients report relief of their vestibular symptoms following canal plugging.

Labyrinthine Concussion and Temporal Bone Fractures

Following a head injury with a concussion, patients may experience position- and motion-induced vertigo and unsteadiness, in addition to high-frequency sensorineural hearing loss.[19] This can occur even in the absence of visible temporal bone fractures on CT scans. These patients have findings that are characterized as a labyrinthine concussion, and are thought to be due to damage to the membranous labyrinth through shearing forces.

A more severe head injury may result in a temporal bone fracture, which may produce both immediate and delayed vestibular symptomatology. The two types of temporal bone fractures encountered are capsular and extracapsular.

Capsular fractures run transverse across the petrous ridge, and are most often due to a severe blow to the occiput. A Battle's sign often accompanies this type of fracture, and this sign is indicative of the severity of the injury. Total loss of hearing and the abrupt onset of severe vertigo accompany this type of fracture, which disrupts the cochlea or the semicircular canals. Because these patients are often comatose for several weeks following their injury, the vestibular system may be partly compensated when the problem is first discovered on regaining consciousness. Most of these patients experience unsteadiness and disequilibrium for up to 6 months, as the membranous labyrinth becomes fixated by labyrinthitis ossificans and as vestibular compensation occurs. The hearing loss is permanent.

Extracapsular fractures of the temporal bone usually run longitudinal or vertical to the petrous ridge. These fractures are more common, and occur in association with a blow to the temporoparietal region of the skull. The vestibular complaints and findings with this fracture are much less severe than those found with capsular fractures. If severe vertigo occurs, a PLF due to ossicular disruption should be suspected. The hearing loss associated with this fracture is usually conductive in nature, although high-frequency sensorineural loss can occasionally be seen. The usual vestibular complaints with this type of fracture are positional vertigo, motion-induced vertigo, and disequilibrium. Most of these symptoms resolve spontaneously, although vestibular rehabilitation and particle repositioning maneuvers may be indicated in some cases. A more complete discussion of temporal bone trauma can be found in Chapter 21.

Syphilitic Labyrinthitis

With the spread of the human immunodeficiency virus, the incidence of syphilis and syphilitic labyrinthitis has increased. Therefore, it is imperative to consider syphilis as the possible etiology of any rapidly progressive hearing loss, with or without vertigo. In the early stages of syphilitic labyrinthitis, vestibular symptoms are uncommon and these cases may be characterized by progressive sensorineural hearing loss only. Steckelberg and McDonald[67] found in 38 cases of syphilitic labyrinthitis that the hearing loss was bilateral in 82% of cases and unilateral in 18%. Episodic vertigo was present in 42% of these cases.

As the patient ages into the forties and fifties, syphilitic labyrinthitis is characterized not only by progressive hearing loss but also by episodic disequilibrium and vertigo. Wilson and Zoller[68] found that that 80% of these patients had vestibular disturbances. Many of these patients have symptoms indistinguishable from Meniere's syndrome.

The pathophysiology in these cases is related to the progression of vasculitis and obliterative endarteritis of the otic capsule.[69] If the bone overlying the semicircular canal is necrosed and sequestered, the patient develops signs indicative of a fistula of the lateral canal. These symptoms include a positive *Hennebert's sign* as well as a positive *Tullio's sign*. If the endarteritis involves the endolymphatic duct, a gumma or reactive fibrosis can block the duct with resultant symptoms of ELH.

The diagnosis of syphilitic labyrinthitis should be considered in any case of episodic vertigo with progressive hearing loss. Either the fluorescent treponemal antibody absorption test (FTA-Abs) or the MHA-TP test should be obtained during the initial evaluation. If either of these tests is positive, the patient should be treated for syphilis. The treatment in syphilitic labyrinthitis includes a combination of intramuscular and oral penicillin and corticosteroids. Because the spirochete replicates very slowly, prolonged therapy is necessary. Initially, benzathine penicillin 2.4 million units IM is given weekly for 3 weeks.[15] This dose is then followed with oral Pen VK 500 mg four times a day for 3 months. Alternatively, intravenous penicillin G in high doses can be used in place of the benzathine penicillin. To this antibiotic regimen is added prednisone 40 to 60 mg per day. Surprising recovery of hearing can accompany this treatment. After 3 months, the prednisone can be tapered, depending on the stability of the hearing threshold. Vestibular symptoms are also improved in the vast majority of these patients.

Vascular Occlusion of the Labyrinthine Artery

Occlusion of the labyrinthine artery leads to sudden profound loss of both cochlear and vestibular function. Although this condition tends to occur in older patients, it can also be seen in younger individuals with atherosclerotic vascular disease or with a hypercoagulation disorder. Prior to the occlusion, patients often complain of episodic vertigo, which can herald the onset of transient ischemic attacks (TIAs). Baloh[70] reported that 62% of TIA patients experience episodic vertigo, and for 18% an isolated episode of vertigo was the initial symptom. TIAs are manifested by a variety of neurologic findings, including visual difficulties or amaurosis fugax, syncope, ataxia, extremity weakness, slurred speech or aphasia, and confusion. Early recognition of this possibility may allow preventive measures to prevent a stroke.

Once the labyrinthine artery is occluded, the hearing loss is usually total and permanent. The acute vertigo episode subsides, leaving the patient with residual unsteadiness and disequilibrium. Over 4 to 6 months, the patient typically improves as the vestibular system undergoes compensation. Pathologic studies[70] of these cases reveal widespread necrosis of the membranous structures as well as labyrinthitis ossificans. As the inner ear ossifies, the membranous structures become fixated, further aiding the compensation of these cases. If labyrinthine artery occlusion is suspected, these patients should be referred for consultation with their internist, as this condition might represent a sentinel event in the development of atherosclerotic vascular disease. Medical management of suspected TIAs and stroke usually includes controlling risk factors, antiplatelet drugs such as aspirin and dipyridamole, and anticoagulants drugs such as Coumadin. Vestibular suppressives, antiemetics, and vestibular rehabilitation can be prescribed to further aid in recovery.

Occlusion of the anterior vestibular artery also causes hearing loss and vertigo. Occlusion of the anterior vestibular artery usually results in the loss of hearing in the higher frequencies. Because the posterior vestibular circulation remains intact, these patients can experience benign paroxysmal positional vertigo (BPPV). After these patients are started on a management plan for their vestibular complaints, they should also be referred for evaluation and further therapy to their internist.

Labyrinthine Fistulas and Labyrinthitis

Erosion of the bony labyrinth by a cholesteatoma leads to the development of a labyrinthine fistula. Fistulas can develop over the lateral, superior, or posterior semicircular canal, as well as over the stapes footplate and cochlea. The symptoms that occur depend on the location and rate of growth of the fistula. If the fistula develops over the stapes footplate or the cochlea, the patient usually experiences mild unsteadiness or vertigo with a sensorineural hearing loss. If the fistula develops over a semicircular canal, vertigo and a positive fistula test are the predominant symptoms, although a mild sensorineural loss is often found. Ear drainage, conductive hearing loss, inflammation, and pain are superimposed on both conditions in the majority of cases. Evaluation of these patients should include microscopic examination and cleaning of the ear to identify the pathology, audiometric examination, and CT scans of the temporal bones. Labyrinthine fistula is a strong indication for surgery in these cases.

Labyrinthitis can develop if bacterial toxins, tissue fluids, or bacteria enter the labyrinthine fluid compartments. Labyrinthitis can be further subdivided into serous labyrinthitis and suppurative labyrinthitis.

Serous labyrinthitis occurs during the course of an episode of acute otitis media or mastoiditis. These patients present with vertigo of varying degrees as well as sensorineural hearing loss. Prompt treatment results in rapid recovery to normal status. In serous labyrinthitis, only bacterial toxins enter the fluid compartments, so that damage is usually not permanent, and therefore serous labyrinthitis is only diagnosed retrospectively, when there is recovery following treatment. Evaluation of serous and suppurative labyrinthitis is essentially the same as that described for labyrinthine fistula.

Suppurative labyrinthitis, on the other hand, presents with more severe vertigo and severe hearing loss in association with the acute otitis media. Suppurative labyrinthitis seems to occur in patients who have extremely intense pain and pressure in the ear. Following bacterial invasion of the inner ear, white blood cell invasion, fibrous exudate formation, membranous destruction, and labyrinthitis ossificans occur in the inner ear. Bacterial invasion usually occurs through the round or oval window, and can follow surgical procedures such as stapedectomy. Unlike serous labyrinthitis, the hearing loss does not recover following suppurative labyrinthitis, although the vertigo improves with the development of labyrinthitis ossificans and with vestibular compensation. Treatment for both serous and suppurative labyrinthitis is aimed at drainage of the inflammatory focus, which might include myringotomy, mastoidectomy, or tympanomastoidectomy. Proper antibiotic coverage with corticosteroids is also indicated in these conditions.

Acoustic Tumors

Acoustic tumors most often present with unilateral progressive sensorineural hearing loss, tinnitus, and disequilibrium. Rarely these patients present with true episodic vertigo, which may be a reflection of either ELH or possibly a sudden change in the tumor size. These considerations are discussed in Chapter 22.

◆ Episodic Vertigo Without Hearing Loss

The differential diagnosis of episodic vertigo without hearing loss includes vestibular neuritis, BPPV, vestibulotoxicity due to drugs, and recurrent vestibulopathy/vascular loop compression syndrome. To rapidly differentiate these entities, vestibular neuritis presents as sudden-onset acute vertigo without hearing loss, usually as a single episode; BPPV presents as multiple brief episodes of vertigo brought on by changing head positions; vestibulotoxicity is a chronic unsteadiness and ataxia that follow the intravenous administration of antibiotics; recurrent vestibulopathy presents with multiple episodes of vertigo without hearing change, and is often accompanied by chronic disequilibrium and positional vertigo.

Vestibular Neuritis

Vestibular neuritis presents as a sudden episode of vertigo without hearing loss in an otherwise healthy patient. It can occur in a single-attack form as well as a multiple-attack form, and can affect one or both ears.

Clinical Presentation

It has been referred to as viral labyrinthitis, epidemic vertigo, neurolabyrinthitis epidemica, acute labyrinthitis, acute vestibular deficit syndrome, vestibular neuronitis, and Scarpa's ganglionitis.[71] It occurs most often in the spring and early summer months. As a result, vestibular neuritis is often associated with upper respiratory infections, occurring 2 to 3 weeks afterward. Vestibular neuritis shows no specific sex predilection, but it is noted more often in patients in their thirties and forties.

Three forms of vestibular neuritis can be differentiated: superior nerve, inferior nerve, and combined superior and inferior nerve. This differentiation is based on utilizing both ENG and VEMP data, because the ENG measures the integrity of the superior nerve and the VEMP measures the integrity of the inferior nerve.

Superior vestibular neuritis is characterized by the sudden onset of vertigo accompanied by nausea and vomiting. The vertigo can be prolonged, the severe episode lasting for several days and gradually improving over several weeks. The hearing is not usually affected by vestibular neuritis, but when it is, it is a high-frequency sensorineural loss that occurs. Vestibular neuritis is sometimes followed by positional vertigo and even BPPV. Recurrent irregular episodes of severe vertigo can also occur with this disorder, a circumstance that may be confused with vestibular Meniere's disease, recurrent vestibulopathy, and vascular loop syndrome. The vertigo and disequilibrium gradually resolve over the first month or two after the initial episode.

Inferior vestibular neuritis is much more subtle in onset. Most patients complain of floating sensation, rocking motion, or a pulling sensation. BPPV from the posterior canal is very rare following inferior vestibular neuritis, as the reflex arc is disrupted. Movement triggered symptoms and visual sensitivity to movement are also frequent complaints. According to Murofushi,[72] inferior vestibular neuritis represents one third of all cases of vestibular neuritis. Because many patients do not seek treatment, the actual course of this illness is uncertain, but in most cases gradual improvement occurs with physical therapy and vestibular supplements.

Combined superior and inferior vestibular neuritis is characterized by severe, catastrophic vertigo ("vestibular crisis). These patients are extremely ill with nausea, vomiting, and dehydration. Even after significant dosages of vestibular suppressives, these patients may be incapacitated by the acute vertigo. Gradually, over the next few months, they improve and are able to resume work, driving, and other activities. The management of these patients is similar to those undergoing a TML, including vestibular rehabilitation therapy and systematic vestibular suppressives.

Histopathology and Pathophysiology

Histopathologic studies have been performed on the temporal bones of patients with clinical histories consistent with vestibular neuritis. The vestibular nerves in these cases have axonal loss, endoneurial fibrosis, and atrophy.[71] These findings suggest that vestibular neuritis is due to a viral infection in the vestibular nerve, rather than to an inflammation of the labyrinth. The pathophysiology of this condition suggests that the acute vertigo accompanies the acute viral inflammation of the vestibular nerve, and may involve one or both ears, either simultaneously or sequentially. If only part of the vestibular nerve is fibrosed following an episode of vestibular neuritis, the remaining axons can be affected again and cause significant symptoms. On the other hand, if most of a vestibular nerve is fibrosed, only minimal symptoms would occur if the nerve were affected again. Several human viruses have been shown to affect the vestibular nerve and the membranous labyrinth, including rubeola, herpes simplex, reovirus, cytomegalovirus, and neurotropic strains of influenza and mumps virus.[73]

Evaluation

The clinician is often asked to see a patient with vestibular neuritis in the emergency department. At that time, the history should focus on the presence or absence of hearing loss, tinnitus, ear fullness or pain, or ear drainage. Other neurologic symptoms should be sought also, including other cranial nerve deficits, weakness, visual deficits, and ataxia or lack of coordination, as well as a history of prior otologic surgery.

The ear, nose, and throat examination and the neurologic examination are then performed. Usually with acute vestibular neuritis, spontaneous nystagmus away from the affected side can be seen without Frenzel glasses. The symptoms and nystagmus worsen with the affected ear in the down position. The seated Romberg test, also known as the Quix test, demonstrates a drift or rotation toward the affected side.

The evaluation of these patients includes audiogram, ENG, rotary chair testing, VEMP, and MRI scans. Audiograms are most often normal, although occasionally they do show a unilateral high-frequency sensorineural hearing loss. The patient in "vestibular crisis" will not tolerate caloric testing. The crisis must first be treated. ENG, if performed shortly after the onset of symptoms, will show spontaneous nystagmus and usually a caloric weakness. ENGs performed after the acute episode has subsided often show a unilateral or a bilateral decrease in caloric excitability, as well as a directional preponderance. Rotational testing usually shows a phase shift and loss of velocity storage, as well as an asymmetry in the VOR gain. The VEMP may show a decrease in amplitude. MRI scans with gadolinium contrast are usually unremarkable, although occasionally an acoustic tumor or a cerebellar infarction can present in an unusual fashion, and these will be detected.

Medical Treatment

Vestibular neuritis is treated initially with vestibular suppressives, such as diazepam 5 to 10 mg IV or p.o. To this regimen is added an antiemetic such as diphenhydramine 25 mg IM every 6 to 8 hours until symptoms subside. A short course of steroid therapy is also begun in these patients, specifically using prednisone 60 mg per day for 7 to 10 days or using a methylprednisolone dose pack. Vestibular rehabilitation is also recommended for these cases.

Rarely, vestibular nerve section might be indicated in a case in which debilitating, episodic vertigo continues to occur.

Benign Paroxysmal Positional Vertigo

BPPV is the most common cause of vertigo of peripheral origin, accounting for nearly 20% of all vestibular complaints.

Clinical Presentation

Patients with this condition typically complain of brief episodes of vertigo brought on by head positioning, especially on getting in and out of bed. The condition is usually worse in the mornings and evenings and it is also characterized by symptomatic and asymptomatic episodes. The average age of onset is 54 years, and the condition typically takes one of three forms[74]: (1) the acute form typically resolves spontaneously over 3 months, (2) the intermittent form has active and inactive periods that may span several years, and (3) the chronic form has continuous symptoms over long durations. In addition to the BPPV, many of these patients also complain of prolonged unsteadiness and lightheadedness.

The specific characteristics of BPPV[75] are critical provocative positioning with the affected ear dependent, rotary nystagmus toward the dependent ear, a brief 1- to 5-second latency prior to onset, limited duration of 10 to 30 seconds, reversal on assuming an upright position, and fatigability of the response.[75] The presence of these findings essentially confirms the diagnosis.

Pathophysiology

BPPV can be seen following head injury, vestibular neuritis, stapes surgery, or Meniere's disease, and without any antecedent event BBPV due to idiopathic causes appears to be the most common. The pathophysiology of BPPV is thought to be due to two proposed mechanisms.[75] The first, called canalolithiasis, proposes that the movement of endolymphatic densities or otoconia during positional testing subsequently causes displacement of the cupula of the posterior semicircular canal. The second, called cupulolithiasis, proposes that otoconia are bound into the cupula, the so-called cupulolithiasis, and with position testing the cupula is deflected. These mechanisms are based on temporal bone histopathology that reveals an agglomeration of basophilic material on the surface of the cupula in BPPV cases, as well as the response of patients to deafferentation of the posterior semicircular canal. Furthermore, Parnes and McClure[75] have noted free-floating particles on opening the posterior semicircular canal for an occlusion procedure.

Evaluation

The evaluation of patients with suspected BPPV includes a history and an ear, nose, and throat examination. The neurotologic examination should also be performed, including the Dix-Hallpike maneuver. An audiogram should be obtained to evaluate for other disorders of the inner ear. In the early phase of BPPV, an ENG probably adds very little information. However, if symptoms persist, the ENG should be obtained to determine if a vestibular weakness exists and to document the presence of positional vertigo.

Also, the VEMP can be used to document that the inferior vestibular nerve is indeed intact. If the VEMP is absent in the affected ear, the posterior canal is probably not the canal causing the symptoms.

MRI scans should also be obtained if the condition persists after therapy or lasts longer than 2 to 3 months.

Management

Management of BPPV begins with a careful explanation to the patient of the nature of the illness. Not only does this alleviate anxiety, but also it provides background information to the patient prior to the inception of various treatments. Vestibular suppressives do not have a significant effect in this condition, although antiemetics can be useful. If the patient has significant symptom-free intervals, fatiguing exercises can be useful as initial therapy. These are performed by asking the patient to sit on the side of the bed and to quickly assume the position that will trigger the vertigo. This should be repeated until the response fatigues.

If the symptoms of BPPV have lasted more than 1 to 2 weeks, the patient should undergo the particle positioning maneuver.[77] In this maneuver, the patient is moved through a sequence of head positions that are thought to cause the movement of the free-floating particles from the posterior canal into the utricle. On completing the particle positioning maneuver, the patient is placed into a soft cervical collar and is advised to avoid bending or moving into a horizontal position for 48 hours. The maneuver is easy to perform, and resolves the BPPV in more than 90% of cases with one to two treatments.[77] A mastoid vibrator or oscillator can also be used in an effort to encourage the movement of the particles into the utricle.

Cases of horizontal canal BPPV have also been recognized. The main differentiating feature is that the provocative position triggers horizontal nystagmus toward the affected ear, as opposed to rotary nystagmus. These cases are treated by a "log rolling" maneuver, which is very similar to the particle positioning maneuver.

An alternative to the particle positioning maneuver is an exercise program that the patient performs, such as the Brandt-Daroff exercise. The objective to this exercise is the same, that is, to reposition the otoconia, and the results are by and large the same as for the office-based maneuvers.

If the symptoms of BPPV do not relent with the particle positioning maneuver and if they are particularly troublesome, two surgical procedures have been used to control the vertigo.

The first procedure that has been used successfully is the middle fossa or retrosigmoid vestibular nerve section. This procedure does control the vertigo in the vast majority of cases, without entailing hearing loss. However, very few patients choose to have an intracranial procedure for BPPV. A second procedure has been successfully employed to control the vertigo in BPPV, the posterior canal occlusion.[76] In this procedure, the posterior canal is identified through a transmastoid approach. The posterior canal is carefully opened (**Fig. 27–11**), the perilymph wicked away, and the canal filled with bone dust and a fascial plug. The procedure does seem to stop the vertigo of BPPV, although a sensorineural hearing loss does occur in 5% of cases. Because of the simplicity and effectiveness of the procedure as well as the low incidence of hearing loss, posterior canal occlusion is currently the procedure of choice for BPPV.

Vestibulotoxicity

Patients who receive ototoxic drugs often suffer from debilitating illnesses that leave them bedridden for prolonged periods of time.[19] Vestibulotoxicity is usually not appreciated until the patient attempts to ambulate, and then notices a severe loss of balance. Vestibulotoxicity, or bilateral vestibular deficits, causes severe ataxia and oscillopsia and usually develops after a long course of intravenous aminoglycoside antibiotic therapy. In these cases, the diagnosis can be easily made by reviewing the medical record to determine if a potentially vestibulotoxic drug has been administered. If a bilateral vestibular deficit is suspected, it is necessary to obtain an audiogram and ENG with ice water calorics. Rotary chair testing can confirm the bilateral vestibular weakness as well as evaluate the higher frequency range. Some regeneration of vestibular sensory neuroepithelia likely will occur, and that, coupled with vestibular rehabilitation, can improve the

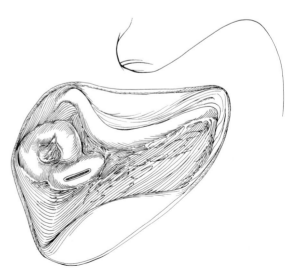

Figure 27–11 Posterior canal occlusion, right ear, surgical position. Fenestra in the bony canal reveals the membranous duct.

daily function of these patients. (For additional information concerning ototoxicity, see Chapter 21.)

Recurrent Vestibulopathy/Vascular Loop Syndrome

Patients who have multiple episodes of vertigo without a hearing loss present a difficult diagnostic problem for the clinician. The symptom complex includes recurrent vertigo, disequilibrium, motion intolerance, and visually induced nausea and instability. Depending on the clinician, these patients are thought to have vestibular Meniere's disease, recurrent vestibular neuritis, vestibular migraine, recurrent vestibulopathy, or vascular loop compression syndrome.

Clinical Presentation

Schwaber and Hall[77] reported a series of 63 patients with this symptom complex. These patients represented 7% of vertigo patients, and females predominated by 2:1. Most patients were between 35 and 55 years old. Symptoms had an average duration of 3.3 years. Approximately 80% had episodic vertigo within the previous year. Ten percent had predominantly positional vertigo. Audiometric studies revealed a high-frequency loss in half, and a middle-frequency loss in 20%. Minor auditory brainstem response (ABR) abnormalities were observed in 80% of cases, including slight prolongation of the wave I–III interval. The vast majority of ENG examinations showed spontaneous nystagmus, and 30% had a caloric weakness. In 42% of cases, vascular enhancement or a widened internal auditory canal was noted on the affected side. In following this series of patients over a 3-year period, 25% improved, 50% remain unchanged, and 25% were worse over time.

Histopathology

Schwaber and Whetsell[64] reported histopathologic studies performed on six vestibular nerves harvested from patients with recurrent vestibulopathy. These nerves were found to have axonal loss and endoneural fibrosis, regardless of whether a vascular loop was present or not. Schwaber and Whetsell noted that the findings in these nerves were most consistent with vestibular neuritis.

The evaluation of patients with recurrent vestibulopathy begins with the ear, nose, and throat examination. The only unusual features seen with this condition are spontaneous nystagmus and a nonclassical Dix-Hallpike test. These patients usually need a complete audiovestibular evaluation, including audiogram, ABR testing, ENG, platform posturography, and MRI and MRA scans. Medical treatment begins with the use of vestibular suppressives in this disorder. Clonazepam 0.5 to 1 mg two to three times per day will control most of the disequilibrium, and alternatively, alprazolam 0.5 to 1 mg twice daily will control the vertigo and optokinetic symptoms. Antinauseants are also helpful in this condition. Most patients benefit from a course of vestibular rehabilitation. Surgery for severe incapacitating disequilibrium and vertigo may be considered for patients with prolongation of interwave latencies on ABR testing. If the wave I–V interval exceeds 0.4 ms, these patients are considered for microvascular decompression of the cochleovestibular nerve. In cases where this has been performed, most patients experience some improvement in their symptoms.

References

1. Committee on Hearing and Equilibrium. Committee on Hearing and Equilibrium guidelines for the diagnosis and evaluation of therapy in Meniere's disease. Otolaryngol Head Neck Surg 1995; 113:181–185
2. Friberg U, Bagger-Sjoback D, Rask-Andersen H. Human endolymphatic duct. An ultrastructural study. Arch Otolaryngol 1984;110:421–428
3. Rassekh CH, Harker LA. The prevalence of migraine in Meniere's disease. Laryngoscope 1992;102:135–138
4. Parker W. Meniere's disease. Etiologic considerations. Arch Otolaryngol Head Neck Surg 1995;121:377–382
5. Paparella M, Mancini F. Vestibular Meniere's. Otolaryngol Head Neck Surg 1985;93:148–151
6. Schuknecht HF, Suzuka Y, Zimmermann C. Delayed endolymphatic hydrops and its relationship to Meniere's disease. Ann Otol Rhinol Laryngol 1990;99:843–862
7. Wladislovsky-Waserman P, Facer GW, Mokri G, Kurland LT. Meniere's disease: a 30-year epidemiologic and clinical study in Rochester, MN 1951–1980. Laryngoscope 1984;94:1098–1102
8. Futaki T, Semba T, Kudo Y, Treatment of hydropic patients by immunoglobin with methyl B12. Am J Otol 1988;9:131–135
9. Derebery MJ, Rao VS, Siglock TJ, Linthicum FH, Nelson RA. Meniere's disease: an immune complex-mediated illness? Laryngoscope 1991; 101:225–229
10. Morrison AW, Mowbray JF, Williamson R, Sheeka S, Sodha N, Koskinen N. On genetic and environmental factors in Meniere's disease. Am J Otol 1994;15:35–39
11. Ylikoski J. Delayed endolymphatic hydrops syndrome after heavy exposure to impulse noise. Am J Otol 1988;9:282–285
12. Derebery MJ, Valenzuela S. Meniere's syndrome and allergy. Otolaryngol Clin North Am 1992;25:213–224
13. Hallpike CS, Cairns H. Observations on the pathology of Meniere's syndrome. J Laryngol Otol 1938;53:625–655
14. Yamakawa K. Ueber die pathologische Veraenderung bei einem Meniere Krnaken. J Otolaryngol Soc Jpn 1938;44:2310–2312
15. Schuknecht HF. Pathology of the Ear, 2nd ed. Philadelphia: Lea & Febiger, 1993:449–529
16. Altmann F, Kornfield M. Histological studies of Meniere's disease. Ann Otol Rhinol Laryngol 1965;74:915–943
17. Ichimiya I, Adams JC, Kimura RS. Changes in immunostaining of cochleas with experimentally induced endolymphatic hydrops. Ann Otol Rhinol Laryngol 1994;103:457–468
18. Masutani H, Takahashi H, Sando I. Stria vascularis in Meniere's disease: a quantitative histopathological study. Auris Nasus Larynx 1992;19:145–152
19. Borjab DI, Bhansali SA, Battista RA. Peripheral Vestibular Disorders. In: Jackler RK, Brackmann DE, eds. Neurotology. St. Louis: Mosby, 1994: 629–650
20. Rauch SD, Merchant SM, Thedinger BA. Meniere's syndrome and endolymphatic hydrops-double blind temporal bone study. Ann Otol Rhinol Laryngol 1989;98:873–883
21. Swart JG, Schuknecht HF. Long-term effects of destruction of the endolymphatic sac in a primate species. Laryngoscope 1988;98:1183–1189
22. Arenberg IK, Marovitz WF, Shambaugh GE. The role of the endolymphatic sac in the pathogenesis of the endolymphatic hydrops in man. Acta Otolaryngol Suppl 1970;275:1–49
23. Arenberg IK, Norback DH, Shambaugh GE. Distribution and density of subepithelial collagen in the endolymphatic sac in patients with Meniere's disease. Am J Otol 1985;6:449–454
24. Gussen R. Meniere syndrome. Compensatory collateral venous drainage with endolymphatic sac fibrosis. Arch Otolaryngol 1974;99:414–418
25. Bagger-Sjoback D, Friberg U, Rask-Andersen H. Human endolymphatic sac: an ultrastructural study. Arch Otolaryngol Head Neck Surg 1986;112:398–409
26. Paparella MM. Pathogenesis of Meniere's disease and Meniere's syndrome. Acta Otolaryngol Suppl 1984;406:10–25
27. Ikeda M, Sando I. The endolymphatic duct and sac in patients with Meniere's disease. A temporal bone histopathological investigation. Ann Otol Rhinol Laryngol 1984;93:540–546
28. Erwall C, Friberg U, Bagger-Sjoback D, Rask-Andersen H. Degradation of the homogenous substance in the endolymphatic sac. Acta Otolaryngol 1988;105:209–217
29. Wackym PA. Histopathologic findings in Meniere's disease. Otolaryngol Head Neck Surg 1995;112:90–100
30. Welling DB, Daniels RL, Brainard J, Western LM, Prior TW. Detection of viral DNA in endolymphatic sac tissue from Meniere's disease patients. Am J Otol 1994;15:639–643

31. Dornhoffer JL, Waner M, Arenberg IK, Montague D. Immunoperoxidase study of the endolymphatic sac in Meniere's disease. Laryngoscope 1993;103:1027–1034

32. Lee FP, Ho TL, Huang TS. Endolymphatic hydrops in animal experiments. A confirmation of mechanical and immunological methods of inducement. Acta Otolaryngol Suppl 1991;485:18–25

33. Masutani H, Takahashi H, Sando I, Sato H. Vestibular aqueduct in Meniere's disease and non-Meniere's disease with endolymphatic hydrops: a computer aided volumetric study. Auris Nasus Larynx 1991;18:351–357

34. Andrews JC, Strelioff D. Modulation of inner ear pressure in experimental endolymphatic hydrops. Otolaryngol Head Neck Surg 1995;112:78–83

35. Horner KC. Auditory and vestibular function in experimental hydrops. Otolaryngol Head Neck Surg 1995;112:84–89

36. Zenner HP, Reuter G, Zimmermann U, Gitter AH, Fermin C, LePage EL. Transitory endolymph leakage induced hearing loss and tinnitus: depolarization, biphasic shortening and loss of electromotility of outer hair cells. Eur Arch Otorhinolaryngol 1994;251:143–153

37. Long C, Morizono T. Hydrostatic pressure measurements of endolymph and perilymph in a guinea pig model of endolymphatic hydrops. Otolaryngol Head Neck Surg 1987;96:83–95

38. Kitahara M, Takeda T, Yazawa Y, Matsubara H, Kitano H. Pathophysiology of Meniere's disease and its subvarieties. Acta Otolaryngol Suppl 1984;406:52–55

39. Juhn SK, Ikeda K, Morizono T, Murphy M. Pathophysiology of inner ear fluid imbalance. Acta Otolaryngol Suppl 1991;485:9–14

40. Cohen J, Morizono T. Changes in EP and inner ear ionic concentrations in experimental endolymphatic hydrops. Acta Otolaryngol 1984;98:398–402

41. Salt AN, DeMott JE. Endolymph calcium increases with time in hydropic guinea pigs. In: Abstracts of the Fifteenth Midwinter Meeting. St. Petersburg Beach, FL: Association for Research in Otolaryngology, 1992:128

42. Ikeda K, Morizono T. Ionic activities of the inner ear fluid and ionic permeabilities of the cochlear duct in endolymphatic hydrops of the guinea pig. Hear Res 1991;51:185–192

43. Morgenstern C, Mori N, Amano H. Pathogenesis of experimental endolymphatic hydrops. Acta Otolaryngol Suppl 1984;406:56–58

44. Van de Water SM, Arenberg IK, Balkany TJ. Auditory dehydration testing: glycerol versus urea. Am J Otol 1986;7:200–203

45. Schwaber MK, Hall JW, Zealear DL. Intraoperative monitoring of the facial and cochleovestibular nerves in otologic surgery: part II. Insights Otolaryngol 1991;6:108

46. Margolis RH, Rieks D, Fournier EM, Levine SE. Tympanic electrocochleography for diagnosis of Meniere's disease. Arch Otolaryngol Head Neck Surg 1995;121:44–55

47. Moffat DA, Baguley DM, Harries MLL, Atlas M, Lynch CA. Bilateral electrocochleographic findings in unilateral Meniere's disease. Otolaryngol Head Neck Surg 1992;107:370–373

48. Keim RJ. Clinical comparison of posturography and electronystagmography. Laryngoscope 1993;103:713–716

49. O'Leary DP, Davis LL. Vestibular autorotation testing of Meniere's disease. Otolaryngol Head Neck Surg 1990;103:66–71

50. de Waele C, Huy PT, Diard JP, et al. Saccular dysfunction in Meniere's disease. Am J Otol 1999;20:223–232

51. Seo T, Yoshida K, Shibano A, Sakagami M. A possible case of saccular endolymphomatic hydrops. ORL J Otorhinolaryngol Relat Spec 1999;61: 215–218

52. Ruckenstein MJ, Rutka JA, Hawke M. The treatment of Meniere's disease: Torol revisited. Laryngoscope 1991;101:211–218

53. Gates GA, Green JD, Tucci DL, Telian SA. The effects of transtympanic micropressure treatment in people with unilateral Meniere's disease. Arch Otolaryngol Head Neck Surg 2004;130:718–723

54. Graham MD, Sataloff RT, Kemnik JL. Titration streptomycin therapy for bilateral Meniere's disease: a preliminary report. Otolaryngol Head Neck Surg 1984;92:440–444

55. Nedzelski JM, Schessel DA, Bryce GE, Pfeiderer AG. Chemical labyrinthectomy: local application of gentamicin for the treatment of unilateral Meniere's disease. Am J Otol 1992;13:18–22

56. Pyykko I, Ishizaki H, Kaasinen S, Aalto H. Intratympanic gentamicin in bilateral Meniere's disease. Otolaryngol Head Neck Surg 1994;110:162–167

57. Telischi FF, Luxford WM. Long-term efficacy of endolymphatic sac surgery for vertigo in Meniere's disease. Otolaryngol Head Neck Surg 1993;109:83–87

58. Goldenberg RA, Justus MA. Endolymphatic mastoid shunt for Meniere's disease: do results must change over time? Laryngoscope 1990;100:141–145

59. Bretlau P, Thomsen J, Tos M, Johnson NJ. Placebo effect in surgery for Meniere's disease: nine year follow-up. Am J Otol 1989;10:259–261

60. Silverstein H, Smouha E, Jones R. Natural history vs. surgery for Meniere's disease. Otolaryngol Head Neck Surg 1989;100:6–16

61. Silverstein H, Norrell H. Retrolabyrinthine vestibular neurectomy. Otolaryngol Head Neck Surg 1982;90:778–782

62. Kemink JL, Telian SE, El-Kashlan H, Langman AW. Retrolabyrinthine vestibular nerve section: efficacy in disorders other than Meniere's disease. Laryngoscope 1991;101:523–529

63. Giddings NA, Shelton C, O'Leary MJ, Brackmann DE. Cochleosacculotomy revisited long term results poorer than expected. Arch Otolaryngol Head Neck Surg 1991;117:1150–1152

64. Schwaber MK, Whetsell WO. Cochleovestibular nerve compression syndrome. II. Vestibular nerve histopathology and theory of pathophysiology. Laryngoscope 1992;102:1030–1036

65. Weider DJ. Treatment and management of perilymph fistula: a New Hampshire experience. Am J Otol 1992;13:158–166

66. Minor LB. Clinical manifestations of superior semicircular canal dehiscence. Laryngoscope 2005;115:1717–1727

67. Steckelberg JM, McDonald TJ. Otologic involvement in late syphilis. Laryngoscope 1984;94:753–757

68. Wilson WR, Zoller M. Electronystagmography in congenital and acquired syphilitic otitis. Ann Otol Rhinol Laryngol 1981;90:21–24

69. Shih L, McElveen JT, Linthicum FH. Management of vertigo in patients with syphilis: Is endolymphatic shunt surgery appropriate? Otolaryngol Head Neck Surg 1988;99:574–577

70. Baloh RW. Vertebrobasilar insufficiency and stroke. Otolaryngol Head Neck Surg 1995;112:114–117

71. Schuknecht HF, Kitamura K. Vestibular neuritis. Ann Otol Rhinol Laryngol Suppl 1981;90:1–19

72. Murofushi T, Halmagyi GM, Javor RA, Cofebatch VG. Absent vestibular-evoked myogenic potentials in vestibular neurolabyrinthitis. An indicator of inferior vestibular nerve involvement? Arch Otolaryngol Head Neck Surg 1996;122:845–848

73. Gacek R. Further observations on posterior ampullary nerve transection for positional vertigo. Ann Otol Rhinol Laryngol 1978;87: 300–305

74. Parnes LS, Price-Jones RG. Particle positioning maneuver for benign paroxysmal positional vertigo. Ann Otol Rhinol Laryngol 1993;102: 325–331

75. Parnes LS, McClure J. Posterior semicircular canal occlusion in the normal hearing ear. Otolaryngol Head Neck Surg 1991;104:52–57

76. Epley JM. The canalith repositioning procedure: for treatment of benign paroxysmal positional vertigo. Otolaryngol Head Neck Surg 1992; 107:399–404

77. Schwaber MK, Hall JW. Cochleovestibular nerve compression syndrome I. Clinical features and audiovestibular findings. Laryngoscope 1992; 102:1020–1029

28

Facial Nerve Disorders

Pamela C. Roehm, Jay T. Rubenstein, and Bruce J. Gantz

Proper management of facial nerve disorders requires an appreciation for the wealth of knowledge about this cranial nerve and for the gaps in our understanding of its pathophysiology. Many facial nerve disorders are extremely rare and their natural history is poorly documented. Other disorders, such as Bell's palsy, are common and the natural history well known. Unfortunately, this knowledge does little to decrease the controversy regarding appropriate management of the disease. It is unlikely that there will be a consensus regarding management of all the disorders described in this chapter. However, when a patient presents with a disorder of the facial nerve, the clinician must advise and provide treatment. In many cases it is appropriate to offer more than one treatment plan and allow the patient to choose, based on the known risks and benefits of that plan. In these situations the patient must be aware of the unknowns inherent in any approach.

◆ Anatomy of the Facial Nerve

The facial nerve has a complex three-dimensional course from its motor nucleus in the anterior pons to its insertion into the muscles of facial expression. After exiting posteriorly from the motor nucleus, fibers of the facial nerve turn abruptly around the abducens nucleus and exit from the brainstem at the pontomedullary junction. At its exit from the brainstem, the facial nerve lies 1.5 mm anterior to the eighth cranial nerve. The nervus intermedius, which is composed of parasympathetic fibers that become the greater superficial petrosal and chorda tympani nerves, exits the brainstem between cranial nerves VII and VIII. The facial nerve is about 1.8 mm in diameter at its root entry zone. After leaving the brainstem, it has a 15- to 17-mm course through the cerebellopontine angle (CPA) prior to entering the porus of the internal auditory canal (IAC). Within the CPA the facial nerve is in close proximity to the anterior inferior cerebellar artery (AICA), which provides the vascular supply to this segment of the nerve. The AICA may lie anterior to or between cranial nerves VII and VIII. Occasionally, a loop of AICA may course laterally to the fundus of the IAC.

After entering the IAC, the facial nerve travels 8 to 10 mm prior to entering the meatal foramen (**Fig. 28–1**). In the IAC it occupies the anterior-superior quadrant and at the fundus it is separated from the superior vestibular nerve by the vertical crest (Bill's bar) and from the cochlear nerve by the transverse crest. On entering the meatal foramen, the facial nerve narrows to its smallest diameter, 0.61 to 0.68 mm. The ratio of the fallopian canal diameter to facial nerve diameter is at its lowest as well. Adour[1] has questioned the concept of meatal entrapment as a mechanism for facial nerve injury, but there are now substantial data demonstrating that entrapment at the meatal foramen and labyrinthine segment plays a role in the pathogenesis of at least some facial nerve disorders as detailed below.[2–13]

The labyrinthine segment is 4 mm in length between the meatal foramen and the geniculate ganglion. It is located immediately posterior and slightly superior to the basal turn of the cochlea. The labyrinthine segment is just anterior to the ampulla of the superior semicircular canal and courses superiorly as it travels laterally, a position of importance for middle fossa surgery. At the geniculate ganglion, the nerve takes a 75-degree turn posteriorly into the tympanic segment. The greater superficial petrosal nerve (GSPN) exits the fallopian canal via the facial hiatus with the superficial petrosal artery (a branch of the middle meningeal artery), which is the vascular supply to this region of the nerve.

The tympanic segment is about 11 mm long and lies between the takeoff of the GSPN and the second genu. It forms the superior aspect of the oval window niche and is readily injured by pathologic processes and unwary middle ear surgeons, due to its frequently occurring dehiscences.[14,15]

After passing between the stapes and the lateral semicircular canal, the nerve turns inferiorly into the mastoid segment. This measures 13 mm in length down to the stylomastoid foramen. The stylomastoid artery, a branch of the postauricular artery, supplies this portion of the nerve. Dense connective tissue envelops the nerve as it exits the stylomastoid foramen. During procedures that require mobilization of this portion of the facial nerve, nerve injury can be avoided by including a margin of the connective tissue with the nerve during mobilization.[16]

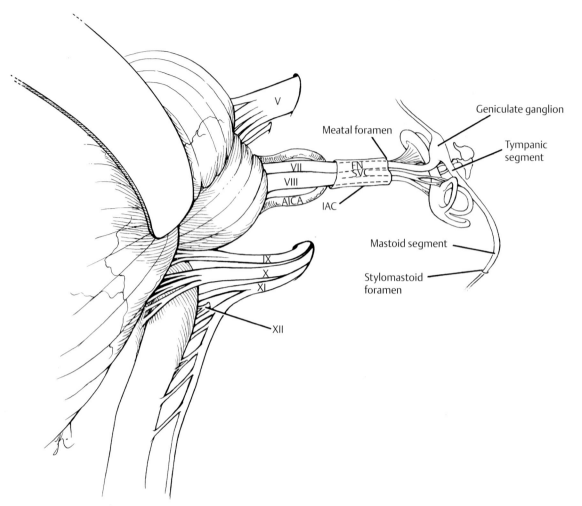

Figure 28–1   Course and relationships of the left facial nerve from the pontomedullary junction to the stylomastoid foramen. AICA, anterior inferior cerebellar artery; IAC, internal auditory canal; FN, facial nerve; SVN, superior vestibular nerve.

◆ Grading of Facial Weakness

Assessment of treatment efficacy requires a consistent system for grading facial weakness. The House-Brackmann scale[17] was originally developed for assessment of outcome in Bell's palsy but has proven useful in management of all acute facial nerve disorders. It is listed in **Table 28–1**.

◆ Facial Nerve Disorders in Adults

Bell's Palsy

One should expect that any fairly common disorder with a well-described natural history, multiple placebo-controlled treatment trials, a wealth of intraoperative observation, and morphologic, histopathologic, electrophysiologic, and molecular data would be treatable with a minimum of controversy. This is far from true in the case of the acute facial paralysis first described by Sir Charles Bell. The debate over the efficacy of any medical or surgical therapy has changed its focus over time, but the fundamental disagreements have not changed in 30 years. Nevertheless, much is known about the natural history, possible etiologies, pathogenesis, and clinical evaluation of the patient with Bell's palsy, so that a treatment algorithm

may be formed and allows for unknown and debatable issues. An excellent review of these issues is available.[18]

Diagnosis

Although Bell's palsy may not be idiopathic,[1] it remains a diagnosis of exclusion. The clinician must exclude all identifiable causes of facial paralysis that may be determined by history, physical examination, or radiologic study. It is not uncommon for CPA tumors, skull base neoplasms, otitis media, or parotid lesions to be misdiagnosed as Bell's palsy. These errors should be rare, as history and physical examination point to the correct diagnosis the vast majority of the time. A partial or total unilateral facial paralysis with onset over a 48-hour period without hearing loss, vertigo, or other cranial neuropathy and with a normal head and neck examination is likely to be Bell's palsy. Other than audiometric evaluation, it does not require further diagnostic workup except for HIV testing or Lyme titers in appropriate circumstances. Some recovery should be noted within 3 to 6 months in all patients.

Occasionally, a sudden total facial paralysis occurs that does not resolve in 6 months. This situation requires thorough imaging and possibly surgical exploration prior to any attempt at reanimation. Parotid malignancy has been reported as long as 10 years after acute facial palsy.[19] A case of fluctuating facial

Table 28–1 The House-Brackmann Scale

Grade	Description	Characteristics
I	Normal	Normal facial function in all areas
II	Mild dysfunction	Gross: slight weakness noticeable on close inspection; may have very slight synkinesis
		At rest: normal symmetry and tone
		Motion
		Forehead: moderate to good
		Eye: complete closure with minimum effort
		Mouth: slight asymmetry
III	Moderate dysfunction	Gross: obvious but not disfiguring difference between two sides; noticeable but not severe synkinesis, contracture, and/or hemifacial spasm
		At rest: normal symmetry and tone
		Motion
		Forehead: slight to moderate movement
		Eye: complete closure with effort
		Mouth: slightly weak with maximum effort
IV	Moderately severe dysfunction	Gross: obvious weakness and/or disfiguring asymmetry
		At rest: normal symmetry and tone
		Motion
		Forehead: none
		Eye: incomplete closure
		Mouth: asymmetric with maximum effort
V	Severe dysfunction	Gross: only barely perceptible motion
		At rest: asymmetry
		Motion
		Forehead: none
		Eye: incomplete closure
		Mouth: slight movement
VI	Total paralysis	No movement

Source: Adapted from House JW, Brackmann DE. Facial nerve grading system. Otolaryngol Head Neck Surg 1985;93:146–147. Reprinted with permission.

paralysis has been seen in our institution in association with negative enhanced magnetic resonance imaging (MRI) and high-resolution temporal bone computed tomography (CT). An occult parotid malignancy was diagnosed 6 months later. Another case of acute facial paralysis 6 months after excision of a squamous cell carcinoma of the cheek skin proved to be metastatic carcinoma despite multiple negative imaging studies. These cases are unusual but point to the necessity of aggressive evaluation of all progressive facial pareses, segmental pareses, pareses associated with facial twitching prior to onset, pareses associated with other cranial neuropathies, and those acute palsies that do not show some recovery within 6 months.

Pathogenesis

May[20] suggested that Bell's palsy begins with involvement of the sensory fibers of the facial nerve and subsequently involves the motor fibers. This process is consistent with the notion that the disease begins as a viral ganglionitis of the geniculate ganglion.[21] Nasopharyngeal cultures,[22] circulating antibodies,[23] biopsy,[24] polymerase chain reaction (PCR) of the geniculate ganglion from archived temporal bone,[25] and PCR of intraoperative washings of the facial nerve[26] from patients with Bell's palsy all point to herpes simplex virus as the main etiologic agent. Ischemic and autoimmune injury have been proposed as the subsequent means of nerve degeneration, but it is now clear that entrapment at the meatal foramen and labyrinthine segment is critical in this process as originally described by Fisch and Esslen.[27] The evidence for this includes the following:

1. Temporal bone histopathologic demonstration of a sharp demarcation between a normal nerve in the IAC and a severely degenerated nerve beyond the meatal foramen in a case of herpes zoster oticus[6]
2. Clear and convincing electrophysiologic evidence[3,5] of conduction block at the meatal foramen and labyrinthine segment
3. Dramatic improvement in conduction across the labyrinthine segment after decompression[3]
4. Intraoperative observation at this institution and others[10] of an edematous-appearing nerve in the IAC and a cadaveric-appearing nerve distally
5. Return of some facial movement in a small number of patients immediately after middle cranial fossa (MCF) decompression[2]
6. Clinical series demonstrating the efficacy of MCF decompression in cases of recurrent facial paralysis[4,12]
7. Gadolinium enhancement of the labyrinthine segment in Bell's palsy and herpes zoster oticus (HZO)[7–9,11,13]

None of these data imply that MCF decompression is indicated for Bell's palsy, but it has convincingly implicated the meatal foramen and labyrinthine segment in the pathologic process. Temporal bone morphometric evidence that the facial nerve is not as tightly constrained at the meatal foramen in young children may account for the lower incidence and better prognosis in this population.[28]

Prognosis

Several large studies have outlined the natural history of Bell's palsy.[29,30] Generally, patients older than age 65 at onset of idiopathic facial paralysis have a worse recovery of facial function than younger patients.[29–31] Likewise, patients with diabetes not only have an increased incidence of Bell's palsy but also have a poorer prognosis.[30,31]

The majority of patients have good recovery of facial function within 3 to 6 months without medical or surgical intervention (except, of course, eye care as needed). Identification of those patients who will not recover grade I or II function therefore should be the next goal after a diagnosis is made. Several important prognostic factors have been noted. Patients who never progress to complete paralysis and those with signs of recovery within the first 2 months have an excellent prognosis, with almost all returning to normal function. Electromyographic (EMG) evidence of voluntary activity[32,33] or an intact stapedial reflex[34] also portends an excellent prognosis. Finally, electroneurography (ENoG) findings of less than 90% degeneration of the electrically evoked compound muscle action potential during the first 2 weeks after onset of paralysis indicate almost certain near-normal or normal recovery. Patients with greater than 90% degeneration in the first 2 weeks have less than a 50% chance of good recovery.[32,33,35] These patients should be the focus of aggressive treatment efforts.

Unfortunately, there is no electrophysiologic test that discriminates between nerve fibers that have undergone axonotmesis,[36,37] which should recover fully, and those that have more severe injury.[21] Further complicating this issue is intraoperative evidence of nerve fibers that are not stimulable distal to a pathologic process, but which become stimulable shortly after removal of the pathology. This represents injury more severe than neuropraxia, but clearly is not axonotmesis because the recovery is too fast to allow time for regeneration. This phenomenon may explain the rapid recovery reported after some MCF decompressions[2] in which response to electrical stimulation was absent preoperatively. It is hoped that laboratory study of this process will improve clinical prognostication. For detailed discussion of prognostic electrical testing, see Chapter 9.

Eye Care

Eye care is the single most important treatment for any patient with grade II or worse facial function. Drying of the eye secondary to decreased eye closure and lacrimation rapidly leads to exposure keratopathy with breakdown of the cornea.[38,39] To prevent this complication, artificial tears are applied at least every 2 hours during the day. At bedtime, ophthalmic ointment is applied and a moisture chamber of plastic wrap is used to cover the eye. Use of a temporary tarsorrhaphy, gold weight, or other oculoplastic techniques provides better eye protection when either facial nerve function is not expected to return or when exposure keratopathy cannot be prevented by medical treatment alone.[38,39] Gold weights have almost entirely replaced tarsorrhapies.

Medical Treatment

Multiple placebo-controlled trials of glucocorticoid therapy for Bell's palsy have demonstrated mixed results, with some studies demonstrating benefit and others showing none. For summaries of these studies with conflicting conclusions see Limb and Niparko,[18] Selesnick and Patwardhan,[40] and Salinas et al.[41] For patients presenting within 3 weeks of onset of paralysis, we currently use prednisone 1 mg/kg/day for 14 days. Patients who have a medical contraindication to oral steroids are treated with weekly transtympanic injections of solumedrol 0.3 to 0.4 cc 40 mg/cc. Acyclovir treatment for Bell's palsy is actively promoted by Adour et al,[42] who claim a statistically significant benefit. However, a systematic review of this study and two other randomized controlled trials revealed a lack of consistent evidence for improved recovery from Bell's palsy in patients treated with antivirals.[43] Acyclovir has low toxicity and, as noted above, there are good theoretical reasons for its use. We currently treat patients with a 2-week course of valacyclovir in addition to steroids. A study by Murakami strongly supports antiviral treatments.[26]

Surgical Treatment

Surgical management of Bell's palsy has evolved along with our understanding of the pathophysiology of the disease. May et al[44] clearly demonstrated the futility of transmastoid decompression. Only MCF decompression of the meatal foramen, labyrinthine segment, and geniculate ganglion can be expected to offer any benefit. Although we perform the MCF approach frequently for acoustic neuroma and vestibular nerve section with minimal morbidity, it is technically challenging even for experienced temporal bone surgeons and has significant potential for complications. Thus, even with proof of the efficacy of decompression, we would only advocate its performance in centers experienced with the MCF approach.

Fisch's[45] landmark study of MCF decompression demonstrated statistically significant improvements in outcome with surgery, but it is difficult to assess the degree of improvement in this study. Use of the House-Brackmann scale in subsequent reports makes this much easier. All patients had >90% degeneration on ENoG within 14 days of onset of total paralysis and no voluntary EMG potentials. Fisch's[32] prognostic studies show at best a 50% rate of spontaneous "satisfactory" recovery when degeneration exceeds 90%. Sillman and coworkers[33] studied ENoG prognostication using the House-Brackmann scale and verified Fisch's result, demonstrating less than 50% recovery to grade I or II function when ENoG degeneration exceeded 90%. Thus the patients who would be expected to spontaneously return to grade I or II less than 50% of the time were treated with MCF decompression.

A multicenter prospective clinical trial of patients with Bell's palsy showed that patients who did not reach 90% degeneration on ENoG within 14 days of paralysis ($n = 54$) all had return of function to House-Brackmann grade I or II (**Table 28–2**). Patients with ≥90% degeneration on ENoG and no EMG motor unit potentials were offered surgical decompression of the facial nerve through an MCF approach. Thirty-four elected to have the decompression, whereas 36 were managed with steroids only. The results of the comparison were statistically significant in favor of decompression ($p < .0002$ stratified exact permutation test). The surgical decompression group exhibited House-Brackmann grade I or II results in 91% of those undergoing MCF decompression within 14 days of onset of acute paralysis. Of the 36 patients who chose not to undergo surgical decompression and were treated solely with steroids, 58% had a poor outcome at 7 months follow-up (House-Brackmann grade III or IV). Only 9% of the patients who did have MCF facial nerve compression had a poor outcome (**Table 28–2**).[46]

Facial nerve decompression for Bell's palsy is rarely necessary as severe degeneration is uncommon. However, when severe degeneration does occur within 14 days of the onset of acute paralysis, and there are no voluntary EMG motor units active, MCF surgical decompression is worthwhile.

Table 28–2 Bell's Palsy Management

ENoG: ≥90% degeneration by 14 days EMG: no voluntary motor unit potentials		
House-Brackmann Grade	**MCF Decompression n**	**Steroids Only n**
I	14	5
II	17	10
III	2	19
IV	1	2
I/II	31(91%)*	15(42%)
III/IV	3(9%)	21(58%)

* p < .0002 stratified exact permutation test
MCF, middle cranial fossa.

Management Algorithm

Our approach to management of Bell's palsy is displayed in **Fig. 28–2**. We perform an ENoG when the patient has a total paralysis and is seen within the first 14 days. If the patient has nearly 90% degeneration or is degenerating quickly, frequent follow-up ENoGs are performed.[32] If the 90% threshold is reached within 14 days and no voluntary EMG activity is seen, MCF decompression of the labyrinthine segment and geniculate ganglion is advised. Contraindications to MCF decompression would include general medical contraindications to surgery and age greater than 65. Beyond this age, the middle fossa dura is thinner and more tightly adherent to the tegmen, making elevation of the temporal lobe substantially more difficult. Some groups use the MCF approach for patients over this age limit for attempted hearing preservation in acoustic neuroma surgery. One group has reported a trend toward lower hearing preservation and increased cerebrospinal fluid (CSF) leak rates in patients over the age of 60 with the MCF approach.[47]

Surgical Technique

Facial nerve monitoring is performed routinely, as the facial nerve may be electrically stimulable with direct contact even when percutaneous stimulation suggests total absence of electrical response. EMG and visual monitoring of facial function require that the anesthesia team avoid use of paralytic agents. A Foley catheter is inserted. Mannitol is given and hyperventilation is performed to reduce intracranial pressure. The hair is shaved above the ear and a posteriorly based 6×6 cm skin flap is elevated as shown in **Fig. 28–3**. An anteriorly based temporalis flap is raised after harvesting a large piece of temporalis fascia for use in closing. A 4×5 cm bone flap centered over the zygomatic root is drilled. Carefully raising the bone flap prevents dural tears, which must be closed to prevent CSF leaks. Bleeding from branches of the middle meningeal artery is controlled with bone wax and bipolar cautery. The vertical cuts must be parallel to facilitate subsequent placement of the middle fossa retractor. The bone flap is wrapped in moist gauze, and the skin and muscle flaps are

Acute Facial Paresis/Paralysis

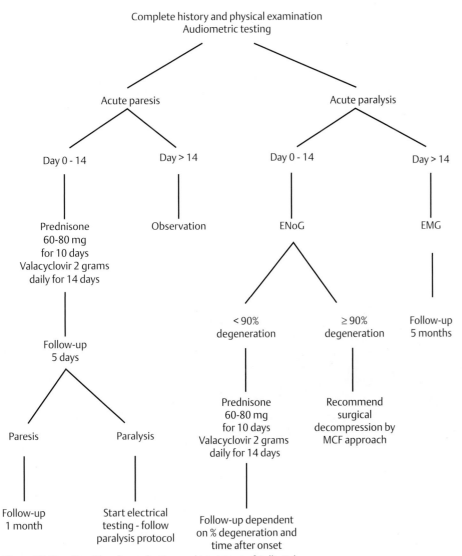

Figure 28–2 Algorithm for evaluation and treatment of Bell's Palsy.

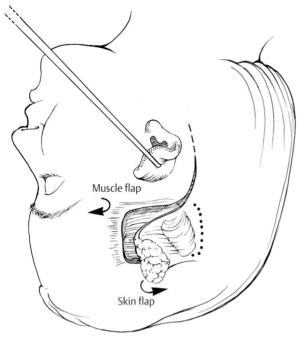

Figure 28–3 Surgical position illustrating the skin incision (solid line) for the MCF approach. Dashed line: mastoid extension if transmastoid exposure is planned. Dotted line: temporalis muscle, fascia, and periosteal flap.

retracted with care to avoid injury to the frontal branch of the extratemporal facial nerve.

The middle fossa dura is elevated off the tegmen using a combination of blunt and sharp dissection, and bipolar cautery. Elevation proceeds from posterior to anterior to avoid injuring an exposed GSPN or geniculate ganglion. The scrub technician watches for facial movement while working near the facial hiatus. The petrous ridge is identified posteriorly and the GSPN anteriorly. Elevation of the dura superiorly, posteriorly, and anteriorly from the surrounding cranium more evenly distributes pressure from the retractor and makes retractor placement significantly easier. The House-Urban retractor is placed with its tip at the petrous ridge medial to the arcuate eminence once sufficient exposure has been gained. Identification of the arcuate eminence can be one of the most difficult aspects of the procedure. Preoperative Stenver's views can be helpful, but experience is the ultimate guide to the location of the superior semicircular canal. Until this critical landmark has been precisely located, slow bone removal broadly over the arcuate eminence and tegmen mastoideum is performed until the yellow-ivory bone of the otic capsule is uncovered. The superior canal is always perpendicular to the petrous ridge. The superior canal is blue-lined, and the IAC is then easily found at a 60-degree angle from the superior canal (**Fig. 28–4**). The GSPN will also be at a 60-degree angle from the IAC, but frequently is covered with bone, limiting its usefulness as a landmark. Unlike MCF surgery for acoustic neuromas, the medial aspect of the IAC should not be widely opened, as this unnecessarily increases the risk of CSF leak. Approximately 120 degrees of the lateral IAC is blue-lined with diamond burs and the facial nerve is identified anterior to the vertical crest. It is then traced laterally to the geniculate ganglion and the tympanic segment. The fallopian canal is thinned with diamond burs and copious irrigation. The final layer of bone is removed with blunt elevators or picks. On exposing the middle ear, care must be taken to avoid injury to the ossicles.

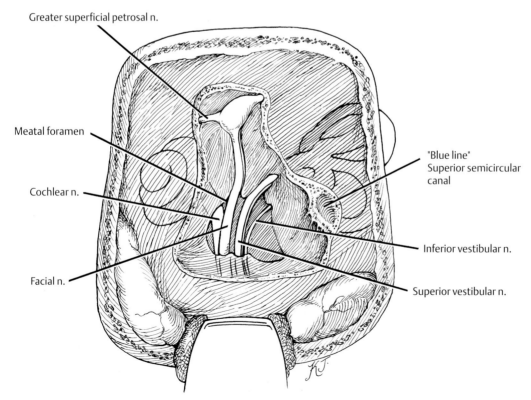

Figure 28–4 Surgical view of the left middle cranial fossa exposure after craniotomy, temporal lobe retraction, and bony exposure are complete.

III Management

380

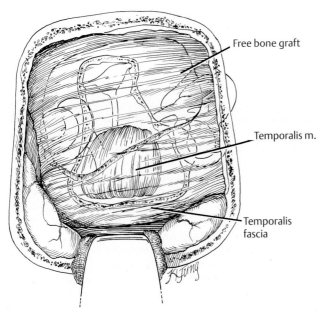

Figure 28–5 Temporalis muscle is placed within the IAC defect at the conclusion of decompression. A free bone graft is placed perpendicular to the axis of the IAC to prevent herniation of the temporal lobe into the middle ear or IAC. Temporalis fascia is then used to seal the temporal lobe dura and IAC.

The final step of the procedure is neurolysis with a 59–10 Beaver disposable microscalpel. Possible surgical findings include a nerve that is so edematous proximal to the meatal foramen that it obscures the superior vestibular nerve. Sometimes fibers "billow" out after the epineurium is split.[10] In cases where intraoperative electrical responses can be obtained, it is not unusual to see substantial decreases in threshold to electrical stimulation in the IAC after bony decompression, with further decreases after neurolysis.

Closure is accomplished by placing a free muscle graft in the IAC and repairing the tegmen tympani with a small bone graft harvested from the bone flap (**Fig. 28–5**). This must be placed to prevent herniation of the temporal lobe into the middle ear and must be positioned to avoid interference with ossicular motion. The temporalis fascia graft is placed under the bone to seal the IAC defect. All exposed air cells are plugged with bone wax. Hyperventilation is stopped, and the temporal lobe is allowed to settle into anatomic position. Two 4–0 Neuralon sutures are used to tack the dura to the pericranium inferiorly to prevent epidural hematoma. The bone flap is replaced and a watertight closure of the temporalis, galea, and skin is performed. A mastoid dressing is applied and the patient is observed in surgical intensive care overnight. At least 48 hours of perioperative steroids, antibiotics, and fluid restriction are routine. If there are no complications, the patient may be discharged as early as postoperative day 3. Potential complications include all of those associated with middle fossa surgery.

The most important management guidelines for "idiopathic" acute facial (Bell's) paralysis are: (1) give eye care to all patients; (2) give high-dose oral glucocorticoids (prednisone) to all patients unless there is a contraindication; (3) give valacyclovir at least one gram orally twice a day. Duration and benefit of this treatment regimen depends on when the patient is first seen, with day 1 defined as the first day of observed weakness. Obviously, the sooner treatment is begun, the more likely it is to help. This latter point is especially true for antiviral medication which works best when started within the first three days and somewhat also if started in the first seven days. After seven days, prednisone still might be helpful, but antivirals might or might not be helpful. (4) When the patient develops total facial paralysis, electrophysiologic testing (ENoG) should be initiated on day 3 or 4 following the onset of total paralysis. The electrophysiologic testing should guide further surgical intervention. The criteria that appears to be the most appropriate are greater than 90% degeneration on ENoG before 15 days of total paralysis and there are no voluntary motor unit potentials on EMG. If surgical intervention is required, the approach should be through the middle fossa for decompression of the tympanic, geniculate ganglion and meatal foramen portions of the facial nerve.

Assume a patient with "idiopathic" acute facial palsy (not Ramsay Hunt) presents on day 2. The landmark study of natural history by Peitersen proved that eye care alone achieved 71% grade I results and a total of 84% grade I-II results. A grade II result is very acceptable. If a patient is treated promptly and aggressively with prednisone-valcyclovir, the grade I-II outcome rises even higher. Obviously, specialty clinics with qualified neurootologists see these "worse case scenario" patients in whom surgery can be very appropriate. However, when emergency physicians, family doctors, internists, and neurologists learn that the standard of initial care is eye care, prednisone, and valacyclovir, the need for surgical intervention will be significantly reduced.[48,49]

Herpes Zoster Oticus

HZO, or Ramsay Hunt syndrome, is characterized by severe pain, vesicles in the conchal bowl and sensory distribution of the facial nerve, and facial paralysis that tends to be more severe than that found in Bell's palsy (**Figs. 28–6** and **28–7**). It is caused by the varicella zoster virus and not infrequently involves the vestibular and cochlear nerves causing hearing loss and vertigo. Involvement of cranial nerves V, IX, X, XI, and XII can also occur, prompting the alternative name "herpes zoster cephalicus."[50] The frequency of complete electrical degeneration of the facial nerve is much higher than with Bell's palsy, and the prognosis for spontaneous, complete recovery is much lower (22 to 31%).[29,51,52] Even with the administration of steroids, facial nerve recovery rates are low.[52,53]

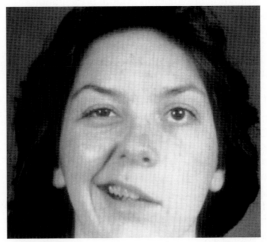

Figure 28–6 Grade IV left facial paralysis from herpes zoster oticus.

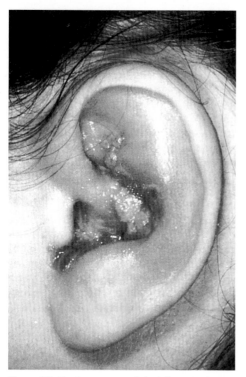

Figure 28–7 Appearance of the left ear in the same patient as in **Fig. 28–6.** Note the vesicles characteristic of herpes zoster oticus.

Two uncontrolled studies of intravenous acyclovir therapy involving a total of 12 patients have demonstrated dramatic improvement of facial function as compared with historical controls.[54,55] Nine of 12 had grade I or II recoveries. Of the three who had grade III recoveries, one had only 1-month follow-up, one was elderly and missed multiple doses, and one began treatment 5 days following onset of paralysis. Other uncontrolled studies have looked at either intravenous or oral acyclovir therapy combined with steroids.[56–59] In the third study, of 91 patients who were treated within 7 days of onset of paralysis, 93% recovered to a grade I or II. In this study, a group of patients treated with steroids alone due to late onset of vesicles showed 68% recovered to a grade I or II.[56] Recovery to grade I or II in the remaining three studies was 36%, 74%, and 82.6%.[56,57,59] These differences appear to reflect both variation in treatment protocols and duration of symptoms prior to presentation.

Although there are good theoretical reasons to perform MCF decompression for this disease, the outcome appears to be so improved by medical therapy alone that this does not appear to be justified. Other studies have shown that HZO is characterized by multiple "skip" lesions throughout the course of the nerve, and so MCF decompression would be inadequate to address all areas of facial nerve compression.[60–65] Finally, ENoG prognostication appears unreliable in HZO. We have had a patient with grade VI facial movement and no response on ENoG recover function after 7 days of IV acyclovir. Again, this may occur because the nerve is more diffusely affected in HZO than in Bell's palsy. A couple of recent articles still advocate surgical decompression, whether through the mastoid alone[60] or through a combined mastoid-MCF approach.[66]

For patients presenting within 3 weeks of onset of paralysis, we treat with a 2-week course of valacyclovir at zoster dosages 1.5 gm twice daily and 1 mg/kg/day prednisone for 14 days. Patients who have a medical contraindication to oral steroids are treated with weekly transtympanic injections of solumedrol 0.3 to 0.4 cc of 40 mg/cc solution.

Facial Neuroma

Typically a schwannoma of the facial nerve, facial neuroma is a rare problem. Treatment decisions are hampered by an incomplete understanding of the disease's natural history. In their review, Lipkin and coworkers[67] were able to identify 248 cases in the world literature and discussed seven cases managed at Baylor over a 20-year period. In a survey of 1400 temporal bones at the University of Minnesota, metastatic and contiguous malignant tumor involvement of the facial nerve was 16 times more common than primary neurogenic tumors, of which there was only one case.[68]

In the Baylor review,[67] facial weakness was a presenting symptom in about two thirds of cases. Approximately one in seven of these experienced sudden facial paresis, with the remainder having a gradual or unspecified onset. Hearing loss was present in half of patients at presentation, with tinnitus, ear canal mass, pain, vestibular symptoms, and otorrhea each occurring in 10 to 15% of cases. Tumor location was also variable, with 19% in the CPA, 30% in the IAC, 42% in the labyrinthine segment and geniculate, 58% in the tympanic segment, 48% in the vertical segment, and 14% peripheral to the stylomastoid foramen. Many tumors involved multiple segments of the nerve. Some cases of tympanic segment neuroma may reflect a reparative response to chronic inflammation.[69]

When the facial neuroma is confined to the IAC or CPA and no facial nerve symptoms are present, misdiagnosis as acoustic neuroma is not uncommon. Fagan et al[70] reported that an MRI showing the bulk of the tumor mass projecting posteriorly into the CPA, rather than concentric within the IAC, is highly suggestive of a facial neuroma. Unfortunately, this relationship is not present in all cases of facial neuroma, especially when the tumors are small.[71,72] Brackmann[72,73] suggests using a combination of ENoG and auditory brainstem response (ABR) to help determine whether a tumor is an acoustic neuroma or a facial neuroma. However, tumors located primarily within the CPA may not affect facial function or ENoG even if quite large.[74]

Management options for facial neuromas include observation, microsurgery, and radiotherapy. Observation is recommended by many authors while the patient continues to have good facial nerve function (grade I or II) due to the risk of definitive treatment to nerve function and the certainty that a graft will yield a grade III or worse outcome.[71,75,76] Others[72] recommend decompression without resection to allow the facial neuroma "room to grow" without compression of the nerve or its blood supply. Using this technique in four patients with intraoperatively discovered facial schwannomas, three patients retained their preoperative facial nerve function and one showed improved function from grade V to grade II.[72] Pulec[77] first showed that some tumors can be dissected off facial nerve fascicles with preservation of facial nerve function at levels better than those expected after facial nerve grafting, and these findings have been confirmed by others, the most recent of which are cited here.[74,78,79] Unfortunately, there is no current preoperative method to determine which facial neuromas would be amenable to fascicle preservation. Some authors have recommended resection soon after diagnosis, regardless of facial nerve function, because they feel

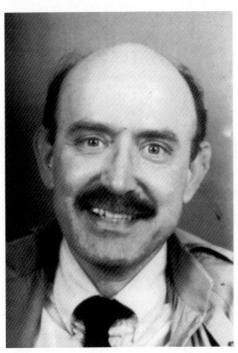

Figure 28–8 Normal facial function in patient known to have a neuroma of the right tympanic segment for 18 years. This was identified on exploratory tympanotomy for conductive hearing loss.

that continued compression of the nerve by the tumor will cause damage to the uninvolved ends of the nerve, yielding poorer results during nerve grafting.[80] Radiotherapy has also been used in the primary treatment of these rare tumors in at least two cases.[81] One patient had a decrease in her tumor size following radiotherapy but no improvement in her facial function, and the second showed improvement in facial function without a decrease in tumor size.[81]

Until there is some means to predict which tumors will grow quickly and which can be treated without increased facial nerve dysfunction, the controversy regarding treatment

of small facial schwannomas is unlikely to be resolved. Brainstem compression from a large CPA mass would mandate immediate resection, but within the temporal bone a facial neuroma could become quite sizable without threatening life. Decisions must be made based on the patient's age, degree of facial function, tumor locations, hearing status, and his or her own desires. **Fig. 28–8** shows normal facial function of a 48-year-old man who had a tympanic facial neuroma diagnosed at exploratory tympanotomy 18 years earlier. **Fig. 28–9** shows an enhanced MRI demonstrating no growth of the tumor. Cases such as this make it difficult to recommend surgery for a nonthreatening facial neuroma until at least grade III weakness is present.

The MRI scan in **Figs. 28–10** and **28–11** demonstrates a contrasting case of a large facial neuroma of the descending segment in a 50-year-old woman with a 6-month history of slowly progressive facial weakness. She had grade III weakness and was not willing to undergo resection and grafting. It is often unwise to biopsy facial neuromas as noted by O'Donoghue et al,[80] but it would have been imprudent to leave a mass of this size in the patient without biopsy. She underwent a transmastoid decompression and biopsy of this mass, which proved to be a facial schwannoma from the second genu through the stylomastoid foramen. She awoke with grade IV facial function, and after 6 months was back to her preoperative grade III function. She was subsequently followed with serial MRI scans.

We have seen five cases of facial neuromas coexisting with vestibular schwannomas in patients with neurofibromatosis type II. In three patients, MCF excision of the acoustic neuroma was planned and the facial neuroma was identified intraoperatively. In the other two patients, who had no residual hearing and larger tumors compressing the brainstem, translabyrinthine excision was performed. The vestibular schwannoma was excised in all cases and the facial neuromas were left in place. In the patients receiving MCF excisions, facial nerve function was preserved in all three. Hearing was initially preserved in two of these patients. In one of the two, hearing was noted to be lost at 6 months and the facial neuroma had enlarged on follow-up MRI. In the patients who had

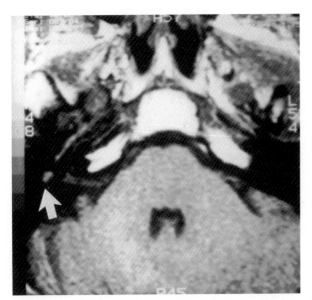
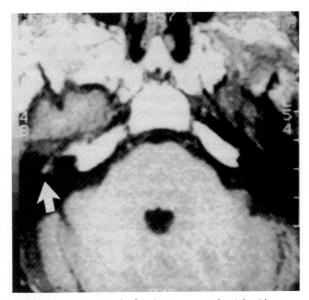

Figure 28–9 Axial MRI with gadolinium on the same patient as in **Fig. 28–8.** The white arrows point to the facial neuroma on the right side.

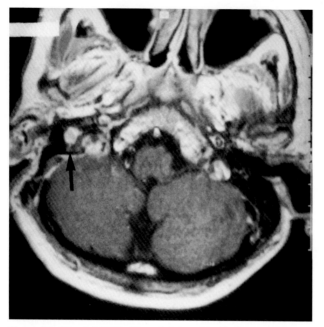

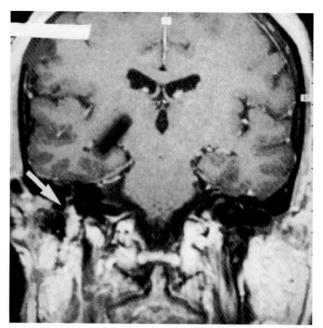

Figure 28–10 Axial MRI with gadolinium. The black arrow points to a large facial neuroma of the descending segment of the right facial nerve.

Figure 28–11 Coronal MRI with gadolinium. Same case as in **Fig. 28–10**. The white arrow points to a massively enlarged right facial nerve.

III Management

translabyrinthine excisions of their tumors, facial nerve function was lost postoperatively despite preservation of the facial neuroma. Obviously, decision making in such cases remains a complex problem.

◆ Facial Nerve Disorders in Children

Orobello[82] has divided pediatric facial nerve disorders into three categories: congenital paralysis, prenatal acquired paralysis, and postnatal acquired paralysis. Congenital facial paralysis consists of developmental errors occurring during embryogenesis. Prenatal acquired paralysis is due to factors extrinsic to the fetus such as intrauterine trauma and maternal exposure to teratogens. Postnatal acquired paralysis includes many of the same diseases that affect adults as well as congenital disorders that manifest later in life. The incidence of newborn facial paralysis is 0.2% of all live births.[83]

Congenital Disorders

Möbius Syndrome

This rare syndrome (**Fig. 28–12**) is characterized by congenital facial diplegia in association with unilateral or bilateral sixth nerve paralysis. Multiple modes of inheritance have been proposed, and there are three known loci for the syndrome.[84] Exposure of the fetus in utero to cocaine,[85] ergotamine,[86] or misoprostol (a synthetic analog of prostaglandin E₁)[85] has been associated with the development of Möbius syndrome as well. There may be associated deformities of the extremities, other cranial nerve deficits, musculoskeletal deficiencies, and mental retardation.[84] The exact site of the lesion is disputed; see Orobello[82] or Gantz and Wackym[88] for summaries. Some studies have noted nuclear abnormalities of cranial nerve VI

and VII; others have noted normal facial nuclei and failure of muscle development. One temporal bone study of an affected patient demonstrated normal facial nerve anatomy to the tympanic segment, where the nerve terminated in a manner consistent with an intrauterine "necrotic lesion" of the temporal bone.[87]

Treatment of these patients mandates ophthalmologic consultation. If motor end plates are absent, XII to VII hypoglossal-to-facial nerve anastomosis or cross-facial reinnervation procedures would not be expected to be of benefit. It motor end plates are present, the above-mentioned temporal bone findings would suggest exploration to identify the termination of the horizontal segment and subsequent grafting. Temporalis transposition may be helpful regardless of muscle status, as it implants a new neuromuscular system. More recent studies have shown that bilateral gracilis free muscle transfers with innervation from a branch of the trigeminal can restore smiling[90] and improve speech intelligibility,[91] even in the absence of biting in some patients.[92]

Hemifacial Microsomia

This term implies unilateral hypoplasia of the first and second branchial arches with resultant microtia, microstomia, and hypoplasia of the mandible. Neurogenic facial paresis is not uncommonly associated with this disorder, and has been reported in 22% of these patients.[93,94] Other congenital syndromes, particularly those with first and second arch abnormalities, may be associated with facial paresis or paralysis.

Congenital Unilateral Lower Lip Palsy

This disorder is characterized by autosomal dominant inheritance of congenital hypoplasia of the depressor anguli

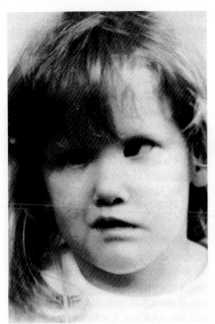 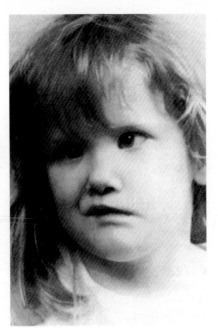

Figure 28–12 Möbius syndrome. **(A)** Left facial paralysis and right facial paresis photographed at rest. **(B)** With smiling and rightward gaze, the right facial paresis and sixth nerve paralysis are apparent.

oris muscle and is manifested by "asymmetric crying facies" and asymmetry with smiling. Other congenital otologic and cardiovascular anomalies may be associated with this syndrome.[95] Facial symmetry and function almost always recover spontaneously.

Prenatal Acquired Paralysis

This category includes intrauterine trauma typically associated with difficult delivery. Cephalopelvic disproportion and high-forceps delivery are typically the cause with the site of lesion in the extratemporal facial nerve, unless temporal bone fracture or intracranial injury have occurred. The trauma may be caused by forceps, but also can occur without forceps presumably from pressure from the maternal sacrum.[96] ENoG within the first 3 days of life should show no degeneration, with the subsequent degree of degeneration depending on the degree of injury. The absence of an evoked response within the first 3 days suggests either a congenital abnormality or earlier intrauterine trauma. EMG can help distinguish the latter two possibilities with the absence of fibrillations or of an evoked response suggesting congenital absence of the nerve-muscle unit. These are important distinctions because facial paralysis associated with delivery has an excellent prognosis with 90% incidence of spontaneous recovery.[96]

Teratogenic causes of facial paralysis include maternal thalidomide exposure and maternal rubella.

Postnatal Acquired Paralysis

This category includes all facial nerve disorders found in adults, but specific mention is made of two disorders that typically manifest in childhood, one hereditary and the other idiopathic.

Osteopetrosis

This disorder, also known as Albers-Schönberg disease, has dominant and recessive forms of varying severity. It is a bony dysplasia that can cause multiple cranial neuropathies secondary to entrapment at neural foramina. Progressive or fluctuating involvement of cranial nerve II, V, VII, and VIII are common. Complete intratemporal facial nerve decompression should be considered if there is radiologic evidence of facial nerve entrapment by osteopetrosis associated with facial dysfunction (see Chapter 22).

Melkersson-Rosenthal Syndrome

This is a triad consisting of recurrent facial or labial edema, fissured tongue (lingua plicata), and recurrent facial paralysis.[97] One or two components of the triad may be present without complete manifestation of the disease. The disease is inherited as an autosomal dominant trait with variable penetrance. The pathophysiology is unknown. Pathologically the disease is characterized by noncaseating granulomas.[98] Clinically, facial paralysis is seen in less than 40% of patients with the disorder. Typically episodes of paralysis become more severe and frequent over time, leading to synkinesis and incomplete recovery.[98] Graham and Kartush[4] reported MCF decompression of six patients for frequently recurring facial paralysis. None had recurrent attacks, including the one patient with Melkersson-Rosenthal syndrome who continued to have attacks of facial edema without weakness. In a second report, a patient had recurrent episodic facial paralysis following a transmastoid decompression. Following MCF decompression, this patient continued to have episodic transient paresis associated with facial edema on the operated side. However, these episodes lasted less than 24 hours, compared with preoperative episodes of facial paresis that would last 6 months at each occurrence.[12]

◆ Facial Paralysis Secondary to Inflammatory Middle Ear Disease

Chronic Otitis Media

The management of facial paralysis secondary to chronic otitis media is perhaps the only topic of this chapter that does not evoke controversy. Facial paralysis or paresis can be a complication of chronic ear disease with or without cholesteatoma. It presents an urgent indication for surgical intervention. In Takahashi and coworkers'[100] series of 1600 patients with facial paralysis, only 50 were secondary to inflammatory middle ear disease. A mastoidectomy appropriate for the type of chronic ear disease present, followed by decompression of the involved portion of the facial nerve, must be performed promptly. Cholesteatoma adherent to the nerve is preferably removed, but it can be exteriorized if this cannot be done safely. Few would argue against a canal-wall-down technique in the setting of cholesteatomatous involvement of the facial nerve.

Acute Otitis Media

Facial paresis secondary to acute otitis media is not uncommon, although its exact incidence is uncertain. Standard treatment consists of myringotomy, intravenous antibiotics, and a high-resolution temporal bone CT to rule out coalescent mastoiditis. If there is no coalescence or other indications for mastoidectomy, the role of surgery for the facial paralysis is poorly defined. Niparko[18] advocates mastoidectomy without nerve decompression if facial function does not return in 1 week. Hughes and Pensak[101] advocate mastoidectomy and decompression from the cochleariform process to the stylomastoid foramen "if nerve dysfunction persists or progresses." Glasscock et al[102] suggest simple mastoidectomy if facial paralysis lasts 2 weeks. Harris[103] advocates mastoidectomy and nerve decompression if significant degeneration is apparent on ENoG.[103] Selesnick and Patwardhan[40] argue against surgical intervention at all. None of these sources relies on any case series because myringotomy and medical therapy are usually effective. In these cases we perform an ENoG if total paralysis is present for 3 days and perform mastoidectomy and nerve decompression from the cochleariform process to the stylomastoid foramen if degeneration exceeds 90%. If degeneration does not reach 90% and no other surgical indication is present, intravenous antibiotics and steroids are continued.

Fig. 28–13 demonstrates the CT scan of a 40-year-old woman who presented with acute otitis media and facial paralysis. Myringotomy and intravenous antibiotics were begun, but an ENoG at 72 hours following paralysis showed no response. Canal-wall-up mastoidectomy demonstrated a granuloma compressed between the stapes and a widely dehiscent tympanic segment. Intraoperative electrical stimulation at 1 V prior to removing the granuloma demonstrated no response from the tympanic segment proximal to the granuloma and small EMG potentials without observable facial movement from the distal mastoid segment. After removing the granuloma and decompressing vertical and tympanic segments, EMG potentials and facial motion were obtained with proximal stimulation at 0.25 V. A neurolysis was not performed. The patient was continued on intravenous antibiotics and discharged on postoperative day 4 with some detectable movement of the midface. Follow-up at 10 days showed grade IV

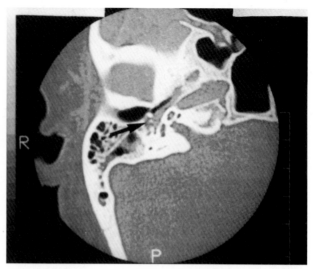

Figure 28–13 Acute otitis media and facial paralysis with complete degeneration on ENoG. Note absence of coalescence. Arrow points to soft tissue mass enveloping stapes. At surgery this was found to be a granuloma compressing the dehiscent tympanic segment. Intraoperative electrophysiologic findings are described in the text.

movement; 1-month follow-up revealed a grade II result. Although we cannot be certain that she would not have had this same result without decompression, the pressure of the granuloma on the dehiscent nerve was sufficient to indent it halfway into the fallopian canal. The intraoperative electrophysiologic changes after decompression were impressive. This case demonstrates that there is clearly a degree of facial nerve injury between neuropraxia and axonotmesis where a focal pathologic process causes a rapidly reversible interference with distal conduction. For more discussion of facial nerve pathology from inflammatory middle ear disease, see Chapter 17.

◆ Hemifacial Spasm and Essential Blepharospasm

Hemifacial spasm (HFS) is unilateral involuntary contraction of the facial musculature,[104] most commonly associated with a vessel contacting the root exit zone of the facial nerve.[105,106] Many studies suggest that HFS results not only from compression of root exit zone by the nerve but also from increased excitability of the facial nucleus.[107] HFS has also been found in several families, and so may be inherited with low penetrance.[108] Patients presenting with HFS rarely (<1%) have a variety of other compressive lesions, including CPA lipomas,[109,110] meningiomas,[111] epidermoids,[112] arachnoid cysts,[113] and aneurysms.[114] Infrequently, these mass lesions may be located on the contralateral side.[115] Thus use of MRI to detect potential mass lesions is necessary in the evaluation of HFS.

Treatment options for HFS include serial Botox injections to affected musculature and microvascular decompression. Elston[116] first used Botox injections for treatment of this disorder and reported relief of involuntary eye contractions in six patients for 15 weeks. In a prospective randomized crossover controlled study of 11 patients with HFS, Yoshimura et al[117] found objective improvement following 84% of injections with

Botox, and no objective improvement in patients who received placebo injections. The main complication was facial weakness, although bruising, diplopia, and ptosis were also reported. Over time, decreased responsiveness to Botox can develop. In a series of 45 patients treated for a mean of 15.8 years with serial Botox A injections, 49% eventually showed a decreased response.[118] The majority of these patients responded to dose adjustment; however, 27% did not respond to increased dosage and 18% had blocking antibodies to Botox A. These patients were treated successfully with Botox B.[118] Microvascular decompression (MVD), typically via suboccipital approach, is also effective in the treatment of HFS, with long-term cure rates in several large studies ranging from 80 to 90.5%.[119–123] Complications of MVD include CSF leak, hearing loss, cerebellar injury, and, rarely, brainstem infarct and death.[119,124]

Although not a disorder of the peripheral facial nerve, essential blepharospasm (EB) may be seen in patients referred for facial nerve disorders and should be distinguished from HFS. EB is a focal dystonia characterized by involuntary bilateral orbicularis oculi closure that can be severe enough to interfere with vision. EB may present along with other focal dystonias or as a component of Meige syndrome (EB plus dystonia of the lower face and jaw). Although the cause of EB is unknown, this condition is sometimes associated with traumatic injury in the area of the eye. The cornerstone of treatment is serial Botox injections[125] with oculoplastic procedures reserved for patients whose EB is resistant to this therapy.[126]

◆ Nerve Repair

Nerve grafting is frequently required when facial neuromas are excised. It is commonly necessary in cases of facial paralysis following penetrating trauma to the facial nerve as well, and is less commonly needed in acoustic neuroma surgery. When a tension-free end-to-end anastomosis can be performed, this is the preferred technique. Most cases require an interposition graft. Either the greater auricular nerve or the sural nerve may be used for this purpose. Whenever there is a proximal and distal facial nerve stump, grafting is much preferred over any other reanimation technique. This is as true in the CPA as it is in the parotid. Suture anastomosis in the CPA is technically challenging, but yields gratifying results with excellent facial tone and good oral sphincter function returning after 6 to 8 months, albeit with significant synkinesis. If no proximal stump is available, a split XII-to-VII anastomosis is our preferred approach. Three 10–0 nylon epineural sutures are placed at anastomoses in the CPA and four are used in the temporal bone or parotid (see Chapter 20). Alternatively, collagen splints can be used to establish the anastomosis in the CPA,[127,128] and tissue glue can be used to anastomose the nerve more distally within the temporal bone or in the periphery.[129]

References

1. Adour KK. Medical management of idiopathic (Bell's) palsy. Otolaryngol Clin North Am 1991;24:663–673
2. McCabe BF. Some evidence for the efficacy of decompression for Bell's palsy: immediate motion postoperatively. Laryngoscope 1977;87:246–249
3. Gantz BJ, Gmur A, Fisch U. Intraoperative evoked electromyography in Bell's palsy. Am J Otolaryngol 1982;3:273–278
4. Graham MD, Kartush JM. Total facial nerve decompression for recurrent facial paralysis: an update. Otolaryngol Head Neck Surg 1989;101:442–444
5. Niparko JK, Kileny PR, Kemink JL, et al. Neurophysiologic intraoperative monitoring: II. Facial nerve function. Am J Otol 1989;10:55–61
6. Jackson CG, Johnson GD, Hyams VJ, Poe DS. Pathologic findings in the labyrinthine segment of the facial nerve in a case of facial paralysis. Ann Otol Rhinol Laryngol 1990;99:327–329
7. Tien R, Dillon WP, Jackler RK. Contrast-enhanced MR imaging of the facial nerve in 11 patients with Bell's palsy. AJNR Am J Neuroradiol 1990;11:735–741
8. Schwaber MK, Larson TC III, Zealear DL, Creasy J. Gadolinium-enhanced magnetic resonance imaging in Bell's palsy. Laryngoscope 1990;100:1264–1269
9. Korzec K, Sobol SM, Kubal W, et al. Gadolinium-enhanced magnetic resonance imaging of the facial nerve in herpes zoster oticus and Bell's palsy: clinical implications. Am J Otol 1991;12:163–168
10. Marsh MA, Coker NJ. Surgical decompression of idiopathic facial palsy. Otolaryngol Clin North Am 1991;24:675–689
11. Girard N, Poncet M, Chays A, et al. MRI exploration of the intrapetrous facial nerve. J Neuroradiol 1993;20:226–238
12. Dutt SN, Mirza S, Irving RM, Donaldson I. Total decompression of facial nerve for Melkersson-Rosenthal syndrome. J Laryngol Otol 2000;114:870–873
13. Kinoshita T, Ishii K, Okitsu T, et al. Facial nerve palsy: evaluation by contrast-enhanced MR imaging. Clin Radiol 2001;56:926–932
14. Schuknecht HF, Gulya AJ. Anatomy of the Temporal Bone with Surgical Implications. Philadelphia: Lea & Febiger, 1986
15. Takahashi H, Sando I. Facial canal dehiscence: histologic study and computer reconstruction. Ann Otol Rhinol Laryngol 1992;101:925–930
16. Brackmann DE, Arriaga MA. Surgery for glomus and jugular foramen tumors. In: Brackmann DE, ed. Otologic Surgery, 2nd ed. Philadelphia: WB Saunders, 2001
17. House JW, Brackmann DE. Facial nerve grading system. Otolaryngol Head Neck Surg 1985;93:146–147
18. Limb CJ, Niparko JK. The acute facial palsies. In: Jackler RK, Brackmann DE, eds. Neurotology, 2nd ed. Philadelphia: Elsevier Mosby, 2005
19. Sclafani AP, Conley JJ. Occult parotid malignancy discovered 10 years after acute onset of complete facial paralysis. Otolaryngol Head Neck Surg 1994;110:235–238
20. May M. Facial nerve disorders. Update 1982. Am J Otol 1982;4:77–88
21. May M, Schaitkin BM. The Facial Nerve, 2nd ed. New York: Thieme, 2000
22. Djupesland G, Berdal P, Johannessen TA, et al. Viral infection as a cause of acute peripheral facial palsy. Arch Otolaryngol 1976;102:403–406
23. Vahlne A, Edstrom S, Arstila P, et al. Bell's palsy and herpes simplex virus. Arch Otolaryngol 1981;107:79–81
24. Mulkens PS, Bleeker JD, Schroder FP. Acute facial paralysis: a virological study. Clin Otolaryngol Allied Sci 1980;5:303–310
25. Burgess RC, Michaels L, Bale JF Jr, Smith RJ. Polymerase chain reaction amplification of herpes simplex viral DNA from the geniculate ganglion of a patient with Bell's palsy. Ann Otol Rhinol Laryngol 1994; 103:775–779
26. Murakami S, Mizobuchi M, Nakashiro Y, et al. Bell palsy and herpes simplex virus: identification of viral DNA in endoneurial fluid and muscle. Ann Intern Med 1996;124:27–30
27. Fisch U, Esslen E. Total intratemporal exposure of the facial nerve. Pathologic findings in Bell's palsy. Arch Otolaryngol 1972;95:335–341
28. Eicher SA, Coker NJ, Alford BR, et al. A comparative study of the fallopian canal at the meatal foramen and labyrinthine segment in young children and adults. Arch Otolaryngol Head Neck Surg 1990;116:1030–1035
29. Peitersen E. The natural history of Bell's Palsy. Am J Otol 1982;4:107–111
30. Adour KK, Byl FM, Hilsinger RL Jr, et al. The true nature of Bell's palsy: analysis of 1,000 consecutive patients. Laryngoscope 1978;88:787–801
31. Devriese PP, Schumacher T, Scheide A, et al. Incidence, prognosis and recovery of Bell's palsy. A survey of about 1000 patients (1974–1983). Clin Otolaryngol Allied Sci 1990;15:15–27
32. Fisch U. Prognostic value of electrical tests in acute facial paralysis. Am J Otol 1984;5:494–498
33. Sillman JS, Niparko JK, Lee SS, Kileny PR. Prognostic value of evoked and standard electromyography in acute facial paralysis. Otolaryngol Head Neck Surg 1992;107:377–381
34. Citron D III, Adour KK. Acoustic reflex and loudness discomfort in acute facial paralysis. Arch Otolaryngol 1978;104:303–306
35. May M, Blumenthal F, Klein SR. Acute Bell's palsy: prognostic value of evoked electromyography, maximal stimulation, and other electrical tests. Am J Otol 1983;5:1–7
36. Seddon H. Three types of nerve injury. Brain 1943;66:237
37. Sunderland S. Nerves and Nerve Injuries. Edinburgh: E & S Livingstone, 1968

38. Seiff SR, Chang J. Management of ophthalmic complications of facial nerve palsy. Otolaryngol Clin North Am 1992;25:669–690

39. Kinney SE, Seeley BM, Seeley MZ, Foster JA. Oculoplastic surgical techniques for protection of the eye in facial nerve paralysis. Am J Otol 2000;21:275–283

40. Selesnick SH, Patwardhan A. Acute facial paralysis: evaluation and early management. Am J Otolaryngol 1994;15:387–408

41. Salinas RA, Alvarez G, Ferreira J. Corticosteroids for Bell's palsy (idiopathic facial paralysis). Cochrane Database Syst Rev 2004;4 CD001942

42. Adour KK, Ruboyianes JM, Von Doersten PG, et al. Bell's palsy treatment with acyclovir and prednisone compared with prednisone alone: a double-blind, randomized, controlled trial. Ann Otol Rhinol Laryngol 1996;105:371–378

43. Allen D, Dunn L. Acyclovir or valaciclovir for Bell's palsy (idiopathic facial paralysis). Cochrane Database Syst Rev 2004;3:CD001869

44. May M, Klein SR, Taylor FH. Idiopathic (Bell's) facial palsy: natural history defies steroid or surgical treatment. Laryngoscope 1985;95:406–409

45. Fisch U. Surgery for Bell's palsy. Arch Otolaryngol 1981;107:1–11

46. Gantz BJ, Rubenstein JT, Gidley P, Woodworth GG. Surgical management of Bell's palsy. Laryngoscope 1999;109:1177–1188

47. Oghalai JS, Buxbaum JL, Pitts LH, Jackler RK. The effect of age on acoustic neuroma surgery outcomes. Otol Neurotol 2003;24:473–477

48. Peitersen E. The natural history of Bell's palsy. Am J Otology 9182:4:107-111

49. Murakami S. Yamano K. Hamajima Y. Evidence-based practical treatments for Bell's palsy. Presented at the annual meeting of the Academy of American Otolaryngology–Head and Neck Surgery, Toronto, Canada, September 19, 2006.

50. Adour KK. Otological complications of herpes zoster. Ann Neurol 1994;35(suppl):S62–S64

51. Devriese P. Herpes zoster causing facial paralysis. In: Fisch U, ed. Facial Nerve Surgery. Amstelveen, Netherlands: Kugler, 1976

52. Robillard RB, Hilsinger RL Jr, Adour KK. Ramsay Hunt facial paralysis: clinical analyses of 185 patients. Otolaryngol Head Neck Surg 1986;95:292–297

53. Kinishi M, Hosomi H, Amatsu M, et al. [Conservative treatment of Hunt syndrome] Nippon Jibiinkoka Gakkai Kaiho 1992;95:65–70

54. Dickins JR, Smith JT, Graham SS. Herpes zoster oticus: treatment with intravenous acyclovir. Laryngoscope 1988;98:776–779

55. Uri N, Greenberg E, Meyer W, Kitzes-Cohen R. Herpes zoster oticus: treatment with acyclovir. Ann Otol Rhinol Laryngol 1992;101:161–162

56. Murakami S, Hato N, Horiuchi J, et al. Treatment of Ramsay Hunt syndrome with acyclovir-prednisone: significance of early diagnosis and treatment. Ann Neurol 1997;41:353–357

57. Ko JY, Sheen TS, Hsu MM. Herpes zoster oticus treated with acyclovir and prednisolone: clinical manifestations and analysis of prognostic factors. Clin Otolaryngol Allied Sci 2000;25:139–142

58. Kinishi M, Amatsu M, Mohri M, et al. Acyclovir improves recovery rate of facial nerve palsy in Ramsay Hunt syndrome. Auris Nasus Larynx 2001;28:223–226

59. Uri N, Greenberg E, Kitzes-Cohen R, Doweck I. Acyclovir in the treatment of Ramsay Hunt syndrome. Otolaryngol Head Neck Surg 2003;129:379–381

60. Honda N, Yanagihara N, Hato N, et al. Swelling of the intratemporal facial nerve in Ramsay Hunt syndrome. Acta Otolaryngol 2002;122:348–352

61. Maybaum JL, Druss JG. Geniculate ganglionitis (Hunt's syndome). Clinical features and histopathology. Arch Otolaryngol 1934;19:574–581

62. Aleksic SN, Budzilovich GN, Lieberman AN. Herpes zoster oticus and facial paralysis (Ramsay Hunt syndrome). Clinico-pathologic study and review of literature. J Neurol Sci 1973;20:149–159

63. Guldberg-Moller J, Olsen S, Kettel K. Histopathology of the facial nerve in herpes zoster oticus. AMA Arch Otolaryngol 1959;69:266–275

64. Blackley B, Freidmann I, Wright I. Herpes zoster auris associated with facial nerve palsy and auditory nerve symptoms. A case report with histopathological findings. Acta Otolaryngol 1967;63:533–550

65. Etholm B, Schuknecht HF. Pathological findings and surgical implications in herpes zoster oticus. Adv Otorhinolaryngol 1983;31:184–190

66. Pulec JL. Total facial nerve decompression: technique to avoid complications. Ear Nose Throat J 1996;75:410–416

67. Lipkin AF, Coker NJ, Jenkins HA, Alford BR. Intracranial and intratemporal facial neuroma. Otolaryngol Head Neck Surg 1987;96:71–79

68. Jung TT, Jun BH, Shea D, Paparella MM. Primary and secondary tumors of the facial nerve. A temporal bone study. Arch Otolaryngol Head Neck Surg 1986;112:1269–1273

69. Babin RW, Harker LA, Kavanaugh KT. Traumatic intratympanic facial neuroma. A clinical report. Am J Otol 1984;5:365–367

70. Fagan PA, Misra SN, Doust B. Facial neuroma of the cerebellopontine angle and the internal auditory canal. Laryngoscope 1993;103:442–446

71. Kania RE, Herman P, Tran Ba Huy P. Vestibular-like facial nerve schwannoma. Auris Nasus Larynx 2004;31:212–219

72. Angeli SI, Brackmann DE. Is surgical excision of facial nerve schwannomas always indicated? Otolaryngol Head Neck Surg 1997;117:S144–S147

73. Brackmann DE, House JW, Selters W. Auditory brainstem responses in facial nerve neurinoma diagnosis. In: Graham MD, House WF, eds. Disorders of the Facial Nerve: Anatomy, Diagnosis, and Management. New York: Raven Press, 1982

74. Nadeau DP, Sataloff RT. Fascicle preservation surgery for facial nerve neuromas involving the posterior cranial fossa. Otol Neurotol 2003;24:317–325

75. Liu R, Fagan P. Facial nerve schwannoma: surgical excision versus conservative management. Ann Otol Rhinol Laryngol 2001;110:1025–1029

76. Kim CS, Chang SO, Oh SH, et al. Management of intratemporal facial nerve schwannoma. Otol Neurotol 2003;24:312–316

77. Pulec JL. Facial nerve neuroma. Laryngoscope 1972;82:1160–1176

78. Perez R, Chen JM, Nedzelski JM. Intratemporal facial nerve schwannoma: a management dilemma. Otol Neurotol 2005;26:121–126

79. Sherman JD, Dagnew E, Pensak ML, et al. Facial nerve neuromas: report of 10 cases and review of the literature. Neurosurgery 2002;50:450–456

80. O'Donoghue GM, Brackmann DE, House JW, Jackler RK. Neuromas of the facial nerve. Am J Otol 1989;10:49–54

81. Hasegawa T, Kobayashi T, Kida Y, et al. Two cases of facial neurinoma successfully treated with gamma knife radiosurgery. No Shinkei Geka 1999;27:171–175

82. Orobello P. Congenital and acquired facial nerve paralysis in children. Otolaryngol Clin North Am 1991;24:647–652

83. Falco NA, Eriksson E. Facial nerve palsy in the newborn: incidence and outcome. Plast Reconstr Surg 1990;85:1–4

84. Kniffen CL, McCusick VA. Moebius syndrome 1. In: McCusick V, ed. Online Mendelian Inheritance in Man. Baltimore: Johns Hopkins University, 2005:157900

85. Kankirawatana P, Tennison MB, D'Cruz O, Greenwood RS. Mobius syndrome in an infant exposed to cocaine in utero. Pediatr Neurol 1993;9:71–72

86. Graf WD, Shepard TH. Uterine contraction in the development of Mobius syndrome. J Child Neurol 1997;12:225–227

87. Gonzalez CH, Vargas FR, Perez AB, et al. Limb deficiency with or without Mobius sequence in seven Brazilian children associated with misoprostol use in the first trimester of pregnancy. Am J Med Genet 1993;47:59–64

88. Gantz BJ, Wackym PA. Facial nerve abnormalities. In: Smith JD, Bumsted RM, eds. Pediatric Facial Plastic and Reconstructive Surgery. New York: Raven Press, 1993

89. Saito H, Takeda T, Kishimoto S. Neonatal facial nerve defect. Acta Otolaryngol Suppl 1994;510:77–81

90. Terzis JK, Noah EM. Dynamic restoration in Mobius and Mobius-like patients. Plast Reconstr Surg 2003;111:40–55

91. Goldberg C, DeLorie R, Zuker RM, Manktelow RT. The effects of gracilis muscle transplantation on speech in children with Moebius syndrome. J Craniofac Surg 2003;14:687–690

92. Lifchez SD, Matloub HS, Gosain AK. Cortical adaptation to restoration of smiling after free muscle transfer innervated by the nerve to the masseter. Plast Reconstr Surg 2005;115:1472–1479

93. Carvalho GJ, Song CS, Vargervik K, Lalwani AK. Auditory and facial nerve dysfunction in patients with hemifacial microsomia. Arch Otolaryngol Head Neck Surg 1999;125:209–212

94. Bassila MK, Goldberg R. The association of facial palsy and/or sensorineural hearing loss in patients with hemifacial microsomia. Cleft Palate J 1989;26:287–291

95. McCusick VA. Depressor anguli oris muscle, hypoplasia of. In: McCusick VA, ed. Online Mendelian Inheritance in Man. Baltimore: Johns Hopkins University, 2005:125520

96. Smith JD, Crumley RL, Harker LA. Facial paralysis in the newborn. Otolaryngol Head Neck Surg 1981;89:1021–1024

97. Kelley J, McCusick VA. Melkersson-Rosenthal syndrome. In: McCusick VA, ed. Online Mendelian Inheritance in Man. Baltimore: Johns Hopkins University, 2005:155900.

98. Hornstein OP. Melkersson Rosenthal syndrome: a neuro-muco-cutaneous disease of complex origin. Curr Probl Dermatol 1973;5:117–156

99. Greene RM, Rogers RS 3rd. Melkersson-Rosenthal syndrome: a review of 36 patients. J Am Acad Dermatol 1989;21:1263–1270

100. Takahashi H, Nakamura H, Yui M, Mori H. Analysis of fifty cases of facial palsy due to otitis media. Arch Otorhinolaryngol 1985;241:163–168

101. Hughes GB, Pensak ML, eds. Clinical Otology, 2nd ed. New York: Thieme, 1997

102. Glasscock ME, Shambaugh GE Jr, Johnson GD, eds. Surgery of the Ear. Philadelphia: WB Saunders, 1990

103. Harris JP, Kim DP, Darrow DH. Complications of chronic otitis media. In: Nadol JB Jr, McKenna, MJ, eds. Surgery of the Ear and Temporal Bone, 2nd ed. Philadelphia: Lippincott Williams & Wilkins, 2004

104. Costa J, Espirito-Santo C, Borges A, et al. Botulinum toxin type A therapy for hemifacial spasm. Cochrane Database Syst Rev 2005;1:CD004899

105. Bernardi B, Zimmerman RA, Savino PJ, Adler C. Magnetic resonance tomographic angiography in the investigation of hemifacial spasm. Neuroradiology 1993;35:606–611

106. Hosoya T, Watanabe N, Yamaguchi K, et al. Three-dimensional-MRI of neurovascular compression in patients with hemifacial spasm. Neuroradiology 1995;37:350–352

107. Moller AR. Vascular compression of cranial nerves: II: pathophysiology. Neurol Res 1999;21:439–443

108. Miwa H, Mizuno Y, Kondo T. Familial hemifacial spasm: report of cases and review of literature. J Neurol Sci 2002;193:97–102

109. Sade B, Mohr G, Dufour JJ. Cerebellopontine angle lipoma presenting with hemifacial spasm: case report and review of the literature. J Otolaryngol 2005;34:270–273

110. Sprik C, Wirtschafter JD. Hemifacial spasm due to intracranial tumor. An international survey of botulinum toxin investigators. Ophthalmology 1988;95:1042–1045

111. Gomez-Perals LF, Ortega-Martinez M, Fernandez-Portales I, Cabezudo-Artero JM. [Hemifacial spasm as clinical presentation of intracranial meningiomas. Report of three cases and review of the literature.] Neurocirugia (Astur) 2005;16:21–25

112. Kobata H, Kondo A, Iwasaki K. Cerebellopontine angle epidermoids presenting with cranial nerve hyperactive dysfunction: pathogenesis and long-term surgical results in 30 patients. Neurosurgery 2002;50:276–285

113. Takano S, Maruno T, Shirai S, Nose T. Facial spasm and paroxysmal tinnitus associated with an arachnoid cyst of the cerebellopontine angle–case report. Neurol Med Chir (Tokyo) 1998;38:100–103

114. Nagata S, Matsushima T, Fujii K, et al. Hemifacial spasm due to tumor, aneurysm, or arteriovenous malformation. Surg Neurol 1992;38:204–209

115. Matsuura N, Kondo A. Trigeminal neuralgia and hemifacial spasm as false localizing signs in patients with a contralateral mass of the posterior cranial fossa. Report of three cases. J Neurosurg 1996;84:1067–1071

116. Elston JS. Botulinum toxin treatment of hemifacial spasm. J Neurol Neurosurg Psychiatry 1986;49:827–829

117. Yoshimura DM, Aminoff MJ, Tami TA, Scott AB. Treatment of hemifacial spasm with botulinum toxin. Muscle Nerve 1992;15:1045–1049

118. Mejia NI, Vuong KD, Jankovic J. Long-term botulinum toxin efficacy, safety, and immunogenicity. Mov Disord 2005;20:592–597

119. Barker FG II, Jannetta PJ, Bissonette DJ, et al. Microvascular decompression for hemifacial spasm. J Neurosurg 1995;82:201–210

120. Illingworth RD, Porter DG, Jakubowski J. Hemifacial spasm: a prospective long-term follow-up of 83 cases treated by microvascular decompression at two neurosurgical centres in the United Kingdom. J Neurol Neurosurg Psychiatry 1996;60:72–77

121. Chung SS, Chang JH, Choi JY, et al. Microvascular decompression for hemifacial spasm: a long-term follow-up of 1,169 consecutive cases. Stereotact Funct Neurosurg 2001;77:190–193

122. Yuan Y, Wang Y, Zhang SX, et al. Microvascular decompression in patients with hemifacial spasm: report of 1200 cases. Chin Med J (Engl) 2005;118:833–836

123. Moffat DA, Durvasula VS, Stevens King A, et al. Outcome following retrosigmoid microvascular decompression of the facial nerve for hemifacial spasm. J Laryngol Otol 2005;119:779–783

124. McLaughlin MR, Jannetta PJ, Clyde BL, et al. Microvascular decompression of cranial nerves: lessons learned after 4400 operations. J Neurosurg 1999;90:1–8

125. Hallett M. Blepharospasm: recent advances. Neurology 2002;59:1306–1312

126. Patel BC. Surgical management of essential blepharospasm. Otolaryngol Clin North Am 2005;38:1075–1098

127. Fisch U, Dobie RA, Gmur A, Felix H. Intracranial facial nerve anastomosis. Am J Otol 1987;8:23–29

128. Arriaga MA, Brackmann DE. Facial nerve repair techniques in cerebellopontine angle tumor surgery. Am J Otol 1992;13:356–359

129. Murray JA, Willins M, Mountain RE. A comparison of glue and a tube as an anastomotic agent to repair the divided buccal branch of the rat facial nerve. Clin Otolaryngol Allied Sci 1994;19:190–192

28 Facial Nerve Disorders

389

29

Immunologic Disorders of the Inner Ear

C. Arturo Solares, Gordon B. Hughes, and Vincent K. Tuohy

The concept that the inner ear is able to initiate an immune response that may lead to otologic dysfunction is relatively recent. There is also reasonable evidence that supports the role of organ-specific autoimmunity in a subset of patients with rapidly progressive sensorineural hearing loss (SNHL). Autoimmune sensorineural hearing loss (ASNHL) has been defined largely on clinical parameters. It typically produces a bilateral, sometimes fluctuating, hearing loss that progresses rapidly over weeks or months.[1] The diagnosis is made by excluding ototoxicity, systemic disease, and other factors that may induce rapidly progressive hearing loss, and by showing a therapeutic response to corticosteroid treatment.

Although autoantibodies and autoreactive T cells have been implicated in the etiopathogenesis of ASNHL, several central issues remain unresolved, including the relative prominence of B-cell or T-cell autoimmunity in the initiation and progression of ASNHL, and the identity of the putative inner ear self-antigen(s) that target ASNHL. The importance of these concepts is that if detected early enough, hearing loss, once thought to be progressive and irreversible, can be restored through appropriate and judicious use of immunosuppressive drugs. This chapter discusses seminal evidence that has led to our current understanding of inner ear immune responses and their relationship to clinical disease. In addition, a summary of the clinical aspects and therapeutic options for ASNHL is presented.

◆ Immunology of the Inner Ear

The blood–brain and blood–labyrinthine barriers are important determinants of the immune responses in the brain and the inner ear, respectively.[2] Due to the blood–brain barrier, the brain is largely isolated from the systemic immune responses under normal conditions. This relative isolation led to the suggestion that the brain is an immunoprivileged site.[3] However, it is now known that isolation of the brain from systemic immune system is far from complete because immune responses can be elicited in the brain under the right circumstances.[4] Due to similarities between the blood–brain and blood–labyrinthine barriers, there was a traditional belief that the inner ear also was immunoprivileged, but this concept has been widely disproved by many authors.[5–7]

Under normal conditions the inner ear contains immunoglobulins and immunocompetent cells.[5,8–10] Immunoglobulins can cross the blood–labyrinthine barrier and are present in inner ear fluids at higher concentrations relative to levels in the central nervous system (CNS).[5,8] Discolo et al,[10] using CD45 immunolabeling, identified a small population of resident monocytes in mouse cochleas in the inferior spiral ligament. Other authors have identified the endolymphatic sac as a source of immunocompetent cells in the inner ear.[11] Thus, the inner ear not only derives its protection through diffusion of immunoglobulin from the systemic circulation and the CNS, but also contains a full array of immunocompetent cells.

Harris[6] performed intracochlear keyhole limpet hemocyanin (KLH) immunization in guinea pigs previously primed to bovine serum albumen (BSA). He subsequently observed increased anti-KLH antibody levels in the inner ear perilymph without a corresponding increase in anti-BSA levels and without an increase in anti-KLH levels in the cerebrospinal fluid (CSF). Harris concluded that the inner ear was fully capable of initiating a local immune response to an antigen by a resident population of immunocompetent T cells.[6] Several subsequent studies involving obliteration of the endolymphatic sac indicated that this inner ear structure known to be involved in endolymph drainage and absorption was also critical for maintaining local memory responses to antigens and initiating the efferent limb of the inner ear immune response.[11–15] Memory responses to inner ear KLH inoculation produced a hearing deficit and cochlear histopathology only when guinea pigs were immunized to KLH.[16] This series of studies clearly showed that the inner ear was immunocompetent.

The molecular basis of the immune response has been extensively studied. Several mediators such as interleukins, interferons, and tumor necrosis factors have been shown to be present in the inner ear. Studies by Gloddek and Harris have helped elucidate the roles of interleukin-2 (IL-2) and transforming growth factor-β (TGF-β) in the cascade of events that takes place. IL-2 cannot be detected in the perilymph under unstimulated conditions, but is a component of the inner-ear immune response. Following inner-ear challenge of the scala tympani with KLH, IL-2 was measurable at 6 hours, peaked at 18 hours, and declined over 5 days. These same investigators also reported an early egress of polymorphonuclear leukocytes and the appearance of fewer monocytes and lymphocytes, and hypothesized that it could be secondary to the actions of IL-2.[15] Yeo and Ryan[17] studied the role of TGF-β in the inner ear. Leukocytes within the scala tympani and scala vestibuli were labeled with mRNA probes to TGF-β1. Following scala tympani challenge with KLH, this label was detected at 1 day, peaked at 3 days, and decreased by 1 week.[17] TGF-β is a chemoattractant for monocytes, T cells, and neutrophils. It also increases the levels of IL-1, IL-6, and platelet-derived growth factor. TGF-β also interferes with the IL-2 response, deactivates macrophages, and inhibits production of interferon-γ (IFN-γ) and tumor necrosis factor-α (TNF-α). More recently, Hirose and Keasler[18] reported that after acoustic injury, there was a substantial increase in inner ear expression of monocyte chemoattractant protein (MCP-1), TNF-α, and IL-1, suggesting that inflammation may have a role in repair after acoustic trauma. Thus, it has become increasingly clear that immune responses may occur in the inner ear and that these responses involve a complex cascade of events potentially activated by any of several mechanisms.

◆ The Role of Autoimmunity in Hearing Loss

In addition to the damage incurred during responses to invading pathogens, the inner ear also may incur damage from autoimmune-mediated inflammation. There is evidence that the inner ear can be affected in a variety of non–organ-specific autoimmune diseases. Hearing loss is a rare complication of polyarteritis nodosa.[19] Wegener's granulomatosis has been associated with both middle and inner ear pathology.[20] Systemic lupus erythematosus can produce necrotizing vasculitis and progressive SNHL or disequilibrium.[1] Some literature reports have implicated rheumatoid arthritis in otologic pathology.[21] Cogan's syndrome, characterized by interstitial keratitis and vestibuloauditory dysfunction,[22] may result from hypersensitivity response to one or more inflammatory agents associated with vasculitis.[23] However, lymphocyte proliferation on exposure to corneal antigen[24,25] and inner ear antigen,[26] suggests organ-specific autoimmunity.

ASNHL is a clinical entity characterized by bilateral, rapidly progressive hearing loss occurring over weeks to months in the absence of systemic immunologic disease. Although its name implies an autoimmune etiopathogenesis, data implicating self-recognition events in the development and progression of ASNHL until recently have been limited to its therapeutic response to immunosuppressive treatment, to detection of serum antibody to heat shock protein 70 kD (HSP70), and to recall responses of peripheral blood mononuclear cells (PBMCs) to crude inner ear homogenate. Its contemporary clinical definition is derived from a seminal study by McCabe,[1] whosesuspicions began when immunosuppressive therapy with corticosteroids and cyclophosphamide not only cleared up a patient's nonhealing mastoid infection but coincidentally improved her rapidly progressive SNHL. Although some of McCabe's earliest reported patients may have had Wegener's granulomatosis, others clearly had

isolated progressive SNHL and benefited from treatment with corticosteroids or cyclophosphamide. He proposed that inner ear–specific autoreactive T cells may mediate ASNHL, and several recent studies have provided support for T-cell–mediated ASNHL.[27,28] However, others have proposed that ASNHL may be the result of autoantibody-mediated injury to the inner ear.[29,30] As described below, our laboratory has recently developed a T-cell–mediated inner ear–specific autoimmune mouse model that mimics the clinical features of ASNHL.[31] We hope that this murine model will facilitate identifying the stages leading to ASNHL and provide a venue for discovering new diagnostic markers and novel treatments for this disorder.

◆ Autoimmune Sensorineural Hearing Loss

Autoreactive T Cells in Autoimmune Sensorineural Hearing Loss

The first compelling evidence that autoreactive T cells may be implicated in ASNHL was provided by McCabe and McCormick who observed leukocyte migration inhibition (LMI) in response to homogenized inner ear membranes in activated PBMC from all 54 of their ASNHL study subjects.[32] The study did not incorporate normal control subjects or a non–inner-ear control antigen in the experimental design. Hughes and colleagues[27] further implicated T-cell autoreactivity in ASNHL by showing that PBMC from ASNHL patients elicited recall proliferative responses to human inner ear homogenate. PBMC from 13/58 (22%) ASNHL subjects with unilateral or bilateral asymmetric SNHL responded to human inner ear antigens. In comparison, only 1/15 (7%) of normal control subjects showed PBMC proliferation to inner ear homogenate. Although the positive predictive value of these proliferation studies was suggested to be 79%, proliferation may best be viewed as a functional IL-2 assay and as such provides limited ability to detect much of the autoreactive T-cell repertoire notoriously known to have cryptic features with low antigen affinity and low precursor frequencies.[33]

Lorenz et al[28] used the enzyme-linked immunosorbent spot (ELISPOT) assay to measure secretion of specific cytokines by individual cells, thereby providing 10- to 200-fold increased sensitivity over conventional proliferation and enzyme-linked immunosorbent assay (ELISA) for detecting T-cell immunoreactivity.[34,35] They found that the PBMC frequencies of IFN-γ–producing T cells specifically responsive to human inner ear homogenate were elevated significantly in 25% (3/12) of ASNHL patients but in none (0/12) of the age- and sex-matched normal control study subjects.[28] These findings indicated that proinflammatory effector T cells specific for inner ear antigens may play a pivotal role in the development and progression of ASNHL.

Although ELISPOT analysis showed autoreactivity in only 25% of ASNHL patients, the true incidence of self-recognition is likely much higher for several reasons: (1) Assessment of self-recognition at a single time point reduces the likelihood of detection, as autoreactivity is better detected when the analysis is performed serially.[36] (2) The use of IFN-γ or any single cytokine for evaluating precursor frequencies of antigen-specific T cells prevents identification of autoreactive T cells that produce other cytokines.[37] (3) Antigen-specific autoreactive T cells may not produce IFN-γ because they may instead make regulatory cytokines such as IL-10 and TGF-β. (4) In humans and mice, the autoreactive repertoire may be compartmentalized in such a way that T cells making IFN-γ are underrepresented in the PBMC.[38] (5) Despite the high sensitivity of the ELISPOT assay, there is still enough "noise" in the assay to prevent detection of low-affinity autoreactive T-cell clones. Thus, ELISPOT detection of self-recognition in 25% of ASNHL patients may be viewed as a minimum rather than actual incidence of inner ear autoreactivity.

Although the ELISPOT provides enhanced sensitivity over LMI and proliferation for detecting T-cell autoreactivity, inner ear homogenate, although useful in determining autoreactivity, provides little help in identifying candidate self-antigens. An epitope-mapping peptide series derived from inner ear–specific proteins may represent a more ideal experimental design. Such overlapping peptides have been most useful in identifying T-cell epitopes that target human autoimmune diseases such as multiple sclerosis[36,39] and insulin-dependent diabetes mellitus.[40,41] Proteins such as cochlin[42] represent promising candidates for generating epitope-mapping peptides because their expression appears to be confined exclusively to the inner ear. Ideally, the ELISPOT assay should detect changes over time in the precursor frequencies of T cells producing a variety of proinflammatory (IFN-γ, IL-2, TNF-α, TNF-β) and antiinflammatory (IL-4, IL-5, IL-10) cytokines in response to overlapping peptides derived from candidate inner ear-specific proteins. Such studies are currently ongoing in our laboratory and may help clarify the development of self-recognition and identify candidate peptides for developing antigen-specific immunotherapies for ASNHL.[43]

Autoantibodies in Autoimmune Sensorineural Hearing Loss

In addition to evidence supporting the involvement of autoreactive T cells in ASNHL, several studies have implicated autoantibodies as potential mediators of inner ear injury. Arnold and colleagues[44] showed that sera from 15/21 (71%) patients with bilateral SNHL of unknown etiology contained antibodies capable of immunostaining human inner ear tissues. Although this study did not include normal control subjects, a later report from the same group confirmed the initial findings by showing immunostaining of human inner ear tissues with serum from 64/119 (54%) subjects with hearing loss compared with 1/25 (4%) normal control subjects.[45] The single normal control subject who showed positive serum immunostaining was subsequently diagnosed with rheumatoid arthritis (RA). These studies, however, did not show a strong correlation between the presence of inner ear–specific serum antibodies and a therapeutic response to corticosteroid treatment, a clinical hallmark of ASNHL.

In more recent studies, Western blot analysis has been used to study reactivity from patients with ASNLH against bovine inner ear material, and it appears that a 68-kD protein is the likely putative antigen.[46] Moscicki and colleagues[47] used Western blot analysis to show that sera from 89% of patients with actively progressing bilateral hearing loss reacted with a 68-kD protein constituent of inner ear extract, whereas patients with inactive disease showed no immunoreactivity. Moreover, patients who were antibody-positive showed a significantly increased incidence of responsiveness to corticosteroid treatment compared with antibody-negative patients. Similar results were subsequently obtained by Gottschlich and colleagues,[48] whose compiled data showed that 90/279 (32%) patients with bilateral rapidly progressive SNHL had elevated anti–68-kD titers, whereas only 5% of control subjects were seropositive. Thus, these studies correlated immunoreactivity directed against a 68-kD antigen with actively progressing bilateral hearing loss.

Considerable evidence indicates that the 68-kD antigen targeted by autoantibody in ASNHL is HSP70, a heat shock protein whose synthesis is greatly enhanced in a variety of tissues following exposure to various stressors, including autoimmunity.[49–53] Monoclonal antibody specific for HSP70 binds the 68-kD antigen, and anti–68-kD sera from ASNHL subjects predominantly target the C-terminal p427–461 region of HSP70.[54,55] Moreover, evidence indicates that a positive Western blot for HSP70 may correlate with corticosteroid responsiveness in ASNHL subjects in a manner similar to seropositive 68-kD immunoreactivity.[47,48,52,56,57] Indeed, it has been postulated that autoantibodies against HSP70 may be implicated directly in the pathogenesis of ASNHL[52,53]; however, immunization of BALB/c or CBA/J mice with bovine HSP70 induced high titer antibody responses to HSP70 without any subsequent changes in auditory brainstem responses (ABRs).[58] Thus, there is no direct proof that HSP70 antibodies are immunopathogenic or cochleopathic in ASNHL. Although the pathogenicity of anti-HSP70 antibodies remains in question, Western blot detection of anti-HSP70 antibodies still provides a useful laboratory marker for supporting the diagnosis of ASNHL with a specificity of 90% and a positive predictive value of 91%.[56] However, with a sensitivity of only 42%, the need to develop a more sensitive assay is obvious.

Boulassel and colleagues[59] showed that ASNHL patients often have elevated immunoglobulin G (IgG) antibody titers to cochlin, an inner ear–specific protein.[59] Cochlin (formerly known as coch-5B2) is a product of the *COCH* gene mapped in humans to chromosome 14q12-q13, and its mutations are associated with an autosomal dominant, nonsyndromic, progressive SNHL with vestibular pathology (DFNA9).[42,60,61] Cochlin is an integral part of the inner ear extracellular matrix and is expressed in the regions of the fibrocytes of the spiral limbus and of the spiral ligament—inner ear regions showing histologic abnormalities in humans with *COCH* mutations.[42,62] Cochlin appears to be the most abundant protein expressed in inner ear tissues,[63] and as such is likely to have a high level of constitutive presentation by local professional antigen-presenting cells, thereby making it a probable target in autoimmune disease of the inner ear and a prime candidate for developing diagnostic markers.

Animal Models for Autoimmune Sensorineural Hearing Loss

The inability to examine temporal bone histopathology in humans during the active phase of disease has impaired identification of inner ear–specific antigens that target ASNHL, elucidation of the sequence of inflammatory and immune events leading to the development of ASNHL, and development of novel therapeutic strategies for preventing progressive hearing loss. Several animal models have been described for the study of ASNHL. In this section we review some of the most relevant model systems used in ASNHL studies not included in other sections of this chapter.

Despite its lack of inner ear–specific expression and its ubiquitous presence in a variety of organs, collagen type II (CII) has been proposed as a potential target antigen in ASNHL. Yoo and colleagues[64] observed significantly decreased amplitudes and delayed latencies in ABR recordings following immunization of female Lewis rats with either bovine or ovine CII. Because hearing loss did not occur in rats immunized with type I collagen, the authors proposed that CII autoreactivity played a key role in the pathogenesis of ASNHL. In subsequent studies, this same group showed that CII-immunized rats, guinea pigs, and chinchillas underwent otospongiotic changes in the osseous labyrinth of the inner ear as well as degeneration of spiral ganglion cells and atrophy of the cochlear nerve, organ of Corti, and stria vascularis. In addition, endolymphatic hydrops, hearing loss, and vestibular dysfunction were observed in all CII-immunized animals:[64,65] Although the observed CII-induced inner ear abnormalities were quite striking, the results have not been reproduced. Using the same CII immunization protocol to prime Wistar-Furth rats, Harris and colleagues[30] were unable to induce hearing loss within 11 months after immunization; CII-associated inner ear pathology was not observed despite high titers of serum and perilymph anti-CII antibodies.

MRL/MpJ-*lpr/lpr* (MRL/*lpr*) and C3H/*lpr* mice have been used recently in ASNHL studies because they develop spontaneous hearing loss secondary to a systemic lymphoproliferative disorder. The *lpr* gene is an autosomal-recessive Fas deletion mutant responsible for failure of Fas-mediated apoptosis, which produces a nonspecific lymphoproliferative disorder associated with spontaneous development of various autoimmune disorders, including systemic lupus erythematosus, glomerulonephritis, polyarteritis, RA, and sialoadenitis.[66-68] Several authors have reported hearing disorders associated with expression of the *lpr* gene.[69-72] Affected animals have circulating antibodies directed against blood vessels in the stria vascularis,[73] breakdown of endothelial tight junctions that make up the stria blood–labyrinth barrier,[69] and corticosteroid-responsive auditory dysfunction.[74]

Recent studies have indicated that the NZB/kl substrain of the autoimmune-prone NZB mouse strain spontaneously develops high-frequency hearing loss with age as determined by elevated ABR thresholds. Hearing loss appears to be due to thickening of the capillary basement membrane of the stria vascularis as a result of IgM and IgG immune complex deposition.[75,76] The similarly derived NZB/san substrain failed to develop spontaneous hearing loss.[76] The hearing loss observed in NZB/kl mice is the result of a systemic disorder that involves accompanying renal pathology.[77] Thus, despite its usefulness as an immune inflammatory model for inner ear pathology, there is no evidence of organ-specific autoimmunity in the hearing loss that occurs in NZB/kl mice.

Autoimmune SNHL is likely mediated by autoreactivity targeted against antigens that are inner ear–specific rather than systemically expressed. Harris[78] induced cochlear lesions in guinea pigs following immunization with either autologous or bovine inner ear homogenates. Although hearing loss occurred in 12/38 (32%) total ears, there was no correlation between degree of hearing loss, histologic changes, and serum antibody titers to inner ear homogenate. Soliman[79,80] also immunized guinea pigs with bovine inner ear homogenate and showed that 36% of the animals developed endolymphatic hydrops, whereas 20% showed ABR documented hearing loss. In addition, immunoglobulin deposition was evident in inner ear structures including the basilar membrane, endolymphatic sac, and midmodiolar blood vessels. Similarly, Yamanobe and Harris[81] induced labyrinthitis in guinea pigs after immunization with bovine inner ear homogenate. Animals developed hearing loss by day 7 and were shown to have cellular infiltration of the inner ear that regressed by 4 weeks postimmunization.

Guinea pigs and mice immunized with chicken and guinea pig inner ear tissues developed hearing loss associated with production of serum antibodies to hair cell stereocilia. However, hearing loss was transient.[82] A pathogenic role for T-cell–dependent immunoglobulins was clearly apparent in studies showing hearing loss in guinea pigs injected with mouse monoclonal antibody (MAb) KHRI-3, an IgG1 generated against guinea pig cochlear hair cells.[83-85] In addition, hearing loss occurred in mice carrying the KHRI-3 hybridoma. This antibody prominently stains cochlear cells bordering the tunnel of Corti and supporting cells of the second and third row of outer hair cells. Recent studies by Nair and colleagues[86] have identified choline transporter-like protein 2 (CTL2), an inner ear glycoprotein with 68- and 72-kD isoforms, as the target of KHRI-3. These investigators reported that sera from patients with autoimmune hearing loss bind to guinea pig inner ear with the same pattern as CTL2 antibodies and concluded that CTL2 is a possible target of autoimmune hearing loss in humans. However, inner ear–specificity of KHRI-3 remains rather questionable because the antibody reacts with several non–inner ear tissues. Furthermore, Western blot analysis showed that KHRI-3 immunostains several bands in cochlear extracts including a 64-kD, 78-kD, and a broad 70- to 75-kD band as well as an additional 68- to 70-kD band in tongue and brain extracts.

Gloddek and colleagues[87,88] induced labyrinthitis in naive Lewis rats following adoptive transfer of activated T-cell lines specific for bovine inner ear homogenate. These experiments support a role for T cells in the initiation and pathogenesis of ASNHL; however, use of inner ear homogenates precludes characterization of the specific self-antigens involved in disease initiation and progression. We recently reported that the inner ear–specific proteins cochlin and β-tectorin were capable of targeting experimental autoimmune hearing loss (EAHL) in mice.[31,89] Five weeks after immunization of SWXJ mice with either Coch 131–150 or β-tectorin 71–90, ABR showed significant hearing loss at all frequencies tested between 4 and 60 kHz. Flow cytometry analysis showed that each peptide selectively activated CD4$^+$ T cells shown by ELISA to be proinflammatory Th1-like T cells expressing an IFN-γ^{high}/IL-4^{low} phenotype. T-cell mediation of EAHL was determined by showing significantly increased ABR thresholds 6 weeks after adoptive transfer of peptide-activated T cells into naive SWXJ recipient mice.[31] Our study provides a contemporary mouse model for clarifying our understanding of ASNHL and should eventually facilitate the development of novel effective treatments for this clinical entity. Moreover, our data provide experimental confirmation that ASNHL may be a T-cell–mediated organ-specific autoimmune disorder of the inner ear.

◆ Clinical Evaluation and Management of Autoimmune Sensorineural Hearing Loss

Most current clinical management guidelines were developed within a decade of McCabe's initial report[1] and have not changed much since then. The mainstay of treatment is high-dose oral prednisone for at least 1 month followed by a slow tapering dose, and maintenance prednisone as needed to control symptoms. Intratympanic steroids may help when systemic steroids are contraindicated or poorly tolerated. A national multicenter trial of methotrexate found no significant difference between experimental and control cohorts.[90] Anecdotal experience suggests that occasional individuals may benefit from methotrexate. Cyclophosphamide, lymphocytoplamapheresis, and other immunosuppressive therapies also may have some benefit but have not been studied carefully. Future prospective clinical trials eventually should provide better treatment guidelines.

Immunologic Disorders of the Inner Ear

Classification of immunologic disorders of the inner ear, some known, others theoretical, remains essentially unchanged since its publication in 1993 (**Table 29–1**).[91] Immunologic inner ear disorders can be primary (originating within the inner ear) or secondary (originating outside the inner ear). Primary inner ear disease can result from autoimmunity or host defense against infections, tumors, and toxins. In theory, primary inner ear disease can be localized to the inner ear or can create immune complexes that cross-react with antigens of distant organs.

Secondary inner ear disease can result from direct or indirect effects of systemic immune disease (**Table 29–2**). Direct pathways may allow autoantibodies from distant organs to cross-react with inner ear antigens. Indirect pathways might trap circulating immune complexes in the inner ear. The stria vascularis might be an innocent bystander attacked by virtue of its rich blood supply, similar to immune-complex glomerulonephritis. Perhaps systemic immune vasculitis impairs circulation to the labyrinthine artery.

Diagnosis of Autoimmune Sensorineural Hearing Loss

Clinical features of ASNHL help differentiate it from other disorders. The recommended clinical and laboratory workup for patients with suspected ASNHL is summarized in **Table 29–3**. The hallmark is rapidly progressive (within 3 months) bilateral

Table 29–1   Immunologic Disorders of the Inner Ear*

Primary (originating within the inner ear)
Localized (without systemic features)
Autoimmunity (ASNHL)
Host defense against tumor, infection, toxins
Generalized (with systemic features)
Immune complexes cross-react with antigens of other organs
Secondary (originating outside the inner ear)
Direct effect of systemic immune disease
Immune complexes cross-react with inner ear antigens
Syndromes (Cogan's, Behçet's)
Indirect effect of systemic immune disease
Circulating immune complexes trapped in stria vascularis
CSF immune complexes trapped in perilymph
Impaired circulation from vasculitis
Biochemical alteration

Source: From Hughes GB, Barna BP, Calabrese LH, Koo A. Immunologic disorders of the inner ear. In: Bailey BJ, ed. Head and Neck Surgery–Otolaryngology. Philadelphia: JB Lippincott, 1993:1833–1842. Reprinted with permission.
*Some remain theoretical and must be proved.

Table 29–2   Some Systemic Immune Diseases that Can Produce Otologic Symptoms

Connective tissue diseases (collagen vascular disorders)
Cogan's syndrome
Polyarteritis nodosa
Aortitis syndrome (Takayasu's disease)
Behçet's disease
Rheumatoid arthritis
Systemic lupus erythematosus
Polymyositis/dermatomyositis
Relapsing polychondritis
Sjögren's syndrome
Other diseases
Hashimoto's thyroiditis
Ulcerative colitis
Glomerulonephritis
Demyelinating disease
Wegener's granulomatosis

Source: From Hughes GB, Barna BP, Calabrese LH, Koo A. Immunologic disorders of the inner ear. In: Bailey BJ, ed. Head and Neck Surgery–Otolaryngology. Philadelphia: JB Lippincott, 1993:1833–1842. Reprinted with permission.

Table 29–3   Recommended Clinical and Laboratory Workup*

1. History
2. Examination (usually normal except for hearing loss and occasional systemic immune disease)
3. FTA-abs or MHA-TP to exclude syphilis
4. Enhanced MRI to exclude vestibular schwannoma
5. Western blot testing if desired (see **Table 29–4**)
6. One month treatment trial of high dose steroids
7. A cochlin cellular test is being developed

Source: From Hughes GB, Barna BP, Calabrese LH, Koo A. Immunologic disorders of the inner ear. In: Bailey BJ, ed. Head and Neck Surgery–Otolaryngology. Philadelphia: JB Lippincott, 1993:1833–1842. Reprinted with permission.
*COCH-activated T-cell testing will be available through IMMCO Diagnostics, Buffalo, New York, in 2007.

SNHL. This time frame helps distinguish ASNHL from ototoxicity with sudden bilateral loss, or age-related presbycusis and noise-induced hearing loss over many months or years. The most common age group is 20 to 50 years at onset of symptoms. Pediatric cases are possible but uncommon. Many older patients present with disease that, in retrospect, may have been present for many years. Disease can affect both sexes, but a female preponderance is noted when reports include both primary and secondary/systemic immune disease. About 50% of patients report dizziness at some time or another, usually lightheadedness if disease is early or ataxia if late. Vertigo from bilateral immune Meniere's syndrome can occur, but is less common. Dizzy symptoms usually parallel hearing loss as activity waxes and wanes.

Physical examination of the ear usually is normal; in a sense, a normal otoscopic exam is another hallmark of ASNHL. In secondary systemic disease, the external or middle ear can be abnormal, for example, involvement of auricular cartilage in relapsing polychondritis, auricular skin in lupus erythematosus, and middle ear in Wegener's granulomatosis. Systemic immune disease, such as RA and polyarteritis nodosa, can produce abnormalities at distant sites, including the ear.

Radiographic and Serologic Studies

Bilateral vestibular schwannomas rarely cause rapidly progressive SNHL; nevertheless, magnetic resonance imaging (MRI) of the brain with attention to the internal auditory canals, with and without gadolinium contrast enhancement, should be obtained even if ASNHL is suspected. Serologic testing for ASNHL is helpful but not essential: clinical hallmarks plus beneficial response to corticosteroids are sufficient. If desired, a serum sample can be sent to IMMCO Diagnostics, Inc. (Buffalo, NY) for Western blot testing (**Table 29–4**) if not available locally.[92] A positive 68-kD band in Western blot supports the diagnosis. Results are more likely to be abnormal when disease is active and in the absence of immunosuppression.

Bilateral progressive SNHL also is the hallmark of otologic syphilis. Meniere's syndrome with vertigo also can occur from luetic disease. Because most patients with late-onset or acquired otologic syphilis have a negative history for syphilis and otherwise normal physical examination, great reliance is based on serologic tests for diagnosis. Treponemal tests have higher predictive value than nontreponemal tests. Either the fluorescent treponemal antibody absorption (FTA-abs) or microhemagglutination assay for *Treponema pallidum* (MHA-TP) should be obtained to rule out otologic syphilis in patients with suspected ASNHL.

Lyme disease and human immunodeficiency virus (HIV-1) infection are rare but possible causes of rapidly progressive SNHL. Lyme disease is caused by infection with *Borrelia burgdorferi* and is transmitted by several species of tick.[93] Initial manifestations consist of a rash at the tick bite, followed much later by arthralgia, neuropathy, meningitis, and myocarditis. Diagnosis of Lyme disease is based on history, tick bite (often unnoticed), and elevated serum or CSF antibodies to the organism. HIV testing also can be obtained if clinically indicated. In a prospective, controlled study, Hausler et al[94] found that HIV-infected patients frequently had abnormal neuro-otologic findings. In advanced stages, both CNS and inner ear deficits were noted, including SNHL and vertigo.

Table 29–4   Procedure for Western Blot Immunoassay*

1. Call IMMCO Diagnostics, Inc. (Buffalo, NY) 1-800-537-TEST.
2. Draw 5–10 mL of blood.
3. Separate serum from clot if possible.
4. Transfer serum into provided plastic tube. If separation facilities are not available, whole blood can be shipped.
5. Label tube with patient's and doctor's names.
6. Complete test request form and check "anti–68-kD (hsp) 70 antibody."
7. Place serum tube into Styrofoam case, and position absorbent paper pad above and below tube.
8. Slip Styrofoam case into sealable plastic bag and place together with completed test request form into shipping container.
9. Tape shut end flaps and ship container by your preferred method.

Source: From Hughes GB. Serologic studies. In: Goebel JA, ed. Practical Management of the Dizzy Patient. Philadelphia: Lippincott Williams & Wilkins, 2001:205–210. Reprinted with permission.
*COCH-activated T-cell testing will be available through IMMCO Diagnostics, Buffalo, New York, in 2007.

Treatment

Systemic Steroids

Systemic administration of steroids is the mainstay of treatment: prednisone 1 mg/kg/day (60 mg in an adult) for 30 days followed by a repeat audiogram. A beneficial treatment response supports ASNHL diagnosis. Low-dose and short-term treatments may not provide any benefit; such incomplete treatment may not provide valid outcome on which to base subsequent therapy. If the 1-month audiogram documents improvement, the steroids are tapered slowly to preserve the gain. The rate of taper varies from patient to patient depending on rate and degree of improvement and toleration of side effects. One suggested tapering course consists of prednisone 40 mg daily for the second month, 30 mg for the third, 20 mg for the fourth, 15 mg for the fifth, 10 mg for the sixth, and even less as needed. Below 20 mg daily, the drug effect transitions from high-dose to low-dose: side effects are less noticeable but hearing may drop or fluctuate. If hearing drops and drug tapering continues, re-treatment with second-course high-dose prednisone may not be as helpful; therefore, once the initial benefit has been gained, the taper should be deliberately slow over many months in most patients, and even slower if symptoms recur as the drug is reduced below 20 mg daily.

Niparko and colleagues[95] analyzed pure-tone and speech audiometric results from a prospective trial of prednisone treatment of subjects with active autoimmune inner ear disease (AIED). This multisite study sought to characterize the pattern and size of the treatment effect as reflected in clinical audiometry and to identify audiometric predictors of response to steroid treatment of AIED.

Adult participants demonstrated clinically established criteria for AIED ($n = 116$). Eligibility required audiometric evidence of active AIED as indicated by idiopathic SNHL with threshold elevations within 3 months of enrollment. The study evaluated audiometric changes after 4 weeks of treatment with pharmacologic doses (60 mg/day) of prednisone, examining the relationship between audiometric pure-tone thresholds at baseline and changes in word recognition scores.

Overall mean pure-tone averages improved from baseline to closeout of prednisone treatment in better-hearing ears from 52.4 to 48.3 dB ($p < .0001$) (**Fig. 29–1**). Mean Word Identification Score (WIS) improved in the better ear from 71.4 to 78.1% ($p < .0001$). In 69 (59.5%) of 116 subjects WIS improved (range: 2 to 80%) in the better ear. In these subjects, the baseline pure-tone thresholds and pure-tone averages (PTAs) correlated significantly and positively with improvement in WIS. **Fig. 29–2** demonstrates the relationship between the PTA at baseline and the percent improvement in speech recognition score that was achievable. The investigators observed that there is a range of baseline hearing that appears most amenable to prednisone treatment when AIED is suspected, between the 35- and 65-dB range of PTAs at baseline.

The investigators concluded that steroid treatment in AIED-mediated hearing loss produces variable but significant hearing gains. Neither a focal, cochleotopic region of greatest vulnerability to AIED nor a frequency-specific amenability to treatment was evident. The study also suggested that analysis of predictors and the degree of treatment effect varies with different approaches to measuring change in the WIS.

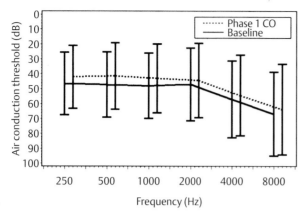

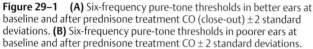

Figure 29–1 **(A)** Six-frequency pure-tone thresholds in better ears at baseline and after prednisone treatment CO (close-out) ±2 standard deviations. **(B)** Six-frequency pure-tone thresholds in poorer ears at baseline and after prednisone treatment CO ± 2 standard deviations.

CO, close out. (From Niparko JK, Wang NY, Rauch SD, et al. Serial audiometry in a clinical trial of AIED treatment. Otol Neurotol 2005;26:908–917. Reprinted by permission.)

At this time, therefore, the three guiding principles of treatment are (1) systemic steroids, usually prednisone; (2) high-dose for at least 30 days; and (3) slow taper over many months to maintain the gain. Some patients require 5, 10, or 15 mg prednisone daily or equivalent alternate-day therapy to maintain hearing. Many patients need to adjust their maintenance dose up or down depending on disease activity. Some eventually can stop therapy if ASNHL is in remission, only to resume high-dose therapy if disease recurs.

Intratympanic Steroids

Intratympanic steroids can be given to the affected ear(s) if systemic therapy is contraindicated or poorly tolerated. Contraindications may include brittle diabetes, uncontrolled hypertension, severe glaucoma, active tuberculosis, partial aseptic necrosis of the femoral head, severe osteoporosis, and psychosis. Most contraindications to systemic steroids are relative and can be controlled and monitored closely. Prospective

study is needed to verify that repeated intratympanic steroid injections have no systemic effect; however, at this time intratympanic steroids appear safe in these clinical settings. Typical dosage is decadron 24 mg% or methylprednisolone 40 mg% over 30 minutes for each treatment. Repeat treatments usually are given weekly, perhaps over 3 to 4 weeks, although the duration of the benefit has not been studied. Intratympanic steroids also can be given to patients who cannot tolerate the side effects of systemic therapy, such as extreme agitation and insomnia, depression, or euphoria; in patients who simply do not like the way they appear with prolonged treatment, such as flushed complexion, weight gain, and facial swelling; and in patients who have tried systemic steroids previously and refuse to take them again.

Anesthetizing the tympanic membrane with phenol or lidocaine is fast and simple. Both cause momentary stinging (phenol) or burning (lidocaine) but then provide excellent anesthesia for anterior and posterior myringotomies without lingering side effects. An occasional patient may experience temporary lightheadedness. Most patients are very comfortable in the reclined chair with a pillow beneath their head, the treated ear kept upward for 30 minutes. The steroid then can be suctioned from the middle ear if desired and the patient sent home.

Disadvantages of intratympanic steroids are obvious: (1) treatment is given to one ear at a time but disease activity usually is bilateral; (2) persistent disease activity over months would require many office visits, usually weekly; (3) underlying systemic disease in secondary SNHL will not be controlled; and (4) beneficial results may treat the disease outcome but may or may not control disease initiation. Nevertheless, because of ease of administration and lack of apparent systemic effects, intratympanic steroids can be offered to selected patients in place of or in addition to systemic therapy.

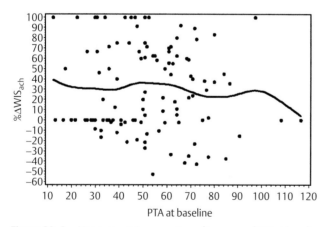

Figure 29–2 Nonparametric regression spline curve of PTA at baseline plotted against %Δ WIS$_{ach}$ (percentage of maximal achievable change in WIS) for better ears. %ΔWIS$_{ach}$ reflects the observed change in WIS expressed as a percentage of the greatest potential change in either direction. A positive %ΔWIS$_{ach}$ is evident across the range of pure-tone averages (PTAs) at baseline. The greatest treatment effects achieved with steroids were observed in the intermediate ranges of PTA at baseline, from a moderate loss at baseline (about 35 dB) up to about 65 dB. (From Niparko JK, Wang NY, Rauch SD, et al. Serial audiometry in a clinical trial of AIED treatment. Otol Neurotol 2005;26:908–917. Reprinted by permission.)

Methotrexate, Etanercept Cyclophosphamide, Diuretics, and Low-Salt Diet

As stated earlier, in primary ASNHL prospective controlled study of prednisone-methotrexate versus prednisone-placebo did not find any benefit of methotrexate, although methotrexate was very well tolerated with rare major adverse effects.[89] An occasional patient with ASNHL may benefit from methotrexate, or may have already tried methotrexate and be convinced that it helps. When bone marrow and liver functions are normal, the patient agrees to use contraception and abstain from alcohol, and understands the risks, such as rare pulmonary fibrosis, methotrexate 7.5 mg weekly can be given for the first month, 15 mg weekly for the second month, and 20 mg weekly thereafter if blood studies remain normal. Some patients then can taper the dose to lower maintenance levels if symptoms are controlled. Folic acid 1 mg daily should be given to minimize risk of bone marrow suppression.

Cyclophosphamide is a powerful immunosuppressive agent with fast therapeutic activity but with more risks than steroids and methotrexate. This drug may be particularly helpful in secondary SNHL from Wegener's granulomatosis, usually together with high-dose prednisone. Because of increased risk of toxicity, cyclophosphamide probably should be prescribed and followed by an immunologist in conjunction with the otologist.

Weekly injections of Enorel™ (Etanercept, Amgen, Immunex Corp., Thousand Oaks, CA) can be given if SNHL is to felt be secondary to rheumatoid arthritis.

Since 1983, autoimmune Meniere's syndrome has been reported and now is well accepted as a clinical variant of ASNHL.[96] Many of these patients have fluctuating hearing, aural pressure, tinnitus, and episodic dizziness or vertigo, which are typical for endolymphatic hydrops.[97] Another similar variant of ASNHL is delayed contralateral endolymphatic hydrops: the first ear is deaf for many years, then the second develops rapidly progressive SNHL. Analogous to treating idiopathic endolymphatic hydrops (Meniere's disease), a low-salt diet and a diuretic can be used to treat immune-mediated hydrops (Meniere's syndrome). The treatment seems best for patients with fluctuating hearing and aural pressure, and can sometimes avoid steroids in mild cases or minimize steroids in more advanced cases. The cornerstone of a low-salt diet and diuretic therapy is the low-salt diet. Patients should not add salt to the food when it is being prepared or when it is on the table. Most patients accept this readily. The more difficult requirement is to limit daily sodium intake to about 2000 mg. The patient must avoid salty foods and read the labels of foods and at the end of the day, estimate daily sodium intake.

The diuretic usually is hydrochlorothiazide 25 mg with triamterene 37.5 mg daily. If the patient is allergic to sulfa medicines, spironolactone 25 mg daily should be used instead. Thiazide diuretics can aggravate renal disease. Also, patients who take daily nonsteroidal antiinflammatory agents (e.g., ibuprophen) should avoid triamterene as the combination can increase the risk of kidney disease. Generally, stronger diuretics do not help much more than hydrochlorothiazide-triamterene, nor does doubling its dose. The objective of a low-salt diet and diuretic is to minimize the dose of systemic steroids required to maintain hearing and avoid dizziness. The combination of glucocorticoid and diuretic can increase risk of serum potassium depletion, which should be monitored.

Lymphocytoplasmapheresis

Plasmapheresis removes immune complexes from the circulation; lymphocytoplasmapheresis removes both humoral and cellular immunopathogens from the circulation. In 1989, Luetje[98] published detailed results of treatment of eight patients with ASNHL with average follow-up of 26 months (range 9 to 54 months). Six patients experienced improved hearing; four of them no longer required steroids or cytotoxic drugs. These preliminary results were very encouraging. Apheresis can be considered when hearing loss progresses despite steroids and cytotoxic drugs, or when medication is not tolerated. In this procedure, about 2 L of blood are filtered three times weekly for 2 weeks, with 5% albumin used for replacement fluid. The procedure does not require hospitalization, takes 3 hours, and is remarkably free of adverse effects; however, it is very expensive and its possible benefit is relatively short-term. Therefore, plasmapheresis should be considered as adjunctive therapy in acute, fulminant disease with no benefit to more traditional therapy.

Hearing Aids and Cochlear Implants

Not infrequently a patient must weigh the side effects of maintenance prednisone against its benefit to hearing. If the patient increases the dosage, hearing is stable and good but side effects and potential risks increase; if the patient reduces the dosage, side effects and potential risks are negligible but hearing declines. Very often this drop in hearing determines the need for a hearing aid in one or both ears. Because ASNHL often fluctuates up and down, a hearing aid with broad dynamic range is recommended.

Rarely, despite aggressive medical management, a patient with primary or secondary immune SNHL experiences a drop in binaural hearing to a level that hearing aids cannot help. These patients are excellent candidates for cochlear implantation. Typically they are postlingual, have relatively recent onset of deafness, and have discrete cochlear pathology that preserves good auditory neural function for stimulation. Frequently these patients have excellent outcomes after cochlear implantation.

◆ Conclusion

It is clear that the inner ear is not an "immunologically privileged" site and may mount an immune response against both foreign- and self-antigens. Autoimmunity may have a central role in otologic dysfunction. Hearing loss has been described in the context of non–organ-specific autoimmune diseases. Furthermore, cochlear damage may be the result of an organ-specific autoimmune event. The progressive hearing loss that occurs in ASNHL may likely be autoimmune in nature, and as such may be amenable to treatment with contemporary immunomodulatory regimens. These immunomodulatory treatments potentially may overcome the limitations inherent in the broadly immunosuppressive corticosteroid regimen currently used for treating ASNHL.

Progress in understanding the inflammatory events involved in ASNHL is clearly hampered by the inherent inability to obtain human temporal bone histopathology during active ASNHL. However, the recent development by our laboratory of a traditional antigen-specific mouse model that targets inner ear antigens in an organ-specific manner should dramatically advance our understanding of autoimmune inflammatory events involved in ASNHL and should facilitate development of contemporary treatment protocols.

Clinically, it is important to recognize this condition early because current treatment modalities may be quite effective in a large number of patients. Hearing loss can be restored through appropriate and judicious use of immunosuppressive drugs. Thus far, the Western blot anti–68-kD immunoassay has been shown to be a specific test to predict therapeutic responsiveness in patients with ASNHL. With further studies, more specific diagnostic methods will be developed and even more effective and less toxic treatments should emerge.

Future research should focus on identifying inner ear–specific proteins as potential targets for ASNHL. By using our animal model, a group of autoantigens, selected from known inner ear proteins, could be identified as potential targets for the human disease. In future research, patients with ASNHL could be screened for T-cell reactivity with a variety of peptides derived from inner ear–specific proteins to determine which peptides are involved in the development of human disease. Identification of target antigens in human disease will allow for the development of targeted immunomodulatory therapies that may improve the prognosis of patients who are currently treated with nonspecific immunosuppressive therapies.

◆ Acknowledgments

This work was supported primarily by grants from the Deafness Research Foundation, New York, NY; the Samuel Rosenthal Foundation and the Milton and Charlotte Kramer Foundation, Cleveland, OH; and the Triple-T Foundation, Chardon, OH. Additional support came from National Institutes of Health grant DC-006422.

◆ Disclosure

The senior authors (G.B.H. and V.K.T.) have a financial relationship with IMMCO Diagnostics, Buffalo, New York, for COCH-activated T-cell diagnostic testing of ASNHL.

References

1. McCabe BF. Autoimmune sensorineural hearing loss. Ann Otol Rhinol Laryngol 1979;88:585–589
2. Harris JP, Ryan AF. Fundamental immune mechanisms of the brain and inner ear. Otolaryngol Head Neck Surg 1995;112:639–653
3. Barker CF, Billingham RE. Immunologically privileged sites. Adv Immunol 1977;25:1–54
4. Harling-Berg CJ, Knopf PM, Cserr HF. Myelin basic protein infused into cerebrospinal fluid suppresses experimental autoimmune encephalomyelitis. J Neuroimmunol 1991;35:45–51
5. Mogi G, Lim DJ, Watanabe N. Immunologic study on the inner ear. Immunoglobulins in perilymph. Arch Otolaryngol 1982;108:270–275
6. Harris JP. Immunology of the inner ear: evidence of local antibody production. Ann Otol Rhinol Laryngol 1984;93:157–162
7. Tomiyama S, Harris JP. Evaluation of the inner ear antibody levels following direct antigen challenge of the endolymphatic sac. Acta Otolaryngol 1989;107:202–209
8. Harris JP. Immunology of the inner ear: response of the inner ear to antigen challenge. Otolaryngol Head Neck Surg 1983;91:18–32
9. Palva T, Raunio V. Disc electrophoretic studies of human perilymph. Ann Otol Rhinol Laryngol 1967;76:23–36
10. Discolo C, Keasler J, Hirose K. Inflammatory cells in the mouse cochlea after acoustic trauma. Paper presented at the annual meeting of the Association for Research in Otolaryngology (ARO), February 21–26, 2004, Daytona Beach, FL, abstract 392
11. Takahashi M, Harris JP. Anatomic distribution and localization of immunocompetent cells in normal mouse endolymphatic sac. Acta Otolaryngol 1988;106:409–416
12. Tomiyama S, Harris JP. The endolymphatic sac: its importance in inner ear immune responses. Laryngoscope 1986;96:685–691
13. Tomiyama S, Harris JP. The role of the endolymphatic sac in inner ear immunity. Acta Otolaryngol 1987;103:182–188
14. Tomiyama S, Keithley EM, Harris JP. Antigen-specific immune response in the inner ear. Ann Otol Rhinol Laryngol 1989;98:447–450
15. Gloddek B, Harris JP. Role of lymphokines in the immune response of the inner ear. Acta Otolaryngol 1989;108:68–75
16. Woolf NK, Harris JP. Cochlear pathophysiology associated with inner ear immune responses. Acta Otolaryngol 1986;102:353–364
17. Yeo SW, Ryan AF. Transforming growth factor-b mRNA expression in the rat cochlea during experimental immune labyrinthitis. In: Mogi G, Veldman J, Kawauchi H, eds. Immunobiology in Otorhinolaryngology–Progress of a Decade. Amsterdam: Kugler, 1994:181–188
18. Hirose K, Keasler J. Proinflammatory cytokine and chemokine expression in the noise-exposed murine cochlea. Paper presented at the annual meeting of the Association for Research in Otolaryngology (ARO), February 21–26, 2004, Daytona Beach, FL, abstract 390
19. Wolf M, Kronenberg J, Engelberg S, Leventon G. Rapidly progressive hearing loss as a symptom of polyarteritis nodosa. Am J Otolaryngol 1987;8:105–108
20. Kempf HG. Ear involvement in Wegener's granulomatosis. Clin Otolaryngol 1989;14:451–456
21. Moffat DA, Ramsden RT, Rosenberg JN, Booth JB, Gibson WPR. Oto-admittance measurements in patients with rheumatoid arthritis. J Laryngol Otol 1977;91:917–927
22. Cogan DG. Syndrome of nonsyphilitic interstitial keratitis and vestibuloauditory symptoms. Arch Ophthalmol 1945;33:144–150
23. Cheson BD, Bluming AZ, Alroy J. Cogan's syndrome: a systemic vasculitis. Am J Med 1976;60:549–555
24. Brinkman CJ, Broekhuyse RM. Cell-mediated immunity after retinal detachment as determined by lymphocyte stimulation. Am J Ophthalmol 1978;86:260–265
25. Cogan DG, Sullivan WR Jr. Immunologic study of nonsyphilitic interstitial keratitis with vestibuloauditory symptoms. Am J Ophthalmol 1975;80:491–494
26. Hughes GB, Kinney SE, Barna BP, Tomsak RL, Calabrese LH. Autoimmune reactivity in Cogan's syndrome: a preliminary report. Otolaryngol Head Neck Surg 1983;91:24–32
27. Hughes GB, Barna BP, Kinney SE, Calabrese LH, Nalepa NL. Predictive value of laboratory tests in "autoimmune" inner ear disease: preliminary report. Laryngoscope 1986;96:502–505
28. Lorenz RR, Solares CA, Williams PM, et al. Interferon-gamma production to inner ear antigens by T cells from patients with autoimmune sensorineural hearing loss. J Neuroimmunol 2002;130:173–178
29. Yoo TJ. Etiopathogenesis of Meniere's disease: a hypothesis. Ann Otol Rhinol Laryngol Suppl 1984;113:6–12
30. Harris JP, Woolf NK, Ryan AF. A reexamination of experimental type II collagen autoimmunity: middle and inner ear morphology and function. Ann Otol Rhinol Laryngol 1986;95:176–180
31. Solares CA, Edling AE, Johnson JM, et al. Murine autoimmune hearing loss mediated by CD4+ T cells specific for inner ear peptides. J Clin Invest 2004;113:1210–1217
32. McCabe BF, McCormick KJ. Tests for autoimmune disease in otology. Am J Otol 1984;5:447–449
33. Sercarz EE, Lehmann PV, Ametani A, Benichou G, Miller A, Moudgil K. Dominance and crypticity of T cell antigenic determinants. Annu Rev Immunol 1993;11:729–766
34. Tanguay S, Killion JJ. Direct comparison of ELISPOT and ELISA-based assays for detection of individual cytokine-secreting cells. Lymphokine Cytokine Res 1994;13:259–263
35. Forsthuber T, Yip HC, Lehmann PV. Induction of TH1 and TH2 immunity in neonatal mice. Science 1996;271:1728–1730
36. Tuohy VK, Yu M, Weinstock-Guttman B, Kinkel RP. Diversity and plasticity of self recognition during the development of multiple sclerosis. J Clin Invest 1997;99:1682–1690
37. Karulin AY, Hesse MD, Tary-Lehmann M, Lehmann PV. Single-cytokine-producing CD4 memory cells predominate in type 1 and type 2 immunity. J Immunol 2000;164:1862–1872
38. Reinhardt RL, Khoruts A, Merica R, Zell T, Jenkins MK. Visualizing the generation of memory CD4 T cells in the whole body. Nature 2001;410:101–105
39. Markovic-Plese S, Fukaura H, Zhang J, et al. T cell recognition of immunodominant and cryptic proteolipid protein epitopes in humans. J Immunol 1995;155:982–992
40. Atkinson MA, Bowman MA, Campbell L, Darrow BL, Kaufman DL, Maclaren NK. Cellular immunity to a determinant common to glutamate decarboxylase and coxsackie virus in insulin-dependent diabetes. J Clin Invest 1994;94:2125–2129
41. Patel SD, Cope AP, Congia M, et al. Identification of immunodominant T cell epitopes of human glutamic acid decarboxylase 65 by using HLA-DR(alpha1*0101,beta1*0401) transgenic mice. Proc Natl Acad Sci U S A 1997;94:8082–8087
42. Robertson NG, Resendes BL, Lin JS, et al. Inner ear localization of mRNA and protein products of COCH, mutated in the sensorineural deafness and vestibular disorder, DFNA9. Hum Mol Genet 2001;10:2493–2500

43. Baek M-J, Park H-M, Johnson JM, Altuntas CZ, Jane-wit D, Jaini R, Solares CA, Thomas DM, Ball EJ, Robertson NG, Morton CC, Hughes GB, Tuohy VK: Increased frequencies of cochlin-specific T cells in patients with autoimmune sensorineural hearing loss. J Immunol 2006;177:4203–4210

44. Arnold W, Pfaltz R, Altermatt HJ. Evidence of serum antibodies against inner ear tissues in the blood of patients with certain sensorineural hearing disorders. Acta Otolaryngol 1985;99:437–444

45. Arnold W, Pfaltz CR. Critical evaluation of the immunofluorescence microscopic test for identification of serum antibodies against human inner ear tissue. Acta Otolaryngol 1987;103:373–378

46. Harris JP, Sharp P. Inner ear autoantibodies in patients with rapidly progressive sensorineural hearing loss. Laryngoscope 1990;100:516–524

47. Moscicki RA, San Martin JE, Quintero CH, Rauch SD, Nadol JB Jr, Bloch KJ. Serum antibody to inner ear proteins in patients with progressive hearing loss. Correlation with disease activity and response to corticosteroid treatment. JAMA 1994;272:611–616

48. Gottschlich S, Billings PB, Keithley EM, Weisman MH, Harris JP. Assessment of serum antibodies in patients with rapidly progressive sensorineural hearing loss and Meniere's disease. Laryngoscope 1995;105:1347–1352

49. Lindquist S, Craig EA. The heat-shock proteins. Annu Rev Genet 1988;22:631–677

50. Welch WJ. Mammalian stress response: cell physiology, structure/function of stress proteins, and implications for medicine and disease. Physiol Rev 1992;72:1063–1081

51. Winfield JB, Jarjour WN. Stress proteins, autoimmunity, and autoimmune disease. Curr Top Microbiol Immunol 1991;167:161–189

52. Billings PB, Keithley EM, Harris JP. Evidence linking the 68 kilodalton antigen identified in progressive sensorineural hearing loss patient sera with heat shock protein 70. Ann Otol Rhinol Laryngol 1995;104:181–188

53. Billings PB, Shin SO, Harris JP. Assessing the role of anti-hsp70 in cochlear impairment. Hear Res 1998;126:210–213

54. Bloch DB, San Martin JE, Rauch SD, Moscicki RA, Bloch KJ. Serum antibodies to heat shock protein 70 in sensorineural hearing loss. Arch Otolaryngol Head Neck Surg 1995;121:1167–1171

55. Bloch DB, Gutierrez JA, Guerriero V Jr, Rauch SD, Bloch KJ. Recognition of a dominant epitope in bovine heat-shock protein 70 in inner ear disease. Laryngoscope 1999;109:621–625

56. Shin SO, Billings PB, Keithley EM, Harris JP. Comparison of anti-heat shock protein 70 (anti-hsp70) and anti-68-kDa inner ear protein in the sera of patients with Meniere's disease. Laryngoscope 1997;107:222–227

57. Hirose K, Wener MH, Duckert LG. Utility of laboratory testing in autoimmune inner ear disease. Laryngoscope 1999;109:1749–1754

58. Trune DR, Kempton JB, Mitchell CR, Hefeneider SH. Failure of elevated heat shock protein 70 antibodies to alter cochlear function in mice. Hear Res 1998;116:65–70

59. Boulassel MR, Tomasi JP, Deggouj N, Gersdorff M. COCH5B2 is target antigen of anti-inner ear antibodies in autoimmune inner ear diseases. Otol Neurotol 2001;22:614–618

60. Robertson NG, Skvorak AB, Yin Y, et al. Mapping and characterization of a novel cochlear gene in human and in mouse: a positional candidate gene for a deafness disorder, DFNA9. Genomics 1997;46:345–354

61. Robertson NG, Lu L, Heller S, et al. Mutations in a novel cochlear gene cause DFNA9, a human nonsyndromic deafness with vestibular dysfunction. Nat Genet 1998;20:299–303

62. Grabski R, Szul T, Sasaki T, et al. Mutations in COCH that result in nonsyndromic autosomal dominant deafness (DFNA9) affect matrix deposition of cochlin. Hum Genet 2003;113:406–416

63. Ikezono T, Omori A, Ichinose S, Pawankar R, Watanabe A, Yagi T. Identification of the protein product of the Coch gene (hereditary deafness gene) as the major component of bovine inner ear protein. Biochim Biophys Acta 2001;1535:258–265

64. Yoo TJ, Tomoda K, Stuart JM, Cremer MA, Townes AS, Kang AH. Type II collagen-induced autoimmune sensorineural hearing loss and vestibular dysfunction in rats. Ann Otol Rhinol Laryngol 1983;92:267–271

65. Yoo TJ, Yazawa Y, Tomoda K, Floyd R. Type II collagen-induced autoimmune endolymphatic hydrops in guinea pig. Science 1983;222:65–67

66. Theofilopoulos AN, Dixon FJ. Murine models of systemic lupus erythematosus. Adv Immunol 1985;37:269–390

67. Kyogoku M, Nose M, Sawai T, Miyazawa M, Tachiwaki O, Kawashima M. Immunopathology of murine lupus-overview, SL/Ni and MRL/Mp-lpr/lpr-. Prog Clin Biol Res 1987;229:95–130

68. Nagata S, Suda T. Fas and Fas ligand: lpr and gld mutations. Immunol Today 1995;16:39–43

69. Lin DW, Trune DR. Breakdown of stria vascularis blood-labyrinth barrier in C3H/lpr autoimmune disease mice. Otolaryngol Head Neck Surg 1997;117:530–534

70. Kusakari C, Hozawa K, Koike S, Kyogoku M, Takasaba T. MRL/MP-lpr/lpr mouse as a model of immune-induced sensorineural hearing loss. Ann Otol Rhinol Laryngol Suppl 1992;157:82–86

71. Ruckenstein MJ, Milburn M, Hu L. Strial dysfunction in the MRL-Fas mouse. Otolaryngol Head Neck Surg 1999;121:452–456

72. Wobig RJ, Kempton J, Trune DR. Steroid-responsive cochlear dysfunction in the MRL/lpr autoimmune mouse. Otolaryngol Head Neck Surg 1999;121:344–347

73. Trune DR. Cochlear immunoglobulin in the C3H/lpr mouse model for autoimmune hearing loss. Otolaryngol Head Neck Surg 1997;117:504–508

74. Trune DR, Wobig RJ, Kempton JB, Hefeneider SH. Steroid treatment improves cochlear function in the MRL.MpJ-Fas(lpr) autoimmune mouse. Hear Res 1999;137:160–166

75. Nariuchi H, Sone M, Tago C, Kurata T, Saito K. Mechanisms of hearing disturbance in an autoimmune model mouse NZB/kl. Acta Otolaryngol Suppl 1994;514:127–131

76. Sone M, Nariuchi H, Saito K, Yanagita N. A substrain of NZB mouse as an animal model of autoimmune inner ear disease. Hear Res 1995;83:26–36

77. Tago C, Yanagita N. Cochlear and renal pathology in the autoimmune strain mouse. Ann Otol Rhinol Laryngol Suppl 1992;157:87–91

78. Harris JP. Experimental autoimmune sensorineural hearing loss. Laryngoscope 1987;97:63–76

79. Soliman AM. The use of immunofluorescence in the non-decalcified frozen guinea pig cochlea to detect autoantibodies in inner ear disorders. Arch Otorhinolaryngol 1987;244:241–245

80. Soliman AM. Experimental autoimmune inner ear disease. Laryngoscope 1989;99:188–193

81. Yamanobe S, Harris JP. Spontaneous remission in experimental autoimmune labyrinthitis. Ann Otol Rhinol Laryngol 1992;101:1007–1014

82. Orozco CR, Niparko JK, Richardson BC, Dolan DF, Ptok MU, Altschuler RA. Experimental model of immune-mediated hearing loss using cross-species immunization. Laryngoscope 1990;100:941–947

83. Nair TS, Raphael Y, Dolan DF, et al. Monoclonal antibody induced hearing loss. Hear Res 1995;83:101–113

84. Nair TS, Prieskorn DM, Miller JM, Dolan DF, Raphael Y, Carey TE. KHRI-3 monoclonal antibody-induced damage to the inner ear: antibody staining of nascent scars. Hear Res 1999;129:50–60

85. Zajic G, Nair TS, Ptok M, et al. Monoclonal antibodies to inner ear antigens: I. Antigens expressed by supporting cells of the guinea pig cochlea. Hear Res 1991;52:59–71

86. Nair TS, Kozma KE, Hoefling NL, et al. Identification and characterization of choline transporter-like protein 2, an inner ear glycoprotein of 68 and 72 kDa that is the target of antibody-induced hearing loss. J Neurosci 2004;24:1772–1779

87. Gloddek B, Gloddek J, Arnold W. Induction of an inner-ear-specific autoreactive T-cell line for the diagnostic evaluation of an autoimmune disease of the inner ear. Ann N Y Acad Sci 1997;830:266–276

88. Gloddek B, Gloddek J, Arnold W. A rat T-cell line that mediates autoimmune disease of the inner ear in the Lewis rat. ORL J Otorhinolaryngol Relat Spec 1999;61:181–187

89. Billings P. Experimental autoimmune hearing loss. J Clin Invest 2004;113:1114–1117

90. Harris JP, Weisman MH, Derebery JM, et al. Treatment of corticosteroid-responsive autoimmune inner ear disease with methotrexate: a randomized controlled trial. JAMA 2003;290:1875–1883

91. Hughes GB, Barna BP, Calabrese LH, Koo A. Immunologic disorders of the inner ear. In: Bailey BJ, ed. Head and Neck Surgery–Otolaryngology. Philadelphia: JB Lippincott, 1993:1833–1842

92. Hughes GB. Serologic studies. In: Goebel JA, ed. Practical Management of the Dizzy Patient. Philadelphia: Lippincott Williams & Wilkins, 2001:205–210

93. Hanner P, Rosenhall U, Edstrom S, Kaijser B. Hearing impairment in patients with antibody production against Borrelia burgdorferi antigen. Lancet 1989;1:13–15

94. Hausler R, Vibert D, Koralnik IJ, Hirschel B. Neuro-otological manifestations in different stages of HIV infection. Acta Otolaryngol Suppl 1991;481:515–521

95. Niparko JK, Wang NY, Rauch SD, et al. Serial audiometry in a clinical trial of AIED treatment. Otol Neurotol 2005;26:908–917

96. Hughes GB, Kinney SE, Barna B, Calabrese LH. Autoimmune reactivity in Meniere's disease. Laryngoscope 1983;93:410–417

97. Hughes GB, Kinney SE, Barna BP. Autoimmune Meniere's syndrome. In: Veldman JE, ed. Immunobiology, Autoimmunity and Transplantation in Otorhinolaryngology. Amsterdam: Kugler, 1985:119–129

98. Luetje CM. Theoretical and practical implications for plasmapheresis in autoimmune inner ear disease. Laryngoscope 1989;99:1137–1146

IV

Rehabilitation

30

Audiologic Rehabilitation

Sharon A. Sandridge and Craig W. Newman

The primary goal of audiologic rehabilitation (AR) is to help patients overcome the communication and psychosocial consequences of hearing loss. In routine clinical practice, hearing aid (HA) dispensing often represents the beginning and end of audiologic intervention. Yet the fitting of amplification is just one step in the process. Included in the process is a complete audiologic evaluation, assessment of individual listening needs, determination of appropriate amplification devices (i.e., HAs, assistive listening devices [ALD], a bone-anchored hearing aid [Baha®] system, or cochlear implants) and follow-up services (i.e., communication strategy training, auditory listening training, or more intensive speech and language therapy). This chapter describes a service delivery model of AR (**Fig. 30–1**) primarily for patients with adult-onset sensorineural hearing loss (SNHL). Given the majority of individuals with conductive hearing loss are treated successfully through medical intervention, this population will not be addressed. Likewise, infants and children with congenital or acquired SNHL will not be addressed, although the main difference in the AR model between children and adults is the need for more intensive follow-up. Before discussing the AR model shown in **Fig. 30–1**, an overview of the psychosocial impact of hearing loss is presented.

◆ Consequences of Hearing Loss

Within the framework of the most recent World Health Organization (WHO)[1] model, health conditions are examined under three domains: body or body condition (impairment), whole person (activity limitations), and person in society (participation restrictions). Using this systems approach, the impact of a hearing loss on the psychosocial functioning can be assessed.

Following is a brief description of each component of the WHO[1] model as it relates to auditory function. *Impairment* is the measurable loss of hearing function. For example, the loss of hair cell function at the basal end of the cochlea causes a high-frequency hearing loss. *Activity limitation* (formerly referred to as disability), on the other hand, is the impact of the hearing loss on the person's ability to communicate or hear

sounds. For example, high-frequency hearing impairment decreases the ability to perceive consonant sounds (e.g., /t/, /s/, /v/, /f/) important for speech understanding. In addition to decreased audibility, SNHL loss produces alterations in (1) dynamic range (i.e., the level difference between uncomfortable listening levels and threshold of audibility); (2) frequency resolution (i.e., separating sounds of different frequencies); and (3) temporal resolution (i.e., intense sounds masking weaker sounds that immediately proceed or follow). The result of each of the aforementioned aspects of hearing loss is reduced speech intelligibility especially in background noise. *Participation restriction* (formally referred to as handicap) represents the nonauditory problems faced by the patient in everyday situations. For example, the individual with high-frequency SNHL no longer attends social functions because it is too difficult to follow conversations. Accordingly, participation restriction represents the social (e.g., withdrawal from communication situations) and emotional (e.g., frustration) manifestations resulting from hearing impairment and activity limitation.

In general, individuals do not seek audiologic services when their hearing loss exists within the impairment domain only. Individuals seek audiologic services when their hearing impairment moves into the participation domain. That is, individuals get medical and audiologic help when hearing loss causes significant difficulty in their day-to-day activities.

◆ Communication Needs Assessment

The first step in the AR process, as shown in **Fig. 30–1**, is to document hearing *impairment* through the audiometric evaluation (see Chapter 8). The results from the audiologic assessment serve as the basis for defining the patient's hearing loss (degree, type, and configuration), establishing the need for medical intervention, assisting in the decisions regarding specific amplification devices (i.e., the electroacoustic parameters of the devices), planning appropriate treatment intervention, setting realistic expectations from amplification, and evaluating improvements following intervention.

Although pure-tone and speech audiometric tests provide information regarding maximum auditory function in optimal

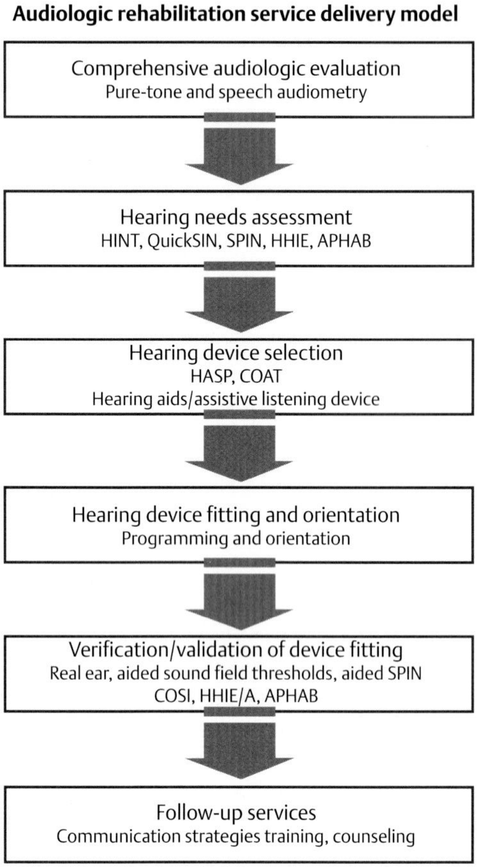

Audiologic rehabilitation service delivery model

Figure 30–1 A flow chart representing the audiologic rehabilitation (AR) model proposed in this chapter.

listening situations, these tests do not assess how well the patient performs in everyday life. Patients' communication needs must be assessed using more ecologically valid tools. A few such tools, as described briefly here, should be included in the hearing needs assessment:

- *Speech Perception in Noise (SPIN)*[2] involves the presentation of 50 sentences in which patients repeat the last word of each sentence. Twenty-five of the sentences are considered high-predictability sentences, that is, the last word is predictable from the context of the sentence (e.g., "The baby slept in the *crib*"). In contrast, the last word for the remaining 25 sentences cannot be predicted from the sentence context (e.g., "She has known about the *drug*") and are considered low-predictability sentences. The test sentences can be presented in quiet or in the presence of multitalker speech babble at various signal-to-noise ratios (SNRs). For example, sentences can be presented at 50 dB HL, and the multitalker babble presented 8 dB less intensely, yielding a +8 SNR.
- *Quick Speech in Noise (QuickSIN)*[3] is a speech-in-noise test that measures the ability to understand sentences in a background noise by presenting six sentences at different SNRs. The test is quick (it takes less than 1 minute), easy to administer and score, has high face validity, and can be useful for patient counseling.
- *Hearing in Noise Test (HINT)*[4] uses sentence-length material to obtain a sentence reception threshold obtained in quiet and again in background noise. An SNR is computed and can be used to demonstrate the effectiveness of amplification

by comparing aided and unaided HINT sentence reception thresholds as well as SNRs.

In addition to objective measures, self-report questionnaires have gained widespread use for quantifying activity limitation and participation restriction. These tools are especially useful when administered in a pre- and posttest format to document AR benefit. Here are a few of the more commonly used psychometrically robust questionnaires:

- *Abbreviated Profile of Hearing Aid Benefit (APHAB)*[5] quantifies the level of difficulty/activity limitation caused by the hearing impairment in given situations as well as documents the reduction in the difficulty through the use of amplification. The questionnaire consists of 24 questions that are divided into four subscales: Ease of Communication, Background Noise, Reverberation, and Aversiveness to Sounds. Patients quantify the level of difficulty on a 7-point scale ranging from "always" (99%) to "never" (1%).
- *Hearing Handicap Inventory for the Elderly/Adult (HHIE/A)*[6,7] assesses self-perceived hearing handicap (participation restriction) for older (HHIE; ≥65 years old) and younger (HHIA; <65 years old) adults. These instruments are 25-item questionnaires measuring social and emotional consequences of hearing loss. Patients respond to each statement with "yes," "sometimes," or "no."

In addition to assessing the patient's communication needs, several biopsychosocial factors require consideration when determining HA candidacy. Among the primary physical variables are the patient's visual status, manual dexterity, shape and dimension of the pinna and external auditory canal, and overall health. Important psychological factors affecting HA candidacy and benefit include motivation, cognitive status, and personality. In fact, motivation is critical to the success of the HA fitting and is a multivariate process incorporating acknowledgment of hearing loss, communication needs, self-image, and expected benefit. The relationship between patients' acknowledgment of hearing loss and motivation has been found to be strongly correlated with HA use and satisfaction.[8] From a social perspective, key variables to consider when evaluating HA candidacy include the patient's lifestyle, family support, and financial factors.

Hearing Device Selection

During this phase (**Fig. 30–1**), the audiologist engages in a complex decision-making process of determining which hearing devices will be the most appropriate. The devices could include HAs, ALDs, or a combination of technology. Self-assessment questionnaires allow the audiologist to best determine which device (or devices) is the most appropriate for the patient.

- *Client Oriented Scale of Improvement (COSI)*[9] allows patients along with the audiologist to isolate up to five specific areas of listening difficulties. The situations are listed and prioritized and can be compared with established norms.
- *Hearing Aid Selection Profile (HASP)*[10] is a 40-item instrument assessing patient's motivation for using amplification, expectations for amplification use, communicative needs, manual dexterity, cosmesis as well as attitudes toward cost and technology. The HASP was designed to be used as a prefitting tool at the outset of AR services to provide the clinician with a

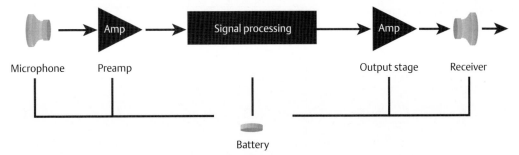

Figure 30–2 A block diagram representing the basic components of an HA. Signal processing could be either analog or digital. Amp, amplifier.

general sense of the patient's expectations and perceptions toward technology, in general, and hearing aids, specifically. A profile is generated from the eight categories useful in specific device selection, counseling for realistic expectations, and as an outcome tool for documenting quality improvements.

- *Characteristics of Amplication Tool (COAT)*, which we developed, is an eight-item questionnaire that assesses eight key areas (see Appendix 30–1). Responses to each item assist the audiologist in selecting the most appropriate HA style, options, and level of technology for a given patient.

Hearing Aids

Choosing the most appropriate HA involves selecting an instrument with the particular combination of characteristics (electroacoustic and nonelectroacoustic) that will meet the needs (listening, communicative, cosmetic, and financial) of the patient. Before discussing those characteristics, **Fig. 30–2** diagrams the basic components of the HA.

Basic Components

Microphone: The microphone is a transducer that converts the acoustic sound entering the HA into an electrical signal. Several types of microphones can be found in HAs. *Omnidirectional* microphones are equally sensitive to sounds from all directions (**Fig. 30–3**). *Directional* microphones, on the other hand, are more sensitive to sounds originating from specific angles, as seen in **Fig. 30–3**. Utilizing more than one microphone within the same device is referred to as *multimicrophone* technology. Combining multiple omnidirectional microphones or an omnidirectional and a directional microphone has been shown to increase speech intelligibility by increasing the SNR.[11,12]

Amplifier: The amplifier is responsible for modifying and increasing the gain of the incoming signal. There are two types of signal processing amplifiers: analog signal processing (ASP) and digital signal processing (DSP). The electrical signal from the microphone in the ASP system is altered through the use of filters. In the DSP system, the electrical signal is converted to a binary code and modified through a set of mathematical algorithms. The incorporation of DSP technology into hearing devices over the past 10 years has expanded the clinical efficacy of amplification through increased fitting flexibility, improved fidelity, feedback management schemes, advanced noise reduction, and use of artificial intelligence. In just 10 years, DSP instruments essentially took over the market going from 0% in 1995 to more than 80% in 2005.[13] It is predicted that in a few years, ASP instruments will command less than 1% of the market share.

Receiver: The receiver functions to convert the amplified electrical signal to an acoustic signal heard by the ear. It is a microphone in reverse.

Battery: Five sizes of batteries are available ranging from a size 5 (5.7 mm in diameter) to a size 675 (11.4 mm in diameter). Generally, as seen in **Table 30-1**, as the size of the HA increases, so does the size of the battery. The larger battery sizes have more battery capacity so they last longer (220 to 350 hours). Regardless of the size, the majority of the batteries today are zinc air. Zinc air batteries use air as the oxidizing agent and remain inactive until the paper tab is removed from the top of the battery.

Additional Hearing Aid Features

- *Telecoil (t-coil):* Some HAs contain a coil of wire that, when activated, creates an electromagnetic field. When the HA electromagnetic field crosses the electromagnetic field emitted by the telephone receiver, the signal from the

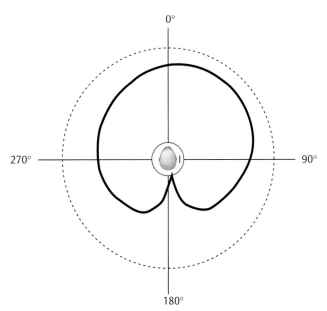

Figure 30–3 Polar plots of omnidirectional and directional microphones are illustrated. Note that the omnidirectional microphone, represented by the dotted line, is equally sensitive to sounds originating from the entire 360-degree plot. The directional microphone, represented by the solid line, shows greater sensitivity to sounds originating from 0-degree azimuth (sounds coming from the front of the listener) and least sensitive to sounds at 180-degree azimuth (sounds coming from the back of the listener). The solid line to the right of the head represents the placement of the HA.

Table 30–1 Description of Size, Dimensions (in millimeters), and Capacity (in milliamps per hour) for Commonly Used Batteries in Different Hearing Aid Styles

Size	Dimensions (Height by Width in mm)	Capacity (mAH)	Hearing Aid Style
5	2.0 by 5.7	35	CIC
10/230	3.5 by 5.7	70	ITC, CIC
312	3.5 by 7.7	140	ITE, CIC
13	5.2 by 7.7	260	ITE, BTE
675	5.2 by 11.4	575	BTE

CIC, completely-in-canal; ITC, in-the-canal; ITE, in-the-ear; BTE, behind-the-ear.

telephone is transferred to the HA. The advantage of using a telecoil is the elimination of feedback when the telephone receiver is placed close to the HA.

- *Channels:* If the frequency response (i.e., the response of the HA across low to high frequencies) is divided into smaller units, the HA is considered to have multiple channels or bands. The division of the entire frequency response into smaller units allows more precise adjustment of the frequency response. As the number of bands/channels increases, theoretically, so does the programming precision.

- *Programs:* Many HAs have multiprograms, that is, they offer different programs for different listening situations. For example, an HA can be programmed to maximize listening in quiet situations, whereas an alternative program provides maximum benefit in noisy situations. Changing programs can be accomplished through the use of remote controls, HA switches, or in some cases the programs change automatically dependent on the listening situation.

Electroacoustic Terminology

Gain refers to the amount or magnitude of amplification. It is the difference between the input and output level of the device. For example, if a 50-dB signal is picked up by the HA and is delivered to the patient's ear at 80 dB, then the gain would be 30 dB. This is graphically illustrated in **Fig. 30–4**.

Frequency response curve is a graphic representation of the amount of gain (in dB) as a function of frequency (**Fig. 30–4**). The characteristics of the HA are often described as a function

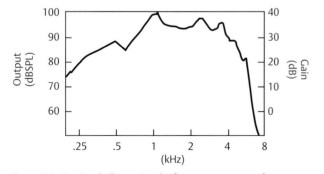

Figure 30–4 Graph illustrating the frequency response from a behind-the-ear HA with an input signal of 60 dB (60 dB as sound pressure level [SPL]). On the left axis are output values. On the right axis are gain values (difference between the input and the output). The solid line represents the frequency-response curve—a graphic display of output of the HA as a function of frequency.

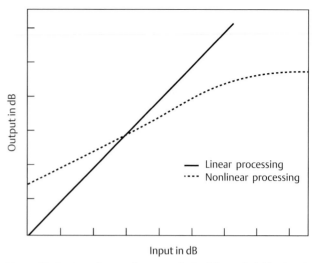

Figure 30–5 Input/output functions for both linear (solid line) and nonlinear processing (dashed line) HAs. Note that the linear processing is a straight line with a 45-degree slope representing equivalent output for given input. For example, for every 5 dB of input there is a corresponding 5 dB increase in HA output. For nonlinear processing, there is not a direct 1-to-1 input/output relationship. The gain for soft input levels is greater proportionally compared with loud input levels.

of the frequency response. For example, an HA may have a high-frequency emphasis, a broadband (relatively flat) response, or a low-frequency emphasis.

Output sound pressure level (OSPL) refers to the maximum output of the device. The OSPL is measured with a 90-dB sound pressure level (SPL) input signal and is referred to as OSPL90. The value of the OSPL90 indicates the maximum output of the device.

Linear and nonlinear processing describes the input/output function of the HA. The input/output function for a linear HA is shown in **Fig. 30–5**. Note that the function is a straight line with a 45-degree slope, indicating that for every decibel increase in input, there is an equal decibel increase in output. Therefore, soft and loud sounds are amplified to the same degree. The input/output function for a nonlinear system, on the other hand, has less output as input increases, resulting in greater amplification for softer sounds (i.e., sounds below the patient's hearing threshold) and less gain for louder sounds (i.e., sounds audible to the patient even without HAs). Nonlinear processing more appropriately mimics the needs of a SNHL than linear processing.

Hearing Aid Styles

There are two basic HA styles: behind the ear (BTE) or custom-molded (**Fig. 30–6**). Briefly, the BTE is a device that sits on or behind the ear and is attached to tubing and an earpiece in the patient's ear. Recently, technological advancements have miniaturized the BTE. Mini and micro BTEs now exist and are coupled to noncustom preformed tubes and domes allowing very open ear fits. In addition, some BTEs now place the receiver in the ear canal rather than in the BTE case. These devices are a new class of BTEs. For custom hearing instruments all the components are housed within a shell that fits in the ear to a greater or lesser extent. Generally, as the hearing loss increases so does the size of the device. As more gain is needed, a greater separation of the receiver and microphone is needed to prevent feedback (whistling of the HA

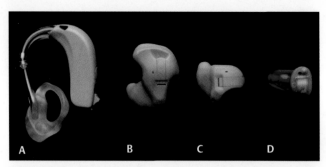

Figure 30–6 Photograph of four major HA styles: **(A)** behind-the-ear (BTE); **(B)** in-the-ear (ITE); **(C)** in-the-canal (ITC); and **(D)** completely-in-the-canal (CIC).

produced by the amplified sound being reamplified). The in-the-ear (ITE) model is the largest of the custom products and completely fills the concha bowl. The ITE can be modified from a full concha to a low profile (LP) to a half-shell (HS). The in-the-canal (ITC) model fills the ear canal but only extends slightly into the concha bowl. The completely-in-the-canal (CIC) model is the smallest of the custom products and fits deep in the ear canal, flush with the meatal opening and is often preferred for its cosmetic appearance. The selection of a specific HA style is dictated by several factors such as physical fit, condition of the ear canal, degree of hearing loss, listening needs, and patient preference. It should be noted that custom products are contraindicated for draining ears, severe to profound hearing losses, or special needs such as direct audio input.

Earmolds

Earmolds for BTE HA/s are custom-made inserts that serve several important functions including (1) coupling the BTE HA to the ear in a comfortable manner, (2) providing an acoustic seal to reduce feedback, (3) directing the sound from the receiver to the eardrum via a sound bore, and (4) acoustically modifying signals produced by the HA.

Fig. 30–7 illustrates several examples of earmold styles. Selection of a particular style is based on HA gain, the shape and size of the pinna and ear canal, and patient preference. In general, higher gain instruments require the selection of more occluding style earmolds. Nonoccluding styles are appropriate to reduce the *occlusion effect* (i.e., increased sound pressure level in the ear canal that causes the HA user's voice to sound louder and hollow), for use with patients having chronic drainage, and for contralateral routing of offside signal (CROS) fittings.

Earmolds are available in several different materials. These range from hard acrylic to soft silicone plastics. Selection of a particular material for a given patient is based on age, facial flex issues, HA gain, allergic reactions, and ear stiffness.

The style and, to some extent, the material of the earmold can alter the frequency response of the amplified signal, affect the perceived quality of the patient's voice, and modify the potential for feedback. There are three primary earmold alterations that can affect the overall acoustic aspects of the coupling system. **Fig. 30–8** illustrates the consequence of *venting*, *damping*, and *horn effects* on the HA frequency response. Venting, a channel drilled through the body of the earmold, reduces feelings of fullness, prevents moisture, and alters low-frequency response. The combination of the location, diameter, and length of the vent has different effects on the low-frequency signal. In general, the shorter and wider the vent is, the greater the attenuation of low frequency. Dampers, a type of resistor placed in the HA earhook or tubing, alter the midfrequency response. Dampers cause acoustic resistance to the amplified signal to reduce resonant peaks in the frequency response, thus smoothing the response. To enhance the high-frequency region, "horn-shaped" tubing or "belled" bores (sound bores that widen at the end of the tube) are used. In contrast, a reverse-horn (sound bores that narrow at the end of the tube) decreases high-frequency output. It is important to understand the complex interaction of the earmold acoustics and the HA output when fitting HAs.

Monaural Versus Binaural

Unless it is medically or audiologically contraindicated, a bilateral hearing loss should be fit with binaural amplification. The major advantages of using two HAs include elimination of head shadow effect (attenuation of high frequencies by as much as 12 to 16 dB when sounds originate from the non-aided side), loudness summation (natural gain of 3 dB), binaural squelch (a 2- to 3-dB improvement in SNR, resulting in a 20 to 30% improvement in speech intelligibility), and localization. **Fig. 30–9** illustrates the benefits of binaural over monaural amplification for speech intelligibility in several different listening situations.[14] Note that speech intelligibility is progressively compromised as listening conditions become more difficult, even for normal-hearing individuals, but significantly more so for monaural amplification use only.

There are certain situations, however, when conventional binaural configurations are inappropriate. For example, patients with unilateral hearing loss or single-sided deafness (SSD) are not candidates for binaural amplification and are unable to take advantage of binaural hearing. SSD patients, however, experience a variety of perceptual difficulties including (1) understanding speech in the presence of background noise, (2) reduced sound localization ability, (3) hearing on the deaf side, and (4) elimination of binaural summation. For these

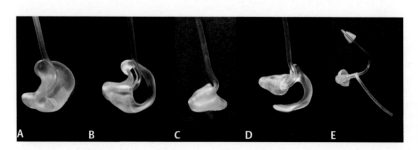

Figure 30–7 Photograph of five major types of earmolds: **(A)** shell; (B) skeleton; **(C)** canal; **(D)** open or CROS; and **(E)** noncustom.

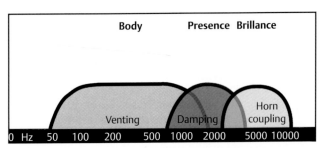

Figure 30–8 Region of the frequency response affected by earmold venting, damping, and horn coupling.

patients, or when a draining ear prohibits the use of a HA on that side, CROS fittings are an appropriate alternative. There are several CROS designs:

- *CROS:* CROS HAs assist patients who have no aidable hearing in one ear but have normal or near normal hearing in the opposite ear. **Fig. 30–10A** displays the CROS configuration and associated audiogram. As shown, the signal is picked up by a microphone located on the poor side and is transmitted to the opposite, better-hearing ear. Sound is transferred via a small cord running behind the head or through wireless transmission.

- *BiCROS* (bilateral CROS)*:* Candidates for BiCROS systems are those patients with asymmetric bilateral hearing loss where the poorer ear is unaidable (e.g., profound hearing loss or very poor word recognition ability). **Fig. 30–10B** displays the BiCROS configuration and associated audiogram. As shown, a microphone is located on each side of the head with the signal delivered (i.e., hardwired or wireless transmission) to a single amplifier and receiver in the better hearing ear. It is noteworthy that both the CROS and BiCROS systems assist with bilateral hearing but do not provide the patient with a true binaural listening experience.

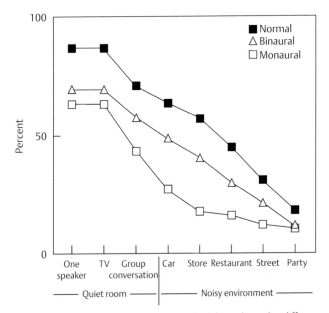

Figure 30–9 Percentage of speech intelligibility achieved in different listening situations for normal hearing and for users of binaural versus monaural amplification. (Adapted from Markides A. Binaural Hearing Aids. New York: Academic Press, 1977. Reprinted with permission.)

- *Transcranial CROS:* Transcranial CROS (**Fig. 30–10C**) is also referred to as a power CROS. Candidacy is similar to that for CROS fittings. In the transcranial CROS configuration, however, the patient is typically fit with a power in-the-ear HA in the nonfunctioning ear, and the vibrations created by the intense sound pressure level cross over the skull and stimulate the opposite cochlea.

Nonstandard Hearing Aid Fittings

- *Bone-conduction hearing aids:* These are appropriate for patients who (1) cannot wear conventional HAs that occlude the ear because doing so may exacerbate outer or middle ear pathology, or (2) have congenitally malformed or absent external or middle ears. In contrast to air-conducted signals, bone-conduction HAs use the vibration of a bone-conduction oscillator to stimulate the cochlea. To achieve adequate coupling of the oscillator to the head, the bone vibrator is typically mounted on one side of a headband, which uses spring tension to hold the bone vibrator against the head. Drawbacks of bone-conduction HAs include significant discomfort caused by the tension of the headband, attenuation of the bone-conducted signal caused by skin and muscle, and unacceptable cosmesis. Two alternatives, the Baha® hearing system and TransEAR™, are now available to alleviate many of the problems associated with both the CROS and bone conduction HAs. The Baha® hearing system involves the attachment of a vibrator to a surgically-place abutement and is appropriate for not only conductive hearing losses but also for patients with SSD. The Baha® hearing system will be discussed in detail in Chapter 31. The TransEAR™, is designed specifically for patients with SSD and places the bone vibrator in the nonfunctional ear to stimulate the contralateral cochlea, similar to the principle of the transcranial CROS.

- *Transposition hearing aids:* These are used on a very limited basis. Candidates include patients with no usable high-frequency hearing. These devices are intended to shift high-frequency signals to a frequency range where the patient has functional hearing. Although transposition HAs provide the listener with the perception of sound, a marked disadvantage is a significantly different sound quality. With advancement in technology, individuals who were previous candidates for transposition HAs may now be candidates for a hybrid cochlear implant system. This hybrid device is designed to activate the high-frequency region of the cochlea through the use of a cochlear implant while stimulating the low-frequency regions of the cochlea through the use of a low-frequency emphasis HA. The cochlear implant/HA combination may prove to be a superior alternative to the transposition HA.

Assistive Listening Device

For the majority of people with hearing loss, HAs are invaluable tools for improving quality of life. Yet even the best HAs cannot solve all of the communication problems faced by a person with hearing loss. Even with the most recent improvements in HA technology, it remains common for individuals with hearing impairment to experience difficulty in listening situations such as a noisy room, large auditorium, or on the telephone. These difficulties occur when noise is present in a listening situation, when the distance between the speaker and listener is greater

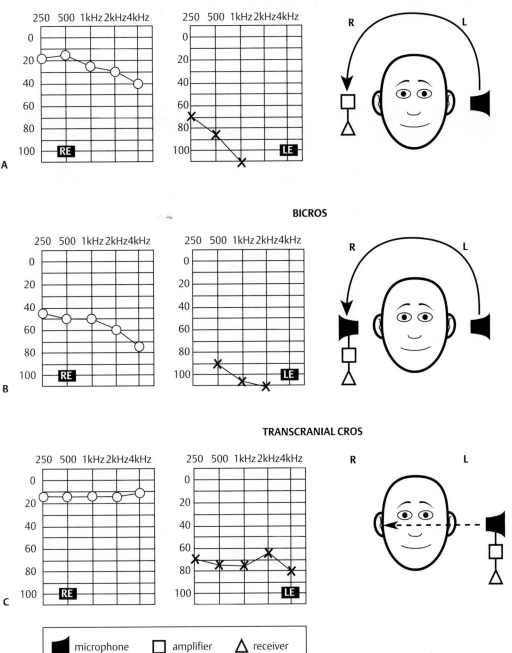

Figure 30–10 Examples of CROS types of HA fittings and associated audiogram: **(A)** CROS; **(B)** BiCROS; and **(C)** transcranial CROS. Note that the sound is picked up on the poorer side (in these examples, the left ear) and routed to the better ear (in these examples, the right ear).

than 3 feet, when the listening environment is reverberant (i.e., with echoes), or when speech quality is poor. Further, some individuals with hearing impairment are poor candidates for HAs because of cognitive (e.g., disorientation, decreased processing speed), physical (e.g., poor manual dexterity), or hearing limitations. Accordingly, the limited performance of HAs can be extended through the use of devices that aid in listening. With the addition of an ALD, the listening distance can be decreased, the speech level compared with the background noise level (SNR) can be improved, and poor room acoustics minimized. For example, FM (frequency modulated) systems

allow the talker's voice to be transmitted across the room directly to the listener, bridging the distance gap and reducing the effects of unwanted competing noise during listening situations.

Another class of devices, known as alerting devices, is available to alert the patient to sounds. The ability to be aware of background sounds and warning signals through the use of smoke/fire alarms, doorbell/telephone signalers (e.g., flashing light devices), and even alarm clocks (e.g., pillow vibrators) restores or maintains a patient's sense of security and independence.

◆ Hearing Device Fitting and Orientation

The next step in the AR model (**Fig. 30–1**) involves the fitting of the HA, which is a multistep process. During the initial appointment, the clinician verifies that the device fits comfortably in the patient's ear. Modifications to the earmold or shell may need to be made to maximize comfort. The HA is programmed to meet the listening needs of the individual. Several specific methods are available to program the device but are beyond the scope of this chapter. Regardless of the fitting protocol, care must be taken to ensure naturalness of the patient's voice, that output does not exceed loudness discomfort level, and that feedback is managed. Following the programming, the use and care of the devices/earmold is explained and demonstrated. The patient must demonstrate a good command of insertion/removal of the battery, manipulating the on/off switch of the device, switching programs, insertion/removal of the device from the ear, and anything unique in the use of the particular instrument. The use of the telecoil, if applicable, should also be reviewed. The initial orientation should be kept as simple as possible, postponing review of nonessential items to a follow-up appointment to avoid overwhelming the patient with too much information.

Hearing Device Verification/Validation

The fitting process is not complete until it has been determined that the HAs are performing as expected and providing the expected benefit (**Fig. 30–1**). The process of assessing the adequacy of the HA fitting is referred to as *verification*. Presently, clinicians have an ever-growing number of options to verify the HA fitting, including electroacoustic analyses, real ear measurements, aided sound field testing, and speech assessments (e.g., aided HINT, aided SPIN). Ultimately, though, we need to know if patients are perceiving improvement in their listening/hearing needs as a result of the intervention. This is documented through *validation* tools. Many tools are available to quantify the self-perceived reduction of activity limitation and participation restriction and improved communication success. Administering the COSI, HHIE/A, and APHAB, for example, in a pre- and posttest paradigm serves to validate intervention. In the current climate of health care, documenting outcome is a necessity rather than a preference.

Communication Improvement Training Follow-Up Services

Audiologic rehabilitation programs should be viewed as a solution-centered problem-solving process aimed at improving communication function at home, in social situations, and in the workplace. With the acknowledgment that HAs alone solve only a portion of the patient's everyday listening difficulties, audiologists routinely counsel patients about a variety of communication improvement techniques aimed at enhancing personal and social interactions. The ultimate goal of this training is to facilitate communication performance to improve the patient's quality of life.

Historically, AR programs for adults provided services emphasizing auditory training, speech reading (i.e., lipreading), or combined auditory-visual speech-perception training. Today, many AR programs focus on developing strategies geared at improving the patient's communication function and recognizing that the communication partner (e.g., spouse, child) is an integral component of the AR process. Accordingly, rehabilitation programs are designed to assist the individual with hearing loss as well as help the partner to communicate more effectively. **Table 30–2** summarizes sample intervention strategies aimed at reducing communication breakdown between hearing-impaired people and those persons with whom they interact (e.g., family, friends, coworkers).

◆ Treatment Effectiveness

The use of an AR model as previously presented is effective in reducing the psychosocial consequences of hearing impairment. Evaluating the effectiveness of HAs alone, Mulrow et al[15] administered the HHIE and the Denver Scale of Communication Function (DSCF)[16] to individuals who were seen for an HA evaluation. In this randomized, controlled clinical trial, half the subjects received HAs and half were assigned to a waiting list (i.e., control group). Both groups

Table 30–2 Sample Communication Improvement Training Techniques

Technique	Definition
Communication strategies	*Anticipatory* strategies are used before the communication situation arises in an attempt to minimize communication breakdown (e.g., anticipate possible dialogue or environmental problems).
	Repair strategies are used to overcome and rectify communication breakdown between the person with hearing impairment and partner (e.g., simplifying statements, summarizing comments, rephrasing sentences, providing key words).
	Facilitative strategies are used to optimize the communication environment (e.g., reduce background noise) and the communication partner's presentation of the message (e.g., slowing rate of speech).
Conversational fluency	Techniques used to improve the flow of conversation between individuals including such factors as turn-taking, and time-sharing (i.e., the proportion of time each communication partner talks during a given conversation). Viewing and analyzing videotaped conversations are used to monitor conversational fluency and improve performance.
Stress management	Individuals are shown how to recognize stressful reactions relating to communication breakdown. Relaxation techniques are taught to assist the patient cope with the physical and psychological responses to stressful situations.
Assertiveness training	Neutral and nonaggressive communication strategies used to promote improved communication performance by communication partners (e.g., "I am having difficulty understanding you, please slow down and speak up slightly") and requests to improve the communication environment (e.g., "I have a hearing loss and have difficulty hearing in this restaurant. Could I please be seated in a booth away from the kitchen and bar area?").

completed the HHIE and DSCF initially (pre–HA fitting for the HA group) as well as at 6 weeks and 4 months after the initial administration (post–HA fitting for the HA group). The findings reported comparable mean values between groups for each measure at the prefitting assessment. Yet the HA group showed significant improvements in social and emotional function (HHIE) and communication function (DSCF) for the 6-week and 4-month administrations, whereas the control group showed no changes in mean values across all three administrations. Other studies have demonstrated short-term (up to 6 months),[17–19] medium-term (7–12 months),[20,21] and long-term (greater than 12 months)[22] HA benefit. Together, these studies suggest that the HAs are beneficial for reducing the psychosocial consequences of the hearing impairment for years.

In addition to hearing-related benefits, the use of HAs has been shown to be related to functional health status and general psychological state. Crandall[23] administered the Sickness Impact Profile (SIP)[24] to a sample of new HA users and found improvements in both the physical and psychosocial domains of function following HA use. In a large survey study conducted by the National Council on Aging, 2069 individuals with hearing loss and 1710 family members provided compelling evidence that benefits from HA use included improvements in emotional stability, interpersonal relationships, overall health, and cognitive function, as well as reductions in anger, frustration, anxiety, social phobias, and depression.[25]

Coupling postfitting counseling-oriented AR programs with the fitting of HAs further assists patients to overcome residual communication difficulties. For example, Abrams et al[26] administered the HHIE as a measure of perceived change in social and emotional domains as a function of intervention strategy to three groups of individuals with hearing impairment: group I was fitted with HAs and participated in a 90-minute group counseling program that met once a week for 3 consecutive weeks; group 2 was fitted with HAs but did not participate in the group counseling program; and group 3 served as a control, receiving no HAs or counseling. For groups 1 and 2, the experimental groups, a reduction in self-perceived handicap was observed. An even greater reduction in self-perceived handicap was shown for group 1, those individuals who also participated in the postfitting counseling sessions, in comparison with group 2, which did not receive additional counseling. Other studies[18,27,28] have shown postfitting counseling to be beneficial in the AR process.

Finally, the cost-effectiveness of HA usage and the impact of an AR program have been examined.[29,30] Such studies are important in this era of cost-containment and justification to third-party payers showing the value of HA intervention. In this connection, Yueh et al[29] conducted a randomized control trial in a sample of veterans with bilaterally sloping moderate to severe SNHL. Individuals in the experimental arm of the study were fit bilaterally with ITE ASP HAs. Instruments fitted were either nonprogrammable, nondirectional HAs or programmable HAs with a switchable directional microphone. To conduct the economic analysis, each subject was asked the following question at the last experimental session: "If you lost your hearing device, how much would you be willing to pay to replace it?" Monthly incomes were adjusted for variations in each subject's income. Interestingly, patients were willing to commit 29% of their monthly income for the conventional and 78% for programmable HAs. These data suggest that patients not only see the value of HAs in general, but also

recognize improved performance of the more advanced HAs employing directional technology in particular. Using a different cost-effectiveness analysis method, namely dollar cost per quality-adjusted life-year (QALY) gained, Abrams et al[30] demonstrated that the cost of effecting change through the use of HAs alone ($60.00 per QALY) was reduced ($31.91) by the addition of a counseling-based postfitting AR program. Accordingly, the inclusion of such an AR program not only improves patient benefit but also is a cost-effective approach in the overall management of hearing loss.

Together, these findings demonstrate that fitting HAs as part of an ongoing process involving follow-up informational and adjustment counseling promotes increased benefit and satisfaction and reduced communication handicap associated with hearing impairment. Further, these studies demonstrate that the benefit derived from amplification and the AR process extends well beyond simply improving audibility, and has a major positive consequence on the person's overall quality of life.

◆ Conclusion

AR should be viewed from a biopsychosocial perspective. That is, the primary goal of the AR process is to help patients overcome the communication and psychosocial consequences of hearing loss. Accordingly, this chapter discussed the importance of amplification within a rehabilitative model that focuses on solving the everyday communication problems faced by patients with hearing loss and their communication partners, including family, friends, and coworkers. Thus, a more contemporary view of AR emphasizes the need to employ management strategies, one of which is the fitting of amplification, that help to restore the patient's functional ability, independence, social and professional interactions, and overall quality of life.

References

1. World Health Organization. The International Classification of Functioning, Disability and Health-IFC. Switzerland: World Health Organization Marketing and Dissemination, 2001
2. Kalikow DN, Stevens KN, Elliot LL. Development of a test of speech intelligibility in noise using sentence materials with controlled word predictability. J Acoust Soc Am 1977;61:1337–1351
3. Killion MC, Niquette PA, Gudmundsen GI, Revit LJ, Banerjee S. Development of a quick speech-in-noise test for measuring signal-to-noise ratio loss in normal hearing and hearing-impaired listeners. J Acoust Soc Am 2004;116:2395–2405
4. Nilsson M, Soli SD, Sullivan JA. Development of the Hearing in Noise Test for the measurement of speech reception thresholds in quiet and in noise. J Acoust Soc Am 1994;95:1085–1099
5. Cox RM, Alexander GC. The abbreviated profile of hearing aid benefit. Ear Hear 1995;16:176–186
6. Weinstein BE, Spitzer JB, Ventry IM. Test-retest reliability of the Hearing Handicap Inventory for the Elderly. Ear Hear 1986;7:295–299
7. Newman CW, Weinstein BE, Jacobson GP, Hug G. Test-retest reliability of the Hearing Handicap Inventory for Adults. Ear Hear 1991;12:355–357
8. Hickson L, Timm M, Worrall L, Bishop K. Hearing aid fitting: outcomes for older adults. Aust J Audiol 1999;21:9–21
9. Dillon H, James A, Ginis J. Client Oriented Scale of Improvement (COSI) and its relationship to several other measures of benefit and satisfaction provided by hearing aids. J Am Acad Audiol 1997;8:27–43
10. Jacobson GP, Newman CW, Fabry DA, Sandridge SA. Development of the three-clinic Hearing Aid Selection Profile (HASP). J Am Acad Audiol 2001;12:128–141
11. Ricketts T. Impact of noise source configuration on directional hearing aid benefit and performance. Ear Hear 2000;21:194–205

12. Ricketts T, Dhar S. Comparison of performance across three directional hearing aids. J Am Acad Audiol 1999;10:180–189

13. Strom KE. The HR 2005 Dispenser Survey. Hear Rev 2005;12(6):18–19, 22, 24–31, 34–36, 72

14. Markides A. Binaural Hearing Aids. New York: Academic Press, 1997

15. Mulrow CD, Aguilar C, Endicott J, et al. Quality-of-life changes and hearing impairment: a randomized trial. Ann Intern Med 1990;113: 188–194

16. Alpiner J, Chevrett W, Gascoe O, Metz M, Olsen R. The Denver Score of Communication Function [unpublished study]. Denver, CO: University of Denver, 1974

17. Malinoff RL, Weinstein BE. Changes in self-assessment of hearing handicap over the first year of hearing aid use by older adults. J Acad Rehab Audiol 1989;22:54–60

18. Primeau R. Hearing aid benefits in adults and older adults. Sem Hear 1997;18:29–36

19. Newman CW, Sandridge SA. Benefit from, satisfaction with, and cost-effectiveness of three different hearing aid technologies. Am J Audiol 1998;7:115–128

20. Taylor K. Self-perceived and audiometric evaluations of hearing aid benefit in the elderly. Ear Hear 1993;14:390–394

21. Tesch-Romer C. Psychological effects of hearing aid use in older adults. J Gerontol B Psychol Sci Soc Sci 1997;52:P127–138

22. Henrichsen J, Noring E, Lindemann L, Christensen B, Parving A. The use and benefit of in-the-ear hearing aids. A four-year follow-up examination. Scand Audiol 1991;20:55–59

23. Crandall C. Hearing aids: their effects on functional health status. Hear J 1988;51:22–30

24. Bergner M, Bobbitt RA, Carter WB, Gilson BS. The Sickness Impact Profile: development and final revision of a health status measure. Med Care 1981;19:787–805

25. Kochkin S, Rogin CM. Quantifying the obvious: the impact of hearing instruments on quality of life. Hear Rev 2000;70:6–34

26. Abrams H, Hnath-Chisolm T, Guerreiro S, Ritterman S. The effects of intervention strategy on self-perception of hearing handicap. Ear Hear 1992;13:371–377

27. Taylor KS, Jurma WE. Patients' task-orientation and perceived benefit of amplification in hearing-impaired elderly persons. Psychol Rep 1997;81: 735–738

28. Chisolm TH, Abrams HB, McArdle R. Short- and long-term outcomes of adult audiological rehabilitation. Ear Hear 2004;25:464–477

29. Yueh B, Souza P, McDowell J, et al. Randomized trial of amplification strategies. Arch Otolaryngol Head Neck Surg 2001;127:1197–1204

30. Abrams HB, Anath Chisolm T, McArdle R. A cost utility analysis of adult group audiologic rehabilitation: Are the benefits worth the cost? J Rehabil Res Dev 2002;39:549–558

Appendix 30–1 Characteristics of Amplification Tool (COAT)

Name: _____   Date: _____

MRN #: _____   Audiologist: _____

Our goal is to maximize your ability to hear so that you can more easily communicate with others. To reach this goal, it is important that we understand your communication needs, your personal preferences, and your expectations. By having a better understanding of your needs, we can use our expertise to recommend the hearing aids that are most appropriate for **you**. By working together **we** will find the best solution for you.

Please complete the following questions. Be as honest as possible. Be as precise as possible.

1. Please list the top three situations where you would most like to hear better. Be as specific as possible.

    _____

    _____

    _____

2. How important is it for you to hear better? Mark an X on the line.

    Not Very Important _____ *Very Important*

3. How motivated are you to wear and use hearing aids? Mark an X on the line.

    Not Very Motivated _____ *Very Motivated*

4. How well do you think modern hearing aids will improve your hearing? I expect them to:

    Not be helpful at all _____ *Greatly improve my hearing*

5. What is your most important consideration regarding hearing aids? Rank order the following factors with **1** as the most important and **4** as the least important. Place an **X** on the line if the item has no importance to you at all.

    _____ Hearing aid size and the ability of others not to see the hearing aids

    _____ Improved ability to hear and understand speech

    _____ Improved ability to understand speech in noisy situations (e.g., restaurants, parties)

    _____ Cost of the hearing aids

Hearing Aid Assessment

6. Do you prefer hearing aids that: (check one)

    _____ are totally automatic so that you do not have to make any adjustments to them.

    _____ allow you to adjust the volume and change the listening programs as you see fit.

    _____ no preference

7. Look at the pictures of the hearing aids. Please place an X on the picture or pictures of the style you would **NOT** be willing to use. Your audiologist will discuss with you if your choices are appropriate for you, given your hearing loss and physical shape of your ear.

8. There is a wide range in hearing aid prices. The cost of hearing aids depends on a variety of factors including the sophistication of the circuitry (for example, higher level technology is more expensive than the more basic hearing aids) and size/style (for example, the CIC hearing aids are more expensive than the BTE instruments). The price ranges listed below are for *two* hearing aids. Please check the cost category that represents the maximum amount you are willing to spend. Please understand that you are not locked into that price range. It is just very helpful for us to know your budget so that we can provide you with the most appropriate hearing aids.

    _____ Level 1 digital hearing aids: Estimated range: $U.S. to $U.S.

    _____ Level 2 digital hearing aids: Estimated range: $U.S. to $U.S.

    _____ Level 3 digital hearing aids: Estimated range: $U.S. to $U.S.

    _____ Level 4 digital hearing aids: Estimated range: $U.S. to $U.S.

Thank you for answering these questions. Your responses will assist us in providing you with the best hearing health care.

31

Implantable Hearing Devices

Charles C. Della Santina, Ryan M. Carpenter, Debara L. Tucci, and John K. Niparko

Advances in signal processing and implantable devices for the auditory system have led to a wide range of treatment opportunities for individuals with sensorineural hearing loss (SNHL). This chapter examines the neurobiology of SNHL, the development of technologies that enable a restored perception of sound, and the clinical application of implantable hearing technologies. We describe in detail practices related to cochlear implantation, including selection of candidates, techniques of device placement and activation, and the use of cochlear implants as a communication tool.

◆ Cochlear Implants

Cochlear implants are neural prostheses that convey sound information to the auditory nervous system via electrical stimulation of the auditory nerve, bypassing hair cells that are dysfunctional in deaf individuals. In a typical device, sound signals detected by a microphone are decomposed into spectral components that each vary in intensity with time. These variations are encoded by the intensity and timing of electrical current pulses delivered via multiple electrodes inserted into the cochlea, with each spectral component represented by the one or more electrodes positioned near the subset of auditory nerve fibers that are normally sensitive to the corresponding range of frequencies (**Fig. 31–1**).

Electrical currents delivered by cochlear implants activate the auditory pathway in deaf individuals through stimulation of the robust population of surviving auditory neurons that subserve the principal speech frequencies. A significant proportion of auditory nerve axons survives even when deafness is profound and early in onset, and these neurons retain their responsiveness to electrical stimulation (**Fig. 31–2**). Auditory neurons activated by the electrical stimulation convey via spike trains the physiologic code that can support the detection and discrimination of complex stimuli.

Cochlear implants support language acquisition by providing auditory informational cues that complement the visual cues available to individuals with profound hearing loss. For most young recipients, developmental learning in the early, formative years enables processing of information from the implant to facilitate speech comprehension and oral language development. As the developmental effects of profound hearing loss are multiple, cochlear implants have been applied to ever younger children in an attempt to mitigate delays in developmental learning, particularly with respect to oral language development, the outcome of primary interest in most cases.

The outcomes associated with cochlear implantation span a range and depend heavily on patient factors. Many patients see dramatic benefit from the implant and demonstrate remarkable functional performance, whereas others may not reach the levels of speech recognition or sound perception to which they aspire. In either case, hearing via a cochlear implant is not the same as normal hearing. Optimal outcomes rarely occur without careful assessment of candidacy to guide surgical and postoperative care. Establishing appropriate patient (or parent) expectations prior to implantation is an important adjunctive goal of candidacy assessment because unrealistic expectations can negatively impact patient participation in essential postoperative rehabilitative care.

Assessing Candidates for a Cochlear Implant

Comprehensive assessment of candidacy is essential to minimize risks and realize benefits of cochlear implantation. To ensure complete assessment of candidacy, clinicians should consider the many factors likely to affect performance with a cochlear implant, including audiologic, medical, surgical, developmental, cognitive, and psychosocial factors. Candidates (or parents) should understand that the cochlear implant is a communication tool and is not curative because expectations largely shape postoperative satisfaction with any form of auditory rehabilitation.[1]

Hearing History and Audiologic Testing

Candidacy should be considered in the context of current functional status and likely outcome with and without cochlear implantation. Patient age, etiology of hearing loss, unaided and aided audition, duration of deafness, and the circumstances of social support surrounding the candidate carry predictive value. Environments that enrich and promote spoken language are likely to exert a favorable influence over use of the device and contribute to maximal benefit from it.

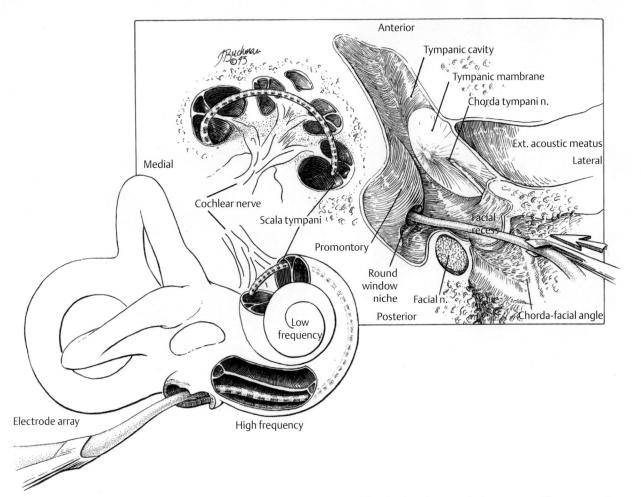

Figure 31–1 A cochlear implant is inserted into the scala tympani of the cochlea via the facial recess and a cochleostomy near the round window. The device's multiple electrodes rest near endings of the cochlear (auditory) nerve, which are arranged from apex to base according to the frequency of sounds to which they are normally sensitive. (Courtesy of J. Buchman, 1993.)

Tyler and Summerfield[2] observed evidence of the influence of auditory plasticity in adults with hearing loss of postlingual onset. Speech perception ability and the duration of profound/total deafness before implantation were negatively and significantly correlated. Performance improved over time after implantation. For adult patients, the level of performance measured shortly after implantation was, on average, about half the level measured eventually. Performance tended to reach an asymptote after about 3 years of implant use.

Such observations suggest that an established pathway for auditory processing is present even in profound SNHL and that refined processing develops over time. Though there are additional negative correlations between duration of deafness and performance,[2–5] such correlations do not apply to every case. Even a prolonged period of deafness does not rule out prospects for open-set speech understanding with a cochlear implant, provided that basic foundations of communicating through audition (e.g., prior hearing aid use, use of lip-reading, and the production of speech) are in place. The greatest contrast in performance of open-set speech recognition exists between adults who acquired deafness postlingually versus those with prelingual deafness.[6] Accordingly, the effect of prelingual deafness on the integrity of the central auditory pathway is an active area of investigation.[7–9] In children, clinical evidence of improved performance with earlier implantation[10] and the greater benefit with length of use in children[11] suggests that the effects of experience can have large effects on speech comprehension with longer implant use.

Preliminary consideration of implant candidacy in deafness is based on an individual's baseline hearing and experience with amplification. As a first approximation of SNHL severity, unaided, pure-tone thresholds are measured using age-appropriate behavioral testing or auditory-evoked potentials. Other objective testing may include measurement of otoacoustic emissions and the acoustic reflex. Although such tests are a useful adjunct in adults and a proxy for speech audiometry in young children, results should be viewed in light of the variability of speech discrimination that can occur with conventional amplification for a given level of SNHL on pure-tone audiometry.

Except in young children, criteria for implantation depend mainly on preoperative speech discrimination, rather than pure-tone audiometry. Currently, criteria vary somewhat across different manufacturers and health care payers but generally include an upper threshold of 40 to 50% words correct (with sentence presentation) for the poorer hearing ear, with up to 60% in the better ear and pure-tone average hearing loss (for 500, 1000, and 2000 Hz) of 70 dB or greater in both ears. As experience with cochlear implants has grown, outcomes have continued to improve, and candidacy criteria

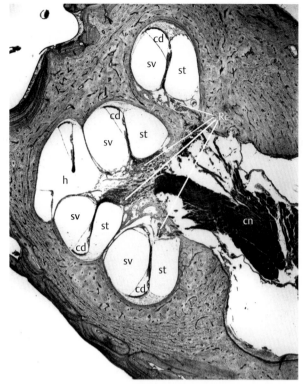

A

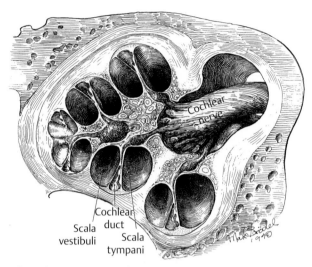

B

Figure 31–2 **(A)** Histologic section through the modiolus of a human cochlea (hematoxylin and eosin stain), and **(B)** corresponding artist's rendition, showing the spiral staircase arrangement of cochlear nerve cell bodies and distal sensory dendrites. Although distal processes may recede in deafness due to hair cell loss, viable cell bodies in Rosenthal's canal remain close to the stimulating electrodes of a cochlear implant in the scala tympani. St, scala tympani; cd, cochlear duct (scala media); sv, scala vestibule; Rc, Rosenthal's canal; cn, cochlear nerve; h, helicotrema. [**(A)** From Niparko JK, ed. Cochlear Implants: Principles and Practices. Philadelphia: Lippincott-Williams & Wilkins, 2000, with permission. **(B)** Courtesy of Max Brödel, Max Brödel Archives, Johns Hopkins School of Medicine, Baltimore, MD. Reprinted with permission.]

based on speech discrimination have continued to evolve toward higher levels of function over the past 25 years.[12,13] Mean recognition scores for words in isolation after implantation now far exceed the 40% level, and individuals with some preserved speech-recognition ability preoperatively often score substantially higher postoperatively than prior to implantation.[3,14] Residual hearing as reflected in aided speech-recognition levels is an important predictor of implant success.[4,5] When combined with duration of deafness, preoperative scores on tests of sentence recognition provide a predictive composite that accounts for approximately 80% of the variance in postoperative word recognition.[13]

An alternative approach to discrimination data in infants and toddlers employs criteria-referenced measures. The Meaningful Auditory Integration Scale (MAIS) consists of 10 questions directed to caregivers. The questions assess device (hearing aid or implant) bonding, spontaneous alerting to sound, and the ability to derive meaning from auditory events.[15] Osberger[16] found that MAIS scores of children with profoundly elevated baseline thresholds improved dramatically with cochlear implantation to levels that matched or exceeded those demonstrated by "gold" category hearing-aid users (i.e., those who achieved favorable outcomes through hearing aid use).

Selected pathologies present a unique challenge in the assessment of implant candidacy from an audiologic viewpoint. Starr and colleagues[17] described auditory neuropathy (AN), a distinctive type of hearing deficit in which the level of speech recognition impairment relates poorly to pure-tone audiometry. Patients with presumed AN have normal outer hair cell function (as revealed by the presence of oto-acoustic emissions, OAEs). Inner hair cell or eighth nerve impairment is suggested by an absent or abnormal auditory brainstem response (ABR). Other findings include absent acoustic stapedial reflexes and word recognition abilities that are disproportionately poorer than predicted from thresholds. Experience with cochlear implantation in children with AN remains largely anecdotal, with published findings varying between observations of high[18,19] to no[20] implant benefit. Interestingly, in children with AN who benefited with implantation, ABRs were generated with implant-mediated stimulation. This suggests that electrical stimulation achieved greater neural synchrony than occurred with conventional amplification.

Auditory-driven behaviors should also be assessed. The auditory skills assessment evaluates the child's ability to attend to and integrate sound with use of conventional amplification. A child may demonstrate residual hearing on audiologic evaluation, yet fail to show the skills needed to make use of that hearing in verbal communication. An auditory skills assessment determines a candidate's ability to attend to sound, to integrate auditory perception with speech production, to make meaningful associations with sounds, and to integrate hearing in social interaction. A speech-language pathologist can determine how a child communicates with others, the candidate's level of communicative intent, and the strategies used to support the intent to communicate.

The candidate's skills in nonverbal problem-solving, attention, and memory affect the postimplant rehabilitation process and may provide predictive information regarding potential use and benefit. Baseline cognitive and psychological assessment of candidates includes measurement of verbal and nonverbal intelligence, visual-motor integration, attention, motor development, behavior, and candidate/family stress. The evaluator counsels candidates or parents about expectations and notes whether these expectations reflect a realistic view of what an implant can provide. Unrealistic expectations are addressed early, to reduce the risk of later patient frustration and consequent device nonuse.

Optimal performance with a cochlear implant requires continued long-term use of the device. Observations that speech-recognition performance asymptotes only after at least 3 years of use, on average, for young children[21] and for adult users[2] underscore the importance of patient engagement with the intervention.

Placement in an appropriate school environment is a key factor in optimizing benefit from the implant in children, and arrangements for this should be put in place before implantation. The school experience should provide opportunity for flexibility as the auditory skills of an implanted child develop and requirements for communication support evolve.[22] An appropriate school environment provides stimulation of audition, maximum attention to language development, encouragement of spoken language, opportunities to interact verbally with adults and peers, and appropriate support services.

Otologic and Medical Assessment

Medical examination yields essential information about the health status of the candidate by identifying potential health concerns and determining suitability for general anesthesia. An otologic evaluation, including history and physical examination, is essential to identifying structural changes in the temporal bone that may affect surgical approach and feasibility. Clinical evaluation of the vestibular system may help to guide the choice of which ear is implanted, and may help predict whether implantation will produce vestibular sequelae.

Establishing the precise etiology of deafness may affect strategies for surgical implantation and postoperative rehabilitation. Meningitis may induce cochlear ossification, and cochlear dysplasia may require special consideration of the surgical plan.[23,24] Cochlear otosclerosis and temporal bone fractures may be more likely to manifest adventitial facial nerve stimulation with activation of the implant,[25] thereby necessitating a considered choice of implant system.

Eustachian tube dysfunction is commonly encountered in childhood candidates. Early management of eustachian tube dysfunction can facilitate accuracy in assessing the level of SNHL and response to amplification.

Tympanic membrane perforations may require treatment before implant surgery. Patients with chronic suppurative otitis media resistant to treatment or poor pneumatization may be treated with obliteration of the mastoid cavity and external canal closure, followed by cochlear implantation at a second operation 3 to 6 months later.[26,27]

Luntz et al[28] found that 74% of children had one or more episodes of acute otitis media before implantation, whereas only 16% had the same diagnosis after implantation. Reduced infection rates were thought to be due to the natural tendency for otitis media to diminish with age, the use of intraoperative

and perioperative antibiotics, and the effect of air cell removal as part of the mastoidectomy.

Vestibular Assessment

The main goal of vestibular function assessment prior to cochlear implantation is to identify significant asymmetry in labyrinthine function, so that cochlear implantation may be directed when possible to the ear with the weaker labyrinth. Although 50% of candidates tested with standard calorics[29] and 40% of those tested using head impulse testing[30] have bilateral vestibular hypofunction to some degree, significant asymmetry is common. When measured using caloric exams, 23% of 43 cochlear implant candidates exhibited ≥20% asymmetry of vestibular function.[29] In another study, ice water caloric testing identified unilateral profound vestibular loss in 11% of 47 candidates.[31] When measured using the quantitative head impulse test, 13% of 16 candidates had significant asymmetry.[30]

Cochlear implantation carries a 38% risk of some loss and approximately a 10% risk of severe or profound loss of vestibular function in the implanted ear as measured by caloric tests.[31] When measured using quantitative head impulse testing, the risk of significant loss is approximately 10%.[30] Because preexisting profound unilateral vestibular loss may be a marker for reduced tolerance of vestibular injury, the risk of implanting an "only balancing ear" may be even greater. Of five patients who received cochlear implants contralateral to an ear with profound vestibular loss, two developed bilateral vestibular hypofunction (BVH) and one of the two suffered complete failure of vestibular reflexes.[31] Given this risk, cochlear implantation of an "only balancing ear" should only be performed after educating patients (or parents) about the possibility of inducing or exacerbating BVH, which can cause disabling postural instability, disequilibrium, and oscillopsia (degradation of visual acuity during head movement). At the same time, one should note that auditory input delivered by a cochlear implant can be essential to language development in young children, and that young patients generally compensate for the loss of vestibular function much more readily and completely than do adults.

At a minimum, vestibular assessment prior to cochlear implantation should include a focused history, a screening vestibular physical examination, and review of labyrinthine anatomy on computed tomography (CT) or magnetic resonance imaging (MRI) obtained for surgical planning. Inconclusive evidence of asymmetric vestibular function should prompt further investigation, including quantitative testing to clarify and document baseline function and to help guide choice of ear to implant.

Imaging Studies

High-resolution CT scans of the temporal bone define surgical anatomy and provide information about cochlear abnormalities that can aid the surgeon in surgical planning and patient counseling. Temporal bone CT scans should be obtained and reviewed for evaluation of temporal bone anatomy with attention to mastoid pneumatization, ossicular anatomy, position of great vessels, position of the facial nerve, caliber of the internal auditory canal (IAC), and labyrinthine anatomy.[32] Scans are examined for evidence of cochlear malformation and ossification, enlarged vestibular aqueduct, and other inner ear and skull base anomalies that can affect implant surgery (**Fig. 31–3**). CT findings of cochlear patency generally correlate with surgical findings,[33] but significant discrepancies can occur as a result of volume averaging.[34,35]

MRI may be a useful adjunct to CT for assessment of implant candidacy.[36–38] Whereas CT is the procedure of choice for detailing bony anatomy, MRI is ideal for imaging soft tissues such as the membranous labyrinth, nerves in the internal auditory canal, and soft tissue within a cochlea en route to cochlear ossification after meningitis. High-resolution T2-weighted MRI is especially helpful for determining cochlear patency (by revealing the presence or absence of fluid within the scalae) and the presence of absence of nerves within the IAC in cases of otic capsule dysplasia (**Fig. 31–4**).

Fast spin-echo (FSE) imaging and fast imaging employing steady-state acquisition (FIESTA) have an advantage over both conventional spin-echo T1-weighted images and conventional T2-weighted images, which require longer scan time. The speed advantage of FSE allows the radiologist to obtain thin-section (2-mm) high-resolution T2-weighted images with excellent contrast in a fraction of the time needed for conventional spin-echo techniques.[39] Arriaga and Carrier[40] compared FSE T2-weighted MRI sequences with CT. In four of 13 patients evaluated with this protocol and CT, the MRI provided information not available from the CT.

Consideration should be given to conditions for which a patient may need future assessment with MRI. Implantation of a magnet in the internal device may be contraindicated in these patients. A nonmagnetic modification of one commercially available device can be made for patients whose medical or neurologic condition mandates future MR studies.[41] Baumgartner et al,[42] however, found that MRI applied to cochlear implant patients using different devices, imaged at 1 Tesla, did not cause implant malfunction or patient injury.

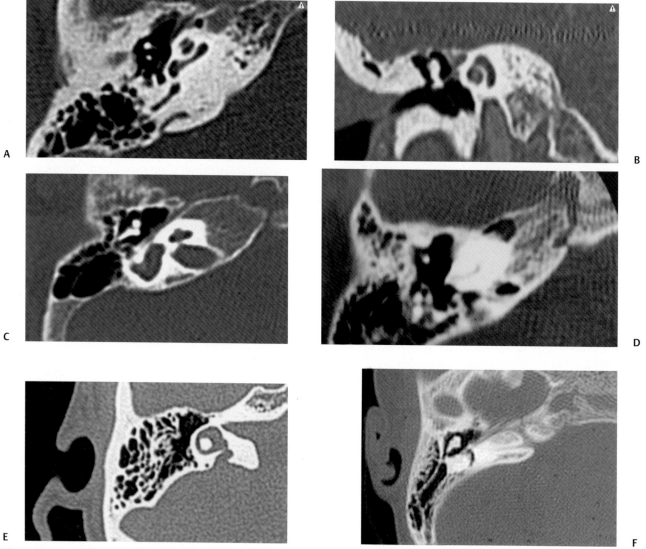

Figure 31–3   Axial **(A)** and coronal **(B)** CT scans of a normal right cochlea. **(C–F)** CT scans of the right ear in several cases of cochlear abnormality, including Mondini dysplasia **(C)**, cochlear ossification after meningitis **(D)**, enlarged vestibular aqueduct **(E)**, and absence of the internal auditory canal **(F)**.

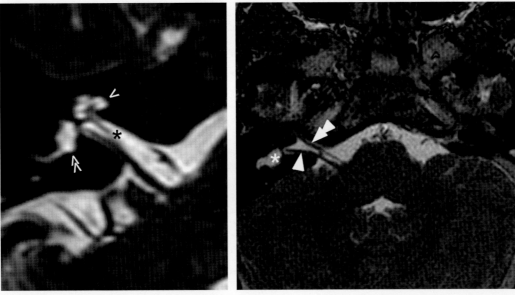

A

B

Figure 31–4 (A) Axial T2-weighted MRI through modiolus of the cochlea of a normal right ear. The cochlea (single arrowhead) is clearly patent, and the scala tympani and scale vestibuli are just distinguishable. The cochlear nerve is visible as a dark linear void in the bright cerebrospinal fluid (CSF) signal of the internal auditory canal (*), as is one branch of the vestibular nerve en route to the vestibule (double arrowhead). **(B)** Axial FIESTA MRI image of a 4-year-old girl undergoing evaluation for cochlear implant candidacy. CT revealed cochlear agenesis on the right and absence of the internal auditory canal on the left. The MRI was obtained to ascertain whether stimulable tissue existed in the right side, and shows a facial nerve (double arrow) and single branch of the eighth cranial nerve going to the vestibule. (Courtesy of C. C. Della Santina.)

Cochlear Implant Surgery

The need for stable interactions between the implant and target neurons underscores the importance of careful, atraumatic device insertion. Traumatic array placement has been associated with poorer outcomes in clinical trials of adults[43] and children.[44] The trauma of inserting the device is minimized through appropriate design and careful surgical technique. With normal cochlear anatomy, the scala tympani offers an easily accessed, mechanically shielded site for electrode placement near the dendrites and cell bodies of auditory nerve afferent fibers. Anatomically based design of electrodes arrays with preformed curvature, stabilized silicone carriers, and anisotropic stiffness helps minimize the risk of injury to the basilar membrane as the device slides within the turns of the scala tympani.

Contemporary cochlear implantation procedures represent modifications of surgical procedures historically employed in managing chronic infections of the mastoid and middle ear. Prophylactic antibiotics are routinely administered to provide coverage for the placement of a prosthetic device; however, the necessity for this measure has not been established. General anesthesia is employed, paralytic agents are avoided, and a facial nerve monitor is often employed. An extended postauricular incision is made (**Fig. 31–5**), and the mastoid cortex and surrounding squamosa portion of the temporal bone are exposed by raising a "flap" of mastoid periosteum pedicled anteroinferiorly. Soft tissue flaps should accommodate stable placement of the implant at a safe margin from overlying incisions and enable internal device placement sufficiently away from the pinna to leave room for an ear-level processor.

A simple mastoidectomy is performed, preserving a slight overhang at the superior and posterior cortical margins (**Fig. 31–6A,B**). This provides protection for the connecting leads. The facial recess is opened to maximize visualization of the incudostapedial joint and cochlear promontory after adequate thinning of the bony canal wall, opening of the antrum, and removal of adequate air cells to enable systematic exposure of the horizontal semicircular canal, fossa incudus, and chorda-facial angle (**Fig. 31–6C,D**).

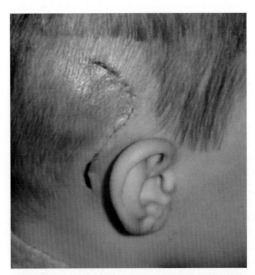

Figure 31–5 An extended postauricular incision (shown approximately 3 weeks postoperatively) used for transmastoid cochlear implantation. Many other incisions can be used. (Courtesy of John Niparko.)

419

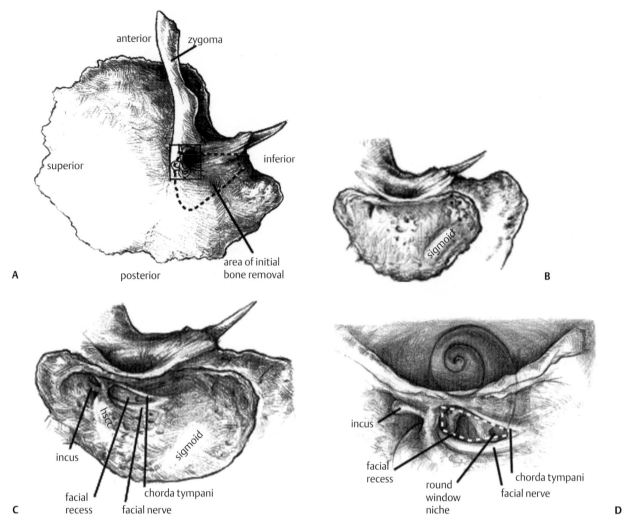

Figure 31–6 Surgical procedures for transmastoid cochlear implantation. **(A,B)** A cortical mastoidectomy is performed, identifying the incus and horizontal semicircular canal eminence (hscc) and keeping the mastoid tegmen, sigmoid sinus, and posterior ear canal wall (peacw) intact. The facial recess is opened **(C)**, the round window niche is identified **(D)**, a well for later placement of the device case is created, a cochleostomy is made anteroinferior to the center of the round window niche, and the electrode array is inserted along a trajectory tangent to the center of the basal turn of the scala tympani (*Continued*)

Before insertion of the electrode array, a well is created behind the mastoid to accommodate the receiver-stimulator portion of the internal device (**Fig. 31–6E**). The receiver-stimulator placement strategy should minimize protrusion, thereby reducing vulnerability to external trauma and restricting device movement, which can shear connecting leads and produce device exposure. If necessary, the overlying scalp is thinned to less than 7 mm in thickness to enable stable, magnetic retention of the external antenna. Hemostasis is confirmed prior to bringing the device into the surgical field, because use of monopolar electrocautery should be avoided once the implant is on the field.

Thinning of the bone anterior to the vertical segment of the facial nerve maximizes visualization of the round window niche via the facial recess (**Fig. 31–6D;** also see **Fig. 31–1**). As the dimensions of the tympanic cavity are established at birth and completed by 6 months of age, the risk associated with the facial recess approach is no greater in children than in adults.[45] However, anecdotal experience suggests that facial recess aeration may be less in children younger than 12 months of age. The chorda tympani nerve may be sacrificed if the facial recess is small or if the array to be implanted requires a generous exposure.[46] Permanent taste disturbance after chorda tympani sacrifice is rare. The round window niche should be exposed, and its tegmen and the round window membrane should be identified.[47] Inspection of the posterior promontory allows for identification of the round window niche if it is bridged with bone; the niche is never more than 2 mm from the inferior margin of the oval window. A cochleostomy accesses the scala tympani, either directly through the round window membrane or indirectly through the promontory anteroinferior to the center of the round window niche. The preferred approach is debatable, but the priority should be to access the scala tympani without inducing direct drilling-injury to the basilar membrane, while providing adequate space for unimpeded insertion of the array carrier.[48] The electrode array is advanced under direct visualization along a trajectory tangential to the basal turn of the scala tympani (**Fig. 31–6F,G**). Resistance to array insertion suggests the risk of buckling of the carrier. Because buckling of the implant can injure the spiral ligament, basilar membrane or cochlear nerve endings, aggressive

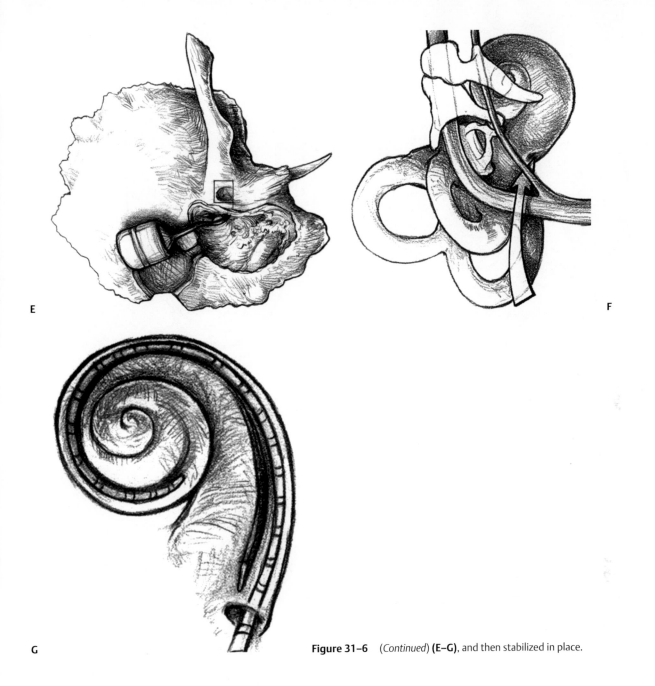

E

F

G

Figure 31–6 *(Continued)* **(E–G)**, and then stabilized in place.

insertion is avoided. Full insertion of the array within the basal turn of the cochlea requires an insertion depth of 25 to 30 mm, depending on array length. After insertion of the array the cochleostomy should be sealed gently with a small piece of fascia. The connecting lead should be stabilized within the facial recess to reduce the likelihood of the array extruding from the cochlea. Drilling a notch in the bridge of bone that defines the superior end of the facial recess provides a convenient slot in which the array lead can be stabilized.

Proximity of electrodes to targeted neuronal populations may influence channel selectivity. With closer approximation of electrodes to the modiolar wall, more focused stimulation of spiral ganglion cells may be achieved.[49] Prior designs of electrode arrays that achieved closer position of electrodes to modiolar neurons using shim-like positioners were abandoned due to suspicions of predisposition to meningitis.[50] Enhanced curvature of the carrier of the array is now favored as a strategy

to achieve closer positioning. **Fig. 31–7** shows examples of cochlear implant internal processors and electrodes that are currently available for clinical use in the United States.

Current electrode carriers are typically inserted over a distance of up to 25 or 30 mm (**Fig. 31–8**). Insertion along this length of the cochlea places electrodes of the array adjacent to fibers of the auditory nerve that normally subserve the entire range of speech frequencies.[51] The aim is to simulate the frequency analysis normally provided by basilar membrane mechanics and the tonotopic pattern of fiber activation within the cochlea. Is deep insertion necessary to achieve optimal performance? Certainly insertion beyond the first portion of the basal (first) turn of the cochlea intuitively seems necessary to approach midfrequency neurons. There is some evidence that speech perception improves with deeper insertion.[52] However, the need for insertion beyond 20 mm into the cochlea is as yet uncertain.

421

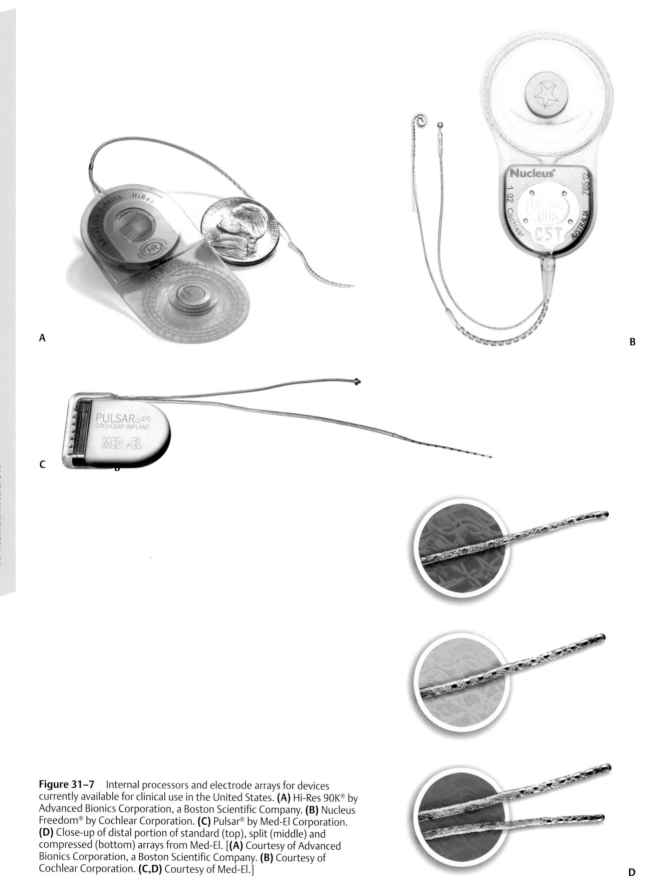

Figure 31–7 Internal processors and electrode arrays for devices currently available for clinical use in the United States. **(A)** Hi-Res 90K® by Advanced Bionics Corporation, a Boston Scientific Company. **(B)** Nucleus Freedom® by Cochlear Corporation. **(C)** Pulsar® by Med-El Corporation. **(D)** Close-up of distal portion of standard (top), split (middle) and compressed (bottom) arrays from Med-El. [**(A)** Courtesy of Advanced Bionics Corporation, a Boston Scientific Company. **(B)** Courtesy of Cochlear Corporation. **(C,D)** Courtesy of Med-El.]

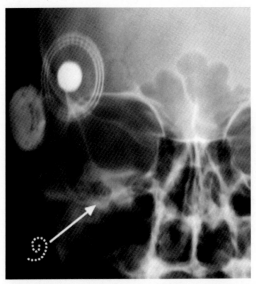

Figure 31–8 Anteroposterior view x-ray of a cochlear implant in place in the right ear, with the curved portion revealing the depth of insertion into the cochlea (see offset dashed line tracing of intracochlear portion). Postoperative acoustic-only audiometry confirmed no change from preoperative pure-tone thresholds, confirming atraumatic placement. (Courtesy of C. C. Della Santina.)

Once the electrode array is in place, the receiver-stimulator is stabilized with sutures to the bony cortex or by virtue of a tight-fit subjacent to the pericranium and deep fascia of the temporalis muscle. As the incision is closed, the implanted device is covered with the skin of the scalp.

Revision Surgery

The feasibility of revision implant surgery, including single-channel to multiple-channel conversion to enhance perception of spectral cues, is now well recognized.[53] However, patients facing reimplantation must be aware of the possibility of differences in sound quality and speech recognition after revision as occurs in roughly 10% of revision cases.[54,55] Revision surgery often entails the need for revising the cochleostomy so as to avoid impediment of the replaced array by the existing scar within the scala tympani.

Implantation of Young Children

Implantation of infants and toddlers can be achieved with no greater risk of complication than that observed for adults.[56–58] Experience with surgical implantation of young children has been reported by several centers, and results are encouraging.[58–60] The most significant developmental changes take place in the size and configuration of the mastoid cavity, which expands in width, length, and depth from birth into the teenage years. Studies with nonhuman primates have shown that because cochlear implantation does not affect growth around bony suture lines, there is no adverse effect on skull growth.[61] On the basis of measurements of skull expansion, Eby and Nadol[62] recommended allowing 2.5 cm of electrode lead redundancy in the mastoid to accommodate head growth and to avoid electrode extrusion. Redundancy of the connecting lead actually does not appear to stabilize the electrode carrier unless it is protected from the tethering effects of connective tissue within the mastoid cavity.

Implantation in Children with Cochlear Ossification and Obstruction

Obstruction of each of the scalae may occur due to inflammatory changes (associated with meningitis, Cogan's syndrome, syphilis, chronic otitis media, and malignant otitis externa), otosclerosis, and trauma.[63] Labyrinthitis ossificans results in the formation of fibrous tissue, with the possibility of subsequent dystrophic calcifications deposited in the normally fluid-filled scalae. The scala tympani, especially in the basal turn, is the most common site of fibrous tissue and new bone growth, regardless of the etiology. However, near-total ossification of the cochlea as shown in **Fig. 31–3D** is unusual. Green et al[64] reported only two cases of total ossification of 24 specimens with some degree of ossification. Balkany et al[65] found that electrode insertion was possible in more than 90% of ossified cochleae. Fayad et al[66] found ossification of the scala tympani that required drilling in 30% of 20 patients with cochlear otosclerosis, but the extent of ossification did not exceed 5 mm in any patient. Performance with the implant was found to be similar to that of patients without ossification.

Because many patients with cochlear ossification receive only partially inserted electrode arrays, performance may suffer either because of smaller numbers of available channels or spiral ganglion cell depletion. However, studies of implant performance with ossified cochleae have shown that general levels of auditory performance are similar to those of patients with patent cochleas.[67,68] In a group of children with postmeningitic deafness (PMD), Francis and colleagues[69] found no significant delays in cognitive performance or speech perception, with the exception of those children who exhibited evidence of meningitis-related hydrocephalus. Thirty-three percent of the children in the PMD group required drill-out of the scala tympani to at least the first turn of the cochlea, and 7% of the group had an incomplete electrode insertion. Data from this case series of 30 children suggest that central factors hold sway in predicting audiologic performance and that ossification does not preclude open-set speech recognition. At this time, however, no performance data are available to guide the surgeon in the choice between an extensive drill-out procedure[70] that may allow complete electrode insertion or a more limited, less invasive procedure likely to allow only partial insertion of the electrode array.

Modified electrode designs may be used when ossification is suspected prior to operation. Compressed arrays include the same number of electrode contacts over a shorter length than conventional arrays (**Fig. 31–7D**). The split electrode offers the same number of electrode contacts on two carriers; one can be inserted through the conventional cochleostomy and another through an apical cochleostomy created distal to the obstruction.[71]

Implantation in Children with Cochlear Dysgenesis

A significant percentage of children with deafness of congenital onset exhibit cochlear malformation, typically manifested as cochlear hypoplasia (**Fig. 31–3C**) or a common cavity.[72] Hypoplastic cochleas are associated with poor definition of cochlear turns and partitions between the modiolus and IAC and relatively low spiral ganglion cell populations.[73] When associated with a narrow or absent IAC on preoperative CT scanning (**Fig. 31–3F**), innervation may be completely absent[74] as supported by electrical evidence of lack of excitability with preoperative testing by means of a transtympanic electrode.[75] Implantation of an ear with a severely narrowed IAC is thus contraindicated in the absence of evidence of peripheral auditory function. Preoperative electrical testing may help in determining this.

Mondini malformation (hypoplasia of the cochlea) is associated with shorter length and relatively low spiral ganglion cell populations, and often has a thin bony partition between the modiolus and a widened IAC.[74] The latter anomaly accounts for the cerebrospinal fluid leak that can occur during a cochleostomy for electrode insertion. Other anomalies involving the round window niche and facial nerve have been observed in association with cochlear malformations.[75,76] Despite associated anomalies, implantation of a sufficient number of electrodes within a malformed cochlea is feasible and can provide a surprising degree of speech perception in many subjects.[75]

Complications of Cochlear Implants

Cochlear implantation entails risks inherent in extended mastoid surgery and those associated with the implanted device. Cohen and colleagues[77] characterized implant-related complications as *major* if they required revision surgery, and *minor* if they resolved with minimal or no treatment. A survey reported 55 major (12%) and 32 minor (7%) complications. Webb et al,[78] reporting their experience with 153 patients, found 13.7% major complications and 13.7% minor complications. Hoffman and Cohen[79] noted that in later follow-up 220 (8%) major and 119 (4.3%) minor complications occurred among 2751 implantations. Direct comparisons of complication rates between reports fail to include information on duration of device use, and studies vary in length and frequency of follow-up. Notwithstanding these limitations, longitudinal tracking indicates a substantial reduction in the incidence of major complications in the past 10 years.[79]

Major complications include facial nerve paralysis and implant exposure due to flap loss. Facial nerve injury is uncommon and, when recognized promptly, unlikely to produce permanent, complete paralysis. Loss of flap viability can lead to wound infection and device extrusion, necessitating scalp flap revision and when intractable infection is present, device removal with or without replacement.

Device Failure

Major complications that are strictly device-related involve partial or complete device failure. As the materials used to fabricate the internal device are expected to maintain a hermetic seal for beyond 100 years, use-related failure per se is not expected. Device failure is attributed to either flaws in manufacturing or trauma. Device failure as a result of loss of electrical function in the external processor commonly produces a sudden loss of function and, therefore, hearing. Intermittency and rarely "popping" sensations occur before processor failure. External processor function may be lost with direct trauma, exposure to water, and, most frequently, normal wear and tear of connecting lead-wires linking the processor unit with the magnetically retained antenna that relays information to the internal device.

Although much less prevalent, device failure as a result of loss of electrical function in the internal device is of considerably greater concern. An internal device failure typically presents as either an immediate cessation of function or intermittency associated with reduced quality of sound and a period of diminishing function over days to weeks. Reports of painful stimulation have been noted, but are rare.

Diagnosis of the mode of failure of an internal device is hampered when the implant lacks telemetry to enable electrical assessment of all contained circuits. When telemetry is available, removing select channels from the "map" of stimulated circuits may allow for continued function. In the absence of telemetry, revision surgery may be the only alternative.

Explanted devices are sent to the manufacturer for assessment of circuit integrity. Formal data on analyses of explanted devices have yet to be reported. However, for the purposes of this review the senior author interviewed manufacturers' engineers and found general trends in patterns of failure across manufacturers. Of devices with a recognizable fault, the general pattern of failure mode occurs with a relative incidence of:

- Hermeticity or moisture: 75%
- Electronic/hybrid failure: 16%
- Electrode/connecting lead: 9%

Cochlear implants have maintained a historical reliability of 99% at 1 year. Reported trends suggest that device reliability has improved over the past 30 years.[80] For example, the failure rate for the third-generation Cochlear Corporation (Lane Cove, New South Wales, Australia) device released in 2001 (0.3% per year) is approximately one third of that associated with their first-generation device (0.8%) used from 1985 to 1998. The United States Food and Drug Administration (FDA) has examined manufacturing processes at all three major manufacturers with public disclosure of concerns relating to two of the three companies.[81,82]

Device failure is the most common indication for revision surgery and cochlear reimplantation. "Upgrades" to more advanced models are rarely indicated, as the level of performance enhancement achievable is subject to individual case consideration. Infection and flap breakdown require reimplantation less frequently.[83]

Luetje and Jackson[84] reported a 9% rate of device failure in a review of 55 children. Their findings matched results found by Parisier et al.[85] The most common failures included fracture of the central pin feed-through for the antenna coil, damaged integrated circuits in the internal receiver from electrostatic discharges (occasionally associated with contact and friction with playground-grade polyethylene), damaged electrodes at the point of exit from the internal receiver, capacitor failure, and electrode-array damage.

Detection of device failure is imperative in the implanted child. The analysis of Parisier et al identified four major risk factors that point to failure: fluctuations in threshold and comfort levels of nine units for more than six electrodes, performance incompatible with age and duration of deafness, complaints of extraneous noises and intermittent shocks, and a high number of external equipment changes. Tests on the device showing an absence of recorded output, abnormal pulse configuration, or lack of amplitude increase in response to increased stimulation can verify failure. Weise et al[86] found evidence of head trauma contributing to a greater risk of device failure in children relative to adults.

Prevention of device failure begins with proper securing of the implant, particularly the connecting lead between the receiver/stimulator and the electrode array, where the device is vulnerable to shearing. Surgeons should secure the device by embedding it in a well drilled in bone and fixing it in place with permanent suture material. Although the evolution of implant design has diminished the rate of device failure, these precautions may help to shield the device from traumatic events.

Implant Infection and Meningitis

The risk of bacterial infection of an implanted device producing labyrinthitis or meningitis and associated reactive fibrosis and destruction of neural elements appears to be low. Franz et al[87] inoculated the bullae of implanted cats with streptococci to evaluate the risk of infection spreading from the middle ear into the implanted cochlea. Despite resulting inflammation of the round window niche, cochlear inflammation was absent. This finding was attributed to a seal that had formed around the electrode at the entrance to either the round window or the cochleostomy, thus forming a protective barrier against implant-surface colonization and bacterial biofilm.[88]

In 2002, an increase in the number of postimplantation meningitis cases was noted anecdotally. Initial reports suggested a higher risk of meningitis in patients implanted with a particular device design and particularly when placed with an intracochlear shim (electrode positioner) and the manufacturer ultimately recalled unimplanted devices utilizing the positioner. The level of risk did not suggest the need for positioner removal unless repeated infections occurred. Since then, continued studies have revealed a higher risk for the disease in patients with all cochlear implants compared with the general population. Children appear to be particularly affected: of the 52 cases originally reported by the FDA, 33 (63%) were under the age of 7.

Reefhuis et al[50] conducted a study of 4264 children implanted between 1997 and 2002 and found 29 cases of bacterial meningitis in 26 children. This rate of meningitis (caused by *Streptococcus pneumoniae*) was 30 times the incidence in the general population. Although the use of a positioner increased the likelihood of contracting meningitis, even children implanted without a positioner had rates of meningitis 16 times higher than the general population. Case-control analysis found the following risk factors: a history of placement of a ventriculoperitoneal cerebrospinal fluid (CSF) shunt, a history of otitis media prior to implantation, the presence of CSF leaks alone or inner-ear malformations with CSF leak, the use of a positioner, incomplete insertion of the electrode, signs of middle-ear inflammation at the time of implantation, and exposure to smoking in the household. Although the incidence of meningitis decreased considerably after the perioperative period, cases still appeared even 2 years after implantation.

The design of the study conducted by Reefhuis et al, as noted by the authors, did not permit the comparison of meningitis risk between deaf children with and without a cochlear implant. That is, there is no comprehensive epidemiologic analysis of the risk of meningitis in deaf children in general. It is biologically plausible that deafness itself poses greater risk of meningitis given the strong association of deafness with skull base anomalies that predispose individuals to the disease. It is also possible that any surgical implant placed in or near the skull base of toddlers and young children (e.g., CSF shunts) does indeed carry a prolonged risk of meningitis.

Cochlear Implant Programming

Initial activation of the cochlear implant typically takes place 3 to 6 weeks after implantation to allow sufficient time for healing of the surgical incision and resolution of the accompanying edema. During routine use of the cochlear implant system the implanted device receives input from an external battery powered speech processor housed in a behind-the-ear unit similar to a hearing aid or in a "body" style encasement worn at the waist, in a pocket, or otherwise harnessed to the body. A microphone captures acoustic input and delivers it to the speech processor, which, in turn, encodes the signal. An external antenna magnetically retained behind the ear transmits the encoded signal across the scalp via radio frequency to the antenna of the internal device. Examples of external equipment are shown in **Fig. 31–9.**

The object of device programming is to establish a set of parameters that will result in optimized access to and perception of auditory input for a given patient. The input and output characteristics of the program or "map" depend on factors such as the microphone response pattern and sensitivity, compression, channel gain, frequency allocation, and feature extraction. The electrode array can stimulate the auditory nerve using pulsatile or analog currents with presentation options from fully simultaneous across electrodes to one or more pairs to sequential. Physiologic measures, behavioral methods, sound-field audiometry, standardized tests, feedback from rehabilitation and educational professionals, and patient report contribute to considerations made in the programming process. In most cases programming decisions revolve around maximizing speech recognition and achieving audibility of all critical components of the speech signal. However, in some cases—for example prelingual hearing loss in an older child without a history of spoken language experience or with multiple sensory deficits—the target outcome may be improved awareness of environmental sounds, speech-reading support, or better functional communication through a combination of manual and oral language.

Dynamic Range

Among the first and most important steps prior to activating the cochlear implant is to determine appropriate stimulation levels. After establishing a connection between a computer and the implant and measuring electrode impedances via back telemetry, the clinician can begin to demarcate the dynamic ranges of individual electrodes in the implanted array. Maximizing the dynamic range is important because it is typically much smaller for electrical stimulation via a cochlear implant than for acoustic stimulation of the normal ear. Normal behavioral responses to acoustic stimulation span approximately 120 dB with corresponding individual fiber dynamic ranges of 20 to 40 dB, whereas corresponding dynamic ranges in electrical stimulation span only 10 to 40 dB and 7 to 10 dB, respectively.[89,90] Compression schemes are required to compact the wide range of sound intensities in the normal acoustic environment into the relatively narrow electrical range between threshold of audibility and the maximum stimulus intensity tolerated by a patient.

Setting individual electrode stimulation levels appropriately carries great importance in establishing an optimally functional program, as failure to do so may result in reduced audibility or discomfort and adversely effect speech recognition.[91,92]

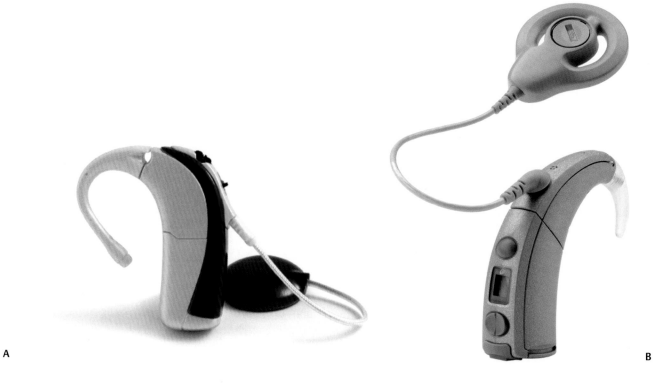

A

B

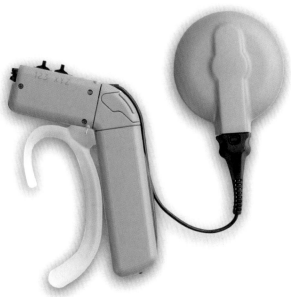

C

Figure 31–9 External behind-the-ear speech processors for Advanced Bionics, a Boston Scientific Company **(A)**, Cochlear Corporation **(B)**, and Med-El **(C)** cochlear implant systems. [**(A)** Courtesy of Advanced Bionics: a Boston Scientific Company, **(B)** Courtesy of Cochlear Corporation. **(C)** Courtesy of Med-El.]

Programming levels vary based on etiology of hearing loss,[93] spiral ganglion cell survival,[94] electrode positioning,[95] and listener experience with the implant. Minimum and maximum programming levels typically increase in the first 3 to 6 months and dynamic range widens due to a greater rate of increase in the upper limits than in minimum or threshold levels.[96,97] These levels typically begin to plateau and stabilize beyond 1 year after initial activation.[98] Electrode arrays with perimodiolar intracochlear placement tend to require lower programming levels[95] and may enable stimulation of more discrete subpopulations of nerve fibers.[99] Stimulation levels at the upper programming limit typically range from 8 to 24 nanocoulomb (nC)/phase.[100] Clinicians should take care not only to set electrode dynamic ranges accurately, but also to balance for equal loudness across electrodes at the extremes of their dynamic ranges.[92] With appropriate programming the patient can generally gain audibility thresholds as good as 20 to 30 dB HL across the speech frequencies (250–8000 Hz).

Objective Measures of Neural Response

Behavioral methods used in device programming require patient responses and sophisticated psychophysical judgments that may be difficult and time-consuming. Young children, older children with limited auditory experience, prelingual hearing loss, or language delay, and even some adults may not offer sufficiently reliable responses to enable optimal programming by behavioral techniques alone. As the minimum age of implantation has declined, the need for objective programming methods has increased. This need has prompted the investigation of several physiologically based methods to facilitate programming in very young children.

Back Telemetry of Neural Responses

Current cochlear implant technology includes back telemetry capabilities, meaning that the intracochlear stimulating electrodes may also serve as recording electrodes. An amplifier in the cochlear implant measures electrical activity detected at the electrode array and relays it back to the external computer for analysis. Commercially available software from two major cochlear implant manufacturers utilizes this capability to allow measurement of the electrically evoked compound action potential (ECAP) from within the cochlea. This is referred to as neural response telemetry (NRT) by Cochlear Corporation or neural response imaging (NRI) by Advanced Bionics (a Boston Scientific Company). Med-El (Innsbruck, Austria) is also developing this capability.[101]

The ECAP is characterized by a negative peak (N1) 200 to 400 microseconds (μs) after the stimulus onset[102–104] followed by a smaller positive peak (P1) around 700 ms[104] and a response amplitude (N1-P1) of up to 0.2 μV.[102] Response amplitudes are larger[105] and thresholds lower[104] toward the apex of the cochlea and responses may not show a "tuning" around the stimulating electrode.[105] **Fig. 31–10** shows an example of a single NRT response recorded with a Nucleus Freedom cochlear implant. **Fig. 31–11** shows similar results for a series of NRI responses recorded with an Advanced Bionics HiRes 90K device.

Although ECAP response thresholds predict the *contour* of behavioral threshold levels fairly well, and to a lesser extent comfort levels, they do not predict *absolute* behavioral levels. ECAP thresholds almost always lie above the threshold of audibility and usually within tolerance limits, but they may exceed maximum comfort levels.[104,106] Typically, response thresholds vary from approximately 53 to 71% of the behavioral

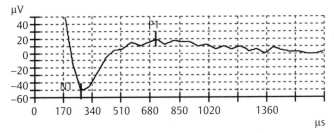

Figure 31–10 Electrically evoked compound action potential in a 14-year-old child showing typical response morphology with peaks N1 and P1. This response was recorded with a Nucleus Freedom cochlear implant using Neural Response Telemetry software (CustomSoundEP 1.2.5). Recording parameters were active electrode, 14 clinical units; recording electrode, 16 clinical units; stimulus level, 174 clinical units. (Courtesy of Cochlear Corporation.)

dynamic range[107–110] depending in part on duration of listener experience with electrical hearing, electrode proximity to the modiolus, and electrode insertion depth (**Fig. 31–12**). In general, ECAP response thresholds show moderate-to-strong correlations with behavioral responses. These correlations are strongest when ECAP-based predictions of programming levels incorporate data from behavioral measurements on at least one electrode.[106,107,111] Correlation coefficients between NRI/NRT and maximum and minimum programming levels range from 0.35 to 0.89 and 0.55 to 0.94, respectively.[104,106–109,111–113]

Electrically Evoked Auditory Brainstem Responses

Unlike the ECAP, electrically evoked auditory brainstem responses (EABR; **Fig. 31–13**) are measured with surface electrodes. Like ECAPs, EABR thresholds correlate with behavioral programming levels.[103,104,106,114] However, EABR has the disadvantages of susceptibility to muscle artifact, small response amplitude, inconvenience of applying electrodes, and a mismatch between the typical rate of stimulation used to elicit the EABR and that used in cochlear implant programming. If used intraoperatively, EABR measurements can extend surgery time, and if used postoperatively sedation may be required. These disadvantages have led to a decline in clinical use of the EABR for programming purposes, with a corresponding rise in use of ECAPs.

One important difference between ECAP responses and EABR is that EABR represents neural activity higher in the brainstem than do ECAPs. Thus, response rates and the significance of responses may differ between the tests. For example, Morita et al[104] described a patient who had ECAP responses but showed no response to EABR. The authors attributed absence of the EABR to speculated metabolic neuropathy in the brain (due to mucopolysaccharidosis). Another study reported fewer "no response" results for EABR (5%) than for ECAP (12–16%).[103]

Electrically Evoked Stapedius Reflex Threshold

A third physiologic programming method involves the electrically evoked stapedius reflex threshold (ESRT). A response threshold is determined by varying the stimulus level delivered to the cochlear implant while observing stimulation-related compliance changes at the tympanic membrane (**Fig. 31–14**). ESRTs correlate with upper programming (comfort) levels with correlation coefficient values ranging from 0.91 to 0.95.[111,115] Threshold responses correspond almost equally to absolute maximum comfort levels.[111,112] ESRT thresholds tend to be higher in the apex than ECAP thresholds in the same region.[103] Due to abnormal tympanometry, lack of patient cooperation, or other reasons, ESRTs were not measurable in 32% of 25 adults[115] and in 28% of 68 children.[103]

Objective Measures as Adjuncts to Programming

Most if not all published research to date (as of September 2005) has used behavioral programming levels as the gold standard against which physiologic methods are measured. However, in practice, these measures complement one another and even reverse roles at times. For example, Overstreet[116] reported cases of poor speech perception when behaviorally measured levels were unusually high or low and

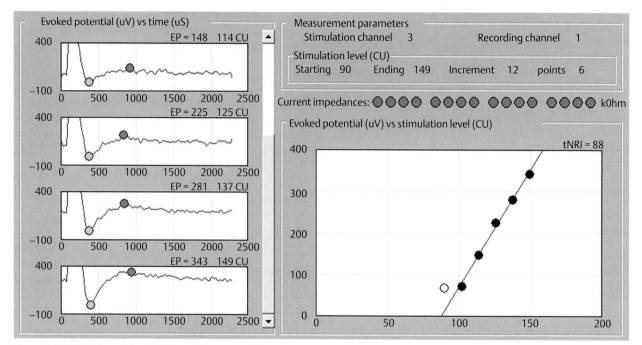

Figure 31–11 Series of electrically evoked compound action potentials recorded with an Advanced Bionic HiRes 90K cochlear implant using neural response imaging (NRI; Soundwave Professional Suite 1.1.38). Shown in the left panel are also plotted graphically in the right panel as a function of stimulus level. Note the linear amplitude growth function. The X intercept, in this case at 88 clinical units marks the calculated NRI response threshold. Recording parameters were as follows: active electrode, 3 clinical units; recording electrode, 1 clinical units (apical); stimulus level, 90 to 149 clinical units. (Courtesy of Advanced Bionics, a Boston Scientific Company.)

did not agree with physiologic data. Programming levels were adjusted to more closely resemble the physiologic responses and speech perception and sound quality improved. In some cases NRI showed adaptation following prolonged use of excessive programming levels. Consequently, a period of cochlear implant disuse was required before NRI threshold levels returned to baseline. Similar cases have been observed by the authors and have been reported anecdotally.[117]

On average, speech perception with programming based on physiologically derived levels is equal to or nearly equal to that achieved with behaviorally based programming.[105,118] However, experience suggests that, where possible, physiologic measures should not be used in isolation and that optimal outcomes are most likely to result from a combination approach that considers the results of behavioral and objective measures. Whatever the technique utilized to set them, stimulation levels and other programming parameters should be verified and validated through functional outcomes and objective data.

Results and Outcomes of Cochlear Implants

Cochlear Implant Results in Adults

Evaluation of the benefit of cochlear implantation in adults has largely focused on measuring gains in speech perception. Multivariate analysis, a statistical technique that determines the role of individual factors contributing to variation in performance, is most commonly employed.[3–5,119–121] The following are among the factors that have been evaluated:

- Subject variables: age of onset, age of implantation, deafness duration, etiology, preoperative hearing, survival and location of spiral ganglion cells, patency of the scala tympani, cognitive skills, personality, visual attention, motivation, engagement, communication mode, and auditory memory.
- Device variables: processor, implant, electrode geometry, electrode number, duration and pattern of implant use, and the strategy employed by the speech processing unit.

Of all identifiable variables, Rubinstein et al[4] found that duration of deafness and preoperative Central Institute for the Deaf sentence understanding scores carry the most significant predictive validity and account for a majority of the variability in results. Friedland et al[5] also found duration of deafness to be the strongest predictor of outcome and noted that implantation of the poorer ear was associated with results

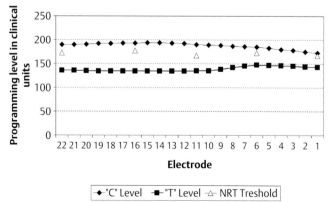

Figure 31–12 Threshold ("T") and maximum comfort ("C") levels with a Nucleus Freedom implant. In these data, measured 1 week after initial activation of the cochlear implant, NRT thresholds fall within 70 to 80% of the dynamic range. (Courtesy of Ryan Carpenter.)

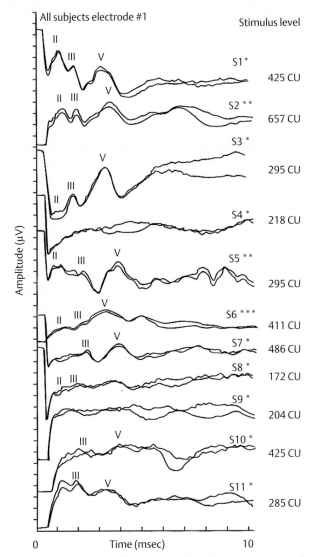

Figure 31–13 Electrically evoked auditory brainstem response from 11 adult subjects with a Clarion cochlear implant. The asterisk(s) next to each subject number denote amplitude in microvolts (μV) per division on the y-axis. *0.76 μV/division; **1.52 μV/division; ***6.10 μV/ division. (From Firszt JB, Chambers RD, Kraus N. Neurophysiology of cochlear implant users. II: comparison among speech perception, dynamic range, and physiological measures. Ear Hear 2002;23:516–531. Reprinted with permission.)

within 2% of those observed in studies of implantation of the better ear. Regression analyses from Rubinstein et al and Friedland et al demonstrate a model for predicting results:

Postimplantation word score
$$= A - B*(dur) + C*(cid) - D*[dur/(1 + cid)]$$

where *dur* is the duration of deafness in years and *cid* is the preoperative Central Institute for the Deaf sentence understanding scores (in percentage points). A, B, C, and D are positive constants that were fit by regression analysis to data from cohorts of cochlear implant recipients. Greater duration of deafness and lower preoperative sentence understanding scores predict lower postimplantation word score, although there is considerable variation in outcomes above and below predicted. In both studies, duration of deafness carried greater predictive value than did preoperative CID scores.

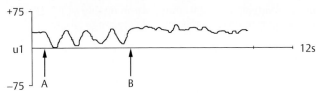

Figure 31–14 Electrically evoked stapedius reflex. The response was elicited using 20-μs pulses presented at 180 clinical units via a Cochlear Freedom implant and recorded using standard clinical immittance equipment (Madsen Zodiac 901). Note the stimulus onset **(A)** followed by four negative peaks corresponding to the stimulus pulses, and the stimulus offset **(B)** followed by no response. (Courtesy of Ryan Carpenter.)

Clinical observations in patients with current processors indicate that for patients with implant experience beyond 6 months, mean scores on word testing approximate 40%, with a range of 0% to 100%.[4] Results achieved with the most recently developed speech processing strategies reveal mean scores above 75% correct on words-in-sentence testing, again with a wide range of scores from 0 to 100%. Subjects perform substantially less well on single-word testing, although mean scores have continued to improve as speech-processing strategies have evolved. For example, **Fig. 31–15** shows the mean preoperative and postoperative speech recognition scores of 106 postlingually deafened adult patients implanted with a Clarion, Nucleus, or Med-El device using consonant-nucleus-consonant (CNC) words and Hearing in Noise Test (HINT) sentences presented in quiet (C. C. Della Santina, unpublished data). After implantation, speech recognition by telephone[122] and music appreciation[123] are observed at increasingly higher rates.

The high prevalence of SNHL among the elderly has prompted evaluations of the benefit of cochlear implantation in this age group.[124–126] For patients undergoing implantation after the age of 65 years, implant usage is high and nonuse (which suggests lack of perceived benefit) is rare.

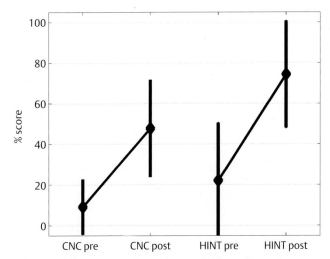

Figure 31–15 Mean ± standard deviation (SD) preoperative and 12-month postoperative speech discrimination scores for CNC monosyllabic words and HINT sentences presented in quiet, for 106 adult cochlear implant recipients with postlingually acquired hearing loss. (Courtesy of C.C. Della Santina.)

Questionnaire assessment of impact on quality of life reveals gains similar to those achieved in younger age groups.

Cochlear Implant Results in Children

Tests of speech perception used for childhood assessment have been described in detail[127] and typically consist of closed-set tests that assess word identification among a limited set of options with auditory cues only, and open-set tests scored by percentage of words correctly repeated, and structured interviews of parents.

Variability in speech-perception performance across subjects is widely recognized.[128-130] Factors implicated in speech-recognition variability include the amount of residual hearing,[131,132] age of implantation,[21,128,133] mode of communication,[134,135] family support,[128] and length of deafness.[132]

Steady gains in speech recognition and perception are found in young deaf children using multichannel cochlear implants.[3,20,59,105,129,130,135-138] For example, Miyamoto et al[139] noted that in 29 children with 1 to 4 years of experience with a cochlear implant, roughly half achieved at least some open-set speech recognition. Waltzman et al[135] found that 14 children implanted before the age of 3 years attained high levels of speech perception performance with only 2 years of experience. Fryauf-Bertschy et al[128] examined speech perception in cochlear-implanted children over 4 years and noted significant increases in pattern perception and results of closed-set speech perception tests.

Another variable that influences speech perception is the generation of technology incorporated in the cochlear implant system. Steady improvements in speech perception have been associated with improvements in signal processing strategies, speech processors, and electrode arrays.[140] Identification of monosyllabic words for individuals using early generations of the Nucleus multichannel cochlear implant averaged 16% early in the pediatric cochlear implant experience,[59] whereas performance averaged greater than 50% on similar measures with later technology.[141] Prior studies have contrasted performance across different manufacturers of devices. However, differences in performance appear more closely related to general demographic differences across patient populations, tests used, and length of experience with the devices than to differences in characteristics of like-generation devices per se.[142-144]

Children implanted prior to age 2 to 3 years[145,146] exhibit better speech recognition outcomes than do children implanted at older ages, and data from McConkey Robbins[10] and Manrique et al[147] indicate that implantation performance of children implanted under the age of 2 years is significantly better than that of children implanted between age 2 and 3 years. Osberger et al[148] noted that children undergoing earlier implantation are more likely to utilize an oral mode of communication, which by itself may be a predictor of higher implant performance—an observation borne out in early studies.[44] Osberger et al also found that children with more residual hearing are undergoing implantation. Gantz and colleagues[149] compiled data from across centers that indicate children with some degree of preoperative open-set speech recognition obtain substantially higher levels of speech comprehension. Taken together, these studies suggest a clear potential for benefit with implantation of younger children, when intervention is provided early or before access to auditory input is lost completely.

Cheng et al[21] performed a meta-analysis of published reports on speech recognition in children with cochlear implants. Of 1916 reports on cochlear implants published since 1966, 44 provided sufficient patient data to compare speech recognition results between published ($n = 1904$ children) and unpublished ($n = 261$) trials. In this analysis the diversity of tests deemed necessary to address the full spectrum of speech recognition skills in implanted children posed a challenge to the task of pooling study results. An expanded format of the Speech Perception Categories[150] was used to combine results across studies. Although this conversion introduced statistical constraints, it allowed comparison of multiple studies and determination of the impact of selected variables (e.g., age at implantation, duration of use, etiology, and age at onset of deafness). The main conclusions of this meta-analysis were that (1) earlier implantation is associated with a greater gain in speech recognition, (2) differences in performance between those with congenital and acquired etiologies diminish in time, and (3) there is no discernible plateau in speech-recognition benefits over 3 years of follow-up. More than 75% of the children with cochlear implants described in peer-reviewed publications achieved substantial open-set speech recognition after 3 years of implant use. Examination of published versus unpublished data failed to show evidence of a publication bias, indicating that outcomes appeared generally equivalent between published and unpublished series.

Language Acquisition in Children with Cochlear Implants

The primary goal of implantation in children is to facilitate comprehension and expression of spoken language. Language is defined as a vehicle for shaping and relating abstractions for communication. Information exchange via spoken language involves a conversion of thought into speech. This conversion relies on mental representations of phonologic (word) structure and syntactic (phrase) structure.[151] Given improved auditory access, sound and phrase structure may be augmented by the cochlear implant. Although challenging to characterize, effects on receptive language skills and language production after implantation represent a critical measure of impact.

The Reynell Developmental Language Scale evaluates both receptive and expressive skills independently.[152] These scales have been normalized on the basis of performance levels of hearing children and have been used in deaf child studies. Whereas deaf children without cochlear implants achieved language competence at half the rate of their hearing peers, implanted subjects exhibited language-learning rates that matched, on average, those of their normal-hearing peers.[152,153] Though an improved rate of language learning was achieved with implantation, a gap in language level between cochlear-implanted children and their normal-hearing peers persisted, presumably due to delayed acquisition of prelinguistic skills prior to intervention.

Robbins and colleagues[152] noted that implantation improved language-learning rates for children in both oral and "total communication" settings based on the Reynell Developmental Language Scale. Geers and colleagues,[44] assessing language skills in implanted children enrolled in oral and total communication settings, found that the groups did not differ in language level, though the oral group demonstrated significantly better speech production.

Correlation studies conducted by Pisoni[154] have yielded statistically significant correlations among results observed in a select group of implanted children who demonstrate superior speech-recognition abilities. Pisoni has speculated that high-performing implanted children are able to process spoken language by encoding, storing, and retrieving the phonologic representations of spoken words.

Language learning also requires the acquisition of communicative behaviors. Substantial gains in linguistic behaviors, including eye contact and turn-taking,[155] and in verbal spontaneity[156] develop within 6 months of implantation. Participation in the hearing world using spoken language is one of the main reasons parents choose to have their child receive a cochlear implant. Language and reading skills are important to learn and maintain at an age-appropriate level to successfully function in the hearing world.

Age at time of implantation is an important factor in predicting language outcomes for prelingually deafened children. Geers[157] revealed that after 5 to 6 years of implant use 43% of congenitally deafened children who were implanted at age 2 had similar speech and language skills to those of normal hearing children. However, only 16% of congenitally deafened children who underwent cochlear implantation at 4 years of age had language skills that were similar to normal-hearing children 5 to 6 years after implant use. Included in the same study were implanted children who became profoundly hearing impaired after birth but were implanted within 1 year of the onset of profound hearing loss. Eighty percent had speech and language skills in the normal range 5 to 6 years postimplantation.[157]

Prelingually deafened children can acquire language skills that are similar to normal-hearing peers with appropriate intervention. Oral education placement versus a total communication education placement leads to greater achievement in expressive language skills, whereas neither communication method seems to have an advantage with regard to fostering receptive language skills.[134] Other factors that predict higher language skills include a higher socioeconomic status, smaller family size, greater nonverbal intelligence, female gender, and the time spent in rehabilitation that is devoted to speech and language.[134]

Although the rate of language development in cochlear implant users varies widely, the language growth rate in cochlear implant users is greater than what is expected of children with profound SNHL without an implant. In fact, Svirsky et al[153] found that prelingually deafened cochlear implant users have a language growth rate that is similar to the language growth rate seen in normal hearing children.

Postimplant Rehabilitation

A language-rich home and school environment supports development of optimal language and literacy skills. Rehabilitative strategies should seek to achieve overall communicative competence as they relate to auditory, speech, and language skills.[158] Ideally, rehabilitative strategies do not aim to teach specific, isolated auditory, speech, or language subskills. Rather, rehabilitative programs should take an integrated approach to rehabilitation. Clinicians should interweave various aspects of communicative competence, listening, speaking, language, and pragmatics. This approach is theorized to lend greater salience in developing spoken language after cochlear implantation. Artificial isolation of these components may impair the normal cascade of skill development and there may be risks of overtraining one aspect of communication to the detriment of other communicative skills. This phenomenon,

referred to as "greenhousing,"[159] may lead to disorders in communicative development when different subskills of communication fail to progress in synchrony. Components of cochlear implant rehabilitation should foster the development of auditory and speech skills in a manner that simulates a hearing child's acquisition of spoken language, while simultaneously addressing remedial needs consequent to auditory deprivation in the child's early development.[158]

The hearing-impaired child is at substantial risk for educational underachievement.[160,161] Educational achievement by the hearing-impaired child can be enhanced by verbal communication if auditory access is achievable.[162] Improved speech perception and production provided by cochlear implants offer the possibility of increased access to oral-based education and enhanced educational independence.

Koch et al[22] and Francis et al[163] tracked the educational progress of implanted children by using an educational resource matrix to map educational and rehabilitative resource utilization. The matrix was developed on the basis of observations that changes in classroom settings (e.g., into a mainstream classroom) are often compensated by an initial increase in interpreter and speech-language therapy. After implantation there is observable movement toward educational independence, but this effect is not immediate and appears to require adjunctive rehabilitative support to be achieved. Within 5 years after implantation, the rate of full-time assignment to a mainstream classroom increases from 12 to 75%.

Bilateral Cochlear Implantation

In an effort to expand the benefits obtained with unilateral cochlear implantation, bilateral implantation has been offered to increasing numbers of patients. Implantation of the second ear some time after implantation of the first ear and bilateral, simultaneous implantations have been described. The potential benefit of bilateral implantation relies on the capacity for patients to integrate bilateral electrical stimulation within the central auditory system. Laboratory trials have focused on an examination of whether the advantages of binaural acoustic hearing extend to those with bilateral implants. Binaural advantages include (1) increased auditory sensitivity (i.e., improved pure-tone thresholds) as a result of summation effects, (2) improved sound source localization, and (3) improved speech recognition in noise. The latter can occur through acoustic effects when the second ear is away from the noise or by neurologic effects when the second ear is closer to the noise source. In the first scenario distance and "head shadow" establish a favorable signal-to-noise ratio for the ear farthest from the noise. In the second, neural integration of bilateral inputs results in "binaural squelch," whereby suppression of the noise enhances speech perception.

Tyler and colleagues[164] have noted that bilateral cochlear implantation generally enables head shadow effects in discerning speech in noise. However, only some patients benefit from summation and squelch effects. Most, but not all, adult bilateral recipients have shown improved horizontal plane localization. Similarly, Litovsky et al[165] and Schoen et al[166] have observed general trends toward additional benefit with the use of a second implant. However, different binaural benefits were obtained in different subjects, and these studies document cases wherein no additional benefit with bilateral implantation was achieved.

Though the era of bilateral implantation has been introduced, there are few controlled trials to date. Preliminary results show promise in enabling the use of the head shadow, an expanded sound field, and some sound localization ability to the majority of bilateral recipients.[167,168] Moreover, some observed benefits are attributable to improved summation and squelch. These findings have demonstrated that the brain can integrate electrical stimulation from the two ears. However, systems that enable integrated, bilateral sound field processing have not yet been introduced clinically, possibly limiting the potential benefits of bilateral implantation.

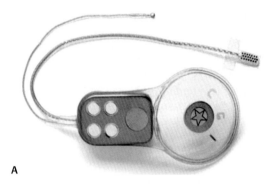

A

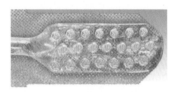

B

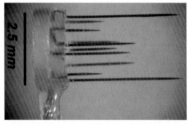

C

◆ Auditory Brainstem Implants

Patients with bilateral hearing loss due to bilateral acoustic tumors [e.g., in neurofibromatosis type 2 (NF2)] experience a devastation of their spoken communication abilities. In such patients, inadequate auditory nerve survival due to tumor progression or tumor removal may render cochlear implantation ineffective. Instead, electrical hearing can be achieved with a multielectrode device placed on the cochlear nucleus of the pontomedullary brainstem, albeit at a level of benefit that so far has not reached open-set speech recognition without visual or contextual cues.[169,170] Newer designs employing multi-tined penetrating microelectrodes may permit access to deeper and more discrete populations of cochlear nucleus neurons, and may offer improved spectral and dynamic range[171] (**Fig. 3–16**).

Surgical technique for auditory brainstem implants (ABIs) involves translabyrinthine approach extended to include additional bone removal posteroinferior of the sigmoid sinus to facilitate sinus compression and consequently increase exposure for both tumor removal and access to the foramen of Luschka (lateral opening of the fourth ventricle) and lateral recess.[172] Cranial nerves V, VII, VIII, IX, and X and the anterior inferior cerebellar artery are identified and used to locate the area in which the cochlear nuclei reside in the superolateral aspect of the floor of the fourth ventricle. Anatomic landmarks may be obscured by choroid plexus and displaced by effects of tumor growth. A well for the processor is created in cortical bone posterosuperior of the mastoid, like that for a cochlear implant. The processor is placed in the well, then the electrode array (which may contain up to 21 electrodes in current-generation devices) is placed on the surface of the brainstem overlying the ventral cochlear nuclei, in the anterosuperolateral aspect of the lateral recess. Placement is adjusted based on intraoperative ABR waveforms elicited by stimulation via the implant, and then the implant is stabilized with a fat graft of piece of Teflon felt.

◆ Implantable Hearing Aids

The majority of cases of SNHL require only acoustic amplification to address communication skills. This is generally accomplished with conventional air conduction hearing aids. Despite improvements in conventional hearing aid technology, only 15% of the 20 million hearing-impaired people in the United States who could benefit from amplification utilize these devices.[173] The development of semi-implantable and totally implantable hearing aids has in part been an attempt to compensate for limitations of conventional hearing aids.

Figure 31–16 **(A)** Auditory brainstem implant (ABI) designed for use in patients without cochlear nerves (e.g., after resection of bilateral acoustic neuromas due to neurofibromatosis type 2). The device is modified from a Cochlear Corporation Nucleus cochlear implant, with electrodes **(B)** designed to sit on the surface of the cochlear nucleus. **(C)** Electrodes for a penetrating ABI designed by McCreery et al at the Huntington Medical Research Institutes. [**(A)** and **(B)** from Cummings CW, ed. Otolaryngology Head and Neck Surgery, vol 4. St. Louis: Elsevier-Mosby, 2005, with permission. **(C)** From McCreery D. et al. Final Report on NIDCD contract N01-DC-1–2105, A cochlear nucleus auditory prosthesis based on microstimulation, http://www.nidcd.nih.gov/funding/programs/npp/pdf/N01-DC-1-2105QPRFF.pdf. Reprinted with permission.]

Implantable hearing aids comprise two types: middle ear aids and bone-anchored devices.

Middle Ear Implantable Hearing Aids

Given the costs and risks of surgical placement, an implantable hearing aid (IHA) should ideally provide significant advantages over conventional hearing aids, including better appearance, improved fidelity, broader frequency response, less distortion, reduction or elimination of feedback, and better speech understanding. The devices should not interfere with residual hearing, limit patient activities, or predispose patients to infection.[174] Several IHA designs are currently under investigation, with at least one already receiving approval by the FDA for clinical use in the United States. However, despite many potential advantages over conventional aids, IHAs have met with limited success to date.

Conventional hearing aids work by amplifying airborne sound prior to its reaching the middle ear. A microphone converts an incoming acoustic signal into an electrical signal that is amplified, filtered, processed to adjust dynamic range, and then transduced by a speaker back into airborne sound waves that then drive the middle ear and inner ear in the normal physiologic manner. Though usually adequate, this approach has several inherent limitations. First, nonlinearities in the transduction process cause distortion and limit the useful dynamic range of the aid. Second, because the impedance mismatch between the air-filled external auditory canal and fluid-filled cochlea is only partly compensated by the middle ear mechanism, much of the amplified airborne sound is reflected back from the tympanic membrane. This limits the acoustic power and perceptual loudness a hearing aid can generate, and increases problems with hearing aid "squeal" due to feedback of sounds reaching the hearing aid's microphone. The potential for feedback limits the useful amplification of a conventional hearing aid, and mandates a tight hearing aid mold fit in the ear canal or placement of the microphone outside the canal, resulting in discomfort, otitis externa, autophony, ear fullness (the occlusion effect), and visibility of the hearing aid. All of these factors conspire to reduce patient acceptance of conventional aids.

In contrast to conventional air-conducting hearing aids, middle ear IHAs are designed to directly drive the ossicular chain, reducing impedance mismatch, feedback, autophony, and distortion of the amplified signal while offering increased functional gain. Some IHA designs require no ear canal components, averting the risk of otitis externa and reducing autophony and ear fullness. There is also a cosmetic advantage to not having a visible apparatus within the ear, though most IHAs do require an external processor that is visible behind the ear.

Product Design

Middle ear IHAs may be completely or partially implantable. Partially implantable devices consist of an external microphone and speech processor, which is connected to an inductive transmitter with an external coil that transmits electrical energy transcutaneously to the internal device. Batteries to power the system are contained within the external device. The internal device consists of a receiving coil, processing electronics, and mechanical driver. A fully implantable system houses all of these components within the implanted portion of the device, and is periodically recharged via a transcutaneous inductive link.

Most IHAs employ either piezoelectric or electromagnetic actuators for converting electrical signals to mechanical

movement of the ossicular chain. Yanagihara and coworkers[175] developed a piezoelectric ceramic bimorph rod that vibrates when driven with an electric voltage and is attached directly to the head of the stapes. This partially implanted device is indicated for patients with mixed hearing loss, with a pure-tone average that does not exceed 50 dB HL.[176]

Implex AG Hearing Technology (Ismaning, Germany) developed a fully implantable middle ear implant (the Totally Implantable Communication Assistance aid, or TICA®) (**Fig. 31–17**). In this device there is a piezoceramic disk over a gas-filled chamber in a titanium casing that is connected to the body of the incus using a titanium rod.[177] The microphone is implanted under the skin in the ear canal via a small opening made in the bone of the posterior external auditory canal wall. Zenner and Leysieffer[178] reported that this totally implantable hearing device has good transfer of power and low-energy consumption, with values at the probe tip corresponding to approximately 100 dB sound pressure level (SPL) at 1 kHz, and can reach greater than 130 dB SPL at high frequencies with minimal distortion. The power consumption for the fully implanted device is approximately 1% of that needed by most electromagnetic systems. The lack of an internal magnet and the use of titanium casing for the TICA offer a significant advantage over magnetic middle ear IHAs with regard to MRI compatibility. A disadvantage is the need to surgically transect the malleus neck to reduce feedback via the ossicular chain and tympanic membrane to the ear canal microphone. Although potentially reversible, this maneuver interferes with normal sound conduction. The device gained regulatory approval in Europe, but it is not yet approved for human clinical trials in the United States. In 2001, Cochlear Corporation (Sydney, Australia) announced the acquisition of core technology from Implex AG, and declared an intent to apply the technology toward development of a fully implantable cochlear implant.

Another fully implantable piezoelectric device under development is the Envoy™ (**Fig. 31–18**) by Envoy Medical Corporation (formerly St. Croix Medical, Minneapolis, MN). This is a fully implanted hearing aid system that comprises a piezoelectric sensor connected to the head of the malleus, an amplifier, and piezoelectric driver that connects to the stapes. The system uses the tympanic membrane as the microphone and then amplifies the mechanical vibration that would otherwise normally occur at the stapes. Javel et al[179] described the piezoelectric bimorph sensor (a crystal that produces an electric current when deformed) used in this system as an alternative to a

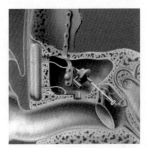
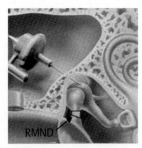
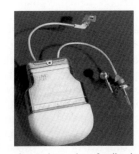

A **B** RMND **C**

Figure 31–17 The TICA, totally implantable middle ear aid developed by Zenner et al and initially marketed by Implex AG Hearing Technology.[78] **(A)** Artist's rendition showing implanted device, with microphone beneath ear canal skin and actuator stabilized in mastoid cavity and abutting head of malleus. **(B)** Malleus neck dissection (RMND) performed to reduce feedback to microphone. **(C)** Device used in clinical trials. (Adapted from Zenner HP, Leysieffer H. Total implantation of the Implex TICA hearing amplifier implant for high frequency sensorineural hearing loss: the Tubingen University experience. Otolaryngol Clin North Am 2001;34:417–446. Reprinted with permission.)

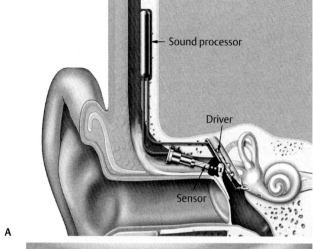

A

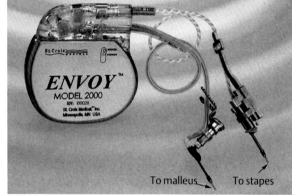

B

Figure 31–18 Envoy™ totally implantable hearing aid. **(A)** Artist's rendition of device in place, with sensor and actuator interfacing with malleus and stapes, respectively, and incus removed. **(B)** Device used in clinical trials. (From Cummings CW, ed. Otolaryngology Head and Neck Surgery, vol 4. St. Louis: Elsevier-Mosby, 2005. Reprinted with permission.)

subcutaneously implanted microphone as an input stage. When surgically placed on the stapes capitulum in cats, the piezoelectric actuator (essentially a sensor run in reverse, so that an applied current evokes mechanical movement) exhibited a sufficiently wide frequency response for use as a hearing aid transducer and yielded output levels ranging from 62 to 108 dB SPL at 4 kHz, 51 to 98 dB SPL at 2 kHz, and 55 to 80 dB SPL at 1 kHz.

Like the TICA, a disadvantage of this device is that it requires resection of part of the ossicular chain (the incus) to prevent feedback from the driver to the sensor; therefore, implantation necessarily interferes with the normal path of conductive hearing. Although the device has not yet gained regulatory approval for routine clinical use, phase II clinical trials are scheduled for completion in 2006. Phase I clinical trial results in seven subjects showed subjectively improved ease of listening and functional gain comparable with that obtained with traditional hearing aids, with the exception of reduced gain at 3 kHz or higher and mean improvement in word recognition of 17% over scores with traditional hearing aids.[180] Four subjects experienced no benefit at activation of the device. This was attributed to hermeticity failure. Three of the four patients underwent revision surgery, and two of those subsequently showed benefit. Thus, five of seven devices were functioning and in use 4 to 6 months following activation. The complete implantability (i.e., cosmetic advantage) of the system generated enthusiasm from subjects in the study.

In electromagnetic implants, sound enters a microphone and is transduced into an electric current that is passed through a wire coil, generating a magnetic field that vibrates a permanent magnet. Vibration is coupled to the ossicular chain, which transfers the vibrations to the inner ear. The Vibrant Soundbridge (now marketed by Vibrant-Med-El, Innsbruck, Austria) (**Fig. 31–19**), Middle Ear Transducer (MET, marketed by Otologics, Inc., Boulder, CO), and the Direct Drive hearing Systems (DDHS, by Soundtec Inc., Oklahoma City, OK) fall into this category.[174] These partially implantable IHAs are under clinical trials in the United States, and one, the Med-El Vibrant® (formerly Vibrant Soundbridge®) has received FDA approval.

The Vibrant Soundbridge is a semi-implantable IHA approved by the FDA for use in patients with moderate/severe SNHL. In this system, an external microphone and processor transmit power and data via a transcutaneous telemetry link to an internal processor, which generates a current in a wire coil of a "floating mass" transducer affixed to the long process of the incus, causing it to vibrate. The transducer is surgically implanted via a transmastoid approach. The floating mass transducer comprises the wire coil (which acts as an electromagnet) around a small permanent magnet.[177,181]

An initial study by Tjellström et al[182] showed that acutely implanted patients undergoing routine stapedotomy surgery reported that sound quality with a floating mass transducer temporarily attached to the incus was "crisp" and "clean" and that thresholds mirrored the bone line of the preoperative audiogram. One study of five subjects[183] showed functional gain equal to or improved over that obtained with air-conduction hearing aids, no significant change in residual hearing, and improvement in perceived benefit compared with air-conduction hearing aids. A phase III clinical trial[184] using a prospective single-subject, repeated measures design showed similar results in a group of 53 subjects. The authors of the clinical trial report asserted that the Vibrant Soundbridge was safe and effective, based on a comparison of preoperative and postoperative unaided pure-tone thresholds in the implanted ear. Mean postoperative change in thresholds was less than 5 dB on a frequency-specific basis, and 2.7 dB for the three frequency pure-tone average. Most patients did not exhibit a clinically significant change in sensitivity (i.e., threshold shift of 10 dB or greater). The study also reported that 86% of patients with the Soundbridge reported satisfaction in clearness and tone compared with 31% with their air conduction hearing aid; 60% reported feedback with their hearing aid; 97% of those who experienced feedback with their hearing aid did not have feedback with the Soundbridge. Three percent (1 subject) did report in feedback with the Soundbridge at 3 months poststimulation. The same study also reported a significant increase in functional gain from 500 to 6000 Hz compared with traditional (air-conduction) hearing aids, indicating increased audibility with the Soundbridge implant. Finally, there was a mean improvement of speech recognition in noise by at least 33 percentage points in 92% of patients compared with scores in the unaided condition. However, it is unclear from that report how patients performed on speech recognition tests in noise compared with air-conduction hearing aids. Note also that only 34% of the subjects wore programmable hearing aids whereas 66% wore analogue, nonprogrammable instruments. Although these authors asserted long-term stability of the Vibrant device, further independent assessment beyond shorter term, retrospective assessments[185,186] remains to be performed.

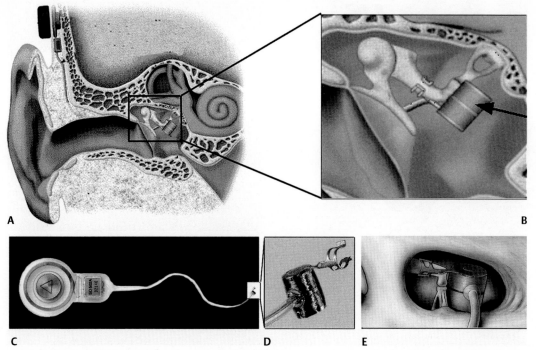

Figure 31–19　Vibrant Med-El (formerly Vibrant Soundbridge) semi-implantable hearing aid. **(A)** External device and power source magnetically coupled to implanted portion, which leads to a magnetic transducer affixed to the long process of the incus **(B**, arrow**).** Implanted portion of the device **(C)** includes an inductive coil for power and signal transmission. Magnetic actuator **(D)** includes a magnet within a wire coil, through which current flows to encode sound and induce incus motion. **(E)** Surgical view of transducer attached to the incus, seen from the mastoid cavity through the facial recess. (Adapted from Cummings CW, ed. Otolaryngology Head and Neck Surgery, vol 4. St. Louis: Elsevier-Mosby, 2005. Reprinted with permission.)

Another electromechanical device currently under development is the Otologics Middle Ear Transducer MET™ (**Fig. 31–20**) Ossicular Stimulator. This partially implanted device incorporates a metal stage affixed in the mastoid to stabilize a linear electromagnetic actuator that abuts and vibrates the incus body. In preclinical studies, in vitro measurements of maximum output, frequency response, distortion and response to loading forces were analyzed, demonstrating that the device produced significant output levels to address the needs of moderately severe-to-severe levels of SNHL. Additionally, the transducer frequency response was found to be relatively flat, varying only approximately 10 dB up to 10 kHz, providing good frequency characteristics for the reproduction of speech. Although not yet approved by the FDA for noninvestigational use, this device is currently undergoing clinical trials.[181]

Other IHAs employing an electromechanical or electromagnetic drive have been described.[174,177,187,188] The Soundtec Direct Drive Hearing System is an FDA-approved IHA that uses an electromagnetic coil in an in-the-ear external device to move a magnet that is surgically implanted on the stapes. The electromagnetic coil is housed in a custom-made earmold. This approach has the benefit of requiring only a minimal, transcanal approach to surgical implantation. Silverstein and colleagues[189] reported generally favorable results with the use of the Soundtec device. However, magnet instability and noise were frequent complaints requiring surgical modifications to address these symptoms.

Although initially positive results have been noted, it remains unclear whether any of the above designs will succeed in realizing the apparent potential of IHAs. Inadequate device durability related to mechanical fatigue of materials is a common and significant challenge, as all IHAs used clinically require vibration of implanted mechanical elements to provide ossicular motion.

Bone-Anchored Hearing Devices

Conductive and mixed hearing losses are highly prevalent disorders that often may be addressed with standard tympanoplasty techniques or rehabilitated with traditional hearing aids. However, there remains a large subset of these patients who are unsuitable surgical candidates for correction of their deficit, or who are unable to tolerate a traditional hearing aid. This group includes patients with chronically draining ears, those with discomfort from the sound levels required from a traditional hearing aid, and patients unable to tolerate a hearing aid because of a large mastoid bowl or meatoplasty following chronic ear surgery. Additionally, patients with otosclerosis, tympanosclerosis, or canal atresia and who have a contraindication to surgical repair may defy traditional approaches. Patients who have undergone external auditory canal closure following extensive skull base surgery also are not amenable to traditional hearing aids. This group of patients may benefit from a device that offers bone-anchored hearing.[190] Patients with single-sided deafness also are candidates.

Osseointegrated implants were first introduced into clinical practice in Scandinavia in the late 1960s, ostensibly for intraoral rehabilitation.[191] Since this time, osseointegrated implants have gained widespread acceptance in the fields of dental, oral/maxillofacial, craniofacial, and orthopedic surgery. Application of this technology to bone-anchored hearing aids represents a refinement of conventional bone-conducting hearing aids. The utility of conventional bone-conducting

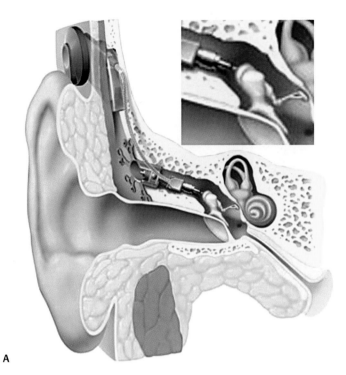

A

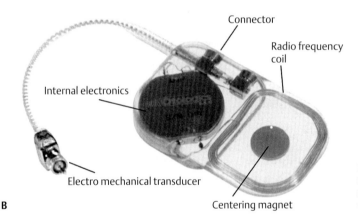

B

Connector

Radio frequency
coil

Internal electronics

Electro mechanical transducer

Centering magnet

Figure 31–20 Otologic MET™ semi-implantable hearing aid.
(A) Schematic of device in place, with inset showing transducer in small well laser-drilled in body of the incus. **(B)** Device as used in clinical trials. (Courtesy of Otologics Corporation.)

devices is now considered limited. The bone conductor must be applied with steady pressure to the mastoid cortex (usually via a headband or eyeglasses). Patients often experience pain, headache, and skin irritation at the contact site. Furrowing of the skull due to pressure is not unusual in children who use bone conductors. Further, sound fidelity is limited by soft tissue attenuation, variable placement of the vibrator, and flaccidity of the securing device (e.g., eyeglass frames).[192] Coupling the bone vibrator to an osseointegrated implant, as originally performed by Tjellström[193] and his team at the Institute of Applied Biotechnology in Sweden in 1977, averts many of these limitations of conventional bone conducting devices.

The success of this technology relies on two basic principles: the creation of a permanent percutaneous connection, and the placement of an osseointegrated titanium abutment upon which a transducer is coupled. The cutaneous-implant interface as originally conceived by Brånemark and Labrektsson[194] is based on biologic principles observed throughout nature. Teeth and nails (as well as talons, tusks, or claws as found in other species) all interface with a thin,

firmly attached cutaneous or mucosal border, with little to no hair. This tissue architecture limits tissue mobility and preserves stability of tissue planes, while inhibiting the penetration of microbes and subsequent inflammation or infection.[195,196] By mimicking these attributes in the skull, the surgeon creates a permanent cutaneous-implant border that the patient may easily maintain.

Advances in metallic biomaterials facilitate the creation of permanent, well-tolerated implant fixtures on which the transducer is placed. Titanium is the most notable among several materials that have found clinical application in anchoring dental prostheses. This is because of its ability to create a corrosion-resistant oxide layer on the surface of the implant that confers osseointegration potential.[197,198] Because the implant may be worn for several decades or longer, the toxicity and carcinogenicity of the oxide coating takes on particular importance.[199] Reports have shown that titanium is superior to stainless steel, lacking steel's high potential for corrosion, or the toxicity of its components.[200,201] To date, pure titanium appears free of the adverse sequelae seen with other metals, and thus continues to represent an ideal implant material.[198]

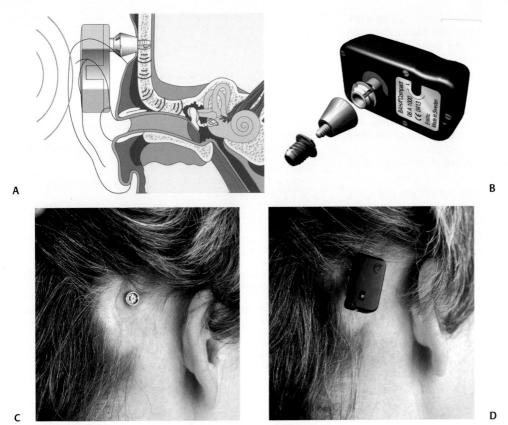

A

B

C

D

Figure 31–21 Bone-anchored hearing aid (BAHA®) by Cochlear Corporation (formerly Entific Corp.). **(A)** Schematic of device in situ. Subcutaneous tissue is removed around a site 50 to 55 mm posterosuperior to the ear canal, to improve coupling of vibration between the external hearing aid and osseointegrated titanium implant embedded in the squamous portion of the temporal bone. **(B)** Enlarged view of device, showing BAHA aid, abutment, and titanium fixture. **(C)** Abutment visible after implantation. **(D)** BAHA aid attached. (Courtesy of Entific Corp.)

Currently, the only commercially available osseointegrated hearing aid is the Bone-Anchored Hearing Aid (the BAHA™, manufactured by Cochlear Corporation, formerly by Entific and NobelBiocare), shown in **Fig. 31–21.** The BAHA™ consists of a pure titanium implant and a sound processor. The processor couples directly to the titanium implant via a skin penetrating abutment, utilizing a force-fit, plastic coupling). Another implantable, magnetically driven osseointegrated hearing aid was also in use (Xomed's Audiant Bone Conductor™); however, technical difficulties with that transcutaneous device led to its recent withdrawal from the marketplace.

In the largest series to date studying the BAHA™, Håkansson et al[192] reported results from 147 patients over 10 years. Patients were divided into three groups based on their pure-tone average (PTA) bone-conduction thresholds: 0–45 dB, 46–60 dB, and >60 dB HL. The authors noted a strong relationship between PTA and successful rehabilitation. In the group with the best cochlear reserve (PTA <45 dB), 89% of patients' hearing was subjectively improved by the implant, whereas 8% felt their hearing was worse. Conversely, in the groups with progressively less cochlear function, 46 to 60 dB and >60 dB, 61% and 22% of patients reported subjective hearing improvement, respectively. Further, speech discrimination scores improved on average from 14% unaided, and 67% with a traditional hearing aid, to 81% with the BAHA. This number increased to 85% if persons with a sensorineural loss greater than 60 dB HL were excluded and to 89% if subjects with PTA worse than 45 dB were excluded. Based on these results, the authors recommended that to be in consideration for a "high success rate" with the BAHA, patients should have a PTA by bone conduction of less than 45 dB HL, though improvements in hearing should still be expected for a PTA of up to 60 dB.

Lustig et al[202] performed a review of the United States experience with the BAHA. The most common indications for implantation included chronic otitis media or draining ears and external auditory canal stenosis or aural atresia. Patients who had undergone skull base surgery and had complete closure of the external auditory canal were also included. Overall, each patient had an average improvement of 32 dB ± 19 dB with the use of the BAHA. Closure of the air–bone gap to within 10 dB of the preoperative bone conduction thresholds occurred in 80% of patients, whereas closure to within 5 dB occurred in 60%. Nearly one third of patients demonstrated "overclosure" of the preoperative bone-conduction threshold of the better hearing ear. Complications were limited to local infection and inflammation at the implant site in three of 40 patients, and failure to osseointegrate in one patient. Patient response to the implant was uniformly satisfactory.

In addition to implantation for purely conductive or mixed hearing losses, emerging data indicate the value of BAHA amplification for patients with unilateral profound SNHL. The BAHA on the deafened ear effectively expanded the sound field for the patient and improved the patient's speech understanding in noise, much like a contralateral routing of sound

(CROS) hearing aid or transcranial CROS system.[203,204] However, in contrast to CROS, BAHA does not require the placement of an earmold in the better hearing ear. As the better hearing ear functions normally, the acoustic "head shadow" can be used to isolate sounds incident to the deafened side, but heard in the better ear through transcranial bone conduction from the BAHA. This avoids the potential discomfort and perceptual costs of wearing an earmold on the better hearing ear. Preliminary results show subjective improvement in both sound quality and speech understanding in noise.[205]

It is possible for the implant to dislodge from the skull after apparent successful, complete osseointegration, unrelated to trauma or other obvious cause. Tjellström (personal communication, September 2005) reported the rate was 6.0% in adults and 5.7% in children. He recommended placing a new implant 7 mm above or below the first site as a short outpatient procedure under a local anesthesia, removing only a small circle of skin and leaving the former surgical site otherwise intact.

◆ Disclosure

Editor Gordon B. Hughes, M.D., is a Co-investigator for phase II clinical trial of the MED-EL Vibrant Soundbridge round window implant.

References

1. Ross M, Levitt H. Consumer satisfaction is not enough: hearing aids are still about hearing. Sem Hear 1997;18:7–11

2. Tyler RS, Summerfield AQ. Cochlear implantation: relationships with research on auditory deprivation and acclimatization. Ear Hear 1996;17(3 suppl):38S–50S

3. Waltzman SB, Fisher SG, Niparko JK, Cohen NL. Predictors of postoperative performance with cochlear implants. Ann Otol Rhinol Laryngol Suppl 1995;165:15–18

4. Rubinstein JT, Parkinson WS, Tyler RS, Gantz BJ. Residual speech recognition and cochlear implant performance: effects of implantation criteria. Am J Otol 1999;20:445–452

5. Friedland DR, Venick HS, Niparko JK. Choice of ear for cochlear implantation: the effect of history and residual hearing on predicted postoperative performance. Otol Neurotol 2003;24:582–589

6. Waltzman SB, Roland JT Jr, Cohen NL. Delayed implantation in congenitally deaf children and adults. Otol Neurotol 2002;23:333–340

7. Pruszewicz A, Demenko G, Wika T. Variability analysis of Fo parameter in the voice of individuals with hearing disturbances. Acta Otolaryngol 1993;113:450–454

8. Teoh SW, Pisoni DB, Miyamoto RT. Cochlear implantation in adults with prelingual deafness. Part I. Clinical results. Laryngoscope 2004; 114:1536–1540

9. Teoh SW, Pisoni DB, Miyamoto RT. Cochlear implantation in adults with prelingual deafness. Part II. Underlying constraints that affect audiological outcomes. Laryngoscope 2004;114:1714–1719 Review

10. McConkey Robbins A, Koch DB, Osberger MJ, Zimmerman-Phillips S, Kishon-Rabin L. Effect of age at cochlear implantation on auditory skill development in infants and toddlers. Arch Otolaryngol Head Neck Surg 2004;130:570–574

11. Cheng AK, Rubin HR, Powe NR, Mellon NK, Francis HW, Niparko JK. A cost-utility analysis of the cochlear implant in children. JAMA 2000;284:850–856

12. NIH consensus conference. Cochlear implants in adults and children. JAMA 1995;274:1955–1961

13. NIH Consensus Development Statement. Cochlear Implants. NIH Consens Statement 1988;7:1–25

14. Tyler RS, Moore BC, Kuk FK. Performance of some of the better cochlear-implant patients. J Speech Hear Res 1989;32:887–911

15. Robbins AM, Renshaw JJ, Berry SW. Evaluating meaningful auditory integration in profoundly hearing-impaired children. Am J Otol 1991;12(suppl):144–150

16. Osberger MJ. Cochlear implantation in children under the age of two years: candidacy considerations. Otolaryngol Head Neck Surg 1997; 117(3 pt 1):145–149

17. Starr A, Picton TW, Sininger Y, Hood LJ, Berlin CI. Auditory neuropathy. Brain 1996;119(pt 3):741–753

18. Trautwein PG, Sininger YS, Nelson R. Cochlear implantation of auditory neuropathy. J Am Acad Audiol 2000;11:309–315

19. Shallop JK, Peterson A, Facer GW, Fabry LB, Driscoll CL. Cochlear implants in five cases of auditory neuropathy: postoperative findings and progress. Laryngoscope 2001;111(4 pt 1):555–562

20. Miyamoto RT, Kirk KI, Svirsky MA, Sehgal ST. Communication skills in pediatric cochlear implant recipients. Acta Otolaryngol 1999; 119:219–224

21. Cheng AK, Grant GD, Niparko JK. A meta-analysis of the pediatric cochlear implant literature. Ann Otol Rhinol Laryngol Suppl 1999;177:124–128

22. Koch ME, Wyatt JR, Francis HW, Niparko JK. A model of educational resource use by children with cochlear implants. Otolaryngol Head Neck Surg 1997;117(3 pt 1):174–179

23. Balkany T, Gantz B, Nadol JB Jr. Multichannel cochlear implants in obstructed and obliterated cochleas. Otolaryngol Head Neck Surg 1988;98:72–81

24. Balkany T, Gantz BJ, Steenerson RL, Cohen NL. Systematic approach to electrode insertion in the ossified cochlea. Otolaryngol Head Neck Surg 1996;114:4–11

25. Niparko JK, Oviatt DL, Coker NJ, Sutton L, Waltzman SB, Cohen NL. Facial nerve stimulation with cochlear implantation. VA Cooperative Study Group on Cochlear Implantation. Otolaryngol Head Neck Surg 1991;104:826–830

26. Gray RF, Irving RM. Cochlear implants in chronic suppurative otitis media. Am J Otol 1995;16:682–686

27. Parnes LS, Gagne JP, Hassan R Cochlear implants and otitis media: considerations in two cleft palate patients. J Otolaryngol 1993;22:345–348

28. Luntz M, Hodges AV, Balkany T, et al. Otitis media in children with cochlear implants. Laryngoscope 1996;106:1403–1405

29. Fina M, Skinner M, Goebel JA, Piccirillo JF, Neely JG, Black O. Vestibular dysfunction after cochlear implantation. Otol Neurotol 2003; 24:234–242

30. Migliaccio AA, Della Santina CC, Carey JP, Niparko JK, Minor LB. The vestibulo-ocular reflex response to head impulses rarely decreases after cochlear implantation. Otol Neurotol 2005;26:655–660

31. Buchman CA, Joy J, Hodges A, Telischi FF, Balkany TJ. Vestibular effects of cochlear implantation. Laryngoscope 2004;114(10 pt 2 suppl 103):1–22

32. Woolley AL, Oser AB, Lusk RP, et al. Preoperative temporal bone computed tomography scan and its use in evaluating the pediatric cochlear implant candidate. Laryngoscope 1997;107:1100–1106

33. Langman AW, Quigley SM. Accuracy of high-resolution computed tomography in cochlear implantation. Otolaryngol Head Neck Surg 1996;114:38–43

34. Wiet RJ, Pyle GM, O'Connor CA, Russell E, Schramm DR. Computed tomography: how accurate a predictor for cochlear implantation? Laryngoscope 1990;100:687–692

35. Frau GN, Luxford WM, Lo WW, Berliner KI, Telischi FF. High-resolution computed tomography in evaluation of cochlear patency in implant candidates: a comparison with surgical findings. J Laryngol Otol 1994;108:743–748

36. Harnsberger HR, Dart DJ, Parkin JL, Smoker WR, Osborn AG. Cochlear implant candidates: assessment with CT and MR imaging. Radiology 1987;164:53–57

37. Casselman JW, Kuhweide R, Deimling M, Ampe W, Dehaene I, Meeus L. Constructive interference in steady state-3DFT MR imaging of the inner ear and cerebellopontine angle. AJNR Am J Neuroradiol 1993;14: 47–57

38. Bettman R, Beek E, Van Olphen A, Zonneveld F, Huizing E. MRI versus CT in assessment of cochlear patency in cochlear implant candidates. Acta Otolaryngol 2004;124:577–581

39. Tien RD, Felsberg GJ, Macfall J. Fast spin-echo high-resolution MR imaging of the inner ear. AJR Am J Roentgenol 1992;159:395–398

40. Arriaga MA, Carrier D. MRI and clinical decisions in cochlear implantation. Am J Otol 1996;17:547–553

41. Heller JW, Brackmann DE, Tucci DL, Nyenhuis JA, Chou CK. Evaluation of MRI compatibility of the modified nucleus multichannel auditory brainstem and cochlear implants. Am J Otol 1996;17:724–729

42. Baumgartner WD, Youssefzadeh S, Hamzavi J, Czerny C, Gstoettner W. Clinical application of magnetic resonance imaging in 30 cochlear implant patients. Otol Neurotol 2001;22:818–822

43. Cohen NL, Waltzman SB, Fisher SG. A prospective, randomized study of cochlear implants. The Department of Veterans Affairs Cochlear Implant Study Group. N Engl J Med 1993;328:233–237

44. Geers AE, Nicholas J, Tye-Murray N, et al. Effects of communication mode on skills of long-term cochlear implant users. Ann Otol Rhinol Laryngol Suppl 2000;185:89–92

45. Bielamowicz SA, Coker NJ, Jenkins HA, Igarashi M. Surgical dimensions of the facial recess in adults and children. Arch Otolaryngol Head Neck Surg 1988;114:534–537

46. Lalwani AK, Larky JB, Wareing MJ, Kwast K, Schindler RA. The Clarion Multi-Strategy Cochlear Implant–surgical technique, complications, and results: a single institutional experience. Am J Otol 1998;19:66–70

47. Proctor B, Bollobas B, Niparko JK. Anatomy of the round window niche. Ann Otol Rhinol Laryngol 1986;95(5 pt 1):444–446

48. Adunka O, Gstoettner W, Hambek M, Unkelbach MH, Radeloff A, Kiefer J. Preservation of basal inner ear structures in cochlear implantation. ORL J Otorhinolaryngol Relat Spec 2004;66:306–312

49. Lenarz T, Kuzma J, Weber BP, et al. New Clarion electrode with positioner: insertion studies. Ann Otol Rhinol Laryngol Suppl 2000;185:16–18

50. Reefhuis J, Honein MA, Whitney CG, et al. Risk of bacterial meningitis in children with cochlear implants. N Engl J Med 2003;349:435–445

51. Greenwood DD. Critical bandwidth and the frequency coordinates of the basilar membrane. J Acoust Soc Am 1961;33:1344–1355

52. Yukawa K, Cohen L, Blamey P, Pyman B, Tungvachirakul V, O'Leary S. Effects of insertion depth of cochlear implant electrodes upon speech perception. Audiol Neurootol 2004;9:163–172

53. Rubinstein JT, Parkinson WS, Lowder MW, Gantz BJ, Nadol JB Jr, Tyler RS. Single-channel to multichannel conversions in adult cochlear implant subjects. Am J Otol 1998;19:461–466

54. Fayad JN, Baino T, Parisier SC. Revision cochlear implant surgery: causes and outcome. Otolaryngol Head Neck Surg 2004;131:429–432

55. Buchman CA, Higgins CA, Cullen R, Pillsbury HC. Revision cochlear implant surgery in adult patients with suspected device malfunction. Otol Neurotol 2004;25:504–510

56. Hoffman RA. Cochlear implant in the child under two years of age: skull growth, otitis media, and selection. Otolaryngol Head Neck Surg 1997;117(3 pt 1):217–219

57. Parisier SC, Chute PM, Popp AL, et al. Surgical techniques for cochlear implantation in the very young child. Otolaryngol Head Neck Surg 1997;117:248–254

58. Waltzman SB, Cohen NL. Cochlear implantation in children younger than 2 years old. Am J Otol 1998;19:158–162

59. Gantz BJ, Tyler RS, Woodworth GG, Tye-Murray N, Fryauf-Bertschy H. Results of multichannel cochlear implants in congenital and acquired prelingual deafness in children: five-year follow-up. Am J Otol 1994;15(suppl 2):1–7

60. Spencer LJ, Gantz BJ, Knutson JF. Outcomes and achievement of students who grew up with access to cochlear implants. Laryngoscope 2004;114:1576–1581

61. Burton MJ, Shepherd RK, Xu SA, Xu J, Franz BK, Clark GM. Cochlear implantation in young children: histological studies on head growth, leadwire design, and electrode fixation in the monkey model. Laryngoscope 1994;104:167–175

62. Eby TL, Nadol JB Jr. Postnatal growth of the human temporal bone. Implications for cochlear implants in children. Ann Otol Rhinol Laryngol 1986;95(4 pt 1):356–382

63. Jackler RK, Luxford WM, Schindler RA, McKerrow WS. Cochlear patency problems in cochlear implantation. Laryngoscope 1987;97(7 pt 1):801–805

64. Green JD Jr, Marion MS, Hinojosa R. Labyrinthitis ossificans: histopathologic consideration for cochlear implantation. Otolaryngol Head Neck Surg 1991;104:320–326

65. Balkany T, Gantz B, Nadol JB. Multi-channel cochlear implants in partially ossified cochleas. Ann Otol Rhinol Laryngol Suppl 1988;135:3–7

66. Fayad J, Moloy P, Linthicum FH Jr. Cochlear otosclerosis: does bone formation affect cochlear implant surgery? (Review) Am J Otol 1990;11:196–200

67. Kemink JL, Zimmerman-Phillips S, Kileny PR, Firszt JB, Novak MA. Auditory performance of children with cochlear ossification and partial implant insertion. Laryngoscope 1992;102:1001–1005

68. Cohen NL, Waltzman SB. Partial insertion of the nucleus multichannel cochlear implant: technique and results. Am J Otol 1993;14:357–361

69. Francis HW, Pulsifer MB, Chinnici J, et al. Effects of central nervous system residua on cochlear implant results in children deafened by meningitis. Arch Otolaryngol Head Neck Surg 2004;130:604–611

70. Gantz BJ, McCabe BF, Tyler RS. Use of multichannel cochlear implants in obstructed and obliterated cochleas. Otolaryngol Head Neck Surg 1988;98:72–81

71. Bredberg G, Lindstrom B, Lopponen H, Skarzynski H, Hyodo M, Sato H. Electrodes for ossified cochleas. Am J Otol 1997;18(suppl 6):S42–S43

72. Jackler RK, Luxford WM, House WF. Congenital malformations of the inner ear: a classification based on embryogenesis. Laryngoscope 1987;97(suppl 40):15–17

73. Schmidt JM. Cochlear neuronal populations in developmental defects of the inner ear. Implications for cochlear implantation. Acta Otolaryngol 1985;99:14–20

74. Jackler R, Luxford W, House W. Sound detection with the cochlear implant in five ears of four children with congenital malformations of the cochlea. Laryngoscope 1987;97(suppl 40):15–17

75. Tucci DL, Telian SA, Zimmerman-Phillips S, Zwolan TA, Kileny PR. Cochlear implantation in patients with cochlear malformations. Arch Otolaryngol Head Neck Surg 1995;121:833–838

76. House JR III, Luxford WM. Facial nerve injury in cochlear implantation. Otolaryngol Head Neck Surg 1993;109:1078–1082

77. Cohen NL, Hoffman RA, Stroschein M. Medical or surgical complications related to the Nucleus multichannel cochlear implant. Ann Otol Rhinol Laryngol Suppl 1988;135:8–13

78. Webb RL, Lehnhardt E, Clark GM, Laszig R, Pyman BC, Franz BK. Surgical complications with the cochlear multiple-channel intracochlear implant: experience at Hannover and Melbourne. Ann Otol Rhinol Laryngol 1991;100:131–136

79. Hoffman RA, Cohen NL. Surgical pitfalls in cochlear implantation. Laryngoscope 1993;103:741–744

80. Cochlear Americas. Nucleus Report. 2004 November/December. http://www.cochlearamericas.com/professional/PDFs/N30791_Nucleus_Report_AQM.pdf. Accessed August 7, 2005

81. United States Food and Drug Administration. Electronic Freedom of Information Reading Room-Warning Letters and Responses. http://www.fda.gov/foi/warning_letters/g5265d.htm. Accessed August 3, 2005

82. United States Food and Drug Administration. Electronic Freedom of Information Reading Room-Warning Letters and Responses. http://www.fda.gov/foi/warning_letters/g5089d.htm. Accessed August 3, 2005

83. Alexiades G, Roland JT Jr, Fishman AJ, Shapiro W, Waltzman SB, Cohen NL. Cochlear reimplantation: surgical techniques and functional results. Laryngoscope 2001;111:1608–1613

84. Luetje CM, Jackson K. Cochlear implants in children: what constitutes a complication. Otolaryngol Head Neck Surg 1997;117:243–247

85. Parisier SC, Chute PM, Popp AL. Cochlear implant mechanical failures. Am J Otol 1996;17:730–734

86. Weise JB, Muller-Deile J, Brademann G, Meyer JE, Ambrosch P, Maune S. Impact to the head increases cochlear implant reimplantation rate in children. Auris Nasus Larynx 2005;32:339–43. Epub May 31, 2005

87. Franz BK, Clark GM, Bloom DM. Effect of experimentally induced otitis media on cochlear implants. Ann Otol Rhinol Laryngol 1987;96(2 pt 1):174–177

88. Antonelli PJ, Lee JC, Burne RA. Bacterial biofilms may contribute to persistent cochlear implant infection. Otol Neurotol 2004;25:953–957

89. Parkins CW, Colombo J. Auditory-nerve single-neuron thresholds to electrical stimulation from scala tympani electrodes. Hear Res 1987;31:267–285

90. Javel E, Tong Y, Shepherd R, Clark G. Responses of cat auditory nerve fibers to biphasic electrical current pulses. Ann Otol Rhinol Laryngol 1987;96(suppl 128):26–30

91. Franck KH, Xu L, Pfingst BE. Effects of stimulus level on speech perception with cochlear prostheses. J Assoc Res Otolaryngol 2003;4:49–59. Epub July 16, 2002

92. Sainz M, de la Torre A, Roldan C, Ruiz JM, Vargas JL. Analysis of programming maps and its application for balancing multichannel cochlear implants. Int J Audiol 2003;42:43–51

93. Papsin BC. Cochlear implantation in children with anomalous cochleovestibular anatomy. Laryngoscope 2005;115(1 pt 2 suppl 106):1–26

94. Kiang N, Moxon E. Physiological considerations in artificial stimulation of the inner ear. Ann Otol Rhinol Laryngol 1972;81:714–730

95. Franck KH, Shah UK, Marsh RR, Potsic WP. Effects of Clarion electrode design on mapping levels in children. Ann Otol Rhinol Laryngol 2002;111(12 pt 1):1128–1132

96. Henkin Y, Kaplan-Neeman R, Muchnik C, Kronenberg J, Hildesheimer M. Changes over time in electrical stimulation levels and electrode impedance values in children using the Nucleus 24M cochlear implant. Int J Pediatr Otorhinolaryngol 2003;67:873–880

97. Butts SL, Hodges AV, Dolan-Ash S, Balkany TJ. Changes in stimulation levels over time in nucleus 22 cochlear implant users. Ann Otol Rhinol Laryngol Suppl 2000;185:53–56

98. Hughes ML, Vander Werff KR, Brown CJ, et al. A longitudinal study of electrode impedance, the electrically evoked compound action potential, and behavioral measures in nucleus 24 cochlear implant users. Ear Hear 2001;22:471–486

99. Cohen LT, Saunders E, Clark GM. Psychophysics of a prototype perimodiolar cochlear implant electrode array. Hear Res 2001;155:63–81

100. Overstreet EH, Belagaje SR, Kirl KI, Lormore K, Zwolan T. Analysis of programming levels as a possible outcome predictor: a cross-device study of pediatric and adult cochlear implant users. Paper presented at the 27th Midwinter Meeting of the Association for Research in Otolaryngology, February 22, 2004, Daytona Beach, FL

101. Veekmans K. Clinical implications of auditory nerve response telemetry with the ART system. Paper presented at the 10th symposium on cochlear implants in children, March 17, 2005, Dallas, TX

102. Brown CJ, Abbas PJ, Gantz BJ. Electrically evoked whole nerve action potentials in Ineraid cochlear implant users: responses to different stimulating electrode configurations and comparison to psychophysical responses. J Acoust Soc Am 1990;88:1385–1391

103. Gordon K, Papsin BC, Harrison RV. Programming cochlear implant stimulation levels in infants and children with a combination of objective measures. Int J Audiol 2004;43(suppl 1):S28–S32

104. Morita T, Naito Y, Nakamura T, Yamaguchi S, Tsuji J, Ito J. Chronological changes of stimulation levels in prelingually deafened children with cochlear implant. Acta Otolaryngol Suppl 2004;551:60–64

105. Frijns JH, Briaire JJ, de Laat JA, Grote JJ. Initial evaluation of the Clarion CII cochlear implant: speech perception and neural response imaging. Ear Hear 2002;23:184–197

106. Brown CJ, Hughes ML, Luk B, Abbas PJ, Wolaver A, Gervais J. The relationship between EAP and EABR thresholds and levels used to program the nucleus 24 speech processor: data from adults. Ear Hear 2000;21:151–163

107. Hughes ML, Brown CJ, Abbas PJ, Wolaver AA, Gervais JP. Comparison of EAP thresholds with MAP levels in the nucleus 24 cochlear implant: data from children. Ear Hear 2000;21:164–174

108. Franck KH, Norton SJ. Estimation of psychophysical levels using the electrically evoked compound action potential measured with the neural response telemetry capabilities of Cochlear Corporation's CI24M device. Ear Hear 2001;22:289–299

109. Polak M, Hodges A, Balkany T. ECAP, ESR and subjective levels for two different nucleus 24 electrode arrays. Otol Neurotol 2005;26:639–645

110. Gordon KA, Ebinger KA, Gilden JE, Shapiro WH. Neural response telemetry in 12- to 24-month-old children. Ann Otol Rhinol Laryngol Suppl 2002;189:42–48

111. Thai-Van H, Truy E, Charasse B, et al. Modeling the relationship between psychophysical perception and electrically evoked compound action potential threshold in young cochlear implant recipients: clinical implications for implant fitting. Clin Neurophysiol 2004;115:2811–2824

112. Thai-Van H, Chanal JM, Coudert C, Veuillet E, Truy E, Collet L. Relationship between NRT measurements and behavioral levels in children with the Nucleus 24 cochlear implant may change over time: preliminary report. Int J Pediatr Otorhinolaryngol 2001;58:153–162

113. Han DM, Chen XQ, Zhao XT, et al. Comparisons between neural response imaging thresholds, electrically evoked auditory reflex thresholds and most comfortable loudness levels in CII bionic ear users with HiResolution trade mark sound processing strategies. Acta Otolaryngol 2005;125:732–735

114. Brown CJ, Abbas PJ, Fryauf-Bertschy H, Kelsay D, Gantz BJ. Intraoperative and postoperative electrically evoked auditory brain stem responses in nucleus cochlear implant users: implications for the fitting process. Ear Hear 1994;15:168–176

115. Hodges AV, Balkany TJ, Ruth RA, Lambert PR, Dolan-Ash S, Schloffman JJ. Electrical middle ear muscle reflex: use in cochlear implant programming. Otolaryngol Head Neck Surg 1997;117(3 pt 1):255–261

116. Overstreet E. Objective measures and program levels: important lessons from simple measures. Paper presented at the 2005 Conference on implantable auditory prostheses, August 3, 2005, Asilomar, CA

117. Mertes J. Effects of overstimulation in the pediatric CI population. Poster presented at the 10th Symposium on Cochlear Implants in Children, March 18, 2005, Dallas, TX

118. Seyle K, Brown CJ. Speech perception using maps based on neural response telemetry measures. Ear Hear 2002;23(1 suppl):72S–79S

119. Gantz BJ, Tyler RS, Knutson JF, et al. Evaluation of five different cochlear implant designs: audiologic assessment and predictors of performance. Laryngoscope 1988;98:1100–1106

120. Kileny P, Zimmerman-Phillips S, Kemink J, Schmaltz S. Effects of preoperative electrical stimulability and historical factors on performance with multichannel cochlear implants. Ann Otol Rhinol Laryngol 1991;100:563–568

121. Miyamoto RT, Osberger MJ, Todd SL, et al. Variables affecting implant performance in children. Laryngoscope 1994;104:1120–1124

122. Cohen NL, Waltzman SB, Shapiro WH. Telephone speech comprehension with use of the nucleus cochlear implant. Ann Otol Rhinol Laryngol Suppl 1989;142:8–11

123. McDermott HJ. Music perception with cochlear implants: a review. Trends Amplif 2004;8:49–82

124. Horn KL, McMahon NB, McMahon DC, Lewis JS, Barker M, Gherini S. Functional use of the Nucleus 22-channel cochlear implant in the elderly. Laryngoscope 1991;101:284–288

125. Facer GW, Peterson AM, Brey RH. Cochlear implantation in the senior citizen age group using the Nucleus 22-channel device. Ann Otol Rhinol Laryngol Suppl;1995;166:187–190

126. Francis HW, Chee N, Yeagle J, Cheng A, Niparko JK. Impact of cochlear implants on the functional health status of older adults. Laryngoscope 2002;112(8 pt 1):1482–1488

127. Kirk K. Challenges in the clinical investigation of cochlear implant outcomes. In: Niparko JK, ed. Cochlear Implants: Principles and Practices. Philadelphia: Lippincott-Williams & Wilkins, 2000:225–259

128. Fryauf-Bertschy H, Tyler RS, Kelsay DM, Gantz BJ, Woodworth GG. Cochlear implant use by prelingually deafened children: the influences of age at implant and length of device use. J Speech Lang Hear Res 1997;40:183–199

129. Tobey E, Geers A, Brenner C. Speech production results: speech feature acquisition. Volta Review 1994;106:109–129

130. Kirk KI, Pisoni DB, Osberger MJ. Lexical effects on spoken word recognition by pediatric cochlear implant users. Ear Hear 1995;16:470–481

131. Zwolan TA, Zimmerman-Phillips S, Ashbaugh CJ, Hieber SJ, Kileny PR, Telian SA. Cochlear implantation of children with minimal open-set speech recognition skills. Ear Hear 1997;18:240–251

132. Meyer TA, Svirsky MA, Kirk KI, Miyamoto RT. Improvements in speech perception by children with profound prelingual hearing loss: effects of device, communication mode, and chronological age. J Speech Lang Hear Res 1998;41:846–858

133. Shea JJ III, Domico EH, Orchik DJ. Speech recognition ability as a function of duration of deafness in multichannel cochlear implant patients. Laryngoscope 1990;100:223–226

134. Geers AE, Nicholas JG, Sedey AL. Language skills of children with early cochlear implantation. Ear Hear 2003;24(1 suppl):46S–58S

135. Waltzman SB, Cohen NL, Gomolin RH, Shapiro WH, Ozdamar SR, Hoffman RA. Long-term results of early cochlear implantation in congenitally and prelingually deafened children. Am J Otol 1994;15(suppl 2):9–13

136. Fryauf-Bertschy H, Tyler RS, Kelsay DM, Gantz BJ. Performance over time of congenitally deaf and postlingually deafened children using a multichannel cochlear implant. J Speech Hear Res 1992;35:913–920

137. Staller SJ. Perceptual and production abilities in profoundly deaf children with multichannel cochlear implants. J Am Acad Audiol 1990;1:1–3

138. Staller SJ, Beiter AL, Brimacombe JA, Mecklenburg DJ, Arndt P. Pediatric performance with the Nucleus 22-channel cochlear implant system. Am J Otol 1991;12(suppl):126–136

139. Miyamoto RT, Osberger MJ, Robbins AM, Myres WA, Kessler K. Prelingually deafened children's performance with the nucleus multichannel cochlear implant. Am J Otol 1993;14:437–445

140. Wilson B. Cochlear implant technology. In: Niparko J, Kirk K, Mellon N, Robbins A, Tucci D, Wilson B, eds. Cochlear Implants: Principles and Practices. Philadelphia: Lippincott Williams & Wilkins, 2000:109–127

141. Skinner MW, Fourakis MS, Holden TA, Holden LK, Demorest ME. Identification of speech by cochlear implant recipients with the multipeak (MPEAK) and spectral peak (SPEAK) speech coding strategies. II: Consonants. Ear Hear 1999;20:443–460

142. Kiefer J, Muller J, Pfenningdorff T, et al. Speech understanding in quiet and in noise with the CIS speech-coding strategy (MED EL Combi-40) compared to the MPEAK and SPEAK strategies (Nucleus). Adv Otorhinolaryngol 1997;52:286–290

143. Helms J, Muller J, Schon F, et al. Evaluation of performance with the COMBI40 cochlear implant in adults: a multicentric clinical study. ORL J Otorhinolaryngol Relat Spec 1997;59:23–35

144. Taitelbaum-Swead R, Kishon-Rabin L, Kaplan-Neeman R, Muchnik C, Kronenberg J, Hildesheimer M. Speech perception of children using Nucleus, Clarion or Med-El cochlear implants. Int J Pediatr Otorhinolaryngol 2005;69:1675–1683. Epub June 13, 2005

145. Waltzman SB, Cohen NL, Shapiro WH. Use of a multichannel cochlear implant in the congenitally and prelingually deaf population. Laryngoscope 1992;102:395–399

146. Brackett D, Zara C. Communication outcomes related to early implantation. Am J Otol 1998;19:453–460

147. Manrique MJ, Huarte A, Amor JC, Baptista P, Garcia-Tapia R. Results in patients with congenital profound hearing loss with intracochlear multichannel implants. Adv Otorhinolaryngol 1993;48:222–230

148. Osberger MJ, Zimmerman-Phillips S, Koch DB. Cochlear implant candidacy and performance trends in children. Ann Otol Rhinol Laryngol Suppl 2002;189:62–65

149. Gantz BJ, Rubinstein JT, Tyler RS, et al. Long-term results of cochlear implants in children with residual hearing. Ann Otol Rhinol Laryngol Suppl 2000;185:33–36

150. Geers AE, Moog JS. Predicting spoken language acquisition of profoundly hearing-impaired children. J Speech Hear Disord 1987;52:84–94

151. Jackendorf RS. Phonological structure. In: Patterns in the Mind: Language and Human Nature. New York: Basic Book, 1994:53–65

152. Robbins AM, Svirsky M, Kirk KI. Children with implants can speak, but can they communicate? Otolaryngol Head Neck Surg 1997;117(3 pt 1):155–160

153. Svirsky MA, Robbins AM, Kirk KI, Pisoni DB, Miyamoto RT. Language development in profoundly deaf children with cochlear implants. Psychol Sci 2000;11:153–158

154. Pisoni D. Individual differences in effectiveness of cochlear implants in prelingually deaf children: some new process measures of performance. Research on Spoken Language Processing Progress Report No. 23. Bloomington, IN: Speech Research Laboratory, 199x

155. Tait M, Lutman ME. Comparison of early communicative behavior in young children with cochlear implants and with hearing aids. Ear Hear 1994;15:352–361

156. Kane MO, Schopmeyer B, Mellon NK, Wang NY, Niparko JK. Prelinguistic communication and subsequent language acquisition in children with cochlear implants. Arch Otolaryngol Head Neck Surg 2004; 130:619–623

157. Geers AE. Speech, language, and reading skills after early cochlear implantation. Arch Otolaryngol Head Neck Surg 2004;130:634–638

158. Robbins AM, Green J, Bollard P. Language development in children following one year of Clarion implant use. Ann Otol Rhinol Laryngol Suppl 2000;185:94–95

159. Robbins AM. Guidelines for the developing oral communication skills in children with cochlear implants. Volta Review 1994;96:75–86

160. Trybus RJ, Karchmer MA. School achievement scores of hearing impaired children: national data on achievement status and growth patterns. Am Ann Deaf 1977;122:62–69

161. Holt JA. Efficiency of screening procedures for assigning levels of the Stanford Achievement Test (eighth edition) to students who are deaf or hard of hearing. Am Ann Deaf 1995;140:23–27

162. Geers AE, Moog JS. Evaluating the benefits of cochlear implants in an education setting. Am J Otol 1991;12(suppl):116–125

163. Francis HW, Koch ME, Wyatt JR, Niparko JK. Trends in educational placement and cost-benefit considerations in children with cochlear implants. Arch Otolaryngol Head Neck Surg 1999;125:499–505

164. Tyler RS, Dunn CC, Witt SA, Preece JP. Residual speech perception and cochlear implant performance in postlingually deafened adults. Ear Hear 2003;24:539–544

165. Litovsky RY, Parkinson A, Arcaroli J, et al. Bilateral cochlear implants in adults and children. Arch Otolaryngol Head Neck Surg 2004; 130:648–655

166. Schoen F, Mueller J, Helms J, Nopp P. Sound localization and sensitivity to interaural cues in bilateral users of the Med-El Combi 40/40+cochlear implant system. Otol Neurotol 2005;26:429–437

167. Laszig R, Aschendorff A, Stecker M, et al. Benefits of bilateral electrical stimulation with the nucleus cochlear implant in adults: 6-month postoperative results. Otol Neurotol 2004;25:958–968

168. Schleich P, Nopp P, D'Haese P. Head shadow, squelch, and summation effects in bilateral users of the MED-EL COMBI 40/40+ cochlear implant. Ear Hear 2004;25:197–204

169. Schwartz MS, Otto SR, Brackmann DE, Hitselberger WE, Shannon RV. Use of a multichannel auditory brainstem implant for neurofibromatosis type 2. Stereotact Funct Neurosurg 2003;81:110–114

170. Otto SR, Brackmann DE, Hitselberger W. Auditory brainstem implantation in 12- to 18-year-olds. Arch Otolaryngol Head Neck Surg 2004;130:656–659

171. Rauschecker JP, Shannon RV. Sending sound to the brain. Science 2002;295:1025–1029

172. Brackmann DE. Auditory brainstem implant: I. Issues in surgical implantation. Otolaryngol Head Neck Surg 1993;108:624–633

173. Esselman GH, Coticchia JM, Wippold FJ 2nd, Fredrickson JM, Vannier MW, Neely JG. Computer-stimulated test fitting of an implantable hearing aid using three-dimensional CT scans of the temporal bone: preliminary study. Am J Otol 1994;15:702–709

174. Goode RL, Rosenbaum ML, Maniglia AJ. The history and development of the implantable hearing aid. Otolaryngol Clin North Am 1995;28:1–16

175. Yanagihara N, Gyo K, Hinohira Y. Partially implantable hearing aid using piezoelectric ceramic ossicular vibrator. Results of the implant operation and assessment of the hearing afforded by the device. Otolaryngol Clin North Am 1995;28:85–97

176. Suzuki J, Kodera K, Nagai K, Yabe T. Partially implantable piezoelectric middle ear hearing device. Long-term results. Otolaryngol Clin North Am 1995;28:99–106

177. Huttenbrink KB. Current status and critical reflections on implantable hearing aids. Am J Otol 1999;20:409–415

178. Zenner HP, Leysieffer H. Total implantation of the Implex TICA hearing amplifier implant for high frequency sensorineural hearing loss: the Tubingen University experience. Otolaryngol Clin North Am 2001;34:417–446

179. Javel E, Grant IL, Kroll K. In vivo characterization of piezoelectric transducers for implantable hearing AIDS. Otol Neurotol 2003;24:784–795

180. Chen DA, Backous DD, Arriaga MA, et al. Phase 1 clinical trial results of the Envoy System: a totally implantable middle ear device for sensorineural hearing loss. Otolaryngol Head Neck Surg 2004;131:904–916

181. Jenkins HA, Niparko JK, Slattery WH, Neely JG, Fredrickson JM. Otologics middle ear transducer ossicular stimulator: performance results with varying degrees of sensorineural hearing loss. Acta Otolaryngol 2004;124:391–394

182. Tjellström A, Luetje CM, Hough JV, et al. Acute human trial of the floating mass transducer. Ear Nose Throat J 1997;76:204–206,209–210

183. Todt I, Seidl RO, Gross M, Ernst A. Comparison of different vibrant soundbridge audioprocessors with conventional hearing AIDS. Otol Neurotol 2002;23:669–673

184. Luetje CM, Brackmann DE, Balkany TJ, et al. Phase III clinical trial results with the Vibrant Soundbridge implantable middle ear hearing device: a prospective controlled multicenter study. Otolaryngol Head Neck Surg 2002;126:97–107

185. Sterkers O, Boucarra D, Labassi S, et al. A middle ear implant, the Symphonix Vibrant Soundbridge: retrospective study of the first 125 patients implanted in France. Otol Neurotol 2003;24:427–436

186. Vincent C, Fraysse B, Lavieille J-P, Truy E, Sterkers O, Vaneecloo: A longitudinal study on postoperative hearing thresholds with the Vibrant Soundbridge device. Eur Arch Otorhino Laryngol 2004;261:493–496

187. Perkins R. Earlens tympanic contact transducer: a new method of sound transduction to the human ear. Otolaryngol Head Neck Surg 1996;114:720–728

188. Maniglia AJ, Ko WH, Garverick SL, et al. Semi-implantable middle ear electromagnetic hearing device for sensorineural hearing loss. Ear Nose Throat J 1997;76:333–338, 340–341

189. Silverstein H, Atkins J, Thompson JH Jr, Gilman N. Experience with the SOUNDTEC implantable hearing aid. Otol Neurotol 2005;26:211–217

190. Lustig L, Niparko J. Osseointegrated implants in otology. Adv Otolaryngol Head Neck Surg 1999;13:105–126

191. Brånemark P, Breine U, Lindstrom J, Doobe W, Doobe W, Doobie W. Intra-osseous anchorage of dental prostheses. I: Experimental studies. Scand J Plast Reconstr Surg 1969;3:81–100

192. Håkansson B, Liden G, Tjellstrom A, et al. Ten years of experience with the Swedish bone-anchored hearing system. Ann Otol Rhinol Laryngol Suppl 1990;151:1–16

193. Tjellström A, Lindstrom J, Hallen O, Albrektsson T, Branemark PI. Osseointegrated titanium implants in the temporal bone. A clinical study on bone-anchored hearing aids. Am J Otol 1981;2:304–310

194. Brånemark P, Labrektsson T. Titanium implants permanently penetrating human skin. Scand J Plast Reconstr Surg 1982;16:17–21

195. Adell R, Lekholm U, Rockler B, et al. Marginal tissue reactions as osseointegrated titanium fixtures: I. A three year longitudinal prospective study. Int J Oral Surg 1986;15:53–61

196. Lekholm U, Adell R, Lindhe J, et al. Marginal tissue reactions at osseointegrated titanium fixtures. (II) A cross-sectional retrospective study. Int J Oral Maxillofac Surg 1986;15:53–61

197. Zarb G. Impact of Osseointegration on Prosthodontics. In: Laney W, Tolman D, eds. Tissue Integration in Oral, Orthopedic and Maxillofacial Reconstruction. Carol Stream, IL: Quintessence, 1992:166–173

198. Johansson CB. On tissue reactions to metal implants. Ph.D. Thesis, Biomaterials/Handicap Research, University of Göteborg, Göteborg, 1991

199. Eriksson E, Brånemark P. Osseointegration from the perspective of the plastic surgeon. Plast Reconstr Surg 1994;93:626–637

200. von Ludinghausen M, Meister P, Probst J. Metallosis after osteosynthesis. Pathol Eur 1970;5:307–314

201. Pazzaglia UE, Minoia C, Ceciliani L, Riccardi C. Metal determination in organic fluids of patients with stainless steel hip arthroplasty. Acta Orthop Scand 1983;54:574–579

202. Lustig LR, Arts HA, Brackmann DE, et al. Hearing rehabilitation using the BAHA bone-anchored hearing aid: results in 40 patients. Otol Neurotol 2001;22:328–334

203. Vaneecloo FM, Ruzza I, Hanson JN, et al. The monaural pseudo-stereophonic hearing aid (BAHA) in unilateral total deafness: a study of 29 patients. Rev Laryngol Otol Rhinol (Bord) 2001;122:343–350

204. Niparko JK, Cox KM, Lustig LR. Comparison of the bone anchored hearing aid implantable hearing device with contralateral routing of offside signal amplification in the rehabilitation of unilateral deafness. Otol Neurotol 2003;24:73–78

205. Wazen JJ, Spitzer JB, Ghossaini SN, et al. Transcranial contralateral cochlear stimulation in unilateral deafness. Otolaryngol Head Neck Surg 2003;129:248–254

32

Rehabilitation of Peripheral Vestibular Disorders

Kelly S. Beaudoin, Kathleen D. Coale, and Judith A. White

◆ Impairments Resulting from Peripheral Vestibular Disorders

Physical and occupational therapists who treat vestibular disorders often have extensive knowledge about treating patients with balance/gait dysfunction and deficits in gaze stability. Common impairments accompanying vestibular dysfunction include decreased gaze stability secondary to abnormal vestibulo-ocular reflex, abnormal motion perception caused by mismatch of sensory inputs affecting sensory integration necessary for balance, abnormal postural control (distorted labyrinthine and otolithic inputs causing impaired equilibrium and body alignment), decreased static and dynamic balance/gait secondary to vestibulospinal outputs responding incorrectly to mismatched sensory inputs, decreased sensory integration for balance (the balance system requires robust inputs from visual, vestibular, and sensory systems to make proper balance reactions), and anxiety. Movement increases instability in a vestibulopathic patient and yet is the absolute requirement for recovery. Physical deconditioning may develop when patients become fearful of movement and severely limit all mobility.

Patients with peripheral vestibular dysfunction present to rehabilitation with the following problems[1]: decreased vestibulo-ocular reflex (VOR) gain,[2] abnormal sensory integration for balance,[3] abnormal vestibulospinal reflex (VSR)/balance/gait,[4] vertigo provoked by position change,[5] limited community mobility,[6] and lack of knowledge regarding their diagnosis and prognosis.

Diagnoses seen by vestibular therapists commonly include both unilateral and bilateral disorders such as labyrinthitis/neuronitis, temporal bone fracture with concussion or benign paroxysmal positional vertigo (BPPV), Meniere's syndrome (acute and chronic), acoustic neuroma (both resected and unresected), herpes zoster oticus/Ramsay Hunt syndrome, labyrinthine infarct, anterior-inferior or posterior-inferior cerebellar stroke, cervicogenic vertigo, BPPV, phobic postural vertigo, aminoglycoside ototoxicity, and hereditary insidious vestibular loss. Central vestibular disorders are not addressed in this chapter.

◆ Evaluation of Peripheral Vestibular Disorders

Clinical evaluation performed by the vestibular therapist consists of tests of gaze stability (**Table 32–1**), static balance/sensory integration for balance (**Table 32–2**), gait, postural control, and positional and positioning testing (see Benign Paroxysmal Positional Vertigo, later in chapter).

Findings from the initial vestibular assessment, along with vestibular laboratory testing results when available, assist the therapist with determining if the deficit is central or peripheral, unilateral or bilateral, or acute or chronic. Once impairments are identified, treatment planning and outcome prediction begin.

The static and dynamic balance tests are intertwined with the sensory integration examination, and information is gleaned about strategies used (ankle, hip, stepping) as well as ability to regain the center of mass over the base of support.[1] Determining which strategies the patient has available for balance recovery aids the therapist in treatment planning to facilitate safe community mobility and prevent falls. Computerized dynamic platform posturography (CDP) is used in tertiary care centers to evaluate sensory integration for balance, center of mass, and sway information. These machines can also measure motor latencies for translational platform movements. Clinical gait examinations commonly employ the Dynamic Gait Index,[2] the Berg Balance Scale,[3] the Timed Up and Go test,[4] and more recently the Functional Gait Assessment.[5] Many of these tests have been shown to be specific for predicting fall risk and assessing outcomes in this patient population.[6–8]

Positional and positioning testing is performed using infrared video-oculography or Frenzel goggles to eliminate visual fixation and allow the examiner to directly visualize torsional nystagmus. The examiner must be knowledgeable in recognizing which nystagmus patterns indicate BPPV (**Table 32–3**) and which patterns indicate other pathophysiology within or outside the peripheral vestibular system.

Other components of the clinical examination include strength, flexibility, and sensory testing of the lower extremities

Table 32–1 Oculomotor Exam

Room light
    VOR to slow head movement
    Head impulse test[5]
    Dynamic (with 2-Hz head movement) versus static visual acuity
    Pursuit eye movements
    Saccade eye movements
    VOR cancellation
Infrared goggles
    Gaze holding: horizontal and vertical
    Head shaking–induced nystagmus horizontal and vertical
    Tragal pressure–induced nystagmus
    Positional testing

and careful consideration of cervical contributions. Manual segmental testing of the cervical spine can provide insight into the patient's problem when peripheral vestibular testing is nonlocalizing.[9] Careful attention to the patient's comorbidities must be given for both treatment planning and outcome prediction. Knowledge of normal age-related changes in visual, sensory, and vestibular function should be employed when treating this population.

Self-perception of dizziness and resultant handicap is commonly measured with the Dizziness Handicap Inventory,[10] the Activities Specific Balance Control Questionnaire,[11] or the Vestibular Activities of Daily Living scale.[12] These questionnaires can be used pre-, mid-, and posttreatment to evaluate results of rehabilitation intervention.

◆ Treatment of Peripheral Vestibular Disorders

Once impairments and functional limitations are identified, research indicates that treatment should begin promptly for optimal outcomes.[13] Recovery of function after vestibular loss involves three different mechanisms[1]: spontaneous recovery,[2] vestibular adaptation/plasticity,[3] and substitution of other strategies.[14]

Much of the static imbalance of vestibular dysfunction resolves spontaneously prior to the initiation of vestibular therapy. Vestibular rehabilitation usually takes place in the subacute stage and utilizes both adaptation and substitution to regain gaze and gait stability as well as community mobility recovery. An error signal is needed to stimulate compensation.[13] Therapists strive to elicit the error signal while treating patients by utilizing active head motion to present the brain with a reduced gain situation causing retinal slip of the foveal visual image. Developing strategies for varied environments found in the community adds context specificity and improves outcome.[13] Utilizing a variety of inputs—visual, vestibular, and somatosensory—enables the patient to develop new strategies for balance control and gaze stability in varying environments. Unilateral vestibular deficits recover gaze and gait stability quite well. Bilateral vestibular loss patients do not return to premorbid activity levels. Bilateral vestibular loss requires more substitution strategies, such as preprogrammed saccades, to facilitate gaze stability while the patient is in motion. Assistive devices, such as canes and walkers, are not often required long-term for the unilateral peripheral vestibular patients. Bilateral vestibular patients have greater loss of vestibular input for balance, and therefore commonly require an assistive device for

Table 32–2 Static Balance Exam

Modified clinical test of sensory integration and balance[1]

1. Eyes open on firm surface, feet together, timed trial of 30 seconds
2. Eyes closed on firm surface, feet together, timed trial of 30 seconds
3. Eyes open on foam surface, feet together, timed trial of 30 seconds
4. Eyes closed on foam surface, feet together, timed trial of 30 seconds
5. Eyes open on firm surface, feet in tandem stance, timed trial of 30 seconds
6. Eyes closed on firm surface, feet in tandem stance, timed trial of 30 seconds

Other static tests of balance

7. Single limb stance, firm surface, eyes open
8. Single limb stance, firm surface, eyes closed
9. Eyes open, firm surface, head pitched up or down 45 degrees
10. Eyes closed, firm surface, head pitched up or down 45 degrees

Table 32–3 Extraocular Muscles and Nystagmus Direction in BPPV Affecting Various Canals

Canal	Ipsilateral Extraocular Muscle	Contralateral Extraocular Muscle	Direction of Nystagmus
Posterior canal	Superior oblique (depression, in-torsion)	Inferior rectus (depression, out-torsion)	Upbeat torsional
Anterior canal	Superior rectus (elevation, in-torsion)	Inferior oblique (elevation, out-torsion)	Downbeat torsional
Horizontal canal	Medial rectus (adduction)	Lateral rectus (abduction)	Geotropic (toward ground)
			Ageotropic (away from ground)

Table 32–4 Vestibular Rehabilitation Plan for Vestibulo-ocular Gain Deficit

Impairment	Goal	Treatment Options
Decreased gaze stability, decreased gain of vestibulo-ocular reflex (VOR), greater than 2 line drop from static visual acuity to dynamic visual acuity on Snellen chart	Allow clear vision when head is in motion	Treatment options: ×1, ×2 viewing exercises, full field ×1, ×2 exercises, preprogrammed saccades, begin with static positions on level progressing to unstable surfaces

Table 32–5 Vestibular Rehabilitation Plan for Static Postural Control Deficits

Impairment	Goal	Treatment Options
Decreased static balance/decreased sensory integration for balance, <30 sec. Timed trials on CTSIB, 5-6 pattern on CDP	Redistribute weighting of preferred balance strategy to use remaining vestibular function, ability to use ankle/hip/stepping strategy as necessary to regain balance without a fall, static balance performance to match age-related norms	Vary surface: firm, foam, uneven, inside, outside; vary lighting/visual inputs, busy environments; vary base of support; vary head position

Table 32–6 Vestibular Rehabilitation Plan for Decreased Dynamic Balance

Impairment	Goal	Treatment Options
Decreased dynamic balance/gait	Safe community ambulation with least restrictive device	Initiate gait without assistive device where safe as early as possible
<45/56 on Berg Balance Scale, <19 on DGI	Fall risk reduction/prevention	Vary surface: firm, foam, uneven, inside, outside, incline, decline
		Incorporate horizontal and vertical head turns
		Incorporate turns, pivots, circles
		Incorporate eyes opened/closed/dim lighting
		Increase visual flow/complexity: walk in closed mall, open mall, sidewalk with and against traffic
		Incorporate Tai Chi exercise[16,17]

Table 32–7 Vestibular Rehabilitation Plan for General Deconditioning

Impairment	Goal	Treatment Options
General deconditioning	Normalize community mobility, increase aerobic capacity	Initiate aerobic exercise: walking, stationary bike as early as possible; progressive strengthening exercises
Decreased strength		
Decreased cardiovascular conditioning		

Table 32–8 Vestibular Rehabilitation Plan for Decreased Cervical Mobility

Impairment	Goal	Treatment Options
Decreased cervical mobility	Normalize cervical segmental mobility to enhance proprioceptive input from the cervical receptors	Soft tissue massage, cervical manual therapy (joint mobilizations/neuromuscular reeducation), postural reeducation, proprioceptive retraining exercises

safe mobility. Recent research in the area of virtual reality is promising to promote treatment in multimodal sensory situations to facilitate better sensory integration for balance.[15]

Based on identified impairments and goals, treatments are provided one or two times per week for 4 to 6 weeks as outlined in **Tables 32–4** to **32–8**.

◆ Benign Paroxysmal Positional Vertigo

Etiology and Presentation

BPPV is the most common peripheral vestibular disorder resulting in complaints of vertigo.[18–20] A study performed in which the patients were considered to have BPPV only if they presented with nystagmus during a Dix-Hallpike test, established an incidence of 10.7 per 100,000 population per year.[18] A study performed by Oghalai et al[21] found that 9% of community-dwelling elderly randomly tested were found to have undiagnosed BPPV, suggesting that BPPV may be more common than estimated. In approximately one third of individuals, BPPV will spontaneously resolve. Many individuals may experience chronic or recurrent BPPV lasting for weeks, sometimes years. New research developments, as well as an increased understanding of vestibular physiology and the pathophysiology of BPPV, have directed new treatment protocols and maneuvers for the specific semicircular canals involved.

BPPV is usually idiopathic and occurs spontaneously; however, it may occur following head trauma or in conjunction with vestibular neuritis or labyrinthitis.[22–24] It is characterized by a brief episode of vertigo associated with a change in position of the head relative to gravity. Common changes in head position that may provoke BPPV include rolling over in bed, sitting up, lying down, looking up, and bending over. Functional activities that may provoke vertigo include the head positioning required at the dentist or the hair salon, gardening, and bending forward. Subjective complaints associated with BPPV include nausea, lightheadedness, and disequilibrium. BPPV is often associated with decreased balance and postural control.[25–27] Individuals may experience decreased balance lasting for hours to days following an episode of BPPV. In a study performed by Ruckenstein,[28] residual symptoms of lightheadedness or imbalance were found to persist 2 weeks after resolution of vertigo in 47% of cases.

General Treatment Considerations

Intervention is directed at restoring the normal mechanisms of the inner ear and resolving symptoms associated with BPPV. It is also important to regard the complications related to single or recurrent episodes of BPPV. BPPV may be benign; however, the secondary comorbidities may be devastating to an individual. The patient's lack of understanding of the cause of his or her symptoms often results in anxiety and depression, which in turn may result in social isolation, which further leads to generalized weakness and deconditioning, which contribute to faulty gait mechanics, decreased balance strategies, and fear of falling, which increases his or her risk for falls. Indirectly, BPPV may result in a greater occurrence of falls than reported.

Consideration should be given to patient education, static and dynamic balance assessment, safety education, and fall-risk prevention. Proper education may significantly reduce the patients' level of anxiety, as well as increase their safety. Understanding the mechanism of BPPV will also enable patients to better self-manage their condition. Falls are one of the leading causes of injury and morbidity in individuals over age 65. Proper balance assessment assists in identifying factors contributing to an individual's risk for falls, which will aid in fall prevention.

Decreased postural stability has been documented in BPPV with the use of CDP.[25–27] Posterior canal BPPV (PC-BPPV) results in an impairment of the vestibular system to maintain postural control and balance.[27] Modification of the posterior canal dynamics, secondary to free-floating otoconia, may affect proper excitation of vestibular afferents, resulting in abnormal vestibulospinal output.[29] Lateral semi-circular canal BPPV (LSC-BPPV) has not been found to make significant deficits in postural control compared with that of PC-BPPV.[30,31] However, a study performed by White et al[31] showed postural abnormalities in 80% of patients with apogeotropic LSC-BPPV.

Postural instability in the elderly may result in falls, especially when combined with secondary comorbidities such as neuropathy, visual impairments, and generalized weakness. Treatment of BPPV using the canalith repositioning maneuver and liberatory maneuver results in improved postural stability in patients with posterior canal BPPV.[25,26] Not all patients immediately revert to normal postural stability after resolving BPPV. Younger individuals are more likely to present with increased stability immediately posttreatment.[26] Assessment and treatment of balance deficits may be necessary to restore balance in the elderly population, as underlying comorbidities may complicate recovery.

Posterior Canal Benign Paroxysmal Positional Vertigo

Posterior canal BPPV is the most common variant; it is estimated that 94% of BPPV cases involve the posterior canal.[32] An episode of PC-BPPV is precipitated by a change in head position relative to gravity such as lying down, looking up, and bending forward. Nystagmus can be evoked by performing the Dix-Hallpike positional maneuver. Identifying the mechanism (cupulolithiasis versus canalithiasis) as well as the involved canal is the first step in selecting the appropriate treatment maneuver.

Schuknecht[33] was the first to suggest that deposits adhering to the cupula of the posterior canal caused the canal to become sensitive to gravity, resulting in BPPV (cupulolithiasis). Changes in head position result in deflection of the cupula and stimulation of the receptors. Cupulolithiasis is characterized by a sensation of vertigo accompanied by upbeat ipsidirectional (toward the downward ear) torsional nystagmus in the Dix-Hallpike test position. The characteristic nystagmus has a short latency with prolonged duration (>60 seconds) and should diminish somewhat with repeated testing. The prolonged duration of positional nystagmus suggests cupulolithiasis as the mechanism. However, we now know that cupulolithiasis is the less frequent type of BPPV encountered.

Further research suggested that otoconia detach from the utricle and fall into the posterior canal where they are free-floating in the endolymph.[34,35] Changes in head position result in movement of the otoconia through the canal, consequentially exciting the receptors and causing the canal to become gravity-sensitive (canalithiasis). Canalithiasis is characterized by a brief sensation of vertigo accompanied by upbeat ipsidirectional (toward the downward ear) torsional nystagmus in the Dix-Hallpike test position. The characteristic nystagmus may occur after a latency of several seconds, which then fatigues rapidly after 10 to 45 seconds. The paroxysmal, short duration of nystagmus suggests canalithiasis as the pathologic mechanism. Typically, reversal of nystagmus is seen when the patient returns to sitting position. Nystagmus should diminish markedly with repeated testing.

If the nystagmus does not fatigue with repeated testing but remains constant in the affected position or if the nystagmus and symptoms do not diminish with repeated testing, the patient should be tested for a central etiology.

Dix-Hallpike Test

The Dix-Hallpike maneuver is the standard test for diagnosis of BPPV.[36] If it fails to reproduce vertigo and nystagmus, it should be repeated. Otoconial debris may collect in the lateral head-hanging position, resulting in a positive test on the second trial.[37] If there is no success at eliciting vertigo or nystagmus in the posterior semicircular canals, the horizontal semicircular canals should be tested. Lest positional testing fail to reveal nystagmus and associated symptoms at the time of examination, BPPV should not be ruled out, as it may have fatigued. The patient should be instructed on self-testing as well as home repositioning therapy.

To perform the Dix-Hallpike test the patient is positioned sitting on the examination table. The head is rotated 45 degrees. The patient is rapidly brought straight back with the head extended approximately 20 degrees. Nystagmus is recorded as well as the patient's subjective complaints.

The patient is then brought back into the sitting position with the head maintained at 45-degree rotation. Reversal of nystagmus is noted[36] (**Fig. 32–1**).

Treatment

The canalith repositioning procedure (CRP) was initially described by Epley to treat BPPV. This procedure was designed to stimulate the migration of free-moving otoconia in the endolymph of the semicircular canal back into the utricle. This procedure is effective in the treatment of PC-BPPV, and was achieved by the use of timed head maneuvers as well as applied vibration.[35] This procedure has been modified to exclude routine vibration. Studies suggest that the modified canalith repositioning procedure is as effective in the treatment of PC-BPPV, and that vibration applied during the maneuver provides no additional benefit and does not affect outcomes.[38–40]

During the CRP (**Fig. 32–2**) the patient is moved rapidly into the Dix-Hallpike position toward the direction of the affected ear. The patient's head is then kept in extension and rotated in

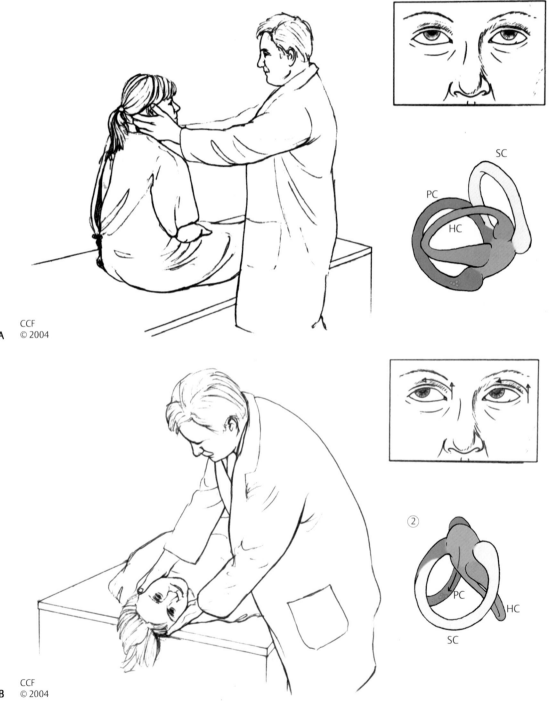

CCF
A © 2004

CCF
B © 2004

Figure 32–1   Dix-Hallpike positioning. **(A)**. Starting position (seated, head turned 45 degrees to the right). Position of the eyes and canalith material in the posterior semicircular canal is shown on the right. **(B)**. Lying position (head turned 45 degrees to the right). Characteristic upbeat and right torsional nystagmus is illustrated; canalith material has traveled down the long arm of the posterior semicircular canal, causing ampullofugal endolymph flow and stimulation of the cupula. (From the Cleveland Clinic Foundation. Reprinted with permission.)

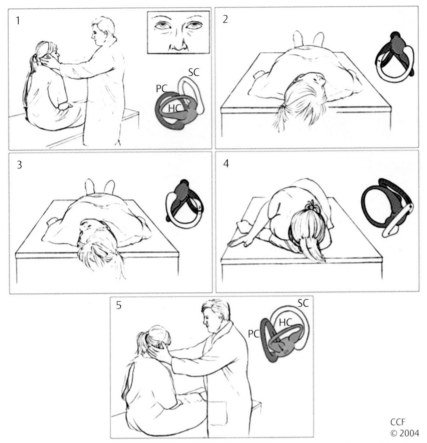

Figure 32–2 Canalith repositioning procedure for right posterior semicircular canal benign paroxysmal positional vertigo. The patient begins in the seated position with the head turned 45 degrees towards the examiner (rightwards, see Box 1). The patient is placed in the right Dix-Hallpike position and the characteristic nystagmus may be observed (Box 2). The patient remains supine and the head is slowly rotated towards the opposite ear (Box 3). The patient rolls onto the opposite shoulder and directs the head into a nose-down position (Box 4). After any nystagmus subsides, the patient is assisted in returning to the original position (Box 5). (From the Cleveland Clinic Foundation. Reprinted with permission.)

the opposite direction 45 degrees toward the unaffected ear. The patient is then rolled into a side-lying position with the head turned 45 degrees downward toward the floor. Keeping the head rotated toward the unaffected ear with the chin tucked in 20 degrees, the patient slowly returns to a seated position.

The Semont liberatory maneuver is also successful in treatment of BPPV.[41] The patient is sitting. The head is turned 45 degrees toward the unaffected side. The patient is then moved rapidly into a side-lying position on the affected side. After 1 to 2 minutes the patient is rapidly moved to the opposite side, maintaining the head in 45 degrees of rotation. This position is maintained for 1 to 2 minutes. The patient is then slowly brought back to a sitting position.

The Brandt-Daroff exercise is aimed at habituation. The patient is sitting. The head is maintained in 45 degrees of rotation. The patient moves quickly into a side-lying position, face up, and holds for 30 seconds. If vertigo is induced, the patient must wait until vertigo subsides plus an additional 30 seconds. The patient then returns to a seated position for 30 seconds. The procedure is then repeated on the opposite side.[42]

A recent evidence-based review by White et al[43] reports that the treatment efficacy for a single canalith repositioning session for posterior semicircular canal BPPV is 78%. Treatment efficacy increases with repetition of the maneuver and reaches an average of 90%.

Lateral Semicircular Canal Benign Paroxysmal Positional Vertigo

Lateral semicircular canal BPPV (LSC-BPPV) is thought to be rarer than posterior canal involvement. It is estimated that 2 to 15% of BPPV cases involve the lateral canal.[42] An episode of LSC-BPPV is precipitated primarily by rolling over in bed, and can be evoked by right and left positional maneuvers performed by rolling the patient's head from side to side in the supine position. Performing supine positional testing, as an adjunct to the standard Dix-Hallpike test, improves the sensitivity in the identification and diagnosis of LSC-BPPV.[31] If the LSC is not tested, BPPV may not be diagnosed and appropriately treated.

Geotropic LSC-BPPV was documented by McClure[44] in 1985. In geotropic LSC-BPPV, ampullopedal flow is stimulated, resulting in nystagmus beating toward the undermost ear when the head is turned from supine to a lateral position (**Fig. 32–3**). Nystagmus is induced by otoconial debris from the utricular macula moving through the LSC, exciting the receptors. It is characterized by a brief sensation of vertigo with short latency and prolonged duration, accompanied by purely horizontal nystagmus. Reversal of nystagmus is seen when the patient is turned to the opposite side and typically does not diminish with repeated testing. Nystagmus and associated symptoms are typically worse when the head is turned toward the affected ear.

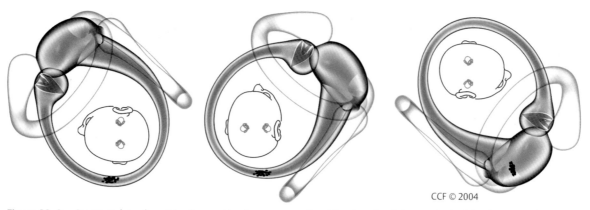

CCF © 2004

Figure 32–3 Geotropic lateral semicircular canal benign paroxysmal positional vertigo (LSC-BPPV). The left ear is viewed from above as the patient lies supine. Head position is indicated. In the central figure, the patient is supine and canalith material is in the distal lateral semicircular canal. On the left side of the figure, the patient has rolled onto the left ear and the canalith material moves towards the left LSC cupula, causing an ampullopetal endolymph current that is excitatory. On the right of the figure, the patient has rolled onto the right ear and the canalith material moves away from the cupula, causing an ampullofugal endolymph flow that is inhibitory. Nystagmus beats towards the undermost ear. (From the Cleveland Clinic Foundation. Reprinted with permission.)

Apogeotropic LSC-BPPV was later documented by Baloh et al[45] in 1995. In apogeotropic nystagmus, ampullofugal flow is stimulated, resulting in nystagmus beating away from the undermost ear when the head is turned from supine to a lateral position. Nystagmus is induced by otoconial debris adhering to the cupula, resulting in the cupula becoming gravity-sensitive (**Fig. 32–4**). Apogeotropic nystagmus also may be induced by the otoconial debris being trapped near the cupula, or proximal segment of the horizontal canal. The characteristics of apogeotropic LSC-BPPV are similar to those of geotropic LSC-BPPV; however, nystagmus is long lasting and beats away from the undermost ear. Nystagmus and associated symptoms are typically worse when the head is turned away from the affected ear. The apogeotropic variant is also more resistant to repositioning maneuvers. A study performed by White et al[43] utilized a combination of techniques for the treatment of apogeotropic LSC-BPPV with only a 50% success rate.

Identifying the involved ear is the first step in choosing the appropriate treatment for LSC-BPPV. Patient is lying supine with the head placed in approximately 20 degrees of flexion. The head is then turned to a lateral position. The direction and degree of nystagmus is noted. The patient's head is then turned to the opposite side and reversal of nystagmus is noted. If the patient lacks appropriate cervical mobility, the patient should be rolled into a side-lying position to increase the sensitivity of the test.

Treatment

Baloh-Lempert 360-Degree Roll
The treatment of choice for geotropic LSC-BPPV is the 360-degree barbecue roll maneuver. The maneuver starts with the patient in the supine position with the head flexed 0 to 30 degrees and consists of three 90-degree head rotations toward the unaffected ear. Each position is held for 30 to 60 seconds. The procedure may be repeated several times to promote the migration of free-moving otoconia in the endolymph of the horizontal canal back into the utricle. This procedure is effective in the treatment of LSC-BPPV and often results in the rapid cessation of positional vertigo and nystagmus.[31,46–48]

Vannucchi-Asprella Maneuver
The patient begins in the sitting position on the examination table and is quickly moved into the supine position. Then the patient's head is quickly rotated toward the unaffected side. Maintaining cervical rotation, the patient is returned to the

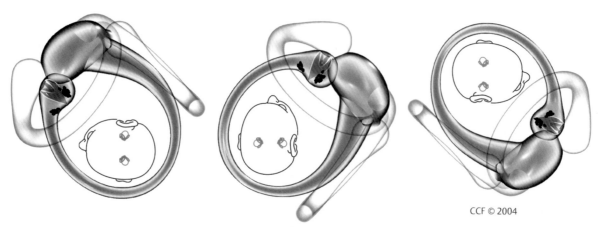

CCF © 2004

Figure 32–4 Apogeotropic lateral semicircular canal benign paroxysmal positional vertigo (LSC-BPPV). The left ear is viewed from above, as the patient lies supine. Head position is indicated. In the central figure, the patient is supine and canalith material is in the proximal lateral semicircular canal, possibly adherent to the cupula. On the left side of the figure, the patient has rolled onto the left ear, causing an ampullofugal endolymph current that is inhibitory. On the right of the figure, the patient has rolled onto the right ear, causing an ampullopetal endolymph flow that is excitatiry. Nystagmus beats away from the undermost ear. (From the Cleveland Clinic Foundation. Reprinted with permission.)

sitting position and the head is returned to midline. This is rapidly repeated five to eight times.[28] This procedure has been reported to be effective in relieving symptoms in 75 to 90% of patients with geotropic LSC-BPPV.[47,49–51]

The Vannucchi-Asprella maneuver is also used in converting apogeotropic to geotropic LSC-BPPV. The procedure is utilized to attempt to detach or mobilize the otoconia from the near-cupula in the posterior portion of the lateral canal.[50,51] Quick head thrusts away from the affected ear may also mobilize the otoconia to the posterior portion of the canal.

Guffoni Maneuver

The patient begins in the sitting position and is rapidly brought into the side-lying position toward the affected side. The patient's head is then rotated 45 degrees downward for the treatment of geotropic LSC-BPPV or 45 degrees upward for the treatment of apogeotropic LSC-BPPV. This position is maintained for 2 to 3 minutes. Ciniglio Appiani et al[52] reported a success rate of 78% on the first trial and 100% with a repeated maneuver in patients with geotropic LSC-BPPV. This maneuver has also been found to be effective in the conversion of apogeotropic LSC-BPPV to geotropic.[50,53]

Modified Brandt Daroff Exercises

Habituation exercise is utilized if there is failure to resolve LSC-BPPV with canalith repositioning maneuver. The patient begins in the sitting position keeping the head straight throughout the procedure, and rapidly lies down toward the affected ear. The patient remains in this position for 30 seconds after the vertigo stops and then repeats this procedure toward the opposite ear.[42]

Forced Prolonged Positioning

The patient is positioned in the side-lying position on the unaffected side. This position is maintained for 12 hours to rid the horizontal semicircular canal of otoconial debris. A study performed by Vannucchi et al[54] found this to be effective in 90% of the patients.

Anterior Semicircular Canal Benign Paroxysmal Positional Vertigo

Anterior canal BPPV is a rare, little-known entity. There may be strong paroxysmal downbeat nystagmus in the head-hanging positioning.[55,56] However, 75% of patients with this finding have explanatory central pathology, so this remains a diagnosis of exclusion. Paroxysmal downbeat nystagmus with a torsional component toward the affected side has been described in both contralateral[32] and ipsilateral[57,58] Dix-Hallpike positioning. This is explained by the gravitational movement of canaliths away from the ampula during positioning that stimulates paroxysmal torsional downbeat nystagmus toward the affected ear. However, fluid dynamics may be complicated by the shared common crus, and some authors suggest considering the vertical canals (anterior and posterior) as a conjoint entity.

Numerous therapeutic maneuvers have been described for anterior canal BPPV, including a deep Dix-Hallpike to the ipsilateral or contralateral side with a return to the sitting position,[59,60] a modified Semont maneuver beginning nose down on the affected side,[58] and an Epley maneuver performed on the contralateral side.[32,37] Because the left anterior and right posterior semicircular canals are coplanar (and similarly the

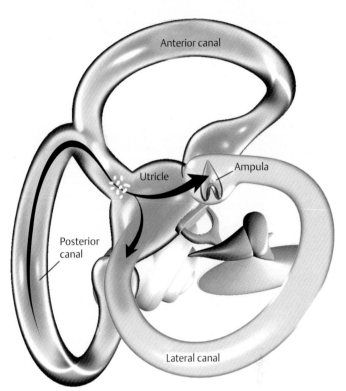

Figure 32–5 Conversion of posterior to lateral canal BPPV. Canalith material leaves the posterior semicircular canal and can move onto the cupula of the lateral semicircular canal, or into the long arm of the lateral semicircular canal. In the first instance the nystagmus on supine positioning is apogeotropic horizontal; in the latter instance it is geotropic horizontal. (From the Cleveland Clinic Foundation. Reprinted by permission.)

right anterior and left posterior), the Dix-Hallpike and canalith repositioning maneuvers are performed on the right side for left anterior canal involvement and vice versa.

◆ Complications and Recurrence

Complications associated with treatment of BPPV include the conversion of otoconial debris from one canal to another[57,61] (**Fig. 32–5**), combined posterior and horizontal canal BPPV, as well as recurrence of BPPV.

The evidence basis of vestibular assessment and outcomes of vestibular rehabilitation is rapidly expanding.[5–8,62] Recent publications substantiate a decreased fall risk and improved dynamic visual acuity after vestibular rehabilitation.[7,62–64] Newer treatment approaches are attempting to enhance dynamic balance strategies in life-like situations.[15] Although research in the area of dynamic balance recovery after vestibular insult is ongoing, challenges remain due to the complex multisystem contributions to balance.[16,65]

References

1. Shumway-Cook A, Horak FB. Assessing the influence of sensory interaction on balance: suggestion from the field. Phys Ther 1986;66:1548–1550
2. Shumway-Cook A, Woollacot M. Motor Control Theory and Practical Applications. Baltimore: Williams & Wilkins, 1995
3. Berg KO, Wood-Dauphinee SL, Williams JI, Gayton DB. Measuring balance in the elderly. Physiotherapy Canada 1989;41:304–311
4. Podsiadlo D, Richardson S. The timed "Up & Go": a test of basic functional mobility for frail elderly persons. J Am Geriatr Soc 1991;39:142–148

5. Wrisley D, Marchetti G, Kuharsky D, Whitney S. Reliability, internal consistency, and validity of data obtained with the functional gait assessment. Phys Ther 2004;84:906–918

6. Hall CD, Schubert MC, Herdman SJ. Prediction of all risk reduction as measured by dynamic gait index in individuals with unilateral vestibular hypofunction. Otol Neurotol 2004;25:746–751

7. Macias JD, Masingale S, Gerkin RD. Efficacy of vestibular rehabilitation therapy in reducing falls. Otolaryngol Head Neck Surg 2005;133:323–325

8. Whitney SL, Marchetti GF, Schade A, Wrisley DM. The sensitivity and specificity of the timed "Up and Go" and the dynamic gait index for self-reported falls in persons with vestibular disorders. J Vestib Res 2004;14:397–409

9. Fitz-Ritson D. Assessments of cervicogenic vertigo. J Manipulative Physio Ther. 1991;14:487–488

10. Jacobson GP, Newman CW. The development of the Dizziness Handicap Inventory. Arch Otolaryngol Head Neck Surg 1990;116:424–427

11. Powell LE, Meyers AM. The Activities-Specific Balance Confidence (ABC) Scale. J Gerontol A Bil Sci Med Sci 1995;50:M28–M34

12. Cohen HS, Kimball KT, Adams AS. Application of the vestibular disorders activities of daily living scale. Laryngoscope 2000;110:1204–1209

13. Zee DS. Adaptation to vestibular disturbances: some clinical implications. Acta Neurol Belg 1991;91:97–104

14. Herdman SJ. Vestibular Rehabilitation. Philadelphia: FA Davis 1994

15. Sparto PJ, Whitney SL, Hodges LF, Furman JM, Redfern MS. Simulator sickness when performing gaze shifts within a wide field of view optic flow environment: preliminary evidence for using virtual reality in vestibular rehabilitation. J Neuroengineering Rehabil 2004;1:14

16. McGibbon CA, Krebs DE, Wolf SL, et al. Tai Chi and vestibular rehabilitation improve vestibulopathic gait via different neuromuscular mechanisms. Preliminary report. BMC Neurol 2005;5:3

17. McGibbon CA, Krebs DE, Wolf SL, Wayne PM, Scarborough DM, Parker SW. Tai Chi and vestibular rehabilitation effects on gaze and whole body stability. J Vestib Res 2004;14:467–478

18. Mizukoshi K, Watanabe Y, Shojaku H, et al. Epidemiological studies on benign paroxysmal positional vertigo in Japan. Acta Otolaryngol Suppl 1988;447:67–72

19. Hotson JR, Baloh RW. Acute vestibular syndrome. N Engl J Med 1998;339:680–685

20. Froehling DA, Silverstein MD, Mohr DN, et al. BPPV: incidence and prognosis in a population based study in Olmsted County, Minnesota. Mayo Clin Proc 1991;66:596–601

21. Oghalai JS, Manolidis S, Barth JL, et al. Unrecognized benign paroxysmal positional vertigo in elderly patients. Otolaryngol Head Neck Surg 2000;122:630–634

22. Bertholon P, Chelikh L, Timoshenko A, et al. Combined horizontal and posterior canal benign paroxysmal positional vertigo in three patients with head trauma. Ann Otol Rhinol Laryngol 2005;114:105–110

23. Baloh RW, Honrubia V, Jacobson K. Benign positional vertigo: clinical and oculographic features in 240 cases. Neurology 1987;37:371–378

24. Pagnini P, Nuti D, Vannucchi P. Benign paroxysmal vertigo of the horizontal canal. ORL J Otorhinolaryngol Relat Spec 1989;51:161–170

25. Di Girolamo S, Paludetti G, Briglia G, et al. Postural control in benign paroxysmal positional vertigo before and after recovery. Acta Otolaryngol 1998;118:289–293

26. Blatt PJ, Georgakakis GA, Herdman SJ, et al. The effect of the canalith repositioning maneuver on resolving postural instability in patients with benign paroxysmal positional vertigo. Am J Otol 2000;21:356–363

27. Black FO, Nashner LM. Postural disturbances in patients with benign paroxysmal positional nystagmus. Ann Otol Rhinol Laryngol 1984;93:595–599

28. Ruckenstein MJ. Therapeutic efficacy of the Epley canalith repositioning maneuver. Laryngoscope 2001;111:940–945

29. Katsarkas A, Kearney R. Postural disturbances in paroxysmal positional vertigo. Am J Otol 1990;11:444–446

30. Di Girolamo S, Ottaviani F, Scarano E, et al. Postural control in horizontal benign paroxysmal positional vertigo. Eur Arch Otorhinolaryngol. 2000;257:372–375

31. White J, Coale K, Catalano P, et al. Diagnosis and management of lateral semicircular canal benign paroxysmal positional vertigo. Otolaryngol Head Neck Surg 2005;133:278–284

32. Honrubia V, Baloh RW, Harris MR, et al. Paroxysmal positional vertigo syndrome. Am J Otol 1999;20:465–470

33. Schuknecht HF. Cupulolithiasis. Arch Otolaryngol 1969;90:765–778

34. Hall SF, Ruby RR, McClure JA. The mechanism of benign paroxysmal vertigo. J Otolaryngol 1979;8:151–158

35. Epley J. The canalith repositioning procedure: for treatment of benign paroxysmal positional vertigo. Otolaryngol Head Neck Surg 1992;107:399–404

36. Dix MR, Hallpike CS. Pathology, symptoms and diagnosis of certain disorders of the vestibular system. Proc R Soc Med 1952;45:341–354

37. Viirre E, Purcell I, Baloh RW. The Dix Hallpike test and the canalith repositioning manever. Laryngoscope 2005;115:184–187

38. Hain TC, Helminski JO, Ries IL, Uddin MK. Vibration does not improve results of the canalith repositioning procedure. Arch Otolaryngol Head Neck Surg 2000;126:617–622

39. Wolf JS, Boyev KP, Manokey BJ, Mattox DE. Success of the modified Epley maneuver in treating benign paroxysmal positional vertigo. Laryngoscope 1999;109:900–903

40. Macias JD, Ellensohn A, Massingale S, Gerkin R. Vibration with the canalith repositioning maneuver: a prospective randomized study to determine efficacy. Laryngoscope 2004;114:1011–1014

41. Semont A, Freyss G, Vitte E. Curing the BPPV with a liberative maneuver. Adv Otorhinolaryngol 1998;42:290–293

42. Herdman SJ, Tusa RJ. Assessment and treatment of patients with benign paroxysmal positional vertigo. In: Vestibular Rehabilitation. Philadelphia: FA Davis, 2000;451–475

43. White J, Savvides P, Cherian N, et al. Canalith repositioning for benign paroxysmal positional vertigo. Otol Neurotol 2005;26:704–710

44. McClure JA. Horizontal canal BPV. J Otolaryngol 1985;14:30–35

45. Baloh RW, Yue Q, Jacobson K, et al. Persistent direction changing positional nystagmus. Neurology 1995;45:1297–1301

46. Lempert T, Tiel-Wilck K. A positional maneuver for treatment of horizontal canal benign positional vertigo. Laryngoscope 1996;106:476–478

47. Ciniglio Appiani G, Gagliardi M, Magliulo G. Physical treatment of horizontal canal benign positional vertigo. Eur Arch Otorhinolaryngol 1997;254:326–328

48. Baloh RW. Horizontal benign positional vertigo. Neurology 1994;44:2214

49. Asprella Libonati G, Gagliardi G, Cifarelli D, Larotonda G. Step by step treatment of lateral semicircular canal canalithiasis under videonystagmoscopic examination. Acta Otorhinolaryngol Ital 2003;23:10–15

50. Casani AP, Vannucci G, Fattori B, Berrettini S. The treatment of horizontal canal positional vertigo: our experience in 66 cases. Laryngoscope 2002;112:172–178

51. Vannucchi P, Asprella Libonati G, Gufoni M. Therapy of lateral semicircular canal canalithiasis. Audiological Medicine 2005;3:52–56

52. Appiani GC, Catania G, Gargliardi M. A liberatory maneuver for the treatment of horizontal canal paroxysmal positional vertigo. Otol Neurotol 2001;22:66–69

53. Appiani GC, Catania G, Gagliardi M, et al. Repositioning maneuver for the treatment of the apogeotropic variant of horizontal canal benign paroxysmal positional vertigo. Otol Neurotol 2005;26:257–260

54. Vannucchi P, Giannoni B, Pagnini P. Treatment of horizontal semicircular canal benign paroxysmal positional vertigo. J Vestib Res 1997;7:1–6

55. Bertholon P, Bronstein AM, Davies RA, Rudge P, Thilo KV. Positional down beating nystagmus in 50 patients: cerebellar disorders and possible anterior semicircular canalithiasis. J Neurol Neurosurg Psychiatry 2002;72:366–372

56. Crevits L. Treatment of anterior canal benign paroxysmal positional vertigo by a prolonged forced position procedure. J Neurol Neurosurg Psychiatry 2004;75:779–781

57. Herdman SJ, Tusa RJ. Complications of the canalith repositioning procedure. Arch Otolaryngol Head Neck Surg 1996;122:281–286

58. Brantberg K, Bergenius J. Treatment of anterior benign paroxysmal positional vertigo by canal plugging: a case report. Acta Otolaryngol 2002;122:28–30

59. Semont A. BPPV, the liberatory maneuvers. In: Guidetti G, Pagnini P, eds. Labyrintholithiasis-Related Paroxysmal Positional Vertigo. Milan: Elsevier (Excerpta Medica), 2002

60. Kim YK, Shin JE, Chung JW. The effect of canalith repositioning for anterior semicircular canal canalithiasis. ORL J Otorhinolaryngol Relat Spec 2005;67:56–60

61. White JA, Oas JG. Diagnosis and management of lateral semicircular canal conversions during particle repositioning therapy. Laryngoscope 2005;115:1895–1897

62. Herdman SJ, Schubert MC, Tusa RJ. Strategies for balance rehabilitation: fall risk and treatment. Ann N Y Acad Sci 2001;942:394–412

63. Badke MB, Shea TH, Miedaner JA, Grove CR. Outcomes after rehabilitation for adults with balance dysfunction. Arch Phys Med Rehabil 2004;85(2):227–233

64. Herdman SJ, Schubert MC, Das VE, Tusa RJ. Recovery of dynamic visual acuity in unilateral vestibular hypofunction. Arch Otolaryngol Head Neck Surg 2003;129(8):819–824

65. Cavanaugh JT, Goldvasser D, McGibbon CA, Krebs DE. Comparison of head and body velocity trajectories during locomotion among healthy and vestibulopathic subjects. J Rehabil Res Dev 2005;42:191–198

33

Rehabilitation and Reanimation of the Paralyzed Face

Kevin A. Shumrick

The human face is unique across the animal kingdom in its ability to express a wide range of emotions and intent. Facial expressions in lower animals are used primarily to express anger or aggression, whereas the human face is capable of clearly signaling to other humans the four major emotions (fear, anger, happiness, and sadness) as well as more subtle nuances such as sympathy, disgust, amusement, disbelief, and surprise. These facial expressions have clearly evolved to aid in the social interaction of humans, and paralysis of the face significantly compromises an individual's ability to function effectively in society. Patients with facial paralysis present an alien countenance that others find disquieting. There is the unspoken fear that whatever is affecting the face is contagious, and many of the basics of social interaction (handshaking, cheek kissing) are approached with trepidation by both the patient and acquaintances. Patients with facial paralysis avoid having photos taken and thus drop out of the photographic record of a family. Similarly, patients begin to avoid social functions and family gatherings because they feel embarrassed and worry that they will make others uncomfortable. All these factors combine to isolate patients socially and are compounded when they try to reenter the work force. At the workplace patients with facial paralysis may face not only social isolation but also subtle discrimination that may prevent them from obtaining jobs or advancing in jobs.

In addition to their socializing functions, the muscles of facial expression are important for proper functioning of the face. The orbicularis oris and oculi are critical for maintaining the sphincteric effect of the lips and eyelids, and without them the affected side loses competency. With loss of the ipsilateral orbicularis oris the affected side of the mouth droops, and drooling of liquids and food results. It is difficult to use a straw and puff the cheek. Without the buccal muscle, food accumulates in the buccal space, contributing to halitosis and dental caries. The orbicularis oculi is responsible for the ability to actively blink the eye and squint. Loss of the ability to effectively blink predisposes the eye to desiccation and corneal ulcers as well as injury by foreign bodies that would normally be blocked by blinking or squinting.

Even though this chapter is devoted to rehabilitation of the paralyzed face, an understanding of the basics of facial nerve anatomy, physiology, and function is essential to plan the timing and method of repair. Additionally, a basic understanding of the fundamentals of nerve degeneration and regeneration helps the surgeon recognize when success of a facial nerve repair is not likely and plan for an alternative method of reanimation.

◆ Facial Nerve Anatomy

The facial nerve is composed of both sensory and motor nerve fibers. Distal to the geniculate ganglion the facial nerve consists of 10,000 fibers of which 7000 are myelinated and innervate the muscles of facial expression.[1] The remaining 3000 fibers supply secretomotor fibers to the salivary and lacrimal glands, and sensory fibers to the lingual taste buds. By the time the facial nerve has exited the stylomastoid foramen, most of the sensory nerve fibers have left the main trunk, and the remaining portion of the nerve is composed almost entirely of myelinated fibers to the facial muscles.

Each motor neuron consists of a cell body located at the brainstem with a myelinated axon that travels to a motor endplate located on a facial muscle. The axons have Schwann cells on their surface, which produce myelin. The myelin is present throughout the length of the axon except at the nodes of Ranvier, which are approximately 2 mm apart (**Fig. 33–1**). Outside the Schwann cell of each axon is the endoneurium, which is a loose connective tissue layer. The facial nerve axons, with their enclosing endoneurium, are grouped into fascicles of varying numbers of axons. These fascicles are distinguished by being surrounded by a layer of connective tissue referred to as perineurium. Finally, the fascicles are bundled together, along with venules and arterioles, by the epineurium into what is formally called a nerve. The epineurium is also referred to as the nerve sheath (**Fig. 33–1**). The facial nerve does not begin as a multifascicular

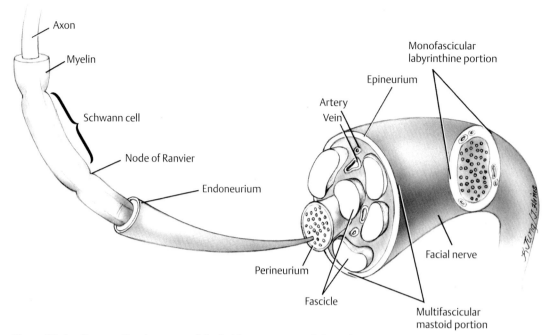

Axon

Myelin

Schwann cell

Node of Ranvier

Endoneurium

Perineurium

Fascicle

Monofascicular
labyrinthine portion

Epineurium

Artery

Vein

Facial nerve

Multifascicular
mastoid portion

Figure 33–1   Cross-sectional anatomy of the facial nerve as it travels from the temporal bone to the facial muscles. Note that in the internal auditory canal it is monofascicular and in the mastoid portion of the facial canal it is divided into multiple fascicles by perineurium.

nerve; when it exits the brainstem and enters the internal auditory canal, it consists of a single fascicle. This monofascicular arrangement continues through the labyrinthine and tympanic segments of the nerve. Distally, in the mastoid portion, the nerve begins to divide into several fascicles, with each fascicle surrounded by perineurium (**Fig. 33–1**). At the level of the stylomastoid foramen the nerve has divided into six to ten fascicles.[2] There has been a lively debate in the literature as to whether the main trunk of the facial nerve has a topographic distribution, which could be useful when performing nerve repairs or nerve grafting.[3–5] This is discussed further in the section on nerve repair, but at present the topographic distribution of the facial nerve has not proven to be clinically useful.

Because several methods of facial reanimation require grafting or nerve transfer to the intraparotid facial nerve, a brief discussion of the extratemporal bone facial nerve anatomy is in order. The facial nerve exits the temporal bone at the stylomastoid foramen. It then travels anteriorly through the substance of the parotid as a single nerve for approximately 2 cm, at which point it consistently bifurcates into an upper and lower division (**Fig. 33–2**). The facial nerve divisions continue anteriorly for several millimeters and then divide into a total of five branches, giving rise to the pes anserinus. The typical branches of the facial nerve are the temporal, zygomatic, buccal, mandibular, and cervical, and these branches can have significant variation in their subsequent course and subdivisions.[6–8] Davis et al[6] identified six different patterns of facial nerve branching with no one type occurring more than 28% of the time.

Even with this variability there are several anatomic landmarks that can facilitate locating various key portions of the extratemporal facial nerve, as noted by Crumley and Scott[9] (**Fig. 33–3**):

1. The pes anserinus is consistently located at a point 1 cm anterior and 2 cm inferior to the tragal cartilage.

2. The superior division of the facial nerve travels on a line from the pes anserinus to approximately the lateral corner of the eyebrow.

3. The buccal branch leaves the pes anserinus and travels anteriorly and slightly superiorly passing 1 cm inferior to the bottom of the zygomatic arch.

4. The marginal mandibular branch leaves the pes and travels inferiorly and anteriorly, passing down over the angle of the mandible and then proceeding inferior to the rim of the mandible for 3 cm before ascending back over the rim of the mandible at its junction with the facial vessels.

Despite the variability of these facial nerve branching patterns, there is consistently found to be cross-innervation between the various branches and even between the upper and lower divisions. This cross-innervation between divisions and branches of the facial nerve is most pronounced between the zygomatic and buccal branches and least for the marginal mandibular branch. This explains why significant deficits of the midfacial muscles are rarely seen from a peripheral facial nerve injury and relatively common from a marginal mandibular nerve injury. This interconnection of branches and divisions also helps explain the phenomenon of synkinesis following injury of the main trunk of the facial nerve because with regeneration the neuronal sprouts not only have free access to reinnervate their original muscle fibers, but also take aberrant routes to facial muscles of different branches and even different divisions. It is not surprising, therefore, that the midface (which has the most interconnections) is also the site of most prominent synkinesis, with the eye and upper lip moving in synchrony.

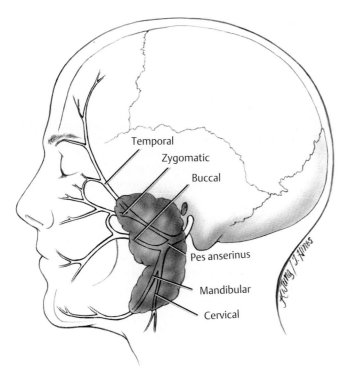

Figure 33–2 Branching of intraparotid facial nerve into upper and lower divisions with five main branches. There is considerable cross-innervation between the zygomatic and buccal branches, which makes these branches most resistant to peripheral injuries, but also most susceptible to synkinesis.

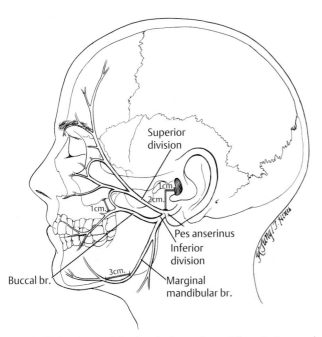

Figure 33–3 Anatomic landmarks for portions of the extratemporal facial nerve. The pes anserinus is located approximately 1 cm anterior and 2 cm inferior to the tragus. The marginal branch dips inferior to the margin of the mandible at the angle and then reemerges above it approximately 3 cm anterior to the angle. The buccal branch runs approximately 1 cm inferior to the zygomatic arch.

◆ Physiology of Nerve Repair

The facial nerve, like other motor nerves, is composed of central nervous system (CNS) axons, which have synaptic connections with several adjacent muscle fibers (referred to as a motor unit). There are estimates that each of the 7000 neuron cell bodies supplies innervation for approximately 25 muscle fibers. It is recognized in muscle physiology that the smaller the ratio of muscle fibers to neuron cell bodies, the more specialized the movement possible. As an example, the gastrocnemius muscle has a ratio of 2000 muscle cells for each neuron cell body, whereas in the larynx the ratio is one to one.[8] The nerve cell body, located in the pons, manufactures functionally important substances, such as neurotransmitters and enzymes, which are transported via the axoplasmic transport system to the motor end-plate.[10,11] Additionally, trophic substances produced at the distal end of the nerve are transmitted back to the cell body and allow central monitoring of the distal nerve via these molecules. Thus, we see that the individual nerve fibers are in a dynamic state with regard to monitoring the health status of the entire nerve and adjusting to changing conditions. When a nerve is injured, distinct histologic and biochemical changes take place in the proximal cell body, distal injured nerve, motor end-plate, and motor unit (muscle fibers). The degree and severity of these changes are due to a variety of factors, which include type of injury (i.e., crush versus transection), age of patient, nutritional status, and distance from injury to cell body.[10] Sunderland[12,13] has developed a classification of facial nerve injury, based on the degree of disruption, which accounts for the observed physiology of nerve repair and predicts the degree of functional recovery. With the fourth- and fifth-degree nerve injuries, commonly seen with facial paralysis patients, all components of the nerve fiber (endoneurium, perineurium, and epineurium) are disrupted.

The neuron cell body undergoes marked metabolic changes following transection of an axon. Protein synthesis and RNA increase steadily for approximately 3 weeks, at which time their levels reach a steady state that persists until the nerve has reestablished connections with a motor end plate. The observation that it takes approximately 3 weeks for a nerve fiber to fully convert to a regenerative state has led some authors to advocate waiting 3 weeks before performing a nerve repair or nerve grafting; however, it has now been well established that the optimum time for repair is as soon after the injury as possible. In the proximal stump of the injured nerve, axonal sprouts begin to form within 3 days of transection. These axonal sprouts grow peripherally at a rate of approximately 1 mm per day. Thus, for a facial nerve injury in the temporal bone to regenerate 14 cm to the facial muscles would take approximately 140 days.[8]

In the nerve segment distal to the site of injury, Wallerian degeneration begins rapidly. The Schwann cells proliferate and convert into macrophages, which phagocytose the myelin, axoplasm, and other products of degeneration. The motor end-plates retract, and if they are not reinnervated within a reasonable amount of time (the exact time is not known but appears to be several years), the synaptic clefts will eventually be obliterated by collagen deposition.

It should be noted that with a facial nerve injury in which the nerve has been transected, the distal nerve end will still conduct impulses via a nerve stimulator and cause facial motion for up to 72 hours after the injury. This is a crucial time period for nerve repair because it allows the surgeon to employ the nerve stimulator to accurately and definitively identify the distal end of the nerve and perform a primary repair or nerve graft. Delay of repair beyond the 72-hour time period means that the nerve must be dissected much more extensively to ensure that the distal end has been accurately identified. Additionally, scarring and fibrosis will begin making the dissection even more difficult. All these factors argue for early exploration of an injury when transection is suspected, and performing a repair in as timely a fashion as possible.

Facial Muscle Degeneration

Although specific data on the degeneration of human facial muscles is lacking, it appears that facial muscles follow a comparable course to other muscles that are denervated. Namely, following denervation there is a progressive diminution of muscle fiber diameter to approximately one-half the original diameter within 1 month of denervation. Following this acute phase of degeneration the muscle fiber appears to stabilize and remains unchanged for a variable period of time. The eventual degree of muscle degeneration is related to the completeness of the original neuronal lesion and whether or not the muscle obtains some degree of reinnervation (from the facial nerve, adjacent facial muscles, or aberrant reinnervation from an alternate nerve such as the trigeminal). During this time it appears that the muscle fiber is susceptible to reinnervation, although with reinnervation it does not regain its original bulk.

A crucial issue in performing a nerve graft or nerve transfer is whether or not there are receptive, viable muscle fibers available for reinnervation; if not, then an alternative method of reanimation should be chosen. This concept is critical to avoid the tragic scenario of performing a hypoglossal-facial anastomosis in a patient with irreversibly atrophied facial muscles who will not regain facial movement and will have the additional disability of a hemitongue deficit. The only way to accurately and expeditiously determine the status of the facial muscles is through electromyography (EMG). EMG can provide four types of information with regard to the status of the facial muscles[9]: (1) EMG can show normal voluntary action potentials, which indicate that the muscles have connections with nerves and are being stimulated to voluntarily contract (indicating that the facial muscles are innervated and not receptive to reinnervation). (2) Polyphasic potentials may be detected, which indicate that reinnervation is proceeding even if there has not been return of voluntary function. The implication is that with simple observation there should be return of innervation and surgery should be delayed and the patient observed for an additional period of time. (3) Denervation or fibrillation potentials indicate the presence of viable but denervated muscle fibers that should be receptive to an attempt at reinnervation. (4) A final possible EMG finding is electrical silence, which indicates the absence of viable, functioning muscle fibers. This could be due to atrophy or congenital absence; in either event a reinnervation attempt would be unsuccessful due to a lack of viable, receptive muscle fibers for the nerve to reinnervate.

Facial Nerve and Muscle Regeneration

When the Schwann cells begin to phagocytose the myelin surrounding the axons, they form tubes referred to as Büngner bands. With regeneration the sprouting axons find their way (probably via chemotaxis factors) into these Büngner tubes

and thereby to the denervated muscle fibers. As axonal sprouts form at the proximal end of the neuron cell body, there may be multiple individual sprouts. However, only one sprout is retained once one reaches a denervated muscle; the rest of the sprouts are then resorbed. There appears to be a time limit within which an axon needs to reestablish a connection with a muscle cell via the Büngner bands or it will undergo degeneration. The exact time course for this degeneration is variable but has been noted to occur within as little as 4 months. Thus, if a nerve is injured and requires a primary repair or nerve graft, the sooner the reparative surgery is performed the better the chances of eventual recovery.

◆ Anatomy and Function of the Facial Muscles

The major disability of facial nerve paralysis is loss of motion of the facial muscles. Therefore, to restore some semblance of normal facial function, it is important to understand the arrangement and function of the facial musculature. The major physiologic function of the facial musculature is to provide competent sphincters of the mouth and eye. Ancillary functions would include aiding mastication and expressing emotions. The ability to express facial emotions through the manipulation of soft tissue by the facial muscles arises from the fact that facial muscles have extensive connections with the overlying facial skin. These attachments of muscle to skin are somewhat unique in the human body; the usual situation for voluntary, skeletal muscle is for it to connect bone to bone or bone to tendon.

Muscles of the Periorbital Region

The major functional muscle of the periorbital region is the orbicularis oculi, which constitutes the majority of the soft tissue of the eyelids (**Fig. 33–4**). The orbicularis oculi run longitudinally along the eyelids with connections to the medial and lateral canthal ligaments, frontal bone, maxilla, zygoma, and skin. When the orbicularis oculi contracts, the eyelids are foreshortened and closed. It is important to note that, as will be

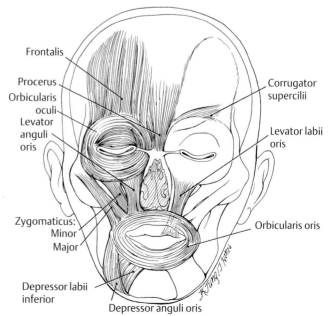

Figure 33–4 The major muscles of facial expression.

seen in the section on eyelid reanimation, the major movement during eyelid closure comes from the upper eyelid with the lower eyelid moving only slightly.

The importance of the ability to close the eye rapidly and forcefully cannot be overemphasized. The blink is a major protective mechanism from foreign bodies as well as for lubricating the eye and removing any debris that may have accumulated on the surface of the cornea. Additionally, the ability to squint or narrow the eye aperture is important to protect the eye from too much light or blowing objects (e.g., sand, rain, etc.).

Other muscles of the forehead region function primarily to move the eyebrows and these are the frontalis, corrugator supercilii, and procerus (**Fig. 33–4**). Although these muscles are much less important for protecting the eye than the orbicularis oculi, they are quite significant for maintenance of normal facial expression. A major consequence of forehead paralysis is pronounced drooping of the eyebrow, which is frequently so severe that, in conjunction with a hypotonic orbicularis oculi, it will droop over the eye and cause visual field obstruction.

Perioral Muscles

The perioral muscles function primarily to control the lips and provide the sphincteric action necessary for mastication and speech. They also provide the motion to bring about the smile and its variations, which are, in all likelihood, the most important of facial expressions. The major perioral muscle is the orbicularis oris, which encircles the mouth and provides the bulk of soft tissue comprising the lips (**Fig. 33–4**). With contraction of the orbicularis oris the lips are compressed together, the deep fibers press the lips against the teeth, and the superficial fibers pull the lip into a pout due to the purse-string effect.[14]

Although the orbicularis oris is the most important muscle for controlling the oral aperture, several other muscles affect the configuration and positioning of the lips. These muscles may be grouped into elevators of the upper lip, elevators of the corner of the mouth, depressors of the lower lip, and depressors of the corner of the mouth (**Fig. 33–4**). However, the major muscles affecting the positioning of the corner of the mouth, for practical purposes, are the zygomaticus major and, to a lesser degree, the zygomaticus minor (**Fig. 33–4**). The zygomaticus muscles arise from the inferior body of the zygoma and insert at the corner of the mouth in the region of the oral commissure by insinuating themselves with the orbicularis oris and depressors of the commissure. Additionally, the zygomaticus muscles send fibers to the overlying skin, which contribute to the formation of the nasolabial fold. The primary function of the zygomaticus muscles is to provide tone and support to the corner of the mouth (with maintenance of the nasolabial fold) and with active contraction elevation of the corner of the mouth into the primary position of the smile. The smile can be modified by the ancillary perioral muscles to add the subtleties of facial expression such as a sneer, grimace, etc.

◆ Methods of Facial Reanimation

Reinnervation Techniques

Primary Anastomosis

If a facial paralysis results from trauma to the facial nerve, the most successful outcome will occur if the nerve is able to regenerate back through its original fascicles. This may be possible when there has been a crush-type injury to the nerve

without actual transection. Once the integrity of the nerve has been disrupted, the best result will be obtained if the two ends of the nerve can be accurately reapproximated. It has been advocated that intrafascicular (using the perineurium) repair of neuron fascicles gives the best return of nerve function, and this method of repair has been proposed for repair of facial nerve injuries, to lessen the synkinesis that can significantly mar an otherwise successful neural repair. However, for intrafascicular repair to decrease synkinesis requires that the nerve has a distinct topographic distribution with nerves in each fascicle going primarily to specific muscles or muscle groups. There is some evidence that there may, in fact, be a distinct topographic orientation of the facial nerve. May[4] had noted clinically that certain types of facial nerve injuries seemed to be reflected in specific deficits of facial movement. Kempe[3] performed topographic stimulation of the facial nerve in patients undergoing resection of glomus jugulare tumors and noted a topographic representation of fibers within the main nerve trunk. However, a very detailed anatomic study by Gacek and Radpour[2] showed that small fascicles of the facial nerve at the level of the internal auditory meatus carry motor fibers to all the distal branches of the facial nerve and that the facial nerve is, at best, only loosely topographically organized. Thus, although an intrafascicular repair does indeed ensure a more accurate reapproximation of individual fascicles, within each fascicle there are nerve fibers going to multiple, different muscles and synkinesis may still result.[8,15] A further concern with intrafascicular repair is that several authors have raised the possibility that the additional dissection required for an intrafascicular repair could enhance scarring and injure the blood supply with significant diminution of functional results.[16,17] If there is a clean laceration of the trunk with the two ends easily available and it is possible to clearly identify corresponding fascicles in each end, then it would be reasonable to attempt an intrafascicular repair of comparable portions of the nerve. Otherwise, most authors now advocate a meticulous epineurial repair with no attempt to reestablish a topographic intrafascicular repair.[8,9,15] The suture method of choice is five to seven sutures of 9-0 monofilament used in a epineurial repair.[18,19]

The location of the transection of the nerve dictates, to some degree, the method of repair. Lesions of the facial nerve at the brainstem or in its temporal portion have been notoriously difficult to suture-repair a primary end-to-end anastomosis. At the brainstem the nerve lacks mobility and it is very difficult to suture deep in the wound. Kanzaki et al[20] reported a series of nine patients who had repair of the facial nerve at the brainstem, four of whom regained facial motion. The authors noted that although the nerve repair is technically demanding, the four patients who regained motion had results superior to those found with any other technique, and the authors felt that it was worth trying if a nerve transection was noted during a skull base procedure. The temporal portion of the nerve is encased in bone and cannot be mobilized without a complete facial nerve decompression. Several studies looked at various conduits as alternatives to facial nerve decompression and mobilization to help guide the regenerating neuronal sprouts from the proximal nerve end to the distal nerve end when a primary repair cannot be attained. The proposed materials for these tubes have ranged from silicone wrapping to vein grafts to polyglycolic acid tubes.[19,21,22] However, there is no convincing evidence that these tubes offer significant advantages over epineurial repair or an interpositional nerve graft.

Given the difficulties with suture approximation of the facial nerve in various locations, it is little wonder that a variety of methods for sutureless repair of the facial nerve have been advocated. The two most prominent techniques for sutureless nerve repair are fibrin glue and laser neurorrhaphy. Although both of these techniques enjoyed high enthusiasm when initially introduced, they have not withstood the test of time and are now generally considered to offer no significant advantage over standard suture repair of the nerve and may very well provide inferior results.[19,23,24]

Interpositional Nerve Grafting

If primary repair of a severed facial nerve is not possible due to a loss of a portion of the nerve or insufficient mobility to approximate the nerve ends, then the next best result is obtained by an interpositional nerve graft, which directs regenerating axons from the proximal nerve stump to the recipient fascicles of the distal nerve stump via the graft's own axon tubes. A variety of materials have been employed to act as replacement conduits for interpositional nerve grafts including gold foil, collagen tubes, and freeze-thawed skeletal muscle. The freeze-thawed muscle works on the principle that after freezing the muscle in liquid nitrogen, when the muscle thaws, the resulting cellular lysis will leave a large number of empty microtubules through which the nerve may regenerate.[25] Although there was considerable initial enthusiasm for the use of freeze-thawed muscle as an interpositional conduit for nerve regeneration, it now appears to be successful only over limited lengths of absent nerve. Mountain et al[26] found that interpositional nerve grafts were superior to freeze-thawed muscle, especially over gaps greater than 0.5 cm. There has also been a considerable amount of research into developing other conduits for regenerating nerves and various trophic factors to stimulate regeneration, but the best evidence at present is that the most successful replacement for a segment of missing facial nerve is an interpositional nerve graft carefully sutured to the cut ends of the nerve with fine monofilament epineurial sutures.[19] The most commonly employed donor nerve for grafting the trunk of the facial nerve proximal to the pes is the great auricular nerve because of its proximity and size similarities (**Fig. 33–5**). However, if a graft must be extended from the main trunk past the pes to individual branches of the facial nerve, then it is preferable to use a nerve with natural branches rather than trying to split the donor nerve into artifical branches. A donor nerve that has a naturally occurring branching similar to the facial nerve is the sural nerve and it is probably the most commonly used graft for replacement of the facial nerve trunk and branches (**Fig. 33–5**). Recently Ng et al[27] reported on the use of endoscopes to decrease the morbidity of sural nerve harvesting.

If during the course of a surgical procedure it becomes necessary to resect a portion of the facial nerve, most authors now recommend some attempt at reestablishing continuity of the nerve with a nerve graft if at all possible. When just a portion of the trunk is missing, a greater auricular cable graft is satisfactory. If a portion of the trunk and pes are missing, then one should use a sural nerve graft that has branches. Although it is recognized that these grafts result in significant synkinesis, they do provide some degree of voluntary motion and the most natural resting tone. Furthermore, it appears that an interpositional nerve graft may be successfully used to replace

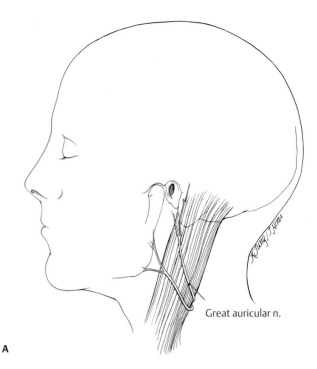

Great auricular n.

A

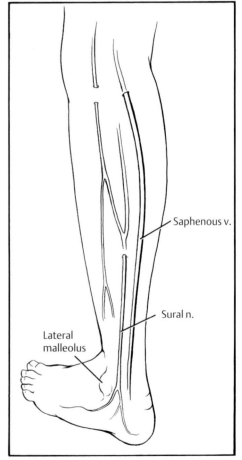

Saphenous v.

Sural n.

Lateral malleolus

B

Figure 33–5 **(A)** Route of the greater auricular nerve, which is frequently used as a replacement graft for facial nerve defect. It is identified running over the anterior border of the sternocleidomastoid (SCM) just superior to the external jugular vein. **(B)** When longer facial nerve grafts are required or the ipsilateral greater auricular (inset) nerve is not available, then a sural nerve graft is harvested. The sural nerve is located just posterior to the lateral malleolus of the fibula and anterior to the saphenous vein. It is then traced superiorly for the desired length.

a missing portion of the facial nerve even if postoperative radiation is to be employed.[28]

Several factors determine whether the proximal nerve is viable and capable of regenerating through a primary anastomosis or a cable graft, but, unfortunately, there are no reliable electrical tests to confirm the viability of the proximal nerve when it is discontinuous with its distal portion. A major factor determining if a proximal nerve will be capable of regenerating is time from injury. Ideally, the reanastomosis should take place as soon as possible following transection, within 30 days if at all possible and probably should not be performed if longer than 1 year from the date of injury because of the high likelihood of neural degeneration and poor chance of success.[29]

A variant on interpositional nerve grafting is the cross-facial nerve graft, in which a jump graft (from either the greater auricular or sural) is anastomosed to a redundant (usually the buccal or orbicularis) branch of the functional facial nerve and then tunneled across the face and anastomosed to the comparable branch of the paralyzed nerve (**Fig. 33–6**). The theory is that with regeneration of the contralateral, functional nerve it will reinnervate the opposite side of the face with similar nervous impulses and provide simultaneous control of discrete regions of the face. Unfortunately, clinical trials with cross-facial nerve grafting have not lived up to expectations, with several patients not developing any facial movement or very weak movement. The results seem to be somewhat better if performed within 6 months of injury, but the major problem appears to be a lack of sufficient neurons growing through the graft with which to provide a substantial muscular contraction.[9,30] At present cross-facial nerve grafting is used primarily to provide innervation for free muscle transfers and is not recommended for isolated reinnervation of the paralyzed face.

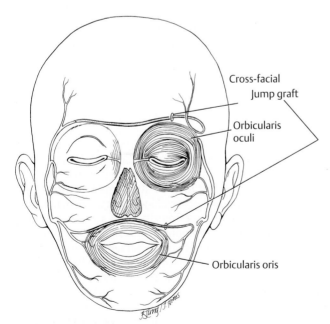

Figure 33–6 Schematic illustration of the use of cross-facial nerve grafts from the functioning facial nerve to distal branches of the paralyzed side. Note that cross-facial nerve grafts require sacrificing branches of the normal nerve. See text for a discussion of the success rate of these grafts.

Labels in figure:
Cross-facial Jump graft
Orbicularis oculi
Orbicularis oris

Hypoglossal-to-Facial Nerve Transfer

If the proximal facial nerve is not available for generating impulses to the facial muscles, but the distal nerve and muscles are intact, then it is possible to establish nervous impulses to the facial musculature by anastomosing the facial nerve to another functioning cranial nerve. However, before sacrificing another cranial nerve, it is advisable to investigate the status of the distal facial nerve and facial musculature to determine whether or not a cross-nerve (substitution) anastomosis has any chance of success. For a cross-nerve graft to be successful, it must have an adequate distal nerve to regenerate along and receptive, viable facial muscles. There is no reliable test to determine the status of the distal nerve or even to help identify it to perform the anastomosis. Crumley and Scott[9] listed several distal nerve-related factors that negatively affect the chances of a successful cross-nerve anastomosis: (1) nature of injury and surgical bed (scarred), (2) location of injury to nerve (distal does better than proximal), (3) age of patient (younger is better), (4) nutritional status of patient, and (5) history of radiation (impedes neural regeneration). It is also important to determine whether the facial muscles are viable, and an EMG can give very valuable information with regard to this. In particular, the surgeon is looking for evidence of functioning, excitable muscle tissue. If no potentials are noted, then the chances of a successful reinnervation are low due to presumed muscular atrophy, and another reanimation modality should be chosen. However, if the EMG is done within 12 months and shows polyphasic action potentials, then this may represent ongoing reinnervation, and surgery should be delayed until it is clear that no return of function occurs. When considering cross-nerve grafting, the ideal EMG finding is fibrillation or denervation potentials, which signify a complete lack of functioning neuronal input but viable muscle fibers.

If it is determined that there is a suitable distal nerve and viable facial muscles, then an anastomosis with another cranial nerve is a possibility. Various nerves have been considered for crossover including the phrenic and spinal accessory, but the largest experience is with the hypoglossal nerve.[31–34] The reasons for choosing the hypoglossal nerve include its surgical proximity, the fact that it shares anatomic and functional relationships with the facial nerve, and the relatively minor donor site morbidity. Before considering sacrificing a hypoglossal nerve, as has been mentioned the integrity of the distal nerve and facial muscles should be investigated. Additionally, the hypoglossal nerve should not be sacrificed if there is the potential for other ipsilateral, vagal, or glossopharyngeal or contralateral hypoglossal deficits, the combination of which could turn the patient into an oral cripple. Additional contraindications to performing a hypoglossal-facial anastomosis would include developmental facial paralysis patients who lack a sufficient population of extracranial facial nerve fibers and muscles, patients who are status post–massive resections of facial nerve and muscle, and patients with neurofibromatosis (type 2) who are at risk for bilateral and multiple cranial nerve tumors.[35]

Surgical Technique

The classic procedure for a hypoglossal/facial crossover is performed through a parotidectomy incision with an extension anteriorly to the tip of the hyoid. The parotid is elevated off the sternocleidomastoid muscle and the facial nerve is

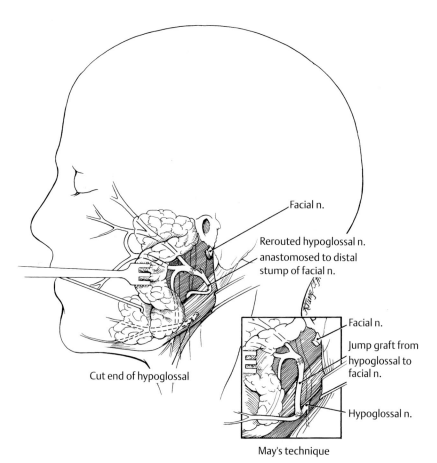

Facial n.

Rerouted hypoglossal n. anastomosed to distal stump of facial n.

Facial n.

Jump graft from hypoglossal to facial n.

Hypoglossal n.

Cut end of hypoglossal

May's technique

Figure 33–7 Classic hypoglossal facial anastomosis. Inset: May's technique of making a partial transection of the hypoglossal nerve and running a jump graft from the hypoglossal to the facial nerve. See text for details.

identified at the stylomastoid foramen and traced anteriorly to the pes. Next the posterior belly of the digastric is identified and the submandibular gland is elevated anteriorly. The hypoglossal nerve is identified deep to the digastric in the bed of the submandibular gland. It is dissected as far anteriorly as possible and the ansa hypoglossal branch identified. In the classic hypoglossal-facial transfer procedure the entire hypoglossal is transected as far anteriorly (distally) as possible and then rerouted to the region of the facial nerve trunk/pes junction. The facial nerve is then divided several millimeters proximal to the pes and the trunk of the hypoglossal anastomosed to the distal end of the facial nerve with 10–0 epineurial sutures (**Fig. 33–7**).

May et al[36] reported an interesting variant on the hypoglossal-facial nerve transfer where just a portion of the hypoglossal nerve is transected and then a jump graft, from either the greater auricular or sural nerve, is sewn from the partially transected hypoglossal to the trunk of the facial nerve (**Fig. 33–7** inset). Using this approach avoids complete loss of the ipsilateral hypoglossal. An additional benefit is that when the entire hypoglossal nerve is anastomosed to the facial nerve the resulting facial tone and movement are exaggerated from the normal side and the grafted side often actually appears hyperfunctional, but with using only a portion of the hypoglossal nerve the resulting tone and movement appear much more normal.

Results

Several factors determine the surgical success and ultimate patient satisfaction with hypoglossal-facial nerve transfers. The procedure appears to have a high success rate with regard

to reestablishing nervous impulses through the facial nerve. Most series report greater than 90% of patients regaining or improving their resting facial tone and regaining some degree of facial motion.[32–35,37,38] Improvement in facial tone starts at approximately 4 to 6 months postoperatively, with voluntary motion starting several months later. Both tone and movement improve for 18 to 24 months. However, simply regaining tone and some facial motion does not ensure a successful outcome. It is very rare for a patient to regain any movement that could be construed as spontaneous or emotive. In fact, it is rare to achieve voluntary movement of discrete regions of the face. Those patients likely to regain control of individual regions of the face are those who are highly motivated, undergo extensive training, and, most importantly, had the crossover performed early after injury to the facial nerve.[34,35] Reviews of several large series of hypoglossal-facial anastomosis report patients obtaining excellent results only approximately 40 to 50% of the time.[33,34,37,38] The major reasons for a less than excellent result are synkinesis, facial movement on eating or talking, and hypertonicity with excessive resting tone and exaggerated voluntary movement. Additionally, when sacrificing the entire hypoglossal nerve, there is a certain degree of morbidity due to the hemitongue flaccidity and eventual atrophy, which may cause difficulty with speaking, eating, and swallowing. The actual incidence of significant postoperative morbidity varies from series to series but may be as high as 74% of patients.[38] The hypoglossal-facial nerve jump graft described by May appears to alleviate many of these shortcomings by intentionally limiting the strength of the hypoglossal regeneration and preserving a majority of the hypoglossal connections to the tongue. Hammerschlag[39] echoes many of May's findings with regard to the hypoglossal jump graft. He was able to achieve House-Brackmann scores of 3 or better in 83% of his patients with very low morbidity. He also noted that his patients required gold weights to achieve acceptable eye closure.

Sobol and May[35,36] have noted that a significant number of patients undergoing a hypoglossal-facial anastomosis continue to have insufficient eye closure. In these cases the authors recommend the addition of an ancillary procedure to improve eye closure. As will be discussed, the current procedures of choice for eyelid reanimation are the insertion of an eyelid gold weight and, if necessary, a lid-tightening procedure. In fact, the gold weight and lid tightening work so well that it has even been suggested to hook up the hypoglossal to just the lower branches of the facial nerve and reanimate the eye with a gold weight, and thereby avoid the synkinesis and hypertonicity, which have plagued the classic hypoglossal-facial anastomosis procedure.[35,36]

Contiguous Muscle for Facial Reanimation

If it is not possible to reestablish nervous impulses through the facial nerve to the facial muscles, then the next step in facial rehabilitation is to replicate the most important facial nerve functions. The three most important functions of the facial nerve are (1) resting tone of the face, which prevents facial drooping; (2) closure of the eye for protection and lubrication; and (3) elevation of the corner of the mouth. Restoration of eye closure will be considered in the section on eyelid reanimation. Restoration of resting facial tone and elevation of the corner of the mouth may be partially restored with transposition of accessory muscles of the face, most commonly the temporalis or masseter. These muscles and their nerve supply (the trigeminal) must be intact. It is not uncommon that during resection of large acoustic neuromas not only the facial nerve but also the trigeminal may be compromised. Additionally, in large resections of the temporal bone or parotid these accessory muscles may be compromised due to actual resection, postoperative scarring, and postoperative radiation.

Temporalis Muscle Transposition

The temporalis is the most commonly employed ancillary muscle for facial rehabilitation. It is a fan-shaped muscle that arises from the temporal line of the temporal bone and passes under the zygomatic arch to insert on the coronoid process of the mandible. The most common application of the temporalis is to detach it from its origin along the temporal crest of the temporal bone and fold it inferiorly over the zygomatic arch. The muscle is then attached to either the perioral or periorbital musculature. With its innervation and blood supply intact, and the insertion on the condyle as an anchoring point, the temporalis may be used as an active animator of the face with some degree of voluntary control.

Anatomy of the Temporalis Muscle

The temporalis muscle is innervated by the motor division of the trigeminal nerve. It is a wide, flat muscle that arises from the temporal crest of the temporal bone where it is attached to both the bone and adjacent periosteum. The muscle fibers converge to form a thick tendon that passes under the zygomatic arch to insert on the coronoid process of the mandible. The temporalis functions as an accessory muscle of mastication and its main action is to elevate the mandible when contracted. The temporalis is covered by a dense fascia that attaches to the zygomatic arch inferiorly and superiorly at the temporal line where it also merges with the pericranium. The nerve to the temporalis enters the infratemporal fossa on the deep (medial) surface of the muscle and then divides into three branches that innervate the anterior, middle, and posterior portions of the muscle.[40] This divided innervation of the temporalis is convenient because it theoretically allows the muscle to be separated into distinct functional units that may be used to perform multiple tasks, or for the use of just a portion of the muscle without having to sacrifice the entire muscle.

To employ the temporalis muscle for facial reanimation the following requirements must be met: (1) intact temporalis muscle, (2) intact nerve supply to the temporalis, (3) intact blood supply to the temporalis, (4) intact zygoma for the temporalis to be folded over to act as a fulcrum against which the temporalis can contract and elevate the face, and (5) intact temporalis fascia.

Surgical Technique

The basic concept behind the use of the temporalis muscle in facial reanimation is to establish a superior-lateral pull that will provide resting tone to the cheek–upper lip complex and, with contraction, a semblance of a smile. The surgical technique of temporalis transfer has undergone several modifications over the past three decades with three principal authors' citations (Rubin,[40] Conley,[41] and May and Drucker[42]) reporting the largest series. May and Drucker's most recent series seems to represent the state of the art with regard to the use of the temporalis for facial reanimation and is corroborated by Conley in the following discussion.

Preoperatively, with the patient awake and sitting, the proposed position of the nasolabial crease is marked by taking measurements from the normal side (a convenient site is the midportion of the normal nasolabial crease to the oral commissure). Once the patient has been appropriately marked and prepped, the temporalis muscle is exposed through a vertical temporal incision running from just above the temporal crest to the level of the zygomatic arch. A plane of dissection is established just on top of the temporalis fascia and extended over the central two thirds of the muscle. In the past the entire muscle was harvested and portions used for ocular reanimation as well as the lower face. However, today most authors advocate harvesting just the central portion of the muscle, based on the nervous anatomy previously discussed, which avoids the prominent temporal depression left by harvesting the entire muscle (**Fig. 33–8**). The muscle flap is outlined with a superior extension of periosteum. It is then incised down to the level of the zygoma and elevated with the deep periosteum attached. The previously marked line for the nasolabial crease is incised and a dissection performed to identify the orbicularis oris muscle; if no muscle is identified, the dissection is continued to the submucosa of the lip. A tunnel is then created from the cheek incision to the temporal incision staying as deep (just above the body of the zygoma) as possible. The temporalis muscle is then split for 2 cm at its distal portion, folded over the zygomatic arch, and passed through the subcutaneous tunnel to the cheek incision. Once at the cheek incision, the muscle is sutured to the orbicularis oris (if available) with 2-0 nonabsorbable sutures under considerable tension (**Fig. 33–8**). If the orbicularis is not

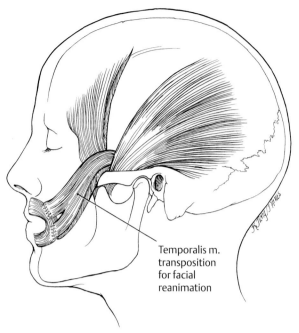

Figure 33–8 Temporalis muscle transposition for facial reanimation. The middle third of the muscle is utilized to minimize bulk over the zygoma and keep donor-site morbidity to a minimum.

identifiable, the muscle is sutured to the submucosal or subcutaneous tissue. Not uncommonly the muscle has insufficient length to reach the corner of the mouth, and a means of extending the muscle is required. Rubin[40] has described a method of using the temporalis fascia but this seems somewhat cumbersome. May and Drucker[42] used Gore-Tex for a time but noted an unacceptable long-term infection and extrusion rate. They now recommend using autogenous fascia lata.[42] It is recommended by all authors writing on this subject that the elevation of the corner of the mouth achieved at the time of surgery should be much more than the desired resting tone in anticipation of some degree of loosening. The temporal defect at the donor site may be filled by a variety of methods including Silastic blocks or a superficial temporalis fascia flap.[41,42]

A major advantage of using the temporalis muscle for facial reanimation is the fact that it should provide some degree of voluntary elevation of the corner of the mouth by having patients bite their posterior teeth together. With practice a surprising degree of voluntary motion of the corner of the mouth may be achieved. However, this motion rarely approaches spontaneous, emotive expression.

Limitations and Complications

Use of the temporalis muscle for facial reanimation is relatively straightforward; possible complications are usually minor. The major shortcoming or complication is failure to regain motion of the corner of the mouth. Failure of reanimation may be due to either the loss of functioning neuronal input or loosening and lengthening of the attachment of the muscle to the corner of the mouth. Other complications or shortcomings of the temporalis transposition are a pronounced bulge of the temporalis over the zygoma, hematoma in the cheek tunnel, extrusion of the perioral sutures, lengthening of material (i.e., Gore-Tex), and infection of the implant placed in the temporal depression.

Masseter Transposition

Previously, the masseter was frequently used to aid in facial reanimation, being innervated by the trigeminal and situated close to the orbicularis oris. However, use of the masseter for facial reanimation is compromised because its origin from the inferior portion of the zygomatic arch gives a posterior pull that is too horizontal to effectively elevate the corner of the mouth. Most authors have stopped recommending the use of the masseter as a primary modality in facial reanimation although it may be considered when the temporalis has been compromised. Rubin[40] describes a technique in which he uses the anterior portion of the masseter in conjunction with the temporalis to improve control of the corner of the mouth and lower lip.

Static Suspension for Restoration of Facial Tone

The ideal goal, restoration of voluntary facial motion with good resting tone, is not always achievable. The most common reasons are lack of usable distal facial nerve to hook up a jump-graft or crossover graft, degeneration or loss of facial muscles, loss or denervation of contiguous facial muscles, and a patient who does not wish to undergo extensive or complicated procedures.

For such patients a reasonable second choice is to provide the illusion of facial tone with static suspension. In fact, static suspension, well done, may go a long way toward ameliorating much of the morbidity and deformity of facial paralysis without imparting any particular morbidity. The major goal of static suspension is to elevate the corner of the mouth and change the expression from anger or sorrow to happiness. Static suspension also helps control drooling and keeps the cheek against the teeth so that food does not become trapped in the buccal space.

In the past, static suspensions were primarily performed with fascia lata as the suspending material. However, fascia lata has a certain donor-site morbidity and tends to stretch out over time with loss of facial tone. To compensate for this loss of tightness, the initial suspension can be overcorrected, but in the immediate postoperative period the patient looks unnaturally tight. Later, after there had been some loosening, the flaccid state associated with facial paralysis would return. An additional difficulty was the fact that there was no easy way to attach the fascia lata to the zygoma, often requiring suturing around the zygoma, which was cumbersome. Within the last several years it appears that the material of choice for performing facial suspensions has become Gore-Tex strips (**Fig. 33–9**).[43–45] Gore-Tex is obtained in sheets of 1- or 2-mm thickness and cut into strips 3 to 4 mm in diameter. There are several different methods of performing facial suspension with Gore-Tex. A very simple, quick, and effective way is to make a small incision over the body of the zygoma and another along the melolabial crease and expose the zygoma and orbicularis oris muscle. Tunnels are then created between the two incisions, and the 2-mm Gore-Tex strip passed between the two. The inferior end of the strip is then sutured to the orbicularis with 4-0 or 5-0 permanent sutures (Mersilene, Ethibond, nylon, Gore-Tex, etc.). The superior end of the strip is then put on tension and the corner of the mouth elevated to the desired position. It is recommended that some overcorrection be included in the original positioning. The strip is then secured to the zygoma with a single 1.5-mm titanium

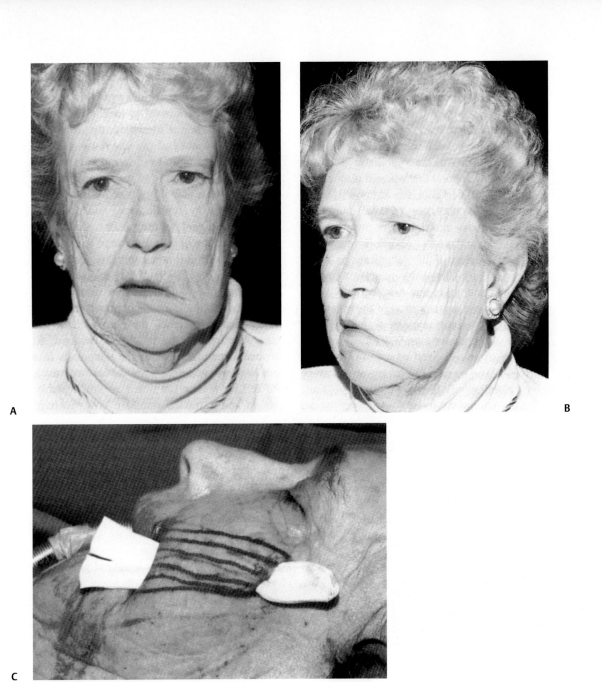

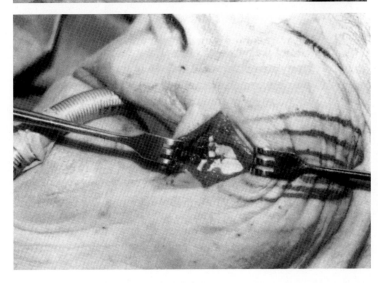

Figure 33–9   (A,B) A 60-year-old woman with long-standing left-sided facial paralysis who was not a candidate for a reinnervation procedure and did not want a temporalis transposition. **(C)** Photo demonstrating 2-mm-thick Gore-Tex strip passing through a tunnel from the body of the zygoma to the melolabial crease. **(D)** The Gore-Tex is sutured to the orbicularis with multiple 4-0 Mersilene sutures.

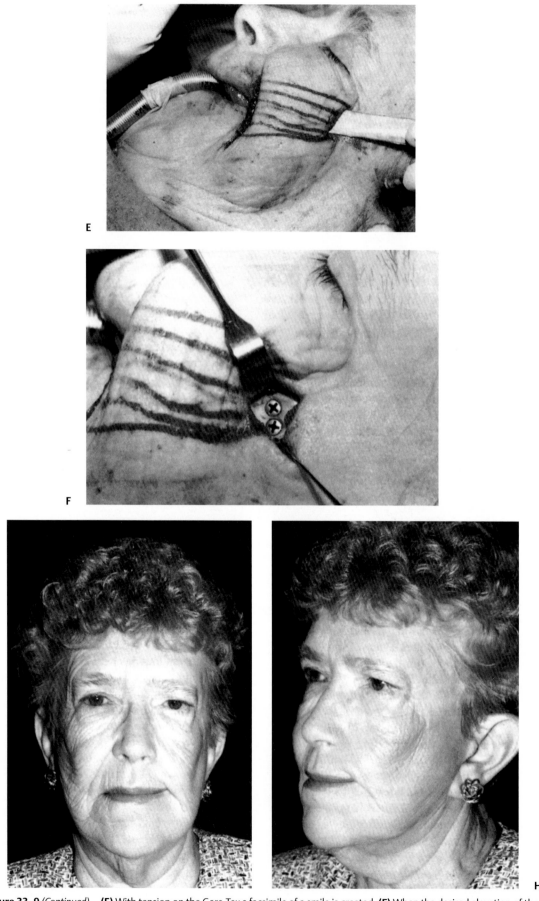

Figure 33–9 *(Continued)* **(E)** With tension on the Gore-Tex a facsimile of a smile is created. **(F)** When the desired elevation of the melolabial crease is obtained, the Gore-Tex is secured to the zygoma with several titanium screws. **(G,H)** Six-month follow-up photo showing stable elevation of the left melolabial crease with Gore-Tex suspension.

screw passed through the Gore-Tex and bone after both are drilled with a 1.0-mm drill bit. This simple technique can give dramatic results, can be done on an outpatient basis with local anesthesia, does not have any donor-site morbidity, is reversible, and may have the potential for even easier revision if there is some loosening over time (by simply removing the screw and advancing the strip and applying a new screw).

Ancillary Procedures for Improving Static Facial Tone

A significant component of the stigmata of facial paralysis results from the abnormal facial appearance at rest. This abnormal appearance is the result of the loss of resting facial muscle tone and the sagging of the facial soft tissues. As a patient ages this abnormal sagging is accentuated giving the patient a very angry, unhappy, severe look. With movement the abnormal appearance is heightened by the innervated muscles pulling the paralyzed soft tissues to the contralateral side. Significant improvement in appearance and function may be achieved by removing the sagging atonic component of the paralyzed face. The paralyzed eyebrow almost never recovers with any reinnervation technique and often does not recover from severe idiopathic (Bell's) paralysis. Endoscopic forehead lifting techniques offer an effective, low-morbidity method for repositioning the eyebrow.[46–48] The incisions are concealed in the hairline, and the ipsilateral forehead is elevated in a subperiosteal plane and then held in position with sutures secured to an absorbable screw or bone tunnel.

Additionally, improvement of resting facial tone may be achieved by the simple technique of excising tissue along the melolabial crease, elevating and lateralizing the ipsilateral lip. For the lower lip, taking a wedge excision of the lateral third of the lip, with careful repair, will reposition the lip and significantly improve both appearance and function.

Finally, botulinum toxin has been used to help restore some degree of facial symmetry by weakening the contralateral muscles.[49,50]

Free Muscle Transfer and Free Microvascular Muscle Transfer

There have been several attempts to bring in new muscle to help restore facial motion. The earliest attempts at bringing new muscle to the paralyzed face involved transferring free muscle grafts sewn to the paralyzed facial muscles with an extension to the contralateral side. The theory was that a certain percentage of the free muscle grafts would survive and draw innervation from the innervated side. However, the results of this technique, although intriguing, have been inconsistent and, at best, supplied weak motion.

A more promising technique is the advent of free microvascular transfer of a muscle and its neurovascular unit. Several different muscles have been used including the gracilis, pectoralis major, pectoralis minor, latissimus dorsi, and serratus anterior. Taylor et al[51] recently championed the use of the coracobrachialis muscle, which they feel is superior to the gracilis. The accompanying nerve to the transplanted muscle is anastomosed to either the contralateral facial nerve via a cross-facial nerve jump graft or to an adjacent cranial motor nerve such as the hypoglossal or deep temporal nerve of the trigeminal.[52–54] A most ambitious microvascular reanimation of the paralyzed face by Ueda et al[55] uses dual muscle (latissimus dorsi and

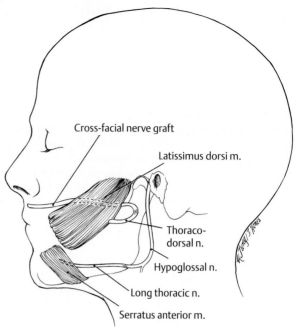

Figure 33–10 Schematic of Ueda et al's[55] report describing a procedure to provide two independently functioning muscles to animate the mouth. Both muscles are transferred via microvascular anastomosis. The latissimus dorsi is innervated via a cross-facial nerve graft, whereas the serratus anterior is anastomosed to the hypoglossal nerve (see text).

serratus anterior) with separate nerve anastomosis to a cross-facial nerve graft and a jump graft to the hypoglossal (**Fig. 33–10**). They use the temporalis for eyelid reanimation and a brow lift for the forehead. The concept is to provide several different motor units under different neuronal input to help avoid synkinesis. However, the authors note that the opposite situation can occur where the patient is unable to coordinate the different transplanted muscle units, resulting in bizarre facial movement. Although Ueda et al's procedure is certainly a remarkable surgical feat, the numbers reported are small and the results shown are not overwhelmingly better than conventional techniques.[56]

As with any new technique, microvascular transplantation of muscle and cross-facial nerve grafting has been evolving.[54,55,57–61] At present it is the only alternative for true facial reanimation in patients in whom the distal facial nerve or facial muscles have been compromised. However, it should be reserved for younger patients who have no other alternative because the success rate diminishes with advancing age.

Eyelid Reanimation

Aside from the cosmetic and social aspects of facial paralysis, one of the major adverse consequences is the ocular sequelae. With facial paralysis the ability to contract the orbicularis oculi is lost and with it the ability to blink. The blink reflex is essential for a healthy eye because with its 0.02-second response time it shields the eye from approaching foreign bodies or objects. Additionally the blink reflex facilitates the distribution of tears over the eye to prevent desiccation and cleans the surface of any debris. Loss of the blink reflex puts the eye at significant risk for exposure keratitis, corneal abrasion, and, ultimately, corneal ulcers. This risk to the eye is compounded if facial paralysis occurs in association with loss of sensation from a trigeminal lesion (which is not uncommon in large acoustic neuromas and skull base tumors) because not only is the ability of the eye to protect and lubricate itself by blinking diminished, but sensory input, which would normally alert the patient to a problem, is also lost. In these cases of combined motor and sensory deficits, the eye can be quickly lost, and proper treatment of the eye must be instituted on an emergent basis. In this regard it is probably best to have an ophthalmologist monitor the status of the globe and cornea.

The major goal of periocular rehabilitation in the patient with facial paralysis is to provide the eye with the ability to lubricate and protect itself, some degree of spontaneous movement, and, if possible, emotive expression. However, the single most important function to provide is the ability to consistently, forcefully, and rapidly close the eye. Opening the eye is not a problem because this is under control of the levator, which is innervated by the third cranial nerve. A variety of techniques have been employed to protect the eye. For many years a partial tarsorrhaphy was the mainstay of managing the paralyzed eye. However, a tarsorrhaphy has several shortcomings including a reduced field of vision, poor cosmesis, inability to protect the eye with blinking, and failure to clean the surface of the eye as the normal blink would. Following tarsorrhaphy came several attempts to provide active reanimation of the eyelid. The temporalis muscle was split and passed around the eye in the hope that with contraction of the temporalis it would simulate the sphincteric effect of the orbicularis and close the eyelid. Unfortunately, splitting and transposition of the temporalis rarely seemed to function with sufficient strength to consistently produce a satisfactory blink. Next came attempts to fashion various types of eyelid springs, which would tend to keep the eyelid closed and would then be opposed by the levator muscle, which would open the eye voluntarily. Eyelid springs were plagued by difficulties with maintaining the proper position and implant extrusion.

An interesting early attempt at reanimating the eyelid was the Arion prosthesis, a silicone band placed in the subcutaneous tissue of both the upper and lower lids. The theory was that with opening the eye (through the use of the levator) the silicone band would be placed on stretch and with relaxation the eyelid would close.[62] However, this technique has been largely abandoned because of difficulty with obtaining the proper tension with the silicone band and cases of prosthesis extrusion.[63]

Illig[64] proposed in 1958 to restore some semblance of a blink with upper eyelid loading. He based this theory on the observation that with normal eyelid closure the lower eyelid has only 1 mm of movement and the upper eyelid is responsible for the rest of eyelid closure. In the following years several authors pursued the concept of lid loading to correct lagophthalmos and gradually evolved the present-day gold implants.

The present-day use of gold weights for reanimation of the eye proceeds as follows. First, the patient is subjected to a thorough ophthalmologic examination with particular emphasis on the status of the cornea to ensure that exposure keratitis has not occurred. Next the eyelids are assessed with regard to tone; if the lower lid is felt to be too lax, a lid-tightening procedure is also planned. The proper size of the gold weight is then determined by taping varying sizes externally to the upper lid and comparing the results. The ideal weight allows fairly rapid closure of the eye without ptosis.

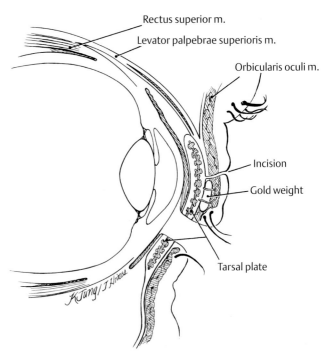

Figure 33–11 Positioning of a gold weight for upper eyelid reanimation. Note that the levator (which is not innervated by the facial nerve) opens the lid and with relaxation gravity closes the weighted lid.

Surgical implantation is straightforward and may be performed under local anesthesia. A skin incision is made in the tarsal crease and carried down through the orbicularis. The tarsal plate is identified, and dissection continued inferiorly and anteriorly over the tarsal plate. Once a suitable pocket has been created the gold weight is slipped into the pocket to lie over the anterior portion of the tarsal plate, just lateral to the center of the eyelid. The weight is then fixed to the tarsal plate with permanent suture (**Fig. 33–11**).

The advantages of the gold weight for eyelid reanimation are the ease of performance, the ease of adjustment and reversibility, and the high percentage of success. Several recent reviews of gold weights for eyelid reanimation report success rates greater than 93%. The disadvantages of gold weights are relatively minor when the alternatives are considered, but include the need for a surgical procedure, the possibility of implant infection or extrusion, ptosis caused by too heavy an implant, the expense of the implant, the visibility of the implant if placed too superficially, and a blink that is not as fast or forceful as a regular blink.[63,65] These disadvantages notwithstanding, it is my opinion that if reinnervation of the eye cannot be accomplished, then lid-loading with gold weights, in conjunction with a lower lid–tightening procedure if necessary, is the current procedure of choice for reanimation of the paralyzed eye.

◆ **Conclusion**

Facial paralysis is a devastating neurologic deficit. Not only is the patient subjected to substantial functional limitations such as difficulty with eating and drinking and severe sight threatening ocular dysfunction, but the patient is also isolated socially. Due to the complexity and subtlety of facial movement and the nuances of facial expressions, the complete rehabilitation of the paralyzed face has remained an elusive goal. However, improvements in technology and surgical techniques have progressed to the point that we now can offer to virtually every patient with facial paralysis some degree of improvement in function and appearance.

References

1. VanBuskirk C. The seventh nerve complex. J Comp Neurol 1945;82: 303–333
2. Gacek RR, Radpour S. Fiber orientation of the facial nerve: an experimental study in the cat. Laryngoscope 1982;92:547–556
3. Kempe LG. Topographic orginization of the distal portion of the facial nerve. J Neurosurg 1980;52:671–673
4. May M. Anatomy of the facial nerve (spatial orientation of fibers in the temporal bone). Laryngoscope 1973;83:1311–1329
5. Millesi H. Facial nerve suture. In: Fisch U, ed. Facial Nerve Surgery. Birmingham, AL: Aesculapius, 1977:209–215
6. Davis RA, Anson BJ, Budinger JM, Kurth LR. Surgical anatomy of the facial nerve and parotid gland based upon a study of 350 cervical facial halves. Surg Gynecol Obstet 1956;102:385–412
7. Bernstein L, Nelson RH. Surgical anatomy of the extraparotid distribution of the facial nerve. Arch Otolaryngol 1984;110:177–182
8. May M. Microanatomy and pathophysiology of the facial nerve. In: May M, ed. The Facial Nerve. New York: Thieme, 1986:63–74
9. Crumley RL, Scott TA. Rehabilitation of facial paralysis. In: Cummings CW, ed. Otolaryngology–Head and Neck Surgery. St. Louis: Mosby Year Book, 1993:1079–1098
10. Johns ME, Crumley RL. Pathophysiology of injury and repair. In: Johns ME, Crumley RL, eds. Facial Nerve Injury, Repair and Rehabilitation. Alexandria, VA: AAO-HNS, 1984:20–25
11. Selzer ME. Nerve regeneration. Sem Neurol 1987;7:88–96
12. Sunderland S. Nerve and Nerve Injuries, 2nd ed. London: Churchill-Livingstone, 1978
13. Sunderland S, Cossar DF. The structure of the facial nerve. Anat Rec 1953; 116:147–162
14. Rubin LR. Expressions of emotions: the role of the nasolabial fold and the anatomy of the smile. In: Rubin LR, ed. The Paralyzed Face. St. Louis: Mosby Year Book, 1991:11–15
15. May M. Anatomy of the facial nerve for the clinician. In: May M, ed. The Facial Nerve. New York: Thieme, 1986:21–62
16. Levinthal R. Comparison of fascicular, interfascicular, and epineurial suture techniques in the repair of simple nerve lacerations. J Neurosurg 1977;47:744–750
17. Tupper JW, Crick JC, Mattleck LR. Fascicular nerve repairs: a comparative study of epineurial and fascicular (perineurial) techniques. Orthop Clin North Am 1988;19:57–69
18. Giddins GE, Wade PJ, Amis AA. Primary nerve repair: strength of repair with different guages of nylon suture material. J Hand Surg (Br) 1989;14: 301–302
19. Terris DJ, Fee WE. Current issues in nerve repair. Arch Otolaryngol Head Neck Surg 1993;119:725–731
20. Kanzaki J, Kunihiro T, O-Uchi T, Ogawa K, Shiobara R, Toya S. Intracranial reconstruction of the facial nerve: clinical observation. Acta Otolaryngol Suppl 1991;487:85–90
21. Walton RL, Brown RE, Matory WE Jr, et al. Autogenous vein graft repair of digital nerve defects in the finger: a retrospective clinical study. Plast Reconstr Surg 1989;84:944–949
22. Hentz VR, Rosen JM, Xiao SJ, McGill KC, Abraham G. A comparison of suture and tubulization nerve repair techniques in a primate. J Hand Surg Am 1991;16:251–261
23. Medders G, Mattox DE, Lyles A. Effects of fibrin glue on rat facial nerve regeneration. Otolaryngol Head Neck Surg 1989;100:106–109
24. Nishihira S, McCaffrey TV. Repair of motor nerve defects: comparison of suture and fibrin adhesive techniques. Otolaryngol Head Neck Surg 1989;100:17–21
25. Glasby MA, Mountain RE, Murray JAM. Repair of the facial nerve using freeze-thawed muscle autografts. A surgical model in the sheep. Arch Otolaryngol Head Neck Surg 1993;119:461–465
26. Mountain RE, et al. A morphological comparison of interposed freeze-thawed skeletal muscle autografts and interposed nerve autografts in the repair of the rat facial nerve. Clin Otolaryngol Allied Sci 1993;18: 171–177
27. Ng RW, Koh AJ, Ho WK. Endoscopic sural nerve harvesting for facial nerve reconstruction. Laryngoscope 2005;115:925–927
28. McGuirt WF, Welling B, McCabe BF. Facial nerve function following irradiated cable grafts. Laryngoscope 1989;99:27–34
29. May M. Surgical rehabilitation of facial palsy: total approach. In: May M, ed. The Facial Nerve. New York: Thieme, 1986:695–777
30. Ferreira M. Cross-facial nerve grafting. Clin Plast Surg 1984;11:211–214
31. Ebersold MJ, Quast LM. Long-term results of spinal accessory nerve-facial nerve anastomosis. J. Neurosurg. 1992;77:51–54
32. Poe DS, Scher N, Panje WR. Facial reanimation by XI–VII anastomosis without shoulder paralysis. Laryngoscope 1989;99:1040–1047
33. Pitty LF, Tator CH. Hypoglossal-facial nerve anastomosis for facial nerve palsy following surgery for cerebellopontine angle tumors. J Neurosurg 1992;77:724–731
34. Conley J, Baker D. Hypoglossal-facial nerve anastomosis for reinnervation of the paralyzed face. Plast Reconstr Surg 1979;63:63–72
35. Sobol SM, May M. Hypoglossal-facial anastomosis: It's role in contemporary facial reanimation. In: Rubin LR, ed. The Paralyzed Face. St. Louis: Mosby Year Book, 1991:137–143
36. May M, Sobol SM, Mester SJ. Hypoglossal-facial nerve interpositional-jump graft for facial reanimation without tongue atrophy. Otolaryngol Head Neck Surg 1991;104:818–825
37. Kunihiro TJ, Kanzaki, Uchi TO. Hypoglossal-facial nerve anastomosis. Acta Otolaryngol Stockh 1991;487:80–84
38. Pensak ML, Jackson CG, Glasscock ME 3rd, Gulya AJ. Facial reanimation with the VII–XII anastomosis: analysis of the functional and psychologic results. Otolaryngol Head Neck Surg 1986;94:305–310
39. Hammerschlag PE. Facial reanimation with jump interpositional graft hypoglossal facial anastomosis and hypoglossal facial anastomosis: evolution in management of facial paralysis. Laryngoscope 1999;109(2 pt 2 suppl 90):1–23
40. Rubin LR. Reanimation of total unilateral facial paralysis by the contiguous facial muscle technique. In: Rubin LR, ed. The Paralyzed Face. St. Louis: Mosby Year Book, 1991:156–177
41. Conley J. Discussion: temporalis muscle for facial reanimation. By M. May and C. Drucker. Arch Otolaryngol Head Neck Surg 1993;119: 383–384
42. May M, Drucker C. Temporalis muscle for facial reanimation. Arch Otolaryngol Head Neck Surg 1993;119:378–382
43. Iwahira Y, Maruyama Y. The use of Gore-Tex soft tissue patch to assist temporal muscle transfer in the treatment of facial nerve palsy. Ann Plast Surg 1992;29:274–277
44. Konior RJ. Facial paralysis reconstruction with Gore-Tex soft tissue patch. Arch Otolaryngol Head Neck Surg 1992;118:1188–1194
45. Petroff MA, Goode RL, Levet Y. Gore-Tex implants: applications in facial paralysis rehabilitation and soft-tissue augmentation. Laryngoscope 1992;102:1185–1189
46. Costantino PD, Hiltzik DH, Moche J, Preminger A. Minimally invasive brow suspension for facial paralysis. Arch Facial Plast Surg 2003;5:171–174
47. Ducic Y, Adelson R. Use of the endoscopic forehead-lift to improve brow position in persistent facial paralysis. Arch Facial Plast Surg 2005;7: 51–54
48. Takushima A, Harii K, Asato H. Endoscopic dissection of recipient facial nerve for vascularized muscle transfer in the treatment of facial paralysis. Br J Plast Surg 2003;56:110–113
49. Clark RP, Berris CE. Botulinum toxin: a treatment for facial asymmetry caused by facial nerve paralysis. Plast Reconstr Surg 2005;115: 573–574
50. Rohrich RJ, Janis JE, Fagien S, Stuzin JM. The cosmetic use of botulinum toxin. Plast Reconstr Surg 2003;112(5 suppl):177S–191S
51. Taylor GI, Cichowitz A, Ang SG, et al. Comparative anatomical study of the gracilis and coracobrachialis muscles: implications for facial reanimation. Plast Reconstr Surg 2003;112:20–30
52. Bradford C. Facial Reanimation. Curr Opin Otolaryngol Head Neck Surg 1994;2:369–374
53. McO'Brien B, Kumar PAV. Cross-face nerve grafting with free vascularized muscle grafts. In: Rubin LR, ed. The Paralyzed Face. St. Louis: Mosby Year Book, 1991:201–212
54. Harii K. Microneurovascular free muscle transplantation. In: Rubin LR, ed. The Paralyzed Face. St. Louis: Mosby Year Book, 1991:178–200
55. Ueda K, Harii K, Yamada A. Free vascularized double muscle transplantation for the treatment of facial paralysis. Plast Reconstr Surg 1995;95: 1288–1296
56. Rubin LR, Discussion of: Free vascularized double muscle transplantation for the treatment of facial paralysis by Ueda et al. Plast Reconstr Surg 1995;95:1297–1298
57. Cuccia G, Shelley O, d'Alcontres FS, et al. A comparison of temporalis transfer and free latissimus dorsi transfer in lower facial reanimation following unilateral longstanding facial palsy. Ann Plast Surg 2005;54: 66–70

58. Harrison DH. The treatment of unilateral and bilateral facial palsy using free muscle transfers. Clin Plast Surg 2002;29:539–549, vi.

59. Terzis JK, Noah EM. Dynamic restoration in Mobius and Mobius-like patients. Plast Reconstr Surg 2003;111:40–55

60. Wei W, Zuoliang Q, Xiaoxi L, et al. Free split and segmental latissimus dorsi muscle transfer in one stage for facial reanimation. Plast Reconstr Surg 1999;103:473–480 discussion 481–2

61. Yla-Kotola TM, Kauhanen MS, Asko-Seljavaara SL. Facial reanimation by transplantation of a microneurovascular muscle: long-term follow-up. Scand J Plast Reconstr Surg Hand Surg 2004;38:272–276

62. Arion HG. Dynamic closure of the lids in paralysis of the orbicularis muscle. Int Surg 1972;57:48–50

63. Townsend DJ. Eyelid reanimation for the treatment of paralytic lagophthalmos: historical perspectives and current applications of the gold weight implant. Ophthal Plast Reconstr Surg 1992;8:196–201

64. Illig KM. Eine neue operationsmethode gegen lagophthalmos. Klin Monatsbl Augenheilkd 1958;132:410

65. Kartush JM, Linstrom CJ, McCann PM, Graham MD. Early gold weight eyelid implantation for facial paralysis. Otolaryngol Head Neck Surg 1990;103:1016–1023

34

Otalgia

John S. McDonald

Otalgia may be primary, with the source being the ear or temporal bone, or it may be secondary, referred to the ear with or without signs or symptoms of the primary source of the pain. In 50% or more of patients who complain of otalgia, the pain emanates from a source other than the ear.[1] Otalgia may be described as aching, boring, sharp, throbbing, burning, itching, or pressure-like with a sensation of fullness. Concomitant complaints of vertigo, tinnitus, and even the subjective sense of hearing degradation may be part of the clinical spectrum of either primary or referred otalgia and cannot be used as differentiating factors.

◆ Nociception and Pain

Bonica[3] defined pain as an unpleasant sensory and emotional experience associated with actual or potential tissue damage or described in terms of such damage. Tissue injury, whether caused by trauma or disease, constitutes a noxious stimulus that will activate nociceptors (receptors preferentially sensitive to a noxious stimulus or to a stimulus that would become noxious if prolonged).[2] The noxious stimulus or tissue damage activates nociceptors at the termination of thinly myelinated Aδ (group III) and unmyelinated C (group IV) afferent nerve fibers in the skin, muscles, joints, fascia, and other deep somatic structures.[3,4] Cutaneous nociceptors may be activated by mechanical, thermal, chemical, or other algesic stimuli, and nociceptors in the deep somatic structures may be activated by disease, inflammatory processes, contraction, ischemia, rapid distention, or other visceral stimuli.

Central to the theme of understanding the mechanism by which pain may be referred to the ear is the concept of central convergence. Sessle et al[5,6] have shown extensive convergence of cutaneous, tooth pulp, visceral, neck, and muscle afferents onto nociceptive and nonnociceptive neurons in the trigeminal subnucleus caudalis or medullary dorsal horn (MDH) and suggested a role for these neurons in mediating pain, its spread, and referral.

The sensory innervation to the ear and periaural region is derived from cranial nerves V, VII, IX, and X as well as cervical nerves II and III. Nociceptive impulses from cranial nerves V, VII, IX, and X have all been shown to synapse with second-order neurons in the trigeminal subnucleus caudalis or the MDH.[4] Nociceptive impulses from cervical nerves 2 and 3 activate neurons in the spinal dorsal horn. There is a high degree of nociceptive convergence of the upper cervical nerves and the trigeminal system, providing overlap of peripheral C2 and C3 nociceptive fibers with other cephalic nociceptive nerves V, VII, IX, and X.[7]

There are three types of neurons in the MDH: low-threshold mechanoreceptors (LTMs), which respond to nonnoxious stimuli; wide dynamic range (WDR) neurons, which respond to both noxious and nonnoxious stimuli; and high-threshold nociceptive-specific (NS) neurons, which respond exclusively to noxious stimuli. A substantial number of the WDR and NS neurons show extensive convergence and can be excited by peripheral afferents from skin, mucosa, viscera (i.e., laryngeal), temporomandibular joint (TMJ), jaw and tongue muscle, tooth pulp, and neck, provoking the spread and referral of pain.[9] Convergence of nociceptive fibers from C2 and C3 with WDR and NS neurons in the MDH may explain referral of pain from noxious stimuli from the C2, C3 region not only to the ear but to the preauricular region and other areas in the face.

◆ Anatomy

The auriculotemporal branch of the mandibular or third division of the fifth cranial nerve (CN V₃) provides sensory innervation for the tragus, anterior and superior aspects of the auricle, and external auditory canal, as well as the anterosuperior portion of the lateral external canal wall and tympanic membrane. The tensor tympani muscle, derived from the mandibular or first branchial arch, is innervated by a small nerve derived from the medial pterygoid branch of CN V₃. Although primarily motor in function, skeletal muscles receive sensory innervation from thinly myelinated Aδ (group III) and unmyelinated C (group IV) afferent nociceptive nerve endings in muscle fascia, in tight spatial connection to muscle arterioles and capillaries, and in tendons, acting as muscle nociceptors.[3,9,10] Electromyographic studies of the tensor tympani and stapedius muscles have demonstrated contraction of both muscles concomitantly with several complex facial movements including tight closure of the eyes, opening and closing of the jaws, speaking, and swallowing.[11] It has been pointed out that tonic contraction of the tensor tympani muscle may be accompanied by otalgia, a sense of pressure and fullness in the ear(s), and tinnitus, or other transient acoustic sensations.[11] Mechanical injury to muscle, which may be derived from repetitive situations such as overcontraction or overstretching muscle may produce pain. Chronic contraction of the masticatory muscles in cases of temporomandibular dysfunction (TMD), worsened by bruxism, may result in tensor tympani-mediated otalgia.

The facial nerve (CN VII) supplies sensory innervation to a portion of the posterior and posterosuperior auricle and to adjacent portions of the external auditory canal and lateral aspect of the tympanic membrane, as well as to a small area of skin in the postauricular area.[1] CN VII also supplies innervation to the stapedius muscle in the middle ear.

The glossopharyngeal nerve (CN IX) provides sensory innervation to part of the posterior portion of the external auditory canal and meatus as well as an adjacent portion of the lateral surface of the tympanic membrane, the majority of the mastoid air cells, and the eustachian tube.[1] The tympanic plexus, which is composed of the tympanic branch of the glossopharyngeal nerve (Jacobson's nerve) and the superior and inferior caroticotympanic branches of the sympathetic plexus surrounding the carotid artery, provides sensory innervation to the middle ear, including the medial aspect of the tympanic membrane.[1] The auricular branch (Arnold's nerve) of the vagus nerve (CN X) innervates a portion of the posterior wall and the floor of the external canal and the corresponding external surface of the tympanic membrane.[1] The upper cervical nerves (C2, C3) also supply sensory innervation to the ear or periauricular structures. The posterior branch of the greater auricular nerve supplies sensory innervation to the majority of the posterior portion of the auricle as well as a portion of the skin over the mastoid region, which also receives some overlapping communication with the lesser occipital nerve (C2) in the mastoid region.

Although pain may be referred to the ear by way of any of the cranial or cervical nerves just mentioned, the most common source of referred pain to the ear is through the trigeminal nerve, the longest cranial nerve with the most extensive distribution in the head and neck region.[12,13]

◆ Mechanism of Referred Pain

The mechanism by which pain may be referred to the ear from distant anatomic sites can be found in the concept of central convergence wherein nociceptive neurons in lower centers such as the MDH receive convergent inputs from various tissues, with the result that higher centers within the brain cannot identify the actual input source.[5,14] These convergent inputs may also be involved in so-called central sensitization or neuroplasticity of nociceptive neurons, a process thought to contribute (along with peripheral sensitization) to hyperalgesia.[15] It is thought that as a result of this nociceptive input, some of the afferent inputs to the nociceptive neurons may be "unmasked" and become more effective in exciting these second-order neurons, with the result that pain is perceived as coming from the tissue that the afferents supply.[16] For example, pain may be experienced in the external ear including part of the external auditory canal and the tympanic membrane by convergence of

primary Aδ or C afferent nociceptive fibers from the auriculotemporal branch of CN V$_3$ with primary Aδ or C nociceptive afferent trigeminal nerve fibers, most commonly other branches of CN V$_3$, at WDR or NS neurons in the MDH. Also, under the influence of nociceptive input from muscle, many cells acquire new receptive fields in deep tissues away from the site of stimulation, with the result that following muscle injury the neurons can be stimulated from body regions somatotypically appropriate for that neuron.[17] Thus, it is also possible that pain may be referred to the middle ear or eustachian tube by convergence of primary afferent nociceptors from the tensor tympani and tensor palati muscles with other primary nociceptive afferents at WDR or NS neurons in the MDH.

It is likely, then, as illustrated in the preceding example of pain sensed in the ear through the auriculotemporal branch of CN V$_3$, that convergence of primary nociceptive afferent fibers from CNs V, VII, IX, and X with WDR and NS neurons in the MDH (trigeminal subnucleus caudalis) may be the means by which pain may be referred to the ear.[8] It is also thought that pain referred to the preauricular region from C3 may be facilitated through overlap of C2 and C3 nociceptive fibers with afferent nociceptive fibers from cranial nerve CN V$_3$.[7]

◆ Primary Otalgia

Pain in the ear or earache may be either primary or referred (secondary otalgia). When the source of the pain and the site to which it is localized are the same, then the patient is said to have primary otalgia. When the source of the pain is distant from the site in which it is perceived (e.g., the ear), then the pain is said to be referred. The differential diagnosis of pathologic causes is enumerated in **Table 34–1**.

Although in most cases the cause of primary otalgia will be readily obvious, potentially the most ominous disorder, primary malignancy of the external canal, may not be at all obvious in its

Table 34–1   Primary Otalgia

Otitis externa (bacterial or fungal)
Myringitis
Cerumen impaction
Foreign body in the ear canal
Perichondritis or chondritis of the auricle
Relapsing polychondritis
Carbuncle or furuncle
Frostbite or burn of auricle
Trauma to the external canal
Traumatic perforation of the tympanic membrane
Hemotympanum
Herpes simplex
Herpes zoster oticus
Eustachian tube dysfunction
Eustachian tube obstruction
Otitis media and mastoiditis, which may be complicated by:
Petrositis
Subperiosteal abscess
Extradural/subdural abscess
Venous sinus thrombosis
Brain abscess
External canal, middle ear, or skull base neoplasms including metastatic disease

early stage and may be overlooked. Conversely, mild erythema of the tympanic membrane or erythema or mild swelling in the external auditory canal should not preclude a thorough head and neck examination to rule out pathology that may refer to the ear and be the true cause of the patient's symptoms. A classic example is the patient with TMD or a TMJ with referred otalgia who may rub the external ear canal with a finger or foreign object in attempts to alleviate the pain, resulting in the appearance of bacterial or fungal otitis externa.

◆ Referred Otalgia

The underlying cause of pain referred to the ear may be either acute or chronic in nature. For the purposes of this chapter, acute causes of referred otalgia are conditions that may be readily diagnosed with well-defined treatment parameters. The majority of these cases will be inflammatory or traumatic in their origin. **Table 34–2** lists the most frequently encountered acute disorders that may produce the feeling of pain in the ear. Those disorders that more frequently present as chronic ongoing pain complaints are illustrated in **Table 34–3** (disorders that will typically have continued to persist beyond the usual course of an acute disease or a reasonable time for an injury to heal, or are associated with some chronic pathologic process causing continuous pain or recurrence of pain at intervals for months or years).[2]

Acute Referred Otalgia

Painful disorders arising in the orofacial region, innervated by the second and third divisions of CN V, are the most common cause of referred pain to the ear.[12,18] Common causes of dental pain in this region include inflammation and pulpal necrosis with or without periapical pathosis and inflammation or infection of the supporting periodontal structures (e.g., the periodontal ligament) including superficial or deep periodontal infections or periodontal abscess. Other dental factors such as unerupted or impacted teeth, traumatic occlusion, ill-fitting dental appliances, or recently adjusted archwires in patients undergoing orthodontic therapy may also be causative factors. Referred pain to the ear may also arise from a variety of nondental, painful, oral inflammatory disorders including recurrent herpetic gingivostomatitis, acute herpes zoster, recurrent aphthous stomatitis (primarily the major scarring form), mucocutaneous disorders such as erosive lichen planus, inflammatory lesions of the tongue such as geographic tongue, and less well understood processes such as burning tongue or burning mouth.

Other painful disorders of the orofacial region that may be the cause of referred pain to the ear include maxillary sinusitis, nasal infections, and parotitis caused by infection or obstruction of Stensen's duct by a stone. Although CN V provides the majority of the sensory trigeminal vascular innervation, some of the dural blood vessels are innervated by fibers from CN V_3. As pain is the only sensation that may be evoked by inflammatory or traction stimuli to the cerebrovascular blood supply, then disease in this area will nonselectively present as pain.

Table 34–2   Referred Otalgia (Acute): Common Causes by Region of Referral

Orofacial region
Exposed root surfaces
Pulpitis or pulpal necrosis
Periapical infection
Periodontal infection (superficial or deep)
Unerupted or impacted teeth
Traumatic occlusion
Ill-fitting dental appliance
Recent adjustment of arch wires (orthodontic therapy)
Primary or recurrent herpetic infection
Acute herpes zoster
Recurrent aphthous stomatitis
Mucocutaneous disorders (i.e., lichen planus)
Geographic tongue
Burning mouth or burning tongue
Maxillary sinusitis
Nasal infections
Parotitis
Pharynx
Inflammatory disorder hypo-oro-nasopharynx
Tonsillitis and peritonsillar abscess
Posttonsillectomy pain
Eagle's syndrome
Larynx and esophagus
Laryngitis
Perichondritis or chondritis
Arthritis of cricoarytenoid joint
Hiatal hernia
Gastroesophageal reflux
Infection or foreign body in esophagus
Other sources
Traction or inflammation involving cerebrovascular blood supply (carotidynia)
Thyroiditis
Angina
Aneurysm of great vessels
Cervical myalgia-fibromyalgia

Table 34–3   Referred Otalgia (Disorders More Typically Chronic in Nature)

Orofacial pain (chronic)
Temporomandibular disorders (TMD, TMJ); includes myofascial pain dysfunction (MPD) and intraarticular TMJ pain
Atypical facial pain
Neurologic disorders
Trigeminal neuralgia
Glossopharyngeal neuralgia
Postherpetic neuralgia
Vagal and superior laryngeal neuralgia
Headaches (ICHD-2 classification)
Primary headache disorders
Tension-type headache now including cervical myalgia
Chronic paroxysmal hemicrania
Temporal arteritis
Secondary headache disorders
Headache or facial pain attributed to disorders of cranium, neck, eyes, ears, nose, sinuses, teeth, mouth, or other facial or cranial structures
Neoplastic disease
Carcinoma, sarcomas (including Hodgkin's and non-Hodgkin's lymphomas), and metastatic disease

Even though the pathogenesis of carotidynia is not clear, the disorder may represent a variant of inflammatory/traction stimuli. Tenderness, particularly near the bifurcation, is present on carotid artery palpation. Otalgia typically is referred to the ipsilateral side. Treatment usually consists of nonsteroidal-antiinflammatory agents. Also, although TMD has an acute phase, it is most notable for its chronic nature, and hence it is included in this chapter in the differential diagnosis of chronic referred otalgia.

Disorders of the pharynx may also present with referred pain to the ear, with inflammatory disorders of the oro-, naso-, or hypopharynx, tonsillitis, peritonsillar abscesses, and post-tonsillectomy pain being common causes of referred otalgia. Eagle's syndrome, caused by an elongated styloid process, may present as referred pain to the ear and also may be confused with, or mimic, glossopharyngeal neuralgia.

Inflammatory disorders of the larynx and esophagus may be referred to the ear through the vagus nerve. Laryngeal causes of referred otalgia include laryngitis, perichondritis, chondritis, and arthritis of the cricoarytenoid joint. Esophageal disorders that may refer to the ear include gastroesophageal reflux, hiatal hernia and inflammation, infection, or foreign body in the esophagus.[19,20] Inflammatory processes arising from visceral sources such as the thyroid gland may be a source of referred pain to the ear as may disorders such as angina and aneurysms of the great vessels.

Chronic Referred Otalgia

When considering the expansive range of innervation of the ear and periaural structures through cranial nerves V, VII, IX, and X in light of the differential diagnosis of chronic pain conditions in the head and neck, then it becomes immediately obvious that the majority of them have at least the potential to refer pain to the ear. Also, taking into consideration the fact that the primary complaint of pain may be in the ear, regardless of the source of the pain, and the fact that chronic pain conditions are frequently of mixed fiber origin, then the potential enormity of the diagnostic challenge becomes obvious.

The differential diagnosis of conditions that may produce chronic pain in the head and neck is a broad one and includes orofacial pain, neurologic disorders, primary and secondary headache disorders, and pain due to cancer.

Orofacial Pain

Chronic orofacial pain conditions that may result in referred pain to the ear include the temporomandibular disorders (TMD, TMJ pain) and atypical facial pain (AFP), with TMD being the more common of the two.

Temporomandibular Disorders

Temporomandibular disorders comprise a multifarious conundrum from the standpoint of both diagnosis and management. Within the differential diagnosis of TMD are nonarticular conditions mimicking this disorder, extraarticular causes of limitation of jaw movement, articular derangement of the TMJ where the disorder in question begins primarily in the joint and remains limited to it, and finally, myofascial pain dysfunction (MPD) with or without intraarticular dysfunction. MPD is far and away the most common cause of TMD and hence one of the most common causes of referred pain from the orofacial region to the ear. Bernstein[12] estimates, for

example, that approximately 40% of patients with referred otalgia have hyperactivity of the muscles of mastication.

In 1952 Travell and Rinzler[21] used the term *myofascial* to refer to pain in a muscle or muscles. Myofascial pain is defined as pain or autonomic phenomena referred from active myofascial trigger points with associated dysfunction.[22] Myofascial pain is the most frequently encountered type of chronic facial, head, and neck pain, and the most controversial. According to Laskin,[23] MPD accounts for as many as 90% of cases of TMD. Although regarded by many as a specific disease entity, others term it a wastebasket diagnosis for soft tissue complaints, and still others simply deny its existence.[24] MPD has been characterized as a regional pain syndrome, often with sudden onset and with trigger points causing locally referred pain.[25] It has been defined as pain, tenderness, or other referred phenomena, with the dysfunction attributed to myofascial trigger points.[22] The sine qua non of MPD is a tender muscle trigger point. Trigger points may be latent or active. Active trigger points produce a pain complaint or other abnormal sensory symptoms. Palpation of an active trigger point may produce or reproduce the complaint of pain or dysfunction. Latent trigger points present with tenderness on palpation but to a lesser extent and without referral of pain.[26,27] Both active and passive trigger points can cause significant motor dysfunction.[27]

Trigger points have been noted to occur primarily in the deep midportion of the muscle and are best located by examining a muscle or muscle group while it is relaxed and being passively stretched by the examiner.[25] To identify a tender muscle trigger point, the examiner must first establish the sensation of finger pressure as a point of reference by palpating a nonpainful area and instructing the patient to respond when pain or tenderness other than the pressure from finger palpation is noted. When a tender muscle trigger point is present, there is usually a nodule or taut band to be felt.[27] Identification of the trigger point is then best done by rolling the nodule or taut band transversely under the fingers. Frequently, a verbal response from the patient is unnecessary as the patient will exhibit an involuntary "jump sign" when a tender muscle trigger point is located.

Myofascial pain appears to occur most commonly in the third, fourth, and fifth decades of life, with women being affected more frequently than men. This is as true for patients with TMD whose pain is of myofascial origin as for patients with tension-type headache produced by active tender muscle trigger points. TMD patients with pain of myofascial origin may present with muscle tenderness, popping or clicking in one or both TMJs, limitation or deflection of jaw movement, and otologic manifestations. They may have jaw pain; frontal, frontotemporal, or occipital headache pain; toothache; sinus pain; earache; pre- or postauricular pain; sore throat; dysphagia; a sense of an object in the throat; or periorbital pain.

Referred or secondary otalgia is a frequent consequence of both acute and chronic orofacial pain conditions with approximately 45% of patients with such pain having diseases of the teeth, periodontium, or suffering from TMD.[18] Pharmacotherapy is usually initiated early to palliate some of the patients' symptoms but should not be the primary treatment in most cases. The nonsteroidal antiinflammatory analgesic group of medications is most frequently used, and there is seldom if ever an indication for the use of narcotic analgesics. Muscle relaxants such as chlorzoxazone, methocarbamol, metaxalone, baclofen, and tizanidine can be used on a relatively long-term basis. Additionally, tricyclic antidepressants are frequently effective analgesic agents in chronic facial pain as they are in tension-type headache. Physical therapy is usually employed and may be accompanied with myoneural block therapy on an adjunctive basis. Frequently, splint therapy using flat plane passive appliances is employed, although this is not indicated in every case. In many cases of severe chronic facial pain, as in other forms of chronic head and neck pain, behavioral medicine evaluation and therapy are indicated and are often as essential as pharmacotherapy and physical therapy in managing the patient's pain.

Atypical Facial Pain

The term *atypical facial pain* (AFP) is characterized as a continuous, or nearly continuous, unilateral, poorly defined, diffuse, aching, boring or burning pain not limited to the distribution of the fifth or ninth cranial nerves. It may overlay the distribution of the cervical nerves. The term *atypical odontalgia* (AO) applies when the pain is said to emanate from a tooth or from several adjacent teeth. Patients with AFP or AO may experience referred otalgia or its diffuse nature may approximate the ear in the preauricular facial region. Although trigger zones are absent, physical examination may reveal hyperalgesia, allodynia, and sympathetic hyperfunction. Attacks of AFP may be set off by mechanical stimulation including percussion or chewing.

Atypical facial pain is one of several neuropathic orofacial pain states. Neuropathic pain is defined as pain initiated or caused by a primary lesion or dysfunction in the nervous system. In addition to mechanisms associated specifically with nerve injury, factors such as peripheral sensitization of nociceptors or central sensitization, which can occur after sufficient nociceptive input, can lead to neuropathic pain.[28,29] Potential etiologic factors include trauma (such as chronic irritation or inflammatory stimuli, endodontic, surgical or other traumatic events), hormonal factors, psychological factors, and local irritation.[29,30] Loss of segmental inhibition from deafferentation following nerve injury or impairment or loss of inhibitory interneurons may also be possible pathogenetic factors in AFP.

A neuropsychiatric assessment of patients with AFP or AO should be pursued as a number of patients with this disorder may be found to have a specific psychiatric diagnosis as classified by the *Diagnostic and Statistical Manual* (DSM-IV) criteria. In a study of 68 patients with AFP, 46 (68%) were found to have a specific diagnosis by DSM-IV criteria, covering a wide variety of disorders, predominantly somatoform, affective, adjustment, or personality disorders.[30]

Although AFP (including AO) is often refractory to both medical and dental therapies, including analgesic therapy, some patients may respond to antidepressants, anticonvulsants, or both in combination. Antidepressant therapy often includes the use of tricyclic antidepressants such as amitriptyline, nortriptyline, and desipramine as well as trazodone, which is classified as an antidepressant and antineuralgic. Anticonvulsant therapy primarily includes the use of gabapentin, although others, such as topiramate and tiagabine, have been used.

Neurologic Disorders

The classification of neuralgias of the face, head, and neck is confounding to many practitioners. Although not encountered as commonly as TMD, trigeminal neuralgia is the most frequently occurring neuralgic condition in the head and neck.

Attacks of pain frequently occur in close proximity to the ear and are the cause of referred pain to the ear in some patients. Because of the relative frequency of occurrence, the etiology, pathogenesis, and management of trigeminal neuralgia have been studied extensively.

Trigeminal Neuralgia

Trigeminal neuralgia, or tic douloureux, is characterized by episodic attacks of agonizingly intense sharp, stabbing, burning, or electric shock–like pain in the trigeminal distribution. Painful episodes may last from a few seconds to a few minutes and are triggered by light touch to a trigger zone on the face or intraorally, including such light stimulus as a breeze or vibration. Trigger zones are particularly common around the mouth and nose, with pain often being exacerbated by such simple acts as washing the face, applying makeup, brushing the teeth, and eating or drinking. Paradoxically, pinching or pressing the trigger area is unlikely to provoke an attack of pain.[31] In the absence of other concomitant disease, physical examination is unremarkable, with the absence of any detectable neurologic deficit within the distribution of the involved branch of the trigeminal nerve. Although in the majority of cases no identifying etiology may be evident at the time of examination, in as many as 15% of patients there may be an underlying cause such as a benign or malignant neoplasm in the posterior fossa or multiple sclerosis that will make its presence known at a later point in time.[33] Thus it is recommended that when the diagnosis of trigeminal neuralgia is considered, a magnetic resonance imaging (MRI) study be performed paying particular attention to the posterior cranial fossa.

Diagnostically, trigeminal neuralgia is most commonly confused with TMD of myofascial origin. The chief differentiating factor here is that the primary pain in trigeminal neuralgia will be limited to a single branch of CN V, whereas pain of myofascial origin is typically diffuse. Other disorders that must be considered when making the diagnosis of trigeminal neuralgia include dental causes such as pulpal pathology, dental infection or cracked teeth, periodontal pathology, pain from pressure of a denture on the mental nerve, AFP including atypical odontalgia, glossopharyngeal neuralgia, postherpetic neuralgia, cluster headache, paroxysmal hemicrania, and temporal arteritis.

It is thought that 80 to 90% of cases of trigeminal neuralgia may arise from specific abnormalities of trigeminal afferent neurons in the trigeminal root or ganglion, resulting in hyperexcitable afferents that give rise to paroxysmal episodes of pain as a result of synchronized after-discharge activity.[29,34]

Both medical and surgical modalities of therapy have been used to treat trigeminal neuralgia. Although trigeminal neuralgia may be an excruciatingly painful disorder, in the absence of a neoplasm as its primary cause it is a nonfatal one, and therefore the primary approach to treatment should be medical intervention with surgery being reserved for patients who become refractory to or are unable to tolerate available medications. Various antineuralgic medications are available for use singly or in combination and include baclofen, carbamazepine, gabapentin, lamotrigine, sodium valproate, clonazepam, and phenytoin. In view of its greater safety, it has been recommended that baclofen should be the initial drug of choice for treating glossopharyngeal or trigeminal neuralgia.[34–36] In those cases where baclofen is ineffective or not tolerated, carbamazepine or gabapentin are the next drugs of choice. For patients who do not respond to therapy with a single medication, the combination of two or more of them may be needed and titrated on an individual basis as tolerated and needed to manage the symptoms. Tricyclic antidepressants such as amitriptyline, nortriptyline or desipramine, trazodone, and nonsteroidal antiinflammatory analgesic medications are frequently helpful when used in combination with antineuralgic drugs. In the author's experience, neural blockade with local anesthetic may also be effective in breaking the cycle of pain when used in combination with antineuralgic medications. In those cases where medications are no longer effective, surgical intervention may then be indicated. Although invasive neurosurgical procedures may provide pain relief, they carry significant risks, potentially permanent sequelae, the potential for failure, and recurrence of pain. Gamma knife radiosurgery is a potential option with low morbidity compared with other interventions and a good to excellent outcome in 77% or more of patients.[37] It should be stressed here that not all patients with trigeminal neuralgia will respond to medical intervention, just as not all patients will respond to surgical treatment, and unfortunately, some patients may not respond well to either modality of treatment.

Glossopharyngeal Neuralgia

Glossopharyngeal neuralgia is a relatively uncommon disorder characterized by unilateral paroxysmal attacks of sharp, stabbing, burning, or electric shock–like pain that may be felt in the posterior tongue, tonsil, lateral pharyngeal wall, nasopharynx, and ear. As with trigeminal neuralgia, a trigger zone is present, usually located in the lateral pharyngeal wall, tonsillar fossa area, or in the area of the external ear posterior to the ramus of the mandible with pain referring outward from the trigger point. Painful episodes may be provoked by stimulation of the trigger zone during swallowing, yawning, or coughing, with some patients experiencing bradycardia, syncope, and seizure during an attack of pain.[38] Other than the presence of a trigger zone, physical examination is essentially unremarkable with the absence of any detectable neurologic deficits. Before making the diagnosis of glossopharyngeal neuralgia, care should be taken to rule out the presence of neoplasm in the oro-, hypo-, or nasopharynx or at the cerebellopontine angle. A technique useful in making the diagnosis of true glossopharyngeal neuralgia is to perform a local anesthetic block of the trigger point. The etiopathogenesis for glossopharyngeal neuralgia is thought to be the same as trigeminal neuralgia, with involvement of the ninth cranial nerve instead of the fifth. Medical intervention for the treatment of glossopharyngeal is also the same as for trigeminal neuralgia.

Postherpetic Neuralgia

The varicella zoster virus (VZV) can remain latent in the dorsal root or cranial nerve ganglion for many years following the original infection and in later life reactivate to cause herpes zoster (shingles). The orofacial region is a relatively common site of involvement for herpes zoster infections. Although the pain and vesicular eruption usually resolve within 2 to 3 weeks, pain in the form of postherpetic neuralgia (PHN) may persist beyond resolution of these initial symptoms. Pain may be referred to the ear from involvement of the cranial and cervical nerves and may mimic geniculate or nervus intermedius neuralgia. Conversely, herpes zoster involving the external ear is a relatively frequent occurrence with referral of pain to the face, mastoid, and occipital regions as well as the neck.

Although the primary goal in the treatment of acute herpes zoster is to palliate the patient's pain and to effect early resolution of the acute stage of the disease, it is believed that in patients 50 years of age or older treatment for the prevention of PHN is essential, because of its frequency of occurrence in this age group and its potentially debilitating nature.[40] PHN may present with allodynia, hyperalgesia, and hyperesthesia. There may be a persistent, severe burning pain or a paroxysmal lancinating pain in the effected area that is often debilitating in nature. It is essential that when the symptoms of postherpetic neuralgia are first noted, a regimen of early aggressive intervention be initiated. Although there is no universally accepted treatment regimen to prophylax against or effect resolution of early cases of postherpetic neuralgia, a variety of treatment approaches have been pursued, and antiviral medications may prove helpful if given early in high dose.[39] In addition to pharmacotherapy, these may include invasive procedures such as the use of sympathetic nerve blocks, somatic nerve blocks, and subcutaneous infiltration of local anesthetic and steroid beneath the areas of acute vesicular eruption, with sympathetic nerve block therapy often being useful in the early phases of postherpetic neuralgia. Pharmacotherapeutic approaches may include the use of antiviral medication such as valacyclovir, corticosteroids, analgesics, antidepressants, or topical therapy. Nonsteroidal antiinflammatory analgesics may be used for controlling mild pain in acute herpes zoster, with opioid therapy being reserved for severe pain exacerbations. Tricyclic antidepressant medications such as amitriptyline, nortriptyline, or desipramine may be used for both their potential pain-relieving and sedative properties. Anxiolytic agents such as lorazepam, alprazolam, or diazepam may also be used on a short-term basis.[39]

A reasonable approach to treating PHN is the use of tricyclic antidepressants (amitriptyline or nortriptyline) or the anticonvulsant gabapentin.[41] Alternative agents, should these not be effective, include desipramine or maprotiline, with serotonergic drugs such as trazodone, clomipramine, or fluoxetine being of possible help with refractory patients; a trial-and-error approach using anticonvulsants such as carbamazepine, phenytoin, clonazepam, and valproic acid may be used. Long-acting oral forms of oxycodone, morphine, and the fentanyl skin patch may be of help.[40] A variety of topical agents, such as capsaicin, and local anesthetic agents, such as the lidocaine skin patch, may be useful adjuncts to other therapies in some patients.[41] Transcutaneous electrical nerve stimulation (TENS) may also be a useful adjunct.

It should be emphasized that time is of the absolute essence, and sympathetic blockade in the form of a series of stellate ganglion blocks should be performed at the first sign of PHN, which should be treated within 6 months of onset, as the likelihood of achieving satisfactory pain relief after this time is considerably diminished.[39]

Vagal and Superior Laryngeal Neuralgia

Vagal and superior laryngeal neuralgia is an uncommon disorder characterized by sudden severe episodic attacks of brief lancinating electric shock–like pain involving the thyroid cartilage, pyriform sinus, and angle of the mandible, but rarely involving in the ear. Attacks of pain may be precipitated by swallowing, yawning, or coughing, and usually occur in combination with glossopharyngeal neuralgia.[41,42] As with the other neuralgias, physical examination is essentially unremarkable with no neurologic deficit being noted within the distribution of the vagus nerve. The diagnosis is established by clinical history and by identifying a trigger zone. Laryngeal topical anesthesia or blockade of the superior laryngeal nerve is said to alleviate the pain and is a useful diagnostic and prognostic procedure.[43]

Pharmacologic therapy as described for trigeminal neuralgia is indicated for the management of this disorder, with surgical management being reserved for those cases in which pharmacotherapy has been unsuccessful.

Headaches

The classification of headache is complex and often controversial. In 1988 the International Headache Society (IHS) published the first-ever classification of headache establishing uniform terminology and consistent operational diagnostic criteria covering the entire range of headache disorders.[44] In 2004 the second edition of the International Classification of Headache Disorders (ICHD-2) was published, providing a foundation for clinical practice and research.[45] The reader is referred to the new ICHD-2 classification for an in-depth look into the current classification of headaches, as only those headache disorders commonly known to present with referred pain to the ear will be discussed here.

Tension-Type Headache

Tension-type headache is the most common type of primary headache, with 80% of all patients who seek medical care for their headaches falling into this category.[32] As currently classified, tension-type headache (TTH) is broken down primarily into infrequent episodic tension-type headache, frequent episodic tension-type headache, and chronic tension-type headache. All three forms are further subclassified as being associated with pericranial tenderness or not. Episodic TTH usually responds to over-the-counter analgesics.[48] For a TTH to be classified as chronic, it must have been present for at least 15 days a month on average, greater than 3 months (180 days per year or more) with the following criteria: lasting hours or may be continuous, and two of these characteristics: bilateral location, pressing/tightening nonpulsatile quality, mild or moderate intensity, and aggravated by routine physical activity such as walking or climbing stairs.[46]

TTH is usually described as a steady nonpulsatile ache that may be localized unilaterally or bilaterally to a single region in the head or it may be generalized. Pain may be felt in the frontotemporal region including the face, occipital region, parietal region, or any combination of these sites, with patients often describing a feeling of tightness, a drawing sensation, or band-like pressure. The pain from TTH, especially headache involving the frontotemporal region, may refer to the ear, presenting as otalgia. As in TMD, the resulting ear pain may be the precipitating agent in causing the patient to seek medical attention. The severity of the headache pain may vary from soreness to gnawing or a dull ache to a sharp episodic or continuous stabbing pain. The patient frequently complains of a feeling of tightness or cramping in the neck or shoulder regions (cervical myalgia). Tension-type headache may begin as either unilateral or bilateral headache pain and may progress from a localized to a generalized headache pain and may be accompanied by symptoms such as photophobia, periorbital pain, lacrimation, tinnitus, vertigo, and referred otalgia.

It should be emphasized that although the pathogenesis of TTH may vary from individual to individual, in the end the primary underlying cause in those patients with pericranial tenderness is myofascial in origin. Hence, it may be difficult to differentiate TTH that includes occipital, parietal, or frontotemporal pain from TMD of myofascial origin. All of these may present as frontotemporal, temporal, or occipital pain often with neck or shoulder tightness and all may be a source of referred pain to the ear or periaural region.

It is also important to understand that patients with myofascial facial pain will relate a history of TTHs, just as patients with TTHs frequently mention a previous or concomitant history of facial pain. Another confounding issue is the frequent bias and lack of global perspective on the part of the clinician. Some physicians fail to examine the orofacial structures and musculature and overdiagnose TTH, and some dentists do not examine beyond the orofacial region and overdiagnose TMD. Musculoskeletal examination of a patient with TTH or TMD of myofascial origin will demonstrate nodular or band-like tender muscle trigger points as previously described, which reproduce or exacerbate the patient's pain complaint. The appropriate diagnosis should be made based on the region from which the primary pain or dysfunction emanates.

Cluster Headache and Other Trigeminal Autonomic Cephalalgias

As a group the autonomic cephalalgias share the clinical features of headache and prominent cranial parasympathetic autonomic features. Although cluster headache is not known to present with secondary otalgia as one of its features, chronic paroxysmal hemicrania, one of the other trigeminal autonomic cephalalgias listed in the ICHD-2, has been reported to present with otalgia with the sensation of external acoustic meatus obstruction.[47]

Temporal Arteritis

Temporal arteritis is a form of primary headache under the moniker of headache attributed to giant cell arteritis. It is characterized by an intense, deep, persistent, throbbing, aching, and burning pain that may be accompanied by hyperalgesia of the scalp and extreme tenderness of the involved arteries. Patients with this disorder may experience pain on mastication and referred pain to the teeth, ear, jaw, zygoma, and nuchal and occipital regions. The initial presenting complaint may be ocular in nature with partial or complete loss of vision. Diagnosis usually requires biopsy, and treatment consists of corticosteroids to prevent blindness.

Secondary Headaches

Secondary headaches include headache or facial pain attributed to disorder of cranium, neck, eyes, ears, nose, sinuses, teeth, mouth, or other facial or cranial structures. The common denominator in headache from this diverse spectrum of disorders is stretching, compression, or inflammation of pain-sensitive structures in the skull, including the brain, meninges, arteries, veins, eyes, ears, teeth, nose, and paranasal sinuses. The underlying cause may be a mass lesion, hemorrhage, or inflammatory disease. For example, as the cerebrovascular innervation (which is selectively nociceptive specific) is supplied by CN V_1 and some CN V_3 fibers, pain may be referred to the ear by any event that produces traction or inflammation in these nerves.

Cervicogenic pain as originally described was a headache form deriving its origin from one of several structures in the neck or back of the head (including nerves, ganglia, nerve roots, uncovertebral joints, intervertebral joints, disks, bone, periosteum, muscle, and ligaments).[48] Headache associated with myofascial tenderness in the cervical musculature is now coded as infrequent episodic TTH, frequent episodic TTH, or chronic TTH, all associated with pericranial tenderness and is no longer included as a form of cervicogenic pain. As its name implies, cervicogenic headache originates in the neck with a referral pattern to the head, frequently the ophthalmic division of the trigeminal nerve, presenting as retro-orbital and frontotemporal headache pain or preauricular pain. This pain referral pattern is explained by close proximity of the cervical spinal and medullary dorsal horn with apparent convergence of some cervical nociceptive afferent fibers in the MDH.[40] Through this pattern of convergence, pain may also be referred to the vertex along the midline, periaural region, pinna, and jaw, including occasionally the teeth.[8]

◆ Discussion

When the otologic examination is normal but the patient complains of ear pain, the general otolaryngologic examination should be extended to include additional areas. If not already obtained, careful mirror or fiberoptic examinations of the nasopharynx and laryngopharynx should be performed. The TMJ, temporal arteries, tonsillar fossae, base of tongue, carotid artery, and neck muscles should be carefully palpated. The teeth and cervical spine can be percussed. Radiographic studies of the skull, sinuses, teeth, TMJs, and cervical spine can be obtained in selected patients.

Two diseases cited in this chapter that require prompt diagnosis and management are temporal arteritis and head and neck malignancy. Although temporal arteritis is uncommon, recognition is vital to initiate corticosteroid treatment and prevent blindness. Classically the artery pulse may be absent and erythrocyte sedimentation rate (ESR) elevated, but on occasion the pulse may be normal, tenderness to palpation minimal, and laboratory tests normal. The physician should maintain a high index of suspicion and initiate corticosteroid therapy promptly.

Recognition of head and neck malignancy is not as urgent as temporal arteritis, but some of these masses can easily be missed, with disastrous results. Particularly, neoplasms in the nasopharynx, sinus, tonsil, base of tongue, and hypopharynx can spread dramatically and quickly if not treated promptly. Ear pain can be the only manifestation of these malignancies. Suspicious soft tissue lesions should be biopsied.

Many different causes of referred otalgia were reviewed in this chapter, and the clinician should be familiar with all of them. For practical purposes, however, the most common causes are TMD (primarily myofascial-pain dysfunction), cervical myalgia, and dental disease. TMD usually refers pain to the preauricular area over the joint and also to the angle of the jaw just behind and deep to the ramus of the mandible. There may be a history of teeth clenching, bruxism, and prolonged dental work. The TMJ may be tender to palpation, and the examiner may feel crepitus; the jaw may deviate or sublux on wide opening. Cervical myalgia usually refers pain to the

postauricular area where the muscles attach to the mastoid tip. The sternocleidomastoid or trapezius muscles may be tender to palpation or may be in spasm on the involved side. Dental abscess may cause tenderness with percussion of the tooth. A dentist can best manage TMD and dental disease, and a physical therapist can help manage temporomandibular and cervical myalgia.

When a patient with persistent ear pain has no identifiable primary or secondary source of the pain, a contrasted MRI of the head (brain) should be obtained with special attention to the base of skull on the involved side, including coronal views of the infratemporal fossa. Although MRI results usually are normal, the patient and physician are reassured that there is no serious intracranial disease. Following an extensive evaluation, if no etiology is found for the otalgia and if there is no response to empiric trials of therapy, the patient should be referred to a pain management clinic, which offers medical therapy as well as behavioral medicine evaluation and counseling.

References

1. Paparella MM, Jung TTK, Gluckman JC, Meyerhoff WL, eds. Otolaryngology, vol 2, 3rd ed. Philadelphia: WB Saunders, 1991:1237–1242
2. Bonica JJ. Definitions and taxonomy of pain. In: Bonica JJ, ed. The Management of Pain, vol 1, 2nd ed. Philadelphia: Lea & Febiger, 1990:18–27
3. Bonica JJ. Anatomic and physiologic basis of nociception and pain. In: Bonica JJ, ed. The Management of Pain, vol 1, 2nd ed. Philadelphia: Lea & Febiger, 1990:28–94
4. Cross SA. Pathophysiology of pain. Mayo Clin Proc 1994;69:375–383
5. Sessle BJ, Hu JW, Amano N, Zhon G. Convergence of cutaneous, tooth pulp, visceral, neck and muscle afferent onto nociceptive and non-nociceptive neurones in trigeminal sub-nucleus caudalis medullary dorsal horn (MDH) and its implications for referred pain. Pain 1986;27:219–235
6. Sessle BJ. The neurobiology of facial and dental pain: present knowledge, future directions. J Dent Res 1987;66:962–981
7. Poletti CE. C-2 and C-3 radiculopathies: anatomy, patterns of cephalic pain and pathology. APS 1992;1:272–275
8. Fromm GH, Sessle BJ. Trigeminal Neuralgia: Current Concepts Regarding Pathogenesis and Treatment. Boston: Butterworth-Heinemann, 1991: 71–104
9. Stacey MJ. Free nerve endings and skeletal muscle of the cat. J Anat 1969; 105:231–254
10. Gerwin RD. Neurobiology of the myofascial trigger point. Baillieres Clin Rheumatol 1994;8:747–762
11. Jerger J. Handbook of Clinical Impedance Audiometry. Dobbs Ferry, NY: American Electromedics, 1975:85–126
12. Bernstein JM. Otalgia: its not always what it seems to be. J Respir Dis 1987;8:71–82
13. Thaller SR, De Silva A. Otalgia with a normal ear. AFP 1987;36:129–136
14. Mense S. Nociception from skeletal muscle in relation to clinical muscle pain. Pain 1993;54:241–289
15. Sessle BJ. Masticatory muscle disorders: basic science perspectives. In: Sessle BJ, Bryant PS, Dionne RA, eds. Temporomandibular Disorders and Related Pain Conditions: Progress in Pain Research and Management, vol 4. Seattle: IASP Press, 1995:47–61
16. Sessle BJ. Recent insights into brainstem mechanisms underlying craniofacial pain. J Dent Educ 2002;66:108–112
17. Mense S. Mechanisms of pain in hind limb muscles: experimental findings and open questions. In: Sessle BJ, Bryant PS, Dionne RA, eds. Temporomandibular Disorders and Related Pain Conditions: Progress and Pain Research and Management, vol 4. Seattle: IASP Press, 1995:63–69
18. Bernstein JM, Mohl ND, Spiller H. Temporomandibular joint dysfunction masquerading as disease of the ear, nose and throat. Trans Am Acad Ophthalmol Otolaryngol 1969;73:1208–1217
19. Gaynor EB. Otolaryngologic manifestations of gastroesophageal reflux. Am J Gastroenterol 1991;86:801–808
20. Gibson WS, Cochran W. Otalgia in infants and children—a manifestation of gastroesophageal reflux. Int J Pediatr Otorhinolaryngol 1994;28: 213–218

21. Travell J, Rinzler SH. The myofascial genesis of pain. Postgrad Med 1952; 11:425–434

22. Travell JG, Simons DG. Myofascial Pain and Dysfunction: The Trigger Point Manual. Baltimore: Williams & Wilkins, 1983

23. Laskin DM. Current concepts in the management of temporomandibular joint disorders. Continuing Education Course presented at Annual Meeting of the American Academy of Oral Pathology, 1982

24. Friction JR, et al. Myofascial pain syndrome of the head and neck: a review of clinical characteristics of 164 patients. Oral Surg Oral Med Oral Pathol 1985;60:615–623

25. Campbell SM. Regional myofascial pain syndromes. Rheum Dis Clin North Am 1989;15:31–44

26. Friction JL. Myofascial pain syndrome. Neurol Clin 1989;7: 413–427

27. Menses, Simons DG. Myofascial pain caused by trigger points. In: Muscle Pain: Understanding Its Nature, Diagnosis, and Treatment. Philadelphia: Lippincott Williams & Wilkins, 2001:205–288

28. Woda A. Mechanisms of neuropathic pain. In: Lund JP, Lavigne GH, Dubner R, Sessle BJ, eds. Orofacial Pain: From Basic Science to Clinical Management. Chicago: Quintessence, 2001:67–78

29. Lavigne G, Woda A, Truelove E, Ship JA, Dao T, Goulet JP. Mechanisms associated with unusual orofacial pain. J Orofac Pain 2005;19:9–21

30. Remick RA, Blasberg B, Campos PE, Miles JE. Psychiatric disorders associated with atypical facial pain. Can J Psychiatry 1983;28:178–181

31. Fromm GH. Trigeminal neuralgia and related disorders. Neurol Clin 1989;7:305–319

32. Headache Classification Committee of the International Headache Society. The International Classification of Headache Disorders. Cephalalgia 2004;24:175–182

33. Devor M, Amir R, Rappaport H. Pathophysiology of trigeminal neuralgia: The ignition hypothesis. Clin J Pain 2002;18:4–13

34. Bullitt E, Tew JM, Boyd J. Intracranial tumors in patients with facial pain. J Neurosurg 1986;64:865–871

35. Fromm GH, Terrence CF, Maroon JC. Trigeminal neuralgia: current concepts regarding etiology and pathogenesis. Arch Neurol 1984;41:1204–1207

36. Fromm GH, Terrence CF, Chattha AS. Baclofen in the treatment of trigeminal neuralgia: double-blind study and long-term follow up. Ann Neurol 1984;15:240–244

37. Petit JH, Herman JM, Nagda S, DiBiase SJ, Chin LS. Radiosurgical treatment of trigeminal neuralgia: evaluating quality of life and treatment outcomes. Int J Radiat Oncol Biol Phys 2003;56:1147–1153

38. Chalmers AC, Olson JL. Glossopharyngeal neuralgia with syncope and cervical mass. Otolaryngol Head Neck Surg 1989;100:252–255

39. Katz JA, Phero JC, McDonald JS, Green DB. Herpes zoster management. Anesth Prog 1989;36:35–40

40. Watson CPN. Management issues of neuropathic trigeminal pain from a medical perspective. J Orofac Pain 2004;18:366–373

41. Loeser JD. Cranial neuralgias. In: Bonica JJ, ed. The Management of Pain, vol 1, 2nd ed. Philadelphia: Lea & Febiger, 1990:676–686

42. Chawla JC, Falconer MA. Glossopharyngeal and vagal neuralgia. BMJ 1967;3:529–531

43. Bonica JJ, ed. The Management of Pain, vol 1. Philadelphia: Lea & Febiger, 1953:790–797

44. Headache Classification Committee of the International Headache Society. Classification and diagnostic criteria for headache disorders, cranial neuralgias and facial pain. Cephalalgia 1988;8(suppl 7):1–96

45. Dalessio DJ. Wolff's Headache and Other Head Pain, 5th ed. New York: Oxford University Press, 1987

46. Lipton RB, Bigal ME, Steiner TH, Silberstein SD, Olesen J. Classification of primary headaches. Neurology 2004;63:427–435

47. Boes CJ, Swanson JW, Dodick DW. Chronic paroxysmal hemicrania presenting as otalgia with a sensation of external acoustic meatus obstruction: two cases and a pathophysiologic hypothesis. Headache 1998; 38:787–791

48. Sjaastad O, Fredriksen TA, Pfaffenrath V. Cervicogenic headache: diagnostic criteria. Headache 1990;30:725–726

35

Evaluation and Management of Pulsatile Tinnitus

Aristides Sismanis

Pulsatile tinnitus (PT) is an uncommon type of tinnitus which often presents a diagnostic and management dilemma to the clinician. Correct diagnosis is essential because many patients with this symptom have a treatable underlying cause. Furthermore, failure to establish the appropriate diagnosis may have disastrous consequences because in some patients an associated life-threatening pathology may be present.

◆ Pathophysiology and Classification

PT most often originates from vascular structures within the cranial cavity, head and neck region, or even the thoracic cavity, and is transmitted to the cochlea by bony or vascular structures. PT arises either from increased flow volume or stenosis of a vascular lumen and according to the vessel of origin it can be classified as *arterial* or *venous*. The venous type can originate not only from primary venous pathologies, but also from conditions causing increased intracranial pressure (ICP) by transmission of arterial pulsations to the dural venous sinuses.[1] In rare instances, PT originates from other nonarterial structures and is classified as *nonvascular*.

PT is classified as *objective* if it is audible to both the patient and examiner, or as *subjective* if it is audible only to the patient.

High-pitched tinnitus, often bilateral, with a pulsatile component should not be confused with arterial PT. This type of tinnitus is usually associated with high-frequency sensorineural hearing loss and is subjective (See Chapter 36).

◆ Arterial Etiologies

Atherosclerotic Carotid Artery Disease

In our experience atherosclerotic carotid artery disease (ACAD) has been the most common cause of PT in patients older than 50 years, especially when associated risk factors such as hypertension, angina, hyperlipidemia, diabetes mellitus, and smoking are present. Objective PT can be the first manifestation of ACAD in some of these patients.[2] PT in ACAD is secondary to bruit(s) produced by turbulent blood flow at stenotic segment(s) of the carotid artery. In a series of 12 patients with PT secondary to ACAD, ipsilateral carotid bruit was present in all of them. Atherosclerotic subclavian artery disease and atherosclerotic occlusion of the contralateral common carotid artery also have been reported in association with PT.[3,4] Diagnosis is confirmed by duplex ultrasound studies.[2]

Vascular Neoplasms of Skull Base and Temporal Bone

Glomus jugulare and tympanicum are the most common vascular tumors of the temporal bone presenting with PT.[5] Other rare middle ear neoplasms associated with PT include hemangiomas,[6] angiomatous meningiomas,[7] and metastatic breast carcinomas.[8]

Intracranial Vascular Abnormalities

Intracranial vascular abnormalities are uncommon etiologies of PT; however, misdiagnosis may lead to catastrophic consequences for patients. At our institution the most common vascular intracranial abnormality presenting with PT is dural arteriovenous fistula (AVF).

Dural AVFs comprise approximately 15% of intracranial arteriovenous malformations (AVMs) and usually become symptomatic during the fifth or sixth decades of life.[9,10] PT is the most common manifestation of these lesions. The transverse and sigmoid dural sinuses are most commonly involved, followed by the cavernous sinus. In contrast to AVMs, AVFs are usually acquired and thought to result from spontaneous dural venous sinus thrombosis, or secondary to trauma, obstructing neoplasm, surgery, or infection. As the thrombosed segment recanalizes, ingrowth of dural arteries takes place and arterial-to-sinus anastomoses are formed.[9]

Pulsatile tinnitus in these patients is of the arterial type and is associated with a bruit over the involved dural sinus (usually audible in the retroauricular area) as well as objective PT (audible in the ear canal). **Fig. 35–1** depicts a carotid angiogram of a patient with an AVF between a posterior meningeal branch of the middle meningeal artery and the transverse sinus.

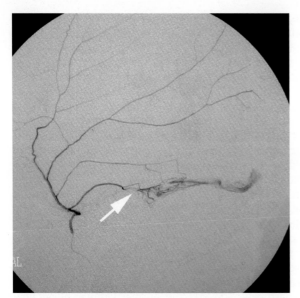

Figure 35–1 Carotid angiography, lateral projection. An arteriovenous fistula (AVF) is shown (arrow) between a posterior meningeal branch of the middle meningeal artery and the transverse sinus.

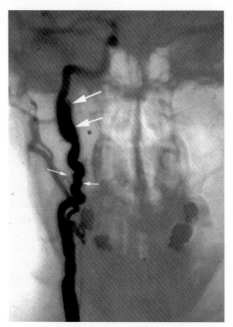

Figure 35–2 Carotid angiography, anterior-posterior view, of a 36-year-old woman with fibromuscular dysplasia. The "string of beads" is a pathognomonic finding (arrows).

The mortality rate from hemorrhage of dural AVFs has been reported to be between 10 and 20%.[9] In cases with retrograde drainage into the cortical veins, the chance of subarachnoid or parenchymal hemorrhage is much higher.[9]

Dissecting aneurysms are also rare, and more often involve the internal carotid arteries and less often the vertebral arteries.[11] Besides objective PT and cervical bruit, manifestations include cervical pain, headache, cerebral ischemic symptoms, cranial neuropathies, vertigo, dysgeusia, and Horner's syndrome.[9,11] The most common angiographic finding is that of irregular stenosis.[11]

Sudden head rotation, especially when accompanied by extension (i.e., the tennis "ace serve"), is a common precipitating event.[12] Fibromuscular dysplasia (FMD) and various arteriopathies such as Marfan syndrome can be predisposing factors.[13] Aneurysms of the intrapetrous carotid artery,[14–16] and of the anterior communicating artery[17] are very rare causes of PT.

Fibromuscular Dysplasia

Fibromuscular dysplasia is a nonatherosclerotic, noninflammatory stenosing vascular disease, which affects younger females and most commonly involves the renal and internal carotid arteries.[18]

Carotid artery FMD is frequently associated with PT. Other symptoms such as vertigo, headache, cervicofacial hypoesthesia, and transient ischemic attacks have been reported.[19,20] The typical angiographic finding is that of a "string of beads."[20] The prevalence of intracranial aneurysms in these patients is approximately 7%.[21] **Fig. 35–2** is a carotid angiogram of a 36-year old woman with FMD.

Tortuous Carotid Artery

These are usually middle-aged patients with audible bruits in the skull base. Diagnosis can be made with computed tomography (CT) angiography. It is likely that aging results in

tortuous carotid vessels with associated turbulent blood flow and PT. In our experience PT subsides spontaneously with time in most of these cases. **Table 35–1** summarizes the less common arterial etiologies of PT.[5,22–36]

◆ Venous Etiologies

Idiopathic Intracranial Hypertension Syndrome

Idiopathic intracranial hypertension (IIH) syndrome is a common cause of venous PT in obese female patients. This syndrome is of unknown etiology in most cases, and is characterized by increased intracranial pressure, normal cerebrospinal fluid (CSF) content, and absent neurologic signs except for occasional V, VI, and VII cranial nerve palsies.[37,38] Other synonyms of this disorder are pseudotumor cerebri and benign intracranial hypertension syndrome; the latter term is recently used less often because the

Table 35–1 Arterial Etiologies of Pulsatile Tinnitus (Less Common)

Intrapetrous carotid artery dissection[34]
Brachiocephalic artery stenosis[23]
External carotid artery stenosis[27]
Ectopic intratympanic carotid artery[22,29,35]
Persistent stapedial artery[32]
Aberrant artery in the stria vascularis[30]
Vascular compression of the eighth nerve[31]
Increased cardiac output (anemia, thyrotoxicosis, pregnancy)[24,25]
Paget's disease[26,28,33]
Aortic murmurs[36]
Otosclerosis[5]
Hypertension; antihypertensive agents[5]

risk of visual loss is not "benign." Etiologies of this entity are summarized in **Table 35–2**.[38–42]

The annual incidence of IIH hypertension is 0.9 per 100,000 people in the general population. This entity is more common in young African-American females who are 20% percent or more above their ideal body weight.[1,43,44] In males this disorder is very rare, and in 25% of patients it may become chronic.[37]

Although the classic presentation of IIH consists of headaches or visual disturbances, PT alone or in association with hearing loss, dizziness, and aural fullness has been reported as the main manifestation(s) of this syndrome.[45–47] Many of these patients are morbidly obese (body weight more than 100 lbs above ideal weight) and have associated papilledema. Absence of papilledema, however, does not exclude this entity.[48–50]

Significant uncertainty exists regarding the pathophysiology of IIH. Many studies have tried to elucidate the underlying cause, often with conflicting results. Proposed theories include increased CSF production, cerebral edema, decreased CSF absorption, and elevated cerebral venous pressure.[38,39,43,51,52] The pathophysiology of IIH in morbidly obese patients most likely results from increased intraabdominal and intrathoracic pressure, cardiac filling, and intracranial venous pressures.[53] This pathophysiologic mechanism is further supported by an animal study demonstrating increased CSF pressure when intraabdominal pressure was acutely raised.[54] Increased cerebral blood flow secondary to cerebrovascular resistance changes and CSF hypersecretion induced by elevated estrogen levels also have been reported as pathophysiologic mechanisms of IIH.[55]

PT in IIH syndrome results from the systolic pulsations of the CSF, which originate mainly from the arteries of the circle of Willis. These pulsations, which are increased in magnitude in the presence of intracranial hypertension, are transmitted to the exposed medial aspect of the dural venous sinuses (transverse and sigmoid) and compress their walls synchronously with the arterial pulsations.[1,56] The resulting periodic lumen narrowing converts the normal laminar blood flow to turbulent, thus producing a low-frequency PT.[1] The low-frequency sensorineural hearing loss seen in many of these patients is believed to result from the masking effect of the PT. This is supported by the fact that light digital compression over the ipsilateral internal jugular vein (IJV) results in cessation of the tinnitus and immediate improvement or normalization of hearing.[1] Stretching or compression of the cochlear nerve and brainstem, caused by the intracranial hypertension or possible edema, may also play a role in the hearing loss and dizziness encountered in these patients. This is supported by the abnormal auditory brainstem response (ABR) present in one third of these patients.[57]

Magnetic resonance venography (MRV) can be very helpful in identifying cerebral venous thrombosis and has been recommended for IIH patients.[58,59] In a recent study, autotriggered elliptic-centric-ordered (ATECO) three-dimensional gadolinium-enhanced MRV identified bilateral sinovenous stenosis in 27 of 29 patients with IIH and only in 4 of 59 controls. It was not clear whether the stenosis was a cause or effect of intracranial hypertension.[60] Anatomic obstruction of the venous transverse sinuses has recently been reported in IIH patients, and direct retrograde cerebral venography (DRCV) with manometry has been recommended to establish the diagnosis.[61,62]

Diagnosis is made by exclusion of other causes of intracranial hypertension and is established by lumbar puncture with confirmation of CSF pressure of more than 200 mm of water with normal CSF constituents.

Jugular Bulb Abnormalities

High-placed and dehiscent jugular bulbs are the most common reported jugular bulb abnormalities.[63–66] **Fig. 35–3** shows a CT angiogram of a patient with an enlarged dehiscent jugular bulb and an associated diverticulum. A bluish and inferiorly based retrotympanic lesion is the typical otoscopic finding.

Idiopathic or Essential Pulsatile Tinnitus

Idiopathic or *essential PT* and *venous hum* are terms used interchangeably in the literature to describe patients with PT of unclear etiology.[67,68] The most common age group of

Table 35–2 Etiologies of Idiopathic Intracranial Hypertension Syndrome[38–42]

Medications	*Obstruction to Venous Drainage*
Amiodarone	Cerebral venous thrombosis
Anabolic steroids	Hypercoagulable states
Chlordecone	Antiphospholipid antibody syndrome
Corticosteroids	Polycythemia
Cyclosporine	Mastoiditis
Diphenylhydantoin	Superior vena cava syndrome
Divalproate	Increased right heart pressure
Growth hormone	Bilateral radical neck dissection
Indomethacin	
Leuprorelin acetate	*Circulatory and Hematologic*
Levothyroxine	Iron-deficiency anemia
Lithium carbonate	Sickle cell anemia
Minocycline	Pernicious anemia
Nalidixic acid	Gastrointestinal hemorrhage
Norplant	Cryofibrinogenemia
Penicillin	
Sulfa antibiotics	*Systemic Disorders*
Tetracyclines and related compounds	Lupus erythematosus
Vitamin A	Sickle cell anemia
All-trans-retinoic acid	Sarcoidosis
	Sleep apnea
Endocrine Disorders	Turner's syndrome
Adrenal insufficiency	Human immunodeficiency virus infection
Hypoparathyroidism	Paget's disease
Hyperthyroidism	Galactosemia
Obesity	Head trauma
Menarche	Nephrotic syndrome
Menstrual irregularities	Uremia
Pregnancy	
Polycystic ovary syndrome	*Infectious*
	Lyme Disease
Nutritional Disorders	Infectious mononucleosis
Hypervitaminosis A	
Hypovitaminosis A	
Hyperalimentation in nutritional deficiency	

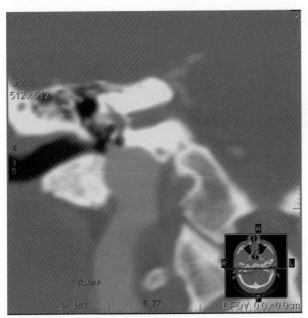

Figure 35–3 Coronal computed tomography (CT) angiogram, venous phase, shows an enlarged dehiscent jugular bulb with an associated diverticulum.

patients with idiopathic PT is between 20 and 40 years and there is a marked female preponderance.[1] A possible cause of idiopathic PT is believed to be turbulent blood flow produced in the IJV as it curves around the lateral process of the atlas.[69]

Diagnosis of this condition should be made only after appropriate evaluation and elimination of other disorders, such as IIH syndrome. Because it is possible that many of the patients reported in the literature with idiopathic PT had an incomplete evaluation to rule out IIH syndrome, it is possible that at least in some of these cases, PT was secondary to this syndrome. Associated symptoms of headaches and blurred vision, especially in morbidly obese female patients, should alert the physician to IIH syndrome. **Table 35–3** summarizes the venous etiologies of PT.[1,63–73]

◆ Nonvascular Etiologies

Palatal, Stapedial, and Tensor Tympani Muscle Myoclonus

Myoclonic contractions of the tensor veli palatini, levator veli palatini, salpingopharyngeus, and superior constrictor muscles can result in objective PT. These contractions can range between 10 and 240 per minute and occasionally may be confused with the arterial pulse. This disorder is usually seen in young patients, usually within the first three decades of life, although it may be seen in older individuals as well.[74,75] Brainstem infarctions, multiple sclerosis, trauma, syphilis, and cerebellar tumors have been reported as etiologies. Involvement of the olivary tracts, posterior longitudinal bundle, dentate nucleus, and reticular formation has been described in these patients.[76,77]

Myoclonic contractions of the stapedial and tensor tympani muscles also have been reported as a cause of PT.[78–80]

Table 35–3 Venous Etiologies of Pulsatile Tinnitus

IIH syndrome[1]
Jugular bulb abnormalities[63–66]
Hydrocephalus associated with stenosis of the sylvian aqueduct[70]
Increased intracranial pressure associated with Arnold-Chiari syndrome[70]
Abnormal condylar and mastoid emissary veins[72,73]
Idiopathic or essential tinnitus[67–69,71]

◆ Evaluation

History

The history is one of the most important aspects in evaluating patients with PT. Typically these patients describe their symptom as hearing their own heartbeat or hearing a "thumping noise," making diagnosis obvious. Occasionally, however, patients do not volunteer the pulsatile component of their tinnitus and this may lead to overlooking this important information.

Associated symptoms of hearing loss, aural fullness, dizziness, headaches, visual loss, transient visual obscurations, retrobulbar pain, and diplopia are highly suggestive of IIH syndrome.[1,46]

Older patients with history of cerebrovascular accident, transient ischemic attacks, myocardial infarction, hyperlipidemia, hypertension, diabetes mellitus, and history of smoking should be suspected of ACAD.[2]

Females with associated headaches, dizzy spells, fatigue, syncopal attacks, and presence of lateralizing neurologic deficits should be evaluated for FMD.[81]

Sudden onset of PT in association with cervical or facial pain, headache, and symptoms of cerebral ischemia is highly suggestive of extracranial or intrapetrous carotid artery dissection.[34,82]

Examination

Young and morbidly obese females should be strongly suspected of IIH syndrome. The body habitus of a morbidly obese patient with IIH syndrome is depicted in **Fig. 35–4.** Otoscopy is essential for the detection of any middle ear pathology such as a high or dehiscent jugular bulb, aberrant carotid artery, glomus tumor, and Schwartze's sign. Rhythmic movements of the tympanic membrane can be present in patients with tensor tympani myoclonus.

A head and neck examination is also important. A palpable thrill can be present in cervical arteriovenous malformations.[33] Myoclonic contractions of the soft palate can be identified in patients with palatal myoclonus. Wide opening of the oral cavity during examination may result in elimination of the soft palate contractions.[71] Inspection with a flexible scope introduced through the nose may facilitate detection of myoclonic movements of the soft palate.

Auscultation of the ear canal, periauricular region, orbits, cervical region, and chest is of utmost importance for detecting objective PT, bruits, and heart murmurs. This should be performed preferably with a modified electronic stethoscope in an audiologic soundproof booth. Auscultation with an electronic stethoscope has been found more sensitive than traditional auscultation.[83,84] **Fig. 35–5** shows such a stethoscope. Should objective PT be detected, its rate should be compared with the patient's arterial pulse. The effect of light digital pressure over the ipsilateral IJV should be checked.

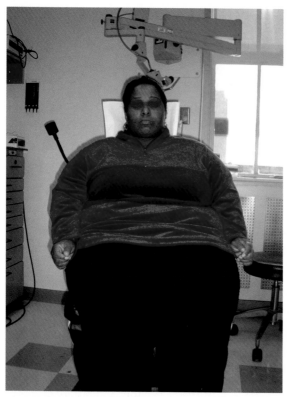

Figure 35–4 Patient with idiopathic intracranial hypertension (IIH) syndrome.

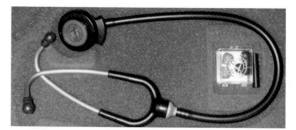

Figure 35–5 Electronic stethoscope (Littmann, model 2000, 3M, St. Paul, MN).

(greater than 200 mm of water).[88] The characteristics of PT in various pathologic conditions are summarized in **Table 35–4**.

Audiologic and Electrophysiologic Testing

Pure-tone (air and bone conduction) and speech audiometry should be performed in all patients. When hearing loss of 20 dB or more is detected in the low frequencies, a repeat audiogram should be obtained while the patient is applying light digital pressure over the ipsilateral IJV. This maneuver typically results in improvement or normalization of pure tones in patients with venous PT, such as in IIH syndrome, because of elimination of the masking effect of the tinnitus.[1] Discrimination is typically excellent in these patients. **Fig. 35–6** depicts characteristic audiograms of a patient with IIH syndrome. Impedance audiometry can be useful in the diagnosis of patients suspected of tensor tympani myoclonus.

Auditory evoked responses should be considered in patients suspected of IIH syndrome. Abnormalities of this test, consisting mainly of prolonged interpeak latencies, have been detected in one third of patients with this syndrome.[57] Normalization or improvement of these abnormalities has been noticed in most of these patients following successful management.[57] Electronystagmography (ENG) should be considered in patients with associated dizziness.[1]

PT of venous origin, often present in patients with IIH syndrome, decreases or is completely eliminated with this maneuver.[146] In patients with arterial PT this maneuver is ineffective. The effect of head rotation on tinnitus intensity should also be tested because venous PT often decreases or completely subsides upon head rotation toward the ipsilateral side, probably because of compression of the IJV between the contracting sternocleidomastoid muscle and the transverse process of the atlas.[146] In selected cases, a complete neurologic examination also should be included.

Neurology consultation should be obtained for patients suspected of IIH syndrome. Papilledema is compatible with this syndrome; its absence, however, does not exclude this entity.[85–87] Diagnosis of this condition is established by lumbar puncture and documentation of elevated CSF pressure

Metabolic Workup

The metabolic workup should be individualized. Serum vitamin A level should be considered in patients with IIH syndrome. Complete blood count and thyroid function test should be obtained in patients with increased cardiac output syndrome to exclude anemia and hyperthyroidism respectively.

Table 35–4 Characteristics of Pulsatile Tinnitus

	IIH Syndrome	ACAD	Glomus Tumors	AVM/AVF
Age	<40 years	>50 years	40 years, average	40 years, average
Sex	Females mainly	More common in females	More common in females	NR
Weight	Obese	NR	NR	NR
Retrotympanic mass	–	–	+	–
Objective PT	+	+	–	–
Arterial PT	–	+	+	+
Venous PT	+	–	–	–
Head bruit	–	–	–	+
Neck bruit	–	+	–	–
Papilledema	Common	–	–	–

IIH, idiopathic intracranial hypertension; ACAD, atherosclerotic carotid artery disease; AVM, arteriovenous malformation; AVF, arteriovenous fistula; NR not related; +, present; –, absent.

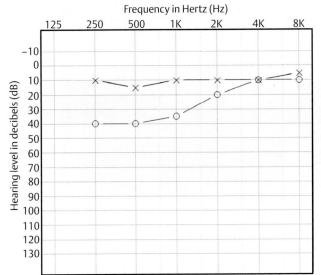

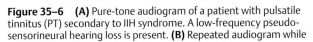

A

Figure 35–6 **(A)** Pure-tone audiogram of a patient with pulsatile tinnitus (PT) secondary to IIH syndrome. A low-frequency pseudo-sensorineural hearing loss is present. **(B)** Repeated audiogram while

B

the masking effect of the PT has been eliminated by digital pressure over the ipsilateral jugular vein reveals normalization of hearing.

Serum lipid profile and fasting blood sugar should be considered in patients undergoing workup for ACAD.

Ultrasound Studies

Duplex ultrasound studies of the carotid arteries and echocardiogram should be considered in patients suspected of ACAD and valvular disease, respectively. These studies should be performed prior to any radiologic evaluation because they may be the only tests required to establish diagnosis.[89]

◆ Radiologic Evaluation

Radiologic evaluation needs to be individualized according to the characteristics of the PT (arterial/venous, subjective/objective) and other clinical findings such as obesity, papilledema, retrotympanic pathology, and the presence of a head/neck bruit.

The recently introduced CT angiography seems to be more sensitive than magnetic resonance angiography/venography (MRA/MRV) in evaluating vascular lesions and it is likely that it will replace the latter in the near future.[90–93] This is a faster imaging technique, and because the upper neck is included, cervical vascular pathology can be detected in the same study. At present many neuroradiologists prefer CT angiography as a substitute for MRA; however, further studies are needed to document the superiority of this very promising radiologic test. The following subsections present the author's current radiologic evaluation approach for patients with PT.

Patients with Normal Otoscopic Findings

Patients suspicious for IIH syndrome (young, obese females with venous type of PT) should have a brain magnetic resonance imaging (MRI) combined with an MRV at the initial evaluation. Although in the literature MRI findings of IIH syndrome, with the exception of an empty sella or small ventricles, have been reported as normal in the majority of

patients,[5] a controlled study of 20 such patients disclosed flattening of the posterior sclera in 80% of patients, empty sella in 70%, distention of the perioptic subarachnoid space in 45%, enhancement of the prelaminar optic nerve in 50%, vertical tortuosity of the orbital optic nerve in 40%, and intraocular protrusion of the prelaminar optic nerve in 30%.[94] **Fig. 35–7** is an MRI of a IIH syndrome patient depicting an empty sella. Head MRV is obtained in conjunction with the MRI, because stenosis/obstruction of the transverse sinus have been reported in IIH syndrome.[59–62] CT angiography with attention to the venous phase is another study to be considered in these patients.

Other rare congenital central nervous system abnormalities such as Chiari I malformation and stenosis of the sylvian aqueduct, which can be associated with intracranial hypertension/PT, can easily be detected with brain MRI.[70] Occlusion

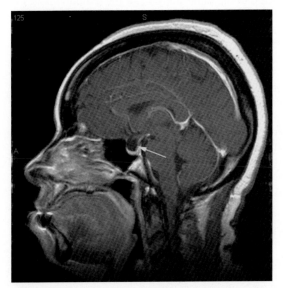

Figure 35–7 Sagittal T1-weighted with gadolinium magnetic resonance imaging shows an empty sella (arrow).

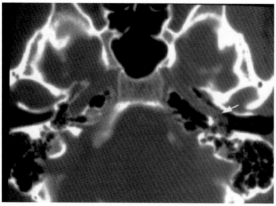 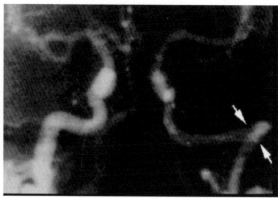

A   B

Figure 35–8 **(A)** Axial CT of a patient with left middle ear aberrant internal carotid artery (arrow). **(B)** Same patient, anteroposterior skull view of an aortic arch injection, reveals the aberrant course of the left internal carotid (arrows) as compared with the normal right internal carotid artery.

of the dural sinuses as well as deformities such as stenosis and hypoplasia can be detected with MRV.

Patients suspicious for arterial pathology (older, nonobese men with arterial type of PT or a head bruit) should be considered for a CT angiogram at the initial evaluation. Tortuous carotid vessels, AVF/AVM, carotid artery dissections/aneurysms, cervical/intracranial ACAD, and FMD can be diagnosed with this study. As mentioned previously, because CT angiography is a relatively new technique and significant experience is still lacking, cases with strong clinical suspicion of an AVF (presence of a bruit in the postauricular region) should be considered for carotid angiography if this study is normal.

Patients with isolated cervical carotid bruits should be considered for a carotid duplex ultrasound prior to CT angiography or MRA. If ACAD is confirmed, in most cases, no other imaging study is necessary.[95]

Patients with Retrotympanic Pathology

These patients should be considered for a CT angiography at the initial evaluation. For glomus tumors (jugulare/tympanicum), the presence of any synchronous carotid body tumor(s) can be easily detected in the same study. CT of the temporal bones is another alternative study. **Fig. 35–8A** shows an axial CT of a patient with left middle ear aberrant internal carotid artery, and **Fig. 35–8B** shows an angiogram of the same patient.

Carotid angiography is indicated only for prospective surgical cases to evaluate the collateral circulation of the brain (arterial and venous) in anticipation of possible vessel ligation or preoperative tumor embolization.[96] For cases with abnormalities of the jugular bulb (high jugular bulb, megabulb, diverticulum), associated deformities of the dural venous sinuses (hypoplasia or aplasia) can be detected in the same study. Cases of aberrant internal carotid artery need no further evaluation. **Fig. 35–9** depicts an algorithm for evaluating PT patients.

◆ Management

Management of patients with PT should be directed toward treating any underlying etiology. The following subsections describe management of the most common PT etiologies.

Idiopathic Intracranial Hypertension Syndrome

These patients often present to an otolaryngologist because of disturbing PT and should be evaluated and treated for any possible associated disorders. Because the majority of these patients are obese and many are even morbidly obese (100 pounds above ideal body weight), it is very important for them to understand the relation between their body weight and PT. Associated comorbidities such as obstructive sleep apnea, hypertension, diabetes mellitus, and gastroesophageal reflux are very common in these patients and should be detected and treated properly. Weight reduction is the most important aspect of management and can reduce or even eliminate PT in the majority of patients.

Administration of acetazolamide (Diamox), 250 mg three times a day, is thought to reduce CSF production and can be helpful in decreasing tinnitus intensity, although it rarely eliminates this symptom.[97]

Lumbar-peritoneal shunt should be considered for pseudotumor cerebri syndrome patients with progressive deterioration of vision, persistent headaches, and disabling PT.[1,5,46,97] In morbidly obese patients, however, this procedure is often complicated by occlusion of the shunt secondary to increased intraabdominal pressure.[98] Optic nerve sheath fenestration is helpful for progressive visual loss and headaches.[97,99]

Weight reduction surgery in morbidly obese patients is very effective in eliminating PT. Thirteen out of 16 patients who underwent this procedure experienced complete resolution of this symptom.[100] Resolution of symptoms has recently been reported following retrograde venography and stenting of the transverse sinus in IIH patients with associated stenosis/obstruction of this structure.[59,61,62]

Fig. 35–10 is the venous phase of a CT angiogram of a female patient with IIH syndrome. A right hypoplastic transverse sinus and a stenotic left transverse sinus are present. This patient might be a candidate for sinus stenting.

Vascular Lesions

Patients with ACAD and more than 60% percent obstruction benefit from carotid endarterectomy.[101] Angioplasty has been reported to relieve PT secondary to atherosclerotic obstruction of the subclavian and intracranial carotid

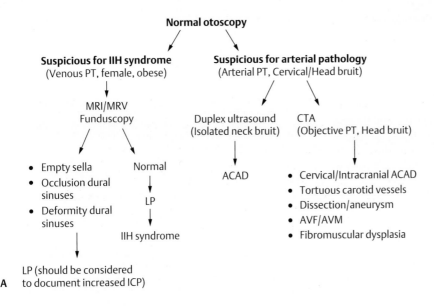

Normal otoscopy

Suspicious for IIH syndrome
(Venous PT, female, obese)

Suspicious for arterial pathology
(Arterial PT, Cervical/Head bruit)

MRI/MRV
Funduscopy

Duplex ultrasound
(Isolated neck bruit)

CTA
(Objective PT, Head bruit)

- Empty sella
- Occlusion dural sinuses
- Deformity dural sinuses

Normal

LP

ACAD

- Cervical/Intracranial ACAD
- Tortuous carotid vessels
- Dissection/aneurysm
- AVF/AVM
- Fibromuscular dysplasia

IIH syndrome

LP (should be considered
A   to document increased ICP)

Retrotympanic pathology

CTA

Glomus tumors (Tympanicum/jugulare
Jugular bulb/Dural venous sinuses abnormalities (Mega bulb, high location, diverticulum)
Aberrant internal carotid artery
B   Carotid body tumor

Figure 35–9   Pulsatile tinnitus evaluation with a **(A)** normal otoscopy and **(B)** retrotympanic pathology. MRI, magnetic resonance imaging; MRV, magnetic resonance venography; LP, lumbar puncture; IIH, idiopathic intracranial hypertension; ACAD, atherosclerotic carotid artery disease; CTA, computed tomography angiography; AVF, arteriovenous fistula; AVM, arteriovenous malformation; ICP, intracranial pressure.

arteries.[3,102] Glomus tympanicum tumors can be treated surgically with minimal complications.[103] Treatment options for glomus jugulare tumors include stereotactic radiosurgery and surgical excision.[104,105] A recently published meta-analysis study of these two modalities of treatment revealed that both are safe and efficacious. Morbidity and recurrences were infrequent in both groups; however, the incidence of late recurrences (after 10 to 20 years) in the radiosurgery group is unknown.[106]

Familiarity with drainage patterns, risk of aggressive symptoms, and recent technical advances is important in decision making for treating intracranial dural AVFs.[107] The majority of patients can be treated with selective embolization.[108,109] Stereotactic radiation therapy has also demonstrated good results in an increasing number of cases.[107]

Fibromuscular dysplasia of the internal carotid is a rare cause of cerebral ischemia, and the majority of patients show no progression. For asymptomatic lesions, a conservative approach is appropriate. Surgical dilatation and standard endarterectomy, although safe and efficient procedures, are seldom indicated.[20,81] Repair of symptomatic high-dehisced jugular bulb has been reported by using pieces of mastoid cortical bone and septal, conchal, tragal cartilage, and bone wax.[29,110–112]

Other Etiologies

Sectioning of the levator veli palatini muscle has been reported for treating palatal myoclonus.[71] Tensor tympani and stapedial myoclonus respond well to sectioning of the respective tendons via tympanotomy.[79,113,114] Botulinum toxin injections have been reported to be effective for palatal myoclonus.[115–117] Pulsatile tinnitus secondary to antihypertensive medications such as enalapril maleate or

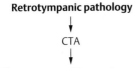

Figure 35–10   CT angio/venous phase of a female patient with IIH syndrome, with a right hypoplastic transverse sinus (short arrow) and a stenotic left transverse sinus (long arrow).

verapamil hydrochloride subsides after discontinuation of these agents.[5] PT secondary to otosclerosis may respond to stapedectomy.[5]

Ligation of the ipsilateral to the tinnitus IJV has been recommended in the literature for patients with idiopathic PT. The results of this procedure, however, have been very inconsistent and overall poor. In a series of 13 patients with essential tinnitus, three underwent ligation of the ipsilateral IJV and only one benefited permanently. The other two patients experienced return of their PT within a few days.[69] Therefore, there is rarely, if ever, an indication for this procedure solely for the purpose of alleviating PT.[118]

References

1. Sismanis A. Otologic manifestations of benign intracranial hypertension syndrome: diagnosis and management. Laryngoscope 1987;97(8 pt 2 suppl 42):1–17

2. Sismanis A, Stamm MA, Sobel M. Objective tinnitus in patients with atherosclerotic carotid artery disease. Am J Otol 1994;15:404–407

3. Donald JJ, Raphael MJ. Pulsatile tinnitus relieved by angioplasty. Clin Radiol 1991;43:132–134

4. Nishikawa M, Handa H, Hirai O, et al. Intolerable pulse-synchronous tinnitus caused by occlusion of the contralateral common carotid artery. A successful treatment by aorto-carotid bypass surgery. Acta Neurochir (Wien) 1989;101:80–83

5. Sismanis A, Smoker WR. Pulsatile tinnitus: recent advances in diagnosis. Laryngoscope 1994;104(6 pt 1):681–688

6. Tokyol C, Yilmaz MD. Middle ear hemangioma: a case report. Am J Otolaryngol 2003;24:405–407

7. Zenke K, Sasaki U, Ohta M, et al. [A case of angiomatous meningioma near the geniculate ganglion] No Shinkei Geka 1991;19:755–759

8. Vasama JP, Pitkaranta A, Piilonen A. Pulsatile audible tinnitus and metastatic breast carcinoma of the temporal bone. ORL J Otorhinolaryngol Relat Spec 2001;63:56–57

9. Carmody RF. Vascular malformations. In: Zimmerman RA, Gibby WA, Carmody RF, ed. Neuroimaging Clinical and Physical Principles. New York: Springer-Verlag, 2000:833–862

10. Hoang TA, Hasso AN. Intracranial vascular malformations. Neuroimaging Clin N Am 1994;4:823–847

11. Pelkonen O, Tikkakoski T, Luotonen J, Sotaniemi K. Pulsatile tinnitus as a symptom of cervicocephalic arterial dissection. J Laryngol Otol 2004;118:193–198

12. Medina DM, Stroke. In: Zimmerman RA, Gibby WA, Carmody RF, ed. Neuroimaging Clinical and Physical Principles. New York: Springer-Verlag, 2000:833–863

13. Schievink WI, Bjornsson J, Piepgras DG. Coexistence of fibromuscular dysplasia and cystic medial necrosis in a patient with Marfan's syndrome and bilateral carotid artery dissections. Stroke 1994; 25:2492–2496

14. Depauw P, Defreyne L, Dewaele F, Caemaert J. Endovascular treatment of a giant petrous internal carotid artery aneurysm. Case report and review of the literature. Minim Invasive Neurosurg 2003;46:250–253

15. Reece PH, Higgins N, Hardy DG, Moffat DA. An aneurysm of the petrous internal carotid artery. J Laryngol Otol 1999;113:55–57

16. McGrail KM, Heros RC, Debrun G, Beyerl BD. Aneurysm of the ICA petrous segment treated by balloon entrapment after EC-IC bypass. Case report. J Neurosurg 1986;65:249–252

17. Austin JR, Maceri DR. Anterior communicating artery aneurysm presenting as pulsatile tinnitus. ORL J Otorhinolaryngol Relat Spec 1993; 55:54–57

18. Slovut DP, Olin JW. Fibromuscular dysplasia. N Engl J Med 2004;350:1862–1871

19. Dufour JJ, Lavigne F, Plante R, Caouette H. Pulsatile tinnitus and fibromuscular dysplasia of the internal carotid. J Otolaryngol 1985;14:293–295

20. Van Damme H, Sakalihasan N, Limet R. Fibromuscular dysplasia of the internal carotid artery. Personal experience with 13 cases and literature review. Acta Chir Belg 1999;99:163–168

21. Cloft HJ, Kallmes DF, Kallmes MH, Goldstein JH, Jensen ME, Dion JE. Prevalence of cerebral aneurysms in patients with fibromuscular dysplasia: a reassessment. J Neurosurg 1998;88:436–440

22. Bold EL, Wanamaker HH, Hughes GB, et al. Magnetic resonance angiography of vascular anomalies of the middle ear. Laryngoscope 1994;104(11 pt 1):1404–1411

23. Campbell JB, Simons RM. Brachiocephalic artery stenosis presenting with objective tinnitus. J Laryngol Otol 1987;101:718–720

24. Cary FH. Symptomatic venous hum. Report of a case. N Engl J Med 1961;264:869–870

25. Cochran JH Jr, Kosmicki PW. Tinnitus as a presenting symptom in pernicious anemia. Ann Otol Rhinol Laryngol 1979;88(2 pt 1):297

26. Davies DG. Paget's disease of the temporal bone. A clinical and histopathological survey. Acta Otolaryngol 1968;Suppl 242:3

27. Fernandez AO. Objective tinnitus: a case report. Am J Otol 1983;4:312–314

28. Gibson R. Tinnitus in Paget's disease with external carotid ligation. J Laryngol Otol 1973;87:299–301

29. Glasscock ME III, Dickins JR, Jackson CG, Wiet RJ. Vascular anomalies of the middle ear. Laryngoscope 1980;90:77–88

30. Gulya AJ, Shuknecht HF. A large artery in the apical region of the cochlea of a man with pulsatile tinnitus. Am J Otol 1984;5:262

31. Lesinski SG, Chambers AA, Komray R, Keiser M, Khodadad G. Why not the eighth nerve? Neurovascular compression–probable cause for pulsatile tinnitus. Otolaryngol Head Neck Surg 1979;87:89–94

32. Leveque H, Bialostozky F, Blanchard CL, Suter CM. Tympanometry in the evaluation of vascular lesions of the middle ear and tinnitus of vascular origin. Laryngoscope 1979;89:1197–1218

33. Levine SB, Snow JB Jr. Pulsatile tinnitus. Laryngoscope 1987;97:401–406

34. Saeed SR, Hinton AE, Ramsden RT, Lye RH. Spontaneous dissection of the intrapetrous internal carotid artery. J Laryngol Otol 1990;104:491–493

35. Steffen TN. Vascular anomalies of the middle ear. Laryngoscope 1968;78:171–197

36. Remley KB, Coit WE, Harnsberger HR, Smoker WR, Jacobs JM, McIff EB. Pulsatile tinnitus and the vascular tympanic membrane: CT, MR, and angiographic findings. Radiology 1990;174:383–389

37. Sorensen PS, Krogsaa B, Gjerris F. Clinical course and prognosis of pseudotumor cerebri. A prospective study of 24 patients. Acta Neurol Scand 1988;77:164–172

38. Fishman RA. Benign intracranial hypertension. In: Fishman RA, ed. Cerebrospinal Fluid in Disease of the Nervous System. Philadelphia: WB Saunders, 1980:128–139

39. Malm J, Kristensen B, Markgren P, Ekstedt J. CSF hydrodynamics in idiopathic intracranial hypertension: a long-term study. Neurology 1992;42:851–858

40. Henry M, Driscoll MC, Miller M, Chang T, Minniti CP. Pseudotumor cerebri in children with sickle cell disease: a case series. Pediatrics 2004;113(3 pt 1):e265–e269

41. Oswald J, Meier K, Reinhart WH, Kuhn M. Pseudotumor cerebri in minocyline treatment. Schweiz Rundsch Med Prax 2001;90:1691–1693

42. Uddin AB. Drug-induced pseudotumor cerebri. Clin Neuropharmacol 2003;26:236–238

43. Friedman DI. Pseudotumor cerebri. Neurosurg Clin North Am 1999;10:609–621, viii.

44. Galvin JA, Van Stavern GP. Clinical characterization of idiopathic intracranial hypertension at the Detroit Medical Center. J Neurol Sci 2004;223:157–160

45. Sismanis A, Hughes GB, Abedi E, Williams GH, Isrow LA. Otologic symptoms and findings of the pseudotumor cerebri syndrome: a preliminary report. Otolaryngol Head Neck Surg 1985;93:398–402

46. Sismanis A, Butts FM, Hughes GB. Objective tinnitus in benign intracranial hypertension: an update. Laryngoscope 1990;100:33–36

47. Weisberg LA. Benign intracranial hypertension. Medicine (Baltimore) 1975;54:197–207

48. Spence JD, Amacher AL, Willis NR. Benign intracranial hypertension without papilledema: role of 24-hour cerebrospinal fluid pressure monitoring in diagnosis and management. Neurosurgery 1980;7:326–336

49. Marcelis J, Silberstein SD. Idiopathic intracranial hypertension without papilledema. Arch Neurol 1991;48:392–399

50. Lipton HL, Michelson PE. Pseudotumor cerebri syndrome without papilledema. JAMA 1972;220:1591–1592

51. Karahalios DG, Rekate HL, Khayata MH, Apostolides PJ. Elevated intracranial venous pressure as a universal mechanism in pseudotumor cerebri of varying etiologies. Neurology 1996;46:198–202

52. King JO, Mitchell PJ, Thomson KR, Tress BM. Cerebral venography and manometry in idiopathic intracranial hypertension. Neurology 1995;45:2224–2228

53. Sugerman HJ, DeMaria EJ, Felton WL III, Nakatsuka M, Sismanis A. Increased intra-abdominal pressure and cardiac filling pressures

in obesity-associated pseudotumor cerebri. Neurology 1997;49:507–511

54. Josephs LG, Este-McDonald JR, Birkett DH, Hirsch EF. Diagnostic laparoscopy increases intracranial pressure. J Trauma 1994;36:815–818

55. Gross CE, Tranmer BI, Adey G, Kohut J. Increased cerebral blood flow in idiopathic pseudotumour cerebri. Neurol Res 1990;12:226–230

56. Langfitt TW. Clinical methods for monitoring intracranial pressure and measuring cerebral blood flow. Clin Neurosurg 1975;22:302–320

57. Sismanis A, Callari RH, Slomka WS, Butts FM. Auditory-evoked responses in benign intracranial hypertension syndrome. Laryngoscope 1990;100:1152–1155

58. Biousse V, Ameri A, Bousser MG. Isolated intracranial hypertension as the only sign of cerebral venous thrombosis. Neurology 1999;53:1537–1542

59. Ogungbo B, Roy D, Gholkar A, Mendelow AD. Endovascular stenting of the transverse sinus in a patient presenting with benign intracranial hypertension. Br J Neurosurg 2003;17:565–568

60. Farb RI, Vanek I, Scott JN, et al. Idiopathic intracranial hypertension: the prevalence and morphology of sinovenous stenosis. Neurology 2003;60:1418–1424

61. Higgins JN, Cousins C, Owler BK, Sarkies N, Pickard JD. Idiopathic intracranial hypertension: 12 cases treated by venous sinus stenting. J Neurol Neurosurg Psychiatry 2003;74:1662–1666

62. Owler BK, Parker G, Halmagyi GM, et al. Pseudotumor cerebri syndrome: venous sinus obstruction and its treatment with stent placement. J Neurosurg 2003;98:1045–1055

63. Buckwalter JA, Sasaki CT, Virapongse C, Kier EL, Bauman N. Pulsatile tinnitus arising from jugular megabulb deformity: a treatment rationale. Laryngoscope 1983;93:1534–1539

64. Overton SB, Ritter FN. A high placed jugular bulb in the middle ear: a clinical and temporal bone study. Laryngoscope 1973;83:1986–1991

65. Robin PE. A case of upwardly situated jugular bulb in left middle ear. J Laryngol Otol 1972;86:1241–1246

66. Smythe GO. A case of protruding jugular bulb. Laryngoscope 1975;75:669–672

67. Chandler JR. Diagnosis and cure of venous hum tinnitus. Laryngoscope 1983;93:892–895

68. Engstrom H, Graf W. On objective tinnitus and its recording. Acta Otolaryngol Suppl 1950;95:127–137

69. Hentzer E. Objective tinnitus of the vascular type. A follow-up study. Acta Otolaryngol 1968;66:273–281

70. Wiggs WJ Jr, Sismanis A, Laine FJ. Pulsatile tinnitus associated with congenital central nervous system malformations. Am J Otol 1996;17:241–244

71. Ward PH, Babin R, Calcaterra TC, Konrad HR. Operative treatment of surgical lesions with objective tinnitus. Ann Otol Rhinol Laryngol 1975;84 (4 pt 1):473–482

72. Lambert PR, Cantrell RW. Objective tinnitus in association with an abnormal posterior condylar emissary vein. Am J Otol 1986;7:204–207

73. Forte V, Turner A, Liu P. Objective tinnitus associated with abnormal mastoid emissary vein. J Otolaryngol 1989;18:232–235

74. Bjork H. Objective tinnitus due to clonus of the soft palate. Acta Otolaryngol Suppl 1954;116:39–45

75. Crandall PH, Fang HC, Herrmann C Jr. Palatal myoclonus; a new approach to the understanding of its production. Neurology 1957;7:37–51

76. Heller MF. Vibratory tinnitus and palatal myoclonus. Acta Otolaryngol 1962;55:292–298

77. Nishigaya K, Kaneko M, Nagaseki Y, Nukui H. Palatal myoclonus induced by extirpation of a cerebellar astrocytoma. Case report. J Neurosurg 1998;88:1107–1110

78. Pulec JL, Hodell SF, Anthony PF. Tinnitus: diagnosis and treatment. Ann Otol Rhinol Laryngol 1978;87(6 pt 1):821–833

79. Golz A, Fradis M, Netzer A, Ridder GJ, Westerman ST, Joachims HZ. Bilateral tinnitus due to middle-ear myoclonus. Int Tinnitus J 2003;9:52–55

80. Bento RF, Sanchez TG, Miniti A, Tedesco-Marchesi AJ. Continuous, high-frequency objective tinnitus caused by middle ear myoclonus. Ear Nose Throat J 1998;77:814–818

81. Wells RP, Smith RR. Fibromuscular dysplasia of the internal carotid artery: a long term follow-up. Neurosurgery 1982;10:39–43

82. Sila CA, Furlan AJ, Little JR. Pulsatile tinnitus. Stroke 1987;18:252–256

83. Sismanis A, Williams GH, King MD. A new electronic device for evaluation of objective tinnitus. Otolaryngol Head Neck Surg 1989;100:644–645

84. Sismanis A, Butts FM. A practical device for detection and recording of objective tinnitus. Otolaryngol Head Neck Surg 1994;110:459–462

85. Lipton HL, Michelson PE. Pseudotumor cerebri syndrome without papilledema. JAMA 1972;220:1591–1592

86. Marcelis J, Silberstein SD. Idiopathic intracranial hypertension without papilledema. Arch Neurol 1991;48:392–399

87. Spence JD, Amacher AL, Willis NR. Benign intracranial hypertension without papilledema: role of 24-hour cerebrospinal fluid pressure monitoring in diagnosis and management. Neurosurgery 1980;7:326–336

88. Wall M, George D. Idiopathic intracranial hypertension. A prospective study of 50 patients. Brain 1991;114(pt 1A):155–180

89. Sismanis A, Stamm MA, Sobel M. Objective tinnitus in patients with atherosclerotic carotid artery disease. Am J Otol 1994;15:404–407

90. De Monti M, Ghilardi G, Caverni L, et al. Multidetector helical angio CT oblique reconstructions orthogonal to internal carotid artery for preoperative evaluation of stenosis. A prospective study of comparison with color Doppler US, digital subtraction angiography and intraoperative data. Minerva Cardioangiol 2003;51:373–385

91. Jayaraman MV, Mayo-Smith WW. Multi-detector CT angiography of the intra-cranial circulation: normal anatomy and pathology with angiographic correlation. Clin Radiol 2004;59:690–698

92. Sanelli PC, Mifsud MJ, Stieg PE. Role of CT angiography in guiding management decisions of newly diagnosed and residual arteriovenous malformations. AJR Am J Roentgenol 2004;183:1123–1126

93. Karamessini MT, Kagadis GC, Petsas T, et al. CT angiography with three-dimensional techniques for the early diagnosis of intracranial aneurysms. Comparison with intra-arterial DSA and the surgical findings. Eur J Radiol 2004;49:212–223

94. Brodsky MC, Vaphiades M. Magnetic resonance imaging in pseudotumor cerebri. Ophthalmology 1998;105:1686–1693

95. Buskens E, Nederkoorn PJ, Buijs-Van Der Woude T, et al. Imaging of carotid arteries in symptomatic patients: cost-effectiveness of diagnostic strategies. Radiology 2004;233:101–112

96. Remley KB, Coit WE, Harnsberger HR, Smoker WR, Jacobs JM, McIff EB. Pulsatile tinnitus and the vascular tympanic membrane: CT, MR, and angiographic findings. Radiology 1990;174:383–389

97. Kesler A, Gadoth N. [Pseudotumor cerebri (PTC–an update).] Harefuah 2002;141:297–300, 312

98. Sugerman HJ, Felton WL III, Salvant JB Jr, Sismanis A, Kellum JM. Effects of surgically induced weight loss on idiopathic intracranial hypertension in morbid obesity. Neurology 1995;45:1655–1659

99. Corbett JJ, Nerad JA, Tse DT, Anderson RL. Results of optic nerve sheath fenestration for pseudotumor cerebri. The lateral orbitotomy approach. Arch Ophthalmol 1988;106:1391–1397

100. Michaelides EM, Sismanis A, Sugerman HJ, Felton WL III. Pulsatile tinnitus in patients with morbid obesity: the effectiveness of weight reduction surgery. Am J Otol 2000;21:682–685

101. Endarterectomy for asymptomatic carotid artery stenosis. Executive Committee for the Asymptomatic Carotid Atherosclerosis Study. JAMA 1995;273:1421–1428

102. Emery DJ, Ferguson RD, Williams JS. Pulsatile tinnitus cured by angioplasty and stenting of petrous carotid artery stenosis. Arch Otolaryngol Head Neck Surg 1998;124:460–461

103. Rohit, Jain Y, Caruso A, Russo A, Sanna M. Glomus tympanicum tumour: an alternative surgical technique. J Laryngol Otol 2003;117:462–466

104. Pollock BE. Stereotactic radiosurgery in patients with glomus jugulare tumors. Neurosurg Focus 2004;17:E10

105. Jackson CG, McGrew BM, Forest JA, Netterville JL, Hampf CF, Glasscock ME III. Lateral skull base surgery for glomus tumors: long-term control. Otol Neurotol 2001;22:377–382

106. Gottfried ON, Liu JK, Couldwell WT. Comparison of radiosurgery and conventional surgery for the treatment of glomus jugulare tumors. Neurosurg Focus 2004;17:E4

107. Kiyosue H, Hori Y, Okahara M, et al. Treatment of intracranial dural arteriovenous fistulas: current strategies based on location and hemodynamics, and alternative techniques of transcatheter embolization. Radiographics 2004;24:1637–1653

108. Urtasun F, Biondi A, Casaco A, et al. Cerebral dural arteriovenous fistulas: percutaneous transvenous embolization. Radiology 1996;199:209–217

109. Viruela F. Update of intravascular functional evaluation and therapy of intracranial arteriovenous malformations. In: Viruela F, Dion J, Duckwiler G, eds. Neuroimaging Clinics of North America. Philadelphia: WB Saunders, 1992:279–289

110. Presutti L, Laudadio P. Jugular bulb diverticula. ORL J Otorhinolaryngol Relat Spec 1991;53:57–60

111. Rouillard R, Leclerc J, Savary P. Pulsatile tinnitus: a dehiscent jugular vein. Laryngoscope 1985;95:188–189

112. Couloigner V, Grayeli AB, Bouccara D, Julien N, Sterkers O. Surgical treatment of the high jugular bulb in patients with Meniere's disease and pulsatile tinnitus. Eur Arch Otorhinolaryngol 1999;256:224–229

113. Golz A, Fradis M, Martzu D, Netzer A, Joachims HZ. Stapedius muscle myoclonus. Ann Otol Rhinol Laryngol 2003;112:522–524

114. Zipfel TE, Kaza SR, Greene JS. Middle-ear myoclonus. J Laryngol Otol 2000;114:207–209

115. Bryce GE, Morrison MD. Botulinum toxin treatment of essential palatal myoclonus tinnitus. J Otolaryngol 1998;27:213–216

116. Jero J, Salmi T. Palatal myoclonus and clicking tinnitus in a 12-year-old girl–case report. Acta Otolaryngol Suppl 2000;543:61–62

117. Srirompotong S, Tiamkao S, Jitpimolmard S. Botulinum toxin injection for objective tinnitus from palatal myoclonus: a case report. J Med Assoc Thai 2002;85:392–395

118. Jackler RK, Brackmann DE, Sismanis A. A warning on venous ligation for pulsatile tinnitus. Otol Neurotol 2001;22:427–428

◆ Editor's (G.B.H.) Note

What a privilege it has been to know Aristides Sismanis, MD, professionally and socially since we were Fellows together at Baptist Hospital, Nashville, Tennessee, with Michael E. Glasscock III, MD, in 1979–1980. By the mid 1980s, Ari had distinguished himself worldwide as the most knowledgeable clinician on pulsatile tinnitus, and more recently as the distinguished G. Douglas Hayden Professor and Chairman of the Virginia Commonwealth University Medical Center Department of Otolaryngology–Head and Neck Surgery. Over the last 27 years, Ari has unselfishly and frequently included me as co-author in many publications. His friendship means a lot to me.

36

Theory and Treatment of Tinnitus and Decreased Sound Tolerance

Pawel J. Jastreboff and Margaret M. Jastreboff

Tinnitus and decreased sound tolerance are challenging topics in the practice of otolaryngology and audiology, as there is no established standard on how to evaluate and treat these conditions. There is ongoing research aimed at investigation of mechanisms underlying these phenomena and at evaluation of emerging treatments. Substantial progress has been achieved during the last decade in understanding tinnitus, and tinnitus and decreased sound tolerance are treated in an effective manner in an increasing number of centers. This chapter provides an overview of the current status of the field.

◆ Definitions and Epidemiology

Tinnitus, commonly described as a ringing in the ears, can actually be perceived as a wide variety of sounds (e.g., ringing, buzzing, crickets, hissing). It is a phantom auditory perception,[1] that is, while the perception is absolutely real, there is no sound or vibratory activity within the cochlea corresponding to the perception.[2,3] The perception of tinnitus results from the presence of tinnitus-related neuronal activity within the auditory pathways. The prevalence of tinnitus is high. About 10 to 20% of people in the general population can perceive it any time that they focus attention on it,[4,5] but interestingly only about 4 to 8% of the general population is bothered by tinnitus to some extent.[6,7] It is difficult to determine the prevalence of clinically significant tinnitus (i.e., tinnitus that affects people to the extent that they need professional help) because many sufferers with troubling tinnitus cease to believe that something can be done to help them and consequently they no longer seek help. Clinical observations indicate that probably at least 1% of the general population suffers from clinically significant tinnitus and 0.5% are profoundly affected by it.[2]

Tinnitus has been linked to several medical problems such as conductive hearing loss (e.g., resulting from otitis media, cerumen impaction, ossicular stiffness/discontinuity, otosclerosis); sensory or neural hearing loss (e.g., related to Meniere's disease, presbycusis, vestibular schwannoma, sudden hearing loss); hormonal changes (e.g., pregnancy, menopause, thyroid dysfunction); and administration of some medications or withdrawal from them.[8,9] Basically, a decrease of the auditory input to higher auditory centers due to any reasons (e.g., medical problem, hearing overprotection, work, or lifestyle) may induce tinnitus.[2] The classic experiment of Heller and Bergman[10] showed that perception of tinnitus was evoked in 94% of normally hearing people without tinnitus who spent a few minutes in an environment with very low sound level. Recent data confirmed the presence of this phenomenon.[11]

The prevalence of bothersome tinnitus is associated with the extent of hearing loss and increases with aging until age 65, when it stabilizes, and then decreases after age of 74.[7] However, when hearing loss is taken into account, the prevalence of tinnitus decreases with age for any given level of hearing loss.[7] Children experience and have problems with tinnitus to a larger extent than was previously assumed.[12–14] They typically do not complain about tinnitus, considering it a natural experience. When they are bothered by tinnitus, they have the same problems as adults. Unrecognized tinnitus may yield incorrect diagnosis of behavioral or learning problems.

In a psychoacoustic evaluation of tinnitus, its pitch-and-loudness match turned out not to be associated with its severity. Except for low pitch or a roaring tinnitus observed in attacks of Meniere's disease, these assessment measures are not helpful for diagnosis or treatment planning. A minimal masking level (i.e., a minimal level of white noise that blocks the perception of tinnitus) might provide some indication of how easy it would be to mask tinnitus, when masking therapy is considered.[15] On the other hand, the results reported by Penner and Bilger[16] showed that to sustain masking of tinnitus for a more than a minute, it might be necessary to increase the sound level substantially (even by 40 to 50 dB over a 30-minute period). This observation demonstrates that a minimal masking level can be used only as an indicator of the effectiveness of masking therapy.

Residual inhibition, that is, a decrease of tinnitus loudness after exposure to intensive sound[17] (recommended as 10 dB above minimal masking level) is another measure promoted as a part of tinnitus evaluation.[18] Although there was considerable expectation, this measure never became useful clinically because residual inhibition, if present, typically lasts only seconds or a minute.[2] Moreover, typically an increase of tinnitus loudness is observed as a result of exposure to loud sound.

Strong somatosensory input to the auditory system has been clearly documented recently.[19,20] It turned out that the input is both excitatory and inhibitory and that it exists at various levels of the auditory system, including the cochlear nuclei complex. This finding might explain why the majority of patients can modulate their tinnitus by manipulating the head/neck area and why it is possible to induce tinnitus by body manipulation in approximately 30% of subjects without prior tinnitus.[21] It has been proposed that in some cases the somatosensory system might be responsible for tinnitus.[22] So far this hypothesis has not yielded a clinically significant treatment, but the modulation of tinnitus with this manipulation has been used for research purposes.[23–25]

In the past, *somatosounds*, that is, perception of the sound generated by the body, such as sound of blood flow, palatal myoclonus, or spontaneous otoacoustic emissions, were labeled as objective tinnitus and differentiated from subjective tinnitus, for which there was no detectable external sound. This categorization has the intrinsic problem of being dependent not on the mechanisms of tinnitus generation but on the technical ability to detect potential real sound, and it is gradually disappearing from the literature in the context of tinnitus. As it is typically difficult to diagnose somatosounds, their prevalence can be only estimated to be in the range of a few percent of all cases. The most common somatosounds are related to the heart beat, as they reflect changes in the speed of blood flow (e.g., great vessel bruits) or fluctuation of blood or cerebrospinal fluid (CSF) pressure. These sounds are typically perceived as pulsation (thus the name *pulsatile tinnitus*). Note that pulsation of loudness of tinnitus does not automatically indicate somatosounds. For example, the tinnitus source—which can be, for example, dependent on functional properties of the outer hair cell (OHC) system[2]—might be affected by CSF pressure, resulting in a fluctuation of tinnitus loudness, still without having any real acoustic signal. There are also nonpulsatile somatosounds, associated for example, with tensor tympani myoclonus, tensor veli palatini myoclonus, eustachian tube dysfunction,[8,26,27] perception of spontaneous oto-acoustic emissions (SOAEs),[28] or temporomandibular joint disorder.[8] Perception of SOAEs is rare, but it is present in a small proportion of patients (typically young women with normal hearing).[29,30] It can be eliminated by administration of aspirin,[31] which attenuates active properties of OHCs.[32,33] Furthermore, hearing loss or aging eliminates SOAEs due to accumulated OHC damage.

Auditory imagery (i.e., perception of distorted speech or music, sometimes labeled as *musical hallucinations*) is an interesting case of central tinnitus.[34] Although this phenomenon is not related to psychiatric problems,[35–38] it is sometimes confused with landmark hallucinations occurring in schizophrenia. It typically affects elderly women with hearing loss.

Tinnitus frequently is accompanied by decreased tolerance to sounds that would not evoke a similar reaction in the average listener.[8,39,40] *Decreased sound tolerance* should be taken into consideration when applying a treatment for tinnitus, as it contributes to enhancement of the tinnitus signal and has an impact on the implementation of sound therapy.[2,41] It has been proposed that two components of decreased sound tolerance should be distinguished: (1) hyperacusis and (2) misophonia.[8,39] In *hyperacusis*, sound-induced neural activity is overamplified within the auditory system, resulting in an abnormally strong reaction to sound occurring within the auditory pathways, and only secondarily affecting the limbic and autonomic nervous systems.[8] This overamplification might occur inside of the cochlea, for example by too high a level of mechanical amplification being provided by OHCs, or by an abnormally high level of sound-evoked neurotransmitters released from inner hair cells (IHCs). Clinical observations suggest that central mechanisms are more prevalent and hyperacusis might result from an increased sensitivity of neurons in the auditory pathways.[39,42–44] The negative reactions to sound and their strength in hyperacusis depend strictly on the physical characterization of the sound, and reactions are independent of the context in which sound is presented.

Epidemiologic data on hyperacusis in the general population are limited. Nevertheless, a questionnaire study of 10,349 randomly selected people found that 15.3% reported decreased sound tolerance.[45] A random sample of 3049 subjects in Germany found that 1.72% reported hyperacusis.[46] Hyperacusis requiring treatment has been reported to accompany tinnitus in approximately 25 to 44%,[40,46,47] and tinnitus was reported to be present in 86% of hyperacusis cases.[48] On the basis of these numbers, it is possible to estimate that at least 1.5% of the general population has hyperacusis requiring treatment.

Hyperacusis has been linked to a number of medical problems, such as Bell's palsy, Lyme disease, Williams syndrome, Ramsay Hunt syndrome, stapedectomy, perilymphatic fistula, head injury, migraine, depression, withdrawal from benzodiazepines, increased CSF pressure, and Addison's disease[48,76–88] Treatments of these medical problems may help with hyperacusis; for example, treating Lyme disease or implementing gradual withdrawal from benzodiazepines can be effective.[2,49]

Misophonia, the dislike of sound, is the second component of decreased sound tolerance and reflects conditioned negative reactions to sound.[8,39] It is a relatively new concept that originated from our observation that many patients were avoiding and disliking sounds, while not necessarily being afraid of them. A variety of negative emotions are involved in misophonia. Phonophobia is considered to be a specific case of misophonia when fear is the dominant emotion.

Considering the mechanisms involved, misophonia can be defined as abnormally strong reactions of the autonomic and limbic systems resulting from enhanced connections between the auditory and limbic systems. These connections encompass both a high cortical level loop with involvement of cognition, as well as subconscious connections, most probably involving the link between the medial geniculate body and amygdala.[50–52] The functions of these connections are governed by the principles of conditioned reflexes. Note that in case of pure misophonia the auditory system is not overactivated and it acts within normal limits.

With misophonia, the strength of a patient's reaction depends to a large extent on the context in which sound appears, and is only partially linked to the physical characteristics of the sound. A patient's previous evaluation, experience with a particular sound, and beliefs linked to it (e.g., a belief that the sound is a potential threat or can be harmful) are very important. One's psychological profile also plays a role in the response to sound.

Misophonia is practically always evoked by significant hyperacusis, but can be present independently as well. Approximately 60% of our patients exhibit misophonia requiring specific treatment.[40] *Note that decreased sound tolerance and its components are related neither to hearing loss nor to recruitment.*[2,39]

◆ Models and Mechanisms

There are a variety of models of tinnitus. The commonly accepted notion that tinnitus is a problem only when it is perceived encouraged a search for mechanisms and development of models of tinnitus generators and strongly focused on the auditory system, particularly the cochlea.[53–59] Within this approach there is lately a shift from focusing on peripheral mechanisms toward mechanisms involving processing information within the central auditory pathways.[60,61] Emphasis is placed on the perception of tinnitus, removing this perception, and achieving silence as an ultimate cure for tinnitus. Attention is focused on potential mechanisms responsible for generating the tinnitus signal, and consequently treatments of tinnitus aim at removing these specific generators.

Various classifications of tinnitus have been introduced. Division of tinnitus into objective and subjective gradually disappear, and objective tinnitus became commonly labeled as a somatosound, whereas the term *tinnitus* is reserved for subjective auditory phantom perception.[2] Another classification was based on anatomy, specifically peripheral versus central auditory pathways. Furosemide, a diuretic acting presumably on the cochlea, was proposed as a test method to determine if tinnitus is peripheral or central. The hypothesis was that if tinnitus improves after furosemide administration, it is peripheral; if it doesn't, it is central.[62]

Another classification assumed specific mechanisms of tinnitus generation. In this respect several mechanisms responsible for the emergence of tinnitus-related neuronal activity have been proposed: (1) abnormal coupling between neurons causing synchronization of neuronal discharges[57]; (2) local decrease of spontaneous activity enhanced by the lateral inhibition[63,64]; (3) unbalanced activation of type I and type II auditory nerve fibers[53]; (4) abnormal neurotransmitter release from IHCs[65]; (5) decreased activity of the efferent system[66]; (6) mechanical displacement within the organ of Corti[67]; (7) abnormalities in transduction processes[65]; (8) abnormal calcium homeostasis[68]; (9) physical or biochemical factors affecting the auditory nerve[57]; (10) enhanced sensitivity of the auditory pathways after decreased auditory input[1]; and (11) discordant damage or dysfunction of OHCs and IHCs.[1,2,2,3] Most of these hypotheses provided an indication of how to treat tinnitus, and some of these methods have been applied in clinical practice, for example, microvascular decompression,[69,70] calcium channel blockers,[71] or infusions of drugs affecting transduction function within the cochlea.[72,73]

Although there is a consensus that a neuronal activity is responsible for tinnitus, there is still no agreement on the type of neuronal activity related to tinnitus. An increase of spontaneous neuronal activity within the nervous system seems to be a dominant theory.[74–76] Synchronization of the activity between neurons as the basis for tinnitus has been suggested as well[77]; however, subsequent research failed to validate this hypothesis.[78,79] Finally, modification in temporal patterns of discharges, including bursting, an epileptic-type of activity, has been proposed,[74] and preliminary data support this hypothesis.[2,74,80,81]

Psychological models of tinnitus represent the other approach. Commonly it is postulated that patients have problems with tinnitus because they have some psychological or psychiatric problem.[82] The auditory system is ignored or its role downplayed and coexistence of hyperacusis with tinnitus is neglected. The brain is typically approached as "A black box" (i.e., a device or theoretical construct with known or specified performance characteristics but unknown or unspecified constituents and means of operation"[83]), and psychological models tend to be oriented toward empirical observation of behavioral reactions, with less attention paid to specific physiological mechanism underlying tinnitus. Treatments based on these models typically focus on improving coping with tinnitus[84,85] and they can provide help in some cases as they are effective in changing the patient's thinking about tinnitus and reversing the consequences of negative counseling. Cognitive-behavioral therapy seems to be the most effective in this category of treatments.[86]

The neurophysiological model of tinnitus, described first in 1990,[1] combines auditory and other systems in the brain that are involved in the perception of, and reactions to, tinnitus, and considers the issue of decreased sound tolerance.[2,3,8,39,41,52,87] This model challenges the common belief that to evoke a reaction to tinnitus it is necessary to perceive it. Although it is obvious that the perception of tinnitus can induce negative reactions, it is possible to develop reactions to tinnitus-related neuronal activity *without* tinnitus perception, just as it is possible to learn to create conditioned reflexes, and to have reactions to stimuli that are not consciously perceived.[88–91] Therefore, reactions to tinnitus can be evoked via conscious and subconscious pathways.[2,41]

Tinnitus-related neuronal activity, referred to later as the *tinnitus signal*, is basically the same in people who only experience tinnitus and those who actually suffer because of it. In the majority of cases, this neuronal activity is a side effect of the attempt of the auditory system to compensate for a dysfunction within the auditory periphery. In people with clinically significant tinnitus, however, this neuronal activity inappropriately activates the limbic and sympathetic part of the autonomic nervous system (**Fig. 36–1**),[1,2,41] resulting in a series of behavioral responses and consequences, such as problems with attention, decreased ability to enjoy one's activities, interference with work, problems with sleep, impaired social interactions (including interactions with family), anxiety, depression, increase of one's general stress level, and panic. It is possible to identify the particular systems in the brain and the specific physiological mechanisms responsible for each of these responses.

The auditory system has direct subcortical and subconscious connections from the medial geniculate body to the lateral nucleus of the amygdala,[50,51] a part of the limbic system, which controls emotional expression, memory storage and recall, motivation and mood, seizure activity, and exerts an important influence on the endocrine and autonomic motor systems.[92]

The limbic system is directly connected with the autonomic nervous system, which consists of two mutually antagonistic parts: the parasympathetic, which prepares the organism for feeding, digestion, rest, and relaxation,[93] and the sympathetic, which has the opposite effect, preparing the body for action (e.g., inhibiting the digestive system, stimulating the heart, dilating the bronchi, contracting the arteries) and, in the extreme, the "fight or flight" reaction. Overactivation of the sympathetic part leads to behavioral reactions that match those reported by patients with clinically significant tinnitus: anxiety, problems with sleep, problems with concentration, panic attacks, and decreased ability to enjoy life activities. It is known that various stimuli can cause overactivation of the limbic and autonomic nervous systems, such as high stress levels, significant problems at work or at home, chronic pain, or the effects of even weak sensory stimuli over which we do not have control. Note that reactions depend on what is being activated (e.g., sympathetic versus parasympathetic nervous system) and are not specific to a type of sensory stimulus (e.g., sound or light).[94] For example, anxiety can be induced by hearing a voice of an enemy or by seeing a gun pointed at us, and relaxation can be induced by hearing a voice of a friend or seeing smiling people around us. A variety of signals (e.g., tinnitus, work environment) could evoke the same reactions.

Exactly the same stimulus can induce diametrically opposite reactions depending on past experience shaping present associations. The same principle applies to tinnitus: if there are not negative associations linked to the perception of tinnitus, then conditioned reflexes linking the auditory with the limbic and autonomic nervous systems do not develop, and the tinnitus signal does not evoke any behavioral reactions. However, *when negative associations develop as a result of a general fear of the unknown, low tolerance to a lack of control over one's environment, or negative counseling, then conditioned reflex arcs are created and the tinnitus signal causes activation of the limbic and autonomic nervous systems, with consequent negative behavioral reactions.*

The functional connections linking the auditory and the limbic and autonomic nervous systems are governed by conditioned reflexes and it is possible to identify two categories of connections: (1) conscious, which involves perception, recognition, evaluation, attention, and other cognitive processes, and occurs at the cortical level; and (2) subconscious (**Fig. 36–1**). Notably, there is no need for a causal link between a stimulus and reactions to create a conditioned reflex, and if tinnitus perception is associated with a high level of emotional distress, the connections are created, causing the tinnitus-related neuronal activity (conditioned stimulus) to evoke activation of the limbic and autonomic nervous systems (conditioned reactions).[2,41]

Reinforcement is necessary to initiate creation of the reflex arc, and several scenarios are observed in the case of tinnitus. Most frequently a negative emotional state is evoked by negative counseling; for example, patients are told unpleasant, threatening news about their tinnitus such as that it might indicate the presence of a tumor, or that something is wrong with the brain, or that tinnitus lasts forever and nothing can be done so "you have to learn to live with it." Such information, particularly coming from a medical professional, frequently has a devastating effect on the patient and leads to strong activation of the limbic and autonomic nervous systems and furthermore evokes survival reflexes. A negative emotional state occurs in cases of the rapid emergence of tinnitus or an increase in preexisting tinnitus (e.g., in the case of sudden hearing loss, exposure to an explosion or gunfire, head trauma etc.). Created reflex arcs undergo further enhancement in a vicious-cycle scenario, which works at the conscious and subconscious levels.[41] Note that this reflex has a strong tendency to become stronger as the signal (tinnitus) is continuously present and the effect of the activation of the limbic and autonomic nervous systems acts as the reinforcement. Thus, both the signal and the reinforcement are continuously present. This situation corresponds to a situation of continuous training, and consequently enhances the strength of the reflex.

At the initial stage of development of tinnitus as a problem, the conscious path is essential and plays a dominant role. Once tinnitus acquires negative connotations, the subconscious conditioned reflex is automatically created and becomes equally important as the conscious path, or even dominant. Sustained enhanced activation of the sympathetic part of the autonomic nervous system is responsible for behaviorally observed problems. *Once the tinnitus signal acquires a high level of negative associations and is classified as creating a potential threat to patients' quality of life, then patients respond by going into an alert mode, with their survival reflexes activated. The dominant, subconscious survival mechanism decreases their ability to enjoy life, pushing patients into anxiety and depression.*[2]

To appreciate the widespread occurrence of the role of habituation, it is important to note certain significant characteristics of brain function that have a major impact on tinnitus patients. It has been firmly established that we cannot perform more than one task involving full cognitive attention at a given time. Performing several tasks can be done by quickly switching from one activity to the other.[95,96] This limitation does not exist for subconscious processing when a large number of stimuli can be processed at the same time. All incoming stimuli (e.g., sounds) are detected and compared with records in memory at the subconscious level without involving cognition, attention, or perception. If the pattern of stimulus is new, then the neuronal activity evoked by it reaches the higher level of the auditory cortex where the sound is always perceived. The limbic and autonomic nervous systems are mildly activated to prepare for potential action, and a conscious decision is made regarding its significance and whether any action is necessary.

When a stimulus has a match in memory, then one of two scenarios occurs. If a stimulus was classified in the past as of low or no significance, then neuronal activity representing this stimulus is blocked from reaching higher cognitive levels and blocked from activating the limbic and autonomic nervous systems. This stimulus undergoes spontaneous habituation of

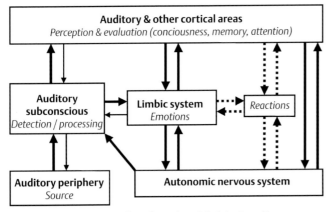

Figure 36–1 The neurophysiological model of tinnitus. (From Jastreboff PJ, Jastreboff MM. Tinnitus and hyperacusis. In: Snow JB Jr, Ballenger JJ, eds. Ballenger's Otorhinolaryngology Head and Neck Surgery, 16th ed. Hamilton, Ontario, Canada: BC Decker, 2003:456–475. Reprinted with permission.)

reaction and perception. As the decision process occurs entirely at the subconscious level, which can process many tasks at the same time, there is no problem with an overload of the system.

The brain spontaneously habituates the tinnitus signal if it has no negative connotations. This is what happens spontaneously in more than 80% of people with tinnitus. If, however, a signal has been classified as having some importance, requiring attention or action, then it is passed to the conscious level and automatically to the limbic and autonomic nervous systems to assure readiness for action that might be needed. These reactions are particularly strong to any stimulus that has negative, threatening implications. For example, if tinnitus was classified as indicating some health problem or as interfering with life, then it is perceived and it further activates the sympathetic part of autonomic nervous system, resulting in feelings of annoyance, anxiety, panic, and so on.

Because only one task requiring full attention can be performed at a given time, all stimuli are classified in a hierarchic manner with an ongoing competition among the various stimuli and activities for having the highest importance and consequently taking hold of the attention. If tinnitus achieves a high level of significance, then it seriously affects attention, interfering with the patient's activities and work. If tinnitus has moderate severity, then other activities are of greater importance and tinnitus is perceived only a fraction of the time. *This explains why people are typically less bothered by mild tinnitus at work, when they are forced to perform other tasks, but tinnitus becomes a significant problem at home, particularly at night, when there are no other competing activities.*

The crucial question for tinnitus treatment is how to remove or change functional connections between the auditory and the limbic and autonomic nervous systems. The hypothesis that these connections are governed by the principles of conditioned reflexes has several profound theoretical and clinical implications.[2,41]

There are a variety of animal models of tinnitus[97–101] that offer the possibility of investigating specific mechanisms involved in generating the tinnitus signal and its perception. These models are typically based on a procedure in which animals are trained using silence as conditioned stimulus (by switching off continuous auditory background) and then tinnitus is introduced hindering detection of silence.[102] At the moment, all these models have the limitation of detecting tinnitus perception only. However, for clinically significant tinnitus the reactions evoked by tinnitus are actually of crucial importance. Studying only perception does not allow differentiating the subjects who experience tinnitus from those who suffer from it.

◆ Treatment

To date there is no method to cure tinnitus, that is, to remove totally its perception. Therefore, the goal of any treatment of clinically significant tinnitus is to remove the effects of tinnitus on the patient's life. A wide variety of treatments have been tried, with mixed results. It is important to recognize the impact of the placebo effect while critically evaluating the results of tinnitus treatment. The placebo effect in cases of tinnitus is high, in the range of 40%[103]; consequently, all open studies are a subject of concern if the reported results

are indeed presenting an improvement over the placebo effect. Many clinicians readily recommend a treatment even if it has mild negative side effects, even when it does not offer real improvement and its action can be most probably explained by the placebo effect (e.g., herbal medications, some alternative medicine therapies). Unfortunately, these treatments may worsen the tinnitus problem, as unsuccessful attempts to achieve improvement enhances patients' conviction that nothing can be done for their tinnitus and increases their stress and frustration. *The critical overview of a wide spectrum of treatments has been published,*[2,104,105] *with the final conclusion that there are no well-documented methods that could be recommended as the standard for tinnitus treatment.*

Tinnitus frequently evokes reactions similar to those of other conditions (e.g., depression, sleep deprivation), or sometimes coexists with treatable health problems (e.g., Meniere's disease). Interventions implemented for these medical conditions do not change tinnitus per se. Inaccurate interpretation of these treatments' outcome led to their specific use for tinnitus even when tinnitus is not accompanied by additional medical problems. For example, antidepressants are frequently prescribed to tinnitus patients even though it has been shown that even effective treatment of depression did not directly improve tinnitus.[105,106]

The automatic assumption that tinnitus can cause problems only when perceived results in focusing on the auditory pathways and on mechanisms of tinnitus generation, putting tinnitus into the realm of otolaryngology. Based on the belief that eliminating tinnitus perception is sufficient and necessary to eliminating tinnitus-induced reactions, many treatments aim at suppression of tinnitus perception. Several specific approaches such as acoustic masking and electrical stimulation, which aim at suppression of the tinnitus signal, gained widespread recognition.

Acoustic masking, first recommended by Jones and Knudsen[107] in 1928 and later by Saltzman and Ersner[108] in 1947, was propagated by Vernon and Schleuning[109] since the late 1970s. Its goal is the elimination of the tinnitus perception by introducing an external sound that is more easily accepted by the patient than the tinnitus. This approach did not involve counseling other than the recommendation of using any sound source to cover the tinnitus. Typically, ear level maskers (i.e., noise generators) or tinnitus instruments (i.e., a combination of noise generator and hearing aid) were utilized to achieve this goal. Mixed results ranging from masking being no better than a placebo device[110] to 64% of success, measured as a percentage of patients who purchased some ear-level device for masking and used them for at least 6 months,[111] were reported over time. For many patients it was very difficult to sustain the masking of the tinnitus, as the sound level that is needed to keep tinnitus masked may increase in a span of minutes to unacceptable levels.[16] Some patients used instruments to achieve partial relief from tinnitus by weakening its signal by external sound.[112] *Recently, masking has been redefined as the use of any sound that provides immediate relief without the necessity of elimination of the tinnitus perception.*[15,113] This approach has been shown to be helpful, particularly in cases of mild tinnitus.[113] Note that if the brain cannot detect the tinnitus signal, as in cases of classic masking, then tinnitus habituation cannot occur, as habituation is an active process and the brain needs to be able to detect a signal to retrain the reaction to it.[2] This prediction has been confirmed by clinical observation[114]; a group of patients, implementing a masking protocol for more than 10 years without any changes in their tinnitus, rapidly habituated once they were put on the habitation-oriented TRT protocol (discussed later in the chapter).

In a small percentage of patients who are using hearing aids, an amplified background sound is sufficient to mask tinnitus.[115] Although patients may obtain relief while using hearing aids, tinnitus becomes audible and bothersome once they remove the aids. Hearing aids are frequently the first approach to be tried for tinnitus, when there is the need to correct hearing loss, and they provide some improvement in 7 to 16% of cases, depending on the extent of counseling.[15,116,117] They provide enhanced input to the auditory system by amplifying environmental sounds and, furthermore, decrease the "strain to hear" phenomenon, which tends to enhance tinnitus. *Without proper background sound enhancement and specific counseling, the usefulness of hearing aids for tinnitus is limited,*[115] *but they are very effective when used according to the neurophysiological model of tinnitus.*[2,87,115]

Electrical stimulation of the periphery of the auditory system has been used, similarly as for acoustic masking, with the goal of suppressing tinnitus perception.[118] Stimulation via a cochlear implant seems to be most efficient and provides relief in approximately 50% of cases.[119,120] Extracochlear stimulation on the promontory can be effective as well.[118] On the other hand, the attempts of stimulation of the external ear, or the skull, yielded mixed results.[8] Recently, a new approach has been proposed with electrical stimulation of the cochlea or auditory nerve by high-frequency electrical pulses (at a rate close to 5 kHz) via a modified cochlear implant or an electrode placed on the promontory.[120,121] Preliminary results indicated an effectiveness of 45%.[121] Interestingly, in some cases it was possible to observe the suppression of the tinnitus without evoking the perception of sound. It was necessary to wait 10 to 15 minutes to observe the full effects of stimulation, which indicates that the effect is central and it does not directly involve restoring random activity within the auditory nerve, as initially postulated.[121]

Recognition of the role of the central auditory system in tinnitus[1,122–124] and the potential involvement of the reorganization of receptive fields within the auditory cortex[125–127] yield methods with direct electric or magnetic stimulation of cortical areas.[128–130] In this respect transcranial magnetic stimulation is particularly interesting as it is noninvasive, and if applied carefully it seems to be without side effects. The proponents of this method localized cortical areas to be stimulated with functional magnetic resonance imaging (fMRI).[130] Preliminary results indicated the potential usefulness of these methods, but the ability to induce prolonged suppression of tinnitus, which is crucial in clinical practice, has not been shown. Otherwise, once tinnitus reappears (e.g., due to discontinuing electrical/magnetic stimulation), it tends to be more bothersome than before suppression.

A wide spectrum of medications has been used to treat tinnitus. Drugs were proposed to attenuate the source of tinnitus within the cochlea.[73,131–133] Typically drugs are proposed based on vague assumptions or anecdotal evidence. Ginkgo biloba is one of the most common remedies taken by patients. A variety of studies yielded mixed results, with a double-blind randomized trial showing its effectiveness to be no better than that of placebo.[134] Similarly, neither caroverine nor gabapentin (Neurontin), which recently gained some interest,[135] has been proven useful for tinnitus.

Treatments based on psychological models typically aim at improving the patient's coping with tinnitus using a variety of tools (e.g., distraction of attention, or change of thinking about tinnitus[85]). These treatments are not attempting to change tinnitus or the reaction evoked by it but rather to improve acceptance of tinnitus-induced reactions. Although some initial improvement could be observed, neither the tinnitus signal nor the reactions are being changed for a prolonged time. Consequently, the positive effects of these methods are difficult to sustain, and without attenuation of tinnitus-induced reactions, focusing on coping methods has limited effectiveness.[2] Nevertheless, improved coping with tinnitus is helpful and it is included in counseling accompanying the majority of treatments.

Another approach to tinnitus aims at changing the emotions associated with tinnitus. Cognitive behavioral therapy is based on the principle that thoughts evoke emotions, and it aims at changing the thoughts related to tinnitus in the attempt to remove negative emotions associated with tinnitus.[86] Its main goal is to modify part of the mechanisms that yield tinnitus distress at the cognitive level. This therapy has been shown to be effective for some patients.[136] The cognitive-behavioral approach has an advantage over the use of psychotropic medications in that it works on specific tinnitus-related thoughts and emotions without affecting emotions not related to tinnitus. Even though cognitive-behavioral therapy influences to some degree the conditioned reflexes, the main focus of all psychological approaches is on cognition, verbalization, and thinking about tinnitus. The literature clearly supports the opposite postulate, as it is possible to learn to create conditioned reflexes and have reactions to stimuli that are not consciously perceived.[137,138]

Stress is a well-recognized factor enhancing tinnitus,[114,139] and it is reasonable to expect that a decrease of the stress level should be helpful in reducing tinnitus as a problem. Unfortunately, past investigations of yoga, biofeedback, relaxation, and music therapies did not provide significant, long-lasting improvement when they were used as an exclusive treatment for tinnitus.[2]

The psychotropic medications, particularly antidepressants and antianxiety drugs, are used to improve the general emotional status of tinnitus patients and through this indirectly improve tinnitus as a problem. Clinical studies have shown that although antidepressants can affect depression in a positive manner, they do not provide help directly for tinnitus.[105,106] A recent study with Paxil (paroxetine) showed some positive effect on tinnitus as well, but only when the drug was used in a very high dose.[140] A majority of medications prescribed to tinnitus patients attempt to eliminate or decrease the reactions evoked by the tinnitus. A variety of psychotropic medications that act on the limbic and autonomic nervous systems have been tested but so far none has been shown to be effective for tinnitus without evoking profound side effects.[2,105]

Tinnitus retraining therapy (TRT), the method based on the neurophysiological model of tinnitus, introduced a new view on tinnitus treatment by incorporating knowledge of how various systems of the brain function and interact with each other in relation to tinnitus. TRT consists of counseling and sound therapy, both strictly following the neurophysiological model. Many elements that were implemented intuitively, or not sufficiently considered in the past, are integral parts of

TRT. TRT aims to induce changes in the mechanisms responsible for transferring tinnitus-related neuronal activity from the auditory system to the limbic and autonomic nervous systems. Note that *TRT attempts neither to eliminate or change the source of the tinnitus signal nor to affect directly the neuronal systems responsible for reactions, but rather at retraining functional connections that transfer tinnitus-related neuronal activity from the auditory pathways to the limbic and autonomic nervous systems.* When these connections are attenuated, reactions disappear and tinnitus ceases to be a problem, even when it is perceived. This process is called *habituation of reactions or passive extinction of conditioned reflexes*[141] *and it is the primary goal of TRT* (**Fig. 36–2**). Once habituation of reaction is partially achieved, habituation of perception (i.e., disappearance of the tinnitus awareness) follows automatically as to all other neutral stimuli.[2] Consequently, as this process acts on the tinnitus signal, disregarding the specifics of neuronal activity responsible for tinnitus, TRT is effective for any type of tinnitus regardless of its etiology.

Spontaneous habituation of tinnitus was first pointed out by Stephens at al[142] as a part of psychological attempts to help tinnitus patients. This process was presented as a passive decline of responses to tinnitus, similarly as to many other stimuli that people are acclimating to. The authors did not propose any specific effective protocol for inducing and sustaining habituation. Coping strategies and attention control techniques were proposed to ease the process of natural habituation.[143] However, no significant, sustained improvement was observed, and clinical results argue against the Hallam model of natural habituation.[144]

The retraining of conditioned reflexes associated with tinnitus cannot be done at the cognitive level. Importantly, for the retraining to occur the stimulus has to be detectable, but not necessary at the cognitive level. Note that psychological methods can work only when the cognitive loop is strongly dominant (**Fig. 36–1**), because these methods cannot change the lower, subconscious conditioned reflex arc. Moreover, as psychological approaches involve frequent (e.g., weekly) visits, and significant time devoted to talking about tinnitus, they tend to increase attention paid to tinnitus, potentially making recovery more difficult.

Sound used in TRT is never masking tinnitus, as this will prevent habituation from occurring. It is necessary for the brain to detect the tinnitus signal to retrain the conditioned reflex arc. Although it is easy to create even a strong conditioned reflex by a single association, the extinguishing of a reflex takes both time and the repetitive association of the tinnitus signal with decreased reinforcement.

The classic approach to passive extinction of conditioned reflexes involves removal of the reinforcement while the unchanged stimulus is presented receptively.[141] This approach cannot be followed directly in the case of tinnitus because reactions of the limbic and autonomic nervous systems act as reinforcement, and they cannot be removed. Therefore, *TRT utilizes a modified approach in which both the reinforcement and the signal are weakened. The decrease of reinforcement is achieved by attenuation of the activation provided from the cognitive level* (**Fig. 36–1**). *This is initiated during the first counseling session* and further sustained and enhanced by subsequent counseling performed during follow-up visits. All counseling sessions are teaching sessions with information passed to patients in an interactive manner, and with the use of illustration, analogies, and parables.[2,87] It is noteworthy that counseling is highly individualized and adapted to the specific patient's case with general guidance related to treatment categories summarized in **Table 36–1.**

Counseling provided throughout the treatment has multiple objectives, with the main goal being to reclassify tinnitus into a category of neutral signals. It is aimed at minimizing activation of the limbic and autonomic nervous systems from the cognitive level. During counseling tinnitus is demystified, and presented as a compensatory action of the auditory system to (typically) peripheral damage in the cochlea. Discordant damage (dysfunction) theory is used to explain how even minor disturbances in function of the outer hair cell system might yield tinnitus.[1,2] Counseling teaches patients about the mechanisms of tinnitus and the way to control it. It is crucial that negative counseling be avoided.

The use of sound is discussed in detail with the patient, as well as the issues of hearing loss, decreased sound tolerance, sleep problems, stress, and other tinnitus-related problems, always considering the specific needs of the individual patient. Sound therapy helps in providing auditory stimulation to decrease the difference between the tinnitus signal and the background neuronal activity to weaken the tinnitus signal and through this promote habituation. This is the reason that ear overprotection is discouraged, and all patients are advised to enrich the background sound (avoid silence). Tinnitus masking is avoided, as the brain has to detect the tinnitus signal to be able to habituate to it. Patients are taught that tinnitus evokes problems as a consequence of the conditioned reflex-based activation of the limbic and autonomic nervous systems by the tinnitus signal, and the perception of tinnitus and what is happening in the auditory system are only secondary. *The tabletop sound machines and ear-level sound generators provide additional sound, which can be further amplified by hearing aids. These devices are very useful in most cases, but they should not be identified with TRT.* TRT can be in theory performed without any type of instrumentation; however, it is not the optimal way. Sound generators are a convenient method of sound delivery and help with compliance but should not be used in patients with hearing loss. In these cases combination instruments (hearing aids and sound generators in one shell) are preferable, but properly chosen and

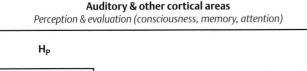

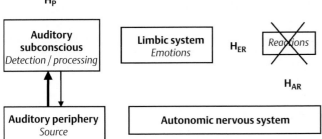

Figure 36–2 Habituation of autonomic (HAR) and emotional reactions (HER) and habituation of perception (HP). (Modified from Jastreboff PJ, Jastreboff MM. Tinnitus and hyperacusis. In: Snow JB Jr, Ballenger JJ, eds. Ballenger's Otorhinolaryngology Head and Neck Surgery. 16th ed. Hamilton, Ontario, Canada: BC Decker, 2003:456–475. Reprinted with permission.)

Table 36–1 Categories of Tinnitus and Hyperacusis Patients

Category	Impact on Life[a]	Tinnitus	Significant Hearing Loss[b]	Hyperacusis	Prolonged Sound-Induced Exacerbation[c]	Counseling[d]	Instrumentation
0	Low	Present	–	–	–	Abbreviated, with emphasis that tinnitus may always be mild and benign	No wearable devices necessary
1	high	Present	–	–	–	Extensive, focused on mechanisms involved in tinnitus generation and in inducing reactions	SG set, if possible, at a mixing point
2	High	Present	Present	–	–	Extensive, focused on mechanisms linking tinnitus and hearing loss	Combi or HA with stress on enrichment of the auditory background
3	High	Not relevant	Not relevant	Present	–	Extensive, focused on mechanisms of decreased sound tolerance; when hearing loss is present as well, mechanisms linking it with decreased sound tolerance and tinnitus are discussed	SG only in cases of normal hearing; combi (or HA) when significant hearing loss present
4	High	Not relevant	Not relevant	Present	Present	Extensive, highly individualized with discussion of potential medical problems	SG set at the threshold; very slow increase of sound level

[a]Impact on life is the extent to which tinnitus or hyperacusis affects the patient's life.

[b]Significant hearing loss has a significant impact on the patient's life.

[c]Prolonged sound-induced exacerbation of tinnitus/hyperacusis is when the effects persist to the following day or longer.

[d]Common treatment for each category involves counseling and the use of enriched auditory background. Sound used in sound therapy is always set below annoyance level. Details of tinnitus retraining therapy implementation are presented elsewhere.[2,87]

SG, sound generators; combi, combination instruments; HA, hearing aids.

set hearing aids, used with enriched background sound, are very successful as well. Although the sound setting of sound generators at the optimal level (i.e., the mixing point, when the external sound starts to mix or blend with tinnitus, but patients can still perceive separately external sound and unchanged tinnitus) is helpful, it frequently cannot be achieved, as the first rule of sound setting in TRT is that sounds used as part of sound therapy should never induce annoyance or discomfort of any type.

As in other treatments TRT aims at achieving a state in which tinnitus is not interfering with the patient's life. Furthermore, *the goal of TRT is that tinnitus, when perceived, does not evoke annoyance*. Note that as in the case with any method that includes counseling as essential part of therapy, it is impossible to conduct a double-blind study on TRT. In the past, the effects of tinnitus treatments were evaluated mainly on the basis of clinical observation. Several clinical studies have been published,[47,145–151] reporting consistently a success rate above 80%. Recently the results of a 3-year well-controlled study of masking treatment and TRT were reported.[152,153] After 18 months, 88% of subjects treated with TRT showed overall improvement classified as at least a five-point improvement in the Tinnitus Severity Index (J. A. Henry, personal communication) and highly statistically significant

overall improvement.[113] Recent results from Spain are in agreement with previously reported success rate.[154] In our clinical experience, the effectiveness of TRT is approximately 80% as well.[2,40,155–159] Moreover, in the majority of cases, it is possible to eliminate decreased sound tolerance.

Over the past 15 years significant progress has been achieved in understanding tinnitus. A variety of mechanisms have been proposed,[1,78,122] a number of animal models have been created,[101,102] and a new method for tinnitus treatment has been introduced.[157,160] Testing and improving already existing methods (e.g., electrical stimulation, new drugs) will continue. Although there are many unanswered questions, it is recognized that much can be done to help tinnitus patients, and currently a number of centers offer comprehensive services for tinnitus patients.

References

1. Jastreboff PJ. Phantom auditory perception (tinnitus): mechanisms of generation and perception. Neurosci Res 1990;8:221–254
2. Jastreboff PJ, Hazell JWP. Tinnitus Retraining Therapy: Implementing the Neurophysiological Model. Cambridge: Cambridge University Press, 2004
3. Jastreboff PJ. Tinnitus as a phantom perception: theories and clinical implications. In: Vernon J, Moller AR, eds. Mechanisms of Tinnitus. Boston, London: Allyn & Bacon, 1995:73–94

4. Davis A, El Refaie A. Epidemiology of Tinnitus. In: Tyler R, ed. Tinnitus Handbook. San Diego: Singular, Thomson Learning, 2000:1–23

5. Axelsson A, Ringdahl A. Tinnitus—a study of its prevalence and characteristics. Br J Audiol 1989;23:53–62

6. Coles RRA. Epidemiology, aetiology and classification. In: Vernon JA, Reich G, eds. Proceedings of the Fifth International Tinnitus Seminar, 1995, Portland, Oregon. Portland: American Tinnitus Association, 1996:25–30

7. Hoffman HJ, Reed GW. Epidemiology of Tinnitus. In: Snow JB, ed. Tinnitus: Theory and Management. Hamilton, London: BC Decker, 2004:16–41

8. Jastreboff PJ, Jastreboff MM. Tinnitus and hyperacusis. In: Snow JB Jr, Ballenger JJ, eds. Ballenger's Otorhinolaryngology Head and Neck Surgery, 16th ed. Hamilton, Ontario, Canada: BC Decker, 2003: 456–475

9. Perry BP, Gantz BJ. Medical and surgical evaluation and management of tinnitus. In: Tyler R, ed. Tinnitus Handbook. San Diego: Singular, Thomson Learning, 2000:221–241

10. Heller MF, Bergman M. Tinnitus aurium in normally hearing persons. Ann Otol Rhinol Laryngol 1953;62:73–93

11. Tucker DA, Phillips SL, Ruth RA, Clayton WA, Royster E, Todd AD. The effect of silence on tinnitus perception. Otolaryngol Head Neck Surg 2005;132:20–24

12. Nodar RH. Tinnitus aurium in school age children: a survey. J Aud Res 1972;12:133–135

13. Martin K, Snashall S. Children presenting with tinnitus: a retrospective study. Br J Audiol 1994;28:111–115

14. Baguley DM, McFerran DJ. Tinnitus in childhood. Int J Pediatr Otorhinolaryngol 1999;49:99–105

15. Vernon JA, Meikle MB. Tinnitus masking. In: Tyler R, ed. Tinnitus Handbook. San Diego: Singular, Thomson Learning, 2000:313–356

16. Penner MJ, Bilger RC. Adaptation and the masking of tinnitus. J Speech Hear Res 1989;32:339–346

17. Feldmann H. Homolateral and contralateral masking of tinnitus by noise-bands and by pure tones. Audiology 1971;10:138–144

18. Vernon JA, Meikle MB. Tinnitus: clinical measurement. Otolaryngol Clin North Am 2003;36:293–305, vi.

19. Zhou J, Shore S. Projections from the trigeminal nuclear complex to the cochlear nuclei: a retrograde and anterograde tracing study in the guinea pig. J Neurosci Res 2004;78:901–907

20. Shore SE. Sensory nuclei in tinnitus. In: Snow JB, ed. Tinnitus: Theory and Management. Hamilton, London: BC Decker, 2004:125–139

21. Sanchez TG, Guerra GCY, Lorenzi MC, Brandao AL, Bento RF. The influence of voluntary muscle contractions upon the onset and modulation of tinnitus. Audiol Neurootol 2002;7:370–375

22. Levine RA. Somatic (craniocervical) tinnitus and the dorsal cochlear nucleus hypothesis. Am J Otolaryngol 1999;20:351–362

23. Cacace AT, Lovely TJ, Parnes SM, Winter DF, McFarland DJ. Gaze-evoked tinnitus following unilateral peripheral auditory deafferentation: a case for anomalous crossmodal plasticity. In: Salvi RJ, Henderson D, Fiorino F, Colletti V, eds. Auditory System Plasticity and Regeneration. New York: Thieme, 1996:354–358

24. Lockwood AH, Wack DS, Burkard RF, et al. The functional anatomy of gaze-evoked tinnitus and sustained lateral gaze. Neurology 2001; 56:472–480

25. Lockwood AH, Salvi RJ, Burkard RF. Tinnitus. N Engl J Med 2002; 347:904–910

26. Oliveira CA, Negreiros JJ, Cavalcante IC, Bahmad JF, Venosa AR. Palatal and middle-ear myoclonus: a cause for objective tinnitus. Int Tinnitus J 2003;9:37–41

27. Ensink RJ, Vingerhoets HM, Schmidt CW, Cremers CW. Treatment for severe palatoclonus by occlusion of the eustachian tube. Otol Neurotol 2003;24:714–716

28. Penner MJ. An estimate of the prevalence of tinnitus caused by spontaneous otoacoustic emissions. Arch Otolaryngol Head Neck Surg 1990;116:418–423

29. Penner MJ. Linking spontaneous otoacoustic emissions and tinnitus. Br J Audiol 1992;26:115–123

30. Lonsbury-Martin BL, Martin GK. Otoacoustic emissions and tinnitus. In: Snow JB, ed. Tinnitus: Theory and Management. Hamilton, London: BC Decker, 2004:69–78

31. Penner MJ, Coles RR. Indications for aspirin as a palliative for tinnitus caused by SOAEs: a case study. Br J Audiol 1992;26:91–96

32. Kujawa SG, Fallon M, Bobbin RP. Intracochlear salicylate reduces low-intensity acoustic and cochlear microphonic distortion products. Hear Res 1992;64:73–80

33. Shehata WE, Brownell WE, Dieler R. Effects of salicylate on shape, electromotility and membrane characteristics of isolated outer hair cells from guinea pig cochlea. Acta Otolaryngol 1991;111:707–718

34. Goodwin PE. Tinnitus and auditory imagery. Am J Otol 1980;2:5–9

35. Berrios GE, Rose GS. Psychiatry of subjective tinnitus: conceptual, historical and clinical aspects. Neurology, Psychiatry and Brain Research 1992;1:76–82

36. Berrios GE. Musical hallucinations: a statistical analysis of 46 cases. Psychopathology 1991;24:356–360

37. Johns LC, Hemsley D, Kuipers E. A comparison of auditory hallucinations in a psychiatric and non-psychiatric group. Br J Clin Psychol 2002;41(pt 1):81–86

38. Nam EC. Is it necessary to differentiate tinnitus from auditory hallucination in schizophrenic patients? J Laryngol Otol 2005;119:352–355

39. Jastreboff PJ, Jastreboff MM. Decreased sound tolerance. In: Snow JB, ed. Tinnitus: Theory and Management. Hamilton, London: BC Decker, 2004:8–15

40. Jastreboff MM, Jastreboff PJ. Decreased sound tolerance and Tinnitus Retraining Therapy (TRT). Australian and New Zealand Journal of Audiology 2002;21:74–81

41. Jastreboff PJ. The neurophysiological model of tinnitus. In: Snow JB, ed. Tinnitus: Theory and Management. Hamilton, London: BC Decker, 2004:96–106

42. Gerken GM. Alteration of central auditory processing of brief stimuli: a review and a neural model. J Acoust Soc Am 1993;93:2038–2049

43. Gerken GM. Central auditory temporal processing: Alterations produced by factors involving the cochlea. In: Dancer A, Henderson D, Salvi R, Hamernik R, eds. Effect of Noise on the Auditory System, 1st ed. Philadelphia: Mosby, 1992:146–155

44. Boettcher FA, Salvi RJ. Functional changes in the ventral cochlear nucleus following acute acoustic overstimulation. J Acoust Soc Am 1993;94:2123–2134

45. Fabijanska A, Rogowski M, Bartnik G, Skarzynski H. Epidemiology of tinnitus and hyperacusis in Poland. In: Hazell JWP, ed. Proceedings of the Sixth International Tinnitus Seminar, 1999, Cambridge, UK. London: Tinnitus and Hyperacusis Center, 1999:569–571

46. Pilgramm M, Rychlick R, Lebisch H, Siedentop H, Goebel G, Kirchhoff D. Tinnitus in the Federal Republic of Germany: a representative epidemiological study. In: Hazell JWP, ed. Proceedings of the Sixth International Tinnitus Seminar, 1999. Cambridge, UK. London, UK: Tinnitus and Hyperacusis Center, 1999:64–67

47. Sheldrake JB, Hazell JWP, Graham RL. Results of tinnitus retraining therapy. In: Hazell JWP, ed. Proceedings of the Sixth International Tinnitus Seminar, 1999, Cambridge, UK. London, UK: Tinnitus and Hyperacusis Center, 1999:292–296

48. Anari M, Axelsson A, Elies W, Magnusson L. Hypersensitivity to sound—questionnaire data, audiometry and classification. Scand Audiol 1999;28:219–230

49. Nields JA, Fallon BA, Jastreboff PJ. Carbamazepine in the treatment of Lyme disease-induced hyperacusis. J Neuropsychiatry Clin Neurosci 1999;11:97–99

50. Farb CR, LeDoux JE. NMDA and AMPA receptors in the lateral nucleus of the amygdala are postsynaptic to auditory thalamic afferents. Synapse 1997;27:106–121

51. Li XF, Phillips R, LeDoux JE. NMDA and non-NMDA receptors contribute to synaptic transmission between the medial geniculate body and the lateral nucleus of the amygdala. Exp Brain Res 1995;105:87–100

52. Jastreboff PJ. Tinnitus habituation therapy (THT) and tinnitus retraining therapy (TRT). In: Tyler R, ed. Tinnitus Handbook. San Diego: Singular, Thomson Learning, 2000:357–376

53. Tonndorf J. The analogy between tinnitus and pain: a suggestion for a physiological basis of chronic tinnitus. Hear Res 1987;28:271–275

54. Kiang NYS, Moxon EC, Levine RA. Auditory-nerve activity in cats with normal and abnormal cochleas. In: Wolstenholme GEW, Knight J, eds. Ciba Foundation Symposium on Sensorineural Hearing Loss. London: Churchill, 1970:241–273

55. Salvi RJ, Ahroon WA. Tinnitus and neural activity. J Speech Hear Res 1983;26:629–632

56. Penner MJ. Two-tone forward masking patterns and tinnitus. J Speech Hear Res 1980;23:779–786

57. Moller AR. Pathophysiology of tinnitus. Ann Otol Rhinol Laryngol 1984;93:39–44

58. Eggermont JJ. On the pathophysiology of tinnitus; a review and a peripheral model. Hear Res 1990;48:111–123

59. Zenner HP, Ernst A. Cochlear-motor, transduction and signal-transfer tinnitus. Eur Arch Otorhinolaryngol 1993;249:447–454

60. Moller AR. Pathophysiology of severe tinnitus and chronic pain. In: Hazell JWP, ed. Proceedings of the Sixth International Tinnitus Seminar, 1999, Cambridge, UK. London, UK: Tinnitus and Hyperacusis Center, 1999:26–31

61. Muhlnickel W, Elbert T, Taub E, Flor H. Reorganization of auditory cortex in tinnitus. Proc Natl Acad Sci U S A 1998;95:10340–10343

62. Guth PS, Risey J, Amedee R, Norris CH. A pharmacological approach to the treatment of tinnitus. In: Aran J-M, Dauman R, eds. Tinnitus 91. Proceedings IV International Tinnitus Seminar, Bordeaux, France, 1991. Amsterdam: Kugler, 1992:115–118

63. Liberman MC, Kiang NY. Acoustic trauma in cats. Acta Otolaryngol Suppl 1978;358:1–63

64. Gerken GM. Central tinnitus and lateral inhibition: an auditory brainstem model. Hear Res 1996;97:75–83

65. Pujol R. Neuropharmacology of the cochlea and tinnitus. In: Aran J-M, Dauman R, eds. Tinnitus 91. Proceedings IV International Tinnitus Seminar, Bordeaux, France, 1991. Amsterdam: Kugler Publications, 1992:103–107

66. Hazell JWP. A cochlear model for tinnitus. In: Feldmann H, ed. Proceedings III International Tinnitus Seminar, Muenster 1987. Karlsruhe: Harsch Verlag, 1987:121–128

67. Tonndorf J. Stereociliary dysfunction, a case of sensory hearing loss, recruitment, poor speech discrimination and tinnitus. Acta Otolaryngol 1981;91:469–479

68. Jastreboff PJ, Nguyen Q, Brennan JF, Sasaki CT. Calcium and calcium channel involvement in tinnitus. In: Aran J-M, Dauman R, eds. Tinnitus 91. Proceedings IV International Tinnitus Seminar, Bordeaux, France, 1991. Amsterdam: Kugler, 1992:109–114

69. Moller AR. The cranial nerve vascular compression syndrome: I. A review of treatment. Acta Neurochir (Wien) 1991;113:18–23

70. Jannetta PJ. Microvascular decompression of the cochlear nerve as treatment of tinnitus. In: Feldmann H, ed. Proceedings III International Tinnitus Seminar, Muenster 1987. Karlsruhe: Harsch Verlag, 1987:348–352

71. Davies E, Knox E, Donaldson I. The usefulness of nimodipine, an L-calcium channel antagonist, in the treatment of tinnitus. Br J Audiol 1994;28:125–129

72. Oestreicher E, Arnold W, Ehrenberger K, Felix D. New approaches for inner ear therapy with glutamate antagonists. Acta Otolaryngol 1999;119:174–178

73. Denk DM, Heinzl H, Franz P, Ehrenberger K. Caroverine in tinnitus treatment. A placebo-controlled blind study. Acta Otolaryngol 1997;117:825–830

74. Jastreboff PJ, Sasaki CT. Salicylate-induced changes in spontaneous activity of single units in the inferior colliculus of the guinea pig. J Acoust Soc Am 1986;80:1384–1391

75. Kaltenbach JA, Rachel JD, Mathog TA, Zhang J, Falzarano PR, Lewandowski M. Cisplatin-induced hyperactivity in the dorsal cochlear nucleus and its relation to outer hair cell loss: relevance to tinnitus. J Neurophysiol 2002;88:699–714

76. Kaltenbach JA, Afman CE. Hyperactivity in the dorsal cochlear nucleus after intense sound exposure and its resemblance to tone-evoked activity: a physiological model for tinnitus. Hear Res 2000;140:165–172

77. Moller AR. Pathophysiology of tinnitus. Ann Otol Rhinol Laryngol 1984;93:39–44

78. Eggermont JJ, Roberts LE. The neuroscience of tinnitus. Trends Neurosci 2004;27:676–682

79. Eggermont JJ, Kenmochi M. Salicylate and quinine selectively increase spontaneous firing rates in secondary auditory cortex. Hear Res 1998;117:149–160

80. Kwon O, Jastreboff MM, Hu S, Shi J, Jastreboff PJ. Modification of single-unit activity related to noise-induced tinnitus in rats. In: Hazell JWP, ed. Proceedings of the Sixth International Tinnitus Seminar, 1999, Cambridge, UK. London, UK: Tinnitus and Hyperacusis Center, 1999:459–462

81. Eggermont JJ, Smith GM, Bowman D. Spontaneous burst firing in cat primary auditory cortex: age and depth dependence and its effect on neural interaction measures. J Neurophysiol 1993;69:1292–1313

82. Hiller W, Goebel G. A psychometric study of complaints in chronic tinnitus. J Psychosom Res 1992;36:337–348

83. The American Heritage Dictionary, 3rd ed. SoftKey International, 1994

84. Henry JL, Wilson PH. Coping with tinnitus: two studies of psychological and audiological characteristics of patients with high and low tinnitus-related distress. Int Tinnitus J 1995;1:85–92

85. Wilson PH, Henry JL. Psychological management of tinnitus. In: Tyler R, ed. Tinnitus Handbook. San Diego: Singular, Thomson Learning, 2000:263–279

86. Henry JL, Wilson PH. Psychological Management of Chronic Tinnitus: A Cognitive-Behavioral Approach. Boston: Allyn & Bacon, 2001.

87. Jastreboff PJ. Tinnitus Retraining Therapy. In: Snow JB, ed. Tinnitus: Theory and Management. Hamilton, London: BC Decker, 2004:295–309.

88. Hoshiyama M, Kakigi R, Watanabe S, Miki K, Takeshima Y. Brain responses for the subconscious recognition of faces. Neurosci Res 2003;46:435–442

89. Klapp ST, Hinkley LB. The negative compatibility effect: unconscious inhibition influences reaction time and response selection. J Exp Psychol Gen 2002;131:255–269

90. Bargh JA, Gollwitzer PM, Lee-Chai A, Barndollar K, Trotschel R. The automated will: nonconscious activation and pursuit of behavioral goals. J Pers Soc Psychol 2001;81:1014–1027

91. Esteves F, Parra C, Dimberg U, Ohman A. Nonconscious associative learning: Pavlovian conditioning of skin conductance responses to masked fear-relevant facial stimuli. Psychophysiology 1994;31:375–385

92. Swanson LW. Limbic System. In: Adelman G, ed. Encyclopedia of Neuroscience. Boston: Birkhauser, 1987:589–591

93. Brooks CM. Autonomic nervous system, nature and functional role. In: Adelman G, ed. Encyclopedia of Neuroscience. Boston: Birkhauser, 1987:96–98

94. Konorski J. Conditioned Reflexes and Neuronal Organization. Cambridge: Cambridge University Press, 1948

95. Kimberg DY, Aguirre GK, D'Esposito M. Modulation of task-related neural activity in task-switching: an fMRI study. Brain Res Cogn Brain Res 2000;10:189–196

96. Sylvester CY, Wager TD, Lacey SC, et al. Switching attention and resolving interference: fMRI measures of executive functions. Neuropsychologia 2003;41:357–370

97. Jastreboff PJ, Brennan JF, Coleman JK, Sasaki CT. Phantom auditory sensation in rats: an animal model for tinnitus. Behav Neurosci 1988;102:811–822

98. Jastreboff PJ, Jastreboff MM, Kwon O, Shi J, Hu S. An animal model of noise induced tinnitus. In: Hazell JWP, ed. Proceedings of the Sixth International Tinnitus Seminar, 1999, Cambridge, UK. London, UK: Tinnitus and Hyperacusis Center, 1999:198–202

99. Bauer CA, Brozoski TJ, Rojas R, Boley J, Wyder M. Behavioral model of chronic tinnitus in rats. Otolaryngol Head Neck Surg 1999;121:457–462

100. Heffner HE, Harrington IA. Tinnitus in hamsters following exposure to intense sound. Hear Res 2002;170:83–95

101. Moody DB. Animal Models of Tinnitus. In: Snow JB, ed. Tinnitus: Theory and Management. Hamilton, London: BC Decker, 2004:80–95

102. Jastreboff PJ, Brennan JF, Coleman JK, Sasaki CT. Phantom auditory sensation in rats: an animal model for tinnitus. Behav Neurosci 1988;102:811–822

103. Duckert LG, Rees TS. Placebo effect in tinnitus management. Otolaryngol Head Neck Surg 1984;92:697–699

104. Dobie RA. A review of randomized clinical trials in tinnitus. Laryngoscope 1999;109:1202–1211

105. Dobie RA. Clinical Trials and Drug Therapy for Tinnitus. In: Snow JB, ed. Tinnitus: Theory and Management. Hamilton, London: BC Decker; 2004:266–277

106. Sullivan MD, Dobie RA, Sakai CS, Katon WJ. Treatment of depressed tinnitus patients with nortriptyline. Ann Otol Rhinol Laryngol 1989;98:867–872

107. Jones IH, Knudsen VO. Certain aspects of tinnitus particularly treatment. Laryngoscope 1928;38:597–611

108. Saltzman M, Ersner MS. A hearing aid for the relief of tinnitus aurium. Laryngoscope 1947;57:358–366

109. Vernon J, Schleuning A. Tinnitus: a new management. Laryngoscope 1978;88:413–419

110. Erlandsson S, Ringdahl A, Hutchins T, Carlsson SG. Treatment of tinnitus: a controlled comparison of masking and placebo. Br J Audiol 1987;21:37–44

111. Johnson RM. The masking of tinnitus. In: Vernon JA, ed. Tinnitus Treatment and Relief, 1st ed. Boston: Allyn and Bacon, 1998:164–186

112. Hazell JW, Wood SM, Cooper HR, et al. A clinical study of tinnitus maskers. Br J Audiol 1985;19:65–146

113. Henry JA, Schechter MA, Zaugg TL, et al. Outcomes of Clinical Trial: Tinnitus Masking versus Tinnitus Retraining Therapy. J Am Acad Audiol 2006;17:104–132

114. Hazell JWP, McKinney CJ. Support for a neurophysiological model of tinnitus. In: Vernon JA, Reich G, eds. Proceedings of the Fifth International Tinnitus Seminar, 1995, Portland, Oregon. Portland: American Tinnitus Association, 1996:51–77

115. Sheldrake JB, Jastreboff MM. Role of hearing aids in management of tinnitus. In: Snow JB, ed. Tinnitus: Theory and Management. Hamilton, London: BC Decker, 2004:312–315

116. Schleuning AJ, Johnson RM, Vernon JA. Evaluation of a tinnitus masking program: a follow-up study of 598 patients. Ear Hear 1980;1:71–74

117. von Wedel H, von Wedel U, Walger M. Tinnitus masking with tinnitus-maskers and hearing aids. In: Vernon J, Moller AR, eds. Mechanisms of Tinnitus. Boston, London: Allyn & Bacon, 1995:187–192

118. Hazell JW, Jastreboff PJ, Meerton LE, Conway MJ. Electrical tinnitus suppression: frequency dependence of effects. Audiology 1993;32:68–77

119. Hazell JW, McKinney CJ, Aleksy W. Mechanisms of tinnitus in profound deafness. Ann Otol Rhinol Laryngol Suppl 1995;166:418–420

120. Rubinstein JT, Tyler RS. Electrical Suppression of Tinnitus. In: Snow JB, ed. Tinnitus: Theory and Management. Hamilton, London: BC Decker, 2004:326–335

121. Rubinstein JT, Tyler RS, Johnson A, Brown CJ. Electrical suppression of tinnitus with high-rate pulse trains. Otol Neurotol 2003;24:478–485

122. Moller AR. Pathophysiology of tinnitus. Otolaryngol Clin North Am 2003;36:249–266, v–vi

123. Reyes SA, Salvi RJ, Burkard RF, et al. Brain imaging of the effects of lidocaine on tinnitus. Hear Res 2002;171:43–50

124. Mirz F, Gjedde A, Ishizu K, Pedersen CB. Cortical networks subserving the perception of tinnitus—a PET study. Acta Otolaryngol Suppl 2000;543:241–243

125. Muhlnickel W, Elbert T, Taub E, Flor H. Reorganization of auditory cortex in tinnitus. Proc Natl Acad Sci U S A 1998;95:10340–10343

126. Muhlau M, Rauschecker JP, Oestreicher E et al. Structural Brain Changes in Tinnitus. Cereb Cortex 2006;16:1283–1288. Epub 2005 Nov 9`

127. Rauschecker JP. Auditory cortical plasticity: a comparison with other sensory systems. Trends Neurosci 1999;22:74–80

128. Kleinjung T, Eichhammer P, Langguth B, et al. Long-term effects of repetitive transcranial magnetic stimulation (rTMS) in patients with chronic tinnitus. Otolaryngol Head Neck Surg 2005;132:566–569

129. Eichhammer P, Langguth B, Marienhagen J, Kleinjung T, Hajak G. Neuronavigated repetitive transcranial magnetic stimulation in patients with tinnitus: a short case series. Biol Psychiatry 2003;54:862–865

130. De Ridder D, Verstraeten E, Van der Kelen K et al. Transcranial magnetic stimulation for tinnitus: influence of tinnitus duration on stimulation parameter choice and maximal tinnitus suppression. Otol Neurotol 2005;26:616–619

131. Risey JA, Guth PS, Amedee RG. Furosemide distinguishes central and peripheral tinnitus. Int Tinnitus J 1995;1:99–103

132. Oestreicher E, Arnold W, Ehrenberger K, Felix D. Memantine suppresses the glutamatergic neurotransmission of mammalian inner hair cells. ORL J Otorhinolaryngol Relat Spec 1998;60:18–21

133. Oliver D, Ludwig J, Reisinger E, Zoellner W, Ruppersberg JP, Fakler B. Memantine inhibits efferent cholinergic transmission in the cochlea by blocking nicotinic acetylcholine receptors of outer hair cells. Mol Pharmacol 2001;60:183–189

134. Drew S, Davies E. Effectiveness of Ginkgo biloba in treating tinnitus: double blind, placebo controlled trial. BMJ 2001;322:73

135. Zapp JJ. Gabapentin for the treatment of tinnitus: a case report. Ear Nose Throat J 2001;80:114–116

136. Andersson G. Psychological aspects of tinnitus and the application of cognitive-behavioral therapy. Clin Psychol Rev 2002;22:977–990

137. Killgore WD, Yurgelun-Todd DA. Activation of the amygdala and anterior cingulate during nonconscious processing of sad versus happy faces. Neuroimage 2004;21:1215–1223

138. Klapp ST, Haas BW. Nonconscious influence of masked stimuli on response selection is limited to concrete stimulus-response associations. J Exp Psychol Hum Percept Perform 2005;31:193–209

139. Sahley TL, Nodar RH. A biochemical model of peripheral tinnitus. Hear Res 2001;152:43–54

140. Robinson SK, Virre ES, Stein MB. Antidepressant therapy for tinnitus. In: Snow JB, ed. Tinnitus: Theory and Management. Hamilton, London: BC Decker, 2004:278–293

141. Konorski J. Integrative Activity of the Brain. Chicago: University of Chicago Press, 1967

142. Stephens SD, Hallam RS, Jakes SC. Tinnitus: a management model. Clin Otolaryngol 1986;11:227–238

143. Jakes SC, Hallam RS, Rachman S, Hinchcliffe R. The effects of reassurance, relaxation training and distraction on chronic tinnitus sufferers. Behav Res Ther 1986;24:497–507

144. Carlsson SG, Erlandsson SI. Habituation and tinnitus: an experimental study. J Psychosom Res 1991;35:509–514

145. Lux-Wellenhof G, Hellweg FC. Longterm follow up study of TRT in Frankfurt. In: Patuzzi R, ed. Proceedings of the Seventh International Tinnitus Seminar. Perth, Australia: University of Western Australia, 2002:277–279

146. Lux-Wellenhof G. Treatment history of incoming patients to the Tinnitus and Hyperacusis Centre in Frankfurt/Main. In: Hazell JWP, ed. Proceedings of the Sixth International Tinnitus Seminar, 1999, Cambridge, UK. London, UK: Tinnitus and Hyperacusis Center, 1999:502–506

147. Bartnik G, Fabijanska A, Rogowski M. Our experience in treatment of patients with tinnitus and/or hyperacusis using the habituation method. In: Hazell JWP, ed. Proceedings of the Sixth International Tinnitus Seminar, 1999, Cambridge, UK. London, UK: Tinnitus and Hyperacusis Center, 1999:415–417

148. Heitzmann T, Rubio L, Cardenas MR, Zofio E. The importance of continuity in TRT patients: Results at 18 months. In: Hazell JWP, ed. Proceedings of the Sixth International Tinnitus Seminar, 1999, Cambridge, UK. London, UK: Tinnitus and Hyperacusis Center, 1999:509–511

149. Herraiz C, Hernandez FJ, Machado A, De Lucas P, Tapia MC. Tinnitus retraining therapy: Our experience. In: Hazell JWP, ed. Proceedings of the Sixth International Tinnitus Seminar, 1999, Cambridge, UK. London, UK: Tinnitus and Hyperacusis Center, 1999:483–484

150. McKinney CJ, Hazell JWP, Graham RL. An evaluation of the TRT method. In: Hazell JWP, ed. Proceedings of the Sixth International Tinnitus Seminar, 1999, Cambridge, UK. London, UK: Tinnitus and Hyperacusis Center, 1999:99–105

151. Berry JA, Gold SL, Frederick EA, Gray WC, Staecker H. Patient-based outcomes in patients with primary tinnitus undergoing tinnitus retraining therapy. Arch Otolaryngol Head Neck Surg 2002;128:1153–1157

152. Henry JA. Tinnitus retraining therapy: description and clinical efficacy. ENT News 2004;13:48–50

153. Henry JA, Jastreboff MM, Jastreboff PJ, Schechter MA, Fausti SA. Assessment of patients for treatment with Tinnitus Retraining Therapy. J Am Acad Audiol 2002;13:523–544

154. Herraiz C, Hernandez FJ, Plaza G, De los Santos G. Long term clinical trial of tinnitus retraining therapy. Otolaryngol Head Neck Surg 2005;133:774–779

155. Jastreboff MM, Jastreboff PJ, Mattox DE. Statistical analysis of the progress of tinnitus treatment during Tinnitus Retraining Therapy (TRT). Association for Research in Otolaryngology Midwinter Meeting, St. Petersburg Beach, Florida, 2001

156. Jastreboff PJ, Jastreboff MM. Tinnitus Retraining Therapy. In: Baguley D, ed. Perspectives in Tinnitus Management. New York, Stuttgart: Thieme, 2001:51–63

157. Jastreboff PJ, Jastreboff MM. Tinnitus Retraining Therapy (TRT) as a method for treatment of tinnitus and hyperacusis patients. J Am Acad Audiol 2000;11:162–177

158. Jastreboff PJ. Categories of the patients and the treatment outcome. In: Hazell JWP, ed. Proceedings of the Sixth International Tinnitus Seminar, 1999, Cambridge, UK. London, UK: Tinnitus and Hyperacusis Center, 1999:394–398

159. Jastreboff PJ, Gray WC, Gold SL. Neurophysiological approach to tinnitus patients. Am J Otol 1996;17:236–240

160. Jastreboff PJ. Clinical implication of the neurophysiological model of tinnitus. In: Vernon JA, Reich G, eds. Proceedings of the Fifth International Tinnitus Seminar, 1995, Portland, Oregon. Portland: American Tinnitus Association, 1996:500–507

Index

Page numbers followed by *f* and *t* indicate figures and tables, respectively.

Index

Index

Index

527

Assurance and Related Services Guidelines

Assurance Handbook Prior to the Issuance of CASs

(The following Guidelines are referred to in this text, though no longer in the current standards collection)

Public Sector [Sections PS 5000–PS 6420]

*Available online at knotia.ca by subscription through most college and university libraries.

INTERNATIONAL FEDERATION OF ACCOUNTANTS
HANDBOOK OF THE CODE OF ETHICS FOR PROFESSIONAL ACCOUNTANTS
2015 EDITION

This handbook brings together for continuing reference background information about the International Federation of Accountants (IFAC) and the official text of the *Code of Ethics for Professional Accountants* (the Code) issued by the International Ethics Standards Board for Accountants (IESBA).

CONTENTS

Source: The full code can be downloaded at www.ifac.org/publications-resources/2012-handbook-code-ethics-professional-accountants.

Seventh Edition

Auditing

AN INTERNATIONAL APPROACH

Wally J. Smieliauskas, Ph.D., C.P.A., C.F.E.
Joseph L. Rotman School of Management
University of Toronto

Kathryn Bewley, Ph.D., C.P.A., C.A.
Ted Rogers School of Business Management
Ryerson University

Mc
Graw
Hill
Education

Auditing: An International Approach
Seventh Edition

The Internet addresses listed in the text were accurate at the time of publication. The inclusion of a website does not indicate an endorsement by the authors or McGraw-Hill Ryerson, and McGraw-Hill Ryerson does not guarantee the accuracy of information presented at these sites.

For all CPA Canada exhibits: Reprinted (or adapted) with permission of Chartered Professional Accountants of Canada, Toronto, Canada. Any changes to the original material are the sole responsibility of the author (and/or publisher) and have not been reviewed or endorsed by CPA Canada.

ISBN-13: 978-1-25-908746-2
ISBN-10: 1-25-908746-8

1 2 3 4 5 6 7 8 9 0 TCP 1 9 8 7 6 5

Printed and bound in Canada.

Care has been taken to trace ownership of copyright material contained in this text; however, the publisher will welcome any information that enables it to rectify any reference or credit for subsequent editions.

Director of Product Management: Rhondda McNabb
Product Manager: Keara Emmett
Executive Marketing Manager: Joy Armitage Taylor
Product Developer: Amy Rydzanicz
Photo/Permissions Research: Tracy Leonard
Product Team Associate: Stephanie Giles
Supervising Editor: Joanne Limebeer
Copy Editor: Julia Cochrane
Plant Production Coordinator: Michelle Saddler
Manufacturing Production Coordinator: Emily Hickey
Cover Design: Dave Murphy
Cover Image: Jose Luis Pelaez/Getty Images
Interior Design: Dave Murphy
Page Layout: SPi Global
Printer: Transcontinental Printing Group

Wally Smieliauskas dedicates this book to
Reid and Lucas.

Kathryn Bewley dedicates this book to all the auditing students,
educators, and practitioners who work so hard to keep auditing essential.

About the Authors

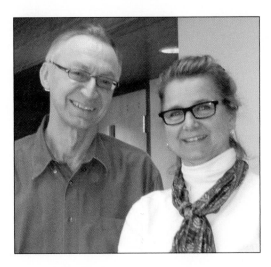

Wally J. Smieliauskas is a professor of accounting at the University of Toronto, where he has been a member of the faculty since 1979. He has published articles on a variety of auditing, accounting, and education issues.

At the University of Toronto, Professor Smieliauskas developed the first degree-credit introductory auditing course (in 1981) and the first advanced auditing course (in 1990). In 1988 he was the first director of the MBA Co-op Program in Professional Accounting, a position he held until 1993. The program is designed to facilitate the entry of undergraduates from various fields into the profession and to provide a broader management education as well as specialized training in accounting, auditing, and tax topics. It has evolved to become the Master of Management & Professional Accounting (MMPA) program now offered through the University of Toronto's Mississauga campus.

Kathryn Bewley has been a professor of accounting and auditing at Ryerson University since 2010 and had previously taught at York University since 1991. She is a member of CPA Ontario and began her career in auditing with Clarkson Gordon in Toronto.

Professor Bewley received her Ph.D. from the University of Waterloo. Her main research focus is on the impact of regulations, including auditing standards, on the information companies report and how people use that information, with a particular interest in environmental reporting. Her work has been published in several professional and academic journals.

BRIEF CONTENTS

CONTENTS

CHAPTER 6   **Assessing Risks in an Audit Engagement**   **243**

CHAPTER 7   **Internal Control over Financial Reporting**   **315**

CHAPTER 8   Audit Evidence and Assurance   361

CHAPTER 9   Control Assessment and Testing   423

PART 3   Performing the Audit

PART 4 Advanced Issues in Professional Public Accounting Practice (on Connect)

PREFACE TO THE SEVENTH EDITION

This seventh edition incorporates the many professional developments that have taken place since the sixth edition (2013). We continue our approach of providing in-depth coverage of fundamental auditing concepts and techniques in the context of current developments affecting the audit profession and practice in Canada and internationally. These developments include the roll-out of the new audit report expected to go into effect December 15, 2016; a new emphasis on ethical reporting; a continuing emphasis on risk-based auditing, auditor independence, and engagement quality standards; and the further maturation of public accountability boards and their monitoring activities.

Since the sixth edition, the auditing profession in Canada has been transformed by the merger of the three previous accounting bodies, CMA, CGA, and CA, into one new association now called CPA Canada (Chartered Professional Accountants of Canada), with parallel changes taking place at the provincial level. This merger is accompanied by changes to the education and certification requirements for professional accountants (PAs) and auditors. Also, the authoritative material previously published by the CICA (Canadian Institute of Chartered Accountants) is now published by CPA Canada. This seventh edition reflects these changes to the extent they have been implemented or finalized up to the time of writing.

Starting in 2011, financial reporting in Canada has been greatly altered by the introduction of two separate sets of Canadian generally accepted accounting principles (GAAP): International Financial Reporting Standards (IFRS) for public companies and Accounting Standards for Private Enterprises (ASPE). The implications of these changes on financial statement audits are reflected in this edition. One important implication is the expanding use of fair value accounting estimates. Further, the increasing complexity and speed of change in business and the economy have greatly increased the need to make many kinds of estimates in financial statements. These changes are placing greater focus on the considerable uncertainty embedded in such accounting numbers, as illustrated in the continuing financial crises that have rippled through the global economy since 2008. This seventh edition provides new, unique coverage of the auditing and assurance issues related to the new audit report, and use of estimates in financial statements, important areas for research and development in current audit practice. The implications for this on risk assessment, evidence gathering, and forming an audit opinion on fair presentation are key challenges we have presented in our discussions of the audit process. Fraud, corporate governance, ethical reporting, independence risk, the role of audit committees, global convergence of audit and accounting standards, and information technology (IT) remain highly relevant to the auditing profession, and information on all of these issues has been updated for the seventh edition.

This edition reflects these developments through early 2015, offering our perspective on their significance. In this current audit environment, we see not only radical changes in audit standards and the regulatory environment but also significantly revised expectations of the auditor's role in corporate governance and capital markets. This environment is characterized by more risks for auditors and their clients than ever before, as well as more restrictions on non-audit services for audit clients. We hope our coverage of these challenging new developments will help students appreciate the dynamic nature of the audit function in our economy, bring up to date the role of auditing in the current financial reporting environment, and provide opportunities to develop the critical thinking skills needed for the next generation of auditors.

WHAT'S NEW IN THE SEVENTH EDITION?

This seventh edition has been developed to make the learning experience enjoyable and straightforward for students, while still fostering essential critical thinking skills that challenge students as they learn. Key updates and ongoing approaches are as follows:

- An Essentials section has been added at the beginning of each chapter to summarize the most important concepts.

- Multiple-choice questions have been added to all chapters.

- Chapter material has been reorganized to facilitate the study of auditing in those universities, colleges, and programs that offer one audit course as well as those that offer two or more audit courses. Introductory material on professional ethics and liability is presented in Part 1, with more in-depth coverage later in Part 4. The coverage of risk and control has been reorganized to cover understanding and assessment of risks in Chapter 6, and then internal controls over financial reporting, risk of material misstatement, and fraud risk in Chapter 7. We are confident this approach will provide students and instructors with more choice in how they engage with the material. The organization of the seventh edition is elaborated on in the section below, where we describe the coverage provided in each of the 4 parts and 21 chapters.

- The innovative introduction of critical thinking concepts that integrate ethical, accounting, and auditing theory to help structure professional audit decision making and analysis in financial reporting has been supplemented by the revised Appendix 3A on the ethics and natural-language reasoning that underlie auditor judgments and the justifications of decisions documented in audit work.

- A streamlined overview of the audit process has been added to Chapter 5, serving as a road map to the procedural topics covered in the text.

- References to specifics of the Canadian Auditing Standards (CASs), based on International Standards on Auditing (ISAs), have been retained in the "Standards Check" boxes located at key points of the discussion as a quick link to the specific paragraphs of the CAS that are relevant to applying the concepts. These are an efficient way to introduce students to how they can use the standards as a resource for understanding and implementing generally accepted auditing standards (GAAS) in practice. *CPA Canada Assurance Handbook* changes through mid-2015 have been incorporated.

- Several new exhibits and tables have been added to summarize concepts and techniques and to help students understand and apply key auditing practices.

- The chapter on auditing accounting estimates (Chapter 19, available on Connect) has been enhanced with an accounting analytics case study. This chapter explains the concepts of CAS 540 and builds on the accounting risk concept introduced in earlier editions, as a way of helping implement critical thinking in audited financial reporting.

- Updated online appendices on the more technical aspects of statistical sampling in auditing, corporate governance, IT, internal control, and critical thinking are provided to help integrate auditing, accounting, and ethical reasoning.

- Various updated anecdotes, asides, short cases, and Application Cases with suggested solutions and analysis in each chapter enrich the text material.

- Several new critical thinking and Internet assignment questions complement the preceding changes, and a number of new cases, including some from the professional accounting exams, have been added.

- Online assessment is now available on Connect, McGraw-Hill's teaching and learning platform.

KEY FEATURES

CPA Canada Handbook Assurance Recommendation Updates: Canadian Auditing Standards and the Convergence to International Auditing

This edition provides complete referencing to CASs. It thus provides essential guidance for auditors in the 21st century. CASs introduce new fundamental concepts, such as ethical reporting frameworks in the form of compliance and fair presentation frameworks. CASs continue the incorporation of international standards started in earlier editions of this text. The inside front cover provides a complete listing of the CASs and the *CPA Canada Handbook* assurance sections. Students and practitioners may find this listing useful for quick reference. At the time of writing (July 2015), CPA Canada plans to continue to use the old *Handbook* sections for other assurance engagements and association rules.

References to U.S. auditing standards, issued by the Public Company Accounting Oversight Board (PCAOB) for public companies and the American Institute of CPAs (AICPA) for non-public companies, are also included where these are relevant in the Canadian environment. This brings students to the leading edge of auditing and responds to the increasing focus on international auditing and accounting standards in the real world of business management.

Risk-Based Auditing

The approach in this text is risk-based auditing. The risk-based audit approach builds on the idea of the strategic systems approach to auditing, developed in the 1990s, stressing that the auditor needs to understand the auditee's business as management runs it to conduct an effective audit. By formally placing these business risk assessment requirements into the standards, the CASs link these requirements clearly to GAAS, which outline the required procedures and judgments supporting the auditor's opinion on whether the financial statements are materially misstated.

This edition continues to build on and further develop a unique feature of the previous edition's concept of accounting risk. Accounting risk extends the risk-based approach to financial reporting issues to estimation uncertainties of accounting estimates, including the fair value accounting of IFRS. This approach clarifies the reasonable range, point estimates, and significant risk concepts introduced in CAS 540 and helps make operational the assessment of estimation uncertainties. This approach also provides a more complete explanation of auditee information risks, a clearer link between audit and accounting theory, and thus an improved basis for making operational the words *present fairly* and ethical reporting in the audit report. Under our critical thinking approach, auditing and accounting standards are increasingly viewed as an integrated framework. We believe that such or related approaches represent the future of 21st-century audited financial reporting.

Fraud Auditing

This text was the first to contain full-chapter coverage of fraud awareness auditing, a crucial topic in the new millennium. With the rapid global growth in white-collar crime, especially that of fraudulent financial reporting, auditors have had to take more responsibility for fraud detection, particularly in the area of premature revenue recognition. We now devote two chapters to this increasingly important topic. Chapter 7 introduces students to the requirements of CAS 240 and CAS 250 as part of basic audit concepts. The purpose of the advanced fraud chapter (Chapter 21, available on Connect) is to create awareness of, and sensitivity to, the signs of potential errors, irregularities, frauds, and corruption. The chapter contains some unique insights into extended auditing, investigation procedures, and detection of fraudulent accounting estimates using the accounting risk concept. In addition, fraud coverage is integrated throughout the text, consistent with the increased need for auditors to detect fraud and other unethical reporting.

Current Audit Environment

A continuation from the previous edition, the current audit environment perspective includes the changes to the auditing standards, the regulatory environment, and society's expectations, as well as an analysis of the significance of these changes. Specific new-millennium topics include the new audit report, increased monitoring of the profession by accountability boards such as the Canadian Public Accountability Board (CPAB), increased emphasis on good corporate governance, the increased importance of audit committees, independence guidance, fraud risk assessments, the risk-based audit approach, increased liability due to statutory law, and increased risks associated with more extensive use of fair value estimates and accounting estimates in general.

Critical Thinking for Ethical Reporting

The pioneering coverage of skepticism and logical argumentation in auditing has been expanded to the broader concept of critical thinking for ethical reporting. Such an expanded approach to a more formalized skepticism incorporates assessments of the character of individuals with whom the auditor deals, the language used in the reasoning, and the logic of the reasoning. Such an approach to skepticism and ethical reasoning is increasingly important in detecting fraudulent financial reporting. Critical thinking provides an improved framework for tackling issues that require integration of ethical, accounting, and audit reasoning. Critical thinking concepts are first introduced in Chapter 3 and then are found integrated throughout the text where appropriate, as well as in new critical thinking discussion and Application Case questions. The revised Appendix 3A coverage of ethics and natural-language reasoning used by auditors to document justification for their conclusions will help students to better understand accountability for their decisions. The accounting risk concept is a major innovation to help make critical thinking for the detection of unethical reporting more operational in a financial reporting setting. The critical thinking material is intended to better prepare students for the realities of a world in which CPAB, PCAOB, and other regulators are taking a harsher view of auditor performance in today's auditing environment.

Learning Aids

Each chapter and section in *Auditing: An International Approach* contains a number of pedagogical features that both enhance and support the learning experience. They include the following:

- **Learning Objectives.** Each chapter opens with a list of pertinent learning objectives for the ensuing chapter material. These are repeated throughout the chapters. In addition, all Multiple Choice Questions, Exercises and Problems, and Discussion Cases are cross-referenced to their corresponding Learning Objectives to assist student learning.

- **Essentials.** At the start of each chapter, we provide a concise overview of the entire topic coverage of the chapter, with a selection of related review questions. The Essentials section can provide a detailed introduction before tackling the details of the chapter, or it might be used for brief coverage of a topic that an instructor may wish to cover at a high level only.

- **Standards Checks.** Excerpts from the CASs are provided to enrich the discussion of key concepts by demonstrating how the standards require them to be applied by auditors in practice.

- **Professional Standards References.** Each chapter references the relevant professional standards for the chapter topics.

- **Anecdotes and Asides.** Illustrative anecdotes and asides are found throughout the text and have been updated considerably in this new edition. Some are located within the chapter text, while others stand alone (in boxes) to add realism and interest for students. A continuing fictional case is provided for the EcoPak company, with an episode of the case appearing at the start of each chapter. In each episode, many of the concepts and issues to be presented in the chapter arise in a realistic audit setting. The result is a real-world flavour of the treatment of auditing.

- **Exhibits.** To assist in the learning process, we have included several more exhibits in this edition to visually illustrate teaching concepts.

- **Icons for Critical Thinking, Fraud/Ethics, International Standards, and Internet Assignments.** For quick and easy identification purposes, we have included these icons to flag the text material dealing with these major issues.

Application Cases with Solution & Analysis

Most chapters include an Application Case with Solution & Analysis illustrating the application of concepts introduced in the chapter. The purpose of the Application Cases is to enliven the study of auditing by introducing the professional judgments involved in the practice of auditing. They supplement the exposition of auditing fundamentals with illustrative situations based on real events. The Application Cases in the chapters of Parts 2 and 3 follow the experiences of a new auditor joining a firm of PAs. Many of the Application Cases deal with what might be considered advanced material by many. Nevertheless, they can serve as a useful basis for class discussion. The solutions provided are not the only ones possible; consequently, they provide an opportunity to develop the critical perspectives that are an important element of professional judgment in auditing.

Key Terms

Throughout the text, key terms are highlighted in boldface print, with definitions conveniently located at the bottom of the page containing the bolded term. Understanding these terms is crucial to success in auditing. An alphabetical glossary is also provided at the end of the text.

ORGANIZATION

Part I: Introduction to Auditing, Public Practice, and Professional Responsibilities

Part 1 consists of four chapters covering the basic orientation to auditing as a profession. Chapter 1 introduces the concept of auditing and the role of the public accounting profession. Chapter 2 introduces GAAS, assurance standards, and quality control standards, providing an overview of the audit process. Chapter 3 introduces professional ethics and professional legal responsibilities, including a technical appendix on critical thinking incorporating the auditor's social role and social expectations. Chapter 4 covers audit reports with emphasis on the new audit report to go into effect at the end of 2016.

Part 2: Basic Auditing Concepts and Techniques

Part 2 is organized to present financial statement audit planning from a business risk perspective. Chapter 5 introduces the most basic concepts of an independent financial statement audit engagement, including the acceptance decision, the auditor's need to understand an auditee's business and its risks, preliminary analytical procedures, and materiality. Chapter 6 explains how auditors' understanding of the business, its environment, and its risks is used to assess the risk that the financial statements are materially misstated. It explains the key concept of financial statement assertions, and the business processes and the related accounting cycles that create the financial statements. Chapter 7 expands on the business understanding and risk assessment by providing an overview of information systems controls used by management to reduce risks of materially misstating this information. Chapter 7 also discusses the auditor's awareness of fraud risk; it explains the nature and signs of fraud and the procedures used to detect it. Chapter 8 presents the fundamental concepts of audit evidence and the evidence-gathering procedures used to develop the detailed audit plan and programs, as well as describing working paper documentation. Chapter 9 elaborates on internal control consideration in an audit engagement, describing the auditor's procedures for evaluating the auditee's internal control, and control risk assessment and control testing in performing the audit.

The topics presented in Chapters 5 through 9 provide a basis for developing an appropriate overall strategy for the audit, the detailed audit plan, and specific programs used to perform the audit. Chapter 10 covers the pervasive concept of audit testing, the major categories of risk that arise in a sampling context and how these relate to audit risk, how testing is affected by the audit risk model, and how representative testing can be implemented using the most simple formulas and tables from statistical sampling. An extensive appendix to Chapter 10 (Appendix 10B, available on Connect) provides more details on the technical aspects of statistical sampling. Application Cases are used to provide practical perspectives on the planning issues covered in Part 2.

Part 3: Performing the Audit

Part 3 contains four chapters that address performing the work set out in a detailed audit plan for the main business processes that will need to be managed in every organization, a fifth chapter that wraps it all up with audit completion considerations, and a sixth chapter that covers applying professional judgment. The processes covered are as follows: the Revenues, Receivables, and Receipts Process (Chapter 11); the Purchases, Payables, and Payments Process (Chapter 12); the Payroll and Production Processes (Chapter 13); and the Finance and Investment Process (Chapter 14). Each of these chapters provides an overview of the transactions, balances, and risks of misstatement in the business process, the relevant controls, and auditing procedures. Application Cases are used to illustrate the application of concepts and techniques in practice, and examples of audit programs are provided to demonstrate the kinds of audit procedures that can be used. Each of these chapters also provides an overview of the balance sheet approach as a basis for the overall analysis of the financial statements. Chapter 15 presents various activities involved in completing the audit work, such as the audit of the revenue and expense accounts, overall analytical review, lawyer's letters, management representation letters, and subsequent events. Chapter 16 provides an overview of issues to consider in the opinion formulation process, including accumulation of misstatements discovered in the audit, adjustments to the financial statements, and the auditor's formation of the opinion to be expressed in the audit report. This chapter includes a summary of the recently issued ISAs that will require expansion of the specific details auditors will report related to their audit opinions.

Part 4: Advanced Issues in Professional Public Accounting Practice

The five chapters in Part 4 (all available on Connect) are designed to stand alone or be integrated piecemeal with the preceding chapters as part of a first course in auditing. However, there is enough material in Part 4 that, when combined with some of the earlier chapters and some readings, such as those indicated in the text, can be the basis for a second, advanced, audit course. Such a course could focus, for example, on auditor problems and judgments in evaluating the quality of financial reporting.

Chapter 17 deals with other assurance and some non-assurance services offered by public accounting firms. Chapter 18 covers the more detailed aspects of professional ethics. Chapter 19 is a new chapter devoted to the increasingly important topic of the audit of accounting estimates. The chapter has two parts. Part I clarifies the difficult concepts of CAS 540 using the idea of accounting risk that can be associated with the point estimate concept of CAS 540. Part II deals with the more complex issues of estimation uncertainty associated with reasonable ranges of CAS 540. Estimation uncertainty is analyzed and integrated with the IFRS conceptual framework for financial reporting with the help of the accounting risk concept. This integration guides auditor judgments with respect to appropriate financial reporting. New analytical tools in the form of accounting analytics using market information and Monte Carlo simulations to help verify accounting estimates have been added to the discussion. These tools help make operational critical thinking about the ethics of accounting estimates. Chapter 20 covers auditor legal liability issues in more detail, extending the coverage of this topic beyond the introductory level of Chapter 3. Finally, Chapter 21 covers the conceptual framework for assurance engagements and some specialized assurance engagements. The second half of Chapter 21 covers fraud awareness auditing in more detail. It gives students a better understanding of the mindset and specialized procedures needed to more effectively detect frauds. This chapter has benefited from our association with the Association of Certified Fraud Examiners (ACFE).

PROFESSIONAL STANDARDS

This text contains numerous references to, and excerpts from, authoritative statements on auditing standards and to standards governing other areas of practice. Even so, it goes beyond the mere repetition of passages from the standards, concentrating on explaining their substance and operational meaning in the context of making auditing decisions. Instructors and students may wish to supplement the text with current editions of pronouncements published by the International Federation of Accountants (IFAC), CPA Canada, and the Institute of Internal Auditors.

MARKET-LEADING TECHNOLOGY

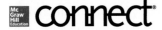

Learn without Limits

McGraw-Hill Connect® is an award-winning digital teaching and learning platform that gives students the means to better connect with their coursework, with their instructors, and with the important concepts that they will need to know for success now and in the future. With Connect, instructors can take advantage of McGraw-Hill's trusted content to seamlessly deliver assignments, quizzes, and tests online. McGraw-Hill Connect is the only learning platform that continuously adapts to each student, delivering precisely what they need, when they need it, so class time is more engaging and effective. Connect makes teaching and learning personal, easy, and proven.

Connect Key Features

SmartBook® As the first and only adaptive reading experience, SmartBook is changing the way students read and learn. SmartBook creates a personalized reading experience by highlighting the most important concepts a student needs to learn at that moment in time. As a student engages with SmartBook, the reading experience continuously adapts by highlighting content based on what each student knows and doesn't know. This ensures that he or she is focused on the content needed to close specific knowledge gaps, while it simultaneously promotes long-term learning.

Connect Insight® Connect Insight is Connect's new one-of-a-kind visual analytics dashboard—now available for both instructors and students—that provides at-a-glance information regarding student performance, which is immediately actionable. By presenting assignment, assessment, and topical performance results together with a time metric that is easily visible for aggregate or individual results, Connect Insight gives the user the ability to take a just-in-time approach to teaching and learning, which was never before available. Connect Insight presents data that empower students and help instructors improve class performance efficiently and effectively.

Simple Assignment Management With Connect, creating assignments is easier than ever, so instructors can spend more time teaching and less time managing. Instructors can

- Assign SmartBook learning modules
- Edit existing questions and create their own questions
- Draw from a variety of text-specific questions, resources, and test bank material to assign online
- Streamline lesson planning, student progress reporting, and assignment grading to make classroom management more efficient than ever

Smart Grading When it comes to studying, time is precious. Connect helps students learn more efficiently by providing feedback and practice material when they need it, where they need it. Instructors can

- Automatically score assignments, giving students immediate feedback on their work and comparisons with correct answers
- Access and review each response; manually change grades or leave comments for students to review
- Track individual student performance—by question or assignment or in relation to the class overall—with detailed grade reports
- Reinforce classroom concepts with practice tests and instant quizzes
- Integrate grade reports easily with Learning Management Systems including Blackboard, D2L, and Moodle

Instructor Library The Connect Instructor Library is a repository for additional resources to improve student engagement in and out of the class. It provides all the critical resources instructors need to build their course. Instructors can

- Access instructor resources
- View assignments and resources created for past sections
- Post their own resources for students to use

Instructor Resources

The instructor area of Connect includes a variety of resources for faculty:

- *Instructor's Solutions Manual.* The solutions manual, created by the authors, provides the answers to problem and assignment material that is featured throughout the text.
- *Computerized Test Bank.* The computerized test bank contains numerous multiple-choice, short-answer, and essay questions.
- *Microsoft® PowerPoint® Lecture Slides.* The PowerPoint slides offer a summary of chapter concepts for lecture purposes.
- *Image Library*

Superior Learning Solutions and Support

The McGraw-Hill Education team is ready to help you assess and integrate any of our products, technology, and services into your course for optimal teaching and learning performance. Whether it's helping your students improve their grades, or putting your entire course online, the McGraw-Hill Education team is here to help you do it. Contact your Learning Solutions Consultant today to learn how to maximize all of the resources!

For more information on the latest technology and Learning Solutions offered by McGraw-Hill Education and its partners, please visit us online: **http://www.mheducation.ca/highereducation/educators/digital-solutions/**.

ACKNOWLEDGMENTS

IFAC and CPA Canada have generously given permission for liberal quotations from official pronouncements and other publications, all of which lend authoritative sources to the text. In addition, several publishing houses, professional associations, and accounting firms have granted permission to quote and extract from their copyrighted material. Their cooperation is much appreciated because a great amount of significant auditing thought exists in this wide variety of sources.

We are also very grateful to the staff at McGraw-Hill Education, who provided their support, management skills, and ideas—especially our editorial team, whose hard work and attention to detail kept us on track and transformed what we wrote into a book.

A special acknowledgment is due to Stephen Spector, CGA, Simon Fraser University, who gave very insightful and thorough feedback on early drafts of the sixth and seventh editions. Many of you know Stephen from manning the CGA booth at CAAA conferences over many years. We finally got a chance to work closely with Stephen, and we must say he contributed greatly to improving the textbook and the instructor's manual. Many thanks, Stephen! Of course, any remaining errors are our responsibility.

A special acknowledgment is also due to Joseph T. Wells, former chairman of ACFE. He created the Certified Fraud Examiner (CFE) designation. Mr. Wells is a well-known authority in the field of fraud examination education, and his entrepreneurial spirit has captured the interest of fraud examination professionals throughout North America.

Special acknowledgment is also due to Steven E. Salterio of Queen's University. Steven contributed greatly to the strategic systems approach to auditing used in this text. Special thanks go to Enola Stoyle for material that was adapted in various forms in this text.

We are grateful to many people involved in the auditing profession in various roles who generously shared their time and ideas with us over the years as the new materials for the book took shape in our minds and on paper, including Keith Bowman, Gary Peall, Rebecca Yosipovich, Dawn McGeachy-Colby, Jim McCarter, Terri McKinnon, Dinh N. Tran, Murad Bhimani, Phil Cowperthwaite, Brian Leader, Susan Cox, participants at the auditing educators' workshop sessions held at the Ted Rogers School and the CAAA during 2011, Joanne Jones, Martha Tory, Luke Baxter, Borden Rhodes, Zak Bensiddick, Sunmin Groot, Jean Bédard, Janne Chung, Susan McCracken, Steve Fortin, Geneviève Turcotte, John Carchrae, James Sylph Alan Willis, Robert Langford, Andre de Haan, Joy Keenan, Sylvia Smith, Dianne Hillier, Jan Munro, Greg Shields and the AASB staff, Karen Duggan, Rand Rowlands, Mark Davies, Mark Lam, and Vaani Maharaj. Thank you very much to Catherine Barrette for providing a number of challenging new end-of-chapter questions for this edition.

We would like to acknowledge our appreciation for the great academics and practitioners who influenced us in various ways as we developed this text, including Ron Gage, Al Rosen, Randy Keller, Don Cockburn, Dagmar Rinne (rest in peace, Dagmar), Morley Lemon, Ingrid Splettstoesser-Hogeterp, Don Leslie, Larry Yarmolinsky, Bill Scott, Efrim Boritz, Joel Amernic, Donna Losell, Ulrich Menzefricke, Russell Craig, Kevin Lam, Yoshihide Toba, Takatoshi Hayashi, Ping Zhang, Hung Chan, Len Brooks, Manfred Schneider, and Irene Wiecek. Also, we have been inspired often by Rod Anderson's 1984 text, *The External Audit*, which set out a logical, conceptual framework for auditing that still stands the test of time.

This text could not have been completed without the cooperation and input of our many auditing students who have shared their perspectives with us over the years. We thank them greatly for their contributions and for encouraging us to make the text ever clearer.

And, lastly, our sincere thanks go out to the reviewers of this seventh edition for their careful review and many detailed and candid comments. We are deeply grateful to all the reviewers who have so diligently read our early chapter drafts and taken so much time to share their experience and wonderful, inspiring examples of how they teach auditing concepts. In each edition, we try to incorporate as many of these excellent ideas and suggestions as our publication page constraints allow:

Shiraz Charania, *Langara College*

Susan Deakin, *Fanshawe College*

Mohamed Dirira, *University of New Brunswick*

Shelley Donald, *University of Waterloo*

Amanda Flint, *Trinity Western University*

Ernie Kerst, *Sheridan Institute of Technology*

Camillo Lento, *Lakehead University*

Erin Marshall, *University of Alberta*

Jagdish Pathak, *University of Windsor*

Wendy Popowich, *Northern Alberta Institute of Technology*

Linda Robinson, *University of Waterloo*

Alla Volodina, *York University*

Cheryl Wilson, *Durham College*

Brad Witt, *Humber College*

Wally Smieliauskas and Kate Bewley
July 2015

Introduction to Auditing

Chapter 1 is an introduction to auditing, especially financial statement auditing. Other accounting courses helped you learn the principles and methods of accounting, but here you will begin to study the ways and means of auditing—the verification of accounting and other information.

LEARNING OBJECTIVES

After completing this chapter, you will be able to do the following:

LO1 Explain the importance of auditing.

LO2 Distinguish auditing from accounting.

LO3 Explain the role of auditing in information risk reduction.

LO4 Describe the other major types of audits and auditors.

LO5 Provide an overview of international auditing and its impact on Canadian Auditing Standards.

LO6 (Appendix 1A) Explain how to become a professional accountant in Canada.

LO7 (Appendix 1B) Distinguish alternative theories of the role of auditing in a society.

CHAPTER APPENDICES

APPENDIX 1A How to Become a Professional Accountant in Canada (on Connect)

APPENDIX 1B Alternative Theories of the Role of Auditing in Society (on Connect)

EcoPak Inc.

Throughout this text, each chapter will open with an episode of the EcoPak Inc. case study. This case study will provide you with a practical context to examine perspectives on how audits are actually performed and to study the important role of the financial statement audit. The EcoPak Inc. case study is a fictional case based on a composite of real events and issues that arise in financial reporting for a growing business.

Kam and Mike have been best friends since high school. While at university, Kam studied business, and Mike studied environmental engineering, but they both ended up finding jobs with Waterfalls Inc., a large 100-year-old public company in the paper and packaging industry. After a few years spent working their way up Waterfalls' corporate ladder, both Kam and Mike are doing quite well. Often, though, when they meet up for lunch, the two of them reminisce about all the ideas they had had years before for businesses they could start up. Kam's aunt, Zhang, is a very successful entrepreneur in the recycled-paper industry, and Kam had always hoped to follow her path.

One day while golfing with Georgina, Waterfalls' chief financial officer, Kam learns that Waterfalls' board has decided to sell off the poorly performing manufacturing division, StyreneTech Inc., Waterfalls' 100%-owned subsidiary producing polystyrene-foam packaging products for the food services industry. According to Georgina, Styrene-Tech's poor performance is due to changes in demand for polystyrene-foam packaging; environmental regulations favouring other materials; and a major fraud in which a purchasing manager was diverting shipments of ethylene raw material to another factory, of which he was part owner. Georgina hints to Kam that Waterfalls' board would favour a management buyout "to avoid having a lot of venture capitalists sniffing around."

Kam tells Mike about this right away, and the wheels start turning. Mike meets with StyreneTech's operations manager and, from their conversation, sees a huge opportunity to move the StyreneTech packaging business into the 21st century by converting its production over to new biomass-based materials, which are biodegradable and made from renewable resources. This would address the environmental concerns and costs that have been dragging StyreneTech's performance down. Once Kam gets his Aunt Zhang interested in the investment, things move quickly. Kam and Mike start looking into the financial side of buying out the StyreneTech business. A large investment from Zhang is needed to come up with the amount Waterfalls wants for the StyreneTech shares.

Since Waterfalls owns 100% of StyreneTech, it must present its shareholders with audited consolidated financial statements (i.e., statements that include the accounts of StyreneTech). Waterfalls' auditors, Grand & Quatre, Public Accountants (G&Q), provided an opinion that Waterfalls' consolidated financial statements were fairly presented at its last fiscal year-end. Georgina gives Kam a copy of StyreneTech's most recent stand-alone–entity financial statements and tells him that while these financial statements have been "reviewed for accuracy" by Waterfalls' internal auditor, they are only needed for tax purposes, so Waterfalls does not pay to have G&Q audit them.

Zhang, however, demands audited financial statements for StyreneTech before she will invest. Kam took just a couple of accounting courses in business school, and Mike does not know anything about financial statements at all, so they are beginning to feel overwhelmed, not really understanding why Zhang wants audited financial statements or how they would get them. Luckily, Mike's sister Nina is a professional accountant working for a mid-sized public accounting firm as an audit manager. Nina agrees to come in on weekends to help them with their finance and accounting, in exchange for shares in the company if they ever get it going. They ask Nina about the audited financial statements. Mike knows about Canada Revenue Agency (CRA) tax auditors—if the StyreneTech financial statements were done for tax reasons, wouldn't that mean they have been audited by a government auditor, someone famous like the Auditor General of Canada, maybe? And what about the internal auditor—why isn't Zhang satisfied with the internal auditor's review of the StyreneTech financial statements?

Nina explains that the StyreneTech financial statements should be audited by independent public accountants (PAs), such as G&Q, because this will give all the prospective investors assurance that the most reliable information about StyreneTech's financial condition and performance is presented. Because G&Q will be independent of Waterfalls' management, and it will perform an examination of Waterfalls' records to support their opinion that the financial information is reliable, this can lessen the investors' concerns that management may be biasing the results upward to get a higher selling price. While Zhang, Kam, and Mike do not have access to StyreneTech's financial information, nor do they have the expertise to assess its reliability, the auditor will do it on their behalf and thus reduce the risk that they are getting biased or inaccurate information.

This makes sense to Kam and Mike—it would be too risky to buy the shares of StyreneTech without getting the audited financial statements. Kam relays this to Georgina, who sighs and says, "Okay, we were going to have to do that eventually anyway, to sell it to venture capitalists, so we will get G&Q to audit the StyreneTech financial statements and get them to you within four weeks."

The Essentials of Auditing, Public Practice, and Professional Responsibilities

Auditing is the verification of information by someone other than the one providing that information. While many types of information can be audited, this text focuses on audits of an entity's financial statements, which summarize the entity's transactions and business events over a period.

Auditing is important in our society because many economic activities are set up as three-party accountability arrangements. In a three-party accountability structure, one party has to rely on the actions and information provided by another party, who may not share the same interests. For example, if the owner of a business (principal) hires a manager (agent) to operate the business, the owner may have a long-term perspective on the sustainability of the business, and the manager may have much shorter term goals. The owner could have concerns that the manager will provide overstated reports of profit to hide poor performance, or take out higher executive compensation than the business can sustain for the long run. There is a risk, which we call information risk, that financial statement information will not be a full, true, and fair representation of the transactions and events that occurred and hence will not be reliable for economic decision making. Unreliable financial statements mean that the financial statements are so full of errors and omissions that the information risk is sufficiently high to mislead users of the financial statements. In other words, financial statements with high information risk result in unethical reporting.

Information risk can be reduced by having another party, the independent auditor, verify how well the information reflects the underlying realities of the entity's operations. The auditor should have no conflict of interest regarding the financial reporting and should be objective, so that the auditor's opinion has value in providing assurance to users of financial statements that the information can be relied on. Unfortunately, auditors sometimes fail to reduce information risk because they lack independence or don't do an effective job of verification, which has resulted in some highly publicized financial calamities, such as Enron, Parmalat, and Sino-Forest. Events such as these have increased the responsibilities of auditors to detect unethical reporting of all kinds—a very big challenge facing auditors today.

How exactly does an independent audit reduce information risk? First, note that auditors are professionals who can offer their accounting and auditing services to the public. Professionals are expected to be competent in their area of specialty and to put the interests of public users of their services ahead of their own interests. The accounting/auditing profession issues standards for quality control in accounting firms, education and qualification of members who will provide public accounting services such as audits, and ethical conduct codes. For auditing, the profession issues standards and guidelines for how to perform an examination that will give the auditor reasonable assurance that financial statements are fairly presented (i.e., not materially misstated), and for how to communicate the conclusions drawn to others. The concept of reasonable assurance describes a mental attitude that the auditor gains from the conclusions drawn from audit examination findings. Based on the examination, if the auditor believes the financial statements to be fairly stated, the auditor will communicate this belief to financial statement users as an opinion in the Auditor's Report. This opinion, in essence, provides a high level of assurance to the user that the auditor believes that the information risk is low and has evidence to support that belief.

An important insight from the three-party accountability perspective is that preparing financial accountability information is not the same thing as auditing it. In fact, the person who prepares financial information cannot audit it because they could never really be objective about it. As a result, the use of an auditing function is seen in a wide range of accountability situations besides financial reporting, such as government spending, taxation, operational audits, assessing environmental contamination, and fraud investigations.

Many members of the auditing profession are not involved in offering audit or other assurance services to the public, and may work in related areas such as general accounting, tax, and consulting. They are still required to adhere to all the professional standards relevant to their work. Over time, the development of professional standards for accounting and auditing has been shifting toward international bodies, leading to more global convergence in accounting and auditing practices.

Review Checkpoints

1-1   Using the example of a business with an owner, a hired manager, and an independent financial statement auditor, apply the three-party accountability structure: Which party would be the first, the second, and the third party in the model? For what is each party accountable?

1-2   What does the concept "reasonable assurance" refer to? How does it relate to information risk reduction?

Introduction: The Concept of Auditing

LO1   Explain the importance of auditing.

Auditing is a field of study that has received considerable media attention lately. In the business press, audit-related issues are mentioned daily. Headlines such as "The Dozy Watchdogs," "The Betrayed Investor," "Dirty Rotten Numbers," and "Accounting in Crisis" indicate that the attention has not all been positive. This reality arises from the fact that auditing is critical to the proper functioning of capital markets, and if audits are perceived to fail, then capital markets can do the same. Without effective audits, modern capital markets cannot fulfill their role as efficient economic systems leading to high living standards. A European Commission Green Paper[1] has concluded that auditors, regulators, and corporate governance are key contributors to financial stability and economic growth. An example of an effective auditor is shown in the box below.

An Effective Auditor

Molex Incorporated is a $2.2 billion electronics manufacturer headquartered in Chicago. In late 2004 Molex's auditor, Deloitte & Touche, complained that CEO J. Joseph King and his CFO had not disclosed that they allowed a bookkeeping error worth 1% of net income into the audited results. When the auditor demanded on November 13 that King be removed from office, the board initially stood behind the CEO with a unanimous vote.

Then Deloitte did something unexpected: It quit. Two weeks later the firm wrote a blistering and detailed account of the affair for public disclosure at the U.S. Securities and Exchange Commission (SEC). That virtually assured that no auditor would work for Molex again as long as King was in charge. Within 10 days the directors had eaten crow: They ousted King, promised to hire a new director with financial expertise for their audit committee, and agreed to take training classes in proper financial reporting.

Source: "The Boss on the Sidelines," *BusinessWeek*, April 25, 2005, p. 94.

The preceding example illustrates the work of effective auditors in the business environment of the 21st century. In modern business, the role of auditing is so critical that references can be made to **audit societies**. In audit societies, economic activities (and other politically important ones) are extensively monitored to ensure market efficiency. In these societies, auditors also monitor the effectiveness and efficiency of government. For example, the political uproar surrounding Canada's Gomery commission inquiry in 2005 was the result of an audit of questionable sponsorship payments that yielded "no value" for taxpayer money spent. As a result of this and similar events, auditing is increasingly recognized as part of a broader process of social control. This expanding role is at the heart of the audit society concept.[2]

But what is auditing, exactly? Simply put, **auditing** is the verification of information by someone other than the one providing that information. Since there are many types of information, there are many types of audits. Most of this text focuses on audits of financial statement information, or *financial statement auditing* for short. Before describing auditing in more detail, we will try to make financial statement auditing more intuitive through a simple illustration.

A Simple Illustration of the Importance of Auditing

Assume you have always wanted to run your own business—say, a Thai food restaurant. After some searching, you find an owner who wants to retire and is willing to sell his busy restaurant in a choice location of a major metropolitan area for $3 million. One of the first things you ask yourself is whether the business is worth the $3 million asking price. How can you answer that?

You could find out the price of similar properties—comparison shop. But, ultimately, you must decide on the value of this particular business. Accounting information is useful in answering these types of questions: What is the business's net worth (Assets – Liabilities)? What is its profitability?

The owner of the restaurant may claim annual profits of $600,000. First, you want to reach an agreement on how that profit is calculated: on a cash basis? before tax? after tax? under generally accepted accounting principles (GAAP)? These are the criteria you might use in measuring the profitability (earnings) of the business.

Having decided on the criteria for measurement, you need to use a decision rule with your measurement. Businesses are frequently valued on some multiple of earnings. For example, if you are willing to pay five times current earnings (calculated using your agreed-upon criteria) and the current owner reports $600,000 in earnings annually, you would be paying five times $600,000 or $3 million for the business. You need accounting information to establish that $600,000 is the current earnings number.

But the owner prepares the accounting records. How do you know they are accurate? There may be errors or, worse, the owner might inflate earnings to get a higher price than the business is worth. For example, if the owner is overstating the earnings and they are only $500,000, the most the business is worth to you is five times $500,000, or $2.5 million, rather than $3 million. In other words, you are concerned about the risk of overpaying for your investment.

What can you do to minimize this risk and give yourself assurance? Hire an auditor! The auditor can help you by verifying that the $600,000 figure reported by the current owner is accurate. The earnings can be calculated

---

audit societies:
the term coined by Michael Power for societies in which there is extensive examination by auditors of economic and other politically important activities

auditing:
the verification of information by someone other than the one providing that information

on whatever basis you agree to, usually **generally accepted accounting principles (GAAP)**, such as International Financial Reporting Standards (IFRS) for publicly accountable enterprises and Accounting Standards for Private Enterprises (ASPE) for private enterprises, which you have studied in your financial accounting courses. The auditor can independently and competently verify the earnings so that you will have more confidence (assurance) in the numbers upon which you base your decision. The auditor increases the reliability, or reduces the risk, of using inaccurate information in your decision making (i.e., the auditor reduces information risk). For example, if the auditor finds that earnings are really $400,000, you should be unwilling to pay more than five times $400,000, or $2 million, for the restaurant. The difference between the original asking price ($3 million) and what you should actually pay ($2 million) is the value of the audit—in this case $1 million. If the audit fee is less than $1 million, you are, therefore, better off having an audit.

This simplified example illustrates the value of auditing in investment decision making. But it also shows how auditing can provide other, more general, social services. For example, the restaurant owner can retire with a fair price for his business, and you can achieve your dreams of owning a restaurant and being your own boss. These are accomplished by using a fair exchange price based on reliable (accurate, trustworthy) information.

The transaction entries that you learn in your accounting courses are part of the raw data auditors deal with. All of the transactions over a period are summarized in financial statements. When auditors verify the reliability of this information, they reduce the information risk associated with financial statements. Now, imagine this illustration extended to all investors contemplating even partial ownership of a business—for example, investors in the stock market—and you will have some idea of how auditing can facilitate efficient economic activities by reducing financial information risk. And when auditors fail to do a proper job of verification (i.e., fail to reduce information risk), the type of headlines noted at the beginning of this section can result.

When you make an investment, you agree to enter into a contract to purchase from another party. The auditor can be called the first party and the seller the second party. Notice, however, that there is a third party—you, the investor. The auditor is an independent party hired to verify information provided by the second party. The auditor is hired because you, the third party, do not trust the information provided by the second party. You feel the information risk is too high; therefore, the first party will provide you with independent verification. We refer to this relationship throughout the text as **three-party accountability**. Note that in the EcoPak Inc. example at the beginning of this chapter, Aunt Zhang is the one demanding the audited financial statements for StyreneTech. She wants reliable, trustworthy information on the prospects for StyreneTech before she is willing to make an investment in it. She wants the information risk on StyreneTech to be sufficiently low (meaning the information has a higher chance of being complete and true) before she is willing to act on that information. Information risk is discussed in more detail later in this chapter.

In an audit society, three-party accountability is so institutionalized that regulators require certain second parties to pay for the audit. In particular, companies whose shares are traded on regulated stock exchanges (public companies) are required to hire an independent auditor to verify the annual financial statements. The accountability is still three party because the audit's purpose is to reduce information risk for the third party, but the public company, the second party, pays the audit fee. It is important to remember that three-party accountability is not determined by who pays the fee.

Exhibit 1–1 indicates how three-party accountability applies to the Molex and Thai restaurant examples. In the exhibit, accountability is represented as a triangle with the auditor of the financial information, the

---

generally accepted accounting principles (GAAP):
those accounting methods that have been established in a particular jurisdiction through formal recognition by a standard-setting body, or by authoritative support or precedent, such as the accounting recommendations of the *CPA Canada Handbook*

three-party accountability:
an accountability relationship in which there are three distinct parties (individuals): an asserter, an assurer, and a user of the asserted information

EXHIBIT 1–1

Three Parties Involved in an Auditing Engagement (Three-Party Accountability)

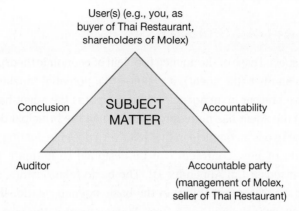

management preparing the financial information, and the users of the financial information at the vertices. The triangle reflects an **accountability relationship** because management is accountable to the users. However, the users cannot rely on financial statements, as they do not trust management sufficiently; they demand that financial statements be verified by a competent, independent auditor. Thus, the auditor is also accountable to the user. Three-party accountability is an important distinguishing feature of auditing.

Note that the concept of three-party accountability means that the auditor is expected to act in the interests of the user of financial statements. If the owner of the Thai restaurant gives you an audited set of financial statements, you are entitled to assume that the auditor has not misled you. This is an important point because if you could not assume the auditor is trustworthy, the relevance of the audit would largely disappear, leaving little, if any, role for the audit in society. Thus, it is extremely important to the audit profession that the auditor be perceived as acting in the interests of the financial statement users (i.e., the third parties), also referred to as **acting in the public interest**. Later in this text, you will see how the public interest is reflected in the objectives of the audit engagement, in auditors' legal liability, and in the professional rules of conduct that determine the auditor's professional role.

Three-party accountability is also important because it distinguishes the type of services that only certified or licensed practitioners can provide (depending on the province) from other services, such as tax work and business-advisory services, which anyone can provide. Audits are part of a broader class of services called *assurance engagements* that are restricted to qualified chartered or licensed accounting professionals (licensed CPAs). This licensing or certification is required to protect the public interest that arises from three-party accountability. *Public accounting* is the term given to services that give rise to three-party accountability and the requirement to act in the public interest. Examples of third parties to which chartered or certified public accountants are accountable include the reporting firm's shareholders, lenders, regulators, employees, customers, suppliers, various levels of government, and the general public. Three-party accountability applies to all assurance engagements. We will clarify these important concepts throughout the rest of the text. For now, think

accountability relationship:
a relationship in which at least one of the parties needs to be able to justify its actions or claims to another party in the relationship

acting in the public interest:
acting in the interests of the users of the financial statements; also, more generally, fulfilling the social role expected of the professional accountant

of three-party accountability as reducing the risk on information created by the second party, the preparer of the information, to foreseeable third parties who use the information. Reducing information risk is synonymous with improving the credibility of, or providing assurance on, information produced by the second party.

Agency Theory and Accountability

Three-party accountability is a special case of the agency problem of economic theory. Whenever a task is delegated by one party (the principal) to another (the agent), it can create a potential "agency problem." Agency problems occur when three conditions are present in an agency relationship: (a) the agent has objectives that are different from those of the principal, (b) the agent has more information than the principal does (information asymmetry), and (c) the contract between the two is incomplete in that not every possible contingency can be anticipated.

Agency theory is the study of how contracts can be designed to mitigate the agency problem. Various solutions to this problem are discussed in Appendix 1B. The basic relationships are illustrated in Exhibit 1–2. The arrows indicate the direction of accountability in the basic agency relationship between the management (agent) and the shareholder/owner (principal) of a firm. Management is the party accountable to the owners, and one way it satisfies this accountability is by preparing financial statements. Financial statements are one way of monitoring how well management is running the firm. However, there is a potential problem in that management may bias its statements, making financial statements less credible. The auditor comes in as an outside, independent accounting expert to verify the accuracy of financial statements, thereby adding credibility to the statements. The auditor, thus, helps monitor management.

EXHIBIT 1–2

Agency Theory and Accountability

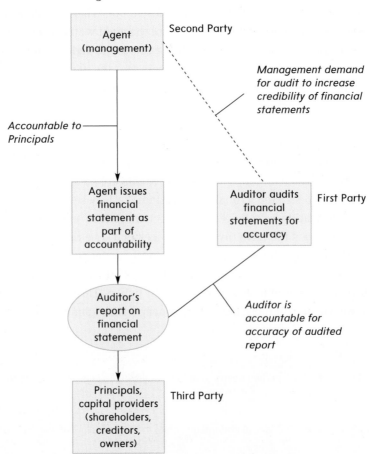

The important thing to note about Exhibit 1–2 is that the auditor is primarily accountable to the principal (owner or capital provider) and not to management, which, acting on behalf of the company, has historically hired and authorized payment for audit services. This fact can create a **conflict of interest** problem for the auditor that affects the auditor's independence in verifying the accuracy of management's statements. The auditor cannot help monitor management if the auditor is not independent of management. This helps explain the importance of auditor independence that is stressed throughout this text, an importance that arises from the objective of meeting third-party needs. Auditor independence and third-party needs also greatly shape ethical reasoning in an audit context, as we will see in Chapter 3. Later in this text, you will learn how corporate governance changes have strengthened three-party accountability by separating various functions that used to be centralized in top management. For now, the important point is that third-party capital providers do not have access to the same information as management, something referred to in the next section as the "remoteness" of accounting information to third-party users.

We hope you have found the preceding illustrations useful. Next, we further clarify the roles of accounting and auditing in the financial reporting environment.

User Demand for Reliable Information

LO2   Distinguish auditing from accounting.

Accounting

The following three underlying conditions affect users' demand for accounting information:

1. *Complexity.* A company's transactions can be numerous and complicated. Users of financial information are not trained to collect and compile it themselves. They need the services of professional accountants.

2. *Remoteness.* Users of financial information are usually separated from a company's accounting records by distance and time, as well as by lack of expertise. They need to employ full-time professional accountants to do the work they cannot do for themselves.

3. *Consequences.* Financial decisions are important to the state of investors' and other users' wealth. Decisions can involve large dollar amounts and massive efforts. The consequences are so important that good information, obtained through the financial reports prepared by accountants, is an absolute necessity.

Accounting is the process of recording, classifying, and summarizing into financial statements a company's transactions that create assets, liabilities, equities, revenues, and expenses. It is the means of satisfying users' demands for financial information that arise from the forces of complexity, remoteness, and consequences. The function of **financial reporting** is to provide statements of financial position (balance sheets), statements

---

conflict of interest:
a situation faced by a professional accountant in which there may be a divergence between the interests of two (or more) parties (e.g., clients) for whom the professional accountant undertakes a professional activity, or between the interests of the professional accountant and the interests of such parties, that could create a threat to the professional accountant's objectivity or other fundamental ethical principles

accounting:
the process of recording, classifying, and summarizing into financial statements a company's transactions that create assets, liabilities, equities, revenues, and expenses

financial reporting:
the broad-based process of providing statements of financial position (balance sheets), statements of results of operations (income statements), statements of results of changes in financial position (cash flow statements), and accompanying disclosure notes (footnotes) to outside decision makers who have no internal source of information such as the management of the company has

of results of operations (income statements), statements of results of changes in financial position (cash flow statements), and accompanying disclosure notes (footnotes) to outside decision makers. A company's accountants are the producers of such financial reports. In short, accounting tries to record and summarize economic reality for the benefit of economic decision makers (the users).

Because of advances in **information technology (IT)**, the form and location in which accounting records are stored has changed dramatically over the past few decades. Although these changes have affected the form of audit evidence, the basic role of verification for users and their decision-making needs has not changed.

The goal of GAAP, which you study in your financial accounting courses, is to yield financial statements that represent as faithfully as possible the economic conditions and performance of a company. This is why GAAP are the most common criteria used in preparing financial statements. However, as illustrated in the introduction, auditors are independent financial reporting experts who are frequently asked to verify that these goals are met.

Review Checkpoints

1-3   Explain how the auditor can help you in your investment decision making.

1-4   Why would Aunt Zhang in the EcoPak Inc. case want audited financial statements even if she has to pay extra for them?

More on Auditing

Financial decision makers usually obtain their accounting information from companies wanting loans or selling stock. This is a potential conflict of interest, a condition that leads to society's demand for audit services. Users need more than just information; they need reliable, error-free information. Preparers and issuers (directors, managers, accountants, and others employed in a business) might benefit from giving false, misleading, or overly optimistic information. The potential conflict is real enough to generate a natural skepticism on the part of users. Thus, users depend on **external auditors**, professional accountants who serve as objective intermediaries and add credibility to financial information. This "adding of credibility" is also known as **providing assurance**, and external auditing of financial statements is described as an **assurance engagement**.

Auditing does not include financial report production. That function is performed by a company's accountants under the direction of management. Auditors determine whether the information in the financial statements is reliable, and they communicate this conclusion to the users by reporting that the company's presentation of financial position, results of operations, and cash flow statement are in accordance with GAAP, or some other disclosed basis of accounting. This is the assurance provided by the assurance function, as it relates to the traditional financial statements. Assurance requires three-party accountability, as discussed previously. To achieve three-party accountability, auditors must not be involved in producing the information audited. Auditors can provide a range of services in addition to audits, and so they are frequently referred to as *public accounting firms*.

information technology (IT):
the hardware and software needed to process data

external auditors:
auditors who are outsiders and independent of the entity being audited

providing assurance:
the adding of credibility to financial information by objective intermediaries

assurance engagement:
an engagement in which the auditor adds either reasonable (high) or moderate (negative) levels of assurance

External auditors work for clients. A **client** is the person (company, board of directors, agency, or some other person or group) who retains the auditor and pays the fee. In financial statement audits, the client and the auditee are usually the same economic entity. The **auditee** is the company or entity whose financial statements are being audited. Occasionally, the client and the auditee are different entities. For example, if Conglomerate Corporation hires and pays the auditors to audit Newtek Company in connection with a proposed acquisition, Conglomerate is the client and Newtek is the auditee. In practice, these two terms are used interchangeably, possibly because the auditee is usually the one paying the auditor.

As explained previously, reliable financial information helps make capital markets efficient and helps people understand the consequences of a wide variety of economic decisions. External auditors practising the assurance function are not, however, the only auditors at work in the economy. Bank examiners, CRA auditors, provincial regulatory agency auditors (e.g., auditors with a province's Commissioner of Insurance), internal auditors employed by a company, and the Office of the Auditor General of Canada (OAG) (or a provincial equivalent) all practise auditing in one form or another. Many acronyms are associated with various auditing associations and auditors. The acronyms are part of the jargon of the profession.

Professional judgment is a widely used concept in accounting and auditing. It is defined in Canadian Auditing Standard (CAS) 200, paragraph 13(k), as "the application of relevant training, knowledge, and experience, within the context provided by auditing, accounting, and ethical standards, in making informed decisions about the courses of action that are appropriate in the circumstances of the audit engagement." Professional judgment is a process used to reach a well-reasoned conclusion. Professional judgment is based on the relevant facts and circumstances at the time the audit decision is made. Professional judgment is critical to effectively performing an audit. Auditors use professional judgment to focus on the most important aspects of an audit. These include determining the nature, timing, and extent of audit procedures and evaluating the appropriateness of the application of GAAP by management.

Professional judgment also involves identifying reasonable alternatives. Careful and objective consideration of information that may seem contradictory to a conclusion is critical to the appropriate application of professional judgment, which is essential to the appropriate application of accounting and auditing standards.

Documentation of professional judgment at the time the judgments are made is also very important. Documentation demonstrates that a sound process was followed and helps the development of a well-reasoned conclusion. This improvement of professional judgment by documentation helps explain why the expression "not documented, not done" is effectively a standard of audit practice. When professional judgment is challenged, contemporaneous documentation shows the analysis of the facts, circumstances, and alternatives considered as well as the basis for conclusions reached. The extent of documentation and effort used in the process will vary with the significance and complexity of an issue. When the professional judgment process is appropriately applied and contemporaneously documented, it is much easier to support and defend the conclusion reached. On the other hand, decisions that appear to be arbitrary; not supported by the facts, evidence, or professional literature; or not well reasoned or well documented are difficult to support.

client:
the person or company who retains the auditor and pays the fee

auditee:
the entity (company, proprietorship, organization, department, etc.) being audited; usually it refers to the entity whose financial statements are being audited

professional judgment:
the application of relevant training, knowledge, and experience, within the context provided by auditing, accounting, and ethical standards, in making informed decisions about the courses of action that are appropriate under the circumstances of the audit engagement

All the above attributes of professional judgment require the involvement of individuals with sufficient knowledge and experience. In addition, an attitude of professional skepticism is essential to the professional judgment process.

Professional skepticism, a term that appears frequently in auditing literature and speech, is an auditor's tendency not to believe management assertions but, instead, to find sufficient support for the assertions through appropriate audit evidence. Professional skepticism is an important aspect of professional judgment. Specifically, professional skepticism means recognizing that circumstances causing the financial statements to be materially misstated may exist (CAS 200.15). Note that to implement this concept of skepticism, the auditor first needs to define "misstatement" and "materiality" and then implement them in practice. You will see that doing this appropriately will present its own challenges.

The word *skepticism* is derived from the Greek word *skeptesthai*, meaning "to reflect, look, or view." It has evolved from ancient Greek philosophy over 2,300 years old to represent the application of reason and critical analysis in supporting a conclusion. Skepticism as adopted by auditors is an important attitude for fulfilling their duties. A skeptical mindset is the key to detecting fraud or other unethical behaviour. The auditor should always consider whether his or her approach is sufficiently skeptical.

Professional skepticism is inherent in applying due care in accordance with professional standards. The business environment that has seen errors and fraud in financial reports dictates this basic level of professional skepticism: A potential conflict of interest always exists between the auditor and the management of the enterprise under audit. This follows from the fact that auditors must add credibility to the financial statements by gathering their own evidence to support their conclusions on the truthfulness and completeness of the financial statements. The belief that the potential for conflict of interest always exists causes auditors to perform procedures in search of misstatements and omissions that would have a material effect on financial statements. This is the primary reason that auditors are demanded and that we have three-party accountability. Professional skepticism tends to make audits more extensive and expensive. The extra work is not needed in the vast majority of audits where there are no material errors, irregularities, frauds, or ethical reporting issues.

Still, due audit care does call for a degree of professional skepticism—an inclination to question all material assertions made by management, whether oral, written, or contained in the accounting records. However, this attitude must be balanced by a willingness to respect the integrity of management. Auditors should neither blindly expect that every management is dishonest nor thoughtlessly assume management to be totally honest. The key lies in auditors' objectivity and in the audit requirement of gathering sufficient appropriate evidence and evaluating financial statement disclosures to reach reasonable and supportable audit decisions.

The checklist below summarizes the preceding discussion. Throughout this book you will learn more about how professional judgment, skepticism, and appropriate evidential support for a conclusion all combine to help achieve audits that result in sufficiently low information risk and ethical financial reporting.

Overview of Key Aspects of Professional Judgment in Auditing

✓ Is well reasoned
✓ Determines the nature, timing, and extent of audit procedures
✓ Evaluates the appropriateness of applicable GAAP
✓ Identifies other reasonable alternative accounting treatments
✓ Is performed with a mindset of professional skepticism: an inclination to question management assertions
✓ Is "not documented, not done": contemporaneous documentation of evidence and reasoning is needed

professional skepticism:
an auditor's tendency to question management representations and look for corroborating evidence before accepting these representations

Review Checkpoints

1-5   What is auditing? What condition creates demand for audits of financial reports?

1-6   What is the difference between a client and an auditee? What are the three parties in three-party accountability?

1-7   What is the difference between auditing and accounting?

1-8   What conditions create demand for financial reports, and who produces financial reports for external users?

Definitions of Auditing

Definitions of Auditing

In 1971, the American Accounting Association (AAA) Committee on Basic Auditing Concepts prepared a comprehensive definition of auditing as follows:

> Auditing is a systematic process of objectively obtaining and evaluating evidence regarding assertions about economic actions and events to ascertain the degree of correspondence between the assertions and established or suitable criteria and communicating the results to interested users.

This definition contains several ideas important in a wide variety of audit practices. The first and most important concept is the perception of auditing as a systematic process that is purposeful, logical, and based on the discipline of a structured approach to decision making. Auditing is not haphazard, unplanned, or unstructured.

The audit process, according to this definition, involves obtaining and evaluating evidence consisting of all the influences that ultimately guide auditors' decisions, and it relates to assertions about economic actions and events. When beginning an audit engagement, an external auditor receives financial statements and other disclosures by management that are management's assertions about economic actions and events (assets, liabilities, revenues, expenses). Evidence is then gathered to either substantiate or contradict these management assertions.

External auditors generally begin work with explicit representations from management—assertions of financial statement numbers and information disclosed in the notes to financial statements. When these assertions are made explicit in writing by the accountable party (the asserter), the resulting audit engagement is referred to as an **attest engagement**. Financial statements are an example of written assertions, and thus the audit of financial statements is an attest engagement. Not all auditors are provided with such explicit representations. An internal auditor, for example, may be assigned to evaluate the cost-effectiveness of the company's policy to lease rather than purchase equipment. A government auditor may be assigned to determine whether the goal of creating an environmental protection agency has been met by the agency's activities. Often, these latter types of auditors must develop the explicit standards of performance for themselves. This type of engagement is called a **direct reporting engagement**.

The purpose of obtaining and evaluating evidence is to determine the degree of correspondence between the assertions and suitable criteria. The findings will ultimately be communicated to interested users. To

attest engagement:
when a public accountant is hired to perform procedures and issue a report resulting from those procedures that affirms the validity of an assertion; also known as an *attestation engagement*

direct reporting engagement:
a type of assurance engagement in which the assertions are implied and not written down in some form

---

EXHIBIT 1–3

Overview of Financial Statement Auditing

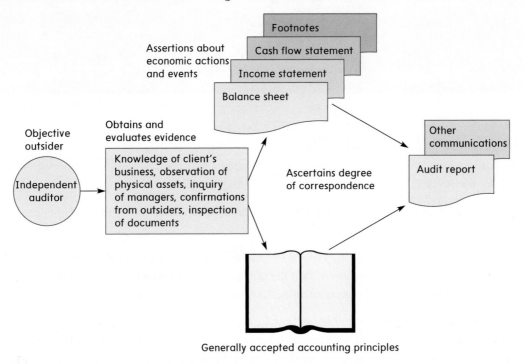

Generally accepted accounting principles

---

communicate in an efficient and understandable manner, there must be a common basis, or suitable criteria, for measuring and describing financial information. These suitable criteria appear in a variety of sources. For external auditors, government auditors, and CRA inspectors, the criteria largely consist of GAAP. CRA inspectors also rely heavily on criteria specified in federal tax acts. Government auditors may rely on criteria established in legislation or regulatory agency rules. Bank examiners and provincial insurance board auditors look to definitions and rules of law. Internal and government auditors rely extensively on financial and managerial models of efficiency and economy, as well as on GAAP. All auditors rely to some extent on the elusive criteria of general truth and fairness.

Exhibit 1–3 depicts an overview of financial statement auditing.

Audit Objective and the Auditor's Report

The AAA definition of auditing is broad and general enough to encompass external, internal, and governmental auditing. In Canada, the CASs, as issued by **Chartered Professional Accountants of Canada (CPA Canada)**, set forth the main objective of a financial statement audit as follows:

> The purpose of an audit is to enhance the degree of confidence of intended users in the financial statements. This is achieved by the expression of an opinion by the auditor on whether the financial statements are prepared, in all material respects, in accordance with an applicable financial reporting framework.[3]

Chartered Professional Accountants of Canada (CPA Canada):
the professional body of chartered professional accountants in Canada

The CPA Canada statement of objective restricts auditing interest to external auditors' audit of the traditional financial statements and accompanying notes. However, as the needs of users change, new audit objectives and reports are created to meet them. Thus, the *CPA Canada Handbook* also offers guidance on such divergent topics as reporting on control procedures at service organizations, solvency issues, and examining a financial forecast in a prospectus. A set of evolving "assurance standards" provides a framework governing a wide range of assurance services, including audit services. These expanding standards indicate a corresponding demand for new types of audits and an expanded social role for auditing. This is consistent with an evolving audit society. Historically, the demand for an expanded role for auditing has grown faster than standard setters' ability to meet the public's expectations of audits. As a result, an **expectations gap** has developed between what the public expects of auditors and what auditors can actually deliver. For example, historically, the public has expected auditors to take on more responsibility for fraud detection and ethical reporting than the standards required. In addition, many people assume that audited financial statements are exact to the nearest penny and that there are no uncertainties associated with financial statements. The expectations gap is discussed further in the context of ethical reporting in Appendix 1B.

The auditor's opinion on financial statements is expressed in the second paragraph of the audit report. This is the culmination of the auditor's work, and almost everything that you will be studying in this text is geared to supporting this conclusion. Hence it is very important!

A standard report is shown in Exhibit 1–4. This is the report that will be required on audits after December 15, 2016. The report to be used before that date is given in Exhibit 1–5. Chapter 4 explains this and other audit reports in more detail. For now, we highlight some key features of it, beginning with the second paragraph. The key words in the second paragraph, the opinion paragraph of the opinion section, are "financial statements present fairly, in all material respects. . . ." This is the auditor's conclusion, and it is intended for the users of financial statements. The third paragraph, the one that ends with "We believe . . . ," tells the user on what basis the auditor reached the conclusion. It tells the user of financial statements that there is a link between the opinion and the audit evidence, something that you will be covering in most of this book. The link supports the conclusion, and it explains why you gather audit evidence. What do you think "independent" means in the third paragraph? See the discussion in the Application Case at the end of the chapter. The fourth paragraph describes key audit matters that were considered significant in a particular audit. The fifth, sixth, and seventh paragraphs summarize the responsibilities of management and corporate governance. The eighth paragraph summarizes auditor responsibilities. There is a reference to additional description of responsibilities, which are discussed in Chapter 4. All this is made public to the user of the report so that the issuing auditor should be willing to stand by the claims in the report. To prove that the auditor is not lying about these claims, audit standards require the auditor to document their work during the audit engagement and to demonstrate the basis of their conclusions. In this book, we refer to one of the **Canadian Auditing Standards (CASs)** as a CAS. Unless otherwise indicated, the equivalent International Standard on Auditing (ISA) is the same number as the CAS number. For example, CAS 700 and ISA 700 refer to the same standard, except for some minor variations, explained later. We refer to each CAS by the number associated with it, such as CAS 700.

Exhibit 1–5 is the standard audit report that can be used before December 15, 2016. It is provided here for completeness. In this text we will focus on the report given in Exhibit 1–4.

expectations gap:
the difference that can arise between what the public expects of the auditor's social role and what the professional standards and practices deliver

Canadian Auditing Standards (CASs):
the auditing standards in Canada using the equivalent International Standards on Auditing (ISAs) and the same numbering system as the ISAs; the subset of assurance standards dealing with "high" or "reasonable" levels of assurance in assurance engagements

EXHIBIT 1–4

Independent Auditor's Report (for audits beginning after December 15, 2016—see Exhibit 1–5 for a standard audit report before this date)

INDEPENDENT AUDITOR'S REPORT

To the Shareholders of ABC Company (or Other Appropriate Addressee)

Report on the Audit of the Financial Statements

Opinion

We have audited the financial statements of ABC Company (the Company), which comprise the statement of financial position as at December 31, 20X1, and the statement of comprehensive income, statement of changes in equity, and statement of cash flows for the year then ended, and notes to the financial statements, including a summary of significant accounting policies.

In our opinion, the accompanying financial statements present fairly, in all material respects (*or give a true and fair view of*), the financial position of the Company as at December 31, 20X1, and (*of*) its financial performance and its cash flows for the year then ended in accordance with International Financial Reporting Standards (IFRS).

Basis for Opinion

We conducted our audit in accordance with Canadian Auditing Standards (CASs). Our responsibilities under those standards are further described in the *Auditor's Responsibilities for the Audit of the Financial Statements* section of our report. We are independent of the Company in accordance with the Provincial Ethics Standards Board for Accountants' *Code of Ethics for Professional Accountants* together with the ethical requirements that are relevant to our audit of the financial statements in [*jurisdiction*], and we have fulfilled our other ethical responsibilities in accordance with these requirements and the Code. We believe that the audit evidence we have obtained is sufficient and appropriate to provide a basis for our opinion.

Key Audit Matters

Key audit matters are those matters that, in our professional judgment, were of most significance in our audit of the financial statements of the current period. These matters were addressed in the context of our audit of the financial statements as a whole, and in forming our opinion, thereon, and we do not provide a separate opinion on these matters.

[Description of each key audit matter in accordance with CAS 701]

Responsibilities of Management and Those Charged with Governance for the Financial Statements *

Management is responsible for the preparation and fair presentation of the financial statements in accordance with IFRS, ** and for such internal control as management determines is necessary to enable the preparation of financial statements that are free from material misstatement, whether due to fraud or error.

In preparing the financial statements, management is responsible for assessing the Company's ability to continue as a going concern, disclosing, as applicable, matters related to going concern and using the going-concern basis of accounting unless management either intends to liquidate the Company or to cease operations, or has no realistic alternative but to do so.

Those charged with governance are responsible for overseeing the Company's financial reporting process.

Auditor's Responsibilities for the Audit of the Financial Statements

Our objectives are to obtain reasonable assurance about whether the financial statements as a whole are free from material misstatement, whether due to fraud or error, and to issue an auditor's report that includes our opinion. Reasonable assurance is a high level of assurance, but it is not a guarantee that an audit conducted in accordance with CASs will always detect a material misstatement when it exists. Misstatements can arise from fraud or error and are considered material if, individually or in the aggregate, they could reasonably be expected to influence the economic decisions of users taken on the basis of these financial statements.

[Additional description of auditor responsibilities is required here, or referenced to an appendix to the report, or reference can be made to a website of an appropriate authority that contains the description of the auditor's responsibilities—the additional description of responsibilities is discussed in Chapter 4 of this textbook.]

The engagement partner on the audit resulting in this independent auditor's report is [name].

[Signature in the name of the audit firm, the personal name of the auditor, or both, as appropriate for the particular jurisdiction]

[Auditor Address]

[Date]

---

* Throughout these illustrative auditor's reports, the terms management and those charged with governance may need to be replaced by another term that is appropriate in the context of the legal framework in the particular jurisdiction.

** Where management's responsibility is to prepare financial statements that give a true and fair view, this may read, "Management is responsible for the preparation of financial statements that give a true and fair view in accordance with IFRS, and for such . . ."

Source: *CPA Canada Handbook—Assurance*, CAS 700, "Forming an Opinion and Reporting on Financial Statements."

EXHIBIT 1–5

Auditor's Standard Report (until December 15, 2016)

To the Shareholders of . . . . .

Report on the Financial Statements

We have audited the accompanying financial statements of ABC Company, which comprise the balance sheet as at December 31, 20X1, and the income statement, statement of changes in equity, and cash flow statement for the year then ended, and a summary of significant accounting policies and other explanatory notes.

Management's Responsibility for the Financial Statements

Management is responsible for the preparation and fair presentation of these financial statements in accordance with Canadian generally accepted accounting principles; this includes the design, implementation, and maintenance of internal control relevant to the preparation and fair presentation of financial statements that are free from material misstatement, whether due to fraud or error.

Auditor's Responsibility

Our responsibility is to express an opinion on these financial statements based on our audit. We conducted our audit in accordance with Canadian generally accepted auditing standards. Those standards require that we comply with ethical requirements and plan and perform the audit to obtain reasonable assurance whether the financial statements are free from material misstatement.

An audit involves performing procedures to obtain audit evidence about the amounts and disclosures in the financial statements. The procedures selected depend on the auditor's judgment, including the assessment of the risks of material misstatement of the financial statements, whether due to fraud or error. In making those risk assessments, the auditor considers internal control relevant to the entity's preparation and fair presentation of the financial statements in order to design audit procedures that are appropriate in the circumstances, but not for the purpose of expressing an opinion on the effectiveness of the entity's internal control. An audit also includes evaluating the appropriateness of accounting policies used and the reasonableness of accounting estimates made by management, as well as evaluating the overall presentation of financial statements.

We believe that the audit evidence we have obtained is sufficient and appropriate to provide a basis for our audit opinion.

Opinion

In our opinion, the financial statements present fairly, in all material respects, the financial position of ABC Company as of December 31, 20X1, and of its financial performance and its cash flows for the year then ended in accordance with Canadian generally accepted accounting principles.

[Auditor's signature]

[Date of auditor's report]

[Auditor's address]

Source: *CPA Canada Handbook—Assurance*, CAS 700, "Forming an Opinion and Reporting on Financial Statements."

A Definition of Auditing Relating to "Risk Reduction"

LO3   Explain the role of auditing in information risk reduction.

Although it is sometimes difficult to distinguish between a definition and a theory, most statements of theory begin with a definition. The theory that auditing is a "risk reduction activity" is gaining popularity, and the following definition supports this view:

> Auditing in financial reporting is a process of reducing (to a socially acceptable level) the information risk to users of financial statements.

Economic activity takes place in an atmosphere of **business risk**. Business risks result from significant conditions, events, circumstances, or actions that might adversely affect the entity's ability to achieve its objectives and execute its strategies (*CPA Canada Handbook—Assurance*, CAS 700, "Forming an Opinion and Reporting on Financial Statements"). Auditors do not directly influence a company's business risk, but they are responsible for ensuring proper disclosure of these risks by the auditee in the financial statements. As the business world becomes more complex, auditors are finding that they must increasingly focus on understanding the client's business risks in order to judge whether the financial statements reflect them properly. It is emphasized in auditing that risk is an important part of economic substance that should be reflected in financial reporting. A good illustration of the effects of business risks related to the economic crisis that began in 2008 is given in the "Accounting Blamed for Global Credit Crisis" box below.

Accounting Blamed for Global Credit Crisis

Wall Street executives and lobbyists say they know what helped push the nation's largest financial institutions over the edge in recent months. The culprit, they say, is accounting.

Companies including American International Group Inc., the insurer that accepted $85 billion in a U.S. takeover, have said the rule by the U.S. Financial Accounting Standards Board requires them to record losses they don't expect to incur. Financial service companies have reported more than $520 billion in write-downs and credit losses since last year [2007]. Supporters of the rule say companies seeking the exemption are citing fair value as a way to cover their poor performance.

Fair value "is an accounting issue that's too important to be left just to accountants," former SEC Chairman Harvey Pitt said in an interview today. Economists, academics and regulators from outside FASB, in addition to accountants, should be involved in considering a new approach to fair value, he said.

"What the banks are telling everyone is that the accounting has caused the problem," former SEC chief accountant Lynn Turner said. "The only thing fair-value accounting did is force you to tell investors you made a bunch of very bad loans."

". . . The banking lobby is also confusing the role of accounts. These should simply be a true and fair record of management's stewardship of the business. How the owners, regulators, and tax authorities that read accounts choose to interpret them is their choice. Complaining about what the accounts show, when we're talking about a system supported by such users of accounts as investors and regulators, is akin to blaming a torch for shining a light on the mess in your cupboard."

As an example of recent accounting challenges, analysts cite Merrill Lynch's sale of $30.6 billion of collateralized debt obligations, or pools of mortgage-linked assets, to the investment company Lone Star Funds for only 22 cents on the dollar in July [2008]. Jessica Oppenheim, a spokeswoman for Merrill, which this month [September 2008] agreed to be purchased by Bank of America, declined to comment.

Advocates for leading financial institutions, including the Financial Services Roundtable and the American Bankers Association, have been raising the issue with government officials in Washington and New York for months. Arizona Sen. John McCain, the GOP presidential candidate, mentioned fair-value accounting as a problem in a recent stump speech.

Lobbyists have been seeking temporary relief from the accounting measure, which they say establishes bargain-basement prices for assets that would be valued far higher during more normal trading conditions. The events of last week raised fresh concerns among industry executives who fear that investments sold to the government as part of the $700 billion bailout plan will set a bargain-basement precedent for the rest of the market.

Banks also have been fighting their auditors, some of which have reasoned that downmarket conditions have persisted for so long that assets are no longer "temporarily impaired" but now require write-downs and capital infusions. Banking trade association officials are scheduled to meet with SEC regulators this week to discuss the issue, which could prompt some banks to attract new capital to meet regulatory requirements.

"The accounting rules and their implications have made this crisis much, much worse than it needed to be," said Ed Yingling, president of the bankers' association. "Instead of measuring the flame, they're pouring fuel on the fire."

Sources: Excerpts from *Washington Post*, Sept. 23, 2008: D01 (Carrie Johnson); Bloomberg.com, Ian Katz, Sept. 23, 2008; and jennifer.hughes@ft.com, www.ft.com/accountancy, *The Financial Times* Limited, 2008.

business risk:
the probability that significant conditions, events, circumstances, or actions might arise that will adversely affect the entity's ability to achieve its objectives and execute its strategies

Information risk refers to the possible failure of financial statements to appropriately reflect the economic substance of business activities and related risks and uncertainties. It thus includes failure to properly disclose business risk. For example, if a company fails to disclose that it plans to file for bankruptcy, the risk of bankruptcy is a business risk, and failure to disclose it is an information risk. Note that information risk is influenced by the evidence of bankruptcy gathered by the auditor and by the accounting principles and rules (i.e., GAAP) for appropriately disclosing the bankruptcy risk. It is useful to remind yourself at this point that information risk arises from the agency relationship described above as part of the three-party accountability concept. Specifically, information risk arises from the information asymmetry and the conflicts of interest inherent in the agency relationship. Note that it is management (the agent) that must produce the information that is audited by the auditor. Thus it is management, not the auditor, that must accept responsibility for the kind of information provided. The auditor in turn accepts the responsibility for performing an appropriate audit of the information provided by management.

Information risk gives rise to the misstatements and omissions in information that auditors are hired to detect and suggest that management correct. That way, auditors reduce information risk, providing assurance that the information is more accurate with the auditor's involvement. This is why you, investing in the Thai restaurant scenario described earlier, or Aunt Zhang, in the EcoPak Inc. case study, may find it worthwhile to have management-prepared financial statements audited by an external auditor independent of management. The "Accounting Blamed for Global Credit Crisis" box illustrates the consequences of having too much information risk in financial reporting due to changes in accounting measurement concepts such as fair value accounting.

Information risk from the auditor's perspective is the risk (probability) that the financial statements distributed by a company will be materially false or misleading. **Materiality**, as used in auditing, means the same thing as it does in your accounting courses. Basically, a material misstatement is one that would affect user decision making. For example, in the Thai restaurant illustration, we saw that an investor might invest much less without an audit because the risk of material misstatement in the unaudited financial statements was very high.

Financial analysts and investors depend on financial reports for stock purchase and sale decisions; creditors (suppliers, banks, and so on) use them to decide whether to give trade credit and bank loans; labour organizations use them to help determine a company's ability to pay wages; and government agencies and Parliament use them in preparing analyses of the economy and making laws concerning taxes, subsidies, and the like. All these users cannot determine whether financial reports are reliable and, therefore, low on the information risk scale. They do not have the expertise, resources, or time to enter thousands of companies to satisfy themselves about the veracity of financial reports. Auditors assume the social role of attesting to published financial information, offering users the valuable service of assurance that the information risk is low. This role of auditors has been institutionalized through laws and regulations.

It is important to be aware that, from the auditor's perspective, there are two major categories of information risk. One is the risk of insufficient evidence being gathered on the facts concerning the client's (auditee's) economic circumstances. This is referred to as **audit risk (account level)**. The other category is the risk that errors associated with forecasts used in GAAP accounting estimates are not properly disclosed. We refer to this

---

information risk:
the possible failure of financial statements to appropriately reflect the economic substance of business activities

materiality:
an audit concept related to an auditor's judgment about matters, such as errors or omissions in the preparation and presentation of financial statements, that could reasonably be expected to influence economic decisions of people using those financial statements, i.e., matters that would be material to those decisions

audit risk (account level):
the probability that an auditor will fail to find a material misstatement that exists in an account balance

second category of information risk as **accounting risk (account level)**. Forecasts are the distinguishing feature of GAAP that separates GAAP accounting from cash basis accounting. Accounting risk is primarily the responsibility of accounting standards. Accounting risk is becoming more important with the increasing use of fair value accounting and the adoption of IFRS. You can see the challenges for auditors in deciding whether fair value accounting "presents fairly" in particular circumstances from the box "Accounting Blamed for Global Credit Crisis"! However, while the term *audit risk* is a key part of auditing standards, accounting risk is dealt with only indirectly in accounting standards. You likely did not encounter the accounting risk concept in your financial accounting courses because accounting theory is not as risk oriented as auditing theory is. This makes controlling information risk in financial reporting a major challenge for auditors. The accounting risk concept used in the more advanced parts of this text, especially Chapter 19, Part II (available on Connect), dealing with the audit of accounting estimates, helps address this key challenge of professional judgment in auditing.

The risk reduction definition may appear very general. As your study of auditing continues, you will find that the primary objective of many auditing tasks is reducing the risk of giving an inappropriate opinion on financial statements. Auditors are careful to work for trustworthy clients, to gather and analyze evidence about the data in financial statements, and to take steps to ensure audit personnel report properly on the statements when adverse information is known. Subsequent chapters will have more to say about these activities. We begin the process with the Application Case discussion at the end of this chapter. The table below summarizes the different aspects of information risk discussed in this chapter.

DIFFERENT DIMENSIONS OF INFORMATION RISK	
CONTRIBUTING FACTORS	**TYPES OF MISSTATEMENT**
Remoteness	Misstatement arising from audit risk
Complexity	
Three-party accountability	Misstatement arising from accounting risk
Conflict of interest	
Information asymmetry	

For now, consider the following box for a current illustration of a call for an audit that may have global repercussions.

Is There Any Gold Inside Fort Knox? An Example of a Burgeoning Demand for an Independent External Audit

Protected by a 109,000-acre [44,000-hectare] U.S. Army post in Kentucky sits one of the Federal Reserve's most secure assets and its only gold depository: the 73-year-old Fort Knox vault. Its glittering gold bricks, totalling 147.3 million ounces [4.176 million kilograms] (that's about US$265 billion as of August 10, 2011), are stacked inside massive granite walls topped with a bombproof roof. Or are they?

For several prominent investors and at least one senior U.S. congressman it is not the security of the facility in Kentucky that is a cause of concern: it is the matter of how much gold remains stored there—and who owns it.

They are worried that no independent auditors appear to have had access to the reported US$265 billion stockpile of brick-shaped gold bars in Fort Knox since the era of President Eisenhower. After the risky trading activities at supposedly

(continued)

accounting risk (account level):
the part of information risk due to incorrectly predicting events, especially in accounting estimates

safe institutions such as AIG, they want to be reassured that the gold reserves are still the exclusive property of the United States. and have not been used to fund risky transactions.

"It has been several decades since the gold in Fort Knox was independently audited or properly accounted for," said Ron Paul, the Texas congressman and former Republican presidential candidate, in an email interview with *The Times*. "The American people deserve to know the truth."

"We're taking the President at his word," said Chris Powell, of the Gold Anti-Trust Action Committee (GATA). "If you go online you can find out how to build a nuclear weapon but you won't find any detailed records on central gold reserves."

A month after President Nixon resigned over the Watergate affair, Congress demanded to inspect the contents of Fort Knox but the trip to Kentucky was dismissed by critics as a photo opportunity. Three years earlier Mr. Nixon brought an end to the gold standard when France and Switzerland demanded to redeem their dollar holdings for gold amid the soaring cost of the Vietnam War.

Many gold investors suspect that the United States has periodically attempted to flood the market with Fort Knox gold to keep prices low and the dollar high—perhaps through international swap agreements with other central banks—but facts remain scarce and the U.S. Treasury denies that any such meddling has gone on for at least the past decade.

Pressure for more openness is mounting after the collapse of the global banking system and renewed interest in a return to the simpler era of the gold standard—a subject that is likely to be raised at the G20 summit next week [April 2009]. China and Russia are calling for the creation of a new world reserve currency amid fears that the Federal Reserve's quantitative easing policy—essentially printing money—might cause hyperinflation, then collapse.

Sources: Excerpts from Chris Ayres in Los Angeles, from *The Times*, March 28, 2009, http://www.timesonline.co.uk/tol/news/world/us_and_americas/article5989271.ece, reprinted at http://www.gata.org/node/7309; and Constance Gustke, January 20, 2010, cbsnews.com/news/is-there-gold-in-fort-knox/#ixzz1RqjMgxrG.

The preceding box illustrates how demand for an audit can arise. Basically, people stop believing the reporting by the report preparer, in this case a government's assertions about the quantity of gold at Fort Knox. So an independent audit is demanded to add credibility. On the other hand, the Royal Canadian Mint announced in June 2009 that 17,500 ounces of Mint gold had been lost or stolen. This disappearance was confirmed during an audit of the Mint by Deloitte & Touche, CAs, under the direction of the Auditor General of Canada. The question asked by U.S. commentators is, if Canada audits its gold, why doesn't the United States? This lack of an independent audit, especially over lengthy periods of time, can raise credibility questions, as you can see from the box.

A related issue to consider at this point is how might you audit something like the quantity of gold? The obvious answer is to go see if it exists! That means actually going to Fort Knox and counting the gold bars. In fact, in auditing, the existence assertion that you will learn about later in this text specifies the need to verify the accuracy of the actual count. Not exactly rocket science! Somebody has to do it, and that somebody is the independent external auditor.

What other things would you need to do? Think of the questions being raised by the doubters of the contents of Fort Knox. It is important for you as an auditor to be aware of the concerns that users of your report may have. First, you would need to count the gold bars and check the accuracy of what is recorded at Fort Knox. Further tests could include checking serial numbers against records for accuracy, determining who owns the gold, and perhaps randomly testing the gold bars for purity. (One conspiracy theory is that the gold in Fort Knox is fake. Search "Is the gold in Fort Knox fake?" on Google to see what we mean.) While some of the conspiracy theories are far-fetched, an independent external audit would likely end much of the speculation. This is an example of how the demand for audits can grow spontaneously and why we are evolving toward an audit society.

Review Checkpoints

1-9 What would you say if asked by an anthropology major, "What do auditors do?"

1-10 What is the essence of the risk reduction definition of auditing?

Kinds of Audits and Auditors

LO4   Describe the other major types of audits and auditors.

The AAA, CPA Canada, and the risk reduction definitions apply to the financial statement audit practice of independent external auditors who practise in public accounting firms. The word *audit*, however, is used in other contexts to describe broader kinds of work.

The variety of audit work performed by different kinds of auditors causes problems with terminology. Hereafter in this text, the terms *independent auditor, external auditor, Chartered Professional Accountant (CPA),* and **public accountant (PA)** refer to people doing audit work with public accounting firms. In governmental and internal contexts, auditors are identified as governmental auditors, operational auditors, and internal auditors. While many of these are chartered accountants or certified general accountants, in this text, the initials PA will refer to CPAs in public practice.

Internal and Operational Auditing

The Institute of Internal Auditors (IIA) defines **internal auditing** and its purpose as follows:

> Internal auditing is an independent, objective assurance and consulting activity designed to add value and improve an organization's operations. It helps an organization accomplish its objectives by bringing a systematic, disciplined approach to evaluate and improve the effectiveness of risk management, control, and governance processes.[4]

Internal auditing is practised by auditors employed by organizations such as banks, hospitals, city governments, and industrial companies. Some internal auditing activity is known as operational auditing. **Operational auditing (performance auditing or management auditing)** is the study of business operations in order to make recommendations about the economic and efficient use of resources, effective achievement of business objectives, and compliance with company policies. The goal of operational auditing is to help managers discharge their management responsibilities and improve profitability.

Internal and operational auditors also perform audits of financial reports for internal use, much as external auditors audit financial statements distributed to outside users. Thus, some internal auditing work is similar to the auditing described elsewhere in this text. In addition, the expanded-scope services provided by internal auditors include (1) reviews of control systems for ensuring compliance with company policies, plans, procedures, and laws and regulations; (2) appraisals of the economy and efficiency of operations; and (3) reviews of program results in comparison with their objectives and goals.

Internal auditors need to be independent of the organization's line managers, much like the external auditors need to be independent of the company management. Independence helps internal auditors be objective and achieve three-party accountability. As noted earlier, you, as a user of audited information, expect the auditor to be unbiased and impartial, as well as competent, in verifying the accuracy of the information you rely on in

public accountant (PA):
an individual doing audit work with a public accounting firm; includes Chartered Professional Accountants (CPAs)

internal auditing:
verification work performed by company employees who are trained in auditing procedures; mainly used for internal control purposes, but external auditors can rely on internal audit work if certain criteria are met

operational auditing (performance auditing or management auditing):
auditors' study of business operations for the purpose of making recommendations about economic and efficient use of resources, effective achievement of business objectives, and compliance with company policies

making your decision. Internal auditors can recommend correction of poor business decisions and practices, and they can praise good decisions and practices. If they were responsible for making the decisions or carrying out the practices themselves, they would hardly be credible in the eyes of the upper-management officers they report to. Consequently, the ideal arrangement is to have internal auditors whose only responsibilities are to audit and report to a higher level in the organization, such as a financial vice-president and the audit committee of the board of directors. This arrangement offers an independence that enhances the appraisal function (internal audit) within a company.

Internal audit can be an important aspect of auditee internal controls, as they monitor auditee operations year round. When such internal independence exists, external auditors may also be able to rely quite a bit on internal audit work as a valuable source of evidence. In the environment of the influential *Sarbanes-Oxley Act* (SOX) legislation passed in the United States, internal auditor reports to independent audit committees are increasingly viewed as indispensable for good corporate governance. In addition, in the SOX world, if an external auditor performs internal audit functions, he or she is deemed to be insufficiently independent and prohibited from auditing for external reporting. Again, this helps preserve external auditor independence.

Public Sector (Governmental) Auditing

The Office of the Auditor General of Canada (OAG) is an accounting, auditing, and investigating agency of Parliament, headed by the Auditor General. In one sense, OAG auditors are the highest level of internal auditors for the federal government. Many provinces have audit agencies similar to the OAG, answering to provincial legislatures and performing the same types of work as we describe in this section. In another sense, the OAG and equivalent provincial auditors are really external auditors with respect to government agencies they audit, because they are organizationally independent.

Many government agencies have their own internal auditors and inspectors, for example, federal ministries such as the Department of National Defence or CRA and provincial education, welfare, and controller agencies. Well-managed local governments (cities, regions, townships) also have internal audit staff. Activities of all levels of government are frequently referred to as the **public sector**.

Internal and public sector auditors have much in common. The OAG and internal auditors share elements of expanded-scope services. The OAG, however, emphasizes the accountability of public officials for the efficient, economical, and effective use of public funds and other resources. CPA Canada sets accounting and auditing standards for all public sector audit engagements, including those of the federal, provincial, and local levels of government.

In the public sector, you can see the audit function applied to financial reports, and a compliance audit function applied to laws and regulations. All government organizations, programs, activities, and functions were created by law and are surrounded by regulations governing the things they can and cannot do. For example, in some provinces, there are serious problems of health card fraud by ineligible persons. A hospital cannot simply provide free services to anyone due to regulations about eligibility of tourists and visitors from other countries. A compliance audit of services involves a study of the hospital's procedures and performance in determining eligibility and treatment of patients. Nationwide, such programs involve millions of people and billions of taxpayers' dollars.

Also, in the public sector you see **value-for-money (VFM) audits**, a category that includes economy, efficiency, and effectiveness audits. Government is always concerned about accountability for taxpayers' resources,

public sector:
activities of all levels of government

value-for-money (VFM) audit:
an audit concept from the public sector that incorporates audits of economy, efficiency, and effectiveness

and VFM audits are a means of improving accountability for the efficient and economical use of resources and the achievement of program goals. VFM audits, like internal auditors' operational audits, involve studies of the management of government organizations, programs, activities, and functions. The following box indicates the range of activities that VFM audits can cover.

Some Examples of Recommendations Based on Value-for-Money Audits Conducted by the Ontario Office of the Provincial Auditor

Health care. Stronger efforts are needed in using available data to identify pharmacies overcharging the Ontario Drug Benefit Plan. Ontario is unprepared for a flu pandemic despite 44 deaths from the 2003 SARS crisis.

Archives. Hundreds of historically significant items, including a valuable Group of Seven painting, have gone missing. Inventory control practices need to be strengthened.

Education. Ontario university buildings are in need of $1.6 billion in repairs. Capital asset management systems need to be enforced.

Environment. Monitoring of hazardous waste shipment has been lax. Hundreds of tonnes of hazardous waste have gone missing. The ministry's own standards need to be better enforced.

Transportation. New drivers are more likely to be involved in collisions if they take the province's beginning driver education course than if they do not. Inappropriate handling of driver education certificates by unscrupulous driving schools is suspected. Systems and procedures for assuring the public's money is properly spent are inadequate.

Criminal law. Several hundred names are missing from the sex offender registry. Amendments to legislation are needed.

Source: 2007 annual report by the Office of the Provincial Auditor of Ontario, as summarized by the authors. More recent reports have similar content but not as varied.

The above list of audits illustrates the huge range of activities that can be audited and important areas of society that are affected. Audits can go well beyond financial statement reporting.

Comprehensive governmental auditing involves financial statement auditing, compliance auditing, and VFM auditing. It goes beyond an audit of financial reports and compliance with laws and regulations to include economy, efficiency, and effectiveness audits. The public sector standard on the elements of comprehensive auditing is similar to the internal auditors' view. Public sector standards do not require all engagements to include all types of audits. The scope of the work is supposed to be determined by the needs of those who use the audit results. Auditors' reputations are highest when they meet these needs.

Judging by the favourable media attention they receive, Canadian public sector auditors probably have the best reputation of any auditors in the world. For example, Christina Blizzard, a columnist for *The Toronto Sun*, stated in a 2002 column discussing a provincial auditor's report, "How come this province is run by politicians, and not by people who can add, subtract, and oh yes, negotiate a deal with the private sector that doesn't rip off taxpayers? What a pity politicians aren't better auditors—and auditors don't run the province."[5] Also, see below for an interview with former Auditor General of Canada Sheila Fraser. Awareness of the value of public sector audits has now spread to countries such as China, where the National Audit Office of the People's Republic of China has become increasingly active in monitoring China's financial system and exposing bribery, corruption,

---

comprehensive governmental auditing:
auditing that goes beyond an audit of financial reports to include economy, efficiency, and effectiveness audits

fraud, capital embezzlement, and inappropriate accounting in state-owned or state-controlled enterprises. Public sector auditors are helping make state capitalism a viable option in China. These public sector auditor roles are outstanding examples of evolving audit societies.

Sheila Fraser: Patron Saint of Auditors?

Auditor General Sheila Fraser laughs heartily when asked what it's like to be a celebrity.

"I've never really thought of myself as a celebrity, quite honestly. I mean, I'm an accountant. So accountants don't expect to get a lot of public recognition." Still, she adds, as her voice quietly trails off, "It has been an amazing time."

Indeed, it has.

In a decade during which Canadians have had three prime ministers—Jean Chrétien, Paul Martin and Stephen Harper—one thing in Ottawa has always been constant. Fraser, the country's top spending watchdog, was there to keep an eye on the politicians and their bureaucrats. To keep them honest.

She has been—odd as it may sound for an auditor general—a rock star to the Canadian people. Her non-partisan credibility is unimpeachable. Her audits have been fair but uncompromising. The media love her. The bureaucrats respect and fear her. The politicians don't dare criticize her. And now she is leaving. Her 10-year term is up. Monday is her last day on the job.

In a wide-ranging and candid interview with *Postmedia News,* Fraser discussed her tenure and whether bureaucrats trembled when they heard she was headed their way. "Quite frankly, no one likes to be audited. None of us. It's like when Revenue Canada phones you and says they're going to audit your tax return. None of us jump up with joy. I'm sure there is a bit of apprehension, but I would hope that they recognize that we are fair and we have a very rigorous process that we go through to ensure that our audits' conclusions are balanced and based on fact."

Fraser's office has conducted hundreds of audits—some routine, others headline-grabbing. She put a spotlight on the cost of the firearms registry, questionable spending by privacy commissioner George Radwanski and prisons ombudsman Ron Stewart, rebate cheques sent to thousands of dead people for home heating costs, shoddy background checks for passport applications, inadequate national emergency response plans, and the shortcomings of public sector integrity commissioner Christiane Ouimet.

But the two audits for which she will be remembered relate to the Quebec sponsorship program. The first was released in May of 2002. She reviewed $1.6 million in contracts awarded by Public Works to a Montreal-based firm, Groupaction, and found the government "did not obtain all of the services for which it paid."

Then came the quote for which she is famous. Fraser blasted senior public servants for breaking "just about every rule in the book." There was an "appalling lack of documentation" and a violation of rules and policies on financial transactions. "This is a completely unacceptable way for government to do business," she said at the time. "Canadian taxpayers deserve better." Strong words for an auditor general. The Mounties began an investigation for possible criminal violations.

It didn't end there. Fraser's instincts were razor sharp. She began a broader audit of all government advertising and sponsorship programs. In February 2004, that audit was released. It was a bombshell. She found Liberal-friendly communications firms collected millions of dollars in commissions for little, if any, work. "This is such a blatant misuse of public funds," said Fraser. "It is shocking." It was the catalyst for a string of events that would change Canadian history. It led to the Gomery commission of inquiry into political kickbacks and, eventually, criminal convictions against some involved in the sponsorship scheme. Ultimately, it contributed to a souring of public support for the governing Liberals and their defeat in the 2006 election by Stephen Harper's Conservatives.

Auditor General Sheila Fraser is leaving her post with a blunt warning for the federal government: Canadians need to be told much more about the looming costs of the aging population, climate change and this country's deteriorating infrastructure. . . .

On Wednesday, she acknowledged that the sponsorship audit was the most heavily covered by media and perhaps the most "sensational of the audits that we did." She said it led to an increase in her office's independence and an expansion of its mandate. The Quebec-born accountant is considered one of the most trustworthy and respected public officials—elected or otherwise—in Ottawa. Fraser was the third "most trusted Canadian" in a *Reader's Digest* poll published this month (behind environmentalist David Suzuki and building contractor Mike Holmes).

Sources: Excerpts from Mark Kennedy (*Natioanl Post,* May 25, 2011, news.nationalpost.com/news/canada/outgoing-ag-sheila-fraser-calls-for-focus-on-climate-health-care); Bruce Cheadle (*Canadian Press,* May 25, 2011); *HuffPost Canada Politics,* "Sheila Fraser as Auditor General: Her Greatest Hits and Reports," August 9, 2011, huffingtonpost.ca/2011/06/09/sheila-fraser-the-auditor-general_n_871980.html.

Regulatory Auditors

For the sake of clarity, other kinds of auditors deserve separate mention. You are probably aware of tax auditors employed by CRA. These auditors take the "economic assertions" of taxable income made by taxpayers in their tax returns and audit these returns to determine their correspondence to the standards found in the *Income Tax Act*. They also audit for fraud and tax evasion. Their reports can either clear a taxpayer's return or claim that additional taxes are due.

Federal and provincial bank examiners audit banks, trust companies, and other financial institutions for evidence of solvency and compliance with banking and other related laws and regulations. In 1985, these examiners as well as external auditors made news with the failures of two Alberta banks—the first Canadian bank failures in over 60 years.

Fraud Auditing and Forensic Accounting

Fraud is an attempt by one party (the fraudster) to deceive someone (the victim) for gain. Fraud falls under the Criminal Code and includes deception based on manipulation of accounting records and financial statements. Recently, auditor responsibilities to detect fraud have significantly increased. Financial statement auditors are now responsible for detecting material financial reporting fraud. They can no longer presume that management is honest. The PA needs to look for fraud risk factors. Some firms are beginning to screen clients before any wrongdoing is even suspected. The screening is done by specialist auditors who may do sensitive interviews or review unusual transactions and suspicious circumstances. In a normal audit, the procedures are diagnostic, not investigative. This is a distinction we will make clear later in the text.

Fraud auditing is a separate engagement that might be done on behalf of the audit committee—a special in-depth investigation of suspected fraud by those with specialized training, and often involving a specialist auditor. It is a proactive approach to detecting financial statement deception using accounting records and information, analytical relations, and awareness of fraud perpetration and concealment in developing investigative procedures.

Fraud auditing and forensic accounting are huge growth areas for public accounting firms in today's world. The main reason for this is that white-collar crime is one of the fastest-growing areas of crime, and police and regulators need the expertise of auditors to carry out these investigations. But there are other factors, and these relate to the broader category of forensic accounting. **Forensic accounting** includes fraud auditing and uses accounting and/or auditing skills in investigations involving legal issues. The legal issues might be criminal (e.g., fraud) or civil (e.g., commercial disputes). Common examples of civil legal disputes are insurance claims for business losses of various types and valuation of spousal business assets in a divorce proceeding.

Two specialist designations are available for investigative engagements. One for CPAs is referred to as CPA-IFA, for investigative and forensic accounting. See the website at difa.utoronto.ca for details. There is also an Association of Certified Fraud Examiners (ACFE), providing training for an internationally recognized designation that does not require any other accounting designation. See its website at acfe.com for details.

fraud:
in financial statement auditing, an intentional act by one or more individuals (the fraudsters) among management, those charged with governance, employees, or third parties, involving the use of deception to obtain an unjust or illegal advantage over someone (the victim)

fraud auditing:
a proactive approach to detect financial frauds using accounting records and information, analytical relationships, and an awareness of fraud perpetration and concealment efforts

forensic accounting:
the application of accounting and auditing skills to legal problems, both civil and criminal

Some people feel all PAs should take more responsibility for detecting fraud, especially financial statement fraud, and that this may be the main reason for the existence of the profession. The controversies generated by the economic crisis of 2008/2009 may strengthen this perspective. Appendix 1B on Connect discusses this increasingly influential view in more detail. Chapter 21 (available on Connect) also gives more details on forensic accounting and fraud auditing.

Review Checkpoints

1-11   Distinguish between forensic accounting and fraud auditing.

1-12   What is fraud?

1-13   What is operational auditing?

1-14   What are the elements of comprehensive auditing?

1-15   What is compliance auditing?

1-16   Name some other types of auditors in addition to external, internal, and governmental auditors.

1-17   Are financial statement audits intended to detect fraud?

Public Accounting

The Accounting Profession

By 2015 all of Canada's professional accounting bodies representing Chartered Accountants (CAs), Certified General Accountants (CGAs) and Certified Management Accountants (CMAs) at the national and provincial levels were unified to create a single designation for professional accountants, the Chartered Professional Accountant (CPA) designation. CPA Canada is now the national umbrella organization, and there are CPA provincial counterpart organizations (e.g., CPA Ontario) for all the provinces.

The vision of the new CPA designation is to be "the pre-eminent internationally recognized Canadian accounting and business credential that best protects and serves the public interest." CPA Canada aims to create professional accounting education requirements that meet or exceed the requirements of the leading global accounting bodies to facilitate a CPA's ability to practise anywhere in the world. See cpacanada.ca for more information.

The CPA education program is developed nationally but delivered provincially. Since regulation of professionals is a provincial matter, each province must pass its own legislation regulating who is allowed to practise public accounting. For example, the *Public Accounting Act of Saskatchewan*, passed in April 2014, united the three accounting bodies in that province.

Detailed requirements for becoming a CPA are given at the CPA certification program website at cpacanada. ca/en/become-a-cpa/why-become-a-cpa/the-cpa-certification-program.

The following is a brief outline of the requirements. All CPAs must have a university degree and meet the prerequisites for the various modules (courses). The CPA Prerequisite Program (CPA PREP) is designed for those who do not have an undergraduate degree in accounting. The PREP consists of two modules in the six technical competency areas of financial reporting, strategy-governance, management accounting, audit and assurance, finance, and tax. The CPA Professional Education Program (CPA PEP) is a graduate-level program that builds on the knowledge of PREP material. The PEP involves two core modules that everyone must take and two elective modules. Public accounting candidates must take the assurance and tax modules as electives. In addition, there are two capstone integrated modules to prepare students for the final professional-level exam. Practical experience requirements must also be satisfied.

The CPA program offers considerable flexibility to pursue various areas of interest and careers. Candidates with a primary interest in public accounting will be required to follow a specific path within CPA certification with a focus on assurance and tax. This textbook gives you most of what you will need to know for assurance.

The goal is to give CPAs a professional credential that is a competitive advantage to accountants on the job market and in their careers. The CPA requires lifelong learning, adherence to a code of conduct, and uniform standards of exit or entry to the profession. Indeed, what distinguishes a CPA from a business degree is that it is a professional credential similar to that of a doctor or lawyer. However, CPA Canada also recognizes that there are accounting careers that do not require qualified CPAs, so they are also offering the Advanced Certificate in Accounting and Finance as an intermediate-level certificate for accountants. At least one auditing course will be required for all of these credentials, and in-depth knowledge of auditing and assurance must be demonstrated on the Common Final Exam for all public accounting candidates.

Public Accounting Firms

Many people think of public accounting in terms of the "big" accounting firms. There are four such firms, often referred to as the "Big Four": Ernst & Young, Deloitte & Touche, KPMG, and PricewaterhouseCoopers. Notwithstanding this perception, public accounting is carried out in hundreds of practice units ranging in size from sole proprietorships (individuals who "hang out a shingle") to international firms employing thousands of professionals. Many students look upon public accounting as the place to begin a career; they gain intimate knowledge of many different business enterprises for the first three to ten years, and then they select an industry segment in which to pursue their interests. Public accounting experience is an excellent background to almost any business career.

Public accountants do business in a competitive environment. They perform audit services in the public interest, but they also need to make a living at it, so they have a profit motive just like other professionals. This duality—profit motive and professional responsibility—creates tensions in their work. As a result of increased litigation against them in the 1990s, the profession lobbied for legislation making it harder to sue professional accounting firms. In 1995, in the United States, legislation was passed allowing public accounting firms to take on the **limited liability partnership (LLP)** form of organization. The LLP structure, which will be covered in Chapter 3, is now common in Canada and around the world.

Throughout the last few decades the non-audit services provided by CPA firms have grown enormously. This growth has led to concerns about the independence of audit services provided by accounting firms that also engaged in extensive, possibly conflicting non-audit services for the same client, or even different clients. Many cite this lack of independence as the primary cause of the profession's problems in today's world.

Public accounting services involve many PAs employed in assurance, tax, and consulting work. Although structures will differ, Exhibit 1–6 shows the organization of a typical larger public accounting firm. Some firms include additional departments, such as small-business advisory or compensation consulting departments, while others might have different names for their staff and management positions.

In Exhibit 1–6, you see the various staffing levels within a public accounting firm. A recent graduate will most likely start work as a staff accountant. This typical entry-level position involves working under the supervision of more-senior people. As auditors need to verify virtually everything the auditee claims in its financial reporting, there is much mundane work to be done in verifying the math and the extensions of financial data and reconciling the physical amounts with recorded amounts. How does a user know the balance sheet balances? Someone needs to verify the seemingly obvious, and that someone is the auditor. You should look upon this experience as a form of apprenticeship. In most firms, your responsibilities will increase quickly once you demonstrate your reliability.

---

limited liability partnership (LLP):
a company whose partners' liability is limited to the capital they have invested in the business

EXHIBIT 1-6

Typical Organization of a Public Accounting Firm

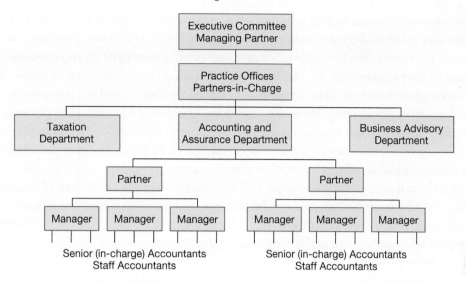

Depending on the firm, there may be several levels of staff accountants. Individuals who have just passed the professional exams are usually the most senior staff accountants and are ready to be promoted to manager once they have had a few years of experience and demonstrated leadership potential. Leadership means having people-management skills that are successful with both clients and staff accountants. Technical skills alone are usually not sufficient for a manager. The ability to expand the firm's practice becomes increasingly important. Getting along comfortably with client personnel is a high priority because otherwise it is difficult to get the information an auditor needs. These personal dynamics become more important at the higher levels in a public accounting firm. Keep this context in mind as you read descriptions of the various procedures in subsequent chapters. Managers supervise most of the details of the audit engagement, as explained throughout this text. They are the backbone of the audit at the technical level.

Partners, working closely with managers, take overall responsibility for the audit and lead meetings with auditees' management and audit committee. Partners usually have at least 10 years' experience and are the only permanent employees in a public accounting firm. About 5% of those with a PA designation become partners, while the rest go into industry or other public accounting firms. For more information on these positions, career opportunities, and the latest salary trends for PAs in North America, see the websites at mcintyre-smith.com and roberthalf.com/finance.

Assurance Services

Audits of traditional financial statements are the most frequent type of assurance services for public companies and for most large and medium-size non-public companies. Auditing amounts to 20–40% of the business of larger public accounting firms. Audit fees make up about 10% of revenues for smaller public accounting firms, and the reporting standards tend to be based on either private entity GAAP or public sector GAAP. Most of this text is about the audit of traditional financial statements using some form of GAAP.

Accounting and review services are the "non-audit" or other services performed frequently for medium-size and small businesses and not-for-profit organizations. A great deal of non-audit work is done by small public accounting practice units. PAs can be associated with clients' financial statements without giving the standard audit report. They can perform compilations, which consist of writing up the financial statements from a client's books and records, without performing any evidence-gathering work. They can perform reviews, which are lesser in scope than audits but include some evidence-gathering work. (Compilation and review standards are explained in more detail in Chapter 17, available on Connect.)

Assurance services are also performed on information in presentations other than traditional financial statements. Since assurance is the adding of credibility by an independent party (assurer, auditor) to representations made by one person or organization to another, demand for a greater variety of PA engagements has grown. PAs provide assurance to vote counts (e.g., for the Academy Awards), to dollar amounts of prizes claimed to have been given in lottery advertisements, to investment performance statistics, and to claims made about the capabilities of computer software programs. These non-traditional services are governed by professional standards.

In this text, we reference three sets of professional standards—Canadian; international; and, to a lesser extent, American—which all influence each other. For example, CPA Canada's Auditing and Assurance Standards Board influences international standards by providing commentary on exposure drafts of new international standards. Once a new international standard is adopted, CPA Canada issues an exposure draft of any unique-to-Canada modifications that must be made before they can be incorporated into CPA Canada standards. Other countries follow similar processes, and, increasingly, the trend is convergence to a common set of standards. For example, CPA Canada adopted international standards with minor modifications in 2011. The CASs are the main professional standards we refer to in this text.

Convergence is a defining characteristic of today's auditing and makes it more important to be aware of the similarities as well as the differences among the standards. International standards reference the International Federation of Accountants' (IFAC's) **International Standards on Auditing (ISAs)**. U.S. Public Company Accounting Oversight Board (PCAOB) standards are referenced to the PCAOB's **auditing standards**. There are also separate audit standards in the United States for non-public companies promulgated by the American Institute of CPAs (AICPA).

Taxation Services

Local, provincial, national, and international tax laws are often called "full-employment acts" for accountants and lawyers; they are complex, and PAs perform tax planning and tax return preparation services in the areas of income, sales, property, and other taxation. A large proportion of small accounting firm work is tax practice. Tax laws change frequently, and tax practitioners have to spend considerable time in continuing education and self-study to keep current.

Consulting or Management Advisory Services

All accounting firms handle a great deal of consulting and management advisory services (some firms refer to these as *management ancillary services*). These are the great "open end" of public accounting practice that puts accountants in direct competition with the non-public accounting consulting firms. The field is virtually limitless, and no list of consulting activities could possibly include all of them. Indeed, accounting firms have created consulting units with professionals from other fields—lawyers, actuaries, engineers, and advertising executives, to name a few. Until the Enron scandal in 2001/2002, many of the large accounting firms had tried to become one-stop shopping centres for clients' auditing, taxation, and business advice needs. However, through the chilling effect of corporate scandals at the beginning of the century, these activities have been greatly restricted whenever the engagement includes assurance services.

International Standards on Auditing (ISAs):
the auditing standards of the International Federation of Accountants

auditing standards:
the subset of assurance standards dealing with "high" or "reasonable" levels of assurance in assurance engagements

Nevertheless, consulting work for non-audit clients may continue to expand to new non-conflicting areas such as eldercare, where PAs provide a package of services ranging from assurance to consulting, bill paying, and financial planning for the elderly. In large public accounting firms, the consulting department is quite often independent from the auditing and accounting departments, performing engagements that do not directly interact with the audits. Public accounting firms are greatly restricted in the types of consulting or business advisory services they can provide to audit clients, particularly for publicly listed companies, but there are no such restrictions for non-audit clients.

International Auditing

LO5 Provide an overview of international auditing and its impact on Canadian Auditing Standards.

Many of the large public accounting firms are worldwide organizations that have grown rapidly in the last few decades, in parallel with the increased economic integration of their global clientele. Developments such as the North American Free Trade Agreement (NAFTA), the evolution of the European Economic Union and other free trade zones, and the pervasive effects of technological change are all contributing to increased global harmonization of auditing and accounting standards. Following this trend, the **International Federation of Accountants (IFAC)**, formed in 1977, is creating, through its independent standard setting board, the International Auditing and Assurance Standards Board (IAASB), international standards by publishing its own handbook on auditing standards that recommends ISAs. ISAs cover basic principles of auditing, auditor's reports, professional independence, reliance on other auditors abroad, and professional qualifications.

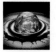 ISAs are becoming the dominant standards worldwide. CPA Canada's policy is to adopt ISAs as is, unless Canadian conditions require a different standard. The sources of auditing standards in Canada are the *CPA Canada Handbook*, whose standards were traditionally referred to as *Handbook* Recommendations, and the Audit Guidelines (AuGs), which provide additional guidance on implementing the standards. CPA Canada adopted the revised and redrafted ISAs as well as the International Standard on Quality Control on December 15, 2009, effective for fiscal periods after December 14, 2010. In 2011, CPA Canada adopted IFRS. It will decide at a future date what, if any, other international standards it will adopt. We provide more details in later chapters. The goal of convergence, or **international harmonization** as it is frequently called, is a key focus of Canadian standard setters in the 21st century. As discussed above, a major reason for the creation of the CPA designation in Canada was to bring Canadian PAs to the forefront of the evolving global CPA profession.

As the world becomes more interdependent, many concepts and terms used in other countries will become increasingly accepted in Canadian practice. Indeed, many large firms already use manuals and training materials reflecting international practice. This text makes use of those terms and concepts and does not restrict itself to those used in the *CPA Canada Handbook* or CASs.

Review Checkpoint

1-18 What is the IAASB, and how do its standards affect auditing standards in Canada?

International Federation of Accountants (IFAC):
an organization dedicated to developing international auditing standards

international harmonization:
international convergence of national accounting and auditing standards with IFRS and ISAs, including going concern, fraud, and the audit risk model

APPLICATION CASE WITH SOLUTION & ANALYSIS

The Auditor's Most Important Quality

DISCUSSION CASE

Review the box titled "Is There Any Gold Inside Fort Knox?" This box illustrates the fundamental social role of the auditor and how it arises. Based on this box, what do you think is the most important personal characteristic of the auditor?

SOLUTION & ANALYSIS

You might think that the most important characteristics of the auditor are to be able to count and to perform other audit procedures. But it should be clear in this case that virtually anybody could figure out the most basic procedures that need to be performed. In fact, let us assume that the U.S. government has performed these and all necessary procedures to keep an accurate record of the gold at Fort Knox, and yet there is still a demand for an independent external audit. So there must be something even more important than just having the knowledge and skill to perform audit procedures competently. The issue here is one of who effectively performs the audit procedures; it is not a government audit that is being demanded, it is an *independent external* audit that is independent of the government.

The key words are *independent* and *external*. The external auditor is expected to be more objective than the government auditor, and the independence criterion is necessary to ensure that there is no conflict of interest—in this case, a bias toward the government. There should not be the appearance of a conflict of interest, but neither should there be in the auditor's actual thought processes. If the external auditor were not independent, or perceived to not be independent, then the purpose of having an external auditor would be defeated. The auditor's lack of independence from the government would not result in the assurance that users expect. Lack of independence prevents the auditor from being effective to third-party users—users are no better off than if there had been no audit.

The need for independence arises from third-party accountability. If the third-party users are to trust the auditor's work, then the auditor must preserve independence. A further complication for the auditor is that this preservation of independence needs to be toward parties who do not pay the auditor. The party who pays the auditor is the auditee (in this case, the U.S. government). The auditor must be especially concerned about independence from the auditee since it is the auditee who is demanding the audit (see Appendix 1B). This importance of independence extends to managing the image of the auditor so that there is not even the appearance of lack of independence.

The significance of independence, essentially an aspect of the auditor's character, is reflected in its extensive coverage in the rules of professional ethics for auditors (Chapter 3) and in the quality control practices of the auditing firms (i.e., public accounting firms) (Chapter 2).

SUMMARY

- This chapter began by illustrating and defining auditing, distinguishing it from accounting. Accounting is the recording and summarizing of information about an entity, whereas auditing is the verification of the accuracy of the accounting by an independent expert, the external auditor. In modern capital markets where the owner is far removed from the management hired to run the company for the benefit of the owners, independent external auditors are crucial to the functioning of the markets.

The practice of public accounting is rooted in the history of auditing. The accounting profession has been undergoing radical changes since the bankruptcy of Enron in December 2001. These changes are being accompanied by broad corporate governance and regulatory reforms. **LO1, 2**

- Auditors contribute to well-functioning capital markets by reducing information risk associated with the financial statements prepared by management. In order to achieve the objective of providing assurance (= reducing information risk), auditors need to use professional judgment and to have a skeptical mindset. Skepticism is required because of the potential conflict of interest that exists between management and the owners, and the accountability that management needs to provide to owners and other capital providers. The addition of the independent external auditor to verify the accuracy of the financial statements creates the three-party accountability concept introduced in the chapter. **LO3**

- Auditing is practised in numerous forms by various practice units, including public accounting firms, the Canada Revenue Agency (CRA), the Office of the Auditor General of Canada (OAG), companies' internal audit departments, and several types of regulatory auditors. Fraud examiners, many of whom are internal auditors and inspectors, have found a niche in auditing-related activities. **LO4**

- Many auditors aspire to become Chartered Professional Accountants (CPAs), Certified Internal Auditors (CIAs), or certified fraud examiners (CFEs); this involves passing rigorous examinations, obtaining practical experience, and maintaining competence through continuing professional education. Each of these groups has a large professional organization that governs the professional standards and quality of practice of its members. **LO4**

- Auditors in Canada use International Standards on Auditing (ISAs) modified for Canadian laws and regulations. These are referred to as Canadian Auditing Standards (CASs). Auditors must be CPAs, registered or licensed in their province, to practise auditing and related services. **LO5**

This chapter has given you a broad overview of auditing. Being aware of the bigger picture of the context of auditing is increasingly important for effective auditing. This is the main reason the concept of critical thinking in professional judgment is being introduced in this text. We end this introduction with a brief overview of what you can expect from this text. Part I, consisting of the first four chapters, introduces you to the most fundamental concepts you will need to consider as an auditor. Part II introduces you to evidence-based concepts of auditing and refines the important concept of internal control. In Part III, you will learn to apply the concepts studied thus far to the various accounts in the financial statements. This part concludes with the opinion that ends the audit report and reflects an evaluation of financial statements as a whole. Part IV covers other assurance engagements and specialized types of auditors and auditing. **LO3, 5**

When you begin the study of auditing, you may be eager to attack the nitty-gritty of financial statement audit work. Although this text will enable you to learn about auditing, instructors are seldom able to duplicate a practice environment in a classroom setting. You may feel frustrated about not knowing "how to do it." This frustration is natural, because auditing is done in the field under pressure of time limits and in the surroundings of client personnel, paperwork, and accounting information systems. Part IV covers at a more-advanced level professional ethics, legal liability, audit of accounting estimates, and specialized assurance and related services. **LO3, 5**

KEY TERMS

accountability relationship	acting in the public interest	audit risk (account level)
accounting	assurance engagement	audit societies
accounting risk (account level)	attest engagement	auditee

auditing	forensic accounting	limited liability partnership
auditing standards	fraud	(LLP)
business risk	fraud auditing	materiality
Canadian Auditing Standard (CAS)	generally accepted accounting	operational auditing (performance
Chartered Professional Accountants of	principles (GAAP)	auditing or management
Canada (CPA Canada)	information risk	auditing)
client	information technology (IT)	professional judgment
comprehensive governmental auditing	internal auditing	professional skepticism
conflict of interest	International Federation of	providing assurance
direct reporting engagement	Accountants (IFAC)	public accountant (PA)
expectations gap	international harmonization	public sector
external auditors	International Standards on Auditing	three-party accountability
financial reporting	(ISAs)	value-for-money (VFM) audit

MULTIPLE-CHOICE QUESTIONS FOR PRACTICE AND REVIEW

MC 1-1 `LO1` When people speak of the assurance function, they are referring to the work of auditors in

a. lending credibility to a client's financial statements.
b. detecting fraud and embezzlement in a company.
c. lending credibility to an auditee's financial statements.
d. performing a program-results audit in a government agency.

MC 1-2 `LO1` Company A hired Sampson & Delila, CPAs, to audit the financial statements of Company B and deliver the audit report to Megabank. Which is the client?

a. Megabank
b. Sampson & Delila
c. Company A
d. Company B

MC 1-3 `LO1` According to CPA Canada, the objective of an audit of financial statements is

a. an expression of opinion on the fairness with which they present financial position, results of operations, and cash flows in conformity with GAAP.
b. an expression of opinion on the fairness with which they present financial position, results of operations, and cash flows in conformity with accounting standards promulgated by the Financial Accounting Standards Board.
c. an expression of opinion on the fairness with which they present financial position, results of operations, and cash flows in conformity with accounting standards promulgated by the CPA Canada Accounting Standards Committee.
d. to obtain systematic and objective evidence about financial assertions and report the results to interested users.

MC 1-4 `LO1` Bankers who are processing loan applications from companies seeking large loans will probably ask for financial statements audited by an independent PA because

a. financial statements are too complex for them to analyze themselves.
b. they are too far away from company headquarters to perform accounting and auditing themselves.
c. the consequences of making a bad loan are very undesirable.

    d. they generally see a potential conflict of interest between company managers who want to get loans and their needs for reliable financial statements.

MC 1-5 `LO4` Operational audits of a company's efficiency and economy of managing projects and of the results of programs are conducted by whom?

    a. Financial statement auditors
    b. The company's internal auditors
    c. Tax auditors employed by the federal government
    d. Fraud auditors

MC 1-6 `LO3` Independent auditors of financial statements perform audits that reduce and control

    a. the business risks faced by investors.
    b. the information risk faced by investors.
    c. the complexity of financial statements.
    d. quality reviews performed by other public accounting firms.

MC 1-7 `LO4` The primary objective of compliance auditing is to

    a. give an opinion on financial statements.
    b. develop a basis for a report on internal control.
    c. perform a study of effective and efficient use of resources.
    d. determine whether auditee personnel are following laws, rules, regulations, and policies.

EXERCISES AND PROBLEMS

EP 1-1 Controller as Auditor. `LO2` The chair of the board of Hughes Corporation proposed that the board hire as controller a PA who had been the manager on the corporation's audit performed by a firm of independent accountants. The chair thought that hiring this person would make the annual audit unnecessary and consequently save the company the fee paid to the auditors. The chair proposed giving this new controller a full staff to conduct such investigations of accounting and operating data as necessary. Evaluate this proposal.

EP 1-2 Controller as Auditor. `LO2` Put yourself in the position of the person hired as controller in the above situation. Suppose the chair of the board moves to discontinue the annual audit because Hughes Corporation now has your services on a full-time basis. You are invited to express your views to the board. Explain how you would discuss the nature of your job as controller and your views on the discontinuance of the annual audit.

EP 1-3 Logic and Method. `LO3` Identify four major factors affecting information risk that make the need for independent audits important in today's business world. Give two examples for each.

EP 1-4 Logic and Method. `LO3` Auditors must have a thorough knowledge of GAAP if they are to properly perform an audit of the financial statements of a company. Explain why this is so. Use capital leases as an example of the need for this knowledge.

EP 1-5 Operational Auditing. `LO4` Bigdeal Corporation manufactures paper and paper products and is trying to decide whether to purchase and merge Smalltek Company. Smalltek has developed a process for manufacturing boxes that can replace other containers, which use fluorocarbons for expelling a liquid product. The price may be as high as $45 million. Bigdeal prefers to buy Smalltek and integrate its products, while leaving the Smalltek management in charge of day-to-day operations. A major consideration is the efficiency and effectiveness of the Smalltek management. Bigdeal wants to obtain a report on the operational efficiency and effectiveness of the Smalltek sales, production, and research and development departments.

Required:

Whom can Bigdeal engage to produce this operational audit report? Several possibilities exist. Are there any particular advantages or disadvantages in choosing among them?

EP 1-6 Auditor as Guarantor. LO1 Your neighbour invited you to lunch yesterday. Sure enough, it was no "free lunch," because he wanted to discuss the annual report of the Dodge Corporation. He owns Dodge shares and has just received the report. He says, "PricewaterhouseCoopers prepared the audited financial statements and gave an unqualified opinion, so my investment must be safe."

Required:

What misconceptions does your neighbour seem to have about the auditor's role with respect to Dodge Corporation?

EP 1-7 Identification of Audits and Auditors. LO4 Audits may be characterized as (a) financial statement audits, (b) compliance audits—audits of compliance with control policies and procedures and with laws and regulations, (c) economy and efficiency audits, or (d) program results audits. The work can be done by independent (external) auditors, internal auditors, or governmental auditors. Below is a list of the purposes or products of various audit engagements.

1. Render a public report on the assumptions and compilation of a revenue forecast by a sports stadium/racetrack complex.
2. Determine the fair presentation in conformity with GAAP of an advertising agency's financial statements.
3. Report on how better care and disposal of vehicles confiscated by drug enforcement agents might save money and benefit law enforcement.
4. Determine the costs of municipal garbage pickup services compared with the same service subcontracted to a private business.
5. Audit tax shelter partnership financing terms.
6. Study a private aircraft manufacturer's test pilot performance in reporting on the results of test flights.
7. Conduct periodic examination of a bank for solvency.
8. Evaluate the promptness of materials inspection in a manufacturer's receiving department.

Required:

Prepare a three-column schedule showing (1) each of the engagements listed above, (2) the type of audit (financial statement, compliance, economy and efficiency, or program results), and (3) the kind of auditors you would expect to be involved.

EP 1-8 Analysis and Judgment. LO3 As part of your regular year-end audit of a publicly held client, you must estimate the probability of success of its proposed new product line. The client has experienced financial difficulty during the last few years and, in your judgment, a successful introduction of the new product line is necessary for the client to remain a going concern.

There are five steps, all of which are necessary for successful introduction of the product: (1) successful labour negotiations between the building trades unions and the construction firms contracted to build the necessary addition to the present plant, (2) successful defence of patent rights, (3) product approval by the Health Branch, (4) successful negotiation of a long-term raw material contract with a foreign supplier, and (5) successful conclusion of distribution contract talks with a large national retail distributor.

In view of the circumstances, you contact experts who have provided your firm with reliable estimates in the past. The labour relations expert estimates that there is an 80% chance of successfully concluding labour negotiations before the strike deadline. Legal counsel advises that there is a 90% chance of successfully defending patent rights. The expert on Health Branch product approvals estimates a 95% chance of approval. The experts in the remaining two areas estimate the probability of successfully resolving the raw materials contract and the distribution contract talks to be 90% in each case. Assume these estimates are reliable.

Required:

What is your assessment of the probability of successful product introduction? (*Hint:* You can assume the five steps are independent of each other.)

EP 1-9 Information Risk Questions. **LO3** Give several examples of misstatements that contribute to audit risk. Give several examples of misstatements that contribute to accounting risk. How can you distinguish between the two types of misstatements? Discuss in class.

EP 1-10 The Audit Society. **LO3** Identify a major finding from the auditor general of your province in 2014 or later. How extensively was it reported in the news media? Identify the three-party accountability in these engagements. Do you think that the media reports reflect well on the auditor? Discuss in class.

EP 1-11 The Audit Society. **LO3** Identify a report on a major investigation of the Auditor General of Canada in 2012 that led to a major embarrassment for the federal government. How extensively was this reported in the media? Identify the three-party accountability in these engagements. Do you think that the media reports reflect well on the auditor? Discuss in class.

Appendix 1A: How to Become a Professional Accountant in Canada (on Connect)
Appendix 1B: Alternative Theories of the Role of Auditing in Society (on Connect)

ENDNOTES

1   European Commission, "Green Paper: Audit Policy: Lessons from the Crisis," October 2010, p. 3, eur-lex.europa.eu/LexUriServ/LexUriServ.do?uri=COM:2010:0561:FIN:EN:PDF.

2   M.P. Power, The Audit Society (New York: Oxford University Press, 1997).

3   Canadian Auditing Standard (CAS) 200.03, "General Objective of the Independent Auditor." The Canadian Auditing Standards of the *CPA Canada Handbook* are the authoritative CPA Canada pronouncements on auditing theory and practice.

4   See theiia.org.

5   Christina Blizzard, The Toronto Sun, December 4, 2002.

Auditors' Professional Roles and Responsibilities

Chapter 2 describes the audit environment, layers of standardization, and professional self-regulation that have evolved to uphold the quality of audits. These layers of control over auditors' work can be viewed as a reflection of the importance of auditing to society and our economy, and of auditors' responsibility in protecting the public interest. It is important to understand that all these layers of control ultimately relate to controlling information risk for users of financial statements.

LEARNING OBJECTIVES

After completing this chapter, you will be able to do the following:

LO1 Describe the current audit environment, including developments in regulatory oversight and provincial regulation of public accountants in Canada.

LO2 List the various practice standards for independent audits of financial statements.

LO3 Summarize the ethical, examination, and reporting standards that make up generally accepted auditing standards as set out in CPA Canada's Canadian Auditing Standards.

LO4 Explain the importance of general assurance standards using examples of assurance matters.

LO5 Explain how requirements of quality control standards are monitored for public accounting firms.

LO6 (Appendix 2A) List the generally accepted auditing standards of the United States.

LO7 (Appendix 2B) Summarize audit quality control monitoring in Canada.

CHAPTER APPENDICES

APPENDIX 2A Generally Accepted Auditing Standards of the United States (on Connect)

APPENDIX 2B Implementation of Quality Control Standards in Canada (on Connect)

EcoPak Inc.

While they are waiting for StyreneTech's audited financial statements, Kam and Mike start looking over Waterfalls Inc.'s consolidated financial statements with Nina. The statements are in a big, glossy document titled "The Annual Report," which also includes the auditor's report, a report on internal control effectiveness and corporate governance, a managements' discussion and analysis report (MD&A), and a corporate environmental and social responsibility report. Nina explains that Waterfalls Inc. is a large public company, so it has to provide a lot more details about its management and governance than a smaller entity like StyreneTech does.

When the audited StyreneTech financial statements are received, Kam and Mike note the auditor's report has exactly the same wording as the Waterfalls one, which makes them a bit suspicious. Both reports say the audits were done in accordance with "standards" and that they provide reasonable assurance. How do they know the PAs at Grand & Quatre LLP (G&Q) did good-quality work? Nina tells them that as PAs, the auditors at G&Q must follow generally accepted auditing standards (GAAS) to ensure that their work is of high quality. As an auditor of public companies, G&Q is also subject to securities regulations and inspections of the quality of their audit work, so Kam and Mike can expect the same quality level for the StyreneTech audit.

When they pass the audited StyreneTech financial statements along to Zhang, who has looked over hundreds of audited financial statements, she is, initially, satisfied with the auditor's report because it is "unmodified." Then, however, her eyes zoom right to the disclosures in the notes, where she finds a note about a contingent liability to some former employees who have developed serious health problems. These former employees have launched a lawsuit against StyreneTech claiming that StyreneTech did not provide adequate protection from the fumes in the factory, which led to their illness. This contingency did not appear in the unaudited financial statements, and in Waterfalls' notes it was combined with some other legal claims but not specifically identified. Based on these audited statements, Zhang tells Kam and Mike that she is not willing to invest in the StyreneTech shares because of that contingent liability. She is only willing to invest in shares of a new corporation that will buy the operating assets of StyreneTech rather than its shares.

When Nina hears about Zhang's decision, she tells Kam and Mike, "Now you see why Zhang wanted those audited statements—they are much more complete because the auditors look for things like contingent liabilities and make sure that all the requirements of generally accepted accounting principles (GAAP) are followed. Zhang is very wise!"

Kam and Mike are very impressed, and they continue to consider things. They have heard that StyreneTech's petroleum-based polystyrene-foam production process releases pollutants that are controlled substances, meaning that the emissions volumes need to be measured and reported to a government agency. They ask Nina if it is possible to have G&Q audit StyreneTech's pollution emissions to see if they comply with the government's limits. Nina says it is possible, since big accounting firms such as G&Q often have environmental auditors on staff, or there are other consulting firms that provide assurance on information other than financial statements, such as pollution volumes. But it could be costly, and it's unlikely that Waterfalls would pay for it, so Kam and Mike would need to really think about why they want that information audited and how much they are willing to pay for it.

Kam and Mike decide to take the plunge and become packaging entrepreneurs. When they tell Nina, she responds by saying, "Congratulations! I know you will both succeed brilliantly! But for now, you really need to get a lawyer to help you start up the new corporation and get you going on acquiring StyreneTech's assets. I can recommend a few good ones."

The Essentials of Auditors' Professional Roles and Responsibilities

Since auditing is a critical function in the economy, it is extensively regulated to ensure it remains effective. In Canada, the regulation of professional accountants and auditors is a provincial responsibility, varying somewhat depending on the legislation in different provinces. The profession also has a national umbrella organization that all provincial organizations are associated with.

The collapse of Enron and the failure of Arthur Andersen, the largest accounting firm at the time, some 15 years ago was a major turning point for the accounting profession, and it has repercussions to this day.

At the time of writing, the profession is being streamlined at both the national and provincial levels by uniting three formerly separate accounting designations (CA, CGA, CMA) into a single designation for Canadian professional accountants, the CPA (Chartered Professional Accountant). The national umbrella organization is now CPA Canada, and there are counterpart CPA associations in each province (e.g., CPA Saskatchewan). CPA Canada is authorized by legislation to set all accounting and auditing practice standards for Canada, and it also sets the education and examination requirements for students interested in obtaining the CPA designation. The provincial associations deliver the CPA Canada educational program and also set a code of ethical conduct that members must follow (e.g., CPA Ontario's "Rules of Professional Conduct"). They are responsible for the admission of members, as well as inspection of accountants' practices and disciplinary actions to enforce the professional ethics code.

The regulation of an individual accountant will depend on what kind of work the person is engaged in. A lot of accounting-related work, such as bookkeeping and financial statement and tax preparation for individuals or private companies, can be done by people who don't have a CPA designation. The CPA designation requires specific higher education and experience, so it can allow accountants to do more complex professional work, and this can be as employees of businesses, as entrepreneurs operating their own consulting service business, or as associates of professional accounting firms.

An important distinction arises when an accountant wants to provide auditing and assurance services for use by the general public; this is referred to as *public accounting*. Since the general public may not be able to assess whether an accountant is properly qualified and regulated to act in their best interest, the intent of the CPA regulations is to protect the interests of the public. Generally, to practise public accounting a person must have a CPA designation, and in many (most) provinces (e.g., Ontario, Alberta, Quebec, Saskatchewan) must obtain further qualification and licensing (e.g., from the Public Accountants Council for the Province of Ontario, PAC). CPA members in public practice will have their work and office procedures inspected periodically by the provincial association to ensure they are in compliance. Further, if a public accounting firm wants to be engaged to audit publicly traded companies, this falls under securities laws, adding an extra layer of regulation. The firm must register with the Canadian Public Accountability Board (CPAB). CPAB will inspect their financial statement audit work on public companies annually to provide the highest level of public protection, since the companies audited can sell their securities directly to the public.

In addition to being highly regulated, financial statement audits themselves are used as an instrument of regulation on corporate reporting. Corporation laws require companies to produce audited annual financial statements (though private and smaller companies can sometimes waive this requirement), and securities laws require public companies to file audited financial statements within 90 days of their year-end.

What do all these regulations require of professional accountants, specifically? To summarize, members of a CPA association are required to comply with the professional ethics code of their provincial association. Every ethics code has five similar components, requiring the member to act with *integrity*, to remain *objective*, to maintain the *professional competencies* their work requires and to do their work with appropriate *due care*, to keep *confidential* all information they acquire through their professional work, and to *behave professionally* in a way that befits a well-respected profession.

These requirements apply to CPAs in private employment or in public accounting practice, though there are more rigorous requirements for CPAs in public accounting engagements. They must also demonstrate they can be objective by remaining independent of any potentially conflicting interests, and must maintain *independence in fact* and also *independence in appearance* to outsiders. While independence in fact is absolutely essential, it is not sufficient unless outsiders can also see evidence that the CPA has no financial or other interest that would cause him or her to act in a biased way rather than in the outside user's best interest. For further guidance, the ethics codes identify five situations that can arise in a three-party accountability relationship and, if they exist, can threaten an auditor's independence: self-review, self-interest, advocacy, familiarity, and intimidation.

CPA members meet the requirement of professional competency and due care in performing their work by complying with requirements of the CPA Canada standards for accounting (GAAP—Accounting Standards for Private Enterprises (ASPE) or International Financial Reporting Standards (IFRS)) and auditing (GAAS—Canadian Auditing Standards (CASs)). Thus, the professional ethics code incorporates the professional accounting and auditing standards, making compliance with them the bottom-line professional responsibility of professional accountants.

For auditing, GAAS are set out in the CASs in the *CPA Canada Assurance Handbook*. CAS 200 is entitled "Overall Objective of the Independent Auditor, and the Conduct of the Audit in Accordance with Canadian Auditing Standards." It states the financial statement auditors' overall objectives as follows:

(a) To obtain reasonable assurance about whether the financial statements as a whole are free from material misstatement, whether due to fraud or error, thereby enabling the auditor to express an opinion on whether the financial statements are prepared, in all material respects, in accordance with an applicable financial reporting framework; and

(b) To report on the financial statements, and communicate as required by the International Standards on Auditing (ISAs), in accordance with the auditor's findings.

CAS 200 also provides principles and fundamental concepts that underlie the auditing function.

The other CASs relate to different aspects of an audit, such as planning and assessing risks of misstatements. Each CAS states its objectives and sets out the requirements an auditor must meet to achieve them. To claim to comply with GAAS, an auditor must comply with every CAS that is relevant in the audit. If a relevant CAS objective cannot be achieved, the auditor has to consider whether an audit conclusion can be reached at all and may have to withdraw from the engagement if not. Any financial statement auditor who does not follow *all the relevant* CASs has not used due care as required by the ethical code and can be judged as having performed a deficient audit.

Review Checkpoints

2-1   How is the accounting profession in Canada regulated?

2-2   What distinguishes public accounting from other types of work professional accountants might perform, such as bookkeeping, financial statement preparation, or tax return preparation?

2-3   Describe the five essential components of a professional ethics code for accountants.

2-4   For what types of work does a professional accountant require independence?

2-5   How does independence in fact differ from independence in appearance? Why, and to whom, does the distinction matter?

2-6   What are five situations that can threaten an auditor's independence? Explain each situation in terms of the three-party accountability model.

2-7   Explain the mechanism by which financial statement audits serve as an instrument of financial regulation.

2-8   Why are professional accountants required to comply with GAAP and GAAS?

2-9   What are the overall objectives of a financial statement audit?

The Current Environment of Auditing

LO1   Describe the current audit environment, including developments in regulatory oversight and provincial regulation of public accountants in Canada.

The audit environment has undergone profound changes as a result of corporate failures such as Enron and WorldCom, starting in 2001. Until 2002, the accounting profession was largely self-regulating. By **self-regulation** we mean that the profession itself established the rules governing audit practice and monitored compliance with them. This reliance on self-regulation changed with the perceived failure of the profession to detect the problems leading to the corporate scandals of 2002/2003. The crucial role of auditing in well-functioning capital markets became clear as never before. This process of rapid change continued with the economic crisis of 2008/2009 as the integrity of capital markets was being questioned all over the world. These developments highlight the importance of controlling information risk and agency problems introduced in Chapter 1.

One important mechanism for controlling information risk is through GAAS, which apply to financial statement audits, and the broader assurance standards, which apply to all audits. These audit standards are formal requirements auditors must meet in carrying out an audit. These standards can be summarized via the five categories in Exhibit 2–1, which we discuss in more detail later. Another way of controlling information risk is through quality control standards of audit practice. To help ensure that all these standards are actually implemented in practice, the accounting profession is monitored externally by CPAB in Canada and through self-regulation. Appendix 2B discusses in more detail the implementation of quality control standards.

The next section briefly summarizes the recent changes in the current audit environment. Later chapters explain the significance of these changes in more detail.

The *Sarbanes-Oxley Act*

"The greed and corruption of top executives at Enron, WorldCom, Global Crossing, Adelphia and numerous other major companies has jeopardized the retirement savings of a generation and unleashed a crisis of confidence that continues to drain values from America's markets.

"There is no question in my mind that trusted executives who betray their workers and shareholders are capable of doing far greater and more lasting damage to our nation, our economy and our way of life than any external attacker" (quote by Walter Shorenstein in "Crackdown on business fraud urged at conference," Jim Christie, November 1, 2002, San Francisco).

The above quote indicates the depths to which the accounting profession's esteem and that of business in general had sunk by the end of 2002. The period roughly from October 2001 through November 2002 had seen the most dramatic changes in the accounting profession since at least the 1930s. There had been more stories on the profession in the mainstream and business media than ever before. Enron, Arthur Andersen, and WorldCom had become household names. The reputation of North American businesses and their auditors had sunk to new lows. For example, in 2002 Tyco International executives were accused of "looting" their company to the tune of US$600 million and treating its assets as their piggy bank. Similar accusations had been made about executives at Adelphia Communications, Global Crossing, WorldCom, Enron and many other companies.

This dramatic shift in attitudes toward capitalism in general and auditors in particular can be assigned to a specific watershed event—the bankruptcy of the energy company Enron on December 2, 2001. The changes

self-regulation:
a situation where the government gives a professional group the power to monitor and discipline its members

since then have been so substantial that the term *post-Enron world* has been used to signify the completely altered corporate landscape that has developed since then.

One of the reasons Enron had such a shock effect was that it was considered a "new-economy" company that pointed the way for the rest of the energy industry as it headed into the 21st century. Enron was the poster child of the new-economy company. It had been considered a highly innovative energy company that had branched out into exotic areas of financial engineering related to energy usage, such as weather derivatives. Some of these innovations were successful and have continued. But the majority appeared to have been little more in substance than manipulation of energy prices (leading to widespread blackouts in California in 2000), or shell games with related parties that deceptively hid liabilities and losses on speculation in the direction of energy prices. Rather than an innovative energy company or new-age hedge fund, Enron turned out to be more like a classic Ponzi scheme, relying on attracting ever more investors to continue bidding up the price of the company's shares.

The aspect of Enron that appeared to enrage the public most was that lower-level employees and others were strongly encouraged, even forced, to invest their retirement savings in Enron stock while top management were selling their shares based on insider knowledge of the disastrous state of affairs. Total losses to shareholders amounted to over US$60 billion, and over 6,000 Enron employees lost their jobs along with their retirement savings. As a result of Enron's bankruptcy, numerous lawsuits have been filed by the shareholders and creditors against Enron's management; its board of directors; its auditor, Arthur Andersen; and numerous financial institutions, including America's biggest banks, which were suspected of arranging the sham transactions. In addition to the U.S. Securities and Exchange Commission (SEC), various state regulators launched investigative probes against these same institutions.

Another casualty of Enron has been the accounting profession itself. Of course, the most immediate impact fell on Arthur Andersen, one of the Big Five accounting firms at the time. Right after Enron's bankruptcy, questions were raised about the effectiveness of its auditor, Arthur Andersen, since there were no official indications of serious problems at Enron until mid-October 2001, when it had to restate previously reported earnings. (Another characteristic of the post-Enron world is that the number of such restatements skyrocketed across North America soon after the failure of Enron.) Joe Berardino, managing partner of Arthur Andersen, tried to explain the apparent audit failure by attributing the problems to the vagueness of accounting standards and the complexity of Andersen's financial statements. This explanation might have been more plausible had not Andersen been involved in designing these very same transactions as part of their consulting work for Enron. The real problem seems to have been that Arthur Andersen lacked independence because it was auditing its own work.

The accounting profession and the public were shocked by revelations in January 2002 that Andersen was engaged in the shredding of many of its Enron audit documents. This shredding began soon after the SEC announced its investigation of Enron's accounting in October 2001, soon after Enron's first announcement of its restatements. Early in January 2002, the shredding practice was made public, and on January 15, 2002, the partner in charge of the Enron audit, David Duncan, was fired by Arthur Andersen. He was later found guilty of obstruction of justice and testified against his former firm. On June 15, 2002, Arthur Andersen itself was convicted of obstruction of justice as a result of what the jury felt was a systematic effort within the firm to destroy relevant evidence about the true condition of Enron.

This conviction of a prominent auditing firm and its subsequent demise was unprecedented in the history of the profession. The entire profession was tarnished by this fiasco involving one of its most reputable firms.

Arthur Andersen was fined $500,000 and placed on a five-year probation. By then it was already destroyed as an auditing firm. Its clients left, concerned that they would be tainted by Arthur Andersen's falling reputation. In a matter of months Arthur Andersen was reduced to a shell of its former self. A firm that at the beginning of 2002 employed 85,000 people worldwide and had built an 89-year-old reputation of high integrity and excellence was essentially destroyed by the time of its sentencing on October 26, 2002. Even though the U.S. Supreme Court later overturned Andersen's conviction, Arthur Anderson was no longer a viable business. There are now only the "Big Four" instead of the "Big Five" accounting firms, and these "Final Four" are now redefining their roles in the post-Enron world.

Unfortunately, it was not only Enron that reshaped the auditing world. Enron was the United States' seventh-largest firm when it went bankrupt. It was the biggest bankruptcy ever at the time. But it was soon followed by yet another, even bigger bankruptcy—that of WorldCom on June 25, 2002. WorldCom was the backbone of the Internet, until its bankruptcy carrying about half of all Internet traffic, and was the United States' fifth-largest firm at the time of its bankruptcy. Total estimated losses to shareholders were US$180 billion, and 17,000 employees lost their jobs. Arthur Andersen was WorldCom's auditor as well.

Enron and WorldCom were not Arthur Andersen's only problem audits. Throughout 2002 every week seemed to reveal a new corporate scandal involving deceptions in audited financial reporting. Although Arthur Andersen was not the only one involved, it accounted for a disproportionate number of these companies, including Global Crossing, Waste Management, Sunbeam, and the Baptist Foundation of North America (the largest non-profit bankruptcy ever—US$570 million in losses).

As result of these and other corporate scandals, there was a worldwide questioning of the integrity of North American capital markets. The WorldCom failure was the most dramatic illustration of this. WorldCom acted as the final straw in prompting the passage of the most drastic legislation affecting the accounting profession since 1933—the *Sarbanes-Oxley Act* (SOX) in 2002.

Key features of SOX include the following:

- Increased oversight of auditors, including audit standard setting by the newly created Public Company Accounting Oversight Board (PCAOB)
- Increased penalties for corporate wrongdoers
- More timely and extensive financial disclosures
- More timely and extensive disclosure of the way the firm is governed
- New options of recourse for aggrieved shareholders, including increased legal liability for auditors

For auditors of public companies, SOX created a five-member **Public Company Accounting Oversight Board (PCAOB)** with the authority to tighten quality control of audit practices and report on inspections of audit firm practices.

Canadian companies listed on U.S. stock exchanges, as well as their auditors, are subject to these SOX rules. SOX and the financial disasters that preceded it have had a huge impact on corporate governance and the regulation of accounting and auditing around the world. For example, in Canada, a predecessor of CPA Canada, the Canadian Institute of Chartered Accountants (CICA), helped organize the creation of its own **Canadian Public Accountability Board (CPAB)** to oversee the auditors of public companies. The CPAB also tightened quality control of audit practice and reports on inspections of audit firm practices. In addition, several of Canada's largest pension and mutual funds banded together in 2002 to form the **Canadian Coalition for Good Governance**. This organization controls hundreds of billions of dollars in assets and monitors executives, audit committees, auditors, and boards of directors in corporate Canada for compliance with what they consider good corporate governance and financial reporting practices. Finally, CPA education and practice are monitored by outside agencies in some provinces. For example, the Public Accountants Council (PAC) was created in 2006, and it determined that only licensed CPAs would be allowed to practise public accounting

Public Company Accounting Oversight Board (PCAOB):
a five-member board created through the *Sarbanes-Oxley Act* (SOX) to oversee the auditors of public companies in the United States

Canadian Public Accountability Board (CPAB):
the board organized to monitor the auditors of public companies in Canada

Canadian Coalition for Good Governance:
a group of the largest pension and mutual funds, whose purpose is to monitor executives and boards of directors to see whether they comply with good corporate governance and financial reporting practices

in Ontario. See pacont.org for PAC's standards, regulations, and handbook regarding education and licensing of CPAs in Ontario. A similar system exists in Quebec.

Despite these changes, the accounting profession in Canada is still largely self-regulating. For example, CPAB does not create audit standards. CPAB's monitoring of auditors is described in more detail in Appendix 2B.

The corporate failures, the fall of Arthur Andersen, and the resulting passage of SOX dramatically changed the corporate environment not only in the United States but also in Canada and the rest of the world. CPAB's and PCAOB's activities reflect the increased regulation of the profession. The Canadian, U.S., and other accountability boards around the world will likely make increased second-guessing of professional judgment a fixture of the post-Enron world. That world is now more complicated for auditors and the profession, and the implications will become clearer over time. However, auditing will likely become more important to accounting firms and to society. The use of more ethical reasoning in reporting will also likely be the result of this increased importance. Specific effects evident through 2015 are included in this text.

The increasing importance of auditing has come at a price; the extensive impact on the markets of the profession's perceived failures means it is no longer acceptable to leave monitoring of the profession to the professionals themselves. The monitoring process now involves groups representing the broader public interest as well as government, but the exact mix of monitors depends on the country. Since most of the corporate failures prompting the changes took place in the United States, the PCAOB has so far led the way in promoting new ways of providing oversight of auditors, and the main instrument of change has been the powers delegated to PCAOB by SOX.

SOX's impact on auditors can be seen throughout the world, but it also had consequences for broader areas of corporate activities. Following is a quick overview of its main impact on auditors:

- Management certification of all its publicly issued financial statements
- Evaluation of internal control in statements made by management
- Closer regulation of the profession, including regular monitoring of its activities
- Greater responsibilities assigned to client audit committees
- Increased importance of the role of the internal auditor

Internal control statements deal with the reliability of the system or process that creates the financial statements.[1]

Audit committees monitor management's financial reporting responsibilities, including meeting with the external auditors and dealing with various audit and accounting matters that may arise during an audit. In Canada, we have weaker and less costly requirements regarding disclosures, which some have dubbed SOX North. Under SOX North, client firms disclose as part of management discussion and analysis (MD&A) only any weaknesses in the design of internal control systems. There is no requirement that the internal controls be tested for effectiveness. There is also no requirement that these disclosures be certified by management, or that the disclosures be audited. Nevertheless, there is some evidence that these less-costly, self-reported disclosures are credible in capital markets.[2] We will discuss audit committees and the evolving concept of internal control in much greater detail throughout the rest of this text.

Perhaps the most important result of SOX for the auditor has been the increased monitoring of the profession, in the form of accountability boards. The board in Canada has authority and responsibilities that are different from those of its U.S. counterpart, as the legal systems and political institutions of the two countries are different.

internal control:
the system of policies and procedures needed to maintain adherence to a company's objectives; especially, the accuracy of recordkeeping and safeguarding of assets

audit committees:
groups that monitor management's financial reporting responsibilities, including meeting with the external auditors and dealing with various audit and accounting matters that may arise

CPAB was created in July 2002 to monitor the auditors of public companies in Canada. However, CPAB is directly funded by the audit firms, leading to questions about its independence from the profession itself. In contrast, the PCAOB is directly funded by the SEC. Another difference is that CPAB uses the profession's auditing, ethics, independence, and quality control standards in performing its monitoring, whereas PCAOB uses its own standards. CPAB, like PCAOB, issues reports on its monitoring that are made public at cpab-ccrc.ca.

The first two consequences of SOX identified above relate to management's increased responsibility for financial reporting and the requirement of an external audit of management's internal control statement. Management's certification of financial reporting means that it must state in writing that it is not aware of any factual errors or omissions of facts that would make the financial and internal control statements misleading. These are best summarized as attempts to strengthen the system of corporate governance. **Corporate governance** describes how well a company is run in the interests of shareholders and other stakeholders. Corporate governance principles are covered in Chapter 6, Appendix 6B (available on Connect). Audit committees and internal auditing are also covered in more detail later.

Other Canadian regulations, especially those in Ontario, have been influenced by the SOX requirements. There is now greater emphasis on more timely disclosures of material information and more disclosure of corporate governance practices. Management is now required to disclose its conclusions about the effectiveness of internal control in the MD&A section of the annual report. In Canada, it is not required that this disclosure on internal control be audited. In contrast, the SEC requires audits of internal control disclosures by registrant companies. In Ontario, the Toronto Stock Exchange (TSX) companies do not need to follow best corporate governance practices, but failure to do so by the largest companies must be disclosed. The Ontario Securities Commission (OSC) specifies the duties and authority of audit committees, including providing a definition of independence of its members.

Review Checkpoints

2-10   What is meant by self-regulation? What are the effects of self-regulation on the profession in the post-Enron environment?

2-11   What are the differences between Canadian and U.S. accountability boards? Compare the differences in their monitoring reports. Which ones do you think are better?

Regulation of Public Accounting

Regulation of public accounting in Canada, as with most professional groups, is a provincial matter. Most provinces have laws, public accountancy acts, that specify who is allowed to practise public accounting in the province. For example, Ontario's *Public Accounting Act* licenses only CPAs who meet the PAC's educational and experience standards to perform what they describe as public accounting functions that meet the public interest. (See their website at pacont.org for more details on their activities and requirements.) For PAC, the public interest is effectively represented by the third-party users of the financial statements. These reforms were linked to the creation of CPAB, incorporated under the *Canada Corporations Act*, which provides oversight of all PAs auditing public companies in Canada.

corporate governance:
the ways in which the suppliers of capital to corporations assure themselves of getting a return on their investment; more generally, under the corporate social responsibility view, corporate governance is the system set up to hold a corporation accountable to employees, communities, the environment, and similar broader social concerns, in addition to being accountable to the capital providers

CPAs who meet provincial requirements are allowed to practise public accounting in their provinces. Public interests, particularly those of vulnerable third parties, must be protected. Quality control standards, and CPAB monitoring implemented in recent years, helps to ensure this protection, as further explained in Appendix 2B.

In addition to the system of regulation outlined previously, other factors greatly influence the profession. These include the legal system the profession operates under (discussed in Chapter 3) and the impact of regulators on practising auditors. Regulators include, at the federal level, the Superintendent of Financial Institutions, whose prime responsibility is regulating the financial services industry under the jurisdiction of the *Federal Bank Act*. At the provincial level, there are the securities commissions with responsibility for investor protection and for ensuring the fairness and efficiency of the province's capital markets. There are securities commissions in every province and territory, but because of the division of powers between the provinces and the federal government, there is no national-level securities commission in Canada comparable with the SEC in the United States. However, since 1999, the Joint Forum of Financial Market Regulators, consisting of provincial securities commissioners and various national regulators, has coordinated and streamlined the regulation of services in Canadian financial markets through voluntary agreement between participants.

The OSC is responsible for the biggest and most-developed capital markets in Canada. We will use it here to illustrate the impact a regulator can have on public accounting. Three principal activities of the OSC ensure the orderly functioning of capital markets within its jurisdiction, such as the TSX:

1. Registering issuers, dealers, and advisers trading in securities and commodity futures contracts

2. Monitoring the full extent of reporting requirements, including those related to prospectuses, takeovers, and continuous disclosure of material information

3. Enforcing the provisions of the *Securities Act* and the *Commodity Futures Act*

A **prospectus** is the information, usually including financial information, about a firm that accompanies any new issuance of shares in a regulated securities market. The staff of the OSC includes a chief accountant and a chief forensic accountant, who work under the director of enforcement. The Office of the Chief Accountant is responsible for formulating financial reporting policy and for monitoring the application of accounting principles and auditing standards by report issuers and their auditors. Financial statements are reviewed on a selective basis, and up to one-quarter of companies reviewed receive comment letters relating to inadequacies in their financial reports. The companies' auditors are also informed of problems. If the financial reporting problems are severe enough, the Enforcement Branch is notified. In 2001, the OSC found revenue recognition to be a significant problem area for high-tech firms.

An example of an Enforcement Branch action affecting an auditor who will testify as a witness is given in the following box. This OSC action followed an investigation of Nortel's accounting launched in April 2004 by the SEC and the OSC. Nortel, then one of Canada's premier high-tech companies in the telecommunications industry, had to restate its financial results for quarterly periods going back through 2003, 2002, and 2001. The restated 2003 results reduced earnings by 41%. By January 2005, Nortel's stock price had dropped to the $4 range from a July 2000 high of $124. Over 90,000 Nortel employees lost their jobs during this period. The earlier 2003 earnings had triggered millions of dollars of bonus payments to management. Twelve senior executives agreed to return $10.4 million of these bonuses, but Nortel filed for bankruptcy in 2009 and the trustees in bankruptcy are still seeking repayment of 2003 bonuses from managers fired in April 2004.

In an attempt to demonstrate that Canada was serious in prosecuting white-collar crime, the RCMP began a criminal investigation into Nortel's accounting on August 16, 2004. The trial did not begin until 2012 and ended early in 2013, as indicated in the next box.

prospectus:
set of financial statements and disclosures distributed to all purchasers in an offering registered under Securities Law

Nortel Fraud Trial Launches with Not-Guilty Pleas, Allegations of a Cookie Jar Culture

The fraud trial of former Nortel Networks Corp. executives began Monday with the prosecution alleging a "cookie jar" culture in which accounting reserves were repeatedly manipulated to meet thresholds and trigger bonus payouts.

"They set their targets," chief prosecutor Robert Hubbard said in his opening remarks before Superior Court Justice Frank Marrocco. "Then they went about doing whatever needed to be done to meet those targets."

The accused, former Nortel chief executive Frank Dunn, former chief financial officer Douglas Beatty, and ex-Nortel corporate controller Michael Gollogly, were fired by Nortel for cause in 2004 amid allegations of financial mismanagement. The RCMP laid fraud charges against the three men in 2008. They are accused of manipulating Nortel's financial reporting to trigger multi-million-dollar bonus payouts linked to the networking company's return to profitability. All three men entered pleas of not guilty at the start of the trial that a spokesman for the Ontario Ministry of the Attorney General said could last more than six months.

The trial ended on January 15, 2013, with the acquittal of all three executives. This acquittal was viewed by some accountants as a disaster for ethical financial reporting in Canada: "The acquittal of Nortel senior executives, many will argue, has all but granted a free legal pass to any company that wants to massage its financial reports to present better numbers to an unknowing public. . . . With the Nortel verdict as precedent, an awful lot of accounting games may now have a stamp of legal legitimacy."

Source: Excerpts from Michael Lewis, "Nortel fraud trial launches with not guilty pleas, allegations of a cookie jar culture," *The Toronto Star*, January 16, 2012, reprinted with permission of Torstar Syndication Services; D. Parkinson, "Nortel judgment won't discourage accounting games," *The Globe and Mail, Report on Business*, January 15, 2013, B5; and Janet McFarland and Richard Blackwell, "Three former Nortel executives found not guilty of fraud," *The Globe and Mail*, January 14, 2013.

What Nortel perhaps best illustrates is the distinction between fraudulent and unethical reporting, and that auditors and regulators should be concerned with both. An independent review by Nortel's audit committee concluded that the corporate culture encouraged financial manipulation through weak internal controls. In January 2005, the board of directors went through a major reorganization, with half of the board members leaving. In addition, a high-profile ethics watchdog and compliance officer was hired to help change the corporate culture. This example illustrates why good corporate governance principles need to be followed. (Corporate governance principles are explored in more detail in Appendix 6B.) Nevertheless, the ultimate failure of Nortel suggests that more can be done by auditors and using accounting standards to deter unethical reporting before it leads to fraud or the failure of a company, or both. Nortel-type reporting issues and their significance for auditors are covered in more detail in subsequent chapters. It's through questionable reporting like Nortel's that the audit report is being modified to encourage auditors to publicize the difficult areas of the audit engagement in their reports.

Getting back to the OSC, it also monitors the setting of auditing and accounting standards by CPA Canada, and it provides input on emerging issues as well as commentary on proposed standards. In addition, since 1989, the OSC has issued Staff Accounting Communiqués (SACs) intended to explain the OSC staff's views on specific reporting issues. Although the SACs have no official OSC approval, OSC staff are likely to challenge any treatment that is inconsistent with an SAC. By publishing the results of its monitoring program, by filing complaints to provincial disciplinary committees, and through its representation on CPA Canada standard-setting boards, in recent years the OSC has had a significant, ongoing impact on the profession.

Other regulators also affect the profession. For example, the Canadian Investor Protection Fund— sponsored by the Toronto and the Montreal stock exchanges, the Canadian Venture Exchange, the Toronto Futures Exchange, and the Investment Dealers Association of Canada—is a trust established to protect customers from the financial failure of a member firm (any member of a sponsoring organization and some U.S. bond dealers that trade in Canada). In recent years, Fund staff have taken a more active supervisory role by overseeing regular monthly, quarterly, and annual reporting; paying surprise visits to offices of member firms; and conducting at least one financial questionnaire per year. The Fund can fine or set sanctions against a member firm that violates capital, reporting, or other requirements. It develops policy statements that address standards for internal control within member firms. Auditors must be aware of these standards when auditing member firms. Internal control reports are discussed in more detail in Chapter 21 (available on Connect).

Another regulator, the **Securities and Exchange Commission (SEC)**, affects Canadian auditors whose client firms have dealings with U.S. securities markets. In recent years, many Canadian companies have gone to U.S. and other international markets to raise cash through an **initial public offering (IPO)**. Because they need to file regulatory documents in each province, which increases the cost of financing, many Canadian companies are finding it cheaper to raise money through public markets in other countries. Canada's Department of Finance has for a number of years explored the idea of creating a national securities regulator (such as the SEC in the United States) or some national coordinator of provincial securities commissions, to improve the quality and competitiveness of Canadian securities markets.[3] The impact of the SEC on auditors is discussed in more detail in Chapter 20 (available on Connect).

An important development in the regulation of the Canadian accounting profession was the creation of the CPAB on July 17, 2002. The Board represents the public interest through being dominated by non-CPA members (seven of the eleven Board members are to be non-CPAs). The Board monitors audit practice and conducts annual inspections of accounting firms to assess their ability to protect the public interest. It has the power to sanction any auditor that fails to protect the public interest, and it is viewed as the first in a series of major structural reforms to protect the integrity of Canada's financial accounting systems. However, CPAB does not create audit standards. That is left to CPA Canada, which as a matter of policy has adopted the international standards that we cover in this text. Other steps include the CPA Canada evolving standard for auditor independence and the creation of provincial boards to oversee the professional conduct and peer-review systems at the provincial level. These activities are discussed in more detail in Appendix 2B.

Finally, regulators, such as provincial ministries of the environment and natural resources, indirectly affect the profession by restricting which activities the clients themselves may need to disclose as part of the clients' business risk.

It should be clear from this brief review that the profession is facing an increasingly complex regulatory environment and that auditors must be sensitized to regulatory concerns in order to do a proper audit. Auditors also need to be concerned with meeting the demands of regulators in different countries. One part of the solution is using worldwide standards whenever feasible.

Review Checkpoints

2-12 Identify several types of professional accountants and their organizations.

2-13 What are some examples of assurance services rendered on representations other than traditional financial statements?

2-14 What are the three major areas of public accounting services?

2-15 Locate Nortel's audit committee report on the Internet. Is the OSC or the SEC website more user-friendly for investors?

Securities and Exchange Commission (SEC):
the main U.S. government agency regulating the securities markets in the United States

initial public offering (IPO):
first-time offering of a corporation's shares to the public

Practice Standards

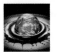
LO2   List the various practice standards for independent audits of financial statements.

Practice standards are general guides for the quality of professional work, and the accounting and auditing profession has many sets of standards to choose from. The remainder of this chapter deals directly with four sets: (1) generally accepted auditing standards (GAAS), issued by CPA Canada's Auditing and Assurance Standards Board (in the *CPA Canada Handbook*); (2) assurance standards, as promulgated by section 5025 of the *CPA Canada Handbook;* (3) CPA Canada's General Standards of Quality Control for Firms Performing Assurance Engagements (CSQC-1); and (4) quality control standards as reflected in firm peer reviews and provincial institutes' practice inspection manuals (covered in Appendix 2B). Several countries have created accountability boards in the post-Enron world. These boards can influence standards through monitoring public company audits and identifying weaknesses in them. In most countries, public companies are those listed on stock exchanges. The rules of professional ethics are also briefly introduced in this chapter and covered in more depth in Chapters 3 and 18 (available on Connect). The CPA Canada Recommendations for compilation and review services are explained in Chapter 17 (available on Connect). In the rest of this text, we may refer to CPA Canada Recommendations as *CPA Canada Handbook* Standards on Assurance or, most commonly, Canadian Auditing Standards (CASs).

You will find relatively few references to the accounting recommendations in this text. CPA Canada issues accounting standards, but this text concentrates on auditing and the practice of accounting, not on the accounting rules themselves. An overview of GAAS is provided in the next section.

Generally Accepted Auditing Standards

LO3   Summarize the ethical, examination, and reporting standards that make up generally accepted auditing standards as set out in CPA Canada's Canadian Auditing Standards.

CPA Canada's **generally accepted auditing standards (GAAS)** were first written as a short statement of eight standards. Since 1975, these eight have been augmented by additional explanations and requirements in the assurance Recommendations of the *CPA Canada Handbook*. Beginning in 2010, *Handbook* section 5100 was largely replaced by CAS 200 (5100, 5021, 5090, and 5095), and professional ethical requirements of the relevant professional accounting organizations were added. These changes are in line with convergence to international standards. CAS 200 is titled "Overall Objective of the Independent Auditor, and the Conduct of the Audit in Accordance with Canadian Auditing Standards." CAS 200 establishes auditors' overall responsibilities when conducting an audit in accordance with CASs. It lists the objectives of the audit and a series of principles and concepts fundamental to financial statement auditing, as shown in Exhibit 2–1.

The importance of GAAS is that they identify the objectives and key principles of the financial statement audit. Every CAS is written so that it identifies the subject and objectives of the standard, provides new definitions wherever applicable, states the requirements for meeting the objective, and provides further explanation for carrying out these requirements. This may include examples of procedures that are appropriate in specific contexts. As we will see in Chapter 3, organizing the standards in this way more closely parallels the concepts of critical thinking within professional judgment. The goal is to have a more logically organized set of standards and to communicate the reasoning behind these standards to the auditor.

generally accepted auditing standards (GAAS):
those auditing recommendations that have been established in a particular jurisdiction by formal recognition by a standard-setting body, or by authoritative support or precedent such as the auditing and assurance recommendations of the *CPA Canada Handbook*

If a relevant CAS objective cannot be achieved in an audit, the auditor has to consider whether the overall objectives of the audit, as stated in CAS 200, can be met. The CASs are issued from time to time, and the objective of each is consistent with the overall objective of CAS 200. You should view CAS 200 as the conceptual framework of financial statement auditing that provides the fundamental principles and objectives of the financial statement audit. For all practical purposes, this consistency of objectives makes all CASs part of GAAS. Any financial statement auditor who does not follow *CPA Canada Handbook* CASs can be judged as performing a deficient audit.

The auditing standards literature also includes a series of Canadian Audit Practice Notes (CAPNs) and **Audit Guidelines (AuGs)**. For the most part, the guidelines give technical help.

Appendix 2A (available on Connect) lists the GAAS used in the United States. Note the similarities to GAAS of Exhibit 2–1.

Canadian Auditing Standards (CASs) are audit-quality recommendations that remain the same over time and for all audits. Auditing procedures, on the other hand, are quite different and include the particular and specialized actions auditors take to obtain evidence in a specific audit engagement. Audit procedures may vary, depending on the complexity of an accounting system (whether

---

EXHIBIT 2–1

Generally Accepted Auditing Standards (Summary of CAS 200, 300, and 315)

Objective of an Audit of Financial Statements

The overall objective of the audit is to enable the auditor to express an opinion on whether the financial statements are prepared, in all material respects, within an applicable (acceptable) financial reporting framework. Most of this text deals with fair presentation frameworks.

General Standard

The auditor should comply with relevant professional ethical requirements relating to audit engagements.

Examination Standards

1. The auditor should conduct an audit in accordance with Canadian Auditing Standards (CASs).
2. In determining the audit procedures to perform in accord with CASs' "scope of an audit," the auditor should comply with each CAS relevant to the audit.
3. The auditor should obtain reasonable assurance that the financial statements taken as a whole are free from material misstatement, whether due to fraud or error.
4. The auditor should plan and perform an audit to reduce audit risk to an acceptably low level that is consistent with the objective of an audit.

Reporting Standards

1. The report should identify the financial statements and distinguish between the responsibilities of management and the responsibilities of the auditor.
2. The auditor should determine whether the financial reporting framework adopted by management in preparing the financial statements is acceptable.
3. The auditor should refer to CAS 700, 701, 705, and 706 when expressing an opinion on a complete set of general purpose financial statements prepared in accordance with a financial reporting framework that is designed to achieve fair presentation.

Skepticism

The auditor should plan and perform an audit with an attitude of professional skepticism, recognizing that circumstances may exist that cause the financial statements to be materially misstated or misleading to third parties.

Source: Adapted from the *CPA Canada Handbook—Assurance*, CAS 200, 300, and 315.

Audit Guidelines (AuGs):
the part of the *CPA Canada Handbook* that provides procedural guidance on implementing generally accepted auditing standards

manual or computerized), the type of company, and other situation-specific factors. These differences explain why audit reports refer to an audit "conducted in accordance with generally accepted auditing standards," rather than "in accordance with auditing procedures." As such, considerable judgment is required to apply audit procedures in specific situations.

Generally Accepted Auditing Standards: Objectives of the Audit of Financial Statements

The overall objective of a financial statement audit is to enable the auditor to express an opinion as to whether the financial statements are prepared, in all material respects, in conformity with an applicable framework. Note how this objective implies three-party accountability. Statements are prepared, and an auditor expresses an opinion on whether the statements conform to an *applicable*, also known as *acceptable, framework*. CPA Canada and international standards view the terms "applicable" and "acceptable" as equivalent, but "acceptable" better reflects both the need for the reporting to be appropriate to third parties and the evaluative component in auditor professional judgment.

CAS 200 offers a very broad financial reporting framework. In this book, we focus primarily on Canadian GAAP as the reporting framework. This reporting includes a balance sheet, income statement, cash flow statement, statement of retained earnings, and notes made up of a summary of significant accounting policies as well as any other explanations.

Generally Accepted Auditing Standards: Ethical Requirements Relating to an Audit of Financial Statements

The ethical requirements section of GAAS relates to the personal integrity and professional qualifications of auditors. Until 2009, section 5100 included what was called a *general standard*. This general standard has been replaced by the rules of professional ethics that are covered in Chapter 3. For now, we will summarize these under three headings.

Competence

The rules of professional ethics require competence—adequate technical training and proficiency—in auditors. This competence begins with an education in accounting, since auditors hold themselves out as experts in accounting standards and financial reporting. It continues with on-the-job training in developing and applying professional judgment in real-world audit situations. This stage provides practice in performing the assurance function, in which auditors learn to (1) recognize the underlying assertions being made by management in each element (account) in the financial statements, (2) decide which evidence is relevant for supporting or refuting the assertions, (3) select and perform procedures for obtaining the evidence, and (4) evaluate the evidence and decide whether management assertions correspond to reality and GAAP. Auditors must be thoughtfully prepared to encounter a wide range of judgments on the part of management accountants—judgments varying from the truly objective to the subjective, and occasional deliberate misstatement within either extreme.

Objectivity and Independence

The ethics rules also require that auditors have an objective state of mind—that is, intellectual honesty and impartiality. Auditors must be unbiased with respect to the financial statements and other information they audit. They are expected to be fair not only to the companies and executives who issue financial information, but also to the outside persons who use it. This type of objectivity in assurance services is achieved by maintaining professional independence, in appearance as well as in fact. The appearance of independence—avoiding financial and managerial relationships with auditees—is important because this is what public users of audit reports can see. They cannot see an auditor's state of mind or attitude. Independence must be carefully guarded because the public will only recognize the professional status of auditors if they perceive them to be independent. Note that this emphasis on independence arises primarily from the need to get the trust of the third-party users of the financial statements. Independence in appearance is addressed in more detail in Chapters 3 and 18.

Some critics of the public accounting profession find it undesirable that auditors are paid by their auditees. They argue that it is impossible to be independent from the party paying the fee. The alternative would be some form of public or government control of accounting fees, and very few PAs want government involvement. Auditing is unique in that, although a company pays the auditor, the real clients are the third-party users of financial statements. This concept of public interest increasingly guides standard setting and regulators in all aspects of the audit environment. An auditor, therefore, needs to differentiate between responsibilities to the company and responsibilities to third parties. Addressing such ethical conflicts in a competent manner is part of what makes public accounting a profession (see Chapter 3 for more details).

Due Professional Care

The exercise of due professional care requires observance of the rules of professional ethics and GAAS. Auditors must be competent and independent, exercising proper care in planning and supervising the audit, in understanding the auditee's control structure, and in obtaining sufficient appropriate evidence. Their training should include computer auditing techniques because of the importance and pervasiveness of computers in the business world.

Many social science theories incorporate the idea of a prudent professional practitioner, for example, the "economic person" of economic theory and the "reasonable person" in law. The qualities of a "prudent auditor," as summarized by Mautz and Sharaf, might be used to demonstrate the concept of due care in an audit:

> A prudent practitioner [auditor] is assumed to have a knowledge of the philosophy and practice of auditing, to have the degree of training, experience, and skill common to the average independent auditor, to have the ability to recognize indications of irregularities, and to keep abreast of developments in the perpetration and detection of irregularities. Due audit care requires the auditor to acquaint himself with the company under examination, the accounting and financial problems of the company . . . to be responsive to unusual events and unfamiliar circumstances, to persist until he has eliminated from his own mind any reasonable doubts he may have about the existence of material irregularities, and to exercise caution in instructing his assistants and reviewing their work.[4]

Due professional care is a matter of what auditors do and how well they do it. A determination of proper care must be reached based on all facts and circumstances in a particular case. When an audit firm's work becomes the subject of a lawsuit, the question of due audit care is frequently at issue (as you will see in Chapter 3).

Review Checkpoints

2-16 What is the difference between auditing standards and auditing procedures?

2-17 By what standard would a judge determine the quality of due professional care? Explain.

Generally Accepted Auditing Standards: Examination Standards

The examination standards are covered by CAS 315 and CAS 300, as well as by CAS 200. These standards set general quality criteria for conducting an audit and also relate to the sufficiency and appropriateness of evidence gathered to support the audit opinion. Auditors cannot effectively satisfy the general standard requiring due professional care if they have not also satisfied the examination standards.

The CAS 200 concepts and principles that influence the examination standards include conduct of an audit, scope of an audit, reasonable assurance, audit risk and materiality, planning and supervision, internal control assessment, and sufficient appropriate evidential matter. All of these are extensively covered in later chapters. Here we will only provide an overview.

Conduct of an Audit of Financial Statements

In order to meet the overall objective of the audit of financial statements, the auditor in Canada must comply with the CASs and the CAPNs. While this might seem to state the obvious, it serves to make the requirement explicit so that there are no excuses for failing to comply.

Scope of an Audit of Financial Statements

The principle of scope in auditing financial statements refers to exercising professional judgment when deciding, based on CASs, on the type and extent of audit procedures to perform under the particular circumstances. The procedures performed must be documented during the audit engagement.

Reasonable Assurance

The evidence gathered during the audit procedures should allow the auditor to have reasonable assurance that the financial statements as a whole are free of material misstatements, whether due to fraud or error. Reasonable assurance means the same as high assurance; that is, assurance should not be too low for an audit engagement. On the other hand, it does not mean certainty or absolute assurance. If assurance were represented as the degree of confidence in the audit opinion, then a range of 90–99% confidence, with 95% being the most common, would be normal. Reasonable assurance is closely related to the concepts of audit risk and materiality.

Audit Risk and Materiality

The risk that an auditor expresses an inappropriate audit opinion when the financial statements are materially misstated is audit risk. As introduced in Chapter 1, this risk relates to evidence gathering. The most serious form of audit risk is failing to detect a material misstatement. These misstatements affect the decisions of third-party users of the financial statements. Reasonable or high audit assurance can only be obtained when audit risk is acceptably low. Thus, the objective of the audit is only achieved when audit risk is reduced to an acceptably low level. This is done through performing effective audit procedures—the means auditors use to obtain evidence for their opinion. The audit opinion must be supported by sufficient appropriate evidence. This is the only acceptable way to meet the overall audit objective. An important means of controlling audit risk is through proper training, planning, and supervision. As noted in Chapter 1, the focus of audit standards is controlling audit risk, whereas how the accounting standards are applied affects the accounting risk.

Planning and Supervision

CAS 300 of the *CPA Canada Handbook* contains several considerations for planning and supervising an audit. They are all concerned with (1) preparing an **audit plan** and supervising the audit work, (2) obtaining knowledge of the auditee's business, and (3) dealing with differences of opinion among the audit firm's own personnel.

Written audit programs are required. An **audit program** lists the audit procedures the auditors will perform to produce the evidence needed for good audit decisions. The procedures in an audit program should include

audit plan:
a document containing all the detailed audit programs listing the procedures to be performed in response to the assessed risk of material misstatement on an audit, guided by the decisions made in the overall audit strategy

audit program:
a document listing the specific detailed audit procedures to be performed in each accounting process to gather sufficient appropriate evidence through control tests, analytical procedures, and other tests of balances to address the audit objectives set out in the program; includes the risk assessment program, the internal control program, and the balance audit program

enough detail to instruct the assistants about the work to be done. (You will see detailed audit programs later in this text.)

An understanding of the auditee's business is an absolute necessity. An auditor must be able to understand the events, transactions, and practices that are characteristic of the business and its management and that may have a significant effect on the financial statements. This knowledge helps auditors identify areas for special attention (the places where errors, irregularities, or frauds might exist), evaluate the reasonableness of accounting estimates made by management, evaluate management's representations and answers to inquiries, and make judgments about the appropriateness of the accounting principles chosen.

Where does an auditor get this understanding of a business? By being there; working in other companies in the same industry; conducting interviews with management and other auditee personnel; reading extensively—accounting and audit guides of various accounting bodies, the practice manuals of the various accounting organizations, industry publications, other companies' financial statements, business periodicals, and textbooks; getting a thorough familiarization presentation from the partner in charge of the audit before beginning the engagement; and being observant and letting on-the-job experience sink into long-term memory. Auditors are increasingly building their understanding of the auditee's business through knowledge-acquisition frameworks from strategic management. These frameworks (covered in more detail in Chapters 5 and 6) provide a structured approach to gaining deep knowledge of the auditee's business and industry.

There is no guarantee that the auditors on an audit team will always agree among themselves on audit decisions, which range from inclusion or omission of procedures to conclusions about the fair presentation of an account or the financial statements as a whole. When differences of opinion arise, audit personnel should consult with each other and with experts in the firm to try to resolve the disagreement. If resolution is not achieved, the audit firm should have procedures allowing an audit team member to document the disagreement and to dissociate himself or herself from the matter. Particularly where there are disagreements, the basis for the final audit decision on the matter should be documented in the working papers for later reference.

Each audit should have a complete audit file of working papers documenting the evidence obtained that supports the audit opinion. Without such evidential support, the audit opinion is not valid. As noted in Chapter 1, "not documented, not done." For example, if you were the auditor in the Fort Knox illustration of Chapter 1, then your opinion is meaningless unless you have an audit file documenting when you visited Fort Knox, what you did on your visit, and what the results of the evidence you obtained shows about the amount of gold in Fort Knox. Your conclusion in your audit file must be consistent with what you say in your audit report. Otherwise, you are lying when issuing your audit report. To see why, check what the audit report says in Exhibit 1–4 and especially note what the last sentence under Basis for Opinion says. If you do not have an audit file supporting the truthfulness of these statements, then you cannot issue an audit opinion. The details and planning of the various procedures to document in an audit file are discussed throughout the rest of this book.

Timing is important for audit planning. To have time to plan an audit, auditors should be engaged before the auditee's fiscal year-end. An early appointment benefits both auditor and auditee. The audit team may be able to perform part of the audit at an **interim date**, a date some weeks or months before the fiscal year-end, and thereby make the rest of the audit work more efficient. It could include preliminary analytical procedures, preliminary assessment of internal control risk, testing the controls, and auditing some account balances. Advance knowledge of problems can enable auditors to alter the audit program so that year-end work (performed on and after the fiscal year-end date) can be more efficient. Planning for the observation of physical inventory and for the confirmation of accounts receivable is particularly important.

interim date:
a date before the end of the period under audit when some of the audit procedures might be performed, such as control evaluation and testing

Too Late

FastTrak Corporation was angry with its auditor because the partner in charge of the engagement would not agree to let management use the operating lease accounting treatment for some heavy equipment whose leases met the criteria for capitalization. FastTrak fired the auditors 10 weeks after the company's balance sheet date and then began contacting other audit firms to restart the audit. However, the audit report was due at the OSC in six weeks. Every other audit firm contacted by FastTrak refused the audit because it could not be planned and performed properly with such a tight deadline.

Internal Control Assessment

The examination standard CAS 315, paragraphs 12–23, requires an understanding of the auditee's internal control. This consists of a company's control environment, accounting system, and control procedures. The existence of a satisfactory internal control system reduces the probability of errors and irregularities in the accounts. Auditors need to know enough about the auditee's control system to assess the control risk. Control risk is the probability that a material misstatement (error or irregularity) could occur and not be prevented or detected on a timely basis by the internal control structure, as is discussed in CAS 200.

The primary purpose of control risk assessment is to help the auditors develop the audit program. This standard presumes two necessary relationships: (1) good internal control reduces the control risk, minimizing the extent of subsequent audit procedures; (2) conversely, poor internal control produces greater control risk, increasing the necessary extent of subsequent audit procedures. If auditors saw no relationship between the quality of controls and the accuracy of output, then an assessment of control risk would be pointless. Audit efficiency would be lost in many cases. (Chapters 6 and 9 explain the work involved in control risk assessment.)

Control Lapse Contributes to Duplicate Payments

All Points Trucking processed insurance claims on damages to shipments in transit on its trucks, paying them through a self-insurance plan. After payment, the claim documents were not marked "paid." Later, the same documents were processed again for duplicate payments to customers, who kicked back 50% to a dishonest All Points employee. When the auditors learned that the claims were not marked as paid, they concluded that the specific control risk of duplicate payments was high and extended their procedures to include a search for duplicate payments in the damage expense account. They found the fraudulent claims and traced the problem to the dishonest employee. Embezzlements of $35,000 per year were stopped.

Sufficient Appropriate Evidential Matter

Examination standard CAS 200 recognizes that evidence is the heart of audits of financial statements, and it requires auditors to obtain enough to justify opinions on those statements. Evidence is the influence on auditors that ultimately guides their decisions. It includes the underlying accounting data and all available corroborating information, as discussed in CAS 330 and CAS 500. Appropriate—that is, reliable and relevant—evidence may take many forms: quantitative or qualitative, objective or subjective, absolutely compelling or mildly persuasive. The audit team's task is to collect and evaluate sufficient appropriate evidence in order to afford a reasonable and logical basis for audit decisions.

The standard refers to sufficient rather than absolute evidence. In most cases, not all of a company's transactions and events are audited, and audit decisions are made by inference based on data samples. The standard gives broad outlines for procedures for gathering evidence—inspection, observation, inquiry, and confirmation. Chapter 8 gives a more thorough explanation of audit objectives and procedures.

Review Checkpoints

2-18   What three elements of planning and supervision are considered essential in audit practice?

2-19   Why does the timing of an auditor's appointment matter in the conduct of a financial statement audit?

2-20   Why does an auditor obtain an understanding of the internal control system?

2-21   Define audit evidence.

Generally Accepted Auditing Standards: Reporting Standards

The ultimate objective of independent auditors—the report on the audit—is guided by the GAAS reporting standards. The three that are identified in CAS 200 deal with acceptability of the financial reporting framework, auditor and management responsibilities, and report content. Auditing standards dictate the use of a "standard report" when the auditor is expressing an opinion on a complete set of general purpose financial statements prepared to achieve fair presentation. Detailed guidance on these reports is given in CAS 700 and CAS 705. These standards cover audit reports using a fair presentation reporting framework, as well as audit reports using a compliance financial reporting framework. Special considerations for reporting on special purpose financial statements, or financial information other than a full set of financial statements, are covered in CAS 800 and CAS 805. In this chapter, we provide an overview of the CAS 700 audit report on fair presentation for a set of general purpose financial statements. Chapter 4 gives more in-depth coverage.

An **unmodified opinion report**, or a report without reservation, means that the auditors are not calling attention to anything wrong with the audit work or the financial statements. The standard unmodified opinion audit report is shown in Exhibit 2–2, which you should review in relation to the discussion that follows. A **modified opinion report** means that either the financial statements contain a departure from GAAP or the scope of the audit work was limited. (You will study modified opinion audit reports in Chapter 4.)

All standard unmodified opinion reports contain the following features:

1. **Title.** The title should refer to the independent auditor, thus indicating that the report is based on an audit examination and not on some other types of engagement.

2. **Address.** The report is normally addressed to those it is prepared for; this may be the shareholders or those charged with governance of the auditee organization.

3. **Introductory paragraph in opinion section.** The introductory paragraph should identify the financial statements and declare that they were audited.

4. **Opinion paragraph in the opinion section.** The report's second paragraph should contain an opinion (opinion paragraph), stating whether the financial statements present fairly, in all material respects, . . . in accordance with GAAP.

5. **Key audit matters.** Auditors must identify the most significant issues during the audit, called the key audit matters. This is the biggest change from the audit report before December 15, 2016, and represents a potentially huge extension of auditor responsibilities in financial statement auditing.

---

unmodified opinion report:
an audit report in which the auditor is not calling attention to anything wrong with the audit work or the financial statements

modified opinion report:
an audit report that contains an opinion paragraph that does not give the positive assurance that everything in the financial statements conforms with GAAP; includes qualified opinion, adverse opinion, and disclaimer of opinion reports

EXHIBIT 2-2

Independent Auditor's Report

To the Shareholders of . . . . .

Report on the Audit of the Financial Statements

Opinion

We have audited the financial statements of ABC Company (the Company), which comprise the statement of financial position as at December 31, 20X1, and the statement of comprehensive income, statement of changes in equity, and statement of cash flows for the year then ended, and notes to the financial statements, including a summary of significant accounting policies.

In our opinion, the accompanying financial statements present fairly, in all material respects, (*or give a true and fair view of*) the financial position of the Company as at December 31, 20X1, and (*of*) its financial performance and its cash flows for the year then ended in accordance with International Financial Reporting Standards (IFRS).

Basis for Opinion

We conducted our audit in accordance with International Standards on Auditing (ISAs). Our responsibilities under those standards are further described in the *Auditor's Responsibilities for the Audit of the Financial Statements* section of our report. We are independent of the Company in accordance with the Provincial Ethics Standards Board for Accountants' *Code of Ethics for Professional Accountants* together with the ethical requirements that are relevant to our audit of the financial statements in [*jurisdiction*], and we have fulfilled our other ethical responsibilities in accordance with these requirements and the Code. We believe that the audit evidence we have obtained is sufficient and appropriate to provide a basis for our opinion.

Key Audit Matters

Key audit matters are those matters that, in our professional judgment, were of most significance in our audit of the financial statements of the current period. These matters were addressed in the context of our audit of the financial statements as a whole, and in forming our opinion, thereon, and we do not provide a separate opinion on these matters.

[Description of each key audit matter in accordance with CAS 701.]

Responsibilities of Management and Those Charged with Governance for the Financial Statements*

Management is responsible for the preparation and fair presentation of the financial statements in accordance with IFRS,** and for such internal control as management determines is necessary to enable the preparation of financial statements that are free from material misstatement, whether due to fraud or error.

In preparing the financial statements, management is responsible for assessing the Company's ability to continue as a going concern, disclosing, as applicable, matters related to going concern and using the going-concern basis of accounting unless management either intends to liquidate the Company or to cease operations, or has no realistic alternative but to do so.

Those charged with governance are responsible for overseeing the Company's financial reporting process.

Auditor's Responsibilities for the Audit of the Financial Statements

Our objectives are to obtain reasonable assurance about whether the financial statements as a whole are free from material misstatement, whether due to fraud or error, and to issue an auditor's report that includes our opinion. Reasonable assurance is a high level of assurance, but is not a guarantee that an audit conducted in accordance with CASs will always detect a material misstatement when it exists. Misstatements can arise from fraud or error and are considered material if, individually or in the aggregate, they could reasonably be expected to influence the economic decisions of users taken on the basis of these financial statements.

[Additional description of auditor responsibilities is required here, or referenced to an appendix to the report, or reference can be made to a website of an appropriate authority that contains the description of the auditor's responsibilities—the additional description of responsibilities is discussed in Chapter 4 of this textbook.]

The engagement partner on the audit resulting in this independent auditor's report is [name].

[Signature in the name of the audit firm, the personal name of the auditor, or both, as appropriate for the particular jurisdiction]

[Auditor Address]

[Date]

---

* Throughout these illustrative auditor's reports, the terms *management* and *those charged with governance* may need to be replaced by another term that is appropriate in the context of the legal framework in the particular jurisdiction.

** Where management's responsibility is to prepare financial statements that give a true and fair view, this may read: "Management is responsible for the preparation of financial statements that give a true and fair view in accordance with International Financial Reporting Standards, and for such. . . ."

Source: Copyright © *CPA Canada Handbook—Assurance*, CAS 700.

6. **Management and corporate governance responsibilities.** The fifth, sixth, and seventh paragraphs of the report state management's responsibilities to prepare the financial statements, and corporate governance responsibilities to oversee financial reporting.

7. **Description of the audit.** The eighth (and possibly additional) paragraph covers auditor responsibilities. This covers what is traditionally referred to as the *scope of the audit.* The principal characteristics of an audit can be added in the report itself, as an appendix to the report, or by reference to the website of an appropriate authority. We discuss these responsibilities in more detail throughout this book and especially in Chapter 4.

8. **Signature.** The auditor should sign the report, manually or otherwise.

9. **Date.** The report should be dated no earlier than the date when the auditor obtained sufficient appropriate audit evidence supporting the auditor's opinion on the financial statements; this will be after those with recognized authority (e.g., board of directors) have taken responsibility for (i.e., approved) the financial statements. The engagement quality control review, discussed later in this chapter (CSCQ-1, CAS 220), also needs to be completed before the date of the auditor's report.

10. **Auditor's address.** The report should name the auditor and the location in the country or jurisdiction where the auditor practises.

Generally Accepted Accounting Principles

In the audit report, the opinion sentence shows that the GAAP standard has been met: "In our opinion, the financial statements . . . present fairly, in all material respects, the financial position . . . and statement of cash flows . . . in accordance with" an acceptable reporting framework such as IFRS or other Canadian GAAP. Here, the auditors make a statement about their belief based on their evidence (opinion). In other words, an opinion requires evidence that is documented in the audit file for the engagement.

Determining the appropriate GAAP in a company's circumstances is not always easy. Students often think of the *CPA Canada Handbook* Recommendations on accounting standards as the complete body of GAAP. This is not so. The *Handbook* Recommendations cover many accounting issues and problems, and the standards for these are generally compelling. However, the *Handbook* does not cover all conceivable accounting matters. When a conclusion about GAAP cannot be found in the *Handbook* Recommendations, auditors follow a hierarchy to find the next highest source of support for an entity's accounting solution to a financial reporting problem. Reference can be made to positions taken by provincial securities commissions, international standards, authoritative pronouncements by other countries' standards boards, industry audit and accounting guides, consensus positions of the CPA Canada Emerging Issues Committee, and other accounting literature.

The unmodified opinion sentence contains implicit messages: (a) the accounting principles in the financial statements have general acceptance—that is, authoritative support; (b) the accounting principles used by the company are appropriate under the circumstances; (c) the financial statements and notes are informative of matters that may affect their use, understanding, and interpretation—that is, disclosures are complete; this last feature refers to both materiality and accuracy; (d) the classification and summary in the financial statements is neither too detailed nor too condensed for users; and (e) the financial statements are accurate within practical materiality limits covered in CAS 320. Auditors and users do not expect financial account balances to be absolutely accurate, as accounting is too complicated and includes too many estimates to expect this. After all, many financial reports use numbers rounded to the thousands, even millions, of dollars! Financial figures are "fair" as long as they are not materially misstated—that is, misstated enough to make a difference in users' decisions. All of these issues in applying GAAP involve professional judgment, which can be defined very generally as making a decision using professional standards and other criteria while maintaining professional ethics responsibilities. (Chapter 3 covers auditors' professional ethics responsibilities.)

Consistency

The reporting standards call for explicit reporting in accordance with GAAP, except under special circumstances. Prior to 1991, all audit reports contained a sentence confirming that GAAP had been "consistently applied" when no changes in the application of accounting principles had been made. This sentence referred to a company's use of the same accounting procedures and methods from year to year. However, the *CPA Canada Handbook (Accounting Part II)*, section 1506, governs the accounting and disclosure of a company's change of accounting principles. In 1991 the reporting standards were changed to allow the audit report to be silent—that is, implicit—about consistency when no accounting changes had been made or when any changes that were made were properly disclosed in the financial statements.

Adequate Disclosure

The reporting standards include a second implicit element. They require auditors to use professional judgment in deciding whether the financial statements and related disclosures contain all the important accounting information users need. It may be necessary to disclose information not specified in authoritative support sources, for instance, if there is an unusual fact situation not encountered before. Using this standard, auditors have latitude to determine what is important and what is not. Likewise, users of financial statements also have the right to claim that certain information is necessary for adequate disclosure. In fact, many lawsuits are brought forward on this issue, and auditors must show reasons for the lack of disclosure. As noted in Chapter 1, disclosures are an important means of dealing with accounting risk and a significant aspect of auditor professional judgment, as many aspects of implementing accounting and auditing standards are not covered by them.

When auditors believe that certain information is necessary for adequate disclosure but the company refuses to disclose it, a departure from GAAP exists. Usually, a qualified opinion is written, and the reason for the departure (missing disclosure) is described in the audit report. Sometimes the missing disclosure is added to the audit report itself.

Report Content

The reporting standard of CAS 700 and CAS 705 states the requirements for an opinion. Two types of modifications to the report are relevant: those that affect the audit opinion and those that do not. In this section, we provide an overview of matters that affect the audit opinion. Chapter 4 provides more details on these and other modifications.

CAS 700 provides guidance for the standard audit report, while CAS 705 provides guidance on modifications to the auditor's report and requires that the report contain either the opinion on the financial statements or an assertion that an opinion cannot be given. This means that there are two classes of opinion statements: all opinions on statements (i.e., unmodified, adverse, and qualified opinions) and the disclaimer of opinion. An **adverse opinion** is the opposite of an unmodified opinion. It states that the financial statements are not

adverse opinion:
an auditor's declaration that financial statements are not in accordance with GAAP

in accordance with GAAP. A **disclaimer of opinion** is an auditor's declaration that no opinion is given. The standard applies to financial statements as a whole; that is, the standard applies equally to the set of financial statements and footnotes and to each individual financial statement and footnote. According to CAS 705, an explanation is required whenever there is a report reservation. Thus, when an adverse opinion, qualified opinion, or disclaimer of opinion is rendered, all the substantive reasons for doing so must be given in an additional paragraph or paragraphs.

Other reporting standards relate to auditor responsibilities and identifying the financial statements covered by the opinion. Every time PAs (even when acting as accountants associated with unaudited financial statements) are associated by name or by action with financial statements, they must report on their work and responsibility. The character of the work is usually described by the standard reference to an audit in accordance with GAAS. But if an audit has been restricted in some way or if the statements are simply unaudited, the auditor must say so.

The "degree of responsibility" is indicated by the form of the opinion. Auditors take full responsibility for their opinion about conformity with GAAP when they give either an unmodified or an adverse opinion. They take no responsibility whatsoever when they give a disclaimer of opinion. When they give qualified opinions, they take responsibility for all matters except those that are the reasons for the qualification. (Qualified and adverse opinions and disclaimers of opinion are discussed more fully in Chapter 4.) These are part of the association rules that cover information the PA is associated with. The association rules will be covered in Chapter 4, after you have been introduced to other types of public accounting engagements.

Review Checkpoints

2-22   What are the nine important features of a standard unmodified audit report?

2-23   Identify various authoritative supports for GAAP, with an indication of their ranking.

2-24   Do auditors take any responsibility for auditees' choices of accounting principles?

2-25   What four kinds of audit opinion statements are identified in this chapter? What is the message of each one?

2-26   What messages are usually implicit in a standard audit report?

Assurance Standards

LO4   Explain the importance of general assurance standards, using examples of assurance matters.

A special framework in the International Federation of Accountants (IFAC) *Handbook* covers the international standards for assurance engagements. It was issued in 2005 and was heavily influenced by the *CPA Canada Handbook*, section 5025. However, the International Standards on Auditing (ISA) for some assurance engagements have not yet been integrated with its framework. As a consequence, CPA Canada continues to use its original assurance standard. Thus, the *CPA Canada Handbook* assurance standard section 5025 is not part of CASs.[5]

In March 1997, the CICA (now CPA Canada) issued section 5025, "Standards for Assurance Engagements." This standard, the first of its kind in the world, is significant because it is intended to provide an umbrella for all

disclaimer of opinion:
an auditor's declaration that no opinion is given on financial statements and the reasons this is so, usually due to a scope limitation; also called a *denial of opinion*

existing and future audit-type engagements, including many that do not involve financial statements. Section 5025 also contemplates different levels of assurance.

An *assurance engagement* is defined in paragraphs 5025.03–5025.04 as follows:

> An engagement where, pursuant to an accountability relationship between two or more parties, a practitioner is engaged to issue a written communication expressing a conclusion concerning a subject matter for which the accountable party is responsible. An *accountability relationship* is a prerequisite for an assurance engagement. An *accountability relationship* exists when one party (the "accountable party") is answerable to and/or is responsible to another party (the "user") for a subject matter, or voluntarily chooses to report to another party on a subject matter. The accountability relationship may arise either as a result of an agreement or legislation, or because a user can be expected to have an interest in how the accountable party has discharged its responsibility for a subject matter.

The assurance standard does not supersede audit and review standards, but it is influencing changes to other assurance standards. It is designed to provide guidance for expanding assurance services to subject matters not currently covered in the *Handbook*. For example, it is the assurance standard that introduced the three-party accountability concept. The general relationships in assurance engagements are given in Exhibit 2–3.

An assertion is a statement about some aspect of a subject matter—for example, that a building exists as of a certain point in time. The assurance standards in section 5025 are quite broad in that they can be applied to assertions that are only implied—a direct reporting engagement—as well as to written

---

EXHIBIT 2–3

Universe of Chartered Professional Accountant Engagements

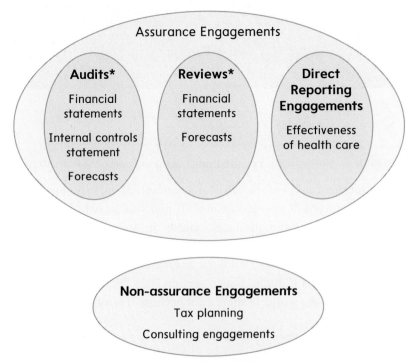

*Audits and reviews are attest engagements.

assertions—an attest (or attestation) engagement. *CPA Canada Handbook* paragraphs 5025.05–5025.06 state the following:

> In an attest engagement, the practitioner's conclusion will be on a written assertion prepared by the accountable party. The assertion evaluates, using suitable criteria, the subject matter for which the accountable party is responsible. In a direct reporting engagement, the practitioner's conclusion will evaluate directly using suitable criteria, the subject matter for which the accountable party is responsible. . . . In these standards, the accountable party is referred to as management. Depending on the circumstance, the user could include a variety of stakeholders such as shareholders, creditors, customers, the board of directors, the audit committee, legislators, or regulators. The practitioner is the person who has overall responsibility for the assurance engagement.

These relationships are illustrated in Exhibit 2–4. For example, the practitioner in paragraph 5025.07 of the exhibit has traditionally been referred to as an *external auditor* in a financial statement assurance engagement. Since most of this text deals with financial statement audits, we will continue using this terminology. After we have become familiar with other assurance services in Chapter 21 (available on Connect), we will explain the assurance standards in more detail.

Reporting is different because assurance engagements on non-financial information do not depend upon GAAP. The assurance standards speak of "evaluation against suitable criteria" and "accordance with generally accepted criteria," and they leave the door open for assurance engagements on a wide variety of assertions. An illustration of how far assurance engagements can go is provided in an article in *The Wall Street Journal* titled "Fore!" (summarized in the box below). Many people appreciate the value of auditors' assurance to historical financial statements, and they have found other representations for PAs to assure, as illustrated in the box "Other Examples of Assurance Engagements."

Fore!

An interesting example of an assurance engagement subject matter is the distance a particular brand of golf balls can be hit on a driving range. This type of assurance engagement was requested by Wilson Sporting Goods Company to prove that amateur golfers could drive Wilson golf balls farther than competing brands of golf balls. The assurance engagement required PAs to measure the average distance of golf drives at 30 driving ranges. The PAs reported that Wilson's brand of golf balls could be hit farther by an average of 5.7 yards per drive. In addition to walking off the distances of the golf drive, the PAs verified that all participants were amateurs, that the participants were not paid by Wilson, and that Wilson's records of the results were accurate.

EXHIBIT 2–4

Three Parties Involved in an Assurance Engagement (Three-Party Accountability)

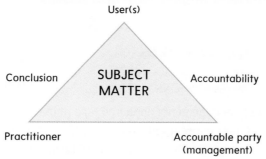

Source: Copyright © *CPA Canada Handbook—Assurance*, paragraph 5025.07.

Other Examples of Assurance Engagements

- Goods and Services Tax (GST), Harmonized Sales Tax (HST), and real estate tax bases
- Political contributions and expenditures
- Financial feasibility of a rapid transit system
- Cost justification for a utility rate increase
- Regulator's questionnaire on business ethics and conduct
- Reliability of drinking water surveillance program
- Quality of nursing home care
- Effectiveness of student loan programs in meeting needs of students
- Effectiveness of research and development activities
- Labour data for union contract negotiation
- Newspaper and magazine audience and circulation data
- Integrity and security of a computer network
- Investment performance statistics
- Insurance claims data
- Pollution emissions data (e.g., greenhouse gas emissions)

An important assurance engagement now required by SOX in the United States is the audit of internal control statements prepared by management. Like audits of financial statements, these internal control audits verify the accuracy of management's internal control statement; the difference is the subject matter.

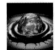 A main objective in developing the assurance standards is to provide a general framework for, and set reasonable boundaries around, the assurance services offered by PAs. Whether these standards actually set boundaries remains to be seen. After all, before the assurance standards were published, CPAs were using the GAAS as a point of departure for other assurance engagements. Now they must use the assurance standards as the point of departure.

Assurance standards are explained in more detail in Chapter 21.

Review Checkpoints

2-27   What are the major differences between assurance standards and GAAS?

2-28   Define assurance engagements.

2-29   What is the theoretical essence of an assurance service?

2-30   **CRITICAL THINKING QUESTION:** In the "Fore!" feature, identify the assertion, the three parties to the engagement, and the criteria being used. Is a high level of assurance being provided? Explain.

Quality Control Standards

LO5   Explain how requirements of quality control standards are monitored for public accounting firms.

GAAS must be observed in each audit engagement conducted by a public accounting firm. Thus, public accounting firms need to observe GAAS in their entire audit practice. While GAAS relate to the conduct of each audit engagement, quality control standards govern the quality of a public accounting firm's audit practice as a whole. Quality control can be defined as actions taken by a public accounting firm to evaluate compliance with professional standards. And a "system of quality control" is designed to provide reasonable assurance of conforming to professional standards. Professional standards include GAAS, as covered in the *CPA Canada Handbook,* as well as provincial rules of ethical conduct.

Elements of Quality Control

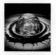 IFAC has identified at least four basic elements of quality control. These are listed and explained briefly in Exhibit 2–5. Various ways the control of the quality of audits have been implemented in practice are discussed in Appendix 2B. The key thing to remember is that the ultimate purpose of all aspects of quality control monitoring and standards is to control the information risk associated with financial statement reporting.

 Both the 1978 Adams Report (*Report of the Special Committee to Examine the Role of the Auditor*) and the 1988 Macdonald Commission Report (*Report of the Commission to Study the Public's Expectations of Audits*) recommended the development of quality control standards to guide public accounting firms. More recently, several regulatory agencies initiated discipline for substandard performance by professional staff in public accounting firms and criticized the individual-level focus of the provincial disciplinary process. In response, provincial institutes are amending their bylaws to bring firms, as well as individuals, within the disciplinary process. This expanded disciplinary process will require new guidelines for evaluating systems of quality control. Increasing litigation is also putting pressure on firms to develop good systems of quality control so that they can demonstrate compliance with professional standards and thus minimize the loss from litigation. In summary, quality control standards exist to increase audit quality. And the purpose of increasing audit quality is to reduce information risk, as discussed in Chapter 1. It is also useful to view the other standards discussed in this chapter as different mechanisms to help reduce information risk. These are summarized in the checklist that follows:

✓ Objectivity and independence
✓ Due care
✓ Competence
✓ Examination standards
✓ Reporting standards
✓ Professional skepticism
✓ Quality control standards
✓ Regulator requirements

EXHIBIT 2–5

Elements of Quality Control

1. Quality control policies and procedures should be implemented both at the level of the audit firm and on individual audits.
2. The audit firm should implement quality control policies and procedures designed to ensure that all audits are conducted in accordance with ISAs or relevant national standards of practice.
3. The firm's general quality control policies and procedures should be communicated to its personnel in a manner that provides reasonable assurance that the policies and procedures are understood and implemented.
4. The auditor should implement those quality control procedures that are, in the context of the policies and procedures of the firm, appropriate to the individual audit. In particular, delegated work should be properly directed, supervised, and reviewed.

Source: Summary of International Standard on Quality Control 1 (ISQC 1) of the International Auditing and Assurance Standards Board, published by the International Federation of Accountants (IFAC), July 17, 2014.

APPLICATION CASE WITH SOLUTION & ANALYSIS

Which Generally Accepted Auditing Standard Is Most Important?

DISCUSSION CASE

This chapter introduced you to GAAS. If you had to pick the one standard that is most important to the profession, which would it be?

SOLUTION & ANALYSIS

A hint to the response for this question was provided to you in the Application Case for Chapter 1. At its most fundamental level, the answer is the need for *independence*. Let us review the independence concept now, using the objective of the audit of financial statements, that is, "to enable the auditor to express an opinion as to whether the financial statements are prepared, in all material respects, in conformity with an applicable framework." Note how this objective implies three-party accountability.

When the standard says "to express an opinion," it does not mean any opinion. It means an opinion that is truthful and, based on the evidence and the evaluation of the evidence, reflects the economic facts of the entity as portrayed by the acceptable framework. By "acceptable" we mean acceptable to the third-party users of financial statements. The second party, the auditee and its management, presumably knows that the framework is acceptable because they take responsibility for having the financial statements prepared. The auditor determines whether the financial statements are acceptable through the gathering of audit evidence and his or her own knowledge of what is acceptable according to the reporting framework. This knowledge is what supports and justifies the audit opinion.

But how does the third-party user know whether the financial reporting is acceptable? The third party is the least knowledgeable and thus relies on the auditor to verify acceptability of the financial reporting. But the auditor cannot just be anybody who is competent. Management, after all, can be very competent in preparing the financial statements and does, in fact, accept responsibility for them. Thus, competence is a necessary condition, but it does not explain why there is a need for an auditor.

As explained in the Application Case and Analysis in Chapter 1, an indispensable characteristic of the auditor is independence. Without independence, the auditor cannot provide the trustworthy opinion that third parties need in order to rely on the financial statements. Thus, to meet the overall objective of generally accepted auditing standards (GAAS), the auditor must be independent. Independence is also what makes the rest of the GAAS relevant, because only with independence will third parties rely sufficiently on the financial reporting by the auditee. The less the third-party financial statement user trusts the first-party financial statement preparer, the more important auditor independence becomes.

The importance of independence extends to the entire accounting firm. Many of the accounting firm quality control standards discussed in this chapter relate to independence. The concept of skepticism requires independence and minimization of conflicts of interest. Some current issues affecting conflicts of interest for accounting firms include mandatory rotation of audit firms every few years and further limits on the type of non-audit services that an audit firm can provide to the auditee.[6] Note that these constraints on audit firm activities all relate to improving at least the appearance of the audit firm's independence from the auditee.

The only way auditors can meet the unique ethical demands of putting the priority of third-party users over the priority of the party who pays for the audit is to be independent of the auditee. This is quite a challenge from the ethical perspective, and is for auditors an ethical issue that is not faced by other professionals. These unique audit challenges are further discussed in Chapter 3, but they are fundamentally based on society's expectations that the auditors need to be independent in fulfilling their social role.

SUMMARY

- The profession is becoming increasingly regulated by outside bodies as a result of perceived audit failures and questionable accounting in the first decade of this century. **LO1**

- Financial statement auditors are most concerned with generally accepted auditing standards (GAAS) because they are the direct guides for the quality of everyday audit practice. The goal of the audit is to provide high assurance that the financial statements present fairly. Or, put another way, the goal of the audit is to reduce information risk associated with the financial statements. The general standard consists of the code of professional ethics, and it sets requirements for auditors' competence, objectivity, and due professional care. The examination standards set requirements for planning and supervising each audit, obtaining an understanding of the auditee's internal controls, and obtaining sufficient appropriate evidence to serve as a basis for an audit report. The reporting standards cover the requirements for an acceptable framework of financial reporting (usually generally accepted accounting principles [GAAP]), auditor and management responsibilities, adequate disclosure, and report content. We briefly reviewed the financial statement audit process to show how GAAS concepts relate to this process. **LO2, 3**

- In all matters relating to financial statement audits, auditors are advised to have a sense of professional skepticism. This attitude is reflected in a "prove it with evidence" response to management representations, to answers for inquiries, and to financial statement assertions themselves. Critical thinking is a broader idea, covered in Chapter 3, that considers not only the evidence, but also related ethical issues and the effects of the reporting framework that should be applied. Critical thinking and skepticism consider how management's reporting may not meet legitimate user needs. Critical thinking helps lead to more ethical reporting. **LO3**

- The assurance standard is the general framework for applying assurance engagements to a wide range of subjects. The standard comprises the quality guides for general assurance work. Theoretically, it could serve as quality guides for independent audits of financial statements. However, it was created long after GAAS for audits of financial statements, and, therefore, GAAS remains the predominant framework for most engagements. **LO4**

- As an auditor, you must have a thorough understanding of these practice standards, especially GAAS. All practical problems can be approached by beginning with a consideration of the practice standards in question. Auditing standards do not exist in a vacuum. They are put to work in numerous practical applications. Practical applications of the standards will be shown in subsequent chapters on audit program planning, execution of auditing procedures, gathering evidence, and auditing decisions. But don't lose sight of the forest for the trees: the ultimate goal of professional standards is to reduce information risk associated with the financial statements. **LO4**

- While assurance standards and GAAS govern the quality of work on each individual engagement, the quality control elements guide a public accounting firm's audit practice as a whole. Quality control is the foundation of the self-regulatory system of peer review, practice inspection, and quality inspection. It also serves as the basis for monitoring by accountability boards. **LO5**

KEY TERMS

adverse opinion

audit committees

Audit Guidelines (AuGs)

audit plan

audit program

Canadian Coalition for Good
 Governance

Canadian Public Accountability
 Board (CPAB)

corporate governance

disclaimer of opinion

generally accepted auditing
 standards (GAAS)

initial public offering (IPO)

interim date

internal control	Public Company Accounting Oversight	self-regulation
modified opinion report	Board (PCAOB)	unmodified opinion report
prospectus	Securities and Exchange	
	Commission (SEC)	

MULTIPLE-CHOICE QUESTIONS FOR PRACTICE AND REVIEW

MC 2-1 **LO3** It is always a good idea for auditors to begin an audit with a professional skepticism characterized by the assumption that

a. a potential conflict of interest always exists between the auditor and the management of the enterprise under audit.
b. in audits of financial statements, the auditor acts exclusively in the capacity of an auditor.
c. the professional status of the independent auditor imposes commensurate professional obligations.
d. financial statements and financial data are verifiable.

MC 2-2 **LO3** When Auditee Company prohibits auditors from visiting selected branch offices of the business, this is an example of interference with

a. reporting independence.
b. investigative independence.
c. auditors' training and proficiency.
d. audit planning and supervision.

MC 2-3 **LO4** After the auditors learned of Auditee Company's failure to record an expense for obsolete inventory, they agreed to a small adjustment to the financial statements because the Auditee president told them the company would violate its debt agreements if the full amount were recorded. This is an example of a lack of

a. auditors' training and proficiency.
b. planning and supervision.
c. audit investigative independence.
d. audit reporting independence.

MC 2-4 **LO3** The primary purpose for obtaining an understanding of the company's internal controls in a financial statement audit is to

a. determine the nature, timing, and extent of auditing procedures to be performed.
b. make consulting suggestions to management.
c. obtain direct, sufficient, and appropriate evidential matter to afford a reasonable basis for an opinion on the financial statements.
d. determine whether the company has changed any accounting principles.

MC 2-5 **LO4** Auditors' activities about which of these generally accepted auditing standards (GAAS) are not affected by the auditee's utilization of a computerized accounting system?

a. The audit report shall state whether the financial statements are presented in accordance with GAAP.
b. The work is to be adequately planned, and assistants, if any, are to be properly supervised.

c. Sufficient appropriate evidential matter is to be obtained . . . to afford a reasonable basis for an opinion regarding the financial statements under audit.

d. The audit is to be performed by a person or persons having adequate technical training and proficiency as an auditor.

MC 2-6 **LO2** Which of the following is not found in the standard unqualified audit report on financial statements?

a. An identification of the financial statements that were audited

b. A general description of an audit

c. An opinion that the financial statements present financial position in conformity with GAAP

d. An emphasis paragraph commenting on the effect of economic conditions on the company

MC 2-7 **LO4** The assurance standards do not contain a requirement that auditors obtain

a. adequate knowledge in the subject matter of the assertions being examined.

b. an understanding of the auditee's internal control structure.

c. sufficient evidence for the conclusions expressed in an attestation report.

d. independence in mental attitude.

MC 2-8 **LO3** Auditor Jones is studying a company's accounting treatment of a series of complicated transactions in exotic financial instruments. She should look for the highest level of authoritative support for proper accounting in

a. provincial securities commissions' staff position statements.

b. CPA Canada industry audit and accounting guides.

c. CPA Canada recommendations in the *Handbook*.

d. Emerging Issues Committee consensus statements.

MC 2-9 **LO5** Which of the following is not an example of a quality control procedure likely to be used by a public accounting firm to meet its professional responsibilities to auditees?

a. Completion of independence questionnaires by all partners and employees

b. Review and approval of audit plan by the partner in charge of the engagement just prior to signing the auditor's report

c. Evaluating professional staff after the conclusion of each engagement

d. Evaluating the integrity of management for each new audit client

MC 2-10 **LO3** Which of the following concepts is not included in the wording of the auditor's standard report?

a. Management's responsibility for the financial statements

b. Auditor's responsibility to assess significant estimates made by management

c. Extent of auditor's reliance on the auditee's internal controls

d. Examination of evidence on a test basis

MC 2-11 **LO3** Which of the following is not mandatory when performing an audit in accordance with GAAS?

a. Proper supervision of assistants

b. Efficient performance of audit procedures

c. Understanding the auditee's system of internal controls

d. Adequate planning of work to be performed

EXERCISES AND PROBLEMS

EP 2-1 Audit Independence and Planning. **LO5** You are meeting with executives of Cooper Cosmetics Corporation to arrange your firm's engagement to audit the corporation's financial statements for the year ending December 31. One executive suggests the audit work be divided among three staff members to minimize audit time, avoid duplication of staff effort, and curtail interference with company operations. One person would examine asset accounts, a second would examine liability accounts, and the third would examine income and expense accounts.

Advertising is the corporation's largest expense, and the advertising manager suggests that a staff member of your firm, whose uncle owns the advertising agency handling the corporation's advertising, be assigned to examine the Advertising Expense account. The staff member has a thorough knowledge of the rather complex contract between Cooper Cosmetics and the advertising agency.

Required:

a. To what extent should a PA follow the auditee management's suggestions for the conduct of an audit? Discuss.
b. List and discuss the reasons why audit work should not be assigned solely according to asset, liability, and income and expense categories.
c. Should the staff member of your public accounting firm whose uncle owns the advertising agency be assigned to examine advertising costs? Discuss.

EP 2-2 Time of Appointment and Planning. **LO3** Your public accounting practice is located in a town of 15,000 people. Your work, conducted by you and two assistants, consists of compiling clients' monthly statements and preparing income tax returns for individuals from cash data and partnership returns from books and records. You have a few corporate clients; however, service to them is limited to preparation of income tax returns and assistance in year-end closings where bookkeeping is deficient.

One of your corporate clients is a retail hardware store. Your work for this company has been limited to preparing the corporation income tax return from a trial balance submitted by the bookkeeper. On December 26, you receive an e-mail from the president of the corporation with the following request:

We have made arrangements with the First National Bank to borrow $500,000 to finance the purchase of a complete line of appliances. The bank has asked us to furnish our auditor's certified statement as of December 31, which is the closing date of our accounting year. The trial balance of the general ledger should be ready by January 10, which should allow ample time to prepare your report for submission to the bank by January 20. In view of the importance of this certified report to our financing program, we trust you will arrange to comply with the foregoing schedule.

Required:

From a theoretical viewpoint, discuss the difficulties that are caused by such a short-notice audit request.

(© 2000, American Institute of CPAs. All Rights Reserved. Adapted by permission.)

EP 2-3 Reporting Standards. **LO3** PA Musgrave and his associates audited the financial statements of North Company, a computer equipment retailer. Musgrave conducted the audit in accordance with the general and field work standards of GAAS and therefore wrote a standard audit description in his audit report. Then he received an emergency call to fill in as a substitute tenor in his barbershop quartet.

No one else was in the office that Saturday afternoon, so he handed you the complete financial statements and footnotes, saying, "Make sure it's OK to write an unmodified opinion on these statements. The working papers are on the table. I'll check with you on Monday morning."

Required:

In general terms, what must you determine in order to write an unmodified opinion paragraph for Musgrave's signature?

EP 2-4 Generally Accepted Auditing Standards in a Computer Environment. `LO2` The Lovett Corporation uses an IBM mainframe computer system with peripheral optical reader and high-speed laser printer equipment. Transaction information is initially recorded on paper documents (e.g., sales invoices) and then read by optical equipment that produces a disk containing the data. These data file disks are processed by a computer program, and printed listings, journals, and general ledger balances are produced on the high-speed printer equipment.

Required:

Explain how the audit standard requiring "adequate technical training and proficiency" is important for satisfying the general and field work standards in the audit of Lovett Corporation's financial statements.

EP 2-5 Audit Report Language. `LO3` The standard unmodified report contains several important sentences and phrases. Explain why each of the following phrases is used instead of the alternative language indicated.

1. Address: "To the Board of Directors and Shareholders" instead of "To Whom It May Concern."
2. "We have audited the balance sheet of Anycompany as of December 31, 20X2, and the related statements of income, retained earnings, and cash flows for the year then ended" instead of "We have audited the attached financial statements."
3. "We conducted our audit in accordance with generally accepted auditing standards" instead of "Our audit was conducted with due audit care appropriate in the circumstances."
4. "In our opinion, the financial statements referred to above present fairly . . . in conformity with generally accepted accounting principles" instead of "The financial statements are true and correct."

EP 2-6 Public Oversight of the Accountancy Profession. `LO7` The CPAB and the PCAOB in the United States provide oversight for PAs who audit public companies. What are the objectives of these boards? What factors should these boards consider in assessing PAs' work?

EP 2-7 Scope of an Audit, Requirement for Specialist Expertise. `LO3` Consider the following two situations:

1. The auditor discovers during the audit that the auditee company has entered a complex legal contract that involves transferring assets to another company if that company performs certain future services by obtaining supplies from a foreign country. The auditor is unable to establish whether the contract imposes any financial liability or has any other financial impact on the auditee company.
2. The auditor learns that the auditee company must comply with environmental standards requiring it to monitor various emissions using complex scientific techniques. The amounts of the financial penalties that can be imposed by the government are determined by the nature and extent of non-compliance with these scientific standards.

Required:

Contrast these two situations in terms of the auditor's responsibility to perform audit procedures and issue a report. Include a recommendation on which form of report would be issued in each case, based on your analysis.

EP 2-8 Assurance Engagements, General Assurance Standards. `LO4` A radio advertisement for a new software management product included the following statement: "According to ITR, Knovel's new software product will pay back in three months."

ITR is an information technology (IT) research firm that is hired by various companies in the IT industry to provide reports on IT usage and sales in the IT market. As soon as ITR's president heard the ad on his car radio, he immediately phoned Knovel and told them to stop using the ad.

Required:

Discuss whether the ad's statement is the result of an assurance engagement. Consider the parties involved, the subject matter, the accountability relationships, the nature of the report, and any other relevant aspects of the situation. Why do you think ITR's president wanted the ad stopped?

EP 2-9 Fair Presentation in Accordance with Generally Accepted Accounting Principles. `LO3` The third reporting standard of GAAS states that the auditor's opinion on the financial statements should indicate whether they present fairly the financial position, results of operations, and changes in financial position in accordance with GAAP. The *CPA Canada Handbook* Recommendations are an important source of GAAP. However, the Recommendations may allow for different interpretations and choices in how they are applied, or they may be silent.

Required:

a. How does the auditor assess whether financial statements are in accordance with GAAP when a conclusion on GAAP is not found in the *CPA Canada Handbook* Recommendations? Give an example of an accounting issue that may not be covered in the Recommendations.

b. How does the auditor assess whether financial statements are in accordance with GAAP when the *CPA Canada Handbook* Recommendations allow for different accounting methods to be acceptable? Give an example of an accounting issue for which alternative acceptable accounting treatments are provided in the Recommendations.

EP 2-10 Missing Disclosure Described in Auditor's Report. `LO3` Bunting Technology Corporation is a large public company that manufactures the IXQ, a telecommunications component that speeds up Internet transmission over fibre-optic cable. Subsequent to its current year-end, but before the audited financial statements are issued, a competitor of Bunting launches a new product that increases transmission speed to one hundred times that of Bunting's IXQ and sells for one-tenth the price. Bunting has approximately 11 months of inventory of the IXQ in inventory, based on the current year's sales levels.

Bunting's auditors, Ditesmoi & Quail (DQ), have determined that this subsequent event warrants a write-down of Bunting's year-end inventory to reflect technological obsolescence. Given that the IXQ is Bunting's main product, the write-down will be highly material. DQ argues that this development will result in a permanent change in Bunting's earnings potential and future cash flows, and it would be misleading users if it is not included in the current-year financial statements.

Bunting's management refuses to record the inventory write-down, arguing that the event occurred after the year-end and therefore does not relate to the current year's results. Also, since the competitor's product is brand new, management argues that there is significant uncertainty about whether it will perform as well in actual use as the competitor claims. Thus, it is premature to assume it will have an impact on IXQ sales, and it is impossible to estimate a dollar amount for the impact. Management is also concerned that, by publicly reporting information about the competing product in Bunting's annual report, DQ will jeopardize several large sales contracts that Bunting is currently negotiating, and this may lower sales even more than if the information were withheld.

DQ issues a qualified audit report that spells out its estimate of the material impact of the technological obsolescence on Bunting's assets, net income, and retained earnings.

Required:

Discuss the issues raised by DQ's decision to issue a qualified report in this situation. Consider the impact of DQ's audit report qualification on Bunting, on users of the audited financial statements, and on DQ as Bunting's auditor.

EP 2-11 Auditors' Professional Skepticism. `LO2` Auditors are required to have professional skepticism, but auditors must also rely on management representations in order to complete the audit. Discuss the inherent conflicts in these two requirements and how they may be resolved.

EP 2-12 Assurance Engagement Other Than Audit or Review. `LO4` During 2002 and 2003, United Nations weapon inspectors entered Iraq to search for "weapons of mass destruction." These include chemical, biological, and nuclear weapons. It had been reported that these weapons and equipment for manufacturing them may have been concealed in public buildings such as schools, hospitals, or apartment buildings.

Required:

Identify the subject matter and design an approach for assessing risks and probabilities of weapons existing, and for implementing the inspection. Use basic audit definitions and approaches from financial statement auditing. For example, compare the weapons inspectors' objectives to the approach to looking for a material understatement of a financial statement liability.

EP 2-13 Audit Weaknesses Found in Canadian Public Accountability Board Inspections. `LO1, 7` Access the CPAB website at cpab-ccrc.ca and find the most common weaknesses in Canadian audit practice as identified in their reports.

EP 2-14 Audit Expectations Gap. `LO1` Some have proposed the idea of an "audit expectations gap," which is the difference between what the auditor accomplishes using GAAS and what third-party users expect from audited financial statements. Do you think there is an expectations gap? Discuss and identify potential sources of the gap.

EP 2-15 Private Sector versus Public Sector Auditing. `LO4` Is there more of an audit expectations gap in private sector auditing or public sector auditing? Discuss. Explain any difference in terms of the independence characteristic. In particular, are public sector auditors more independent than private sector auditors? Discuss.

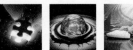

EP 2-16 Audit Expectations Gap. `LO1, 2` Ask a relative or friend what they think auditors do. Are auditors expected to find all errors? Find all intentional errors? Find all unintentional errors (no

matter how small)? Ask them to read the auditor's report in Exhibit 2–1. Then ask whether this report meets their expectations of the auditor's role. Does the auditor's report meet your expectations if you were investing in the Thai restaurant illustration at the beginning of Chapter 1?

Appendix 2A: Generally Accepted Auditing Standards of the United States (on Connect)
Appendix 2B: Implementation of Quality Control Standards in Canada (on Connect)

ENDNOTES

1   We clarify official terminology by always referring to "reports" as auditor-prepared and "statements" as management-prepared communications.

2   H. Lu, G. Richardson, and S. Salterio. "Direct and indirect effects of internal control weaknesses on accrual quality: Evidence from a unique Canadian regulatory setting," *Contemporary Accounting Research*, CAAA, Summer 2011, pp. 675–707.

3   A. Freeman and K. Hawlett, "Keep IPO's at home: Martin," *The Globe and Mail*, March 8, 1996, B1.

4   R. Mautz and H. Sharaf, *The Philosophy of Auditing* (American Accounting Association, 1961), p. 140.

5   Section 5025 is included in the *CPA Canada Assurance Handbook* as an "Other Canadian Standard" or OCS.

6   Tim Kiladze, "Auditors rethink industry rules post-crisis," *The Globe and Mail*, March 9, 2012.

Auditors' Ethical and Legal Responsibilities

Chapter 3 describes the moral, professional, and legal responsibilities that the public expects auditors to meet, further demonstrating the importance society attaches to the auditor's role in protecting the public interest.

LEARNING OBJECTIVES

After completing this chapter, you will be able to do the following:

LO1 Outline the concept of auditor responsibilities.

LO2 Explain the importance of the study of ethics in helping define auditor responsibilities.

LO3 Outline the characteristics of critical thinking.

LO4 Describe the purpose and contents of the codes of professional ethics established by the various professional accounting bodies.

LO5 Explain the importance of an independence framework for auditors.

LO6 Outline auditor legal responsibilities.

LO7 Outline the various types of common law liability for public accountants, citing specific case precedents.

LO8 (Appendix 3A) Explain how professional judgment, critical thinking, and principles-based reasoning are related.

CHAPTER APPENDIX

APPENDIX 3A Framework for Critical Thinking (on Connect)

EcoPak Inc.

Two years ago, Kam and Mike started up a corporation called EcoPak Inc. to purchase the operating assets of the former StyreneTech company. They each own 45% of the EcoPak common shares, and Nina was given 10% of the common shares in return for her help in starting up the company. Zhang has invested in convertible preferred shares that can be converted to a 50% common share interest at any time.

Kam and Mike kept the styrene-foam production business going to generate cash flows and developed the materials and production processes for their new biomass product line. Kam has also been very busy in his role as head of business development, and EcoPak has obtained a big contract to supply hot-food containers to a national restaurant chain. If the food containers perform well, the chain will consider having EcoPak also provide all its coffee cups. Kam has several other large contracts very close to signing, and it is now necessary for EcoPak to expand its production capacity significantly.

Kam has attracted a lot of business media coverage. EcoPak's highly innovative production process, which makes use of agricultural waste by-products, produces zero pollutant emissions and results in a completely biodegradable product. Consequently, an ethical investment management firm has approached Kam about investing in EcoPak to help finance the expansion of its biomass production. This firm has asked EcoPak to provide an environmental report on its operations; it is their policy to invest based on an audited environmental report or by doing its own audit of the company's operations to assess its environmental sustainability and performance. But Kam and Mike are thinking of doing an environmental report solely on the new biomass business, leaving out any mention of the styrene-foam business. They are pretty sure a report on that pollution-emitting, petroleum-based process would send the ethical investors running! But how can they get it audited? Time to call Nina; she's a senior audit manager now, so maybe she can do it.

When Nina hears what Kam and Mike have in mind, she is upset: "First, since I own shares in EcoPak I cannot audit the company—I am not independent! But even if I could, your plan to report on just one-half of your operations is misleading. I am a professional public accountant, and I can't associate myself with information that I know could be misleading to someone making an important decision based on it. *And*, even if you do an environmental report presenting all of your operations, I am not an environmental expert so I have no competence to provide assurance on the report. Remember those professional standards we talked about when you were looking at StyreneTech's audited financial statements? I need to comply with those or my work won't have the quality the public expects. So, basically, what you are asking me to do is totally unethical! And maybe it's time you two started thinking about the ethics of your own situation at EcoPak—taking a lot of credit for being so 'environmentally responsible' when half of your operations and most of your cash flows come from a really toxic process and a product that ends up littering the environment."

Kam and Mike fall over themselves apologizing to Nina. They realize they had not thought things through very well, and what she is saying makes a lot of sense. But they are also in a real bind because without new financing and without the cash flow from the styrene-foam business, they cannot expand the biomass business! Nina suggests they work with the ethical investment firm; Kam should try to sell them on the idea that their investment in EcoPak will allow the company not only to expand the biomass material line but also to shut down the styrene-foam line very soon. They will be getting twice the bang for their ethical buck.

Kam and Mike decide to engage an engineering firm to do an environmental audit of EcoPak's operations. A big surprise is uncovered during the audit—all the land behind the factory has been contaminated by a large spill of a toxic material, benzene, that had occurred a couple of years before they took over StyreneTech's operations! The Ministry of the Environment had issued a cleanup order against StyreneTech, and the company had done the first phase of cleanup to prevent the pollutant from spreading, but then the operating assets were sold to EcoPak. Since this is the land that will be used to expand their factory, EcoPak will need to complete the second cleanup phase— removal of the contaminated soil—before the expansion can occur. The cost of the cleanup is very high.

When Nina hears about this, she realizes that Grand & Quatre (G&Q) missed a huge issue in their audit, since this problem existed at the time of their audit work. She advises Kam and Mike to see a lawyer about suing G&Q for the cost of the cleanup, since it was a known liability of an estimable amount that should have been accrued in the StyreneTech financial statements: "At best, if G&Q was just sloppy and didn't ask the right questions, you should be able to show that their negligence resulted in your loss. But if G&Q knew about it, and let the Waterfalls Inc. management intimidate them into leaving it off the books because StyreneTech was being sold, that is a much more serious issue that will kill G&Q's reputation should it become public!"

The Essentials of Auditors' Ethical and Legal Responsibilities

Audits cannot be effective unless they are performed ethically. The essence of information risk is the possibility that reporting will be done unethically, for example, to conceal fraud or provide a deceptive and misleading impression of the financial performance and condition of a company. The essential role and responsibility of an auditor are to establish and communicate assurance to users that financial statements are fairly presented, implying that unethical reporting has not occurred. In this role an auditor cannot have any conflict of interest. This requirement is explicitly stated in the accountants' professional ethics code.

When you start to read the actual wording of the professional ethics code, you will probably find it all very general and vague, and it may not be easy to imagine how anyone could actually apply it. Professional practice in a three-party accountability situation gives rise to many conflicts and dilemmas. It is usually fairly easy to do the right thing, but it is often very difficult indeed to know what the right thing is. Personal biases can arise for anyone, including auditors, and are, by definition, hard to see from the inside.

As an example, say you are auditing a company's financial statements and find that you really like the company's controller because he has a great sense of humour, finds hilarious videos on the Internet, and always brings you a coffee in the morning. Your audit analysis work suggests that the company's travel expenses look much too high, but the controller explains that it is because some new salespeople hired in the past year had to travel more frequently to establish relations with new customers. Will the fact that you feel positively toward the controller personally make you inclined to take his word for it, even though with a bit of extra effort you could easily corroborate his story? You could do this by asking some other people in the company management (e.g., the sales manager) and by checking the payroll records to see if new sales department employees were added during the year. Say you did look for this corroborating evidence and it showed that there were actually far fewer sales employees during the year, and rather than travelling, they mainly contacted customers by phone and email. Then what would you do? If you put yourself in this situation, you will start to feel what it is like to be responsible for gathering evidence that gives reasonable assurance about whether financial information is misstated or not.

To address the challenges of dealing with potential biases like this, and other conflicts of interest and ethical dilemmas in auditing practice, two crucial interrelated concepts have been developed and incorporated into the auditing standards: *professional skepticism* and *professional judgment.*

Professional skepticism means that an auditor always wants to question the claims made by the management of the enterprise under audit and to look for corroborating evidence. This is not the same as automatically suspecting that everything management says is false; it simply reflects that the auditor has a duty to corroborate management's claims and assertions—this is what the ethics code refers to as using due care. A practical approach to being skeptical is to always be thinking about what could go wrong. Since a potential conflict of interest always exists between the auditor and management, it follows that auditors must gather their own evidence on the financial statements and disclosures to reach a reasonable and supportable decision to provide assurance on the truthfulness of the financial statements. How does an auditor know the decision is reasonable and supportable? The auditor must use a *critical thinking process* of reasoning to assess logically whether the evidence obtained provides reliable reasons that are relevant to supporting the conclusion.

Professional judgment refers to an auditor applying relevant training, knowledge, and experience, in the context provided by auditing, accounting, and ethical standards, to make informed decisions about the most appropriate action to take in the circumstances of an audit engagement. Professional judgment in financial statement auditing requires critical thinking on accounting issues and the evidence related to them. A critical thinking framework can be used to decide when an audit conclusion is sufficiently justified, considering possible conflicts of interest.

In auditing, the goal is often to determine the best (most truthful, fairest) position when there are conflicting positions (e.g., the inventory should be $X, or should be $X less a write-down of $Y). A critical thinking process that can be used in auditing to determine the most truthful claim involves the following steps:

1. As the auditor, define your role in an engagement, and identify the needs and responsibilities of the other parties in the three-party accountability relationship, including any potential conflicts of interest.

2. Identify contentious issues that need to be resolved in the engagement, such as controversial financial reporting issues. For example, the auditor might believe that the company has a large quantity of inventory items that are obsolete and their costs should be written off. Management states that it expects to succeed in selling these items for more than their costs by finding new marketing channels. Is the inventory valuation accounting estimate that management is claiming "reasonable" and "presented fairly"?

3. Explain the reasons and motivations for competing positions to be sure you understand others' positions. For example, what are the consequences for management if a large inventory write-down expense has to be recorded? Will debt covenants be affected, etc.?

4. Evaluate the arguments (assumptions, evidence) that relate to the competing positions and assess whether they are plausible and how strongly they link logically to a conclusion that each alternative position is true or not true. Applying logic essentially means identifying reasons that support a claim or conclusion. Sources of reasons include accounting and auditing concepts, assumptions, and principles. These concepts, along with the words used to state them (rhetoric), will affect the persuasiveness of your reasons as an auditor.

5. Form a conclusion on which position is most likely to be true. The conclusion is based on two conditions: the validity of the reasons and how strongly they support the conclusion.

Note that experience is an essential ingredient of skepticism and good professional judgment, so auditing work is typically organized so that more-junior auditors work under the supervision of more-experienced ones. Still, being independent and objective, taking a skeptical attitude, and thinking carefully and critically are ultimately an individual responsibility. If an individual's own critical reasoning leads to the conclusion that some action or decision is unethical, it is still unethical even if more-experienced people support it, or if "everyone is doing it."

If an audit fails to detect unethical reporting, and the third party believes that auditors have not met their professional responsibilities, auditors can face legal liability. Third-party beliefs may be based on what is referred to in auditing as the *expectations gap*. The gap exists between what users of audit reports expect—that auditors will always detect errors, fraud, theft, and illegal acts and report them publicly—and what auditors take responsibility for—detecting material misstatements. This gap can lead to lawsuits, particularly if a business fails, because even if auditors have performed well, the users may expect them to have done more to warn of the future business failure.

Historically, auditors' liability in Canada has been based on *common law liability*. Under common law, an auditor can be sued successfully if the plaintiff can prove four elements of negligence:

1. There was a legal duty of care to the plaintiff.

2. There was a breach of that duty.

3. There is proof that damages to the plaintiff resulted from the breach.

4. There is a reasonable connection between the breach and the damages.

The auditors' defence in a liability lawsuit is to show that any of the elements is not proven.

Controversies about audit effectiveness in recent years have also expanded the statutory liability of auditors who audit public companies. This type of liability is written into law statutes that specify when auditors can be found liable and the ranges of penalties auditors can be charged if they are liable. The *Sarbanes-Oxley Act* (SOX) in the United States is a well-known example of a law that can affect auditor liability. The development of statute-based regulation of auditors reflects the fact that governments no longer rely on the audit profession to self-regulate, as historically was the case.

Review Checkpoints

3-1   What is a financial statement auditor's responsibility in relation to unethical financial reporting?

3-2   What is the meaning of an auditor's opinion that a set of financial statements is "fairly presented"?

3-3   Give examples of conflicts that could arise between the following parties in a three-party accountability situation: (a) the management and the shareholders of a company, (b) the auditor and the management of a company, (c) the shareholders and the auditor of a company.

3-4   How can an auditor's objectivity be affected by his or her own personal biases?

3-5   What is professional skepticism? How does it relate to an auditor's objectivity? How does it relate to the professional accountant's ethical requirement to use due care?

3-6   What is critical thinking? How is it useful to an auditor?

3-7   What is the relation between professional judgment and critical thinking?

3-8   Why is experience important in using good professional judgment?

3-9   Does professional experience guarantee that auditors will reach ethical decisions in auditing conflict situations? Explain your position.

3-10   What is the expectations gap in auditing? How does it relate to auditor liability?

3-11   What are the elements of negligence that apply in establishing auditor liability under common law?

3-12   What is the difference between common law and statutory laws in relation to determining auditor legal liability?

Introduction

LO1   Outline the concept of auditor responsibilities.

As part of a privileged profession, auditors are responsible to society. This responsibility can be divided into three categories: moral, professional, and legal. Morality deals with character and "doing the right thing," as is determined largely by social norms. Morality deals with distinctions between right and wrong actions or behaviour. Auditors have a responsibility to conform to social norms. Auditors' **moral responsibilities** can be summarized as "public accountants should be upright, not kept upright." Ethics relates to proper conduct in life, and a study of ethics helps the auditor develop a set of principles by which to live.

moral responsibilities:
the rules and principles conforming to broad social norms of behaviour

Professional responsibilities refer to the more formal ethical responsibilities of auditors. Ethics is the philosophical study of morality. The emphasis on philosophy means that ethics is a more formal study and analysis of morality. These responsibilities (or *professional ethics*) are the rules and principles for the proper conduct of an auditor in his or her work. Professional ethics are necessary for a number of reasons: to obtain the respect and confidence of the public, to distinguish the professional from the general public, to achieve order within the profession, and to provide a means of self-policing the profession. All of these are meant to help meet the expectations of society as to the auditor's role. However, social norms and social expectations of auditors change, and a study of ethics is helpful in preparing for lifelong adaptation. For example, auditors are increasingly viewed as a key component of well-functioning capital markets. The first half of this chapter will focus on ethics that are particular to accountants and auditors in relation to their professional responsibilities.

Legal responsibilities are the risks auditors accept in a court of law while practising public accounting. The legal system is a chief means of regulating the social and professional responsibilities of auditors. These include the risks that arise from failing to use due care in the conduct of the audit. There is an interaction between legal and professional responsibilities, and they both relate to significant violations of society's expectations of the social role of the auditor.

General Ethics

LO2   Explain the importance of the study of ethics in helping define auditor responsibilities.

 A pervasive sense of proper ethical conduct is critical for professional accountants. Two aspects of ethics operate in the professional environment: general ethics (the spirit or principles) and professional ethics (the rules). Mautz and Sharaf have contributed the following thoughts to the link between general and professional ethics:

The theory of ethics has been a subject of interest to philosophers since the beginnings of recorded thought. Because philosophers are concerned with the good of all mankind, their discussions have been concerned with what we may call general ethics rather than the ethics of small groups such as the members of a given profession. We cannot look, therefore, to their philosophical theories for direct solutions to our special problems. Nevertheless, their work with general ethics is of primary importance to the development of an appropriate concept in any special field. Ethical behaviour in auditing or in any other activity is no more than a special application of the general notion of ethical conduct devised by philosophy. Ethical conduct in auditing draws its justification and basic nature from the general theory of ethics. Thus, we are well advised to give some attention to the ideas and reasoning of some of the great philosophers on this subject.[1]

Overview

What is ethics? Wheelwright gives a more complete definition of ethics as "that branch of philosophy which is the systematic study of reflective choice, of the standards of right and wrong by which it is to be guided, and of the goods toward which it may ultimately be directed."[2] In this definition, you can detect three key elements

---

professional responsibilities:
the rules and principles for the proper conduct of an auditor in his or her work; necessary to obtain the respect and confidence of the public, achieve order within the profession, and provide a means of self-policing the profession; also known as *professional ethics*

of ethics: (1) it involves questions requiring reflective choice (decision problems), (2) it involves guides to distinguish right from wrong (moral principles), and (3) it is concerned with the consequences of decisions.

What is an ethical problem? A problem exists when you must choose among alternative actions and the right choice is not absolutely clear. It is an ethical problem because the alternative actions affect the well-being of other people. An **ethical dilemma** is a problem that arises when a reason to act in a certain way is offset by a reason to not act in that way. The way to resolve such dilemmas is to rely on the primary ethical principle underlying the action. This can be influenced by the context of the dilemma. The process of identifying the primary ethical principle is a major reason we introduce **critical thinking** in this chapter. The process of identifying the primary accounting, auditing, and ethical principles to be relied upon in a particular situation, with all the principles being consistent, is one way to characterize critical thinking in professional judgment.

What is ethical behaviour? There are two standard philosophical answers to this question: (1) it is behaviour that produces the greatest good, and (2) it is behaviour that conforms to moral rules and principles. Problem situations arise when two or more rules conflict or when a rule and the criterion of "greatest good" conflict. Some examples of these are given later in this chapter.

Why does an individual or group need a code of ethical conduct? While it has been said that a person should be upright and not kept upright, a code serves as a useful reference or benchmark and specifies the criteria for the conduct of a profession. Society changes, and this creates challenges in adhering to general principles. For example, it is not always obvious what constitutes proper professional conduct in social networking sites. Thus, codes of professional ethics provide some solutions that may not be available in general ethics theories, it allows individuals to know what the profession expects, and it publicly declares the profession's principles of conduct so these standards can be enforced.

A Variety of Roles and Conflicts

The decision-maker role does not fully describe a professional person's entire ethical obligation. Each person acts as an individual, a member of a profession, and a member of society. Hence, accountants and auditors are also spectators (observing the decisions of colleagues), advisers (counselling co-workers), instructors (teaching accounting students or new employees on the job), judges (serving on disciplinary committees of provincial associations), and critics (commenting on the ethical decisions of others). All of these roles are important in the practice of professional ethics. In addition, public accountants (PAs) work as consultants, tax advisers, and auditors, and there can be conflicts of interest in serving these professional roles. Also, within the auditing role, there can be conflicts between the preparers and users of financial information. Finally, there can be conflicts between the different users of financial information, and auditors must be ready to act as a type of accounting referee.

An Ethical Decision Process

Your primary goal in considering general ethics is arriving at a set of acceptable methods for making ethical decisions. Consequently, you will only behave according to the rules of professional conduct if you understand the general principles of ethics. Essentially, ethics is principles based.

ethical dilemma:
a problem that arises when a reason to act in a certain way is offset by a reason to not act in that way

critical thinking:
the process of justifying one's conclusion or decision by providing good or acceptable reasons

In the previous definition of ethics, one of the key elements was reflective choice. This involves an important sequence of events, beginning with recognizing decision problems. Collecting evidence, in the ethics context, refers to thinking about rules of behaviour and outcomes of alternative actions. The process ends with analyzing the situation and taking an action. Ethical decision problems almost always involve projecting yourself into the future to live with your decisions. Professional ethical decisions usually turn on two questions: What written and unwritten rules govern my behaviour? What are the possible consequences of my choices? Principles of ethics can help you think about these two questions in real situations.

To Tell or Not to Tell?

 In your work as an auditor, you discover that the cashier, who has custody over the petty cash fund, has forged several payment records in order to cover innocent mistakes and make the fund balance each month when it is replenished. Your investigation reveals that the amount involved during the year is $240. The cashier is a woman, age 55, and the president of the company is a man who tolerates no mistakes, intentional or otherwise, in the accounting records. In fact, he is unyielding in this respect. He asks you about the results of your audit. Not doubting that the cashier would be fired if the forgeries were known, should you remain silent or tell the truth?

Philosophical Principles in Ethics

A discussion of ethical theories would be unnecessary if we accepted a simple rule: "Let your conscience be your guide." Such a rule is appealing because it calls on an individual's own judgment, which may be based on wisdom, insight, or adherence to custom or an authoritative code. However, it might also be based on self-interest, caprice, immaturity, ignorance, stubbornness, or misunderstanding.

In a similar manner, relying on the opinions of others or a social group is not always enough, as they may perpetuate a custom or habit that is wrong (e.g., prejudice). Adhering blindly to custom or group habits is abdicating individual responsibility. Titus and Keeton summarized this point succinctly: "Each person capable of making moral decisions is responsible for making his own decisions. The ultimate locus of moral responsibility is in the individual."[3] Ethical principles provide some guidelines for taking individual decisions and actions. The earlier illustration (To Tell or Not to Tell?) and the one that follows (Conflicting Duties) demonstrate some ethical problems that, for most people, would present difficult choices. Consider them in light of the ethical principles discussed following the box.

Conflicting Duties

 Because of your fine reputation as a PA, you were invited to become a director of a local bank and were pleased to accept the position. While serving on the board, you learned that a bank director is under a duty to use care and prudence in administering the affairs of the bank, and that failure to do so in such a way that the bank suffers a financial loss means that the director(s) may be held liable for damages. This month, in the course of an audit, you discover a seriously weakened financial position in a client who has a large loan from your bank. Prompt disclosure to the other bank directors would minimize the bank's loss, but since the audit report cannot be completed for another three weeks, such disclosure would amount to divulging confidential information gained in the course of an audit engagement (prohibited by confidentiality principles). You can remain silent and honour confidentiality principles (and fail to honour your duty as a bank director), or you can speak up to the other directors (thus violating confidentiality principles). Which should you choose?

Ethical theories can be subdivided into two types: monistic and pluralistic. **Monistic theories** assume that universal principles apply regardless of the specific facts. **Pluralistic theories**, on the other hand, assume that there are no universal principles and that the best approach is to use the principles that are most relevant in a particular case.

There are a number of monistic theories. The most important are deontological (or duty-based) theories dominated by the ideas of Immanuel Kant and utilitarianism. **Deontological (Kantian) ethics** assumes that there are universal principles (**imperatives**) such as the biblical Ten Commandments that must always be followed regardless of the consequences. Kant maintained that motive and duty alone define a moral act, not the consequences of the act.

Some object to the imperative principle because so-called universal rules always turn out to have exceptions. Others respond that if the rule is stated properly to include the exceptional cases, then the principle is still valid. But the human experience is complicated, and the rules would be very complex if they had to cover all possible cases.[4] This problem is not unique to ethics, as identifying the universal or primary principles and concepts of anything is a challenge for anyone trying to justify some action or conclusion. Universal principles are generally easier to identify in mathematics and the physical sciences than they are in social sciences such as accounting and auditing. Nevertheless, auditors must try to give the best reasons they can for their professional judgments and conclusions (claims). These reasons must also be based on the audit evidence.

Another major problem with duty-based ethics is that duties can conflict; one then needs to sort out which duty is most important, depending on the specific context. The professional rules of conduct for accountants have been greatly influenced by duty-based Kantian ethics and can be viewed as duties. But there is also a potential conflict of professional rules, most notably the rules of confidentiality and of not being associated with misleading information. This ethical dilemma was illustrated in the preceding box (Conflicting Duties), and the related rules are discussed later in this chapter and in Chapter 18 (available on Connect).

Another monistic theory is **consequentialism**, that is, basing the decision on the consequences of an action. Utilitarianism indicates that when we have a choice, we pick the one that results in the best outcome (that is, has the highest utility). **Utilitarianism** is a specialized case of consequentialism that chooses the action that maximizes the greatest good for the greatest number of people. A minority, however, might suffer as a consequence of this. Related difficulties with utilitarianism include deciding what is "good" and what is a "fair" distribution of the good. In other words, who decides how to measure utility in the particular circumstances? Addressing such complications requires more refined concepts, and these may be influenced by culture and ideology.

These monistic theories are not sufficient on their own to handle the complexities of most real-life ethical problems, including those of professional accounting ethics. Nevertheless, they can be important principles

monistic theories:
ethical theories that assume universal principles apply regardless of the specific facts of a situation

pluralistic theories:
ethical theories that assume that there are no universal principles and that the best approach is to use the principles that are most relevant in a particular case

deontological (Kantian) ethics:
the moral theory that an action is right if it is based on a sense of duty or obligation

imperatives:
universal principles assumed by monistic moral theories

consequentialism:
a moral theory that the choice of action is made based solely on the consequences, that is, that it maximizes utility; note that economics and business are based on this theory

utilitarianism:
a moral theory that the right choice is the one that results in the greatest good for the greatest number of people

when providing reasons for a claim or decision. For example, standard economic theory is based on utilitarianism, the same theory used in cost-benefit analysis. However, exclusive reliance on one principle in all situations can lead to problems. The cost-benefit analysis approach was used by many public accounting firms in the 1990s when they decided to put more emphasis on developing the management consulting side of their practices rather than on auditing. In some cases, auditing was viewed as a "loss leader" in creating more lucrative consulting practices. At the time, the big public accounting firms were also the largest consulting firms in the world.[5] The resulting increase in consulting revenues was so large that the appearance of independence was affected. Many feel that overreliance on consulting led to Arthur Andersen's demise. This focus on utilitarianism thus caused the profession a great deal of grief. With the passage of SOX and other reforms, the pendulum is now swinging the other way—the focus on quality control emphasizes auditors' duties toward the public interest.

Ethical reasoning is different from other types of reasoning because it considers the perspective of others. A problem is that there can be different dimensions to an ethical dilemma, and monistic theories are usually insufficient to deal with every aspect. Specifically, ethics is very context specific. You will especially note this in the rules for independence discussed later in this chapter. But this should already be evident to you from your study of accounting. The way we account and the disclosure language used in financial reporting are also very context specific (for example, whether or not the going-concern assumption is satisfied).

One of the key assumptions of accounting is the going-concern assumption mentioned above. If this assumption is not true, then you cannot use the accounting standards that rely on it. But the auditor can rarely be certain that a business will continue with certainty. Then the question becomes how certain you must be as an auditor. This illustrates the importance of context in an appropriate accounting for a given situation, and the difficult duty of the auditor to assess the appropriateness of the reporting in words and numbers. It is also common to need to consider several issues at once. Thus, for example, the dimension relating to the duties of an auditor reflects Kantian theories, whereas the dimension of the dilemma relating to outcomes of auditor decisions reflects consequentialist reasoning.

There are other ethical theories, such as virtue ethics, that relate to the personal character of the decision maker. Yet other ethical theories focus on the need for justice in a decision, or the need to preserve certain rights of individuals, or other aspects of the social impact of a decision. More recent ethical theories critically evaluate the social origins of ethical theories and the societies in which the ethical theories evolve. These are referred to as critical theory and post-modernity. Many post-moderns subscribe to the view of Zygmunt Bauman that "Human reality is messy and ambiguous, and so moral decisions, unlike abstract ethical principles, are ambivalent."[6] Nevertheless, by being synthesized to differences in the way people might view things through differences in the way to deal with these complexities, auditors are better prepared to reach an appropriate conclusion. This is now recognized in the Canadian Auditing Standards CAS 200.13 definition of professional judgment as given in Chapter 1, which in part states ". . .uses the application of ethical standards in making informed decisions. . . ."

Note that CAS 200 says nothing about ethical theories, but implicit is that somehow the auditor will manage to do the right thing. We thus introduce the concept of critical thinking to look more deeply at professional judgment beyond that given in auditing standards. You can view this as part of the education and experience needed in fulfilling professional judgment expectations of auditors. Going beyond the standards is especially important when the standards do not cover all of society's expectations of auditors. This is illustrated in the next box.

The consequences of a decision for others and the ability to imagine their feelings about these must be part of ethical reasoning. This ability to imagine is frequently referred to as **moral imagination**. For example, a moral imagination helps in the understanding of user needs in financial reporting. This may be an important way of avoiding litigation, as discussed in the box below. Had the CEO at Molex (the company described at the beginning of Chapter 1) used his moral imagination, he might not have been fired.

moral imagination:
the part of ethical reasoning where one has the ability to imagine others' feelings about the consequences of a decision

The Significance *of United States V. Simon* (Popularly Known as the *Continental Vending* Case), 1969

The circumstances were judged to be evidence of willful violation of Section 32 of the *Exchange Act*. Generally accepted accounting principles (GAAP) were viewed by the judge as persuasive but not necessarily conclusive criteria for financial reporting. Section 32 states the criminal penalties for violation of the *Exchange Act*. Like Section 24 of the *Securities Act*, the critical test is whether the violator acted "willfully and knowingly."

In affirming the conviction, the appeals court stated that it should be the auditor's responsibility to report factually whenever corporate activities are carried out for the benefit of the president of the company and when "looting" has occurred.

The significance of this case is that while the auditor was able to prove that the financial statements were in conformity with GAAP at the time, the auditor was nevertheless found guilty of committing fraud! This is because the accounting standards at the time did not require disclosure of material related party transactions. While the auditor knew that the related party transactions were material and presented in a misleading way, the auditor relied on technical conformity with GAAP to support his opinion. The courts disagreed. The courts concluded that when the auditor uses the words "present fairly" in his report, it means more than mere conformity with GAAP. A higher-level principle comes into play that can be interpreted as meeting the needs of third parties. These needs include being understandable and not misleading to non-accountants. In essence, the courts said that auditors should use more "common sense" in deciding on user needs. An auditor cannot "hide behind GAAP" to avoid making informative disclosures and meeting third-party needs. Technical conformity with GAAP can be irrelevant in meeting user needs because the assumptions of an applicable reporting framework may not apply in particular circumstances. An auditor must look to broader-level principles and objectives of financial reporting in order to decide if the financial statements result in being "presented fairly." Put another way, "present fairly" is more principles based, whereas "in conformity with GAAP" or "in accordance with GAAP" is more rules-based accounting.[7]

The issue of principles-based accounting is becoming even more important with the distinctions made by CAS 200.13 between a "compliance" reporting framework and a "fair presentation framework." The words "present fairly" now mean something. The auditor can use the words "present fairly" in the opinion paragraph only if a fair presentation reporting framework is used, as defined in CAS 200.13. A fair presentation framework is one that is more principles based, allowing disclosures beyond and departures from more-specific reporting requirements. This focus on broader principles, understanding user needs, and related concepts is a major reason for introducing the critical thinking concept in this chapter.

Postscript: The auditors of Continental Vending were found guilty of criminal fraud in misleading investors despite the auditee's compliance (in accordance) with GAAP. The auditors were sentenced to jail but were pardoned by President Nixon. This case set the legal precedent for the importance of principles-based accounting.

More on Critical Thinking

LO3   Outline the characteristics of critical thinking.

With the adoption of international standards and their greater emphasis on the most basic principles of accounting and auditing, the role of critical thinking in professional judgment has become more important. For example, auditors now need to distinguish between "compliance" and "fairness of presentation" with an appropriate financial reporting framework. In addition, critical thinking and skepticism become more important when the auditor takes on more responsibility for detecting fraud and other types of unethical reporting. Critical thinking considers how the financial statements will be used in a particular engagement. This is necessary in evaluating the appropriateness of how the assertions are presented to third parties and how courts might view a situation in litigation. Critical thinking is especially important in evaluating the application of accounting principles using accounting estimates, as covered in Chapter 19 (available on Connect). As noted in Chapter 1, the economic crisis of 2008/2009 created new concerns about the limits of the audit process and the financial reporting that it verifies. When combined with new concepts like accounting risk, critical thinking can be used to help address these concerns. A framework for critical thinking is outlined in this section and more thoroughly discussed in Appendix 3A (available on Connect). Applications of different parts of this framework are illustrated in the exercises throughout the text.

Auditors cannot rely on standards for detailed rules in all possible situations. The international code of professional ethics of the International Federation of Accountants (IFAC) recognizes that every engagement is unique, and, consequently, auditors must tailor their moral imaginations to the specific circumstances of the engagement. This is part of being a professional rather than just a technician mechanically following standards and rules of conduct. It does not work to rely too much on one broad principle of morality, such as utilitarianism, to resolve all ethical conflicts. By the same token, it is not sufficient to merely follow detailed rules of GAAP and generally accepted auditing standards (GAAS) and rules of ethics on an engagement in order to meet audit objectives. The social and moral world is complicated and messy. People will disagree on how to measure utility and how to prioritize rights and duties. Critical thinking is an increasingly important skill for auditors wishing to meet ethical reporting expectations of users of financial statements. A framework for structured thinking will better prepare you to deal with the ethical and other issues of professional judgment in the 21st-century audit environment. A **critical thinking framework** is one that consists of principles, concepts, and their application, and ethics is an important concept within the framework. In the end, the auditor must have good reasons other than that "it feels right" to support a position.

As illustrated in the "Continental Vending" box, reliance on detailed rules of GAAS and GAAP may not be enough for good professional judgment. Standards should not be seen as a recipe to memorize, and true professionalism means being aware of how and why the standards have evolved the way they have. Basic principles underlie all the standards and the standard-setting process. Some of these principles are more obvious than others, and critical thinking helps identify the less obvious ones. For example, Appendix 1B discusses theories related to the important concept of meeting the public interest. Ultimately, the auditor relies on fundamental principles, such as fairness of presentation in the circumstances, meeting the public interest, and maintaining the reputation of the profession. There are no universal rules for achieving these in all situations, and the auditor must think through each case in a systematic way. A critical thinking framework is a guide to helping achieve a well-supported conclusion.

A key step in critical thinking is applying logic to your reasoning. Applying logic essentially means identifying reasons supporting a claim or conclusion. There must be a link between reasons and a conclusion, and on an audit engagement, we want that link to be strong. A second condition, that of truth or substantial truth of the reasons, should be met before we can say that an audit conclusion is justified by the reasons given. If both these conditions are satisfied, then we can say that our conclusion is justified by the reasons. The term *sound reasoning*, the essence of being objective on an issue, can be used when our conclusions are justified this way. Thus, for example, CAS 200, A6–A7, requires the auditor to identify the broad principles and concepts serving as a basis for applying accounting policies to meet the general reporting objectives of a framework, such as the International Financial Reporting Standards (IFRS) conceptual framework. These broad principles and concepts are the basis for sound reasoning regarding fairness of presentation and ethical reporting in particular circumstances.

If sound reasoning is sufficiently documented, then it also provides evidence of how objective and competent the auditor is on a particular engagement. This is why the Canadian Public Accountability Board (CPAB), the regulators, and the courts like to look at audit documentation and why the documentation standards of audit work are important.

Critical thinking involves questioning the application of a standard, the concepts and principles underlying it, and the consistency of standards with one another. Questioning of standards may go back to questions about the goals of financial reporting, as is becoming evident with the CASs' new classification of financial reporting frameworks as general purpose versus special purpose, and fairness of presentation versus compliance

critical thinking framework:
principles and concepts to help structure your thinking for more ethical reporting so that your conclusions will be better justified

objectives. These are difficult tasks! But logical consideration of the differences is what makes the auditor a true professional (instead of merely one who uses the rules-following mentality or "checklist mentality" of a non-professional—the type of drudge work that is increasingly being outsourced by accounting firms to countries with cheaper labour costs).

Whereas logic is concerned with the link between reasons and conclusion, the truthfulness of reasons is determined by the source of the reasons. Sources of reasons include accounting and auditing theory and their underlying concepts, assumptions, and principles. These concepts, along with the words used to state them, affect the persuasiveness of your reasons as an auditor. A critical thinker uses language to clarify, not cloud or bias, the reasoning. For example, an auditor uses the words "present fairly" to persuade the user of the acceptability of the audited financial statements. But these words should have some meaning if they are to go beyond just sounding nice. CAS 200.13 now explicitly distinguishes between "compliance" and "fair presentation" financial reporting frameworks, and we will get into these distinctions later in the text. For now, note from the Continental Vending case that had the auditors used better judgment, including more "common sense," rather than trying to "hide behind GAAP," they might not have been found guilty of committing fraud for issuing a report that they should have known would be misleading or unethical.

Professional judgment in auditing is essentially critical thinking on accounting issues and the evidence related to them. The critical thinking framework can be used to decide when an audit conclusion is sufficiently justified. When this reasoning is documented in an audit, there is no basis for questioning the sufficiency of audit documentation. The continuing problems found by the CPAB in auditor documentation suggest insufficient critical thinking in professional judgment on the part of practising auditors. These CPAB findings are reviewed later in the advanced chapter on auditor responsibilities (Chapter 18). For a more complete discussion of the critical thinking framework, along with illustrations of its application, see Appendix 3A.

This brief review of the principles of ethics and critical thinking provides some background on the way people approach difficult decision problems. The greatest task is to take general ethical principles and apply them to a real decision. Applying them through codes of professional ethics is a challenge. In this book, we suggest that the minimal critical thinking issues auditors should consider are the following. It is important to supply good reasons for conclusions (claims). The most important reasons relate to how to apply ethical, accounting, and auditing principles underlying the professional standards to the particular circumstances of a client's reporting. The reasons should be acceptable to third parties, especially capital providers. And the reasons should ultimately be based on materiality and the various risk concepts introduced in this book. In true critical thinking, however, the auditor should also consider alternative reasons that might support a different conclusion. The type of skepticism that the auditor applies to his or her own reasoning is a key part of critical thinking. It is the type of reflective thinking required in good ethical reasoning combined with the principles of argumentation and logic discussed in Appendix 3A. We thus apply the term *critical thinking* to professional judgment that uses concepts and principles beyond those found in existing professional standards.

Professional judgment in its most basic form involves several key steps:

1. Identifying the crucial issues

2. Gathering information on all the significant assertions

3. Identifying possible alternative courses of action

4. Evaluating the alternative courses of actions

5. Deciding on the best course of action

Note that step 1 especially involves consideration of the broader context of the audit-task environment, such as the type of accountability needed and who is the accountable party. In addition, there are professional judgments on primarily auditing issues (gathering and evaluating the evidence) and professional judgments in evaluating the application of the accounting. Combining these judgments requires yet more judgment, with the critical thinking elements discussed above and in Appendix 3A. To avoid confusion, in the rest of this book we use the term *professional judgment* as defined in CAS 200, and the deeper and more integrative structures of these judgments we refer to as critical thinking. Critical thinking is more of an advanced audit topic.

Later chapters illustrate applying professional judgment and the critical thinking framework to specific audit and accounting issues.

The rest of this chapter is devoted to the more practical rules of professional ethics, related concepts and principles, and their application in relevant situations. These professional rules and principles rely on the various ethical theories discussed in this section, especially duty-based theories, for their justification.

Review Checkpoints

3-13 Why should auditors act as though there is always a potential conflict of interest between the auditor and the management of the enterprise under audit?

3-14 Can the auditor detect deception without being skeptical? Explain.

3-15 What is a professional accountant's role with regard to ethical decision problems?

3-16 When might the rule "Let conscience be your guide" not be a sufficient basis for your personal ethical decisions? for your professional ethical decisions?

3-17 Assume that you accept the following ethical rule: "Failure to tell the whole truth is wrong." In the illustrations about (a) your position as a bank director and (b) your knowledge of the cashier's forgeries, what would this rule require you to do? Why is an unalterable rule, such as this one, considered an element of duty-based ethical theory?

3-18 How do utilitarian ethics differ from duty-based ethics?

3-19 Why are simplified monistic theories of ethics not sufficient for professional decision making?

3-20 Why is critical thinking becoming more important in the CAS and IFRS audit environment?

Codes of Professional Ethics

LO4 Describe the purpose and contents of the codes of professional ethics established by the various professional accounting bodies.

All the Chartered Professional Accountant (CPA) provincial bodies and the IFAC have their own rules of professional conduct for their members and students, either provincially or nationally. Generally, these rules are published as part of a member's handbook identifying the various activities and regulations of the public accounting associations and include a section on professional conduct. Codes of conduct need to develop a balance between detailed rules and more general principles. They also need to be practical, and, as a result, they tend to have similar frameworks, as indicated in the box below.

The codes of professional conduct are usually organized hierarchically, moving from general principles at the beginning, to rules, and then on to specific interpretations of the rules. The general principles are sometimes referred to as "ideal standards" and the more specific rules and related interpretations as "minimum standards."

An example of a code is the CPA Ontario *Member's Handbook*, which identifies the various activities and regulations of CPA Ontario, including a section on professional conduct that is divided into three parts: the Foreword, the Rules of Professional Conduct, and the Interpretation of the Rules. Many people consider the Foreword the most important part of the professional conduct regulations, because it contains principles that provide guidance in the absence of specific rules.[8] See the following link for the website: cpaontario.ca/Resources/Membershandbook/1011page2635.pdf.

International Federation of Accountants Framework for a Code of Ethics for Professional Accountants (as Adapted for This Book)

- Objective: to serve the public interest (this cannot be accomplished by mere conformity to detailed rules—this dedication to serve is more like a state of mind).
- Principles necessary to attain objective:
  - Integrity
  - Objectivity
  - Professional competence and due care
  - Confidentiality
  - Professional behaviour (includes conformity with technical standards)
- Conformity is achieved by identifying, evaluating, and controlling threats to non-conformity to an acceptable level.
- IFAC also provides examples, but these are not exhaustive, as this is impossible. Therefore, a principles approach should be followed (as indicated by the above principles).[9] The various codes of professional conduct are meant to apply to all members, with exceptions for students and members not in public practice. The CPA provincial bodies have substantially harmonized their codes so that the CPA code can be viewed as more of a national one. The CASs do not refer to the IFAC's code of ethics. Instead, Canadian CPAs use the code of the provincial accounting body to which they belong.

The Foreword is essential reading for CPA members and students, as the handbook specifically advises that all the rules in it "are to be read in the light of the Foreword to the rules." In this sense, the Foreword is analogous to the conceptual framework of accounting; for example, there is the conceptual framework of IFRS, and the rules themselves are like the Recommendations in the *CPA Canada Handbook*.

The Foreword has clearly defined sections. The first section sets out the purpose of the rules, which is to guide the profession in serving the public. The second reviews the key characteristics that mark a profession and a professional, concluding that "chartered accountancy is a profession." The third section identifies the five "fundamental statements of accepted conduct" around which all the rules are centred. The five fundamental principles of professional accounting ethics on pages 6–7 of the *Member's Handbook* can be summarized as follows:

1. *Professional Behaviour:* to serve the public interest and maintain the good reputation of the profession [by the way, you may be interested in the definition of a professional and his or her role in society—this is covered on pages 4–5 of the Rules of Professional Conduct]

2. *Integrity and Due Care* in performing professional services.

3. *Professional Competence:* Skills and training you must have, including the importance of maintaining your competence over time through continuing professional education and experience.

4. *Confidentiality*

5. *Objectivity:* Must be maintained in all professional services. This means members' professional judgments must not be impaired or perceived to be impaired. With respect to assurance services (e.g., audits), the special term *independence* is used instead of *objectivity*.

These most general principles of practice that need to be adhered to by every accounting professional are followed by 35 pages of more-detailed rules to help guide the proper implementation of the principles.

Let's focus on a single principle to review how the logic works. On page 7 of the Rules of Professional Conduct, you will find four paragraphs describing objectivity and its independence counterpart in audit engagements. In addition, on pages 18–46 you have 29 more pages describing essentially the principle as it applies to different circumstances. These more-specific applications of the principles are referred to as "rules." Note that the rules related to independence (204) start with six pages of definitions illustrating the importance of specific words used in the rule. A review of the definitions should indicate to you that they are used to describe (specify) situations or contexts that threaten independence. The specific contexts that indicate when independence is impaired can be classified as follows: financial interests, loans and guarantees, close business relationships, family and personal relationships, serving as an officer or director of an audit or review client, long association of senior personnel with a reporting issuer or client, performance of management functions for an assurance client, preparation of journal entries and source documents, provision of valuation services to a reporting issuer audit client, provision of internal audit services to a reporting issuer audit client, and a range of prohibited other services to different types of clients. The rules are very specific as to type of client and prohibitions. Note they are a series of "Thou shalt nots" for accountants, similar in form to the Biblical commandments.

These detailed rules do not exhaust the guidance in the Rules of Professional Conduct. There are almost 80 pages of even more detailed interpretations of Rule 204 in the Interpretations part of the Rules of Professional Conduct, basically giving more-specific guidance about conditions under which independence is impaired. For example, interpretations 39–44 describe specific sources of threats to independence: self-interest threat, self-review threat, advocacy threat, familiarity threat, and intimidation threat. These threats are examples of circumstances or situations in which independence or the appearance of independence may be viewed as impaired. Note that the assessment of the appearance of impairment of independence is one that requires moral imagination on the part of the auditor to understand a third party's viewpoint. So what these rules and interpretations try to do is help the auditor visualize the different conditions that can impair independence. This list is not exhaustive, because there is no way that the rules can anticipate every possible social context that could lead to an impairment of independence. For example, if you start dating someone working for a client, at what point is your independence in auditing the client compromised? There is no hard and fast rule. That's because social relationships in general are complicated and ultimately it's your character that determines if you act professionally. This is an example of the relevance of virtue ethics in auditing.

Page 8 of the Rules of Professional Conduct outlines a reasoning process to resolve ethical conflicts that consists of the following points:

- Relevant facts (data)
- Ethical issues involved (more data, but about the circumstances or context)
- Fundamental principles and rules applicable (warrants)
- Established internal procedures (data)
- Alternative courses of action (moral imagination, data)

Note that this reasoning is not in standard form as discussed in Appendix 3A, with warrants first. This is because to get an understanding of which warrants or principles might be relevant to a situation, the decision-making auditor first has to understand what the issues are, and that understanding is generally a form of data about the context of the situation. Once this is sorted out and an understanding of the issues is reached, then the reasoning can be set up in standard form to make sure that the reasoning supports the conclusion as well as possible. The Rules of Professional Conduct note (page 8) that the action taken should be "consistent with the fundamental principles and rules identified as being pertinent."

An implicit assumption the Rules of Professional Conduct make is that the rules are consistent with the principles, and furthermore the principles are consistent with each other, that is, they don't conflict. If there were such conflicts, then page 13 of the Rules of Professional Conduct indicates that the principles in the Foreword to the rules should take precedence. That's because the principles are designed to make the profession socially useful in protecting the public interest (page 7), and by definition this requires adherence to the professional ethics principles.

These principles are ideals every professional aspires to. The rules themselves are more specific because they are intended as enforceable guides to action. However, adherence to the rules represents only a minimum acceptable level of performance for CPAs. On the other hand, because they are more detailed, the rules are more-specific benchmarks that a member's performance can be measured against.

The Foreword singles out several principles requiring additional guidance: (a) sustaining professional competence (principle 2 above), (b) avoiding conflicts of interest in respect of a client's affairs (principle 5), and (c) practice development based on professional excellence rather than self-promotion (principle 1). It is evident from the space devoted to them that these particular principles require the most-detailed guidance. However, as the Foreword makes clear, as ethical decision making becomes more complex yet indispensable for maintaining the public interest, the absence of specific rules makes the principles that much more important. As a result, some writers have concluded that the five principles should be given much more prominence and be used more frequently.[10]

After the Foreword are the rules of conduct themselves. The CPA Ontario Council also publishes "Council Interpretations" of these rules—detailed explanations to help members understand particular applications of them. Anyone departing from Council interpretations has the burden of justifying that departure in any disciplinary hearing.

The IFAC includes a code of ethics for PAs as part of their standards as well. It avoids preparing detailed rules or interpretations, as these will be influenced by national laws, culture, and the particular circumstances of the engagement. However, a detailed rule should not conflict with a basic principle, for if it did the system of ethical reasoning would be illogical. Instead, detailed rules should clarify the application of a principle yet be consistent with it. The principle has conceptual primacy over a detailed rule. This means that if a rule conflicts with a principle, the principle overrides the rule. This is referred to as principles-based reasoning. Principles-based reasoning has always been important in moral philosophy. Principles-based reasoning is also increasingly important in financial reporting and auditing, especially under IFRS. It can also be referred to as "top-down" reasoning if the reasoning is laid out in standard logical form, as explained in Appendix 3A.

Part A of the IFAC code provides general concepts and a conceptual framework, and part B illustrates how the framework is applied by CPAs in specific situations. IFAC feels that specific rules can be arbitrary and not represent the public interest in all cases, justifying a conceptual approach. The framework identifies threats against conformity to the general principles; evaluates their significance; and, if warranted, applies safeguards eliminating or reducing them to acceptable levels. This framework is summarized in the box below, and the principles are discussed in more detail in the rest of the chapter. Note that serving the public interest can be viewed as the most important principle, since the remaining principles and detailed rules are meant to support this objective. Thus, there can be a hierarchy of principles. As accounting and auditing further evolve you can expect more clarification of the principles. For example, should there be a priority or hierarchy of user needs that have to be met in serving the goal of meeting the public interest? If the professional standards do not specify such a priority, then the auditor must make this decision on each engagement at least implicitly. This is one reason to practise critical thinking—it helps document the reasoning of your professional judgment.

International Federation of Accountants Conceptual Framework for Resolving a Conflict in the Application of Fundamental Principles

- Step 1: Members should consider the following:
  - Identify the relevant facts.
  - Identify ethical issues involved.
  - Identify fundamental principles related to the matters in question.
  - Identify established internal procedure.
  - Identify alternative courses of action.
- Step 2: Identify the appropriate course of action consistent with fundamental principles.
- Step 3: If the conflict cannot be resolved consistent with fundamental principles, then the auditor should refuse to be associated with the conflict whenever possible.

There is much similarity in the concepts of all professional codes. These are reviewed in the next section, along with the related rules.

Rules of Professional Conduct

The rules of professional conduct derive their authority from the bylaws of the various CPA professional bodies (or those that strive to be recognized as such). Members of these groups are responsible for compliance with the rules by all employees and partners associated with them. Further, members may not have other people to carry out prohibited acts on their behalf.

The various CPA bodies have detailed rules of conduct that have much in common, and we cannot list all of them, so those of CPA Ontario are given in the following box and will serve as an illustration. (Full access to the CPA Ontario handbook is at cpaontario.ca/Resources/Membershandbook/1011page2629.pdf.) In terms of the critical-thinking framework, these rules can be viewed as important reasons for taking (or not taking) a particular action. Specifically, the rules follow the logic of Kantian imperatives or duties, although there is also an element of utilitarianism, as is indicated in the discussion following the box.

The rest of this section discusses professional ethical principles, and their related rules, in more detail. However, you should refer to the appropriate provincial members' handbooks for more extensive guidance on rules related to your province or territory.

The CPA Ontario Rules of Professional Conduct

TABLE OF CONTENTS

FIRST BYLAW OF 1973

FOREWORD

Application of the rules of professional conduct
Interpretation of the rules of professional conduct

100—GENERAL

101 Compliance with bylaws, regulations and rules
102 Matters to be reported to CPA Ontario
102.1 Illegal Activities
102.2 Other provincial bodies
102.3 Other professional regulatory bodies
102.4 Other regulatory bodies
103 False or misleading applications
104 Requirement to co-operate
105 Hindrance, inappropriate influence and intimidation

200—STANDARDS OF CONDUCT AFFECTING THE PUBLIC INTEREST

201.1,
.2 & .3 Maintenance of reputation of profession
201.4 Advocacy services
202.1 Integrity and due care
202.2 Objectivity
203.1 Professional competence
203.2 Co-operation with practice inspections and conduct investigations
204 Independence
204.1 Assurance and specified auditing procedures engagements
204.2 Compliance with Rule 204.1

(continued)

204.3 Identification of threats and safeguards

204.4 Specific prohibitions, assurance and specified auditing procedures engagements

204.5 Documentation

204.6 Members must disclose prohibited interests and relationships

204.7 Firms to ensure compliance by partners and professional employees

204.8 Independence: insolvency engagements

204.9 Disclosure of impaired independence

205 False or misleading documents and oral representations

206 Compliance with professional standards

207 Unauthorized benefits

208 Confidentiality of information

209 Borrowing from clients

210 Conflict of interest

211 Duty to report breach of rules of professional conduct

212.1 Handling of trust funds and other property

212.2 Handling property of others

213 Unlawful activity

214 Fee quotations

215 Contingent fees

216 Payment or receipt of commissions

217.1 Advertising and promotion

217.2 Solicitation

217.3 Endorsements

218 Retention of documentation and working papers

300—RELATIONS WITH FELLOW MEMBERS AND WITH NON-MEMBERS ENGAGED IN PUBLIC ACCOUNTING

302 Communication with predecessor

303 Co-operation with successor accountant

304 Joint engagements

305 Communication of special engagements to incumbent

306.1 Responsibilities on accepting engagements

306.2 Responsibilities on referred engagements

400—ORGANIZATION AND CONDUCT OF A PROFESSIONAL PRACTICE

401 Practice names

402 Use of descriptive styles

403 Association with firms

404 Operation of members' offices

405 Office by representation

406 Member responsible for a non-member in practice of public accounting

407 Related business or practice, and member responsible for non-member in such business or practice

408 Association of member with non-members in public practice

409 Practice of public accounting in corporate form

500—RULES OF PROFESSIONAL CONDUCT APPLICABLE ONLY TO FIRMS

501 Firm's maintenance of policies and procedures for compliance with professional standards

502 Firm's maintenance of policies and procedures: competence and conduct of firm members

503 Association with firms

APPENDIX A

Former Rule of Professional Conduct 204 (Objectivity)

Serving the Public Interest

The single most important principle for accountants is to serve the public interest; they can do so only if the profession maintains a good reputation. This is a way of characterizing expectations of the auditor's social role. The auditor cannot be said to meet the public interest unless the auditor fulfills the social role expected. "The phrase 'at all times' is significant because the public will view any serious transgression of a professional accountant, including those outside business or professional activity, as a black mark against the profession as a whole. Consequently, if a professional accountant is convicted of a minimal offense or fraud, his or her certification is usually revoked."[11] The remaining principles all serve to support this first one. In this sense, this principle has primacy over the others, as discussed earlier.

Serving the public interest primarily means to competently fulfill the role expected by the public. This is succinctly captured in Rule 205, which prohibits the PA from being associated with false or misleading information. Note that violation of this rule is illustrated in the Continental Vending case. As stated in the auditor's report, the role of the auditor is to express an opinion based on the audit of the financial statements prepared by management. In fulfilling this responsibility, the auditor reduces the risk of the financial statements being false or misleading to an appropriately low level. Terms such as *present fairly, in all material respects, audit risk, materiality*, and *risk of material misstatement* used throughout the text capture this concept.

If the audit fails to detect a material misstatement, then the audit fails. This can have serious consequences for the accounting firm. The rapid demise of Arthur Andersen as a result of the failure of their Enron audit illustrates this. The profession is now particularly sensitized to the importance of not being associated with misleading information. And Rule 205 now probably represents the most important rule, particularly in light of responsibilities placed on auditors by SOX and the CPAB, as discussed in Chapter 2.

In a financial statement audit, Rule 205 relates to the auditor not being associated with misleading financial information. This rule clarifies what it means to serve the public interest as an auditor. The responsibility to the public is paramount. This primary responsibility is different for auditors than for other professions, such as law or medicine, in which the primary responsibility is to the client or patient. The auditor's responsibility is so important to third parties that it overrides his or her obligations to companies or clients. This creates a unique moral situation in which the auditor is theoretically not working for the person or company that pays him or her. This uniqueness is captured by the independence rule, discussed in the next section, which exists primarily to convince the third parties in three-party accountability that the auditor's primary objective is to meet their financial reporting needs. This is the key responsibility of the auditor's role, thereby serving the public interest and maintaining the reputation of the profession. The rule, therefore, reflects society's expectations of the role of the auditor. As you will see, many audit concepts and standards relate to effectively fulfilling the social role associated with Rule 205.

Integrity

Integrity is the duty to be honest and conscientious in performing professional services. Integrity relates to the basic character of the professional—a PA must be upright, not kept upright. Without integrity among its members, the profession cannot maintain its good reputation and serve the public interest.

Independence and Objectivity

LO5   Explain the importance of an independence framework for auditors.

Rule 204.1 dealing with independence was introduced to you in Chapter 2. *Independence* and *objectivity* are closely related terms; in this case, *independence* is a way of achieving objectivity, and it is the term given to the objectivity required in the special case of assurance engagements. The term *independence* is also used in

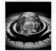 the *Canada Business Corporations Act* (CBCA), in some provincial corporations acts, and in various professional rules of conduct. Canadian legislation requires that the auditor be "independent"— presumably, the fact of independence must be determined by the courts.

CBCA, section 161, defines independence as a key qualification of an auditor, as indicated in the following box.

Canada Business Corporations Act, Section 161

Qualification of auditor

161.(1)   Subject to subsection (5), a person is disqualified from being an auditor of a corporation if the person is not independent of the corporation, any of its affiliates, or the directors or officers of any such corporation or its affiliates.

Independence

(2)   For the purpose of this section,

(a) independence is a question of fact; and

(b) a person is deemed not to be independent if the person or the person's business partner

(i) is a business **partner**, a director, an officer or an employee of the corporation or any of its affiliates, or a business partner of any director, officer or employee of any such corporation or any of its affiliates;

(ii) **beneficially** owns or controls, directly or indirectly, a material interest in the securities of the corporation or any of its affiliates,

(iii) has been a receiver-manager, sequestrator, liquidator or trustee in bankruptcy of the corporation or any of its affiliates within two years of the person's proposed appointment as auditor of the corporation.

Duty to resign

(3)   An auditor who becomes disqualified under this section shall, subject to subsection (5), resign forthwith after becoming aware of the disqualification.

Source: *Canada Business Corporations Act*, section 161.

The term *independence* is internationally recognized. For example, IFAC's *Technical Standard on Ethics*, section 8, specifies that "professional accountants in public practice when undertaking a reporting assignment should be independent in fact and appearance." Similar wording regarding the need for independence is used in the code of conduct of Certified Management Accountants of Ontario (CMA Ontario).

The IFAC and the CPA provincial bodies all have standard frameworks for independence based on the five following threats or risks to a PA's independence:

1.   Self-review—providing assurance on his or her own work

2.   Self-interest—for example, benefiting from a financial interest in a client

3.   Advocacy—promoting a client's position or opinion

4.   Familiarity—becoming too sympathetic to a client's interests

5.   Intimidation—being deterred from acting objectively by actual or perceived threats from a client

Under all the independence standards, the PA must identify and evaluate the significance of any independence threat. If threats are other than clearly insignificant, the PA must apply safeguards to eliminate the threats or take action to reduce them to a level that would pose no real or perceived compromise. If no safeguards are adequate to preserve independence, the PA must eliminate the activity, interest, or relationship that is creating the threat, or refuse to perform or continue the particular engagement.[12]

We refer to the need to control independence threats as the independence principle. Principles like this one assist sound, structured ethical reasoning by auditors. Independence problems and other elements indicating lack of audit quality have been a continuing concern in CPAB's monitoring reports over the years.[13]

The Canadian legislation referred to previously requires independence for financial statement audit services. However, review services of unaudited financial statements, such as engagements to report on prospective financial statements (forecasts and projections) and expressing opinions on representations other than financial statements (e.g., reports on internal control), all require independence as well. The definition of public practice is significant here. A member is considered to be in the public practice of accounting if he or she (1) lets it be known publicly that he or she is a PA, and (2) offers the types of services rendered by other PAs. The latter part of the definition is very broad because PAs perform a wide range of accounting, audit, taxation, and consulting services.[14] This means that most PAs who seek clients from the general public are in the practice of public accounting. For example, the PAs who work for H&R Block, the tax preparation corporation, are in public practice if they let themselves be known as PAs. Non-PAs who perform these same services are, of course, not held to these standards, and this is partly why PAs have a different social status.

Since the purpose of independent financial auditing is to add credibility to financial statements, auditors must be impartial and unbiased with respect to both the client management and the client entity itself. Auditors must be independent in fact and also independent of outside decision makers who rely on their assurance services. Independence is, in fact, a mental condition and difficult to demonstrate by physical or visual means. Thus, some things that give the appearance of lacking independence may be prohibited in specific interpretations of the independence principle. Note how awareness of other perspectives is crucial in correctly assessing the various independence risks.

IFAC's conceptual framework approach to ethics consists of compliance with its fundamental principles, identification of threats to achieving those principles, and safeguarding against these threats. The safeguards include training, professional standards, regulatory monitoring, and corporate governance. They are implemented using a process similar to that outlined for critical thinking earlier in this chapter. In brief, achieving the objective of independence is accomplished through understanding users' perspectives, taking actions that address the risk of threats against their interests, and reducing those risks of threats to acceptable levels. The box below identifies the concepts of programming, investigative, and reporting independence that are useful in avoiding influences that might bias judgment.

Three Aspects of Practical Independence

Programming Independence

Auditors must remain free from interference by client managers who try to restrict, specify, or modify the procedures auditors want to perform, including any attempt to assign personnel or otherwise control the audit work. Occasionally, client managers try to limit the number of auditors permitted in a location.

Investigative Independence

Auditors must have free access to books, records, correspondence, and other evidence. They must have the cooperation of management without any attempt to interpret or screen evidence. Sometimes, client managers refuse auditors' requests for access to necessary information.

Reporting Independence

Auditors must not let any feelings of loyalty to the client or auditee interfere with their obligation to report fully and fairly. Neither should the client management be allowed to overrule auditors' judgments on the appropriate content of an audit report. Disciplinary actions have been taken against auditors who go to a client management conference with a preliminary estimate for a financial adjustment and emerge after agreeing with management to a smaller adjustment.

Detailed Independence Rules

Observing the rules regarding prohibited activities is an important way of maintaining the independence principle. The fact that the rules vary with the circumstances is a complication. A member may divest a prohibited financial interest before the first work on a new client begins, and, if the engagement continues, it is improper to reinvest. Direct or indirect financial interests are allowed up to the point of materiality, that is, until they make significant contributions to the PA's wealth. This provision permits members to hold mutual fund shares and have some limited business transactions with clients.

As noted previously in this text, SOX has been an influence globally in determining which threats to independence are against the public interest. The currently prohibited activities seem to focus on the self-review threat. Other threats will likely be identified, as CPA Canada, CPAB, the U.S. Securities and Exchanges Commission (SEC), and the Public Company Accounting Oversight Board (PCAOB) establish more regulations that are deemed to be in the public interest. Earlier standards and rules of professional conduct were focused on self-interest and intimidation threats through rules on financial interests and those related to conflicts of interest. The more detailed rules are reviewed next.

Permitted Loans

If the client is a bank or other financial institution, the codes of conduct generally allow home mortgages, immaterial loans, and secured loans, all made under a client's normal lending terms. Nor is independence considered impaired if a member obtains the following types of personal loans from assurance service clients: auto loans and leases, insurance policy loans based on policy surrender value, loans collateralized by cash deposits at the same financial institution, and credit card balances and cash advances equivalent to those of other customers in the normal course of business. For insurance company clients, the PA can borrow against the cash surrender value of a life insurance policy. However, the loans should have the same terms as granted to other customers of the institution in the normal course of business. Potentially, these kinds of permitted loans could be abused in spirit, as apparently happened in the United States in the 1990s. The key ethical judgment is in understanding "the normal course of business" and, more basically, in awareness of the types of loans that could lead to even the perception of impairment of auditor independence.

Other Issues Related to the Independence Principle

Broadly defined, the codes of conduct collectively prohibit activities that amount to having the ability to make decisions for the client or to act as management. The appearance of independence is impaired if such a connection existed at any time during the period covered by the financial statements, regardless of whether the association was terminated prior to the beginning of the audit work. The presumption is that members cannot be independent and objective when attesting to decisions they took part in or are connected with.

In terms of ethical principles, these rules may be justified on a utilitarian theory basis as far as direct financial interests are concerned. The logic is something like this: the greatest good is created by making a situation free of any suspicious circumstances, no matter how innocent they may be in truth. The goodwill of public reliance and respect is greater than the PA's sacrifice of the opportunity to invest in securities of clients or participate in their management. Note that this reasoning relies on putting priority on the interests of third parties, which is why we noted in the Chapter 1 Application Case that independence can be argued as the most important personal characteristic of the auditor (this is also stressed in CAS 200, paragraphs 14 and CA14). This increasing emphasis on independence reflects changes in societal norms with respect to the role of the external auditor, and these, in turn, influence the courts, regulators, and regulations affecting auditors.

In addition to the issues previously discussed, there are other rules relevant to the independence principle, now briefly described.

Honorary Positions in Non-profit Organizations

Ordinarily, independence is impaired if a CPA serves on an organization's board of directors. However, members can be honorary directors of charity hospitals, fund drives, symphony orchestra societies, and other non-profit organizations so long as (1) the position is purely honorary, (2) the CPA is identified as an honorary director on letterheads and other literature, (3) the only form of participation is the use of the CPA's name, and (4) the CPA does not vote with the board or participate in management functions. When all these criteria are satisfied, the CPA/board member can perform assurance services because the appearances of independence will have been preserved.

Retired Partners

Independence problems do not end when partners retire, resign, or otherwise leave an accounting firm. A former partner can impair independence by association with a client of the former firm. However, the problems are solved and independence is not impaired if (1) the person's retirement benefits are fixed, (2) the person is no longer active in the accounting firm (some retired partners remain "active"), and (3) the former partner is not held out to be associated with the accounting firm by a reasonable observer. Regulators may have stricter rules relating to former partners.

Accounting and Other Services

If a CPA performs the bookkeeping and makes accounting decisions for a company and the management does not know enough about the financial statements to take primary responsibility for them, the CPA cannot be considered independent for assurance services. It might be perceived that the CPA has both prepared the financial statements or other data and given an audit report or other assurance on his or her own work. The CPA can perform the bookkeeping and counsel the client management about the accounting principle choices, but in the final analysis, management must be able to say, "These are our financial statements (or other data); we made the choices of accounting principles; we take primary responsibility for them." Again, regulators may have stricter rules relating to such bookkeeping services.

SOX prohibits the following services for auditors of publicly traded companies: internal audit services for the client, financial information system design and implementation, and tax services. For other companies, all of these services must be pre-approved by the client's audit committee and disclosed to regulators.

Rotation of Partners and Second Partner Review

The CPAB and SOX require rotation of the lead audit partner and/or concurring review partner (but not the audit firm) every five years. The five-year period includes time spent providing professional services as a non-partner (e.g., manager). The intent of the rule is to prevent auditors from becoming too complacent and not sufficiently skeptical about the client relationship. A second partner review is now mandated by both the CPAB and SOX.

Actual or Threatened Litigation

When a CPA and a client move into an adversarial relationship and away from the cooperative one needed in an assurance engagement, independence is threatened by appearances of the CPA trying to serve his or her own best interests. CPAs are considered not independent when (1) company management threatens or actually starts a lawsuit against them, alleging deficiencies in audit or other assurance work, or (2) the CPA threatens or starts litigation against the company management, alleging fraud or deceit. Such cases may be rare, but auditors get out of such difficult audit situations by ending the assurance engagement. Essentially, the CPA–client relationship ends, and the litigation begins a new relationship.

Investor or Investee Relationships

In this context, the terms *investor* and *investee* have the same meaning as in rules about accounting for investments in the equity method, covered in accounting standard IAS 28 and *CPA Canada Handbook* section 3050. The *investor* is the party that has significant influence over a business, and the *investee* is the business in which the investor has the significant influence.

When the CPA's client is the investor, the CPA's direct or material indirect financial interest in a non-client investee impairs the CPA's independence. The reasoning is that the client investor, through its ability to influence a non-client investee, can materially increase or decrease the CPA's financial stake in the investee. If, on the other hand, the non-client investee is immaterial to the investor, independence is not considered impaired when the CPA's financial interest in a non-client investee is immaterial in relation to the CPA's wealth.

When a CPA has an investment in a non-client investor, (a) this investment may be a direct or material indirect financial interest that will diminish independence with respect to a client investee; (b) independence is not impaired, as long as the CPA does not have significant influence over the actions or financial statements of the non-client investor; but (c) independence is impaired when the CPA's investment gives him or her significant influence over the actions of the non-client investor, which might, in turn, influence the client investee. In any of these relationships, the independence of the CPA is impaired because it puts him or her in a position similar to that of a member of management of the client investee.

Effect of Family Relationships

The codes of conduct and all the interpretations apply to members, but being a member of a professional accounting institute, society, or association should not be confused with the use of the word "member" in the rule. For purposes of independence, the terms *member* and *member's firm* generally include the following:

- All partners in the accounting firm
- All professional employees participating in the engagement, including audit, tax, and management consulting personnel
- All other manager-level employees located in a firm office that does a significant part of the audit
- Any CPA firm personnel formerly employed by or connected with the audit client in a managerial capacity unless the person (a) is disassociated from the client and (b) does not participate in the engagement
- Any CPA firm professional (e.g., partner, manager, staff) who is associated with the client in a managerial capacity and is located in an office of the CPA firm that does a significant part of the engagement

The term *member* excludes students registered under the bylaws of the professional body. However, the codes of conduct can include students, depending on the bylaws of the professional body.

All of this is rather complicated, but the bottom line is that it is rare for any partners or shareholders in the firm to be able to have any of the financial or managerial relationships. It is possible for managers and staff to have such relationships, provided they are far removed from the actual work on the audit engagement.

Financial interests of spouses and dependent persons (whether related or not) and some financial interests of close relatives are attributed to the member. Thus, for example, independence would be impaired if (a) a spouse or dependant of a member had a direct financial interest in an audit client or (b) a member on an engagement knew about a sibling's or non-dependent child's material financial interest in a client.

Employment relationships of spouses, dependent persons, and close relatives can be attributed to a member. Positions that are "audit sensitive" or can exercise significant influence over the operating, financial, or accounting policies of the client (e.g., cashier, internal auditor, accounting supervisor, purchasing agent, inventory warehouse supervisor) are attributed to the member and impair independence. However, such employment poses no problem when it cannot influence the audit work (e.g., secretarial, non-financial positions).

The code of conduct rules are the minimum criteria relating to independence. CPA firms can make more limiting rules. The anecdote in the box below shows some rules given to job applicants of a Big Four accounting firm.

Analysis of Independence Rules

Generally, the rules of professional conduct and corporate legislation imply a fine distinction between independence, integrity, and objectivity. The spirit of the rules is that integrity and objectivity are required in connection with all professional services and, in addition, independence is required for assurance services. In this context, integrity and objectivity are the larger concepts, and independence is a special condition largely defined by the matters of appearance specified in the codes or their interpretations. Conflicts of interest, for

If Employed by "Anonymous Firm," I Understand That . . .

Professional staff members of the firm, their spouses, and dependants are prohibited from owning or controlling investments in any of our clients and certain related non-clients, and I will be required to dispose of any such investments before commencing employment with the firm.

I will be prohibited from disclosing non-public information regarding clients or other entities to anyone, other than for firm business, or using it for any personal purpose.

I will be expected to devote my energies to the firm to the fullest extent possible and refrain from other business interests that might require significant time or that could be considered a conflict of interest.

Neither an offer of employment nor employment itself carries with it a guarantee of tenure of employment, and my employment, compensation, and benefits can be terminated, with or without cause or notice, at any time at the option of the firm or me.

example, as cited in CPA Ontario Rule 204, refer to avoiding business interests in which the accountant's personal financial relationships or relationships with other clients might tempt him or her not to serve the best interests of a client or the public that uses the results of the engagement. Note, however, that the focus of the independence rules in the "Anonymous Firm" box above is on meeting third-party user needs, and that independence is required in performing any kind of assurance service.

The issue of independence gained even more prominence on January 6, 2000, when the SEC published a report citing thousands of violations by one of the Big Four firms of rules requiring PAs to remain independent from companies they audit. This occurred despite concerns about independence that led to the May 1997 creation of a new private sector body, the Independence Standards Board. In 1999, the Board issued its first standard, requiring auditors to confirm their independence annually to audit committees. Other items on the Board's agenda included an official definition of independence as well as a conceptual framework for it. The Board was disbanded and replaced in 2002 by the PCAOB created under SOX. Fully operational since 2003, the PCAOB has even more demanding objectives. It is clear that maintenance of independence is a continuing and growing concern within the profession.

Phrases such as "shall not knowingly misrepresent facts" and "[shall not] subordinate his or her judgment to others" emphasize conditions people ordinarily identify with the concepts of integrity and objectivity. PAs who know about a client's lies on a tax return, false journal entries, material misrepresentations in financial statements, and the like have violated both the spirit and the letter of the rules of conduct.

Review Checkpoint

3-21   What are the three specific aspects of independence that an auditor should carefully guard in the course of a financial statement audit?

Professional Competence and Due Care

The professional competence and due care rules of the codes of conduct can be summarized as follows:

A. *Professional competence.* Undertake only those professional services that the member or the member's firm can reasonably expect to be completed with professional competence.

B. *Due professional care.* Exercise due professional care in the performance of professional services.

C. *Planning and supervision.* Adequately plan and supervise the performance of professional services.

D. *Sufficient relevant data.* Obtain sufficient relevant data to afford a reasonable basis for conclusions or recommendations in relation to any professional services performed.

Analysis of Competence and Due Care Rules

The professional competence and due care principles are a comprehensive statement of general standards that PAs are expected to observe in all areas of practice. These are the principles that enforce the various series of professional standards. For example, there is usually a specific rule relating to compliance with professional standards.

Compliance with Professional Standards

A member or firm engaged in the practice of public accounting shall perform professional services in accordance with generally accepted standards of practice of the profession (from Rule 206 of CPA Ontario).

Analysis of Compliance Rule

This rule may be viewed as an extension and refinement of the due care principle. It implies adherence to technical standards in all areas of professional service, including review and compilation (unaudited financial statements), consulting, tax, and other professional services. The practical effect of this rule is to make non-compliance with all technical standards subject to disciplinary proceedings. Thus, failure to follow auditing, accounting, and review standards, as well as assurance, compilation, and professional conduct standards, is a violation of this rule.

There are many more detailed rules, as you can see from the *CPA Ontario Handbook*'s table of contents. More thorough coverage of the rules and the profession's system of enforcement of them are covered as an advanced topic in Chapter 18. An important part of enforcement is covered in the second half of this chapter as legal liabilities that arise for failing to follow professional standards.

Summary of Professional Ethics Responsibilities

This overview of professional ethics began with considerations of moral philosophy and its relationship to provincial rules of professional conduct.

Professional ethics for PAs is not simply a matter covered by a few rules in a formal code of professional conduct. Concepts of proper professional conduct permeate all areas of practice. Ethics and its accompanying disciplinary potential are the foundation for fulfilling the auditor's social role.

Your knowledge of philosophical principles in ethics will help you make decisions about the provincial rules of professional conduct. This structured approach to thoughtful decisions is important not only when you are employed in public accounting but also when you work in government, industry, or education. The ethics rules may appear to be restrictive, but they are intended for the benefit of the public as well as for the discipline of PAs.

PAs must be careful in all areas of practice. Regulators' views on ethics rules may differ in several aspects from the provincial institute views. As an accountant, you must not lose sight of the non-accountants' perspective. No matter how complex or technical a decision may be, a simplified view of it always tends to cut away the details of special technical issues to get directly to the heart of the matter. A sense of professionalism coupled with sensitivity to the impact of decisions on other people is invaluable in the practice of accounting and auditing. This is the key lesson from the Continental Vending case.

Finally, it should be noted that there is a strong link between codes of conduct and GAAS. In fact, codes of conduct can be viewed as a means of fulfilling auditor responsibilities for GAAS and assurance standards. For example, the first GAAS standard, which relates to the personal attributes of the auditor (see Chapter 2), closely corresponds to the ethical principles of integrity, objectivity, independence, professional competence, and due care. The dominance of ethical issues over accounting or auditing techniques is increasingly being recognized throughout the profession. Most audit failures appear to be attributable to poor professional judgment, at least in hindsight, that arises from improper consideration of conflicts of interest on various disclosure and measurement issues. Critical thinking can help address this problem, at least for the more contentious issues.

The Legal Environment and Auditor Legal Responsibilities

LO6   Outline auditor legal responsibilities.

Legal liability is an important measure of the costs of failing to fulfill professional responsibilities to society. In order to get our bearings on how the law affects auditors, we begin with an overview of the legal system. Law is essentially a social system for resolving conflicts. Conflicts between individuals (and corporations) that are settled in court are part of what is called *private law* or *civil law*. Disputes between an individual and the state, as well as those between states or different levels of government, are settled in the part of the legal system called public law. Public law includes criminal law, administrative law, and constitutional law. All public law is codified by statute passed by some level of government.

Common law refers to the system of law based primarily on previous judicial decisions; unlike public law, its laws have not been codified in statutes via legislation (statutory law). It is a distinctive part of the Anglo-American system of private/civil law used in Canada, the United States, and most former colonies of the British Empire. There are several major categories of civil law: contracts (agreements or promises that create expectations for others), torts (civil wrongs, such as negligent actions, which create obligations for the offending party), and property (rights over goods and land). Common law liabilities for auditors arise from the law of contracts or torts. Statutory law liabilities for auditors arise from administrative law related to economic regulation and from criminal charges.

Because common law has been the main source of auditor liability in the past, most of this section is devoted to introducing the main principles of legal liability under common law. After that, we review some key statutory law responsibilities arising from legislation.

Lawsuit Causes and Frequency

One study of law cases showed that accountants' and auditors' legal troubles arose from five major types of errors. In 129 cases, 334 errors were found, classified as follows: (a) 33% involved misinterpretation of accounting principles, (b) 15% involved misinterpretation of auditing standards, (c) 29% involved faulty implementation of auditing procedures, (d) 13% involved client fraud, and (e) 7% involved fraud by the auditor.[15] These data suggest that accountants and auditors are exposed to liability for failure to report known departures from accounting principles, failure to conduct audits properly, failure to detect management fraud, and actually being party to frauds. Threat of lawsuits has also affected how PAs conduct their work in consulting services and tax practice; about 60% of civil damage suits arise from tax practice disputes. However, lawsuits related to audits tend to be high cost, resulting in much higher claims.[16]

All litigation is serious and results in expenses for defence, but not all cases result in payments for damage. In fact, about 40% of the lawsuits in the period 1960–1985 were dismissed or settled with no payment by the accounting firm. Another 30% were settled by payment of approximately $1 million or less. This leaves about 30% of the cases where the auditors paid significant damage awards. The legal fees for a long-running case can also be huge. For some reason, in Canada such lawsuits can drag out over a long time. Imagine the costs an accounting firm incurs in defending itself from a single lawsuit for over 20 years. All these data relate exclusively to lawsuits over audit services.[17]

Audit Responsibilities

Many users of audit reports expect auditors to detect fraud, theft, and illegal acts and to report them publicly. In the auditor's report, auditors take responsibility for detecting material misstatements in financial statements, whether due to fraud or unintentional misstatements. Fraud and misleading financial statements are large concerns of financial statement users. They are afraid of information risk due to intentional misstatements, and they want it reduced, even eliminated. Some of their expectations are very high, resulting in an expectations gap between the diligence users expect and the diligence auditors are able to accept.

The audit responsibility for detection of fraud in financial statements is a complex topic, as seen in Chapters 7 and 21 (available on Connect). Auditors take some responsibility but not as much as many users expect. For example, see CAS 240 and CAS 250. This disparity leads to lawsuits, even when auditors have performed well.

The next parts of this chapter cover PAs' legal liabilities under common law and statutory law. The principle of *stare decisis,* or to stand by a previous decision, is important to common law. The practical problem in many cases, however, is whether the facts in a given case are similar enough to those in a precedent-setting one. Rarely are the facts exactly the same. Common law is "common knowledge," in the sense that judges tend to follow the collective wisdom of past cases. In contrast, statutory law is prohibitions enacted in statutes by a legislature—for example, the CBCA and related provincial corporations acts. Most countries' laws arise from legislation (statutory law) rather than precedent (common law). Such legal systems are called Code-Law systems.

Review Checkpoints

3-22   What are class-action lawsuits, and why should auditors be concerned about them?

3-23   What are some causes of auditors becoming defendants in lawsuits?

3-24   What proportion of lawsuits against accountants relate to tax practice?

Liability under Common Law

LO7   Outline the various types of common law liability for public accountants, citing specific case precedents.

Legal liabilities of PAs arise from lawsuits brought on the basis of the law of contracts or as tort actions for negligence. Most lawsuits stem from a breach of contract claim that accounting or auditing services were not performed in the manner agreed.

Tort refers to a private or civil wrong or injury (e.g., fraud, deceit, or injury), an action normally initiated by users of financial statements. The rule of the law of torts is to compensate victims for harm suffered from the activities of others. The problem for tort law is to identify the actions creating a right to compensation. The law takes into account the fault or blame of the defendant (breach of duty) and whether the defendant's conduct could be considered the cause of the harm (causation), both of which must be established in order for the defendant to be found liable for damages. However, the burden of proof for tort actions varies depending on social policy. For example, under "no-fault" schemes, the burden of compensation is spread widely to all automobile owners.[18]

Suits for civil damages under common law usually result when someone suffers a financial loss after relying on financial statements later found to be materially misleading. In the popular press, such unfortunate events are called *audit failures.* While a business failure is a bankruptcy or other serious financial difficulty arising from many kinds of adverse economic events, an audit failure is based on an auditor's faulty performance, that is, a failure to conduct an audit in accordance with GAAS so that misleading financial statements get published.

tort:
legal action covering civil complaints other than breach of contract; normally initiated by users of financial statements

Characteristics of Common Law Actions

When injured parties consider themselves damaged by a PA and bring a lawsuit, they generally assert all possible causes of action, including breach of contract, tort, deceit, fraud, or whatever else may be relevant to the claim.

Burden of Proof on the Plaintiff

Actions brought under common law place most of the burdens of affirmative proof on the plaintiff, who must prove that

1. he or she was damaged or suffered a loss,

2. there was a beneficiary relationship with the defendant,

3. the financial statements were materially misleading or the accountant's advice was faulty,

4. he or she relied on the statements or advice,

5. they were the direct cause of the loss, and

6. the accountant was negligent, grossly negligent, deceitful, or otherwise responsible for damages.

Four Elements of Negligence

Clients may bring a lawsuit for breach of contract. The relationship of direct involvement between parties to a contract is also known as *privity*. When privity exists, a plaintiff usually need only show that the defendant accountant was negligent—showed lack of reasonable care in the performance of professional accounting tasks. If negligence is proved, the accountant may be liable, provided the client did not contribute to his or her own harm.

Most auditor **legal responsibilities** arise from the law of negligence, the part of the common law known as the law of torts. Negligence is the failure to perform a duty with the requisite standard care (due care as it relates to one's public calling or profession). Under the common law of torts for negligence, all of the following four elements of negligence must be established by the plaintiff if he or she is to successfully sue the auditor.

1. There must be a legal duty of care to the plaintiff.

2. There must be a breach in that duty (e.g., failure to follow GAAS and/or GAAP).

3. There must be proof that damage resulted (otherwise the plaintiff is limited to the amount of the audit fee).

4. There must be a reasonably proximate connection between the breach of duty and the resulting damage (e.g., losses must occur subsequent to the firm's audit).

The auditor's defence is to demonstrate that at least one of the preceding elements is missing. The auditor may also argue that the plaintiff contributed to his or her own loss by, for example, not correcting accounting weaknesses in the reporting system. However, this defence applies only to parties having a contractual relationship with the auditor. Just to keep things straight, the auditor is the first party, the contractual client (who hires the auditor for the audit engagement and thus has privity of contract with the auditor) is the second party, and other audited financial statement users are third parties.

These three parties are the same as in the three-party accountability discussed in Chapters 1 and 2. The only difference in legal three-party accountability is that the company is viewed as inseparable from management. In the situation of a corporation, the company itself is the legal entity, and the management is acting on behalf of the legal entity. This illustrates how fundamental the legal system is in establishing auditor responsibilities to society. You have seen in Chapter 2 how critical three-party accountability is to the assurance engagement

legal responsibilities:
auditor responsibilities imposed by the legal system

concept. In Chapter 4, you will see that three-party accountability is an important aspect of the broadest set of public accounting standards: association rules.

Limited Liability Partnerships

In Canada and the United States, **joint and several liability** means any of several defendants that have caused part of the damages are liable to the plaintiffs for the entire amount of damages. This system was set up to protect plaintiffs from having to sue several different parties to recover the full amount of damages. Under joint and several liability, the courts can force the defendant with the "deepest pockets" to pay all the damages even though he or she may have contributed, say, only 1% to the losses. It is, of course, then up to the defendant auditor to recover shares of the losses from the others. If the other defendants are in bankruptcy, however, this can leave the auditor with all the losses. The following box, from a *National Post* article, indicates the problems that joint and several liability has caused in Canada.

> **joint and several liability:**
> a legal liability regime in which one party found to be liable can be required to pay the full amount of the damages even if there are other parties that are partially liable but bankrupt or otherwise unable to pay a proportionate share of the damages

Outdated Liability Laws Harming Economy: ICAO

TRANSACTIONS "JUST DON'T GET DONE" AS AUDITORS TURN AWAY BUSINESS

Canada's antiquated liability laws are badly hurting the economy, according to the country's largest accounting body, which is spearheading demands for liability reform.

The Institute of Chartered Accountants of Ontario [now CPA Ontario]—with 35,000 members—said the laws lag behind those in other parts of the world and the failure to make crucial reforms could force an exodus of investment to more attractive jurisdictions.

The ICAO estimates the amount of litigation against the big accounting firms has increased by more than 300% since 1988. The cost of liability insurance for auditors is as much as three times higher than it was in 2001, and the number of firms offering audit services in Canada has dropped by 50% in the past two years, from 400 to just over 200.

Brian Hunt, president and chief executive officer of the ICAO, said failure to fully reform the laws could result in a worst-case scenario where individuals and business ask, "Why would I do business in Canada, when I could get more protection south of the border?"

A recent ICAO survey of more than 500 small and mid-sized accounting firms in Ontario showed that almost three-quarters of the firms surveyed say they have faced a moderate to significant increase in professional liability costs over the past five years. Two-thirds also said liability-related issues are deterring them from taking on client-engagements.

Joel Cohen, executive audit partner at mid-tier Canadian accounting firm RSM Richter LLP, said the current regime also restricts access to the capital markets, even for well-governed companies operating in stable industries, because audit firms are unwilling to take on the risk of providing accounting and auditing services.

"We are at a competitive disadvantage," Mr. Cohen said.

Mr. Cohen said the current liability environment has forced RSM Richter to turn down engagements on five or six transactions in the past six months alone. He said it is doubtful the companies involved will find an audit firm in Canada willing to help them.

"We are limiting liability anyway by limiting access to our service," he said.

In one case, RSM Richter needed to enlist another department auditor for a client of its firm. But, Mr. Cohen said, no one was willing to take on the risk, even though the client was a "solid company, making profits, where the business was not risky."

Canada's liability laws "inhibit the completion of transactions. They just don't get done," he added.

(continued)

Len Crispino, president and chief executive officer of the Ontario Chamber of Commerce, said he has heard anecdotal evidence among his members to support the accountants' position. "It's becoming tougher and tougher to get an accounting firm," he said, "and, in a sense, we all lose."

The key issue is Canada's "joint-and-several" liability laws, which mean an auditor who is only 1% to blame for a corporate bankruptcy can be forced to pay out 100% of the costs associated with any litigation.

Mr. Cohen said the main problem with Canada's joint-and-several liability laws is that they make the risks of providing audit and accounting services "unquantifiable."

That is not the same in other countries. In Australia, legislators recently enacted laws to cap the amount of liability that audit firms could be forced to suffer. In the United States, federal legislators introduced a form of proportionate liability—the costs of losing in litigation are proportionate to the attributed blame—as far back as 1995, and 39 states have eliminated or significantly amended their joint-and-several liability laws. The United Kingdom and the European Union have also indicated plans to move away from joint-and-several liability.

The Ontario government has recognized the issue and has passed legislation to put some limits on professional liability. However, joint-and-several liability continues to apply in many cases, including civil suits involving audited documents, such as prospectuses, take-over bid circulars, and issuer bid circulars, which are generally considered higher risk.

The ICAO is pushing for further changes to fully eliminate joint-and-several liability, Mr. Hunt said. He said he expects resistance from the legal community and from shareholder activists who might perceive reform as something that only favours the big accounting firms. But, he said, these groups do not understand the magnitude of the problem.

Mr. Hunt said not only would the number of firms offering audit services in Canada continue to decline, but there could be a drain of qualified and experienced accountants to countries where the risks of performing audits is much lower. He said this will all add up to audit costs that will be higher in Canada than in other countries.

One sign of the increased risks, Mr. Cohen said, is the cost of professional indemnity insurance for audit firms, which tripled in Canada between 2001 and 2004.

The big accounting firms are also feeling the pinch of rising costs due to Canada's liability regime, said Lou Pagnutti, chairman and chief executive officer for Canada at big four accounting firm Ernst & Young LLP. Since the collapse of Arthur Andersen, the big accounting firms are finding it increasingly difficult to obtain professional indemnity insurance in Canada, he said. "Even if you can get it," he said, "the premiums have increased." Premiums here for the big firms have risen by as much as 30% to 40% a year, forcing them to arrange expensive self-insurance, Mr. Pagnutti said. "Absent liability reform," he said, "there will be further cost increases."

Source: Duncan Mavin, "Outdated liability laws harming economy: ICAO: Transactions 'just don't get done' as auditors turn away business," *The National Post*, Wednesday, June 29, 2005, p. FP7. © 2015 National Post, a division of Postmedia Network Inc.

In light of these potential legal liabilities, the limited liability partnership (LLP) was created. In 1998, Ontario was the first province to enact legislation allowing the use of the LLP form of organization, followed by Alberta in 1999. With the traditional partnership form of organization, the partners themselves are liable for all debts and liabilities incurred by their firm. In an LLP, the negligent partner is still liable to the extent of his or her own personal assets, while the personal assets of non-negligent partners are not threatened.

Thus, the LLP form of organization can generally reduce the risk to partners of legal liability. However, the LLP form of organization did not prevent the demise of Arthur Andersen, so there are now obvious limits to its benefits. In particular, the LLP form may have less impact under a system where the primary source of legal liability is from statutory law via a high-profile regulator, something that can affect the LLP's reputation in the marketplace—a system that looks increasingly likely in the current environment.

Defences of the Accountant

The defendant accountant in a common law action presents evidence to counter the plaintiff's claims and evidence. For example, the accountant might offer evidence that the plaintiff was not in privity, or not foreseen;

that the financial statements were not misleading; or that the plaintiff contributed to the negligence. The primary defence against a negligence claim is to offer evidence that the audit had been conducted in accordance with GAAS with due professional care.

Extent of Liability for Staff of Public Accounting Firms

You may be interested in knowing about who suffers exposure and penalties in lawsuits—accounting firms, partners, managers, senior accountants, staff assistants, or all of these? Most lawsuits centre attention on the accounting firm and on the partners and managers involved in the audit or other accounting work. However, court opinions have cited the work of senior accountants, and there is no reason that the work of new staff assistant accountants should not also come under review. All persons involved in professional accounting are exposed to potential liability.

U.S. auditing standards titled "Planning and Supervision" offer some important thoughts for accountants who question the validity of some of the work being done in an audit. Accountants can express their own positions and let the working paper records show the nature of the disagreement and the resolution of the question. SAS 22 expressed the appropriate action as follows:

"The auditor with final responsibility for the examination [partner in charge of the audit] and assistants should be aware of the procedures to be followed when differences of opinion concerning accounting and auditing issues exist among firm personnel involved in the examination. Such procedures should enable an assistant to document his disagreement with the conclusions reached if, after appropriate consultation, he believes it necessary to disassociate himself from the resolution of the matter. In this situation, the basis for the final resolution should also be documented."

Some courts hold plaintiffs to a strict privity criterion in order to have a standing in court. In New York courts, the general rule is that the accountants must have been aware that the financial reports were to be used for a particular purpose, that a particular third party was going to rely on the reports, and that there is a link between the accountants and the third party demonstrating that the accountants knew of the reliance on the reports. This has prompted some users of financial statements to request a **reliance letter**, in which accountants sign that they have been notified that a particular recipient of the financial statements and audit report intends to rely upon them for particular purposes. The American Institute of CPAs (AICPA) has warned accountants to be careful when signing such letters as they might become an automatic proof of users' actual reliance.

In several Canadian cases, the auditors successfully argued that clients should not have relied on the financial statements to make their investment decision.[19] A good example is banks' claims that they have been misled by the financial statements. The fourth element of negligence is key here: did the banks' losses follow from the auditor's breach of duty with regard to auditing the financial statements? Rowan notes that "the courts carefully review the degree of reliance plaintiff bankers have on misleading financial statements. Banks usually have available to them not only their customers' financial statements but a great deal of other information as well. Their decision to continue a loan is very often based on considerations quite apart from any reliance they may place on the opinion of the customer's auditors. In these circumstances, the auditors ought not to be found liable—or at least not entirely—for the bank's losses." In general, "it's refreshing to see a court carefully reviewing the degree of reliance plaintiff bankers place on misleading financial statements."[20]

reliance letter:
a document that accountants sign showing that they have been notified that a particular recipient of the financial statements and audit report intends to rely upon them for particular purposes

Statutory Law Liability

In addition to liabilities imposed by common law, auditors need to be concerned with statutory law liability. Auditors should not grumble too loudly about this special burden because it is statutory law requirements that drive much of the demand for audit services in the first place! For example, companies beyond a certain size, incorporated under CBCA or provincial corporation acts, are required to hire an external auditor to audit the financial statements. This creates a guaranteed demand for audit services, which some have argued has made the profession less vigilant in maintaining the quality of audits in today's rapidly changing financial reporting environment.[21] The highlights of the CBCA are as follows:

1. The CBCA identifies conditions under which the auditor is not considered independent in section 161.
2. It identifies conditions of appointing and retiring the auditor in sections 162 and 163.
3. It identifies the auditor's rights and responsibilities in section 168:
   (a) to attend shareholder meetings,
   (b) to provide a written statement of reasons for a resignation, and
   (c) to make an audit examination unimpeded and gain access to data the auditor considers necessary.
4. The CBCA identifies the financial statements subject to audit, and specifies that the financial statements must be in conformity with the *CPA Canada Handbook.*
5. Until 1994, the CBCA requirements for audited financial statements applied to all companies incorporated under the Act with revenues in excess of $10 million or assets greater than $5 million. Under amendments to the CBCA made in 1994, privately held companies are no longer required to have their financial statements audited or disclosed. The *Ontario Business Corporations Act* requires audits only for companies having at least $100 million of either assets or revenues; other provincial corporations acts vary in their reporting requirements.

Legislation, such as the CBCA, can also increase auditor legal liability beyond that under common law. The earliest statutory law that increased auditor liability arose from the passage of the SEC Acts in the United States in 1933 and 1934. Canadian auditors are exposed to this liability when they audit companies whose shares are listed on the U.S. stock exchanges (NASDAQ, NYSE, AMEX). The SEC was created in the 1930s to enforce these Acts and subsequent legislation such as SOX. The SEC has the power to prevent auditors from auditing SEC registrants, either temporarily or permanently. In addition, the SEC can decide what the GAAP are.

The ultimate authority on accounting issues for public companies in the United States is the SEC, whereas in Canada, via the *CPA Canada Handbook*, the CBCA mandates that it is CPA Canada. This gives the *CPA Canada Handbook* standards much higher legal status than comparable standards in the United States. But note that this result is due to statutory law, again illustrating how the legal system shapes the auditor's role in society.

In 1995, the American accounting profession was successful in having the U.S. Congress pass (over President Clinton's veto) the *Private Securities Litigation Reform Act*, which changed auditor liability under SEC section 10b (discussed in Chapter 21). There were three objectives to the Act. First, it was intended to "discourage abusive claims of investors' losses due to fraudulent misstatements or omissions by issuers of securities" (and professionals associated with the misstatements or omissions, such as auditors). Second, the Act provided more protection against securities fraud. Third, the Act increased the flow of forward-looking financial information. The Act met these objectives by imposing specific pleading requirements, reducing discovery's effectiveness in coercing settlements, mandating sanctions for frivolous claims, giving the plaintiff class far more control over class actions, providing for proportionate liability except in cases of known fraud, creating a safe harbour for forward-looking information, and codifying auditors' responsibilities to search for and disclose fraud.[22]

For the purposes of this chapter, the most important feature of the Act concerns the reform of joint and several liability, which, under SEC law, now applies only to auditors who knowingly commit a violation of the security law. "A defendant (auditor) whose conduct is less culpable is liable only for a percentage of the total damages corresponding to the percentage of responsibility allocated to the defendant (auditor) by the jury. . . . Thus, for example, if a PA firm is found 10% responsible for an injury and insolvent corporate management is allocated 90%, the PA firm no longer will have to make up all of the management's share (as long as the PA firm did not engage in knowing fraud)."[23] This type of liability is referred to as **proportionate liability**.

The CBCA was amended in 2001 to change the liability associated with financial statement misrepresentations from one of joint and several liability to modified proportionate liability. Auditors in Canada are now liable under the CBCA to the extent of their degree of responsibility for the loss (proportionate liability). However, the proportionate liability is modified in that if other defendants in the lawsuit are unable to pay, the auditor is then liable for additional payments capped at 50% of his or her own original liability. Under some conditions, the courts can revert to the joint and several liability, in which case the auditor may be required to pay up to 100% of the damages.[24]

Another example of legislation that has had widespread impact on auditors is SOX, discussed in Chapter 2. As noted there, SOX created the PCAOB, which is now responsible for creating and enforcing U.S. auditing standards for public companies.

The SEC Act of 1933 regulates disclosure of information in a new public offering of securities for SEC registrants. If there is false or misleading information in the registration statement, auditors (and others associated with this information, such as management) are liable for losses suffered by third parties. The plaintiff does not have to prove negligence or fraud, only that a loss was suffered through investing in the registered security and that there was a material misstatement or omission in the audited statements. Unlike under common law, the plaintiff need not prove that the auditor was negligent, the second item of the list given earlier. Instead, the burden is on the defendant auditor to prove that he or she was not negligent. In other words, there is a shifting of the burden of proof from the plaintiff to the defendant auditor.

This shifting of the burden is important, as the party having the burden must provide evidence that their claim is true. To illustrate how crucial this is in the reasoning process, think of the expression that you have probably heard before, "innocent until proven guilty." In other words, you cannot be locked up by the police arbitrarily unless they have strong evidence against you. You do not have to prove your innocence in criminal law; instead you are presumed innocent unless the prosecutor has met its burden of proof in providing convincing evidence that you are guilty. All this is established within a court of law. So, you can see now that the SEC Act of 1933 imposes an extra burden on the auditor of proving non-negligence in a court of law. This is one good reason to have the audit well documented.

The SEC Act of 1934 relates to auditor liability for periodic filings: annual reports (form 10-K); quarterly reports (form 10-Q); and selected special events (form 8-K), such as a change in auditor. The liability can be imposed on anyone who makes a false or misleading statement in the filings. In order to avoid liability, the burden of proof falls on the auditor to prove he or she had no knowledge of the material misstatement in the filing. This defence is available only to auditors who can demonstrate that they "acted in good faith," meaning that they are not judged to be "grossly negligent" in conducting the audit.

Post-Enron provincial legislation in Canada under the leadership of the **Canadian Securities Administrators (CSA)** is influencing a whole new set of auditor liabilities. These are in response to decreased liabilities resulting from the *Hercules* case that did away with most third-party liability under common law, discussed in Chapter 20 (available on Connect).

The *Hercules* case, along with post-Enron developments, prompted Ontario to pass its Bill 198 in December 2002. Bill 198 (now the *Ontario Securities Act* or OSA) is similar in scope to SEC laws already discussed. The CSA is promoting passage of similar legislation throughout all of Canada's provinces in an effort to demonstrate that Canadian regulators are as concerned with preserving the integrity of their capital markets as the SEC is in the United States.

proportionate liability:
a legal liability regime where a party found to be partly liable is only responsible for paying a part of the damages in proportion to their share of the blame

Canadian Securities Administrators (CSA):
the organization of Canadian provincial securities market administrators and regulators

This legislation creates a statutory law civil liability for PAs and others accused of misleading the public. It allows class-action lawsuits against PAs, placing the burden of proof on the auditor that a drop in the client's share price was not due to a financial statement misrepresentation (this is the "fraud on the market" presumption used by the SEC in the United States). "In short, this is a presumption that the capital markets operate efficiently, such that there are sufficient market participants who in fact do understand and rely on corporate disclosures to affect share price. As a result, although a particular individual may not have been aware of the offending representation, or may not have understood it, his or her share price can be said to have been in reliance on it, as the price at which he or she traded was affected by the misrepresentation." Under the OSA regime, the plaintiff investors can make the case that fraud on the market took place, but the burden is on the plaintiff investors to prove it. If the plaintiff investor meets this burden and a misrepresentation has been identified, it is up to the auditor to show that any losses suffered by investors were not due to the misrepresentation. However, the legislation puts caps on the PA's liability, and it uses the proportionate rule, rather than the joint and several liability rule. These limitations on liability, however, do not apply if the PA knowingly deceived the market.[25] Although the OSA was passed in December 2002, it was not proclaimed (put into force) until late 2004 and went into effect December 2005. The article below discusses the significance of this legislation.

These legislative initiatives seem to be inspired by U.S. statutory law covered in this chapter. It should be noted that PAs in Canada already had similar liabilities for initial public offerings of securities. The newer legislation extended the liability to subsequent financial statements of companies already listed on the Toronto Stock Exchange (TSX), and such an extension exposes the Canadian PA to far more potential legal liability, especially to shareholders of clients who could not previously sue.

Law Makes It Easier for Investors to Sue

"MORE GROUNDS FOR SUITS"

So you lost money on a stock and want to sue the company for misleading statements.

What is already a common practice in the United States is coming to Canada. Canadian public companies are readying themselves for broad new legislation that will greatly increase investors' ability to file civil lawsuits against them.

The new civil liability legislation will come out by the end of the year [2005] and substantially widens the type of disclosure investors can use as a basis for litigation.

This means that false or misleading information in press releases and financial statements will soon be fair game. It can even extend to public oral statements, such as conference calls or speeches, made by authorized company representatives. Currently, investor lawsuits are limited to information in a prospectus.

This new addition to the *Ontario Securities Act* was actually introduced by the provincial government in late 2004. But the clock is now ticking for companies to get their disclosure models in order, since it comes into effect Dec. 31.

. . .

"This may constitute the biggest change to Canadian securities law in the last 25 years," according to a report by law firm Borden Ladner Gervais LLP.

One of the most significant parts of the new law is how plaintiffs will no longer have to prove they relied on the misrepresentation when investing in a company. For example, under the current legislation, an investor would have to say "I bought this stock reliant on XX amount of earnings, and it turns out they were really XXX. . . . I relied on this information and I can prove it," said Paul Findlay, a lawyer at Borden Ladner who co-wrote the report.

This was a significant stumbling block to class-action suits in Ontario, since they typically involve groups of shareholders and it was pretty much impossible to prove that each investor had looked at and relied on the information in question, he added.

With this impediment removed, there is little doubt there will be an increase in securities class-action lawsuits in the province. Plus, it could make it more attractive for shareholders to file suits against cross-listed Canadian companies here, Mr. Findlay said. In the past, these actions have often taken place in the United States, which already has some provisions for materially false and misleading information in continuous disclosure.

The auditors' defence under OSA is to show that they acted with due professional care and they had no reasonable basis for believing the financial statements to be false. To prove due diligence, auditors need to document their work in the audit file—a topic discussed in later chapters.

An additional feature of OSA that is relevant to auditors is the restriction of the amount of liability to the proportionate liability. This amount is also capped at the greater of $1 million or the amount of revenues earned from the client "during the 12 months preceding the misrepresentation."[26]

Legal Liability Implications for Auditor Practice

As a result of the increasingly litigious climate, auditors ought to

(a) Be wary of what kind of clients are accepted.

(b) Know (thoroughly) the client's business (KNOB).

(c) Perform quality audits:

   (i) Use qualified, properly trained and supervised, and motivated personnel.
   (ii) Obtain sufficient appropriate evidence (including proper elicitation of oral evidence and documentation of client's oral evidence).
   (iii) Prepare good working papers.
   (iv) Obtain engagement and representation letters.

Increased litigation has also caused improvements in audit working paper files through use of

(a) Forceful management letters that are "unambiguous and couched in terms of alarm with respect to problematic internal controls or sloppy bookkeeping."

(b) Detailed memos in the working papers describing the conversation with the client and accompanied by a follow-up letter to the client.

(c) A letter to the client or note to the file documenting discussions to reduce audit fees or changing to a review engagement.[27]

The business press provides much anecdotal evidence that there can be serious problems in many auditor-client relationships. For example, according to a vice-president of finance of a major Canadian company, "it's very easy for management to browbeat an auditor at any time in the audit," and "anything goes unless there is a rule to the contrary" (in the *CPA Canada Handbook*).

To combat these problems, auditors should report to a company's audit committee (or equivalent), standard setters should reduce the number of accounting alternatives in GAAP, auditors need more guidance on how to report on a company's ability to continue, and auditors need to better document high-risk clients and be ready to take immediate defensive measures. Some firms now even "fire" their troublesome clients. Some warning signs of potentially troublesome clients are financial or organizational difficulty, involvement in suspicious transactions, uncooperativeness, fee pressures, refusal to sign engagement and representation letters, and frequent involvement in litigation.

Before accepting clients, PAs should ask why a client is changing accountants, visit the client's business, meet its accounting and tax personnel, and check their references. A useful client acceptance checklist could be used that documents whether a client should be accepted for an engagement. This form should be prepared before the engagement letter is submitted. If this screening does not result in rejection of an existing or prospective client, it may also be used to identify engagements that require extra precautions, such as very precise engagement letters and advance collection of fees.[28] In the current environment, these recommendations have become standard practice and will likely be mandatory once the various new accountability boards and newly empowered regulators develop their own tightened requirements.

APPLICATION CASE WITH SOLUTION & ANALYSIS

Burden of Proof Concept in Law and Auditing

DISCUSSION CASE

 In law, the "burden of proof" concept helps decide who wins at trial. The burden is normally on the plaintiff party. The reasoning in law is similar to that of critical thinking used in this book. In fact, legal reasoning has had a great impact on the argumentative aspects of critical thinking. Under critical thinking, auditors have a burden of proof that must be satisfied on every audit engagement in order to be prepared to defend challenges to their decisions. This burden is reflected in auditing standards. What is the burden of proof on an audit engagement?

SOLUTION & ANALYSIS

Auditors claim to provide high or reasonable evidential assurance on an audit engagement. In other words, they gather sufficient evidence to keep the risk of failing to detect material factual misstatements to an acceptable level.

The audit evidence responsibility—to be in conformity with audit evidence standards—is satisfied when evidence risk is acceptably low, and assurance (equals one minus evidence risk) is therefore acceptably high. This responsibility parallels burden of proof in civil law, which looks for "the balance of probabilities" or the "preponderance of evidence" to be acceptably high or reasonable. The meaning of these terms of civil law varies, depending on the context. For example, in commercial disputes, balance of probabilities means that if the evidence makes the plaintiff's position more likely to be true than the defendant's, then the plaintiff wins the case. On the other hand, the auditor's burden of proof is determined by the audit standards.

Civil burdens of proof are in sharp contrast to criminal law procedures, where the state must prove the guilt of the defendant "beyond a reasonable doubt" for a conviction. Applying both the concept of beyond a reasonable doubt and the courts' operating presumption that all are presumed innocent until proven guilty will result in an extremely remote chance of sending an innocent person to jail.

These distinctions can be important in defining auditor responsibility for detecting fraud, since fraud is a criminal act that falls under the criminal code. The O. J. Simpson trials can be used to illustrate the distinction. At his first trial in 1995, a criminal trial, Simpson was found not guilty of the charge of murdering his wife and her friend. That is, the jury was not convinced "beyond a reasonable doubt" that Simpson was guilty. The burden of proof was not met by the prosecution and the presumption of innocence was not overturned by the evidence presented at trial. But, at a civil trial in 1997, Simpson was found responsible for the wrongful deaths of both individuals and was required to pay a settlement of US$33.5 million. The facts and evidence were substantially the same, but the burden of proof is much lower for a plaintiff in a civil trial, so Simpson lost that case.

These cases have implications for auditors; even if they were able to meet the burden of proof of an audit engagement and provide high assurance that fraud took place, it does not mean the auditor can make an accusation of fraud. The fraud must be proved in criminal court. Moreover, auditors must be careful in the language they use to describe suspicions of fraud based on audit evidence. Auditors should always refer to the risks or evidence of fraud, not to proven fraud, lest they be sued for libel or slander. This is an important aspect of the context of audit engagements and the amount of responsibility auditors can take for detecting fraud. These responsibilities are discussed further in Chapter 7.

Burden of proof underlies the concept of audit assertions, which will be introduced in Part II of this text. For these assertions, the auditor must obtain sufficient evidence on each audit that they are all reasonably true. Audit assurance is the same as "high" or "reasonable" assurance. Assurance relates to how sure the auditor is about the audit assertions. Thus, audit theory is closely tied to the burden of proof concept. However, not all possible assertions need to be given high assurance on an audit. The burden of proof for the auditor extends only to the assertions specified by GAAS. There are other assertions in financial reporting, such as the going-concern assumption and monetary-unit assumption of most reporting frameworks. The auditor is not required to prove that these assumptions are true as assertions. Instead, the auditor assumes these assumptions are true unless there is evidence to the contrary during the engagement. If that is the case, then the auditor may need to take fairly drastic action, such as switching to another appropriate reporting framework. For example, if there is sufficient risk that the going-concern assumption is wrong, then the auditor may require that the client switch to a liquidation basis of accounting in order that the financial statements present fairly. This would be a fairly drastic and controversial action but, nevertheless, of increasing importance to auditors, as is reflected in continuing concerns about auditor failure to warn investors and the public about corporate failures and the need for government bailouts during the 2008/2009 financial crisis. The status of the going-concern assumption is discussed further in Chapter 19.

The monetary-unit assumption has not been questioned lately because of low inflation. However, when this assumption is violated by economic events, such as the high inflationary environment of the 1980s, then, again, auditors and accounting standards may require supplementary disclosures (i.e., using a different reporting framework), such as inflation-adjusted reporting, as was common in the 1980s. These examples illustrate that the financial reporting environment is not static and can change rapidly. Users of financial statements expect auditors to be attuned to their needs and to take into account such environmental changes in selecting an acceptable reporting framework. The auditor obligations to (a) consider matching user needs with the financial reporting framework, in the particular circumstances, and (b) match the burden of proof with the relevant assertions help explain why auditors need to be more critical thinkers if they are to maintain effectiveness in the 21st century.

Until Enron, the major source of liability for PAs was under common law, but Enron changed all that. The fatal damage to Arthur Andersen seems to have been caused by the SEC, which had charged the audit firm with securities fraud two years previously over its audit of Waste Management Company. It should be noted that SEC prosecutions are under statutory law. Arthur Andersen ultimately paid a $7 million fine in June 2001. This set the stage for the company's rapid loss of reputation when the Enron audit problems surfaced six months later. The company had already lost most of its big clients by the time of its conviction—which was overturned by the U.S. Supreme Court in 2005—and the accounting world was shocked and dazed by the speed of its disintegration.

Since Enron, the SEC appears to have become much more aggressive in imposing statutory legal liability. For example, on January 29, 2003, the SEC sued one of the Big Four firms for securities fraud, alleging that it let Xerox Corp. inflate pre-tax earnings by over $3 billion from 1997 to 2000. Xerox agreed to a record $10 million penalty to settle the SEC charges. By this point, Xerox had also dropped the public accounting firm as its auditor. After an investigation, this became SEC's first fraud case against a major accounting firm since Enron's collapse. The SEC alleged the following: "Instead of putting a stop to Xerox's fraudulent conduct, the public accounting firm defendants themselves engaged in fraud by falsely representing to the public that they had applied professional auditing standards to their review of Xerox's accounting." The public accounting firm vigorously and publicly defended its work, but the case illustrates that statutory law may become a bigger threat to the profession than common law liability, especially if reputational effects are taken into consideration.

It should be noted that under SEC law, securities fraud puts a greater burden of proof on the defendant PA, as outlined in this chapter, than is generally the case for fraud defendants, also discussed in this chapter. In addition, the SEC doctrine of "fraud on the market," which may be adopted by the Ontario Securities Commission (OSC), increases PA liability to broader classes of potential plaintiffs.

In Ontario, Bill 198 was passed December 9, 2002, giving the OSC potentially greater power in setting rules for appointing auditors than even SOX does. These events also suggest that statutory law liability may become a greater threat to the profession than common law liability.

However, there are few precedents to go by other than those already outlined. So, other than noting the potential changes in future liability in this introduction, this chapter focuses on the more traditional common law source of auditors' legal liability.

SUMMARY

- Your knowledge of philosophical principles in ethics will help you make decisions about the provincial rules of professional conduct. This structured approach to thoughtful decisions is important not only when you are employed in public accounting but also when you work in government, industry, and education. The ethics rules may appear to be restrictive, but they are intended for the benefit of the public as well as for the discipline of PAs. **LO1, 2**

- PAs must be careful in all areas of practice. Regulators' views on ethics rules may differ in several aspects from the provincial institute views. As an accountant, you must not lose sight of the non-accountant's perspective. No matter how complex or technical a decision may be, a simplified view of it always tends to cut away the details of special technical issues to get directly to the heart of the matter. A sense of professionalism coupled with sensitivity to the impact of decisions on other people is invaluable in the practice of accounting and auditing. **LO3**

- Finally, with respect to ethics it should be noted that there is a strong link between codes of conduct and generally accepted auditing standards (GAAS). In fact, codes of conduct can be viewed as a means of fulfilling auditor responsibilities for GAAS and assurance standards. For example, the first GAAS standard, which relates to the personal attributes of the auditor (see Chapter 2), closely corresponds to the ethical principles of integrity, objectivity, independence, professional competence, and due care discussed previously. The dominance of ethical issues over accounting or auditing techniques is increasingly being recognized throughout the profession. Most audit failures appear to be attributable to poor professional judgment, at least in hindsight, that arises from improper consideration of conflicts of interest on various disclosure and measurement issues.[29] Critical thinking is intended to help address this problem, at least for the most contentious issues. **LO4, 5**

- Litigation against accountants has greatly increased in Canada, mirroring developments in the United States. **LO6**

- Damage claims of hundreds of millions of dollars have been paid by public accounting firms and their insurers. Insurance is expensive and hard to obtain. The SEC has sued several of the largest accounting firms for securities fraud within the last decade. One of these firms, Arthur Andersen, paid fines of $7 million and later was convicted of "obstructing justice" and forced into bankruptcy. Accountants are not alone in this rash of litigation, which affects manufacturers, architects, doctors, and people in many other walks of life. **LO6**

- The professional accounting organizations have joined with other interest groups pushing for "tort reform" of various types (e.g., limitation of damages, identification of liability) in an effort to stem the tide. **LO6**

- Other effects of this climate take the form of changing the nature of organizations in which PAs practice (such as to LLPs). **LO6**

- Accountants' liability to clients and third parties under common law has expanded. Fifty years ago, a strict privity doctrine required other parties to be in a contract with and known to the accountant before they could sue for damages based on negligence. Of course, if an accountant was grossly negligent in such a way that his or her actions amounted to constructive fraud, liability exists as it would for anyone who committed a fraud. **LO7**

- Over the years, the privity doctrine was modified in many jurisdictions, leading to liability for ordinary negligence to primary beneficiaries (known users) of the accountants' work product, and then to liability based on ordinary negligence to foreseen and foreseeable beneficiaries (users not so easily known). **LO7**

- While the general movement has been to expand accountants' liability for ordinary negligence, some jurisdictions have held closer to the privity doctrine of the past. The treatment can vary from province to province. **LO7**

- The last decade has brought increased risk of litigation arising from statutory law, especially in Ontario. **LO6**

- Increased liability and loss of reputation arises from laws against bribery, money laundering, and terrorist financing. **LO6**

- The sources of liability and burdens of proof are summarized in Exhibit 3–1 below. **LO6**

EXHIBIT 3–1

Summary of Auditor Liabilities

SOURCE OF LAW	LIABILITY ARISING FROM	BURDEN OF PROOF
Common law—contractual clients; corporate entity, not shareholders	Breach of contract negligence	On client
	Gross negligence or fraud	On client
		On client
Common law—third parties	Negligence	On third-party non-shareholder
	Gross negligence or fraud	On third parties including shareholders
Civil liability under statutory law (e.g., OSC)	Negligence	On shareholder
	Gross negligence or fraud on the market	On shareholder
		On auditor in the United States, possibly in Canada
Criminal liability (i.e., auditor can be imprisoned)	Gross negligence or fraud	On Crown

KEY TERMS

Canadian Securities
   Administrators (CSA)

consequentialism

critical thinking

critical thinking framework

deontological (Kantian) ethics

ethical dilemma

imperatives

joint and several liability

legal responsibilities

monistic theories

moral imagination

moral responsibilities	proportionate liability	utilitarianism
pluralistic theories	reliance letter	
professional responsibilities	tort	

MULTIPLE-CHOICE QUESTIONS FOR PRACTICE AND REVIEW

MC 3-1 `LO5` Auditors are interested in having independence in appearance because

a. they want to impress the public with their independence in fact.

b. they want the public at large to have confidence in the profession.

c. they need to comply with the standards of field work of GAAS.

d. audits should be planned, and assistants, if any, need to be properly supervised.

MC 3-2 `LO1` If a PA says she always follows the rule that requires adherence to CPA pronouncements in order to give a standard unqualified audit report, she is following a philosophy characterized by

a. the imperative principle in ethics.

b. the utilitarian principle in ethics.

c. the generalization principle in ethics.

d. reliance on one's inner conscience.

MC 3-3 `LO4` Which of the following committees have been authorized to discipline members in violation of the rules of professional conduct?

a. CPA Canada Committee on Professional Ethics

b. Appeals Committee

c. Discipline Committee

d. Professional Conduct Committee

MC 3-4 `LO4` Which of the following bodies does not have any power to punish individual members for violations of the rules of professional conduct?

a. CPA Canada

b. Canada Revenue Agency

c. OSC

d. CPA Ontario

MC 3-5 `LO4` Phil Greb has a thriving practice in which he assists lawyers in preparing litigation dealing with accounting and auditing matters. Phil is "practising public accounting" if he

a. uses his PA designation on his letterhead and business card.

b. is in partnership with another PA.

c. practises in a limited partnership with other PAs.

d. never lets his clients know that he is a PA.

MC 3-6 `LO4` CPA Ontario should remove its general prohibition against PAs taking commissions and contingent fees because

a. CPAs prefer more price competition to less.

b. commissions and contingent fees enhance audit independence.

c. the Charter of Rights will force the change anyway.

d. objectivity is not always necessary in accounting and auditing services.

MC 3-7 `LO5` PA Smith is the auditor of Ajax Corporation. Her audit independence will not be considered impaired if she

a. owns $1,000 worth of Ajax shares.

b. has a husband who owns $2,000 worth of Ajax shares.

c. has a sister who is the financial vice-president of Ajax.

d. owns $1,000 worth of the shares of Pericles Corporation, which is controlled by Ajax as a result of Ajax's ownership of 40 percent of Pericles's shares, and Pericles contributes 3 percent of the total assets and income in Ajax's financial statements.

MC 3-8 `LO4` When a client's financial statements contain a material departure from a *CPA Canada Handbook* Accounting Recommendation and the PA believes that disclosure is necessary to make the statements not misleading, the PA

a. must qualify the audit report for a departure from GAAP.

b. can explain why the departure is necessary, and then give an unqualified opinion paragraph in the audit report.

c. must give an adverse audit report.

d. can give the standard unqualified audit report with an unqualified opinion paragraph.

MC 3-9 `LO4` Which of the following would not be considered confidential information obtained in the course of an engagement and for which the client's consent would be needed for disclosure?

a. Information about whether a consulting client has paid the PA's fees on time

b. The actuarial assumptions used by a tax client in calculating pension expense

c. Management's strategic plan for next year's labour negotiations

d. Information about material contingent liabilities relevant for audited financial statements

MC 3-10 `LO4` Which of the following would probably not be considered an "act discreditable to the profession"?

a. Numerous moving traffic violations

b. Failing to file the PA's own tax return

c. Filing a fraudulent tax return for a client in severe financial difficulty

d. Refusing to hire Asian Canadians in an accounting practice

MC 3-11 `LO4` A group of investors sued Anderson, Olds & Watershed, PAs, for alleged damages suffered when the company they held common shares in went bankrupt. In order to avoid liability under the common law, AOW must prove which of the following?

a. The investors actually suffered a loss.

b. The investors relied on the financial statements audited by AOW.

c. The investors' loss was a direct result of their reliance on the audited financial statements.

d. The audit was conducted in accordance with GAAS and with due professional care.

MC 3-12 `LO6` A PA's legal licence to practise public accounting can be revoked by which organization?

a. CPA Canada

b. Provincial body of PAs

c. Auditing Standards Board

d. Provincial securities commissions

MC 3-13 `LO5` A PA's independence would not be considered impaired if he had

a. owned common shares of the audit client but sold them before the company became a client.

b. sold short his common shares of an audit client while working on the audit engagement.

c. served as the company's treasurer for six months during the year covered by the audit but resigned before the company became a client.

d. performed the bookkeeping and financial statement preparation for the company, which had no accounting personnel, and a president with no understanding of accounting principles.

MC 3-14 `LO4` When a PA knows that a tax client has skimmed cash receipts and not reported the income in his federal income tax return, but she signs the return as a PA who prepared the return, that PA has violated which rule of professional conduct?

a. Confidential Client Information

b. Integrity and Objectivity

c. Independence

d. Accounting Principles

MC 3-15 `LO6` Under the *Foreign Corrupt Practices Act,*

a. companies must refrain from bribing foreign politicians for commercial advantage.

b. independent auditors must audit all elements of a company's internal control system.

c. independent auditors must establish control systems to keep books, records, and accounts properly.

d. independent auditors must prepare the financial statements.

MC 3-16 `LO7` The management accountants employed by Robbins Inc. wrongly charged executives' personal expenses to the overhead on a government contract. Their activities can be characterized as

a. errors in the application of accounting principles.

b. irregularities of the type independent auditors should plan an audit to detect.

c. irregularities of the type independent auditors have no responsibility to plan an audit to detect.

d. illegal acts of a type independent auditors should be aware might occur in government contract business.

EXERCISES AND PROBLEMS

EP 3-1 Independence, Integrity, and Objectivity Cases. `LO3, 5` Knowledge of the rules of conduct and related interpretations on independence, integrity, and objectivity will help you respond to the following cases.

Required:

For each case, state whether or not the action or situation violates the rules of professional conduct, explain why, and cite the relevant rule or interpretation.

a. R. Stout, PA, performs the audit of the local symphony society. Because of her good work, she was elected an honorary member of the board of directors.

b. N. Wolfe, a retired partner of your public accounting firm, has just been appointed to the board of directors of Palmer Corporation, your firm's client. Wolfe is also an ex officio member of your firm's income tax advisory committee, which meets monthly to discuss income tax problems of the partnership's clients, some of which are competitors of Palmer Corporation. The partnership pays Wolfe $100 for each committee meeting attended and a monthly retirement benefit, fixed by a retirement plan policy, of $1,000.

  c. Archie Goodwin, PA, performs significant day-to-day bookkeeping services for Harper Corporation and supervises the work of the one part-time bookkeeper employed by Marvin Harper. This year, Marvin wants to engage PA Goodwin to perform an audit.

  d. PA Fritz's wife owns 20% of the common shares of Botacel Company, which wants Fritz to perform the audit for the calendar year ended December 31, 20X4.

  e. Fritz's wife gave her shares to their 10-year-old daughter on July 1, 20X4.

  f. Fritz's daughter, acting through an appropriate custodian, sold the shares to her grandfather on August 1, 20X7. His purchase, as an accommodation, took one-half of his retirement savings.

  g. Fritz's father managed to sell the shares on August 15, 20X7, to his brother, who lives in Brazil. The brother moved there 20 years ago and has not returned.

  h. Clyde Brenner is a manager in the Waterloo office of a large national public accounting firm. His wife, Bonnie, is assistant controller in ATC Corporation, a client of the firm whose audit is performed by the Toronto office. Bonnie and Clyde live in Guelph and commute to their respective workplaces.

  i. Clyde Brenner just received word that he has been admitted to the partnership.

  j. The Rockhard Trust Company, a client of your firm, privately told your local managing partner that a block of funds would be set aside for home loans for qualified new employees. Rockhard's president is well aware that your firm experiences some difficulty hiring good people in the mid-size but growing community and is willing to do what he can to help while mortgage money is so tight. Several new assistant accountants obtained home loans under this arrangement.

(© 2000, American Institute of CPAs. All Rights Reserved. Adapted by permission.)

EP 3-2 Independence, Integrity, and Objectivity Cases. `LO3, 5` Knowledge of the rules of conduct; interpretations thereof; and related rulings on independence, integrity, and objectivity will help you respond to the following cases.

Required:

For each case, state whether or not the action or situation violates the rules of professional conduct, explain why, and cite the relevant rule or interpretation.

  a. Your client, Contrary Corporation, is very upset over the fact that your audit last year failed to detect an $800,000 inventory overstatement caused by employee theft and falsification of the records. The board discussed the matter and authorized its lawyers to explore the possibility of a lawsuit for damages.

  b. Contrary Corporation filed a lawsuit alleging negligent audit work, seeking $1 million in damages.

  c. In response to the lawsuit by Contrary, you decided to start litigation against certain officers of the company, alleging management fraud and deceit. You are asking for a damages judgment of $500,000.

  d. The Allright Insurance company paid Contrary Corporation $700,000 under fidelity bonds covering the employees involved in the inventory theft. Both you and Contrary Corporation have dropped your lawsuits. However, under subrogation rights, Allright has sued your audit firm for damages on the grounds of negligent performance of the audit.

  e. Colt & Associates, PAs, audit Gore Company. Alice Colt (CEO) and Bill Gore (president) discovered a limited real estate partnership deal that looked too good to pass up. Colt purchased limited partnership interests amounting to 23% of all such interests, and Gore personally purchased 31%. Unrelated investors held the remaining 46%. Colt and Gore congratulated themselves on the opportunity and agreed to be passive investors with respect to the partnership.

  f. A group of dissident shareholders filed a class-action lawsuit against both you and your client, Amalgamated Inc., for $30 million. They allege there was a conspiracy to present misleading financial statements in connection with a recent merger.

g. PA Anderson, a partner in the firm of Anderson, Olds & Watershed (a professional accounting corporation), owns 25% of the common shares of Dove Corporation (not a client of AOW). This year Dove purchased a 32% interest in Tale Company and is accounting for the investment using the equity method of accounting. The investment amounts to 11% of Dove's consolidated net assets. Tale Company has been an audit client of AOW for 12 years.

h. Durkin & Panzer, PAs, regularly perform the audit of the North Country Bank, and the firm is preparing for the audit of the financial statements for the year ended December 31, 20X4.

i. Two directors of the North Country Bank became partners in D&P, PAs, on July 1, 20X4, resigning their directorship on that date. They will not participate in the audit.

j. During 20X4, the former controller of the North Country Bank, now a partner of D&P, was frequently called on for assistance regarding loan approvals and the bank's minimum chequing account policy. In addition, he conducted a computer feasibility study for North Country.

(© 2000, American Institute of CPAs. All Rights Reserved. Adapted by permission.)

k. The Cather Corporation is indebted to a PA for unpaid fees and has offered to give the PA unsecured interest-bearing notes. Alternatively, Cather Corporation offered to give two shares of its common stock, after which 10,002 shares would be outstanding.

(© 2000, American Institute of CPAs. All Rights Reserved. Adapted by permission.)

l. Johnny Keems is not yet a PA but is doing quite well in his first employment with a large public accounting firm. He has been on the job two years and has become a "heavy junior." If he passes the PA exam in September, he will be promoted to senior accountant. This month, during the audit of Row Lumber Company, Johnny told the controller about how he is remodelling an old house. The controller likes Johnny and has a load of needed materials delivered to the house, billing Johnny at a 70% discount—a savings over the normal cash discount of about $300. Johnny paid the bill and was happy to have the materials, which he otherwise would not have been able to afford on his meagre salary.

m. PA Lily Rowan inherited $1 million from her grandfather, $100,000 of which was the value of shares in the North Country Bank. Lily practises accounting in Hamilton, and several of her audit clients have loans from the bank.

n. Groaner Corporation is in financial difficulty. You are about to sign the report on the current audit when your firm's office manager informs you that the audit fee for last year has not yet been paid.

o. Your audit client, Glow Company, is opening a plant in a distant city. Glow's president asks that your firm's office in that city recruit and hire a new plant controller and a cost accountant.

EP 3-3 Common Law Liability Exposure. `LO7` Smith, PA, is the auditor for Juniper Manufacturing Corporation, a privately owned company that has a June 30 fiscal year-end. Juniper arranged for a substantial bank loan, which was dependent on the bank's receiving, by September 30, audited financial statements showing a current ratio of at least 2 to 1. On September 25, just before the audit report was to be issued, Smith received an anonymous letter on Juniper's stationery indicating that a five-year lease by Juniper, as lessee, of a factory building that was accounted for in the financial statements as an operating lease was in fact a capital lease. The letter stated that there was a secret written agreement with the lessor modifying the lease and creating a capital lease.

Smith confronted the president of Juniper, who admitted that a secret agreement existed but said it was necessary to treat the lease as an operating lease to meet the current ratio requirement of the pending loan and that nobody would ever discover the secret agreement with the lessor. The president said that if Smith did not issue his report by September 30, Juniper would sue Smith for substantial damages that would result from not getting the loan. Under this pressure and because the working papers contained a copy of the five-year lease agreement supporting the operating lease treatment, Smith issued his report with an unqualified opinion on September 29. In spite of the fact that the loan was received, Juniper went bankrupt. The bank is suing Smith to recover its losses on the loan and the lessor is suing Smith to recover uncollected rents.

Required:

Answer the following, setting forth reasons for any conclusions stated.

a. Is Smith liable to the bank?

b. Is Smith liable to the lessor?

c. Was Smith independent?

(© 2000, American Institute of CPAs. All Rights Reserved. Adapted by permission.)

DISCUSSION CASES

DC 3-1 General Ethics.   **LO1, 2**   Is there any moral difference between a disapproved action in which you are caught and the same action that never becomes known to anyone else? Do many persons in business and professional society distinguish between these two circumstances? If you respond that you do (or do not) perceive a difference while persons in business and professional society do not (or do), then how do you explain the differences in attitudes?

DC 3-2 Ethics Decision Problem.   **LO2**   You are treasurer of a church. A member approaches you with the following proposition: "I will donate shares to the church on December 31, if, on January 1, you will sell them back to me. All you will need to do is convey the certificate with your signature to me in return for my cheque, which will be for the asking price of the shares quoted that day without reduction for commissions."

The member's objective, of course, is to obtain the income tax deduction as of December 31, but he wants to maintain his ownership interest. The policy of the church board is not to hold any shares but to sell shares within a reasonably short time.

Required:

a. Should the treasurer accommodate the member? Would you if you were treasurer?

b. Would your considerations and conclusions be any different if the church

1. was financially secure and the gift was small?

2. was financially secure and the gift was large?

3. would be in deficit position for the year were it not for the gift?

DC 3-3 Competition and Audit Proposals.   **LO1**   Accounting firms are often asked to present "proposals" to companies' boards of directors. These proposals are comprehensive booklets, accompanied by oral presentations, telling about the firm's personnel, technology, special qualifications, and expertise in hope of convincing the board to award the work to the firm.

Dena has a new job as staff assistant to Michael, chairman of the board of Granof Grain Company. The company has a policy of engaging new auditors every seven years. The board will hear oral proposals from 12 accounting firms. This is the second day of the three-day meeting. Dena's job is to help evaluate the proposals. Yesterday, the proposal by Anderson, Olds & Watershed was clearly the best.

Then Dena sees Michael's staff chief, Mindy, a brash go-getter, slip a copy of the AOW written proposal into an envelope. Mindy tells Dena to take it to a friend who works for Hunt and Hunt, a public accounting firm scheduled to make its presentation tomorrow. Mindy says, "I told him we'd let him glance at the best proposal." Michael is absent from the meeting and will not return for two hours.

What should Dena do? What should PA Hunt do if he receives the AOW proposal, assuming he has time to modify the Hunt and Hunt proposal before tomorrow's presentation?

DC 3-4 Engagement Timekeeping Records. **LO1** A time budget is always prepared for audit engagements. Numbers of hours are estimated for various segments of the work—for example, internal control evaluation, cash, inventory, and report review. Audit supervisors expect the work segments to be completed within budget, and staff accountants' performance is evaluated in part on ability to perform audit work efficiently within budget.

Sarah is an audit manager who has worked hard to get promoted. She hopes to become a partner in two or three years. Finishing audits on time weighs heavily on her performance evaluation. She assigned the cash audit work to Craig, who has worked for the firm for 10 months. Craig hopes to get a promotion and salary raise this year. Twenty hours were budgeted for the cash work. Craig is efficient, but it took 30 hours to finish because the company had added seven new bank accounts. Craig was worried about his performance evaluation, so he recorded 20 hours for the cash work and put the other 10 hours under the internal control evaluation budget.

What do you think about Craig's resolution of his problem? Was his action a form of lying? What would you think of his action if the internal control evaluation work was presented "under budget" because it was not yet complete, and another assistant was assigned to finish that work segment later?

DC 3-5 Audit Overtime. **LO1, 2** All accountants' performance evaluations are based in part on their ability to do audit work efficiently and within the time budget planned for the engagement. New staff accountants, in particular, usually have some early difficulty learning speedy work habits, which demand that no time be wasted.

Elizabeth started work for Anderson, Olds & Watershed in September. After attending the staff training school, she was assigned to the Rising Sun Company audit. Her first work assignment was to complete the extensive recalculation of the inventory compilation, using the audit test counts and audited unit prices for several hundred inventory items. Her time budget for the work was six hours. She started at 4 p.m. and was not finished when everyone left the office at 6 p.m. Not wanting to stay downtown alone, she took all the necessary working papers home. She resumed work at 8 p.m. and finished at 3 a.m. The next day, she returned to the Rising Sun offices, put the completed working papers in the file, and recorded six hours in the time budget/actual schedule. Her supervisor was pleased, especially about her diligence in taking the work home.

What do you think about Elizabeth's diligence and her understatement of the time she took to finish the work? What if she had received help at home from her husband? What if she had been unable to finish and had left the work at home for her husband to finish while he took off a day from his job interviews?

DC 3-6 Form of Practice, Technical Standards, and Confidentiality. **LO4** Knowledge of the rules of conduct and interpretations thereof will help you respond to this case problem.

Gilbert and Bradley formed a corporation called Financial Services Inc. Each took 50% of the authorized common shares. Gilbert is a PA and a member of the provincial institute. Bradley is a CPCU (Chartered Property Casualty Underwriter). The corporation performs auditing and tax services under Gilbert's direction and insurance services under Bradley's supervision. The opening of the corporation's office was announced in a full-page advertisement in the local newspaper.

One of the corporation's first audit clients was the Grandtime Company. Grandtime had total assets of $600,000 and total liabilities of $270,000. In the course of the audit, Gilbert found that

Grandtime's building with a book value of $240,000 was pledged as a security for a 10-year term note in the amount of $200,000. The client's statement did not mention that the building was pledged as security for the 10-year term note. However, as the failure to disclose the lien did not affect either the value of the assets or the amount of the liabilities, and the audit was satisfactory in all other respects, Gilbert rendered an unqualified opinion on Grandtime's financial statements. About two months after the date of his opinion, Gilbert learned that an insurance company was planning to lend Grandtime $150,000 in the form of a first-mortgage note on the building. Realizing the insurance company was unaware of the existing lien on the building, Gilbert had Bradley notify the insurance company of the fact that Grandtime's building was pledged as security for the term note.

Shortly after the events described above, Gilbert was charged with several violations of professional ethics.

Required:

Identify and discuss the rules of professional conduct violated by Gilbert and the nature of the violations.

(© 2000, American Institute of CPAs. All Rights Reserved. Adapted by permission.)

DC 3-7 Another Milestone Lawsuit against Auditors: The Unexpected Failure of Lehman Brothers. LO7 The failure of Lehman Brothers bank on September 15, 2008, created the largest bankruptcy in U.S. history and the global financial crisis that followed. There was no indication of going-concern problems in Lehman's financial reporting before it filed for bankruptcy. To say that the markets were surprised by its bankruptcy would be an understatement. The state of New York sued the audit firm to recover $150 million in fees earned. Many investors are also suing the audit firm. The audit firm publicly claimed that the financial statements of Lehman were "in accordance with GAAP." The audit firm tried to get legal jurisdiction changed to U.S. federal court in hopes of a better outcome. On March 22, 2012, the case was moved from the federal court back to the New York state court because it was not within federal jurisdiction. In 2015 the charges were settled, with the accounting firm paying a settlement fee of $10 million and not admitting to any wrongdoing.

Required:

With some additional research, discuss the similarities of the Lehman Bros. case with that of Continental Vending, also discussed in this chapter.

Appendix 3A: Framework for Critical Thinking (on Connect)

ENDNOTES

1   R. K. Mautz and H. A. Sharaf, *The Philosophy of Auditing* (American Accounting Association, 1991).

2   P. Wheelwright, *A Critical Introduction to Ethics*, 3rd ed. (Indianapolis, IN: Odyssey Press, 1959).

3   H. H. Titus and M. Keeton, *Ethics for Today*, 4th ed. (New York: American Book-Stratford Press, 1966), p. 131.

4   Several rules of professional conduct to be discussed shortly are explicitly phrased to provide exceptions to the general rules (e.g., Rules 210 and 204 of the CPA Ontario Rules of Professional Conduct). Imperative rules also seem to generate borderline cases, so the ethics divisions of public accounting professional bodies issue interpretations and rulings to explain the applicability of the rules.

5   For a good review of the history of the profession during this period, see A. R. Wyatt, "Accounting professionalism—They just don't get it!" *Accounting Horizons*, March 2004, pp. 45–54.

6   Z. Bauman, *Postmodern Ethics* (Oxford: Blackwell, 1993).

7   See R .M. Mano, M. Moritsen, and R. Pace, "Principles-based accounting," *CPA Journal*, February 2006, pp. 60–63, for more discussion.

8   K. Gunning, "Required reading," *CA Magazine*, November 1992, pp. 38–40.

9   IFAC Handbook, 2005, Code of Ethics for Professional Accountants, pp. 25–26.

10   K. Gunning, *ibid.*

11   L. J. Brooks, *Professional Ethics for Accountants* (Minneapolis/St. Paul: West Publishing, 1995), p. 120.

12   As modified from "Proposed new independence standards for auditors," *CA Magazine*, October 2002, p. 51.

13   See cpab-ccrc.ca/en/topics/Reports/Pages/default.aspx for the CPAB reports.

14   CPA Canada's definition of public accountant in its *Terminology for Accountants*, 4th ed. (1992), is as follows: "1. The performance of services for clients, the purpose of which is to add credibility to financial information that may be relied upon by interested parties. 2. The performance of independent professional accounting and related services for clients. 3. Any service so defined by a particular statute or authority."

15   K. St. Pierre and J. Anderson, "An analysis of audit failures based on documented legal cases," *Journal of Accounting, Auditing, and Finance*, Spring 1982, pp. 236–237.

16   S. Andersen and J. Wolfe, "A perspective on audit malpractice claims," *Journal of Accountancy*, September 2002, p. 59.

17   Z. Palmrose, "An analysis of auditor litigation and audit service quality," *Accounting Review*, January 1988, pp. 55–73.

18   J. E. Smyth, D. A. Soberman, and A. J. Easson, *The Law and Business Administration in Canada*, 7th ed. (Prentice Hall, 1995), pp. 76–79.

19   "Auditing in crisis," *The Bottom Line*, March 1990.

20   H. Rowan, "Are banks looking to pin the blame?" *CA Magazine*, June 1988.

21   For example, see A. Rosen and M. Rosen, *Swindlers* (Toronto: Madison Press Books, 2010), p. 17.

22   A. R. Andrews and G. Simonette Jr., "Tort reform revolution," *Journal of Accountancy*, September 1996, p. 54.

23   *Ibid.*, p. 50.

24   See M. Paskell-Mede, "Fair shares," *CA Magazine*, November 2001, pp. 31–32; G. McLennan, "Trust not," *CA Magazine*, June/July, 1993, pp. 40–43; and M. Paskell-Mede, "Adviser relationships," *CA Magazine*, May 1995, pp. 27–32.

25   G. McLennan, "Trust Not," *CA Magazine*, June/July 1993, pp. 40–43.

26   *Ibid.*, p. 35.

27   M. Paskell-Mede, "So sue me," *CA Magazine*, February 1991, pp. 36–38; M. Paskell-Mede, "What liability crisis," *CA Magazine*, May 1994, pp. 42–43.

28   M. F. Murray, "When a client is a liability," *Journal of Accountancy*, September 1992, pp. 54–58.

29   L. J. Brooks, *Professional Ethics for Accountants* (Minneapolis/St. Paul: West Publishing Company, 1995), p. 69; also see S. Gunz and J. McCutcheon, "Some unresolved ethical issues in auditing," *Journal of Business Ethics*, October 1991, pp. 777–785.

CHAPTER 4

Reports on Audited Financial Statements

This chapter covers the most frequent variations in audit reports. Management is primarily responsible for the fair presentation of financial statements in conformity with generally accepted accounting principles (GAAP). Auditors are primarily responsible for their own audit reports of the financial statements. As a starting point, this chapter explains the standard unmodified opinion audit report. Then the changes necessary to the standard language when auditors cannot give a "clean opinion" are discussed.

LEARNING OBJECTIVES

After completing this chapter, you will be able to do the following:

LO1 Describe the association framework.

LO2 Determine whether a public accountant is associated with financial statements.

LO3 Describe the three levels of assurance.

LO4 Compare and contrast the scope and opinion paragraphs in an independent auditor's report.

LO5 For a given set of accounting facts and audit circumstances, analyze qualified, adverse, and disclaimer audit reports.

LO6 Determine the effects of materiality and uncertainty on audit report choices.

LO7 Explain the purpose of significant matter paragraphs.

LO8 (Appendix 4A) Describe the Standard Unqualified Report of the Public Company Accounting Oversight Board/ American Institute of CPAs.

LO9 (Appendix 4B) Describe the auditor's standard report for use before December 15, 2016.

LO10 (Appendix 4C) Explain the reporting on the application of accounting principles.

CHAPTER APPENDICES

APPENDIX 4A The Standard Unqualified Report of the Public Company Accounting Oversight Board/American Institute of CPAs

APPENDIX 4B The Auditor's Standard Report for Use before December 15, 2016

APPENDIX 4C Reporting on the Application of Accounting Principles

EcoPak Inc.

A few years have passed, and EcoPak's biomass-based food packaging business is doing very well and looking to further expand. Kam and Mike are considering taking EcoPak public, and Nina suggests they start by finding an auditor, since they will need several years of audited financial statements for their initial public offering (IPO). Nina recommends an acquaintance, Ella Foure, an audit partner from the firm Pettit and Foure (P&F).

Ella meets with Kam and Mike. They are very impressed by her expertise. She is very knowledgeable about their products and industry, as she has been on the Environmental Stewardship Board and has other audit clients in startup biotechnology businesses. Kam is so impressed that he asks Ella if she could appear in one of EcoPak's promotional videos to endorse the profit potential of their new product line: "If you are our auditor and also promote our products, it will send a really powerful message to prospective customers and investors!" Ella explains that if she were to do that she could not also be their auditor as she is then associated with EcoPak and its information. Under the ethics rules, she should not "advocate" for audit clients because it would impair her independence. For example, if she made a claim about a new product and that product turned out to be a failure, it would be hard for her to be unbiased about reporting that she was wrong.

Ella gets back to talking about an audit engagement by asking about the company's information systems. Mike tells Ella about some problems they experienced in the past year. Their inventory system became corrupted, and records for three months of transactions were lost. But the inventory and profit numbers are up, so Mike doesn't think there's any need to investigate or try to recreate those records. Ella finds this troubling, since she doesn't know Mike well and it sounds like he might be trying to manipulate the financial records. But she sets that suspicion aside until she gets more familiar with things.

If EcoPak's system problem was unintentional and she cannot find an alternative means of getting audit evidence, Ella explains to Kam and Mike that they will probably get a qualified audit opinion because this is a scope limitation. If there is some way she can find alternative evidence to support the year-end numbers, however, an unmodified audit opinion might be given. Now Mike is really starting to get confused: "What would be wrong with a 'qualified opinion'? Isn't that a good thing—what we would want from a licensed auditor like you?" Ella explains that the term *qualified* is used in a special way by auditors. To auditors, it means that the auditor's opinion on the reliability of the financial statements is restricted or limited in some way. In this case, it is restricted by an inability to find all the records that the auditor may need to be reasonably sure a material misstatement is not present in the inventory account or transactions.

On further questioning, Ella realizes that EcoPak's systems are really inadequate for the volume of business, and that the company is probably not auditable at this time. She suggests that EcoPak consider bringing in some information technology (IT) consultants to set up appropriate business processes, a reliable information system, and internal controls. It may be feasible and beneficial to have P&F perform a different type of assurance engagement this year, such as a review engagement. A review type of engagement provides only moderate assurance, not high assurance, like an audit, so it requires less evidence than an audit. The IT system deficiency may allow the negative assurance opinion provided by a review engagement, as long as EcoPak's year-end numbers make sense. That will also give Ella a good basis for starting the audit in the following year, since she will already have a good knowledge of EcoPak's business, and its systems and internal control will be more reliable. Kam and Mike think this is a good plan to help them continue to grow their business. They decide to go ahead with her suggestions and are grateful for her advice.

The Essentials of Reports on Audited Financial Statements

The independent auditor's report on an company's financial statements is a standardized public statement that an auditor must provide when he or she has completed the financial statement audit engagement. When the financial statements are prepared in accordance with generally accepted accounting principles (GAAP), they are expected to fairly present the financial position, financial performance, and cash flows of a company. This means the financial statements should give users a full and unbiased understanding of these aspects of the economic realities of the company. The auditor's report is the most public output of a financial statement audit and states the auditor's opinion on whether the financial statements are fairly presented. Forming this opinion is the ultimate goal of the whole process of planning and performing a financial statement audit engagement. The audit profession has traditionally preferred that all audit reports use very similar wording; this is so people using an audit report are less likely to interpret it in ways the auditor didn't intend. This standardized wording is set out in the generally accepted auditing standards (GAAS) reporting standards, CAS 700, 701, 705, and 706.

Often the report will tell users that the auditors believe the financial statements do indeed present the financial information fairly; this is sometimes called an unmodified auditor's opinion or, with the same meaning, a "clean" audit opinion. In the past it has also been called an "unqualified" opinion, but this term is falling out of use in GAAS because it is so ambiguous: the word *unqualified* sounds "bad" but really it means it's a "good" type of report. Clean opinion audit reports are the most commonly observed type, because they are generally desired by companies that engage a financial statement auditor. Further, securities regulations require that a publicly listed company obtain a clean audit opinion on its annual financial statements to maintain its stock market listing. So most of the audit reports we see in public will be of the clean opinion type.

In some cases, the audit engagement might lead the auditor to conclude that a clean opinion is not appropriate for some reason(s). Then the auditor will have to communicate a different message by reporting a modified audit opinion, which is also called a qualified audit opinion. Since many possible situations can result in a modified opinion, there are standardized approaches in GAAS for categorizing these problems and reporting on them. The two main categories of problems that can lead to a modified opinion are (i) GAAP violations that affect fair presentation and (ii) audit scope limitations that impair the auditor's ability to fully comply with GAAS. Note that the first type relates to management's responsibility to provide fairly presented financial statements, while the second relates to the auditor's responsibility to conduct an audit that complies with GAAS.

How do GAAS say to report problems of these kinds? It depends on how severely the problems could affect users of the financial statements. If the problem is or could be significant to people using the financial statements, but applies to only one or more isolated aspects of the fair presentation of financial statements, the auditor would issue a qualified opinion that describes the isolated impacts of the reservations he or she has, but otherwise provides a clean opinion on the rest of the financial statements. If the problems are so severe and pervasive that they could affect the fair presentation of the financial statements as a whole, the auditor must go further than just qualifying the opinion. In the case of a pervasive GAAP violation, the auditor must give an adverse opinion. With an adverse opinion, the report says that auditor believes the financial statements are *not* fairly presented in accordance with GAAP. In the case of a pervasive scope limitation, a disclaimer of opinion must be issued. With a disclaimer of opinion, the report says that the auditor is unable to provide any opinion because it was impossible to get the audit evidence required to establish reasonable assurance regarding fair presentation for the financial statements as a whole.

Here are some examples to illustrate and clarify these types of opinions. If management refuses to record a provision for obsolete inventory, and the auditor believes a significant amount of inventory is unlikely to be sellable, but the rest of the financial statements are fairly presented, the auditor qualifies the opinion for a GAAP violation regarding inventory valuation and related accounts such as cost of sales and gross profit. If management refuses to consolidate a number of large controlled subsidiaries, and the auditor believes financial statements as a whole are not fairly presented, an adverse opinion is issued for this GAAP violation. If the inventory records were destroyed by a warehouse fire and there is no basis to assess whether inventory has been accounted for properly, the auditor would give a qualified opinion due to a scope limitation for inventory and related accounts. If the entire accounting system was destroyed by a flood and there was no information available to support the financial statements, the auditor would issue a disclaimer of opinion, as there is no way to meet the requirements of GAAS in this situation.

The auditors' report is addressed to the main stakeholders, usually the corporation's shareholders, and is dated and signed by the auditors at the end of the audit engagement. The reporting standards of GAAS set out four main segments that the auditors' report must present:

- An introductory paragraph stating the company name and the set of financial statements that were audited.
- A management responsibility paragraph, listing management's responsibilities for fair presentation of financial statements and for internal control as necessary to ensure financial statements are free of material misstatements due to fraud or error.
- A description of auditor responsibility in three paragraphs outlining (i) the auditors' responsibility to express an opinion based on conducting an audit in compliance with GAAS and ethical requirements, (ii) a summary of what an audit examination involves, and (iii) a statement of the auditors' belief that their procedures provided a sufficient and appropriate basis for their audit opinion.
- An opinion paragraph on the fair presentation of the financial statements.

If a modified opinion is required, the GAAS reporting standards also set out guidelines for how the auditor should explain this situation in the report, as well as the additional paragraphs of information the report must include.

Currently the boilerplate nature of the standardized audit report wording is under some scrutiny and there is ongoing discussion about expanding GAAS reporting standards to allow an auditor to include more company-specific audit information in the auditor's report, in the form of Auditor's Comments.

Some additional, more advanced considerations related to audit reports will be briefly noted here. First, a fundamental concept related to auditor reporting is *association*, which refers to the situation when a professional accountant has performed some work or agreed to have his or her name connected to a company or its information. This association situation could lead the public to believe the accountant has been involved in some independent capacity and to place more trust in the company and its information than otherwise. To protect the public's best interests, the accounting profession has developed protocols for how accountants can identify when they are associated and has set out requirements they must then follow. These protocols are an important way for accountants to meet the ethical standard of *integrity*, by helping them to avoid being involved with the public's use of misleading information. The essential requirements when associated are to ensure that any professional standards related to the work are followed, and to communicate clearly the nature and extent of the work done and the accountant's responsibility to possible users. So, we can view the auditor's report on financial statements as a special, but very common, example of the communication responsibility that arises because a professional accountant is associated with an entity and its information.

Also, note that an auditor's opinion is based on obtaining reasonable assurance, also referred to as a *high level of assurance,* about the fair presentation of the financial statements. In practice, public accountants (PAs) may offer engagements that provide a lower level of assurance that is based primarily on analysis rather than gathering independent evidence. These are referred to as *review engagements* or *moderate assurance engagements.* If users are satisfied with moderate assurance, a review engagement may be chosen rather than an audit, since the review engagement procedures are less time-consuming and costly than getting the high level of assurance required to issue an audit opinion. Professional accountants may also provide a range of other non-assurance related services for financial statements. One common example is when a professional accountant simply prepares financial statements from information in the company's books and records, without doing any independent verification or analysis. This type of *compilation engagement* offers no assurance, but association exists, so the accountant must still attach a report called a "Notice to Reader" to inform users of the very limited nature of the accountant's involvement.

Review Checkpoints

4-1   What does an independent auditor's report on financial statements state? When does the auditor provide this report?

4-2   What does it mean to say that the financial statements "present fairly" in accordance with GAAP?

4-3   Why does the auditor's report traditionally have standardized wording?

4-4   Does the requirement for standardized audit report wording relate to the "expectations gap" in some way? Explain.

4-5   What standards are followed for writing an auditor's report?

4-6   What does the term *unmodified audit opinion* mean? What simpler term for this type of opinion is often used in practice?

4-7   What information is the auditor communicating to financial statement users when he or she issues an unmodified audit opinion?

4-8   Why do most of the public company audit reports we see include unmodified audit opinions?

4-9   What is a modified (or qualified) audit opinion? How does it differ from an unmodified audit opinion?

4-10 What are two main categories of problems that can prevent an auditor from issuing an unmodified audit opinion on GAAP financial statements? Which type relates to management's responsibilities and which type relates to auditors' responsibilities?

4-11 What kind of audit opinion is used if there are GAAP violations but they only affect isolated information in the financial statements? What kind of opinion is given if the GAAP violations severely undermine the usefulness of the financial statements overall?

4-12 What kind of audit opinion is given if the scope of the audit engagement was limited but the problems would only affect isolated information in the financial statements? What kind of report is used if there are audit scope limitations that made it impossible for the auditor to determine if the financial statements as a whole are fairly presented for users?

4-13 What are the main components that GAAS require to be included in an auditor's report on financial statements?

4-14 Explain why there is some discussion now in the auditing profession of expanding the standard auditor's report wording to include more customized Auditor's Comments.

4-15 What does the term *association* mean in the accounting profession? What responsibilities arise for a professional accountant who is considered to be associated with a company's financial information?

4-16 What does the term *high level of assurance* mean?

4-17 What level of assurance does an audit provide?

4-18 What term is used for a type of assurance engagement that provides a moderate, rather than a high, level of assurance?

4-19 What is the difference between the accountant's work when issuing an audit opinion, and the work when issuing a review engagement report?

4-20 What term is used when a professional accountant simply prepares financial statements for a company, but does not do any work that could support giving assurance to users about the fair presentation of these financial statements?

4-21 What does a professional accountant's Notice to Reader report on financial statements indicate to financial statement users?

4-22 Why does association exist if a professional accountant is only providing a Notice to Reader report on a company's financial statements?

The Association Framework

LO1 Describe the association framework.

The public accounting services covered in this chapter are part of the broadest concept of auditor involvement with a business enterprise's information—that of association. **Association** is a term used within the profession to indicate a PA's involvement with an enterprise or with information issued by that enterprise. General standards for association are covered in the *CPA Canada Handbook*. At the time of writing, there were comparable international standards on association, but they are not in the Canadian Auditing Standards (CASs).

Association can arise in three ways:

1. Through some action, the PA associates himself or herself with information issued by the enterprise.
2. Without the PA's knowledge or consent, the enterprise indicates that the PA was involved with information issued by it.
3. A third party assumes the PA is involved with information issued by an enterprise.

According to paragraph 5020.04 of the *Handbook,* a PA associates himself or herself with information when they either perform services or consent to the use of their name in connection with that information. When associated with information, a PA's professional responsibilities include the following:

1. Applicable standards in the *CPA Canada Handbook* must be met.
2. The PA complies with the appropriate rules of professional conduct.
3. There is appropriate communication of the extent of the PA's involvement with the information.

association:
a term used within the profession to indicate a public accountant's involvement with an enterprise or with information issued by that enterprise

The PA should ensure that the information they are associated with is accurate, accurately reproduced, and not misleading. If the client attempts to make inappropriate use of his or her name, the PA should amend the information or get legal advice.

Exhibit 4–1 provides a framework illustrating the relationships between various types of engagements and *CPA Canada Handbook* sections, including CASs. As a result of the changes to public accounting brought on by section 5025, the concept of association had to be revised to incorporate the assurance framework. Further revisions were required with adoption of CASs. CASs are for now viewed outside the association framework. The association responsibilities are illustrated in section 5020.A.

Revising the concept of association meant that changes to PAs' responses to various client actions were also necessary. Their responsibilities concerning information or subject matters they are inappropriately associated with are summarized on the decision tree in the second box below relating to section 5020.A.

Exhibit 4–1 provides a preliminary version of the evolving association framework for all assurance engagements. The CASs are also part of an assurance framework like that covered in section 5025. Many of the other types of engagements are covered in Chapter 21 of this text (available on Connect). In the next section, we deal with determination and obligations of association.

EXHIBIT 4–1

Overview of the *CPA Canada Assurance Handbook*

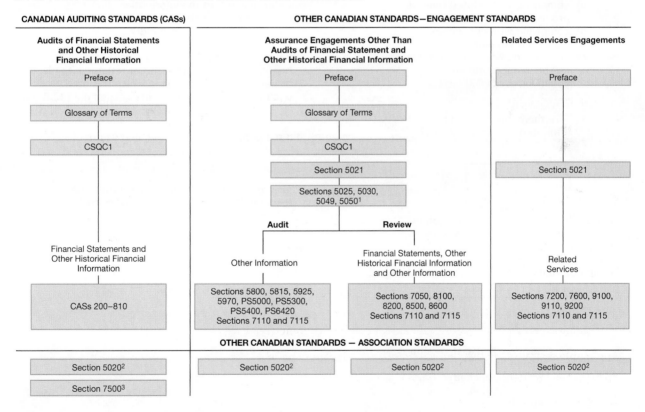

[1] USING THE WORK OF INTERNAL AUDIT IN ASSURANCE ENGAGEMENTS OTHER THAN AUDITS OF FINANCIAL STATEMENTS AND OTHER HISTORICAL FINANCIAL INFORMATION. Section 5050, provides guidance on using the work of internal audit in carrying out an audit engagement other than an audit of financial statements and other historical financial information. The guidance may be useful for other types of engagements.

[2] ASSOCIATION, Section 5020, provides guidance on the public accountant's association with information, which may occur irrespective of the type of engagement.

[3] AUDITOR ASSOCIATION WITH ANNUAL REPORTS, INTERIM REPORTS, AND OTHER PUBLIC DOCUMENTS. Section 7500, provides guidance on the auditor's responsibilities, after the completion of the audit of the entity's financial statements, when the auditor agrees to consent to the use of the auditor's report in connection with a designated document.

Source: Preface to *CPA Canada Handbook—Assurance*, Appendix 4, 2014.

Association with Financial Statements

LO2 Determine whether a public accountant is associated with financial statements.

Auditing standards require a report in all cases where a PA's name is **associated with financial statements**. As a PA, you are associated with financial statements when (1) you have consented to the use of your name in connection with them, or (2) you have prepared or performed some other services with respect to them, even if your name is not used in any written report. This is covered in the *CPA Canada Handbook*, paragraph 5020.04.

The concept of association is far reaching with respect to financial statements. A PA is associated with the financial statements when (1) these are merely reproduced on the PA's letterhead, (2) they are produced by the

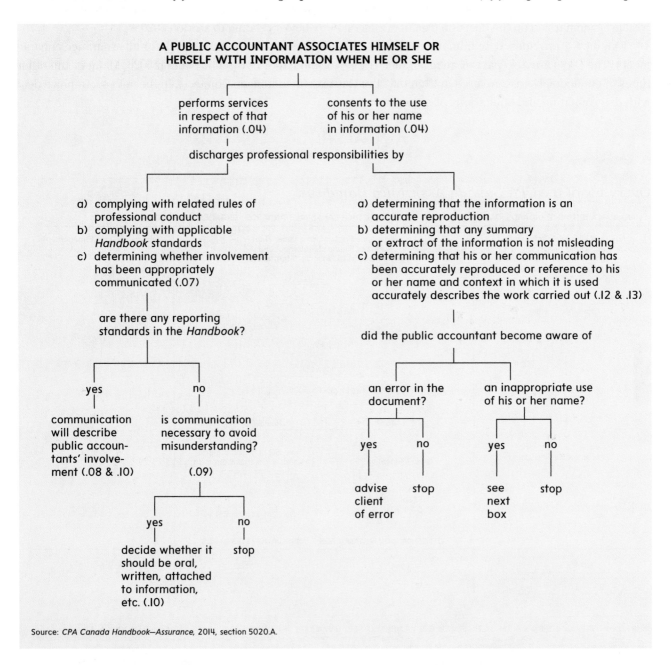

Source: *CPA Canada Handbook—Assurance,* 2014, section 5020.A.

associated with financial statements:
any involvement of a public accountant with financial statements issued by a client

PA's computer as part of a bookkeeping service, or (3) a document containing financial statements merely identifies him or her as the PA or auditor for the company. A report is required in these cases of association because most users of financial statements will assume that an audit has been conducted and that "everything is OK" on the basis of the involvement. Consequently, an obligation exists to inform the users about the nature of the work performed, if any, and the conclusions the PA has made about the financial statements. These responsibilities are summarized in the preceding and following boxes. Note that these responsibilities arise from potential legal liability due to misunderstandings of the nature of a PA's engagement. Many users, including the client, tend to assume that the PA's involvement with financial information constitutes an audit. A good illustration is to talk to your friends who have not taken an auditing course and ask them what they think "association" with a PA means. Association rules exist to clarify the role of a PA in an engagement, especially to third parties. Also, note that the focus of association rules is to reduce the risk that third parties will be misled by the nature of the PA's involvement. This reflects the unique obligation PAs have to third-party users of their work discussed in Chapter 3. The existence of these rules indicates the overriding importance of PA responsibilities to third parties that dominates much of the reasoning of audit engagements.

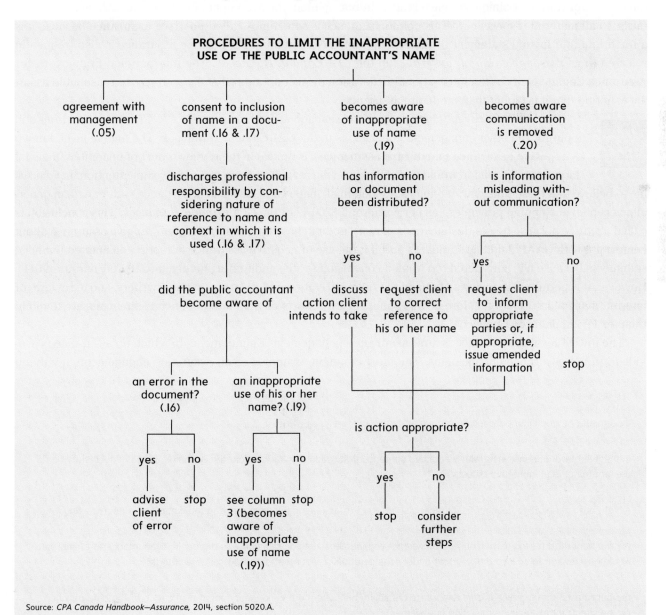

PROCEDURES TO LIMIT THE INAPPROPRIATE USE OF THE PUBLIC ACCOUNTANT'S NAME

Source: *CPA Canada Handbook—Assurance*, 2014, section 5020.A.

The next section outlines the various levels of assurance that are possible in public accounting engagements. We then discuss the audit reports that result from an audit of financial statements—the main audit covered in this text.

Review Checkpoint

4-23   Why should PAs issue a report whenever they are associated with financial statements?

Levels of Assurance

LO3   Describe the three levels of assurance.

In practice, accountants and auditors can render three types of conclusions, or **levels of assurance**, about financial statements. The highest level of assurance is the standard unmodified report, sometimes referred to as the **clean opinion**. Its opinion sentence reads, "In our opinion, the accompanying financial statements present fairly, in all material respects. . . ." This opinion sentence is sometimes called **positive assurance** because it is a forthright and factual statement of the PA's opinion based on an audit. Positive assurance is also frequently referred to as *reasonable* or *high assurance* in the *CPA Canada Handbook*. The International Framework for Assurance Engagements of the International Federation of Accountants (IFAC) also refers to reasonable assurance, noting that it is higher than moderate assurance.

 Current CASs cover only high-assurance engagements; hence the old *CICA Handbook* sections still apply for the other engagement conclusions in the *CPA Canada Handbook*. The middle level, known as **negative assurance (moderate assurance)**, is typical in the review report of unaudited financial statements. Its opinion would read, "Based on my review, nothing has come to my attention that causes me to believe that these financial statements are not, in all material respects, in accordance with Canadian generally accepted accounting principles," as per paragraph 8200.42 of the *CPA Canada Handbook*. This conclusion is called *negative* because it uses the backdoor phrase "nothing has come to my attention" to give assurance about conformity with GAAP. Auditing standards prohibit the use of negative assurance in reports on audited financial statements because it is considered too weak a conclusion for the audit effort involved (CAS 700, paragraph 11). However, it is permitted in reviews of unaudited financial statements, in letters to underwriters, and in reviews of interim financial information. (More details about review reports on unaudited financial statements are found in Chapter 17, available on Connect.)

The lowest level of assurance is a **no assurance** engagement. Engagements in which no assurance is provided are not assurance engagements. The most common examples of no assurance engagements involving

levels of assurance:
the amount of credibility provided by accountants and auditors

clean opinion:
the highest level of assurance, with an opinion sentence that reads, "In our opinion, the accompanying financial statements present fairly, in all material respects . . ."

positive assurance:
a high, but not absolute, level of assurance; also referred to as reasonable assurance in the context of audit reporting

negative assurance (moderate assurance):
a statement that, having carried out a professional engagement, nothing has come to the public accountant's attention that would give reason to believe that matters under consideration do not meet specified suitable criteria

no assurance:
the public accountant provides zero assurance credibility because there is no independent verification of the data provided by the client; for example, compilation engagement

Standards Check

CAS 700 Forming an Opinion and Reporting on Financial Statements

35. When expressing an unmodified opinion on financial statements prepared in accordance with a fair presentation framework, the auditor's opinion shall, unless otherwise required by law or regulation, use one of the following phrases, which are regarded as being equivalent:
    (a) The financial statements present fairly, in all material respects, . . . in accordance with [the applicable financial reporting framework]; or
    (b) The financial statements give a true and fair view of . . . in accordance with [the applicable financial reporting framework]. (Ref: Para. A27–A33)

Source: *CPA Canada Handbook—Assurance,* 2014.

financial statement information are compilation engagements and specified procedures engagements. The practitioner is, therefore, not expressing a conclusion on the reliability of the statements. His or her involvement presumably adds accounting credibility to the financial statements even though there is no supporting evidence or audit assurance provided. For example, accounting credibility includes the use of correct account titles and format in the financial statements, but there is no verification of the accuracy of the underlying accounting records. (More details about compilation reports on unaudited financial statements are provided in Chapter 17.)

The professional credibility in accounting and tax services provided by PAs is the main reason for the rules of association. These rules provide guidance on avoiding association with misleading information and, thereby, assist in maintaining the reputation of the public accounting profession. The levels of assurance are shown in Exhibit 4–2. It should be noted that audit, review, and compilation engagements are intended to provide the specified assurance levels given in Exhibit 4–2. As we will see when discussing the disclaimer of opinion, under some conditions not even an audit engagement can provide much assurance.

The most important aspect of the concept of assurance levels is that it reflects the separate levels of evidence the PA has gathered to support the conclusions in the various types of assurance engagements. Compilation engagements provide no assurance because the PA is required to gather less evidence. The reason compilations are considered a no assurance engagement is because PAs are not required to gather any evidence

EXHIBIT 4-2

Levels of Assurance

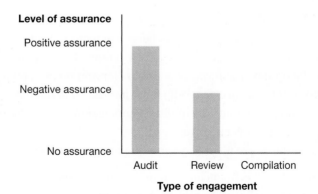

on the financial information. In any of these engagements, however, a PA's responsibility is to not be associated if they become aware that there is a reporting deficiency associated with the financial information. We cover PA responsibilities for review and compilations in more detail in Chapter 17.

Review Checkpoints

4-24   What is the most important distinction between an auditor's opinion on financial statements and other PA communications?

4-25   What is negative assurance? When is negative assurance permitted?

4-26   What is the difference between assurance and accounting credibility?

Auditor's Reports and Variations

LO4   Compare and contrast the scope and opinion paragraphs in an independent auditor's report.

In this section, we cover the various audit reports on management's financial statements. There are two broad categories: the standard unmodified report covered in CAS 700 and report reservations.

The standard unmodified report contains five basic segments: (1) the opinion segment, (2) the basis for opinion segment, (3) the key audit matters segment, (4) the management (or other preparer) and governance responsibility segment, and (5) the auditor responsibility paragraphs. An example is given in Exhibit 4–3. The technical details of this report were introduced in Chapter 2. The equivalent report used in the United States is given in Appendix 4A and is quite similar to the report used in Canada for audits before December 14, 2010, when Canada switched to CASs based on international audit standards. Appendix 4B gives an example unmodified report to be used before December 15, 2016. The before and after December 15, 2016, reports have many features in common, with the after December 15, 2016, report adding significant new paragraphs and related responsibilities. This expansion in auditor responsibilities can be viewed as attempts by the profession to reduce the expectations gap and to be more cooperative with users by providing more information on important matters identified in an audit.

Meaning of the Introductory, Opinion, Key Audit Matters, Scope, and Opinion Paragraphs

Many users understand the audit report by counting the paragraphs! Crude as this may seem, it makes some sense because each of the six standard paragraphs is supposed to convey the same message on all audits. The first place most analysts look in the client's annual report is the audit report, as any major problems in using the financial statements should be identified there.

Introductory and Opinion Paragraphs

The introductory paragraph declares that an audit has been conducted and identifies the financial statements. These identifications are important, because if a financial statement is not identified in this introductory paragraph, the opinion paragraph does not offer any opinion on it.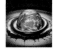

Users of audited financial statements are generally most interested in the opinion paragraph, which is actually one long sentence. This sentence contains the auditors' conclusions about the financial statements. It is the public manifestation of the private audit decision process.

The following reporting standards are incorporated in the opinion sentence:

1. The standard report states that the financial statements are presented fairly in all material respects in accordance with GAAP, such as IFRS or Canadian Accounting Standards for Private Enterprises (ASPE). Under CAS 700, general purpose financial statements using such GAAP are deemed capable of achieving

EXHIBIT 4-3

Independent Auditor's Report

To the Shareholders of . . .
Report on the Audit of the Financial Statements
Opinion

We have audited the financial statements of ABC Company (the Company), which comprise the statement of financial position as at December 31, 20X0, and the statement of comprehensive income, statement of changes in equity, and statement of cash flows for the year then ended, and notes to the financial statements, including a summary of significant accounting policies.

In our opinion, the accompanying financial statements present fairly, in all material respects, [*or give a true and fair view of*] the financial position of the Company as at December 31, 20X0, and [*of*] its financial performance and its cash flows for the year then ended in accordance with International Financial Reporting Standards (IFRS).

Basis for Opinion

We conducted our audit in accordance with CASs. Our responsibilities under those standards are further described in the *Auditor's Responsibilities for the Audit of the Financial Statements* section of our report. We are independent of the Company in accordance with the Provincial Ethics Standards Board for Accountants' *Code of Ethics for Professional Accountants* together with the ethical requirements that are relevant to our audit of the financial statements in [*jurisdiction*], and we have fulfilled our other ethical responsibilities in accordance with these requirements and the Code. We believe that the audit evidence we have obtained is sufficient and appropriate to provide a basis for our opinion.

Key Audit Matters

Key audit matters are those matters that, in our professional judgment, were of most significance in our audit of the financial statements of the current period. These matters were addressed in the context of our audit of the financial statements as a whole, and in forming our opinion, thereon, and we do not provide a separate opinion on these matters.

[*Description of each key audit matter in accordance with CAS 701.*]

Responsibilities of Management and Those Charged with Governance for the Financial Statements[1]

Management is responsible for the preparation and fair presentation of the financial statements in accordance with IFRS,[2] and for such internal control as management determines is necessary to enable the preparation of financial statements that are free from material misstatement, whether due to fraud or error.

In preparing the financial statements, management is responsible for assessing the Company's ability to continue as a going concern, disclosing, as applicable, matters related to going concern and using the going-concern basis of accounting unless management intends to liquidate the Company or to cease operations, or has no realistic alternative but to do so.

Those charged with governance are responsible for overseeing the Company's financial reporting process.

Auditors' Responsibilities for the Audit of the Financial Statements

Our objectives are to obtain reasonable assurance about whether the financial statements as a whole are free from material misstatement, whether due to fraud or error, and to issue an auditor's report that includes our opinion. Reasonable assurance is a high level of assurance but is not a guarantee that an audit conducted in accordance with CASs will always detect a material misstatement when it exists. Misstatements can arise from fraud or error and are considered material if, individually or in the aggregate, they could reasonably be expected to influence the economic decisions of users taken on the basis of these financial statements.

[*Additional description of auditor responsibilities is required here, or referenced to an appendix to the report, or reference can be made to a website of an appropriate authority that contains the description of the auditor's responsibilities.*]

The engagement partner on the audit resulting in this independent auditor's report is [name].

[*Signature in the name of the audit firm, the personal name of the auditor, or both, as appropriate for the particular jurisdiction*]

[*Auditor Address*]

[*Date*]

Source: *CPA Canada Handbook—Assurance*, 2015, CAS 700 (adapted from Appendix, Illustration 1).

fairness of presentation under certain conditions. General purpose financial reporting implies broad principles that are a basis for developing and applying policies consistent with the concepts underlying the requirements of the framework. Such a framework is also referred to as an "acceptable financial reporting framework," and it provides a proper context for evaluating fairness of presentation (CAS 210). Note that in the Exhibit 4–3 version of the report, the opinion paragraph has two options regarding fairness of presentation—the traditional one (present fairly) and the "true and fair" wording common in Europe.

2.   The standard report, by its silence, regards the financial statement disclosures as reasonably adequate. This is part of the fairness criteria noted in item 1.

3.   The standard report contains an expression of opinion regarding the financial statements.

4.   An overall opinion is expressed in the standard report, so reasons for not expressing an opinion need not be stated.

Key Audit Matters Paragraph

As noted in Chapter 2, this new paragraph could greatly increase auditor responsibilities. Here the auditor is required to identify key audit matters in the engagement, such as difficulties in auditing going-concern issues; accounting estimates with significant risks; and issues of significant public interest, such as financial institutions and charities. In the United Kingdom, where this requirement has been in place for a few years, key matters of interest that are frequently disclosed in the auditor's report include materiality and basis for its calculation, the level of unadjusted audit differences, and the auditors' most significant assessments of risks of material misstatement and how they were dealt with. These include material uncertainties with respect to going concern and inherent limitations on the auditor's ability to detect material misstatements due to future events (CAS 570, para. 6). They may also include disclosures of key assumptions, such the disclosure of the range of possible outcomes and other qualitative and quantitative disclosures relating to key sources of estimation uncertainty or critical accounting estimates, as part of addressing why the matter was one of significance in the audit and how the matter was addressed in the audit (CAS 701, para. A41). See the box below for illustrative excerpts of key matters by U.K. auditors. Such key matter disclosures could greatly assist users in understanding the risks facing the reporting entity's business and could potentially represent an important new source of information to analysts in interpreting the financial statements. This way, auditing standards attempt to close the expectations gap. But such disclosure of audit matters could also greatly expand auditor responsibilities and require auditors to get more training in analytical techniques useful to users and to learn to more effectively communicate risks and uncertainties. The key matters paragraph requirements may also help auditors better address questionable or unethical reporting of the type used by Nortel, as discussed in Chapter 2.

Illustrative Excerpts of Key Matters from U.K. Audits

From Audit Report on the 2013 Annual Report of Rolls-Royce Holdings PLC

Findings on the valuation of Daimler AG's put option: "We found that the resulting estimate was acceptable but mildly optimistic resulting in a somewhat lower liability being recorded than might otherwise have been the case."

From Audit Report on the 2014 Annual Report of Vodafone Group PLC

Verizon disposal and changes to materiality: "Profit before tax has been adjusted for separately disclosed items, notably impairment charges and trading results of Verizon Wireless prior to its classification as a discontinued operation. We consider this adjusted measure to be a key driver of business value and a focus for shareholders. Materiality is lower for the year ended 31 March 2013 primarily as a result of the disposal of Verizon Wireless."

Management's and Governance Responsibility Paragraphs

The fifth and sixth paragraphs of the auditor's report give notice of management's (or other preparer's) responsibility to prepare the financial statements in conformity with a fair presentation reporting framework. This includes designing, implementing, and maintaining internal control; selecting and applying appropriate accounting policies; making accounting estimates that are reasonable in the circumstances; and primary responsibility for avoiding fraudulent financial reporting. The seventh paragraph emphasizes corporate governance's role in overseeing the financial reporting process.

Standards Check

CAS 210 Agreeing the Terms of Audit Engagements

CA8a. In Canada, incorporating or other governing legislation often specifies that GAAP be used when preparing general purpose financial statements. Such legislation usually indicates that GAAP means "the standards set out in the *CPA Canada Handbook.*" The *Handbook* contains the accounting standards promulgated by the Accounting Standards Board and the Public Sector Accounting Standards Board. In Canada, these standards are generally accepted and are relevant in determining the acceptability of the applicable financial reporting framework even when incorporating or other governing legislation does not specify that GAAP be used when preparing general purpose financial statements. [This is a Canadian-only paragraph. There is no equivalent paragraph in corresponding ISA 210.]

CA8b. Some legislation and regulation also permits certain reporting issuers to use International Financial Reporting Standards, promulgated by the International Accounting Standards Board, or U.S. GAAP, promulgated by the U.S. Financial Accounting Standards Board.

Source: *CPA Canada Handbook—Assurance,* 2014.

Auditor's Responsibility Paragraphs

Auditors must render a fair presentation of their own work, as well as an opinion on the financial statements. These paragraphs of the report, also referred to as the scope paragraphs, are the auditor's report of the character of the work in the audit. This portion of the report is vitally important for disclosure of the quality and extent of the audit itself. Note that it makes explicit the auditor's responsibility to detect fraudulent reporting, abide by ethical standards, and appropriately support the opinion with audit evidence.

The sentence "We conducted our audit in accordance with Canadian generally accepted auditing standards" refers primarily to the general and the examination standards. Its message is that (1) the auditors were trained and proficient, (2) the auditors were independent, (3) due professional care was exercised, (4) the work was planned and supervised, (5) a sufficient understanding of the internal control structure was obtained, and (6) sufficient appropriate evidential matter was obtained. To the extent that one or more of these standards is not actually satisfied during an audit, the scope paragraphs must be qualified. A qualification means that an explanation of exactly which standard was not satisfied is added. In practice, auditors always change the standard opinion paragraph language when the scope paragraph is qualified.

The scope paragraphs contain general descriptions of the audit work in addition to the reference to Canadian auditing standards. They make special mention of the auditors' assessment of the choice of accounting principles and the evaluation of the overall financial statement presentation. It also lists any conditions that prevented the auditor from getting sufficient appropriate evidence, things that might also be areas for improvement in the client's system of recordkeeping.

The new audit reporting standard also requires the disclosure of the following detailed responsibilities either in the report itself, referenced in an appendix to the report, or by reference to an official website listing the responsibilities:

As part of an audit in accordance with CASs, we exercise professional judgment and maintain professional skepticism throughout the audit. We also

- Identify and assess the risks of material misstatement of the financial statements, whether due to fraud or error; design and perform audit procedures responsive to those risks; and obtain audit evidence that is sufficient and appropriate to provide a basis for our opinion. The risk of not detecting a material misstatement resulting from fraud is higher than for one resulting from error, as fraud may involve collusion, forgery, intentional omissions, misrepresentations, or the override of internal control.
- Obtain an understanding of internal control relevant to the audit in order to design audit procedures that are appropriate in the circumstances, but not for the purpose of expressing an opinion on the effectiveness of the Company's internal control.[3]
- Evaluate the appropriateness of accounting policies used and the reasonableness of accounting estimates and related disclosures made by management.
- Conclude on the appropriateness of management's use of the going-concern basis of accounting and, based on the audit evidence obtained, whether a material uncertainty exists related to events or conditions that may cast significant doubt on the Company's ability to continue as a going concern. If we conclude that a material uncertainty exists, we are required to draw attention in our auditor's report to the related disclosures in the financial statements or, if such disclosures are inadequate, to modify our opinion. Our conclusions are based on the audit evidence obtained up to the date of our auditor's report. However, future events or conditions may cause the Company to cease to continue as a going concern.
- Evaluate the overall presentation, structure, and content of the financial statements, including the disclosures, and whether the financial statements represent the underlying transactions and events in a manner that achieves fair presentation.

We communicate with those charged with governance regarding, among other matters, the planned scope and timing of the audit and significant audit findings, including any significant deficiencies in internal control that we identify during our audit.

We also provide those charged with governance with a statement that we have complied with relevant ethical requirements regarding independence, and to communicate with them all relationships and other matters that may reasonably be thought to bear on our independence, and where applicable, related safeguards.

From the matters communicated with those charged with governance, we determine those matters that were of most significance in the audit of the financial statements of the current period and are therefore the key audit matters. We describe these matters in our auditor's report unless law or regulation precludes public disclosure about the matter or when, in extremely rare circumstances, we determine that a matter should not be communicated in our report because the adverse consequences of doing so would reasonably be expected to outweigh the public interest benefits of such communication.

Source: *CPA Canada Handbook—Assurance*, 2015, CAS 700 (adapted from Appendix, Illustration 1).

The above points illustrate the importance of critical thinking and professional judgment in determining the acceptability of a financial reporting framework. Essentially, auditors are expected to be familiar with both the detailed accounting rules and the basic principles and concepts underlying them. These allow the auditor to determine if the rules are applicable in a specific auditee context. In particular, auditors must be sure that the particular rule applied is appropriate and not misleading in the context. This is the essence of the fairness of presentation framework of CAS 700.

Standards Check

CAS 210 Agreeing the Terms of Audit Engagements

6. In order to establish whether the preconditions for an audit are present, the auditor shall

(a) Determine whether the financial reporting framework to be applied in the preparation of the financial statements is acceptable; and (Ref: Para. A2–A10)

A2. For purposes of the CASs, the applicable financial reporting framework provides the criteria the auditor uses to audit the financial statements, including, where relevant, their fair presentation.

A3. Without an acceptable financial reporting framework, management does not have an appropriate basis for the preparation of the financial statements and the auditor does not have suitable criteria for auditing the financial statements.

A4. Factors that are relevant to the auditor's determination of the acceptability of the financial reporting framework to be applied in the preparation of the financial statements include

• The nature of the entity (for example, whether it is a business enterprise, a public sector entity, or a not-for-profit organization);

• The purpose of the financial statements (for example, whether they are prepared to meet the common financial information needs of a wide range of users or the financial information needs of specific users); [*Note: These are called "general purpose frameworks" and "special purpose frameworks," respectively.*]

• The nature of the financial statements (for example, whether the financial statements are a complete set of financial statements or a single financial statement); and

• Whether law or regulation prescribes the applicable financial reporting framework.

A8. At present, there is no objective and authoritative basis that has been generally recognized globally for judging the acceptability of general purpose frameworks. In the absence of such a basis, financial reporting standards established by organizations that are authorized or recognized to promulgate standards to be used by certain types of entities are presumed to be acceptable for general purpose financial statements prepared by such entities. . . . Examples of such financial reporting standards include

• International Financial Reporting Standards, and

• Accounting principles promulgated by an authorized or recognized standards setting organization in a particular jurisdiction, provided the organization follows an established and transparent process involving deliberation and consideration of the views of a wide range of stakeholders. [*Note: CPA Canada's ASPE is one of these acceptable frameworks.*]

Source: *CPA Canada Handbook–Assurance,* 2015.

With regard to the opinion reservations of CAS 705, other examples later in this chapter will show how auditors assert that an opinion cannot be expressed (disclaimer of opinion) or how audit responsibility can be limited (qualified opinion).

In the reporting standards, the term *financial statements* includes not only the traditional balance sheet, income statement, and cash flow statement but also all the footnote disclosures and additional information (e.g., earnings per share calculations) that are integral to the basic financial presentation required by GAAP. The report comments on consistency only when accounting principles have been changed and disclosures are considered inadequate. The adequacy of disclosures may be judged by GAAP requirements, but auditors must also be sensitive to the information needs of investors, creditors, and other users when considering information that is not explicitly required by GAAP. Disgruntled investors often use the "lack of informative disclosure" criterion as a basis for lawsuits. Users feel they have been misled in that case, and auditors need to be sensitized to these expectations. This is part of the context of financial reporting in a

Standards Check

CAS 210 Agreeing the Terms of Audit Engagements

3. Acceptable financial reporting frameworks normally exhibit the following attributes that result in information provided in financial statements that is useful to the intended users:

   (a) Relevance, in that the information provided in the financial statements is relevant to the nature of the entity and the purpose of the financial statements. For example, in the case of a business enterprise that prepares general purpose financial statements, relevance is assessed in terms of the information necessary to meet the common financial information needs of a wide range of users in making economic decisions. These needs are ordinarily met by presenting the financial position, financial performance, and cash flows of the business enterprise.

   (b) Completeness, in that transactions and events, account balances, and disclosures that could affect conclusions based on the financial statements are not omitted.

   (c) Reliability, in that the information provided in the financial statements

      (i) Where applicable, reflects the economic substance of events and transactions and not merely their legal form; and

      (ii) Results in reasonably consistent evaluation, measurement, presentation, and disclosure, when used in similar circumstances.

   (d) Neutrality, in that it contributes to information in the financial statements that is free from bias.

   (e) Understandability, in that the information in the financial statements is clear and comprehensive and not subject to significantly different interpretation.

Source: *CPA Canada Handbook—Assurance*, 2015.

particular engagement discussed in CAS 700. Critical thinking can aid in this understanding of the unique features of specific engagements, and moral imagination is an example of anticipating user needs for the engagement.

Standards Check

CAS 700 Forming an Opinion and Reporting on Financial Statements

13. In particular, the auditor shall evaluate whether, in view of the requirements of the applicable financial reporting framework,

   (a) The financial statements adequately disclose the significant accounting policies selected and applied;

   (b) The accounting policies selected and applied are consistent with the applicable financial reporting framework and are appropriate;

   (c) The accounting estimates made by management are reasonable;

   (d) The information presented in the financial statements is relevant, reliable, comparable, and understandable;

   (e) The financial statements provide adequate disclosures to enable the intended users to understand the effect of material transactions and events on the information conveyed in the financial statements; and (Ref: Para. A4)

   (f) The terminology used in the financial statements, including the title of each financial statement, is appropriate.

Source: *CPA Canada Handbook—Assurance*, 2015.

The context of financial reporting usually affects the audit report decision in two ways. First, additional disclosures beyond those required by specific accounting rules may be needed in order for the financial reporting not to be misleading. Second, mechanical application of a specific accounting rule may give misleading results in some circumstances, causing the auditor to insist on deviating from that rule in order to get a presentation that is not misleading. In both cases, the aim is to be consistent with the fairness of presentation framework.

Standards Check

CAS 700 Forming an Opinion and Reporting on Financial Statements

Definitions

7. For purposes of the CASs, the following terms have the meanings attributed below:

   (a) General purpose financial statements—Financial statements prepared in accordance with a general purpose framework. *[Note: CAS 800 deals with audit reports for "special purpose" frameworks.]*

   (b) General purpose framework—A financial reporting framework designed to meet the common financial information needs of a wide range of users. The financial reporting framework may be a fair presentation framework or a compliance framework. The term *fair presentation framework* is used to refer to a financial reporting framework that requires compliance with the requirements of the framework and

   (i) Acknowledges explicitly or implicitly that, to achieve fair presentation of the financial statements, it may be necessary for management to provide disclosures beyond those specifically required by the framework; or

   (ii) Acknowledges explicitly that it may be necessary for management to depart from a requirement of the framework to achieve fair presentation of the financial statements. Such departures are expected to be necessary only in extremely rare circumstances.

   The term *compliance framework* is used to refer to a financial reporting framework that requires compliance with the requirements of the framework, but does not contain the acknowledgements in (i) or (ii) above.

Source: *CPA Canada Handbook—Assurance*, 2015.

Reservation in the Audit Report

The following sections of this chapter explain major variations on the standard report, often referred to as **reservations**. There are two basic reasons for giving a report that contains other than the standard, unmodified audit opinion.

When the financial statements contain a departure from GAAP, including inadequate disclosure, the auditors must choose between a qualified opinion and an adverse opinion. The choice depends on the materiality (significance) and pervasiveness of the effect of the GAAP departure. This is frequently referred to as an **accounting deficiency reservation**. When there is a scope limitation (extent of audit work has been limited), and the auditors have not been able to obtain sufficient appropriate evidence on a particular account balance or disclosure, the auditors must choose between a qualified opinion and a disclaimer of opinion. The choice depends on the materiality of the matter for which evidence is not sufficient. A scope limitation reservation is also frequently referred to as an **audit deficiency reservation**.

The chart below summarizes the types of audit opinions introduced in this chapter: the unmodified, or "clean" audit report under CAS 700, and three main types of modified reports under CAS 705.

TYPES OF AUDIT OPINIONS IN CAS 700, 705			
	SEVERITY OF PROBLEM		
	NOT MATERIAL	MATERIAL BUT NOT PERVASIVE	MATERIAL AND PERVASIVE
Nature of Audit Problem			
GAAP departure	Unmodified	Qualified for GAAP	Adverse opinion
Scope limitation	Unmodified	Qualified for scope	Disclaimer of opinion

reservations:
major variations on the standard audit report

accounting deficiency reservation:
a reservation based on a known GAAP departure

audit deficiency reservation:
a reservation based on insufficient audit evidence (scope restriction)

Standards Check

CAS 700 Forming an Opinion and Reporting on Financial Statements

Definitions

7. (c) Unmodified opinion—The opinion expressed by the auditor when the auditor concludes that the financial statements are prepared, in all material respects, in accordance with the applicable financial reporting framework.

CAS 705 Modifications to the Opinion in the Independent Auditor's Report

Definitions

5. (b) Modified opinion—A qualified opinion, an adverse opinion, or a disclaimer of opinion.

Source: *CPA Canada Handbook—Assurance*, 2014.

Effects of Lack of Independence

 Independence is the foundation of the audit function. When independence is lacking, an audit in accordance with GAAS is impossible, and the auditors should resign or not accept an audit engagement. An audit does not simply require the application of the tools, techniques, and procedures of auditing; it also requires independence in mental attitude of the auditors. This idea is reflected in the general standard and codes of professional ethics, an example of which is Rule 204, entitled "Independence."

204.1 (Independence In) Assurance and Specified Auditing Procedures Engagements

A member or firm who engages or participates in an engagement (a) to issue a written communication under the terms of an assurance engagement, or (b) to issue a report on the results of applying specified auditing procedures, shall be and remain independent such that the member, firm, and members of the firm shall be and remain free of any influence, interest, or relationship that, in respect of the engagement, impairs the professional judgment or objectivity of the member, firm, or member of the firm or that, in the view of a reasonable observer, would impair the professional judgment or objectivity of the member, firm, or member of the firm.

This rule applies to the auditors of financial statements. The criteria for determining independence are discussed in Chapter 4.

Source: CPA Ontario.

Review Checkpoints

4-27   Think about the standard unmodified introductory and scope paragraphs. What do they identify as the objects of the audit? What is meant by the sentence, "We conducted our audit in accordance with Canadian generally accepted auditing standards"?

4-28   What are the major reasons for departures from the unmodified audit opinion?

4-29   If an auditor is not independent with respect to an auditee company, what should he or she do?

4-30   Why is independence important for auditors?

Audit Report Reservations

LO5   For a given set of accounting facts and audit circumstances, analyze qualified, adverse, and disclaimer audit reports.

LO6   Determine the effects of materiality and uncertainty on audit report choices.

Audit reports containing other than the standard unmodified audit opinion are called audit report reservations. The most common report reservations are called **qualified reports** because they contain an opinion paragraph that does not give the positive assurance that everything in the financial statements is in conformity with GAAP. There are two basic types of qualified reports: GAAP departure reports and scope limitation reports.

Generally Accepted Accounting Principles Departure Reports

For various reasons, a company's management can decide to present financial statements containing an accounting treatment or disclosure that is not in conformity with GAAP. They may not wish to capitalize leases and show the related debt, may calculate earnings per share incorrectly, may not accrue unbilled revenue at the end of a period, may make unreasonable accounting estimates, or may be reluctant to disclose all the known details of a contingency. Whatever the reason for the departure from GAAP, the auditor must decide on the type of opinion to render.

If the departure is immaterial or insignificant, it can be treated as if it did not exist and the audit opinion can be unmodified. What is considered immaterial under the circumstances is a matter of the auditor's professional judgment. Critical thinking can help structure this decision.

If, in the auditor's judgment, the departure is material enough to potentially affect users' decisions based on the financial statements, the opinion must be qualified. In this case, the qualification takes the "except for" language form. The opinion sentence begins, "In my opinion, except for the [nature of the GAAP departure], the financial statements present fairly, in all material respects . . . in accordance with Canadian generally accepted accounting principles." This style of qualification identifies the particular departure but says that the financial statements are otherwise in conformity with GAAP. The nature of the GAAP departure must be explained in a separate paragraph (called the *basis of modification paragraph*) placed immediately after the opinion paragraph, as covered by CAS 705, paragraphs 16–18. The introductory and auditor responsibilities (scope) paragraphs are the same as in the standard unmodified report. After all, the audit was performed without limitation, and the auditors have sufficient appropriate evidence about the financial statements, including the GAAP departure.

GAAP departure report examples are hard to find in published financial statements. Most published statements come under the jurisdiction of the provincial securities commissions, which require public companies to file financial statements without any departures from GAAP. Exhibit 4–4 shows a GAAP departure due to a failure to record depreciation.

If the GAAP departures are either (1) much more material, or "so significant that they overshadow the financial statements," or (2) pervasive, affecting numerous accounts and financial statement relationships, there is a condition of **pervasive materiality**, and an adverse opinion should be given. An adverse opinion is exactly

qualified reports:
audit reports that contain an opinion paragraph that does not give the positive assurance that everything in the financial statements is in conformity with generally accepted accounting principles

pervasive materiality:
departures from generally accepted accounting principles that are so significant that they overshadow the financial statements or affect numerous accounts and financial statement relationships

---

EXHIBIT 4–4

Departure from Generally Accepted Accounting Principles Due to a Failure to Record Depreciation

Departure from generally accepted accounting principles—no depreciation recorded. When the auditor has determined that a qualification is the type of reservation required, the following wording may be appropriate.

AUDITOR'S REPORT

To the Shareholders of ....

[The introductory, management responsibility, and auditor responsibility paragraphs are the same as in the unmodified report (see Exhibit 4–3). A basis of modification paragraph is added to provide more details immediately following the opinion paragraph as follows.]

Qualified Opinion

In my opinion, except for the effects of the failure to record depreciation as described in the Basis for Qualified Opinion paragraph, these financial statements present fairly, in all material respects, the financial position of the company as at ...., 20...., and the results of its operations and the cash flows for the year then ended in accordance with International Financial Reporting Standards.

Basis for Qualified Opinion

Note .... describes the depreciation policy with respect to the company's manufacturing plants and equipment. The note also indicates that the company is not depreciating its head office building, which it acquired 5 years ago, on the grounds that it is not a producing asset and is maintaining its value as a potential rental or resale property. In this respect the financial statements are not in accordance with generally accepted accounting principles. The estimated useful life of similar buildings is usually considered to be between 30 and 40 years. If depreciation had been provided on the basis of an estimated useful life of, say, 35 years, depreciation for the current year would have been increased by $.......... (20....$..........), net income after taxes would have been decreased by $..........(20....$..........), accumulated depreciation would have been increased by $..........(20....$..........), and the balance of deferred income taxes and the closing balance of retained earnings would have been reduced by $..........(20....$..........) and $..........(20....$..........), respectively.

(signed)....................

PUBLIC ACCOUNTANT

Source: *CPA Canada Handbook—Assurance*, 2014, CAS 705 (adapted from Appendix Illustration 1).

---

the opposite of the unmodified opinion. In this type of opinion, auditors say the financial statements do not fairly present the financial position, results of operations, and changes in financial position in conformity with GAAP. When this opinion is given, all the substantive reasons for it must be disclosed in the basis of modification paragraph(s), as covered by *CPA Canada Handbook* CAS 705. The introductory and scope paragraphs should not be modified because, in order to decide to use the adverse opinion, the audit team must possess all evidence necessary to reach the decision. Pervasive materiality is closely related to the overall materiality of CAS 320. Specifically, pervasive materiality can greatly exceed overall materiality and may affect many line items in the financial statements. Pervasive materiality of misstatement in the financial statements results in a virtually guaranteed adverse opinion. For many auditors, misstatements in excess of overall materiality warrant an adverse opinion. This is another area of professional judgment. At the end of the chapter we summarize the effects of materiality concepts on the audit report.

Because of the securities commission requirements, adverse opinions are hard to find. The example in Exhibit 4–5 is due to a disagreement between the auditor and management on the carrying value of a long-term investment. That departure from GAAP is considered to be highly or pervasively material, or well in excess of what would be considered material for an "except for" qualification.

Practically speaking, auditors require more evidence to support an adverse opinion than to support an unmodified opinion. Perhaps this can be attributed to auditors' reluctance to be bearers of bad news. However, audit standards are quite clear that if an auditor has a basis for an adverse opinion, the uncomfortable position cannot be relieved by giving a disclaimer of opinion. GAAP departure reports cover those situations where the auditor knows the true state of affairs—there is or there is not an accounting deficiency. The next section will outline situations where the auditor does not know the true state of affairs. These are situations where there are limitations on the scope of the auditors' work.

EXHIBIT 4–5

Adverse Report

Departure from generally accepted accounting principles—disagreement on carrying value of a long-term investment.

[When the auditor has determined that an adverse opinion is the type of reservation required, the following wording may be appropriate. (For an adverse opinion, "present fairly" in the opinion paragraph need not be modified with the phrase "in all material respects.")]

INDEPENDENT AUDITOR'S REPORT

To the Shareholders of....................

[The introductory, management, governance responsibility, and auditor responsibilities paragraphs are the same as in the unmodified report (see Exhibit 4–3). A new basis of modification paragraph is added after the scope paragraphs to provide more details immediately following the opinion paragraph as follows.]

Adverse Opinion

In my opinion, because the write-down has not been made for the significant decline in value of the investment described in the preceding paragraph, these financial statements do not present fairly the financial position of the company as at ...., 20...., and the results of its operations and the cash flows for the year then ended in accordance with International Financial Reporting Standards.

Basis for Adverse Opinion

The company's investment in X Company Ltd., its only asset, which is carried at a cost of $10,000,000, has declined in value to an amount of $5,850,000. The loss in the value of this investment, in my opinion, is other than a temporary decline and in such circumstances generally accepted accounting principles require that the investment be written down to recognize the loss. If this decline in value had been recognized, the investment, net income for the year, and retained earnings would have been reduced by $4,150,000.

City   **(signed)**....................

Date   **PUBLIC ACCOUNTANT**

Source: *CPA Canada Handbook—Assurance*, 2015, CAS 705 (adapted from Appendix Illustration 2).

Review Checkpoints

4-31   What extent of evidence is required as a basis for the unmodified opinion? for an adverse opinion? for an opinion qualified for GAAP departure?

4-32   What effect does the materiality of a GAAP departure have on the auditor's reporting decision?

Scope Limitation Reports

Auditors are in the most comfortable position when they have all the evidence needed to make a report decision—whether the opinion is to be unmodified, adverse, or qualified. There are two kinds of situations, however, that can result in a **scope limitation**—a condition where the auditors are unable to obtain sufficient appropriate evidence: (1) management deliberately refuses to let auditors perform some procedures, or (2) circumstances, such as late appointment of the auditor, make it impossible for some procedures to be performed.

If management's refusal or the circumstances affect the audit in a minor, immaterial way, or if sufficient appropriate evidence can be obtained by other means, the audit can be considered to be unaffected, and the opinion can be unmodified as if the limitation had never occurred. Management's deliberate refusal to give access to documents or to otherwise limit audit procedures is the most serious condition. It casts doubt on management's integrity. (Why is management refusing access or limiting the work?) In most such cases, the audit report is qualified or an opinion is disclaimed, depending upon the materiality of the financial items affected.

scope limitation:

a condition where auditors are unable to obtain sufficient appropriate evidence

Exhibit 4–6 (A and B) shows two reports that illustrate the auditors' alternatives. The failure to take physical counts of inventory, as shown, might have been a deliberate management action, or it might have resulted from other circumstances, such as the company's not anticipating the need for an audit and appointing the auditor after the latest year-end.

In Exhibit 4–6A, the opinion is modified. Here, the lack of evidence is considered material, but not pervasively or highly material enough (i.e., exceeding overall materiality) to overwhelm the meaning of modified audit opinion and the usefulness of the remainder of the financial statements. The proper qualification meaning here is: "In our opinion, except for the effects of adjustments, if any, as might have been determined to be necessary had we been able to examine evidence regarding the inventories, the financial statements present fairly, in all material respects, . . . in conformity with generally accepted accounting principles." This report "carves out" the inventory from the audit reporting responsibility, thus taking no audit responsibility for this part of the financial statements.

Note that the introductory, management, governance responsibilities, and key audit matters paragraphs in Exhibit 4–6A are the same as for an unmodified report. However, the last auditor's responsibility paragraph is modified because the audit was not completed entirely in accordance with GAAS. Specifically, sufficient appropriate evidence about the inventories was not obtained. Whenever the scope has been affected by an important omission of audit work, the opinion paragraph should also be qualified.

The situation in Exhibit 4–6B is considered fatal to the audit opinion. In this case, the inventories are too large and too important to say "except for adjustments, if any." The audit report must then be a disclaimer of opinion.

It is important to remember that scope limitation reservations arise only when it is not possible to obtain compensating assurance from alternative audit procedures. If, for example, in Exhibits 4–6A and B the auditor had been able to satisfy himself or herself through alternative procedures that the inventory was materially accurate, then an unmodified opinion could have been issued for both exhibits. Thus, scope limitation reports are issued only if, in the auditor's judgment, the alternative procedures do not compensate for the restriction.

To summarize, we can view audit reservations as arising from two types of circumstances: audit deficiencies, due to scope limitations, and accounting deficiencies, resulting from a GAAP departure. Audit deficiencies can result in either a qualification or a disclaimer of opinion, depending on the significance of the scope limitation. In an audit deficiency reservation, both the scope and opinion paragraphs are affected. When there is an audit deficiency, the auditor does not have enough evidence or does not know the true state of affairs. An accounting deficiency, on the other hand, can result in either a qualification or an adverse opinion, depending on the significance of the GAAP departure. In an accounting deficiency reservation, only the opinion paragraph is affected. To reach a conclusion about an accounting deficiency, the auditor must have sufficient appropriate evidence to support the conclusion. In the situation of an accounting deficiency report modification, the auditor is in a position to know the true state of affairs and presents that truth in as fair a manner as possible. This may require additional disclosures in the notes to the financial statements going beyond GAAP requirements, as illustrated in the Continental Vending case of Chapter 3. These types of judgments can be very difficult and complex, and they may go beyond the standards. This sensitivity to user needs, and clear communication in response to these needs, are an important reason that ethical issues are becoming more prominent in auditing and financial reporting. To help address these increased auditor responsibilities, we introduced critical thinking and principles-based reasoning in Chapter 3.

Other Responsibilities with a Disclaimer

A disclaimer of opinion because of severe scope limitation or because of association with unaudited financial statements carries some additional reporting responsibilities. In addition to the disclaimer, these rules should be followed:

- If the PA should learn that the statements are not in conformity with generally accepted accounting principles (including adequate disclosures), the departures should be explained in the disclaimer.
- If prior years' unaudited statements are presented, the disclaimer should cover them as well as the current-year statement.

EXHIBIT 4-6A

Scope Limitation Reports

QUALIFIED OPINION

Scope limitation—The auditor is appointed during the year and is unable to observe the inventory count at the beginning of the year. (It is assumed that the prior year's figures were unaudited and that the auditor was satisfied with respect to all other aspects of inventories and all other opening figures.) When the auditor has determined that a qualification is the type of reservation required, the following wording may be appropriate.

INDEPENDENT AUDITOR'S REPORT

[The introductory, management, governance, and audit responsibilities paragraphs are the same as in the unmodified report (see Exhibit 4–3). But the qualified opinion and the basis for the qualified opinion have been changed.]

Qualified Opinion

In our opinion, except for the possible effects of the matter described in the Basis for Qualified Opinion paragraph, the financial statements present fairly, in all material respects, the financial position of ABC Company as at December 31, 20XX, and its financial performance and its cash flows for the year then ended in accordance with International Financial Reporting Standards

Basis for Qualified Opinion

Because we were appointed auditor of ABC Company during the current year, we were not able to observe the counting of physical inventories at the beginning of the year nor satisfy ourselves concerning those inventory quantities by alternative means. Since opening inventories enter into the determination of the results of operations and cash flows, we were unable to determine whether adjustments to cost of sales, income taxes, net income for the year, opening retained earnings, and cash provided from operations might be necessary.

We conducted our audit in accordance with CASs. Our responsibilities under those standards are further described in the *Auditor's Responsibilities for the Audit of the Financial Statements* section of our report. We are independent of the Company in accordance with the Provincial Ethics Standards Board for Accountants' *Code of Ethics for Professional Accountants* together with the ethical requirements that are relevant to our audit of the financial statements in *[jurisdiction]*, and we have fulfilled our other ethical responsibilities in accordance with these requirements and the Code. We believe that the audit evidence we have obtained is sufficient and appropriate to provide a basis for our qualified opinion.

Key Audit Matters

Key audit matters are those matters that, in our professional judgment, were of most significance in our audit of the financial statements of the current period. These matters were addressed in the context of our audit of the financial statements as a whole, and in forming our opinion, thereon, and we do not provide a separate opinion on these matters. In addition to the matter described in the Basis for Qualified Opinion section, we have determined matters described below to be the key matters to be communicated in our report.

[Description of each key audit matter in accordance with CAS 701.]

City   **(signed).....................**

Date   **PUBLIC ACCOUNTANT**

Source: *CPA Canada Handbook—Assurance*, 2014, CAS 705 (adapted from Appendix Illustration 3).

It should be stressed that both auditor and client work to avoid a report reservation. It may take much discussion and negotiation between the auditor and client management to do this. This negotiation is discussed in more detail in Chapter 16, after we have considered the topic of available evidence at the end of the engagement.

Exhibit 4–7 summarizes the audit decision process in arriving at either some type of reservation (far right column) or an unqualified opinion (far left column). Make sure you understand the reasoning behind the paths shown in this exhibit.

EXHIBIT 4–6B

Scope Limitation Reports

DISCLAIMER OF OPINION

Scope limitation—the physical inventory count was not observed by the auditor and there are serious deficiencies in the accounting records and in the system of internal control over inventory.

[When the auditor has determined that a denial of opinion is the type of reservation required, the following wording may be appropriate. (For a disclaimer of opinion, "presented fairly" in the opinion paragraph need not be modified with the phrase "in all material respects.")]

INDEPENDENT AUDITOR'S REPORT

To the Shareholders of.....................

[The introductory, management, and governance responsibility paragraphs are the same as in the unmodified report (see Exhibit 4–3). The Auditor Responsibility and opinion paragraphs are modified, and a Basis for Disclaimer of Opinion paragraph is added after providing the disclaimer of opinion.]

Disclaimer of Opinion

We do not express an opinion on the financial statements. Because of the significance of the matter described in the Basis for Disclaimer of Opinion paragraph, we have not been able to obtain sufficient appropriate audit evidence to provide a basis for an audit opinion.

Basis for Disclaimer of Opinion

The company's investment in inventory is carried at XXX on the company's statement of financial position, which represents over 90% of the company's net assets as at December 31, 20XX. We were not able to observe all physical inventories due to limitations placed on the scope of our work by the company's management. As a result, we were unable to determine whether any adjustments were necessary in respect of the company's assets at year-end, expenses and net income for the year, and retained earnings at year-end.

Auditor's Responsibilities

Our responsibility is to express an opinion on these financial statements based on conducting the audit in accordance with Canadian generally accepted auditing standards. Because of the matter described in the Basis for Disclaimer of Opinion paragraph, however, we were not able to obtain sufficient appropriate audit evidence to provide a basis for an audit opinion.

We are independent of the Company in accordance with the Provincial Ethics Standards Board for Accountants' *Code of Ethics for Professional Accountants* together with the ethical requirements that are relevant to our audit of the financial statements in *[jurisdiction]*, and we have fulfilled our other ethical responsibilities in accordance with these requirements and the Code.

City   **(signed)**.....................

Date   **PUBLIC ACCOUNTANT**

Source: *CPA Canada Handbook—Assurance*, 2014, CAS 705 (adapted from Appendix Illustration 4).

Review Checkpoints

4-33 What are the differences between a report qualified for a scope limitation and a standard unmodified report?

4-34 What are the differences between a report in which the opinion is disclaimed because of scope limitation and a standard unmodified report?

4-35 The auditor knows about the client's situation for which opinions? Explain.

4-36 Explain the effect of materiality or pervasive materiality on an auditor report when the client uses an accounting method that departs from GAAP.

4-37 Explain the effect of pervasive materiality on an auditor report when there is a scope limitation.

4-38 Explain the effect of pervasive materiality on an auditor report when there is a material uncertainty associated with the financial statements.

4-39 Identify the levels of assurance associated with auditor reports.

4-40 Under what conditions would an auditor use an emphasis of matter paragraph?

EXHIBIT 4-7

Audit Report Decision Process

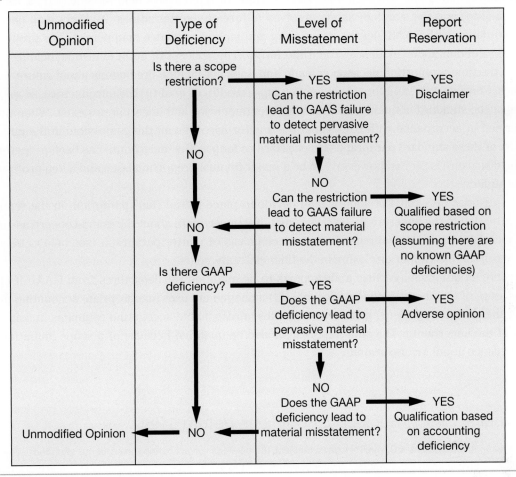

Significant Matter Paragraphs

LO7   Explain the purpose of significant matter paragraphs.

In previous sections of this chapter, you studied scope limitations in which either management or circumstances prevented the auditors from obtaining sufficient appropriate evidence about a part of the financial statements. A different type of problem arises when client uncertainties exist. We will refer to these as accounting uncertainties because they do not arise from scope limitations. Instead, they are related to inexact measurements of accounting values or **accounting measurement uncertainties** of accounting standards. In the IFRS conceptual framework, measurement uncertainty characterizes the reliability of the measurement. A good example of an accounting uncertainty is an accounting contingency, which is defined in the *Handbook,* paragraph 3290.02 (ASPE, or IFRS/IAS 37):

A contingency is . . . an existing condition, or situation, involving uncertainty as to possible gain ("gain contingency") or loss ("loss contingency") to an enterprise that will ultimately be resolved when one or more future events occur or fail to occur. Resolution of the uncertainty may confirm the acquisition of an asset or the reduction of a liability or the loss or impairment of an asset or the incurrence of a liability.

accounting measurement uncertainties:
similar to estimation uncertainty, which is defined in CAS 540.07 as "the susceptibility of an accounting estimate and related disclosures to an inherent lack of precision in its measurement," except that accounting measurement uncertainties apply to all accounting measurements, not just accounting estimates

Handbook section 3290 sets forth accounting and disclosure standards for contingencies. One of the most common involves the uncertain outcome of litigation pending against a company. Accounting uncertainties include not only lawsuits but also such things as the value of fixed assets held for sale (e.g., a whole plant or warehouse facility) and the status of assets involved in foreign expropriations. Auditors may perform procedures in accordance with GAAS, yet the uncertainty and lack of evidence may persist. The problem is that it is impossible to obtain audit "evidence" about the future. The concept of audit evidence includes information knowable at the time a reporting decision is made and does not include predictions about future resolution of uncertainties. Consequently, auditors should not change (modify or qualify) the introductory, scope, or opinion paragraphs of the standard unqualified report when contingencies and uncertainties exist. When the audit has been performed in accordance with GAAS, and the auditor has done all things possible in the circumstances, no alteration of these standard paragraphs is necessary as long as the uncertainty has been properly disclosed. Whether the disclosure is proper, however, can be a major financial reporting issue and a key professional judgment of the auditor.

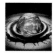 Under CAS 706, the auditor may decide to place a "red flag" paragraph in the report to draw attention to the uncertainty. If there is material uncertainty about the going-concern assumption, for example, then CAS 706 requires that an emphasis of matter paragraph (see below) be added even when there is proper disclosure in the financial statements.

Uncertainty situations may cause audit reports to be qualified for departures from GAAP if (1) management's disclosure of the uncertainty is inadequate, (2) management uses inappropriate accounting principles to account for the uncertainty, or (3) management makes unreasonable accounting estimates in connection with the effects of the uncertainty. The audit report may also be qualified because of a scope limitation regarding available evidence about an uncertainty.

A Historical Note: "Subject to" Opinions before 1980

From the early 1960s until 1980, auditors gave "subject to" opinions for accounting uncertainty situations. The opinion sentence was qualified with these words: "In our opinion, subject to the effects of such adjustments, if any, as might have been determined had the outcome of the uncertainty discussed in the preceding paragraph been known . . . ." The explanatory paragraph was placed before the opinion paragraph, and the opinion was considered qualified. You may see this form of "subject to" opinion when you use reports issued in 1980 and earlier. However, the audit standards were changed in 1980, and now the "subject to" wording is prohibited, the explanatory paragraph is no longer used, and the opinion sentence itself is unqualified.

The inclusion of significant matter paragraphs, discussed below, appears to be one way that the basic red-flagging objective of "subject to" opinions may be resurrected.

Significant Matter Paragraph(s): Modifications That Do Not Affect the Audit Opinion

Sometimes auditors opt to add additional information to the audit report. Two types of additions are possible under CAS 706: emphasis of matter (EOM) paragraphs and other matter (OM) paragraphs. These are used to enrich the information content beyond the standard unqualified report wording. Under CAS 706, the EOM paragraph can be used for a much broader range of issues than allowed previously. One or more paragraphs can be added in the audit report regarding something the auditor believes readers should consider important or useful, or when the auditor intends to write an unqualified opinion paragraph. Indeed, the matter emphasized is not supposed to be mentioned in the standard unqualified opinion sentence. EOM paragraphs are required when there is material uncertainty regarding the going-concern assumption. Exhibit 4–8 illustrates an EOM paragraph.

EXHIBIT 4–8

Example of an Emphasis of Matter Paragraph

Without qualifying our opinion we draw attention to Note X to the financial statements. The Company is the defendant in a lawsuit alleging infringement of certain patent rights and claiming royalties and punitive damages. The Company has filed a counter action, and preliminary hearings and discovery proceedings on both actions are in progress. The ultimate outcome of the matter cannot presently be determined and no provision for any liability that may result has been made in the financial statements.

Source: © *CPA Canada Handbook*, CAS 706.

OM paragraphs are distinguished from EOM paragraphs by the information they reference. EOM paragraphs refer only to information presented or disclosed in the financial statements, whereas OM paragraphs relate to information that is not required to be disclosed in the financial statements. For example, OM paragraphs can refer to other information, such as Management Discussion and Analysis (MD&A) or comparative information from other periods, especially when there appear to be discrepancies between the two. OM paragraphs also matter in a situation where the prior-year financial statements were audited by a different audit firm.

APPLICATION CASE WITH SOLUTION & ANALYSIS

Meaning of the Words "Present Fairly" in the Auditor's Report

DISCUSSION CASE

Your client, Margo, has prepared financial statements that she feels are in conformity with Canadian GAAP, but she notes that in your report you use the words "present fairly, in all material respects . . . in accordance with Canadian GAAP." She asks you to explain what these words mean so that she can fulfill her responsibilities to prepare the financial statements appropriately.

SOLUTION & ANALYSIS

"Present fairly" is one of those widely used accounting terms that is never defined in any standard. As auditor, you must provide an intuitive and reasonable, if not authoritative, explanation of its meaning. A good starting point is telling Margo that the statements must not mislead users. They must tell the truth about economic reality, including appropriate disclosures of business risks, using an acceptable reporting framework. Failure to appropriately disclose business risks and economic reality leads to information risk in financial reporting. Defining fairness of presentation in financial reporting so that it includes a risk orientation will lead to acceptable levels of information risk.

But what is "economic reality," then? Obviously, there should be no deliberate errors concerning the economic facts of Margo's reporting entity. This is implicit in both GAAP and your studies of financial accounting, and it is worth remembering as an auditor. By verifying those facts, as an auditor, you will determine which ones are correct and which are misleading. Hence, fair presentation includes an understanding that an auditor will be able to verify the facts through records kept by Margo's accounting system. The system should allow the auditor to gather independent corroborating evidence of the information. This way, the risk of errors in that information will be reduced to a level that you as auditor find acceptable for financial reporting. This is the low audit risk component of information risk that auditors aim to achieve. However, auditors also need to keep track of the accounting risks associated with forecasting in GAAP estimates. Forecasts are based on assumptions, and if those assumptions are unrealistic or unreasonable, the accounting risks associated with the accounting estimates increase. And increased accounting risks, in turn, lead to increased information risks in financial reporting. Thus, fair presentation also includes appropriately disclosing business risks through accounting entries and perhaps through appropriate note disclosures as well.

A specific example of this is the proper accounting for accounts receivable that you studied in your financial accounting course. To determine the appropriateness of the presentation of accounts receivable in the balance sheet, it must be verified that the receivables exist, that they are owed to Margo's company, and that they have been properly recorded and classified, per GAAP, as of the balance sheet date. All of this is factual information based on past events that can be verified by various audit procedures that you will be studying in this book. Verification is, therefore, the process of assuring yourself and others that these facts are accurately recorded. As an auditor, you will gather evidence from Margo's accounting system that the facts regarding receivables are accurate.

However, auditors, in fact, rarely find it an economical use of their time to exhaustively gather evidence on accounts receivable. So, they do less than that and, instead, accept that the less-than-perfect evidence creates a risk of undetected material factual errors regarding receivables. It is important to remember that audit risk for receivables is the risk of failing to detect material factual errors in the records for receivables. Audit risk is, therefore, an evidence-gathering risk.

The other component of information risk is accounting risk. This risk considers the question of whether all the receivables will be collected at their face amounts, regardless of how accurately the amounts were recorded. This uncertainty is unavoidable because it relates to the future and there is little that is certain about the future. Neither you (the auditor) nor Margo can predict with certainty, as of the balance sheet date, which receivables will be collected at face value. You might recall from your accounting course that there are techniques for calculating bad debt expense that do not seem to involve forecasting. However, such techniques are based on assumptions from experience. If these assumptions are wrong, the resulting estimate will be wrong as well. Some common assumptions are that percentage collection experienced in the past will continue to apply, that interest rates won't change, or that other economic factors will remain the same. Only the passage of time and actual collection of payments on the receivables can eliminate the uncertainty around these things. But, in the meantime, under the periodic reporting system of GAAP accounting you do not have the luxury of waiting for these future events to take place; you need an estimate of these future events now! An estimate of amounts to be realized as future cash flows is made by estimating the amount that will be uncollectible. The forecast of uncollectible amounts is the basis for adjustments to the allowance for doubtful accounts that will help you estimate the realizable value of receivables. This is necessary for proper valuation of receivables and also for proper matching.

Because there is no guarantee that the estimates will be accurate, it is likely that there will be a deviation between the estimate for bad debt expense and what will actually be realized as uncollectible. We call this the forecast error. A forecast error has the same impact on financial reporting as a recorded factual error—it is the difference between what is recorded and what is ultimately realized. Thus, material forecast errors have the same impact as material factual errors in financial reporting. This means that accounting risk should be as important as audit risk to users of financial statements. The problem, as we will see later, is that GAAP are largely silent on the acceptability of accounting risks for various accounts. GAAP do not normally consider the reasonableness of specific assumptions in making some forecasts. This forecast evaluation task is left to the professional judgment of the auditor. We introduce subjective concepts, such as accounting risk, to facilitate the decision making that goes into them. Thus, a logical aspect of fairness of presentation within GAAP is that accounting risk is kept to some "acceptable" level—at least as it concerns the amounts recorded as line items in the financial statements. This helps determine which assumptions to treat as reasonable. By keeping accounting risks appropriately low, we help keep information risk low and thereby make operational the concept of fair presentation. The question of note disclosures in the financial statements also affects fair presentation, as you saw in the Continental Vending case of Chapter 3.

Unless otherwise indicated, in this textbook we use the term *GAAP* to mean "presented fairly within Canadian GAAP." In the auditor's report, this wording can be viewed as a reminder to auditors that in applying GAAP they need to consider the reasonableness of assumptions for making accounting estimates (leading to acceptable accounting risk), as well as the importance of an acceptably low level of risk of factual errors in financial statements. (If we assume that auditors demand that management correct all material factual errors upon detection, then the latter risk corresponds to audit risk.) With both conditions satisfied, a more comprehensive risk-oriented approach to achieving "fairness of presentation in conformity with GAAP" is possible. This is the approach we follow throughout this text.

SUMMARY

- This chapter began with setting forth the requirement that auditors must report whenever they are associated with financial statements. This report can take different forms in different circumstances—audit assurance, negative assurance, and no assurance. These levels of assurance are further explained in terms of (1) reports qualified for scope limitations and departures from GAAP, (2) adverse reports resulting from GAAP departures, and (3) disclaimers of opinion resulting from lack of independence and lack of sufficient appropriate evidence.   **LO1, 2, 3, 4**

- Auditing standards refer to several basic circumstances that cause departures from the standard unqualified audit report. These circumstances are shown in Exhibit 4–9 in relation to the influence of materiality. You can see that each report is qualified when the situation involves materiality, but becomes a disclaimer or an adverse report when the situation involves misstatements much greater than overall materiality. The exception is the lack of independence issue, where materiality does not make a difference. It should also be noted that materiality by itself cannot be used to distinguish between fair presentation and compliance reporting frameworks of CAS 200.13. That distinction is primarily a function of the quality and form of information disclosure, as discussed in the application case of this chapter. For example, significant matter paragraphs, key audit matter paragraphs, and a more complete description of auditor responsibilities are different ways the auditor can help close the expectations gap and achieve fair presentation for users. Note how important clearer and more complete communications are to achieving this objective. In Exhibit 4–9, note the importance of disclosures in dealing with uncertainty and materiality. Further discussion is provided in subsequent chapters.   **LO5, 6**

- Throughout this chapter's explanation of the auditors' choices of reports, the materiality dimension played an important role. When an auditor makes decisions about the audit report, immaterial or unimportant information can be ignored and treated as if it does not exist. However, when inaccuracies, departures from GAAP, accounting changes, and uncertainties have a large enough financial impact, the standard audit report must be changed. In practice, when an auditor decides a matter is material enough to make a difference, a further distinction must be made between misstatements of "specific materiality" and those of "overall materiality" of CAS 320. Overall materiality is for financial statements as a whole. Specific materiality is smaller than overall materiality and relates to specific user needs for specific classes of transactions, account balances, or disclosures. These are further discussed in Chapter 5, but the main point about specific and overall materialities is that they relate directly to user needs. This is what affects the audit report when the auditee refuses to adjust for its material misstatement.

    You might wonder why auditees would not correct material misstatements. They may have their own reasons, and so critical thinking is needed to decide if those reasons are good enough! This is also part of the report decision.   **LO6**

- Materiality means that the item in question is important and needs to be disclosed or that the opinion for it needs to be qualified—the information cannot simply be ignored. Overall materiality means that the item is important and has a significant impact on the reporting decision. The biggest distinction between the two materialities is the number of users affected by the potential misstatements: overall materiality affects many more users than does specific materiality. In the current environment, the amount of misstatement that is considered acceptable has been reduced in many audits so that both materialities have also been reduced. As you will see in later chapters, this effectively increases the amount of audit work in the engagement.   **LO6**

- Audit reports can also be modified and expanded with additional paragraphs. Such additions to the audit report arise from the need for emphasis of matter (EOM) and other matter (OM) paragraphs in certain situations. These are explained in the last section of this chapter. Appendix 4C of this chapter covers "shopping" for accounting principles and auditors. Standards exist to raise the public perception that auditors are careful about competing with each other on the basis of professional opinions.   **LO7**

EXHIBIT 4–9

Influence of Materiality on Audit Reports

CIRCUMSTANCES FOR DEPARTURE FROM STANDARD REPORT	USUAL TYPE OF REPORT IF MISSTATEMENTS EXCEED THE GIVEN MATERIALITY	
	SPECIFIC MATERIALITY	OVERALL MATERIALITY
Departure from GAAP	Qualified opinion "except for": separate paragraph discloses reasons and effects*	Adverse opinion: separate paragraph discloses reasons and effects
Scope limitation (lack of evidence)	Qualified opinion: refers to possible effects on financials	Disclaimer of opinion: separate paragraph explains limitations
Uncertainty	Unmodified opinion**	Unmodified opinion**

*Where the departure is necessary to make the financials not misleading, an unqualified opinion is issued with an explanation of the circumstances.

**Unless there is a failure to properly disclose an uncertainty, such as an accounting contingency or going-concern problem.

KEY TERMS

accounting deficiency
   reservation
accounting measurement
   uncertainties
associated with financial
   statements

association
audit deficiency reservation
clean opinion
levels of assurance
negative assurance
   (moderate assurance)

no assurance
pervasive materiality
positive assurance
qualified reports
reservations
scope limitation

MULTIPLE-CHOICE QUESTIONS FOR PRACTICE AND REVIEW

MC 4-1 **LO5** A PA developed a system for clients to enter transaction data by remote terminal into the PA's computer. The PA's system processes the data and prints monthly financial statements. When delivered to the clients, these financial statements should include

a. a standard unqualified audit report.

b. an adverse audit report.

c. a report describing the character of the engagement and the degree of responsibility the PA is taking.

d. a description of the remote terminal system and of the controls for ensuring accurate data processing.

MC 4-2 **LO3** According to CPA Canada, what is the objective of an audit of financial statements?

a. An expression of opinion on the fairness with which they present financial position, results of operations, and cash flows in conformity with GAAP

b. An expression of opinion on the fairness with which they present financial position, results of operations, and cash flows in conformity with FASB

c. An expression of opinion on the fairness with which they present financial position, results of operations, and cash flows in conformity with GAAS

d. To obtain systematic and objective evidence about financial assertions and report the results to interested users

MC 4-3 **LO5** Some of the GAAS require certain statements in all audit reports ("explicit"), and others require statements only under certain conditions ("implicit"). Which of the following is always an explicit feature of the reporting standards?

Standards

a. GAAP

b. Consistency

c. Disclosure

d. GAAS

MC 4-4 **LO5** A PA finds that the client has not capitalized a material amount of leases in the financial statements. When considering the materiality of this departure from GAAP, the PA's reporting options are

a. unqualified opinion or disclaimer of opinion.

b. unqualified opinion or qualified opinion.

c. EOM paragraph with unqualified opinion or adverse opinion.

d. qualified opinion or adverse opinion.

MC 4-5 **LO5, 6** An auditor has found that the client is suffering financial difficulty and that the going-concern status is seriously in doubt. The client has not placed good disclosures in the financial statements. Which of the following audit report alternatives must the PA choose?

a. Unqualified report with a going-concern explanatory (EOM) paragraph

b. Disclaimer of opinion

c. Qualified opinion or adverse opinion

d. Standard unqualified report

MC 4-6 **LO5, 6** A company accomplished an early extinguishment of debt, and the auditors believe that recognition of a huge loss distorts the financial statements and causes them to be misleading. The auditors' reporting choices are to

a. explain the situation and give an adverse opinion.

b. explain the situation and give a disclaimer of opinion.

c. explain the situation and give an unqualified opinion, relying on rules of professional conduct not to be associated with misleading financial statements.

d. give the standard unqualified audit report.

MC 4-7 `LO7` Which of these situations would require an auditor to insert an explanatory paragraph about consistency in an unqualified audit report?

a. Client changed its estimated allowance for uncollectible accounts receivable
b. Client corrected a prior mistake in accounting for interest capitalization
c. Client sold one of its subsidiaries and consolidated six this year compared with seven last year
d. Client switched to early adoption of IFRS changes

MC 4-8 `LO6` Phil became the new auditor for Royal Corporation, succeeding Liz, who audited the financial statements last year. Phil needs to report on Royal's comparative financial statements and should write in his report an explanation about another auditor having audited the prior year

a. only if Liz's opinion last year was qualified.
b. describing the prior audit and the opinion, but not naming Liz as the predecessor auditor.
c. describing the audit but not revealing the type of opinion Liz gave.
d. describing the audit and the opinion, and naming Liz as the predecessor auditor.

MC 4-9 `LO5` When other independent auditors are involved in the current audit on parts of the client's business, the principal auditor can write an audit report that

a. mentions the other auditors but fails to describe the extent of the other auditors' work, and gives an unqualified opinion.
b. does not mention the other auditors and gives an unqualified opinion in a standard unqualified report.
c. places primary responsibility for the audit report on the other auditors.
d. names the other auditors, describes their work, and presents only the principal auditor's report.

MC 4-10 `LO7` An EOM paragraph inserted in an audit report causes the report to be characterized as

a. an unqualified opinion report.
b. a divided responsibility.
c. an adverse opinion report.
d. a denial of opinion.

MC 4-11 `LO5` When will an auditor express an opinion containing the phrase "except for"?

a. The client refuses to provide for a probable income tax liability that is very material, or super-material.
b. There is a high degree of uncertainty associated with the client company's future.
c. He or she did not perform procedures sufficient to form an opinion on the valuation of accounts receivable that are material.
d. The auditor is basing his or her opinion in part on work done by another auditor.

EXERCISES AND PROBLEMS

EP 4-1 Association with Financial Statements. `LO1`

Required:

For each of the situations described below, state whether the PA is or is not associated with the financial statements. What is the consequence of being associated with financial statements?

a. The PA audits financial statements and his or her name is in the corporate annual report containing them.

b. The PA prepares the financial statements in the partnership tax return.

c. The PA uses the computer to process client-submitted data and deliver financial statement output.

d. The PA uses the computer to process client-submitted data and deliver a general ledger printout.

e. The PA lets the client copy client-prepared financial statements on the PA's letterhead.

f. The client issues quarterly financial statements and mentions the PA's review procedures but does not list the PA's name in the document.

g. The PA renders consulting advice about the system to prepare interim financial statements but does not review the statements prior to their release.

EP 4-2 Reports and the Effect of Materiality. `LO6` The concept of materiality is important to PAs in audits of financial statements and expressions of opinion on these statements.

Required:

How will materiality influence an auditor's reporting decision in the following circumstances?

a. The client prohibits confirmation of accounts receivable, and sufficient appropriate evidence cannot be obtained using alternative procedures.

b. The client is a gas and electric utility company that follows the practice of recognizing revenue when it is billed to customers. At the end of the year, amounts earned but not yet billed are not recorded in the accounts or reported in the financial statements.

c. The client leases buildings for its chain of transmission repair shops under terms that qualify as capital leases. These leases are not capitalized as leased property assets and lease obligations.

d. The client company has lost a lawsuit. The case is on appeal in an attempt to reduce the amount of damages awarded to the plaintiffs.

EP 4-3 Scope Limitation, Auditor Independence. `LO4` Crow Corporation, a public company, has set up a number of limited partnerships to pursue some risky development projects. The limited partnerships borrow money from various financial institutions to support the development projects, and Crow guarantees these loans. Crow's interest in each limited partnership is set at a level just below the percentage that would require the partnerships, and their debts, to be included in Crow's consolidated financial statements. These percentages are set out specifically in the professional accounting recommendations that form the basis of GAAP for the purpose of Crow's financial reporting.

Zilch Zulch LLP (ZZ) has been the auditor of Crow since Crow's incorporation 30 years ago. The current CFO of Crow was formerly an audit partner in ZZ and was in charge of the Crow audit for five years before Crow hired her as its CFO. Because of her familiarity with ZZ's approach to setting materiality for its audits, the CFO was able to suggest the amount of a loan that could be guaranteed in each limited partnership without being material. If an individual loan were material, it would need to be disclosed as a contingency in Crow's consolidated financial statements even if the partnership was not required to be consolidated. Approximately 1,000 limited partnerships were set up, since a large sum of money was required to fund Crow's development activities. Because of the way the limited partnerships were structured, none of them were consolidated and no disclosure of Crow's loan guarantees to the partnerships was made in Crow's 20X0 financial statements, despite the fact that in total they exceeded the reported long-term debt and shareholders' equity of Crow.

Zero Mustbe, the audit partner in charge of the audit of Crow's 20X0 consolidated financial statements, was somewhat puzzled as to why there were so many limited partnerships, since only one development project was being undertaken. However, he was assured by Crow's CFO that the structure was appropriate and in accordance with GAAP because, in her words, "It was all set up by financial engineers with PhDs in ZZ's consulting group. These people know all about GAAP and are much smarter that you are, Zero, so there is nothing to be concerned about."

As a result of his audit work, Zero provided a clean audit opinion on Crow's 20X0 consolidated financial statements. During 20X1, adverse events resulted in Crow's being unable to meet its obligations under the loan guarantees and it went bankrupt.

Required:

Comment on the adequacy of Zero's audit, the independence and scope issues raised, and the appropriateness of issuing a clean audit report in this scenario.

EP 4-4 Negative and Positive Assurance and Users' Needs. `LO3` Ellen Eagle is a banker in a small town. Her customers, Dave and Dot Dauber, are the owners of a franchised candy store in town. They have an opportunity to buy a second franchised store in a nearby town and are requesting that Ellen increase their bank loan from $300,000 to $2,000,000 to finance this acquisition. The Daubers are two of Ellen's best customers and have always made their loan payments on time during the 10 years they have been customers of her bank. Currently, Ellen is requiring the Daubers to provide annual financial statements with a review report of a PA. To approve the requested loan increase, the bank's head office will require them to provide audited annual financial statements.

Required:

Distinguish between a review report and an audit report. Why would the bank require an audit instead of a review in this case? Do you think the bank's policy is reasonable?

EP 4-5 Arguments with Auditors. `LO5` Officers of the Kingston Company do not want to disclose information about the product liability lawsuit filed by a customer asking $500,000 in damages. They believe the suit is frivolous and without merit. Outside counsel is more cautious. The auditors insist upon disclosure. Angered, the Kingston Company chairman of the board threatens to sue the auditors if a standard unmodified report is not issued within three days.

Required:

Explain the issues raised in the preceding situation. What actions do you recommend to the company's auditor?

EP 4-6 Errors in a Comparative Report with Change from Prior Year. `LO5` The following audit report was drafted by an assistant at the completion of the audit of Cramdon Inc., on March 1, 20X5. The partner in charge of the engagement has decided the opinion on the 20X4 financial statements should be modified only with reference to the change in the method of computing sales. Also, because of a litigation uncertainty, an uncertainty paragraph was included in the audit report on the 20X3 financial statements, which are included for comparative purposes. The 20X3 audit report (same audit firm) was dated March 5, 20X4, and on October 15, 20X4, the litigation was resolved in favour of Cramdon Inc.

Auditor's Draft Report
To the Board of Directors of Cramdon Inc.:
We have audited the accompanying financial statements of Cramdon Inc., as of December 31, 20X4 and 20X3. These financial statements are the responsibility of the Company's Management. Our responsibility is to express an opinion on these financial statements based on our audits.

We conducted our audits in accordance with generally accepted auditing standards. Those standards require that we plan and perform the audit to obtain reasonable assurance about whether the financial statements are free of material misstatement. An audit includes examining, on a test basis, evidence supporting the amounts and disclosures in the financial statements. An audit also includes assessing the accounting principles used and significant estimates made by management, as well as evaluating the overall financial statement presentation. We believe that our audit provides a reasonable basis for our opinion.

As discussed in Note 7 to the financial statements, our previous report on the 20X3 financial statements contained an explanatory paragraph regarding a particular litigation uncertainty. Because of our lawyer's meritorious defence in this litigation, our current report on these financial statements does not include such an explanatory paragraph.

In our opinion, based on the preceding, the financial statements referred to above present fairly, in all material respects, the financial position of Cramdon Inc. as of December 31, 20X4, and the results of its operations and its cash flows for the period then ended in conformity with generally accepted accounting principles consistently applied, except for the changes in the method of computing sales as described in Note 14 to the financial statements.

/s/ PA Firm
March 5, 20X5

Required:

Identify the deficiencies and errors in the draft report and write an explanation of the reasons they are errors and deficiencies. Do not rewrite the report.

EP 4-7 Negative and Positive Assurance and Users' Needs.   `LO3`   One of your neighbours, Hans House, is a minority shareholder of Grackle Corporation, a private company. Grackle is also the company that employs Hans. Recently Hans and the other Grackle Corporation shareholders were asked to approve a resolution that would waive the requirement for the company to have its financial statements audited. The company has been audited in past years but will have a review instead of an audit if the resolution is passed unanimously by the shareholders. Hans knows that you are an advanced accounting student and has asked for your advice on whether he should vote for or against the audit waiver.

Required:

List the factors that Hans should consider in making this decision. What fact situations would support voting for the audit waiver, and what fact situations would indicate he should vote against the waiver?

EP 4-8 Distinguishing Forms of Assurance.   `LO3`

Required:

Explain the difference between "negative assurance" and an "adverse opinion."

EP 4-9 Generally Accepted Auditing Standards General Standard, Audit Scope.   `LO4`

Required:

Give three examples of fact situations in which the General Standards of GAAS are not met. For each example, explain the impact of the violation on the scope of the audit and the audit report.

EP 4-10 Generally Accepted Auditing Standards Examination Standard, Audit Scope.   `LO5`

Required:

Give one example of a fact situation in which each of the three Examination Standards of GAAS are not met. For each example, explain the impact of the violation on the scope of the audit and the audit report.

EP 4-11 Audit Opinion on Financial Statements. `LO5` The unmodified audit opinion states that the financial statements ". . . present fairly . . . in accordance with Canadian generally accepted accounting principles."

Required:

a. Explain, from the perspective of the auditing profession, why the auditor's opinion on fair presentation of financial statements is given in reference to Canadian GAAP.

b. Explain, from the perspective of financial statement users, the contrasting view that the auditor's responsibility to assess the fair presentation goes beyond a literal interpretation of whether the statements meet the requirements of Canadian GAAP.

c. Which position, (a) or (b), do you agree with? Why?

EP 4-12 Audit Scope Limitations—Auditor Appointed Late. `LO4`

Required:

a. What alternative procedures can an auditor perform to determine whether the inventory balance is not materially misstated when he or she is appointed in the middle of the year and did not observe the inventory count at the end of the prior year?

b. What alternative procedures can an auditor perform to determine whether the inventory balance is not materially misstated when he or she was appointed after the year-end under audit and was not able to observe the count of either the opening or the ending inventory?

c. What are the reporting implications if alternative procedures can be performed and provide sufficient audit evidence in situations (a) and (b) above?

d. What are the reporting implications if alternative procedures cannot be used to satisfy audit evidence requirements in situations (a) and (b) above?

EP 4-13 Audit Scope Limitations—Client Imposed. `LO4`

Required:

a. What alternative procedures can an auditor perform to determine whether the accounts receivable balance is not materially misstated when client management will not permit audit confirmations to be used?

b. What are the reporting implications if alternative procedures can be performed and provide sufficient audit evidence in situation (a)?

c. What are the reporting implications if alternative procedures cannot be used to satisfy audit evidence requirements in situation (a)?

EP 4-14 Reporting on Contingencies. `LO6`

Required:

Describe the pre-2011 requirements of Canadian GAAS for reporting for contingencies and uncertainties. Identify the pros and cons of the current approach, contrasting these with the pros and cons of the "subject to" opinions that were used in Canada prior to 1980.

EP 4-15 Reporting Going-Concern Uncertainties. `LO6` Current Canadian GAAS through 2015 do not permit the auditor to refer to a going-concern uncertainty in the audit report when the uncertainty is properly disclosed in the financial statement notes.

Required:

a. Describe the strengths and weaknesses of this approach, taking into consideration the perspectives of the company, its financial statement users, and its auditor.

b. Identify one or more alternative reporting methods that may be more beneficial to financial statement users.

c. You have been invited to comment to the Canadian assurance standards-setting board on its current audit reporting standards. What comment would you make to the standard setters on the issue of audit reporting when there is substantial doubt about a company's ability to continue as a going concern?

EP 4-16 Going-Concern Assumption—One-Year Limitation. `LO6` For the purpose of assessing the going-concern assumption, it is presumed that the auditor will consider whether the company will continue in existence for a "reasonable time" that does not exceed one year beyond the date of the financial statements.

Required:

Give reasons that auditors are not required to consider the entity's ability to continue as a going concern for a period longer than one year. In your opinion, is this one-year limitation reasonable? Explain and evaluate possible alternative approaches to support your opinion.

EP 4-17 Standards-Setting Research. `LO6`

Required:

Investigate the history and current status of the CPA Canada Exposure Draft on the going-concern assumption that was originally issued in 1996. Use the CPA Canada website, *CA Magazine*, and other professional publications to conduct this research. Explain how the due process involved in setting Canadian auditing standards is illustrated by the history of this Exposure Draft.

EP 4-18 Going-Concern Issue. `LO6` PA is the auditor of Jayhawk Inc. Jayhawk's revenues and profitability have decreased in each of the past three years and, as of this year-end, 20X3, its retained earnings will fall into a deficit balance. Jayhawk's long-term debt comes due in 20X4, and its management is currently renegotiating the repayment date and terms with its bondholders. According to PA's discussions with management, the renegotiation is not going well and there is a significant risk that the bondholders will put Jayhawk into receivership and liquidate its assets. Jayhawk's CFO has provided draft 20X3 financial statements to PA that are prepared in accordance with GAAP.

Required:

a. Discuss the audit reporting implications of the preceding situation.

b. Assume the long-term debt repayment date was not until 20X5. Would your response differ?

EP 4-19 Going-Concern Audit Reporting. `LO6` Before 2011, the old *CICA Handbook*, paragraph 5510.53, provided guidance for audit reporting when there is a going-concern problem.

Required:

a. Critique the audit reporting required by paragraph 5510.53 from the perspective of a financial statement user who owns shares of the auditee company.

b. Assume the role of the company's auditor. How would you respond to the criticisms raised in (a)?

EP 4-20 Report on the Application of Accounting Principles. `LO9` *CPA Canada Handbook* section 7600 sets out procedures relating to requests for advice from a PA from parties other than the PA's audit clients.

Required:

a. What are the purposes of section 7600?

b. Describe the requirements of section 7600, and explain how effective they are in achieving the purposes described in part (a).

EP 4-21 Report on the Application of Accounting Principles. `LO9` Kite Corporation's auditor, PA1, formed the opinion that Kite should accrue for estimated future costs to clean up an environmental problem on one of Kite's properties in its 20X3 financial statements. Kite requested a second opinion from PA2 on this issue. PA2 gave an opinion that the estimated liability amount is contingent on various future events that are highly uncertain, such as changes in environmental regulations and environmental cleanup technologies. Thus it is a contingency that is too uncertain to accrue and, in accordance with GAAP, it should only be disclosed. Kite's management sides with the opinion of PA2 because it prevents the company from reporting a loss; it allows Kite's management to receive bonuses for 20X3; and, in their view, it is a more appropriate application of GAAP.

Required:

a. Assume that Kite is a public company and PA1 and PA2 are Big Four audit firms. What public perception of auditors may arise if disputes on the application of GAAP can be resolved by the public company's obtaining an opinion from another auditor?

b. Take the role of PA1. What issues arise by Kite's taking this action in your dispute over the accrual of the contingent liability?

c. Take the role of PA2. What considerations should you make before issuing your opinion?

d. Take the role of one of Kite's directors. What issues arise by Kite's management's taking this action in resolving its dispute with PA1 over the accrual of the contingent liability?

EP 4-22 Audit Evidence from Specialists. `LO5` Lark Limited reports a material balance of deferred development costs in its current financial statements. The cost relates to the development of a mobile robot that can be used to monitor temperature, humidity, and security in large warehouses. Lark's auditor obtained an engineers' report to support the technological feasibility of the robotics project and a market research consultant's report to determine the selling prices and volumes likely to be achieved over the first 10 years that the product is marketed.

Required:

Explain the nature of audit evidence obtained in this case. How would this audit evidence affect the auditor's report? Compare the use of these specialists' reports in the audit with using the reports of other auditors.

EP 4-23 Nortel Accounting and Consequence. `LO6`

Required:

Find Nortel's 2004 annual report on its website or in SEC filings, and review the audit reports for 2001–2004. In light of Nortel's history (as indicated in Chapter 2), do you think these reports are appropriate? Discuss.

EP 4-24 Going-Concern Disclosures. `LO6`

Required:

Explain auditor responsibilities regarding going-concern disclosures under GAAS. Contrast these with GAAP requirements, and discuss ways of reconciling the two.

The Standard Unmodified Report of the Public Company Accounting Oversight Board/ American Institute of CPAs

LO8 Describe the Standard Unmodified Report of the Public Company Accounting Oversight Board/American Institute of CPAs.

AU Section 508 (paragraph .08) Reports on Audited Financial Statements

Independent Auditor's Report

We have audited the accompanying balance sheet of X Company as of December 31, 20X1, and the related statements of income, retained earnings, and cash flows for the year then ended. These financial statements are the responsibility of the Company's management. Our responsibility is to express an opinion on these financial statements based on our audit.

We conducted our audit in accordance with auditing standards generally accepted in the United States of America. Those standards require that we plan and perform the audit to obtain reasonable assurance about whether the financial statements are free of material misstatement. An audit includes examining, on a test basis, evidence supporting the amounts and disclosures in the financial statements. An audit also includes assessing the accounting principles used and significant estimates made by management, as well as evaluating the overall financial statement presentation. We believe that our audit provides a reasonable basis for our opinion.

In our opinion, the financial statements referred to above present fairly, in all material respects, the financial position of X Company as of [at] December 31, 20X1, and the results of its operations and its cash flows for the year then ended in conformity with accounting principles generally accepted in the United States of America.

Signed,

Date,

The Auditor's Standard Report for Use before December 15, 2016

LO9 Describe the auditor's standard report for use before December 15, 2016.

To the Shareholders of . . . . .

Report on the Financial Statements

We have audited the accompanying financial statements of ABC Company, which comprise the balance sheet as at December 31, 20X1, and the income statement, statement of changes in equity, and cash flow statement for the year then ended, and a summary of significant accounting policies and other explanatory notes.

Management's Responsibility for the Financial Statements

Management is responsible for the preparation and fair presentation of these financial statements in accordance with Canadian generally accepted accounting principles; this includes the design, implementation, and maintenance of internal control relevant to the preparation and fair presentation of financial statements that are free from material misstatement, whether due to fraud or error.

Auditor's Responsibility

Our responsibility is to express an opinion on these financial statements based on our audit. We conducted our audit in accordance with Canadian generally accepted auditing standards. Those standards require that we comply with ethical requirements and plan and perform the audit to obtain reasonable assurance whether the financial statements are free from material misstatement.

An audit involves performing procedures to obtain audit evidence about the amounts and disclosures in the financial statements. The procedures selected depend on the auditor's judgment, including the assessment of the risks of material misstatement of the financial statements, whether due to fraud or error. In making those risk assessments, the auditor considers internal control relevant to the entity's preparation and fair presentation of the financial statements in order to design audit procedures that are appropriate in the circumstances, but not for the purpose of expressing an opinion on the effectiveness of the entity's internal control. An audit also includes evaluating the appropriateness of accounting policies used and the reasonableness of accounting estimates made by management, as well as evaluating the overall presentation of financial statements.

We believe that the audit evidence we have obtained is sufficient and appropriate to provide a basis for our audit opinion.

Opinion

In our opinion, the financial statements present fairly, in all material respects, the financial position of ABC Company as of December 31, 20X1, and of its financial performance and its cash flows for the year then ended in accordance with Canadian generally accepted accounting principles.

[Auditor's signature]

[Date of auditor's report]

[Auditor's address]

Source: CPA Canada *Handbook—Assurance*, CAS 700, "Forming an Opinion and Reporting on Financial Statements."

Reporting on the Application of Accounting Principles

LO10 Explain the reporting on the application of accounting principles.

The subject of reporting on the application of accounting principles touches a sensitive nerve in the public accounting profession. It arose from clients' "shopping" for an auditor who would agree to give an unmodified audit report on a questionable accounting treatment. Shopping often involved auditor–client disagreements, after which the client said, "If you won't agree with my accounting treatment, then I'll find an auditor who will." These disagreements often involved early revenue recognition and unwarranted expense or loss deferral. A few cases of misleading financial statements occurred after the shopping resulted in clients' switching to more agreeable auditors. However, the practice is not entirely undesirable, because complex accounting matters often benefit from consultation with other PAs. Note that these situations illustrate the importance of a variety of perspectives on a financial reporting issue—a key aspect of critical thinking in professional judgment. It is clear from such situations that the application of accounting standards in specific circumstances is not always straightforward. Critical thinking helps to deal with such situations in a systematic, more defensible way.

The *CPA Canada Handbook* section 7600 established procedures for dealing with requests for consultation from parties other than an auditor's own clients. These parties can include other companies (non-clients who are shopping), lawyers, investment bankers, and perhaps other people. Section 7600 is applicable in the following situations:

- When preparing a written report or giving oral advice on specific transactions, either completed or proposed
- When preparing a written report or giving oral advice on the type of audit opinion that might be rendered on specific financial statements
- When preparing a written report on hypothetical transactions

The standard does not apply to conclusions about accounting principles offered in connection with litigation support engagements or expert witness work, nor does it apply to advice given to another PA in public practice. It also does not apply to an accounting firm's expressions of positions in newsletters, articles, speeches, lectures, and the like, provided that the positions do not give advice on a specific transaction or apply to a specific company.

The basic requirements are to consider the circumstances of the request for advice, its purpose, and the intended use of the report of the advice; to obtain an understanding of the form and substance of the transaction in question; to review applicable GAAP; to consult with other professionals, if necessary; and to perform research to determine the existence of creditable analogies and precedents (i.e., find the authoritative support). When the request for advice comes from a business that already has another auditor, the consulting PA should consult with the other auditor to learn all the facts and circumstances.

Written reports are required and should include these elements:

- A description of the nature of the engagement and a statement that it was performed in accordance with standards for such engagements
- A statement of relevant facts and assumptions, and the sources of information
- A statement of the advice—the conclusion about appropriate accounting principles or the type of audit report, including reasons for the conclusions, if appropriate
- A statement that a company's management is responsible for proper accounting treatments, in consultation with its own auditors
- A statement that any differences in facts, circumstances, or assumptions might change the conclusions

The purpose of the section 7600 standards is to impose some discipline on the process of shopping/consultation and to make it more difficult for companies to seek out a "willing" auditor.

ENDNOTES

1. Throughout these illustrative auditor's reports, the terms *management* and *those charged with governance* may need to be replaced by another term that is appropriate in the context of the legal framework in the particular jurisdiction.

2. Where management's responsibility is to prepare financial statements that give a true and fair view, this may read: "Management is responsible for the preparation of financial statements that give a true and fair view in accordance with IFRS, and for such. . . ."

3. This sentence would be modified, as appropriate, in circumstances where the auditor also has a responsibility to issue an opinion on the effectiveness of internal control in conjunction with the audit of the financial statements.

Gust
the ¡
audit
enga

Pre

and

This pre
ered anc
    Buil
Part 2 w
engager
risks of
support
    Cha
stateme
a roadn
accepte
text. Ne
or she r
that hel
audit ca
    Loo
your kr
audit w
ing proc
of the a
ical pro
manage
ing frar
and the
    To ?
stateme
or Acce
GAAP..
ent its f
dance v
While tl
coverec
    Aft
appreci
shows?

Basic Auditing Concepts and Techniques

Preliminary Audit Planning: Understanding the Auditee's Business

Chapter 5 will take you through the startup activities of the audit of an organization's general purpose financial statements. You will study the activities, concepts, and tools seen in a typical audit engagement.

LEARNING OBJECTIVES

After completing this chapter, you will be able to do the following:

LO1 Summarize the financial statement audit process.

LO2 Explain the main characteristics of an independent audit engagement.

LO3 Describe the activities auditors undertake to decide whether to accept a financial statement audit engagement, and the first tasks performed once an audit engagement is accepted.

LO4 Explain why auditors need to understand the auditee organization's business and environment and its risks and controls at the start of a financial statement audit.

LO5 Use preliminary analytical procedures on management's draft financial statements to identify areas where misstatements are most likely.

LO6 Explain the materiality levels used for planning the audit and how these amounts are determined.

LO7 List the preliminary planning decisions set out in the overall audit strategy.

LO8 (Appendix 5A) Know the types of ratios typically applied to financial statements to identify potential risks of misstatement.

LO9 (Appendix 5B) Describe the contents of an audit engagement letter.

Ethics codes for professional accountants require a successor auditor to initiate contact and attempt to obtain basic information directly from the predecessor. The former auditor knows a great deal about the auditee and can give information that will be useful in (1) deciding whether to accept the new auditee and (2) planning the audit. The rules of conduct require a predecessor auditor to respond promptly to communications from a successor and, at a minimum, report whether the predecessor knows of any reason that the successor should not accept the engagement. How detailed this communication is will depend on whether the client has given consent to the predecessor to release confidential auditee information to the successor.

It is common practice for the successor to explain the situation and the rules to the auditee's management, asking them to give the predecessor consent to speak to the successor and allow the successor to review the prior year's audit files. This consent will determine the amount of auditee information conveyed to the successor. If consent is given to speak freely, it is not unusual to have a cordial changeover, with the successor interviewing the predecessor's staff and obtaining copies of the predecessor's working papers, thus greatly facilitating the successor's first-time audit.[2]

Note that the audit files belong to the auditor, not the auditee, but confidentiality must be respected, even after the auditor–auditee relationship ends. The prospective auditee management's refusal to consent would raise serious concerns about its integrity, and the successor may decide it is too risky to accept this engagement.

Auditor's Risk from Accepting an Audit Engagement

There will always be some risk in taking on an audit, but, ultimately, the auditor must decide whether the risk is manageable, prior to accepting a particular engagement. Some of the key factors that go into this decision are presented in Exhibit 5–2.

EXHIBIT 5–2

The Auditor's Risk from Accepting an Audit Engagement

FACTORS AFFECTING THE AUDITOR'S RISK FROM ACCEPTING THE ENGAGEMENT	IMPLICATIONS FOR THE AUDITOR'S ASSESSMENT
How widely distributed are the audited financial statements?	If widely distributed to the public, such as for a publicly listed company, the risk from accepting the engagement is higher (reputation risk). If the distribution is limited, the risk is lower.
How strong is the financial condition of the auditee?	If the financial condition is poor, the risk from accepting the engagement is higher because financial failure can lead to investor losses and lawsuits against the auditor to recover them (legal liability risk). Another concern could be that the audit fees cannot be collected to cover the costs of doing the audit. If the financial condition is strong, the risk is lower.
How trustworthy is the auditee's management?	If the auditor has reason to doubt management's integrity, the risk from accepting the engagement is higher (misstated financial reporting risk). If the auditor has reasons to believe management is trustworthy, the risk is lower.
How complex is the financial reporting required?	If the auditee has complicated or unusual accounting requirements, such as derivatives use or foreign operations, and/or engages in unusual transactions, such as related party or inter-corporate investments, the accounting will be very challenging and the risk from accepting the engagement will be higher (misstated financial reporting risk). If the auditee has relatively straightforward activities and transactions, the risk will be lower.
How knowledgeable are the people likely to be using the financial statements?	If the users are relatively naive, and/or completely reliant on the audited financial statements for their decision needs, the risk from accepting the engagement will be higher (legal liability risk). If the users are relatively sophisticated and/or have direct access to relevant information other than the audited financial statements for their decisions, the risk will be lower.

We can envision the auditor's assessment of his or her risk from an audit engagement along a continuum. An auditor may decide to take on a low-, a moderate-, or even a high-risk engagement, as long as the auditor is confident that this risk can be managed down to an acceptable level through careful performance of high-quality audit work. But at very high levels, just like the "revs" of a car engine, at some point the risk crosses the "red line" and the auditor will have to decline the engagement. Where is the red line? It depends on the judgment of each auditor, which is based on their capacity to manage the risks and their personal tolerance for risk.

Review Checkpoints

5-37   What sources of information can an auditor use in deciding whether to accept an audit engagement? What risks must the auditor assess using this information before accepting the engagement?

5-38   Why does the successor auditor need to obtain the auditee's consent in order for the predecessor auditor to provide the successor with information about the auditee?

5-39   High Roller Inc. needs an audit and has asked two different audit firms to bid on the engagement. Both auditors assess the engagement risk to be high. Auditor A declines the engagement, but Auditor B agrees to accept it. Why could the two auditors reach different conclusions in this situation?

Engagement Letters

When a new audit is accepted, the auditor must obtain an **engagement letter**. Auditing standards provide a template for an engagement letter. Every letter needs to be adapted to the circumstances of the auditee organization and the audit; an example is provided in Appendix 5B. Auditing standards require that the auditor and auditee management understand and agree upon the terms of the engagement.[3] The agreement is documented to reduce the risk that either the auditor or the auditee misinterprets the needs or expectations of the other party. For continuing auditees, the auditor confirms the terms of the engagement annually, in writing. Every year, the auditor must take into account whether there are any new circumstances that would require the terms to be revised, such as a significant change in the nature or size of the entity's business.

The engagement letter is, in effect, the contract. The letter should cover the objective, scope, and limitations of the audit as well as respective responsibilities of both parties. It should specify the applicable financial reporting framework to be used, explain the form of audit report expected to be given, and indicate that the form of report may change if circumstances require that. The letter may list special requests and assignments the auditors will undertake, or it may be a standard letter stating that an audit of financial statements will be performed in accordance with GAAS. An engagement letter can head off claims that the auditors did not perform the work promised; for example, agreeing on a completion date can reduce disappointments later on. The engagement letter may also set forth the auditor's fee, which is normally based on the time required to perform the services. Such time estimates require some familiarity with the accounting system. Also, changes in services from the previous year will be communicated.

Staff Assignment and Time Budgets

The availability of staff with appropriate skills to conduct the audit is a key consideration in the engagement acceptance decision. If a new audit engagement is accepted, most public accounting firms will assign a full-service team to it. For audits of larger organizations, this team usually consists of the audit engagement partner

engagement letter:
a document that sets out the terms of the engagement forming a contract between the auditor and the client when a new audit engagement is accepted

Standards Check

CAS 210 Agreeing on the Terms of Audit Engagements (partial)

10. . . . the agreed terms of the audit engagement shall be recorded in an audit engagement letter or other suitable form of written agreement and shall include (Ref: Para. A22–A25)

(a) The objective and scope of the audit of the financial statements;

(b) The responsibilities of the auditor;

(c) The responsibilities of management;

(d) Identification of the applicable financial reporting framework for the preparation of the financial statements; and

(e) Reference to the expected form and content of any reports to be issued by the auditor and a statement that there may be circumstances in which a report may differ from its expected form and content.

Source: *CPA Canada Handbook—Assurance,* 2014.

(the person with final responsibility for the audit), the audit manager, one or more senior audit staff members, staff assistants or public accounting students, information systems or industry experts (if needed), and a tax partner. For smaller auditees, the team may consist of only one or two people, for example, the partner and one staff assistant. For larger auditees and public company audits, the audit firm policies may require that a second audit partner review the work of the audit team to ensure that audit quality standards are met. This partner is expected to have a detached professional point of view because he or she is not directly responsible for keeping friendly relations with the auditee's personnel.

The partner and manager in charge of the audit prepare a time budget as a plan for the timing of the work and the number of hours each segment of the audit is expected to take. The budget is based on last year's performance for continuing auditees, taking into account any changes in the auditee's business. In a first-time audit, it may be based on a predecessor auditor's experience or on general experience with similar companies. A simple time budget is shown in Exhibit 5–3. This particular budget is illustrative only and not complete. Real time budgets are much more detailed, but the exhibit shows a typical assignment of work to audit team members at different experience levels, such as partner, manager, senior auditor in charge of field work, and intermediate and junior staff assistants. This table shows time at interim and at year-end.

Interim audit work covers procedures performed several weeks or months before the balance sheet date and includes the bulk of the audit planning work. The exact timing of the interim work depends on the circumstances, such as when enough transaction data will be available to make it efficient for the auditor to start performing procedures, when auditee reconciliations or count procedures are available for audit purposes, and when auditee staff has time to accommodate and assist the auditors.

Year-end audit work refers to procedures performed at and shortly after the balance sheet date. As many auditees have year-ends on the same date (December 31 is common), audit firms typically ensure they will have time and people available by spreading the workload over the year. For many audit firms, the busy season runs from October through June of the following year. The interim work can consist of both internal control risk assessment and auditing balances as they exist at an early date, or examination of documents or electronic information only available for a certain period during the year.

The time taken to perform procedures for each segment of the audit work is recorded by budget category so that (1) there is a record for billing the auditee, (2) the efficiency of the audit team members can be evaluated,

Interim audit work:

covers procedures performed several weeks or months before the balance sheet date

year-end audit work:

audit procedures performed at and shortly after the balance sheet date and (3) there is a record for planning the next audit. This may cause some staff members to feel pressured to meet the budget. Beginning auditors, in particular, can get frustrated before they learn how to work efficiently. They may be tempted to understate the actual time they spent, with the result that not enough time is budgeted for future audits. Firms can lessen the problem by building learning time for less-experienced staff into the budgets.

EXHIBIT 5-3

Illustration of a Simple Time Budget

	STAFF ASSIGNED	AUDIT TIME BUDGET (HOURS)	
		INTERIM	YEAR-END
Knowledge of the business	Whole team	15	
Assessment of risk of material misstatement	Partner, Manager, and Senior	10	
Control testing	Senior and Junior	30	10
Audit planning	Partner and Manager	22	3
Related parties investigation	Manager	5	15
Auditor-auditee conferences	Whole team	10	18
Cash	Junior	10	15
Accounts receivable	Intermediate	15	5
Inventory	Senior	35	20
Accounts payable	Intermediate	5	35
Other accounts	Senior		10
Representation letters	Manager and Senior		10
Financial statement review	Partner and Manager		25
Report preparation	Partner		12
Total		157	178

Review Checkpoints

5-40   What benefits are obtained by having an engagement letter?

5-41   What is the purpose of a time budget, and what information does it contain?

5-42   What is interim audit work? year-end audit work?

Understanding the Auditee's Business, Environment, and Risks

LO4   Explain why auditors need to understand the auditee organization's business and environment and its risks and controls at the start of a financial statement audit.

Understanding the Business and Its Environment and Risks

The objective of a financial statement audit is to render an opinion on whether the financial statements, taken as a whole, are fairly presented in accordance with GAAP. Understanding the auditee's business and its operating environment is very important in starting out the audit, as it helps to assess the risk that the auditee's financial statements might contain material misstatements and therefore not be fairly presented. The term *material* in the preceding sentence refers to the key accounting and auditing concept of materiality—a misstatement significant enough to affect an important decision someone might make on the basis of that information.

Early in the engagement, the auditor sets out to understand the auditee's business, its environment, and its internal controls, in order to identify and assess the risks of material misstatement in the financial statements. This understanding is the basis of establishing an **overall audit strategy** for the engagement and guiding the design of a detailed audit plan containing a set of audit programs that effectively address all the significant risks of financial statement misstatements. An audit program is a list of the specific procedures to be performed to obtain sufficient appropriate evidence about significant components of the financial statements. This evidence is the basis on which the auditor obtains reasonable assurance that the financial statements are fairly presented and supports the opinion stated in the auditor's report.

Standards Check

CAS 320 Materiality in Planning and Performing an Audit

2. Financial reporting frameworks often discuss the concept of materiality in the context of the preparation and presentation of financial statements. Although financial reporting frameworks may discuss materiality in different terms, they generally explain that
   - Misstatements, including omissions, are considered to be material if they, individually or in the aggregate, could reasonably be expected to influence the economic decisions of users taken on the basis of the financial statements;
   - Judgments about materiality are made in light of surrounding circumstances and are affected by the size or nature of a misstatement or a combination of both; and
   - Judgments about matters that are material to users of the financial statements are based on a consideration of the common financial information needs of users as a group. The possible effect of misstatements on specific individual users, whose needs may vary widely, is not considered.

Source: *CPA Canada Handbook—Assurance*, 2014.

Auditing standards require the auditor to document the overall strategy, audit plan, audit programs, and evidence that support the report.[4] A program "in my head" is not sufficient. Audit programs are explained more fully in the remaining chapters of Part 2, and detailed examples are provided in Part 3.

To ascertain the auditee's business risks, first the auditor investigates management's understanding of its business risks, and then he or she independently assesses both the business risk and management's risk assessment process to determine how likely a material misstatement of the financial statements is. The auditing standards explain the risk assessment procedures for obtaining an understanding of the auditee as well as sources of information about the auditee entity and its environment, including its internal control.

The standards also require the audit team to discuss the susceptibility of the auditee's financial statements to material misstatement. Based on its shared understanding, the audit team can identify what can go wrong at

overall audit strategy:
an audit planning document that sets the scope, timing, and direction of the audit, and that guides the development of the audit plan, including the reporting objectives; the nature, timing, and extent of resources necessary to perform the engagement; and the nature of the communications required

Standards Check

CAS 315 Identifying and Assessing the Risks of Material Misstatement through Understanding the Entity and Its Environment

3. The objective of the auditor is to identify and assess the risks of material misstatement, whether due to fraud or error, at the financial statement and assertion levels, through understanding the entity and its environment, including the entity's internal control, thereby providing a basis for designing and implementing responses to the assessed risks of material misstatement.

5. The auditor shall perform risk assessment procedures to provide a basis for the identification and assessment of risks of material misstatement at the financial statement and assertion levels. Risk assessment procedures by themselves, however, do not provide sufficient appropriate audit evidence on which to base the audit opinion. (Ref: Para. A1–A5)

Source: *CPA Canada Handbook—Assurance,* 2014.

the financial statement level.[5] Assessing the **risk of material misstatement at the financial statement level** requires the audit team to identify any factors that create significant business and fraud risks that could have a pervasive effect on many elements of the financial statements.

Standards Check

CAS 315 Identifying and Assessing the Risks of Material Misstatement through Understanding the Entity and Its Environment

11. The auditor shall obtain an understanding of the following:
    (a) Relevant industry, regulatory, and other external factors including the applicable financial reporting framework. (Ref: Para. A17–A22)
    (b) The nature of the entity, including
        (i) Its operations;
        (ii) Its ownership and governance structures;
        (iii) The types of investments that the entity is making and plans to make, including investments in special purpose entities; and
        (iv) The way that the entity is structured and how it is financed, to enable the auditor to understand the classes of transactions, account balances, and disclosures to be expected in the financial statements. (Ref: Para. A23–A27)
    (c) The entity's selection and application of accounting policies, including the reasons for changes thereto. The auditor shall evaluate whether the entity's accounting policies are appropriate for its business and consistent with the applicable financial reporting framework and accounting policies used in the relevant industry. (Ref: Para. A28)
    (d) The entity's objectives and strategies, and those related business risks that may result in risks of material misstatement. (Ref: Para. A29–A35)
    (e) The measurement and review of the entity's financial performance. (Ref: Para. A36–A41)

Source: *CPA Canada Handbook—Assurance,* 2014.

risk of material misstatement at the financial statement level:
the auditor's assessment, based on pervasive factors such as fraud, going concern, or other significant business-level risks, of the probability that errors or fraud have affected the financial statements overall such that financial statement users may be misled

Standards Check

CAS 315 Identifying and Assessing the Risks of Material Misstatement through Understanding the Entity and Its Environment

10. The engagement partner and other key engagement team members shall discuss the susceptibility of the entity's financial statements to material misstatement, and the application of the applicable financial reporting framework to the entity's facts and circumstances. The engagement partner shall determine which matters are to be communicated to engagement team members not involved in the discussion. (Ref: Para. A14–A16)

Source: *CPA Canada Handbook—Assurance*, 2014.

Later, the audit team will perform more-detailed risk assessments of the individual elements of the financial statements: the classes of transactions, account balances, and disclosures. These financial statement elements are made up of specific "assertions" or fundamental claims by management. There are five principal assertions: existence, completeness, ownership, valuation, and presentation. As will be explained in Chapter 6, these terms mean management is claiming that, for each element of the financial statements, the element exists or has occurred; it is complete; it is a right owned or an obligation owed by the entity; its value is measured appropriately in accordance with the financial reporting framework; and it is presented appropriately in terms of classification, description, and disclosure. The auditor assesses risk in the financial statement elements assertion by assertion.[6]

Standards Check

CAS 315 Identifying and Assessing the Risks of Material Misstatement through Understanding the Entity and Its Environment

25. The auditor shall identify and assess the risks of material misstatement at
    (a) The financial statement level; and (Ref: Para. A105–A108)
    (b) The assertion level for classes of transactions, account balances, and disclosures (Ref: Para. A109–A113), to provide a basis for designing and performing further audit procedures.
26. For this purpose, the auditor shall
    (a) Identify risks throughout the process of obtaining an understanding of the entity and its environment, including relevant controls that relate to the risks, and by considering the classes of transactions, account balances, and disclosures in the financial statements; (Ref: Para. A114–A115)
    (b) Assess the identified risks, and evaluate whether they relate more pervasively to the financial statements as a whole and potentially affect many assertions;
    (c) Relate the identified risks to what can go wrong at the assertion level, taking account of relevant controls that the auditor intends to test; and (Ref: Para. A116–A118)
    (d) Consider the likelihood of misstatement, including the possibility of multiple misstatements, and whether the potential misstatement is of a magnitude that could result in a material misstatement.

Source: *CPA Canada Handbook—Assurance*, 2014.

We will begin with a discussion of the risk assessment at the financial statement level. Exhibit 5–4 summarizes the auditor's considerations in this risk assessment process and the role these considerations play in the thought process of assessing risk. The exhibit then gives some specific examples of the kinds of risk factors the auditor will investigate to learn if risks exist and how significant they might be. To plan an effective audit, the auditor needs to assess the most significant ways that the financial statements might have become misstated. The audit needs to be performed with significant risks in mind to make sure the auditors look at the right things in enough depth when they do their audit work.

As set out in the examples in Exhibit 5–4, some risks are inherent in the auditee's normal business operations. All businesses operate in a risky environment, and their managers need to have good strategies and processes to survive and succeed. Risks also arise from internal characteristics of the entity, such as the quality of its governance and management structure and the strength of its accounting systems and controls. **Significant risks** generally arise when the business risks are not adequately managed and controlled, or when the business's strategy involves taking on more risk that it can handle. Risks tend to become significant through business environment and operational risks in combination with entity risk factors.

EXHIBIT 5–4

An Overview of the Auditor's Assessment of Risk of Material Misstatement at the Financial Statement Level

AUDITOR RISK ASSESSMENT	IMPLICATIONS	EXAMPLES
WHAT NEEDS TO BE CONSIDERED?	WHY IS THIS CONSIDERED?	WHAT DO AUDITORS NEED TO LOOK FOR AND DO?
• What is the underlying economic reality of the entity's financial condition and performance?	This is what the financial statements should capture and communicate to users.	Business environment risks related to • Industry, regulatory, economy-related, and other external factors Business operational risks related to • Strategy and related business processes, investments, financing, and performance measures
• What could have gone wrong in preparing the financial statements?	This will lead to misstating the financial statements.	Entity risks related to • Corporate governance, management quality, related parties, internal control, accounting policies, information systems, etc.
• Is there any significant risk that any of these things have, in fact, gone wrong?	This is the auditor's assessment of risk of material misstatement at the financial statement level.	Significant risks arise due to • Fraud • Weak governance • Questionable management integrity and competence • Risky business strategy fitting poorly with business's risks • Questionable going-concern assumption • Weak internal controls • Management override of controls • Management bias in accounting policy choices and estimates • Manipulation of financial statements through inappropriate closing entries • Complex accounting principles and policies • Complex information systems and information technology • Unusual related party transactions
• If there are one or more significant risks, what evidence can auditors obtain to confirm or dispel suspicions that the events occurred/exist?	This will guide the auditors' overall audit strategy and planned audit procedures.	**The whole audit process needs to be designed to address these risks!**

---

significant risks:
identified and assessed risks of material misstatement that, in the auditor's judgment, require special audit consideration

Standards Check

CAS 315 Identifying and Assessing the Risks of Material Misstatement through Understanding the Entity and Its Environment

28. In exercising judgment as to which risks are significant risks, the auditor shall consider at least the following:
    (a) Whether the risk is a risk of fraud;
    (b) Whether the risk is related to recent significant economic, accounting, or other developments and, therefore, requires specific attention;
    (c) The complexity of transactions;
    (d) Whether the risk involves significant transactions with related parties;
    (e) The degree of subjectivity in the measurement of financial information related to the risk, especially those measurements involving a wide range of measurement uncertainty; and
    (f) Whether the risk involves significant transactions that are outside the normal course of business for the entity, or that otherwise appear to be unusual. (Ref: Para. A119–A123)

Source: *CPA Canada Handbook—Assurance,* 2014.

Standards Check

CAS 330 The Auditor's Responses to Assessed Risks

Substantive Procedures Related to the Financial Statement Closing Process
20. The auditor's substantive procedures shall include the following audit procedures related to the financial statement closing process:
    (a) Agreeing or reconciling the financial statements with the underlying accounting records; and
    (b) Examining material journal entries and other adjustments made during the course of preparing the financial statements. (Ref: Para. A52)

Source: *CPA Canada Handbook—Assurance,* 2014.

Special Note: Managing Risks in the Audit Profession and Practice, and in Audit Engagements

At this point in the discussion, you may be wondering, "Just how many kinds of risk do auditors have to deal with? There seem to be too many to keep track of!" You are right—the risks that need to be managed in the auditor's role are varied and complex, and this certainly is a challenge in learning, and practising, auditing! This special note will try to organize and classify these risks to help you understand why there are so many different types.

Earlier under LO3, we discussed the idea of the "auditor's risk from accepting the engagement" as a key element in the decision to become an organization's auditor in the first place. You may have noted that this type of risk is from the auditor's own personal perspective, as a professional person running a public accounting practice as a business. While it may seem somewhat self-interested for auditors to care about these more personal risks, auditors need to do this to ensure they succeed personally and also to ensure the whole auditing profession stays viable and strong. Consider what could happen if lots of auditors tried to do audits that were too risky; many of them would fail and the quality of financial statements would decline.

Now, under LO4, note that our perspective has shifted away from thinking about an auditor's personal perspective on his or her own risks; now we are thinking instead about risks in the auditee's business from the perspective of the auditor's professional responsibility to reduce *information risk* for financial statement users. Once they accept the audit engagement and start to perform it, auditors have to focus on risks in the auditee's business and how these risks might lead to material misstatement of the information in the financial statements. These are the audit risks that need to be managed to provide an opinion on whether a set of financial statements is fairly presented to users. The remaining discussions on risk will focus on this perspective, that is, auditors meeting their professional duties through performing audits that reduce the risk of material misstatement to an acceptably low level. But it may be helpful to keep in mind this 180-degree swing in our perspective on risk as we proceed to look at how auditors assess and respond to risk of material misstatement in the auditee's financial statements.

One additional perspective on risk should also be noted. All businesses face risks in their operating environment. As the saying goes: no risk, no reward. How big these business risks are, and how good the managers are at keeping things under control, are the underlying factors that may, or may not, lead to the material misstatements an auditor is concerned about. So it is also important to keep in mind that the auditor's perspective on assessing the risk of material misstatement integrates both the auditee's business-level risks and the risk that these may have led to materially misstated financial statements.

Business Environment Risks

In order to design the audit, auditors must understand the broad economic environment the auditee operates in, including such things as the effects of national economic policies (e.g., price regulations and import/export restrictions), the geographic location and its economy (e.g., Alberta's resource-based economy, or Ontario's manufacturing-based economy), and developments in taxation and regulatory areas (e.g., deregulation in agriculture and telecommunications, approval processes in the drug and chemical industries). For example, an increase in the Canadian dollar relative to the U.S. dollar negatively affects Canadian firms that rely on exports to the United States because their products become more expensive and thus less competitive in the U.S. market. A rapid, unexpected decrease in energy prices, as occurred during 2014, negatively impacts businesses in the resource sector but may be favourable to businesses such as manufacturing through decreased costs, or retail or tourism through increasing disposable income of consumers. In response to climate change concerns, a global initiative to reduce carbon emissions by imposing carbon taxes or emissions caps creates uncertainty and risk affecting many business models, particularly those whose energy needs result in high levels of carbon emissions.

In 2008, a credit crisis in the global financial system resulted in a deep, worldwide economic recession affecting many sectors of the economy. Such economic events can require business managers to make drastic changes to operating plans in order to survive and succeed. Some businesses benefit from economic turmoil, but many are not able to continue as going concerns. Clearly, auditors must have a strong grasp of the potential impact of economic events on a company's business in order to ensure its financial information fairly presents its underlying economic condition.

Industry characteristics also affect business risks. There are great differences in production and marketing in banking, insurance, mutual funds, retail food, hospitality, oil and gas, agriculture, manufacturing, and so forth. No auditors are experts in all these businesses. Audit firms typically have people who are expert in one or two industries and rely on them to manage audits in those industries. Indeed, some public accounting firms have a reputation for having many auditees in particular industries.

Risk In the Forestry Industry

During the 2000s, the Canadian forestry industry became subject to countervailing and anti-dumping duties of 27% on all lumber exported to the United States, its major buyer. In a poll of its members taken in June 2003, the Canadian Federation of Independent Business found that 70% of British Columbia's small forestry businesses reported being significantly or somewhat harmed by the lumber dispute. This is an example of a strategic risk faced by businesses in industries that depend on foreign sales where high, unexpected duties could put some companies into financial distress if profits fall. Auditors need to be aware of such risk to understand the business performance and how it affects the financial statements. Alternatively, financial statements indicating growth in profitability while heavy duties were being imposed go against expectations and need to be investigated carefully. It may suggest a misstatement.

(continued)

While the duty crisis described above was resolved by an agreement between Canada and the United States in 2006, in late 2008 another risk for the forestry industry appeared when AbitibiBowater Inc. decided to shut a money-losing newsprint mill in Newfoundland. The provincial government took action to expropriate the company's timber cutting rights. These rights had been granted in 1905 to a company that eventually became AbitibiBowater in exchange for creating jobs and investing in Newfoundland. The government also took steps to expropriate the company's hydroelectricity rights, which are even more valuable. Taking the view that the company had reneged on its side of the agreement by throwing the newsprint workers out of their jobs, the government's position was that the deal was no longer valid. As AbitibiBowater was planning to sell these rights to try to turn its struggling business around, this extraordinary event could have a significant impact on results in its financial position and future prospects. The company's auditors needed a good understanding of this situation involving the ownership of these rights to ensure the financial statements presented it fairly to users. This type of risk can also arise in oil-producing businesses operating in countries such as Venezuela, where the government has introduced laws to nationalize all oil properties regardless of ownership.

A later development affecting the Canadian forestry industry was a dramatic global shift in demand from its traditional trading partner, the United States, to China's booming economy. In May 2011, British Columbia's softwood lumber exports to China were 746,000 cubic metres, triple what they were a year earlier and surpassing the U.S. sales by $3 million. The shift was in part attributable to a significant slump in U.S. housing starts, but opening up to a huge new market has given Canadian producers a lot more leverage in negotiating duties with the United States, since there is less basis to accuse Canada of "dumping." And other Asian countries, such as Japan and India, also present enticing new markets. How predictable is this volume of sales, and at what prices, depends on many future factors, such as growth in housing starts in Asia, types of wood demanded, and competition from other global lumber producers like Europe—all factors an auditor will need to track to understand the business risks in any forestry company!

Sources: Ministry of Forests and Range, Province of British Columbia website, www.mit.gov.bc.ca/softwood/; "NL government to expropriate most AbitibiBowater assets," *Fort McMurray Today,* December 16, 2008, p. 2; "Premier Williams takes on pulp giant; but AbitibiBowater threatens legal action as Newfoundland seizes hydro and timber assets," *The Toronto Star,* December 17, 2008, p. B01; "AbitibiBowater calls expropriation 'hostile,'" *Waterloo Region Record,* December 20, 2008, p. F3; CBC News, "B.C. lumber exports to China soar," July 17, 2011, cbc.ca/news/canada/british-columbia/b-c-lumber-exports-to-china-soar-1.1073899; woodmarkets.com/canadian-exports-china-increase/; Frank Jack Daniel, "Venezuela to nationalize U.S. firm's oil rigs," Reuters US Edition, June 24, 2010, reuters.com/article/2010/06/24/us-venezuela-nationalizations-idUSTRE65N0UM20100624.

These events illustrate why in-depth knowledge of business is required to plan an audit. Auditors are expected to use integrative reasoning to draw together many complex and rapidly changing factors in reaching their conclusions. Accounting is supposed to reflect the economic substance of an entity's transactions, events, and conditions. Auditing in this dynamic world requires asking management the right questions, which calls for strong understanding of the auditee's business, environment, and risks.

The following box illustrates the kinds of risks a high-technology business faces. Intellectual property rights and patents raise a possibility that certain liabilities might be understated in the financial statements. In this case, the company faced significant risks related to development and patenting of its technology and the existence of other, similar patents. Management needs a process for managing these risks, and auditors need to assess whether these risks and liabilities have been reported fully in the statements.

Microsoft Loses Patent Battle with Canada's i4i

A Win for Intellectual Property Rights, or "Patent Trolls"?

Microsoft has lost an appeal to the U.S. Supreme Court over a $290 million award made against it in a patent dispute with the Canadian company i4i, which claimed a version of Microsoft Word infringed a patented method for editing documents.

The case began in 2007 when i4i sued Microsoft for infringing a patent covering a technology that lets users manipulate the architecture and content of a document. It said that Microsoft infringed the patent by allowing Word users to create custom XML documents. In 2009, the U.S. District Court for the Eastern District of Texas ruled in i4i's favour and ordered Microsoft to stop selling Word products in the United States in their current form. Microsoft removed the feature in order to keep selling its software.

Microsoft then appealed to the Supreme Court, saying the trial court's requirements had put an "overly demanding" standard to its invalidity defence: requiring it to prove its defence by "clear and convincing" evidence, rather than the more relaxed "preponderance of evidence." The difference would be similar to a criminal versus civil standard of proof, between "beyond all reasonable doubt" and "balance of probability."

Currently, when a patent holder accuses someone of infringing a patent, the burden is on the infringer to prove with "clear and convincing evidence" that the patent is invalid, said Sarah Columbia, head of the intellectual-property litigation practice at McDermott Will & Emery LLP. The decision means companies challenging patents being used in court battles will have to provide convincing proof that a patent is invalid if they want to have it set aside. Microsoft had sought to weaken the level of proof needed.

Microsoft argued that when new evidence is presented that could invalidate a patent, the burden of proof should be lowered to a preponderance of the evidence, considered a less-strict burden than clear and convincing evidence. The U.S. Supreme Court, however, upheld the lower court decisions that the burden of proof should continue to be applied.

Microsoft and others in the technology sector are likely to be unhappy with the ruling. While such companies have plenty of their own patents, they are more likely to be the subject of lawsuits, often lodged by so-called patent trolls, than to be defending their own patents. Patent trolls are companies that buy patents with the primary goal of asserting them for financial gain.

i4i, set up in 1993 by Michel Vulpe, has provided systems for the U.S. Patent Office ("Ironic, in the circumstances" remarked Loudon Owen, chairman of i4i); the U.S. Air Force; and a number of pharmaceutical companies, including Novo Nordisk and Bayer. Basically, it takes huge amounts of unstructured data and puts XML wrappers around it, making it useful and usable. The company has repeatedly insisted that it is not a "patent troll" and that it creates real value through the application of its systems for clients.

Microsoft and i4i held discussions in 2000 and 2001 about XML and custom XML, but no business emerged. Microsoft subsequently began using structured XML in Word, infuriating i4i.

Mr. Owen said, "Microsoft tried to gut the value of patents by introducing a lower standard for invalidating patents. It is now 100% clear that you can only invalidate a patent based on 'clear and convincing' evidence." He called the ruling "one of the most significant business cases the court has decided in decades. Affirmation of the federal circuit on a ruling in favour of patent holders is virtually unprecedented. While this ruling maintains the prevailing standard, the innovation community must be ever-vigilant to defend its property rights."

The decision will have repercussions in cases where patents are the key element of the case—which will affect everyone from smartphone manufacturers to app developers.

Organizations including Apple, Google, EMC, Cisco Systems, and the Electronic Frontier Foundation had all filed documents with the court in support of Microsoft's argument.

Doug Cawley of the law firm McKool Smith worked as lead trial counsel for i4i. He says today's ruling is an important victory for patent holders everywhere. "We are very pleased that the High Court agreed with our position that Congress intended a heightened standard of evidence to invalidate a patent," said Mr. Cawley. "Today's ruling, which enforces the Federal Circuit's historical reliance on 'clear and convincing evidence,' will have a sweeping impact on how patents are protected." Pharmaceutical companies, however, are likely to applaud the decision, Ackerman said. "They haven't seen these troll suits and they rely very heavily on patent protection to keep [generic brands] out," he said. "They invest lots of money and want their patents to be strong."

Sources: Nancy Gohring, "Supreme Court ruling seen as a win for patent trolls," IDG News, June 9, 2011 at pcworld.com/article/229968/article. html; "McKool Smith helps i4i win $290 million Supreme Court ruling," PR Newswire, June 9, 2011, at prnewswire.com/news-releases/mckool-smith-helps-i4i-win-290-million-supreme-court-ruling-123571679.html; Charles Arthur, "Microsoft loses patent battle with Canada's i4i: Supreme Court decision means firms will have to provide proof a patent is invalid," *The Guardian* (UK), June 10, 2011, at guardian.co.uk/technology/2011/jun/10/microsoft-canada-i4i-patent.

Review Checkpoints

5-43   Why does the auditor need a good understanding of the auditee's business and environment?

5-44   How do changes in the economic environment affect a business's risks?

5-45   How do changes in the industry environment affect a business's risks?

5-46   What specific risks exist in high-tech companies? in the forestry industry?

Preliminary Analytical Procedures for Audit Planning

Preliminary Analytical Procedures

 Use preliminary analytical procedures on management's draft financial statements to identify areas where misstatements are most likely.

Auditors use the planning tools of business risk assessment, analytical procedures, materiality decisions, overall audit strategy, audit risk assessment, and audit plans to guide and direct their work. Based on the preliminary analysis and on understanding the auditee's financial reporting and its business risks, auditors establish the overall audit strategy for the engagement; set out the basic scope, nature, and timing of the work to be performed; and identify any key risk areas requiring special attention by the audit team.[7]

GAAS require that analytical procedures be applied at two points in an audit, at the beginning and at the end. At the beginning, the planning stage risk assessment discussed in this chapter (CAS 315) involves analysis. At the end, the partner in charge of the audit must review the overall quality of the audit work and look for problems by analyzing the financial statements (CAS 520). Auditors may also decide to use analytical procedures in a third way, to provide substantive evidence about specific financial statement assertions (CAS 520 and 330).[8] The auditing standards do not specify which particular analytical procedures are required, as this is left to the auditors' professional judgment based on the circumstances of each audit.

Standards Check

CAS 315 Identifying and Assessing the Risks of Material Misstatement through Understanding the Entity and Its Environment

6. The risk assessment procedures shall include the following:

(a) Inquiries of management and of others within the entity who in the auditor's judgment may have information that is likely to assist in identifying risks of material misstatement due to fraud or error. (Ref: Para. A6)

(b) Analytical procedures. (Ref: Para. A7–A10)

(c) Observation and inspection. (Ref: Para. A11)

CAS 520 Analytical Procedures

6. The auditor shall design and perform analytical procedures near the end of the audit that assist the auditor when forming an overall conclusion as to whether the financial statements are consistent with the auditor's understanding of the entity. (Ref: Para. A17–A19)

Source: *CPA Canada Handbook—Assurance*, 2014.

Analytical procedures are powerful techniques for identifying unusual changes and relations in financial statement data. The purpose of doing **analysis** at the beginning of the engagement is "attention directing"—to alert the audit team to problems (errors, fraud) that may exist in the account balances, transactions, and disclosures and to guide the design of further audit work.[9] The auditor's understanding of the business risks is

analytical procedures:
specific methods and tests used to perform analysis on client account balances

analysis:
a process of examining a complex item to better understand it by using techniques such as breaking it down into finer aspects and comparing it to other items

important in identifying the changes and relations expected based on how the business performed during the audited period and what might indicate that the financial information is misstated.

Five types of general analytical procedures that may be performed on financial statement data are listed below. The first three types involve comparisons with other relevant data, and the last two involve studying relationships.

1. Compare current-year account balances with balances for one or more comparable periods.

2. Compare current-year account balances and financial relationships (e.g., ratios) with similar information for the industry the company operates in.

3. Compare the current-year account balances with the company's anticipated results as found in the budgets and forecasts.

4. Evaluate the relationships of current-year account balances to other current-year balances for conformity to predictable patterns based on the company's experience.

5. Study the relationships of current-year account balances to relevant non-financial information (e.g., physical production statistics or capacity constraints).

Two procedures often used as a starting point are **horizontal analysis** (type 1), which is the comparison of changes of financial statement amounts across two or more years, and **vertical analysis** (type 4), which is the comparison of financial statement amounts expressed each year as proportions of a base (e.g., sales for the income statement accounts and total assets for the balance sheet accounts, or ratios such as debt-to-equity or working capital). In the sections that follow, these procedures are emphasized. In particular, type 1 is implemented by comparison of current-year account balances with balances for one or more comparable periods, and type 4 by analysis of the relationships of individual account balances with other current-year total balances as the base. A combination of types 1 and 4, implemented by examining the trends in various ratios over time, is very effective as well.

Research finds that analytical procedures are most effective when integrated with other sources of information, especially when accompanied by a strong knowledge of the auditee's business. "Auditors must combine different types of knowledge (accounting, general business, industry, and auditee-specific) and issues (operating, financing, and investing) into a whole. This skill is needed whether analytical procedures are used for planning, substantive testing, or overall review purposes, but it appears to be most critical at overall review, where the auditor's goal is to examine the financial statements to determine whether they make sense taken as a whole."[10]

Analytical procedures can also take other forms, ranging from simple to complex. A wide range of early information-gathering activities can be defined as "analytical procedures," including the following:

- Review of accounting misstatements discovered in prior-year audits and any adjustments proposed to management
- Conversations with auditee personnel regarding developments affecting the organization, such as changes in strategy, business processes, information technology, key management, ownership, industry conditions, economic conditions, and legal environment
- Review of the corporate charter and bylaws or partnership agreement
- Review of contracts, agreements, and legal proceedings
- Reading and study of the **minutes** of meetings of the board of directors, the group charged with governance of the organization, and any subcommittees of the board (e.g., executive committee, finance committee, compensation committee, audit committee)

horizontal analysis:
a comparison of changes of financial statement numbers and ratios across two or more years

vertical analysis:
the analytical procedure of comparing all financial statement items to a common base, for example, total assets or total sales

minutes:
formal written records of key events and decisions made in a formal meeting, such as a corporate board meeting

The box below outlines some of the key knowledge that auditors obtain from reading minutes.

What's in the Minutes of Meetings?

Boards of directors are responsible for monitoring the auditee's business. The minutes of both their meetings and their committees (e.g., executive committee, finance committee, compensation committee, audit committee) contain information of vital interest to the independent auditors. Some examples are as follows:

- Declared amount of dividends
- Authorization of officers' salaries and bonuses
- Authorization of stock options and other "perq" compensation
- Acceptance of contracts, agreements, and lawsuit settlements
- Approval of major purchases of property, plant, and equipment and of investments
- Discussions of any acquisitions, mergers, and divestitures in progress
- Authorization of financing by share issues, long-term debt, and leases
- Approval to pledge assets as security for debts
- Discussion of negotiations on bank loans and payment waivers
- Approval of accounting policies and accounting for estimates and unusual transactions
- Authorizations for individuals to sign bank cheques

Auditors take notes on or make copies of important parts of the minutes and compare them with information in the accounting records, financial statements, and note disclosures (e.g., compare the amount of dividends declared with the amount paid and reported in the financial statements). Because the minutes are so important in determining what needs to be reported in order to obtain fair presentation, denying access to the board of directors meeting minutes constitutes a major scope restriction by an auditee. In such a case, because of the pervasive impact that boards of directors' decisions can have on financial statement measurements and disclosures, a disclaimer of audit opinion is likely. When the auditor expects to issue a disclaimer of opinion, the audit firm will usually resign from the audit engagement since the audit would add little value.

Other types of analytical procedures can be complex, including mathematical time series and regression calculations, comparisons of multi-year data, and trend and ratio analyses. Exhibit 5–5 later on illustrates an approach that combines analysis of relationships (financial ratios) and trends (current year versus prior year).

Review Checkpoints

5-47   What is the purpose of performing analytical procedures at the beginning of the audit engagement?

5-48   What is the role of the auditor's understanding of the business and its risks in performing analytical procedures?

5-49   What are five types of general analytical procedures?

5-50   What official documents and authorizations should an auditor read when performing preliminary analytical procedures?

5-51   What important information can be found in directors' minutes about officers' compensation, business operations, corporate finance, accounting policies, and control?

5-52   What is the role of business risk analysis in the audit planning process?

Applying Analytical Procedures to Management's Draft Financial Statements

One of the first things the auditor receives is **management's draft financial statements**. Depending on the organization, these financial statements may be virtually complete and final (e.g., in a large company with many professionally qualified accountants on staff) or preliminary statements that still require adjustments for items such as bonuses and income taxes (e.g., in a small company with few in-house accountants). Even when the audit begins with a set of draft statements still requiring final adjustments, the auditor must remember that all financial reporting decisions are management's responsibility. Particularly in smaller organizations, an auditor may identify appropriate adjustments or accounting entries, but, to maintain independence, the auditor must ensure that management approves and takes responsibility for all the accounting choices made.

Analysis Procedures for Attention Directing

Auditors perform analytical procedures on the draft statements looking for relationships that do not make sense, as these may indicate problem areas where the accounts do not faithfully represent the underlying economic substance. **Representational faithfulness** is a fundamental accounting concept relating to the quality of the claims, or assertions, that management makes in fairly presenting its financial statements. Analysis of the financial statements' assertions is very important in the business risk approach to auditing, as we will discuss throughout the stages of the audit process. Here in the planning stage, analytical procedures are primarily **attention directing**: they do not provide direct evidence about the numbers in the financial statements, but their main purpose is to help the audit team plan effective audit programs, maximizing the probability of finding any material misstatements. They identify potential problem areas so that the subsequent work can be designed to reduce the risk of missing something important. The analysis application explained here illustrates this attention-directing aspect—the pointing out of accounts that may contain misstatements.

Use an Organized Approach

By following an organized approach—using a standard starting place—preliminary analytical procedures can provide considerable familiarity with the auditee's business. Many auditors start with comparative financial statements and calculate common-size statements (vertical analysis) and year-to-year change in balance sheet and income statement accounts (horizontal analysis). This is the start of describing the financial activities for the current year under audit.

Exhibit 5–5 contains financial balances for the prior year (consider them audited) and the current year (consider them draft numbers not yet audited) for the EcoPak Inc. company in the chapter-opening audit story. Common-size statements (vertical) are shown in parallel columns, and the dollar amount and percentage change (horizontal) are shown in the last two columns. These analytical procedures generate basic analytical data that are the starting point for the auditors' further evaluation and inquiry.

---

management's draft financial statements:
the set of financial statements an auditor receives from the auditee's management at the start of the year-end audit work, containing the management assertions (claims) that will be subject to verification by the auditor

representational faithfulness:
when information presented in an entity's financial statements closely corresponds to the actual underlying transactions and events affecting it, conveying their economic substance rather than simply their legal form

attention directing:
refers to the main purpose of analytical procedures when they are performed for risk assessment procedures early in the audit engagement, which is to focus the auditor's assessment on unusual changes or conditions

Describe the Financial Activities

After generating these basic financial data, the next step is to describe the financial changes and relationships visible in them. According to the draft financial statements in Exhibit 5–5, the company increased net income through increasing sales by 10%, reducing cost of goods sold as a proportion of sales, and controlling other expenses. At least some of the sales growth appears to have been prompted by easier credit (larger accounts receivable) and more service (more equipment in use). The company also used much of its cash and borrowed to purchase the equipment, make its payment on the long-term debt, and pay dividends.

EXHIBIT 5–5

EcoPak Inc.: Preliminary Analytical Procedures Data

	PRIOR YEAR		CURRENT YEAR		CHANGE	
	BALANCE	COMMON-SIZE ANALYSIS	BALANCE	COMMON-SIZE ANALYSIS	AMOUNT	PERCENT CHANGE ANALYSIS
Assets						
Cash	$ 600,000	14.78%	$ 200,000	4.12%	($ 400,000)	−66.67%
Accounts receivable	500,000	12.32	900,000	18.56	400,000	80.00
Allowance for doubtful accounts	(40,000)	−0.99	(50,000)	−1.03	(10,000)	25.00
Inventories	1,500,000	36.95	1,600,000	32.99	100,000	6.67
Total current assets	2,560,000	63.05	2,650,000	54.63	90,000	3.52
Property, plant, & equipment	3,000,000	73.89	4,000,000	82.47	1,000,000	33.33
Accumulated amortization	(1,500,000)	−36.95	(1,800,000)	−37.11	(300,000)	20.00
Total assets	$4,060,000	100.00%	$4,850,000	100.00%	$ 790,000	19.46%
Liabilities and Equity						
Accounts payable	$ 500,000	12.32%	$ 400,000	8.25%	($ 100,000)	−20.00%
Bank loans, 11%	0	0.00	750,000	15.46	750,000	
Accrued interest	60,000	1.48	40,000	0.82	(20,000)	−33.33
Total current liabilities	560,000	13.79	1,190,000	24.53	630,000	112.50
Long-term debt, 10%	600,000	14.78	400,000	8.25	(200,000)	−33.33
Total liabilities	1,160,000	28.57	1,590,000	32.78	430,000	37.07
Share capital	2,000,000	49.26	2,000,000	41.24	0	0.00
Retained earnings	900,000	22.17	1,260,000	25.98	360,000	40.00
Total liabilities and equity	$4,060,000	100.00%	$4,850,000	100.00%	$ 790,000	19.46%
Income						
Sales (net)	$9,000,000	100.00%	$9,900,000	100.00%	$ 900,000	10.00%
Cost of goods sold	6,750,000	75.00	7,200,000	72.73	450,000	6.67
Gross margin	2,250,000	25.00	2,700,000	27.27	450,000	20.00
General expense	1,590,000	17.67	1,734,000	17.52	144,000	9.06
Amortization	300,000	3.33	300,000	3.03	0	0.00
Operating income	360,000	4.00	666,000	6.46	306,000	85.00
Interest expense	60,000	0.67	40,000	0.40	(20,000)	−33.33
Income taxes (40%)	120,000	1.33	256,000	2.59	136,000	113.33
Net income	$ 180,000	2.00%	$ 370,000	3.74%	$ 190,000	105.56%

Ask Relevant Questions

The next step is to ask, "What could be wrong?" and "What errors, fraud, or legitimate explanations might account for these financial results?" For this explanation we will limit our attention to the accounts receivable and inventory, while other ratios can help support the analysis. Exhibit 5–6 contains several familiar ratios, and Appendix 5A includes a list of commonly used ratios with their formulas.

EXHIBIT 5–6

EcoPak Inc.: Selected Financial Ratios

	PRIOR YEAR	CURRENT YEAR	PERCENT CHANGE
Balance Sheet Ratios			
Current ratio	4.57	2.23	−51.29%
Days' sales in receivables	18.40	30.91	67.98
Doubtful accounts ratio	0.0800	0.0556	−30.56
Days' sales in inventory	80.00	80.00	0.00
Debt/equity ratio	0.40	0.49	21.93
Operations Ratios			
Receivables turnover	19.57	11.65	−40.47
Inventory turnover	4.50	4.50	0.00
Cost of goods sold/sales	75.00%	72.73%	−3.03
Gross margin percentage	25.00%	27.27%	9.09
Return on beginning equity	6.62%	12.76%	92.80
Financial Distress Ratios[11]			
Working capital/total assets	0.49	0.30	−38.89
Retained earnings/total assets	0.22	0.26	17.20
EBIT/total assets	0.09	0.14	54.87
Market value of equity/total debt	2.59	1.89	−27.04
Net sales/total assets	2.22	2.04	−7.92
Discriminant Z score	4.96	4.35	−12.32

Review Checkpoints

5-53   What are management's draft financial statements?

5-54   What methods can auditors use to apply comparison and ratio analysis to management's financial statements?

5-55   What can the auditor learn from a vertical analysis?

5-56   What can the auditor learn from a horizontal analysis?

5-57   What are some of the ratios that can be used in preliminary analytical procedures?

Here are two examples of the kinds of questions auditors should ask about these financial statements.

- *Are the accounts receivable collectible?* (Or, is the allowance for doubtful accounts large enough?) Easier credit can lead to more bad debts. The company has a much larger amount of receivables (see Exhibit 5–5), days' sales in receivables has increased significantly (see Exhibit 5–6), receivables turnover has decreased (see Exhibit 5–6), and allowance for doubtful accounts is smaller in proportion to the receivables (see Exhibit 5–6). If the prior-year allowance for bad debts at 8% of receivables was appropriate, and conditions have not worsened, perhaps the allowance should be closer to $72,000 than to $50,000. The auditors should work carefully on the evidence related to accounts receivable valuation.

- *Could the inventory be overstated?* (Or, could the cost of the goods sold be understated?) Overstatement of the ending inventory would cause the cost of goods sold to be understated. The percentage of cost of goods sold to sales shows a decrease (see Exhibits 5–5 and 5–6). If the 75% of the prior year represents a more accurate cost of goods sold, the income before taxes may be overstated by $225,000 (75% of $9.9 million minus $7.2 million unaudited cost of goods sold). The days' sales in inventory and the inventory turnover remained the same (see Exhibit 5–6), but you might expect them to change in light of the larger volume of sales. Careful work on the physical count and valuation of inventory is needed.

Other questions can be asked and other relationships derived when industry statistics are available. Industry statistics from services such as Statistics Canada, FPinformart.ca, Dun & Bradstreet, Thomson Research, and Mergent Online typically include industry averages for important financial yardsticks, such as gross profit margin, return on sales, current ratio, and debt/net worth. A comparison with auditee data may reveal out-of-line statistics indicating company strength, a weak financial position, or possibly an error or misstatement in the statements. However, remember that averages may not be representative of a particular company.

Comparing reported financial results with internal budgets and forecasts can also be useful. If a budget or forecast represents management's estimate of probable future outcomes, items that fall short of or exceed the estimates become audit-relevant questions. If a company expected to sell 10,000 units of a product but sold only 5,000, the auditors would plan a careful lower-of-cost-and-market study of the inventory of unsold units. If 15,000 were sold, they would plan a careful audit for sales validity. Comparisons can be tricky, however. Some companies use budgets and forecasts as goals rather than as expressions of probable outcomes. Also, the avoidance of shortfall or excess might be the result of managers manipulating the numbers to "meet the budget." Auditors must be careful to learn about a company's business conditions from sources other than the internal records when analyzing comparisons with budgets and forecasts.

Look at the Cash Flows

The analysis of changes in cash flows from operating, investment, and financing activities is a very informative tool. A cash flow deficit from operations may signal financial difficulty. Companies fail when they run out of cash (no surprise) and are unable to pay their debts when they become due. In a small business audit, the auditee

Review Checkpoints

5-58 How can computing the accounts receivable turnover ratio indicate potential misstatement in the accounts receivable balance?

5-59 How can computing the number of days of sales in inventory indicate potential misstatement in the inventory balance?

5-60 What conclusion can you draw by analyzing the relationship between retained earnings and income for the EcoPak Inc. data shown in Exhibit 5–5?

5-61 What is the net cash flow for the current year for EcoPak Inc., shown in Exhibit 5–5?

5-62 Why don't preliminary analytical procedures provide direct evidence about financial statement misstatements? What then is their purpose in an audit?

may not have prepared a cash flow statement. In that case, the auditors can use the comparative financial statements to prepare one, providing this important part of their preliminary analysis.

Materiality Levels for Audit Planning

LO6 Explain the materiality levels used for planning the audit and how these amounts are determined.

Materiality is one of the first important judgments the auditor must make, since it affects every other planning, examination, and reporting decision. The auditor's materiality decisions are an important application of professional judgment and involve both qualitative and quantitative considerations. In planning an audit, the materiality level decisions are based on the auditor's knowledge about the organization's business risks, identification of the likely users and uses of its audited general purpose financial statements, preliminary analysis of its draft financial statements, and experience in prior audits.

Materiality Decisions in the Context of the Whole Audit Process

It is important to note that audit materiality concepts apply throughout all the steps of the audit process shown in Exhibit 5–1. To provide you with this larger context, we will introduce our discussion of materiality with a brief overview of the materiality decisions that must be made throughout an audit. Then, in this chapter we will focus on the planning step, looking at the first materiality decisions made to assess the key risk areas and to plan how to perform the audit to respond to those key risks. As we work through how to design audit procedures and use sampling procedures throughout Parts 2 and 3 of the text, we will see examples of how the materiality concept is applied in practice. Finally, in Chapter 16 we will discuss how the materiality decisions are applied at the very end of the audit to form a conclusion about what opinion to give in the auditor's report. Ultimately, the overall materiality level sets the ceiling for what accumulated misstatements can be accepted to be able to conclude that the financial statements are not materially misstated. Exhibit 5–7 summarizes the key materiality decisions throughout the audit and gives examples of the auditors' qualitative and quantitative judgments related to each.

Standards Check

CAS 320 Materiality in Planning and Performing an Audit

5. The concept of materiality is applied by the auditor both in planning and performing the audit, and in evaluating the effect of identified misstatements on the audit and of uncorrected misstatements, if any, on the financial statements and in forming the opinion in the auditor's report. (Ref: Para. A1)

6. In planning the audit, the auditor makes judgments about the size of misstatements that will be considered material. These judgments provide a basis for
   (a) Determining the nature, timing, and extent of risk assessment procedures;
   (b) Identifying and assessing the risks of material misstatement; and
   (c) Determining the nature, timing, and extent of further audit procedures.

Source: *CPA Canada Handbook—Assurance,* 2014.

Materiality Decisions throughout the Audit Process

AUDIT PROCESS STEPS	EXAMPLES OF AUDITOR CONSIDERATIONS TO DECIDE ON MATERIALITY LEVELS	
	QUANTITATIVE FACTORS	QUALITATIVE FACTORS
Assessing Risks of Material Misstatement • Planning the audit engagement	CONSIDER: • What rules of thumb (e.g., 5% of normal pre-tax income, 1/2 to 1% of revenue) are most appropriate to the engagement?	CONSIDER: • Who are the key financial statement users and their decisions based on the financial statements? • What are the key accounts and relations in the financial statements?
Responding to Assessed Risks • Performing audit procedures that provide sufficient appropriate audit evidence	CONSIDER: • What are the sizes of account balances and transactions to be audited? • For large amounts (e.g., "populations") to be tested, are sample sizes based on performance materiality? • Are there any smaller amounts that may only need minimal audit procedures? • Any suspected fraud is always material!	CONSIDER: • Have any unexpected events or conditions affected risks of material misstatement and/or initial planning materiality decisions? • Are there any suspicions raised of fraud or illegal acts?
Concluding • Forming an opinion on whether financial statements are materially misstated (i.e., not fairly presented)	CONSIDER: • Has the audit team found misstatements that, if not corrected by management, will add up to an amount close to or greater than overall materiality? • If any misstatements extrapolated from errors found in sampling tests are included with identified accumulated misstatements, does this exceed overall materiality? • Is there a need to modify the audit opinion?	CONSIDER: • What is the nature of misstatements identified (are they masking important trends or affecting key covenants and contracts based on financial information)? • Are management's justifications for not correcting valid? • Is the impact of misstatements on financial statements and key user decisions expected to be significant? • Is there a need to modify the audit opinion?

When planning a financial statement audit, auditors first decide on a level of **materiality for the financial statements as a whole (overall materiality),** which they consider as the largest amount of uncorrected monetary misstatement that might exist in published financial statements that still **present fairly (fairly present)** the company's financial position and results of operations in conformity with GAAP. The concept of fair presentation comes from the accounting standards and generally means that the financial statements do not contain misstatements or omissions significant enough to mislead users into making inappropriate economic decisions based on those financial statements.

materiality for the financial statements as a whole (overall materiality):
an auditor's judgment regarding what is the largest amount of uncorrected monetary misstatement that might exist in financial statements that still fairly presents the auditee's financial position and results of operations under an acceptable financial reporting framework

present fairly (fairly present):
in financial reporting, that management's financial statements achieve the properties of being a faithful representation of the economic realities they purport to portray, and of not being misleading to users

CAS 320 Materiality in Planning and Performing an Audit

10. When establishing the overall audit strategy, the auditor shall determine materiality for the financial statements as a whole. *[Note: In this text we use the term* overall materiality *for this amount.]*

Source: *CPA Canada Handbook—Assurance,* 2014.

Financial Statement Materiality

So what is materiality, and how can you deal with it? In financial accounting and reporting, information is material and should be disclosed if it is likely to influence the economic decisions of financial statement users. Auditing standards provide guidance intended to help auditors with these judgments.[12] The emphasis is on the users' point of view, not that of accountants or managers. Thus, "material" means important or significant.

An analogy placing the materiality concept in a more everyday context may be helpful. Imagine you are planning to get your computer repaired, and the technician tells you it will most likely cost $500, but the actual amount could be between $490 and $510. Would you decide to go ahead with the repairs, given the range in estimates? Most people probably would not let a $10 difference on $500 affect their decision; that is to say, $10 is not "material" to their decision. If the technician said the actual price could be between $100 and $900, most people would find that range too big to accept. The possible $400 variation (in either direction) from the likely cost of $500 is an amount that does affect the decision: it is highly material. If a technician said the repair would be $500 and it ended up being $900, most people would say that the $500 number was materially misstated! What if the technician gave a range of $450 to $550? Some people might be okay with this range, while others would find another technician who could give a more precise amount. This analogy illustrates how materiality is viewed as an amount that a typical user of the information finds significant to their decision making. It also illustrates how materiality is a judgment call because the exact amount cannot be specified and it can vary from user to user.

It is a challenge for an auditor to judge what amount is material to users. To some extent, the auditor guesses what a typical financial statement user would consider significant to his or her decisions. It is even more challenging to apply materiality in performing the audit and evaluating the audit results. Financial statement measurements and information in disclosures are not perfectly accurate. However, do not conclude that financial reports are inherently imprecise and inaccurate. Some numbers will contain mistakes, and some are imprecise because they are based on estimates. Everyone knows that people make mistakes (e.g., billing a customer the wrong amount or using the wrong price to value inventory), and many financial measurements are based on estimates (e.g., the estimated depreciable lives of fixed assets or the estimated amount of uncollectible accounts receivable). However, this is not an excuse to be sloppy about clerical accuracy or negligent in accounting judgments. As an example of applying materiality to auditing accounting numbers that involve a high degree of management judgment, the box below illustrates the auditor's approach for assessing management's estimates.

Audit Considerations for Accounting Estimates

An accounting estimate is an approximation of a financial statement number, and estimates are often included in financial statements (see CAS 540). Examples are net realizable value of accounts receivable, fair values of assets and liabilities, amortization expense, lease capitalization criteria, percentage-of-completion contract revenues, pension expense, and warranty liabilities.

Management is responsible for making accounting estimates. Auditors are responsible for determining that all appropriate estimates have been made, that they are reasonable, and that they are presented and disclosed in conformity with GAAP.

As part of the audit process, the auditors produce their own estimate and compare it with management's. Often, a range for an amount is considered. For example, management may estimate an allowance for doubtful accounts at $50,000, and

(continued)

the auditors may estimate it at $40,000 to $55,000. In this case, management's estimate is within the auditor's range of reasonableness. However, the auditors should take note that the management estimate leans toward the conservative side (more than the auditors' $40,000 lower estimate, but not much less than the auditors' higher $55,000 estimate). If other estimates exhibit the same conservatism and the aggregate effect is material, the auditors will need to evaluate the overall reasonableness of the effect of all estimates taken together.

If the auditors develop an estimate that differs (e.g., a range of $55,000 to $70,000 for the allowance that management estimated at $50,000), the difference between management's estimate and the closest end of the auditors' range is considered a misstatement (in this case, misstatement = $5,000 = auditors' $55,000 minus management's $50,000). The remaining difference to the farthest end of the range ($15,000 = $70,000 − $55,000) is noted and reconsidered in combination with the findings on all management's estimates.

Some evidence of the reasonableness of estimates is the actual experience of the company with financial amounts estimated at an earlier date. Tracking the accuracy of management's earlier estimates can provide the auditor with information on the expected accuracy of future estimates.

Auditors are limited by the nature of accounting. Some amount of inaccuracy is unavoidable in financial statements for the following reasons:

1. Unimportant inaccuracies do not affect users' decisions and hence are not material.

2. The cost of finding and correcting small errors is too great.

3. The time taken to find them would delay issuance of financial statements.

Accounting numbers are never perfectly accurate, but public accountants (PAs) and auditors want to ensure that financial reports do not contain material misstatements that could make them misleading.

Standards Check

CAS 320 Materiality in Planning and Performing an Audit

4. The auditor's determination of materiality is a matter of professional judgment and is affected by the auditor's perception of the financial information needs of users of the financial statements. In this context, it is reasonable for the auditor to assume that users

   (a) Have a reasonable knowledge of business and economic activities and accounting and a willingness to study the information in the financial statements with reasonable diligence;

   (b) Understand that financial statements are prepared, presented, and audited to levels of materiality;

   (c) Recognize the uncertainties inherent in the measurement of amounts based on the use of estimates, judgment, and the consideration of future events; and

   (d) Make reasonable economic decisions on the basis of the information in the financial statements.

Source: CPA Canada Handbook—Assurance, 2014.

Review Checkpoints

5-63   Why is the materiality decision one of the first decisions made in the audit?

5-64   What is material information in accounting and auditing?

5-65   What limitations of accounting affect auditors?

5-66   How is the materiality level applied in auditing an accounting estimate?

5-67   What do you think is the best objective evidence of the reasonableness of an accounting estimate? Use the allowance for doubtful accounts receivable as an example.

Performance Materiality

When setting out the overall audit strategy, the auditor first determines a materiality level for the financial statements as a whole (overall materiality). However, just as accounting may have limitations, there are also limitations in performing an audit. Since not every item can be tested, and totally conclusive evidence is never available, auditors might misinterpret or overlook evidence that could reveal misstatements. To leave room for the possibility that their audit work might miss some errors in the financial statements, auditors will determine an amount referred to as **performance materiality**, which is somewhat less than the materiality for the financial statements as a whole. By designing their audit work to search out this smaller amount of misstatement, auditors can reduce the risk that the total of uncorrected and undetected misstatements exceeds the materiality level for the financial statements as a whole. In other words, even if the auditors do miss some misstatement, they have an allowance set aside that can be used up before the total misstatements exceed the overall materiality level. To illustrate, imagine you are going on a four-day holiday. You have $700 to spend and know your hotel will be $100 per night. You could spend all your remaining $300 on meals and entertainment, but if you are cautious, you will keep some of it aside for unexpected events such as a lost phone or a medical emergency.

The difference between the overall materiality level and the performance materiality level can be seen as a cushion against misstatements, unknown to the auditor, that could make the financial statements materially misstated, just as holiday cash is kept aside for unexpected events. The smaller performance materiality is used to identify and assess risks, to design audit procedures to be done in response to the assessed risks, and to evaluate the results of sampling procedures. How much smaller should it be? Again, we see the need for auditors to use their judgment. Hints for making your decision can be found in the amount of misstatements found in previous audits, in the average in similar organizations if it is a new audit, or in practical application guidance rules of thumb.

Standards Check

CAS 320 Materiality in Planning and Performing an Audit

9. For purposes of the CASs, performance materiality means the amount or amounts set by the auditor at less than materiality for the financial statements as a whole to reduce to an appropriately low level the probability that the aggregate of uncorrected and undetected misstatements exceeds materiality for the financial statements as a whole. . . .

11. The auditor shall determine performance materiality for purposes of assessing the risks of material misstatement and determining the nature, timing, and extent of further audit procedures. (Ref: Para. A12)

Source: *CPA Canada Handbook–Assurance*, 2014.

Since the materiality decisions are made early in the audit, auditors must reconsider their decisions whenever new information that might affect the materiality decision surfaces during the audit. If the auditor decides the materiality should be revised to a smaller amount, the auditor will probably have to extend any testing that was done based on the larger materiality level. Note an important relationship illustrated here: as the audit materiality level gets smaller, the auditor must do more work to find any material misstatements. As an analogy, imagine you drive your car to the shopping centre one day, and park in the parking lot just as a snowstorm is starting. When you go back outside after shopping, everything is covered in a deep blanket of snow. Imagine that your car is "material"—you need to find it so you can drive home. You will probably have a little bit of work to do to identify which bump in the snow has your car under it, maybe brushing off one or two others in the general area before you find the right one. But say you realize that you dropped your car keys in

performance materiality:
an amount set by the auditor at less than materiality for the financial statements as a whole, to reduce to an appropriately low level the probability that the aggregate of uncorrected and undetected misstatements exceeds materiality for the financial statements as a whole

the parking lot on the way into the mall, so now your tiny car keys are "material" to being able to drive home. How much more work will you need to do to find your keys under all that snow, compared with finding a big car? A lot more digging![13]

Review Checkpoints

5-68   How does overall materiality for the financial statements as a whole differ from overall performance materiality in the auditing standards?

5-69   What issues arise if an auditor realizes partway through the audit that a smaller materiality level is appropriate?

Materiality Judgment Criteria

Materiality is both a quantitative and a qualitative judgment, made in the context of the auditee's specific circumstances. The importance of the qualitative aspects of materiality is highlighted in the current environment because of a perception that the materiality concept had been "abused"—used as an excuse to do less audit work or not require correction of significant misstatement. For example, under U.S. Securities and Exchange Commission (SEC) regulations, auditors are not allowed to rely exclusively on quantitative benchmarks. In particular, any quantitatively small misstatements resulting from intentional misstatement, intentional violation of the law, or intentional earnings manipulation must be considered material. Generally, a quantitatively immaterial misstatement is now considered material if it

- masks a change in earnings or other trends,
- hides a failure to meet analysts' consensus expectations for the auditee,
- changes a loss into net income or vice versa,
- concerns a segment of the business that is considered significant,
- affects the auditee's compliance with regulatory requirements,
- involves concealment of an unlawful transaction or fraud, or
- has the effect of increasing management compensation—for example, satisfies requirements for the award of bonuses or other forms of incentive compensation.[14]

The next section covers some traditional quantitative materiality guidelines, and it will also show how even these considerations include qualitative aspects. Auditors consider these factors as well as professional judgment in determining materiality levels.

Materiality Judgment Criteria—Quantitative

Accountants might prefer that definitive, quantitative materiality guides could be issued, but understand the drawbacks of having guidelines that are too rigid. Appropriate materiality levels are based on auditor judgment on an audit-by-audit basis. The auditing standards offer some guidance on quantitative measures of materiality that might be appropriate when making a preliminary assessment of what is material to the financial statements.[15]

Some common rules of thumb are as follows:

- 5–10% of income before tax from continuing operations
- 5–10% of income before tax and bonuses (for an owner-managed enterprise with a tax-minimization objective where net income is consistently nominal)
- Industry-specific measures of materiality that have become generally accepted in practice, for example,
  (a) For a not-for-profit entity, 0.5–2% of total expenses or total revenues
  (b) For a mutual fund entity, 0.5–1% of net asset value
  (c) For a real estate business entity that owns income-producing real properties, 1% of revenue

The auditor must use professional judgment in selecting alternative financial statement items when making a quantitative determination of materiality. Depending on circumstances, other items could be total revenues (for startup companies), net assets, total assets, gross profit, and cash flows from operations. An averaging technique based on several items may be useful in some situations.

Standards Check

CAS 320 Materiality in Planning and Performing an Audit

A3. Determining materiality involves the exercise of professional judgment. A percentage is often applied to a chosen benchmark as a starting point in determining materiality for the financial statements as a whole. Factors that may affect the identification of an appropriate benchmark include the following:
- The elements of the financial statements (for example, assets, liabilities, equity, revenue, expenses);
- Whether there are items on which the attention of the users of the particular entity's financial statements tends to be focused (for example, for the purpose of evaluating financial performance users may tend to focus on profit, revenue, or net assets);
- The nature of the entity, where the entity is in its life cycle, and the industry and economic environment in which the entity operates;
- The entity's ownership structure and the way it is financed (for example, if an entity is financed solely by debt rather than equity, users may put more emphasis on assets, and claims on them, than on the entity's earnings); and
- The relative volatility of the benchmark.

A4. Examples of benchmarks that may be appropriate, depending on the circumstances of the entity, include categories of reported income such as profit before tax, total revenue, gross profit and total expenses, and total equity or net asset value. Profit before tax from continuing operations is often used for profit-oriented entities. When profit before tax from continuing operations is volatile, other benchmarks may be more appropriate, such as gross profit or total revenues.

A5. Circumstances that give rise to an exceptional decrease or increase in such profit may lead the auditor to conclude that materiality for the financial statements as a whole is more appropriately determined using a normalized profit before tax from continuing operations figure based on past results.

Source: *CPA Canada Handbook—Assurance*, 2014.

If income is used, it should be adjusted for abnormal or extraordinary items. If it is negative or close to zero, or if it fluctuates significantly from year to year, an average could be used. "Normalizing" income should be done with caution, and if it is difficult to justify normalized income, such as when income is negative or too small relative to other items, then it may be best to use a different basis altogether. Auditors cannot apply the rules of thumb mechanically: other factors, such as those discussed below, must be considered. Note the role of qualitative factors in these, even though the main issue is quantitative in nature.

Absolute Size A potential misstatement may be important because of its size, regardless of any other considerations. Not many auditors use absolute size alone as a criterion, because a given amount may be appropriate in one case but not in another. Yet some auditors have been known to say that $1 million (or some other large number) is material, no matter what. Even in a very large company, people may find it hard to believe that a large dollar amount of error could be missed first by management, and then by auditors!

Relative Size The relationship of potential misstatement to a relevant base number is often used. Potential misstatements in income statement accounts are usually related to net income before taxes. In balance sheet accounts, they may be related to a subtotal number, such as current assets or net working capital. A misstatement in segment information may be small in relation to the total business but important for analysis of the segment.

Particular Transactions, Balances, or Disclosures Requiring Lower Materiality Level In some audits, an auditor may decide that certain classes of transactions, account balances, or disclosures should be audited to a lower amount than the amount being used as the materiality level for the financial statements as a whole. The auditor might expect that users' decisions based on these items will be affected by a lesser amount of misstatement than the level for the financial statements as a whole. This could arise in the case of certain measures or disclosures required by law (for example, executive compensation and related party transactions), for disclosures that are key to a particular industry (such as research and development costs for a pharmaceutical company), or for disclosures that are given special attention by users (such as a newly acquired business, or new program expenditures in a government department). Using an amount lower than whole materiality for a certain accounts affects audit sampling decisions, as it can be the basis for setting a **specific materiality** for that account, and there would also be a **specific performance materiality** level based on it.[16] In this introduction to the materiality concept, we will mainly work with the overall materiality for the financial statements as a whole and the performance materiality level related to it, and treat specific materialities as an advanced topic.

Standards Check

CAS 320 Materiality in Planning and Performing an Audit

10. . . . If, in the specific circumstances of the entity, there is one or more particular classes of transactions, account balances, or disclosures for which misstatements of lesser amounts than materiality for the financial statements as a whole could reasonably be expected to influence the economic decisions of users taken on the basis of the financial statements, the auditor shall also determine the materiality level or levels to be applied to those particular classes of transactions, account balances, or disclosures. *[Note: In this text we use the term* specific materiality *for this amount.]*

Source: *CPA Canada Handbook—Assurance,* 2014.

Materiality Judgment Criteria—Qualitative

The quantitative materiality guidelines are a good starting point for qualitative judgments, as they can be applied fairly objectively in every audit. Having the result of the mechanical quantitative calculation, the auditor then needs to stand back to take a broad perspective and consider other factors that may be informative about the consequences of the materiality level used. New information that causes revision to materiality during the audit is usually a qualitative consideration.

User-Related Factors Certain users may require more-precise financial information. It might be the only information available for a new business or it might contain the profit information that shareholders' dividend income is based on. Some users might scrutinize financial reports to determine whether specific laws or practices, such as anti-competitive practices or environmental protection agreements, are being followed. For audits of public sector entities, the financial statements may be used to make non-economic decisions, for example, whether policies have been complied with and operations have been effective in meeting policy objectives, so what is significant may go beyond just the financial information.

specific materiality:
the materiality level(s) to be applied to those particular classes of transactions, account balances, or disclosures for which misstatements of lesser amounts than materiality for the financial statements as a whole could reasonably be expected to influence the economic decisions of users taken on the basis of the financial statements

specific performance materiality:
the amount(s) set by the auditor at less than the specific materiality level(s) to reduce to an appropriately low level the probability that the aggregate of uncorrected and undetected misstatements exceeds specific materiality

CAS 320 Materiality in Planning and Performing an Audit

Considerations Specific to Public Sector Entities

A2. In the case of a public sector entity, legislators and regulators are often the primary users of its financial statements. Furthermore, the financial statements may be used to make decisions other than economic decisions. The determination of materiality for the financial statements as a whole (and, if applicable, materiality level or levels for particular classes of transactions, account balances, or disclosures) in an audit of the financial statements of a public sector entity is therefore influenced by law, regulation, or other authority, and by the financial information needs of legislators and the public in relation to public sector programs. (Ref: Para. 10)

Source: *CPA Canada Handbook—Assurance,* 2014.

Nature of the Item or Issue　Small items may be considered material because of what they suggest about management's character or how they interact with a specific user decision or evaluation. For example, an illegal payment is important because of what it is, not because of its absolute or relative amount. Other qualitative factors include whether a misstatement affects the trend of earnings, whether analysts' forecasts are met, and whether a loan covenant is violated. Generally, potential errors in the more liquid assets (cash, receivables, and inventory) are considered more important than potential errors in other accounts (such as fixed assets and prepaid expenses) because of their impact on the liquidity ratios that are often included in debt covenants.

Circumstances　Auditors generally use a smaller materiality level, and thus smaller permitted misstatement, for auditees whose financial statements will be widely used (publicly held companies) or used by important outsiders (bank loan officers) than they do for auditees whose financial statement users are closer to management and may have access to other sources of information. Auditors also tend to exercise more care and use a more stringent materiality criterion when management exercises discretion over an accounting treatment, and when important decisions will be based on the financial statement information. Troublesome events, such as the corporate and audit failures that continue to occur, have also led auditors to lower materiality and audit measurement and disclosures with more precision. These matters relate as much to risks as they do to financial statement materiality, as the two concepts are closely related in planning the nature, timing, and extent of the auditor's work.

Summary of Materiality Levels in the Auditing Standards

Exhibit 5–8 summarizes the four main types of materiality levels set out the auditing standards and provides the terms we will use in the text. Although this is a complete listing of all the materiality concepts covered by audit standards and practice, they do not necessarily all need to be used on an audit. One that is absolutely required on every audit engagement is the overall materiality. This is the one we focus on in the text. Performance materiality is also required by CAS 320 and can be viewed as a function of how auditors frame an audit decision problem with the help of a sampling model.[17] The specific materiality amounts are used only when auditors determine that, to meet specific user needs, there are particular classes of transactions, account balances, or disclosures that need to be audited to a lower level than the overall materiality; for example, if one use of the reported revenues is to calculate a net revenue–based royalty owed by the company, the revenues could be audited to a smaller, specific materiality level to ensure the amount is more precise. Thus, specific materiality level(s) are not used in every audit.

While it may seem that the "performance" concept complicates things unnecessarily, you can think about the performance materiality concept as a means to an end. The concept exists to aid auditors in meeting the ultimate objective of addressing user needs as reflected by overall and specific materialities. Performance materialities are used in statistical auditing to control some of the risks associated with auditing procedures. This application is further discussed in Chapter 10.

EXHIBIT 5–8

Materiality Amounts in Generally Accepted Auditing Standards and Terminology Used in this Text

Two Types of Materiality Decisions (audit purpose)	Overall Materiality (amount(s) based on user needs)	Performance Materiality (lesser amount(s) allowing a margin for potential undetected misstatements, e.g., due to sampling risk)
Two levels at which materiality is determined (when GAAS require it to be determined):		
For the financial statements as a whole (required to be determined on every audit)	overall materiality	overall performance materiality
For a particular class of transactions, or account balance, or disclosure (required only when auditor determines users have needs for certain financial statement elements to be more precise)	specific materiality	specific performance materiality (Note: This is similar to "tolerable misstatement," as defined in CAS 530.)

Standards Check

CAS 320 Materiality in Planning and Performing an Audit

Performance Materiality (Ref: Para. 11)

A12. Planning the audit solely to detect individually material misstatements overlooks the fact that the aggregate of individually immaterial misstatements may cause the financial statements to be materially misstated, and leaves no margin for possible undetected misstatements. Performance materiality . . . is set to reduce to an appropriately low level the probability that the aggregate of uncorrected and undetected misstatements in the financial statements exceeds materiality for the financial statements as a whole. . . . The determination of performance materiality is not a simple mechanical calculation and involves the exercise of professional judgment. It is affected by the auditor's understanding of the entity, updated during the performance of the risk assessment procedures, and the nature and extent of misstatements identified in previous audits and thereby the auditor's expectations in relation to misstatements in the current period.

Source: *CPA Canada Handbook–Assurance,* 2014, adapted.

Exhibit 5–9 illustrates a materiality worksheet that could be used to summarize the quantitative and qualitative factors that go into an auditor's decision on both the materiality level for financial statements as a whole and the performance materiality.

The materiality judgment for the current-year financial information of EcoPak Inc. shown in Exhibit 5–5 involves focusing on the most important financial decisions made based on the financial statements. The centre of attention will be different for different audits. For example, the focus may be the current asset–liability position for a company in financial difficulty seeking to renew its bank loans. This company may be experiencing operating losses, and the balance sheet, rather than the income statement, will be the most important information. In other cases, such as when a company is growing and issuing shares to the public, decisions based on income performance are the focus, so the income statement and the net income number may be the most important.

At this point, it is useful to review the purposes of determining materiality. First, materiality levels determined at the planning stage are used to decide how much work to do on each financial statement item. In performing the audit work, they are used for deciding on the extent of testing for control and substantive procedures, including determining the appropriate sample sizes. At the completion stage of the audit, auditors use them to evaluate the cumulative effects of all known or potential misstatements. For example, if the audit work discovered five different $15,000 mistakes that all increase net income, and the net income–based materiality limit is $50,000, it would be appropriate to consider these as material because in total they exceed materiality.

While misstatements may be discovered in auditing an income statement account, the misstatement's materiality must be considered in relation to one or more balance sheet accounts. This is because income misstatements in the double-entry bookkeeping system can leave a **dangling debit (or credit)** somewhere in the balance sheet accounts, and the audit challenge is to find it. (E.g., if fictitious credit sales were recorded, setting up fictitious accounts receivable will balance the accounts.) If there is no dangling debit or credit, the other side of the misstatement transaction has gone through the income statement, probably causing misstatement in two accounts (opposite directions), with no net effect on the net income bottom line. (In the previous example, if the fictitious accounts receivable were written off as bad debt expense, both the revenue and bad debt expense would be overstated, but the income would not be misstated.) The articulation of the balance sheet and income statement shown here supports setting materiality at the financial statement level, since then what is material in the balance sheet is also material in the income statement, and vice versa.

Review Checkpoints

5-70   Why are qualitative criteria important in the auditor's materiality decision?

5-71   Do auditing standards require auditors to use a specific quantitative criterion to determine materiality?

5-72   How do fraud considerations relate to the auditor's materiality decision?

Documenting the Overall Audit Strategy and Audit Plan

Overall Audit Strategy

LO7   List the preliminary planning decisions set out in the overall audit strategy.

As discussed throughout Part 2 of the text, audit planning is an ongoing, iterative process where information gained as the audit is performed may result in refinements to the plan. The preliminary planning activities are the basis for establishing the overall audit strategy, which sets the scope, timing, and direction of the audit engagement, and guides the development of the detailed audit plan. In developing the overall audit strategy, CAS 300 requires the audit partner to consider the following:

- The characteristics of the entity and the engagement that define the engagement's scope
- What reporting is expected to result from the engagement that affects the timing of the audit work and the communications needed between team members and between the audit team and the auditee
- What key factors will be significant in planning and executing the audit work
- What resources the audit firm will need to perform the audit effectively

The overall audit strategy documents information about (1) investigation or review of the prospective or continuing engagement and client relationship, including relevant ethical and independence considerations; (2) staff, and special technical or industry expertise required; (3) preliminary materiality levels; (4) assessment of significant industry or company risks and related audit issues; (5) identification of unusual accounting principles; (6) use of substantive or combined audit approach; (7) nature and extent of resources required; (8) staff assignment and scheduling of team communications and field work; and (9) special considerations for initial or group audit engagements. The auditor is also required to communicate an overview of the planned scope and timing of the audit to those charged with governance, based on this overall audit strategy.[18]

dangling debit (or credit):
a false or erroneous debit (or credit) balance that exists because one or more accounts are misstated

EXHIBIT 5–9

Materiality Assessment: Illustration Using a Practice Form as a Template

Auditee: _EcoPak_   **Year-end:** _20X4_

Materiality Assessment

1. Qualitative Factors   **Comments**

(a) Identify the specific users of the financial statements for this engagement.

> _Board members, current shareholders, potential shareholders (IPO being considered), bank_

(b) Identify what expectations the users may have for the financial statements for this engagement.

> _GAAP (ASPE), fair presentation of current performance, accurate valuation of assets and liabilities_

(c) Identify any possible situations or misstatements that would affect a user now or at some future point, regardless of the materiality level (e.g., consider environmental matters, policies, statutes, safety issues).

> _Potential future site reclamation obligations due to past environmental damage on factory site._

2. Quantitative Factors

(a) Planning data

	This Year Actual (if adjusted)	This Year Anticipated ($000 per draft f/s)	Last Year	2nd Preceding Year
Assets	N/A	4,060	3,850	3,700
Liabilities		1,160	1,103	1,001
Equity		2,900	2,747	2,699
Sales/revenue		9,000	8,100	7,300
Gross profit		2,250	2,130	1,809
Expenses		1,950	1,901	1,607
Income before tax		300	229	202
Overall materiality		14	12	

(b) Normalized pre-tax income

	This Year Actual (if adjusted)	This Year Anticipated	Last Year	2nd Preceding Year
Estimated pre-tax income	$ N/A	300	229	202
Adjustment for non-recurring items or unadjusted errors brought forward				
inventory write-down due to market adjustments not expected to recur		+40	none	none
Normalized pre-tax income	$	340	229	202

	Prepared	Reviewed	Audit File Index
Date & initials	20/03/x4 T.K.	29/03/x4	420

(continued)

EXHIBIT 5–9

Materiality Assessment: Illustration Using a Practice Form as a Template (*continued*)

3. Materiality Considerations

(a) Profit-oriented enterprises

Identify Financial Statement Users	Measurement Base	Factor Applied*	Possible Materiality	Comments
Current and potential shareholders, bank	Normalized pre-tax income	5% × 340	$17	
Bank, board	Assets Equity Revenue Gross profit Other	1/2% × 4060	$20.3	Not used: materiality based on pretax income is most appropriate for this audit.

*Materiality guidelines

Normalized pre-tax income	5–10%	These materiality factors are provided as guidelines only and should be used only as
Assets	1/2–1%	an aid in the development of your professional judgment. The materiality level should
Equity	1/2–5%	represent the largest amount of a misstatement or group of misstatements that would
Revenue	1/2–1%	not, in your judgment, influence or change a decision based on the financial statements.
Gross profit	1/2–5%	Often, normalized pre-tax income is used as an initial reference point for businesses,

although it may not be sufficient for businesses with little or no income. Weighted averages are also used at times. Revenue is often used for NPOs. See CAS 320, paragraphs A3–A9 for more guidance.

(b) Not-for-profit enterprises *N/A—EcoPak is a for-profit business*

Identify Financial Statement Users	Measurement Base Revenue/Expenses	Factor Applied*	Possible Materiality	Comments
Governmental authorities				
Funding organizations				
Directors				
Other				

*Materiality factors for audit of not-for-profit entities
Total expenses or total revenues 1/2 to 2%

(c) Other factors considered in determining overall materiality and performance materiality for this engagement

We have done the audit for three years; generally few errors have been found, all were adjusted by client. Undetected misstatements may exist due to sampling risks and valuation estimations in inventory, A/R, accrued environmental reclamation liability, unlikely to exceed 30% of overall materiality

Overall Materiality Assessment for Financial Statements as a Whole

Based on the anticipated financial statement amounts and on the other factors described above, overall materiality for this engagement is as follows:

$ 17,000   Misstatements below this threshold, if not corrected, will be accumulated on the Possible Adjustments Sheet unless such misstatements are deemed trivial (below $ _____). Note: The auditor may designate an amount below which misstatements are deemed trivial and need not be accumulated because the auditor expects that the accumulation of such amounts clearly will not have a material effect on the financial statements. In so doing, the auditor considers the fact that the determination of materiality involves qualitative as well as quantitative considerations and that misstatements of a relatively small amount could nevertheless have a material effect on the financial statements. The summary of uncorrected misstatements included in or attached to the management representation letter need not include trivial misstatements.

Performance Materiality Assessment

Based on expected misstatements in current-period financial statements of **$5,000**, and on other factors noted above, performance materiality for planning the audit is as follows:
$ 12,000.

	Prepared	Reviewed	Index
Date & initials	20/03/X4 T.K.	29/03/X4	420

Standards Check

CAS 300 Planning an Audit of Financial Statements

7. The auditor shall establish an overall audit strategy that sets the scope, timing, and direction of the audit, and that guides the development of the audit plan.

8. In establishing the overall audit strategy, the auditor shall
   (a) Identify the characteristics of the engagement that define its scope;
   (b) Ascertain the reporting objectives of the engagement to plan the timing of the audit and the nature of the communications required;
   (c) Consider the factors that, in the auditor's professional judgment, are significant in directing the engagement team's efforts;
   (d) Consider the results of preliminary engagement activities and, where applicable, whether knowledge gained on other engagements performed by the engagement partner for the entity is relevant; and
   (e) Ascertain the nature, timing, and extent of resources necessary to perform the engagement. (Ref: Para. A8–A11)

Source: *CPA Canada Handbook—Assurance,* 2014.

Exhibit 5–10 provides a checklist of considerations auditors include in developing the overall audit strategy for a typical continuing audit engagement. The checklist is a questionnaire form that could be used to document the planning, as required by the auditing standards. The first part lists considerations that are usually relevant in ongoing audits, and the following two parts relate to specific circumstances, such as initial engagements or audits of consolidated financial statements. Many of these matters will influence the detailed audit plan, which the auditor will develop after fully assessing the auditee's business risks and related internal control. The list covers a broad range of matters applicable to many engagements and can be adapted to each specific audit situation.

EXHIBIT 5–10

Considerations in Establishing the Overall Audit Strategy

Matters relevant to planning financial statement audits

Document the following information based on inquiries of appropriate auditee personnel:

Response/File
Documentation
Reference

Considerations applicable on most continuing audits of stand-alone financial statements

Engagement Characteristics
- Entity's reporting requirements and deadlines
- Financial reporting framework used in financial information to be audited under a GAAP framework or otherwise acceptable per CAS 210
- Any requirement to reconcile to another financial reporting framework
- Any additional specific reporting requirements, e.g., industry, regulatory, legislated (e.g., in public sector) requirements
- Expected audit coverage, including the number, locations, and nature of business components
- Reporting currency to be used; need for currency translation in the audited financial information
- Existence of related parties and extent of any related party transactions and balances
- Impact of information technology on data available for audit procedures; potential to use computer-assisted audit techniques
- Organizational structure, key auditee personnel, information systems, and availability of data relevant to audit
- Need to use work of others for audit evidence, such as other auditors, experts with specialized knowledge, internal audit work, service organizations, audit reports on effective design or operation of controls performed by them

(continued)

EXHIBIT 5-10

Considerations in Establishing the Overall Audit Strategy (*continued*)

Audit Timing and Communications
- Schedule of meetings with management and those charged with governance to discuss the nature, timing, and extent of the audit work; expected type and timing of auditor's report; management letters; and other communications, both written and oral, throughout the engagement
- Expected nature and timing of communications and meetings among engagement team members
- Expected timing for performing and reviewing audit work
- Plan for communicating to engagement team members the need to question management and exercise professional skepticism in gathering and evaluating audit evidence throughout the audit

Preliminary Audit Activities
- Initial determination of appropriate materiality and performance materiality level for financial statements as a whole for planning purposes (and lower levels for specific financial statement elements, if required)
- Reconsideration of materiality levels based on new information as audit procedures are performed during the course of the audit
- Identification of material business components and financial statement account balances
- Preliminary identification of significant audit issues (areas where there may be a higher risk of material misstatement)
- Consideration of results of previous audits, including evaluation of internal control operating effectiveness, management's commitment to effective internal control, nature and magnitude of misstatements identified by the auditor, any restatements and corrections made by management
- Consideration of volume of transactions, complexity of information systems, availability of records, importance of internal control to successful business operations, and other relevant factors to determine whether it is more efficient for the auditor to test internal control effectiveness to obtain audit assurance
- Preliminary decision on whether a combined approach (using both control testing evidence and substantive evidence) should be used for any aspects of the audit

Identification of Significant Audit Issues
- Consideration of significant business developments, such as changes in information technology and business processes; key management changes; and acquisitions, mergers, and divestments
- Consideration of significant industry developments, such as changes in industry regulations, new reporting requirements, and the legal environment affecting the entity
- Consideration of significant changes in the applicable financial accounting standards

Nature, Timing, and Extent of Required Resources
- Consideration of impact of assessed risk of material misstatement at the overall financial statement level on engagement staffing, direction, supervision, and review
- Selection of, and audit work assignment to, engagement team members; assigning appropriately experienced team members to areas with higher risks of material misstatement
- Engagement time budgeting, including considering adequate time for high-risk areas, supervision, and review of less-experienced team members

Additional Considerations for Specific Circumstances

Initial audits
- Consider
  - if entity previously audited, matters raised in communications with predecessor and accessibility of previous audit working papers
  - impact on engagement and audit report of availability of evidence regarding opening balances, consistency of accounting policies, and comparative figures if these are reported

Group audits of consolidated entities
- Consider
  - the nature of the control relationships between a parent and its components that determine how the group is to be consolidated
  - the extent to which components are audited by other auditors
  - the need for a statutory audit of stand-alone financial statements in addition to an audit for consolidation purposes
  - communication with auditors of components, regarding things such as the expected types and timing of reports to be issued and other communications
  - the setting and communicating of materiality for auditors of components
  - the nature, timing, and extent of resources needed for the engagement team to assess understanding, group-wide risks and controls, and consolidation process

Source: Adapted from CASs 300, 510, 600.

A key purpose of the *overall audit strategy* is to pull together all relevant preliminary planning activities to guide the development of the detailed audit plan. The *audit plan* details the nature, timing, and extent of the risk assessment and further audit procedures planned to address the specific assertions for each component of the audit. The "nature" of audit procedures refers to evidence techniques they will use. The "timing" refers to when they will be performed, whether before (interim date), at, or after the auditee's year-end. Timing may have other aspects, such as surprise procedures (unannounced to auditee personnel) or the need to observe periodic auditee procedures, such as rotating inventory counts during the year. The "extent" usually refers to the sample sizes of data to be selected for examination, such as the number of customer accounts receivable to confirm, or the number of inventory categories/products to count.

The planned procedures are often presented in a set of specific audit programs. An *audit program* is a list of *auditing procedures* focused on a major financial statement component. The programs include specific audit objectives and procedures for determining inherent and control risk, obtaining the sufficient appropriate evidence that is the basis for the audit report, and producing the required documentation. In the following chapters we will examine how auditors develop the detailed audit plan and specific programs.

Standards Check

CAS 230 Audit Documentation

8. The auditor shall prepare audit documentation that is sufficient to enable an experienced auditor, having no previous connection with the audit, to understand (Ref: Para. A2–A5, A16–A17)

    (a) The nature, timing, and extent of the audit procedures performed to comply with the CASs and applicable legal and regulatory requirements; (Ref: Para. A6–A7)

    (b) The results of the audit procedures performed, and the audit evidence obtained; and

    (c) Significant matters arising during the audit, the conclusions reached thereon, and significant professional judgments made in reaching those conclusions. (Ref: Para. A8–A11)

Source: *CPA Canada Handbook—Assurance, 2014.*

Standards Check

CAS 300 Planning an Audit of Financial Statements

9. The auditor shall develop an audit plan that shall include a description of

    (a) The nature, timing, and extent of planned risk assessment procedures, as determined under CAS 315.

    (b) The nature, timing, and extent of planned further audit procedures at the assertion level, as determined under CAS 330.

    (c) Other planned audit procedures that are required to be carried out so that the engagement complies with CASs. (Ref: Para. A12)

Source: *CPA Canada Handbook—Assurance, 2014.*

Review Checkpoints

5-73 What audit planning activities are documented in the overall audit strategy?

5-74 How does the overall audit strategy relate to the audit plan and detailed programs?

APPLICATION CASE WITH SOLUTION & ANALYSIS

Audit Engagement Acceptance Decision

DISCUSSION CASE

About a year ago, Jack joined a medium-sized local public accounting firm as a junior auditor. Early in his first year Jack got the opportunity to work on a new audit client acceptance decision with Hilda, one of the firm's top audit managers. The prospective client is a local company called Sweet Dreams Inc. Hilda had gathered information about Sweet Dreams as required to comply with the firm's quality control standards, and she asked Jack to review it and comment on her recommendation that the firm accept the audit engagement. Hilda saw this as a way for Jack to get familiar with the client as he was the junior member of the Sweet Dreams audit team, but it was also a way for Jack to learn the firm's procedures for new client acceptance decisions. Some of the key points Jack noted in reviewing the information Hilda had gathered follow:

- Sweet Dreams operates a chain of retail mattress stores across the city. It is privately owned by three sisters who inherited the company from their parents, the company's founders. The owners are not involved in managing the business, but it pays quarterly dividends that are their main source of income. The three sisters are all highly involved in local charitable associations and are well respected in the community. The company's board of directors includes the three owners, the company president, a retired audit partner who is now working as a highly regarded business consultant for a number of local private companies, and a university professor who is an expert on sleeping and health research.

- Sweet Dreams' predecessor auditor, a partner in a small local firm, resigned from the audit because she is planning to retire from practice soon. Since all her partners also plan to retire in a few years, she felt it would be in Sweet Dreams' best interest to switch to another firm that could continue the audit for a longer time.

- The predecessor's response letter to Hilda also indicated that Sweet Dreams had been an excellent audit client over 20 years. Management is very competent and control conscious, ensuring employees keep accurate records and follow all control procedures. Misstatements uncovered by the auditor, even immaterial ones, have always been promptly corrected, and they have always paid the audit fees in full, promptly. The predecessor also noted that management has given its permission for her to give its new auditors access to her prior year's audit files to facilitate their familiarization with the company.

- The company is very profitable and the owners receive audited financial statements annually, as well as quarterly profit reports. Management provided Hilda with the company's most recent financial statements, and she notes that it uses an appropriate acceptable basis of accounting. Management and senior employees participate in a profit-sharing plan that gives them above-average earnings.

- The company participates in many community fundraising events, such as supplying new mattresses to homeless shelters. Sweet Dreams was the first business in the city to undertake a comprehensive waste and energy reduction program. Employees are proud to work for Sweet Dreams, and it has won awards from the city for its community and environmental initiatives.

After his review of Hilda's documentation, Jack felt he had a good introduction to Sweet Dreams and that he fully understood why Hilda recommended that the firm accept it as a new audit client.

Later that year, Hilda assigned Jack to assist on another new client acceptance decision, this time for Grouse Mines Limited. She was very impressed with Jack's progress, and decided to give him a little more rope this time by letting him gather some of the background information required. Jack was instructed not to contact Grouse management, as that would have to be done by one of the firm's partners, but to do any other information gathering that could be relevant to the firm's acceptance decision. Jack was happy to have this challenge and set about his work, gathering the following points:

- Grouse is a mining company that owns and operates several mines outside the city. Grouse also owns mining properties in South America and Indonesia, which are operated by local managers. The company's board of directors is made up of the company's CEO; its CFO; its COO; and the CEO of another mining company, who owns 20% of the Grouse common shares.
- Its shares are publicly traded on the over-the-counter market.
- After Jack attempted to contact him three times, Grouse's predecessor auditor finally responded to Jack by telephone. He explained that his firm has resigned from all its public company audits because "we are sick and tired of CPAB breathing down our necks about trivial issues like documentation." Further, he "can't give any reason why your firm shouldn't accept the audit. Grouse always paid its audit fees, and we plan to continue to do consulting work for them on financing, management compensation, and environmental disclosure issues. Now that we don't have CPAB tying our hands, we should be able to provide much more valuable business advice to Grouse's management." When Jack inquired about the possibility of reviewing prior-year working papers, the predecessor said it would not be possible since his firm's staff is "far too busy to spend the time it would take to get those old files ready for your firm to see."
- In reviewing Grouse's regulatory filings on SEDAR, Jack notes Grouse's profitability had been declining until two years ago when it hired a mining veteran as its new CEO to implement serious cost-cutting measures. The company's profits have increased modestly in the last two years, but it is late in filing its most recent quarterly report. The CEO and her management team have stock options that will vest next year.
- Grouse's recent annual report includes several pages of disclosure about its environmental management policies and its compliance with all environment regulations.
- News stories have appeared reporting that residents living near the mines in Canada and the other countries have organized protests after noting an increase in breathing problems as well as several serious fish kills in the rivers downstream of the mines' tailings ponds.
- Grouse recently issued a press release announcing it has preliminary assays indicating that one of the world's largest reserves of platinum exists in one of its South American mining properties. Further testing is being done and more-certain estimates of the platinum reserve quantities are expected to be available sometime next year.

In trying to apply what he learned in his prior experience with Sweet Dreams, Jack is amazed at how different the Grouse situation is in just about every aspect. He is looking forward to a meeting with Hilda to discuss all the information. What do you think are the key points for Jack to consider in this case as he prepares for the meeting?

SOLUTION & ANALYSIS

Let us now consider the key points Jack has learned about these two different prospective audit clients by applying the list of acceptance decision procedures provided in this chapter.

1. *Obtaining and reviewing financial information about the prospective auditee organization to determine purpose, main users, and basis of accounting.* Sweet Dreams provided Jack's firm with relevant reports, indicating its management has a good sense of the role and responsibilities of an auditor. Hilda also learned that the purpose and main users are the three sisters who own the shares, and she determined the basis of accounting appropriate for this purpose and these users. The board of directors includes independent members with relevant expertise in the business and financial matters.

   Grouse is publicly traded and Jack was thus able to obtain relevant information from the regulatory filings, which are available online. But additional information is needed from Grouse management in order to assess all the purposes and users of its financial statements. As a mining company, Grouse's basis of accounting may be complex, and discussions with management are needed to learn more details and establish the appropriateness of its accounting policies for estimates related to mineral reserves, revenue recognition, environmental liability estimates, and so on. Grouse's board of directors is dominated by company managers, with only one independent member with relevant expertise.

2. *Evaluating the public accounting firm and individual auditors' independence from the prospect.* This would be done at the firm level as part of quality control procedures. Hilda and Jack can only know about their own independence: close relatives who are employees of these companies or hold shares or debts that could create a conflict of interest (self-interest threat). These factors need to be considered for all audit staff.

   Other independence threats relating to acceptance decisions need to be considered at the firm level. Examples of these threats are any prior association with these companies involving promoting their position (assisting the company with obtaining a bank loan, a possible advocacy threat), personal or business relations making it difficult to exercise professional skepticism (a former audit partner now being on the prospect's management team, a potential familiarity threat), or any risk for intimidation of an auditor with respect to the financial statements or the conduct of the audit (management seems very aggressive and motivated to manipulate the financial statements, possibly an intimidation threat).

   Jack might have a concern about the likelihood of a Grouse management attempt at intimidation of the auditor, as there are indicators that its cost-cutting actions may have increased its risk of environmental liability (news reports), and there is motivation related to the stock options that will vest next year (reports of a huge platinum find would increase Grouse's share price at the time these options vest, and history has shown that such findings can easily be falsified or overstated). Not enough information is given in this case to go any further on these independence aspects, but remember they are critical to the firm's acceptance decision. Independence threats were explained in more detail in Chapter 3.

3. *Considering whether the public accounting firm has competency, resources, and any special skills required.* Sweet Dreams is a local business in a fairly straightforward industry, and its basis of accounting was appropriate, so it seems reasonable to assume Jack's firm has the staff and competency to do the job. Any specific information systems or tax expertise required would also be typical, so the required competencies would be readily available within the firm.

   Grouse is in a specialized industry with more-complex operations to account for. Jack's firm may have other audits of mining companies in the area, and thus have the expertise to handle the mining-specific accounting issues. Grouse also has operations in foreign countries. If these are material, Jack's firm will need to obtain knowledge of foreign laws and regulations and be able to do audit work in those locations. Using the work of foreign auditors will increase the complexity and risk of this engagement. Jack's mid-size local firm may not be able to manage that aspect of auditing Grouse.

4. *Obtaining information from management as to whether the prospect's management accepts responsibility for the financial statement preparation and implementing adequate controls to reduce risk of errors and fraud.* The case suggests Sweet Dreams' management is aware of and has accepted its responsibilities for (1) preparing financial statements in accordance with an acceptable financial reporting framework and (2) implementing adequate internal control to reduce risk of error and fraud. Their most recent financial statements and information indicate strong control awareness at the management level and throughout the whole organization. Employee pride and community involvement suggest that integrity and responsibility, which are desirable qualities in an auditee, are part of the corporate culture at Sweet Dreams.

   Jack did not meet with Grouse management, so information on these issues is missing, but there are hints in information Jack obtained from other sources, as is seen below.

5. *Considering whether the engagement would require special attention or involve unusual risks.* Sweet Dreams does not appear to present any special concerns, but it is important that the owners depend on the audited financial statements for information about the financial position of the business.

   The preliminary analysis shows that Grouse presents many risks, such that the firm may already find the company and the engagement too risky to accept just on the basis of what Jack has learned.

6. *Searching for news reports and, when possible, asking business associates about the organization.* Some key information about both companies was obtained from news reports. These can be searched quite easily online using a search tool like Google. A firm partner may ask business associates about the prospective client, but this must be done carefully and in compliance with confidentiality rules of the profession or the firm. Partners often have a wide network of business associates where a lot of useful information can be obtained informally, possibly over a game of golf or a dinner, without breaking any confidence.

7. *For new audits, communicating with the previous auditor.* Sweet Dreams' predecessor auditor has provided Hilda with much useful information. The predecessor has good reasons for resigning, and the fact that her partners are not taking over does not reflect badly on the integrity of management or the risk of Sweet Dreams as an auditee. She reports there were no disagreements with management about accounting matters in many years as the company's auditor. We also learn that management will be very cooperative and helpful to the auditor, which is a sign the audit can be done well within a reasonable amount of audit time.

   The information obtained from Grouse's predecessor auditor paints a rather risky picture. The predecessor appears to have lacked competence to do the audit, as evidenced by deficiencies in documentation found by CPAB's inspectors. The fact that it was doing consulting work on executive compensation, financing, and disclosure means it lacked independence. Public company auditors cannot consult on these areas as they will be involved with reporting decisions and, therefore, not be objective in assessing the company's financial statements. The fact that the auditor resigned and was not dismissed by the auditee suggests that management did not object to the predecessor's lack of competence and independence, further bringing management's integrity and competence into question.

   The predecessor's reluctance to respond to Jack's request and failure to do so in writing also cast doubt on the quality of that firm and its audits of Grouse. Since his only reply was by telephone, it is important that Jack make detailed notes right away so there is reliable documentation of the predecessor's responses. The refusal to provide Jack's firm with access to any working papers also suggests a poor-quality audit, increasing the risk that Grouse's opening balance sheet is misstated—creating audit difficulties for the current year and potentially a scope limitation.

   Based on all the factors given, it seems likely that Sweet Dreams will be a great audit client, but Grouse appears at this stage to be a very undesirable one. Jack's firm may want one of its partners to obtain further information by contacting Grouse's management and inquiring in the local community, but it seems likely this will only confirm its undesirability.

   As a further exercise, we briefly give some thought to how these considerations might be different if these were decisions about continuing with existing audit client relationships instead of about new engagements.

- There would be no predecessor.
- Jack's firm would need to consider whether any changes in the economy, operating environment, ownership structure, accounting standards, or other factors could affect the risk of the auditee, the firm's ability to complete the audit, independence, appropriateness of the financial reporting framework, adequacy of internal control, and so on. Such changes could affect the risk of material misstatement at the financial statement level or at the assertion level.

- The information would be obtained from the same sources as those used above: management inquiry, research, and inquiries to associates. The main difference is that now the firm is starting with a high level of knowledge of the auditee and factoring in new information about any significant changes to assess acceptability.

SUMMARY

- An overview of the financial statement audit process as required by Canadian GAAS (CASs) was presented, with links to the text chapters where the topics are covered. A more detailed flow diagram, which appears in the inside back cover of the text, was also discussed. **LO1**

- The main characteristics of an independent audit engagement were reviewed, including various types of entities that require financial statement audits and why, who are the entity's management and those charged with its governance, who are the main stakeholders using financial statements, and the financial reporting frameworks that may be acceptable for management to choose for its financial statements. We noted that many concepts, tools, and activities will be similar for most types of financial statement audits, but that special entities such as public sector organizations or very small businesses may require special considerations. We noted that, for simplicity, most of the text would be based on the assumption that the entity under audit is a reasonably large corporation preparing financial statements for shareholders in accordance with a fair presentation framework, such as IFRS. **LO2**

- The pre-engagement risk management activities auditors perform to decide whether to accept a financial statement audit engagement were discussed. The auditor's concerns for the risks a particular engagement might bring to the auditor and his or her success in practice, through potential impact on reputation, liability, or cost recovery, were presented. **LO3**

- The need for auditors to understand the auditee organization's business, its environment, and its risks at the start of a financial statement audit was explained. The responsibilities of management for presenting financial statements that reflect the underlying economic performance and conditions of the entity were discussed. The key audit step of receiving management's draft financial statements as the subject matter of the audit was pointed out. **LO4**

- The analytical procedures auditors use for their preliminary risk assessment were described. Examples were provided showing the way these are used on management's draft financial statements to identify areas where misstatements are most likely. **LO5**

- The materiality concept and the levels used for planning the audit were explained. These include materiality for the financial statements as a whole and performance materiality. An example of how these amounts are determined was provided by showing a sample form that might be used as a practice aid for calculating materiality levels on an engagement. The advanced topic of specific materialities was also briefly noted, for those situations when an auditor may choose to use amounts smaller than the overall materiality level, based on users' specific requirements related to key account balances, transactions, or disclosure in a particular financial statement audit engagement. **LO6**

- The preliminary planning decisions set out in the overall audit strategy were listed, and the role of the overall audit strategy in developing the audit plan at a more detailed performance level was presented. **LO7**

Finally, an application case with analysis was presented to illustrate an audit engagement acceptance decision in a realistic scenario.

KEY TERMS

analysis	management's draft financial statements	representational faithfulness
analytical procedures	materiality for the financial statements as a whole (overall materiality)	risk of material misstatement at the financial statement level
attention directing		significant risks
audit quality management		specific materiality
auditor's risk from taking the engagement	minutes	specific performance materiality
dangling debit (or credit)	overall audit strategy	successor
engagement letter	performance materiality	those charged with governance
horizontal analysis	pre-audit risk management activities	vertical analysis
interim audit work	predecessor	year-end audit work
	present fairly (fairly present)	

MULTIPLE-CHOICE QUESTIONS FOR PRACTICE AND REVIEW

MC 5-1 **LO3** An audit engagement letter should normally include the following matter of agreement between the auditor and the auditee.

a. Schedules and analyses to be prepared by the auditee's employees
b. Methods of statistical sampling the auditor will use
c. Specification of litigation in progress against the auditee
d. Auditee representations about availability of all minutes of meetings of the board of directors

MC 5-2 **LO3** When a successor auditor initiates communications with a predecessor auditor, under the professional ethics codes the successor is required

a. to take responsibility for obtaining the auditee's consent for the predecessor to give information about prior audits.
b. to conduct interviews with the predecessor audit firm's engagement partner and all audit staff involved in the prior audit.
c. to obtain copies of all of the predecessor auditor's working papers.
d. to assess the predecessor audit engagement partner's integrity and competence.

MC 5-3 **LO3** GAAS require that auditors prepare and use

a. a written engagement letter for all audits.
b. a written engagement letter only for new, first-time audits.
c. a written overall audit representation letter.
d. a written audit representation letter only for new audits.

MC 5-4 **LO1** During the risk assessment step of the overall audit process, the auditor

a. identifies the auditor's own risks from accepting the engagement.
b. accumulates the misstatements discovered during the audit.

c. forms a conclusion on fair presentation of the financial statements and issues the appropriate audit opinion.

d. performs substantive procedures.

MC 5-5 `LO4` Understanding the client's business environment is important to the auditor because

a. it helps distinguish interim audit work from year-end audit work.

b. management's draft financial statements contain assertions about the business environment.

c. it helps the auditor to assess the risks that the financial statements contain misstatements.

d. it eliminates the need for the auditor to understand the auditee's internal controls.

MC 5-6 `LO1` During the response to assessed risks step of the overall audit process, the auditor

a. identifies the auditor's own risks from accepting the engagement.

b. develops the audit plan and detailed audit programs.

c. reviews the overall evidence obtained from the audit.

d. performs substantive procedures.

MC 5-7 `LO6` Auditors are not responsible for accounting estimates with respect to

a. making the estimates.

b. determining the reasonableness of estimates.

c. determining that estimates are presented in conformity with GAAP.

d. determining that estimates are adequately disclosed in the financial statements.

MC 5-8 `LO7` The overall audit strategy required by CAS 300

a. cannot be decided by the audit engagement partner to avoid independence threats.

b. identifies characteristics of the auditee entity and the engagement that define its scope.

c. requires the audit engagement partner to set the scope, timing, and direction of the audit, which cannot be changed until the auditor's report is issued at the end of the engagement.

d. includes detailed plans for gathering audit evidence.

MC 5-9 `LO5` Auditors perform analytical procedures in the planning stage of an audit for the purpose of

a. deciding the matters to cover in an engagement letter.

b. identifying unusual conditions that deserve more auditing effort.

c. determining which of the financial statement balances are the most important for the auditee's financial statements.

d. determining the nature, timing, and extent of audit procedures for auditing the inventory.

MC 5-10 `LO5` Analytical procedures used when planning an audit should concentrate on

a. weaknesses in the company's internal control procedures.

b. predictability of account balances based on individual transactions.

c. five major management assertions in financial statements.

d. accounts and relationships that may represent specific potential problems and risks in the financial statements.

MC 5-11 `LO5` When a company that has $5 million in current assets and $3 million in current liabilities pays $1 million of its accounts payable, its current ratio will

a. increase.

b. decrease.

c. remain unchanged.

d. not enough information is given to answer

MC 5-12 `LO5` When a company that has $3 million in current assets and $5 million in current liabilities pays $1 million of its accounts payable, its current ratio will

a. increase.

b. decrease.

c. remain unchanged.

d. not enough information is given to answer

MC 5-13 `LO5` When a company that has $5 million in current assets and $5 million in current liabilities pays $1 million of its accounts payable, its current ratio will

a. increase.

b. decrease.

c. remain unchanged.

d. not enough information is given to answer

MC 5-14 `LO5` ABC Company sells its products for a (gross) profit. If ABC increases its sales by 15 percent and increases its cost of goods sold by 7 percent, its costs of goods sold ratio will

a. increase.

b. decrease.

c. remain unchanged.

d. not enough information is given to answer

MC 5-15 `LO5` Analytical procedures are generally used to produce evidence from

a. confirmations mailed directly to the auditors by auditee customers.

b. physical observation of inventories.

c. relationships among current financial balances and prior balances, forecasts, and non-financial data.

d. detailed examination of external and internal documents.

MC 5-16 `LO5` Which of the following match-ups of types of analytical procedures and sources of information makes the most sense?

TYPE OF ANALYTICAL PROCEDURE	SOURCE OF INFORMATION
a. Comparison of current account balances with prior-period statistics	Physical production
b. Comparison of current account balances with expected balances	Company's budgets and forecasts
c. Evaluation of current account balances with relation to predictable historical patterns	Published industry ratios
d. Evaluation of current account balances in relation to non-financial information	Company's own comparative financial statements

MC 5-17 `LO5` Analytical procedures can be used in which of the following ways?

a. As a substitute for control testing to assess control effectiveness

b. As attention-directing methods at the end of an audit

c. As substantive audit procedures to obtain evidence when planning an audit

d. As a means of overall review of the financial statements at the end of an audit

MC 5-18 `LO6` Which of the following is not a benefit claimed for the practice of determining materiality in the initial planning stage of starting an audit?

a. Being able to fine-tune the audit work for effectiveness and efficiency

b. Avoiding the problem of doing more work than necessary (over-auditing)

c. Being able to decide early what kind of audit opinion to give

d. Avoiding the problem of doing too little work (under-auditing)

MC 5-19 `LO6` Materiality in the context of audit planning means

a. amounts that should be disclosed if they are likely to influence the economic decisions of financial statement users.

b. the largest amount of uncorrected dollar misstatement that could exist in published financial statements while still fairly presenting the company's financial position and results of operations in conformity with GAAP.

c. part of the overall materiality amount for the financial statements assigned to a particular account.

d. a dollar amount of materiality assigned to an account as required by auditing standards.

MC 5-20 `LO2` According to CAS 200, those charged with governance

a. have the main responsibility for the day-to-day accounting functions of the auditee.

b. must be a part of the most senior management of the auditee.

c. are responsible for the operations of the entity and thus are accountable to its stakeholders.

d. assist the auditor by making key judgments such as materiality and audit risk.

MC 5-21 `LO3` When taking an engagement, the auditor's risk is best described as follows.

a. The risk that negative consequences will arise for the auditor's professional practice as a result of taking on a particular audit engagement

b. The risk that the auditor will uncover fraudulent activities during the engagement

c. The risk that the auditor will need to qualify his or her opinion for the audit engagement

d. The risk that the auditor will find a material misstatement in the financial statements during the course of the audit

MC 5-22 `LO6` When auditors determine financial statement materiality for a given audit engagement, they should primarily base their decisions on

a. the materiality level used by the company's management for internal audits.

b. users of the financial statements and their specific needs.

c. the prior year's materiality level.

d. the risk level determined in the preliminary assessment.

EXERCISES AND PROBLEMS

EP 5-1 Analytical Review Ratio Relationships. `LO5` The following situations represent errors and irregularities that can occur in financial statements.

Required:

State how the ratio in question would compare to what the ratio should have been had the error or irregularity not occurred.

a. The company recorded fictitious sales with credits to sales revenue accounts and debits to accounts receivable. Inventory was reduced and cost of goods sold was increased for the profitable "sales." Is the current ratio greater than, equal to, or less than what it should have been?

b. The company recorded cash disbursements paying trade accounts payable but held the cheques past the year-end date—meaning that the "disbursements" should not have been shown as credits to cash and debits to accounts payable. Is the current ratio greater than, equal to, or less than what it should have been? Consider cases in which the current ratio before the improper "disbursement" recording would have been (1) greater than 1:1, (2) equal to 1:1, and (3) less than 1:1.

c. The company uses a periodic inventory system for determining the balance sheet amount of inventory at year-end. Very near the year-end, merchandise was received, placed in the stockroom, and counted, but the purchase transaction was neither recorded nor paid until the next month. What was the effect on inventory, cost of goods sold, gross profit, and net income? How were these ratios affected, compared with what they would have been without the error: current ratio, return on beginning equity, gross margin ratio, cost of goods sold ratio, inventory turnover, and receivables turnover?

d. The company is loath to write off customer accounts receivable, even though the financial vice-president makes entirely adequate provision for uncollectible amounts in the allowance for bad debts. The gross receivables and the allowance both contain amounts that should have been written off long ago. How are these ratios affected compared with what they would have been if the old receivables were properly written off: current ratio, days' sales in receivables, doubtful account ratio, receivables turnover, return on beginning equity, working capital/total assets?

e. Since last year, the company has reorganized its lines of business and placed more emphasis on its traditional products while selling off some marginal businesses merged by the previous go-go management. Total assets are 10% less than they were last year, but working capital has increased. Retained earnings remain the same because the disposals created no gains, and the net income after taxes is still near zero, the same as last year. Earnings before interest and taxes remain the same, small but positive. The total market value of the company's equity has not increased, but that is better than the declines of the past several years. Proceeds from the disposals have been used to retire long-term debt. Net sales have decreased 5%, because the sales decrease resulting from the disposals has not been overcome by increased sales of the traditional products. Is the discriminant Z score (see Appendix 5A) of the current year higher or lower than that of the prior year?

EP 5-2 Understand the Business—Transactions and Accounts. **LO4** In the table below, the left column names several classes of transactions. The right column names several general ledger accounts.

CLASSES OF TRANSACTIONS	GENERAL LEDGER ACCOUNTS
Cash receipts	Cash
Cash disbursements	Accounts receivable
Credit sales	Allowance for doubtful accounts
Sales returns and allowances	Inventory
Purchases on credit	Fixed assets
Purchase returns	Accounts payable
Uncollectible account write-offs	Long-term debt
	Sales revenue
	Investment income
	Expenses

Required:

Identify the general ledger accounts that are affected by each class of transactions.

Approach:

Match the classes of transactions with the general ledger accounts where their debits and credits are usually entered.

EP 5-3 Auditing an Accounting Estimate. `LO5` Suppose management estimated the lower of cost and net realizable value of some obsolete inventory at $99,000 and wrote it down from $120,000, recognizing a loss of $21,000. The auditors obtained the following information: The inventory in question could be sold for an amount between $78,000 and $92,000. The costs of advertising and shipping could range from $5,000 to $7,000.

Required:

a. Would you propose an audit adjustment to the management estimate? Write the appropriate accounting entry.
b. If management's estimate of inventory market (lower than cost) had been $80,000, would you propose an audit adjustment? Write the appropriate accounting entry.

EP 5-4 Risk of Misstatement in Various Accounts. `LO4, 5`

Required:

Based on information you have available in Chapter 5:

a. Which accounts may be most susceptible to overstatement? to understatement?
b. Why do you think a company might permit asset accounts to be understated?
c. Why do you think a company might permit liability accounts to be overstated?
d. Which direction of misstatement is most likely: income overstatement or income understatement?

EP 5-5 Audit Acceptance and Planning. `LO1, 2, 3, 7` You have just started working as a junior accountant for Suppan & Associates LLP, a mid-size firm specializing in the audit of small retail and service companies. Just as you are finishing your review the firm's Quality Control Policies & Procedures Manual, one of the audit partners calls you into his office to discuss a prospective new audit engagement client:

"Welcome to the firm. I hope you are getting adjusted by now! I just got a call this morning from Devi Devine, the owner of a chain of local dry-cleaning stores. She thinks her company will need an audit of its financial statements because they are seeking to borrow a large amount of money from the bank to upgrade their equipment to use the newer environmentally friendly processes. I have an appointment to meet her tomorrow morning and started making some notes about the points to cover at the meeting, but I have to run out right now to deal with a medical emergency. My son had a fall at soccer and needs to go to the hospital emergency clinic for stitches—we could be waiting around there all day and night!

"Since you haven't yet been assigned to any work yet, can you finish up these notes for me so I'll be ready for tomorrow? Since this company has never been audited before, I want to be sure I explain to them what an independent financial statement audit is, why they may or may not need one, and what it will involve. I also want to make sure that I get all the information our firm needs to make a decision on whether we can accept the engagement. I have met the owner and her husband a few times at the local Chamber of Commerce meetings, and they seem to have a good reputation in the business community. It looks good, too, that they want to move to more environmentally friendly dry cleaning—I know many people are looking for that kind of service now due to allergies and other sensitivities. Here are the notes I've prepared so far (Exhibit EP 5-5), so please expand on these points—I want to be sure to cover everything important at the meeting tomorrow. I know Devi is a very busy businesswoman."

Required:

Complete the "To do" points in the audit partner's draft meeting notes.

Draft Notes for Meeting with Pristine Cleaners Inc. Owner, Devi Devine

1. Discuss the nature of an independent audit; determine whether it is needed.
   To do: List questions to ask Devi.
2. Summarize the audit process.
   To do: List what she can expect if an audit engagement is performed.
3. Determine whether professional and ethics codes will allow our firm to accept.
   To do: List the information we'll need to get from Devi to make this decision, and also other information we need from other sources.
4. Review the points to be covered in the Overall Audit Strategy, if we accept.
   To do: Review CAS 300, paragraph 8—list what it requires.

EP 5-6 Experts' Work as Audit Evidence. `LO4, 7` According to CAS 620, if expertise in a field other than accounting or auditing is required to obtain sufficient appropriate audit evidence, an auditor may need to use the work of an auditor's expert. The need for special expertise may include such matters as

- The valuation of complex financial instruments, land and buildings, plant and machinery, jewellery, works of art, antiques, intangible assets, and business combinations and conducting impairment reviews
- The actuarial calculation of liabilities associated with insurance contracts or employee benefit plans
- The estimation of oil and gas reserves
- The valuation of environmental liabilities and site cleanup costs
- The interpretation of contracts, laws, and regulations
- The analysis of complex or unusual tax compliance issues

Required:

How does an auditor determine the need to use an expert when developing the overall audit strategy? What additional work does an auditor need to perform if planning to use an expert's work as audit evidence to form an audit opinion?

EP 5-7 Applying the Canadian Auditing Standards to an Audit Engagement Acceptance Decision. `LO3, 4`

Required:

As an exercise in using the CASs, see if you can link up the related CAS requirements and application and other explanatory material to the steps Jack has taken in the Analysis section of the Application Case and Analysis in this chapter. Also explain how Jack is applying the standards.

(CPA Canada Handbook—Assurance, 2014)

DISCUSSION CASES

DC 5-1 Communications between Predecessor and Successor Auditors. `LO2, 3` Your firm has been contacted by the president of Lyrac Inc. about becoming the company's auditor. Lyrac was audited last year by PA Diggs and, while generally pleased with the services provided by Diggs, the president of Lyrac thinks the audit work was too detailed and interfered excessively with normal office routines. You have asked Lyrac's president to inform Diggs of the decision to change auditors, but he does not wish to do so.

Required:

List and discuss the steps to follow in dealing with a predecessor auditor and a new audit client before accepting the engagement. (*Hint:* Use the independence rules of conduct for a complete response to this requirement.)

DC 5-2 **Audit Engagement Acceptance.** LO2, 3 You are an auditor in an accounting firm that has 10 offices in three provinces. Sonny Shine has approached you with a request for your firm to audit his company. He is president of Hitech Software and Games Inc., a five-year-old company that has recently grown to $40 million in sales and $20 million in total assets. Shine is thinking about going public with a $17 million issue of common shares, of which $10 million would be a secondary issue of shares he holds. You are very happy about this opportunity because Shine is the new president of the Symphony Society board and has made quite a civic impression since he came to your medium-size city seven years ago. Hitech is one of the growing employers in the city.

Required:

a. Discuss the sources of information and the types of inquiries you and the firm's partners can make in connection with accepting Hitech as a new client.
b. Do professional conduct/ethics codes require any investigation of prospective clients?
c. Suppose Shine also told you that 10 years ago his closely held hamburger franchise business went bankrupt, and you learn from its former auditors (partners in another office of your own firm) that Shine played fast and loose with franchise-fee income recognition rules and presented such difficulties that your office in another city resigned from the audit (before the bankruptcy). Do you think the partner in charge of the audit practice at your firm should accept Hitech as a new client?

DC 5-3 **Pre-engagement and Preliminary Analysis Activities.** LO1, 2, 3, 4, 5, 6 Sunrise Solar Inc. (SSI) is a medium-size company that is developing solar energy systems for private residences and small businesses. It is privately owned, with the majority of the shares held by the company's president, Shu Mingfei. Started up two years ago, to date, it is mostly involved in research and development, but this year it completed its first customer sales and installation. Shu has engaged your firm to do the current year's audit because she plans to obtain $20 million in debt financing from outside investors to allow further commercialization of the SSI systems. You are now reviewing SSI's preliminary general ledger trial balance in order to begin preparing the audit planning.

The following is a summary of the accounts that appear in this trial balance as at year-end:

ACCOUNT	BALANCE DR/(CR)
Cash	$ 101,209
Accounts receivable	85,019
Allowance for bad debts	(15,000)
Inventory, finished goods	900,550
Inventory, work-in-process	44,666
Inventory, raw material	67,890
Deferred development costs	34,445
Property, plant, and equipment	3,700,990
Accumulated amortization, PPE	(901,108)
Patents, at cost	1,010,000
Accounts payable	(198,009)
Warranty provision	(30,000)
Shareholder loan, non–interest bearing	(11,000,000)

(continued)

ACCOUNT	BALANCE DR/(CR)
Share capital, common shares	(1,000)
Retained earnings	1,364,767
Revenue	(812,202)
Cost of goods sold	666,502
General and administration expenses	1,002,500
Research and development expenses	3,990,000
Other expenses	89,990

Required:

a. Identify three factors that your firm should consider before agreeing to conduct the audit.

b. What are the economic and industry risks affecting this business? How would these risks affect the company's financial statements and your overall audit strategy?

c. State the dollar amount you would consider an appropriate materiality level for planning this audit, giving your supporting reasons. Explain why the materiality judgment is one of the first important decisions your team must make in planning this audit.

d. List two analytical procedures you could perform using the trial balance data above (you are not required to calculate any ratios). Explain what each procedure can tell you about the risks in SSI's financial statements. Give one example of additional information you would want to obtain to perform analytical procedures in this audit, and a reason why it would be useful.

DC 5-4   Accepting an Engagement and Risk Analysis.   `LO3, 4`   Miller & Bell (M&B) is a medium-size accounting firm that was recently approached by Mints, a candy company, to take on their year-end audit engagement. The Director of Marketing at Mints, Valerie, suggested M&B since she had heard good things about M&B and her cousin is a staff accountant for M&B. The main partner at M&B has gathered the following information about Mints:

- Mints has eight shareholders. Greg, a creative entrepreneur, started Mints in 2001 and owns 51% of the company, while the remaining 49% is split equally between seven shareholders. Most shareholders are passive investors, but Greg is actively involved in the operations of Mints, as he is currently the CFO.

- Mints' candy is very popular in Europe, so a large part of the sales are made in euros. Mints tries to manage the foreign exchange risk by entering into complex cash flow hedges and purchasing forward contracts in euros.

- Mints is looking for a new auditor, as they disagreed with their previous auditor about their revenue recognition policy. Mints indicated that their previous auditor was too conservative.

- Mints has been showing a profit for the past two years, but it did run into some financial difficulties three years ago. Due to the financial difficulties, Mints had to obtain additional financing from the bank. As a result, Mints is subject to additional debt covenants, and the bank requires an audit of its financial statements to be performed.

Required:

You work as a senior auditor for M&B, and the partner has asked you to prepare a report that discusses what should be considered in M&B's decision to accept or decline Mints' audit engagement. Based on the information provided above, prepare a report to the M&B partner as requested, which discusses each element, explains why it is relevant to the decision, and explains whether the element presents a high/moderate/low risk for accepting the engagement. Use the table below to identify the key elements that should be covered in your report.

ELEMENT TO BE CONSIDERED	RISK FROM ACCEPTING THE ENGAGEMENT	WHY IS THE INFORMATION RELEVANT TO THE DECISION?

DC 5-5 Quantitative and qualitative materiality criteria. [LO6, 7] You are performing the audit of the Pirouette Systems Inc. (PSI) financial statements for its year ended November 30, 20X0. PSI is a private company that sells and installs computer networks for businesses in the Toronto area. PSI has four shareholders, who are all actively involved in the business. PSI's audited financial statements are used mainly by its bank, which has made a large operating loan. The bank requires PSI to maintain a current ratio of at least 1.2 to 1, based on its year-end financial statements; otherwise the bank can require PSI to repay the loan in full immediately.

PSI's accounting policy for recognizing revenue is to recognize 50% of the sales contract amount when the customer signs a sales contract and the balance when the network installation is complete. All sales are on account. During 20X0, PSI hired a new sales manager, who has focused on making sales to larger companies. On November 30, 20X0, the sales manager reported to PSI's accountant that $250,000 should be recorded as sales revenue. This amount is 50% of the revenue on a large sale to a new customer. This is the largest single sale in PSI's history. In January 20X1, while doing the audit, you discovered that the sales manager was premature in reporting this contract as a sale, since the customer did not actually give the final approval of the contract purchase of the network until December 15, 20X0.

Before correcting this error, PSI's draft financial statements show the following:

Net income before taxes: $6,200,000

Accounts receivable, net of allowance for bad debts: $850,000

Total current assets: $1,100,000

Total current liabilities: $860,000

Required:

a. Explain how the accounts in the PSI financial statements will be affected by this error. In your explanation, identify the assertion(s) violated by this error.

b. Calculate the impact of this error on PSI's current ratio (Note: Current ratio = Current assets/Current liabilities.)

c. Would you consider this error material? Justify your response.

DC 5-6 Materiality Level Reduced. [LO6] Your firm has done the audit of Rhea Fashions Inc. for many years. You are in charge of the fieldwork for the current year's audit. Rhea is a manufacturer of high-fashion clothing. Its shares are publicly traded, but a majority of the common shares are held by the members of the family that started the business during the 1950s. During the current year, Rhea's business shrank substantially because it lost a major customer, a countrywide department store chain that went out of business. Rhea has not been able to replace the lost business. Since many of Rhea's long-time employees were happy to take an early retirement offer, Rhea management's strategy now is to continue to operate only a few unique clothing brands that represented about 50% of its sales volume in prior years. The materiality level used in the prior years was $80,000. The audit partner has determined that the appropriate materiality for the current-year financial statement audit is $40,000.

Required:

a. Discuss the factors that the audit partner would have considered in deciding to reduce the materiality level.

b. What impact will the lower materiality level likely have on your audit procedures in the current year?

c. While reviewing the previous year's audit file, you note that last year's staff uncovered one error. Rhea had failed to accrue approximately $50,000 of customer volume discounts because of a calculation error in computing the customer's total sales. Since the error was less than materiality, no adjustment was made to the prior year's financial statements. Explain the impact this error had on the prior year's financial statements; the impact it will have on the current year's financial statements when it reverses; and the impact it will have on your audit, given your new materiality level.

DC 5-7   Materiality Approaches in Audit Practice.   `LO6`   Three former university classmates are meeting for dinner to celebrate completing their first year as junior auditors at three different public accounting firms. After reminiscing about the time they all skipped their auditing class to go to a playoff hockey game, one of them recalls, "It was great the Canucks won that game, even though they didn't make it to the next round. But the auditing class we missed that night was on materiality. I have learned a lot on the job, but materiality is still the one decision we make at work that makes no sense to me. And that makes me nervous because materiality is such a key factor in deciding what accounts to focus our audit work on and how much testing to do."

During the ensuing discussion they realize that their three firms use three different approaches to setting materiality for planning purposes. In Firm 1, the level of materiality is set for the whole audit based on 5–10% of normal earnings, or other benchmarks if earnings are not useful. In Firm 2, a similar method is used to come up with the starting materiality amount but then adjustments are made for anticipated misstatements and prior-year misstatement reversals, resulting in using a smaller amount for the purpose of planning the audit. In Firm 3, a similar starting point is used but the amount is then allocated to different accounts based on their size and any special user-based considerations, such as whether the amount is used in a debt covenant.

Required:

Discuss the implications for audit practice of having so much variability in setting materiality. What is the impact of CAS 320 on the three different approaches described in this scenario?

DC 5-8   Materiality and Misstatements in Estimates.   `LO6`   The auditors of Letron Inc. have set an overall materiality level of $900,000 and a performance materiality level of $800,000 for the current-year audit, 20X2. They used the same materiality levels in their 20X1 audit. Letron is in the telecommunications equipment business, and its inventory value is subject to fluctuations due to changes in supply and demand as well as technological obsolescence, creating considerable measurement uncertainty. Management's point estimate of the inventories' value as of the end of 20X2 is $15.9 million, after reversal of a write-down that was taken in 20X1. The auditors have established a range of estimates for the inventory value of $14–16 million, so management's point estimate is within the auditors' range. In 20X1, poor market conditions prevailed and Letron wrote down its inventory to net realizable value, estimated to be $12.3 million. Management and the auditor had a disagreement regarding inventory valuation for 20X1, because it fell outside of the auditors' range of $13–15 million. However, this difference and the aggregated misstatements for 20X1 were less than the performance materiality, so these misstatements were not corrected. Letron initiated a bonus plan in 20X0 that would reward top management if the company reported positive profits. Letron reported losses in 20X0 and 20X1. In 20X2, Letron reported a small profit, giving rise to a substantial bonus to its management team.

Required:

Assume the role of Letron's auditor, and explain the actions you would take in this situation, based on applying the requirements and guidance in CAS 450 and CAS 540.

DC 5-9 Overall Audit Strategy, Retail Industry. **LO7** Using the SEDAR database (sedar.com), find the most recent annual reports for two Canadian retailers (e.g., Loblaw, Rona, Danier Leather).

Required:

a. Based on the information provided in the companies' audited financial statements and the Management Discussion and Analysis (and, optionally, other Internet research you may wish to do), use the planning document shown in Exhibit 5–10 to identify and list key information items that should be documented in the "Engagement Characteristics" section of the overall audit strategy for each of these companies.

b. What do you think would be the most significant audit issues in each company? Explain issues that would be similar in each audit. For any issues you identify that would differ between the companies, explain why you think these differences would exist.

DC 5-10 Horizontal and Vertical Analysis. **LO5** Horizontal analysis refers to changes in financial statement numbers and ratios across two or more years. Vertical analysis refers to financial statement amounts expressed each year as proportions of a base, such as sales for the income statement accounts, and total assets for the balance sheet accounts. Exhibit DC 5-10–1 contains the Retail Company's prior-year (audited) and current-year (unaudited) financial statements, along with amounts and percentages of change from year to year (horizontal analysis) and common-size percentages (vertical analysis). Exhibit DC5-10–2 contains selected financial ratios based on these financial statements. Analysis of these data may enable auditors to detect relationships that raise questions about misleading financial statements.

Required:

Study the data in Exhibits DC 5-10–1 and DC 5-10–2. Write a memo identifying and explaining potential problem areas where misstatements in the current-year financial statements might exist. Additional information about Retail Company is as follows:

- The new bank loan, obtained on July 1 of the current year, requires maintenance of a 2:1 current ratio.
- Principal of $100,000 plus interest on the 10% long-term note obtained several years ago in the original amount of $800,000 is due each January 1.
- The company has never paid dividends on its common shares and has no plans for a dividend.

EXHIBIT DC 5-10–1

Retail Company Horizontal and Vertical Analysis

	PRIOR YEAR AUDITED		CURRENT YEAR		CHANGE	
	BALANCE	COMMON SIZE	BALANCE	COMMON SIZE	AMOUNT	PERCENT
Assets:						
Cash	$ 600,000	14.78%	$ 484,000	9.69%	(116,000)	−19.33%
Accounts receivable	500,000	12.32	400,000	8.01	(100,000)	−20.00
Allowance for doubtful accounts	(40,000)	−0.99	(30,000)	−0.60	10,000	−25.00
Inventory	1,500,000	−36.95	1,940,000	38.85	440,000	29.33
Total current assets	$2,560,000	63.05	2,794,000	55.95	234,000	9.14
Capital assets	3,000,000	73.89	4,000,000	80.10	1,000,000	33.33
Accumulated depreciation	(1,500,000)	−36.95	(1,800,000)	−36.04	(300,000)	20.00
Total assets	$4,060,000	100.00%	$4,994,000	100.00%	934,000	23.00%

(continued)

Retail Company Horizontal and Vertical Analysis (*continued*)

	PRIOR YEAR AUDITED		CURRENT YEAR		CHANGE	
	BALANCE	COMMON SIZE	BALANCE	COMMON SIZE	AMOUNT	PERCENT
Liabilities and equity:						
Accounts payable	$ 450,000	11.08%	$ 600,000	12.01%	150,000	33.33%
Bank loans, 11%	0	0.00	750,000	15.02	750,000	NA
Accrued interest	50,000	1.23	40,000	0.80	(10,000)	−20.00
Accruals and other	60,000	1.48	10,000	0.20	(50,000)	−83.33
Total current liabilities	560,000	13.79	1,400,000	28.03	840,000	150.00
Long-term debt, 10%	500,000	12.32	400,000	8.01	(100,000)	−20.00
Total liabilities	1,060,000	26.11	1,800,000	36.04	740,000	69.81
Share capital	2,000,000	49.26	2,000,000	40.05	0	0
Retained earnings	1,000,000	24.63	1,194,000	23.91	194,000	19.40
Total liabilities and equity	$4,060,000	100.00%	$4,994,000	100.00%	934,000	23.00%
Statement of operations:						
Sales (net)	$9,000,000	100.00%	$8,100,000	100.00%	(900,000)	−10.00%
Cost of goods sold	6,296,000	69.96	5,265,000	65.00	(1,031,000)	−16.38
Gross margin	2,704,000	30.04	2,835,000	35.00	131,000	4.84
General expense	2,044,000	22.71	2,005,000	24.75	(39,000)	−1.91
Amortization	300,000	3.33	300,000	3.70	0	0
Operating income	360,000	4.00	530,000	6.54	170,000	47.22
Interest expense	50,000	0.56	40,000	0.49	(10,000)	−20.00
Income taxes (40%)	124,000	1.38	196,000	2.42	72,000	58.06
Net income	$ 186,000	2.07%	$294,000	3.63%	108,000	58.06%

NA means not applicable.

Retail Company Comparative Ratio Analysis

	PRIOR YEAR	CURRENT YEAR	PERCENT CHANGE
Balance sheet ratios:			
Current ratio	4.57	2.0	−56.34%
Days' sales in receivables	18.40	16.44	−10.63
Doubtful accounts ratio	0.08	0.075	−6.25
Days' sales in inventory	85.77	132.65	54.66
Debt/equity ratio	0.35	0.56	40.89
Operations ratios:			
Receivables turnover	19.57	21.89	11.89
Inventory turnover	4.20	2.71	−35.34
Cost of goods sold/sales	69.96%	65.00%	−7.08
Gross margin %	30.04%	35.00%	16.49
Return on equity	6.61%	9.80%	48.26

Selected Financial Ratios

LO8 Know the types of ratios typically applied to financial statements to identify potential risks of misstatement.

BALANCE SHEET RATIOS	FORMULA*
Current ratio	$\dfrac{\text{Current assets}}{\text{Current liabilities}}$
Days' sales in receivables	$\dfrac{\text{Ending net receivables}}{\text{Credit sales}} \times 360$
Doubtful account ratio	$\dfrac{\text{Allowance for doubtful accounts}}{\text{Ending gross receivables}}$
Days' sales in inventory	$\dfrac{\text{Ending inventory}}{\text{Cost of goods sold}} \times 360$
Debt ratio	$\dfrac{\text{Current and long-term debt}}{\text{Shareholder equity}}$
Equity multiplier ratio	$\dfrac{\text{Total assets}}{\text{Shareholder equity}}$

OPERATIONS RATIOS

Profit margin	$\dfrac{\text{Net income}}{\text{Total revenues}}$
Total asset turnover	$\dfrac{\text{Total revenues}}{\text{Total assets}}$
Receivables turnover	$\dfrac{\text{Credit sales}}{\text{Ending net receivables}}$
Inventory turnover	$\dfrac{\text{Cost of goods sold}}{\text{Ending inventory}}$
Cost of goods sold ratio	$\dfrac{\text{Cost of goods sold}}{\text{Net sales}}$
Gross margin ratio	$\dfrac{\text{Net sales} - \text{Cost of goods sold}}{\text{Net sales}}$
Operating margin percentage	$\dfrac{\text{Operating revenues} - \text{Operating expenses}}{\text{Operating revenues}}$
Return on beginning equity	$\dfrac{\text{Net income}}{\text{Shareholder equity (beginning)}}$

BALANCE SHEET RATIOS	FORMULA*

FINANCIAL DISTRESS RATIOS[19]

FORMULA*

Discriminant Z score[20],**

$$Z = 1.2X_1 + 1.4X_2 + 3.3X_3 + 0.6X_4 + 1.0X_5$$

where:

(X_1) Working capital ÷ Total assets

$$\frac{\text{Current assets} - \text{Current liabilities}}{\text{Total assets}}$$

(X_2) Retained earnings ÷ Total assets

$$\frac{\text{Retained earnings (ending)}}{\text{Total assets}}$$

(X_3) Earnings before interest and taxes ÷ Total assets

$$\frac{\text{Net income} + \text{Interest expense} + \text{Income tax expense}}{\text{Total assets}}$$

(X_4) Market value of equity ÷ Total debt

$$\frac{\text{Market value of common and preferred shares}}{\text{Total assets}}$$

(X_5) Net sales ÷ Total assets

$$\frac{\text{Net sales}}{\text{Total assets}}$$

*These ratios are shown to be calculated using year-end numbers, rather than year average, for balances, such as accounts receivable and inventory. Other accounting and finance reference books may contain formulas using year-average numbers. As long as no unusual changes have occurred during the year, the year-end numbers can have much audit relevance because they reflect the most current balance data. For comparative purposes, the ratios should be calculated on the same basis for all the years being compared. In the EcoPak example in Exhibits 5–5 and 5–6, the market value of the equity in the calculations is $3 million.

**The discriminant Z score is an index of a company's financial health. The higher the Z-score, the better the financial health of the company. The lower the score, the closer the company is to financial failure. The Z-score that predicts financial failure is a matter of debate. Research suggests that companies with scores above 3.0 never go bankrupt. Generally, companies with scores below 1.0 can be expected to experience financial difficulty of some kind. The score can be a negative number. It should be stressed that these ratios are indicators only and therefore need to be combined with in-depth analysis before any final conclusions can be reached.

APPENDIX 5B

Example of an Audit Engagement Letter

LO9   Describe the contents of an audit engagement letter.

This example shows how an engagement letter could be written for an audit of a privately held real estate development company.

November 6, 20X4

Ms. Harriet Liu, President
Real Estate Development Limited
600 Paree Street
Richmond, BC

(continued)

Dear Ms. Liu:

You have requested that we audit the financial statements of Real Estate Development Limited ("the company"), which comprise the balance sheet as at December 31, 20X4, and the income statement, statement of changes in equity, and cash flow statement for the year then ended, and a summary of significant accounting policies and other explanatory notes. Our audit will be conducted with the objective of expressing an opinion on the financial statements. Our understanding is that the intended purposes of the financial statements are to report to the Real Estate Development Limited shareholders and to satisfy the requirements of Real Estate Development Limited's credit agreement with the Regal Bank of British Columbia. We are pleased to confirm our acceptance and our understanding of this audit engagement by means of this letter.

Our Responsibilities

As auditors, our responsibility is to conduct the audit in accordance with Canadian generally accepted auditing standards. Those standards require that we comply with ethical requirements and plan and perform the audit to obtain reasonable assurance whether the financial statements are free from material misstatement. An audit involves performing procedures to obtain audit evidence about the amounts and disclosures in the financial statements. The procedures selected depend on the auditor's judgment, including the assessment of the risks of material misstatement of the financial statements, whether due to fraud or error. An audit also includes evaluating the appropriateness of accounting policies used and the reasonableness of accounting estimates made by management, as well as evaluating the overall presentation of the financial statements.

Because of the test nature and other inherent limitations of an audit, together with the inherent limitations of any accounting and internal control system, there is an unavoidable risk that even some material misstatements may remain undiscovered.

In making our risk assessments, we consider internal control relevant to the entity's preparation and fair presentation of the financial statements in order to design audit procedures that are appropriate in the circumstances, but not for the purpose of expressing a separate opinion on the effectiveness of the entity's internal control. However, if we identify any of the following matters, they will be communicated to you:

(a) Misstatements, resulting from error, other than trivial errors

(b) Fraud or any information obtained that indicates that a fraud may exist

(c) Evidence obtained that indicates that an illegal or possibly illegal act, other than one considered inconsequential, has occurred

(d) Significant weaknesses in the design or implementation of internal control to prevent and detect fraud or error

(e) Related party transactions identified by our audit team that are not in the normal course of operations and that involve significant judgments made by management concerning measurement or disclosure

The matters communicated will be those that we identify during the course of our audit. Audits do not usually identify all matters that may be of interest to management in discharging its responsibilities. The type and significance of the matter to be communicated will determine the level of management to which the communication is directed.

One of the underlying principles of the profession is a duty of confidentiality with respect to client affairs. Accordingly, except for information that is in or enters the public domain, we will not provide any third party with confidential information concerning the company's affairs without the company's prior consent, unless required to do so by legal authority, or the rules of professional conduct/code of ethics of the provincial public accountancy council.

(continued)

Company Responsibilities

Our audit will be conducted on the basis that you, your management team, and the company's Board of Directors who are charged with governance acknowledge and understand that you are responsible for

(a) Preparation and fair presentation of the financial statements in accordance with Canadian generally accepted accounting principles. This includes the design, implementation, and maintenance of internal control relevant to the preparation and fair presentation of financial statements that are free from material misstatement, whether due to fraud or error.

(b) Providing us with all information, such as records, documentation, and related data; copies of all minutes of meetings of shareholders, directors, and committees of directors; and other matters that are relevant to the preparation and fair presentation of the financial statements.

(c) Providing us with any additional information we may request from the company, such as

- Information relating to any known or probable instances of non-compliance with legislative or regulatory requirements, including financial reporting requirements;
- Information relating to any illegal or possibly illegal acts, and all facts related thereto;
- Information regarding all related parties and related party transactions;
- An assessment of the risk that the financial statements may be materially misstated as a result of fraud;
- Information relating to fraud or suspected fraud affecting the entity involving management, employees who have significant roles in internal control, or others, where the fraud could have a non-trivial effect on the financial statements;
- Information relating to any allegations of fraud or suspected fraud affecting the entity's financial statements communicated by employees, former employees, regulators, or others;
- Significant assumptions underlying fair value measurements and disclosures in the financial statements, and management's assessment of their reasonableness;
- Any plans or intentions that may affect the carrying value or classification of assets or liabilities;
- Information relating to the measurement and disclosure of transactions with related parties;
- An assessment of all areas of measurement uncertainty known to management that are required to be disclosed in accordance with Canadian generally accepted accounting principles;
- Information relating to claims and possible claims, whether or not they have been discussed with Real Estate Development Limited's legal counsel; other liabilities and contingent gains or losses, including those associated with guarantees, whether written or oral, under which Real Estate Development Limited is contingently liable;
- Information on whether Real Estate Development Limited has satisfactory title to assets, whether any liens or encumbrances on assets exist, and whether any assets are pledged as collateral;
- Information relating to compliance with aspects of contractual agreements that may affect the financial statements; and
- Information concerning subsequent events.

(d) Providing us with unrestricted access to those within the company from whom we determine it is necessary to obtain audit evidence

As part of our audit process, we will request from management and, where appropriate, those charged with governance, written confirmation concerning representations provided to us during the audit on matters that are

- Directly related to items that are material, either individually or in the aggregate, to the financial statements;

(continued)

- Not directly related to items that are material to the financial statements but are significant, either individually or in the aggregate, to the engagement; and
- Relevant to your judgments or estimates that are material, either individually or in the aggregate, to the financial statements.

Reporting

Unless unanticipated difficulties are encountered, at the conclusion of our audit we will submit to you a report containing our opinion on the financial statements. We expect to report as shown in the Appendix to this letter:

[The wording of the Standard Audit Report would be included with the engagement letter as an Appendix.]

If during the course of our work it appears for any reason that we will not be in a position to render an unmodified opinion on the financial statements, we will discuss this with you.

Other Matters

We will ask that your personnel, to the extent possible, prepare various schedules and analyses and make various invoices and other documents available to the audit team members. This assistance will facilitate our work and minimize your audit costs. We look forward to full cooperation from your staff during our audit.

We may also submit to you a memorandum containing our comments on the adequacy of existing systems of internal control, accounting policies and procedures, and other related matters that come to our attention during the course of the audit.

We ask that our firm name be used only with our consent, and that any information to which we have attached a communication be issued with that communication unless otherwise agreed to by our firm.

Our charges to the company for the audit services will be made at our regular rates plus out-of-pocket expenses. Bills will be rendered on a regular basis with payment to be made upon presentation.

The above terms of this engagement will be effective from year to year until amended or terminated in writing. If you have any questions about the contents of this letter, please raise them with Mo Kelley, the audit partner assigned to your audit.

If the services outlined are in accordance with your requirements and if the above terms are acceptable to you, **please sign the copy of this letter in the space provided below and return it to us.** We appreciate the opportunity to be of service to your company.

Yours very truly,

Kelley and Randu, LLP, PUBLIC ACCOUNTANTS

Acknowledged and agreed on behalf of Real Estate Development Limited by

_____ _____
Harriet Liu   [date]

Source: Adapted from *CPA Canada Handbook—Assurance,* section 5110 appendix (2006 ed.), and CAS 210 (2014 ed.).

ENDNOTES

1   See, for example, "Briefing: Accounting scandals (The dozy watchdogs)," *The Economist*, December 13, 2014, pp. 24–26.

2   A change of auditors involves the successor reporting on the current year, where the prior-year comparative financial statements were audited by the predecessor. The successor's audit report should disclose this fact in a separate other matters paragraph following the opinion paragraph, as required in CAS 710.

3   CAS 210, paragraphs 3, 6, and 10.

4   CAS 300, paragraphs 7–8; CAS 230, paragraph 8.

5   CAS 315.

6   These more-detailed risk assessment procedures are what the CASs refer to as the "assertion level" risk assessments. Stay tuned: the assertion concept will be explained in Chapter 6, and these more-detailed risk assessments at the assertion level will be discussed in Chapter 7. These different concepts and perspectives illustrate the integrative thinking an audit team has to do to draw together considerations gathered by many different people from different sources and perspectives when they are assessing risks of material misstatement.

7   CAS 300.

8   Stay tuned: examples of this use are provided in Part 3.

9   The use of analytical procedures at the completion step of the audit will be explained in Chapter 15.

10   E. Hirst, L. Koonce, and F. Philipps, "First, know the business," *CA Magazine*, August 1998, p. 41.

11   E. I. Altman, "Financial ratios, discriminant analysis and the prediction of corporate bankruptcy," *The Journal of Finance*, September 1968, pp. 589–609; and Appendix 5A of this chapter.

12   CAS 320, paragraphs 9–11.

13   The authors are grateful to Professor Morley Lemon for inspiring this analogy, and for many other inspiring ways to think about auditing.

14   SEC Staff Accounting Bulletin (SAB) 99.

15   CAS 320, paragraphs A3–A5.

16   CAS 320 (9–10, A10), CAS 530, and further discussion in Chapter 10. Some discussion of the specific materialities is provided in understanding different types of audit report qualifications in Chapter 4.

17   Some sampling models do not require the use of a smaller performance materiality to allow for potential undetected misstatements due to sampling risk. This is explained in Chapter 10.

18   CAS 260, paragraph 15.

19   Altman, 1968.

20   *Ibid.*

Assessing Risks in an Audit Engagement

This chapter looks at how auditors gain an understanding of the auditee's risks and controls to assess the risks of a material misstatement occurring because of error or fraud. Auditors use this understanding to develop a detailed audit plan that addresses the assessed risks and provides reasonable assurance that the financial statements are not materially misstated.

LEARNING OBJECTIVES

After completing this chapter, you will be able to do the following:

LO1 Explain how the auditor's understanding of the business risks is used to assess the risk of material misstatement at the financial statement level.

LO2 Identify the principal assertions in management's financial statements and the related risks of material misstatement.

LO3 Describe the conceptual audit risk model and its components.

LO4 Explain the usefulness and limitations of the audit risk model in conducting the audit.

LO5 Outline the relationships among the business processes and accounting processes (or cycles) that constitute an organization's information system and generate management's general purpose financial statements.

LO6 **(Appendix 6A)** Explain the industry, regulatory, and other external factors that affect an auditee's business risk and related risk of material misstatement in its financial statements.

LO7 **(Appendix 6A)** Explain how an auditor uses an understanding of the auditee's business risk and its management risk assessment processes to assess the risk of material misstatement in the assertions of its financial statements.

LO8 **(Appendix 6B)** Explain corporate governance and developments in corporate governance standards that affect the role of external auditors in conducting audit engagements.

CHAPTER APPENDICES

APPENDIX 6A   Business Risk Factors Used to Assess the Risk of Material Misstatement

APPENDIX 6B   Corporate Governance (on Connect)

EcoPak Inc.

Tariq is looking forward to becoming the engagement partner for the EcoPak audit. He has only recently been promoted to partner at Meyer & Gustav (M&G), and the EcoPak engagement will give him a good starting point to build his practice in the growing sustainable materials industry. He has known Ella for many years and has a lot of respect for her good judgment and integrity, so her recommendation of EcoPak as a good client carries a lot of weight. He is very grateful to Ella for giving him full access to a review of Pettit and Foure (P&F) LLP's prior audit files, as that has given him confidence in EcoPak's management's integrity and willingness to accept responsibility for fair presentation of the company's financial statements. Ella's files also gave Tariq a lot of insight into EcoPak's business, management, and operating environment.

Still, Tariq now needs to make some important judgments of his own in relation to the risks he is taking on with this audit. He needs to make his own inquiries about Kam, Mike, and Nina in the business community, even though Ella's vouching for their integrity is a good start. They have some governance strength—separate chair and CEO—but Zhang also owns another business that sells preprocessed materials to EcoPak, so there are some related party issues to be concerned about. They also lack independent directors with financial expertise, and this may make his job a bit more difficult when he has to explain any complex financial reporting problems to those charged with governance. And while EcoPak has been very successful, recently its growth has involved investing in plant expansions but financing them with fairly short-term bank debts with tight covenants. That situation increases the risk of EcoPak running into some financial difficulties, although at this time there is low risk that it cannot continue as a going concern into next year. The infusion of cash EcoPak hopes to obtain from its initial public offering (IPO) is crucial to strengthening its balance sheet. So an IPO makes business sense, but it also creates a lot more risk for Tariq, since many more users will rely on the audited financial statements to make decisions about buying EcoPak shares.

Fortunately, Tariq can confer with more-senior partners in his firm, some of whom were involved in M&G's decision to accept the EcoPak engagement. One of these partners, Phyllis Amana, helps Tariq reach the conclusion that the risk of material misstatement at the financial statement level appears to be moderate, subject to further analysis that Tariq will be doing himself as part of his audit planning. Phyllis also notes that given EcoPak's plan to go public in three years, the audit should be done to reduce audit risk to a minimum. This means a high level of audit work will need to be done to make sure the staff do a thorough examination and obtain a lot of independent evidence to support the numbers in EcoPak's financial statements.

Tariq starts to analyze EcoPak's monthly financial statements for the current year to date in relation to the audited financial statements of last year, to determine more specifically which accounts have the highest risk of being misstated by an amount large enough to be significant to people who might use these financial statements. His eyes light on the inventory—there are some unusual fluctuations in relation to cost of sales in comparison to last year. This may indicate problems in how the inventory has been valued at year-end. He also notes that the relatively flat trend in the plant and equipment asset account balances does not seem consistent with his knowledge of what happened in the operations during the year. This may indicate that some new plant assets have not been recorded, so the account balances are not complete. His next step is to arrange a visit with Nina to learn more about the results and to make some inquiries to help him understand how effective EcoPak's internal controls were in reducing the risks that misstatements could occur and not be detected and fixed in their accounting records.

When Tariq calls Nina to set up a meeting, she seems a bit agitated, and he asks her if everything is all right. "Tariq, I don't know how to say this, so I'll just spit it out. I am becoming suspicious that there might be some kind of fraud going on in our raw materials purchasing department! We had a good control system set up a few years ago, but things just haven't been adding up in the past few months." Tariq arranges to come out the next week to go over Nina's concerns. He also makes a note that the risk of taking on this audit engagement may have just gone up!

The Essentials of Assessing Risks in an Audit Engagement

A financial statement audit under generally accepted auditing standards (GAAS) is performed from a risk-based perspective. In essence, a risk is the probability of some undesirable thing happening in the future. One of the starting points in a risk-based audit is to understand the business risks that the auditee's management must navigate to keep the business successful. Management is responsible for addressing the risks arising in the company's business environment and operations. Management is also responsible for ensuring the company's financial statements fairly present the business's economic performance and financial position, both good and bad. At the preliminary stage of audit planning, the auditors will take a high-level view, based on the nature of the business and its environment, its financial strength, and its corporate governance, to make an overall assessment of the risk of material misstatement for the financial statements. This allows the auditors to focus on key risk areas that they expect to encounter and set up an overall audit strategy that sets out the main resources required to perform the audit.

Auditors need to identify the sources of the business's risks and learn how management deals with them by gaining an understanding of management's risk assessment processes. For risk arising from the business environment and operations, management's main risk assessment tools involve strategic planning, using appropriate business processes, and implementing reliable information systems. Risks related to financial reporting and disclosure are managed mainly by strong internal controls over financial reporting and over the accounting information system. If management's risk assessment processes are not strong, it becomes more likely that the business risk will not be reduced. This leads to more problems that should be captured in the financial information system. In this way, business risk can contribute to higher risk of material misstatement. If these problems are not picked up by the information system, perhaps because they are not routine or expected situations, it may affect the fair presentation of the financial statements. If the financial information systems and internal control are not strong, this can also result in misstatements in the financial statements. So the auditors' understanding of the business and its management controls must be very deep to allow them to assess how effective the management processes and controls are likely to be in managing these interrelated types of risk.

A useful practical tool auditors apply in the risk assessment exercise is to break down the information contained in financial statements into different assertions, or claims, that management is making to fairly present its financial statement numbers and disclosures. By considering these more narrowly defined aspects of the classes of transactions, account balances, and disclosures in the financial statements, auditors are better able to specify the impact of business risks on the fair presentation. Also, very importantly, these more targeted risk assessments are the basis for the second step of the audit process, responding to the assessed risks. Having a more specific understanding of what could have gone wrong helps auditors identify the kinds of independent evidence they will need to gather to get reasonable assurance about whether the financial statement information is fairly presented. Every financial statement number can be viewed as making five main types of assertions: existence, completeness, ownership, valuation, and presentation. Consider an example like the inventory account balance. By including a balance for inventory in its statement of financial position, management makes the following specific claims:

- The inventory really exists (e.g., someone could go and actually look at it).
- All the inventory that exists is included (e.g., there isn't a separate storage area left out).
- The company owns the inventory (e.g., any consignment inventory held for others is excluded).
- The inventory is appropriately valued in accordance with generally accepted accounting principles (GAAP) (e.g., appropriate costs have been included and consideration given to whether the costs are below the net realizable value).
- The inventory has been classified appropriately, and disclosures required to achieve fair presentation are included (e.g., the inventory is included in current assets, and the financial statement notes explain the valuation policies and break down the major categories included).

The assertions provide a very powerful conceptual tool for performing an audit. They help auditors to think more specifically about what assertions are most difficult to get right in a particular business, and to consider if management's risk assessment processes, business processes, and internal control systems are strong enough to lower the highest-risk assertions. As auditors move on to the second step of the audit process, responding to the assessed risks, assertions can really help them to identify the most relevant evidence they can gather to gain reasonable assurance that the risk of material misstatement is acceptably low.

Essentially, to perform a risk-based audit, the auditor needs to focus on two related factors that create a *risk of material misstatement* at the assertion level. The first factor is the inherent risks arising in the business environment and operations: these can make material misstatements more likely to happen in the first place. The second factor is the control risks arising from a lack of effective internal control over the financial information system: these can allow material misstatements to enter the information system and go uncorrected. The auditor's business knowledge and understanding of management's internal controls are used to visualize which assertions are most vulnerable to misstatements arising from these inherent and/or control risks. The auditor assesses the risk of material misstatement in the assertions in all the main transactions, account balances, and disclosures in the company's financial statements. For example, the auditor might assess a risk as high, medium, or low—but note that this must be based on an auditor's professional judgment—it cannot really be measured precisely. Still, since an assessed risk level is essentially an estimated probability, some auditors may find it useful to think of the risk level in terms of numerical probabilities, or ranges of probabilities.

An auditor's verification work provides assurance that the financial statement information is not materially misstated. Since the auditor's overall objective is to get reasonable assurance to support the audit opinion, it stands to reason that those areas with the highest risks are the ones where the auditor will need to put in the most effort to verify whether a misstatement has occurred. The term *audit risk* is used to express the risk that the auditor gives an opinion that the financial statements are fairly presented when they are actually materially misstated. Essentially, audit risk refers to the risk of audit failure, that is, the risk that the audit has failed to meet its objective. Conceptually, we can look at audit risk and audit assurance as complements: by obtaining a reasonable (i.e., high) level of assurance that there is no material misstatement, the audit risk is lowered. So another way to look at the overall objective of the audit is in terms of audit risk: the auditor wants to make sure the audit risk is acceptably low before issuing a clean audit opinion.

The audit profession has developed a conceptual tool called the *audit risk model* to keep track of these risk assessments and determine the best audit approach for getting the assurance required to achieve a low audit risk level overall. The components of the model are audit risk (AR), risk of material misstatement (RMM) {RMM = inherent risk (IR) × control risk (CR)}, and detection risk (DR), and the formula is AR = IR × CR × DR. The AR level is set for the audit overall, and RMM (or IR and CR) assessments are made at the assertion level.

Audit risk is defined as the probability that the auditor gives an opinion that the financial statements are fairly presented when they are actually materially misstated, as noted above. To use due care, an auditor will always want to reduce audit risk to a very low level. However, some engagements might call for a much lower audit risk than others. If the circumstances of the engagement indicate that the consequences of audit failure would be extremely damaging to the auditor's reputation and would likely create legal liability, the auditor will try to achieve the lowest audit risk possible. Since achieving lower audit risk requires getting more assurance, it requires higher audit effort, and thus a higher cost of doing the audit will be incurred. Factors like the extent to which users rely on the audit opinion, the kinds of decisions they make, the financial health of the business, and the competency of management can affect how much impact an audit failure will have on the auditor's reputation and liability. Auditors consider these kinds of factors to decide how low the audit risk needs to be on a particular engagement. On engagements where there are fewer or no outside users relying on the audited financial statements to make risky financial decisions, the auditor might be willing to accept somewhat more audit risk. In that case the auditor will still do everything required with due care, but can perhaps be more cost efficient in doing the audit work

Risk of material misstatement is the auditor's assessment of the probability that one or more assertions in the elements of the financial statements are materially misstated due to inherent and control risks. It is very important to note that the risk of material misstatement exists due to the nature of the auditee's business and its management. Auditors have no influence over these risks or responsibility to address them. The auditors' responsibility is to understand the business well enough so they can assess how serious these risks are for the purpose of planning auditing procedures that will determine whether material misstatements have, in fact, arisen in management's financial statements.

Inherent risk is defined as the probability that material misstatements affecting one or more financial statement assertions could have occurred in the first place, before any controls were applied. For example, if an equipment manufacturer uses a complex process to calculate the manufacturing cost of a technologically complex product, there is a high inherent risk that an error could occur in the costing calculation. So the auditor would assess a high inherent risk to the valuation assertion of the inventory account balance, and also to the related cost of sales transactions. Auditors use professional judgment to assess inherent risk, using their understanding of the business's risk.

Control risk is the probability that management's internal control policies and procedures will fail to prevent material misstatements from occurring in the first place, or fail to detect and correct them once they have occurred. For example, an essential control procedure is to regularly reconcile the company's cash account balance to the bank balance. If the company issued a large cheque to buy holiday gifts for its customers and forgot to enter it in the books, a bank reconciliation would detect this error and indicate how to correct it. If the bank reconciliation is not done, this kind of error will not be detected and corrected and will result in overstatement of the cash balance. So, if control procedures like this are not done regularly, control risk will be assessed higher for the existence assertion of the cash account (and other related assertions).

Inherent risk and control risk are different, but they interact because controls are designed by management to reduce the types of risks that are inherent in a company's business. For example, if the company has a supervisor who carefully reviews the complex cost calculations, this control can prevent a costing error from getting entered into the inventory account in the first place. So auditors can combine the assessment of inherent and control risk, so that together they capture the risk of material misstatement.

Detection risk is defined as the probability that the auditor's procedures will fail to detect a misstatement that has occurred (due to inherent risk) and has not been corrected by the company's internal controls (due to control risk). It is the auditor's responsibility to keep the detection risk to a low enough level to achieve an acceptably low level of audit risk. The auditor lowers detection risk by performing independent investigation work that gives assurance that material misstatements have not occurred.

To plan the audit work required, the auditor has to determine the detection risk level that will produce an acceptably low audit risk level, given the level of risk of material misstatement that is present in the auditee's financial information. We can relate all these risk factors by rearranging the above formula to solve for DR, as follows:

$$DR = AR \div RMM \qquad \{or\ DR = AR \div (IR \times CR)\}$$

To illustrate how the model works as an aid to audit judgment, consider some possible situations.

Before any audit work is done, there is some possible level of risk of material misstatement, but detection risk is 100%, so AR = RMM. This means the risk of a clean audit opinion being wrong is essentially the risk that the financial statements are materially wrong. Obviously, if an auditor gives a clean opinion without doing anything, this would be very risky.

If the auditor wants to accept only a very low audit risk (say 2%), and the risk of material misstatement of a particular assertion is assessed as being fairly high (say 60%), then the auditor will need to achieve a detection risk of 3%, which is very low. To achieve this the auditor will need to obtain a lot of independent evidence to support a conclusion that there is no material misstatement in the assertion.

If, on another audit, the auditor found it reasonable to accept a higher audit risk (say 10%), and an assertion also has an assessed risk of material misstatement of 60%, in this case the auditor needs to achieve a detection risk of 6%, which would require less evidence than to achieve a detection risk of 3%. Also, in the same audit, if another assertion has a very low risk of material misstatement (say 20%), the auditor could accept a detection risk of 50%—much higher—and still achieve the 10% audit risk, so this could be done with much less audit evidence than would be needed to achieve a very low detection risk.

While recognizing that these risk decisions are all judgments rather than precise probability measures, the audit risk model does provide a useful thinking tool for making very important audit planning decisions, by helping auditors distinguish the financial statement assertions that will require the most audit effort from those that do not require as much time and attention.

Another perspective can be taken on the audit risk model components by considering the various sources of assurance available in an audit. Auditors get assurance about financial statement assertions from three main sources: the inherent nature of the assertion, the effectiveness of management's controls over the assertion, and the relevant evidence obtained through audit investigation work. Using this view, in a particular audit an auditor might get some assurance from the fact that there is an inherently low risk of material misstatement, and more assurance from verifying that there are strong controls over the assertion. In this case, to achieve the high/reasonable assurance required, the assurance needed from audit evidence may be fairly low. Alternatively, if the assertion is inherently risky, very little assurance can be take from this. If the controls over that assertion are strong, however, and the auditor verifies them to be effective, assurance may be taken from that, and a moderate amount of audit evidence is needed to achieve reasonable assurance that there is no material misstatement. But if the controls over this inherently risky assertion are also weak, or the auditor chooses not to verify the controls, a high level of assurance will have to come from audit evidence work to allow the auditor to have reasonable assurance that the financial statements are not materially misstated.

From a practical perspective, to audit a set of financial statements it is essential to understand the information system an organization uses to produce its financial statements. The information system is made up of business processes and the accounting processes related to them. Business processes are each organization's unique ways of coordinating work, information, and knowledge to achieve its strategic goals, such as producing value-added products or services. Most organizations will have key business processes for revenues (customer relations), purchasing (supply management), payroll (human resources), financing, and investing, and for manufacturing businesses there will also be a production process. These business processes each have an embedded accounting process to capture relevant financial information, which then flows through the accounting information system into management's financial statements. An accounting process can be thought of as a cycle because it records transaction information from the same business activity and runs through the same accounting process over and over, in a cycle. Auditors will usually organize their audit plan and staffing in line with the auditee's accounting processes, since this tends to be the most effective way to gain familiarity with the information system that produces the financial statements.

Review Checkpoints

6-1 What does the term *risk* mean?

6-2 Describe what is meant by saying that an audit under GAAS is risk based.

6-3 What do auditors achieve by assessing risk of material misstatement at the financial statement level?

6-4 What are management's responsibilities related to the risk of material misstatement in the financial statements?

6-5 What are business risks? What are management's main tools for managing business risks?

6-6 How are risks related to financial information and disclosure managed?

6-7 Why do auditors need to understand how management assesses risks?

6-8 What does the term *assertion* mean in financial statement auditing? What are the different aspects of financial statements that assertions relate to?

6-9 List five main assertions that can be used in practice, and give an example of each assertion for these accounts/transactions: Cash, Accounts Payable, Revenues.

6-10 How is it helpful to an auditor to apply the assertions to the classes of transactions, account balances, and disclosures in the financial statements? Discuss how assertions are useful in the risk assessment step (step i) and the response to assessed risk step (step ii) of the audit process.

6-11 What two types of risk factors create the risk of material misstatement? What is the auditor's responsibility related to the risk of material misstatement in the auditee's financial statements?

6-12 What does it mean to say that the auditor assesses risk of material misstatement at the assertion level?

6-13 How is the term *audit risk* defined in GAAS?

6-14 How does the concept of reasonable assurance relate to the concept of audit risk?

6-15 How does the level of audit risk an auditor accepts when giving an audit opinion relate to the ethical requirement to use due care?

6-16 What are the components of the audit risk model, and how are they defined?

6-17 Why would an auditor want to accept much lower audit risk on a particular audit compared to another? On what factors would this choice depend?

6-18 State the audit risk model formula, and explain the relations among the factors it includes.

6-19 What does it mean to say detection risk will be low? high? Give an example of an audit scenario where the acceptable detection risk would be high and one where it would be low.

6-20 What is the main use of the audit risk model for audit planning?

6-21 What are the sources of assurance available for an assertion? How do they relate to the audit risk model components?

6-22   What are accounting processes, and how do they relate to business processes?

6-23   Identify the main accounting processes typically found in a manufacturing business.

6-24   Why do auditors need an understanding of the auditee's accounting processes?

Business Risk and the Risk of Material Misstatement of the Financial Statements

LO1   Explain how the auditor's understanding of the business risks is used to assess the risk of material misstatement at the financial statement level.

The risk-based audit approach requires the auditor to understand the auditee's business risks and strategy and its related internal control: first, in order to assess the risks of material misstatement, and then to design and perform procedures that address the assessed risks. Understanding business risks and management's risk assessment processes allows auditors to learn about the risks the business faces, management's strategy for addressing those risks to meet organization goals, and the business processes management uses to implement the strategy. Analyzing business risk can help the auditor answer questions such as the following:

1.   What is the entity's strategy? How does it generate revenues and profits?

2.   Does the strategy appear to be successful now and for the future?

3.   What are the business risks/threats that can prevent the entity from achieving its strategic goals?

4.   What business processes, internal controls, and information systems does the entity management use to manage these risks?

5.   What risks can affect the financial statements?

Answers to these questions allow the auditor to identify significant risks that could result in material misstatements. In particular, the answer to question 4 requires an in-depth evaluation of the design and implementation of internal controls during the audit period—also known as assessing the **entity's risk assessment process**. Management must have a risk assessment process to deal with uncertainty and associated risks and opportunities, thereby allowing the organization to meet its goals. A useful guide to entity risk assessment is COSO's *Enterprise Risk Management—Integrated Framework*, which provides the following definition:

> Enterprise risk management is a process, effected by an entity's board of directors, management, and other personnel, applied in strategy setting and across the enterprise, designed to identify potential events that may affect the entity, and manage risk to be within its risk appetite, to provide reasonable assurance regarding the achievement of entity objectives.[1]

The auditor's first step is understanding the entity management's own process for identifying business risks affecting financial reporting objectives and for deciding on actions to minimize these risks. Organizations approach risk assessment in various ways, and understanding management's assessment process helps the auditor, in turn, to assess the risk that the financial statements could be materially misstated. In this text, the need for

entity's risk assessment process:
management's process for identifying business risks that could affect financial reporting objectives and for deciding on actions to address and minimize these risks; understanding this process helps auditors assess the risk that the financial statements could be materially misstated; see *management's risk assessment process*

the auditor to understand the auditee's business risks and strategy to assess the risk of material misstatement is called the *risk-based approach to auditing.*

In smaller businesses, where management may not have a formal risk assessment process, the auditor should discuss with management how risks to the business are identified and how they are addressed.

Business Processes

Management tries to minimize business risks by designing well-thought-out business processes. Business processes are a structured set of activities designed to produce a specific output that matches a business strategy. Examples are customer relations management in a consumer products distribution firm, or processing income tax returns in the Canada Revenue Agency's operations. If the business process produces value-added output according to the strategy, it is more likely that the business will achieve its objectives and not fall prey to the various risks. Business processes are the source of the transactions and events that need to be captured in the business's information system and its financial statements, so it is important for auditors to understand the business processes that create evidence that can support the validity and accuracy of the information that ends up in the financial statements.

Standards Check

CAS 315 Identifying and Assessing the Risks of Material Misstatement through Understanding the Entity and Its Environment

18. The auditor shall obtain an understanding of the information system, including the related business processes, relevant to financial reporting.

A84. An entity's business processes are the activities designed to
   - Develop, purchase, produce, sell, and distribute an entity's products and services;
   - Ensure compliance with laws and regulations; and
   - Record information, including accounting and financial reporting information.

Business processes result in the transactions that are recorded, processed, and reported by the information system. Obtaining an understanding of the entity's business processes, which include how transactions are originated, assists the auditor to obtain an understanding of the entity's information system relevant to financial reporting in a manner that is appropriate to the entity's circumstances.

Source: *CPA Canada Handbook—Assurance,* 2014.

The business process view of the firm has become an important perspective in management in recent years. Business processes work to create value for customers and thus achieve strategic objectives. Typically, they will cross boundaries between an organization's functional departments, such as sales, marketing, manufacturing, and research and development, and involve groups of employees from the different areas working together to complete the work. Exhibit 6–1 shows examples of some simplified business processes for an airline company and a manufacturing company, illustrating how the different functions combine to achieve the overall goal.

Business processes are each organization's unique ways of coordinating work, information, and knowledge to produce a value-added product or service. This business process–based management approach has been facilitated by the development of powerful information systems, called **enterprise resource planning systems (ERPs)**, that can integrate enterprise-wide resource and accounting information. These information systems

enterprise resource planning systems (ERPs):
information systems in which inputs and outputs from many or all the business processes are processed in an integrated manner, so the accounting component of the information system will be closely related to many other functional areas, such as sales, inventory, human resources, and cash management

EXHIBIT 6–1

Examples of Business Processes

A. BUSINESS PROCESSES IN A PASSENGER AIRLINE COMPANY

Market and sell services
1. Develop a marketing plan.
2. Form and continue alliances with other airlines.
3. Establish positive customer contact.

Provide transportation services
1. Acquire, maintain, and manage assets: airplanes, parts, hangars.
2. Manage safety and risk.

B. BUSINESS PROCESSES IN A MANUFACTURING COMPANY

Production Processes

Planning production
1. Schedule production.
2. Order materials.

Manufacturing product
1. Assemble product.
2. Test product.
3. Record costs of materials, labour, and overhead used.

Shipping product
1. Ship product ordered.
2. Record inventory used.

Order Fulfillment Processes

Process sales orders
1. Receive the order.
2. Enter the order.
3. Clear the order once shipped.

Account for the sale
1. Check and approve credit.
2. Generate invoice upon shipment.
3. Post sales journal entry.

can help organizations achieve efficiencies by automating parts of their business processes, but this still requires careful analysis and planning. The most important strategic decisions involve understanding what business processes need improvement and how information systems can improve them, not simply buying the latest information technology.

The business process view also highlights the fact that business organizations differ in terms of the kinds of activities they perform and the technology they use. Some organizations use mainly routine tasks that can easily be reduced to simple formal rules that require little judgment (e.g., inventory ordering in a grocery business). These types of tasks can easily be programmed, and these organizations are more likely to be run hierarchically. In contrast, organizations with activities that are non-routine and require judgment (e.g., an engineering firm designing specifications for office towers) would have complex functions in their operation and thus would be run less hierarchically.

Review Checkpoints

6-25 Explain the risk-based approach to the audit. What is its purpose?

6-26 What is the goal of business analysis?

6-27   How does understanding the business's strategy help the auditor to assess business risk?

6-28   What is a business process?

6-29   How do business processes relate to the financial statements?

6-30   Give an example of one business risk that affects the airline industry and one that affects a manufacturing business.

Effects of Information Technology on Business Risk

Changes in information technology affect business risks and processes in many organizations. As business information systems become more integrated and complex, the business processes change and new business risks are introduced that could affect the financial statements. Managers responsible for the entity's information technology, such as the chief information officer (CIO), are a useful source of the necessary knowledge. In industries significantly affected by information technology complexity, such as those involved in **e-commerce**, the business risks that can affect the financial statements may be greater.

To understand management's strategy and risk assessment processes for e-commerce, the auditor would consider factors such as the following:

- What are the sources of e-commerce revenue for the entity? Will the entity be acting as a principal or agent for goods or services sold?
- Has management identified e-commerce opportunities and risks in a documented strategy that is supported by appropriate controls, or is e-commerce subject to ad hoc development in response to opportunities and risks as they arise?
- Are the information technology (IT) skills and knowledge of entity personnel appropriate to establish and maintain information systems, including the security infrastructure and related controls, as it affects the financial reporting process? Information security issues arising from the firm's website can provide an access point for unauthorized hacking into the entity's financial and customer records. The security infrastructure and related controls need to be more extensive where the website is used for transacting with business partners and customers, or where systems are highly integrated.[2]

Summary

Understanding business risk and business processes helps the auditor to identify risk areas that may affect the amounts and relations among the numbers recorded in the accounting system and the financial statements. The process analysis may also suggest disclosures that should be present in the notes to the financial statements. Business risks and audit risk assessment are an important consideration in applying the audit risk model components (this will be discussed later in the chapter), in relation to developing the detailed audit plan, and in testing the internal controls.[3]

Review Checkpoints

6-31   How do an organization's business risks relate to its strategies and business processes?

6-32   How do complex IT and e-commerce affect the risks of financial statement misstatements?

6-33   What are the implications of a business using e-commerce on its business risk?

e-commerce:
any trade that takes place by electronic means

Applying an Understanding of the Business to a Critical Assessment of Management's Financial Statements

This section expands on how the auditor applies an understanding of the business, its environment, and risks, as well as management's process for managing those risks, in assessing the risk of material misstatement of the financial statements.

The auditor's concern is that the financial statements will not capture the underlying business reality fairly and in accordance with GAAP because errors or fraud have occurred. The auditor considers whether his or her analysis of business performance is consistent with the performance portrayed in the financial statements. The auditor should also consider how performance measures are used, both externally (e.g., key performance indicators reported to analysts, creditors, and shareholders) and internally (e.g., for personnel review and incentive programs). Performance measurements can place pressures on the business managers that increase the risk of their being motivated to deliberately misstate the financial statements, as illustrated by the audit guidance in the following box and further discussed in Chapter 7.

Potential Trouble Spots

Fraud is usually concealed, making it very challenging for an auditor to detect. Fraud by management, usually in the form of fraudulent financial reporting, is especially difficult for auditors to detect. When planning the audit, the auditor may notice certain events or conditions referred to as "fraud risk factors." These are events or conditions that suggest individuals in management may have had an incentive or have been pressured to commit fraud, have had a perceived opportunity to commit fraud, and have been able to rationalize committing a fraud.

These three factors are often referred to as the **fraud triangle** because fraud becomes very likely when all three are present. Some examples of risk factors often present in situations where frauds have occurred are as follows:

(a) *Incentives* arising from the availability of significant bonuses when profit targets are met, or pressures to meet earnings expectations or existing debt covenants to obtain additional debt financing;

(b) *Opportunities* provided by an ineffective control environment with poor access controls that can allow management override; and

(c) *Rationalization* of committing a fraud due to the individual's attitude, character, or particular set of ethical values (extreme pressures to report or conceal certain financial information can sometimes serve as the rationalization to commit fraud for people who are otherwise honest).

While fraud risk factors may not always lead to fraud, they should be considered in the auditor's assessment of the risks of material misstatement if they are present.

Source: Adapted from CAS 315 (paragraphs 25–27, A116) and CAS 240 (paragraphs 3, A1).

Financial Performance Analysis

Financial performance analysis extends the preliminary analytical procedures discussed in Chapter 5. It includes examining key sets of financial statement ratios (e.g., short-term liquidity ratios—see Appendix 5A for details), examining trends over time in those ratios, and considering the interrelationships among the ratios for consistency. Based on previous audit findings and the business risk assessment, the auditor forms expectations about what the financial analysis should discover.

Financial performance analysis includes a review of management's significant accounting policy choices and benchmarking those with significant industry competitors. Here, the auditor is attempting to gain an understanding of the degree of conservatism of management's accounting policy selection. In particular, the auditor considers the revenue recognition policy, as this has been a key area of abuse when apparently profitable companies suddenly fail.[4] See Exhibit 6–2 for examples. If the accounting policies vary significantly from industry

fraud triangle:
a model of the three factors that make fraud likely: incentive, opportunity, and rationalization (or similar concepts)

EXHIBIT 6–2

Accounting Gimmicks for Earnings Manipulation That Indicate Higher Risk of Material Misstatement of Financial Statements

- Recording revenue before it is earned
- Creating fictitious revenue
- Boosting profits with non-recurring transactions
- Shifting current expenses to a later period
- Failing to record or disclose liabilities
- Shifting current income to a later period
- Shifting future expenses to an earlier period

norms, the auditor can adjust the accounting policies to those normal to the industry and "reperform" the quantitative financial performance analysis to compare with industry benchmarks. This may suggest areas of additional audit work to reduce audit risk to an appropriately low level, or it may suggest that management should modify its accounting policies and practices.

Standards Check

CAS 240 The Auditor's Responsibilities Relating to Fraud in an Audit of Financial Statements

Unusual or Unexpected Relationships Identified

22. The auditor shall evaluate whether unusual or unexpected relationships that have been identified in performing analytical procedures, including those related to revenue accounts, may indicate risks of material misstatement due to fraud.

Source: *CPA Canada Handbook—Assurance*, 2014.

Part of the financial analysis in for-profit companies involves considering the quality of the earnings. **Quality of earnings** refers to the auditee's ability to replicate its earnings, both the amounts and the trends, over relatively long periods. Exhibit 6–3 lists factors indicative of high earnings quality. Indications of low-quality earnings may

EXHIBIT 6–3

High-Quality Earnings for Assessing Risk of Material Misstatement of Financial Statements

1. The following earnings management practices are not used by firms with high-quality earnings:
    (a) Using accounting accruals to smooth income increases over time
    (b) Structuring business transactions to ensure an outcome desired by management on accounting income for the period
    (c) Making management choices based primarily on short-term profitability
2. High-quality earnings have operating cash flows and income recognized close together over time.
3. Indicators of high-quality earnings include
    (a) Consistency of accounting accruals from year to year
    (b) Reduction of income through accounting policy changes
    (c) Short time lag between income recognition and the related cash being received by the business

quality of earnings:
the extent to which the reported earnings number represents actual economic performance, rather than selective accounting policy choices or management manipulation

result in the auditor's performing additional audit procedures to reduce risk to an appropriately low level or suggesting adjustments to management's financial statements.

Auditing standards require the auditor to communicate on a timely basis with the audit committee, or with those charged with governance for the financial reporting process, on matters that are significant qualitative aspects of the entity's accounting practices, including accounting policies, estimates, and disclosures.[5] This communication should consist of open and frank discussions among the auditor, audit committee, and management on all items that have a significant effect on the understandability, relevance, reliability, and comparability of the financial statements, including the following:

- Impact on earnings of implementing changes in accounting policies
- Effect of significant accounting policies in controversial or emerging areas or those unique to an industry
- Estimates, judgments, and uncertainties
- Existence of acceptable alternative policies and methods, the acceptability of the particular policy or method used by management, the financial statement amounts that are affected by the choice of principles, information concerning accounting principles used by peer group companies, and the auditor's views on whether management has chosen the most appropriate practice
- Unusual transactions
- Timing of transactions that affect the recognition of revenues or avoid recognition of expenses

The auditor must also ask management and those charged with governance about any known or suspected frauds affecting the auditee.[6] The auditor has an ongoing responsibility to communicate any suspicions or evidence of fraud to a level of management higher than the employees involved, or to those charged with governance if high-level managers are suspected.

Standards Check

CAS 260 Communication with Those Charged with Governance

Significant Findings from the Audit

16. The auditor shall communicate with those charged with governance (Ref: Para. A16)
   (a) The auditor's views about significant qualitative aspects of the entity's accounting practices, including accounting policies, accounting estimates, and financial statement disclosures. When applicable, the auditor shall explain to those charged with governance why the auditor considers a significant accounting practice, that is acceptable under the applicable financial reporting framework, not to be most appropriate to the particular circumstances of the entity; (Ref: Para. A17)
   (b) Significant difficulties, if any, encountered during the audit; (Ref: Para. A18)
   (c) Unless all of those charged with governance are involved in managing the entity,
      (i) Significant matters, if any, arising from the audit that were discussed, or subject to correspondence with management; and (Ref: Para. A19)
      (ii) Written representations the auditor is requesting; and
   (d) Other matters, if any, arising from the audit that in the auditor's professional judgment are significant to the oversight of the financial reporting process. (Ref: Para. A20)

Source: *CPA Canada Handbook—Assurance,* 2014.

Summary

The risk-based approach to auditing starts with a business risk analysis that provides an understanding of the auditee's business, its environment, and the risks it faces. The auditor considers the strategic goals of the business, the risks of not meeting those goals, and the process the entity's management uses to manage these risks. The auditor then examines the financial and non-financial performance of the entity to assess whether the

CAS 240 The Auditor's Responsibilities Relating to Fraud in an Audit of Financial Statements

41. Unless all of those charged with governance are involved in managing the entity, if the auditor has identified or suspects fraud involving (a) management, (b) employees who have significant roles in internal control, or (c) others where the fraud results in a material misstatement in the financial statements, the auditor shall communicate these matters to those charged with governance on a timely basis. If the auditor suspects fraud involving management, the auditor shall communicate these suspicions to those charged with governance and discuss with them the nature, timing, and extent of audit procedures necessary to complete the audit. (Ref: Para. A61–A63)

Source: *CPA Canada Handbook—Assurance,* 2014.

performance reported in management's financial statements is consistent with the auditor's understanding of the business risk and its performance. The business risk assessment can identify risks that can have a pervasive impact on the financial statements as a whole, such as those arising from fraud, management bias, manipulation of reported results, lack of management competence, or a deficiency in the overall control environment (discussed more in Chapter 7). Significant uncertainties about the company's ability to continue as a going concern may also be discovered during the auditor's business risk analysis. This business risk assessment is also the starting point for identifying the specific nature of misstatements that are most likely in the financial statements. Financial statement assertions are a very important auditing tool that auditors use for performing these more specific risk assessments. Assertions and their use in planning an audit are explained in the next section.

Review Checkpoints

6-34 What are some examples of external and internal business performance measures? How can these performance measures motivate management to misstate the financial statements?

6-35 What are some gimmicks that management can use to manipulate earnings?

6-36 What is earnings quality, and what are some indicators of high-quality earnings?

6-37 What are the auditor's communication responsibilities when he or she suspects or finds evidence of fraud? How do his or her responsibilities differ if the fraud involves low-level employees or high-level managers?

6-38 Why does an auditor review management's significant accounting policy choices and compare them with those of significant industry competitors?

Financial Statement Assertions and Audit Objectives

LO2 Identify the principal assertions in management's financial statements and the related risks of material misstatement.

Assertions in Financial Statements

This section explains the concept of the financial statement **assertions**. Assertions are the claims management makes in presenting its financial statements. The assertions are an essential concept in auditing, as they

assertions:
claims that management makes in financial statements that the auditor needs to verify or refute by obtaining relevant audit evidence

tie together the auditor's assessed risks of misstatements in the elements of the auditee's financial statements (transactions, account balances, and disclosures), and the auditor's objectives regarding the evidence needed to respond to the risks and obtain reasonable assurance about the fair presentation of the financial statements. Keep the following things in mind as you study this key concept:

- Management's accounting system produces a trial balance.
- Management arranges the trial balance and other information into financial statements and thereby makes certain assertions about how the financial statements represent the underlying economic data.
- Auditors use these assertions as focal points assessing specific risks of material misstatement.
- Auditors use the risk assessments at the assertion level to set **audit objectives** and design specific **evidence-gathering procedures** in response to these assessed risks.
- The practical audit objectives are to obtain and evaluate evidence about whether or not the assertions made by management in financial statements hold true.

To introduce the assertions concept, we will start with five principal assertions that, while broadly defined, are distinct and comprehensive conceptual descriptions of the claims in financial statement elements:

1. Existence (occurrence)
2. Completeness
3. Ownership (rights and obligations)
4. Valuation (measurement and allocation)
5. Presentation (classification and disclosure)

Exhibit 6–4 shows these assertions in relation to Inventory, one of the main accounts in a typical balance sheet. These five definitions cover all the claims and are a simple way to start learning about the usefulness of assertions. In practice, auditors may use more-detailed assertion definitions, such as those set out in CAS 315 (see Exhibit 6–6).

The five assertions will be described in more detail below in the context of audit objectives and procedures. For all assertions, the audit objective is to prove with evidence whether or not the assertion holds true.

Existence (Occurrence)

Management's claim is that the reported financial statement amounts are genuine, not fictitious. For revenue and expense transactions, the existence assertion is also described as *occurrence*, as the auditor requires evidence that transactions are valid and actually occurred. An account balance overstatement, for example, is an existence error. To obtain evidence about whether cash, inventory, receivables, and other assets actually exist, auditors will physically count cash and inventory, obtain written confirmation of receivables from the customers, and perform other validation procedures. Beginning students must be careful at this point, however, because finding evidence of existence alone generally proves little about the other four assertions.

audit objectives:
the auditor's goals in relation to obtaining audit evidence that verifies or refutes management's financial statement assertions

evidence-gathering procedures:
the activities auditors perform to obtain independent proof in relating the financial statements to the assertions in order to meet the audit objectives

EXHIBIT 6–4

Management Assertions about Inventory

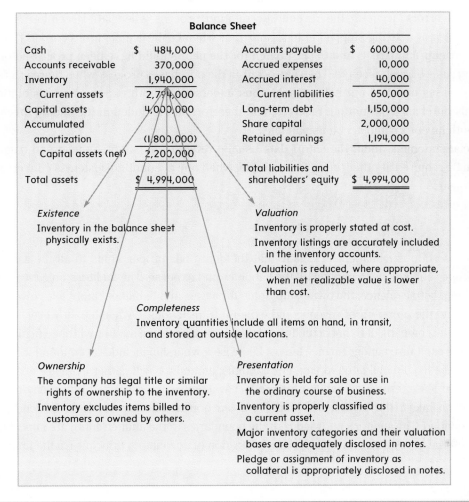

Balance Sheet

Cash	$ 484,000		Accounts payable	$ 600,000
Accounts receivable	370,000		Accrued expenses	10,000
Inventory	1,940,000		Accrued interest	40,000
Current assets	2,794,000		Current liabilities	650,000
Capital assets	4,000,000		Long-term debt	1,150,000
Accumulated			Share capital	2,000,000
amortization	(1,800,000)		Retained earnings	1,194,000
Capital assets (net)	2,200,000			
			Total liabilities and	
Total assets	$ 4,994,000		shareholders' equity	$ 4,994,000

Existence
Inventory in the balance sheet physically exists.

Valuation
Inventory is properly stated at cost.
Inventory listings are accurately included in the inventory accounts.
Valuation is reduced, where appropriate, when net realizable value is lower than cost.

Completeness
Inventory quantities include all items on hand, in transit, and stored at outside locations.

Ownership
The company has legal title or similar rights of ownership to the inventory.
Inventory excludes items billed to customers or owned by others.

Presentation
Inventory is held for sale or use in the ordinary course of business.
Inventory is properly classified as a current asset.
Major inventory categories and their valuation bases are adequately disclosed in notes.
Pledge or assignment of inventory as collateral is appropriately disclosed in notes.

Completeness

Management's claim is that all amounts that should be included in the financial statements have been included. A completeness error exists when a transaction total or account balance is understated; in other words, the accounting is not complete for a transaction that has really occurred. Thus, auditors gather evidence that inventory on hand is included, inventory consigned out is included, sales that occurred have been recorded, and so forth. Auditing this assertion means auditing what is not there, so it creates special difficulties for the auditor. Management's written representation that all transactions are included in the accounts is always obtained by the auditor, but this alone is not sufficient. Auditors also need to gather corroborating evidence, often from several sources.

Cutoff

Proper *cutoff* means accounting for all transactions that occurred during a period without postponing some recordings to the next period or accelerating next-period transactions into the current-year accounts. Cutoff errors result in accounts being overstated or understated and, therefore, relate to either the existence or the completeness assertion. Audit procedures to verify that the cutoff transactions are correctly accounted for provide essential evidence related to the existence and completeness assertions, and some auditors consider cutoff as a separate assertion of its own due to its importance.

Simple cutoff errors occur in the revenue accounting process when late-December sales invoices are recorded for goods not actually shipped until January, or when cash receipts are recorded through the end of the week (e.g., Friday, January 4) and the last batch for the year should have been processed on December 31, thus overstating sales or cash receipts. They can occur in the purchases process when there is a failure to record accruals for expenses incurred but not yet paid, thus understating both expenses and liabilities. A failure to record materials purchased but not yet received, and therefore not included in the ending inventory, results in understating both inventory and accounts payable.

In a financial statement audit, the cutoff date usually refers to the auditee's year-end balance sheet date; however, it can be required at other times, for example, when one accounting system is converted to a new system during the year.

Ownership (Rights and Obligations)

The ownership assertion is management's claim that the entity has proper rights to all the assets and revenues reported and proper obligations to pay out all the liabilities and expense. The auditor's objective related to *ownership* is establishing, with evidence, the ownership rights for assets and liabilities (more like "ower"-ship when they are obligations) and the propriety of revenue and expense transactions. Ownership, however, can include assets (rights) for which the company does not actually hold title. For example, an auditor will specifically gather evidence about the amounts capitalized under finance leases. Likewise, ownership includes accounting liabilities that a company may not yet be legally obligated to pay. For example, an auditor will gather evidence about the obligations under a capitalized lease, estimated liability for product warranties, or estimated future environmental cleanup costs. This assertion links to the fundamental "entity" concept you are familiar with from the conceptual framework of financial accounting. The auditor's knowledge of the boundaries of the auditee entity are important in setting the scope of the audit and in assessing the appropriate application of accounting principles in the financial statements.

Valuation (Measurement and Allocation)

The valuation assertion has several aspects to note. Management's claim for this assertion is that the dollar amounts recorded in the financial statements are correctly calculated and allocated, and the measurement bases used are appropriate in accordance with GAAP. Valuation can involve the measurement approach used (historic cost, fair value, present value) or the method of allocating joint costs. Auditors obtain evidence about specific dollar measurements by procedures such as reconciling bank accounts, comparing vendors' invoices to inventory prices, obtaining lower-of-cost-and-market data, and evaluating collectability of receivables. Many valuation and allocation decisions involve determining the proper application of GAAP.

Presentation (Classification and Disclosure)

Management's claim related to presentation is that the financial statements are presented fairly in accordance with GAAP. To verify this claim, auditors must determine whether accounting principles are properly selected and applied, whether financial information is presented in accordance with the underlying economic reality, whether disclosures are adequate, and whether any GAAP that apply have been followed—all aspects of financial statement *presentation*. Specific objectives of presentation include proper balance sheet classification (e.g., current versus long-term), proper income statement classification (e.g., cost of sales components, discontinued operations items, interest expenses, income taxes), and note disclosure of accounting policies and account details. The presentation assertion is the meeting place between accounting principles and audit reporting standards.

What Is the "Assessed Risk of Material Misstatement at the *Assertion* Level"?

You can think of the assertions as the claims that management is making to outside users in relation to each amount and disclosure in the *entity's general purpose financial statements*. Remember that management is responsible for creating a set of financial statements that tell a true and complete story about the entity's performance and financial position to outside users. If, taken all together, the assertions are all valid, then management's financial statements will likely be "fairly presented"; that is, they will exhibit the required qualities of relevance, completeness, reliability, neutrality, and understandability (CAS 210, Appendix 2) and contain all the disclosures necessary for a fair presentation financial reporting framework (CAS 700, paragraph 13), as discussed in Chapter 4.

In turn, an auditor's responsibility is to provide his or her independent opinion on whether management's financial statements are fairly presented. To achieve this objective, assertions are a very useful analytical tool that helps the auditor identify what types of evidence to get when performing the audit procedures. Assertions break down the claims that need to be proved into logical, focused pieces. This makes the job of planning audit procedures much more manageable because auditors can use the assertions to think specifically about what could go wrong and how likely it is that this could have happened. In the CAS terminology, when auditors think about these questions they are "assessing the risks of material misstatement at the assertion level" (CAS 315). When auditors identify the evidence they need to get to determine whether the assertions hold water, and perform procedures to get that evidence, these are their "responses to the assessed risks" (CAS 330). So you can see that assertions provide a key linkage throughout the audit process. It may be a bit challenging to understand them at first, but once you do it will give you a very strong basis for understanding the whole audit process!

Exhibit 6–4 indicates the specific assertions management is making for one major balance sheet account, Inventory. Exhibit 6–5 expands on this by giving a statement of each assertion for all the main financial statement amounts, plus an example of something that could go wrong for each assertion. It is important to note that

Standards Check

CAS 315 Identifying and Assessing the Risks of Material Misstatement through Understanding the Entity and Its Environment

25. The auditor shall identify and assess the risks of material misstatement at
    (a) The financial statement level; and (Ref: Para. A105– A108)
    (b) The assertion level for classes of transactions, account balances, and disclosures (Ref: Para. A109–A113), to provide a basis for designing and performing further audit procedures.
26. For this purpose, the auditor shall
    (a) Identify risks throughout the process of obtaining an understanding of the entity and its environment, including relevant controls that relate to the risks, and by considering the classes of transactions, account balances, and disclosures in the financial statements; (Ref: Para. A114–A115)
    (b) Assess the identified risks, and evaluate whether they relate more pervasively to the financial statements as a whole and potentially affect many assertions;
    (c) Relate the identified risks to what can go wrong at the assertion level, taking account of relevant controls that the auditor intends to test; and (Ref: Para. A116–A118)
    (d) Consider the likelihood of misstatement, including the possibility of multiple misstatements, and whether the potential misstatement is of a magnitude that could result in a material misstatement.

Source: *CPA Canada Handbook—Assurance*, 2014.

EXHIBIT 6–5

Assertions for Financial Statement Elements in Exhibit 6–4 plus Income Statement Elements, Related Audit Objectives, and Examples of Misstatements

Audit objective: to prove with evidence whether each assertion holds for the information in management's financial statements.

Example of what could go wrong to cause a misstatement for each assertion.

ACCOUNT	AMOUNT (IN CANADIAN DOLLARS)	EXISTENCE	COMPLETENESS	OWNERSHIP	VALUATION	PRESENTATION
Assets						
Cash	$ 484,000	**Audit objective:** There is real cash on hand and in bank accounts of this amount. **What could go wrong:** *The company has failed to record outstanding cheques.*	All the cash that exists is included in the balance. *The company has failed to record outstanding deposits.*	The company has the right to use all this cash. *Use of some of the cash balance is restricted due to the requirement of a bank loan.*	The cash value is calculated in Canadian dollars. *The cash is in U.S. dollars and has not been converted to Canadian dollars.*	The cash is appropriately presented as a current asset. *The net balance in the company's bank accounts is an overdraft (negative) and should be shown as a current liability.*
Accounts receivable	370,000	The amounts are actual debts owing to the company by its customers. *Amounts are still included that have already been paid by customers.*	All the invoices outstanding have been included. *Sales on account for the last day of the year were not recorded until the start of the following year (cutoff error).*	The company has the right to collect the cash for these amounts. *The company has already sold the receivables to a finance company for 75% of face value.*	The amount is the net realizable amount that is likely to be collected. *The company has not made any allowance for possible bad debts.*	The amounts are due to be collected in the current operating period. *Some amounts are not due for two years and should be included in long-term assets.*
Inventory	1,940,000	Inventory in the balance sheet physically exists. *Items of inventory that have already been sold and shipped to customers have not been removed from inventory records.*	Inventory quantities include all items on hand, in transit, and stored at outside locations. *Items of the company's inventory that are being stored offsite in a public warehouse have been omitted from the inventory records.*	The company has legal title or similar rights of ownership to the inventory. Inventory excludes items billed to customers or owned by others. *Items of inventory sold but not yet picked up by the customer have been included in the inventory balance.*	Inventory listings are accurately included in the inventory accounts. Inventory is properly valued at cost. Valuation is reduced where appropriate when net realizable value is lower than cost. *Selling prices for all items in inventory have dropped below cost but no write-down has been recorded.*	Inventory is held for sale or use in the ordinary course of business, properly classified as a current asset, and major categories and their valuation bases are adequately disclosed in notes. Pledge or assignment of inventory as collateral is appropriately disclosed. *The basis of valuation for inventory is not disclosed in the accounting policy note.*

(continued)

EXHIBIT 6-5

Assertions for Financial Statement Elements in Exhibit 6–4 plus Income Statement Elements, Related Audit Objectives, and Examples of Misstatements (*continued*)

ACCOUNT	AMOUNT (IN CANADIAN DOLLARS)	EXISTENCE	COMPLETENESS	OWNERSHIP	VALUATION	PRESENTATION
Capital assets (PPE* and intangibles)	4,000,000	PPE and intangibles included in the balance sheet physically or legally exist. *An old truck has been scrapped but its cost has not been removed from the accounts.*	All PPE and intangibles owned or under capitalized lease by the company are included in the account. *A new truck was purchased but the accountant forgot to record it in the PPE account.*	The company has legal title of ownership or similar ownership rights, or a capitalized lease for all recorded PPE and intangibles. *The company entered a sale and lease-back agreement during the year on a factory building that is still included in PPE, but the lease is an operating type.*	PPE and intangibles are properly valued at cost (or fair value) according to the company's accounting policy. A reasonable allowance for depreciation/ amortization is recorded. *The company did not record amortization on patents it owns that will expire in five years.*	PPE and intangibles are held for use in the ordinary course of business, properly classified as long-term assets, and major categories and their valuation bases are adequately disclosed in notes. Pledge or assignment of PPE for collateral is appropriately disclosed. *The detailed breakdown of the PPE and intangibles categories, cost and accumulated amortization, is not disclosed in the notes.*
Accumulated amortization (AA)	(1,800,000)	AA included in the balance sheet relates to existing PPE and intangibles. *An old truck has been scrapped but its AA has not been removed from the accounts.*	AA is recorded for all PPE and intangibles owned or under capitalized lease. *A new truck was purchased in the year but the accountant failed to record amortization on it for the year.*	AA included in the balance sheet relates to PPE and intangibles owned or properly capitalized by the company. *AA has been included that relates to a building now used under an operating lease.*	AA has been correctly calculated and recorded in accordance with the company's accounting policies. *The company used the wrong declining balance percentage to calculate depreciation on its trucks.*	AA is properly classified as a contra-asset; allocation methods for each major PPE and intangibles category are adequately disclosed in notes. *The amortization method for intangible assets is not disclosed in the notes.*
Liabilities and Equity						
Accounts payable	$ 600,000	All accounts payable included in the balance are existing obligations of the company to its suppliers. *A supplier's invoice that was accrued has been paid, but the amount was debited to office supplies rather than accounts payable.*	No actual obligations to suppliers have been omitted from the balance. *Goods are in transit to the company at year-end with FOB shipping point, but the supplier's invoice was not included in accounts payable.*	All obligations are actually owed by the company to its suppliers. *A supplier invoice was received that was actually for a different company, but it has been recorded in the accounts payable balance.*	Accounts payable are shown at the correct amounts that will ultimately be paid. *The company's accounting policy is to recognize any early payment discounts available at the time the invoice is accrued, but the accountant has not made the proper adjustments at year-end.*	The amounts are due to be paid in the current operating period. *Some amounts are not due for two years and should be included in long-term liabilities.*

(*continued*)

EXHIBIT 6–5

Assertions for Financial Statement Elements in Exhibit 6–4 plus Income Statement Elements, Related Audit Objectives, and Examples of Misstatements (*continued*)

ACCOUNT	AMOUNT (IN CANADIAN DOLLARS)	EXISTENCE	COMPLETENESS	OWNERSHIP	VALUATION	PRESENTATION
Accrued expenses	10,000	All accrued expenses are existing non–trade related obligations of the company. *The company accrued its outstanding utility bill twice in error.*	No actual non-trade obligations have been omitted from the balance. *The company failed to accrue for outstanding employee wages.*	All obligations are actually owed by the company to outside parties. *The company accrued a property insurance premium that is actually owed by the company's president personally.*	All accrued expenses are shown at the correct amounts that will ultimately be paid. *The company miscalculated its accrual for outstanding vacation pay.*	The amounts are due to be paid in the current operating period. *Some amounts are not due for two years and should be included in long-term liabilities.*
Accrued interest	40,000	All accrued interest exists and is related to real obligations of the company. *The company has accrued interest on a bank loan that was repaid early and not outstanding at year-end.*	No actual unpaid interest obligations have been omitted from the balance. *The company failed to accrue for interest outstanding on a new mortgage loan.*	All interest obligations are actually owed by the company to outside parties. *The company accrued mortgage interest that is actually owed by an employee.*	Accrued interest is correctly calculated. *The company miscalculated the number of days' interest accrued prior to year-end and accrued an incorrect amount.*	The amounts are properly presented as interest accruals, and details of interest terms are correctly disclosed. *The company failed to disclose the interest rates on its long-term liabilities.*
Long-term debt	40,000	All long-term debts are real obligations of the company. *The company has included a bank loan that was repaid early and no longer outstanding at year-end.*	No outstanding long-term obligations have been omitted from the balance. *The company failed to record a capitalized lease obligation.*	All long-term obligations are actually owed by the company to outside parties. *The company accrued mortgage interest that is actually owed by an employee.*	Accrued interest is correctly calculated. *The company miscalculated the number of days' interest accrued prior to year-end and accrued an incorrect amount.*	The amounts are properly presented as interest accruals, and details of interest terms are correctly disclosed. *The company failed to disclose the interest rates on its long-term liabilities.*
Share capital	2,000,000	All share capital recorded was properly issued and outstanding at year-end. *The company included subscription shares that were not issued until the following year.*	No outstanding paid-up share capital has been omitted. *The company issued new shares and forgot to record them.*	All shares issued properly represent legal ownership interests in the company. *The company repurchased and cancelled some shares but is still showing them as issued and outstanding.*	Shares are recorded at amounts received or by another appropriate valuation basis. *The fair value of property received in exchange for shares was calculated incorrectly.*	All shares issued are properly classified as equity, and details of amounts and numbers of shares issued for all share classes are properly disclosed in notes. *The detailed breakdown of the PPE and intangibles categories, cost and accumulated amortization, is not disclosed in the notes.*

(continued)

EXHIBIT 6-5

Assertions for Financial Statement Elements in Exhibit 6–4 plus Income Statement Elements, Related Audit Objectives, and Examples of Misstatements (*continued*)

ACCOUNT	AMOUNT (IN CANADIAN DOLLARS)	EXISTENCE	COMPLETENESS	OWNERSHIP	VALUATION	PRESENTATION
Retained earnings	1,194,000	Retained earnings includes only the net earnings retained in the company. *The company paid a dividend and recorded it as an expense rather than as a reduction of retained earnings.*	Retained earnings includes all the net earnings retained in the company. *The company has forgotten to close its current net income into the retained earnings account.*	The company has the right to distribute the amount in its retained earnings account. *The company declared a dividend prior to year-end and did not record a dividend payable or reduce retained earnings.*	Retained earnings is correctly calculated. *A debit to retained earnings that arose on repurchasing some shares at their fair value was incorrectly calculated.*	Retained earnings continuity is properly reported and all changes to retained earnings are adequately described. *The company recorded a large debit to retained earnings that is not described fully in the financial statements or explained in the notes.*
Revenues	1,000,000	All revenue recorded by the company actually occurred and is appropriate to recognize in the current year. *A sales contract was recognized in the current year, but the criteria for revenue recognition were not met until the following year.*	No revenues that should have been recognized in the year have been omitted. *A sale was completed just prior to year-end but was not recorded until the following year. (Note: This is a cutoff error.)*	The company has the right to receive benefits for all revenues recorded in the year. *The company sold consignment inventory on behalf of another company but recorded the entire sale amount instead of just the 5% commission it is entitled to.*	Revenues have been correctly calculated and allocated to the year in which they are earned. *Revenue recognition on a percentage-of-completion basis was calculated using the wrong percentage.*	Revenues are clearly presented in the financial statements, significant categories are shown separately, and revenue recognition accounting policies are adequately explained in the notes. *Revenue recognition policies are not disclosed in the notes.*
Cost of sales	650,000	All costs of sales recorded by the company are appropriate to recognize in the current year. *Cost of sales was overstated due to an understatement error in counting year-end inventory.*	No costs of sales that should have been recognized in the year have been omitted. *Cost of sales was understated due to an overstatement error in counting year-end inventory.*	All the costs of sales recorded in the year were related to generating the company's own sales revenues. *The company included an electricity bill of the next-door factory in its own costs of sales in error.*	Costs of sales have been correctly calculated and allocated to the year in which the related revenues are recognized. *Allocation of fixed overheads to ending inventory was calculated incorrectly.*	Costs of sales are presented appropriately in the financial statements, and significant accounting policies used are adequately explained in the notes. *Accounting policies related to the reported costs of sales are not disclosed in the notes.*
Other expenses	200,000	All other expenses recorded by the company are appropriate to recognize in the current year. *Other expense was overstated due to an over-accrual of management bonuses that were not earned in the year.*	No other expenses that should have been recognized in the year have been omitted. *Other expense was understated due to failure to accrue management bonuses earned in the year.*	All the other expenses recorded in the year were related to the company's own operating, financing, or investing activities. *The company included air fares expenses for employee vacation travel that are not proper expenses of the company.*	Other expenses have all been correctly calculated and allocated to the year to which they relate. *Compensation expense for employee stock options granted in the year was not correctly calculated.*	Other expenses are presented appropriately in the financial statements, and significant accounting policies used are adequately explained in the notes. *Accounting policies related to the reported other expenses were not disclosed in the notes.*

* PPE = property, plant, and equipment.

the exhibit gives just one example; there are usually other things that can go wrong. As you study this exhibit, you might try to think of other things that could go wrong as a good exercise to test your understanding of assertions at the conceptual level. (*Hint:* Try to think about what each account represents in terms of the real economic information it is supposed to communicate about the entity; then think about what management's accounting system is supposed to capture to present that information, and what might not have worked properly to result in a misstatement in the amount in relation to a particular assertion.)

Now that you have an understanding of the main concept of assertions as they relate to the criteria of fair presentation, our next step is to look at how assertions are further refined and focused in the Canadian Auditing Standards (CASs). For example, CAS 315, paragraph A111, defines the assertions in terms of the three main financial reporting categories: account balances, classes of transactions, and disclosures. These finer definitions make it easier for auditors to use the assertion concepts to consider potential misstatements in financial statement information and to design effective auditing procedures. The detailed assertions as set out in the CASs are shown in Exhibit 6–6, with cross-references to the five principal assertions.

Summary: Assertions and Planning the Audit

Financial statement assertions are the fundamental management claims to be audited and the focal points for all audit procedures. In an audit program, the evidence produced by each procedure relates to one or more specific objectives linked to specific assertions about the financial information being audited. If you have obtained a list of audit procedures (e.g., from last year's audit file), you can begin planning by asking the following questions:

- What are the specific assertions management is making by reporting this financial information?
- What are the risks of material misstatement in these assertions?
- Which assertion(s) does this audit procedure produce evidence about?
- Does the list of procedures (the audit program) address the risk of material misstatement in all the assertions?

Qualitative factors, cost of the procedure, risk level associated with each assertion, and materiality determine the extent to which a particular procedure is used.

You can simplify the five major assertions by thinking of them as existence, completeness, ownership, valuation, and presentation (E, C, O, V, P). Each of them has additional aspects, depending on the financial items you are auditing and the audit evidence available. How procedures are linked to assertions is an important topic in understanding audit evidence and the assurance it provides, and this topic is our starting point for developing the audit plan and detailed programs.

Review Checkpoints

6-39   Briefly explain the five principal assertions that can be made in management's financial statements, and then describe the auditors' objectives related to each.

6-40   How do financial statement assertions relate to audit procedures?

6-41   Why is it particularly challenging to obtain audit evidence about the completeness assertion?

6-42   Why should auditors think about what could go wrong in a particular assertion?

6-43   How are assertions used in audit planning?

EXHIBIT 6-6

How the Five Principal Assertions Link to the Detailed Assertion Descriptions Used in CAS 315 for Classes of Transactions, Account Balances, and Presentation and Disclosure

Assertion terms used in CAS 315 are defined at the transaction, account balance, and disclosure levels. Auditing standards require the auditor to assess risk of material misstatement assertion by assertion for the classes of transactions, account balances, and presentation/disclosure that make up the financial statements.

Below we show how these more-detailed definitions are linked to the five principal assertions we are using in the text. In planning and performing the audit, an auditor may use the assertions as described in the standards, or may express them differently, as long as all aspects described in the standards have been covered. Some auditors may prefer to combine assertions about transactions and events with those about account balances, or to cover proper cutoff of transactions and events under occurrence and completeness assertions rather than as a stand-alone assertion.

THE FIVE PRINCIPAL ASSERTIONS	LINKS TO DETAILED ASSERTIONS DESCRIBED IN CAS 315		
	(a) ASSERTIONS ABOUT CLASSES OF TRANSACTIONS AND EVENTS	(b) ASSERTIONS ABOUT BALANCE SHEET ITEMS	(c) ASSERTIONS ABOUT PRESENTATION AND DISCLOSURE
Existence (occurrence)	**(i) Occurrence** Transactions and events that have been recorded have occurred and pertain to the entity. **(iv) Cutoff** Transactions and events have been recorded in the correct accounting period (not too early).	**(i) Existence** Assets, liabilities, and equity interests exist.	**(i) Occurrence and rights and obligations** Disclosed events, transactions, and other matters have occurred and pertain to the entity.
Ownership (rights & obligations)		**(ii) Rights and obligations** The entity holds or controls the rights to assets, and liabilities are the obligations of the entity.	**(i) Occurrence and rights and obligations** Disclosed events, transactions, and other matters have occurred and pertain to the entity.
Completeness	**(ii) Completeness** All transactions and events that should have been recorded have been recorded. **(iv) Cutoff** Transactions and events have been recorded in the correct accounting period (not too late).	**(iii) Completeness** All assets, liabilities, and equity interests that should have been recorded have been recorded.	**(ii) Completeness** All disclosures that should have been included in the financial statements have been included.
Valuation	**(iii) Accuracy** Amounts and other data relating to recorded transactions and events have been recorded appropriately.	**(iv) Valuation and allocation** Assets, liabilities, and equity interests are included in the financial statements at appropriate amounts, and any resulting measurement or allocation adjustments are appropriately recorded.	**(iv) Accuracy and valuation** Financial and other information is disclosed fairly and at appropriate amounts.
Presentation	**(v) Classification** Transactions and events have been recorded in the proper accounts.		**(iii) Classification and understandability** Financial information is appropriately presented and described, and disclosures are clearly expressed.

Source: Adapted from CAS 315, paragraph A124.

The Audit Risk Model and Its Components

LO3 Describe the conceptual audit risk model and its components.

Auditing is fundamentally a risk management process. Audit risk is related to the information risk (discussed in Chapter 1) that audited financial statements that are materially misstated will go out to users. Assurance is the complement of audit risk—the higher the assurance, the lower the audit risk. Auditors strive to lower audit risk by performing audit work that gives a high level of assurance that the statements are fairly presented.

Understanding the auditee's business and performing preliminary analytical procedures help auditors to identify problem areas and make an overall business risk assessment. The organization's management is responsible for addressing business risk by implementing effective internal control. Thus, business risk and internal control are inseparable concepts that exist within an auditee organization. To develop the audit work programs, auditors need to assess inherent risk and control risk specifically in audit-related terms. In this section we will discuss the auditor's decision on what audit risk level needs to be achieved, the conceptual model that relates audit risk to the inherent and control risks of the auditee, and how this model can be used to determine the amount of assurance that needs to be obtained from performing audit detection procedures to lower the level of detection risk that the auditor is accepting. In auditing, the term *risk* should always be used with a modifier (business, engagement, audit, inherent, control, detection, and so on) to specify the one you mean.

Audit Risk: An Essential Audit Planning Decision

In an overall sense, audit risk is the probability that an auditor will fail to express a reservation of opinion on financial statements that are materially misstated. Let us start by reviewing and integrating some of the concepts we've already covered.

Chapter 5 explained how auditors must first consider the engagement's risks to decide whether or not to take it on. We saw that auditors may even take on a fairly high-risk engagement if they believe they can manage the risks down to a tolerable level. Earlier, we also saw that according the CAS 200, a financial statement auditor's overall objective is "to obtain reasonable assurance about whether the financial statements as a whole are free from material misstatement, whether due to fraud or error. . . ."[7] CAS 200 also notes that the term *reasonable assurance* should be taken to mean a high level of assurance.

Standards Check

CAS 200 Overall Objectives of the Independent Auditor and the Conduct of an Audit in Accordance with CASs

5. Reasonable assurance is a high level of assurance. It is obtained when the auditor has obtained sufficient appropriate audit evidence to reduce audit risk (that is, the risk that the auditor expresses an inappropriate opinion when the financial statements are materially misstated) to an acceptably low level.

Source: *CPA Canada Handbook—Assurance*, 2014.

Taking all these ideas together, we see that to provide high enough assurance to support an audit opinion, the auditor needs to manage the audit risk down to a level low enough to offset the engagement's risks. To illustrate the relations between these risks, Exhibit 6–7 sets out the possibilities to consider.

The logic of Exhibit 6–7 is that as the likelihood of negative consequences for the auditor's practice gets larger, the auditor can take less chance of missing a material misstatement and so must plan to achieve a lower

Relating Engagement and Audit Risks

AUDITOR'S ASSESSMENT OF RISK FROM ACCEPTING ENGAGEMENT	AUDIT RISK THAT CAN BE ACCEPTED	AUDITOR DECISION
Extremely high	Extremely low level, near zero	It is probably impossible to achieve a near-zero risk, so do not accept the engagement.
High	Lowest	Accept engagement only if the auditor can achieve a very low audit risk by performing extensive auditing work.
Moderate	Moderate	Accept engagement, plan to achieve a moderate audit risk level, and perform a less extensive level of audit work.
Low	Highest	Accept audit, plan to achieve a somewhat higher audit risk, and perform a relatively lower level of audit work.

audit risk. Since achieving a lower audit risk involves more audit effort than does achieving a higher audit risk, it costs more. Therefore, an auditor's decision on what audit risk level to accept comes down to a cost-benefit analysis. Audit risk can at best be controlled at a low level but not eliminated, even when audits are well planned and carefully performed. The risk of audit failure is much greater in poorly planned and carelessly performed audits. Planned audit risk varies according to engagement circumstances. Generally, the more risky the auditee or the more users rely on the audited financial statements, the lower is the planned audit risk. As the risk of being sued for material misstatement increases, an auditor will decrease planned audit risk to compensate for the increased risk associated with the engagement. Many auditing firms have developed internal guidelines for setting planned levels of audit risk.

The auditing profession has no hard standard for an acceptable level of audit risk, except that it should be "appropriately low" and involve the exercise of professional judgment. At one time, the Canadian auditing guidance suggested that most auditors should strive to limit such risks to no more than 5%. However, auditors would be appalled to think that even 1% of their audits would be bad. For a large auditing firm with 2,000 audits per year, accepting 5% audit risk makes it look as though the firm will have 100 failed audits every year! But that would only be the case if every auditee had financial statements that were materially misstated, and not all do. So, even with using 5% planned audit risk on every engagement, it is likely there will be audit failures much less than 5% of the time. As an example, if we assumed there is a material misstatement in 6% of a firm's audit engagements, then, with 5% audit risk, of the 2,000 audits performed per year, there might be 6 failed audits—a lot less than 100.

The concept of audit risk also applies to individual account balances, transactions, and disclosures. Here, the risk is that material misstatement is not discovered in an account balance (e.g., the inventory total), a transaction stream (e.g., total revenues), or a disclosure (e.g., pension liability). Audit risk is often used in practice with regard to individual balances and disclosures. In summary, audit risk is the same whether applied to financial statements as a whole or to individual accounts. Thus, for example, if audit risk is set at 5%, this level is used for all accounts as well as for financial statements as a whole.

The Audit Risk Model

Why do auditors care about what audit risk level is acceptable? Intuitively, audit risk is the probability that the audit fails to detect a material misstatement. Starting with a target level of acceptable audit risk allows auditors to plan their evidence-gathering work by taking into account various audit-related risks in a systematic way.

CAS 200 Overall Objectives of the Independent Auditor and the Conduct of an Audit in Accordance with CASs

Audit Risk

A32.   Audit risk is a function of the risks of material misstatement and detection risk. The assessment of risks is based on audit procedures to obtain information necessary for that purpose and evidence obtained throughout the audit. The assessment of risks is a matter of professional judgment, rather than a matter capable of precise measurement.

A33.   For purposes of the CASs, audit risk does not include the risk that the auditor might express an opinion that the financial statements are materially misstated when they are not. This risk is ordinarily insignificant. Further, audit risk is a technical term related to the process of auditing; it does not refer to the auditor's business risks, such as loss from litigation, adverse publicity, or other events arising in connection with the audit of financial statements.

Source: *CPA Canada Handbook—Assurance*, 2014.

To aid in planning the audit, the main risk elements can be expressed conceptually by developing a simple model that assumes the elements of audit risk are independent. Thus, the risk elements are related as follows:

$$\text{Audit risk (AR)} = \text{Risk of material misstatement (RMM)} \times \text{Detection risk (DR)}$$

We can make the model more precise by noting that the risk of material misstatement will occur when (1) there is a material misstatement to start with (inherent risk), (2) the internal controls fail to detect and correct the material misstatement (control risk), and (3) the audit procedures also fail to detect the material misstatement (detection risk). The audit fails only if all three events occur. So, in expanded form, the audit risk model is

$$\text{Audit risk (AR)} = \text{Inherent risk (IR)} \times \text{Control risk (CR)} \times \text{Detection risk (DR)}$$

Audit risk is, thus, the probability that the audit fails. The probability of audit success is one minus the probability that it fails; therefore, audit assurance equals one minus audit risk. Thus, reducing acceptable (or planned) audit risk, say from 5% to 1%, is equal to increasing acceptable (or planned) audit assurance from 95% to 99% in this example.

In their work, auditors want to hold the audit risk to a relatively low level (e.g., 0.05, or an average of 5% of audit decisions when there is a material misstatement will be wrong). The auditor first decides what audit risk level must be achieved and then uses the audit risk model to plan the audit work effort required. The auditor accomplishes this by first assessing the levels of inherent risk and control risk that exist in the auditee organization and then solving for the level of detection risk that needs to be achieved to reduce audit risk to the acceptably low level. Rearranging the model to solve for detection risk results in the following:

$$\text{Detection risk (DR)} = \frac{\text{Audit risk (AR)}}{\text{Inherent risk (IR)} \times \text{Control risk (CR)}}$$

In summary, audit risk is a quality criterion based on professional judgment; it is the auditor's choice. In contrast, the other risk assessments are estimates based on professional judgment and evidence, as discussed next.

Review Checkpoints

6-44   What are the four risks included in the audit risk model? How are they related?

6-45   What factors influence the auditor's decision on an acceptable audit risk level?

Inherent Risk

Inherent risk is the probability that material misstatements affecting one or more assertions could have occurred in transactions within the accounting system used to develop financial statements, or in an account balance.[8] Put another way, inherent risk is the risk of material misstatement occurring in the first place. Auditors do not create or affect inherent risk; they can only try to assess its magnitude. It is a characteristic of the auditee's business, the major types of transactions, and the effectiveness of its accountants, so understanding the auditee's business risk is important for assessing inherent risks. It is important to understand that audit care should be greater where inherent risk is greater.

An assessment of inherent risk can be based on a variety of information. If material misstatements were discovered during the last year's audit, inherent risk will be considered higher than it would be if last year's audit had no material misstatements. Auditors may believe that the organization's accounting clerks tend to misunderstand GAAP and the organization's own accounting policies, thus suggesting a significant probability of mistakes in transaction processing. The nature of the auditee's business may produce complicated transactions and calculations known to be susceptible to accounting treatment error (e.g., real estate, franchising, oil and gas transactions). Some kinds of inventories (e.g., coal, grain, cocoa) may be harder to count, value, and keep accurately in perpetual records than are others (e.g., cars, jewellery). Some accounts (e.g., cash and inventory) are more susceptible to embezzlement, theft, or other losses than are other accounts (e.g., land and prepaid expenses). Changes in the economic environment can affect the risk of material misstatement, so auditors should take these changes into account in their risk assessments and audit planning.

Revenue accounting can have high inherent risk. Exhibit 6–8 shows the main results of a survey of 586 businesses that finds revenue recognition is the process most vulnerable to material errors; this is because of the complexity of revenue accounting. Businesses often use information from many sources and compile the revenue numbers in spreadsheets, rather than by an automated system, which increases the inherent risk of material errors and inaccuracies.

EXHIBIT 6–8

Revenue Reporting Risk

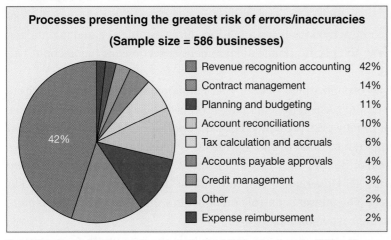

Processes presenting the greatest risk of errors/inaccuracies

(Sample size = 586 businesses)

Revenue recognition accounting	42%
Contract management	14%
Planning and budgeting	11%
Account reconciliations	10%
Tax calculation and accruals	6%
Accounts payable approvals	4%
Credit management	3%
Other	2%
Expense reimbursement	2%

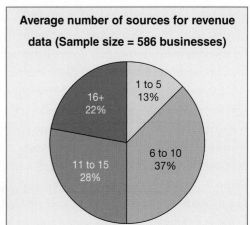

Average number of sources for revenue data (Sample size = 586 businesses)

1 to 5 13%
6 to 10 37%
11 to 15 28%
16+ 22%

Source: Gerry Murray, "Revenue reporting risk remains high," *CA Magazine*, December 2008, p. 10.

---

inherent risk:
the probability that material misstatements could have occurred

Auditor experience has also shown that because of management optimism and bias, asset and revenue accounts tend to have a higher inherent risk of overstatement than understatement, while liability accounts have a higher inherent risk of understatement than overstatement. Because of this, auditors tend to use procedures that are more effective in detecting overstatements for auditing revenues and assets. At the same time, audit procedures that are more effective in detecting understatements are more likely to be used with liability and expense accounts. Thus, the inherent risks determine the importance of various procedures for different accounts.

A summary of some of the key factors that go into the inherent risk assessment are listed below. Consider business factors and events that could lead to a material misstatement in the financial statements:

- Accounting policies requiring complex calculations, valuation estimates, and judgment
- Accounting staff competency, experience
- Assets that are susceptible to theft
- Business involving complicated transactions, assets, or liabilities
- Business subject to complex or changing laws or regulations, including foreign laws
- Changes in technology that can affect operations, product obsolescence
- Complex contracts with customers or suppliers
- Economic conditions that affect business negatively
- Knowledge of actual or suspected or alleged fraud affecting the entity
- Incentives that may induce management to manipulate accounting information
- Management integrity (willingness to override controls)
- Material misstatements of past years, and how they were handled
- Operations in multiple locations
- Organizational changes, especially in accounting personnel and systems
- Other relevant risk factors

Control Risk

Control risk is the probability that the auditee's internal control policies and procedures will fail to detect or prevent material misstatements. Auditors do not create or affect the control risk. They can only evaluate an organization's control system and assess the probability of material misstatements. Auditors are mainly concerned with "internal control relevant to the audit"—those policies and procedures established and maintained by management that affect control risk relating to specific financial statement assertions at the account balance, class of transactions, or disclosure level.

Internal control is a key component of an organization's overall risk management framework. Auditors use the risk management frameworks for assessing risks at the company level, as well as for auditing controls over financial reporting. The risk and control frameworks presented here are the *Internal Control—Integrated Framework* of the Committee of Sponsoring Organizations of the Treadway Commission (COSO); *Guidance on Control* from CPA Canada's Criteria of Control Board (CoCo); and *Control Objectives for Information and Related Technology* (COBIT), published by the IT Governance Institute. These frameworks are all further described in Appendix 7A, available on Connect. The internal control components will be discussed in Chapters 7 and 9. Frameworks are a useful tool to help improve audit quality.[9]

The control frameworks define control broadly. The CoCo framework includes an organization's resources, systems, processes, culture, structure, and tasks that work together to support the organization's objectives.

control risk:
the risk that the client's internal controls will not prevent or detect a material misstatement

Effective management, therefore, needs an integrated structure of control processes—processes for strategic control, management control, and business process control. Strategic and management control processes encompass controls for that entity as a whole. These controls often rely on long-term and strategically relevant criteria to evaluate overall corporate performance at the division or unit level by management. Business process controls operate at the specific process level.

Thus, management control systems are much broader than are "internal controls relevant to the audit." Internal controls relevant to the audit are a subset of this broader view of controls. Auditors are mainly concerned with accounting controls and systems. There are many other controls present in organizations that may not be relevant to the auditor.

Preliminary control effectiveness conclusions and risk assessments are made for audit planning purposes. An auditor's assessment of control risk is based on the study and evaluation of the company's control system. Auditors often carry preconceived notions about control risk when they audit the same organization year after year. Starting with knowledge of last year's conclusions on control risk assessment is known as **anchoring**, and it represents (1) a useful continuity with the auditee, but also (2) a potential pitfall if conditions worsen and the auditor fails to acknowledge the deterioration of control.

Note that control risk assessment provides only an indirect assessment of the monetary amount of misstatement of financial statements. As a result, special labels, such as **control testing (compliance testing)**, are given to the procedures used in the control risk assessment.[10] Control risk should not be assessed so low that auditors place complete reliance on controls and do not perform any other audit work. Many auditors conclude their control risk assessment decisions with descriptive assessments (e.g., high, moderate, low), and some auditors put probability numbers on them (e.g., 1.0, 0.50, 0.30).

Combined Inherent and Control Risk: The Risk of Material Misstatement

As discussed above, inherent risk and control risk are different in nature but related, so auditors can combine their assessment of these two risks into what is called the **risk of material misstatement**. The standards emphasize understanding an auditee's business and assessing the risk of material misstatement in planning the audit.

Inherent and control risks can be difficult to assess separately because some internal controls "work" only when errors, irregularities, and other misstatements occur, while others are preventive in nature and so tend to reduce inherent risk. An auditor may make separate or combined assessments of inherent and control risk, depending on preferred audit procedures and practical considerations.

The risks of material misstatement at the financial statement and assertion levels are a basis for designing further audit procedures. When the auditor's assessment of the risk of material misstatement includes an expectation of the operating effectiveness of controls, the standards state that there must be supporting tests of those controls. Internal control is a complex and critical consideration in every audit.[11]

anchoring:
preconceived notions about control risk that auditors carry over when they perform an audit on a client year after year, a potential pitfall if conditions have changed

control testing (compliance testing):
performing procedures to assess whether controls are operating effectively

risk of material misstatement:
the auditor's assessment of the probability that the financial statements are materially misstated prior to being audited; assessed at the level of the financial statements overall, based on pervasive factors such as fraud, going concern, or other significant business-level risks, to develop the overall audit strategy; and also assessed as the combined inherent and control risk at the assertion level for developing a detailed audit plan and specific procedures

Standards Check

CAS 200 Overall Objectives of the Independent Auditor and the Conduct of an Audit in Accordance with CASs

13(n).   Risk of material misstatement—The risk that the financial statements are materially misstated prior to audit. This consists of two components, described as follows at the assertion level.

(i) Inherent risk—The susceptibility of an assertion about a class of transaction, account balance, or disclosure to a misstatement that could be material, either individually or when aggregated with other misstatements, before consideration of any related controls.

(ii) Control risk—The risk that a misstatement that could occur in an assertion about a class of transaction, account balance, or disclosure and that could be material, either individually or when aggregated with other misstatements, will not be prevented, or detected and corrected, on a timely basis by the entity's internal control.

A40.   The CASs do not ordinarily refer to inherent risk and control risk separately, but rather to a combined assessment of the "risks of material misstatement." However, the auditor may make separate or combined assessments of inherent and control risk depending on preferred audit techniques or methodologies and practical considerations. The assessment of the risks of material misstatement may be expressed in quantitative terms, such as in percentages, or in non-quantitative terms. In any case, the need for the auditor to make appropriate risk assessments is more important than the different approaches by which they may be made.

Source: *CPA Canada Handbook—Assurance*, 2014.

Detection Risk

Detection risk is the risk that any material misstatement that has not been prevented or corrected by the auditee's internal control will not be detected by the auditor. In contrast to the inherent and control risks, it is the auditor's responsibility to reduce detection risk to an acceptably low level by performing evidence-gathering procedures. These **substantive audit procedures** are the auditors' opportunity to detect material misstatements that can cause financial statements to be misleading. Substantive procedures provide a *direct* assessment of the monetary amount of misstatement in the auditee's proposed accounting. In this way, they differ from control testing procedures, which only provide *indirect* evidence about whether material misstatement might have arisen due to control deficiencies. As a result, substantive procedures are highly effective in detecting material misstatements and are therefore considered the most important audit procedures. Thus, at least some substantive procedures must be performed in every audit to comply with the CASs. The two categories of substantive procedures are (1) tests of the details of transactions, balances, and disclosures and (2) analytical procedures applied to produce circumstantial evidence about specific monetary amounts in the accounts. Detection risk is the probability that these substantive procedures will fail to detect material misstatements.

At this point, it may be helpful to use an analogy to compare the auditor's risk assessment to something you are probably more familiar with, like a hockey game, as set out in the following box.

detection risk:
the risk that the auditor's procedures will fail to find a material misstatement that exists in the accounts

substantive audit procedures:
designed to detect material misstatements at the assertion level; comprising tests of details (classes of transactions, account balances, and disclosures) and substantive analytical procedures

Standards Check

CAS 330 The Auditor's Responses to Assessed Risks

18.   Irrespective of the assessed risks of material misstatement, the auditor shall design and perform substantive procedures for each material class of transactions, account balance, and disclosure. (Ref: Para. A42–A47)

Source: *CPA Canada Handbook–Assurance,* 2014.

The Risk of Material Misstatement—They Shoot! They Score!

Think of a "material misstatement" in audited financial statements as the unfortunate event of the opposing team getting the puck into a hockey team's net. The "risk of material misstatement" is the probability of the opposing team's getting a shot on the defending team's net. The "inherent risk" of this happening depends on the skill, effort, and luck of the opposing team's players in shooting the puck toward the net. The defending team cannot affect this inherent risk—it can only try to prevent it. The team's defence provides the "internal control," skating backwards furiously and swinging their sticks to prevent the puck from getting through to the net. The "control risk" is the probability that the defence will fail to stop the puck getting through. If they fail, the goalie is there to detect the incoming puck and stop it. The risk of the goalie's failing to stop the puck after it gets through the defence is like the "detection risk," and if the goalie works effectively this risk is reduced. To be successful, the team needs a goalie that can lower the risk of the puck's getting into the net. The goalie in this analogy is like the auditor, the final line of defence to detect the incoming "puck"—material misstatement—and stop it. If the puck gets past the goalie, the analogy to financial statement auditing is that audited statements go out containing a material misstatement, which is referred to as "audit risk."

Bringing the analogy back to the audit context, we see that audit risk is realized when a material misstatement exists (inherent risk), controls fail to stop it (control risk), and the auditor's work fails to discover it (detection risk). Note that this illustration is based on an objective fact—a goal, or a misstatement—but accounting standards can involve subjectivity due to the need to make estimates based on expectations of future events. Note also that in this analogy the opposing team is deliberately trying to score, but in reality the auditor is concerned about both unintentional and intentional misstatements.

Review Checkpoints

6-46   Give an example of one account with high inherent risk and one with low inherent risk.

6-47   What is the purpose of a control framework?

6-48   Identify two control frameworks that can help in the auditor's preliminary control risk assessment.

6-49   How are auditors' judgments about the quality or effectiveness of internal control affected by anchoring?

6-50   In the hockey game analogy used to explain the audit risk factors, whom do the hockey team's fans represent?

Working with the Audit Risk Model

LO4   Explain the usefulness and limitations of the audit risk model in conducting the audit.

This section works through various examples, using hypothetical numerical values, to illustrate how the relations in the audit risk model work.

First, it is instructive to look at the audit risk model dynamically, by comparing its values at the start of an audit, before any work is done, to its values at the end of an audit, where the auditor has determined that a clean opinion can be given on the financial statements.

Before the audit starts, detection risk is 100% (DR = 1.0), since nothing has been done yet about reducing the risk of not detecting material misstatements. Similarly, the auditor must assume control risk is 1.0 since there is no evidence yet about whether controls are effective enough to reduce the risk of misstatement. The auditor will have done some preliminary risk assessment and may have enough knowledge to assess inherent risk at less than 100%, and let's assume for the illustration it is about 0.50. At this point, then, audit risk essentially equals the inherent risk of a material misstatement being in the financial statements in the first place:

$$AR = IR \times CR \times DR$$

$$AR = 0.50 \times 1.0 \times 1.0 = 0.50 \text{ or } 50\%$$

Clearly, 50% is way too much risk for an auditor to give a clean opinion on the financial statements! The whole objective of the audit is to get this risk down to an acceptably low level as judged by the auditor based on the risks in the engagement. For this illustration, say the auditor wanted the audit risk to be no higher than 0.05. How is that achieved? Well, the auditor will have to do some work! First, the auditor may decide to test the effectiveness of controls to establish evidence that control risk is less than 1.0; say, this work results in an assessed control risk of 0.20. Where are we now? Recalculating the risk model shows that at this point the audit risk achieved is

$$AR = 0.50 \times 0.20 \times 1.0 = 0.10$$

This is still higher than the auditor's goal of AR = 0.05, and now the auditor has to do some substantive work that can detect any material misstatement in the accounts. Using the hypothetical values in the illustration, we can calculate that the auditor needs to do enough detection work to reduce detection risk from 1.0 to a level that leaves only a 5% risk of giving the wrong audit opinion. Note how the audit risk model can be used to plan the required extent of audit work by rearranging it to solve for detection risk:

$$DR = \frac{AR}{IR \times CR}$$

$$= \frac{0.05}{0.50 \times 0.20} = 0.50$$

Conceptually, the model indicates that as long as the auditor feels substantive evidence-gathering procedures have at least a 50% chance of detecting material misstatement, the required audit risk level of 0.05 is achieved—the auditor will be taking only a 5% chance of giving a clean opinion on statements that are materially misstated.

As another illustration at the account level, assume that in another audit the auditor thought the inventory balance had a high inherent risk of material misstatement (say, IR = 0.90) and that the auditee's internal control was only somewhat effective—say, CR = 0.70. If the auditor wanted audit risk at a 5% level (AR = 0.05), planned audit procedures would need to achieve detection risk that did not exceed 0.08 (approximately). In other words, the model indicates that the auditor in this case can only afford to take an 8% chance of missing a misstatement:

$$AR = IR \times CR \times DR$$

$$DR = \frac{AR}{IR \times CR}$$

$$= \frac{0.05}{0.90 \times 0.70} = 0.08$$

In a different audit, say, the auditor has assessed inherent risk to be very low for accounts receivable—for example, IR = 0.20—and, further, has tested the internal controls and found them to be very effective, so control risk is also very low—say, CR = 0.20. Say this auditee is a high-profile public company, so the auditor wants to achieve a very low audit risk of 0.01. Solving for DR in this case yields

$$DR = \frac{AR}{IR \times CR}$$

$$= \frac{0.01}{0.20 \times 0.20} = 0.25$$

These are hypothetical illustrations only. In practice, it is difficult to know if the audit has been planned and performed well enough to hold the detection risk as low as 8%, or 25%, or 50%. Despite its simplicity, the audit risk model is only a conceptual tool, but it is helpful for planning audits. Intuitively, to be 92% confident (1.00 – 0.08) of finding any material misstatement in the inventory seems to require gathering more persuasive evidence than to be only, say, 80% confident. Auditors have few ways to calculate detection risk, however, and this model is more a way to think about audit risks than a way to calculate them. However, some auditors use this model in practice to calculate risks and the related extent of audit testing (sample size). Chapter 10 gives more details on the audit risk model as applied to audit sampling.

The model produces some insights, including these:

1. Auditors cannot rely on an estimate of zero inherent risk without other evidence-gathering procedures, which would appear as follows:

$$AR = IR \ (= 0) \times CR \times DR = 0$$

2. Auditors cannot rely only on internal control, which would appear as follows:

$$AR = IR \times CR \ (= 0) \times DR = 0$$

3. Audits would not be exhibiting due audit care if the risk of failure to detect material misstatements were too high; for example,

$$AR = IR \ (= 0.80) \times CR \ (= 0.80) \times DR \ (= 0.50) = 0.32$$

4. Auditors could rely almost exclusively on evidence produced by substantive procedures, even if they think inherent risk and control risk are high. For example (provided AR = 0.05 is acceptable):

$$AR = IR \ (= 1.00) \times CR \ (= 1.00) \times DR \ (= 0.05) = 0.05$$

Even though the conceptual audit risk model appears to be precise when presented this way, in reality, applying it is difficult and highly subjective. However, it can help auditors decide whether they have obtained sufficient appropriate audit evidence. The objective in an audit is to limit audit risk to a low level, as judged by the auditor. This is done by assessing inherent risk and control risk along a spectrum; often auditors will use two or three broad levels: high, moderate, or low risk. The greater the inherent and control risks are, the lower the detection risk needs to be, resulting in more audit procedures (more in number, effectiveness, and extent). The objective is to limit audit risk to an appropriately low level, thereby achieving reasonably high assurance that the financial statements are free of material misstatement.

To integrate some of these concepts, recall that assurance is the complement of risk. To consider a numerical example, if audit risk of 5% were achieved, then the assurance obtained would be 95%. Put another way, the auditor would be 95% sure that the financial statements do not contain a material misstatement. Essentially, the auditor has obtained this assurance from the three factors in the audit risk model. The sources of assurance are the inherent nature of the item, the control exercised over the item, and the results of the various substantive detection procedures performed. Remember, too, that the audit risk model articulates with the concept of materiality and that materiality is involved throughout the risk assessment process, as further explained in the next section.

How Materiality and Audit Risk Are Related

Materiality refers to the magnitude of a misstatement, while audit risk refers to the level of assurance that material misstatement does not exist in the financial statements. The materiality decision is based on how misstatements will affect financial statement users. Understanding the business and its environment helps the auditor identify financial statement users and assess what is significant to their decisions. For example, the shareholders of a medium-size private company may rely on the audited income number to calculate managers' bonuses. A smaller misstatement might affect them more than would be the case in a large public company where a user's decision is less directly related to the audited income figure. An auditor decides on the materiality level independent of audit risk considerations.

Acceptable audit risk is determined by how much assurance the auditor requires. For example, say venture capital investors are basing their financing decisions on the audited information; if the audit fails to uncover a material misstatement, these investors will lose money and there is a high risk they will sue the auditor, so high assurance is required. High-profile companies such as banks require high assurance, as audit failure affects many people and generates a lot of bad news coverage, seriously damaging an auditor's reputation. As audit risk is the complement of audit assurance, requiring a high level of assurance means setting audit risk low. The auditor is only willing to accept a small risk of missing a material misstatement.

Audit risk and materiality thus both deal with the sufficiency of evidence. If the audit risk is set lower, or materiality is set smaller, the evidence required will increase. Both audit risk and materiality levels will be planned early in the engagement. These planned levels are used throughout the audit for financial statements as a whole, as well as for individual accounts, unless situations discovered during performance of the audit indicate they should be adjusted. Inherent risk, control risk, and detection risk, on the other hand, will vary assertion by assertion for each account balance, transaction stream, and disclosure, depending on the conditions for each assertion. Nonetheless, as long as the risk model is used so that the audit risk for each financial statement assertion is at or below the planned levels, the auditor is reasonably certain that sufficient appropriate evidence has been obtained to support the audit opinion. However, there are practical limits to the evidence decision, so trade-offs have to be made; not all the evidence can be obtained at a reasonable cost or quickly enough to provide a timely audit report, and not all evidence has the same level of reliability. The concepts of materiality and audit risk are important elements in exercising professional judgment about the sufficiency and appropriateness of audit evidence, and both affect the quality of the audit.

The materiality and audit risk decision's main impact is on the extent of audit evidence that needs to be gathered. To be systematic and consistent, auditors try to keep the planning decision for materiality levels separate from the assurance level decision. But when an auditor believes a high level of assurance is needed, choosing a low audit risk level and choosing a low materiality level have the same impact: both will increase the amount of evidence the audit will need to gather. The underlying considerations of materiality and audit risk concepts are, however, different in nature, so it is good practice to keep these decisions separate in planning an audit.

Business Risk and the Audit Risk Model

Now that we have reviewed the risk model auditors use to identify and manage the risk element in an audit engagement, you may be wondering: How does an auditor get a handle on all these different risks? Canadian GAAS set out a **business risk–based audit approach (risk-based audit approach)**, and business risk is a pervasive consideration throughout the audit process. Backing up a bit to the topics in Chapter 5, we saw that the early stages of the audit involve auditors doing a lot of preliminary research to understand the auditee's business and its risks, determine materiality levels, identify significant issues that can affect its financial statements, and set out an overall audit strategy. Business risk is the main driver of the auditor's risk assessments.

Business risk is defined as any event or action adversely affecting an organization's ability to achieve its business objectives and execute its strategies. For examples, the introduction of the automobile replaced horse and buggy in the 1920s, the development of the personal computer and its word-processing capabilities dramatically reduced the market for electric typewriters in the 1980s, digital video discs (DVDs) replaced video cassette tapes in the 2000s, and online streaming is replacing DVDs in the 2010s. Now, the capability for downloading and streaming music and video files over the Internet severely challenges business models of the music and movie industries and their methods of making profits. These examples illustrate why auditing standards emphasize the financial statement auditor's need to understand and respond to business risk.[12]

Standards Check

CAS 315 Identifying and Assessing the Risks of Material Misstatement through Understanding the Entity and Its Environment

4. (b) Business risk—A risk resulting from significant conditions, events, circumstances, actions, or inactions, that could adversely affect an entity's ability to achieve its objectives and execute its strategies, or from the setting of inappropriate objectives and strategies.

Source: *CPA Canada Handbook—Assurance,* 2014.

The current business risk–based audit approach of the auditing standards emerged in the 1990s in response to increasingly complex businesses, operating environments, systems, and financing techniques. In the past, audit partners' personal experience, knowledge, and practice skills were sufficient to perform effective audits for relatively simple businesses. As businesses became more complex, it became evident that auditors, especially less experienced ones, needed more guidance and formalized structure for exercising good auditor judgment. Auditors were not always able to assess the many ways that events and conditions of a business increase the risk that its financial statements do not fairly present the business's financial realities.

Use of a risk-based audit approach in Canadian and international auditing standards places business risk assessment at the heart of the audit process. Appendix 6A provides a summary of the risk factors set out in the auditing standards as an example of the comprehensive aspects of business risk that a financial statement auditor considers when assessing the risk of material misstatement.

business risk–based audit approach (risk-based audit approach):
the requirement for the auditor to understand the client's business risks and strategy in order to assess the risks of material misstatement in the financial statements and design appropriate audit procedures in response to those risks

The remainder of this chapter will focus primarily on the information system an organization uses to produce financial statements. The information system is made up of business processes and the accounting processes related to them. The accounting processes create the financial information that flows into management's financial statements. The following chapter will discuss how understanding internal control and information systems helps to assess control risk. The inherent and control risk assessment procedures are the basis of developing a detailed plan to gather evidence to reduce the risk of material misstatement to an acceptable level given the level of audit risk the auditor has decided is acceptable for the engagement.

Review Checkpoints

6-51   How do bad economic times increase the risks that auditors should be alert to in auditees' financial statements?

6-52   What is the difference between "audit risk in an overall sense" and "audit risk applied to individual account balances"?

6-53   How does the auditor's decision on materiality relate to audit risk?

6-54   What is the relationship between business risk and audit risk?

6-55   How can the risk model be expanded to incorporate limitations to the audit that arise from accounting and other business risks?

Accounting Processes and the Financial Statements

LO5   Outline the relationships among the business processes and accounting processes (or cycles) that constitute an organization's information system and generate management's general purpose financial statements.

After performing preliminary analysis of the financial statements and expanding this with an in-depth analysis of the entity's business risk, we can consider how management's financial statements are created from a more informed perspective. Two points need to be stressed about management's financial statements: (1) they are the responsibility of the organization's management; thus, they contain management's assertions about economic actions and events; and (2) the numbers in them are produced by the organization's information system, which includes the accounting system that generates the trial balance. The relationship between the accounting system and the trial balance is shown in Exhibit 6–9, and the relationship between the trial balance and the financial statements is illustrated in Exhibit 6–10.[13] These exhibits show the trial balance of EcoPak Inc.

The EcoPak trial balance is shortened and simplified; real trial balances are more complex, with hundreds of accounts. To simplify the audit plan, auditors apply one of a fairly standard set of business processes, each of which has a set of accounts and an **accounting process** related to it. There are four basic accounting processes:

1.   Revenue process, dealing with accounting for the sales activities of the firm

2.   Purchasing process, dealing with accounting for purchasing goods and services

accounting process:
transactions streams and related account balances used to capture financial data about a business process in the accounting information system; also referred to as an *accounting cycle*

3. Production process, dealing with accounting for manufacturing and inventory costing

4. Financing process, dealing with the accounting for all the financing activities of the firm

An accounting process can be thought of as a cycle. The accounts go together in the accounting information system because they record transaction information from the same business activity and run through the same accounting process over and over, in a cycle. These routine transactions are recorded by the organization's accountants using journal entries involving the same set of accounts. The cycle perspective looks at accounts grouped according to the routine transactions by which all are normally affected. For example, the revenue cycle starts with a sale and the recording of an account receivable, which is later collected in cash, provided for in an allowance for doubtful accounts, or written off. The typical journal entries used in the revenue cycle are as follows:

> Dr. Accounts Receivable
> Cr. Sales Revenue
> *To record sales made on account*

> Dr. Cash
> Cr. Accounts Receivable
> *To record collection of receivables*

> Dr. Bad Debt Expense
> Cr. Allowance for Bad Debts
> *To provide for accounts receivable likely to be uncollectible*

> Dr. Allowance for Bad Debts
> Cr. Accounts Receivable
> *To write off uncollectible accounts receivable previously provided for*

Auditors find it easier to audit the related accounts with a coordinated set of procedures instead of attacking each account as if it stood alone, as predictable relationships should exist among these accounts. For example, if sales decrease but accounts receivable increase it may be a warning sign of financial difficulties. Also, the audit evidence available for one part of the accounting process often also contains information for other parts; for example, recording collection of a receivable involves recording the invoice information as well as the information about the cash collected. The cycle concept is part of the relation-based analytical procedures discussed in the following section.

In Exhibit 6–9, to illustrate the idea of the accounting processes, the EcoPak accounts are put into an order not normally seen in a trial balance. Some accounts are in more than one process. For example, the cash account is represented in all the processes because (a) cash receipts are involved in cash sales and collections of accounts receivable (revenue process), (b) cash receipts arise from issuing shares and loan proceeds (finance process), (c) cash payments are involved in buying inventory and capital assets and in paying for expenses (purchases process), and (d) cash payments are involved in paying wages (payroll process) and overhead expenses (production process).

When placed in the financial statements, the accounts and their descriptive titles contain the assertions that are the focal points of audit procedures. Exhibit 6–10 carries the accounts forward to the financial statements. Exhibit 6–11 illustrates the relationships among business activities, accounting processes, and the financial statements. These accounting processes will be covered in more detail in Chapters 11 through 14.

To summarize the business process view of an organization, Exhibit 6–12 provides a big-picture overview showing how all the entity's activities and business processes flow through to its financial statements.

EXHIBIT 6-9

EcoPak Trial Balance, December 31, 20X2

Revenue process	Purchasing process	Production process	Financing process		Debit	Credit
X	X	X	X	Cash	484,000	
X	X			Accounts receivable	400,000	
X				Allowance for doubtful accounts		30,000
X				Sales		8,500,000
X				Sales returns	400,000	
X				Bad debt expense	50,000	
	X	X		Inventory	1,940,000	
	X			Capital assets	4,000,000	
	X			Accumulated amortization		1,800,000
	X			Accounts payable		600,000
	X			Accrued expenses		10,000
	X			General expense	1,955,000	
		X		Cost of goods sold	5,265,000	
		X		Amortization expense	300,000	
			X	Bank loans		750,000
			X	Long-term notes		400,000
			X	Accrued interest		40,000
			X	Share capital		2,000,000
			X	Retained earnings		900,000
			X	Dividends declared	0	
			X	Interest expense	40,000	
			X	Income tax expense	196,000	
					15,030,000	15,030,000

Note: The coloured numbers in this exhibit relate to the corresponding coloured numbers in Exhibit 6–10. For example, subtract Sales returns from Sales (in purple) in this exhibit to get Sales (net) in Exhibit 6–10.

Review Checkpoints

6-56 What are four of the major accounting processes? What accounts can be identified with each? Why can an accounting process be described as a cycle?

6-57 Why is the cash account involved in more than one accounting process?

6-58 Why do auditors tend to find it easier to look at accounting processes rather than individual trial balance accounts?

EXHIBIT 6-10

EcoPak Inc. Unaudited Financial Statements

BALANCE SHEET

Cash	$ 484,000	Accounts payable	$ 600,000
Accounts receivable	370,000	Accrued expenses	10,000
Inventory	1,940,000	Accrued interest	40,000
Current assets	$2,794,000	Current liabilities	$ 630,000
Capital assets (gross)	$4,000,000	Long-term debt	$ 1,150,000
Accumulated amortization	(1,800,000)		
		Share capital	$2,000,000
Captial assets (net)	$2,000,000	Retained earnings	1,194,000
		Total liabilities and	
Total assets	$ 4,994,000	shareholders' equity	$ 4,994,000

STATEMENT OF INCOME

Sales (net)	$ 8,100,000
Cost of goods sold	5,265,000
Gross profit	$2,835,000
General expenses	$2,005,000
Amortization expense	300,000
Interest expense	40,000
Operating income before taxes	$ 490,000
Income tax expense	196,000
Net income	$ 294,000

NOTES TO FINANCIAL STATEMENTS
1. Accounting Policies
2. Inventories
3. Plant and Equipment
4. Long-Term Debt
5. Stock Options
6. Income Taxes
7. Contingencies
8. Etc.

CASH FLOWS

Operations:

Net income	$ 294,000
Amortization	300,000
Decrease in accounts receivable	90,000
Increase in inventory	(440,000)
Increase in accounts payable	150,000
Decrease in accrued expenses	(40,000)
Decrease in accrued interest	(20,000)
Cash flow from operations	$ 334,000
Investing activities:	
Purchase capital assets	$ (1,000,000)
Financing activities:	
Bank loan	$ 750,000
Repay notes payable	(200,000)
Financing activities	$550,000
Increase (decrease) in cash	$ (114,000)
Beginning balance	600,000
Ending balance	$ 484,000

Summary

To determine the risk that the financial statements could be materially misstated, the auditor learns about management's understanding of the business and its risk assessment process, and independently considers how the business risk could result in material misstatements of the financial statements. In the risk-based approach to auditing, the auditor must understand the auditee's business risk and its management risk assessment processes and control techniques to assess the risk of material misstatement in the financial statements overall and at the assertion level. The examples in Appendix 6A illustrate how business risk and control are linked, and how auditors develop a full understanding of the auditee's business by considering them together. To provide a better understanding of the procedures companies use to implement control over financial reporting, the next chapter gives an overview of the entity's internal control structure. The auditors' understanding of internal control is key to assessing risks and designing audit work so that it gives reasonable assurance that the financial statements are not materially misstated.

Relationships among Business Processes, Accounting Processes, and Financial Statements

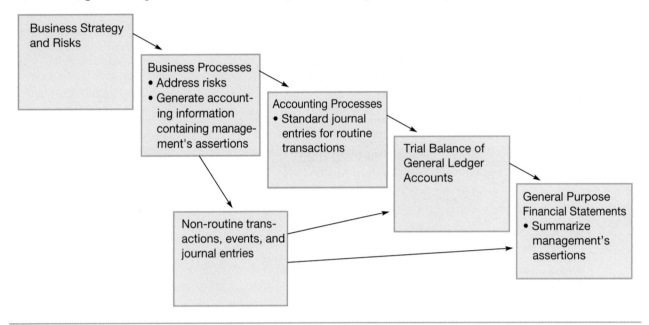

Capturing an Organization's Business Processes in Its Financial Statements

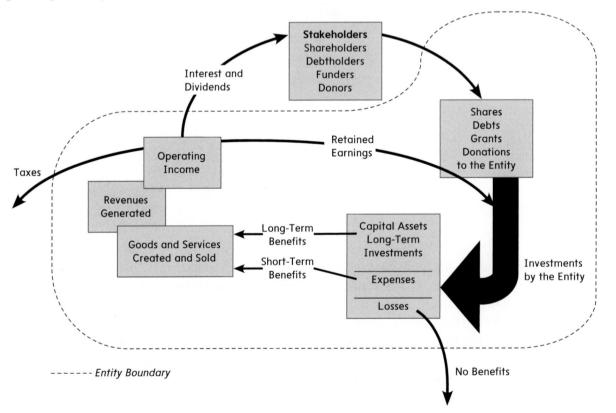

APPLICATION CASE WITH SOLUTION & ANALYSIS

Business Risk Analysis and Audit Implications

DISCUSSION CASE

Jack has recently joined a public accounting firm as a junior auditor and has been assigned to the audit team for SUN Energy Corporation (SUN). Based on a review of previous years' audit working papers and permanent files, SUN's 20X7 quarterly reports, and its draft 20X7 Management Discussion and Analysis, Jack learned the following:

SUN is a Canadian-based solar energy technology company that currently has three distinct operations focusing on (1) development and commercialization of photovoltaic (PV) cell technology, (2) development of a PV silicon processing technology, and (3) sales and installation of PV systems. SUN's goal is to make solar energy a cost-effective, mainstream energy solution. The company was incorporated in October 1993 and began trading on the TSX Technology Exchange in 20X3. In March 20X6, SUN started trading on the Frankfurt Open Market System. Jack's firm has audited the company since 20X2.

Governance

SUN currently has a six-member board of directors. The president and CEO is the only officer or employee of the company on the Board and is also a member of the Audit Committee. In April 20X7, the company hired a chief financial officer (CFO) who had previously worked as chief accountant for another technology company. Prior to this, the company had a limited number of qualified accounting staff and relied mainly on an outside accounting firm to prepare its financial statements. The key employees are scientists and engineers, and most of the financial forecasts have been generated by them, not the accounting staff.

Operations

According to Photon Consulting, a leading solar energy industry research company, the solar energy market is growing at 40% annually with an upward trend that management expects will continue. Details of SUN's three main business lines are as follows:

Photovoltaic Cell Technology

SUN's PV cell technology operation is currently developing a high-efficiency silicon wafer PV solar cell. The company's wholly owned German subsidiary SUN Technologies Deutschland GmbH (SUN Germany) is constructing a PV cell manufacturing plant in Germany with an initial capacity of 80 MW of PV cells per year. The PV cell manufacturing plant is expected to commence operations in the second fiscal quarter of 20X8. The plant is sized for three fully automated process lines that start with silicon wafers and finish with PV cells ready to be sold to PV module manufacturers. SUN's manufacturing strategy is to initially build two production lines. The first line will use turnkey, "off the shelf," technology to produce PV cells with a targeted efficiency of 15%. The second line will produce PV cells based on SUN's proprietary technology with a targeted efficiency of 18%.

Photovoltaic Silicon Processing Technology

SUN's PV silicon operation is developing a new PV silicon processing technology to produce solar-grade silicon (also known as "polysilicon"). PV silicon is currently in tight supply worldwide and is a key input for manufacturing PV cells. In 20X6, SUN received funding from the Canadian government to build and equip a pilot plant on the campus of a top engineering university and formed a consortium with other technology firms to conduct this research and development. Provided the current research and development is completed and funding is sourced, the silicon processing operation is expected to remove a barrier to growth (silicon wafer shortage) for the company's PV technology operation.

Photovoltaic Systems

SUN's systems operation focuses on the design, distribution, installation, and support of PV systems on residential, industrial, commercial, and institutional buildings as well as the installation of PV systems on open land, so-called solar parks. The high cost of electricity in Ontario has increased interest in solar energy generation facilities. SUN's systems operation has entered into six non-binding letters of interest related to supplying PV systems for proposed solar park developments.

Business Strategy

SUN's ability to successfully manufacture PV cells depends on securing silicon wafers, a key raw material input. In the current tight silicon market, well-positioned companies will have an advantage. SUN's strategy is to pay higher prices for silicon and to secure silicon supply in the spot market because of its highly efficient use of it. The larger competitors in the industry are expected to rely on buying power and strong relationships with feedstock suppliers for their supply and, thus, market share.

In the short term, SUN is planning to secure a supply of silicon wafers for 20X8 with a combination of supply contracts, proprietary refining, and spot market purchases. Several industry estimates suggest a significant increase in silicon supply during 20X8. No contracts for silicon supplies are in place at this time, in anticipation of falling prices. In the long term, the company expects to produce its own silicon.

There is a trend toward vertical integration in the solar industry. SUN is targeting the high-efficiency end of the market and believes that it will have a competitive cost advantage. Downstream module manufacturers and system integrators appear to be willing to pay a premium for high-efficiency cells. SUN's management believes that this combination is a unique approach that will generate superior margins once the German plant is operational. SUN's value proposition is the combination of high-efficiency cells produced at a lower cost, with a focus on selling to existing module manufacturers by demonstrating that they can increase their profit with SUN's product. SUN has a thin-film technology approach that reduces risk and provides the potential for a broader product line. It gives SUN the option to produce a lower-efficiency thin-film-only product in the face of continued silicon shortages.

The systems operation functions in a highly competitive market, both in Ontario and in the rest of North America—especially in terms of e-commerce competition. The competitors are very fragmented in both location and size, creating niche opportunities that can be exploited through developing strategic supply and customer relationships.

Intellectual Property

SUN relies on a combination of patents, internally developed know-how, and trade secrets to protect its proprietary technology and PV cell prototypes. Much intellectual property and expertise is being created at the laboratory and manufacturing levels.

Marketing and Distribution Methods

The main distribution channel is a value-added distributor of solar products and solutions with a limited Web presence. Under direction of its new Vice-President of Business Development (hired in 20X7), the company plans to market its own brand of key solar technology components and services (including repairs) on the Internet. The target market is solar professionals (e.g., knowledgeable power end-users, dealers, and tradespeople), commercial customers (e.g., solar farms), and builders of energy-efficient homes.

The SUN name is well-known to customers within its home market of southern Ontario who desire a broad assortment of PV products. The company has an extensive contact database of customers, channel partners, builders, and government bodies.

Financial Performance

SUN has incurred losses since its inception and may be unable to generate net sales that achieve or sustain profitability for the future. For example, the company's cash requirements increased significantly in 20X7, and construction costs of the German plant will increase them again in 20X8. In addition, operating expenses will increase as it expands its operations.

The company's ability to reach and sustain profitability depends on factors such as the growth rate of the solar energy industry, market demand for solar modules, the competitiveness of its products and services, and its ability to increase production volumes. The solar energy market is at a relatively early stage of development, and the extent of its acceptance is uncertain. Many factors may affect the demand for solar modules, including the following:

- Cost-effectiveness, performance, and reliability of solar modules compared with conventional and other non-solar energy sources and products

- Government incentives that support the solar energy industry

- Success of other renewable energy generation technologies, such as hydroelectric, wind, geothermal, solar thermal, concentrated photovoltaic, and biomass

- Economic and market conditions such as change in fossil fuel prices

- Capital expenditures by end-users of solar modules, which tend to decrease when the economy slows and interest rates increase

In September 20X7, SUN issued 21 million additional common shares for cash, raising approximately $28 million in new equity. The net proceeds of the offering will be used primarily to (1) secure additional supplies of silicon wafers, (2) accelerate the research and development on silicon processing, and (3) provide additional working capital to the company's systems operating unit. In the interim, the $28 million will be invested in government securities or other short-term, interest-bearing, investment-grade securities as approved by the company's audit committee.

Regulatory Actions

On May 28, 20X4, and May 9, 20X5, the Ontario Securities Commission (OSC) issued Cease Trade Orders (CTOs) against SUN for failing to file annual statements within the required time frame. The CTOs were lifted in each case within two weeks, once the audited statements were filed.

Auditor's Approach

To analyze SUN's business, environment, and risks, Jack organizes his information using these steps:

(a) Identify the key business factors, explaining why auditors must understand each factor to assess the risks of material misstatements. As a guide, consider

– Industry, regulatory, and other external risk factors;

– The nature of SUN's business (operations, investments, financing); and

– SUN's objectives and strategy to address business risks.

(b) Link these business risk factors to specific risks of material misstatement of the SUN financial statements. Explain clearly how the risks could lead to material misstatements.

(c) A key item in SUN's draft 20X7 balance sheet assets is patents with a cost of $439,000 and accumulated amortization of $310,000. The financial statement notes state that "Patent costs include legal fees incurred to obtain patents for technology developed or acquired by the company, and are being amortized over a period of five years." Assess the inherent risk for the patents balance, basing the assessment on the five principal assertions and giving the reasons supporting the assessment. How does this inherent risk assessment relate to the auditor's expectations regarding management's risk assessment processes and internal controls over patent assets, as well as to the planned approach for obtaining audit evidence for this account?

SOLUTION & ANALYSIS

Note: The following is one way to analyze the case, but other valid approaches and points are possible.

(a) Risk Factors

Governance—The CEO is on the audit committee. There is little financial expertise on the Board and in the accounting department. The new CFO's competency and qualifications are not known yet. The corporate culture is dominated by scientists, so finances may not be well managed.

Controls over financial reporting—There have been two CTOs for late filing; thus, financial reporting control weakness is a major risk factor. Control risk appears high. CFO/CEO certifications on financial statements and internal control effectiveness may be misstated.

Industry, regulatory, other external risk factors—The company operates in a highly competitive technological market. Management must have risk assessment processes in place to address risks such as the following:

1. New product market acceptance risk: Market risk exists for new products, such as the PV cell technology and solar-grade silicon technology. There is no assurance that new products will be accepted, desired volumes will be realized, or product will not become obsolete. In addition, new product offerings will also require significant marketing and sales efforts to gain market acceptance.

2. Competition: Many of SUN's current and potential competitors have greater financial, marketing, technical, and other resources. There can be no assurance that SUN will be able to compete successfully with its existing or new competitors.

3. Availability of solar-grade silicon and manufacturing inputs: Inability to secure raw materials and other inputs to meet sales demands could negatively impact sales and earnings. The current shortage of silicon has increased the price significantly. There may be shortages of solar-grade silicon, wafers, and certain specialized manufacturing tools and fixtures at any time, especially in periods of strong market demand. Few suppliers and quickly changing demand may also limit availability of inputs. With commercialization of the SUN PV cell technology, the inconsistent supply of solar-grade silicon could seriously impact SUN's sales and prospects.

4. Government subsidies for solar products: The solar market is somewhat dependent on government subsidies and programs that change with the political situation, with resultant changes in demand and pricing.

5. Foreign exchange risk: SUN's effort to sell its PV cells and solar-grade silicon in foreign markets will create exposure to exchange rates, primarily the U.S. dollar and the euro, which may negatively impact SUN's future financial performance.

Operations—Risks and uncertainties associated with operations:

1. Product development risk: SUN PV technology and solar-grade silicon technology development are spending research resources but are not yet commercialized. There is no guarantee that the PV technology will achieve the solar cell efficiency necessary for success in the market. Commercializing any product includes the risk that full-scale production may not be at an acceptable cost level. In addition, the solar-grade silicon technology is in early stages of development and there is no guarantee that technical milestones can be achieved.

2. Limited protection of patents and proprietary rights: The company relies on a combination of patents, trademarks, trade secrets, and know-how to protect its proprietary technology and rights. The company might not have resources to repair or protect current or future patents against infringements and challenges. Its trade secrets might be independently developed by competitors.

3. Expansion risk: Bringing the SUN PV cells to market may require SUN to invest in new production equipment and systems and put manufacturing plants on tight time schedules, often without guaranteed revenue volumes. Bringing investments into production quickly may expose SUN to integration risks, depending on the size of the investment, the schedule, the technology involved, and the nature of the products to be produced.

4. Manufacturing risk: SUN's production of PV cell manufacturing operations in Germany will require acquisition of land, development of manufacturing plants and production equipment, hiring of managerial personnel and skilled labour, and adequate financing arrangements. There is no assurance the company will be able to obtain these input factors or meet its implementation timeline.

5. Dependence on key personnel: SUN's success depends on attracting and retaining highly skilled personnel in key areas, including management. Unexpected loss of SUN's key employees could be detrimental to future operations. There is no assurance that the company will be able to engage or retain necessary personnel.

6. Financial position: While SUN has raised additional capital in 20X6 and early 20X7, additional funds are required to complete the commercialization of the SUN PV technology and the SUN solar-grade silicon technology.

7. Dependence on government funding: SUN's short-term business plan is based on securing government funding from the Province of Ontario. Its plan for a manufacturing plant in Germany depends on government funding as well. Failure to finalize the funding agreements would have a materially adverse impact on the company's short-term plans.

(b) Link Business Risks to Risk of Material Misstatement

Industry, regulatory, and other external risk factors:

*   Risk of material misstatement: Commodity prices and currency fluctuations are risk factors that may affect inventory valuation (lower of cost and net realizable value); contingent losses due to regulatory violations are probable and require disclosure (there may be other points linked to industry and external risk factors).

Nature of SUN's business (operations, investments, financing):

*   Risk of material misstatement: Inventory valuation may be affected by changes in costs imposed by suppliers and marketability; valuation of PPE and intangibles may be affected negatively by poor investment management risk or inadequate capitalization to complete construction, or by inability to

protect intellectual property rights; contingent liability disclosures may be incomplete if unreported product liability or patent infringement issues occur (there may be other points linked to operating/investing/financing risk factors).

SUN's objectives and strategy to address business risks:

- Risk of material misstatement: Strategies to address its risks may fail and the company may go bankrupt given the risky nature of its industry; the alternative energy market is at a very early stage; other points may be related to management's strategic risk assessment factors.

(c) Assess the Inherent Risk for the Patents Balance at the Assertion Level

The inherent risk assessments take into consideration the nature of the item and the risk that an error can have occurred in accounting for that item in the first place. The assessment will be at two levels, high and not high.

Patents are a critical asset in solar technology, so development businesses tend to have higher inherent risks. Thus, auditors expect management to have strong risk assessment processes and strong controls in place to offset and reduce these risks.

Referring to the Five Principal Assertions

- *Existence:* Not high inherent risk, because it is unlikely a patent would be set up in the books unless it existed, and this can be verified quite reliably by examining legal documents, cash disbursements, etc.

- *Completeness:* High inherent risk, as management may have patents that it didn't inform accounting staff about; some R&D expenses may have actually been to create patents; little reliable audit evidence is available for this.

- *Valuation:* High inherent risk (very high), because if the technology is not successful it creates high risk that the patent is worthless or overvalued, future earnings potential is very subjective and management could be biased; cost itself has fairly low inherent risk since the payments to create patents are quite objectively determined and clearly linked to creation of legal patent rights.

- *Ownership:* High inherent risk, related to the legal enforceability and protection of patents from infringement by others; relates to the valuation of the patents as well.

- *Presentation:* Not high inherent risk; appropriate accounting policies for Intangibles are set out in IAS 38 so it is clear for auditors to verify that the presentation is acceptable, but appropriate amortization may be an issue as it is subjective (useful life, etc.), increasing inherent risk.

If there are strong controls, it may be feasible and efficient for the auditor to test these controls and obtain some assurance from them that will lower the amount of assurance required from substantive tests. On the other hand, if the controls are not very strong, the risk of material misstatement will be very high for high inherent risk items and the auditor will need extensive substantive evidence to be able to get reasonable assurance to form an opinion about whether the financial statements are fairly stated.

SUMMARY

Chapter 6 extended the preliminary understanding of the auditee's business introduced in Chapter 5.

- How auditors use their understanding of business risks to assess risks of material misstatement at the financial statement level was explained. **LO1**

- A key auditing tool, assertions that describe the claims management makes in its financial statements, was explained. Five principal assertions—existence, completeness, ownership, valuation, and presentation—were described. An example of application of the assertion concept in practice was presented, showing how the five principal assertion concepts are elaborated to correspond to the classes of transactions, account balances, and disclosures in financial statements. The use of assertions as the focal point for designing audit procedures in response to assessed risk was explained. **LO2**

- The concept of audit risk was explained as being the probability that a clean audit opinion is given on financial statements that contain a material misstatement. Audit, inherent, control, and detection risks were described in terms of a conceptual model for managing audit risk in an audit engagement. The relation of business risk to audit risk was explained to show various important judgments that auditors must make and that are supported by a deep understanding of the auditee's business and its risk. **LO3**

- Examples were presented using theoretical risk assessments to demonstrate the usefulness of the audit risk model. Challenges and limitations of using the conceptual audit risk model were also discussed. The relation between materiality and audit risk was also explained in terms of the different nature of these two concepts and their similar impact on the extent of audit work planned. **LO4**

- The chapter ended with a description of businesses processes, how they are used to implement the business strategy, and how auditors can assess the auditee's business risk through strategic analysis and business process analysis. The relationships among business processes, accounting processes (or cycles), and management's general purpose financial statements were presented. **LO5**

- The factors that affect business risk, and the link between business risk and risk of material misstatement at the assertion level, are introduced, and examples of techniques apply these links to risk assessment are given in Appendix 6A. Corporate governance factors that relate to auditors' roles in audit engagements are discussed in Appendix 6B (available on Connect). **LO6, 7, 8**

KEY TERMS

accounting process

anchoring

assertions

audit objectives

business risk–based audit approach
  (risk-based audit approach)

control risk

control testing (compliance testing)

detection risk

e-commerce

enterprise resource planning
  systems (ERPs)

entity's risk assessment process

evidence-gathering procedures

fraud triangle

inherent risk

quality of earnings

risk of material misstatement

substantive audit procedures

MULTIPLE-CHOICE QUESTIONS FOR PRACTICE AND REVIEW

MC 6-1 `LO1` Business risk is related to business strategy because

a. auditors assess business risk so they can provide their auditees with a business strategy.
b. business risks are events or actions that cause changes in technology.
c. managers frequently change their business risks in response to changes in the business strategy.
d. business risks are events or actions that may have a negative effect on the audit client's ability to achieve its strategic objectives.

MC 6-2 `LO1` Information technology changes can affect business risk when

a. they result in a need to change business processes.
b. they do not include e-commerce activities.
c. systems become less complex.
d. systems become less integrated

MC 6-3 `LO1` The auditor assesses a business risk as high when

a. it is unlikely and moderate.
b. it is likely and significant.
c. it is possible and insignificant.
d. it is likely and insignificant.

MC 6-4 `LO1` Which of the following is not likely to be an important source of information the auditor can use to understand a client's business?

a. Geologist's reports on mineral reserves
b. Internal auditors
c. Retail sales statistics
d. Monday night football scores

MC 6-5 `LO2` If the XYZ company reports a $355,000 balance of accounts receivable, the existence assertion means

a. there are no accounts receivable by XYZ that have not been included in the balance.
b. all the amounts making up the $355,000 balance will be collected in full, in cash.
c. all the amounts included in the $355,000 balance represent valid sales on account that are still outstanding and due to the company.
d. the receivables have not been sold to another company.

MC 6-6 `LO3` The risk that the auditors' own work will lead to the decision that material misstatements do not exist in the financial statements, when in fact such misstatements do exist, is

a. audit risk.
b. inherent risk.
c. control risk.
d. detection risk.

MC 6-7 `LO4` Auditors are responsible for the quality of the work related to management and control of

a. inherent risk.
b. relative risk.
c. control risk.
d. detection risk.

MC 6-8 `LO4` The auditors assessed a combined inherent risk and control risk at 0.67 and said they wanted to achieve a 0.15 risk of failing to detect misstatements in an account with a material balance. What audit risk are auditors planning to accept for this audit?

a. 0.20
b. 0.10
c. 0.75
d. 0.05

MC 6-9 `LO5` The cash account is included in more than one accounting process because

a. all the business processes involve either receiving or paying out cash at some point.
b. cash is the most difficult asset to control.
c. cash is the easiest asset to steal.
d. cash can be either an asset or a liability.

MC 6-10 `LO5` The revenue process of a company generally includes these accounts.

a. Inventory, accounts payable, and general expenses
b. Inventory, general expenses, and payroll
c. Cash, accounts receivable, and sales
d. Cash, notes payable, and capital stock

MC 6-11 `LO5` Management's general purpose financial statements

a. are the responsibility of the auditor.
b. include only non-routine transactions.
c. make assertions that are the focal point of audit procedures.
d. can rarely be reconciled to the auditee's trial balance.

MC 6-12 `LO2` Management assertions are

a. stated in the footnotes to the financial statements.
b. implied or expressed representations about the financial statements.
c. explicitly expressed representations about the financial statements.
d. provided to the auditor in the assertions letter, but are not disclosed on the financial statements.

MC 6-13 `LO3` In the audit risk model, audit risk (AR) refers to

a. an uncorrected misstatement that would probably affect users of the financial statements.
b. the probability that a material misstatement occurred in an assertion of a class of transactions, account balance, or disclosure.
c. the probability that management's internal controls do not catch a misstatement once it has occurred.

 d. the probability that audit procedures don't catch a misstatement that has occurred and was not caught by the auditee's internal control.

 e. the risk the auditor is willing to accept of giving a clean audit opinion on financial statements that are materially misstated.

MC 6-14   **LO3**   In the audit risk model, inherent risk (IR) refers to

 a. the probability that management's internal controls do not catch a misstatement once it has occurred.

 b. the probability that a material misstatement occurred in an assertion of a class of transactions, account balance, or disclosure.

 c. the risk the auditor is willing to accept of giving a clean audit opinion on financial statements that are materially misstated.

 d. the probability that audit procedures won't catch a misstatement that has occurred and was not caught by the auditee's internal control.

 e. a misstatement that would probably affect users of the financial statements.

MC 6-15   **LO3**   In the audit risk model, control risk (CR) refers to

 a. the risk the auditor is willing to accept of giving a clean audit opinion on financial statements that are materially misstated.

 b. a misstatement that would probably affect users of the financial statements.

 c. the probability that management's internal controls do not catch a misstatement once it has occurred.

 d. the probability that audit procedures won't catch a misstatement that has occurred and was not caught by the auditee's internal control.

 e. the probability that a material misstatement occurred in an assertion of a class of transactions, account balance, or disclosure.

MC 6-16   **LO3**   In the audit risk model, detection risk (DR) refers to

 a. the risk the auditor is willing to accept of giving a clean audit opinion on financial statements that are materially misstated.

 b. the probability that a material misstatement occurred in an assertion of a class of transactions, account balance, or disclosure.

 c. the probability that management's internal controls do not catch a misstatement once it has occurred.

 d. the probability that audit procedures won't catch a misstatement that has occurred and was not caught by the auditee's internal control.

 e. a misstatement that would probably affect users of the financial statements.

MC 6-17   **LO2**   Assertions are used in financial statement auditing for

 a. defining aspects of the classes of transactions, account balances, and disclosures in the financial statements to help auditors specify the impact of business risks on fair presentation.

 b. providing specific substantive evidence auditors can rely on to indicate material misstatements.

 c. providing auditors with independent evidence and reasonable assurance about whether the financial statement information is fairly presented.

 d. supporting the auditor's conclusions and the opinion in the auditor's report regarding what could have gone wrong in the financial statements.

MC 6-18 `LO2` BDD Co. has a large balance of accounts receivable from many different customers, some of which are more than 60 days overdue. BDD management asserts that it will collect all the accounts eventually by applying pressure on the slow payers. For this reason, BDD's management claims that it would be understating BDD's assets if it were to set up a provision for bad debts. The assertion that may be materially misstated for BDD's accounts receivable balance by this situation is

a. the completeness assertion.
b. the inherent risk assertion.
c. the existence/occurrence assertion.
d. the valuation assertion.
e. the recognition assertion

MC 6-19 `LO2` LMN Co. is holding consignment inventory for another company, which must be excluded from LMN's financial statements to comply with

a. the completeness assertion.
b. the ownership/rights and obligations assertion.
c. the existence/occurrence assertion.
d. the valuation assertion.
e. the recognition assertion.

MC 6-20 `LO2` If XYZ Co. records sales revenues in its current-year financial statements for shipments that were made the first day of its following fiscal year, the assertion affected is

a. valuation (the sales amounts are not correctly calculated).
b. completeness (the sales were not completed at year-end).
c. existence/occurrence (the sales did not occur during the fiscal year).
d. ownership/rights and obligations (XYZ does not have the rights to the sales at year-end).

MC 6-21 `LO2` The sole shareholder of Jade Company had a contractor pave the parking lot at the company building, and also pave the driveway of his home. Both paving jobs were billed to the company on a single invoice. The assertion affected by this activity is

a. accuracy.
b. valuation.
c. completeness.
d. ownership/rights and obligations.
e. existence/occurrence.

MC 6-22 `LO3` Oakland Hills (OH) is a ski resort, and the revenue they report each year is greatly affected by the temperature and snowfall in the winter months. The variation in revenues from year to year is difficult for management, as their bonus is based on increasing income year over year. This situation best describes which kind of risk?

a. Audit risk
b. Inherent risk
c. Control risk
d. Detection risk

MC 6-23 `LO3` Evelyn is the controller of Mylan Connections (MC), a public relations firm with 50 account managers. Travel expenses for the consultants represent one of the largest expenses for MC. Evelyn does a thorough review of each expense report at the end of the month to ensure that all expenses are valid. The expense reports are then passed on to the VP Operations for his approval. When Evelyn is on vacation, the VP Operations simply approves the expense reports to ensure there are no delays in reimbursing the consultants. The situation above best describes what kind of risk?

a. Audit risk
b. Inherent risk
c. Control risk
d. Detection risk

MC 6-24 `LO4` When performing the audit risk assessment, it was determined that the audit risk for GXP's current-year audit increased from moderate to high. As a result, the auditor should

a. proceed with the audit in a similar manner to the prior year as this is a recurring engagement and the auditor is familiar with the client.
b. refuse the mandate for the current year to avoid an audit risk that is too high.
c. adjust the audit work performed in the current year as compared to the prior year to reduce audit risk to an acceptable level.
d. accept the engagement only if GXP agrees to a review-level engagement that would reduce the auditor's liability.

EXERCISES AND PROBLEMS

EP6-1 Understanding Business Risk. `LO1` Super Natural Foods Limited manufactures, distributes, and sells all-natural grocery products.

Required:

Describe three business risks for this company, and explain why they are important considerations for the auditor of its financial statements. Consider the following categories from CAS 315, as listed in Appendix 6A: industry risks, regulatory risks, and operating risks.

EP6-2 Significant Audit Issues; Audit Risk Decision. `LO1, 3` You are the auditor of Royal Health Limited (Royal). Royal is a public company that grows medicinal plants and sells them across North America, Europe, and Asia. Its largest expense is marketing. All its marketing is done by another company that is owned by one of Royal's directors.

Required:

Identify three key audit issues in this company, and explain how these will affect your audit risk, using the audit risk model.

EP6-3 Business Processes; Accounting Processes/Cycles. `LO5`

Required:

Explain what an accounting process/cycle is and how it relates to business processes and to the entity's financial statements. Why is the approach of identifying accounting processes/cycles useful in planning an audit?

EP6-4 Business Processes, Different Industries. LO5

Required:

What business processes would be related to each of the four accounting processes in the following businesses?

a. a bicycle manufacturing business
b. an architectural firm
c. a retail grocery store

EP6-5 Performance Measures in Risk Assessment. LO1, 5

Required:

In assessing the risk of material misstatement in the financial statements as a whole, why should auditors pay particular attention to external and internal performance measures that are used to evaluate the management, and to the impact of material misstatements on the quality of earnings?

EP 6-6 Assertions. LO2 The assertions listed in CAS 315 (see Exhibit 6–6) are each cross-referenced to the five principal assertions.

Required:

Why are these different terms used to describe assertions in different audit guidance materials?

DISCUSSION CASES

DC 6-1 Audit Risk Model. LO3 Audit risks for particular accounts and disclosures can be conceptualized in this model: Audit risk (AR) = Inherent risk (IR) × Internal control risk (CR) × Detection risk (DR).

Required:

Use this model as a framework for considering the following situations and deciding whether the auditor's conclusion is appropriate:

a. Ohlsen, PA, has participated in the audit of Limberg Cheese Company for five years, first as an assistant accountant and the last two years as the senior accountant. He has never seen an accounting adjustment recommended. He believes the inherent risk must be zero.

b. Jones, PA, has just (November 30) completed an exhaustive study and evaluation of the internal control system of Lang's Derfer Foods Inc. (fiscal year ending December 31). She believes the control risk must be zero because no material errors could possibly slip through the many error-checking procedures and review layers used by Lang's Derfer.

c. Fields, PA, is lazy and does not like audit jobs in Toronto, anyway. On the audit of Hogtown Manufacturing Company, he decided to use detail procedures to audit the year-end balances very thoroughly to the extent that his risk of failing to detect material errors and irregularities should be 0.02 or less. He gave no thought to inherent risk and conducted only a very limited review of Hogtown's internal control system.

d. Shad, PA, is nearing the end of a "dirty" audit of Allnight Protection Company. Allnight's accounting personnel all resigned during the year and were replaced by inexperienced people. The controller resigned last month in disgust. The journals and ledgers were a mess because the one computer specialist was hospitalized for three months during the year. Shad thought thankfully, "I've been able to do this audit in less time than last year when everything was operating smoothly."

DC 6-2 Planning, Inherent and Control Risk, Manufacturing Business.   LO1, 2, 3, 4   Darter Ltd. is a medium-size business involved in manufacturing and assembling consumer electronic products, such as DVD players, radios, and satellite receivers. It is privately owned. Its minority shareholders requested that the annual financial statements be audited for the first time this year. Your firm is engaged to do the current year's audit. You are now reviewing Darter's preliminary general ledger trial balance in order to begin preparing the planning memorandum. Consider the following accounts that appear in this trial balance:

> Cash
> Inventory, finished goods
> Inventory, work-in-progress
> Inventory, unassembled components
> Inventory, spare parts
> Property, plant, and equipment
> Deferred development costs
> Goodwill
> Accounts payable
> Warranty provision
> Bank loan, long term
> Share capital, common shares
> Retained earnings
> Revenue
> Cost of goods sold
> General and administration expense

Required:

a. Evaluate the inherent risk for each of the above accounts. List two accounts that you think would have the highest inherent risks, and two that would have the lowest. Indicate whether there are any particular assertions (i.e., existence, completeness, ownership, valuation, presentation) that the risks mainly relate to. Give reasons that support your assessments, and state any assumptions you need to make.

b. For one of the high-risk accounts you identified in (a), explain how the inherent risk level will relate to the types of controls that Darter's management implements for each of these accounts. Consider costs and benefits of implementing effective controls.

c. For one of the high-risk accounts you identified in (a), describe the procedures you would use to assess the control risk.

d. How would you expect the company's accounts to differ, and how would your inherent risk assessment differ, if the company's business were

- An iron mine
- A piano manufacturer
- A bank
- A shipping line

DC 6-3 Business Risk Analysis.   LO1, 5   Assume you have recently been assigned to the audit team working on the financial statement audit of Town Groceries Limited (TGL). As a member of the team, you are now in the process of gaining an understanding of the company's business, environment, and risks.

From the 20X4 Town Groceries Limited Annual Report you have learned the following about this business and its strategy:

TGL is Canada's largest food distributor and a leading provider of general merchandise products and services. TGL is committed to providing Canadians with a one-stop destination in meeting their food and everyday household needs. This goal is pursued through a portfolio of store formats across the country.

It operates across Canada under various operating banners (including Maritime Grocery, Western Groceries, and other banners). These banners are set up as 658 corporate-owned stores, 400 franchised stores, and 519 associated stores. The store network is supported by 32 warehouse facilities located across Canada. Some 130,000 full-time and part-time employees execute its business strategy in more than 1,000 corporate and franchised stores from coast to coast. TGL is known for the quality, innovation, and value of its food offering. It also offers a strong private label program, including the unique Choice of Choice and OurTown brands.

While food remains at the heart of its offering, TGL stores provide a wide, growing range of general merchandise products and services. In addition, their Town Financial Inc. offers personal banking, a popular credit card, auto and home insurance, and the Town Points loyalty program.

TGL seeks to achieve its business objectives through stable, sustainable, and long-term growth. It seeks to provide superior returns to its shareholders through a combination of dividends and share price appreciation. Its willingness to assume prudent operating risks is equalled by its commitment to the maintenance of a strong balance sheet position.

In executing its strategies, TGL allocates the resources needed to invest in and expand its existing markets. It also maintains an active product development program.

TGL is highly selective in its consideration of acquisitions and other business opportunities. Given the competitive nature of its industry, TGL also strives to make its operating environment as stable and as cost effective as possible. It works to ensure that its technology systems and logistics enhance the efficiency of its operations.

It strives to contribute to the communities it serves and to exercise responsible corporate citizenship.

Required:

a. Based on the preceding information, discuss the industry, regulatory, and other external factors that are relevant in understanding TGL's business and its environment. Use the risk factors outlined in Appendix 6A as a guide.

b. Link the risk factors you identified in (a) to the risks in TGL's operations. Link these operating risks to risks of TGL's financial statements being materially misstated.

c. Outline TGL's strategy, and describe, in general terms, the business processes you expect to find the company using to achieve its strategy. Consider the four typical business processes discussed in this chapter to develop your response.

d. While reading through the business section of the newspaper, you came across the following article on TGL's third-quarter results for 20X5 (see box below). What strategic risks are illustrated in the results being described in the article? Speculate on what strategic errors and/or business process deficiencies at TGL have contributed to these woes. What impact do you expect these events to have on TGL's financial results for 20X5?

TGL Profit Slumps, CEO Vows to Continue Retooling the Grocery Operations

July 30, 20X5

TGL Cos. Ltd. will stick to its current retooling strategy, the grocery chain CEO said yesterday, even though its third-quarter profit slumped by 26%. Profit was dragged down by supply-chain hiccups and higher-than-expected costs related to TGL's retooling strategy.

The supermarket operator reported its summer-quarter profit fell to $192 million, or 7 cents a share, from $258 million, or 9.4 cents, a year ago. Analysts were expecting a profit of 10 cents per share, even though the company had previously warned that its planned retooling of supply chains, systems, and administration would likely result in some short-term profit decreases.

TGL's CEO said that retooling the national supply chain and converting to a common-information systems platform has taken longer and been more disruptive than planned, negatively affecting TGL's performance in the short term. The CEO expressed disappointment with the progress to date but vows that the company is taking strong action to resolve the problems and will be a stronger and much more competitive player as a result of these changes.

Another issue affecting profit arose from TGL's new third-party-operated general merchandise warehouse and distribution centre for the western region failing to reach the planned operating efficiency and capacity on schedule.

The profit declines come despite TGL's sales growing 6.4 per cent from a year earlier, to $8.7 billion from $8.1 billion, with growth across all regions. Sales at older stores, and sales of the general and beauty product lines, tended to be flat, however, as they were most affected by the supply chain disruptions.

TGL reported that $30 million of the profit decline was due to the flat sales, restructuring and other charges reduced it by another $27 million, and a special charge relating to a reassessment by the Canada Revenue Agency relating to sales taxes on certain new lines of merchandise brought it down by another $20 million.

DC 6-4 Business Risk and Risk of Material Misstatement. **LO1, 2, 3** You have joined a public accounting firm as a junior auditor and have been assigned to the audit team for one of your firm's largest audit engagements, Cold Beverages Corp. (CB), a large public company. CB was incorporated in Canada several decades ago. Your firm has audited CB for many years. Based on your review of previous years' audit working papers, CB's 20X3 quarterly reports, and its draft 20X3 Management Discussion and Analysis, you have learned the following.

CB is one of the world's largest non-alcoholic beverage producers, providing about 65% of the world's retailer-branded soft drinks, bottled water, juice drinks, and teas. Approximately 90% of its output is sold to retailers for sale under the retailers' brands, with the remainder sold under CB's own brand names. The company operates in Canada, the United States, Mexico, the United Kingdom, and other countries in Europe. In the past four years, CB has expanded its production and distribution capabilities mainly through acquisitions of other businesses. It plans to grow mainly by leveraging existing customer relationships, developing new products and distribution channels, and obtaining new customers in new markets. During 20X1 and 20X2, CB rationalized its business by focusing on its highest-performing production facilities, resulting in plant and warehouse closures in North America.

CB's products are sold primarily to a small group of very large customers, including large grocery and retail chains. One customer, Tram-Mart, accounts for about 40% of CB's total 20X3 revenues, and its nine next-largest customers account for about 30% of 20X3 revenues. Products are delivered by third-party carriers or are picked up by customers at CB's plants.

The main raw material used in production is water. Other materials required are mainly plastic bottles, aluminum cans, packaging materials, sweeteners, and flavourings. CB typically enters into annual arrangements with its suppliers rather than long-term contracts. At the end of each one-year period CB must renegotiate with the suppliers or find new suppliers. The prices of these materials fluctuate on world markets, but generally there are adequate supplies available, and this is expected to continue in the future. During 20X2, the price of aluminum cans increased substantially and CB's management decided to enter a five-year agreement with a supplier at a fixed cost. During 20X3, the price of aluminum fell quite substantially. Because of growing demand for corn-based products, the costs of the main sweeteners used by CB have increased substantially in 20X3. CB does not use derivatives to manage the risks of these price changes.

A key to CB's success is its intellectual property, consisting of trade secrets, beverage formulas, and trademarks for its beverage brands. These intangibles are protected mainly by registration, contractual agreements, employee confidentiality agreements, and rigorous prosecution of any infringements using all available common and statutory laws.

Competition in the soft drinks industry is fierce. Three huge multinationals control about 85% of consumer sales and spend heavily on promotion. Other competitors are local independent producers who sell at aggressively discounted prices, and some large U.S. retail chains that manufacture their own soft drinks and actively seek new customers to expand their sales. CB's management addresses these competitive threats by offering efficient distribution choices, top-quality products, attractive packaging, effective marketing strategies, and superior service.

CB's business is subject to many federal, state, provincial, and local laws and regulations that govern product manufacturing, distribution, labelling, and safety. It is also subject to a number of environmental laws relating to fuel use and storage, water use and treatment, waste disposal, and employee safety. Failure to comply with these laws and regulations can have very negative consequences, including penalties and fines. Currently, CB is not in compliance with the provincial *Environmental Protection Act* requirements that set a minimum percentage of its products that must be sold in refillable containers. At this time, the government is not enforcing this law. CB's management believes that none of its main competitors are in compliance either, and so it could not remain competitive if it attempted to comply.

During 20X3, CB's management identified material weaknesses in the company's internal controls over financial reporting. The main issues are related to controls over periodic inventory counts and credit notes. Inventory-counting procedures were not properly executed because employees were not properly trained and supervised, resulting in an inability to produce a complete and accurate physical count. Lack of segregation of duties in the issuing of credit notes to customers permitted a fraud to occur. An accounts receivable clerk was discovered to be colluding with a warehouse employee to divert cases of high-value beverages from legitimate customer orders and cover up the shortages by issuing phony credit notes. The stolen beverages were sold by the warehouse employee to small local restaurants and variety stores. Both employees have been fired, and management is in the process of redesigning its inventory control and credit note issuing procedures. Another weakness was found in the global material acquisition function, where supplier contracts were not being properly authorized, resulting in improper agreements being entered into, and increased risk of employees in different countries accepting bribes from suppliers or engaging in other illegal acts.

Early in 20X4, CB reported its fourth quarter of 20X3 performance, a large loss that was worse than financial analysts expected and much worse than the fourth quarter of 20X2. CB management blames the poor performance on price competition and on declining soft drink consumption in developed countries. Over the 20X3 year, the company has reported very poor quarterly results, and its share price has fallen dramatically all year. The analysts have also expressed concern that CB is close to violating its debt covenants and may have difficulty obtaining the financing it will require to succeed unless its profitability improves substantially in the early part of 20X4. To try to please investors, CB's new CEO, a respected industry veteran, recently held a press conference to show off the company's new head office in Alberta and its innovative new products, and to explain how it is changing the company culture to focus on a turnaround strategy.

Required:

a. Identify key business factors in the CB case and explain why its auditors must understand each factor to assess the risks of material misstatements. As a guide, consider the following categories:

- Industry, regulatory, and other external risk factors
- Nature of CB's business (operations, investments, financing)
- CB's objectives and strategy to address business risks

b. Link the business risk factors you identified in (a) to some specific risks of material misstatement of the CB financial statements. Explain clearly how the risks could lead to the financial statements being materially misstated.

c. What information relevant to understanding internal control is indicated in the case? Consider control environment and accounting controls relevant to financial reporting. How would you assess the effectiveness of CB's internal control to reduce the risk of material misstatement?

DC 6-5 Obtaining a "Sufficient" Understanding of Internal Control. `LO3, 4` The 12 partners of a regional public accounting firm met in special session to discuss audit engagement efficiency. Jones spoke up, saying:

"We all certainly appreciate the firm-wide policies set up by Martin and Smith, especially in connection with the audits of the large companies that have come our way recently. Their experience with a large national firm has helped build up our practice. But I think the standard policy of conducting reviews and tests of internal control on all audits is raising our costs too much. We can't charge our smaller clients fees for all the time the staff spend on this work. I would like to propose that we give engagement partners discretion to decide whether to do a lot of work on assessing control risk. I may be an old mossback, but I think I can finish a competent audit without it."

Discussion on the subject continued but ended when Martin said, with some emotion: "But we can't disregard generally accepted auditing standards like Jones proposes!"

Required:

What do you think of Jones's proposal and Martin's view of the issue? Discuss.

DC 6-6 Comprehensive Audit Planning Decisions. `LO1, 2, 3, 4` (and from Chapter 5: `LO3, 4, 5, 6`) You have been assigned to the audit of the financial statements of Office Moving and Storage Limited (OMS) for its year ending December 31, 20X2. The company started 10 years ago and is in the business of moving furniture and equipment for company offices across Canada, and also providing storage for companies requiring that service. The company is owned by three shareholders who are all involved in operating the company.

OMS owns four properties outside of major urban centres; this is where it has warehouse buildings for storing customers' furniture and garages for parking its own moving trucks. OMS has a force of salespeople who follow commercial real estate construction and leasing reports to identify sales prospects: large and medium-size companies that are planning to move offices. The prospects are assigned to salespeople who then follow up and try to sell a moving and storage contract to the company, along with other services to facilitate the office move. The salespeople prepare a cost quote for doing the move, which must be approved by the regional sales manager prior to giving it to the prospect company. The regional sales managers have the authority to lower the quoted price if a competing moving company undercuts OMS's quote. Once a move has been started, in many cases the customer requires extra services beyond those contracted for (such as extra boxes, packing, disassembling furniture, or removal of garbage), and these are billed as extra charges. The moving employees on the job record the types of extra services provided in a Customer Moving Job Report. These extras are then priced by the assistant sales managers and added to the amount billed to the customer.

Customers with approved credit ratings are required to pay 25% of the contracted price as a deposit and are billed for the remaining contract cost and any extras after the move is completed. They have 10 days to pay in full. Customers without approved credit ratings are required to pay the full contract price in advance, and if any extra service charges arise during the move, they must pay the moving employees for these in cash at the time of the move.

In the preliminary audit planning done to date, your audit manager has determined that revenues are the class of transactions with the highest risk of material misstatement. You have been assigned to continue the OMS audit planning work by finalizing and documenting various risk assessment and planning decisions so the audit team can move on to developing the detailed audit plans.

It is now January 20X3, and you are at the OMS offices to begin your audit work. In discussion with the company's management, you have learned that OMS typically does about 30–40 moves per month, with 40 being about the maximum number it can handle with its current employees and trucks. About 80% of its sales are on account to customers with good credit ratings; the balance of its sales are paid in advance. Starting in the current year, the company has purchased future contracts to lock in fuel prices, since fuel is a major operating expense. The company's policy is to value these future contracts at fair value in its year-end balance sheet, with unrealized gains included in Revenues, and unrealized losses included in Operating Costs. The company is planning to expand its operations in the next two years by acquiring another established moving company that specializes in smaller company moves. The acquisition and expansion will be financed by issuing shares to other investors who will not be actively involved in the business.

Below is the December 31, 20X2 adjusted trial balance listing that you have obtained from OMS's management:

OFFICE MOVING AND STORAGE LIMITED		
TRIAL BALANCE AS OF DECEMBER 31, 20X2	DEBITS	CREDITS
Cash	275,090	
Accounts receivable	1,596,540	
Allowance for bad debts		167,957
Financial instruments, fuel futures contracts, at fair value	670,329	
Prepaid insurance	293,509	
Land	1,500,000	
Buildings, cost	1,881,356	
Accumulated depreciation, buildings		411,545
Moving trucks, at cost	2,430,230	
Accumulated depreciation, moving trucks		1,175,871
		(continued)

Accounts payable		1,169,191
Income taxes payable		201,104
Estimated damage provisions, uninsured portion		81,549
Bank loan, long term		1,650,000
Share capital, common shares		1,500,000
Retained earnings, beginning of year		1,147,668
Revenue		43,304,071
Operating costs	25,184,877	
General and administration expenses	12,578,787	
Other expenses	3,943,738	
Income tax expense	454,500	
Totals	50,808,956	50,808,956

Required:

Continue audit planning for OMS based on answering the following questions:

a. Identify three factors your audit firm would have had to consider in order to decide to accept the OMS audit engagement for the current year, and explain how each factor affects this acceptance decision.

b. Using the trial balance data above, analyze OMS's financial statements by calculating its current ratio and accounts receivable turnover ratio.

   (*Note:* Current ratio = Current assets/Current liabilities, and Accounts receivable turnover = Credit sales revenue for the year/Net accounts receivable at year-end.)

   Explain what this analysis can tell you about the risks in OMS's financial statements, and what further investigation the analytical results may suggest.

c. What materiality levels would you use to plan this audit? Show your calculations and justify your decision. You can assume your audit firm has the following policy: Performance materiality should be 70% of the overall materiality level for financial statements as a whole, unless specific information indicates a different value should be used.

d. What audit risk level would you be willing to accept for this engagement? Describe your choice in terms of one of these levels: *low, lower, lowest.* Explain the factors that support your decision.

e. Based on the business risk analysis for OMS, your audit manager believes the OMS revenue class of transactions has the highest risk of material misstatement. Identify and explain three business risk factors in OMS that would support your manager's assessment.

f. Your manager has asked you to assess the inherent risk of misstatement at the assertion level for the revenues. Use the level *high* or *not high* to describe your assessments, and explain the factors that support your assessments.

DC 6-7 Financial Performance Analysis. **LO1, 2** On your first day of a summer internship at BSP Auditing Services, you sit in on an introductory meeting between Ben, a partner at BSP, and Jackie, the CEO of Brenda Catering Inc. (BCI). The following conversation occurs:

> Ben: You are showing a 3% increase in profit for this current year. This is very impressive considering most catering businesses are experiencing losses. How did you manage this?

> Jackie: We worked really hard and had a big sale at the end of the year. We had to be creative! For example, I came up with a "stock up your freezer" promotion where I offered a 10% discount on

all frozen food for the month of December so that our clients could save on food that they can purchase now, freeze, and use later. It was so popular that we had trouble keeping up with the deliveries.

Another big part of our business is catering weddings in the summer. Wedding events are usually booked one to two years ahead. A big part of the work related to the wedding is obtaining the contract and discussing menus with the bride and groom. Our VP operations suggested that we book a portion of these revenues when the contract is signed in order to match the revenue to the period where the work is done. We have started to book 20% of the revenue from wedding contracts in the year where the contract is signed. This is fairly conservative as we require a 10% non-refundable deposit with each contract. I don't know why other catering businesses don't do this.

Ben: Ok, we'll have to look into these new policies and promotions during our audit. I also wanted to ask about your "Organic Lunch Box" segment of the business. I saw in the local news that there was some controversy over this as it was proved that not all ingredients used were organic. What is the update on this situation?

Jackie: I expect this controversy to go away very soon. It was mostly started by one of our competitors to hurt our reputation. It's true that we did use some non-organic ingredients even if we had advertised 100% organic. We've changed those ingredients and I can now assure you that the "Organic Lunch Box" is made from 100% organic ingredients. We are being sued by clients for $200,000, but we didn't know the ingredients were non-organic, so we can't be forced to pay anything. That's why I didn't accrue anything in this year's financial statements for this.

Required:

Based on the conversation above, prepare a preliminary financial performance analysis for BCI by

a. identifying questionable accounting policies and potential earnings manipulation.
b. indicating the impact on the risk of material misstatement, noting the assertion(s) mainly affected.

DC 6-8 Preliminary Analysis, Materiality, Assertions. `LO1, 2, 3, 4` (and from Chapter 5: `LO3, 4, 5, 6`) Your firm has been engaged to do the current year's audit of Dawood Ltd., a medium-sized business involved in manufacturing television screens and computer monitors. Dawood is privately owned, and its two shareholders have requested that the annual financial statements be audited for the first time this year. One of the shareholders manages the business; the other is not involved. You are now reviewing Dawood's preliminary general ledger trial balance, shown below, to begin the audit planning.

Required:

a. When planning this audit, explain why it is important for Dawood's auditor to understand its business, its environment, and its risks.
b. Determine an appropriate materiality level for preliminary audit planning purposes. Explain your reasons for selecting this materiality level.
c. List two analytical procedures you could perform using the trial balance data above. Explain what each procedure can tell you about the risks in Dawood's financial statements and what further investigation the analytical results may suggest.
d. Identify two accounts that you feel would have the highest risk of material misstatement and two that you think would have the lowest. Explain the reasons for your risk assessments.
e. Assume you have determined that Dawood's inventory account is a high-risk item. Assess the risk of material misstatement for the inventory account, using the five principal assertions as the basis for your assessment. (You will probably have to make some assumptions, since little information

ACCOUNT	BALANCE DR/(CR)
Cash	$ 10,009
Accounts receivable	167,090
Allowance for bad debts	(25,000)
Inventory, finished goods	200,550
Inventory, work-in-process	94,601
Inventory, purchased components	199,800
Inventory, parts	34,400
Property, plant, and equipment (PPE)	9,700,100
Accumulated amortization, PPE	(3,607,597)
Accounts payable	(222,400)
Warranty provision	(87,000)
Bank loan, long term	(1,000,000)
Share capital, common shares	(1,500,000)
Retained earnings	(1,738,442)
Revenue	(9,005,800)
Cost of goods sold	4,696,600
General and administration expenses	1,902,500
Other expenses	180,589

is available in the case. In a real audit, these assumptions are points you would want to inquire about to obtain the information needed.) Give the reasons supporting your assessment.

Business Risk Factors Used to Assess the Risk of Material Misstatement

LO6 Explain the industry, regulatory, and other external factors that affect an auditee's business risk and related risk of material misstatement in its financial statements.

This appendix lists the business risks that the auditor considers when assessing the risk of material financial statement misstatement and explains how business risk is linked to the assessment of risk of misstatements at the assertion level. Business risk factors include those shown in the following box.

Understanding the Entity and Its Environment, Including Internal Control

Industry, Regulatory, and Other External Factors, Including the Applicable Financial Reporting Framework

Industry conditions

(a) The market and competition, including demand, capacity, and price competition
(b) Cyclical or seasonal activity
(c) Product technology relating to the entity's products
(d) Energy supply and cost

Regulatory environment

(a) Accounting principles and industry-specific practices
(b) Regulatory framework for a regulated industry
(c) Legislation and regulation that significantly affect the entity's operations
  (i) Regulatory requirements
  (ii) Direct supervisory activities
(d) Taxation (corporate and other)
(e) Government policies currently affecting the conduct of the entity's business
  (i) Monetary, including foreign exchange controls
  (ii) Fiscal
  (iii) Financial incentives (e.g., government aid programs)
  (iv) Tariffs, trade restrictions
(f) Environmental requirements affecting the industry and the entity's business

Other external factors currently affecting the entity's business

(a) General level of economic activity (e.g., recession, growth)
(b) Interest rates and availability of financing
(c) Inflation, currency revaluation

(continued)

Nature of the entity

Business operations

(a) Nature of the business
- (i) Profit-oriented organization (e.g., financial or other services, manufacturer, wholesaler, importer, exporter)
- (ii) Government (e.g., federal, provincial, territorial, local)
- (iii) Government organization (e.g., department/ministry, Crown corporation, fund, agency)
- (iv) Not-for-profit organization (e.g., an entity established for social, educational, religious, health, or philanthropic purposes)

(b) Nature of revenue sources (e.g., manufacturer; wholesaler; banking, insurance, or other financial services; import/export trading; utility; transportation; technology products and services)

(c) Products or services and markets (e.g., major customers and contracts, terms of payment, profit margins, market share, competitors, exports, pricing policies, reputation of products, warranties, order book, trends, marketing strategy and objectives, manufacturing processes)

(d) Conduct of operations (e.g., stages and methods of production, business segments, delivery of products and services, details of declining or expanding operations)

(e) Alliances, joint ventures, and outsourcing activities

(f) Involvement in electronic commerce, including Internet sales and marketing activities

(g) Geographic dispersion and industry segmentation

(h) Location of production facilities, warehouses, and offices

(i) Key customers

(j) Important suppliers of goods and services (e.g., long-term contracts, stability of supply, terms of payment, imports, methods of delivery such as "just-in-time")

(k) Employment (e.g., by location, supply, wage levels, union contracts, pension and other post-employment benefits, stock option or incentive bonus arrangements, and government regulation related to employment matters)

(l) Research and development activities and expenditures

(m) Transactions with related parties

(n) Nature of expenditures, including programs and activities of not-for-profit and government entities

Investments

(a) Acquisitions, mergers, or disposals of business activities (planned or recently executed)

(b) Investments and dispositions of securities and loans

(c) Capital investment activities, including investments in plant, equipment, and technology, and any recent or planned changes

(d) Investments in non-consolidated entities, including partnerships, joint ventures, and special purpose entities

Financing

(a) Group structure—major subsidiaries and associated entities, including consolidated and non-consolidated structures

(b) Debt structure, including covenants, restrictions, guarantees, and off–balance sheet financing arrangements

(c) Leasing of property, plant, or equipment for use in the business

(d) Beneficial owners (local, foreign, business reputation, and experience)

(e) Related parties

(f) Use of derivative financial instruments

(g) Form of ownership (e.g., private company, public company, partnership, joint venture, government owned or controlled, member owned)

Financial reporting

(a) Accounting principles and industry-specific practices

(b) Revenue recognition practices

(c) Accounting for fair values

(d) Inventories (e.g., locations, quantities)

(e) Foreign currency assets, liabilities, and transactions

(f) Industry-specific significant categories (e.g., loans and investments for banks, accounts receivable and inventory for manufacturers, research and development for pharmaceuticals)

(g) Accounting for unusual or complex transactions including those in controversial or emerging areas (e.g., accounting for stock-based compensation)

(h) Financial statement presentation and disclosure

(continued)

Objectives and strategies and related business risks

(a) Existence of objectives (e.g., how the entity addresses industry, regulatory, and other external factors) relating to, for example, the following:

   (i) Industry developments (e.g., the entity might not have the personnel or expertise to deal with the changes in the industry)

   (ii) New products and services (e.g., potential for increased product liability)

   (iii) Expansion of the business (e.g., demand might not have been accurately estimated)

   (iv) New accounting requirements (e.g., potential incomplete or improper implementation, or increased costs)

   (v) Regulatory requirements (e.g., there might be increased legal exposure)

   (vi) Current and prospective financing requirements (e.g., potential loss of financing due to the entity's inability to meet requirements)

   (vii) Use of IT (e.g., systems and processes may be incompatible)

(b) Effects of implementing a strategy, particularly any effects that will lead to new accounting requirements (e.g., potential incomplete or improper implementation)

Measurement and review of the entity's financial performance

(a) Key ratios and operating statistics

(b) Key performance indicators

(c) Employee performance measures and incentive compensation policies

(d) Trends

(e) Use of forecasts, budgets, and variance analysis

(f) Analyst reports and credit rating reports

(g) Competitor analysis

(h) Period-on-period financial performance (revenue growth, profitability, leverage)

Internal control components

(a) Control environment

(b) Risk assessment process

(c) Information system, including the related business processes relevant to financial reporting and communication

(d) Control activities

(e) Monitoring of controls

Source: Adapted from CAS 315.

How Business Risk Is Linked To The Risk Of Material Misstatement

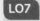 **LO7** Explain how an auditor uses an understanding of the auditee's business risk and its management risk assessment processes to assess the risk of material misstatement in the assertions of its financial statements.

To determine the risk that the financial statements could be materially misstated, the auditor learns about management's understanding of the business and its risk assessment process and independently considers how the business risk could result in material misstatements at the assertion level in the elements of the financial statements. This section describes a process the auditor may use to make this risk assessment.

The auditor knows that management has to take certain risks to achieve rewards in the marketplace. These are the risks management accepts from being in business; in effect, these risks are tolerated on a cost-benefit basis. Risks can be managed in any of four ways:

1. Avoided by not performing those business activities that would cause the risk to occur
2. Monitored to ensure costs continue to be less than benefits
3. Reduced to an acceptable level via management controls embedded in business processes
4. Transferred to another party via a contract (e.g., insurance)

After understanding the business risks, the auditor needs to consider which risks are high. He or she examines two factors in this analysis: the likelihood the risk will occur and the magnitude of the risk. Each risk is qualitatively judged according to a three-point scale on likelihood of occurrence (unlikely, possible, or likely) and magnitude of risk (insignificant, moderate, and significant). When considered together, these two factors allow the auditor to classify a risk as low, medium, or high.

Exhibit 6A–1 is a graphical representation of an auditor's risk assessment process. For example, point A indicates a business risk that will probably occur and, if so, will have a significant effect. Therefore, the auditor would classify point A as a high risk. Using a smartphone company such as Apple as an example, point A could be the risk of technological obsolescence of iPhones. Point E indicates a business risk that is unlikely to occur, and if it did it would be insignificant in size. Hence, the auditor would classify this risk as low. For a smartphone company, point E might be the risk that it will be required to change its packaging materials to comply with new environmental regulations.

Most business risks are managed through an effective risk management process and well-designed business processes, although some fall into the transferred category. The auditor considers any of the risks that might prevent the entity from carrying out its processes effectively and then identifies the risk management techniques in place to ensure efficient and effective functioning of those business processes. The risk management process can be broadly defined as the elements of an organization, including its resources, culture, structure, processes, systems, and tasks, that work together to help its people achieve the organization's objectives. See Exhibit 6A–2 for examples of risk management techniques.

The auditor can consider these risk management techniques by determining if the key performance indicators are effective at controlling the process and if management is actually using these techniques. At this

EXHIBIT 6A–1

Initial Risk Assessment

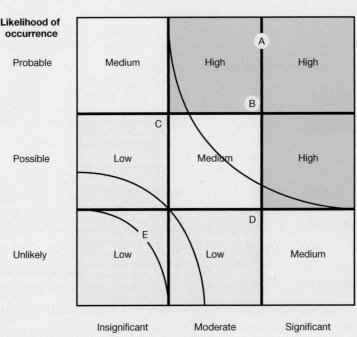

EXHIBIT 6A-2

Examples of Risk Management Techniques

- Budget systems
- Forecasting systems
- Physical measures of process performance (e.g., defect rates)
- Quality enhancement programs
- Performance indicators (both financial and non-financial)
- Process monitoring activities
- Accounting internal controls

---

point, the auditor makes a preliminary assessment of whether the risk management process is appropriate for producing reliable financial statements. The auditor then evaluates the results that effective risk management has had on the original risk analysis. Exhibit 6A–3 shows the auditor reassessing business risk after examining management's risk reduction process. The auditor has reclassified point A from a high risk to a medium-to-high risk. For the smartphone company example, say, the auditor finds the company's product development process is effective in staying ahead of the technological developments in the industry, and its sales forecasting is linked closely to production to ensure slow-moving models are taken out of production quickly. This lowers the assessed risk of obsolescence in the inventory valuation assertion. Note, however, that controls did not reduce the risks associated with point B. Point B might be the risk that smartphone production equipment assets will not last as long as planned. If management has not addressed this risk, it increases the risk that the value of those assets is impaired. Risks that are not moved into the low category by management controls represent categories for which the controls fail to reduce the risks that the financial statements do not portray the actual business performance. These are areas that need to be audited with the greatest care.

To illustrate how risk assessment works in practice, let us consider the case of a business in the food manufacturing industry. The story in the box below illustrates the kinds of risks that a food manufacturing company has to manage, and the potential financial impact.

Business Risk in the Food Industry

On Sunday, August 17, 2008, Canada's largest food processing company announced it was recalling two types of packaged roast beef products because of concerns they may have been contaminated with bacteria known as *Listeria monocytogenes*. By August 29, there were 29 confirmed and 35 suspected cases of Listeriosis, 9 confirmed deaths, another 6 deaths under investigation, and more than 200 different products pulled from store shelves across the country. Ultimately, the deaths of 20 people were attributed to this outbreak.

Consumption of food contaminated with *Listeria monocytogenes* may cause Listeriosis, a food-borne illness that can be fatal in as many as one in three cases. Listeria is very common in the environment, and fortunately it is not dangerous to most people. Very young children, the elderly, pregnant women, and people with weakened immune systems are at the greatest risk. Listeria is a particular concern in refrigerated meat-packing plants because, unlike other types of bacteria, it has adapted to survive in colder temperatures. Using a genetic identification technique called *pulsed field gel electrophoresis*, health officials were able to match the strain of Listeria people got sick from to meat products produced in Maple Leaf's Toronto plant.

Recalls can be disastrous for a company that processes food, potentially damaging its brand equity and sales volumes, but they are not uncommon. The Canadian Food Inspection Agency website lists dozens of recalls and alerts. Maple Leaf's president is credited with saving his company from ruin by responding quickly and candidly. He held news conferences and accepted responsibility for the situation, noting that the company has excellent systems and processes in place, but that in this crisis its best efforts had failed to ensure food safety. He stressed that the company's priority at this time was not

(continued)

cost or market share, its priority was to do the right thing for its customers. The Toronto plant was immediately shut down to be fully sanitized, and all aspects of the processing system were examined by outside experts. It voluntarily expanded the recall of products manufactured in this plant (Establishment No. 97B) as a precautionary measure.

The company reported that its protocol is to test the Toronto plant's surfaces for contamination 3,000 times a year. If any contamination is found, the area is sanitized and then retested until three negatives in a row are found. While positive results for Listeria inside a food plant are common, the president told reporters at the time that nothing out of the ordinary had been reported in the period leading up to the outbreak in the Toronto plant.

Stock market analysts who cover Maple Leaf remained positive about the company in the midst of the crisis, finding the company's transparency and prompt handling of the situation to be consistent with best practices in crisis management and corporate public relations. Reported estimates indicated the company spent around $5 million to deal immediately with the crisis, the company's massive recall is thought to have cost $20 million, and the potential class action suits may have cost even more.

Maple Leaf's trend to consolidate into larger processing plants can be a strength as new efficiencies can be leveraged. On the other hand, it can sometimes create a weakness, especially when something like a Listeria outbreak occurs. Centralization can increase the impact of a bacterial outbreak because any breakdown in control can affect more products. Instead of recalling 20 or 30 products, Maple Leaf had to recall hundreds that may have been affected.

Improvements in information technology that allow products to be tracked through a meat-packing plant have made recalls more effective in the meat industry. A bar code is given to each individual cut, and it can be used to trace back to the animal and the farm it came from. This can help companies manage food safety risks. This can also help reassure the public, as many customers can now be expected to look for greater assurance about where their food originates.

While Maple Leaf was able to weather this storm, future challenges are always waiting. In 2010, the company undertook an ambitious $1 billion plant modernization plan, closing down many old plants and making strategic investments in building new ones, such as the massive bakery opened in Hamilton in September, 2011. A rising Canadian dollar against the U.S. currency had a significant impact on its sales and profitability. In 2011, unprecedented global food inflation resulted in skyrocketing prices for corn and wheat, the main raw materials for many Maple Leaf products. Food prices were up 4.4% in August, including a 5% jump at stores, according to Statistics Canada. Both are a serious concern for the company—one that consumers will have to help bear.

Michael McCain, chief executive with Maple Leaf Foods Inc., said, "We have the ability to pass on that inflation through responsible pricing in the marketplace and we have done that. We do it responsibly. We look for every opportunity to reduce costs first." These issues also serve to emphasize why Maple Leaf needs to spend heavily to modernize its business lines.

Sources: Steve Buist, "From food recall to deadly outbreak," *The Hamilton Spectator*, August 30, 2008, p. A01; Robert Cribb, Record News Service, "Listeriosis reporting rule dropped before deadly outbreak," *Waterloo Region Record*, October 6, 2008, p. A1; "Maple Leaf expands product recall from Toronto Plant as a precautionary measure," *Market News Publishing*, August 25, 2008; Peter Epp, "Food origin questions arise again," *Chatham This Week*, September 3, 2008, p. 6; CP Toronto, "Maple Leaf Foods CEO admits even after intensive sanitization of the plant, 'We will never, never eliminate it . . . ,'" *London Free Press*, October 10, 2008; Eric Lam, "Higher food inflation to force Maple Leaf to raise prices," FinancialPost.com, September 28, 2011, business.financialpost.com/2011/09/28/high-food-inflation-to-force-maple-leaf-to-raise-prices/.

As the story shows, a food manufacturing company's success depends on delivering wholesome, tasty foods at reasonable prices for consumers and at a cost that ensures the company remains profitable. Since food products spoil very easily, if management does not implement effective controls, the risk of delivering spoiled food will be assessed as probable. Since spoiled food can make people ill, and even be fatal, this risk would have a very significant negative impact on the company. In the risk assessment matrix, this risk would be assessed as high. It would affect the financial statements because of the product liability contingency if consumers decide to sue the company; this risk relates to the completeness assertion for liabilities. If the brand reputation is damaged, this could even result in the company's being unable to continue as a going concern; this risk is at the overall financial statement level.

Management's risk assessment needs to ensure appropriate control techniques are embedded in the business processes; in the Maple Leaf case, this includes its safety inspection protocols and its product identification and tracking processes. The company also uses insurance as a risk-transferring management tool, though it is unlikely that all its risks can be fully insured because of the uncertainty of when food contamination or

Risk Assessment after Considering Management Controls

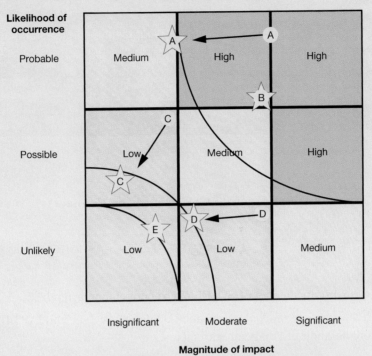

other business risks might occur. The auditor of a food manufacturing company would look for strong management controls related to these risks and would obtain first-hand information to verify them. If strong controls are in place, the assessed risk will be lower. How much lower? This is a judgment call, but there is so much uncertainty about these risks it is unlikely they can be reduced below a moderate level.

Another business risk in this industry, and in many others, arises from the use of commodity products as raw materials. Commodity prices fluctuate significantly, making it difficult to budget accurately. This can result in cost overruns that make inventory costs higher than market values, affecting the financial statement inventory valuation assertion. A risk management technique to reduce this risk is entering forward contracts with fixed prices for commodities, effectively transferring this risk to the other party in the contract.

Summary

To determine the risk that the financial statements could be materially misstated, the auditor learns about management's understanding of the business and its risk assessment process, and independently considers how the business risk could result in material misstatements at the assertion level in the elements of the financial statements. In the risk-based approach to auditing, the auditor must understand the auditee's business risk and its management risk assessment processes and control techniques to assess the risk of material misstatement in the financial statements overall and at the assertion level. The examples above illustrate how business risk and control are linked, and how auditors develop a full understanding of the auditee's business by considering them together. To provide a better understanding of the procedures companies use to implement control over financial reporting, the next chapter gives an overview of the entity's internal control structure. The auditors' understanding of internal control is key to assessing risks and designing audit work so that it gives reasonable assurance that the financial statements are not materially misstated.

Review Checkpoints

6A-1   How can business risks be managed?

6A-2   What is the relationship between business risks and business processes?

6A-3   What are some examples of management controls? What are the purposes of management controls?

6A-4   Why does the auditor consider management's controls of business processes?

6A-5   How does business analysis relate to the auditor's goal of assessing the risk that the financial statements might be materially misstated?

Appendix 6B: Corporate Governance (on Connect)

ENDNOTES

1   COSO website: coso.org/documents/COSO_ERM_ExecutiveSummary.pdf.

2   Adapted from *CPA Canada Handbook*, Assurance Guideline AuG-32, and IAPS 1013, Electronic Commerce—Effect on the Audit of Financial Statements.

3   Stay tuned: the detailed audit plan is discussed more in Chapter 8, and testing internal controls in Chapter 9.

4   CAS 240.

5   CAS 260, paragraph 16(a).

6   CAS 240, paragraphs 40–41.

7   CAS 200, paragraph 11(a).

8   CAS 315, CAS 200.

9   For audits of internal control that are integrated with a financial statement audit, use of a control framework is mandated by Public Company Accounting Oversight Board (PCAOB) Auditing Standard No. 5 and by the *CPA Canada Handbook*—Assurance, OCS 5925.

10   Stay tuned: this process is covered in more detail in Chapter 9.

11   Stay tuned: control evaluation and testing will be explained in more detail in Chapters 9 and 10.

12   CAS 315.

13   The term *amortization* is the general term for allocating capital asset costs over the years benefited. Historically and internationally, specialized names for amortization have evolved in practice. Depreciation is amortization applied to tangible capital assets, such as machinery and buildings, while the term *depletion* tends to be used for natural resources. In practice, amortization tends to be used in the more restricted sense of applying to intangible assets and premium or discount on long-term debt. For simplicity, in Exhibit 6–9 and thereafter, we treat all these allocations as specialized names for amortization.

CHAPTER 7

Internal Control over Financial Reporting

Management's internal control structure is designed and implemented to manage business risks and to produce financial statements and disclosures that are free of misstatement due to error or fraud. Business risk and control are tightly linked, and in the risk-based audit approach the auditors must consider the elements of management's control structure to gain a better understanding of how internal control can affect the audit and the risk that the financial statements will be materially misstated. Financial statement auditors also need to be aware of the risk of fraud and illegal acts and are responsible for communicating any suspicions and findings to those charged with governance.

LEARNING OBJECTIVES

After completing this chapter, you will be able to do the following:

LO1 Describe the five components of the internal control framework: the control environment, management's risk assessment process, information systems and communication, control activities, and monitoring.

LO2 Explain how the auditor's understanding of an organization's internal control helps the auditor to assess and respond to the risk that the organization's financial statements are misstated.

LO3 Differentiate among errors, frauds, and illegal acts that might occur in an organization.

LO4 Describe auditors' responsibilities to detect and report frauds, errors, and illegal acts.

LO5 Describe some of the conditions that lead to fraud risks.

LO6 **(Appendix 7A)** Describe control frameworks used for risk management in organizations, and how auditors use them for understanding an auditee's internal control.

LO7 **(Appendix 7B)** Describe fraud risk assessment and auditing procedures, and the company documents auditors can use to detect fraud.

CHAPTER APPENDICES

APPENDIX 7A   Risk and Internal Control Frameworks (on Connect)

APPENDIX 7B   Procedures and Documents Auditors Use for Fraud Detection (on Connect)

EcoPak Inc.

Mike gets involved right away in investigating EcoPak's suspected fraud, since it relates to the production operations. He and Nina describe to Tariq various changes they implemented during the prior year to make their production much more efficient in terms of the conversion of raw biomass material into finished packaging stock. EcoPak's engineers developed an innovative new process that increases the air component of the final packaging material without increasing its volume or reducing its strength. This process has now been patented. They expected the new process would drastically increase their overall contribution margin but were puzzled about why it seemed to just stick around the same percentage as before. When Mike and Nina started to dig into the production cost records and variances, they noticed that the volume usage of the key raw material had decreased as they had expected, but its costs had increased, thus offsetting any volume gains. On further investigation, they found that the main cost increases were in the raw material that is purchased solely from the plant that Zhang owns.

When they told Zhang about these discrepancies, she immediately launched an investigation that revealed that the accounts receivable manager at her plant had been adding a percentage to the selling prices of the material above the approved price list. Mike and Nina investigated on the EcoPak side and found their accounts payable manager had been approving the payments for these higher amounts. When they asked her why she had been approving what amounted to unauthorized overpayments, she apologized profusely. She had been using her authority to override the controls but never thought it would amount to a big enough difference to hurt EcoPak's profitability. She related how the accounts receivable manager at Zhang's plant had been her boyfriend. When she told him about EcoPak's new process that would lead to them purchasing lower quantities of the material his company supplies to them, it gave him the idea for the scam. A lack of segregation of duties at his company allowed him to inflate the selling prices and then skim off the excess amounts when he received the inflated payments from EcoPak. But for his scam to succeed, he needed his girlfriend to override the controls at EcoPak. She said they used the money at first to do a bit of gambling and take a luxury cruise. Then, about two weeks ago, she confronted him about stopping the whole scheme because it was starting to seem really bad, and they broke up.

Zhang was absolutely outraged when she heard the whole story: "Both these people are stealing from our company. They must be fired instantly, and I will do everything I can to see they never work again in our industry!" While Tariq feels very bad that EcoPak had to experience such a tawdry fraud, he realizes that the incident shows EcoPak does have some strong management level controls: Mike and Nina's monitoring of the costs and variances allowed them to notice right away that their reported results did not mesh with what had been going on in their operation. And there was a control over paying the authorized prices—it had to be overridden by collusion for the fraud to proceed. However, he also realized that even the best controls can be overridden by those given authority, who are trusted to apply them. For Tariq, this is a good reminder that fraud risk always needs to be kept in mind in auditing a company (and managing it, too!).

Tariq took Nina out for lunch soon after the dust settled. They compared stories about their university accounting courses when they first learned about fraud, and Nina exclaimed, "I never thought it would actually happen to my company!" She then told Tariq an amazing story. "A couple of weeks ago, I got a call from a guy who claimed to be an 'IFRS consultant' from one of the big investment firms. He said he'd heard we were planning to do an IPO soon, and he could really help us 'make our financial statements shine.' He said he could help us get significantly higher price for our shares when we first issue them to the public. He said he knew lots of tricks 'to plump up your balance sheet' that he'd learned from companies such as WorldCom and Enron. He said those stories happened so long ago that nobody remembers them any more, not even the auditors, so they will work again. I couldn't believe my ears! I tried to find out more about who he works for, but he cut me off saying he had another important call. I even tried to trace the number but it was blocked. Wow, it takes all kinds, I guess!"

On his way home, Tariq reflected on all these events, and the business relations he has been building with Nina, Mike, Kam, and Zhang. It all made him realize he was getting a good feeling about management's integrity at EcoPak.

The Essentials of Internal Control over Financial Reporting

Management's internal control structure is designed and implemented to manage business risks and to produce fairly presented financial statements and disclosures. Business risk and control are tightly linked, and in the risk-based audit approach the auditors must consider the elements of management's control structure to gain a better understanding of how internal control can affect the audit and the risk that the financial statements will be materially misstated.

To understand internal control that is relevant to the audit, generally accepted auditing standards (GAAS) suggest that auditors use an *internal control framework* to identify different aspects of the structure. This internal control framework has the following five components: (a) *control environment*; (b) *management risk assessment process*; (c) *information system*, including the related business processes relevant to financial reporting and communication; (d) *control activities*; and (e) *monitoring of controls*.

The control environment relates to the tone set by the top people in the organization, which will strongly influence the culture and ethical attitudes of everyone throughout. The control environment, risk assessment process, information system, and control monitoring elements of this framework are all *company-level controls* that have a pervasive and organization-wide impact that can affect the quality of the financial statements, albeit indirectly. The *control activities* are control procedures that relate to specific processes, applications, and transactions that are more directly related to accounting information, so these are very relevant to the audit. The auditor is primarily interested in how these accounting control activities help a company safeguard assets and prepare financial statements that comply with generally accepted accounting principles (GAAP).

Misstatements can arise in financial statements from either error or fraud. Errors are unintentional mistakes in amounts or disclosures in financial statements. Frauds are intentional misstatements or omissions in financial statements with an intent to deceive others, including fraudulent financial reporting and misappropriation of assets. Misappropriation of assets fraud is often called "fraud against the company" because it is usually carried out by lower-level employees, and management and auditors have a common interest in detecting such fraud. In contrast, fraudulent financial reporting (issuing misleading financial statements) is fraud by the company against new investors, so it puts the auditor in a fight against the auditee's management and those charged with governance of the reporting entity.

Management and those charged with governance carry the primary responsibility for prevention and detection of fraud. This responsibility includes designing and implementing internal controls and other corporate governance mechanisms to deter fraud. Since GAAS require auditors to obtain reasonable assurance that financial statements are free of material misstatement due to error or fraud, auditors are responsible for assessing fraud risk. Since fraud involves an intent to deceive, it will be deliberately concealed from auditors, so auditors must always give special consideration to the possibility that fraud has occurred.

Auditors do not determine whether a fraud or illegal act has occurred; only a court of law can make this determination. Auditors assess fraud risk by asking management about fraud and by identifying fraud risk factors noted during the auditor's risk assessment procedures. The auditor should also obtain written management representations about management's suspicions or knowledge of any actual fraud and its extent. If the auditors find factors that raise a suspicion that fraud may be occurring, this possibility needs to be followed up to confirm or dispel the suspicion. Auditors must always assume fraud risk exists for revenue recognition. Any findings that indicate a possible fraud should be discussed among the audit team members, including the audit partner and most-experienced personnel. A suspicion of fraud that an audit team cannot dispel has to be communicated to appropriate levels of management and those charged with governance (e.g., the audit committee). As a general rule, the auditor should communicate any suspicion of fraud to a level of management or governance above the level thought to be involved in the fraud. The auditor may be required to report fraud to outside agencies, and in this case would need to get legal advice because this would conflict with the auditor's professional ethics requirement to keep client information confidential.

When is fraud most likely to occur? The probability of fraud is a function of three factors, known as the fraud triangle: motive, opportunity, and lack of integrity. When one or more of these factors weigh heavily in the direction of fraud, the probability increases. GAAS recommend these factors as a framework for linking sources of these risks to audit procedures. Auditors use these risk factors as guides for evaluating whether the risk of material fraud is at acceptable levels.

Motives refer to incentives or pressures to try to gain from fraud and may include personal financial needs or a strong desire by management to achieve certain profit targets for personal gain (e.g., performance bonuses or stock options). Lack of integrity refers to a person's attitude and ability to rationalize how their fraudulent actions are justified, which can arise when the company's control environment does not set a high-level "tone at the top" and expectation for honest behaviour. Opportunities often arise from poor internal control or when people can collude to circumvent controls. Since management can always override controls (after all, they are responsible for implementing them), the risk of management fraud through misleading financial statements is the most problematic for auditors.

Auditors must also consider whether management has been involved in any illegal acts. The auditors' knowledge of the business and inquiries of management help to identify laws and regulations that, if violated and not reported, could result in material misstatements. In addition, auditors should obtain management representations about awareness and disclosure of possibly illegal acts. The auditor is mainly concerned about non-compliance with laws that directly affect the financial statements, such as tax and pension laws. However, the auditor also needs to consider any non-compliance with other laws that could indirectly affect the financial statements. For example, if the violations could lead to substantial fines or closure of operations, they could affect the company's ability to continue as a going concern. Management's failure to comply with laws and regulations that affect its operations can have a significant negative impact on a company.

Auditors are responsible under GAAS for communicating with those charged with governance when they become aware of any possible fraud or non-compliance with laws or regulations. In some cases, auditors may also communicate about these issues to appropriate levels of management. Generally, suspected fraud and illegal acts will be reported to a level of management above the level suspected to be involved.

Review Checkpoints

7-1   What is the purpose of management's internal control structure? Why do auditors need to understand it?

7-2   What is an internal control framework, and how is it used in a financial statement audit?

7-3   Describe the five components of an internal control framework.

7-4   Distinguish between the internal control elements that are company-level controls and those that are control activities. Which of these types is most directly relevant to a financial statement audit? Why?

7-5   What are management's main purposes in implementing control activities?

7-6   Why do financial statement auditors have a responsibility to consider the risk of fraud?

7-7   What is the essential difference between and error and fraud?

7-8   Distinguish between fraud that involves theft of company assets and fraud that involves presenting misleading financial statements. Who is likely to be responsible for each type? Which is of greater concern to an auditor? Why?

7-9   Who has the primary responsibility for preventing and detecting fraud in a company?

7-10   What procedures do auditors use to assess fraud risk? What are an auditor's responsibilities if a fraud is suspected?

7-11   Identify and explain the three factors that make it more likely that a fraud will occur.

7-12   What are illegal acts? When and why would an independent financial statement auditor be concerned about them?

7-13   What communication responsibilities do auditors have regarding any suspicions or knowledge of fraud or illegal acts in an auditee?

Understanding Internal Control

LO1   Describe the five components of the internal control framework: the control environment, management's risk assessment process, information systems and communication, control activities, and monitoring.

Chapter 6 covered the risk-based approach to auditing by explaining the audit risk model and how auditors analyze the auditee's business risk to assess the risk of material misstatement. This is the most challenging part of financial statement auditing, requiring integration of complex concepts and the application of professional judgment. Congratulations for sticking it out to this point in the text! Chapter 6 also stressed that business risk and internal control are so tightly linked that auditors need to consider them together. At this point in an audit, the audit team would begin considering internal control in relation to their understanding of the business risk in order to assess the risk of material misstatement in the financial statements. Chapter 7 will continue this explanation of risk and control by giving an overview of internal control as it exists in most organizations, and then considering how internal control relates to the risk that the financial statements are materially misstated at the assertion level for the main classes of transactions, account balances, and disclosures. These assertion-level risk assessments are used to design audit procedures that respond appropriately to the assessed risks. This chapter will also specifically consider the risk of misstatement due to fraud (intentional misstatements). In Chapter 8, we will introduce you to some key audit tools: the concepts of evidence and the types of audit procedures used to gather it. These procedures are designed in response to the auditor's assertion-level risk assessments. With these tools in hand, you will be ready for Chapter 9, where we will discuss in more detail how auditors assess control risk and test specific controls.

Internal Control Framework and Its Components

For financial statement audit purposes, internal control is defined as the process designed, implemented, and maintained by management and other auditee personnel to provide reasonable assurance about the reliability of financial reporting, effectiveness and efficiency of operations, and compliance with applicable laws and regulations. The

Standards Check

CAS 315 Identifying and Assessing the Risks of Material Misstatement through Understanding the Entity and Its Environment

A51.   The division of internal control into the following five components, for the purposes of the CASs, provides a useful framework for auditors to consider how different aspects of an entity's internal control may affect the audit:

(a) Control environment;

(b) Entity's risk assessment process;

(c) The information system, including the related business processes relevant to financial reporting and communication;

(d) Control activities; and

(e) Monitoring of controls.

The division does not necessarily reflect how an entity designs, implements, and maintains internal control, or how it may classify any particular component. Auditors may use different terminology or frameworks to describe the various aspects of internal control, and their effect on the audit, than those used in this CAS, provided all the components described in this CAS are addressed.

Source: *CPA Canada Handbook—Assurance*, 2014.

auditing standard CAS 315, paragraph A51 (see above), describes internal control. An overview of COSO's internal control framework is given in Exhibit 7–1; in this text we focus on the financial reporting part of this framework.

These components provide a comprehensive basis for considering how different aspects of an entity's internal control may affect the financial statements. Control components (a), (b), (c), and (e) of CAS 315, paragraph A51, above, constitute the **company-level controls**. These controls permeate the organization and can have a big impact on whether its financial reporting and disclosures objectives are met. As discussed earlier, control component (b) includes the risk assessment processes and management control techniques implemented to assess adherence to management policy, promote operational efficiencies, and address strategic risks. The auditor's examination of these management risk assessment processes and controls is particularly useful for identifying accounting items with the highest risk of material misstatement. As discussed in Chapter 5, these are areas that will be flagged in the overall audit strategy as "significant risks" or "key audit areas" for the purpose of planning the resources required to do the audit.

Component (d), the **control activities**, comprises controls over processes, applications, and transactions more closely related to accounting information; these are the internal controls most relevant to the audit. The auditor is primarily interested in how these accounting control activities help a company safeguard its assets and prepare financial statements that comply with GAAP.[1]

Audits of small entities may require different control considerations than audits of large ones do. In a small entity, there is a concentration of ownership and management in one person or a small number of people. There are likely also few sources of income, unsophisticated recordkeeping, and limited internal controls, together with the potential for management override of controls.[2]

The five control components illustrated in Exhibit 7–1 are further described below, and in Appendix 7A (available on Connect). Special internal control considerations of small entities are also addressed.

company-level controls:
internal control framework components that permeate the organization and affect the quality of its financial reporting and disclosures, consisting of the control environment; the entity's risk assessment process; the information system, including the related business processes, relevant to financial reporting and communication; and monitoring of controls

control activities:
specific company procedures designed to control processes, transactions, and applications that affect accounting information; consisting of general control activities and application-based control activities

EXHIBIT 7–1

Internal Control Framework—Overview

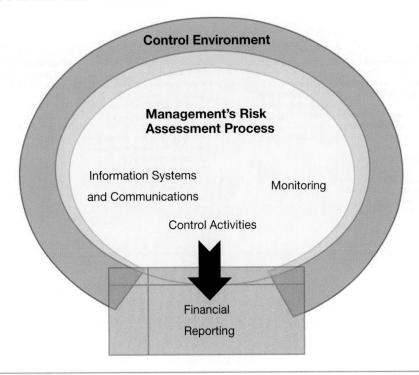

Exhibit 7–2 summarizes the key elements of the company-level controls and illustrates how they influence the effectiveness of the control activities.

Control Environment

Management's and directors' attitudes, awareness, and actions concerning the company's internal controls set the tone for the **control environment**. The way that integrity and ethical values are communicated and enforced in the company is also part of the control environment because the controls cannot be more effective than the integrity levels and ethical values of the people who create, administer, and monitor them. Management must act to remove or reduce incentives and temptations motivating people in the organization to act unethically. It must assess requisite skills and knowledge for particular jobs, ensuring that people in those positions are competent. Directors or others charged with governance of the organization should be independent from management and experienced and knowledgeable enough to pursue difficult questions with management as well as internal and external auditors. They should be responsible for the design and effective operation of whistle-blower procedures, and they should be engaged in a process for assessing internal control effectiveness.

Management's approach to taking and monitoring business risks, attitudes toward financial reporting (conservative or aggressive selection of accounting principles and use of accounting estimates), and controls are critical to the strength of the control environment. To set the right example, management should react immediately and appropriately to control violations. Clear policies relating to appropriate business practices, knowledge and

control environment:
the attitudes, operating styles, capabilities, and actions of an organization's governance and management functions in relation to the organization's internal control that can provide the resources, policies, and discipline to establish a "tone at the top" that is conducive to the organization meeting its strategic objectives, providing reliable internal and external financial reporting, and operating efficiently and ethically; considered to be the foundation for all other components of internal control (i.e., control activities, management's risk assessment process, information system and communication, monitoring)

EXHIBIT 7–2

Control Framework for Risk Assessment

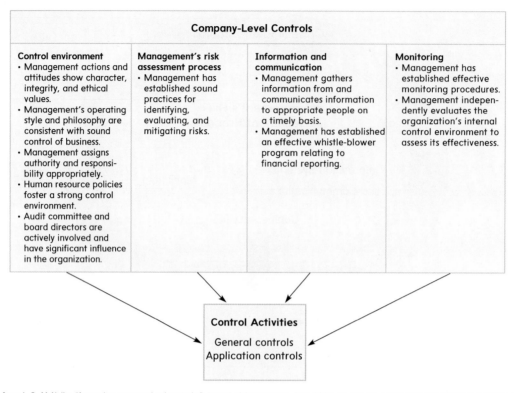

experience of key personnel, and resources for carrying out duties should be in place. Policies should ensure that all personnel understand the entity's objectives, know how their individual actions interrelate, contribute to those objectives, and are aware of what they will be held accountable for.

The control environment is concerned with management attitudes, structure (organization chart), effective communication of control objectives, and supervision of personnel and activities, as noted previously. The elements of internal control environments are summarized in the following box.

Key Elements of the Internal Control Environment

- Management's philosophy and operating style
- Entity's organization structure
- Functioning of the board of directors, particularly its audit committee
- Methods of assigning authority and responsibility
- Management's monitoring methods, including internal auditing
- Personnel policies and practices
- External influences (e.g., examinations by bank regulatory agencies)
- Control environment for information systems, which includes the organizational and logical controls of system development, access to computers and computer files, authorization of changes to program and data files, storage and maintenance of data, and emergency planning for backup and recovery of systems and data

Two categories of controls are **preventive controls** and **detective controls**. Preventive controls are more effective than detective controls, because detective controls only come into play after misstatements have entered the system and must be accompanied by appropriate procedures to correct the misstatement. Corrective accounting procedures are challenging, as you will have seen in your financial accounting courses, so overall it is always more effective (and less risky) if errors can be prevented in the first place. Generally, environmental controls can be characterized as preventive controls, since they are there to prevent misstatements from arising in the first place. Auditors tend to focus their preliminary evaluation on environmental controls for this reason and also because they have such a pervasive impact on the accounting processes affected.

Since the mid-1980s, when existence of management fraud in financial statements became more open to public discussion, "tone at the top" has become a catchphrase for the foundation of good internal control; company tone is virtually identical to control environment. A wide variety of activities characterize the control environment, some of them obvious, such as who has the immediate responsibility to authorize payments in payroll processing. Other aspects of the control environment, such as management's philosophy, are hard for auditors to understand and document. The following box illustrates some criteria to consider in evaluating the human factor in the control environment.

Tone at the Top

All control rests ultimately on people assuming responsibility for their decisions and actions. Organizational values that people find acceptable encourage them to assume responsibility for the continuous improvement of their organization.

Shared ethical values influence all behaviour in an organization. Together with an understanding of mission and vision, they constitute the basic identity that will shape the way an individual, group, organization, or board will operate, and they provide stability over time. Shared values contribute to control because they provide a guide for individual, group, or team decision making, action, and policy.

The values and preferences of senior management and the board of directors greatly influence an organization's objectives and systems. These values and preferences address issues such as the following:

- Good corporate citizenship
- Commitment to truth and fair dealing
- Commitment to quality and competence
- Leadership by example
- Compliance with laws, regulations, rules, and organizational policy
- Respect for the privacy of auditee, organization, and employee information
- Fair treatment of and respect for individuals
- Fair relationships with competitors
- Commitment to ensuring integrity of transactions and records
- A professional approach to financial reporting

Ethical values are part of an organization's culture and provide an unwritten code of conduct against which behaviour is measured. A formal written code of conduct offers a means for consistent communication of the standards of ethical behaviour. People can periodically be asked to confirm their understanding and observance of the code.

Source: *CPA Canada Handbook—Guidance of the Criteria of Control Committee*, 2015, paragraphs 57, 59, 60, and 63..

The board of directors and the audit committee are critical corporate governance elements of high-level internal control. Among the board's key functions is monitoring that traditionally least-monitored group of employees—top management. In the wake of the Enron and other accounting scandals, the role of the board

preventive controls:
control procedures designed primarily to ensure that error or fraud does not occur in the first place in the accounting information system

detective controls:
control procedures designed to detect any error or fraud that has occurred in the accounting information system; must also be accompanied by appropriate procedures designed to effectively correct any errrors

and audit committee in monitoring management and financial reporting rose to unprecedented levels. The audit committee, usually a subcommittee of the board's members, helps the board by overseeing the financial reporting as well as external and internal auditing functions. The audit committee's prime role is to act as intermediary between management and the auditor in the external audit, helping make it function more independently.[3]

Small entities may use the control environment elements differently than larger entities; for example, they may rely on oral communication and personal relations to establish ethical standards, rather than using more-formal methods. Directors of small entities are less likely to be independent of management, and owners are more likely to be involved in managing day-to-day operations.

Management's Risk Assessment Process

As explained earlier, **management's risk assessment process** is used to identify risks relevant to misstatements occurring in the preparation of financial statements and to estimate the risks' significance and likelihood. It helps management to decide how to manage the business risk efficiently and effectively. Risks can arise or change with changing circumstances, so risk assessment is a continuous process. The operating environment, personnel changes, growth, new technologies, new business lines, structural changes in the organization, and new accounting pronouncements can affect the risk assessment.

Even small entities are expected to have a risk assessment process, but it is likely to be quite basic and informal. Management may be aware of risks related to financial reporting mainly through personal involvement with employees and outside parties.

Information Systems, Related Business Processes, and Communication

An **information system** can be broadly defined as a set of interrelated functions that collect, process, store, and distribute information in an organization. It is used to support management decisions and to help people in the organization perform analysis, develop models, collaborate on projects, and create knowledge. An information system has three main activities: input, processing, and output. The input is mainly data, the raw facts collected from the environment. Processing converts data into output in an understandable and useful form referred to as information. Many information systems are highly automated, making extensive use of information technology (IT). The components of an information system are hardware, software, people, procedures, and data.

Information Systems and Business Processes

The information system is related to all of the key business processes. It is important that the auditor understand how the information system relates to financial reporting, and how it is used to communicate information within the organization. In organizations with enterprise resource planning systems (ERPs), the information inputs and outputs from many or all of the business processes will be processed in an integrated manner, so the accounting component of the information system will be closely related to many other functional areas, such as sales, inventory, human resources, and cash management. Within the business process view, logical links exist between information generated in various processes and the accounting component of the information system.

The quality of system-generated information affects management's ability to make appropriate decisions in managing and controlling the entity's activities and in preparing reliable financial reports. The auditor needs to understand how the auditee's information system is used in its financial reporting process and identify the risks associated with IT use. Financial reporting objectives rely on information system procedures and records

management's risk assessment process:
the methods used by an organization's management to identify the risks to be managed, including those that can lead to misstated financial information, and to determine appropriate actions; see *entity's risk assessment process*

information system:
a set of interrelated functions that collect, process, store, and distribute information in an organization; in relation to financial reporting, the manual and technology-based procedures and records used in the accounting system to capture and report an organization's transactions, events, and conditions to maintain accountability for the related assets, liabilities, and equity and ensure information required to be disclosed is appropriately reported in the financial statements

established to initiate, record, process, and report entity transactions (and events and conditions) as well as to maintain accountability for the related assets, liabilities, and equity.[4]

Communication

Communication helps ensure that information system control procedures are implemented correctly and exceptions are reported and acted on appropriately. Good communications procedures help ensure that important tasks do not just fall between the cracks because no one was sure whose job it was to do them.

The auditor must understand how the information system facilitates communications within the organization, in particular those aspects that relate to implementation of internal control. Internal control involves activities, policies, and procedures ensuring that threats that may prevent the business from achieving its strategy are addressed. Control activities occur within both IT and manual processes, have various objectives, and are applied at various organizational and functional levels; thus, effective communication is essential for internal control to work properly.

Open communications enhance internal control effectiveness. Employees involved in financial reporting must understand their individual roles and responsibilities in implementing internal control, as well as how their activities relate to the work. Communications policies show the importance of employees reporting and acting on control exceptions immediately and establish appropriate channels for reporting these to appropriate levels within the organization. Communication media include accounting and financial reporting manuals, policy manuals, and internal memoranda. Communications can be performed electronically, orally, and through management's actions.

Business processes and information systems in small entities are likely to be less formal than in larger organizations, but they are just as important. In small entities, accounting procedures, records, or controls may not be in writing but will exist informally if the organization has a good risk assessment process and related internal controls. If management is highly involved in the business processes, there may be no need for extensive written descriptions of company policies or accounting procedures. Communication may also be less formal and easier to achieve, as fewer people are involved and management tends to be more accessible to other employees than is the case in larger, more hierarchical organizations.

Review Checkpoints

7-14   What are the five basic components of internal control?

7-15   What are the basic functions and components of an information system? How do information system functions relate to financial statement assertions?

7-16   How does the information system facilitate communication within an organization? Why is this communication important?

7-17   What are some of the important characteristics of "tone at the top" and control environment?

7-18   Are environmental controls preventive or detective/corrective? Explain.

Accounting Control Activities

Companies have many policies and procedures that help ensure necessary actions are taken to prevent risks threatening the entity's financial reporting objectives. As explained previously in this chapter, the auditor uses a **control framework (internal control framework, internal control structure)** to understand and evaluate the auditee's internal control. Control policies and procedures make up the control activities component of

communication:
the procedures and channels used to process and share information among people in an organization to enhance understanding and effectiveness, including accounting policies, control activities, and people's roles and responsibilities

control framework (internal control framework, internal control structure):
a model used to present the different elements of an organization's internal control structure and how they fit together, useful to auditors for documenting their understanding of an auditee's internal control over financial reporting; the control framework developed by COSO is commonly used by auditors because it is recommended by generally accepted auditing standards

the company's control framework. All control procedures are directed, one way or another, toward preventing, or detecting and correcting, misstatements that may arise due to error or fraud. Note that detection controls must always be accompanied by corrective actions in order to be effective. The two broad groups of accounting control activities are **general controls** and **application controls**. These will be introduced briefly here and described in more detail in the context of testing controls in Chapter 9.

General Controls

General controls include organizational features, such as capable personnel, segregation of responsibilities, controlled access, and periodic comparison. Like environmental controls, general controls are primarily preventive and have a pervasive impact on the various accounting processes. For these reasons, an auditor's preliminary evaluation of internal controls tends to focus on environmental and general controls.

Application Controls

Application controls are viewed in terms of whether they relate to data input, processing, or output of the accounting system. They help ensure that all recorded transactions really occurred, are authorized, and are completely and accurately entered and processed through the system. The different accounting processes—revenues/receivables/receipts, purchases/payables/payments, production/payroll, and investing/financing—each has its own risks that lead to errors or make the business susceptible to fraud or other illegal acts. Thus, specific application control procedures are designed to address the risks and control objectives for each accounting process.

Examples of application controls are

1. Authorization checks prior to data input

2. Arithmetical checks of the accuracy of records

3. Maintenance and review of accounts and trial balances

4. Automated information processing controls such as validity checks of input data and numerical sequence checks

5. Manual follow-up of exception reports

Application controls are explained in more detail in Chapter 9, where we look at control testing, and in Chapters 11 through 14, where they form part of the detailed audit programs applied to the accounting processes.

Higher-level policies established by management or those charged with governance are the basis for certain control activities. For example, authorization controls may be delegated under established guidelines or under non-routine transactions, such as major acquisitions, which may require specific high-level approval, in some cases that of shareholders. This further illustrates the relationship between the control environment, other company-level controls, and the specific control activities that auditors may test and rely on for audit evidence purposes.

Control activities in small entities are likely to be similar to those in larger entities, but less formal. Certain types of control activities may not be relevant in a small owner-managed entity because of controls applied by management. For example, if the owner-manager retains authority for approving credit sales, significant purchases, and draw-downs on lines of credit, this can provide strong control over those activities, reducing the need for more-structured control activities. Note, however, that in a less structured control system, the risk of management overriding controls is greater, which auditors need to consider when assessing fraud risk. An appropriate segregation of duties often presents difficulties in small entities. Even companies with only a few employees, however, may be able to assign responsibilities so that there is appropriate segregation, or, if that is not possible, management may monitor the incompatible activities to achieve control objectives.

general controls:
organizational features that have a pervasive impact on accounting processes and applications and the effectiveness of application-level control procedures

application controls:
control procedures performed at the application level relating to data input, processing, and output in an accounting information system

Monitoring Controls

An important management responsibility is establishing and maintaining internal control on an ongoing basis. This includes considering whether controls are operating as intended and modifying them as appropriate for changes in conditions. It may include reviews of the timeliness of bank reconciliations, evaluation of sales personnel's compliance with entity policies by internal auditors, and oversight of compliance with entity ethical or business practice policies by the legal department.

Monitoring of controls assesses the quality of internal control performance over time and involves considering the design and operation of controls, including taking necessary corrective actions to ensure the controls' continued effective operation. For example, if the timeliness and accuracy of bank reconciliations are not monitored, personnel are likely to stop preparing them. Monitoring of controls is accomplished through ongoing monitoring activities, separate evaluations, or a combination of the two.

These activities are built into an entity's regular, recurring activities and include regular management and supervisory activities. Managers of sales, purchasing, and production at divisional and corporate levels stay in touch with operations and question reports that differ significantly from what they know of operations. Internal auditors or personnel performing similar functions may contribute to the monitoring of an entity's controls through separate evaluations of the design and operation of internal control. They communicate information about strengths, weaknesses, and recommendations for improving internal control.

Information from external parties may be part of monitoring activities, if it indicates problems or highlights areas in need of improvement. Customers corroborate billing data by either paying their invoices or questioning their charges. Suppliers may raise questions about late or incorrect payments of invoices, indicating problems in the purchasing and payment controls. Management monitoring activities may consider information relating to internal control from external auditors.

Ongoing monitoring activities of smaller entities are likely to be informal and performed as a part of the overall management of the entity's operations. Through close involvement in operations, management might identify significant variances from expectations and inaccuracies in financial data and ensure corrective action is taken.

Review Checkpoints

7-19 What is the auditor's main purpose in understanding the auditee's internal control system?

7-20 What are monitoring controls?

7-21 Describe and distinguish among the control environment, general controls, and application controls.

7-22 What organizational features can act as general controls?

7-23 What is the purpose of application controls? How does it differ from the purpose of general controls?

How Internal Control Relates to the Risk of Material Misstatement

LO2 Explain how the auditor's understanding of an organization's internal control helps the auditor to assess and respond to the risk that the organization's financial statements are misstated.

Audit work related to internal control involves understanding control in the context of the business and its risks, assessing significant risks of financial statement misstatement, and performing tests of controls if needed to

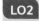

monitoring:
management's ongoing process for reviewing and assessing whether the control procedures in place are adequate to address control risks and are operating effectively as intended, and determining areas that need improvement

further assess risks or provide audit evidence. This section discusses how the auditor's understanding of internal control helps in assessing the overall risk of material misstatement. It reviews the key components of internal control, with a particular focus on the controls that relate to financial reporting and disclosure.

As discussed above, the internal control framework includes company-level controls (control environment, risk assessment process, information systems and communication, and monitoring) and control activities (general and application). Exhibit 7–1 showed how these components are related and work to support each other.

To assess the risk of material misstatement at the financial statement level, the auditor needs a detailed knowledge of internal control components relevant to financial reporting; these components are the control environment elements that affect financial reporting and the information system.

The auditor gains knowledge mainly by making inquiries of auditee personnel. This provides an understanding of the flow of transactions through the accounting information system and the elements of the control environment that affect it. The auditor gathers information about the following features: (a) the organizational structure; (b) the methods used by the auditee to communicate responsibility and authority; (c) the methods used by management to supervise the accounting information systems, including the existence of an internal audit function; and (d) the accounting information system. A questionnaire is sometimes used to guide the inquiries. An example of a questionnaire summarizing some key questions an auditor asks is provided in Exhibit 7–3. It is important to note that while standardized questionnaires and other audit forms are helpful starting points, the auditor must always use care to adapt them to the specific circumstances of the auditee's business and risks by adding any missing considerations and omitting any items that are not applicable to the engagement.

EXHIBIT 7–3

Internal Control Questionnaire

RESPONSE/FILE
DOCUMENTATION
REFERENCE

Purpose: This questionnaire is used to document information gathered through inquiries about the key internal control elements related to financial reporting. This information supports an assessment of the risk of material misstatement at the overall financial statement level.

Consider the effectiveness of the following internal control elements to reduce the risk of material misstatement of the financial statements. Consider the impact of internal control effectiveness on the audit plan to obtain evidence.

The Organizational Structure
The organizational structure defines how the organization plans, executes, controls, and reviews the activities that it undertakes to achieve its strategic objectives.
   Obtain information about the key organizational structure aspects that relate to accounting information systems:
- The corporate structure, whether there are subsidiaries or other components in different locations, and how their information systems are integrated
- Management's attitudes and actions toward financial reporting, information processing, accounting functions, and personnel
- Ownership and relations between owners and other parties; how the information system identifies related party transactions
- How authority and responsibility for information system operating activities are assigned
- How reporting relationships and authorization hierarchies are established
- Policies and practices for hiring, training, evaluation, promotion, and compensation, as well as for remedial actions for accounting and IT personnel
- A description of the company's information system and IT resources, including personnel within the IT department, interaction with personnel in other departments, details of computer equipment used, the use of an outside services centre, if any, and locations from which the computer resources can be accessed

Consider:
- Is access controlled to information systems used to process accounting information? Are the company policies regarding access only by authorized personnel adequate?
- Are responsibilities segregated appropriately between systems and programming staff and operations personnel?
- Is the information systems function integrated with the overall organization structure?

(continued)

EXHIBIT 7–3

Internal Control Questionnaire *(continued)*

Methods Used to Communicate Responsibility and Authority

Obtain information about

- Accounting and other policy manuals, including IT operations and user manuals
- Formal job descriptions for accounting and IT personnel
- Related user personnel job descriptions that may also be helpful
- How information system resources are managed and how priorities are determined
- How other non-accounting departments within the company understand how they must comply with financial information processing, related standards, and procedures

Consider:

- Are communications between user departments and the information systems department open and adequate to determine whether system controls are effective and to detect and correct any processing errors that arise?

Methods Used by Management to Supervise the System

Obtain information about the procedures used to supervise the information system, including

- Existence of systems design and documentation standards and the extent to which they are used
- Existence and quality of procedures for system and program modification, systems acceptance approval, and output modification (such as changes in reports or files)
- Procedures limiting access to authorized information, particularly with respect to sensitive information
- Availability of financial and other reports, such as budget/performance reviews for use by management
- Existence of an internal audit function and the degree of its involvement in reviewing computer-produced accounting records and related controls, and its involvement in systems development control evaluation and testing

Consider:

- Are management supervision procedures adequate to maintain the overall accuracy and authorization of the information processed and reports generated by information systems?

RESPONSE/FILE
DOCUMENTATION
REFERENCE

The Accounting Information System

The accounting information system includes the accounting processes as well as procedures and records that the organization uses to meet its financial reporting objectives. These objectives include reporting financial transactions, events, and conditions; maintaining records needed for accountability for the organization's assets, liabilities, and equity; and compliance with laws and regulations.

Obtain information about the accounting information system and the flow of transactions to understand the information systems relevant to financial reporting, including

- Significant classes of transactions arising from the organization's business processes, such as selling, purchasing, producing goods and services, and recording financial and non-financial information for reporting and management control purposes
- IT and manual procedures that initiate, record, process, and report transactions, including period-end cutoff procedures
- Electronic or manual accounting records and information supporting transactions
- Use of information systems to capture significant events and conditions other than transactions
- Financial reporting processes, significant accounting estimates, and disclosures
- Procedures to transfer information from processing systems (e.g., accounts receivable subledger) to general ledger or financial reporting systems
- Use of standard, recurring journal entries to record transactions, such as sales, purchases, and cash disbursements, in the general ledger (e.g., daily sales journal entries), or to record periodic accounting estimates (e.g., amortization).
- Use of non-standard journal entries to record non-recurring, unusual transactions or adjustments (e.g., changes in estimated uncollectible accounts receivable, asset disposals or asset impairment estimates, consolidating adjustments) for manual, paper-based general ledger systems identified through inspection of ledgers, journals, and supporting documentation or for automated general ledger systems, where such entries may exist only in electronic form identified through the use of computer-assisted audit techniques
- Procedures that ensure information for disclosures required by the applicable financial reporting framework is accumulated, recorded, processed, summarized, and appropriately reported
- How the incorrect processing of transactions is resolved (e.g., a suspense file, how it is cleared on a timely basis)
- How authorized system control overrides are processed and accounted for
- Risks of material misstatement associated with inappropriate override of controls over journal entries and the controls surrounding non-standard journal entries, including automated journal entries that produce no visible evidence of intervention in the information systems

Consider:

- Is the accounting system designed and operated to ensure the organization's financial reporting objectives are met, such that all relevant financial transactions, events, and conditions are captured and reported; accurate records needed for accountability for assets, liabilities, and equity are kept; and compliance with laws and regulations is maintained?

Review Checkpoints

7-24   What kinds of knowledge does the auditor gather to understand internal control and assess the risk of material misstatement?

7-25   Compare and contrast company-level controls and internal controls relevant to the audit.

7-26   What are the two main types of control activities that are used in information systems?

7-27   What aspects of the accounting system are relevant to financial reporting objectives?

7-28   What misstatement risks might not be eliminated by automated control procedures? How does this possibility affect the audit?

7-29   Why do auditors seek information about the use of non-standard journal entries?

Through the inquiries noted in Exhibit 7–3, the audit team gains an understanding of the control environment, the accounting information system, and the flow of transactions. Auditors consider the auditee's methods for processing significant accounting information, including the use of outside organizations such as data-processing service centres. The auditee's methods influence the design of the accounting system, the nature of its control procedures, and the extent to which its internal control effectively reduces its financial reporting risks. This, in turn, affects the auditors' assessment of the risk of material misstatement and how they plan to conduct their audit.

Exhibit 7–4 summarizes the components of the financial reporting process. It illustrates how the auditee's business risk, processes, information systems, and controls result in production of the information reported in management's financial statements. The auditee's business and its environment generate the activities that are captured, monitored, and controlled by the information systems, which include manual and automated processes. The information systems are based on a financial reporting framework, usually GAAP, and internal control elements related to financial reporting. This section concludes the introduction to the business risk–based audit approach and the knowledge-gathering work auditors perform to identify the main risks of material misstatement at the overall financial statement level.

EXHIBIT 7–4

The Financial Reporting Process in an Auditee Company

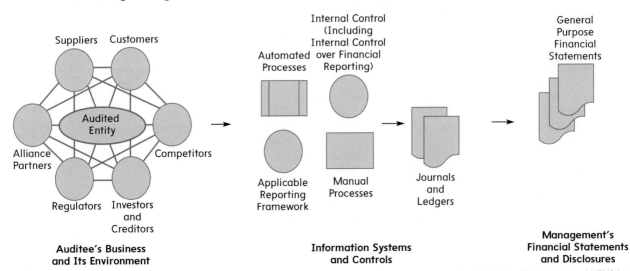

Source: Timothy B. Bell, Mark E. Peecher, and Ira Solomon, *The 21st Century Public Company Audit: Conceptual Elements of KPMG's Global Audit of Methodology*, p. 4 (KPMG International © 2005).

Internal Control and Fraud Detection

Management and those charged with governance are responsible for preventing and detecting fraud. They meet this responsibility by designing and implementing effective internal controls and other corporate governance mechanisms to deter fraud. A 2012 study by the Association of Certified Fraud Examiners showed that over 40% of all frauds are detected through tips from employees. This explains why the *Sarbanes-Oxley Act* (SOX) requires audit committees to encourage anonymous whistle-blowing by employees. Almost 30% of frauds were detected by management review and internal audit, 9% by other internal controls, 7% by accident, and 3% by external auditors.[5] The rest of the chapter discusses the risk of fraud and auditors' responsibilities for detecting and communicating about fraud and illegal acts.

Fraud Risk Assessment

LO3   Differentiate among errors, frauds, and illegal acts that might occur in an organization.

CAS 240 notes that misstatements in the financial statements can arise from either error or fraud.

Errors are unintentional misstatements or omissions of amounts or disclosures in financial statements. Frauds are intentional misstatements.

Fraud is knowingly making material misrepresentations of fact, with the intent of inducing someone to believe the falsehood, act upon it, and thus suffer a loss or damage. This definition includes all the ways in which people can lie, cheat, steal, and dupe others.

There are several kinds of fraud. Some are defined in laws, while others are matters of general understanding. Exhibit 7–5 shows some acts and devices often involved in financial frauds. Collectively, these are known as

---

EXHIBIT 7–5

An Abundance of Frauds

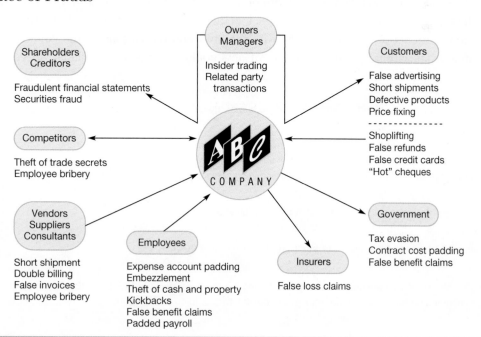

---

errors:

in financial statement auditing, unintentional misstatements or omissions of amounts or disclosures in financial statements

white-collar crime—the misdeeds done by people who wear business suits to work and steal with a pencil or a computer. White-collar crimes involve ink stains instead of blood stains.

Auditors are mainly concerned with two types of fraud: **fraudulent financial reporting** (usually a type of management fraud involving management making false and misleading claims in financial statements), and employees' **misappropriation of assets**. The word *fraud* is used in this chapter, but in practice, the auditor is concerned with a suspected fraud rather than a proven one. Final determination of whether fraud has occurred is a legal matter to be decided by a court of law.

Fraud involves the following:

1. Use of deception such as manipulation, falsification, or alteration of accounting records or documentation;

2. Misrepresentation or intentional omission of events, transactions, or other significant information; or

3. Intentional misapplication of accounting principles relating to amount, classification, or manner of presentation of disclosure.

Employee fraud is dishonestly taking money or other property from an employer. It usually involves falsifications of some kind—falsifying documents, lying, exceeding authority, or violating an employer's policies. It consists of three phases: (1) the fraudulent act, (2) the conversion of the money or property to the fraudster's use, and (3) the cover-up. Perpetrators of this type of fraud against the corporation can be anyone from the lowest-level employee to an executive manager.

Embezzlement is employees or non-employees wrongfully taking money or property entrusted to their care, custody, and control. It is often accompanied by false accounting entries and other forms of lying and cover-up. **Defalcation** is another name for employee fraud and embezzlement. Technically, the term is used when somebody in charge of safekeeping the assets is doing the stealing.

Fraudulent financial reporting is a type of fraud perpetrated by management through exploitation of its authority. The United States National Commission on Fraudulent Financial Reporting (1987) defined it as intentional or reckless conduct, whether by act or omission, that results in materially misleading financial statements. Weaknesses in corporate governance create opportunities for management fraud. The perpetrators are management, the victims are investors and creditors, and the instruments of perpetration are corporations.[6]

An **illegal act** is an act of non-compliance with the laws and regulations of the country or countries in which the auditee organization operates. A range of acts could be considered "illegal" in various countries.

---

white-collar crime:
misdeeds committed by business and government professionals, typically non-violent

fraudulent financial reporting:
intentional manipulation of reported financial results (by manipulation of accounting records or supporting documents, misrepresentation or omission of significant information, or intentional misapplication of accounting principles) to portray a misstated economic picture of the firm by which the perpetrator seeks an increase in personal wealth through a rise in stock price or compensation

misappropriation of assets:
the theft or misuse of an organization's assets (a type of defalcation)

employee fraud:
the use of dishonest means to take money or other property from an employer

embezzlement:
fraud involving employees or non-employees wrongfully taking money or property entrusted to their care, custody, and control; often accompanied by false accounting entries and other forms of lying and cover-up

defalcation:
fraud in which an employee takes assets (money or property) from an organization for personal gain; may be due to corruption or asset misappropriation

illegal act:
in financial statement auditing, non-compliance with a domestic or foreign statutory law or government regulation attributable to the entity under audit, or to management or employees acting on the entity's behalf; this does not include personal misconduct by the entity's management or employees unrelated to the entity's business activities

CAS 240 The Auditor's Responsibilities Relating to Fraud in an Audit of Financial Statements

2. Misstatements in the financial statements can arise from either fraud or error. The distinguishing factor between fraud and error is whether the underlying action that results in the misstatement of the financial statements is intentional or unintentional.

3. Although fraud is a broad legal concept, for purposes of the CASs, the auditor is concerned with fraud that causes a material misstatement in the financial statements. Two types of intentional misstatements are relevant to the auditor—misstatements resulting from fraudulent financial reporting and misstatements resulting from misappropriation of assets. Although the auditor may suspect or, in rare cases, identify the occurrence of fraud, the auditor does not make legal determinations of whether fraud has actually occurred. (Ref: Para. A1–A6)

4. The primary responsibility for the prevention and detection of fraud rests with both those charged with governance of the entity and management. It is important that management, with the oversight of those charged with governance, place a strong emphasis on fraud prevention, which may reduce opportunities for fraud to take place, and fraud deterrence, which could persuade individuals not to commit fraud because of the likelihood of detection and punishment. This involves a commitment to creating a culture of honesty and ethical behaviour that can be reinforced by an active oversight by those charged with governance. Oversight by those charged with governance includes considering the potential for override of controls or other inappropriate influence over the financial reporting process, such as efforts by management to manage earnings in order to influence the perceptions of analysts as to the entity's performance and profitability.

Source: *CPA Canada Handbook—Assurance,* 2014.

Illegal acts may have a direct effect on financial statement amounts, such as understating a tax liability, or an indirect effect, such as not complying with health and safety regulations. Like fraud, in practice, auditors do not determine whether an illegal act has occurred because this can only be decided by a court of law. Auditors are concerned with suspicions of illegal acts that can directly or ultimately affect fair presentation of the company's financial statements and raise questions about management's integrity.

What may turn out to be one of the biggest frauds ever was first made public in December 2008. It was the Madoff fraud described in the box below.

Ponzi Scam Artists Share Charm, Respectability

Why they are called con men? They are smart, have an aura of success about them, exude charm and respectability, and, most of all, they instill "CONfidence." Bernard Madoff, the Wall Street trader convicted for running the biggest Ponzi scheme in history, shares many of the basic qualities of Ponzi swindlers through history, according to law enforcement authorities and others who study scams. Scam artists affect confidence, charm, and a command of finance that makes them appear trustworthy.

The original Ponzi schemer, Charles Ponzi, was an Italian immigrant who worked as a waiter, bank teller, and nurse before he talked investors into sinking their money into his short-lived swindle, a complex but completely bogus scheme involving postal currency. In 1920, Ponzi began advertising that he could make a 50% return for investors in only 45 days. Ponzi began taking in money from all over New England and New Jersey as people mortgaged their homes and handed over their life savings to invest in this bonanza. Some tens of millions of dollars were invested with him before the fraud was discovered. Ponzi's scheme was hugely lucrative for some early investors (he was even lauded as a hero in the Italian community!), but ultimately he cheated thousands of people out of $10 million. He was imprisoned for mail fraud before being deported in 1934.

A Ponzi scheme, also known as a pyramid scheme, is a scam in which people are enticed to invest in a fraudulent operation that falsely promises exceptionally high returns. The earliest investors are paid their big "returns" out of the money put in by later investors, thus giving the false impression of good returns. These schemes collapse once the promoter can no longer bring in enough money to pay existing investors who seek to redeem out their investments. Ponzi's scheme was one of the most famous con games of his time, and his name has been given to similar scams ever since.

(continued)

People who run Ponzis can fall into two types. There are the con artists like Ponzi who set out to cheat investors quickly and run. Then, there are those who started a legitimate investment business but lost money, so they used new investors' money improperly to cover up the losses, which piled up as more new money was used to pay "returns" to earlier investors. (Perhaps if Madoff had not faced $7 billion in redemptions, his Ponzi scheme might not have been discovered.) Some speculate that Madoff was of the second type—once highly respected on Wall Street and a former Nasdaq chairman. While appearing bookish and unassuming, he maintained a lavish lifestyle, with luxurious homes, expensive cars, and exclusive club memberships, and also donated millions to charity. He was widely considered to have the magic touch as an investor.

When Madoff confessed and was arrested in 2008, he told F.B.I. agents that the losses might be $50 billion, according to court filings. Various institutions and individuals have so far reported losses totalling more than $20 billion, but it is unclear how much of that is cash they actually invested and how much represents paper profits based on the falsified returns Mr. Madoff said investors were earning.

Madoff regularly delivered returns of 10–17% to investors, a very good year-in, year-out return but on the low end of the 10–100% a year typically offered in more aggressive Ponzi schemes. Returns such as those Madoff reported should have been a major warning signal, because assets guaranteeing such high returns year after year without risk simply do not exist. Ponzi schemes can pay initial investors these returns by raising more money from new investors instead of the legitimate way of making profitable investments.

Madoff's practices appear to have gone on for many years and involved thousands of clients who invested both directly with him and through third-party hedge funds. Investors across the New York area clamoured to invest with Madoff because of his continuous double-digit returns and the reports of serious wealth creation. Some of those investors never took out a cent of what they invested, while others took out only a fraction, and a few took out more than they put in. His arrest and conviction is seen as a serious black eye for the hedge fund industry and for all non-transparent investment vehicles as the scandal reveals the inner workings of the hedge fund industry, whereby intermediary feeders bring in their clients and take fees for putting clients with an investment manager.

Sources: Denise Lavoie, "Ponzi scam artists through history share charm, respectability," *Pittsburgh Post-Gazette*, December 20, 2008, A8; Alex Berenson, "Even winners may lose with Madoff," *New York Times*, December 19, 2008, nytimes.com/2008/12/19/business/19ponzi.html; and Robert Lenzner, "Bernie Madoff's $50 billion Ponzi scheme," forbes.com, December 12, 2008, forbes.com/2008/12/12/madoff-ponzi-hedge-pf-ii-in_rl_1212croesus_inl.html.

Review Checkpoints

7-30   What are the defining characteristics of white-collar crime, employee fraud, embezzlement, defalcation, management fraud, errors, and illegal acts?

7-31   What does a fraud perpetrator look like? How does he or she act?

Auditors' Responsibilities for Detecting Frauds, Errors, and Illegal Acts

LO4   Describe auditors' responsibilities to detect and report frauds, errors, and illegal acts.

In response to the growing problems of fraud, auditors have taken on increased responsibility for detecting fraud and other illegal acts in recent years. As indicated in the auditor's report (Chapter 4), auditors have the responsibility "to obtain reasonable (i.e., high) assurance as to whether the financial statements are free of material misstatements," including misstatements due to fraud. The Canadian Auditing Standards (CASs) set out rigorous requirements relating to fraud in a financial statement audit.

Standards Check

CAS 240 The Auditor's Responsibilities Relating to Fraud in an Audit of Financial Statements

17. An auditor conducting an audit in accordance with CASs is responsible for obtaining reasonable assurance that the financial statements taken as a whole are free from material misstatement, whether caused by fraud or error. Owing to the inherent limitations of an audit, there is an unavoidable risk that some material misstatements of the financial statements may not be detected, even though the audit is properly planned and performed in accordance with the CASs.

Source: *CPA Canada Handbook—Assurance,* 2014.

Auditors' Responsibility to Consider Fraud and Error in an Audit of Financial Statements

CAS 240 requires the auditor to make inquiries of management about fraud and to consider **fraud risk** on every audit engagement. The auditor should document fraud risk factors identified as being present during the auditor's assessment process and document the auditor's response to the assessed risks of material misstatement due to fraud at the financial statement level. This includes the nature, timing, and extent of audit procedures and how the procedures link with the assessed fraud risks at the assertion level. The auditor should also obtain written management representations about management's suspicions or knowledge of any actual fraud and its extent. Findings should be communicated to management; those charged with governance of the reporting entity, the audit committee or equivalent; and, where required or permitted, outside agencies. CAS 240 also makes clear that the primary responsibility for the prevention and detection of fraud rests with management and those charged with governance of the reporting entity. This responsibility includes designing and implementing internal controls and other corporate governance mechanisms to deter fraud. Misappropriation of assets fraud is frequently termed *fraud against the company* because it is usually carried out by lower-level employees, and management and auditors have a common interest in detecting such fraud. In contrast, fraudulent financial reporting (misreporting fraud) is a fraud *by* the company but against investors that pits the auditor against management and its corporate governance. Ponzi schemes are a misreporting fraud.

Standards Check

CAS 240 The Auditor's Responsibilities Relating to Fraud in an Audit of Financial Statements

5. The auditor shall make inquiries of management regarding
   (a) Management's assessment of the risk that the financial statements may be materially misstated due to fraud, including the nature, extent, and frequency of such assessments; (Ref: Para. A12–A13)
   (b) Management's process for identifying and responding to the risks of fraud in the entity, including any specific risks of fraud that management has identified or that have been brought to its attention, or classes of transactions, account balances, or disclosures for which a risk of fraud is likely to exist; (Ref: Para. A14)
   (c) Management's communication, if any, to those charged with governance regarding its processes for identifying and responding to the risks of fraud in the entity; and
   (d) Management's communication, if any, to employees regarding its views on business practices and ethical behaviour.

Source: *CPA Canada Handbook—Assurance,* 2014.

fraud risk:
in financial statement auditing, the possibility that fraud has resulted in intentional misstatement in the financial statements; two types of intentional misstatements are relevant to the auditor: those resulting from fraudulent financial reporting and those resulting from misappropriation of assets

CAS 240 requires auditors to maintain professional skepticism and make no assumption about management's honesty.[7] CAS 240, paragraph 26, requires auditors to presume there is always a risk of fraudulent revenue recognition, a presumption that is "rebuttable" by the audit evidence. That is, if the auditors can convince themselves that the risk is appropriately low (the Public Company Accounting Oversight Board [PCAOB] suggests it should be "remote"), then the presumption is rejected. This logic is similar to the burden of proof concept in law and critical thinking.

Standards Check

CAS 240 The Auditor's Responsibilities Relating to Fraud in an Audit of Financial Statements

12. In accordance with CAS 200, the auditor shall maintain professional skepticism throughout the audit, recognizing the possibility that a material misstatement due to fraud could exist, notwithstanding the auditor's past experience of the honesty and integrity of the entity's management and those charged with governance. (Ref: Para. A7–A8)

Source: *CPA Canada Handbook—Assurance*, 2014.

How does the auditor justify that the fraud risk is sufficiently low? Under CAS 240, the rebuttable presumption requires auditors to perform analytical procedures on revenues, make inquiries, and scan for unusual entries (especially at year-end), and the audit team should have brainstorming sessions to identify and share information on fraud risk factors during the audit. Auditors also need to identify biases in management accounting estimates and be able to understand the business rationale of transactions. If the auditors cannot reject the rebuttable presumption, then they need to raise the matter with those charged with governance (audit committee or equivalent) and take it from there.

External auditors assess the risk of fraud through warning signs. A study by American researchers provides guidance on these: "The lack of awareness of the warning signs of fraud is a frequently cited cause of audit failure. If auditors better understood the signs and applied professional skepticism, they would decrease their risk of not detecting fraud. Knowing the most important warning signs should help auditors do a better job of assessing fraud risk."[8] A survey of 130 auditors asked them to rank 30 commonly cited fraud warning signals according to their significance. The auditors ranked client dishonesty as the most important factor. The survey revealed that auditors generally perceived "attitude" factors to be more important warning signs of fraud than "situational" factors. The top 15 warning signs are listed in the following box (see also the two boxes that follow).

Auditors' Ranking of the Relative Importance of Fraud Warning Signs

1. Managers have lied to the auditors or have been overly evasive in response to audit inquiries.
2. The auditor's experience with management indicates a degree of dishonesty.
3. Management places undue emphasis on meeting earnings projections or the quantitative targets.
4. Management has engaged in frequent disputes with auditors, particularly about aggressive application of accounting principles that increase earnings.
5. The client has engaged in opinion shopping.
6. Management's attitude toward financial reporting is unduly aggressive.
7. The client has a weak control environment.
8. A substantial portion of management compensation depends on meeting quantified targets.
9. Management displays significant disrespect for regulatory bodies.
10. Management operating and financial decisions are dominated by a single person or a few persons acting in concert.

(continued)

11.   Client managers display a hostile attitude toward the auditors.

12.   Management displays a propensity to take undue risks.

13.   There are frequent and significant difficult-to-audit transactions.

14.   Key managers are considered highly unreasonable.

15.   The client's organization is decentralized without adequate monitoring.

Source: V. B. Heiman-Hoffman, K. P. Morgan, and J. M. Patton, "The warning signs of fraudulent financial reporting," *Journal of Accountancy*, October 1996, pp. 76–77. Copyright 1996. American Institute of Certified Public Accountants, Inc. All rights reserved. Used with permission.

No Separation of Duties

An electronic data processing employee instructed the company's computer to pay his wife rent for land she had allegedly leased to the company by assigning her an alphanumeric code as a lessor and then ordering the payments. The control lesson: never let a data entry clerk who processes payment claims also have access to the approved vendor master file for additions or deletions.

Source: G. J. Bologna and R. J. Lindquist, *Fraud Auditing and Forensic Accounting* (New York: John Wiley & Sons, 1987), pp. 70–71.

Money, Money, Money Case

Brian Molony, a 29-year-old assistant branch manager and lending officer of a large downtown Toronto bank, defrauded the bank of some $10.2 million over a 20-month period. He fabricated loans to real and fictitious customers and gambled away the proceeds at an Atlantic City casino. Molony was such a valued customer that the casino flew its corporate jet to Toronto to pick him up for weekend jaunts.

The defalcation came to light when Canadian law enforcement authorities arrested Molony for a traffic violation on his return from a trip to Atlantic City. He was searched and found to be carrying about $29,000 in currency. That information was passed on to the bank, which then conducted an audit and found the fictional loans and transfers of funds to the casino. The bank sued the casino to recover at least part of its loss.

Molony used a *lapping scheme* to keep auditors off his trail—that is, he paid off earlier loans with subsequent loans so that no delinquencies would show. However, the fictional loan balances grew and grew. Molony's superior at the branch had approved the larger loans because "he had no reason to mistrust him." The branch manager was subsequently suspended, along with the assistant branch manager for administration, a credit officer, and an auditor.

Source: G. J. Bologna and R. J. Lindquist, *Fraud Auditing and Forensic Accounting*, 2nd ed. (New York: John Wiley & Sons, 1995), pp. 230–231. Reprinted by permission of John Wiley & Sons Inc.

The traditional role of the investigative or forensic auditor was to get involved when the risk of fraud was not sufficiently low (i.e., when there was cause for concern because there were too many fraud risk factors, and those charged with governance authorized further investigation). However, forensic auditors are increasingly being used to proactively perform the initial fraud risk assessments in planning the audit. They may be used to screen clients and be involved in the initial meetings with audit committees and management. There are several reasons for this trend. First, it acts as a fraud deterrent and makes the client aware of how seriously the profession takes its fraud detection responsibilities. Second, forensic auditors are specially trained in techniques to indicate when people are lying. Finally, forensic auditors are more familiar with legal requirements regarding documentation of frauds, such as witness statements, confessions, control of the chain of custody of evidence, and preparation of written reports for use as evidence in a court of law.

Illegal Acts by Auditees

ISA 250, on which CAS 250 is based, is written to apply in a wide variety of legal environments around the world. While it notes that some laws and regulations will have a direct effect on the financial statements as they determine the reported amounts and disclosures, others must be complied with to allow the entity to conduct its business but do not have a direct effect on its financial statements. This auditing standard uses a fairly broad term, "non-compliance with laws and regulations," to cover a range of acts that could be considered "illegal" in various countries. We will use the term *illegal acts* in our discussion of this topic. CAS 250 requires auditors to consider the consequences of the illegal acts very broadly, and the best way of disclosing these consequences. If failures to disclose would result in a material misstatement, then the auditor should attempt to reduce this risk to an appropriately low level. CAS 250 acknowledges that illegal acts may be difficult to detect because of (1) efforts made to conceal them and (2) questions about whether an act is illegal, which are complex and may only be resolved by a court of law. For these reasons, the engagement letter should inform management of the audit's limitations in detecting illegal acts.

Standards Check

CAS 250 Consideration of Laws and Regulations in an Audit of Financial Statements

8. The auditor is required by this CAS to remain alert to the possibility that other audit procedures applied for the purpose of forming an opinion on financial statements may bring instances of identified or suspected non-compliance to the auditor's attention. Maintaining professional skepticism throughout the audit, as required by CAS 200, is important in this context, given the extent of laws and regulations that affect the entity.

Source: *CPA Canada Handbook—Assurance*, 2014.

The auditors' knowledge of the business and inquiries of management help to identify laws and regulations that if violated and not reported, could result in material misstatements. In addition, auditors should inquire and obtain representations about awareness and disclosure of possibly illegal acts. Material, possibly illegal, acts should be communicated to those charged with governance (audit committee) and appropriate levels of management.

Standards Check

CAS 250 Consideration of Laws and Regulations in an Audit of Financial Statements

12. As part of obtaining an understanding of the entity and its environment in accordance with CAS 315, the auditor shall obtain a general understanding of
    (a) The legal and regulatory framework applicable to the entity and the industry or sector in which the entity operates; and
    (b) How the entity is complying with that framework. (Ref: Para. A7)
16. The auditor shall request management and, where appropriate, those charged with governance, to provide written representations that all known instances of non-compliance or suspected non-compliance with laws and regulations whose effects should be considered when preparing financial statements have been disclosed to the auditor. (Ref: Para. A12)

Source: *CPA Canada Handbook—Assurance*, 2014.

Summary

From a critical thinking perspective, the most important development regarding the fraud and illegal acts auditing standards was dropping the assumption that management is honest, a change that took place in 2004. For instance, auditors must explicitly address the risks of fraud in revenue recognition in every audit. If risk is present, the auditor must perform further procedures, but even without this risk auditors must now document the reasons (i.e., from a critical thinking perspective, the auditor must use audit evidence to argue that fraud risk is at an acceptable level). If sufficient risk of material fraud exists (i.e., fraud risk is high), then a fraud auditor should be called in, with the approval of the auditee's directors, audit committee, or management. If the risk of material fraud or non-compliance with laws and regulations is not acceptably low, then the auditor cannot issue a clean audit opinion.

Auditing Accounting Estimates and Fair Value Accounting

CAS 540 relates to manipulation of estimates in fraudulent financial reporting. This area is difficult, because accounting estimates are an approximation of a financial statement element, item, or account made by an organization's management, for example, for allowance for bad debts, net realizable value of inventory, impairment write-downs of fixed assets, percentage-of-completion revenue, and fair value accounting estimates.

CAS 540 deals with estimation uncertainty and the need to address significant risks associated with this uncertainty by ensuring that they are adequately disclosed. Disclosure may be through appropriate accounting adjustments, by the notes to the financial statements, or possibly through adding paragraphs in the auditor's report.[9] Critical thinking concepts that make use of conceptual frameworks in accounting and auditing can help guide the appropriate auditor response.

Management is responsible for making the accounting estimates, and auditors are responsible for evaluating the reasonableness of these within the financial statements as a whole. Auditors are supposed to keep track of the differences between management's estimates and the closest reasonable estimates supported by the audit evidence. Uncorrected differences between the two cause increased estimation uncertainty. Auditors are also supposed to evaluate both the total of the differences for indications of a systematic bias and the combination of the differences, along with other likely errors in the financial statements.

Standards Check

CAS 540 Auditing Accounting Estimates, Including Fair Value Accounting Estimates, and Related Disclosures

20. For accounting estimates that give rise to significant risks, the auditor shall also evaluate the adequacy of the disclosure of their estimation uncertainty in the financial statements in the context of the applicable financial reporting framework. (Ref: Para. A122–A123)

Indicators of Possible Management Bias

21. The auditor shall review the judgments and decisions made by management in the making of accounting estimates to identify whether there are indicators of possible management bias. Indicators of possible management bias do not themselves constitute misstatements for the purposes of drawing conclusions on the reasonableness of individual accounting estimates. (Ref: Para. A124–A125)

Source: *CPA Canada Handbook—Assurance*, 2014.

Communication with Those Charged with Governance (Audit Committees or Equivalent)

CAS 260 requires that those charged with governance (audit committees or equivalent) be informed about the scope and results of the independent audit. The auditing standards place great faith in audit committees and boards of directors, although their effectiveness has, at times, been questioned.[10] This CAS requires oral or written communication from the auditors on the following: (a) misstatements other than trivial errors; (b) fraud; (c) misstatements that may cause future financial statements to be materially misstated; (d) illegal or possibly illegal acts, other than ones considered inconsequential; and (e) significant weaknesses in internal control.

Note that there are some differences in the CASs between responsibility for detecting material misstatements due to error and those due to fraud. Specifically, CAS 240 states that an auditor is responsible for obtaining reasonable assurance whether the financial statements are free of material misstatement without qualifying the sources of that misstatement, while later, the same CAS 240, paragraph 6, explains that an auditor is less likely (because of concealment) to detect misstatement due to fraud than he or she is to detect that resulting from error. In addition, CAS 250 suggests that some illegal acts, specifically those that only indirectly affect financial statements, such as building code violations, may have an even lower chance of being detected by an external auditor.

GAAS (CAS 240) require extensive documentation related to the auditors' efforts to detect fraud on a financial statement audit engagement, such as the following:

- The significant decisions reached during audit team discussions about fraud risk
- The identified and assessed risks of material misstatement due to fraud at the financial statement level and at the assertion level
- The overall responses to the assessed fraud risks, including the nature, timing, and extent of audit procedures performed and how they link to the assessed fraud risks at the assertion level
- The results of the audit procedures performed, including those designed to address the risk of management override of controls
- The communications about fraud made to management, those charged with governance, regulators, and others
- The specific reasons for that conclusion if the auditor has rebutted the presumption of fraud risk for revenue recognition in the engagement

Materiality and Fraud or Illegal Acts

Standards of materiality thresholds for external auditors are related to the reporting auditors' knowledge of errors, fraud, and illegal acts. Immaterial errors are supposed to be reported to management at least one level above the people involved. Small matters can be kept in the management family, but errors material to the financial statements must be adjusted and handled by management responsible for the financial statements, to the satisfaction of auditors, or else the audit report will be qualified.

Auditors should inform those charged with governance about all frauds, both suspected and known, except those that are, in the auditor's judgment, "clearly inconsequential." Those involving senior management are never inconsequential. In the CASs, discretion is used to determine whether something is minor enough not to matter or report. However, auditors must be satisfied with how management and directors deal with frauds. If uncertainties persist about the frauds and management's actions, the audit report should be qualified, with reasons, or the auditors may withdraw from the engagement.

The "clearly inconsequential" materiality standard also applies to clients' illegal acts. Ones that are more than inconsequential are reported to the organization's audit committee and disclosed in the financial statements. External auditors always have the option to withdraw from the engagement if management and directors do not take satisfactory action under the circumstances.

Standards Check

CAS 260 Communication with Those Charged with Governance

16. The auditor shall communicate with those charged with governance (Ref: Para. A16)

    (a) The auditor's views about significant qualitative aspects of the entity's accounting practices, including accounting policies, accounting estimates, and financial statement disclosures. When applicable, the auditor shall explain to those charged with governance why the auditor considers a significant accounting practice, that is acceptable under the applicable financial reporting framework, not to be most appropriate to the particular circumstances of the entity; (Ref: Para. A17)

    (b) Significant difficulties, if any, encountered during the audit; (Ref: Para. A18)

    (c) Unless all of those charged with governance are involved in managing the entity,

        (i) Significant matters, if any, arising from the audit that were discussed, or subject to correspondence with management; and (Ref: Para. A19)

        (ii) Written representations the auditor is requesting; and

    (d) Other matters, if any, arising from the audit that, in the auditor's professional judgment, are significant to the oversight of the financial reporting process. (Ref: Para. A20)

A18. Significant difficulties encountered during the audit may include such matters as

- Significant delays in management providing required information;
- An unnecessarily brief time within which to complete the audit;
- Extensive unexpected effort required to obtain sufficient appropriate audit evidence;
- The unavailability of expected information;
- Restrictions imposed on the auditor by management; and
- Management's unwillingness to make or extend its assessment of the entity's ability to continue as a going concern when requested.

In some circumstances, such difficulties may constitute a scope limitation that leads to a modification of the auditor's opinion.

Source: *CPA Canada Handbook—Assurance,* 2014.

Under the CASs, disclosures of irregularities and clients' illegal acts to outside agencies are limited. If the auditors are fired, the provincial securities commission may require an explanation. A fired auditor can inform the successor auditor of any professional matters regarding the firm when the successor makes the inquiries required by professional ethics. Auditors must respond to a subpoena issued by a court or other agency with authority, which will happen in a lawsuit or prosecution. When performing work under public sector audit standards, auditors are required to report irregularities and illegal acts to the client agency under the audit contract, which may be an agency other than the one being audited.

Review Checkpoint

7-32 What are the CAS requirements regarding (a) fraud risk assessment (b) procedural audit work, (c) professional skepticism, and (d) reporting?

Conditions that Make Fraud Possible, Even Easy

LO5 Describe some of the conditions that lead to fraud risks.

When can fraud occur? The probability of fraud is a function of three factors: motive, opportunity, and lack of integrity. When one or two of these factors weigh heavily in the direction of fraud, the probability increases. When three of them lean in the direction of fraud, it will almost certainly occur.[11] As Bologna and

Lindquist put it, some people are honest all the time, some people (fewer than the honest ones) are dishonest all the time, most people are honest some of the time, and some people are honest most of the time.[12] The three fraud risk factors are discussed next.

The importance of the three risk factors—motive, opportunity, and lack of integrity—has also been acknowledged in GAAS. GAAS use these factors as a framework for linking sources of these risks to audit procedures. Motive relates to incentives or pressures and lack of integrity relates to rationalization or attitude. These can also be viewed as social, economic, and moral incentives. The three forms of **fraud incentive** are referred to as the fraud triangle or triangulation. Evidence or signs of these incentives are the fraud risk factors. Fraud is most likely to occur when all three types of factors are present. Hence, auditors use these risk factors as guides for evaluating whether the risk of material fraud is at acceptable levels.

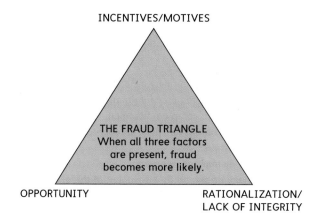

Fraud Incentive

Pressure a person experiences and believes cannot be shared with friends and confidants may lead to committing fraud or can serve as the motive for fraud. *Psychotic* motivation is relatively rare and is experienced by habitual criminals who steal simply for the sake of stealing. *Egocentric* motivations drive people to steal to achieve more personal prestige. *Ideological* motivations are held by people who think that their cause is morally superior and that they are justified in making someone else a victim. *Economic* motive is far more common than the other three in business frauds and is simply a need for money. At times, it can be intertwined with egocentric and ideological motivations. Ordinarily honest people can fall into circumstances where there is a new or unexpected need for money and when the normal options for talking about it or going through legitimate channels seem unavailable. Consider these needs:

- College or university tuition
- Gambling debts
- Drugs
- Alimony and child support
- Expensive lifestyle (homes, cars, boats)
- Business or stock speculation losses
- Taxation on good financial results

fraud incentive:
when management is under pressure, from sources outside or inside the entity, to achieve an expected (perhaps unrealistic) earnings target or financial outcome, particularly as the consequences to management for failing to meet financial goals can be significant; also, when individuals are tempted to misappropriate assets because, for example, they are living beyond their means

Probably the most important motive that external auditors consider is compensation tied to accounting measures of performance. This situation creates incentives to manipulate the accounting measurements.

Fraud Opportunity

A **fraud opportunity** is an open door for solving the unshareable problem by violating a trust. The violation may be a circumvention of internal control policies and procedures, or it may be taking advantage of an absence or lapse of control procedures. Everyone has some degree of trust placed on them in their job, and the higher the position in an organization, the greater the degree of trust, hence, the greater the opportunity for larger frauds. Here are some examples of opportunities:

- Nobody counts the inventory, so losses are not known.
- The petty cash box is often left unattended.
- Supervisors set a bad example by taking supplies home.
- Upper management considered a written statement of ethics but decided not to publish one.
- Another employee was caught and fired, but not prosecuted.
- The finance vice-president has investment authority without any review.
- Frequent emergency jobs leave a lot of excess material just lying around.

I Couldn't Tell Anyone

An unmarried young woman stole $300 from her employer to pay for an abortion. Coming from a family that strongly disdained premarital sex, she felt that her only alternative was to have the secret abortion. Once she realized how easy it was to steal, however, she took another $86,000 before being caught.

Source: W. S. Albrecht, "How CPAs can help clients prevent employee fraud," *Journal of Accountancy*, December 1988, p. 113. Copyright 1988. American Institute of Certified Public Accountants, Inc. All rights reserved. Used with permission.

Probably the most significant opportunity as far as external auditors are concerned is lack of controls at the highest levels (corporate governance) to prevent management from overriding accounting controls.

Fraud Rationalization

Most people in a civilized society can be assumed to know the difference between right and wrong. While unimpeachable integrity is the ability to act according to the highest moral and ethical values all the time, lapses and occasional lack of integrity permit pressure and opportunity to take form as fraud. People normally do not make deliberate decisions to "lack integrity today while I steal some money," but they sometimes do find ways to rationalize their act, by describing it to themselves in a way that makes it acceptable to their self-image. Some common examples of **fraud rationalization** are, "I need it more than they do" (Robin Hood theory), "I'll pay it back," "I'm not hurting anybody," "the company can afford it," and "everybody does it."

fraud opportunity:
when an individual believes internal control can be overridden to allow a fraud to be perpetrated, for example, when the individual is in a position of trust or has knowledge of specific deficiencies in internal control

fraud rationalization:
when individuals possess an attitude, character, or set of ethical values allowing them to knowingly and intentionally commit a dishonest act, or when otherwise honest individuals are in an environment that puts sufficient pressure on them to commit a fraudulent act

As was evident from the auditor survey results presented earlier, lack of integrity appears to be the most important factor affecting the risk of management fraud. This should not be surprising since—given managers' authority, responsibilities, and incentives—the other factors of pressure and opportunity are already largely present, and integrity is the only thing preventing fraud at the top levels of the organization. This may be a reason that "tone at the top" is one of the most important aspects of good internal controls.

She Can Do Everything

Mrs. Lemon was the only bookkeeper for an electrical supply company. She wrote the cheques and reconciled the bank account. In the cash disbursements journal, she coded some cheques as inventory, but she wrote the cheques to herself, using her own name. When the cheques were returned with the bank statement, she simply destroyed them. She stole $416,000 over five years. After being caught and sentenced to prison, she testified to having continuous guilt over doing something she knew was wrong.

Source: "Auditing for internal fraud" training course © 2006 Association of Certified Fraud Examiners.

The Most Common Computer-Related Crimes

Whereas computer hacking (unauthorized breaking into computers) has received most of the recent media attention, the most prevalent computer crime is the fraudulent disbursement of funds, which is generally preceded by the submission of a spurious claim in one of the following forms:
- False vendor, supplier, or contractor invoice
- False governmental benefit claim
- False fringe benefit claim
- False refund or credit claim
- False payroll claim
- False expense claim

Fraudulent disbursement of funds usually requires a data entry clerk in accounts payable, payroll, or the benefits section, acting either alone or in collusion with an insider or outsider (depending on how tight the internal controls are). From an accountant's perspective, the claim is a false debit to an expense so that a corresponding credit can be posted to the cash account for the issuance of a cheque. Auditors assert that such disbursement frauds represent more than half of all frauds by lower-level employees.

At higher management levels, the typical fraud involves overstating profits by the fabrication of such data as sales, which are increased arbitrarily (sales booked before the sales transaction is completed), and the understatement of expenses, which are arbitrarily reduced or disguised as deferrals to the next accounting period. There are numerous variations on these two main themes: overstatement of sales and understatement of expenses. One of the more common ploys to overstate profits is to arbitrarily increase the ending inventory of manufactured goods or merchandise held for sale. That ploy results in understating the cost of goods sold and thereby increasing the net profit.

The executive compensation system often provides the incentive to overstate profits. If bonus awards depend on profits, executives have an economic incentive to fudge the numbers. They may also be tempted to do so if they own a great many company shares, whose value depends on investors' perceptions of profitability. If profits are down, investors are unhappy and may rush to sell, thus causing a lowered share price and depressing the value of the executive's own shares.

Manipulations of this type often require line executives and personnel in accounting and data processing capacities to conspire. Such conspiracies have become a recurring theme in business. The pressure on executives for high performance grows each year. We are therefore likely to see more such frauds in the future.

Source: G. J. Bologna and A. J. Lindquist, *Fraud Auditing and Forensic Accounting*, 2nd ed. (New York: John Wiley & Sons, 1995), pp. 176–179. Reprinted by permission of John Wiley & Sons, Inc.

Standards Check

CAS 240 The Auditor's Responsibilities Relating to Fraud in an Audit of Financial Statements

A1. Fraud, whether fraudulent financial reporting or misappropriation of assets, involves incentive or pressure to commit fraud, perceived opportunity to do so, and some rationalization of the act. For example:

• Incentive or pressure to commit fraudulent financial reporting may exist when management is under pressure, from sources outside or inside the entity, to achieve an expected (and perhaps unrealistic) earnings target or financial outcome—particularly since the consequences to management for failing to meet financial goals can be significant. Similarly, individuals may have an incentive to misappropriate assets, for example, because the individuals are living beyond their means.

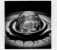

• A perceived opportunity to commit fraud may exist when an individual believes internal control can be overridden, for example, because the individual is in a position of trust or has knowledge of specific deficiencies in internal control.

• Individuals may be able to rationalize committing a fraudulent act. Some individuals possess an attitude, character, or set of ethical values that allows them knowingly and intentionally to commit a dishonest act. However, even otherwise honest individuals can commit fraud in an environment that imposes sufficient pressure on them.

Source: *CPA Canada Handbook—Assurance,* 2014.

Appendix 1 of CAS 240 gives examples of factors relating to the two types of frauds: fraudulent financial reporting and misappropriation of assets. The factors are classified based on the three conditions generally present when material misstatements due to fraud occur: (a) incentives or pressures, (b) opportunities, and (c) attitudes or rationalizations. Appendix 2 of CAS 240 gives examples of audit procedures addressing higher than acceptable risks of fraud. These include revenue recognition procedures, such as confirming relevant contract terms and absence of side agreements with customers; inventory procedures, such as surprise inventory count observations; and procedures related to verifying management estimates by obtaining a comparable estimate from an independent expert. The Application Case in this chapter illustrates some fundamental issues related to acceptability of management estimates.

Review Checkpoints

7-33 What are some of the pressures that can cause honest people to contemplate theft? List some egocentric and ideological pressures, as well as economic ones.

7-34 What kinds of conditions provide opportunities for employee fraud and financial statement fraud?

7-35 Give some examples of some rationalizations to excuse fraud. Would you be able to use them?

Former U.S. Securities and Exchange Commission (SEC) chairman Arthur Levitt was critical of the profession for allowing "hocus-pocus accounting" that facilitates financial statement fraud. The following box summarizes some forms of hocus-pocus accounting that were emerging in the 1990s.

Hocus-Pocus Accounting

Executive Summary

• Public companies that fail to report quarterly earnings that meet or exceed analysts' expectations often experience a drop in their stock prices. This can lead to practices that sometimes include fraudulent overstatement of quarterly revenue.

(continued)

- One of the most common schemes is the bill-and-hold sales transaction. While it is not necessarily a GAAP violation, it is often associated with financial frauds and calls for deeper investigation. The SEC says that all of the following conditions must be met for revenue recognition to be appropriate:

  - The risks of ownership must have passed to the buyer.
  - The customer must have a commitment to purchase, preferably in writing.
  - The buyer must request the bill-and-sale transaction and substantiate a business purpose for it.
  - A fixed delivery date must exist.
  - The seller must not retain any significant specific performance obligations.
  - The goods must be complete and ready for shipment and not subject to being used to fill other orders.

- Deals called sham transactions refer specifically to sales schemes that appear genuine but are actually rigged for the purpose of letting the seller recognize revenue. Other indicators that fraudulent financial reporting might exist are bogus shipping dates, revenue figures that always meet analysts' expectations, and transactions with unusual payment terms.

Auditors with a good understanding of the client, the business, and its products are well prepared to see the warning signs of revenue recognition fraud.

Source: D. R. Carmichael, "Hocus-pocus accounting," *Journal of Accountancy*, October 1999, p. 60. Copyright 1996. American Institute of Certified Public Accountants, Inc. All rights reserved. Used with permission.

Characteristics of Fraudsters

White-collar criminals are not like typical bank robbers, who are often described as "young and dumb" because of comical mistakes like writing the holdup note on the back of a probation identification card, leaving the getaway car keys on the convenience store counter, using a zucchini as a holdup weapon, and timing the holdup to get stuck in rush-hour traffic. Then there is the classic story about the robber who ran into his own mother at the bank (she turned him in!).

Burglars and robbers average about $400–$500 for each hit. Employee frauds average $20,000, or up to $500,000 if a computer is used. Yet employee frauds are not usually the intricate, well-disguised ploys of espionage novels. Who are these thieves? What do they look like? Unfortunately, they look and are like most everybody else, including you and me: likely married, well-educated, between 20 and 60 years old, and long-term employees. They are probably socially conforming, without an arrest record, and possibly even church members. In most instances, the fraudster will act alone.

White-collar criminals do not make themselves obvious, although there may be telltale signs, described in Appendix 10B (available on Connect) as behavioural "red flags." Unfortunately, the largest frauds are committed by people who hold high executive positions, have long tenure with an organization, and are respected and trusted employees. After all, these are the people who have access to the largest amounts of money and have the power to give orders and override controls (see the following boxes).

Who Does it?

 Alex W. was a 47-year-old treasurer of a credit union. Over a seven-year period, he stole $160,000. He was a good husband and the father of six children, and he was a highly reputed official of the credit union. His misappropriations came as a stunning surprise to his associates. He owed significant amounts on his home, cars, university for two children, two side investments, and five different credit cards. His monthly payments significantly exceeded his take-home pay.

The Case of the Extra Checkout

The district grocery store manager could not understand why receipts and profitability had fallen and inventory was hard to manage at one of the largest stores in her area. She hired an investigator who covertly observed the checkout clerks and reported that none of the nine had shown suspicious behaviour at any of the nine checkout counters. Nine? That store has only eight, she exclaimed! The store manager had installed another checkout aisle, not connected to the cash receipts and inventory maintenance central computer, and was pocketing all the receipts from that register.

Free Parking?

Outside the Bristle Zoo, there is a parking lot for 150 cars and 8 buses. For 25 years, its parking fees were managed by a very pleasant attendant. The fees were for $5 for cars and $20 for buses. Then, one day, after 25 solid years of never missing a day of work, he just did not show up, so the Zoo Management called the city council and asked it to send them another parking agent. The council did some research and replied that the parking lot was the zoo's own responsibility. The zoo advised the council that the attendant was a city employee. The city council responded that the lot attendant had never been on the city payroll.

Meanwhile, sitting in his villa somewhere on the coast of Spain or France or Italy is a man who had apparently had a ticket machine installed completely on his own and then simply began to show up every day to collect and keep the parking fees, estimated at about $560 per day—for 25 years. Assuming 7 days a week, this amounts to just over $7 million, and no one even knows his name.

This is one fraud that really "slipped between the cracks" from an internal control perspective!

External and internal auditors get credit for finding about 10–20% of discovered frauds. Voluntary confessions, anonymous tips, and other haphazard means uncover a larger percentage. Fraud examiners have a still higher success rate because they are called in for a specific purpose when fraud is known or highly suspected.

Some aspects of audit methodology make a big difference in fraud discovery success. Financial auditors use inductive reasoning: they sample accounting data, derive audit findings, and project the findings to a conclusion about the population. Fraud examiners use similar reasoning but with a focus on individual responsibility: they identify the suspects from tip-offs, make clinical observations (stakeouts), conduct interviews and interrogations, eliminate dead-end results, and concentrate on running the fraudster to ground. They can conduct covert activities not in the financial auditors' tool kit. The luxury of the forensic approach involves surveying a wide array of information and sources, eliminating the extraneous, and retaining the selection that proves the fraud. However, as critical thinking recognizes, proof is a relative concept. While a signed confession to fraud may be considered the most conclusive evidence one can get, courts are skeptical of evidence that purports to overcome the presumption of innocence until proven guilty in the Anglo-Saxon system of law. This aspect of fraud auditing and critical thinking is discussed in Appendix 7B of this chapter.

APPLICATION CASE WITH SOLUTION & ANALYSIS

Overstate the Inventory; Understate the Cost of Goods Sold

DISCUSSION CASE

A division manager at Doughboy Foods wanted to meet his profit goals and simply submitted overstated quantities in inventory reports. The manager (a) inserted fictitious count sheets in the independent auditors' working papers; (b) handed additional count sheets to the independent auditors after the count was completed, saying "these got left out of your set"; and (c) inserted false data into the computer system that produced a final inventory compilation (even though this ploy caused the computer-generated inventory to not match with the count sheets). Overstated inventory caused understated cost of goods sold; overstated net income and retained earnings; and overstated current assets, working capital, and total assets.

Audit Trail

In general, management reports should correspond to accounting records. The manager's inventory reports showed amounts larger than those in the accounts. He fixed the problem by showing false inventory that was "not recorded on the books." The food products inventory was overstated by $650,000. Through a two-year period, the false reports caused an income overstatement of 15% in the first year and would have caused a 39% overstatement in the second year.

SOLUTION & ANALYSIS

Audit Approach

Audit Objective

Obtain evidence of the existence, completeness, and valuation of inventory.

Controls Relevant to the Process

Inventory counts should be taken under controlled conditions, but not under the control of managers who might benefit from manipulation. (However, if these managers are present, auditors should nevertheless be prepared to perform the audit work.) Inventory takers should be trained and follow instructions for recording quantities and conditions.

Audit Procedures

Tests of Controls

Auditors should attend the inventory-taking training sessions and study the instructions for adequacy. Managers and auditors should observe the inventory taking to ensure compliance with the instructions.

Tests of Details of Balance

For evidence of existence, select a sample of inventory items from the perpetual records and test-count them in the warehouse. For evidence of completeness, select a sample of inventory items in the warehouse, test-count them, and trace them to the final inventory compilation. For evidence of valuation, find the proper prices of inventory for one or both of the samples, calculate the total cost for the items, and compare this with the amounts recorded in the books. Compare book inventory amounts with management reports. Control the working papers so that only members of the audit team have access. Analytical procedures gave some signals. The particular manager's division had the lowest inventory turnover rate (6.3%) among all the company divisions (comparable turnover, about 11.1%), and its inventory had consistently increased from year to year (227% over the two-year period).

Audit Results

In the second year, when the manager handed over the count sheets "that got left out of your set," the auditor thanked him and then went to the warehouse to check them out. Finding them inaccurate, she compared book inventories with his management reports and found an overstatement in the reports. This prompted further comparison of the computer-generated inventory with the count sheets and more evidence of overstated quantities on 22 of the 99 count sheets.

SUMMARY

- The chapter introduced internal control, an important component of the auditor's understanding of the auditee's business: the information systems that management has in place for running the business and meeting its information needs. A conceptual framework useful for understanding internal control was introduced. Understanding internal control is critical to assessing the possibility that management controls have not addressed the business risks that could lead to the financial statements being misstated. This is because the financial statements result from a firm's business processes and information systems, and thus they are vulnerable to any control deficiencies and weaknesses that might exist. This framework consists of company-level controls and specific control activities. Company-level controls include the control environment, management's risk assessment processes, information systems related to business processes and communications policies, and management's monitoring activities. Control activities, a component of internal control that consists of general and application controls, were also briefly introduced here for completeness but will be explained in more detail in Chapter 9.   **LO1**

- The chapter showed how auditors use their internal control understanding to make a preliminary assessment of the risk of material misstatement at the financial statement level, including an integrated overview of the business and its processes, and how these are captured in financial statements through the internal control and information systems.   **LO2**

- The auditor's responsibility for fraud risk assessment was introduced by explaining the types of errors, frauds, and illegal acts that can be perpetrated. Errors are unintentional misstatements or omissions of amounts or disclosures in financial statements. Frauds are intentional misstatements or omissions in financial statements, including fraudulent financial reporting (usually a type of management fraud) and misappropriations of assets (defalcations). Illegal acts are acts of non-compliance with the laws and regulations under which the organization operates.   **LO3**

- Auditors are responsible for assessing the risk of fraud and for performing fraud detection procedures when fraud is suspected. Auditors need to analyze the financial statements to detect unexpected relationships and examine unusual transactions and journal entries to assess these risks. Auditors are concerned with suspicions of fraud and illegal acts that can directly or ultimately affect fair presentation of the company's financial statements and raise questions about management's integrity. Auditors do not determine whether a fraud or illegal act has occurred, as this can only be decided by a court of law. Auditors' responsibilities to communicate with those charged with governance and management and to document their decisions and procedures related to fraud risk and illegal acts were explained.   **LO4**

- Individuals may contemplate fraud when they have a motive, usually a financial need, for stealing money or property. When there is a combination of motive with opportunity and a lapse of integrity, there is a high probability of fraud or theft. Opportunities arise when an organization's management is lax in setting an example of good behaviour and in maintaining a supportive control environment. The fear of getting caught by control procedures deters some fraudsters. Also, attentive management of personnel can ease the pressures people feel and, thus, reduce the incidence of fraud. Fraudulent financial reporting involves a high level of management overriding controls and taking advantage of its authority. It is viewed as fraud by the company against its investors, those who will be misled by the misleading financial statements. There is a higher risk of this occurring when management is faced with challenges and wants to report financial conditions and results better than they actually are, or otherwise manipulate the reported information.   **LO5**

- Appendix 7A describes risk and internal control frameworks as management tools that have been developed to help managers design and implement internal controls, explaining how these tools can be helpful for auditors' understanding and evaluation of internal control.   **LO6**

- Appendix 7B explains how auditors need to know the red flags, the signs and indications that accompany many fraudulent activities. When studying a business operation, auditors need to "think like a crook" to uncover possibilities for theft, as this can help in the planning of procedures designed to determine whether fraud has occurred. Often, imaginative extended procedures will unearth evidence of fraudulent activity. However, technical and personal care must always be exercised because accusations of fraud are always taken very seriously. For this reason, after preliminary findings indicate possible fraud, auditors should enlist the cooperation of management and assist fraud examination professionals in bringing an investigation to a conclusion. Various documents can be examined by auditors for unusual conditions, such as alterations, falsifications, and control overrides. These can indicate an increased risk of fraud.   **LO7**

KEY TERMS

application controls	detective controls	general controls
communication	embezzlement	illegal act
company-level controls	employee fraud	information system
control activities	errors	management's risk assessment
control environment	fraud incentive	process
control framework (internal control	fraud opportunity	misappropriation of assets
framework, internal control	fraud rationalization	monitoring
structure)	fraud risk	preventive controls
defalcation	fraudulent financial reporting	white-collar crime

MULTIPLE-CHOICE QUESTIONS FOR PRACTICE AND REVIEW

MC 7-1   **LO1**   Auditors must obtain an understanding of internal control because

a. the financial statements determine the appropriate business processes and internal control framework.
b. it is critical when assessing the possibility that management controls have not addressed the business risks that could lead to the financial statements being misstated.
c. audit control testing procedures must be focused on any control deficiencies and weaknesses that might exist.
d. they are responsible for implementing company-level controls and specific control activities in the auditee's control framework.

MC 7-2   **LO1**   Company-level controls include

a. systems input, processing, and output controls.
b. general controls, segregation controls, and application control procedures.
c. inherent, preventive, corrective, and detective controls.
d. control environment, management's risk assessment processes, information systems, and monitoring.

MC 7-3 `LO2` The primary purpose for obtaining an understanding of an auditee's internal control structure is to

a. provide a basis for making constructive suggestions in a management letter.
b. determine the nature, timing, and extent of tests to be performed in the audit.
c. obtain sufficient appropriate evidential matter to afford a reasonable basis for an opinion on the financial statements under examination.
d. provide information for a communication of internal control structure–related matters to management.

MC 7-4 `LO2` What do management's internal control responsibilities include?

a. Reducing the amount of testing done by the auditors
b. Allowing the auditors to assess control risk
c. Preventing and detecting fraud
d. Implementing policies and procedures such that auditors can assess control risk as being low

MC 7-5 `LO1` Fabre Travels, a large travel agency, has put in place the following controls. Which of these controls represents a company-level control?

a. Each travel agent must sign a letter at the beginning of each year acknowledging they read and understood the company's code of conduct.
b. Payroll of each travel agent must be approved by the head of their department prior to being processed.
c. A random review of calls made by the agents is made by the VP Operations to monitor the quality of the communication between an agent and the client.
d. If a travel agent wants to award a discount to a customer on a particular trip, they must obtain an authorization from their manager.

MC 7-6 `LO2` Clive Papers Inc. (CPI), a printing company, implemented the following controls over its procurement and inventory process. Which of these controls represents a preventive control?

a. The warehouse manager performs an inventory count at the end of each month to identify any damaged or stolen goods.
b. The VP Operations reviews the purchasing report on a weekly basis to identify any unusual activity.
c. A reconciliation of the inventory level, units purchased, and units sold is performed by the assistant controller on a monthly basis.
d. Access to the purchasing module of the information system is restricted to three purchasing agents who are entitled to make purchases for CPI.

MC 7-7 `LO4` When it comes to fraud, the auditor's responsibility consists of

a. detecting any type of fraud that occurred during the reporting period.
b. detecting fraud only if it is above the planning materiality level.
c. making inquiries with management about fraud and considering fraud risks.
d. The auditor is not responsible for detecting fraud.

MC 7-8 `LO3` Which of the following is characteristic of management fraud?

a. Falsification of documents in order to steal money from an employer
b. Victimization of investors through the use of materially misleading financial statements
c. Illegal acts committed by management to evade laws and regulations
d. Conversion of stolen inventory to cash deposited in a falsified bank account

MC 7-9 **LO3** CASs do not require auditors of financial statements to do which of the following?

a. Understand the nature of errors and fraud
b. Assess the risk of occurrence of errors and fraud
c. Design audits to provide reasonable assurance of detecting errors and fraud
d. Report all finding of errors and suspected fraud to police authorities

MC 7-10 **LO4** Which of the following types of auditors have the highest expectations in their audit standards regarding the detection of fraud?

a. External auditors of financial statements
b. Government auditors of financial statements, programs, activities, and functions
c. Internal auditors employed by companies
d. Management advisory consultants engaged to design a company's information system

MC 7-11 **LO5** When auditing with "fraud awareness," auditors should especially notice and follow up employee activities under which of these conditions?

a. The company always estimates the inventory but never takes a complete physical count.
b. The petty cash box is always locked in the desk of the custodian.
c. Management has published a company code of ethics and sends frequent communication newsletters about it.
d. The board of directors reviews and approves all investment transactions.

MC 7-12 **LO5** Which of the following gives the least indication of fraudulent activity?

a. Numerous cash refunds have been made to different people at the same post office box address.
b. The internal auditor cannot locate several credit memos to support reductions of customers' balances.
c. The bank reconciliation has no outstanding cheques or deposits older than 15 days.
d. Three people were absent the day the auditors handed out the paycheques and have not picked them up four weeks later.

MC 7-13 **LO5** Which of the following combinations is a good means of hiding employee fraud but a poor means of carrying out management (financial reporting) fraud?

a. Overstating sales revenue and overstating customer accounts receivable balances
b. Overstating sales revenue and overstating bad debt expense
c. Understating interest expense and understating accrued interest payable
d. Omitting the disclosure of information about related party sales to the president's relatives at below-market prices

MC 7-14 **LO5** Which of these arrangements of duties could most likely lead to an embezzlement or theft?

a. The inventory warehouse manager is responsible for making the physical inventory observation and reconciling discrepancies to the perpetual inventory records.
b. The cashier prepared the bank deposit, endorsed the cheques with a company stamp, and took the cash and cheques to the bank for deposit (no other bookkeeping duties).
c. The accounts receivable clerk received a list of payments received by the cashier so that he could make entries in the customers' accounts receivable subsidiary accounts.
d. The financial vice-president received cheques made out to suppliers and the supporting invoices, signed the cheques, and put them in the mail to the payees.

MC 7-15 `LO4` If sales and income were overstated by recording a false credit sale at the end of the year, in which account could you find the false "dangling debit"?

a. Inventory
b. Cost of goods sold
c. Bad debt expense
d. Accounts receivable

MC 7-16 `LO5` Where has experience shown that most accounting errors requiring adjustment can be found?

a. Systematic processing of large volumes of day-to-day ordinary transactions
b. Payroll fraudsters' mistakes in using unissued social insurance numbers
c. Petty cash embezzlements
d. Non-routine, non-systematic journal entries

MC 7-17 `LO5` Which of the following situations in the purchasing process creates the highest risk of fraud by making payments to a fictitious supplier?

a. The company has a comprehensive code of ethical conduct that all employees must sign.
b. The system automatically conducts independent credit checks of new suppliers.
c. New supplier authorization in the purchasing system can be set up by anyone in the accounting department.
d. Strong password controls exist so that only authorized purchasing department employees can gain access to the purchasing system.
e. All supplier payments are made by electronic funds transfers.

MC 7-18 `LO4` When an auditor notices evidence of a potential fraud while performing an audit, the auditor should

a. only report it to the company's management if the impact is believed to be material.
b. perform additional procedures to be able to conclude on the existence of the fraud.
c. report their findings to the appropriate level of management and the audit committee and let the court conclude on the existence of a fraud.
d. discuss the evidence with the concerned employee(s) to obtain more information.

MC7-19 `LO4` In accordance with CAS 240, when an auditor is inquiring about the risk of fraud and errors, what would the auditor *not* be required to ask management about?

a. Management's assessment of the risk that the financial statements may be materially misstated due to fraud, including the nature, extent, and frequency of such assessments
b. Management's communication, if any, to those charged with governance regarding its processes for identifying and responding to the risks of fraud in the entity
c. Management's process for identifying and responding to the risks of fraud in the entity, including any specific risks of fraud that management has identified or that have been brought to its attention, or classes of transactions, account balances, or disclosures for which a risk of fraud is likely to exist
d. Management's direct involvement in fraudulent activities during the current reporting period

MC 7-20 [LO3] Buddiez is an increasingly popular social network platform, and Kristy, a junior auditor, is helping with the risk of fraud assessment for this year's audit of the financial statements. She has been asked to identify possible indicators of management bias. What item below could be an indicator of management bias?

a. A new CFO was hired two months before year-end to turn the company around and increase profitability in the next three years.
b. A large variance in revenues was observed due to international sales and the decrease in the value of the local currency.
c. The Senior Financial Analyst computed the fair value of a derivative instrument incorrectly.
d. The VP Marketing's performance rating is based on the increase in the number of users for the network.

MC 7-21 [LO5] François is the manager of a restaurant. He has been noticing that the inventory of wine is decreasing and bottles often go missing, as they frequently cannot reconcile the beginning inventory, sales, and ending inventory. What could be an indicator of a fraud opportunity?

a. His employees always work long hours on weekends and evenings.
b. The cellar contains many expensive and rare bottles.
c. Employees are allowed to purchase wine from the restaurant at a discounted price through their employee privilege program.
d. The cellar is located at the back of the restaurant and remains open during dinner service to allow efficient access for wait staff.

EXERCISES AND PROBLEMS

EP 7-1 Give Examples of Errors and Frauds. [LO1] This is an exercise concerning financial reporting misstatements, not employee theft.

Required:

Give an example of an error or fraud that would misstate financial statements to affect the accounts as follows, taken one case at a time. (*Note:* "Overstate" means the account has a higher value than would be appropriate under GAAP, and "understate" means it has a lower value.)

a. Overstate an asset; understate another asset.
b. Overstate an asset; overstate shareholder equity.
c. Overstate an asset; overstate revenue.
d. Overstate an asset; understate an expense.
e. Overstate a liability; overstate an expense.
f. Understate an asset; overstate an expense.
g. Understate a liability; understate an expense.

EP 7-2 Overall Analysis of Accounting Estimates. [LO1, 5] Oak Industries, a manufacturer of cable TV equipment and an operator of subscription TV systems, had a multitude of problems. Subscription services in a market area, for which $12 million cost had been deferred, were being terminated, and the customers were not paying on time ($4 million receivables in doubt). The chances are 50–50 that the business will survive another two years.

An electronic part turned out to have defects that needed correction. Warranty expenses are estimated to range from $2 million to $6 million. The inventory of the part ($10 million) is obsolete, but $1 million can be recovered as salvage or the parts in inventory can be rebuilt at a cost of $2 million (selling price of the inventory on hand would then be $8 million, with 20% of selling price required to market and ship the products, and the normal profit expected is 5% of the selling price). If the inventory were scrapped, the company would manufacture a replacement inventory at a cost of $6 million, excluding marketing and shipping costs and normal profit.

The company has defaulted on completion of a military contract, and the government is claiming a $2 million refund. Company lawyers think the dispute might be settled for as little as $1 million.

The auditors had previously determined that an overstatement of income before taxes of $7 million would be material to the financial statements. These items were the only ones left for audit decisions about possible adjustment. Management has presented the analysis below for the determination of loss recognition:

Provide for expected warranty expense	2,000,000
Lower of cost and market inventory write-down	2,000,000
Loss on government contract refund	—
Total write-offs and losses	$11,000,000

Required:

Prepare your own analysis of the amount of adjustment to the financial statements. Assume that none of these estimates have been recorded yet, and give the adjusting entry you would recommend. Give any supplementary explanations you believe necessary to support your recommendation.

EP 7-3 Select Effective Procedures Responding to Fraud Risk. `LO3, 4, 6` Below are some "suspicions." You have been requested to select some effective extended procedures designed to confirm or deny the suspicions.

Required:

Write out the procedure you would suggest for each case so that another person would know what to do.

a. The custodian of the petty cash fund may be removing cash on Friday afternoon to pay for his weekend activities.

b. A manager has noticed that eight new vendors have been added to the purchasing department approved list since the assistant purchasing agent was promoted to chief agent three weeks ago. She suspects that all or some of them may be phony companies set up by the new chief purchasing agent.

c. The payroll supervisor may be stealing unclaimed paycheques of people who quit work and don't pick up the last cheque.

d. Although no customers have complained, cash collections on accounts receivable are down, and the counter clerks may have stolen customers' payments.

e. The cashier may have "borrowed" money, covering it by holding each day's deposit until there is enough cash from the daily collection to make up the shortage, before sending the deposit to the bank.

EP 7-4 Assessing Fraud Risk and Audit Procedures to Follow Up. `LO3, 4, 5` The following situations may raise a suspicion of fraud on an audit engagement.

Required:

Explain how each situation could indicate a fraud risk and how the auditor could confirm or dispel it.

a. An employee can authorize medical insurance claims and enter them into the system for payment without supervisory review. What might happen?

b. The inventory warehouse manager was also responsible for making the physical inventory observation and reconciling discrepancies to the perpetual inventory records. What might happen?

c. The petty cash custodian was replaced and the frequency of fund reimbursement decreased from every two days to every four days. What might you suspect?

d. Both sales and income may have been overstated by recording a false cash sale at the end of the year. What "dangling debit" might give the scheme away?

e. A company may have recorded fictitious sales. What account could you audit to determine whether this has happened?

EP 7-5 Fraud Risk Assessment. `LO4, 5`

Required:

Give some examples of control omissions that would make it easy to "think like a crook" and see opportunities for fraud.

EP 7-6 Fraud Risk Assessment. `LO4, 5`

Required:

List three general descriptions of the kinds of accounting and reporting manipulations that are most likely to produce materially misleading financial statements.

DISCUSSION CASES

DC 7-1 Famous Fraud Case Analysis. `LO3, 4, 5`

Required:

Do a Web search on the successful prosecution of the CEO of WorldCom, Tyco, or Adelphia through 2006, and answer the following:

a. How was the fraud detected?

b. How was the fraud perpetrated? Was it a financial statement fraud?

c. What was the weakness in internal control or corporate governance that allowed the fraud to occur?

d. Should a financial statement audit have detected this fraud? Discuss CAS 240 requirements that could have detected the fraud.

e. Would an internal control audit have detected this fraud? Discuss.

DC 7-2 Detecting Fraud. `LO3, 5` Play Green Inc. (PGI) is a public company that operates a number of sports facilities across Canada. Your friend Gildan is a junior auditor with the public accounting firm that has audited PGI for many years. Gildan is auditing the cash balance and has found some discrepancies between the bank records and PGI's accounting records. The discrepancies add up to a total overstatement of $135,000, and materiality for this audit has been set at $150,000. After inquiring of the PGI accounting manager about these discrepancies, Gildan gets a call from the President's secretary—the President has asked to meet with Gildan on this matter.

The President starts off by complimenting Gildan on his good accounting and auditing skills. He says he was very impressed that Gildan was able to discover the problems in the cash accounts. He provides Gildan with a written representation for his audit file stating that the cash discrepancies have been noted by company management, and the cash balance is fairly presented.

The President then tells Gildan that he is starting up a new golf course venture, separate from PGI, and could really use a talented accountant like Gildan to be his business partner in this new venture. Gildan would not be required to make any investment in the new business, but would receive 50% ownership in exchange for providing his accounting services to this business. The President would own the other 50%. Since the work on the new venture would only take Gildan about five hours per week, the President expects Gildan to keep his job with the auditing firm and continue working as the junior auditor on the PGI audit team.

Gildan has come to tell you about this offer from the President because he is very happy about it. At the same time he is a bit concerned that it seems too good to be true, and asks for your advice on what he should do.

Required:

Analyze Gildan's situation and advise him on the best way to proceed.

DC 7-3 Control Environment Evaluation `LO1`   Bruce Barnett Investment (BBI) is a prominent hedge fund on Bay Street in Toronto. Bruce founded the hedge in 2001 and today, BBI has 41 employees and manages close to $1 billion in assets.

Your friend Jenn had an internship at BBI over the summer and she was eager to tell you about her experience:

> I was very lucky to get that job! There was an extensive interview process, as BBI is keen on ensuring they hire the best person for the job. Once I was selected, they checked all my references, did a background check, and finally offered me the job.
>
> At BBI, Bruce is the CEO, chairman of the board, and still the best account manager in this business. Bruce is involved in every aspect of the business and he is everywhere. He constantly oversees what you do and often tells you to change something you've done because he disagrees. Bruce is a legend at the office. No one dares to contradict him.
>
> Bruce is all about maximizing the returns, and he is very good at motivating people. He offers large bonuses based on portfolio profitability and promotes traders that do well. He doesn't seem to care how they make profit, as long as the numbers are good.
>
> It was good work experience overall and I learned a lot. We had to attend many information sessions on regulations for trading as well as panel discussions on ethics in finance. Bruce never came to those, but all employees had to attend.

Required:

Comment on the control environment of BBI. Ensure that you support why a certain element of the control environment is positive or negative.

DC 7-4 J. J. Barnicke Ltd.: Missing Millions and Widow with Lavish Lifestyle.[13] `LO3, 4, 6`
Elizabeth (Liz) Lake lives in a million-dollar mansion in Don Mills. She spends time with her three children at a 1,134-square-metre waterfront "cottage" in central Ontario. She also gets about $22,600 a month—or $270,000 a year—to maintain those properties and cover living expenses.

Prominent realtor Joe Barnicke says it's all possible with money her late husband stole from him, his firm J. J. Barnicke Ltd., and a family trust fund. Liz Lake has kept that lifestyle for almost two years since her husband jumped in front of a train at York Mills subway station. Jim Lake committed suicide on the morning of March 18, 1996, less than an hour after Barnicke confronted him at the firm's downtown office about a lot of missing money. Lake, the firm's star chief financial officer, excused himself and never returned.

Barnicke and his company immediately filed a lawsuit in court against Liz Lake and her husband's estate to recover what was left of $19.8 million Lake allegedly swiped over a decade. But Barnicke, the firm's 74-year-old chairman, has found it isn't easy trying to get any of the alleged stolen money back. The courts are slow and Liz Lake is fighting him all the way for the mansion, country estate, cars, boats, snowmobiles, and life insurance proceeds. Barnicke won't talk publicly about the case but acquaintances say he's bitter and disillusioned over Liz Lake's continuing monthly "allowances" and the lengthy court proceedings. In the battle over the estate, Barnicke figures there's now only about $4 million to $5 million left—including life insurance proceeds—after all the spending.

No wonder. One of Lake's own accounting reports filed with the court reveals the couple spent almost $7 million after tax in the three years before his death. Lake fuelled that spending by jacking up his pay through misappropriation of Barnicke funds, according to documents filed in court. After a brief probe, Barnicke and top-flight forensic accountants Lindquist Avey MacDonald Baskerville Inc. said a paper trail revealed that the likeable Lake moved money from the company's operating funds and the chairman's personal accounts to a payroll system. He then transferred the money into personal bank accounts at the Bank of Nova Scotia.

Lake ran the payroll system, from which he was paid. Investigators found a copy of Lake's T4 form to Revenue Canada in his briefcase showing a gross income of $2,468,938.63 for 1995. But Lake's annual salary never exceeded $110,000, Barnicke said in the claim. Barnicke's lawsuit also alleges Lake, who was 36 when he died, had improperly moved $1.5 million from a trust fund for Barnicke's three children to his own account. Barnicke said his signatures on the transfer requests were forgeries.

Liz Lake denies her husband stole the money. If her husband did, it's Barnicke's own fault and he should suffer the losses, her statement of defence said. If the company had shown a minimal amount of diligence, it could have stopped any alleged losses and Lake might still be alive, she added. "The plaintiffs (Barnicke) by their gross negligence caused or contributed to the death of her husband and the father of her three children," the statement of defence said. She insists that all money received from the company was earned, "and was accurately recorded in J. J. Barnicke Ltd.'s books and records." Those books and records were kept at the company offices and in fact Lake paid taxes on the full amount. As well, Elizabeth Lake points out, the Barnicke books were made available to accountants Ernst & Young "at least annually" and all her husband's earnings were deposited in their joint account at the Bank of Nova Scotia. (The bank is also named in the company's civil suit.)

Joe Barnicke, the blustery patriarch of the company, scoffs at the suggestion they are responsible for any financial loss. "He stole the money," he told *The Toronto Sun* this week. "He stole the money. That's all we can say." Meanwhile, Barnicke's lawyer, Chris Osborne, said the cost of paying for Liz Lake's lifestyle is "bleeding" the estate of hundreds of thousands of dollars. Reports placed on the public record suggest Liz and Jim Lake didn't hold back in the last years of his life. Lake collected annual paycheques ranging from $2.2 million to $4.3 million in gross income from 1990 to 1995. Lake's own printout of "inflows" and "outflows" covering July 1993 to February 1996 disclosed that income from work, interest, and revenue on property sales totalled about $7 million. But the outflows for expenses left them with only $35,000. Furthermore, (the receiver) said at one point the couple regularly rang up credit card charges of more than $43,000 a month. The Lakes had "very lavish spending habits," the receiver noted.

Required:

a. Comment on the apparent control weaknesses at J. J. Barnicke suggested by the events in the above story. Explain how these weaknesses increased the risk of fraud in the company.

b. Assume the role of the judge. Which party's arguments do you think are more convincing? What additional evidence could each party provide to you that would strengthen their case?

c. What audit procedures might have been used to uncover the transfer of company funds to Mr. Lake's bank account?

DC 7-5 Management Controls, Impact on Audit. LO1, 2 Jabiru Inc.'s senior management recently obtained a new decision-support database system that allows the managers to generate standard reports and also customize inquiries that use data from all functional areas of their company. Before this system was in place, reports to senior managers were generated manually by the operations managers in the various departments, such as purchasing, marketing, inventory control, production, human resources, and administration. The senior managers are much happier with the new system because now they can generate reports as soon as the period ends, they can draw the data directly from the company's computer databases, they can control the content and format of the reports, and the operating managers have less opportunity to manipulate the information in the reports. For example, in the first two months of the new system, senior managers were able to identify a discrepancy in the production department that was resulting in significant shrinkage and were able to correct the control weakness quickly. The previous report, which had been designed and produced by the production manager, did not include the data needed to identify the shrinkage problem.

Required:

a. Discuss how the new decision-support database system affects Jabiru's internal control and its risk of material misstatement.

b. Comment on the potential audit planning implications of the new decision-support database system.

Appendix 7A Risk and Internal Control Frameworks (on Connect)
Appendix 7B Procedures and Documents Auditors Use for Fraud Detection (on Connect)

ENDNOTES

1. As noted in previous chapters, the regulations in the *Sarbanes-Oxley Act* (SOX) 404 and Public Company Accounting Oversight Board (PCAOB) Auditing Standard 5 for audits of management's internal control reporting and the similar standards now introduced in Canada for audits of control effectiveness (*CPA Canada Handbook*, "An audit of internal control over financial reporting that is integrated with an audit of financial statements") require an internal control assessment at the company level and the control activity level.

2. CAS 315, paragraphs A46, A49, and A50.

3   Appendix 6B, available on Connect, further explains the traditional responsibilities of the board and audit committee, as well as their expanded corporate governance responsibilities in today's environment.

4   Stay tuned: these functions will be discussed in detail in Chapter 9.

5   Association of Certified Fraud Examiners, *2012 Report to the Nations—Key Findings and Highlights*, available at acfe.com/rttn-highlights.aspx.

6   R. K. Elliott and J. J. Willingham, *Management Fraud: Detection and Deterrence* (New York: Petrocelli Books, Inc., 1980), p. 4.

7   For example, see D. Selley and E. Turner, "Detecting fraud and error," *CA Magazine*, August 2004, p. 38.

8   V. B. Heiman-Hoffman, K. P. Morgan, and J. M. Patton, "The warning signs of fraudulent financial reporting," *Journal of Accountancy*, October 1996, pp. 76–77.

9   For example, using emphasis of matter paragraphs, as described in CAS 706.

10 Wechsler reported the findings of the National Commission on Fraudulent Financial Reporting: of the 120 fraudulent financial reporting cases brought by the U.S. Securities and Exchange Commission (SEC) between 1981 and 1986, two-thirds involved companies that had audit committees. This caused Professor Briloff to remark, "Now I see that they are not functioning as they should" (D. Wechsler, "Giving the watchdog fangs," *Forbes*, November 13, 1989, p. 130.) However, these observations make one wonder about the thousands of companies with and without audit committees that did not get involved in fraudulent financial reporting.

11 For further references, see D. R. Cressey, "Management fraud, accounting controls, and criminological theory," pp. 117–147, and Albrecht et al., "Auditor involvement in the detection of fraud," pp. 207–261, both in R. K. Elliott and J. J. Willingham, *Management Fraud: Detection and Deterrence* (New York: Petrocelli Books Inc., 1980); J. K. Loebbecke, M. M. Eining, and J. J. Willingham, "Auditors' experience with material irregularities: Frequency, nature, and detectability," *Auditing: A Journal of Practice and Theory*, Fall 1989, pp. 1–28.

12 G. J. Bologna and R. J. Lindquist, *Fraud Auditing and Forensic Accounting* (New York: Wiley & Sons, 1987), p. 8.

13 Tony Van Apphen, *The Toronto Star*, December 14, 1997, p. A1; Scott Burnside, *The Toronto Sun*, June 23, 1996, p. 45.

Audit Evidence and Assurance

Chapter 8 expands on the concepts of audit evidence—the auditor's source of reasonable assurance that financial statements are not materially misstated. It covers evidence-gathering procedures and how auditors use them for risk assessment, control testing, and substantive testing.

LEARNING OBJECTIVES

After completing this chapter, you will be able to do the following:

LO1 Outline six general audit techniques for gathering evidence.

LO2 Identify the procedures and sources of information auditors can use to obtain evidence for understanding an auditee's business and industry, assessing risk, and responding to assessed risk.

LO3 Explain audit evidence in terms of its appropriateness and relative strength of persuasiveness.

LO4 Describe the content and purpose of the audit plan as well as the specific audit programs and detailed procedures it contains.

LO5 Evaluate audit working paper documentation for proper form and content.

EcoPak Inc.

Tariq and the audit team he has assembled are going at full speed now, developing their audit plan and audit programs for their first audit of EcoPak. Belinda has been assigned as the audit manager for the EcoPak engagement, Donna is the senior audit assistant, and there will be one junior assistant as well: Caleb. Belinda is a very experienced manager, but Donna is doing her first audit in the senior's role. After a very helpful team meeting, in which Tariq and Belinda presented the main information they have gathered so far, Donna is setting out to prepare the plan for the audit of the revenue, receivables, and receipts (R/R/R) process. Meyer & Gustav (M&G) has standard planning forms that outline a basic audit program for each process in a typical company, and Donna's job today is to adapt it to the circumstances of EcoPak's revenue process. She is also explaining the plan to Caleb, who is in his first year with the firm and has never audited the R/R/R section before.

Most of EcoPak's revenues are generated through long-term contracts with large customers, such as companies operating fast food restaurant chains, or with buying groups for independent restaurants in major urban areas. The contracts provide for volume discounts at various sales levels, so there is some complexity in ensuring the discounts are calculated correctly. Donna's preliminary work indicates they can rely on some controls in this process, so a combined approach is being considered.

Because M&G was able to obtain copies of some of the predecessor auditor's working papers, they have the system description details on file. Donna and Caleb are studying these to get an idea of how it all works before they head over to EcoPak's head office next week to start the interim audit work. They note that there are two classes of transactions in this process, sales and cash receipts, and one main balance, accounts receivable. They set out to assess risk of material misstatement at the assertion level based on their business understanding and preliminary risk assessments. Belinda instructed them to focus only on the most significant inherent risks of material misstatement and bring her their proposed plan by the end of the day.

Donna and Caleb decide that for the accounts receivable balance, there is not much risk of error in the existence or completeness assertions, since the system is automated and generates invoices simultaneously with any delivery. They decide that they should test the information technology (IT) controls over this transaction processing, and if they are effective the risk of errors will be minimal. However, the processing of volume discounts seems complex and involves a large degree of manual calculation, so there could be a risk of measurement errors that will affect the valuation assertion. They also realize that sending letters to customers and getting them to confirm how much they owe EcoPak at year-end would be pretty easy because there are only a few large customers, so only a few letters could verify a large portion of the balance with substantive evidence. That would also provide substantive evidence about whether there were any errors in the volume discount calculations. For the cash receipts, they assess the completeness assertion to be high risk, since there is always a risk that cash could be misappropriated. To test the completeness of cash receipts, they think they should inspect the supporting documentation (remittance advices) for a sample of cash receipts collected from customers, trace each receipt to the bank deposit slip and related bank statement, trace the debit entries to the cash account in the general ledger, and trace the credit entries to the accounts receivable subledger. Donna realizes that if there is a risk that cash receipts are incomplete (understated), this will also flow through to cause an existence (overstatement) risk in the accounts receivable balance, so the confirmation procedure seems like an even better idea, since it will provide some persuasive evidence about both these risks.

Caleb seems to be catching on quickly, so Donna asks him what he thinks is the biggest risk in the sales transactions. Caleb considers that if some fictitious sales were recorded, it would lead to overstatements of both revenues and accounts receivable. Even though the audit team has not seen anything that might indicate EcoPak's management or accounting staff would inflate their sales, Caleb notes that they do have incentives to do it, since it makes the company look a lot more successful (*and* they are considering doing an initial public offering [IPO]!). His gut feeling is that as independent auditors, they should be skeptical about such things and not just assume that everything is okay. So, he feels they need to test whether the sales really occurred by inspecting shipping documents to confirm that the sales recorded are all supported by valid sales transactions with customers.

Donna is pleased: "Nice analysis, Caleb! You are catching on. Let's enter all these assertion-level risk assessments and the evidence-gathering procedures we think we should do to respond to those risks into the R/R/R planning form now. That will document our work, and then we can go over to see what Belinda thinks about our decisions before we start making arrangements to go to EcoPak's offices."

The Essentials of Audit Evidence

An essential feature of a financial statement audit engagement is that the auditor must obtain independent evidence that supports the assertions in the financial statements. Audit procedures provide evidence that can support reasonable assurance. The audit evidence obtained must be persuasive enough for the auditor to reach a well-reasoned conclusion that the financial statements are not materially misstated. The concept of reasonable assurance in auditing is based essentially on logical argumentation, where assertions are the claims to be proven, and various forms of evidence are used to build an argument that could persuade someone that the claims are evident. Recall the critical thinking process we looked at in Chapter 3, and note how it, too, is based on logical argumentation.

Throughout the steps of the audit process, audit procedures are used for four main purposes: risk assessment procedures, control testing procedures, substantive procedures, and analytical procedures.

As we worked with the audit risk model, we saw that to achieve an acceptably low level of audit risk, auditors have to do audit work to lower their risk of not detecting a material misstatement. Auditors assess the risk of materiality at the assertion level, and this is the starting point for planning how to go about gathering evidence that is relevant to assessing whether material misstatements have entered the financial statements. The sources of relevant evidence available include the auditee's personnel, systems and records, procedures, physical assets, internal and external documents, external organizations, external experts, and various industry and economic research data.

Auditors have six main types of evidence-gathering techniques available in their tool kit. These are

- Inspection
- Observation
- Confirmation
- Reperformance/recalculation
- Analysis
- Inquiry

Since these tools are so important for creating audit evidence-gathering procedures, many auditors use an acronym to remember them (e.g., IOCRAI). *Inspection* is performed by the auditor personally examining a physical asset or a document or record of the auditee organization. *Observation* involves the auditor using sight or other senses to assess conditions or activities in the auditee. *Confirmation* is done by requesting that an independent external party verify information about the auditee by providing an oral or written response directly to the auditor. *Reperformance/recalculation* is done by the auditor performing the same procedure, calculation, or process that the auditee staff has done, to check if the result is the same. *Analysis* involves studying comparisons and relationships and comparing results to auditor expectations to determine if financial information is reasonable. *Inquiry* involves the auditor asking questions of auditee personnel and obtaining oral or written information directly from them. Risk assessment procedures mainly use the inquiry and analysis techniques. They give the auditor useful evidence for understanding and insight into the likelihood of material misstatements, but they only provide indirect evidence about whether the financial statements are actually misstated. Control tests mainly use inquiry, observation, inspection, and reperformance techniques and give relevant evidence about internal control effectiveness, i.e., whether management's internal control over financial reporting is being complied with so misstatements are less likely. Control tests only give indirect evidence that the financial statements are not misstated, however. Substantive procedures examine evidence about dollar amounts and details for specific assertions in financial statement items and disclosures, so they can provide direct evidence about whether there are misstatements. Substantive procedures mainly involve confirmation, inspection, reperformance/recalculation, and analysis if specific data is used. Analytical procedures include a broad range of activities that can provide indirect or direct evidence about material misstatement, and since they can be used to corroborate other evidence, they can increase the overall reliability of the auditor's evidence. Thus, analysis is widely used throughout the audit process. Analytical procedures are used for attention-directing purposes in the risk assessment step of the audit process and are used as an overall reasonability evaluation by the engagement partner at the final step of the audit, before forming an opinion on fair presentation. They may also be used for substantive evidence in the second step of the audit process, to respond to assessed risks by testing the reasonability of accounting balances.

To support reasonable assurance, generally accepted auditing standards (GAAS) do not allow auditors to rely only on risk assessment, control effectiveness, and analytical evidence, however. Substantive audit evidence must always be obtained to support the audit opinion.

To provide reasonable assurance, the audit evidence obtained must be convincing. GAAS use the term *sufficient appropriate audit evidence* to describe the quantity and quality of evidence needed to support an audit opinion. Sufficiency of evidence means there is enough evidence so that most people would find it reasonable to support the conclusion. Appropriateness means the evidence is relevant to the assertions and reliable enough to be believable. Relevance refers to the logical connection between the evidence and the assertion. Reliability depends on the source and nature of the evidence. Generally, the most reliable evidence is the direct personal knowledge of the auditor, for example, that obtained from inspecting physical assets or recalculating prepaid expenses, and the least reliable is representations of management, for example, that obtained from inquiries about whether all contingent liabilities have been disclosed.

Four key decisions must be made in designing audit procedures: the nature of the evidence technique to use, how many items should be tested, which items to test, and when the procedures should be performed (i.e., the nature, extent, selection, and timing, or NEST). Audit evidence techniques can be selected from commonly used procedures (e.g., confirm a sample of 30 accounts receivable balances) or might be specially designed to meet audit objectives in unique client situations. In the planning stage, the auditors will have identified the highest-risk assertions to be addressed and the types of evidence sources that exist in the auditee's business. The high-risk assertions are the most important audit objectives, and the available procedures are the means of meeting them (this is "responding to the assessed risks" in the GAAS terminology). Fortunately, most companies have similar financial reporting requirements, and there are auditing procedures that are commonly applicable on most audits. So we don't need to reinvent the wheel for every financial statement audit, but we do need to be aware of unique aspects in each audit and be prepared to develop appropriate responses.

Audit programs are lists of audit procedures to be performed for each area of the financial statement audit. To develop audit programs, auditors need to ask: "What evidence is needed to address the highest-risk assertions? Why is this evidence relevant to the assertion? How can this evidence be obtained?" Audit programs are the instructions that audit team members who are assigned to work on the audit will follow.

Clear and careful documentation of the programs is important to ensure they will be done well. GAAS require documentation of the planned procedures, as well as requiring the findings and conclusions of the audit staff to be retained in files. These audit documentation files are reviewed for quality and completeness by more-senior audit staff. They will ultimately be reviewed by the audit engagement partner, who is responsible for deciding whether the audit evidence obtained supports signing the audit opinion.

The requirement to obtain sufficient appropriate independent evidence is what distinguishes an audit opinion from all other reports accountants give to third parties, such as review engagement reports or compilation reports. Even so, evidence that provides an auditor with reasonable assurance that the financial statement assertions are not materially misstated can allow an auditor to conclude that the risk of material misstatement is very low, but the risk can never be zero due to the inherent limitations of accounting. So professional judgment always plays an essential role in auditing.

Review Checkpoints

8-1 Explain why independent audit evidence needs to be persuasive.

8-2 Explain the logical argumentation approach that underlies how an auditor uses audit evidence to support reasonable assurance.

8-3 List and describe six main techniques used to gather audit evidence.

8-4 Identify four main purposes of auditing procedures used in the three steps of the audit process.

8-5 Explain why risk assessment and control testing procedures give indirect rather than direct audit evidence relevant to the audit opinion.

8-6 Explain why substantive audit procedures provide direct evidence relevant to the audit opinion.

8-7 Explain why analytical procedures are used throughout the audit process.

8-8 Identify two points in the audit process when analytical procedures are required by GAAS, and explain why they are considered necessary.

8-9 Why does corroboration increase the reliability of evidence?

8-10 What are two important qualities of evidence that increase its reliability?

8-11 Explain what sufficient appropriate audit evidence means in GAAS.

8-12 What makes evidence relevant?

8-13 How does an auditor determine that the evidence obtained is sufficient to support the audit conclusion?

8-14 How do the evidence techniques relate to audit procedures?

8-15 What do audit programs contain? How are they used in an audit?

8-16 What is the purpose of audit documentation? How is it created in an audit engagement? Why do GAAS require it to be complete and clear?

8-17 How does the evidence requirement for an audit opinion differ from that of other types of professional accounting engagements?

Evidence-Gathering Audit Procedures

LO1 Outline six general audit techniques for gathering evidence.

Most of the auditor's work involves designing and performing audit procedures to obtain **sufficient appropriate audit evidence** and then evaluating that evidence to draw reasonable conclusions on which to base the audit opinion. This chapter explains how auditors apply judgment to determine the sufficiency and appropriateness of evidence as a source of reasonable assurance and to develop detailed evidence-gathering procedures in the audit plan.

Auditors obtain six basic types of evidence and use six general techniques to gather it. The six techniques are (1) inspection, (2) observation, (3) confirmation, (4) recalculation/reperformance, (5) analysis, and (6) inquiry. One or more of these techniques may be used no matter what account balance, class of transactions, control procedure, or other information is under audit.

sufficient appropriate audit evidence:
information obtained by an auditor in relation to one or more audit objectives (assertions) that is adequately persuasive to support a logical conclusion; "sufficiency" generally refers to the quantity (sample size) and independence of the evidential matter in relation to the level of risk of material misstatement; "appropriateness" generally refers to the level of reliability of the evidential matter and its relevance to the audit objective

Evidence that comes from inspection, observation, or recalculation/reperformance techniques is generally the most reliable because it is based on the auditor's personal knowledge. Evidence in the form of written confirmations from external sources also has high reliability since it is outside the control of auditee management. In Chapters 6 and 7, we showed how inquiry is an important evidence-gathering technique used to obtain information from auditee personnel or external sources for understanding the auditee's business and assessing the risk of material misstatement. Inquiry generates essential audit evidence, but inquiry alone does not provide sufficient audit evidence that there is no material misstatement, or that internal control is effective. Auditors use a combination of evidence-gathering techniques to look for corroborating evidence, since that is more persuasive than a single piece of evidence. Auditors cannot obtain absolute assurance because of the limitations of audit procedures and accounting itself, so professional judgment is required in deciding when the evidence gathered is enough to provide reasonable assurance.

Standards Check

CAS 500 Audit Evidence

6. The auditor shall design and perform audit procedures that are appropriate in the circumstances for the purpose of obtaining sufficient appropriate audit evidence. (Ref: Para. A1–A25)

A2. Most of the auditor's work in forming the auditor's opinion consists of obtaining and evaluating audit evidence. Audit procedures to obtain audit evidence can include inspection, observation, confirmation, recalculation, reperformance, and analytical procedures, often in some combination, in addition to inquiry. Although inquiry may provide important audit evidence, and may even produce evidence of a misstatement, inquiry alone ordinarily does not provide sufficient audit evidence of the absence of a material misstatement at the assertion level, nor of the operating effectiveness of controls.

Source: *CPA Canada Handbook—Assurance*, 2014.

Evidence Techniques and Types of Audit Procedures

In practice, the general techniques form the basis for more specifically defined audit procedures. As we look in more detail at how audits are planned and performed, we will see that the evidence techniques are used in the design of four main types of audit procedures: risk assessment procedures, analytical procedures, control testing procedures, and substantive procedures.

Risk assessment procedures give auditors relevant evidence that is useful for understanding and assessing the likelihood of material misstatements, but they only provide indirect evidence about whether the financial statements are actually misstated. Analytical procedures include a broad range of activities that can provide indirect or direct evidence about material misstatement and can also be used to corroborate other evidence, so they are widely used throughout the steps of the audit process. Control testing procedures give relevant evidence about internal control effectiveness, i.e., whether management's internal control procedures are being complied with so misstatements are less likely, but control tests only give indirect evidence that the financial statements are not misstated. Substantive procedures examine evidence about monetary amounts and details for specific assertions in financial statement items and disclosures, so they can provide direct evidence about whether there are misstatements. Auditors can sometimes design procedures called *dual-purpose audit procedures* that include steps to test the effectiveness of an internal control procedure as well as steps that give substantive evidence about the resulting monetary balance related to the internal control procedure. Dual-purpose procedures use the same sample of transactions or account balances to obtain the evidence, so they can be performed more efficiently than separately performing control tests and substantive procedures.

To support reasonable assurance, GAAS do not allow auditors to rely only on risk assessment, control effectiveness, and analysis. They need to get direct evidence, so some substantive audit procedures must always be performed to support the audit opinion.

Exhibit 8–1 shows the six general techniques matched to the types of evidence each provides and gives some examples of specific procedures that could be included in an audit program.

EXHIBIT 8-1

Audit Techniques and Related Types of Evidence

AUDIT TECHNIQUE	TYPES OF EVIDENCE	EXAMPLES OF SPECIFIC PROCEDURES (AND HOW THEY ARE USED IN AN AUDIT)
1. Inspection	1a. Documents prepared by independent parties 1b. Documents prepared by the auditee 1c. Physical inspection of tangible assets	1a. Read the terms of the lease agreement for the lessee (understanding business). 1b. Review the inventory variance analysis report prepared by the production department (assessing risk). 1c. Test counts of a sample of physical inventory quantities on hand at year-end (substantive verification of account balance). Examine damaged inventory on hand (substantive verification of account balance).
2. Observation	2. Auditor's observations	2. Observe data entry procedures (understanding controls and control testing). Observe petty cash control procedures (understanding controls and control testing). Observe auditee's inventory-counting procedures (understanding controls and control testing).
3. Confirmation	3. Statements by independent parties	3. Obtain written confirmation of accounts receivable balance from a sample of customers (substantive verification of account balance). Obtain written confirmation of loan amount, interest, collateral, and payment dates from lender (substantive verification of account balance).
4. Recalculation/ reperformance	4. Auditor's calculations or performance	4. Recompute amortization expense using declining balance method (substantive verification of account balance). Recompute "price times quantity" on a sample of invoices (substantive verification of account balance). Recompute sales tax as a percentage of total sale amount on a sample of invoices (substantive verification of account balance). Reperform data entry procedure with automated missing data control (control testing).
5. Analysis	5. Data interrelationships	5. Analyze monthly gross margin by product line. Compare inventory turnover rate to previous year (assessing risk and/or corroborating substantive verification findings).
6. Inquiry	6. Statements by auditee personnel	6. Inquire about frequency of bank reconciliation procedures (understanding controls for risk assessment). Inquire about which employee totals cash receipts and deposits them to the bank (understanding controls for risk assessment).

Inspection

Inspection consists of examining records and documents or looking at assets with physical substance. The procedures that can be used have different degrees of thoroughness: examining, perusing, reading, reviewing, scanning, scrutinizing, tracing, and vouching. Physically inspecting tangible assets provides reliable evidence of existence and may give some evidence of condition, and hence valuation, but it does not provide reliable evidence of ownership. Much auditing work involves examining authoritative documents prepared by independent parties and by the auditee. Physical inspection of formal documents with intrinsic value, such as securities certificates, provides reliable evidence about existence. Records and documents that do not have an intrinsic market value, such as invoices, purchase orders, or contracts, have varying degrees of reliability for different assertions, depending mainly on the reliability of their source. Documents held by the auditee and available for auditors' inspection can be classified by whether they originate from external or internal sources, as discussed below.

Inspection:
audit procedures that involve examining an auditee's records or documents, whether internal or external, in paper form, electronic form, or other media, or a physically examining an asset; provides evidence of, for example, the existence of an asset, the occurrence of a transaction, or the appropriate application of GAAP to the item; inspection of documents takes the form of vouching, tracing, and scanning; also called inspection of documents, physical inspection

Documents Prepared by Independent External Parties

A great deal of documentary evidence is "external-internal," that is, convincing documentation prepared or validated by other parties and sent to the auditee, or made available online. The signatures, seals, engravings, secure password-protected websites, and other distinctive aspects of formal authoritative documents make them difficult to alter and, therefore, more reliable than ordinary documents prepared by outsiders. Some examples of formal authoritative documents and ordinary documents are listed below:

EXTERNAL-INTERNAL TYPES OF DOCUMENTARY EVIDENCE	
FORMAL AUTHORITATIVE DOCUMENTS	**ORDINARY DOCUMENTS**
1. Bank statements, secure online banking account access	1. Suppliers' invoices
2. Cancelled cheques	2. Customers' purchase orders
3. Insurance policies	3. Loan applications
4. Notes receivable	4. Credit notes received
5. Securities certificates, secure online investment accounts	5. Expense receipts
6. Loan and collateral agreements	6. Insurance policy applications
7. Elaborate contracts	7. Simple, standard contracts
8. Title papers (e.g., automobiles, real estate)	8. Correspondence
9. Income and payroll tax assessments	

Documents Prepared and Processed within the Entity under Audit

Documents prepared and processed by the auditee are internal evidence. Some of these documents may be quite informal and not very authoritative or reliable. Generally, the reliability of these documents depends on the quality of internal control under which they were produced and processed. Some of the most common of these documents are as follows:

1. Sales invoice copies
2. Sales summary reports
3. Shipping documents
4. Credit notes issued
5. Purchase requisition slips
6. Purchase orders
7. Receiving reports
8. Cost distribution reports
9. Employee payroll information forms
10. Bank deposit listings and slips
11. Budgets and performance reports
12. Documentation of transactions with subsidiary or affiliated companies
13. General journal entry support forms

Inspection of Documents: Vouching, Tracing, and Scanning Procedures

Vouching—Examination of Documents   In **vouching**, an auditor selects a sample of financial information items from an account (e.g., the posting of a sales invoice in a customer's master file) and goes backward through

vouching:
an audit procedure that involves examining documents based on the selection of transactions, entries, or balances that appear in the auditee's general ledger accounts and seeking evidence that supports the validity of the item; sometimes referred to as "grave to cradle" testing

the accounting and control system to find and examine the source documentation supporting the items. For a sales invoice, the auditor examines the journal entry or data input list; sales summary; sales invoice copy and shipping documents; and, finally, customer purchase order. Vouching helps auditors decide if all recorded data are adequately supported (the existence/occurrence assertion), but it does not provide evidence that all events were recorded. This latter problem is covered by tracing.

Tracing—Examination of Documents **Tracing** takes the opposite direction to vouching. In tracing, the auditor selects a sample of basic source documents and goes forward through the accounting and control system (whether computer or manual) to find the final recording of the transaction in the general ledger accounts. For example, samples of payroll payments are traced to cost and expense accounts, sales invoices to the sales accounts, cash receipts to the accounts receivable subsidiary accounts, and cash payments to the accounts payable subsidiary accounts. Using tracing, an auditor can decide whether all events were recorded (the completeness assertion) and complement the evidence obtained by vouching. Auditors must also be alert to significant events that may not have been captured in the source documents or entered into the accounting system.

Scanning—Examination of Documents **Scanning** is performed by reviewing the auditee's files and records, being alert to any unusual items and events. A typical scanning instruction in an audit program is, "Scan all the expense accounts for credit entries; vouch any to source documents."

Scanning involves looking for anything unusual. The procedure usually does not produce direct evidence itself, but it can raise questions for which other evidence must be obtained. Scanning can be accomplished on computer records online, using audit software, or on printed-out reports. Typical items discovered by the scanning effort are debits in revenue accounts, credits in expense accounts, unusually large accounts receivable write-offs, unusually large paycheques, unusually small sales volume in the month following the year-end, and large cash deposits just prior to year-end. Scanning can give some evidence of existence of assets and completeness of accounting records, including proper cutoff of material transactions.

Scanning is valuable when sampling methods are applied in audit decisions. When a sample is the basis for selecting items for audit, there is always the risk of choosing a sample that does not reflect the entire population of items, resulting in a decision error. Auditors subjectively reduce this risk by scanning items not selected in the sample.

Review Checkpoints

8-18 List six audit techniques used to gather evidence and the types of evidence related to them.

8-19 Differentiate between authoritative and ordinary externally produced documents.

8-20 Define the following terms: *vouching*, *tracing*, and *scanning*.

tracing:
an audit procedure that involves examining documents based on the selection of evidence in supporting documents of transactions or other events and then following the information forward through the accounting processing system to find whether it has been included in the auditee's general ledger accounts; sometimes referred to as "cradle to grave" testing

scanning:
an audit procedure in which the auditor quickly reviews a whole report, account, journal, or other listing in the auditee's records to look for any unusual items that require further investigation

Observation

Observation consists of looking at how policy or procedures are applied by others. It provides highly reliable evidence as to performance or conditions at a given point in time, but it does not necessarily reflect performance at other times or over long periods. The technique is used whenever auditors take an inspection tour, watch personnel carry out accounting and control activities, or participate in a surprise petty cash count or payroll distribution. Physical observation also produces a general awareness of events in the auditee's offices.

External Confirmation

Confirmation consists of an inquiry, usually written, to third parties external to the auditee, to verify accounting records. Direct correspondence with independent external parties is a confirmation procedure widely used in auditing. For example, *external confirmation* for accounts receivable is recommended by Canadian Auditing Standard (CAS) 505.

Standards Check

CAS 505 External Confirmations

2. CAS 500 indicates that the reliability of audit evidence is influenced by its source and by its nature and is dependent on the individual circumstances under which it is obtained . . . ; depending on the circumstances of the audit, audit evidence in the form of external confirmations received directly by the auditor from confirming parties may be more reliable than evidence generated internally by the entity.

Source: *CPA Canada Handbook—Assurance*, 2014.

Confirmation can produce evidence of existence, ownership, valuation, and cutoff. Most transactions involve external parties, and, theoretically, confirmation could be conducted even on such items as paycheques. Confirmation is one of the more labour-intensive audit procedures, so auditors often limit its use to major transactions and balances that external parties can provide information about. A selection of confirmation applications follows:

*   Banks—account balances
*   Customers—receivables balances
*   Borrowers—note terms and balances
*   Agents—inventory or consignment in warehouse
*   Lenders—note terms and balances
*   Policyholders—life insurance contracts
*   Suppliers—accounts payable balances
*   Registrar—number of shares outstanding
*   Legal counsel—litigation in progress
*   Trustees—securities held, terms of agreements
*   Lessors—lease terms

observation:
an audit procedure that consists of looking at a process or procedure being performed by others, for example, the auditor's observation of inventory counting by the entity's personnel, or of the performance of control activities

confirmation:
an audit procedure by which auditors obtain evidence in the form of a direct written response to the auditor from a third party (the confirming party), in paper form, or by electronic or other medium, usually the evidence is related to certain account balances or other information such as terms of agreements or transactions with third parties; also called external confirmation

Some important general points about confirmations are as follows:

- Confirmation letters should be printed on the auditee's letterhead and signed by an auditee officer.
- Auditors should be very careful that the recipient's address is reliable and not altered by auditee personnel so that it misdirects the confirmation.
- The request should seek information the recipient can supply, such as the amount of their account balance or the amounts of specified invoices or notes.
- Confirmations should be controlled by the audit firm, not given to auditee personnel for mailing.
- Responses should be returned directly to the audit firm, not to the auditee. To ensure the evidence is independent and highly reliable, there should be no opportunity for auditee personnel to alter the confirmation responses.

Confirmations of receivables and payables can take two forms, namely positive confirmation and negative confirmation. Positive confirmations request replies in all cases, whether the account balance is considered correct or incorrect. Negative confirmations request replies only if the account balance is considered incorrect. Auditors make second and third attempts to non-responders of requests for positive confirmation. If no response to a positive confirmation request appears, or if the response to either type of confirmation varies from the auditee's records, the auditors should investigate with other audit procedures, such as checking whether the customer paid the receivable after year-end, or inspecting internal documents for evidence supporting the recording of the receivable.[1]

Recalculation/Reperformance

Recalculation is redoing calculations already performed by auditee personnel. This produces compelling mathematical evidence since the auditee calculation is either right or wrong. Computer-generated calculations can be recalculated using auditing software, with differences being highlighted for further audit investigation. Mathematical evidence can serve the objectives of both existence and valuation for financial statement amounts that result from calculations, for example, depreciation, pension liabilities, prepaid expenses, accrued interest expense, and/or payroll liabilities. Recalculation, in combination with other procedures, is also used to provide evidence of valuation for all other financial data. It provides highly reliable evidence of mathematical accuracy, but the number generated is only as good as the components; the auditor must audit every significant part of the original computation if recalculation is to provide strong, persuasive evidence.

A related type of evidence is called **reperformance**. Usually applied in control testing, the auditor independently executes one or more of the auditee's internal control procedures. This can provide compelling evidence about the effectiveness of a control procedure.

Review Checkpoints

8-21　What are the strengths and limitations of recalculation-based audit evidence?

8-22　What are the strengths and limitations of observation-based audit evidence?

8-23　Why must the entire confirmation process be controlled by the audit firm?

8-24　What can auditors do to improve the effectiveness of confirmation requests?

recalculation:
an audit procedure that involves redoing computations already performed by auditee personnel to determine if the result is accurate; may be done manually or electronically

reperformance:
an audit procedure in which the auditor executes a procedure that is part of the auditee's internal control to obtain evidence about the effectiveness of controls or the accuracy of the auditor's understanding of the auditee's information system

Analysis

The term **analysis** refers to methods of study and comparison that auditors use to obtain evidence about financial statement accounts. Analysis is the "other" category in the list of six auditing techniques and can include any other verification work an auditor wants to do that does not meet the definition of inspection, observation, confirmation, recalculation/reperformance, or structured inquiry. *Analytical procedures* range from simple comparisons to complex mathematical estimation models. They can be used to obtain evidence on any of the financial statement assertions, but they are most useful for assertions of completeness, valuation, and presentation.[2] Analytical procedures are widely used for auditing the income statement items, such as operating, administration, interest, and other expenses.

Analysis is a flexible and powerful technique for obtaining evidence about whether the financial statements are fairly presented, so auditors use analysis in all three steps of the audit process. As discussed in Chapter 5, GAAS require auditors to use analysis in the risk assessment step, to obtain a preliminary understanding of the audit client and assess the risks of material misstatement. GAAS also require auditors to use analysis at the conclusion step, to support the audit opinion. This final, overall analysis of the financial statements is essential for evaluating whether they are fairly presented. Auditors also often perform analytical procedures in their audit programs to obtain substantive evidence related to the assessed risks of misstatement.

Analysis consists of

1. Identifying the components of a financial statement item so the characteristics of these can be considered in designing the nature, extent, selection, and timing of other audit procedures; and

2. Performing analytical procedures, which are techniques by which the auditor

    (i) Studies and uses meaningful relationships among elements of financial and non-financial information to form expectations about what the amounts recorded in the accounts should be;

    (ii) Compares expected with recorded amounts to identify fluctuations and relationships that are not consistent with other relevant information or that deviate significantly from expected amounts; and

    (iii) Uses the results of this comparison to help determine what, if any, other audit procedures are needed for obtaining sufficient appropriate audit evidence that the recorded amounts are not materially misstated.[3]

The difference between item 1 above and scanning is that analysis relates to a comparison of financial statement components, whereas scanning relates to the detailed records about a particular component.

Analytical procedures can be classified into the five general types discussed in Chapter 5. When analysis is used to provide substantive evidence, auditors need to be careful to use independent, reliable information for comparison purposes. Thus, the sources of information used in analytical procedures need to be assessed for independence and objectivity. Quantitative information must be verified by the auditor if a high level of reliance

---

analysis:
audit procedures that involve identifying the components of financial information and evaluating financial information by studying plausible relationships among both financial and non-financial data to identify fluctuations or relationships that are inconsistent with other relevant information or that differ from expected values by a significant amount and need to be investigated in order to assess risk of material misstatement, obtain substantive evidence, or form an overall opinion at the end of the audit

CAS 520 Analytical Procedures

5. When designing and performing substantive analytical procedures, either alone or in combination with tests of details, as substantive procedures in accordance with CAS 330, paragraph 18, the auditor shall (Ref: Para. A4–A5)

(a) Determine the suitability of particular substantive analytical procedures for given assertions, taking account of the assessed risks of material misstatement and tests of details, if any, for these assertions; (Ref: Para. A6–A11)

(b) Evaluate the reliability of data from which the auditor's expectation of recorded amounts or ratios is developed, taking account of source, comparability, and nature and relevance of information available, and controls over preparation; (Ref: Para. A12–A14)

(c) Develop an expectation of recorded amounts or ratios and evaluate whether the expectation is sufficiently precise to identify a misstatement that, individually or when aggregated with other misstatements, may cause the financial statements to be materially misstated; and (Ref: Para. A15)

(d) Determine the amount of any difference of recorded amounts from expected values that is acceptable without further investigation as required by paragraph 7. (Ref: Para. A16)

Source: *CPA Canada Handbook—Assurance*, 2014.

is placed on the evidence provided by analysis. Examples of the types of independent information sources, and how their reliability can be verified, are as follows:

INFORMATION SOURCE	EVIDENCE OF RELIABILITY OF INFORMATION SOURCE
Financial account information for comparable prior period(s)	The information agrees with audited financial statements, or information in prior-year audit working papers (e.g., monthly results).
Company budgets and forecasts	The budgeting or forecasting process is reviewed by the auditor and found to be based on realistic assumptions and methods, and targets are achievable under normal business conditions. Budget and forecast information is produced by the company's information systems under internal controls monitored by senior management; the auditor has assessed these controls to be strong. Budgets and forecasts are used by the board of directors for decision making.
Financial relationships among accounts in the current period	Account balances used in analysis should be agreed/referenced to audit working papers in the current-year file where they are verified substantively.
Industry statistics	Sources should be well-known industry analysis services (e.g., Moody's, Standard and Poor's), and reports used should be obtained directly by the auditors.
Non-financial information, such as physical production statistics	Non-financial information is prepared by the company's information systems under internal controls monitored by senior management; the auditor has assessed these controls to be effective. The non-financial information is used by senior management and the board for decision making.

Because analytical procedures are loosely defined, it is tempting for auditors, and people in general, to consider the evidence produced to be "soft." Therefore, they may tend to concentrate more on recalculation, observation, confirmation, inspection of assets, and vouching of documents that are perceived to produce "hard" evidence. However, analytical procedures can be very effective, because they integrate evidence from a variety of sources and often provide an independent way of gathering evidence about whether the financial statement assertions hold true. Some examples of using analytical procedures to detect misstatements are given in the following box.

Finding Misstatements with Analytical Procedures

- Auditors noticed large quantities of rolled steel in the company's inventory. Several 30,000-kilogram rolls were entered in the inventory list. The false entries were detected because the auditor knew the company's fork-lift trucks had a 10,000-kilogram lifting capacity.
- Auditors compared the total quantity of vegetable oils the company claimed to have inventoried in its tanks with the storage capacity reported in national export statistics. The company's "quantity on hand" amounted to 90% of the national supply and greatly exceeded its own tank capacity.
- Last year's working papers showed that the company employees had failed to accrue wages payable at the year-end date. A search for the current accrual entry showed it had been forgotten again.
- Auditors programmed a complex regression model to estimate the electric utility company's total revenue. They used empirical relations of fuel consumption, meteorological reports of weather conditions, and population census data in the area. The regression model estimated revenue within close range of the reported revenue.

Auditing research has found that "soft" procedures like analytical procedures and discussion of findings with auditee personnel can lead to detecting a significant proportion of the misstatements discovered in audits.[4] Analytical procedures are a good value since they are usually less costly than the more detailed, document-oriented procedures. Also, the "hard-evidence" procedures have their own pitfalls. Auditors may not be competent to "see" things they are supposed to observe. Auditee personnel can manipulate confirmations. The following box illustrates problems that can arise in evaluating evidence obtained with hard-evidence procedures. An audit program makes use of several different types of procedures, and analytical procedures deserve a prominent place.

Potholes in the Audit Procedure Road

Recalculation:
An auditor calculated inventory valuations (quantities times price) thinking the measuring unit was gross (144 units each), but the auditee had actually recorded counts in dozens (12 units each), thus causing the inventory valuation to be 12 times the proper measure.

Inspection of Assets:
While inspecting the fertilizer tank assets in ranch country, the auditor was fooled when the manager was able to move the tanks to other locations and place new numbers on them. The auditor "inspected" the same tanks many times.

Confirmation:
The auditor sent a bank confirmation letter to verify the existence of $3.2 billion of cash in the company's bank account in New York. Unfortunately, the auditor put the confirmation letter in the client's outgoing mail box, and it was intercepted by management, who copied the signature of an actual bank official from another document and pasted it onto the auditor's confirmation response form. A company employee was sent to New York to mail the letter to add authenticity. When the response confirming $3.2 billion of non-existent cash was received, the auditor did not notice these falsifications.

Inquiry:
Seeking evidence of the collectability of accounts receivable, the auditors "audited by conversation" and took the credit manager's word about the collection probabilities on the over-90-day past-due accounts. They sought no other evidence and did not discover that reported "net realizable value" of accounts receivable was materially overstated.

Inspection by Examination of Documents, Vouching Procedure:
The auditors of a wholesaling company did not notice that the bank statement had been crudely altered by writing over a "3" to make it look like a "9," so the ending balance looked like $930,725 instead of the real balance, $330,725.

Inspection by the Scanning Procedure:
The auditors of a bank extracted a computer list of all the bank's loans over $1,000. They neglected to perform a similar scan for loans with negative balances, a condition that should not occur. The bank had data processing problems that caused many loan balances to be negative, although the trial balance balanced!

Review Checkpoints

8-25   What does analysis consist of?

8-26   What are the three stages in an audit engagement when analysis is used?

8-27   What sources of information are useful for performing analysis?

8-28   If analysis is used to provide substantive audit evidence, what steps must be taken regarding the source information used in the analysis?

8-29   Discuss the effectiveness of analysis for discovering misstatements.

Inquiry

Inquiry generally involves collecting oral evidence from independent parties, auditee officials, and employees. Auditors use inquiry procedures early in the audit when they have an information-gathering meeting with the client management and tour the offices and operating facilities. Evidence gathered by formal and informal inquiry of auditee personnel generally cannot stand alone and must be corroborated by the findings of other procedures. Further inquiries could be made from other appropriate sources within the entity. Consistent responses increase the persuasiveness of the inquiry-based evidence. Sometimes, however, conflicting evidence might come from someone volunteering adverse information, such as an admission of theft, deliberate misstatement, or use of an accounting policy that is misleading. The auditor will have to use considerable judgment to reconcile conflicting evidence or to decide what additional evidence to gather. Skepticism and a critical attitude are, as always, important aspects of professional judgment.

Inquiries, interviews, and other oral evidence are significant within the profession because management's explanations are an important part of obtaining an understanding of the business environment and risk, and the nature of specific transactions.[5] Management's explanations can be compared with those of other auditee employees, industry experts, and other sources of evidence. The explanations auditors obtain through good inquiry procedures can be very effective in detecting fraud and management motives (discussed in Chapter 7), and in assessing the reasonableness of management assumptions for accounting estimates (discussed in Chapter 19, available on Connect). Auditors must obtain statements from management in the written representation letter acknowledging all important inquiries.[6]

The audit standards rely heavily on audit inquiry evidence, and the CPA Canada research report entitled *Audit Enquiry* identifies ways of making it more reliable. For example, assessing the reliability of the auditee's accounting estimates process frequently involves discussions with senior management. The CPA Canada report illustrates inquiries of senior management in customer service, manufacturing, quality control, marketing, and finance to assess the adequacy of an allowance for warranty claims.

Team discussions required by audit standards at the planning and risk assessment stages of the audit enhance integration and synthesis of the whole range of audit evidence obtained by audit team members.[7] Inquiry-based evidence is subject to individual interpretations, so getting different audit team members' perspectives on it can lead to better-reasoned conclusions. Timely, well-organized audit discussions facilitate sharing of inquiry evidence and other corroborating evidence to identify inconsistencies that may indicate material misstatement due to error, and particularly to detect fraud.[8]

inquiry:
audit procedures that involve asking knowledgeable persons within the auditee organization or outside for relevant financial and/or non-financial information; may provide the auditor with information not available otherwise, provide corroboration for other audit evidence obtained, or provide conflicting information that requires additional audit investigation; includes written representations from management that are obtained at the end of an audit engagement

Standards Check

CAS 300 Planning an Audit of Financial Statements

5. The engagement partner and other key members of the engagement team shall be involved in planning the audit, including planning and participating in the discussion among engagement team members. (Ref: Para. A4)

CAS 240 The Auditor's Responsibilities Relating to Fraud in an Audit of Financial Statements

15. CAS 315 requires a discussion among the engagement team members and a determination by the engagement partner of which matters are to be communicated to those team members not involved in the discussion. This discussion shall place particular emphasis on how and where the entity's financial statements may be susceptible to material misstatement due to fraud, including how fraud might occur. The discussion shall occur setting aside beliefs that the engagement team members may have that management and those charged with governance are honest and have integrity. (Ref: Para. A10–A11)

Source: *CPA Canada Handbook–Assurance*, 2014.

A CPA Canada research report makes this note about team meetings: "Debriefings following interviews and site visits should encourage perceptions and intuitive feelings to be brought out, and information challenged to help identify inconsistencies and gaps . . . and answer colleagues' questions about their findings and impressions. . . . The objective, of course, is an integration of findings, capitalizing on the synergy that can come from focused group effort."[9] Junior auditors have the opportunity to learn from more-experienced auditors how to apply judgment in evaluating evidence, and they can also benefit the team by bringing in their own objective viewpoints.

Special Note on Dual-Purpose Audit Procedures

Dual-purpose audit procedures are multi-step procedures that are designed to meet the purpose of a control test and the purpose of a substantive test, thus the name "dual-purpose." By using several different evidence techniques on the same sample of transactions, dual-purpose audit procedures combine steps to test the effectiveness of an internal control procedure with steps that give substantive evidence about the resulting monetary balance. When auditors plan to assess control effectiveness by testing the company's controls for a sample of transactions, it may often be more efficient to use the same sample for both purposes, rather than doing these tests separately. A dual-purpose procedure will follow the same sample of transactions from the control testing through to where they are recorded in the general ledger, to obtain substantive evidence verifying the related account balance.

For example, a control testing audit procedure for sales transactions might include the following steps: observing that a sale cannot be processed until the customer's credit is approved by the credit manager, inspecting the shipping documents to ensure the information has been agreed to the sales order details and approved by the shipping department manager, and inspecting the related invoice to ensure the accounts receivable assistant has verified that the correct quantities and approved selling prices have been used to calculate the invoice totals. These procedures will provide evidence about the effectiveness of these controls to reduce the risk that a material misstatement of sales would not be detected by the company's controls. But they don't test whether the invoice amount is correctly calculated and correctly entered in the revenues and accounts receivables accounts. By extending the test on the controls all the way through to recalculating the invoice total, agreeing the selling price to the approved price list, and tracing the dollar amount of the invoice into the sales journal, the accounts receivable subledger, and the general ledger records, auditors also obtain substantive evidence about whether the monetary amounts have all been included, are valid, and are correctly valued.[10] Since dual-purpose procedures use the same sample of transactions or account balances to obtain the evidence, they may allow the audit work to be completed on a more timely basis.

Business Information Sources and Methods

LO2   Identify the procedures and sources of information auditors can use to obtain evidence for understanding an auditee's business and industry, assessing risk, and responding to assessed risk.

This section summarizes the application of audit procedures to obtain evidence in the risk assessment and risk response steps of the audit process that were set out in Exhibit 5–1. The audit process begins by obtaining an understanding of the auditee and its risks. Then the auditor performs risk assessment procedures to identify the risk of material misstatement at the overall financial statement level and the assertion level. From this, the auditor determines what procedures are necessary to address the assessed risks and reduce the risk of material misstatement to an acceptable level.

These further procedures may include tests of controls if the auditor decides they are appropriate in responding to the risks of material misstatement. The auditor must always perform some substantive procedures so that there are reasonable conclusions on which to base the audit opinion.[11] Substantive procedures give direct evidence about the financial amounts reported in the financial statements, while risk assessment procedures and control tests only provide indirect evidence about monetary misstatements. Substantive procedures can be either tests of details or substantive analytical procedures. Exhibit 8–2 matches up these steps in the audit process with the main procedures used for evidence gathering.

How do auditors obtain evidence? The information sources and methods auditors use to obtain evidence are explained below to show how the evidence-gathering procedures can be performed in practice. These are some examples from the wide variety of information sources auditors use to understand the auditee's business, industry, and environment when they assess risks of material misstatement and respond to them with further auditing procedures.

Obtaining Information from Inquiry, Including Prior Working Papers

Inquiry and interviews with the company's management, directors, and audit committee brings auditors up to date on changes in the business and industry. Interviews with auditee personnel (which include observations about the cooperation and integrity of auditee managers) build personal working relationships and develop auditors' understanding of problem areas in the financial statements. In specialized industries, management may have experts on staff or consultants who are important sources of an understanding of the business and its risks.

Information gathered in prior audits, and documented in the working papers, can also provide relevant and reliable information as follows:

- The nature of the organization, its environment, and its internal control
- Significant changes that the entity or its operations may have undergone since the prior financial period, which help the auditor identify and assess new risks of material misstatement
- Misstatements discovered in past audits and the timeliness of their correction

To use prior-period information in the current year, the auditor has to determine its relevance. For example, changes in the control environment may cause information obtained in the prior year to be irrelevant, so the auditor needs to make inquiries and possibly perform other procedures, such as walk-throughs of relevant systems.

EXHIBIT 8–2

Types of Evidence Procedures Used in the Steps of the Audit Process

STEPS OF THE AUDIT PROCESS AND AUDITOR'S OBJECTIVES	TYPES OF AUDIT EVIDENCE-GATHERING PROCEDURES USED
RISK ASSESSMENT STEP	
Understanding the auditee and its risks	Inquiries of auditee personnel, including study of prior years' audit working paper information Inquiries of external parties, including industry, government, and other research sources
Assessing the risk of material misstatement (inherent and control risks)	Inquiry of auditee personnel Analysis of draft financial statements, including comparisons to prior years Observation, including operation of accounting information system and internal control
RISK RESPONSE STEP	
Tests of control effectiveness: • obtain indirect assurance regarding risk of material misstatements of monetary amounts in financial statements; assess control risk	Inquiry of auditee personnel Observation of controls performed by auditee personnel Recalculation/reperformance of controls Inspection of documents and records in used in the control system
Substantive tests of details of transactions and account balances: • obtain direct evidence regarding material misstatement of monetary amounts in financial statements	Inspections of documents, records, and assets Observation of accounting procedures and practices External confirmation Recalculation/reperformance
Dual-purpose tests of controls and substantive details of transactions and balances: • obtain evidence regarding both control effectiveness and material misstatement of monetary amounts in financial statements	Inquiry of auditee personnel Observation of controls performed by auditee personnel Recalculation/reperformance of controls and recording Inspections of documents and records
Substantive analytical procedures	Analysis of relations to other financial and non-financial information Comparison of actual and expected values
CONCLUDING AND REPORTING STEP	
Overall analysis of financial statements and disclosures: • assess reasonability of overall financial statement amounts, presentation, and related disclosures to ensure fair presentation	Analysis of relations to other financial and non-financial information Analysis of impact of uncorrected misstatements on ratios and key performance indicators

For first-time audits, there is often no prior working paper information, so this can require more work than in a repeat engagement. When it is a company's first audit, but not its first year of operation, additional work includes establishing a starting place with reliable opening account balances for the audit. Inventory, fixed assets, and intangible assets accounts affect the current-year income and cash flow statements. If this information cannot be obtained, the scope of the current-year audit will be limited, and the opening balances and all the income statement amounts affected by them will require an audit report qualification.[12]

Inquiry also gives the auditor a fuller understanding of the needs of the users of the auditee's financial statements than was obtained when assessing whether to accept the engagement. The information obtained from inquiries of management, when combined with analysis of management's draft financial statements, helps the auditor to assess what is significant to users.

Standards Check

CAS 330 The Auditor's Responses to Assessed Risks

14. If the auditor plans to use audit evidence from a previous audit about the operating effectiveness of specific controls, the auditor shall establish the continuing relevance of that evidence by obtaining audit evidence about whether significant changes in those controls have occurred subsequent to the previous audit. The auditor shall obtain this evidence by performing inquiry combined with observation or inspection, to confirm the understanding of those specific controls, and

    (a) If there have been changes that affect the continuing relevance of the audit evidence from the previous audit, the auditor shall test the controls in the current audit; (Ref: Para. A36)

    (b) If there have not been such changes, the auditor shall test the controls at least once in every third audit, and shall test some controls each audit to avoid the possibility of testing all the controls on which the auditor intends to rely in a single audit period with no testing of controls in the subsequent two audit periods. (Ref: Para. A37–A39)

CAS 510 Initial Audit Engagements—Opening Balances

10. If the auditor is unable to obtain sufficient appropriate audit evidence regarding the opening balances, the auditor shall express a qualified opinion or disclaim an opinion on the financial statements, as appropriate, in accordance with CAS 705. (Ref: Para. A8)

Source: *CPA Canada Handbook—Assurance,* 2014.

Obtaining Information from Observation

At the same time that inquiries and interviews take place, the audit team can take a tour of the company's physical facilities to look for activities and things that should be reflected in the accounting records. For example, an auditor might notice a jumbled pile of materials and parts in the warehouse and make a mental note to check how these items are valued in the inventory account balance. The tour is the time for auditors to get personal knowledge by seeing company personnel doing their day-to-day tasks. Later, the auditors will meet these same people in more directed evidence-gathering circumstances.

Obtaining Information from Research Databases

Most industries have specialized trade magazines and journals, which are valuable for acquiring and maintaining industry expertise. Specific information about public companies can be found in registration statements and annual report filings with the provincial securities commissions. CPA Canada, the International Federation of Accountants (IFAC), and the American Institute of Certified Public Accountants (AICPA) industry accounting and auditing guides explain the typical transactions and accounts used by various kinds of businesses and not-for-profit organizations.

General business magazines and newspapers often contribute insights about an industry, a company, and individual corporate officers. Many are available, including *Canadian Business, Report on Business Magazine, Business Week, Forbes, Harvard Business Review, Barron's,* and *The Wall Street Journal,* and the business sections of newspapers such as *The Globe and Mail* and the *National Post.* Practising auditors typically read several of these regularly. A selection of other public information sources is shown in the following box.

The Internet is a very important information source for auditors. An organization's website might have financial statements and other information. Using effective search engines, such as Google, industry information and comparisons can also be obtained, allowing auditors to improve their business knowledge and thus design more

Sources of General Business and Industry Information

Statistics Canada (including economic forecasts)

D&B Principal International Businesses

Hoover's

Standard & Poor's Register of Corporations, Directors, and Executives

CPA Canada *Audit Risk Alert*s

Value Line Investment Survey

Moody's Investors Services (moodys.com)

CFO Magazine

Analysts' reports

D&B Key Business Ratios

Audit firm libraries, universities, dissertations on specialized industry topics

LexisNexis

Auditee websites, trade associations, conferences

effective analytical procedures. For larger companies, analyst and credit rating coverage are invaluable sources of information. Many articles in the business media are based on changes in credit ratings or analyst recommendations concerning specific companies and industries. Brokerage firms' websites contain analysis of publicly traded companies. Investor websites such as Motley Fool (fool.com) can provide valuable clues of potential problems in an auditee's (or potential auditee's) business. Be aware, however, that Internet information may not always be reliable and must be used with caution. A minimum knowledge of the auditee and its industry is necessary to properly interpret such information.

Obtaining Information from Internal Auditors

Audit efficiency can be realized by working in tandem with internal auditors. Independent external auditors should understand a company's internal audit activities as they relate to the internal control system. Internal auditors can also assist by providing information for understanding the business and its systems and controls, and even by performing control or substantive testing under the supervision of the external audit team. It is important to note that the external auditor still has sole responsibility for the audit opinion expressed, and that responsibility is not reduced if the external auditor uses the work of the internal audit function.[13]

Standards Check

CAS 610 Using the Work of Internal Auditors

Evaluating the Internal Audit Function

15. The external auditor shall determine whether the work of the internal audit function can be used for purposes of the audit by evaluating the following:

(a) The extent to which the internal audit function's organizational status and relevant policies and procedures support the objectivity of the internal auditors; (Ref: Para. A5–A9)

(b) The level of competence of the internal audit function; and (Ref: Para. A5–A9)

(c) Whether the internal audit function applies a systematic and disciplined approach, including quality control. (Ref: Para. A10–A11)

Source: *CPA Canada Handbook—Assurance*, 2014.

Use of Auditor's Experts

Auditors are not expected to be experts in all areas that may contribute information to the financial statements. In some cases, the auditor's understanding of the business can signal a need for the audit firm to use experts who have the relevant specialized knowledge. Experts are persons skilled in fields other than accounting and auditing, such as actuaries, appraisers, legal counsel, engineers, chemists, and geologists, who are needed for obtaining the understanding and evidence necessary for a particular account or assertion. For lower-risk assertions, auditors may consult with experts who are employed by, or engaged by, the auditee firm. For higher-risk situations, or where the auditee does not have its own experts, auditors will need to engage external experts who are independent of the auditee. When external experts are engaged, they must have appropriate professional qualifications and good reputations. They are not part of the audit team but still must be unrelated to the auditee, in order to provide objective evidence. Alternatively, auditor's experts may be employees of the audit firm, in which case they are subject to all the firm and engagement quality control standards, like any other audit team member. Auditors must obtain an understanding of the expert's methods, assumptions, and source data and be able to evaluate whether the expert's work is adequate for the purposes of the audit, and whether the findings are reasonable.[14]

Standards Check

CAS 620 Using the Work of an Auditor's Expert

7. If expertise in a field other than accounting or auditing is necessary to obtain sufficient appropriate audit evidence, the auditor shall determine whether to use the work of an auditor's expert. (Ref: Para. A4–A9)

6. (a) Auditor's expert—An individual or organization possessing expertise in a field other than accounting or auditing, whose work in that field is used by the auditor to assist the auditor in obtaining sufficient appropriate audit evidence. An auditor's expert may be either an auditor's internal expert (who is a partner or staff, including temporary staff, of the auditor's firm or a network firm), or an auditor's external expert. (Ref: Para. A1–A3)

Source: *CPA Canada Handbook—Assurance*, 2014.

Review Checkpoints

8-30 What are some of the methods and sources of information the auditor can use to understand an auditee's business?

8-31 When does an auditor need to use the work of an expert? What additional requirements must the auditor meet to use an expert's work as evidence?

Sufficient Appropriate Evidence in Auditing

LO3 Explain audit evidence in terms of its appropriateness and relative strength of persuasiveness.

After assessing the risk of material misstatement in the assertions in management's draft financial statements, auditors proceed to the task of designing specific procedures for gathering evidence related to these assertions. However, before studying how to design these procedures, you need to understand some features of evidence in auditing.

Auditing standards require auditors to obtain sufficient appropriate evidence as the basis for an audit opinion on financial statements.[15] The accounting records (journals, ledgers, accounting policy manuals, computer files, and the like) are evidence of the bookkeeping/accounting process but are not considered sufficient appropriate supporting evidence for the financial statements. The auditor must find independent evidence corroborating these records through direct personal knowledge, such as by inspection of documents, external confirmation, and inquiry of company personnel. Evidence is gathered and analyzed to support an auditor's conclusion on whether the financial statements are fairly presented and conform to generally accepted accounting principles (GAAP).

Identifying audit evidence is a key critical thinking activity in exercising professional audit judgment. To form an opinion on the fair presentation of the financial statements, the auditor requires evidence to (a) judge rationally whether the financial statement assertions are true and (b) provide logical support for the opinion expressed in the audit report.

Appropriateness of Evidence

 Appropriateness of evidence relates to its qualitative aspects: is it relevant and reliable? Evidence that is relevant and highly reliable is persuasive as proof regarding the financial statement assertions. For assertions that have a high risk of material misstatement, auditors need the most persuasive evidence they can get.

Relevant audit evidence means that it must relate logically to at least one of the financial statement assertions; otherwise it is not relevant to the auditor. Relevant evidence allows the auditor to meet the audit objectives.

Standards Check

CAS 500 Audit Evidence

5. (b) Appropriateness (of audit evidence)—The measure of the quality of audit evidence, that is, its relevance and its reliability in providing support for the conclusions on which the auditor's opinion is based.

Source: *CPA Canada Handbook—Assurance,* 2014.

Exhibit 8–3 lists general audit techniques and the financial statement assertion each may provide relevant evidence about. Note that most evidence is not conclusive on its own, so corroborating evidence is often required to provide reasonable assurance, especially when the assessed risk of material misstatement is high. Consequently, the comparison below should be viewed as only a rough guide, subject to the specific considerations in each audit.

The reliability of audit evidence depends on its nature and source. Exhibit 8–4 illustrates a hierarchy of the reliability of different types of audit evidence. The types of evidence considered to be most reliable are those obtained through an auditor's direct, personal knowledge, while the least reliable are those that are based on subjective claims of auditee personnel, as these can be biased. The most reliable evidence comes from procedures such as the auditor's physical inspection of tangible assets, external confirmation or documents obtained from knowledgeable third parties, and the auditor's own mathematical recalculations or reperformance. Documents from external sources obtained from the auditee, auditee-produced documents when internal controls are strong, candid auditor observations, and analytical procedures based on specific verified data are considered moderately reliable. The least reliable types of evidence are spoken or written responses by auditee personnel to auditors' inquiries, overt auditor observations where people may not act as they usually do, auditee-prepared documents when controls are not strong, and analytical procedures based on very general or unverified data. Documentary evidence originating outside the auditee's data processing system but received and processed by the auditee (external-internal evidence) is generally considered reliable. However, the circumstances of internal control quality are important.

Note that the key principle here is how independent the evidence is, and the extent to which the auditor can know personally that it has not been skewed by auditee biases. Evidence consisting of internal documents that are produced, circulated, and stored within the auditee's information system is generally considered low in reliability. However, internal evidence is used extensively if internal control is satisfactory. Internal evidence is also generally easy to obtain and, therefore, tends to be less costly than other evidence. Sometimes, internal

EXHIBIT 8–3

Audit Techniques and Their Relevance to Financial Statement Assertions

GENERAL AUDIT TECHNIQUE	FINANCIAL STATEMENT ASSERTIONS THE EVIDENCE MAY BE RELEVANT TO
Inspection of documents	Existence, Including Cutoff: vouching direction Completeness, Including Cutoff: tracing direction Valuation: partially Ownership/Rights and Obligations Presentation and Disclosure
Inspection of physical assets	Existence Valuation: partially; usually requires corroborating evidence Ownership: partially; usually requires corroborating evidence Presentation and Disclosure
External Confirmation	Existence Ownership/Rights and Obligations Valuation: partially; usually requires corroborating evidence Cutoff: partially; usually requires corroborating evidence
Recalculation	Existence Valuation
Analysis: Scanning	All assertions: partially, perhaps raises questions that may be relevant to all assertions, but may not produce actual "evidence"; when performed on recorded amounts, evidence may be relevant to Existence, Valuation, Ownership, and Presentation/Disclosure; when performed on source documents, evidence may be relevant to Completeness
Analysis: Analytical Procedures on Financial Relationships	Existence: partially; usually requires corroborating evidence Completeness: partially; usually requires corroborating evidence Valuation: partially; usually requires corroborating evidence
Inquiry	All assertions; partially, but responses typically yield more assertions, in turn subject to audit with corroborating evidence

EXHIBIT 8–4

Hierarchy of Audit Evidence Reliability

MOST RELIABLE
Physical inspection
Confirmation
External documentation
Recalculation, reperformance

LESS RELIABLE
External-internal documentation
Internal documentation
 (with good internal controls)
Observation
Analytical procedures with
 specific data

LEAST RELIABLE
Internal documentation
 (if poor internal controls)
Inquiry
Broad analytical procedures

documentation is the only kind of evidence available and can be of some value, but if the related assertion has a high risk, a lack of any corroborating evidence presents an audit scope limitation.[16] Similarly, auditors' own observations can be reliable when they are sure they are observing the way things really happen, not just "for show" because people know an auditor is watching.

Auditors must be careful about the appropriateness of evidence and choose the audit procedure providing the evidence that is the most reliable. If physical observation and mathematical calculation are not relevant to the account, impossible, or too costly, then auditors move down the hierarchy to the procedure that will give the best evidence available—best in the sense of most appropriate or persuasive under the circumstances. It should be the most reliable evidence that can be obtained in a cost-effective manner, relative to a particular audit objective.

There may be situations, however, where no highly reliable source of evidence is available, such as cash donations received by a charity or online sales transactions that leave no visible trail. In these cases, there may be two or more less-reliable pieces of evidence that together may support the assertion. If the pieces of evidence are consistent with each other and are from two independent sources, the evidence may be persuasive enough in the auditor's judgment. For example, to combine evidence sources an auditor might observe employee procedures and test controls of these, plus review summarized sales reports prepared for marketing purposes. Another example is given in the following box.

Related Parties—A Perfect Storm in Auditing

The existence of related parties poses considerable auditing challenges and can increase risks of material misstatement of the financial statements due to error and fraud. It is very important to ensure the audit planning process allows enough time to understand the auditee's business and ownership structure so that related parties can be identified. This note deals with the audit planning and evidence issues created by related parties.

Because the related party may have control or significant influence over the entity's operating, investing, and financing policies, transactions with them might not always be conducted under normal market terms. For example, assets could be transferred from the entity to a related party, such as a shareholder, for either no consideration or for an amount considerably below the assets' fair value, perhaps with no business justification. Related party relationships might also limit an audit, as the relationships may be complex, the entity's information systems may not be designed to flag transactions with related parties (management may not even know about them!), and reliable audit evidence about the transactions may not exist.

The fact that the different financial reporting frameworks have different accounting standards for related party transactions makes things even more complex. For example, in Canadian GAAP, ASPE—section 3840 sets out recommendations for both measurement and disclosure, while IFRS—IAS 24 only deals with disclosure of related party transactions. GAAS (CAS 550) require auditors to understand the entity's related party relationships and transactions well enough to be able to assess the risk of misstatement and to conclude whether the financial statements are fairly presented in accordance with the framework's requirements. For example, selling an asset to a controlling shareholder for far more than its fair value and then reporting the gain as a profit when it was intended as an equity contribution by the shareholder is not fair presentation. Not disclosing that an entity's ability to continue as a going concern depends on continuing financial support from a related party is also misleading.

Finally, related parties can increase fraud risk, as these relationships may present a greater opportunity for collusion, concealment, manipulation, or falsification of evidential records and documents by management.

How do auditors defend against this "perfect storm"? Maintaining professional skepticism throughout the audit is the auditor's strongest weapon in noticing the unusual transactions and relationships that have no apparent business purpose and may not be reflected appropriately in the financial statements. Another key tool is frequent discussion among audit team members, where observations and management inquiry responses are compared so that inconsistencies needing follow-up are highlighted. Inconsistent stories can indicate that the entity's financial statements are more susceptible to material fraud or error because of its related party relationships and transactions, and the auditor has to dig deeper to find them. The audit problem with related parties is that evidence obtained from them should not be considered highly reliable in terms of persuasiveness. The source of the evidence may be biased. Hence, auditors should obtain evidence of the purpose, nature, and extent of related party transactions and their effect on financial statements. Evidence should extend beyond management inquiry, and corroborating evidence should be obtained to increase persuasiveness.

Sources: CAS 550 "Related parties"; *CPA Canada Handbook—Accounting, Part II*, section 3840 "Related party transactions"; IAS 24, "Related party disclosures."

Sufficiency of Evidence

Sufficiency considers how much appropriate evidence is enough. The matter of sufficiency is an important application of auditors' professional judgment, as this will vary from situation to situation. The standards cannot really set out a specific amount of evidence required. Realistically, however, audit decisions must be based on enough evidence to stand the scrutiny of other auditors (supervisors and reviewers) and outsiders (such as critics, judges, practice inspectors, or Canadian Public Accountability Board [CPAB] inspectors).

The real test of sufficiency is whether the body of evidence you have gathered allows someone else to reach the same conclusions you reached. The fact that important evidence is difficult or costly to obtain is not an adequate reason for failing to obtain it. If an auditor has not been able to obtain sufficient appropriate audit evidence about a material financial statement assertion, CAS 330 states that the auditor should express a qualified opinion or a disclaimer of opinion, as was discussed in Chapter 4.

Standards Check

CAS 500 Audit Evidence

5. (e) Sufficiency (of audit evidence)—The measure of the quantity of audit evidence. The quantity of the audit evidence needed is affected by the auditor's assessment of the risks of material misstatement and also by the quality of such audit evidence.

CAS 330 The Auditor's Responses to Assessed Risks

27. If the auditor has not obtained sufficient appropriate audit evidence as to a material financial statement assertion, the auditor shall attempt to obtain further audit evidence. If the auditor is unable to obtain sufficient appropriate audit evidence, the auditor shall express a qualified opinion or disclaim an opinion on the financial statements.

Source: *CPA Canada Handbook—Assurance*, 2014.

With these aspects of evidence in mind, you will be ready to study the general processes for designing specific procedures in the detailed audit plan, which will be covered next.

Review Checkpoints

8-32 What is the relationship between assertions and the relevance of audit evidence?

8-33 What factors determine whether audit evidence is appropriate? What types of audit evidence are most reliable? least reliable?

8-34 How is an auditor's professional judgment applied in assessing the appropriateness of audit evidence?

8-35 Give a general definition of external, external-internal, and internal documentary evidence.

8-36 What is the problem with evidence obtained from related parties?

8-37 Distinguish between the appropriateness of audit evidence and the sufficiency of audit evidence.

8-38 What action is required if an auditor cannot obtain sufficient appropriate audit evidence?

Exhibit 8–5 shows the interrelationships among the auditing concepts discussed in this and earlier chapters, and how these concepts underlie the auditor's judgment about what audit evidence is required to meet the sufficiency and appropriateness criteria. We start with the materiality considerations; these are shown along the left side of the exhibit. The auditor determines materiality levels based on assessments of how precise the financial statements need to be. As we have seen, this involves considering at what point the magnitude of misstatement would be large enough to start to be detrimental to users' decisions based on the financial statements. The audit risk model components are shown in the centre of the diagram. The auditor's assessments of risk determine how much evidence needs to be gathered to increase assurance to a high enough level to bring audit risk to an acceptably low level given the auditor's risks in taking on the engagement.

The right side of the diagram deals with the characteristics of potential audit evidence. Note that the evidence decision must take into account practical limitations—not all evidence can be obtained at a reasonable cost or quickly enough to provide a timely audit report. Not all evidence has the same level of reliability. Trade-offs have to be made because of these limitations. The concepts of materiality and audit risk guide these trade-offs. This diagram shows the kind of complex analysis that is at the heart of professional judgment about the sufficiency and appropriateness of audit evidence. Essentially, the auditor's evidence judgment results from the trade-off among these three decisions: how small a misstatement do we need to find (materiality), how certain do we need to be that we found it (audit risk to be accepted), and what evidence is available and practical to obtain that can provide a high enough level of assurance of finding misstatements that are above the materiality threshold.

EXHIBIT 8–5

Auditor Judgments on Sufficiency and Appropriateness of Evidence

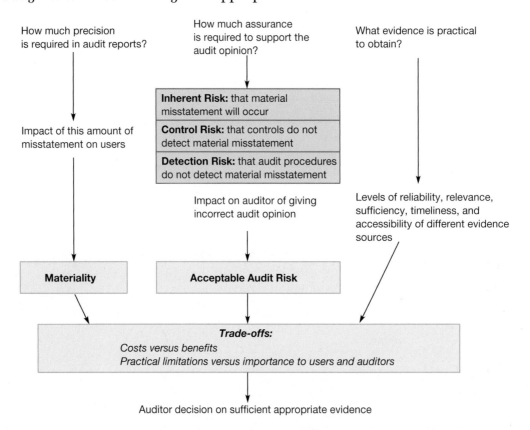

Audit Plan and Detailed Programs

LO4 Describe the content and purpose of the audit plan as well as the specific audit programs and detailed procedures it contains.

As discussed throughout Part 2 of the text, audit planning is an ongoing process. Planning is done at the start of the audit but continues throughout, as new information results in revisions to the plan.

The Planning Documentation

All the planning activities are recorded and summarized in planning documentation, sometimes referred to as a **planning memorandum**. While audit firms can use a variety of planning and documentation practices, the specific planning steps and documents outlined in the auditing standards are likely to be commonly used, so they are discussed here.[17]

Auditors prepare a document, called the overall audit strategy, summarizing the preliminary planning procedures and key decisions, as was introduced in Chapter 5. This document contains the results of analytical review, the decision on materiality levels, and the risk assessment. It gives specific attention to the effect of these on the nature, extent, and timing of audit resources needed to perform the work. The auditor's understanding of the business helps to assess inherent risk, and understanding the information systems and controls helps to assess control risk. These also aid in identifying what kinds of evidence are available and at what cost, the third component of the evidence decision outlined in Exhibit 8–5.

The **audit approach decision** is the next planning decision to be documented. The audit team must decide whether to use a combined approach or a substantive approach. As was introduced in Chapter 5, a combined audit approach involves testing the effectiveness of internal controls. Using the audit risk model relations, if the auditor gets evidence that controls are effective, it reduces the control risk aspect of the risk of material misstatement at the assertion level. When the risk of material misstatement is lower, the desired audit risk level can be achieved without having to reduce the detection risk as much. If more detection risk can be accepted, the extent of substantive testing required is reduced. Depending on the circumstances of the audit, this may be the most cost-effective way to obtain the required audit assurance. Essentially, the auditor is getting some assurance from the evidence that the controls work, so less is required from substantive sources to reach the level of reasonable assurance. In a substantive approach, the auditors will only have to understand controls for the purpose of the overall risk assessment and planning, but will not need to test controls as a component of the audit evidence. All the evidence will come from substantive sources. If the auditors believe they can get reasonable assurance without having evidence about the effectiveness of controls, and if the substantive procedures required would be less costly than combining control testing and substantive procedures, it may be more cost effective to use a substantive approach. These decisions are explained further in Chapter 9.

planning memorandum:
audit documentation where all planning activities are recorded and summarized; usually includes the overall audit strategy, the audit plan, and detailed audit programs

audit approach decision:
an auditor's choice of whether to use a combined audit approach that includes testing internal control effectiveness or a substantive audit approach that obtains all the evidence from substantive sources

The risk assessment and audit approach decisions guide the development of the audit plan, which summarizes the details of how the work is to be done. An audit plan includes all the specific detailed audit programs to be used in the engagement. As shown in Exhibit 8–5, the practical considerations and the trade-offs between the risk components and materiality guide decisions on what and how much evidence to gather through control tests, analytical procedures, and other tests of details of balances, using the evidence-gathering techniques discussed above. These evidence decisions are the basis of the audit programs that make up the audit plan. These procedures are designed to result in sufficient appropriate evidence that addresses the audit objectives set out in the program. The programs usually look like a to-do list for audit staff, some of whom may have little prior audit experience. Also included in the planning documentation are the audit team's understanding of the auditee's business and risks that were relevant in developing the decisions.

Auditors use three main types of audit programs: the **risk assessment program**, the **internal control program**, and the **balance audit program**. The risk assessment program lists the specific procedures for gaining understanding of the auditee's business transaction processing systems and controls, as well as for assessing the inherent risks and the control risks. The risks are assessed for the assertions in financial account balances and transaction streams that result from the information system processes. The internal control program involves documenting the understanding of internal control and specifies the control testing procedures to be performed to assess control effectiveness and control risk—indirect evidence regarding the likelihood of monetary misstatements in the financial statements. It is sometimes called an "interim audit program" since it is mostly performed at an interim time between year-ends. The balance audit program lists the substantive procedures for gathering direct evidence on the assertions (i.e., existence, completeness, valuation, ownership, presentation) about monetary amounts in the account balances, transactions, and related disclosures.

These audit programs combine all the considerations of audit planning discussed up to this point:

- Understanding the auditee's business, its environment and risks, its information systems, and its internal control
- Preliminary materiality decisions
- Assertions and objectives contained in the auditee's financial statements
- Preliminary analytical procedures for identifying specific risk areas in the unaudited financial statements
- Preliminary risk assessments
- Persuasive strengths of evidence
- Audit procedures for obtaining evidence: control testing, substantive detail testing, and substantive analytical procedures

In actual field situations, these audit programs can be very lengthy. Program documents may include separate listings of procedures and questionnaires on the company's business strategies and risk, business processes, internal control environment, management controls, and control procedures. To put the sequence of topics you have read about up until now into perspective, the following two boxes highlight typical components of audit programs.[18]

risk assessment program:
an audit planning document listing the specific procedures for gaining understanding of the auditee's business transaction processing systems and controls, as well as for assessing the inherent risks and the control risk for the assertions in financial account balances and transaction streams

internal control program:
an audit planning document summarizing the auditor's understanding of internal control and the control testing procedures to be performed to assess control risk and control effectiveness; sometimes called the interim audit program

balance audit program:
a list of the substantive procedures for gathering direct evidence on the assertions (i.e., existence, completeness, valuation, ownership, presentation) about dollar amounts in the account balances

Understand the Business Risk, Inherent Risk, and Control Risk

Risk Assessment Program

- Communicate with predecessor auditors (for new engagements).
- Study prior-year audit working papers, professional audit and accounting guides, and industry publications concerning the company and its industry.
- Interview management with regard to business risks, processes and controls, and accounting policies, and any significant changes in the current year.
- Evaluate the competence and independence of the company's internal auditors, if any.
- Determine the need to use the auditor's own experts on the engagement.
- Determine the extent of significant IT applications in the company's accounting system.
- Obtain the draft financial statements and make decisions about the planning materiality appropriate under the circumstances.
- Perform preliminary analytical procedures to identify risk areas in the financial statement accounts.
- Assess the inherent risk in general and also with respect to particular accounts, transactions, and disclosures, at the overall financial statement and the assertion levels.

Internal Control Program

- Obtain an understanding of the company's internal control through interviews, observations, and tests of controls (see Chapter 9).
- Perform detailed tests of control procedures, if necessary (see Chapters 9 and 10).
- Assess the control risk (see Chapters 9 and 10).
- Use the control risk assessment to design the nature, timing, and extent of substantive audit procedures (see Chapters 9 and 10).

The balance audit program consists of several programs, each applicable to a particular account. Auditors first subdivide the financial statements into accounting processes or cycles (as explained in Chapter 6) and then turn their attention to the accounts in each. The procedures in these audit programs are designed to obtain evidence about the existence, completeness, valuation, ownership, and presentation assertions implicit in each account title and balance. The box below contains a partial program for the revenue process, with brief specifications of procedures for auditing the accounts receivable balance. The procedures contain many of the elements of the general techniques that were explained in the previous section (e.g., confirmation, recalculation, inquiry, inspection, and the assertions toward which they are directed).

Example of Balance Audit Program in Revenue, Receivables, Receipts Process

Accounts Receivable

- Obtain an aged trial balance of the receivables and agree it to the general ledger control account.
- Prepare and send confirmations on a sample of customers' accounts receivable. Analyze the responses.
- Calculate and analyze the age status of the accounts and the allowance for uncollectible accounts.
- Interview the credit manager concerning the past-due accounts; review credit reports for analysis of high-risk overdue accounts.
- Vouch receivables balances to cash payments received after the confirmation date.
- Read loan agreements and make note of any pledge of receivables, sales with recourse or other restrictions, or contingencies related to the receivables.
- Read sales contracts for evidence of customers' rights of return or price allowance terms.
- Obtain written representations from the auditee management concerning pledges for collateral, related party receivables, collectability, and other matters related to accounts receivable.

The detailed audit programs of the audit plan should contain descriptions of the specific audit procedures to be performed. Each procedure's description should indicate its nature, extent, and timing, as well as a direct association with one or more financial statement assertions. The **nature of audit procedures** refers to the six general techniques: inspection, observation, confirmation, recalculation/reperformance, analysis, and inquiry. The **extent and selection of audit procedures** refers to the amount of work done and the basis of selection of items, such as the sample size for an audit test procedure (e.g., confirm 30 outstanding accounts receivable balances with customers based on random selection), or the number of reports to be scanned (e.g., review the sales journal entries for three days randomly selected from each month to look for unusual items). The **timing of audit procedures** is when they are performed: at the preliminary planning stage, at an interim point in the year (before the balance sheet date), at year-end, or shortly after the balance sheet date. CAS 330, paragraph 22, explains what procedures the auditor needs to do to cover the remaining period to year-end when substantive procedures are done at the interim date.

Standards Check

CAS 330 The Auditor's Responses to Assessed Risks

22. If substantive procedures are performed at an interim date, the auditor shall cover the remaining period by performing
    (a) Substantive procedures, combined with tests of controls for the intervening period; or
    (b) If the auditor determines that it is sufficient, further substantive procedures only that provide a reasonable basis for extending the audit conclusions from the interim date to the period-end. (Ref: Para. A54–A57)

Source: *CPA Canada Handbook—Assurance*, 2014.

Before, during, and after the fieldwork period, the auditor responsible for an audit engagement constantly monitors events that may affect an auditee's business risk, the client relationship, or the engagement. The box below gives an example of why auditors must read the news and consider the impact of new developments on their audit engagements—significant changes in an auditee's business risk can occur any time!

Money Launderers Spread Their Net

It was reported that automated banking machines (ABMs) located in small retail shops have become a prime vehicle for money laundering by organized crime gangs in the suburban areas around a major city. The shop's revenue is a percentage of the service charge paid by anyone taking cash out of the ABM, with the balance of the service fee going to the bank that provides the ABM. Shop employees are responsible for refilling the machine with cash taken in legitimately from customer sales. It was suspected that some employees would accept "dirty cash" (i.e., proceeds of crime) from criminals and use that to refill the ABMs instead of the clean cash from the cash register, which was given to the criminals. The dishonest employees receive a portion of the cash exchanged as their cut of the deal.

Now put yourself in the shoes of the auditor of a company that owns a chain of small retailers operating ABMs in this area. How does this development affect the business risk of this auditee? The auditor needs to determine if management

(continued)

nature of audit procedures:
the six general techniques of an account balance audit program: recalculation/reperformance, confirmation, inquiry, inspection, observation, and analysis

extent and selection of audit procedures:
the amount of audit work planned, such as sample size for an audit test and the method for selecting sample items

timing of audit procedures:
when the planned audit procedures are to be performed, either before, at, or after period-end

has identified this risk and responded appropriately by ensuring employees are adequately screened before hiring and are trained to be aware of the money-laundering laws and criminal penalties. Are there controls over employee activities, and is management monitoring them to ensure they are working? Even if the auditor discovers this situation six months before the audit is set to start, the information should be documented in the planning file. The auditor should also contact the auditee management as soon as possible to discuss the impact of this development on their business risk and what actions they are taking. Management may be too busy running the day-to-day operations to monitor business risks continuously!

Review Checkpoints

8-39   What information is summarized in the audit planning document or memorandum? How does it relate to the preparation of audit programs?

8-40   What are the kinds of audit programs, and what is the purpose of each?

8-41   What is meant by the terms nature, extent, selection, and timing (NEST) of audit procedures?

Audit Documentation

LO5   Evaluate audit working paper documentation for proper form and content.

No audit is complete without proper documentation. The planning document described above is a key component of the audit documentation, and additional documentation is required for the rest of the audit work. Documentation provides a record of the auditor's work for the purpose of file reviews; practice and regulatory inspections; or, in some cases, defence against a lawsuit. Audit working papers (which may be on paper or in electronic form) are the auditors' record of compliance with GAAS. They should contain support for decisions on procedures deemed necessary and all other important decisions made during the audit.[19] Even though the auditor is the legal owner of the working papers, professional ethics requires that there is auditee consent before transferring them because of the confidential information in them. Audit files must be retained for several years as required by professional accounting association rules and practice inspection procedures. Last year's file is a rich resource for the current year's engagement team on continuing audits. It provides valuable insights into key entity characteristics, likely risk areas, findings, and evidence relevant to the current year's financial statements, such as the audited opening balances.

Standards Check

CAS 230 Audit Documentation

2.   Audit documentation that meets the requirements of this CAS and the specific documentation requirements of other relevant CASs provides
   (a) Evidence of the auditor's basis for a conclusion about the achievement of the overall objectives of the auditor; and
   (b) Evidence that the audit was planned and performed in accordance with CASs/ISAs and applicable legal and regulatory requirements.

Source: *CPA Canada Handbook—Assurance,* 2014.

The following box outlines the impact that destroying audit working papers has on the value of the audit and the reputation of the audit firm. The Andersen document-shredding scandal was a key driver for development of more rigorous auditing standards. It shows why documentation is considered important by audit firms and the auditing standard setters.

Shredded Audit Papers . . . Shredded Auditor Reputation

In 2001, Andersen was the fifth-largest auditing firm in the world, employing 85,000 people in 84 countries and reporting revenues of US$9.3 billion. In a crippling blow, in March 2002, the U.S. Justice Department indicted Andersen on criminal charges of obstruction of justice. The indictment alleged that the audit firm had shredded tons of documents sought by investigators who were probing financial problems at Andersen's client, the energy giant Enron Corp. These criminal charges were the first to come out in the Enron case, and they struck a blow that eventually led to the demise of the nearly 90-year-old auditing firm that had long enjoyed a solid reputation for integrity. The events that led to the destruction of Andersen are related below.

Signs of trouble at Enron first arose in the summer of 2001, when Enron vice-president Sherron Watkins warned chairman Kenneth Lay that the company might be overcome by a wave of accounting scandals unless it took quick action to correct a series of questionable transactions that its auditors, Andersen, had helped it to devise. Despite this warning, Enron's stock price collapsed amid questions about its accounting practices, and in December 2001 it declared bankruptcy. Thousands of employees lost their jobs, and current as well as former employees lost their retirement savings as they had been encouraged to invest them in Enron shares. As rumours began to circulate that Andersen should not have given a clean audit opinion on Enron's financial statements, its reputation fell under suspicion and lawsuits against it began to pour in. Andersen's reputation declined further in January 2002, when it announced publicly that it had shredded documents related to Enron's audit.

The indictment against Andersen, issued by a federal grand jury in Houston, alleged a widespread effort to destroy audit documentation related to questionable transactions at Enron. As the indictment proceeded, prosecutors piled more pressure on Andersen by revealing damaging e-mails between auditors in the middle of the mass destruction of Enron documents, including one that read, "Argh, send more shredding bags."

As stories of the document shredding covered the front pages of newspapers, Andersen began to lose some of its biggest clients, casting doubt on whether the firm would be able to survive the crisis. The jury trial began on May 2, 2002, and on June 15, 2002, a guilty verdict was handed down. Andersen was found guilty of obstruction of justice and was barred from auditing SEC-registered companies after August 31, 2002. By then a large number of Andersen's 2,300 public-company clients had already replaced Andersen. As a result of these events, Andersen's ability to continue as an auditing firm was effectively destroyed, and it ceased operations on August 31, 2002.

Accounting researchers found that, in the days following Andersen's January 2002 announcement that it shredded Enron audit documents, the share prices of Andersen's other clients experienced a significant drop, indicating that investors downgraded the quality of the audits performed by Andersen. These findings show the importance of the auditor's reputation to investors. If investors believe the audit is of low quality, they have less assurance that the company's financial statements reflect its real business performance and financial position. They assess a higher likelihood that its income and net book value are overstated and that the auditor has failed to report this.

On May 31, 2005, the U.S. Supreme Court overturned the 2002 criminal conviction of Andersen on the grounds that the Houston jury was given overly broad instructions by the federal judge who presided at the trial that found it guilty of obstruction of justice. But, by then, Andersen, its reputation, and its business were long gone.

Sources: S. English, "Auditor overtime 'used for shredding,'" *Daily Telegraph*, May 22, 2002, p. 32, © Telegraph Group Limited; C. Mondics and S. M. Hopkins, "Andersen indicted in Enron shredding," *The Record*, March 15, 2002, p. a01, © 2002 North Jersey Media Group Inc. All rights reserved; K. Bewley, J. Chung, and S. McCracken, "An examination of auditor choice using evidence from Andersen's demise," *International Journal of Auditing*, 12 (2008), pp. 89–110; P. Chaney and K. Philipich, "Shredded reputation: The cost of audit failure," *Journal of Accounting Research*, 40 (4), pp. 1221–1245, © 2002, Blackwell Publishing.

Working paper files can be classified into three categories: (1) **permanent file**, (2) audit administrative files, and (3) audit evidence files. The last two categories are often called the **current file** because they relate to the planning and performance of the audit of the current period.

permanent file:
audit working papers that are of continuing interest from year to year, including the client company's articles of incorporation, shareholder agreements, major contracts, and minutes

current file:
the administrative and evidence audit working papers that relate to the audit work for the year being audited

Permanent File

The permanent file contains information of continuing interest over many years' audits of the same auditee. This file can be used year after year, whereas each year's current audit evidence papers are filed away after they have served their purpose. Documents of permanent interest and applicability include (1) copies or excerpts of the corporate charter and bylaws or partnership agreements; (2) copies or excerpts of continuing contracts, such as leases, bond indentures, royalty agreements, and management bonus contracts; (3) a history of the company, its products, and its markets; (4) excerpts of minutes of shareholders' and directors' meetings on matters of lasting interest; and (5) continuing schedules of accounts whose balances are carried forward for several years, such as share capital, retained earnings, and partnership capital. Copies of prior years' financial statements and audit reports may also be included. The permanent file is a ready source of information for new auditors on the engagement who must familiarize themselves with the auditee.

Audit Administrative File

Administrative papers contain the documentation of the early planning phases of the current audit. They usually include the engagement letter, staff assignment notes, conclusions related to understanding the auditee's business, results of preliminary analytical procedures, initial assessments of audit risks, initial assessments of audit materiality, and other decisions set out in the overall audit strategy. Many auditing firms follow the practice of summarizing these data in an engagement planning memorandum.

Audit planning and administration also include work on the preliminary assessment of control risk and preparation of a written audit plan. The following items are usually among the administrative working papers in each year's current file:

1. Engagement letter

2. Staff assignments

3. Auditee organization chart

4. Memoranda of meetings with management and those charged with governance (board of directors, audit committee)

5. Overall audit strategy:

    (a) Preliminary analytical review notes

    (b) Initial risk assessment notes

    (c) Initial materiality assessment notes

    (d) Audit engagement time budget

6. Internal control questionnaire and control analyses:

    (a) Management controls questionnaire

    (b) IT controls questionnaire

    (c) Internal control system flowcharts

7. Audit plan and specific audit programs

8. Working trial balance of general ledger accounts

9. Working paper record of preliminary adjusting and reclassifying entries

10. Review notes and unfinished procedures (all cleared by the end of the field work)

Audit Evidence Files—Current File Organization and Indexing

The current-year audit evidence working papers are typically organized in sections: major accounting processes or cycles and balance sheet accounts. Each section contains a lead sheet that shows the dollar amounts reported in the financial statements, summary of the audit objectives in relation to the account's assertions, procedures performed, evidence obtained, and conclusions reached for that section overall. The lead sheet is like an index, or table of contents, that provides references to all the audit working paper pages relating to the audit work on that section (see Exhibit 8–6 for an example of the Cash section of an audit file). These papers communicate the quality of the audit, so they must be clear, concise, complete, neat, well indexed, and informative.

Auditing firms use different methods of arranging and indexing working papers. Usually, the papers are grouped behind the trial balance, ordered according to balance sheet and income statement captions. The current assets usually appear first, followed by fixed assets, other assets, liabilities, equities, revenue, and expense accounts. A typical arrangement is shown in Exhibit 8–7.

Each separate working paper (or multiple pages that go together) must be complete in the sense that it can be removed from the working paper file and considered on its own, with proper cross-references available to show how the page fits in with the others. Working papers may be hard copy (handwritten, typed, printed from

EXHIBIT 8–6

Example of a Lead Sheet and Related Detailed Audit Working Papers

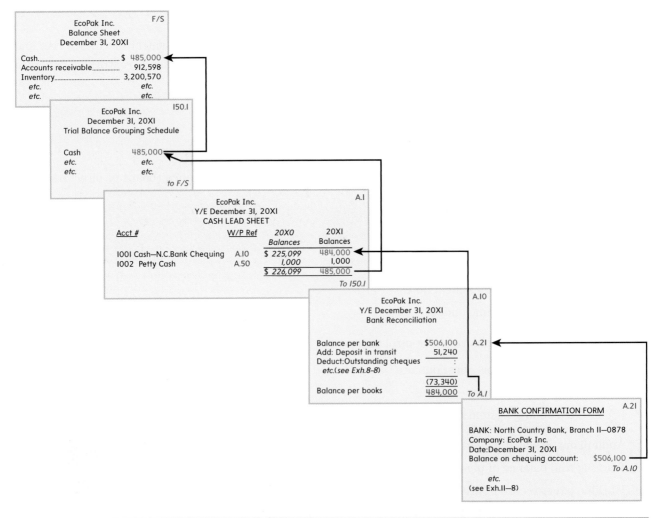

computer files) or stored electronically. Exhibit 8–8 provides an example working paper: a printout of a bank reconciliation from the auditee's accounting system supporting the cash account amount recorded in the company's trial balance. The auditor has used the auditee-prepared report to document audit work results by making handwritten notes on the auditee-prepared document.

The current audit evidence papers must show the auditors' decision problems and conclusions. The papers must record the management assertions that were audited (book values or qualitative disclosures), the evidence gathered about them, and the final decisions. Auditing standards recommend that the working papers show (1) evidence that the work was adequately planned and supervised, (2) a description of audit evidence obtained, (3) evidence of the evaluation and disposition of misstatements, and (4) copies of letters or notes concerning audit matters reported to the auditee. In addition, they contain support for the auditors' conclusions related to whether the financial statements conform to GAAP and whether the disclosures are adequate. The working papers should also explain how exceptions and unusual accounting questions were resolved or treated. (Note in Exhibit 8–8 the auditor's confirmation of the disputed accounts payable liability.) Taken altogether, these features should demonstrate that all the auditing standards were followed.

EXHIBIT 8–7

Current File Documenting the Audit Planning and Evidence for the Period Being Audited

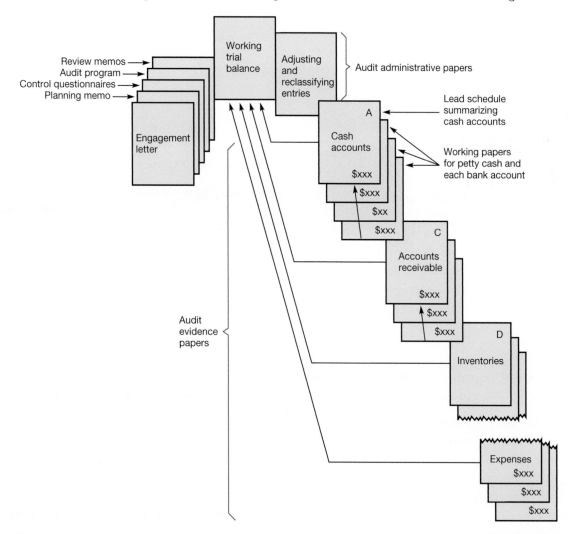

EXHIBIT 8–8

Illustrative Working Paper: Audit of a Bank Reconciliation

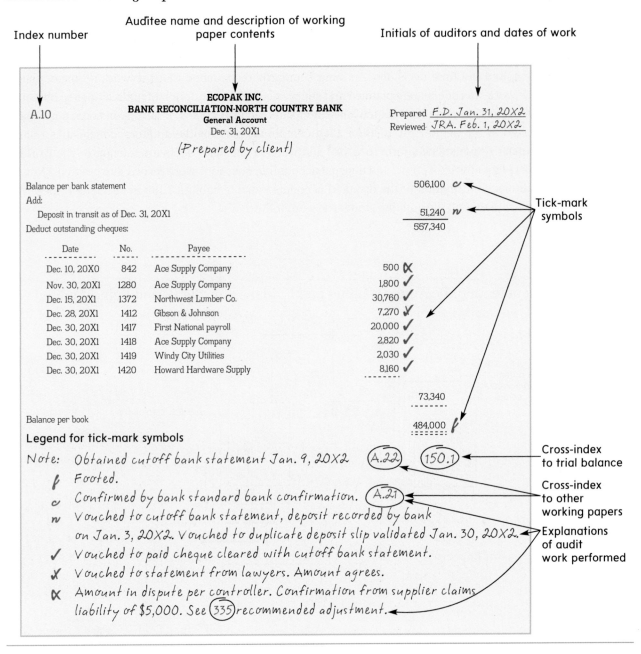

The quality of the audit documentation depends on the working papers being prepared according to specific formats. The following formatting points are also shown in the working paper example in Exhibit 8–8:

- *Indexing.* Each working paper is given an index number, like a book page number, so it can be found, removed, and replaced without loss. An index number might consist of a section letter (e.g., A) and a page number within that section (e.g., A.20). Each section could be given to a different audit team without affecting other sections. (An example of an indexing system used in practice is provided in Appendix 11C, available on Connect.)

- *Cross-indexing.* Numbers or comments related to other working papers should note the index of the other working paper(s) so that the connections can be followed.

- *Heading.* Each working paper is titled with the name of the company, the period of the financial statements being audited, and a descriptive title of the contents of the working paper. If the paper was created by auditee personnel (rather than the auditor), this is noted in the title using a notation such as "Prepared by client," or "PBC" for short.
- *Signatures and initials.* The auditor who performs the work and the supervisor who reviews it must sign the working papers so that persons responsible for the work can be identified.
- *Dates of audit work.* The dates of performance and review are recorded on the working papers so that reviewers can tell when the work was performed.
- *Tick marks and explanations.* Tick marks are the auditor's shorthand for indicating the work performed. They must always be accompanied by a full explanation of the auditing work.

Standards Check

CAS 230 Audit Documentation

9. In documenting the nature, timing, and extent of audit procedures performed, the auditor shall record
   (a) The identifying characteristics of the specific items or matters tested; (Ref: Para. A12)
   (b) Who performed the audit work and the date such work was completed; and
   (c) Who reviewed the audit work performed and the date and extent of such review. (Ref: Para. A13)

Source: *CPA Canada Handbook—Assurance,* 2014.

Audit Working Paper Software

Specialized working paper software is typically used in public practice to prepare audit documentation files. Electronic working "papers" automate many tasks, such as carrying adjustments over to related working paper documents and the financial statements. Good working paper software integrates the audit information and makes it easy to access, review, and change the format, content, or order of the files. Because most organizations' data are already in electronic form, it is simple to integrate the data into electronic audit documentation files. The volume of paper required for file documentation is reduced or eliminated, and with laptop computers there is better communication and information sharing among team members, as well as continuous monitoring and review of the work, even from a distance, by a supervisor. The entire audit process can benefit from software-based efficiencies, such as standard templates and electronic questionnaires.

Audit working paper software also facilitates analysis. Links can be established to other databases or even websites so that data or information can be cross-referenced or transferred to the working papers. Thus, audit staff work and various other sources of information can be integrated to support the auditor's opinion. Quality control considerations related to use of audit documentation software include hardware and software integrity, access security, staff training, document scanning procedures, and continuous upgrades with advances in technology. Some original source documents, such as important contracts, may still need to be kept in hard copy form. An example of a working paper software program used in public practice is CaseWare.

Audit documentation's key role is to provide a record of the work done, to help in revising the audit plan as the work proceeds, to allow for quality control reviews to be done effectively, and to help with planning the subsequent year's audit work. As the discussion in Part 2 up to now has shown, audit planning is a process of learning, feedback, and continuous improvement, as is depicted in Exhibit 8–9.

EXHIBIT 8–9

Audit Planning—A Process of Continuous Improvement

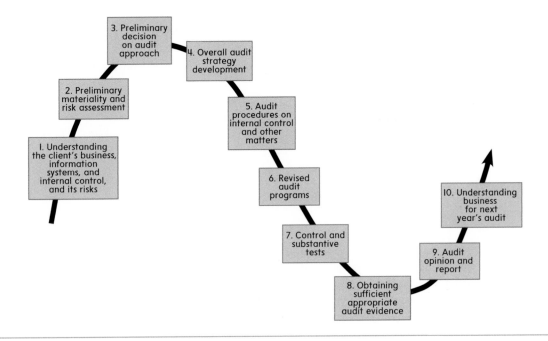

Standards Check

CAS 230 Audit Documentation

14. The auditor shall assemble the audit documentation in an audit file and complete the administrative process of assembling the final audit file on a timely basis after the date of the auditor's report. (Ref: Para. A21–A22)

A21. ... An appropriate time limit within which to complete the assembly of the final audit file is ordinarily not more than 60 days after the date of the auditor's report.

A23. ... The retention period for audit engagements ordinarily is no shorter than five years from the date of the auditor's report.. . .

Source: *CPA Canada Handbook—Assurance*, 2014.

Review Checkpoints

8-42 Why do audit firms and auditing standards require auditors to prepare and retain specific documentation of their audit work?

8-43 What information would you expect to find in a permanent audit file, and how would auditors use this information?

8-44 What audit administration working papers are included in the current audit files?

8-45 What is considered the most important content of the current audit files?

8-46 What is the purpose of indexing and cross-referencing audit working papers?

8-47 What techniques can auditors use to improve the quality of working paper documentation?

8-48 How is software used to prepare audit working papers?

APPLICATION CASE WITH SOLUTION & ANALYSIS

Review of an Audit Plan

DISCUSSION CASE

Toward the end of his first year in public practice, Jack is assigned to the audit team for Foyer Properties Inc. (Foyer). Foyer's main activity is development and leasing of commercial real estate properties, such as shopping malls and office towers. In the past few years, Foyer has developed a niche residential property business: building university residences and nursing homes and leasing them under a head lease with a public sector organization, such as a university or municipal government. The public sector organization handles collection from the individual residents. Foyer is a private company, with the chair holding 60% of the shares and the president and chief operating officer (COO) holding the remaining 40%.

Foyer has been a long-time audit for Jack's firm. The previous audit manager, Hank, just left the firm after 10 years to be the CFO at a local mining company, and Hilda has taken over from him for the 20X8 audit. Hank had been on the Foyer audit since joining the firm and had managed the audit for the past six years. Looking over the previous audit files, Hilda noted that Hank had not changed the audit approach for years: a substantive approach focusing primarily on verifying existence and valuation of all the major real estate properties and all large transactions, such as the major purchase or sale of a property. Since accounts receivable from the universities and governments were always received by the time the audit was being done, they were verified by vouching subsequent receipts, not by confirmation. Revenues and expenses from the property leasing operations were audited entirely by analytical procedures.

Hilda is confident that the past audits obtained sufficient appropriate evidence to support the audit opinion, which has always been unmodified, but Hank left too many important planning judgments "in his head" rather than documenting them. Hilda feels that the audit planning documentation should be updated to follow the risk-based approach. This may identify areas where a more effective audit approach could be applied. Since Jack has had experience using risk-based audit plans in several of his other audits this year, Hilda thought it would be a good learning experience for Jack to apply the risk-based approach in Foyer's audit planning.

Hilda has asked Jack to develop a risk-based overall audit strategy and preliminary audit plan for the current-year audit of Foyer. She would then like him to compare this plan with the plan used in previous years to identify and justify any differences.

The first thing Jack does is get out Foyer's prior-year audit files (for its year ended December 31, 20X7) and study the final financial statements and the planning memorandum that Hank had prepared. Jack notices that Hank's planning memo has been copied and carried forward for several years, with any new information tacked on at the end. Extracts from Foyer's prior-year audited financial statements and planning memorandum are provided below. What steps will Jack go through to create a risk-based audit plan?

FOYER PROPERTIES INC.
CONSOLIDATED BALANCE SHEET AS AT DECEMBER 31, 20X7

	20X7	20X6
	(in thousands of dollars)	
Assets		
Rental properties (note 4)	$32,180	$36,211
Cash and short-term investments	8,296	8,910
Deferred charges (note 7)	2,031	2,052

(continued)

Other (note 8)	929	528
Construction in progress	857	402
Corporate taxes recoverable	28	—
	$44,321	$48,103
Liabilities		
Mortgages and other loans payable (note 10)	$26,362	$31,247
Accounts payable and accrued liabilities	968	870
Pension obligation (note 11)	768	828
Tenant deposits	297	393
	28,395	33,338
Shareholders' equity		
Share capital (note 12)	5,850	5,850
Retained earnings	10,076	8,915
	15,926	14,765
	$44,321	$48,103

STATEMENT OF INCOME AND RETAINED EARNINGS FOR THE YEAR ENDED DECEMBER 31, 20X7

Real estate operations	**20X7**	**20X6**
	(in thousands of dollars)	
Revenue		
Rental income	$ 4,847	$4,600
Property management and other fees	902	1,137
	5,749	5,737
Operating expenses		
Municipal taxes	586	874
Repairs and maintenance	472	411
Utilities	251	356
Property management	201	164
Insurance	44	50
	1,554	1,855
	4,195	3,882
Interest	2,044	1,656
Amortization	999	828
	3,043	2,484
Net income from real estate operations	1,152	1,398
Other income (loss)		
Gain on disposition of real estate assets	1,518	2,806
Interest and other investment income	368	450
	1,886	3,256
General and administrative expenses		
Salaries and benefits	275	290

	20X7	20X6
Office	355	274
Capital taxes	71	99
Professional fees	42	32
	743	695
Net income for the year	2,295	3,959
Dividends paid during the year	(1,134)	(798)
Retained earnings, beginning of the year	8,915	5,754
Retained earnings, end of the year	$10,076	$8,915

NOTE 4. RENTAL PROPERTIES AND OTHER CAPITAL ASSETS (IN THOUSANDS OF DOLLARS)

	20X7			20X6
	Cost	Accumulated amortization	Net book value	Net book value
Buildings	$25,738	$2,763	$22,975	$28,028
Land	8,870	–	8,870	7,826
Parking lots and roadways	192	40	151	161
Furniture, fixtures, and equipment	370	187	183	196
	$35,170	$2,990	$32,180	$36,211

NOTE 10. MORTGAGES AND OTHER LOANS PAYABLE (IN THOUSANDS OF DOLLARS)

	20X7	20X6
Mortgages and loans secured by rental properties and bearing interest at fixed rates ranging from 5.45% to 7.28%, blended monthly payments	$24,404	$30,524
Loan secured by rental property and bearing interest at prime plus 1.25%, blended monthly payments, due on demand	1,958	723
	$26,362	$31,247

Interest paid on this debt during the year totalled $2,043.

Foyer Properties Inc.
Planning Memorandum

Prepared by: Hank Grouse, Senior Manager

Knowledge of the Auditee Business

Private corporation, provincial incorporation on April 1, 20X0. Two shareholders: one (holds 40%) is the general manager of the business; the other (holds 60%) is chair of the corporation's board. Both have access to monthly financial reports and other information they require. Main reason for audit is to support borrowing for construction financing—the shareholders feel audited financial statements show the company is solid. Main operations are developing and leasing commercial shopping malls and office buildings, with focus on high-quality properties and tenants (e.g., banks, pharmacies).

Materiality

Materiality $90,000 (10% normal pretax profit)

Risk Analysis

- Audit risk: Can accept the highest level

  Reasons for conclusion: Private company, few shareholders have access to all financial reports, other users are creditors with property-securing loans, company is profitable and in strong financial position.

- Inherent risk: LOW

  Reasons for conclusion: Operations and accounting not complex, previous audit work good, typically find only small (less than $3,000) misstatements that management always corrects, and low volume of high-value transactions not susceptible to error and easily monitored by management.

- Control risk: HIGH—assumed to be high: we cannot rely on control risk being lower since we don't plan to test controls; we will test substantively only

  Reasons for conclusion: Controls appear strong, management control attitudes good, senior management monitors financial results closely, president is a major shareholder, clear job descriptions and lines of authority, rigorous human resource policies for hiring and evaluation and compensation, and no fraud indicators noted.

- Detection risk: MODERATELY HIGH

  Reasons for conclusion: Substantive evidence will verify key assertions for all significant financial statement amounts.

Other Planning Points

- Commercial real estate market values tend to be stable.
- Environmental liabilities—management is on top of this; no problems to date over 25 purchase deals.
- Management policy is to retain adequate cash reserves to have flexibility to pay for unexpected repairs, or to be able to seize good acquisition opportunities that can arise at any time.
- Communications between shareholders are open; any shareholder loans or other related party transactions are agreed on and approved by both.
- All accounting policies used are acceptable in the real estate industry.
- Management's key performance measure is cash flow from operations (net revenue from properties less debt service, so risk of manipulation of accruals is minimal—only cash is considered)

Systems Notes

- Control environment is strong; will not rely on systems and application controls; substantive approach will be used.
- An industry standard financial reporting package (Yardi) is used—providing reliable monthly operating information (actuals vs. budgets)—summary data automatically update the general ledger accounts.
- Logins used for access; no systems changes required as operation is quite stable.
- The Yardi system is behind a firewall from the office computer network, so the Internet interface has minimal security risk.

Significant Financial Statement Accounts, Audit Approach to Verify to Assertions:

R/R/R Key Assertions—Completeness, Existence, Valuation
- Rent roll (rent revenue journal) is updated regularly, management reviews reports monthly, and rent entries are easily auditable by matching to lease agreements.

P/P/P Key Assertions—Completeness, Existence, Valuation
- Management closely monitors monthly financial reports and follows up discrepancies.

- Expenditures are largely regular and predictable, so variances are easily detected.
- Two signatures (CFO and Operations Manager) required on all cheques.
- Audit will be by analytical procedures: detailed comparison to prior years, by property, by month, and comparison to budgets.

Rental Properties—Existence, Ownership, Valuation

- Purchase agreement and lease agreement terms will be verified. Property tax bills will be inspected to verify Foyer retains ownership of each property. Loans and collateral agreements will be confirmed; analysis of interest and property taxes will be based on these inputs. Lease agreements and lease receipts will be analyzed in relation to properties leased. Management representations will be obtained to ensure no property sales are unrecorded and all purchases and new leases are recorded.

Additions to Planning Memorandum

Note new information for 20X5 audit:

Company has entered a specialized residential real estate leasing business. Residential properties, such as student residences and nursing homes, are developed to order for public sector organizations, such as universities and municipal governments—risks seem low. Foyer's management has capability to handle this type of operation, so no impact on audit for now.

Note for planning 20X6 audit:

Asset sale transactions can be complex. We were asked to review the agreement terms and management's proposed accounting entry prior to finalizing so that there are no surprises when it comes to reporting sale in year-end financial statements; determined a $300,000 adjustment was required to management's proposed entry to account for the stepped-up rent payments over the term of the lease, per GAAP.

Notes for planning 20X7 audit:

Hank met with Foyer president to discuss the audit plan. He noted that construction project cost overruns on the public sector residential property have been a problem, as public sector officials get involved and demand various changes to the agreed plans. Foyer has hired a new construction project manager with experience in the public sector so these demands can be handled better. The construction manager reviews and approves all expenditures, and the two cheque-signing officers will not sign unless this approval is received. Construction changes and cost overruns are a potential risk area, since the lease payments are set prior to construction and may not be adequate to recover a higher investment in the property.

Note for planning 20X8 audit:

Hank had lunch with the Foyer president and learned that 10 public sector residential properties are now leased, and 6 more are under construction. The company's strategy is to grow the public sector residential business, as commercial real estate leasing is mature and harder to grow. Most of Foyer's commercial properties can be sold now for good gains, so the new strategy is to begin to divest the commercial buildings when market conditions are optimal and buyers are found.

SOLUTION & ANALYSIS

After reviewing all the planning notes, Jack realizes that Hank had obtained a very thorough knowledge of the company and its risks and controls, and he had assessed the risks of material misstatement appropriately. He had also developed a reasonable response to the assessed risks by deciding to use a substantive audit approach.

However, the effectiveness of the audit can be improved by implementing a more strategic analysis of the business risk factors, explicitly linking these to risk of material misstatement at the financial statement level and at the assertion level for the significant classes of transactions, account balances, and disclosures. Jack could reorganize the information from the planning notes and preliminary analysis of Foyer's financial statements to follow the risk-based planning steps and develop more fully the links between the business risks and specific risks of material misstatement and the audit responses that should be performed. The risk assessment must also consider fraud risk more explicitly.

Management's related controls to reduce those risks could be considered, and the remaining risks that the audit plan needs to respond to identified. This analysis would more likely draw the audit team's attention to the potential increase in risk from the company's new strategy in the public sector residential leasing business. The audit team will develop appropriate responses by planning further audit procedures related to this business line. The materiality determination and qualitative factors considered should also be more fully explained and documented.

Jack could document the business risk analysis by type of factor, as follows.

Understanding the Entity and Its Business, Environment, Risks, and Controls

Nature of entity

Private corporation, provincial incorporation on April 1, 20X0. Two shareholders: one (holds 40%) is the general manager of the business; the other (holds 60%) is chair of the corporation's board. Both have access to monthly financial reports and other information they require. Main reason for audit is to support borrowing for construction financing; the shareholders feel audited financial statements show potential lenders that the company is solid. Main operations are developing and leasing commercial shopping malls and office buildings, focus on high-quality properties and tenants (e.g., banks, pharmacies).

Industry risk factors

No significant risks: local operation, very minimal and non-complex regulatory environment, and simple valuation measurements.

Legal regulatory risk factors

For land/property purchases need to do due diligence re environmental liabilities. Management is on top of this; no problems to date with over 25 purchase deals closed.

Economic risk factors

Real estate values have stopped increasing in current year but are expected to be stable, not crash, in near term. Fair values exceed carrying values so no impairment expected; no financial instruments or complex financing are used, just standard mortgage loans.

Business relations

No key competitors/suppliers. Key customers are city government and universities involved in residential properties.

Strategy and related processes

Develop and lease profitable buildings.
- Select unique locations for targeted tenants—high-quality businesses, public sector residential.
- Plan construction and monitor project costs closely to keep investment at level where required return can be achieved.
- Structure leases to ensure adequate rate of return on investment and recovery of operating cost and any increases (e.g., energy, property taxes, insurance).
- Implement effective collection procedures to ensure cash flows are on time and as planned.

- Arrange loans from large financial institutions, using specific assets as collateral, to obtain low-cost financing.

- Retain adequate cash reserves to have flexibility in paying for unexpected repairs or seizing good acquisition opportunities that can arise at any time.

Internal Control Factors

Control environment

- Management is experienced and successful in industry.

- Management works as team.

- Clear job descriptions and lines of authority exist.

Management's risk assessment process

- Conservative risk takers, focus on rates of return on investment

- Budgeting for new property developments and ongoing operations

Information system, related business processes, financial reporting, and communication

- Company uses industry-standard information system (Yardi).

- Accounting policies follow real estate industry guidelines re depreciation assumptions and so on.

- Cash and straight line revenue recognition for stepped rent leases (per GAAP) is used.

Control activities

- Access controls, regular reporting

Monitoring of controls

- Top management is actively involved and monitors all aspects of the operation.

Key Financial Statement Accounts and Underlying Business Processes

Revenue process

- The rent roll is updated regularly; system controls are strong; management reviews key reports.

- As long as the company-level controls are adequate, the audit approach can be based on substantive testing alone because the rent transactions can be verified by matching them to lease agreements.

Purchasing process

- Management closely monitors monthly financial reports and follows up discrepancies.

- Expenditures are largely regular and predictable, so variances are easily detected.

- Two signatures are required on all cheques.

Key performance measure

Cash flow operations show net revenue from properties less debt service (so risk of manipulation of accruals is minimal—only cash is considered).

Systems

Industry standard financial reporting package (Yardi) used:

- Provides reliable monthly operating information (actuals vs. budgets)

- Summary data from Yardi manually transferred to general ledger

- Logins used for access; no systems changes required as operation is quite stable

- Yardi system is behind firewall from the office computer network; reduces Internet security risk

Materiality Determination

Users—Shareholders, lenders

Qualitative considerations—very profitable business, well capitalized, well managed, low transaction volume; we have audited it problem-free for many years, no management or operating changes this year.

Worksheet:

	ANTICIPATED CURRENT YEAR	PRIOR YEAR
Net income before taxes (NIBT)	$2.95m	$2.3m*
Total assets	$50m	$44m
Non-recurring items in income		
– Gain on sale	$2m	$1.5m
NIBT—normal, continuing	$.95m	$0.8m
Typical percentage:		
– NIBT 5–10%, use 10% due to qualitative factors	$95,000	$80,000
Comparison with alternative base—Total assets 0.5–1%	$250,000	$220,000
Materiality for financial statement as a whole	$95,000	$80,000
Anticipated misstatements based on previous audits		
– Less than $5,000, most years misstatements negligible	$5,000	$5,000
Performance materiality	$90,000	$75,000

*m = million.

A matrix such as the one below could be used to organize the planning considerations. The key risk revealed by Jack's review is entered as an example, and the other business risks in Foyer can be analyzed and entered similarly.

Describe business risks with financial reporting implications, or fraud risks	Describe related risks of material misstatement by account and assertion	Rate risks as high/ medium/ low	Describe management control(s) addressing the risk	Rate control effectiveness to reduce risk as high/medium/low	Are risks adequately controlled? Yes/No	Audit implications: e.g., control testing required, further audit procedures required to address remaining risk
– Public sector residential projects fix future lease payments prior to construction. – Construction cost overruns can occur to meet public sector officials' demands. – Etc.	– Rental property costs can exceed recoverable values. – Fraud risk of kickbacks to public sector officials exists.	Medium	– Project costs are approved. – Project cost overruns are monitored. – Leasing agreements are structured to provide required return on investment.	Medium	Yes	– Observe and inquire as to monitoring effectiveness. – Examine project costs, approvals. – Analyze lease agreement; verify recovery of investment and operating costs.

Overall Audit Strategy—Other Preliminary Conclusions

- Financial reporting framework is GAAP (Accounting Standards for Private Enterprises [ASPE]), an acceptable, fair presentation framework.
- Preliminary risk assessment at financial statement level: LOW
  - It appears risks of material misstatement are low initially, and management risk assessment is adequate to reduce these. Some further procedures are needed to verify conclusions based on management control effectiveness via observation and inquiry of management.
  - Risk of material misstatement due to fraud is addressed as follows. The close attention of the two shareholders to operating matters and discussion with management and shareholders indicates no employee fraud has been discovered or suspected in recent years. Risk of fraud in revenues must always be considered, especially as the rent receipts are mainly cash. We use a substantive approach: substantive analytical procedures can be highly effective in this business since the lease terms are fixed. Also, indicators of revenue fraud are specifically noted in the planned tests of details for the rental revenue cash receipts transactions. Past audits have not found any fraud indicators. Finally, overall review of the financial statements will play close attention to the possibility of manipulation of revenue recognition procedures by management.
- Preliminary audit strategy to respond to assessed risk at financial statement level:
  - Consider that business processes involve a small number of large transactions for property sales, planned and monitored construction project costs for development process, lease-driven revenue streams, and predictable cost patterns for rental processes. The substantive approach is most effective to obtain sufficient appropriate evidence.
- Preliminary risk assessment at assertion level:
  - Main identified risks affect the following accounts/assertions:
    * Rental property/Valuation (costs incurred and recoverability of investment)
    * Rental revenue/Existence (public sector leases)

Preliminary Audit Plan to Respond to Assessed Risks:

(a) *Timing*

Year-end balance audit—not efficient to do interim work

(b) *Nature*

Rental property valuation—detailed analysis of budget and actual costs, any changes in project costs (overruns), and changes in economic factors that can suggest investment not recoverable

Revenues—detailed analysis based on comparison with lease agreements and verifying cash receipts; for new public sector residential business, external confirmation to be obtained of terms and payments from appropriate counterparty to ensure no fraudulent scheme is occurring

Expenses—predictable: we have a history for comparison, so analysis of reasonability is sufficient; can also indicate any misstatements/fraud in revenues

(c) *Extent*

Plan to confirm all revenue amounts that are material in total from one counterparty

Analysis will cover all significant accounts on balance sheet and income statement

Staffing

Experienced staff should be assigned to perform the bulk of the audit work as the analysis requires careful judgment and preparation. One junior staff member should be assigned to get experience but needs close supervision. A team meeting should be held prior to beginning audit preparations. Daily meetings should be held during field work to cross-reference findings. A final meeting should be held after the files are completed for the partners' review and to clear any outstanding issues, if possible, or ensure they are documented clearly for the partner to follow up.

Summary

Overall, the auditee presents a low risk of misstatement, and the substantive verification of year-end balances of rental property (vouching costs), loan balances and terms (confirmation), and public sector residential lease revenues (confirmation), combined with detailed analytical procedures, will provide sufficient appropriate evidence that material misstatement does not exist in the financial statements.

SUMMARY

This chapter continued the study of audit planning started in Chapters 6 and 7 by explaining the role of sufficient appropriate audit evidence in developing reasonable assurance to support the audit opinion.

- The six general techniques for obtaining audit evidence were explained. **LO1**
- The main sources of evidence were outlined. **LO2**
- The underlying theory of evidence and its persuasiveness was explored by discussing the fundamental auditing concept of sufficient appropriate audit evidence along with the reliability of various techniques for gathering it. This explanation of procedures was enriched with additional notes about the ways in which procedures can be misapplied. **LO3**
- The chapter provided an overview of the audit plan and specific programs for collecting evidence. Programs were categorized as risk assessment programs, internal control programs, and balance audit programs. **LO4**
- The chapter described some key considerations about audit documentation by looking at planning documentation: the form, content, and purpose of audit working papers. **LO5**

The chapter finished with an Application Case that provided an opportunity to review a risk-based audit plan for the audit of a real estate business. Now the stage is set for Chapter 9, where we pursue a more detailed examination of the auditor's review, understanding of the auditee's information systems, and evaluation and testing of internal control.

KEY TERMS

analysis	internal control program	reperformance
audit approach decision	inquiry	risk assessment program
balance audit program	nature of audit procedures	scanning
confirmation	observation	sufficient appropriate audit evidence
current file	permanent file	timing of audit procedures
extent and selection	planning memorandum	tracing
inspection	recalculation	vouching

MULTIPLE-CHOICE QUESTIONS FOR PRACTICE AND REVIEW

MC 8-1 `LO4` An audit program contains

a. specifications of audit standards relevant to the financial statements being audited.
b. specifications of procedures the auditors believe appropriate for the financial statements under audit.
c. documentation of the assertions under audit, the evidence obtained, and the conclusions reached.
d. reconciliation of the account balances in the financial statements with the account balances in the auditee's general ledger.

MC 8-2 `LO2` When auditing the existence assertion for an asset, auditors proceed from the

a. financial statement numbers back to the potentially unrecorded items.
b. potentially unrecorded items forward to the financial statement numbers.
c. general ledger back to the supporting original transaction documents.
d. supporting original transaction documents to the general ledger.

MC 8-3 `LO2` The objective in an auditor's review of credit ratings of an auditee's customers is to obtain evidence related to management's assertion about

a. completeness.
b. existence.
c. ownership.
d. valuation.

MC 8-4 `LO3` Jones, PA, is planning the audit of Rhonda's Company. Rhonda verbally asserts to Jones that all the expenses for the year have been recorded in the accounts. Rhonda's representation in this regard

a. is sufficient evidence for Jones to conclude that the completeness assertion is supported for the expenses.
b. can enable Jones to minimize his work on the assessment of control risk for the completeness of expenses.
c. should be disregarded because it is not in writing.
d. is not considered a sufficient basis for Jones to conclude that all expenses have been recorded.

MC 8-5 `LO3` The evidence considered most reliable by auditors consists of

a. internal documents, such as sales invoice copies produced under conditions of strong internal control.
b. written representations made by the president of the company.
c. documentary evidence obtained directly from independent external sources.
d. direct personal knowledge obtained through physical observation and mathematical recalculation.

MC 8-6 `LO2` Confirmations of accounts receivable provide evidence primarily about these two assertions:

a. Completeness and valuation
b. Valuation and ownership
c. Ownership and existence
d. Existence and completeness

MC 8-7 `LO3` Obtaining sufficient audit evidence about the sales revenues of a given company means that the auditor

a. tested all sales transactions for the given period.
b. tested more than 50% of the sales transactions for the given period.
c. tested a reasonable sample of sales transactions for the given period.
d. tested only the sales transactions with an amount higher than the performance materiality.

MC 8-8 `LO5` An audit working paper that shows the detailed evidence and procedures regarding the balance in the accumulated depreciation account for the year under audit will be found in the

a. current file evidence working papers.
b. permanent file working papers.
c. administrative working papers in the current file.
d. planning memorandum in the current file.

MC 8-9 `LO5` An auditor's permanent file working papers would most likely contain

a. internal control analysis for the current year.
b. the latest engagement letter.
c. memoranda of meetings with management.
d. excerpts of the corporate charter and bylaws.

MC 8-10 `LO1` Tima is working on the audit of Stellar Productions Inc. Today she is touring the factory with the production manager, and she is discussing the procedures for recording the flow of goods through the production process with various factory employees. Tima is applying which kinds of audit evidence techniques?

a. Inquiry and inspection
b. Observation and confirmation
c. Observation and documentation
d. Inquiry and observation

MC 8-11 `LO1` Calvin is performing the following auditing procedures related to revenues: (i) obtaining production records of physical quantities sold and calculating an estimate of total sales dollars based on average selling prices; (ii) comparing revenue dollars and physical quantities with prior-year data and industry economic statistics. Which types of evidence-gathering procedures is Calvin using?

a. (i) Observation; (ii) confirmation
b. (i) Recalculation; (ii) analysis
c. (i) Recalculation; (ii) inspection (vouching)
d. (i) Analysis; (ii) analysis

MC 8-12 `LO1` Bosso Properties Inc. records its real estate investment properties at fair value under IFRS. Sidra is performing the following procedures as part of the audit program for the valuation assertion for this asset: (i) For investment property valued at fair value, examine and verify appraisal reports that Bosso's CFO has obtained from an independent professional real estate valuator. (ii) Summarize the additions and disposals recorded in Bosso's detailed investment property subsidiary records, and agree the balance to the general ledger control account. Which types of evidence-gathering procedures is Sidra using?

a. (i) Confirmation; (ii) inspection (scanning)
b. (i) Recalculation; (ii) analysis
c. (i) Inspection (vouching); (ii) recalculation
d. (i) Confirmation; (ii) recalculation

MC 8-13 **LO1** Marc, a junior auditor, attended the inventory count of Mira's Office Shop, a large retailer of office supplies and electronics. Marc watched Mira's employees doing the count and reported on whether or not the inventory count's directives were followed. The above procedure is an example of

a. inspection.
b. observation.
c. reperformance.
d. analysis.

MC 8-14 **LO1** As part of the review of McMaster Auto Parts, France met with the CEO to obtain an explanation for their decreasing gross margin percent for this year as compared to last year. The above procedure is an example of

a. confirmation.
b. inquiry.
c. observation.
d. reperformance.

EXERCISES AND PROBLEMS

EP 8-1 Audit Procedures. **LO1** Auditors frequently refer to the terms *standards* and *procedures*. Standards deal with measures of the quality of performance. Standards specifically refer to the GAAS expressed in the CASs. Procedures specifically refer to the methods or techniques used by auditors in the conduct of the examination. Procedures are also expressed in the CASs.

Required:

List six different types of procedures auditors can use to obtain evidence during an audit of financial statements, and give an example of each.

EP 8-2 Potential Audit Procedure Failures. **LO1** Some general audit procedures are (*a*) recalculation, (*b*) physical inspections, (*c*) confirmation (accounts receivable, cash, or other assets), (*d*) verbal inquiry, (*e*) inspection of internal documents, and (*f*) scanning.

Required:

For each procedure listed, discuss one way the procedure could be misapplied or the auditors could be misled in such a way as to render the work (audit evidence) misleading or irrelevant. Give examples that are different from the examples presented in Chapter 8.

EP 8-3 Confirmation Procedure. **LO1, 2** An auditor accumulates various kinds of evidence on which to base the opinion on financial statements. Among this evidence are confirmations from third parties.

Required:

a. What is an audit confirmation?
b. What characteristics of the confirmation process and the recipient are important if an auditor is to consider the confirmation evidence reliable and appropriate?

EP 8-4 Audit Procedure Terminology. **LO1, 2**

Required:

Identify one or more types of procedures being employed in each situation described below (vouching, tracing, recalculation, observation, and so on).

1. An auditor uses audit software to select suppliers' accounts payable with debit balances and compares amounts and computation with cash disbursements and supplier credit memos.
2. An auditor examines property insurance policies and checks insurance expense and the prepaid insurance balance for the year. The auditor then reviews the expense in light of changes and ending balances in PPE asset accounts.
3. An auditor uses audit software to test perpetual inventory records for items that have not been used in production for three months or more. The auditee states that the items are obsolete and have already been written down. The auditor checks journal entries to support the auditee's statements.
4. An auditor tests cash remittance advices to see that allowances and discounts given to customers are appropriate and that receipts are posted to the correct customer accounts in the right amounts, and reviews the documents supporting unusual discounts and allowances.
5. An auditor watches the auditee take a physical inventory. A letter is also received from a public warehouse stating the amounts of the auditee's inventory stored in its warehouse. The company's cost flow assumption, FIFO (first in, first out), is then tested by the auditor's computer software program.

EP 8-5 General Audit Procedures and Financial Statement Assertions. **LO3** The six general audit procedures produce evidence about the principal management assertions in financial statements. However, some procedures are useful for producing evidence about certain assertions, while other procedures are useful for producing evidence about other assertions. The assertion being audited may influence the auditors' choice of procedures.

Required:

Prepare a two-column table with the six general procedures listed on the left. Opposite each one, write the financial statement assertions most usefully audited by using each procedure. Then provide a specific example of an account that would be found in the audit of a real estate company, and expand the general procedures to explain specifically how the evidence would be obtained for this auditee.

EP 8-6 Relative Appropriateness of Evidence. **LO3** Generally accepted standards for performing a financial statement audit require that auditors obtain sufficient appropriate evidence that provides a reasonable basis for forming an opinion on the fair presentation of the financial statements they are auditing. In considering what constitutes sufficient appropriate evidence, a distinction should be made between underlying accounting data and all corroborating information available to the auditor.

Required:

Compare and discuss how effectively each of the following sources of evidence provides support for the auditor's opinion on the financial statements.

a. The relative appropriateness of evidence obtained from external and internal sources
b. The role of internal control with respect to internal evidence produced by an auditee's data processing system
c. The relative persuasiveness of auditor observation and recalculation evidence compared with the external, external-internal, and internal documentary evidence

(© 2000, American Institute of CPAs. All Rights Reserved. Adapted by permission.)

EP 8-7 Relative Appropriateness of Evidence. `LO3`

Required:

1. Classify the following evidential items by source (direct knowledge, external, and so on), rank them in order of reliability, and explain the reasons for your ranking.
   a. Amounts shown on monthly statements from creditors
   b. Amounts shown on "paid on account" in the accounts payable register
   c. Amount of "discounts lost expense" computed by the auditor from unaudited supporting documents
   d. Amounts shown in letters received directly from creditors

2. Classify the following evidential items by source (direct knowledge, external, and so on), rank them in order of reliability, and explain the reasons for your ranking.
   a. Amounts shown on a letter received directly from an independent bond trustee
   b. Amounts obtained from minutes of board of directors' meetings
   c. Auditors' recalculation of bond interest and amortized cost when remaining term and status of bond are audited
   d. Amounts shown on cancelled cheques

EP 8-8 Audit Working Paper Documentation. `LO4, 5` The preparation of working papers is an integral part of the auditors' responsibility to document their work in a financial statement audit engagement. On a recurring engagement, auditors review the audit programs and working papers from their prior audit while planning the current audit to determine their usefulness for the current-year work.

Required:

a. (i) What are the purposes or functions of audit working paper documentation? (ii) What records may be included in audit working papers?
b. What factors affect an auditor's judgment of the type and content of the working papers for a particular engagement?
c. To comply with GAAS, an auditor includes certain evidence in his or her working papers, for example, evidence that the audit was planned and work of assistants was supervised and reviewed. What other evidence should an auditor include in audit working papers to comply with GAAS?

d. How can an auditor make the most effective use of the preceding year's audit programs in a recurring audit?

(© 2000, American Institute of CPAs. All Rights Reserved. Adapted by permission.)

EP 8-9 Audit Procedure for Error Detection. `LO5` You are performing the audit of the JZ Limited (JZ) financial statements for its year ended September 30, 20X2. JZ is a private company that provides computer network repair services to businesses in the Greater Toronto Area (GTA). JZ has four shareholders, who are all actively involved in the business in various technical and marketing roles. JZ's audited financial statements are used mainly by its bank to support an ongoing operating loan arrangement. JZ has a general manager who receives a bonus based on 1% of monthly sales, subject to a maximum bonus of $2,000 per month.

JZ's accounting policy is to recognize revenue when each repair job is completed. All sales are on account. At their September 30, 20X2, year-end, JZ had completed a large job, but during your audit you discovered that the company's accountant did not record this sales revenue until October 10, 20X2, when the company issued the customer an invoice for $145,000. The accountant was late in issuing the invoice because the general manager had not finished preparing the supporting documents for the sale in time for his year-end cutoff. The general manager had instructed the accountant to proceed with the cutoff anyway.

Before correcting this error, JZ's draft financial statements show sales revenues of $3,200,000 and accounts receivable, net of allowance for bad debts, of $450,000.

Required:

a. Explain how the accounts in the JZ financial statements will be affected by this error.
b. Explain the assertion that has been violated by this error.
c. Give one example of an audit procedure that would have discovered this error.
d. What is the impact of this error on JZ's accounts receivable turnover? (*Note:* Accounts receivable turnover = Credit sales for the year/Net accounts receivable at year-end)
e. Would you consider this error to be material? Justify your response.

EP 8-10 Identifying the Type of Audit Procedure. `LO1, 2` For each of the procedures in the table below, indicate the type of procedure being performed (inspection, observation, confirmation, reperformance/recalculation, inquiry, analysis).

DESCRIPTION	TYPE OF PROCEDURE
1. Vouch a sample of purchase orders to receiving reports.	
2. Obtain the client's payroll deduction worksheet and perform the computation.	
3. Obtain a letter from the company's external lawyer with regard to the existence and possible outcome of existing claims at year-end.	
4. Talk with the company's management to determine if obsolescence factors are present for the production assets.	
5. Obtain the minutes from the board of directors' meetings to determine if the business acquisition was approved.	
6. Ask a purchasing clerk to enter a purchase order in the accounting system for an amount above their authorized credit limit and verify that the system will block this purchase from being processed.	

(continued)

DESCRIPTION	TYPE OF PROCEDURE
7. Compare the revenues and expenses with those of the prior year to identify any unusual variances.	
8. Ask the in-house legal counsel about the anticipated outcome of the ongoing litigation and the estimated amount of any settlement.	

EP 8-11 Information Sources and Reliability of Evidence. **LO1, 2, 3** The following information is available to Griffin & Fox, the auditors of Melba Inc.

Required:

For each of the following situations, discuss which source information would be considered of higher quality in terms of audit evidence. Ensure you support why a specific source of information would be considered higher quality.

Situation 1: To support the existence, completeness, and accuracy of the inventory, Melba Inc. provided its auditor with a summary of its inventory count. Griffin & Fox also sent a staff accountant to observe the inventory count.

Situation 2: The head of the legal department at Melba met with the partner of Griffin & Fox to discuss a lawsuit Melba is currently facing from one of its clients. The legal counsel of Melba has been involved with the case since it was first filed and has extensive knowledge of the case, so he provided a good estimate for the legal provision. Griffin & Fox also obtained a confirmation letter from Melba's external counsel.

Situation 3: The control environment and internal controls at Melba have been assessed as strong for the current year. To assess the accuracy of the payroll expenses, Melba provided Griffin & Fox with an automated report detailing the various source deductions that are computed by the system when the payroll is processed. Griffin & Fox also did an overall analysis of the payroll deductions to ensure there were no large variances since the prior year.

Situation 4: To verify the accuracy of the sales, Griffin & Fox obtained a sample of *sales invoices* generated by Melba's sales system. Griffin & Fox also looked at Melba's *sales ledger* to trace certain sales.

DISCUSSION CASES

DC 8-1 Financial Assertions and Audit Procedures. **LO2** Assume that your audit firm was engaged to examine the financial statements of Karwan Company for the year ended December 31.

You have learned that on November 1, Karwan borrowed $500,000 from Regional Bank to finance plant expansion. The long-term note agreement provided for the annual payment of principal and interest over five years. The existing plant was pledged as security for the loan.

Because of the unexpected difficulties in acquiring the building site, the plant expansion did not begin on time. To make use of the borrowed funds, management decided to invest in stocks and bonds, and on November 16 the $500,000 was invested in securities.

Required:

Describe a complete audit program for collecting relevant evidence for the audit of investments in securities at December 31.

Approach:

Develop specific assertions related to investments in securities at December 31 based on the five principle assertions.

DC 8-2 Financial Assertions and Audit Procedures.   `LO3, 4`   You were engaged to audit the financial statements of Karachi Company for the year ended December 31, 20X1.

On June 1, 20X1, Karachi initiated a product warranty program to help it stay competitive with other companies in its industry. The warranty covers parts, labour, and shipping to repair any defect within one year of purchase.

During 20X1, Karachi paid $50,000 in warranty costs on product sales of $4,000,000 (approximately 80,000 units). Based on this, management estimates its warranty liability at December 31 is $80,000.

Required:

Design an audit program for collecting relevant evidence for the audit of the estimated warranty liability.

Approach:

Develop specific assertions and audit objectives related to warranty liability based on the five principle assertions. Assess which assertions have a high risk of material misstatement, and which do not have a high risk. Then identify evidence that can be obtained by the auditors to support or refute these assertions.

DC 8-3 Appropriateness of Evidence and Related Parties.   `LO3, 5`   Julio & Johnson, PAs, are engaged to do the audit of the Guaranteed Finance Company. Johnson is performing the audit procedures for evaluating the collectability of real estate loans. Johnson is working on two particular loans: (1) a $4 million loan secured by the Smith Street Apartments and (2) a $5.5 million construction loan on the Baker Street Apartments now being built. The appraisals performed by Guaranteed Appraisal Partners Inc. showed values in excess of the loan amounts. Upon inquiry, Bumpus, the finance company's vice-president for loan acquisition, stated, "I know the Smith Street loan is good because I myself own 40% of the partnership that owns the property and is obligated on the loan."

Johnson then wrote the following in the working papers: (1) the Smith Street loan appears collectible; Bumpus personally attested to knowledge of the collectability as a major owner in the partnership obligated on the loan; (2) the Baker Street loan is assumed to be collectible because it is new and construction is still in progress; and (3) the appraised values all exceed the loan amounts.

Required:

a. Do you perceive any problems with related party involvement in the evidence used by Johnson? Explain.
b. Do you perceive any problems with Johnson's reasoning or the appropriateness of evidence used in that reasoning? Explain.

DC 8-4 Audit Plan with Weaknesses in Revenue Controls, Not-for-Profit Auditee.   `LO1, 4`   Kindness Home (KH) is a not-for-profit organization that operates a nursing home in a town near a major city. You are auditing the revenue and receivables at KH. The nursing home has a reputation for delivering excellent patient services, but its accounting department is understaffed and does not have time for internal verification or other accuracy checks. Your assessment of controls over cash receipts indicates that there are effective management supervision and monitoring procedures in place, and you have found no indication of fraud risk, but past audits have found misstatements in recording the patient invoices and accounts receivable. In confirming the accounts receivable from patients in past audits, you have had a very low response rate. Furthermore, those patients who did respond did not appear to know what information they were being asked to provide or what their correct outstanding balance actually was. You have had the same experience in confirming receivables at other nursing homes. The nursing home has a large bank loan payable, which is up for renewal two months after year-end. The bank's loan officer has told management the bank's head office may not approve a renewal. The bank is concerned about its exposure to not-for-profit nursing homes because many new government-funded nursing homes are expected to open over the next few years. These new long-term care facilities will be more modern and will be located closer to many large hospitals than KH.

Required:

a. Identify the business risks in KH.
b. Assess the risk of material misstatement at the overall financial statement level. Identify the inherent and control risk factors in the organization to support your assessment.
c. In the audit of the revenues, explain the overall audit approach you would use to obtain sufficient appropriate evidence in this situation. Give clear reasons for the mix of control and substantive work you would plan to do. Describe the substantive tests you would perform to audit the revenue transactions in this organization. Be specific, and show how the tests tie in to the relevant assertions.

DC 8-5 Working Paper Review. **LO5** The schedule in Exhibit DC 8-5 was prepared by the controller of World Manufacturing Inc. for use by the independent auditors during their examination of World's financial statements. All procedures performed by the audit assistant were noted in the

EXHIBIT DC 8-5

Marketable Securities (World Manufacturing Inc., year ended December 31, 20X2)

DESCRIPTION OF SECURITY			SERIAL NO.	FACE VALUE OF BONDS	GENERAL LEDGER JAN. 1	PURCHASED IN 20X2	SOLD IN 20X2	COST	GENERAL LEDGER DEC. 31	DEC. 31 MARKET	Dividend and Interest PAY DATE(S)	AMT. RECEIVED	ACCRUALS DEC. 31
CORP. BONDS	%	YR. DUE											
											Jan. 15	300**b,d**	
A	6	09	21-7	10,000	9,400**a**				9,400	9,100	Jul. 15	300**b,d**	275
D	4	03	73-0	30,000	27,500**a**				27,500	26,220	Dec. 1	1,200**b,d**	100
G	9	06	16-4	5,000	4,000**a**				4,000	5,080	Aug. 1	450**b,d**	188
Rc	5	03	08/2	70,000	66,000**a**		57,000**b**	66,000					
Sc	10	07	07-4	100,000		100,000**e**			100,000	101,250	Jul. 1	5,000**b,d**	5,000
					106,900	100,000	57,000	66,000	140,900	141,650		7,250	5,563
					a,f	**f**	**f**	**f**	**f,g**	**f**		**f**	**f**

(continued)

EXHIBIT DC 8-5

Marketable Securities (World Manufacturing Inc., year ended December 31, 20X2) *(continued)*

Stocks

						Mar. 1	750**b,d**	
P 1,000 shs	1,044	75,00**a**		7,500	7,600	Jun. 1	750**b,d**	
Common						Sep. 1	750**b,d**	
						Dec. 1	750**b,d**	250
						Mar. 1	750**b,d**	
U 50 shs	8,530	9,700**a**		9,700	9,800	Feb. 1	800**b,d**	
Common						Aug. 1	800**b,d**	667
		17,200		17,200	17,400		4,600	917
		a,f		**f,g**	**f**		**f**	**f**

Legends and comments relative to above:

a = Beginning balances agreed to 20X1 working papers
b = Traced to cash receipts
c = Minutes examined (purchase and sales approved by the board of directors)
d = Agreed to general ledger entry to income account
e = Confirmed by tracing to broker's advice
f = Totals footed
g = Agreed to general ledger

---

bottom "Legend" section, and it was initialled properly, dated and indexed, and then submitted to a senior member of the audit staff for review. Internal control was reviewed and is considered to be satisfactory.

Required:

a. What information essential to the audit of marketable securities is missing from the schedule?
b. What essential audit procedures were not noted as having been performed by the audit assistant?

(© 2000, American Institute of CPAs. All Rights Reserved. Adapted by permission.)

DC 8-6 Comprehensive Audit Planning Case. `LO1, 2, 4` You have been assigned to the audit of the financial statements of Equality Coffee Roasters Limited (ECR) for its year ending December 31, 20X2. The company started five years ago and is in the business of obtaining coffee beans from around the world under a fair trade policy, roasting the beans locally, and selling them to coffee shops in Ontario. Most of their sales are in the urban centres of the province. ECR's business involves obtaining raw coffee beans from coffee-producing countries around the world. ECR's business model is to only purchase coffee from certified fair trading plantations where the agricultural workers receive a fair wage and share of profits. Investors in ECR's shares are primarily ethical investors and mutual funds that concentrate on investing in companies that have high corporate social responsibility ratings.

In the preliminary audit planning done to date, your audit manager has determined that inventory is the account with the highest risk of material misstatement. Last year, the audit team uncovered an error in the ending inventory balance in the amount of a $65,000 overstatement. You have been assigned to continue the ECR audit planning work by finalizing and documenting various risk assessment and planning decisions so the audit team can move on to developing the detailed audit plans.

It is now January 20X3, and you are at the ECR offices to begin your audit work. In discussion with the company's management, you have learned that ECR currently has about 10% of the coffee bean market in Ontario. Its coffee is considered to be a premium product because of its ethical sources but also because it purchases only the highest quality of Arabica beans and uses a special just-in-time roasting and delivery business process that puts the very best quality product into the stores at the peak of its flavour. About 75% of its sales are to independent neighbourhood coffee shops in urban areas. ECR also sells to one major coffee shop chain and supplies an up-market grocery store chain. Fair trade coffees can sell for 20–25% more than coffee from other sources and have enjoyed increasing popularity over the past few years.

Exhibit DC 8-6 shows the December 31, 20X2, adjusted trial balance listing that you have obtained from ECR management.

EXHIBIT DC 8-6

Equality Coffee Roasters Limited Trial Balance as of December 31, 20X2

	DEBITS	CREDITS
Cash	248,726	
Accounts receivable	946,241	
Allowance for bad debts		61,444
Inventory, finished goods	4,670,992	
Inventory, work-in-process	606,086	
Inventory, raw materials	1,668,580	
Patents, at cost	84,547	
Provision for inventory obsolescence		98,311
Property, plant, and equipment (PPE)	23,842,581	
Accumulated amortization, PPE		9,585,303
Accounts payable		1,961,300
Income taxes payable		46,206
Warranty provision		73,733
Long-term bonds payable, due 20X4		4,915,540
Share capital, common shares		245,777
Retained earnings, beginning of year		11,838,430
Revenue		21,658,361
Cost of goods sold	11,469,184	
General and administration expenses	3,687,884	
Other expenses	2,209,535	
Management bonuses	500,000	
Income tax expense	550,049	
Totals	50,484,406	50,484,405

Required:

Continue the audit planning for ECR by answering the following questions.

  a. List and explain three factors your audit firm would have to consider in order to decide to accept the ECR audit engagement for the current year.

  b. What materiality levels would you use for planning this audit? Show your calculations and justify your decision.

  c. What audit risk level would you be willing to accept for this engagement? Describe your choice in terms of one of these levels: low, lower, lowest. Explain the factors that support your decision.

  d. Describe three business risk factors that could increase the risk of material misstatement in the ECR financial statements. Explain which account(s) each of the business risk factors could affect and the type of misstatement(s) that it might cause.

  e. Based on the business risk analysis for ECR, your audit manager believes the ECR inventory account balance has the highest risk of material misstatement. Your manager has asked you to assess the inherent risk of misstatement at the assertion level for the inventory. Use the level high, medium, or low to describe your assessment, and explain the factors that support your assessment.

  f. Describe two audit evidence-gathering procedures you would perform that would provide relevant evidence regarding one or more of the assessed risks in the inventory assertions. Explain what type of evidence the procedures would provide. Discuss how reliable this audit evidence is.

DC 8-7 Comprehensive Audit Planning Case. `LO1, 2, 4` Silvah Leasing Ltd. (SLL) is a private company founded over 20 years ago. Its main business is providing lease financing to small to medium-size local businesses for financing their operating equipment, store fixtures, and so on. SLL's business is direct lease financing, and the company never takes ownership of any of the leased assets. Leasing is popular with smaller businesses since the economy has been in a recession, and leasing assets rather than buying conserves cash. Many larger financial institutions have become more active in selling leases to the smaller customers that have been SSL's main source of business, to increase their own revenues during the recessionary times. Equipment vendors are also increasingly providing financing with equipment sales to increase their own business.

   D. Silvah owns the majority of the common shares and runs the business with three employees. There are two minority shareholders who are family members, M. Silvah and J. Silvah. Your firm has audited SLL for several years. The company's bank demands annual audited financial statements because of SLL's large outstanding bank loan.

The current year's trial balance has been obtained by your audit team. This is shown below.

Required:

  a. List the preliminary audit procedures that your firm should perform to decide whether to accept the SSL audit engagement for the current year, and explain how each factor affects the acceptance decision.

  b. What *materiality levels* would you use for planning this audit? Show your calculations and justify your decision. You can assume your audit firm has the following policy: Performance materiality should be 70% of the materiality level for financial statements as a whole, unless specific information indicates a different value should be used.

  c. Identify and explain three *business risk factors* in SLL that you would need to understand in order to assess the risk of material misstatement in its financial statements.

d. Apply two analytical procedures (e.g., ratios) to the SSL financial information that may be relevant for understanding SSL's business performance. Explain how your findings can be informative for assessing the risk of material misstatement at the financial statement level for SSL.

e. Based on the business risk analysis for SLL, your audit manager believes the SLL lease receivables balance has a high risk of material misstatement. Your manager has asked you to assess the risk of material misstatement *at the assertion level* for this account. Use the level "high" or "not high" to describe your assessments, and explain the factors that support them.

f. The audit risk model is a conceptual model that auditors use to manage risks in an audit engagement. Describe the components of the audit risk model and how they are related to each other. How would this model help an auditor plan for specific control testing procedures and substantive auditing procedures at SLL?

g. Explain what kinds of fraud risk might exist in a business like SSL. How would you assess the risk of fraud for this audit engagement?

h. Describe two audit evidence-gathering procedures you would perform that would provide relevant evidence regarding one or more of the assessed risks in the lease receivables assertions. Explain what type of evidence the procedures would provide. Discuss how reliable this audit evidence is.

SILVAH LEASING LTD. TRIAL BALANCE AS OF DECEMBER 31, 20X2	DEBITS	CREDITS
Cash	182,500	
Prepaid expenses	40,076	
Finance leases and loans receivable	9,202,900	
Allowance for bad debts		734,980
Due from M. Silvah, related party	2,000,000	
Investments, at fair value through net income	278,903	
Land	118,102	
Building	168,076	
Office furniture and equipment	135,998	
Software, net of amortization	353,395	
Accumulated depreciation, building		100,846
Accumulated depreciation, office furniture & equipment		89,976
Bank loans		4,900,985
Accounts payable		66,934
Income taxes payable		35,414
Customer deposits		766,667
Share capital, common shares		100
Retained earnings, beginning of year		5,381,246
Lease interest revenue		3,643,330
Interest expense	431,171	
Depreciation & amortization	132,050	
Bad debts	1,001,000	

(continued)

SILVAH LEASING LTD.		
TRIAL BALANCE AS OF DECEMBER 31, 20X2	**DEBITS**	**CREDITS**
Collection and credit research	12,250	
Salary expense	554,112	
Management bonuses	500,000	
Other expenses	497,690	
Income tax expense	112,255	
Totals	15,720,478	15,720,478
Check (= Debits − Credits)		0

ENDNOTES

1 Stay tuned: the uses and limitations of confirmations, as well as issues arising from procedures for obtaining them, are explained more fully in Chapter 11.

2 D. G. Smith, *Analytical Review* (CICA, 1983), Chapter 2.

3 CAS 520.

4 R. E. Hylas and R. H. Ashton, "Audit detection of financial statement errors," *The Accounting Review*, October 1982, pp. 751–765.

5 S. Smith, "A matter of evidence," *CA Magazine*, October 1994, pp. 57–58.

6 Stay tuned: representation letters are covered in detail in Chapter 15.

7 CAS 300, CAS 315.

8 CAS 240.

9 CICA, *Audit Enquiry* (CICA, March 2000), p. 24.

10 More examples of dual-purpose tests can seen in some of the Application Cases at the end of Chapters 11 and 12.

11 CAS 330, paragraph 18.

12 CAS 510.

13 CAS 610, paragraph 11.

14 CAS 620.

15 CAS 500, paragraph 6.

16 See discussion of scope limitations and the audit opinion in Chapter 4.

17 CAS 300.

18 Stay tuned: the technical parts of internal control risk assessment programs are explained more fully in Chapter 9.

19 CAS 230.

Control Assessment and Testing

Chapter 9 expands on the auditor's internal control work by describing the activities of internal control evaluation and highlighting the role of control risk assessment and testing in planning the audit.

LEARNING OBJECTIVES

After completing this chapter, you will be able to do the following:

LO1 Distinguish between management's and auditors' responsibilities regarding an auditee organization's internal controls.

LO2 Explain why the auditor evaluates an auditee's internal controls.

LO3 Define management's internal control objectives, and relate them to the financial statement assertions.

LO4 Explain the impact on control risk of general and application control activities in the auditee's accounting information systems.

LO5 Describe how auditors document an accounting system to identify control strengths and weaknesses in order to assess control risk.

LO6 Write control tests for an audit program.

LO7 Outline the auditor's responsibility when internal control evaluation work detects or indicates a significant control weakness or a high risk of fraudulent misstatement.

LO8 (Appendix 9A) Describe the contents and purpose of internal control questionnaires in an auditor's control evaluation.

LO9 (Appendix 9A) Describe the contents of flowcharts and their use to document controls in accounting processes.

LO10 (Appendix 9B) Explain why an auditor must understand the organization's information systems and technology to plan a financial statement audit.

LO11 (Appendix 9B) Describe the characteristics and control risks in basic information technology–based accounting information systems.

LO12 (Appendix 9B) Describe the following approaches to auditing information systems: auditing around the computer, auditing through the computer with computer-assisted audit techniques, and auditing with the computer using generalized audit software.

CHAPTER APPENDICES

APPENDIX 9A   Internal Control Assessment Aids for Audit Planning

APPENDIX 9B   Understanding Information Systems and Technology for Risk and Control Assessment (on Connect)

EcoPak

EcoPak Inc.

Donna and Caleb go to EcoPak to begin the systems part of their work at the company. It is early November and EcoPak has a December 31 year-end. They learn from Nina that because the customers require a fairly predictable supply of their food containers, EcoPak is able to schedule production very close to delivery dates and keep its own inventory to minimal levels. To operate this way, all EcoPak's systems are highly integrated and linked electronically to its customers' systems. Next, Donna and Caleb interview the accounts receivable manager and quickly learn that the sales system description notes they have from last year need to be updated. The system notes explain the flow of documents to process a customer order, record a sale, and set up the related receivable, but they realize that this refers to electronic documents processed within EcoPak's computer system. Since a large volume of sales transactions occurs, and they are all processed automatically, the only evidence available to verify that all the sales recorded are real, authorized, accurately calculated, and posted is electronic. Tariq has assigned one of Meyer & Gustav's (M&G's) information technology (IT) audit experts, Shree, to the EcoPak audit team, and Donna contacts her to let her know she will need to design some IT-based audit procedures to get the evidence they need to audit the sales transactions.

Donna and Caleb also learn how the volume discounts are processed at EcoPak. The system automatically invoices all sales at the full contract prices, and one of the accounting clerks has the job of doing a monthly review of each customer's sales for the year to date, to identify when each volume-discount level is reached. The clerk manually processes a volume-discount credit note to the customer for the amount of volume discount earned. Since the discount rates are sometimes renegotiated during the year, or special arrangements are made, this part of the process is always a manual adjustment and can get somewhat complex. The volume credit notes are all approved by the accounts receivable manager, and a monthly report is also sent to Nina, who monitors the reasonableness of the amounts each customer is receiving.

Donna decides they should try to test controls over this process to lessen the extent of volume credit note transactions that need to be tested substantively. She designs a dual-purpose test that not only tests whether the controls they have identified are being effectively applied but also traces the credit note entry through the accounting system to the general ledger. She also asks Caleb to think about how an analytical procedure could be used to assess whether the year-end sales total is reasonable.

Caleb really likes this kind of mental challenge, and a bit later, he tells Donna about an idea he has: "I think if I review all the customer contracts to get the volume-discount levels and percentages, and then use the reported sales totals by customers from their monthly management sales reports, I should be able to come up with an amount pretty close to what we would expect the total sales less volume credit notes to be for the year. Now, it is possible that the sales force made a lot of special deals that might throw the relationships off, so I will ask the sales manager about that, and then see whether what she says makes sense with what my analysis shows. How does that sound to you, Donna?"

"Brilliant, Caleb. I think that will be pretty strong evidence, even though it is analytical, because it uses a lot of corroborating evidence from other sources. It uses the monthly management sales reports that we will have assessed for reliability through inquiry, analysis, and Shree's systems testing, as well as inquiry evidence independently obtained from the sales manager, plus our inspection of the sales contract terms. Very creative. I think you are going to do well in this job!"

The Essentials of Control Assessment and Testing

Internal control is designed and implemented by a company's management to detect and correct errors that find their way into the accounting information system, to prevent the errors from entering it in the first place, and to prevent fraud. Management is responsible for fair presentation of the financial statements and needs to design and implement internal controls that will be effective in reducing errors and fraud in the accounting system that can lead to misstatements in financial statements. Errors related to the validity, accuracy, completeness, authorization, and proper period-end cutoff of the transactions processed in the accounting system can lead to misstatements in the financial statement assertions. Management will implement control procedures with the objective of reducing the risk of these types of misstatements. Internal control procedures are costly, so management must balance the costs of control against the risks they eliminate. It is not possible to eliminate all risk of misstatement, so financial statement assertions with high inherent risk generally call for implementing a high level of control to offset the risk.

An auditor of the company's financial statements is concerned about potential errors and fraud in accounting systems that can create misstatements in the assertions, so the auditor looks for strong effective controls that will reduce the risk of material misstatement. Evaluation of internal control is an essential, but complex, element of the audit process. Auditors face a number of decision points that require a strong understanding of risks in a business, management controls, and audit procedures for assessing whether controls are strong enough to rely on for assurance and determining which controls auditors need to test to get reasonable assurance that the risk of material misstatement is low. There also may be cost-effectiveness considerations in deciding how to perform the audit.

In planning the audit, the auditor's control evaluation process identifies significant risks and management's internal control related to them, to make a decision on the most effective audit approach to use. Often, a combined audit approach is planned, which includes a combination of testing controls and obtaining substantive evidence. This can be used when it is most effective for the auditors to have evidence that controls are strong, and corroborating substantive evidence about whether any monetary misstatements exist in the financial statement assertions. In some cases, auditors may decide that it is not necessary to test controls, since very persuasive substantive evidence can be obtained to provide high assurance of no material misstatement. In these cases they would use a substantive audit approach and not test the controls. There are several other possible situations to take note of. If controls are essential to reduce the risk of misstatement, and substantive evidence alone cannot provide reasonable assurance, a combined approach must be used. If controls appear to be ineffective, or do not exist, a substantive approach must be used. In all cases, the audit approach needs to be revised to reflect the results of control assessment and testing, which will ensure the most effective audit approach is used. The auditor must communicate findings of significant control weaknesses to management and those charged with governance because maintaining effective internal control is one of management's primary responsibilities. Thus, using a combined approach is more likely to provide valuable information to the audit client as well. If the audit reveals controls over significant risks are ineffective or absent, the company may not be auditable and the auditor will probably have to resign from the engagement.

The auditor's process for evaluating internal control has three general aspects that can be viewed as phases to help us get an overall appreciation for the audit work required.

Phase 1. Understand what could go wrong in the financial statements, identify significant risks that need to be controlled (ask yourself: "What could go wrong in this business that would flow into misstatements in the financial statements?"), and describe management's control procedures by documenting the internal control system in the audit file.

Phase 2. Assess control risk at the assertion level by documenting the general controls and application control procedures in the accounting system and identifying control strengths and weaknesses related to the significant risks.

Phase 3. Perform the control tests required, and determine whether audit programs require revision based on these findings.

The phases can provide a structured way to explain the analytical thinking that auditors follow to decide on the best approach for collecting sufficient appropriate evidence. Note, however, that in practice these phases tend to overlap since, for example, the main reasons auditors need to understand control is so they can assess control risk, and their final risk assessments are based on the results of testing controls.

The auditor's understanding of the internal control framework was introduced in Chapter 7 (Exhibit 7–1) in the context of understanding the entire control framework that management has in place to control the significant risks in the business. The framework considers the overall control environment and other company-level controls. These aspects of control set the tone and create conditions that support the effectiveness of the control activities related to financial reporting, which are the auditor's main interest. This holistic understanding of the control framework helps the auditor assess the overall strength of internal control in the organization and identify significant risks that can lead to material misstatements of the financial statements. For significant risks, the auditor looks for control activities, which are specific procedures performed by the company's accounting personnel at the accounting process level, to assess whether they are adequate to reduce the risks. For each accounting process in the business, general control activities affect the effectiveness of the whole process, and specific application control procedures for detailed transaction processing address management's control objectives in that process. General controls are policies such as segregation of incompatible functions and proper training and supervision of employees; they have a pervasive effect over all the more detailed specific control procedures the employees perform. The specific application control procedures are specific tasks employees perform in an accounting process to ensure the control objectives are met for data input, processing, and output, such as ensuring any transaction data entered into the accounting process are authorized and accurate.

The auditor has to document this understanding of how the accounting system works; this is a requirement of generally accepted auditing standards (GAAS). Various documentation styles are available, such as narratives, process tables, and flowcharts. The auditor chooses the most suitable style. A simple accounting process can usually be described adequately by a narrative, while tables and flowcharts allow for detailed descriptions in more complex processes where a lot of different functions and people are involved. The auditor's internal control documentation is used to identify control strengths and weaknesses that could affect financial statement assertions. An audit analysis approach that can be used to assess control risk is to prepare a bridging working paper that links control findings (strengths or weaknesses) to potential misstatements. The bridging analysis identifies the kinds of control tests and substantive procedures that should be done in response to the risks.

Auditor control testing is required most often for high-volume transaction streams that have a lot of variability in the amounts recorded. These are cash payments transactions, cash receipts transactions, and revenue transactions in most businesses. A control test has two parts: part 1 is to identify the data population (e.g., revenue transactions) from which a sample of items will be selected for testing, and part 2 is a description of the technique the auditor will perform to produce relevant evidence about whether the control objective is being met (e.g., verify that a shipping document was issued for each sales invoice issued). Usually one sample of transaction items can be used for a set of testing procedures that will cover all the objectives.

If auditors identify weaknesses in the controls over significant risks, this needs to be communicated to management. If the weaknesses make the possibility of material misstatement very high, auditors must communicate their findings to those charged with governance (audit committee).

Review Checkpoints

9-1 What are management's responsibilities for internal control? What risks must management control against?

9-2 Why does management need to balance the costs and benefits of implementing internal control?

9-3 What are auditors' responsibilities related to an auditee organization's internal control?

9-4 What is the purpose of the auditor's control evaluation process?

9-5 How is an auditor's understanding of management's internal control over the significant risks in the business used to decide on the most effective audit approach?

9-6 What is the difference between a combined audit approach and a substantive audit approach?

9-7 In what situations would an auditor decide to use a combined audit approach?

9-8 In what situations would an auditor decide to use a substantive audit approach?

9-9 What are the three phases of a control evaluation? How will the auditor's work in these phases overlap in practice?

9-10 How do auditors use their understanding of the auditee's internal control framework?

9-11 Why are the controls over financial reporting the most important part of the internal control framework from the auditor's perspective?

9-12 What are the two types of control activities that make up controls over financial reporting at the accounting process level?

9-13 What are general control activities? Give examples.

9-14 What are specific application control procedures? Why are they different in different accounting processes?

9-15 Why must auditors document their understanding of internal control?

9-16 What styles of accounting system documentation are available for auditors to choose from? What will the choice depend on?

9-17 What is the main purpose of documenting controls in an accounting system?

9-18 What do auditors do if they find strong controls in an accounting system?

9-19 What do auditors do if they find control weaknesses in an accounting system?

9-20 For which type of transaction stream are auditors most likely to test controls?

9-21   What are the two parts of a control test?

9-22   When do auditors need to communicate about their control evaluation findings to management? to those charged with governance?

Internal Control Assessment for Planning the Audit

Chapters 5 to 8 discussed the need to understand internal control before making a preliminary assessment of the risk of material misstatement and designing the overall audit strategy and audit plan. In Chapter 9, these planning activities, concepts, and tools are used to identify and evaluate specific controls that can detect or prevent material misstatements. Financial assertions are applied to identify specific control risks in the auditee's information systems and processes and to indicate the objectives of management's control procedures. Management's control objectives are then used to assess the strengths and weaknesses in the internal control systems. The control strengths and weaknesses guide the auditor's plans on whether to test control procedures.

Internal control evaluation and control risk assessment are essential components of every financial statement audit and must be considered in planning the audit work. GAAS emphasize internal control and the **controls relevant to the audit**.[1] The standards require the auditor to understand the auditee's controls related to significant risks and to assess the risk of material misstatement. When controls must operate effectively for the auditor to lower the assessed risk of material misstatement to an acceptable level, the auditor is required to test the effectiveness of those controls.

Standards Check

CAS 315 Identifying and Assessing the Risks of Material Misstatement through Understanding the Entity and Its Environment

12.   The auditor shall obtain an understanding of internal control relevant to the audit. Although most controls relevant to the audit are likely to relate to financial reporting, not all controls that relate to financial reporting are relevant to the audit. It is a matter of the auditor's professional judgment whether a control, individually or in combination with others, is relevant to the audit. (Ref: Para. A42–A65)

Source: *CPA Canada Handbook—Assurance*, 2014.

Management versus Auditor Responsibility for Control

LO1   Distinguish between management's and auditors' responsibilities regarding an auditee organization's internal controls.

A company's management deals with rapidly shifting economic and competitive conditions, evolving technology, and changes in customer demand, and it must respond to these changes to ensure survival and growth. Internal controls are put in place to keep the company on course toward achieving its goals and to help anticipate

controls relevant to the audit:
elements of an auditee's internal control that directly or indirectly affect the risk of material misstatement of the financial statements being audited

changes that can affect their plans. In this dynamic and risky environment, internal controls help management improve operating efficiency, minimize risks of asset loss, enhance the reliability of financial statements, and monitor compliance with laws and regulations.

Management balances the cost of controls with the benefit of risk reduction. Each successive safeguard costs money, and at some point the costs will exceed the benefits because it is not possible to reduce risks to zero. Managers need to decide what level of risk is acceptable, recognizing that the cost of an entity's internal controls should not exceed the expected benefits. If management understates the risks through ignorance, poor analysis, or an attempt to cut costs, it becomes a source of control risk.

Review Checkpoints

9-23 Explain management's responsibilities regarding its organization's internal control.

9-24 Why does management have to trade off between costs and benefits of internal controls?

9-25 How does management's cost-benefit trade-off decision affect control risk?

9-26 Why do internal controls provide reasonable but not absolute assurance that control objectives are met?

9-27 How can management's cost-benefit judgments lead to internal control deficiencies?

External auditors are not responsible for designing effective internal control for auditees. They are responsible for evaluating existing internal controls and assessing the risk of a material misstatement related to them. They use their assessment to determine the audit work required and develop appropriate audit programs to support their opinion. Public accounting firms may help design internal control systems as consulting engagements for non-audit clients. Such design work must be separate and apart from a financial statement audit engagement because it could impair the auditor's objectivity in assessing those controls in an audit. This would create a self-review threat to the auditor's independence.

Given the realities of reasonable assurance, auditors must carefully determine whether a system contains any internal control weakness. The auditor's primary purpose for this evaluation of internal control is to guide the design of the final audit plan. For this reason, the auditor's understanding of the auditee's internal control and the control risk assessment must be documented.

External auditors' documentation of control weaknesses can help management carry out its responsibility for maintaining effective internal control. However, external auditors' observations and recommendations are usually limited to external financial reporting matters. Their basis for knowing about control weaknesses comes from familiarity with the types of misstatements due to errors and frauds that can occur in an account balance or class of transactions. Clearly, hundreds of innocent errors and not-so-innocent fraud schemes are possible. Rather than discuss hundreds of possible errors and frauds, we show in Exhibit 9–1 six general categories of things that could go wrong in the accounting processes, along with some examples. Management's responsibility is to control against these types of problems. The external auditors' task of control risk assessment involves finding out what the company does to prevent, detect, and correct these potential errors and fraud. You will encounter the flip side of these when you study management's control objectives later in this chapter.[2]

EXHIBIT 9-1

General Categories and Examples of Misstatements

CATEGORY	EXAMPLE OF WHAT COULD GO WRONG	ASSERTION-BASED CONTROL RISK AFFECTED
1. Invalid transactions are recorded.	Fictitious sales are recorded and charged to non-existent customers.	Existence (of accounts receivable)/Occurrence (of sales)
2. Valid transactions are omitted from the accounts.	Shipments to customers never get recorded.	Completeness
3. Unauthorized transactions are executed and recorded.	A customer's order is not approved for credit, yet the goods are shipped, billed, and charged to the customer without requiring payment in advance.	Ownership
4. Transaction amounts are inaccurate.	A customer is billed and the sale is recorded in the wrong amount because the quantity shipped and/or the quantity billed are not the same, and/or the unit price is for a different product.	Valuation
5. Transactions are classified in the wrong accounts.	Proceeds of the sale of an office building are recorded as sales revenue.	Presentation
6. Transactions are recorded in the wrong period.	Shipments made in January are backdated and recorded as sales and charges to customers in December (previous year); shipments in December are recorded as sales and charges to customers in January (next year).	Cutoff errors affecting Existence/Occurrence on one side of transaction and Completeness on the other

Review Checkpoints

9-28   What are auditors' responsibilities in relation to an auditee's internal controls?

9-29   Why is being involved in designing internal controls considered a risk to auditor independence?

9-30   How do external auditors help managers meet their responsibilities for internal control?

9-31   Define control risk, and list six general categories of misstatements that controls are intended to prevent, detect, and correct.

Reasons for Control Evaluation

LO2   Explain why the auditor evaluates an auditee's internal controls.

Control evaluation is the process auditors use to make a decision on which audit approach to use and to determine which specific control activities need to be tested and which control testing is required to achieve reasonable assurance that financial statements are not materially misstated. This is a complex aspect of the audit process that involves many integrated assessments and judgments. To introduce the most important points, it will be helpful to start by "keeping our eyes on the prize," that is, our goal of obtaining reasonable assurance about the fair presentation of the auditee's financial statements. Then we will examine the control evaluation process from the perspective of how it contributes to performing a **highly effective audit**.

highly effective audit:
an audit designed to have a very high chance of detecting material misstatements in the financial statements, which is a major goal of the auditor's control evaluation process

Revisiting the Overall Purpose of the Audit

As you study auditors' control tests and their relation to substantive tests of account balances, it may be helpful for you to think again about the overall purpose of all audit procedures. The purpose of all audit work is to obtain reasonable assurance about whether the financial statements as a whole are free from material misstatement, whether due to fraud or error. Reasonable assurance is required to be able to express an opinion on whether the financial statements are fairly presented, in all material respects, in accordance with generally accepted accounting principles (GAAP). In turn, the purpose of audit procedures is to obtain sufficient appropriate audit evidence about the assessed risks of material misstatement by designing and implementing appropriate procedures in response to these risks. The most effective approach will integrate all aspects of the auditee's business and systems into the overall design of the audit. The choice of control reliance and substantive evidence should maximize the effectiveness of the audit. A secondary goal in designing the audit approach is to make the audit as efficient as possible, without sacrificing effectiveness.

Control Is Evaluated to Make the Audit More Effective

As introduced in Chapters 6 and 7, control risk is the risk that internal control will fail to prevent or detect a material misstatement. The auditor will consider the impact that controls have on safeguarding the company's assets and the accuracy of the accounting records (accounting controls), financial reporting, and disclosures. The primary reason an auditor needs to evaluate a company's internal control and assess control risk is to have a basis for planning the audit and determining the nature, timing, and extent of audit procedures to be performed in the detailed audit plan. Exhibit 9–2 outlines the roles of internal control, risk assessment, and control testing in this process.

By understanding the business and its risks, the auditor's main goal is to identify significant risks of material misstatement, and assessing both inherent and control risk is a key step in performing this assessment. The inherent and control risk assessments can be combined, since they are closely related. For example, consider an item with high inherent risk, such as an inventory of Rolex watches in a jewellery business. The inherent risk is high because these items are easy to pick up and conceal, have a high dollar value, and are easy to sell illegally. The auditor would expect management to have strong controls in place against this significant risk; otherwise, the company could not survive. So, the auditor will expect to observe effective and continuous controls over the Rolex inventory in the internal control system. If this is not found, further substantive procedures need to be planned to address the high risk that the inventory is materially misstated.

As shown in Exhibit 9–2, the auditor identifies control procedures related to the significant risks identified in the auditee's financial statements and prepares a preliminary audit program that includes tests of these controls. This preliminary program might be last year's audit program or a template program that will need to be modified on the basis of auditee-specific preliminary analytical review findings, materiality, and risk assessments.

The results of the control tests will indicate how effective (strong) the controls over significant risks are. If they are found to be strong, control risk can be assessed to be low and the audit program of substantive procedures can be developed to provide sufficient appropriate evidence based on a lower risk of material misstatement. If, however, the tests reveal the controls over significant risks are not effective, these weaknesses increase the risk of material misstatement. In this case, the auditor has several judgments to make related to how severe these weaknesses are.

First, the auditor has to decide whether sufficient appropriate evidence can still be obtained by performing more extensive substantive procedures than would be done if controls were found to be strong. If so, the audit program will be revised accordingly to respond to the assessed risk, and the audit can continue. Second, the auditor must always report significant control weaknesses to management, so it can take action to implement changes to address the weaknesses. The auditor must also decide if the weaknesses are so significant

EXHIBIT 9–2

Role of Control Risk Assessment and Control Testing in the Audit Process

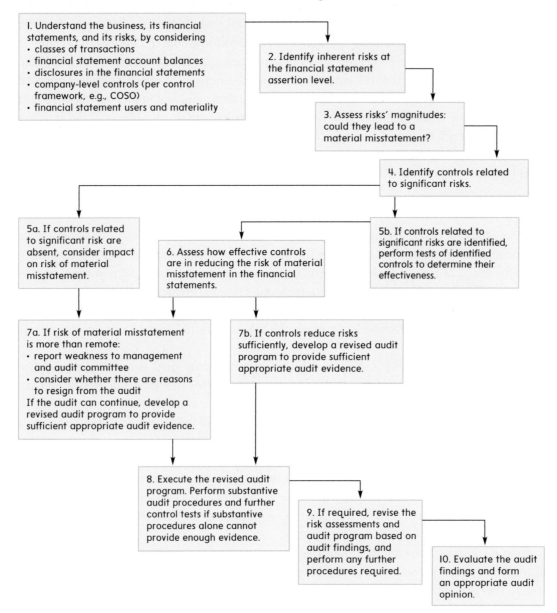

(or if the controls so lacking) that it is highly likely that material misstatements have resulted. In that case, the weaknesses will also need to be reported to those above management, for example, those charged with governance, such as the audit committee of the company, to ensure they are aware of the need for management to correct material internal control weaknesses. Finally, in cases of very high risk of material misstatement due to control weaknesses, the auditor has to consider if there are serious doubts about whether it is possible to get sufficient appropriate evidence to support an audit conclusion. Recall in Chapter 5 we saw that management must take responsibility for implementing effective internal control over financial reporting as part of the preconditions for accepting an audit engagement. Once an auditor discovers this condition is not being met, meaning the company is probably not auditable, the auditor should resign.

If the auditor believes the audit can be done, a substantive program that has been designed in response to the assessed control risk level (high if weak control or low if strong control) should be performed. Note also that there may be risks of misstatements that substantive procedures alone cannot remove. For example, a completeness assertion is virtually impossible to verify without some evaluation of control effectiveness, as that assures auditors that items they might not know about, such as accrued liabilities, get recorded. So control tests on these controls must be done to achieve reasonable assurance. Based on the results of the revised substantive program and the tests of any essential controls, it may be necessary to again revise the risk assessments, adapt the audit programs accordingly, and perform further procedures indicated by these findings.

Once the auditor is satisfied that the procedures performed can provide sufficient appropriate evidence, as shown in the final box in Exhibit 9–2, the findings from the procedures should be evaluated to form an opinion on whether or not the financial information is materially misstated.

Summary

A control evaluation is used to determine the most effective way to do the audit and may also suggest ways to be more efficient without reducing effectiveness. In many cases, if significant controls are found to be strong, efficiencies can be achieved if less-intensive substantive work is required. If controls are weak, in some cases more-extensive substantive procedures can be performed to provide persuasive evidence about whether the financial statements contain a material error. It is possible that the auditor's detailed control evaluation will reveal that management's controls are so weak that it will be difficult, or impossible, to obtain appropriate evidence from the accounting records. If that situation occurs, the auditor will have to conclude that the organization is not auditable and withdraw from the engagement or issue a disclaimer of opinion. This type of audit situation is rare, since with very poor controls a business could not survive for long.

The diagram below illustrates the relations among the auditor's inherent risk and control risk assessments, and the detection risk that needs to be achieved, in terms of the audit risk model discussed in Chapter 6. Recall that the detection risk that must be achieved is inversely proportional to the amount and persuasiveness of the substantive audit evidence that will need to be obtained.

Impact of Assessed Levels of Inherent and Control Risks on Detection Risk and Planned Substantive Evidence Gathering

		ASSESSED CONTROL RISK	
		Risk is high • Controls are weak or auditor decided not to test them.	**Risk is not high** • Controls are effective and auditor confirmed this by testing them.
ASSESSED INHERENT RISK	**Risk is high.**	Accepted detection risk must be low. *Highly persuasive substantive evidence is needed to obtain assurance about material misstatement of financial statements.*	Accepted detection risk will be medium. *Moderately persuasive substantive evidence should be obtained.*
	Risk is not high.	Accepted detection risk will be medium. *Moderately persuasive substantive evidence should be obtained.*	Accepted detection risk can be high. *A relatively low level of substantive evidence can be used to support reasonable assurance.*

Review Checkpoints

9-32 Why does the auditor evaluate the auditee's internal controls?

9-33 Why does an inventory of Rolex watches have a high inherent risk, and why does the auditor expect management to have strong controls over this inventory?

9-34 Why can it be efficient for the auditor to rely on internal controls?

9-35 What is the impact on audit work when auditors find management's controls are very deficient overall?

9-36 Explain how there can be situations when auditors must test a particular control to comply with GAAS.

9-37 If internal controls are weak, in what situations could an audit still be done, and in what situations would it not be possible to do an audit?

Types of Auditing Procedures: How Control Tests, Substantive Tests, and Dual-Purpose Tests Differ

In the discussion of Exhibit 9–2 above, we tend to discuss control tests and substantive procedures as if these are easily distinguishable. But both types make use of the six general evidence techniques described in Chapter 8, so what auditors do to perform each of the types is not all that different. What distinguishes a control test from a substantive procedure is the auditor's purpose in doing the test. With a control test, the auditor wants to obtain evidence about the operating effectiveness of control procedures to provide indirect evidence about the risk of material misstatement of monetary amounts in the financial statements. For substantive procedures, the auditor wants to obtain direct evidence about monetary misstatements.

As discussed earlier, a procedure may be designed that serves both purposes by providing both control and substantive evidence: a **dual-purpose audit procedure**. For example, a selection of recorded sales entries could be used to both vouch sales to supporting shipping documents and calculate the correct monetary amount of sales. The first part of the test provides information about control compliance, while the second is monetary value information that may help measure the amount of misstatement in the general ledger balance of sales. Another example is a test that verifies effectiveness of a control that ensures all payments have been properly authorized and then also traces each payment amount to the cash records and the general ledger for substantive evidence of correct recording in the appropriate account balances. Dual-purpose procedures can provide efficiencies that lower the cost of obtaining sufficient appropriate evidence.

Management's Final Closing Journal Entries Are Always High Risk

Note that even if auditors assess a low control risk by performing control testing on the information system, the potential for **management override of controls** means it is still necessary to perform substantive procedures to evaluate the integrity and accuracy of the **financial statement closing process**. This is because

dual-purpose audit procedure:
an auditing procedure designed to provide both control effectiveness evidence and substantive evidence from the same sample of items; can increase efficiency in obtaining audit evidence

management override of controls:
when management uses its authority and responsibility for the organization's internal control as a means to ignore or circumvent controls; often a facilitator of fraudulent financial reporting

financial statement closing process:
the final adjusting journal entries and other procedures management oversees at the final stage of preparing financial statements

material misstatements can arise from errors or fraud during this final stage of financial statement preparation. As an extreme example, say that at the very last minute management decides it needs to put through a final adjusting entry for a material amount. This journal entry includes a debit to long-term debt and a credit to revenue. This simple two-line journal entry would completely distort the financial statements! Another situation that can occur is if management decides that some of the expenses, such as development of a new product, should be set up as assets: debit assets, credit expenses, increase profits. So auditors always need to check any late entries with detailed substantive procedures. These substantive procedures include reconciling the final financial statements with the general ledger and supporting accounting records. They also include examining the purpose and appropriateness of any material final adjusting and closing journal entries or other adjustments that cause the final financial statement amounts to differ significantly from those in the general ledger. The general ledger was produced from the information system and thus subject to auditor control testing, so any later adjusting entries still need to be examined substantively.

Review Checkpoints

9-38   Explain how using dual-purpose tests can lower audit costs.

9-39   What does it mean if an overall audit plan is said to be cost effective? How do auditors develop a cost-effective overall audit plan?

9-40   Why are the financial statement closing process and final adjusting entries always high risk, even if controls over the information system and general ledger accounts were found to be strong?

9-41   What procedures are auditors required to perform related to the financial statement closing process? What can they find?

An Illustration of How Control Evaluation Affects the Audit Plan

The auditor's control evaluation will affect the procedures included in the detailed audit programs that make up the audit plan. As explained in Chapter 8, an audit program is a list of specific audit procedures designed to produce evidence about the assertions in financial statements. Each procedure's description should indicate its **nature, timing, and extent**, as well as a direct association with one or more financial statement assertions. The nature of procedures refers to which of the six general techniques the procedure will involve, the timing specifies when they will be performed, and the extent refers to the amount of evidence to be obtained, such as the sample size, as well as the selection approach for any samples to be used.

Exhibit 9–3 lists five procedures for auditing two of the accounts receivable assertions as part of the account balance audit program. The existence and completeness subheadings and columns in the exhibit indicate connections to financial statement assertions and to the nature, timing, and extent of the procedures. Some decisions about the timing and extent of work shown in this exhibit suggest the auditor has assessed control risk to be low:

- Confirmation of a sample of customer accounts receivable before year-end, instead of confirmation of all accounts as of December 31

nature, timing, and extent:
the aspects that fully describe a specific audit procedure in an audit program, which indicate the evidence techniques the procedure uses and its objective related to financial statement assertions or control effectiveness; when during the engagement it will be performed; and the sampling approach, sample size, and basis of selecting sample items

- Vouching the last 5 days' recorded sales to bills of lading for cutoff evidence, instead of vouching the last 15 days' sales
- Tracing the last 5 days' shipments to recorded sales invoices for cutoff evidence, instead of tracing the last 15 days' shipments

---

EXHIBIT 9–3

Accounts Receivable Balance Audit Program When Controls Are Tested to Be Strong (Partial Illustration)

ASSERTIONS/PROCEDURES	NATURE	TIMING	EXTENT
Existence/Cutoff: Accounts receivable are authentic obligations owed to the company and represent sales made before December 31.			
1. Obtain a trial balance of customers' accounts. Select 75 for positive confirmation.	Confirmation	November 1 (interim date)	Limited sample
2. Obtain a year-end trial balance of customer accounts. Compare to the November 1 trial balance, and investigate significant changes by vouching large increases to sales invoices and bills of lading.	Analytical procedures Document vouching	December 31 (year-end)	All customer accounts
3. Select all the sales invoices recorded in the last five days of the year, and vouch to bills of lading for December shipping date.	Document vouching	December 31 (year-end)	Last five days' sales
Completeness/Cutoff: Accounts receivable include all amounts owed to the company at December 31.			
4. Send positive confirmations to customers with zero balances.	Confirmation	December 31 (year-end)	All zero-balance accounts
5. Select all the bills of lading dated in the last five days of the year, and trace to sales invoices recorded in December.	Document tracing	December 31 (year-end)	Last five days' shipments

---

The program above is appropriate when the auditors tested the controls and found them to be strong. In that case, the auditors believe the preceding program is effective and efficient. If they found control weaknesses, the risk of material misstatement is increased and a different program would be more appropriate, but it would probably take more time and cost more, too. For example, it might require the auditor to do the following:

- Confirm the customer accounts as of year-end, December 31, rather than an earlier date.
- Confirm a larger sample of customer accounts.
- Select all the sales invoices recorded in the last 15 days for vouching to December shipping documents.
- Select all shipping documents dated in the last 15 days for tracing to December sales invoices.

Note that in this higher-risk situation, more-substantive evidence is needed to provide reasonable assurance about whether or not there is a material financial statement misstatement. If this costs more, so be it. Effectiveness is the primary concern.

The preliminary audit program in Exhibit 9–3, therefore, depends on the auditor having assessed a low control risk related to the company's internal control over accounts receivable. The task is to assess the inherent and internal control risks that there is a material misstatement (error or fraud) in the accounts receivable total. If the risks are too high, procedures are changed to provide for greater extent (larger samples) and closer timing (confirmation moved to December 31). Likewise, if the risk is not high, less work needs to be done (e.g., the confirmation of zero-balance receivables might be omitted). In general, a good system of internal control should result in less audit work than a bad system of internal control. Thus, audit efficiencies, such as less testing and spreading the audit work out over more convenient times, come from good internal controls.

Review Checkpoints

9-42 How does the auditor's control risk assessment affect the preliminary audit program?

9-43 What audit planning activities are performed to lead up to the control risk evaluation?

9-44 Give two reasons controls would be tested.

9-45 In what situation(s) would controls not be tested?

Three Phases of Control Evaluation

The rest of this chapter explains the control evaluation process outlined above in much greater detail. This will introduce more perspectives and considerations that arise in practice to help you better appreciate the judgments auditors will make in different audit situations. We will structure these discussions in terms of the three broad "phases" that describe different aspects of the control evaluation process:

Phase 1. Understanding the control system. This phase expands on the understanding started earlier, in the risk assessment step of the audit process (Chapters 5–7), taking an auditor's perspective on management's control objectives, by considering how these objectives relate to the financial statement assertions and identifying the types of control activities management implements in the business to meet these objectives.

Phase 2. Assessing control risk. This phase involves identifying strengths and weaknesses in the accounting information system. Audit documentation describing the system is prepared to support these assessments.

Phase 3. Testing controls. In this phase we look at how audit procedures are used to ensure control objectives are being met. (The main coverage of control testing is in this chapter, and Chapter 10 covers sampling aspects. Testing controls will also be integrated with the planned substantive audit procedures included in audit programs that will be covered in detail in Part 3.)

Even though the general aspects of each phase are different, there are overlaps and feedback loops between the various parts of the process, as was introduced in discussing Exhibit 9–2 above. For example, we are showing the *understanding* phase and the *control risk assessment* phase as distinct to help you to comprehend the purpose of this part of the audit work. But in practice most auditors do the two together because the purpose of understanding the controls is to assess control risk. Also, the auditor's control risk assessments are based on the control testing results. The three phases described here are a structured way to explain the analytical thinking that auditors follow to decide on the best approach for collecting sufficient appropriate evidence to support their audit opinion.

As the audit work proceeds, new knowledge will allow the audit team to continuously refine and improve the planned audit work, if needed. In many audits, however, the design of the initial plan will be just right and revisions won't be needed. We will now look at the detailed audit work done to understand, assess, and test internal control, noting that the findings of this work may result in some revisions to the original strategy and planned audit approach.

Phase 1—Understanding Controls

Management's Control Objectives and Procedures

LO3 Define management's internal control objectives, and relate them to the financial statement assertions.

This section will look in depth at what auditors need to understand about management internal control. The objective of management's application control procedures is to process transactions correctly. Correctly processed transactions produce accurate account balances, which, in turn, help produce reliable assertions in the financial statements, as shown in Exhibit 9–4. The exhibit gives an example of two revenue transaction streams, sales invoicing and cash receipts, and links these to the control objectives. These control objectives then link to the impact of the transaction streams on increasing (sales) and decreasing (cash receipts) the accounts receivable account balance. If the control objectives over the transaction streams are met, this should ensure that the assertions in the final account balance are true. Note also the general control policies and procedures that apply to the whole accounting process; these determine the overall effectiveness of any specific application control procedures in meeting the control objectives.

EXHIBIT 9–4

Control Objectives and Financial Statement Assertions—An Example for Revenue Transactions

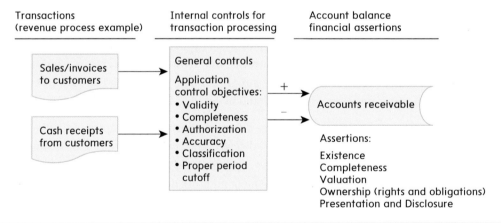

Control Objectives

Note that each control objective is the flip side of one of the six misstatement risks shown in Exhibit 9–1. The six objectives are listed in Exhibit 9–5, with a general statement of each objective along with a specific example for the revenue transaction process. The explanations that follow this exhibit tell you more about these objectives and give examples of auditee procedures designed to accomplish them.

Internal Control Objectives

OBJECTIVE	GENERAL STATEMENT OF CONTROL OBJECTIVE AND EXAMPLES OF RELATED CONTROL RISKS	MAIN RELATED FINANCIAL STATEMENT ASSERTIONS	SPECIFIC EXAMPLE (REVENUE PROCESS)
Validity	Control objective: Recorded transactions are valid and documented. Control risk: Fictitious sales are recorded; sales are recorded before shipment occurs.	Existence Ownership	Recorded sales are supported by invoices, shipping documents, and customer orders.
Completeness	Control objective: All valid transactions are recorded, and none are omitted. Control risk: Goods are shipped but sale is not recorded.	Completeness Ownership	All shipping documents are prenumbered and matched with sales invoices daily.
Authorization	Control objective: Transactions are authorized according to company policy. Control risk: Goods are sold on account to an unauthorized customer with poor credit rating.	Existence Valuation Ownership	Credit sales over $1,000 are given prior approval by the credit manager.
Accuracy	Control objective: Transaction dollar amounts are properly calculated. Control risk: Incorrect prices or tax rates are used; calculation errors are made in extending and totalling the invoice amount.	Valuation	Sales invoices contain correct quantities and are mathematically correct.
Classification	Control objective: Transactions are properly classified in the accounts. Control risk: A sale to a subsidiary company is misclassified as a regular outside sale.	Valuation Presentation/ Disclosure	Sales to subsidiaries and affiliates are classified as intercompany transactions.
Proper period cutoff	Control objective: Transactions are recorded in the proper period. Control risk: The first sales of the new year are included in the current year; the shipments of goods on the last day of the year are not recorded until the next year.	Existence Completeness Ownership Presentation/ Disclosure	Sales of the current period are charged to customers in the current period, and sales of the next period are charged in the next period.

Validity is ensuring that recorded transactions are ones that should be recorded; that is, they really exist. The auditee's procedure might require matching shipping documents with sales invoices before a sale is recorded. This procedure prevents the recording of undocumented (possibly fictitious) sales.

Completeness is ensuring that valid transactions are not missing from the accounting records. If sales are represented by shipments, then every shipment should be matched with a sales invoice. Transaction documents (e.g., shipping documents) are often prenumbered, and accounting for their numerical sequence is a control procedure designed to achieve the completeness objective.

validity:
a management control objective of ensuring that the recorded transactions are ones that should be recorded, that is, that they exist

completeness:
a management control objective of ensuring that valid transactions are not missing from the accounting records

Authorization is ensuring that transactions are approved before they are recorded, that is, they are "owned" by the company. Management establishes criteria for recognizing transactions in the accounting system and for supervisory approval of them, much as credit sales must be preapproved. A control system should stop any unauthorized transactions from entering the accounting records.

The nature of authorization for transactions may vary. For example, authorization is not usually needed to record a cash receipt from a regular customer, since companies are happy to accept payments, but a sales manager may need to approve giving a discount after the end of the discount period. Unauthorized transactions of any kind are a source of risk that the auditor needs to understand. For example, unauthorized cash receipts may be part of a fraud cover-up or an illegal money laundering scheme.

Authorization for routine transactions may be delegated to a fairly low level of management. For example, (1) credit sales with a value of more than $1,000 require credit manager approval, or (2) purchases for more than $500 must be approved by a senior purchasing manager. Some authorizations have to come from a high level of the company's governance structure, such as the board of directors. For example, significant non-routine transactions, such as sales of major assets and acquisition of another business, or signing the company name to a loan agreement, will usually be authorized specifically by the board of directors, with the authorization included in the minutes of that board meeting.

Accuracy is ensuring that monetary amounts are calculated correctly. A manual or computer check that the quantity invoiced equals the quantity shipped and the correct list price is used, with a correctly calculated total, is a control procedure for accuracy.

Classification is ensuring that transactions are recorded in the right accounts, charged or credited to the right customers (including classification of sales to subsidiaries and affiliates, as mentioned in Exhibit 9–5), entered in the correct segment product line or inventory description, and so forth. Classification errors between balance sheet and income statement accounts present the greatest risk of misstatement because they will change the net income. For example, before its bankruptcy WorldCom misstated its income by misclassifying operating expenses as assets, thereby concealing its poor financial performance from financial statement users.

Proper period cutoff refers to ensuring that transactions are accounted for in the period they occurred in. This control objective relates to both the existence and the completeness assertions. The auditee's accountants must be alert to the dates of transactions in relation to month-, quarter-, and year-end. Proper period accounting cutoff is a pervasive problem. It is mentioned in relation to all kinds of transactions—sales, purchases, inventories, expense accruals, income accruals, and others. The risk of errors in cutoff is high because they are complex and non-routine events, but they can also be used to manipulate income, for example, by using accruals to record sales too early or expenses too late.

General control over the accounting process is concerned with ensuring that the accounting process for all transactions is performed completely and in conformity with GAAP. For example, a clerk can perform a reconciliation procedure to balance the total of individual receivables in the subledger with the control account

---

authorization:
a management control objective of ensuring that transactions are approved before they are recorded

accuracy:
a management control objective of ensuring that monetary transaction amounts are calculated correctly during data input, processing, and output

classification:
a management control objective of ensuring that transactions are recorded in the correct accounts in the accounting information system, including general ledger accounts, subledger accounts, and journals

proper period cutoff:
a management control objective of ensuring that transactions occurring near a period-end are recorded in the period in which they correctly belong according to the company's financial reporting framework (e.g., generally accepted accounting principles)

balance in the general ledger, to verify that all entries to the control account have also been entered in individual customers' accounts. Bank reconciliation should be done to agree the cash general ledger balance to the bank account statement, and it should be done by a person who is independent of cash recording. Balancing, verification, and reconciliation procedures like these can meet more than one control objective. These kinds of general control activities over the accounting work are essential to reducing control problems related to any of the control objectives.

Control Objectives and Assertions

The control objectives are closely connected to the assertions in management's financial statements. For example, the accuracy control objective relates to the existence, completeness, and valuation assertions, as mechanical errors will result in overstated, understated, or incorrectly measured balances. However, recognizing that the control objective is to assess accuracy is more helpful in designing appropriate tests, such as tests for errors of billing at too low or too high a price, or for a smaller or larger quantity than shipped, or for using price lists in U.S. dollars when the financial statement information should be in Canadian dollars.

The grid in Exhibit 9–6 shows how the control objectives are related to the assertions, with the X's showing the primary relevance. To interpret Exhibit 9–6, link the achievement of control objectives with the probability that an assertion may be materially misstated. For example, a strong control over the validity of recorded sales and cash receipts transactions, an effective system of credit authorization, and a system ensuring that transactions are recorded in the proper period can allow control risk related to the existence/occurrence assertions for accounts receivable and sales balances to be assessed as low.

EXHIBIT 9–6

How Control Objectives Relate to Financial Statement Assertions

CONTROL OBJECTIVE	FINANCIAL STATEMENT ASSERTIONS				
	EXISTENCE	COMPLETENESS	VALUATION	OWNERSHIP	PRESENTATION AND DISCLOSURE
Validity	X			X	
Completeness		X		X	
Authorization	X		X	X	
Accuracy			X		
Classification			X		X
Proper Period	X	X		X	X

However, an auditor may find that some, but not all, of the control objectives for a particular account balance (i.e., set of assertions) are achieved. For example, the above situation may coexist with failure to achieve control over the completeness of recording sales transactions and accounts receivable amounts. In this case, the preliminary audit program may be revised to require more substantive work related to the completeness of accounts receivable (the assertion that was assessed as having high control risk) and be unchanged for the work on the existence of accounts receivable (which was assessed as low control risk).

The evaluation of a company's internal control involves an assessment of the control risk (CR) related to each assertion. (The audit risk model, $AR = IR \times CR \times DR$, was explained in Chapter 6.) In this assessment, an auditor expresses the effectiveness of the control system for meeting its objectives by preventing, detecting, and correcting specific errors in management's financial statement assertions.

Review Checkpoints

9-49   Why do control procedures affect management's financial statement assertions?

9-50   Explain the importance of general controls over an accounting process.

9-51   List the control objectives and the misstatement risk that each objective relates to.

9-52   Why can some authorization procedures be performed by low-level managers? What kinds of authorizations need to come from the board of directors?

9-53   What are the risks related to cutoff procedures?

9-54   Match the six control objectives to the five principal assertions.

9-55   Can control risk be high for one assertion and low for another assertion for the same account balance? Explain.

9-56   How does the auditor's control risk assessment relate to audit risk?

Understanding General and Application Control Activities

LO4   Explain the impact on control risk of general and application control activities in the auditee's accounting information systems.

Nature and Timing of Phase 1 Work

Understanding controls is a key part of understanding the business and risk of misstatement introduced in Chapters 5 and 6. Done early in the engagement, this work acquaints auditors with the overall control environment and the flow of transactions through the accounting system. We will now apply this understanding to identify significant risks at the assertion level in account balances, transaction streams, and disclosures. These risks will correspond to the key control activities that should be in place to minimize them, as described in the following section.

Standards Check

Cas 315 Identifying and Assessing the Risks of Material Misstatement through Understanding the Entity and Its Environment

14.   The auditor shall obtain an understanding of the control environment. As part of obtaining this understanding, the auditor shall evaluate whether

(a) Management, with the oversight of those charged with governance, has created and maintained a culture of honesty and ethical behaviour; and

(b) The strengths in the control environment elements collectively provide an appropriate foundation for the other components of internal control, and whether those other components are not undermined by deficiencies in the control environment. (Ref: Para. A69–A78)

Source: *CPA Canada Handbook—Assurance*, 2014.

Control Activities: General Controls and Application Control Procedures

The internal control framework presented earlier[3] showed that management implements control activities to achieve the organization's control objectives. Control activities are classified as either general controls or application control procedures. General controls are policies and organizational features that have an overall impact on accounting processes. Applications control procedures are specific employee tasks that address the control objectives relating to input, processing, and output of data in each accounting process. All control activities are directed toward preventing, or detecting and correcting, misstatements in the organization's financial records and reporting. Exhibit 9–7 provides an overview of control activities, which are further explained below.

Overview of Control Activities

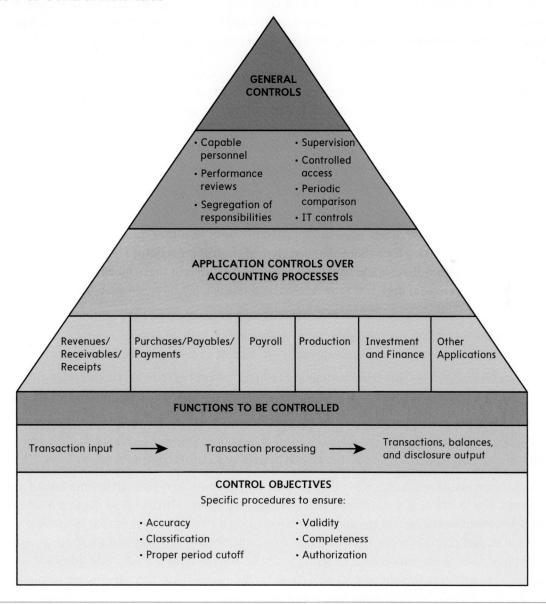

General Controls

General controls are organizational features such as capable personnel, segregation of responsibilities, controlled access, and periodic comparison. Similar to environmental controls, general controls have a pervasive impact on all aspects of the accounting processes. They are primarily preventive in nature. For these reasons, auditors tend to focus on environmental and general controls in the preliminary evaluation of internal controls, as well as in evaluating the specific application controls. Some of the general controls are discussed below.

Capable Personnel   The people who make the system work are the most important aspect of control. Proper training should be provided so people know how to do their work correctly. Personnel problems might result in internal control problems. For example, high turnover in accounting jobs means that inexperienced people are doing the accounting and control tasks, and they generally make more mistakes than experienced people. New accounting officers and managers (e.g., financial vice-president, controller, chief accountant, plant accountant, or data-processing manager) may be unfamiliar with company accounting and may make technical and judgmental errors. Accounting officers and employees may be fired because they refuse to go along with improper accounting procedures desired by a higher level of management. In general, accounting personnel changes may be a warning signal.

Performance Reviews   Management reviews of how reported performance compares with expectations are an effective general control. Comparing reported performance with budgets and prior years is an important part of management's risk assessment process. Management should follow up on any discrepancies and, if errors or other irregularities are uncovered, take appropriate action to implement corrections and solutions. Performance review procedures can be reperformed by auditors as part of their analytical procedures to reveal significant control weaknesses, risks, or actual errors or fraud.

Segregation of Responsibilities   An important characteristic of reliable internal control is the appropriate segregation of functional responsibilities. Sometimes called *division of duties*, proper segregation of incompatible responsibilities is necessary for making detailed clerical control procedures effective. There are four kinds of functional responsibilities that should each be performed by different departments, or at least by different people on the company's accounting staff:

1. *Authorization to execute transactions.* This duty belongs to people who have authority and responsibility for initiating the recordkeeping for transactions. Authorization may be general, referring to a class of transactions (e.g., all purchases), or it may be specific (e.g., sale of a major asset).

2. *Recording of transactions.* This is the accounting and recordkeeping function (bookkeeping).

3. *Custody of assets involved in the transactions.* This is the actual physical possession or effective physical control of property.

4. *Periodic reconciliation of existing assets to recorded amounts.* This duty refers to making comparisons at regular intervals and taking appropriate action with respect to any differences.

Responsibilities are incompatible when they place a single person in a position to both create and conceal errors or fraud. For example, if a warehouse receiver can also approve write-off of damaged inventory, then inventory items could be stolen and the shortages covered up by issuing a report that they were written off. No one person should control two or more functional responsibilities. The first and fourth responsibilities are management functions, the second is an accounting function, and the third is a custodial (physical access) function. If different departments or persons deal with the different transactions, two benefits are obtained: (1) fraud requires collusion of two or more people, and most people hesitate to ask for help when conducting wrongful acts, and (2) innocent errors are more likely to be found and flagged for correction. The saying that two heads are better than one is very true for internal control: the more people assigned to control duties, the better the controls. The costs, however, are higher as well. Any control system will reflect a cost-benefit compromise.

Separation of the duties is also an important IT control. Work performed by analysts, programmers, and operators should be segregated. Anyone who designs a processing system should not do the technical programming work, and anyone who performs either of these tasks should not be the computer operator when "live" data are being processed. People performing each function should not have access to each other's work, and only the computer operators should have access to the equipment. Lack of separation of duties along these lines should be considered a serious weakness in general control. A lack of segregation here could be compensated for by having a separate information control group, or monitoring by the user departments. The following box gives an example of what can happen when incompatible IT functions are performed by the same individual.

Programmer and Operator Combined

A programmer employed by a large U.S. savings and loan association wrote a special subroutine that could be activated by a command from the computer console. The computation of interest on deposits and certificates was programmed to truncate calculations at the third decimal place. The special subroutine instructed the program to accumulate the truncated fractions and, when processing was complete, to credit the amount to the programmer-operator's savings account. Whenever this person was on duty for the interest calculation run, she could "make" several hundred dollars! She had to be on duty to manipulate the control figures "properly" so that the error of paying interest into her account would not be detected by the control group. She was a programmer with computer operation duties.

Supervision Supervision is an important element of control. Management's supervision of the work of clerks and computers carrying out the accounting and control procedures is important. A supervisor could, for example, oversee the credit manager's performance or could periodically compare the sum of customers' balances with the accounts receivable control account total. Supervisors or department heads can correct errors found by the clerical staff and make or approve accounting decisions. Supervision is an important way for management to monitor and maintain a system of internal control.

Controlled Access Access to assets, important records, documents, and blank forms should be limited to authorized personnel. Inventory and cash should not be available to people who have no need to handle them. Likewise, access to cost records and accounts receivable records should be denied to people who do not have a recordkeeping responsibility for them. Access to blank forms is the equivalent of access to, or custody of, an important asset. For example, someone who has access to blank cheques has a type of custody of and access to cash. Blank sales invoices and shipping orders are very important for accounting and control, and their availability should be restricted to those involved in accounting for sales.

In the IT used in the systems, controlled access is achieved through locating hardware, software, and data in secured facilities, and through use of user identity codes and passwords to restrict online access for data and programs to authorized personnel. Who should have access to which IT functions should be determined on the basis of keeping incompatible functions separate.

A physical control's relevance to financial statement reliability and the audit depends on the auditee's accounting system. For example, if management uses periodic physical counts to detect any inventory losses and records all these losses in the financial statements, the physical controls will not be highly relevant to the audit. However, if management relies on perpetual inventory records for financial reporting purposes and inventory is physically counted at a date other than year-end, then the physical security controls will be relevant to the audit. In this case, the auditor needs assurance that controls operated effectively throughout the period between the physical count and the financial statement date to have sufficient appropriate audit evidence about the reported ending inventory balance.

Periodic Comparison and Reconciliation Management is accountable for the organization's assets and liabilities and so is responsible for ensuring that they are properly recorded. The recorded amounts should be periodically compared with independent evidence of existence and valuation, and any differences should be reconciled and explained. This is done by periodic counting of cash, securities, and inventory and then comparing the results with control totals in the accounting records. Internal auditors and others on an accounting staff could do this on a regular basis, but the same people should not also be responsible for authorizing related transactions, accounting, or recordkeeping, or have custodial responsibility for the assets.

Periodic comparisons that management performs include counts of cash on hand, reconciliation of bank statements, confirmation of accounts receivable balances, reconciling customer account balances to the general ledger accounts receivable control balance, reconciling accounts payable to supplier statements, and other comparisons to verify if accounting records represent the real assets and liabilities for which management is accountable. Frequent comparisons give management more opportunities to detect errors in the records than infrequent ones do, and these can also motivate employees to work more accurately. As is the case for all control procedures, how frequently the comparisons are performed is based on the relative costs and benefits. Very frequent comparisons are worthwhile for assets especially susceptible to loss or error, or ones that are highly valuable. In other words, if the inherent risk is high, the controls should be strengthened to compensate and lower the control risk.

Follow-up to correct errors found by periodic comparisons is also important. This lowers the risk that material misstatements will remain in the accounts. Error-checking techniques for accounting data can be categorized as (1) input controls, (2) processing controls, and (3) output controls. The weakest point in computer systems is input—the point at which transaction data are transformed from hard-copy source documents or online order keying into machine-readable form. When undetected errors are entered originally, they may not be detected during processing, and, if detected, they can be costly to correct. For this reason, preventive controls at input are the most cost effective. Processing controls are error-condition check routines written into the computer program. Output control refers primarily to control over the distribution of reports, but it includes feedback on errors and comparison of input totals to output totals. Error-checking techniques are closely related to application controls, but, because errors compound if they are not corrected quickly and appropriately, they have a pervasive impact on the accounting system's integrity. The auditor should consider the overall effectiveness of error correction procedures as a key part of the general IT control activities.

Information Technology Controls   General IT controls are policies and procedures that relate to the IT systems and support the effective functioning of IT application controls by helping to ensure the continued proper operation of information systems. These controls apply to mainframe, server, and end-user environments. General IT controls over computer operations commonly include the following:

- Operating system and application software acquisition, change, and maintenance
- Access security: authorization for access to systems, programs, and data files
- System and application development and maintenance
- Routine data and system backup procedures
- Disaster recovery plans to restore systems and data, or to provide backup-processing capability
- Physical security of the IT assets, including adequate safeguards such as secured facilities; restricted access to assets, media, and records; and appropriate environmental controls such as air conditioning and smoke detectors

Review Checkpoints

9-57   List four duties that should be segregated within an information system. Why does this improve internal control?

9-58   Give some examples of periodic comparisons a company's management can perform. How do they control the accuracy of its financial records?

9-59   List some commonly used general controls related to IT.

9-60   What risks are addressed by controlled access?

Application Control Procedures

Application control procedures are specific control activities used in each accounting process to meet the relevant control objectives. Auditors evaluate the activities in terms of how they address financial reporting risk at the assertion level. The audit approach starts with documenting the information system and its accounting processes. It identifies the application controls related to input, processing, and output within each process. Examples of application control procedures are as follows:

- The sales data input clerk verifies that each sale on account is to a valid customer on the approved credit list.
- The inventory receiver checks that the quantity and description of goods received matches the information on the supplier's packing slip.
- The accounts payable clerk ensures that the supplier invoice is matched with appropriate supporting purchase order documents and approvals prior to processing a payment.
- The payroll clerk verifies that the hours worked by casual labourers are approved by a supervisor and the rate of pay is approved by the payroll manager before processing the hourly wages payroll payments.

   Methods of documenting accounting systems and controls are discussed next.

Phase 2—Assessing Control Risk

Documentation of an Accounting Information System

LO5   Describe how auditors document an accounting system to identify control strengths and weaknesses in order to assess control risk.

Auditors' identification of the strengths and weaknesses of internal controls in the accounting system comes through several sources of information: (1) last year's audit experience with the company, (2) auditee personnel responses to inquiries, (3) documents and records inspection, and (4) walk-through observation of the activities and operations of a single transaction. Such walk-through procedures have traditionally been used to verify the accuracy of the auditor's narrative or flowchart description of the system.

   Working paper documentation should include records showing the audit team's understanding of the internal controls. It can be summarized in the form of questionnaires, narratives, and flowcharts. The decision on how much reliance to place on controls and how much to place on substantive work must also be documented in the audit file, explaining underlying reasons, for instance, to increase effectiveness and efficiency. This is helpful for reference in next year's audit.

Internal Control Questionnaire and Narrative

The most efficient means of gathering evidence about internal control is to conduct formal interviews with knowledgeable managers using a checklist guide such as the **internal control questionnaire**, an example of which is shown in Exhibit 9–8. This questionnaire is organized under headings identifying the questions related to the environment and general controls and those related to each of the six control objectives. Using these six categories helps to ensure the questionnaire will cover all the assertions.

internal control questionnaire:
a checklist used by auditors to gather evidence about the auditee's control environment and its general and application control activities

EXHIBIT 9–8

Example of an Internal Control Questionnaire—Revenue Transaction Processing

Auditee _____   Audit Date _____

Auditee Personnel Interviewed _____

_____

_____

Auditor _____   Date Completed _____

Reviewed by _____   Date Reviewed _____

Question	Answer			
	NA	**Yes**	**No**	**Remarks**
Environment and General Controls Related to Sales Transaction Processing				
1. Is the credit department independent of the marketing department?				
2. Are sales accounting staff properly trained in and subject to supervisory reviews? Are they independent of marketing and credit departments? Are summary journal entries approved before posting?				
3. Are non-routine sales of the following types controlled by the same procedures described below: sales to employees, COD (cash on delivery) sales, disposals of property, cash sales, and scrap sales?				
4. Are policies in place to ensure effective IT management and IT staff supervision?				
5. Are IT systems general controls in place to ensure				
– accurate data and processing of sales transactions?				
– authorized access to data and application software?				
Application Control Assessments:				
Validity Objective				
6. Are procedures in place to				
– prevent fictitious sales being recorded in accounts?				
– ensure approved revenue recognition policies are followed?				
7. Is access to sales invoice blanks, or online order entry, restricted to authorized personnel?				
8. Are prenumbered bills of lading or other shipping documents prepared or completed in the shipping department?				
Completeness Objective				
9. Are procedures in place to ensure				
– all goods shipped/services performed are invoiced?				
– no fictitious sales credits are recorded?				
10. Are sales invoice blanks or online orders numbered sequentially?				
11. Is the sequence checked for missing invoices by appropriate personnel?				
12. Is the shipping document numerical sequence checked for missing bills of lading numbers by appropriate personnel?				

(continued)

EXHIBIT 9–8

Example of an Internal Control Questionnaire—Revenue Transaction Processing *(continued)*

Question	Answer			
	NA	Yes	No	Remarks
Authorization Objective				
13. Are all credit sales approved by the credit department prior to shipment?				
14. Are sales prices and terms based on approved standards?				
15. Are returned sales credits and other credits supported by documentation as to receipt, condition, and quantity and approved by a responsible officer?				
Accuracy Objective				
16. Are shipped quantities compared with invoice quantities by appropriate personnel?				
17. Are sales invoices checked for error in quantities, prices, extensions and footing, and freight allowances, as well as checked with customer's orders?				
18. Is there an overall check on arithmetic accuracy of period sales data by a statistical or product-line analysis?				
19. Are periodic sales data reported directly to general ledger accounting independent of accounts receivable accounting?				
Classification Objective				
20. Does the accounting manual contain instructions for classifying revenues according to the company's revenue recognition policies?				
21. Are accounting supervisors aware of related parties, and are related party transactions flagged in the accounting system?				
Proper Period Objective				
22. Does the accounting manual contain instructions to date sales invoices on the shipment date?				
23. Do accounting staff understand proper period cutoff procedures for sales and cash receipts?				
24. Does the information system correctly age receivables to provide information about doubtful accounts?				

Internal control questionnaires are designed to help the audit team obtain evidence about the control environment as well as about the general and application control activities that can reduce risks of error and fraud. A strength of questionnaires is that they minimize the risk that an important point will be forgotten. Questions are usually worded so that a "yes" answer indicates an appropriate control procedure, and a "no" answer points out some possible weakness or control deficiency, thus making analysis easier. The answers, however, should not be taken as final and definitive evidence about how well control actually functions. Evidence obtained through the interview-questionnaire process is hearsay, as its source is an individual who, while knowledgeable, may not be the person who actually performs the control work. These individuals may give answers reflecting what they believe the system should be rather than what it really is, may be unaware of informal ways that have been changed, or may be innocently ignorant of the system details. Nevertheless, interviews and questionnaires are useful as a starting point. If a manager admits to a weak control, it is important to document and follow up in subsequent audit work.

The questionnaire answers can be used to write up narrative descriptions of each important control subsystem in the company. The description should include all the environmental elements, the accounting process, and the control procedures. A narrative description is often suitable in audits of small businesses or simple accounting processes within larger organizations.

Review Checkpoints

9-61   What does the auditor need to understand about the auditee's control environment?

9-62   What does the auditor need to understand about the flow of transactions in the auditee's information systems?

9-63   What sources of information can auditors use to gain knowledge about the auditee's internal controls?

9-64   What internal control documentation needs to be included in the audit files?

9-65   Why is audit file documentation required for the auditor's decision on whether to rely on controls in the audit planning?

9-66   What is an audit internal control questionnaire?

9-67   What is an internal control system narrative, and what is it used for in an audit?

Control System Flowcharts for Accounting Transaction Processing

Flowcharts are one technique that can be used by auditors to document their understanding of accounting processes and controls. Many control-conscious companies have their own flowcharts, usually prepared by internal auditors, that external auditors can use instead of constructing their own. The advantages of flowcharts can be summarized by an old adage, "A picture is worth a thousand words." They enhance auditors' evaluations and are easy to update—simply add or delete symbols and lines. The audit team may find that the company already has documentation related to the flow of transactions that may be adequate for understanding the accounting system. Early in the audit planning, the internal auditors and other auditee personnel should be consulted to determine whether they have documentation that can be useful.

Flowchart construction takes time, because an auditor must learn about the operating of personnel involved in the system and gather samples of relevant documents. Thus, the information for the flowchart, like the narrative description, involves a lot of legwork and observation. When the flowchart is complete, however, the result is an easily evaluated, informative description of the system. Flowcharting software that saves time and produces more readable output is available. Some simple symbols and styles for preparing flowcharts, and a partial example of a flowchart, are provided in Appendix 9A.[4]

Regardless of the method used to develop the flowchart, its accuracy can be verified by performing a **walk-through procedure** of the documents and procedures to see if they are processed as described in the flowchart. An understanding of the flow of transactions through the accounting system supports the design of substantive audit procedures, and it begins with referring to the auditee's description of the accounting processes. Descriptions could include user manuals and instructions, file descriptions, system flowcharts, and narrative descriptions.

Internal Control Evaluation and Planned Audit Approach

A brief review of how internal controls affect the planned audit approach and detailed audit programs for each significant transaction stream and account balance concludes this section.

1. All audit engagements involve some evaluation of internal controls, even if only on environmental controls affecting all processes (e.g., reconciliation of general ledger to subsidiary ledgers). Under GAAS, auditors are required to understand internal controls in order to assess the risk of material misstatement for all audits (CAS 200 and CAS 315).

walk-through procedure:
an audit procedure that follows one or more transactions through an accounting process to confirm that the documents, procedures, and work flows documented in the auditor's system description narrative or flowcharts are accurate

2. Internal control is documented through narratives, questionnaires, or flowcharts (see Appendix 9A for examples). These are corroborated with walk-through procedures, which include tracing of a representative transaction.

3. In reaching a preliminary evaluation of internal control, the auditor must consider

   (a) Misstatements that may arise.

   (b) Controls that exist to prevent or detect those misstatements.

   Professional judgment is applied to knowledge gained in point (b).

4. The review, preliminary evaluation, and documentation must be applied to specific internal controls within an individual accounting process. The specific controls activities, not the system as a whole, are assessed. Only the specific controls from which auditors intend to obtain audit assurance need to be tested.

5. If the auditor wishes to use internal controls as a component of audit evidence, tests of control need to be planned and executed. The decision to test the controls is a function of

   (a) Evaluation of the design of the system.

   (b) Cost-benefit trade-offs of control testing, assuming the design is adequate.

6. The auditor will choose one of two planned audit approaches.

   (a) If the auditor is unable to rely, or chooses not to rely, on internal control effectiveness, the **substantive audit approach** will be used. All evidence will come from substantive procedures.

   (b) Alternatively, if the auditor decides to test internal controls, and these tests confirm that the controls are operating effectively, then the auditor will choose to use a **combined audit approach**, which may reduce the required extent of substantive audit procedures. Another case where a combined audit approach will be used is when the auditor cannot obtain sufficient appropriate audit evidence on the basis of substantive tests alone; in this case, testing controls and finding them effective can increase the evidence sufficiency to an acceptable level to support the audit opinion (CAS 330).

Standards Check

Cas 200 Overall Objectives of the Independent Auditor and the Conduct of an Audit in Accordance with CASs

A39. Control risk is a function of the effectiveness of the design, implementation, and maintenance of internal control by management to address identified risks that threaten the achievement of the entity's objectives relevant to preparation of the entity's financial statements. However, internal control, no matter how well designed and operated, can only reduce, but not eliminate, risks of material misstatement in the financial statements, because of the inherent limitations of internal control. These include, for example, the possibility of human errors or mistakes, or of controls being circumvented by collusion or inappropriate management override. Accordingly, some control risk will always exist. The CASs provide the conditions under which the auditor is required to, or may choose to, test the operating effectiveness of controls in determining the nature, timing, and extent of substantive procedures to be performed.

Source: *CPA Canada Handbook—Assurance,* 2014.

substantive audit approach:
an approach to performing an audit that involves obtaining assurance only from substantive procedures, with no reliance on internal control effectiveness

combined audit approach:
an approach to performing an audit that involves obtaining assurance from reliance on internal controls based on testing their effectiveness, combined with assurance from substantive procedures

Standards Check

CAS 330 The Auditor's Responses to Assessed Risks

A2.   The assessment of the risks of material misstatement at the financial statement level, and thereby the auditor's overall responses, is affected by the auditor's understanding of the control environment. An effective control environment may allow the auditor to have more confidence in internal control and the reliability of audit evidence generated internally within the entity and thus, for example, allow the auditor to conduct some audit procedures at an interim date rather than at the period-end. Deficiencies in the control environment, however, have the opposite effect; for example, the auditor may respond to an ineffective control environment by

- Conducting more audit procedures as of the period-end rather than at an interim date.
- Obtaining more extensive audit evidence from substantive procedures.
- Increasing the number of locations to be included in the audit scope.

A3.   Such considerations, therefore, have a significant bearing on the auditor's general approach, for example, an emphasis on substantive procedures (substantive approach), or an approach that uses tests of controls as well as substantive procedures (combined approach).

Source: *CPA Canada Handbook—Assurance*, 2014.

Review Checkpoints

9-68   What is the purpose of an internal control systems flowchart? How does it differ from a narrative?

9-69   Why do many organizations document their internal control system?

9-70   What is a walk-through, and why is this procedure used in an audit?

9-71   What role can internal auditors play in internal control system documentation?

9-72   What is a substantive audit approach, and how does it differ from a combined audit approach? Give examples of situations when each type would be used in an audit engagement.

Identifying Strengths and Weaknesses in the Controls to Assess Control Risk

After obtaining an understanding of the internal control and making a preliminary decision on an audit approach, the audit team assesses the control risk at the assertion level. Control risk assessment involves the following:

- Identifying specific control objectives based on the risks of misstatements that may be present in significant accounting applications
- Identifying the points in the flow of transactions where specific types of misstatements could occur
- Identifying specific control procedures designed to prevent or detect misstatements
- Identifying the control procedures that must function to prevent or detect misstatements
- Evaluating the design of control procedures to determine whether it suggests the auditee has strong control procedures in place and whether it may be cost effective to test these controls as part of the audit.

A useful assessment technique is to analyze control strengths and weaknesses. **Control strengths** are specific features of effective control procedures that would prevent, detect, or correct material misstatements.

control strengths:
specific features of effective controls that would prevent, detect, or correct material misstatements

Control weaknesses are a lack of controls in particular areas that would allow material errors to get by undetected. The auditors' findings and preliminary conclusions on control strengths and weaknesses should be written up for the working paper files in a document called a **bridge working paper**—so called because it connects (bridges) the control evaluation to subsequent audit procedures. An example of a bridge working paper summarizing the significant strengths and weaknesses in a Revenue accounting process is shown in Exhibit 9–9 (note that these are the strengths and weaknesses apparent in the flowchart example given in Appendix 9A in Exhibit 9A–3). On the flowchart, the strengths are indicated by S- and the weaknesses by W-. In Exhibit 9–9,

---

EXHIBIT 9–9

Bridge Working Paper

Prepared by _____ Date: _____ File Index: _____

Reviewed by _____ Date: _____

EcoPak Inc.
Credit Approval, Sales Processing, Shipment and Delivery Control
December 31, 20X1

	Strength/Weakness*	Audit Implication	Implications for Audit Program
S-1	Credit approval is done on sales order.	Credit authorization reduces risk of bad debt loss and helps check on validity of customer identification.	*Control testing to evaluate effectiveness:* a. Select a sample of recorded sales invoices, and look for credit manager signature on attached sales order.
S-2	Unit prices are taken from an authorized list.	Prices are in accordance with company policy, minimizing customer disputes.	b. Using the S-1 sample of sales invoices, vouch prices used thereon to the price lists.
S-3	Sales are not recorded until goods are shipped.	Cutoff will be proper and sales will not be recorded too early.	c. Using the S-1 sample of sales invoices, compare the recording date with the shipment date on attached bill of lading or copy 4. d. Also, scan the "pending shipment" file for old invoices that might represent unrecorded shipments.
W-1	Shipping personnel have transaction alteration (initiation) authority to change the quantities on invoices, as well as custody of the goods.	Dishonest shipping personnel can let accomplices receive large quantities and alter the invoice to charge them for small quantities. If this happened, sales and accounts receivable would be understated, and inventory could be overstated.	*Impact of weakness on planned substantive audit procedures:* There is a control weakness related to invoicing completeness and inventory custody. Expand our substantive procedures during our observations and test counts during the client's physical inventory count (extensive work) to detect material overstatement.

*S = strength; W = weakness.

---

control weaknesses:
the lack of effective controls in particular areas that would allow material errors to get by undetected

bridge working paper:
audit documentation that connects (bridges) the control evaluation to subsequent audit procedures by summarizing the major control strengths and weaknesses, listing test of control procedures for auditing the control strengths, and suggesting substantive audit procedures to be performed to respond to the weaknesses

the "Implications for Audit Program" column (the last column in the exhibit) contains control testing audit procedures for evaluating the control strengths, and suggestions about substantive account balance audit procedures that respond to the weaknesses. Auditors do not need to test control weaknesses just to prove they are weak places because this is inefficient. However, auditors do always need to take the implications of control weaknesses into account when assessing the risk of material misstatements in the financial statements. Control weaknesses that present a significant risk of material misstatement must be communicated by the auditor to management and those charged with governance,[5] often with the auditor's recommendation for addressing the weaknesses.

At this stage in the control risk assessment, the control risk related to the inventory balance's existence might be set very high (e.g., 0.8 or 0.9 in probability terms). The three control strengths, however, relate to good control over sales validity and accounts receivable accuracy. The auditors will probably want to rely on these controls to reduce audit work on the accounts receivable balance. Tests of these control procedures would need to be performed to obtain evidence about whether the apparent strengths are actually performed well. The "audit program" segment of Exhibit 9–9 for each of the strengths describes specific control tests of the relevant control procedure. Testing controls (phase 3) consists of tests designed to produce evidence of how well the controls worked in practice. If they pass the auditor's criteria (the required degree of compliance), control risk can be assessed low, but, if they fail the test, a high control risk is assessed and the audit plan must be revised to take the control weakness into account. Control tests only provide indirect evidence of the monetary accuracy of financial statement balances because not all monetary misstatements are caused by control weaknesses. Substantive testing provides more direct evidence about monetary accuracy.

Review Checkpoints

9-73 What steps are involved in a control risk assessment?

9-74 What is a control strength? What is a control weakness? How do control strengths relate to control testing?

9-75 What is the purpose of a bridge working paper, and what information does it contain?

9-76 Why is it not necessary to test control weaknesses? What action does the auditor need to take when control evaluation work indicates a control weakness?

9-77 What are the implications for the audit program if tests of key controls indicate they are operating effectively for the whole period being audited? What are the implications if a key control is tested and a high degree of non-compliance is found?

This section on control risk assessment concludes with a special note on considerations of manual and IT controls in information systems.

Special Note: Manual and Information Technology–Based Controls

Identifying specific control objectives is the same for both manual and IT-based control procedures. However, the points in the flow of transactions where misstatements could occur may be different. The controls associated with prevention, detection, and correction of misstatements are identified in three broad categories: input, processing, and output controls. The points in an IT-based accounting process where misstatements might occur are as follows:

Input

1. Activities related to source data preparation are performed, causing the flow of transactions to include authorization and initial execution.

2. Manual procedures are applied to source data, such as a manual summary of accounting data (preparation of batch totals).

3. Source data are converted into computer-readable form.

4. Input files are identified for use in processing.

Processing

5. Information is transferred from one computer program to another.

6. Computer-readable files are used to supply additional information relating to individual transactions (e.g., customer credit reports).

7. Transactions are initiated by the computer.

Output

8. Output files are created or master files are updated.

9. Master files are changed (records added, deleted, or modified) outside the normal flow of transactions within each cycle through file maintenance procedures.

10. Output reports or files are produced.

11. Errors identified by control procedures are corrected.

Once the audit team has identified the risks, specific control objectives can be related to such points. For example, invoicing customers with incorrect prices if the wrong price-list file has been used would lead to a misstatement. The control objective for this type of misstatement is, "Appropriate price information should be used during the invoicing process."

Control procedures should be related to specific control objectives. For example, for the objective of using appropriate price information, one control procedure might be, "The invoicing program should use the most up-to-date price-list file, and the price-list file date should appear on the invoicing summary management report. The accounts receivable manager should review the invoicing summary report and verify that the correct price list has been used to calculate the invoice amounts prior to issuing and sending the invoices to customers."

Manual control procedures may differ from IT controls that are designed to accomplish the same control objectives. For example, in a manual procedure, credit approval is usually indicated by an authorized person putting their signature on a source document, such as a customer's order or invoice. In an IT-based procedure, approval can be accomplished by the authorized person using an approved password that releases a credit sale transaction by assigning a special code to it. Even though the objectives are the same, the methods used to achieve the objectives and the visible evidence differ, so different audit approaches may be required as well. The following section describes manual and IT control components in detail and discusses the benefits and risks of each type of control.

Manual and Information Technology Controls over Information Processing Almost all entities use IT systems for financial reporting and operational purposes, but even so, there will also be manual elements to the systems. The system of internal control is also likely to contain manual and automated procedures, the characteristics of which will affect the auditor's risk assessment and design of further audit procedures. The methods used to process accounting transactions will affect a company's organizational structure and influence the procedures and techniques used to accomplish the objectives of internal control.

Manual system controls include approvals, management reviews of reports and activities, reconciliations, and follow-up of reconciling items. Controls in IT systems will typically be a combination of automated controls (e.g., controls embedded in computer programs) and manual controls, which may either use information produced by IT or be independent of IT. In order to understand internal control, the auditor has to understand the risks of IT or manual systems and whether management has responded adequately by establishing effective controls. Some of the risks and benefits of manual versus IT procedures in internal control are noted in the following box.

Manual Versus Information Technology Controls: Risks and Benefits

Information Technology Control Benefits	**Information Technology Control Risks**
IT controls can enhance internal control effectiveness and efficiency by	IT can also create specific internal control risks, including
• Consistently processing large volumes of transactions or data by applying predefined business rules and performing complex calculations • Enhancing the timeliness, availability, and accuracy of information • Facilitating further information analysis • Enhancing the entity's performance monitoring • Reducing the risk of controls being overridden • Allowing effective segregation of duties by implementing security controls in applications, databases, and operating systems	• Reliance on inaccurate systems, programs, or data • Unauthorized data access allowing data destruction; improper changes; or recording of unauthorized, inaccurate, or non-existent transactions, particularly when multiple users access a common database • IT personnel gaining inappropriate or unnecessary access privileges that undermine segregation of duties or allow unauthorized changes to master file data, systems, or programs • Failure to make necessary updates to systems or programs • Inappropriate manual intervention • Potential loss of data or inability to access data as required due to unauthorized access or malicious access and activity by outsiders
Manual Control Benefits	**Manual Control Risks**
Manual systems can be beneficial when judgment and discretion are required, such as for	Manual controls tend to raise the following risks:
• Large, unusual, or non-recurring transactions • Circumstances where errors are difficult to define, anticipate, or predict • Changing circumstances that require a control response outside the scope of an existing automated control • Monitoring the effectiveness of automated controls	• Possibility of human error, so mistakes can occur and consistent application cannot be assumed • Relative ease of bypassing, ignoring, or overriding • Lower effectiveness for high-volume or recurring transactions, or other situations where typical errors can be anticipated, prevented, or detected by control parameters that can be automated

Source: Adapted from CAS 315.

Every accounting system must contain procedures, whether manual or IT based, ensuring proper recording of transactions, prevention or detection of errors and fraud, and monitoring of control effectiveness. It is management's responsibility to establish and maintain internal controls, and the information system policies and procedures are part of this. The audit team's responsibility is to assess the control risk in the system. Management can meet its responsibility and also assist auditors by (1) ensuring that documentation of the system is complete and up to date, (2) maintaining a system of transaction processing that includes an audit trail, and (3) making IT resources and knowledgeable personnel available to the auditors. Appendix 9B (available on Connect) provides a detailed description of the characteristics of IT-based information systems, and of the auditors' risk and control assessment, for students who are interested in applying the concepts and techniques from their management information systems courses.

Summary of Phases 1 and 2

According to GAAS, the auditor is required to assess control risk for the different classes of transactions and account balances at the assertion level. The information gathered about the auditee's control environment, the accounting information systems, and the control procedures should enable the auditor to reach one of the following conclusions about control risk and the most effective audit approach to use.

1. *Control risk may be assessed low, and it seems efficient to test controls.* The auditor believes the control procedures designed to prevent or detect misstatements can be audited for compliance in a cost-effective manner, reducing the amount of substantive evidence needed for reasonable assurance. Alternatively, when certain control procedures are essential for reducing risk of material misstatement, and substantive procedures alone won't provide sufficient appropriate evidence about the assertion(s), controls must be tested to support the audit opinion. In this case, the auditor plans an audit approach that combines control testing and substantive evidence gathering.

2. *Control risk may be assessed low, but audit inefficiencies would occur if controls were tested.* Control policies and procedures appear to be good, but testing controls is not cost effective because substantive procedures can provide sufficient appropriate evidence and are more efficient than a combined approach. In this case the auditors would concentrate attention on the substantive audit procedures.

3. *Control risk may be assessed high.* Control policies and procedures do not appear to be sufficient to prevent or detect material misstatements. In this case, the auditors will concentrate on substantive audit procedures. The auditor also has additional responsibilities to report the control weaknesses to management and those charged with governance. If the effective operation of controls is essential to reduce the risk of material misstatement, and substantive procedures alone will not provide sufficient appropriate evidence about the assertion(s), a scope limitation exists that may prevent the auditor from obtaining reasonable assurance that no material misstatement has occurred.

The control risk conclusion determines the approach that will be followed in planning the audit. The first conclusion above will result in the auditor's choosing a combined audit approach using both control and substantive testing, and the second and third conclusions will result in choosing an approach based on obtaining substantive evidence. Since the auditor is required to make the control assessment at the assertion level, it may be possible to identify specific control procedures that provide a low-risk assessment with regard to some but not all assertions, leading the auditor to use a combination of tests of controls and substantive auditing. Other audit objectives may be achieved through substantive procedures alone. Exhibit 9–10 summarizes the possible control risk assessment outcomes and the considerations regarding audit approach.

EXHIBIT 9–10

Implications of Control Risk Assessments on the Audit Approach

CONTROL RISK ASSESSMENT	COST-BENEFIT AND SCOPE CONSIDERATIONS	AUDITOR'S DECISION ON AUDIT APPROACH
Low or moderate (controls effective)	Control reliance reduces required substantive procedures in excess of cost of control testing.	**Combined Audit Approach** – Test controls. – Reduced planned substantive procedures can still provide high assurance.
Low or moderate (controls effective)	Substantive procedures can provide sufficient appropriate evidence at a lower cost than control tests.	**Substantive Audit Approach** – Do not test controls. – Plan substantive procedures to provide high assurance.
Low or moderate (controls effective)	Substantive procedures alone cannot provide sufficient assurance.	**Combined Audit Approach** – Test controls. – Plan substantive procedures to provide high assurance.
High (no controls or control not effective)	Substantive procedures alone can provide sufficient assurance.	**Substantive Audit Approach** – Do not test controls. – Plan substantive procedures to provide high assurance.
High (no controls or control not effective)	Substantive procedures alone *cannot* provide sufficient assurance.	It is unlikely that sufficient evidence can be obtained in this situation. Scope limitation—Modified audit opinion (qualified or disclaimer of opinion) may be required.

To summarize the auditor's control assessment up to this point, phases 1 and 2 can be described as dealing with the evaluation of whether the controls are designed to operate effectively. Now we move on to phase 3, where we test the actual operation of the controls.

Review Checkpoints

9-84   Why are the control objectives the same regardless of whether manual or IT control procedures are used?

9-85   Why might manual control procedures differ from IT control procedures, even if both are directed at the same control objective?

9-86   Describe one manual and one IT control procedure designed to prevent a credit sale being processed without proper authorization by the credit manager.

9-87   What three conclusions about control risk can be reached based on internal control evaluation? What are the implications of each on the audit approach selected?

Phase 3—Control Testing

Development of Control Test Procedures to Include in Audit Programs

LO6   Write control tests for an audit program.

By the third phase of an internal control evaluation, auditors will have assessed individual controls. To reach a conclusion on control risk, auditors must determine (a) what degree of compliance with the control policies and procedures is required, and then (b) what degree of control compliance is actually present. The degree of compliance required is the criterion that control performance is assessed against. Knowing that compliance cannot be perfect, auditors might decide, for example, that using shipping documents to validate sales invoice recordings 96% of the time is sufficient to assess a low control risk for the audit of accounts receivable (controls relating to the existence assertion in receivables and sales). Auditors perform control tests to determine how well the company's control procedures actually worked during the period under audit.

A control test has two parts. Part one is identifying the data population from which to select a sample of items for audit. Part two is describing the action to be taken to produce relevant evidence. Basically, the action determines whether the selected items correspond to a standard (e.g., mathematical accuracy) and agree with information in another data population. Study the control tests in the audit program in Exhibit 9–9, which shows this two-part design.

Review Checkpoints

9-88   What do the terms *required degree of control compliance* and *actual degree of control compliance* mean?

9-89   How does the degree of control reliance relate to the auditor's control risk assessment?

9-90   What is a control test? Why do auditors perform control tests? What audit evidence is produced by control tests?

9-91   What two parts are important in writing out a control test for an audit program?

One other important aspect of these audit procedures is known as the **direction of the test**. The procedures described in Exhibit 9–9 provide evidence about control over the validity of sales transactions. However, they do not provide evidence about control over completeness of recording all shipments. Another data population, the shipping documents, can be sampled to provide evidence about completeness. The direction of the test idea is illustrated in Exhibit 9–11. For example, if the completeness control is found to be strong, the auditors could omit the year-end procedure of confirming customers' zero-balance accounts receivable to search for unrecorded assets (understatements).

EXHIBIT 9–11

Direction of Control Testing

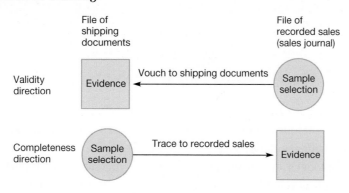

---

direction of the test:

a description of the nature of an audit test procedure in terms of whether it involves vouching from the accounting records back to source documents ("grave to cradle") or tracing from the source documents up to the accounting records ("cradle to grave")

Linking back to the discussion in Chapter 6, recall that auditors identify accounting processes in which the accounts and transactions tend to move together in a cycle for the purpose of designing audit programs. Taking the revenues/receivables/receipts process as an example, two classes of transactions change the accounts receivable balance: the credit sales revenue transactions and the cash receipts transactions. If there is an invalid (non-existent) credit sale recorded, both the revenue transaction total and the accounts receivable balance will be overstated (an existence/occurrence assertion misstatement). These misstatements go in the same direction. So, if controls are strong over validity of recording sales, this means controls lower the risk of misstatement in the existence assertion and the auditor can consider getting less-substantive evidence regarding that assertion for the accounts receivable balance. On the other hand, if an invalid (non-existent) cash collection transaction is recorded, it would result in the accounts receivable balance being understated (a completeness assertion misstatement). These misstatements go in opposite directions. So, if controls over validity of cash collections are found to be strong, there is less risk of a completeness error and less need for substantive evidence in relation to the risk. Conversely, if control weaknesses are found in transactions classes, this will increase the substantive evidence that must be collected for the corresponding assertions in the balance audit program.

If control tests involve recalculation/reperformance, auditors redo the arithmetic calculations and comparisons that employees were supposed to have performed. This control could be tested by inspection alone—looking to see if the documents were marked with an initial, signature, or stamp indicating they had been checked. Recalculation/reperformance provides more reliable, first-hand evidence that the control operates effectively. Merely inspecting the control only provides evidence that it exists, not that it operates effectively. Performing both procedures with dual-purpose tests is very cost effective. Much of the cost of control testing is in designing the procedures and selecting the sample to inspect. The marginal cost of extending the work to reperform the calculation or comparison can often be worthwhile. The additional evidence is also substantive in nature, since it would actually detect any material misstatement—hence the term *dual purpose*, that is, providing evidence of both control effectiveness and whether any monetary errors have occurred.

Review Checkpoints

9-92   How does the direction of a control test relate to control objectives?

9-93   What is the difference between inspection and reperformance in control testing?

9-94   Explain how overstatements in the revenues and cash receipts transactions affect the assertions of the accounts receivable balance.

9-95   What is a dual-purpose test?

Control tests that depend on documentary evidence, such as signatures, initials, checklists, or reconciliation working papers, provide better evidence than procedures that leave no documentary traces. Some control elements, such as segregation of employees' duties, may produce no documents. Since reperformance of these control operations cannot be done, a less reliable procedure, observation, must be used: an auditor performs unobtrusive eyewitness observation of employees at their jobs performing control operations.

Control tests should be applied to samples of transactions and control procedures executed throughout the period being audited. This is required because the auditor's conclusions about whether controls operated effectively must apply to the whole period covered by the financial statements under audit.

Auditor control testing is required most often for high-volume transaction streams that have a lot of variability in the amounts recorded. In many businesses, these will be the cash payments transactions, cash receipts transactions, and revenue transactions. Examples of detailed internal control questionnaires for these transaction streams are provided in Appendices 11A and 12A.

The box below gives an example of a control test that could be included in the internal control program for the sales revenue process. It consists of procedures you could perform to produce evidence about the effectiveness of an auditee's internal control performance. The control tests listed in the box determine how well the control procedures were followed on the transactions affecting accounts receivable. After each action, the parenthetical note tells you the control objective being tested. This program describes the *nature* of the control testing procedures, designed using some of the evidence-gathering techniques discussed in Chapter 8.

Example of a Control Test in an Internal Control Audit Program

1. Select a sample of recorded sales invoice documents, and perform the following inspection and reperformance procedures:
    (a) Determine whether a shipping document was issued for the sale (evidence of validity).
    (b) Determine whether credit was approved (evidence of authorization).
    (c) Determine whether product prices on the invoice agree with the approved price list (evidence of authorization and accuracy).
    (d) Compare the quantity billed with the quantity shipped (evidence of accuracy).
    (e) Recalculate the invoice arithmetic (evidence of accuracy).
    (f) Compare the shipment date with the invoice record date (evidence of proper period cutoff).
    (g) Note the type of product shipped, and determine proper classification in the right product-line revenue account (evidence of classification).
2. Select a sample of shipping orders and perform the following:
    (a) Trace them to recorded sales invoices (evidence of completeness).
    (b) The procedures in 1(b), (c), (d), (e), (f), and (g) could also be performed on the sales invoices produced by this sample. However, the work need not be duplicated.
3. Scan the accounts receivable for postings from sources other than the sales and cash receipts journals (e.g., general journal adjusting entries, credit memos). Vouch a sample of such entries to supporting documents (evidence of validity, authorization, accuracy, and classification).

Review Checkpoints

9-96 How are control procedures with no documentary evidence tested?

9-97 Why would controls be tested for the whole period being audited?

Audit Procedures Planned to Respond to Assessed Risks of Material Misstatement

The auditor's control evaluation links directly to performing further audit procedures. To show this link, the audit standards that result in the auditor's obtaining reasonable assurance on fair presentation of the financial statements are summarized in the box below.

Audit Procedures Responsive to the Assessed Risks of Material Misstatement at the Assertion Level

Overview

The purpose of the auditor's inherent and control risk assessment is to allow the auditor to design and perform appropriate audit procedures that reflect the risks of material misstatement at the assertion level for each class of transaction, account balance, and disclosure.

When the auditor intends to rely on the operating effectiveness of controls in determining the nature, timing, and extent of substantive procedures, the auditor must obtain audit evidence to determine whether the controls are operating effectively. Control testing is also required in situations when substantive procedures alone cannot provide sufficient appropriate audit evidence at the assertion level.

Control Testing

When the auditor plans to rely on controls over a risk the auditor has determined to be significant, the auditor shall test those controls in the current period.

In designing and performing tests of controls, the auditor shall obtain more persuasive audit evidence the greater the reliance the auditor places on the effectiveness of a control.

The auditor shall test controls for the particular time, or throughout the period, for which the auditor intends to rely on those controls.

If the auditor plans to use audit evidence from a previous audit about the operating effectiveness of specific controls, the auditor shall establish the continuing relevance of that evidence by obtaining audit evidence about whether significant changes in those controls have occurred subsequent to the previous audit. The auditor shall obtain this evidence by performing inquiry combined with observation or inspection, to confirm the understanding of those specific controls. In addition:

(a) If there have been changes that affect the continuing relevance of the audit evidence from the previous audit, the auditor shall test the controls in the current audit.

(b) If there have not been such changes, the auditor shall test the controls at least once in every third audit, and shall test some controls in each audit to avoid the possibility of testing all the controls on which the auditor intends to rely in a single audit period with no testing of controls in the subsequent two audit periods.

Evaluating the Operating Effectiveness of Controls

When evaluating the operating effectiveness of relevant controls, the auditor shall evaluate whether misstatements that have been detected by substantive procedures indicate that controls are not operating effectively. The absence of misstatements detected by substantive procedures, however, does not provide audit evidence that controls related to the assertion being tested are effective.

When deviations from controls upon which the auditor intends to rely are detected, the auditor shall make specific inquiries to understand these matters and their potential consequences, and shall determine whether

(a) The tests of controls that have been performed provide an appropriate basis for reliance on the controls;

(b) Additional tests of controls are necessary; or

(c) The potential risks of misstatement need to be addressed using substantive procedures.

Material Control Weaknesses

The auditor shall evaluate whether, on the basis of the audit work performed, the auditor has identified a material weakness in the operating effectiveness of controls.

The auditor shall communicate material weaknesses in internal control identified during the audit on a timely basis to management at an appropriate level of responsibility and, as required by CAS 260, "Communication with Those Charged with Governance," unless all of those charged with governance are involved in managing the entity.

Substantive Procedures

Regardless of the assessed risks of material misstatement, the auditor shall design and perform substantive procedures for each material class of transactions, account balance, and disclosure.

(continued)

When the auditor has determined that an assessed risk of material misstatement at the assertion level is significant the auditor shall perform substantive procedures that are specifically responsive to that risk. When the approach to a significant risk consists only of substantive procedures, those procedures shall include tests of details.

The auditor's substantive procedures shall include the following audit procedures related to the financial statement closing process:

(a) Agreeing or reconciling the financial statements with the underlying accounting records, and

(b) Examining material journal entries and other adjustments made during the course of preparing the financial statements.

Source: Adapted from CAS 330, "The Auditor's Responses to Assessed Risks."

Auditor's Responsibility to Report Internal Control Deficiencies and Fraud Risks

 Outline the auditor's responsibility when internal control evaluation work detects or indicates a significant control weakness or a high risk of fraudulent misstatement.

After the auditors have evaluated and tested internal controls, they are in a strong position to assess the likelihood of material misstatements. This is a good point at which to review auditor responsibilities for detecting and communicating misstatements.

The auditor is responsible for reporting all identified deficiencies in internal control, other than obviously trivial ones, to an appropriate level of management as soon as possible. The appropriate level of management is usually the one at least one level above those responsible for the deficient controls. If the auditor finds that there is a **compensating control**, an alternative effective control that achieves the same purpose as the missing one, then there might not be a deficiency or a need to communicate it. Determining whether a compensating control is effective in reducing financial statement misstatements is an important area of auditor judgment. Management has incentives to try to rationalize that a control is compensating to avoid a control deficiency being reported to those charged with governance, or in its annual management discussion and analysis (MD&A) presented to shareholders.

If the auditor believes an identified control deficiency or combination of deficiencies exposes the entity to a serious risk of material misstatement, it is considered to be a **significant control deficiency**. The auditor is responsible for reporting all significant deficiencies in writing to those charged with governance (audit committee or equivalent). Examples of such deficiencies are a control environment weakness indicating a lack of management competence or integrity, a lack of effective controls over critical accounting processes, a weakness allowing a material misstatement or fraud, or a weakness that increases the entity's susceptibility to fraud. The auditor is required to communicate material weaknesses or other important issues, such as discovery of a

compensating control:
an alternative, effective control that achieves the same purpose as a missing control, such that the missing control is not considered to be a control deficiency that needs to be communicated to management or those charged with governance

significant control deficiency:
an identified control deficiency or combination of deficiencies that the auditor believes exposes the entity to a serious risk of material misstatement

fraud or material misstatement, to management and those charged with governance, at various stages of the audit.[6] These communications are two-way: the auditor provides entity officials with information they need to discharge their responsibilities, and the entity officials provide the auditor with any information they have that is relevant to the audit.

Standards Check

CAS 265 Communicating Deficiencies in Internal Control to Those Charged with Governance and Management

9. The auditor shall communicate in writing significant deficiencies in internal control identified during the audit to those charged with governance on a timely basis. (Ref: Para. A12–A18, A27)

10. The auditor shall also communicate to management at an appropriate level of responsibility on a timely basis (Ref: Para. A19, A27)

    (a) In writing, significant deficiencies in internal control that the auditor has communicated or intends to communicate to those charged with governance, unless it would be inappropriate to communicate directly to management in the circumstances; and (Ref: Para. A14, A20–A21)

    (b) Other deficiencies in internal control identified during the audit that have not been communicated to management by other parties and that, in the auditor's professional judgment, are of sufficient importance to merit management's attention. (Ref: Para. A22–A26)

Source: *CPA Canada Handbook—Assurance*, 2014.

While the auditor's communication to management can be oral rather than written when the control deficiencies are not significant, serious control weaknesses uncovered during the normal performance of the audit are communicated in writing to management in a **management letter (management control letter)**. A copy of the written communication, or a memorandum summarizing the discussion if reported orally, should be included in the auditor's file documentation.

Whenever written communication is made, there is potential for misinterpretation, so it is important for the auditor to include a very clear description of the deficiencies identified, their potential effects, and the reasons for the communication. The auditor should also explain that the audit's objective was to express an opinion on the financial statements as a whole; therefore, other deficiencies may exist and other controls not mentioned may not be effective.

In the United States, audit requirements for listed public companies include an auditor's report on the management's report on internal control effectiveness. In Canada, at the time of writing this type of requirement for audit reporting related to internal control was not in place. CPA Canada has issued a practice standard (*CPA Canada Assurance Handbook*, OCS 5925) based on U.S. Public Company Accounting Oversight Board (PCAOB) Auditing Standard No. 5 for integrated audits of financial statements and internal control effectiveness. This guidance is used by Canadian auditors who need to comply with U.S. auditing standards because they audit companies listed on U.S. stock markets. Otherwise, at this time these internal control audit reports are voluntary in Canada.

management letter (management control letter):
a written communication to management of control deficiencies uncovered by the auditor

These communication responsibilities highlight the need for the audit to be performed with professional skepticism, which means the auditor should

1. Be aware of factors that increase the risk of misstatement and take these into account in performing the audit, and

2. Take appropriate action if there is evidence that contradicts the assumption of management integrity.

Note that many risk factors relate to poor internal controls. If there are enough red flags present, the auditor will assess a higher inherent risk, and, if control risk is also high, these higher assessments will cause the auditor to

- Obtain more reliable evidence;
- Expand the extent of audit procedures performed;
- Apply audit procedures closer to, or as of, the balance sheet date; and
- Require more extensive supervision of assistants and/or assignment of assistants with more experience and training.

In essence, if the auditor suspects that the financial statements are misstated due to error or fraud, he or she should perform procedures to confirm or dispel that suspicion.

To summarize, the auditor should inform the appropriate level of management whenever there is evidence of a non-trivial misstatement and weaknesses in internal control that could allow a material misstatement to occur. The audit committee or board of directors should be informed of all significant misstatements and any that appear to be intentional and fraud related. (Procedures for fraud detection are discussed in more detail in Chapter 7.)

APPLICATION CASE WITH SOLUTION & ANALYSIS

Information Systems and Controls in a Small Business

DISCUSSION CASE

After only a year as an audit manager in a medium-size public accounting firm, Hilda has brought in her first new audit client, Ming Auto Perfection Inc. (Ming). The firm's audit partners are happy that Hilda has shown such initiative so early in her career. Also, the firm recently lost some larger audit clients to the Big Four firms after mergers or buyouts, so the partners now believe their best opportunity for growing their auditing practice is in the small and medium-size enterprise (SME) sector.

Ming Chi started his business 12 years ago as a car wash in a busy part of the city. A few years later, he married Jin and she joined in the business, with Chi keeping 51% of the shares and Jin receiving 49%. Thanks to Jin's outstanding marketing skills and Chi's strength in operating management, Ming soon expanded from individual car washes to operating a full car cleaning and detailing service for several taxi companies and other businesses in the city. Recently, Ming expanded further, designing and applying advertising material to the sides of taxis and buses. The company has grown successfully and now has six full-time employees.

Recently, Jin decided to move away to care for her aging relatives. She will no longer be actively involved in running the business but will retain her 49% interest. Chi and Jin decided that an independent audit of the company's financial statements would be valuable to them both since it would provide Jin with more comfort about the fairness of the reported profits, even though she will be living in another country. Hilda knows the Mings personally because their sons played in the same hockey league. The Mings have an excellent reputation in the business community, so it was an easy decision for the firm to accept Ming as a new auditee.

However, since Hilda's firm is fairly new to SME auditing, and the partners want to develop this area of practice, they have asked Hilda to use the Ming audit as a basis for developing a robust audit methodology that addresses special concerns in audits of smaller enterprises. Hilda has always been impressed by Jack's grasp of audit theory and his ability to apply it practically, and she thinks it would be an excellent learning experience for him to draft up the small business considerations that the firm can use as a general practice guidance and a great opportunity for him to impress the partners right before bonus and promotion time.

Jack meets with Chi to learn about Ming's operations and information systems, and a few key differences from larger organization become apparent. Chi is actively involved, understands all the systems, and can do anyone else's job. Most employees do a number of different accounting tasks, sometimes ones that are incompatible from a control perspective. Most of the accounting information is captured and processed by manual processes and ad hoc computer programs like Microsoft Excel, Word, and Access. An off-the-shelf accounting package called QuickBooks is used to generate the general ledger and draft financial statements. The office PCs are networked, but there are no user access restrictions; however, the PCs are all in plain sight.

Jack's observations raise a number of questions about the differences between Ming and the larger companies Jack has audited. A good way to begin the SME guidance document for the practice is to consider some key questions Jack will try to answer in this case.

SOLUTION & ANALYSIS

Some key questions and related considerations are as follows.

What aspects of good internal control differ between large organizations and small ones?

A company must be large and employ several people (about 10 or more) to have a theoretically appropriate segregation of functional responsibilities and the accompanying high degree of specialization of work. Supervision requires people. There is extensive necessary paperwork and computer control necessary in most large systems. Large organization control theory and practice suggest that people performing in accounting and control roles do not engage in frequent personal interaction across functional responsibility boundaries.

What are the two main features of internal control in a small business?

The small number of people engaged in the accounting and control systems makes segregation of functional responsibilities very difficult. Also, the owner-manager is actively involved in the operation of the accounting and control system, making the owner-manager's competence and integrity important considerations for the auditor.

How does the cost of implementing controls affect large businesses differently than small ones?

The theoretical dimensions of good control tend to fit large, not small, businesses. A large company employs enough people to have appropriate segregation of functional responsibilities along with its high degree of specialization of work. There are also enough people to provide supervision and to prepare the paperwork and perform other controls, such as reviews and reconciliations. The computer control necessary in most large systems is extensive and also requires staff to design and implement it. The theory of large organization control also suggests that people performing accounting and control roles do not engage in frequent personal interaction across functional responsibility boundaries, as they usually do in a small business. Small businesses' costs will be affected because they are unlikely to enjoy economies of scale in implementing controls, whereas large businesses will likely be able to justify the cost of the suggested ideal control policies, procedures, and staffing.

The theory of internal control applies to both large and small businesses as long as the underlying behavioural assumptions are met. However, the fact that small businesses employ only a few people usually means that the required separation of duties is not met, and the entire general theory is less applicable for practical reasons; strict separation of duties, tight authority structure, an extensive system of rules and files, and impersonality are harder to accomplish when there are only a few employees operating in an informal manner. The costs of controls are more easily absorbed in a large business, and the benefits of elaborate control structures are also likely to be greater in a large business. In a small business, communications and observation, particularly by the owner-manager, can be highly effective control components.

What impact do the owner-manager role and the lack of complexity have on the internal control requirements of a small business?

Internal control questionnaires designed specifically for small businesses contain more items related to the owner-manager and other key personnel than do large business questionnaires.

What control risks are related to rapid growth in a small business?

As a small business grows, the transition to more formalized internal control tends to lag behind. For example, the owner-manager may become overburdened with control duties and tacitly delegate these to others but fail to monitor these duties adequately. The need to hire a controller may not be apparent in time to prevent serious and costly breakdowns in the internal controls over financial reporting. The intermediate-size stage represents a turning point where both owner-manager and auditor need to be very careful. At this point, such measures as limited specialization and surety bonding of employees may help make the transition.

What cost-effectiveness considerations tend to be important in planning small business audits?

Most auditors rely primarily on substantive evidence with small business audits. The minimum documentation required in a small business audit is an internal control memorandum with a narrative description of the control system and the results of internal control evaluation. The description should include weaknesses, implications, and recommendations. Generalized audit software applications can be a major advantage, allowing the auditor to obtain a higher degree of audit assurance at little additional cost.

Auditors can also use trial balance and financial statement software, prepare audit programs, and use planning and administration tools to increase efficiency.

Which important duties are generally not segregated in small business computer systems?

Accounting functions—people in user departments may initiate and authorize source documents, enter data, operate the computer, and distribute output reports.

Computer functions—functions of programming and operating the computer might not be separated; programs and data are often resident on disk at all times and accessible by any operator.

What control techniques can a company use to achieve control over the operation of a PC-based accounting system?

- Restricted access to input devices
- Standard screens and computer prompting
- Online editing and sight verification

What control techniques can a company use to achieve control over the computer processing of accounting data in a PC system?

- Transaction logs
- Control totals
- Balancing input to output
- Audit trail

What are the major characteristics and control problems in PC installations?
Characteristics:

- Staff and location of the computer—operated by small staff located within the user department and without physical security
- Programs—supplied by computer manufacturers or software houses
- Processing mode—interactive data entry by users with most of the master files accessible for inquiry and direct update

Control Problems:

- Lack of segregation of duties
- Lack of controls on the operating system and application programs
- Unlimited access to data files and programs
- No record of usage
- No backup of essential files
- No audit trail of processing
- No authorization or record of program changes

SUMMARY

This chapter explained the theory and practice of auditors' involvement with an auditee's internal control.

- The distinction between management's and the auditor's responsibilities with respect to internal control was explained. Elements of the accounting system were described in conjunction with control procedures management has designed and implemented to prevent, detect, and correct misstatements that occur in transactions. These misstatements were systematized in a set of seven categories of misstatements that can occur. **LO1**

- The reasons auditors assess the control risk were discussed. The control understanding and risk assessment allow the auditor to plan a cost-effective audit, including a decision on whether to use a substantive approach or a combined approach. We presented the cost-benefit and reasonable assurance considerations that affect the auditor's choice of audit approach with respect to relying on controls and the extent to which substantive work will be used in forming the audit opinion. It was shown that understanding the auditee's business and information systems is relevant to control understanding. **LO2**

- By identifying six categories of potential misstatements, and looking at the flip side of them, the six control objectives an organization's management needs to achieve were identified. These control objectives were related to the management assertions in the financial statements. **LO3**

- Control activities were organized under the headings of general controls and application controls. The main types of general controls were explained. The control techniques management implements for addressing the control objectives as they relate to input, processing, and output of data in each accounting process were discussed. We explained these integrated IT-based accounting systems with control consideration. **LO4**

- Documentation of an accounting information system and its application control activities includes control questionnaires, flowcharts, and narratives. Questionnaires and flowcharts were demonstrated. This then led to the test of controls decisions and the cost reduction reasons for doing work to obtain a low control risk assessment. The assessed control risk was connected to the control risk component in the audit risk model (covered in Chapter 6). Control evidence was linked to audit programs by presenting a bridge working paper. The chapter also reviewed and compared considerations for auditing IT-based and manual information systems and controls. **LO5**

- The design of control test procedures for an internal control program was presented. The relation between the direction of testing classes of transactions and the control objectives to which the test results are relevant was discussed. The link between the control test findings, control risk assessment, and the impact on risk of material misstatement in the assertions of the related account balance was discussed in terms of the impact on the need to do further substantive procedures. The chapter also summarized key auditing standards requirements related to control risk assessment, control testing, and their relation to substantive procedures. The discussion of control risk assessment provided some basis for the theory and practice of audit sampling, which is covered next, in Chapter 10. **LO6**

- The chapter discussed the auditor's responsibilities for communicating with management and those charged with governance when control work reveals a significant control deficiency, a fraudulent misstatement, or a high risk of one occurring. **LO7**

To be able to summarize the role of information systems and control in (a) capturing relevant information from the organization's business environment and activities and (b) processing it into the financial statements and disclosures that contain management assertions about the organization's performance and financial position, it may be helpful to review the big-picture overview of the financial reporting process presented in Exhibit 7–4 in Chapter 7.

This chapter concluded with an Application Case showing how control theory and evaluations apply to small businesses.

Two appendices provide further details relating to how auditors document internal controls for evaluating the control strength and weaknesses in accounting processes, and issues related to auditing IT elements of the information system. **LO9, 10, 11**

KEY TERMS

accuracy	controls relevant to the audit	nature, timing, and extent
authorization	direction of the test	proper period cutoff
bridge working papers	dual-purpose audit procedure	significant control deficiency
classification	financial statement closing process	substantive audit approach
combined audit approach	highly effective audit	validity
compensating control	internal control questionnaire	walk-through procedure
completeness	management letter (management	
control strengths	control letter)	
control weaknesses	management override of controls	

MULTIPLE-CHOICE QUESTIONS FOR PRACTICE AND REVIEW

MC 9-1 **LO4** Which of the following can an auditor observe as a general control activity used by companies?

a. Segregation of functional responsibilities
b. Management philosophy and operating style
c. Open lines of communication to the audit committee of the board of directors
d. External influences such as federal bank regulator audits

MC 9-2 **LO4** A company's application control procedure is

a. an action taken by auditors to obtain evidence.
b. an action taken by company personnel for the purpose of preventing, detecting, and correcting errors and irregularities in transactions.
c. a method for recording, summarizing, and reporting financial information.
d. the functioning of the board of directors in support of its audit committee.

MC 9-3 **LO3** The control objective intended to reduce the probability that fictitious transactions get recorded in the accounts is

a. completeness. c. proper period.
b. authorization. d. validity.

MC 9-4 **LO3** The control objective intended to reduce the probability that a credit sale transaction will get debited to cash instead of accounts receivable is

a. validity. c. accuracy.
b. classification. d. completeness.

MC 9-5 `LO1` Management's responsibilities for internal control over financial reporting include

a. ensuring the fair presentation of the financial statements.

b. assessing material misstatements in the financial statements due to errors and fraud.

c. designing and implementing effective internal controls.

d. ensuring the costs of control exceed the risks they eliminate.

MC 9-6 `LO1` A customer's order was not approved for credit because the credit manager had not yet finished searching the customer's credit rating information. Yet the goods were shipped, invoiced, and charged to the customer without requiring payment in advance. Which control objective is not being met?

a. Completeness c. Authorization

b. Validity d. Accuracy

MC 9-7 `LO5` When performing an audit, the auditor must obtain an understanding of the internal controls relevant to the audit. Which of the controls below would be considered *the least relevant* to an audit?

a. The front entrance of the building is always locked and can only be unlocked when employees scan their access cards.

b. The company performs monthly inventory counts to identify any missing items in a timely manner.

c. The CFO must approve any disbursements above a $25,000 threshold.

d. The controller performs a review of the amortization computation on a quarterly basis.

MC 9-8 `LO3` In updating a computerized accounts receivable file, which of the following would be used as a batch control to verify the accuracy of the posting of cash receipts remittances?

a. The sum of the cash deposits plus the discounts less the sales returns

b. The sum of the cash deposits

c. The sum of the cash deposits less the discounts taken by customers

d. The sum of the cash deposits plus the discounts taken by customers

MC 9-9 `LO2` In most audits of large companies, internal control risk assessment contributes to audit efficiency, which means

a. the cost of year-end audit work will exceed the cost of control evaluation work.

b. auditors will be able to reduce the cost of year-end audit work by an amount more than the control evaluation costs.

c. the cost of control evaluation work will exceed the cost of year-end audit work.

d. auditors will be able to reduce the cost of year-end audit work by an amount less than the control evaluation costs.

MC 9-10 `LO5` Which of the following is a tool designed to help the audit team obtain evidence about the control environment and the accounting and control procedures of an audit client?

a. A narrative memorandum describing the control system

b. An internal control questionnaire

c. A flowchart of the documents and procedures used by the company

d. A well-indexed file of working papers

MC 9-11 `LO5` A bridge working paper shows the connection between

a. control evaluation findings and subsequent audit procedures.
b. control objectives and accounting system procedures.
c. control objectives and company control procedures.
d. financial statement assertions and tests of control procedures.

MC 9-12 `LO6` Control tests are required for

a. obtaining evidence about the financial statement assertions.
b. accomplishing control over the validity of recorded transactions.
c. analytical review of financial statement balances.
d. obtaining evidence about the operating effectiveness of company control procedures.

MC 9-13 `LO3` Why does GAAS specifically require auditors to examine the adjusting entries made by management as part of the closing process at the end of the accounting period to prepare the financial statements?

a. These should have been included with the routine, systematic journal entries made by accounting personnel.
b. These entries can be used by management to implement fraudulent financial reporting.
c. These entries are often used to cover up employees' misappropriation of assets during the period.
d. These are non-routine, non-systematic journal entries and always have the highest risk.

MC 9-14 `LO2` The auditee's computerized exception-reporting system helps an auditor to conduct a more efficient audit because it

a. condenses data significantly.
b. highlights abnormal conditions.
c. decreases the tests of computer controls requirements.
d. is efficient computer input control.

MC 9-15 `LO6` Mohit Corp. is a manufacturer of specialized diving gear. What internal control could be tested by its auditor to support the objective of proper period cutoff for their Cost of Goods Sold accounts?

a. The operations manager reviews the inventory listing for any outdated gear or slow-moving inventory.
b. An inventory count is performed each quarter.
c. The warehouse manager prepares a detailed shipping document for all inventory items that leave the warehouse.
d. The controller performs a detailed analysis of raw material inventory, work-in-process, and finished goods inventory to detect any unexpected variance.

MC 9-16 `LO6` What internal control could be tested by the auditors of Mohit Corp. to support the objective of authorization for the cash account?

a. A bank reconciliation is performed by a senior accountant on a monthly basis.
b. The bank reconciliation is reviewed by the controller on a monthly basis.
c. All foreign currency transactions are automatically adjusted to the local currency by the information system using Bank of Canada rates.
d. All cheques issued for an amount equal to or greater than $2,500 must have two signatures (CFO and Treasurer).

EXERCISES AND PROBLEMS

EP 9-1 Internal Control Understanding and Assessment. `LO1, 3, 4, 5` Assume that when conducting procedures to obtain an understanding of the internal control structure in the Denton Seed Company, you checked "No" to the following internal control questionnaire items (based on those illustrated in the chapter):

- Does access to online files require specific passwords to be entered to identify and validate the terminal user?
- Are control totals established by the user prior to submitting data for processing? (Order entry application subsystem)
- Are input control totals reconciled to output control totals? (Order entry application subsystem)

Required:

a. Describe the misstatements due to error or fraud that could occur because of the weaknesses indicated by the lack of controls.
b. Explain the impact these control weaknesses would have on the audit approach selected and on the design of the audit programs.

EP 9-2 Approach for Internal Control Assessment. `LO2, 3` One of the things you can do in a logical approach to the assessment of internal control is imagine what types of errors could occur with regard to each significant class of transactions. Assume a company has the significant classes of transactions listed below.

Required:

For each one, identify one or more errors that could occur, and name the accounts that would be affected if proper controls were not specified or followed satisfactorily.

1. Credit sales transactions
2. Raw materials purchase transactions
3. Payroll transactions
4. Equipment acquisition transactions
5. Cash receipts transactions
6. Leasing transactions
7. Dividend transactions
8. Investment transactions (short term)

EP 9-3 Control Evaluation, Control Testing. `LO3, 4, 5, 6` The auditor learns that the auditee has a control procedure in place that addresses the validity of sales and existence of accounts receivable. When a truck driver picks up goods from the warehouse, the warehouse employee has the driver sign a "shipper's receipt" showing the quantities and item numbers shipped, and the customer information. The shipper's receipts are filed in date order in the warehouse office. A copy of the signed shipper's receipt is sent to the accounting office, where it is used to record the reduction in inventory and issue a sales invoice. The invoice number is noted on the shipper's receipt and it is filed by invoice number in the accounting area. Since the auditee has a large number of customers, the auditor decides this is a control that will be tested.

Required:

a. Why would the auditor decide to test this control?
b. What will the auditor achieve by testing this control?

c. Design a control test the auditor could perform for this control procedure. Describe the two parts of the test in detail.

d. Assume the auditor performs a control test and finds the control procedure operated properly 95% of the time. How does this evidence affect the auditor's control risk assessment? What if the control operated properly 60% of the time? 99% of the time?

EP 9-4 Online Sales, Audit Procedures. **LO3, 4, 5, 6** Online retailers, such as Amazon.ca and Grocerygateway.com, make use of online customer order forms to allow customers to input all the required sale, delivery, and payment data.

Required:

a. Identify control procedures that can be used in an online sales order system, and the risk(s) each addresses.

b. How would the revenue control objectives be audited in an online retail sales business?

EP 9-5 Auditee's Control Procedures and Audit Programs. **LO3, 4, 5, 6** To test an organization's internal control procedures, auditors design a test of controls audit program. This audit program is a list of control tests to be performed, and each is directly related to an important auditee control procedure. Auditors perform the tests to obtain evidence about the operating effectiveness of the auditee's control procedures.

Required:

The controls listed below relate to a system for processing sales transactions. Each numbered item indicates an error or irregularity that could occur and specifies a control procedure that could prevent or detect it. Identify the control objective satisfied by the auditee's control procedure. Write the test of controls audit program by specifying an effective control test to produce evidence about the auditee's performance of the control procedure. [*Hint:* A control test is a two-part statement consisting of (1) identification of a data population from which a sample can be drawn and (2) expression of an action to take.]

1. The company wants to avoid selling goods on credit to bad credit risks. Poor credit control could create problems with estimating the allowance for bad debts and a potential error by overstating the realizable value of accounts receivable. Therefore, the control procedure is as follows. Each customer order is to be reviewed and approved for 30-day credit by the credit department supervisor. The supervisor then notes the decision on the customer order, which is eventually attached to copy 2 of the sales invoice and filed by date in the accounts receivable department. The company used sales invoices numbered 20,001 through 30,000 during the period under review.

2. The company considers sales transactions complete when shipment is made. The control procedures are as follows: Shipping department personnel prepare prenumbered shipping documents in duplicate (sending one copy to the customer and filing the other copy in numerical order in the shipping department file). The shipping clerk marks up copy 3 of the invoice, indicating the quantity shipped, the date, and the shipping document number, and sends it to the billing department, where it is taken as authorization to complete the sales recording. Copy 3 is then filed in a daily batch in the billing department. These procedures are designed to prevent the recording of sales (i) for which no shipment is made or (ii) before the date of shipment.

3. The company wants to control unit pricing and mathematical errors that could result in overcharging or undercharging customers, thus producing the errors of overstatement or understatement of sales revenue and accounts receivable. The accounting procedures are as follows: Billing clerks use a catalogue list price to price the shipment on invoice copies 1, 2, and 3. They compute the dollar amount

of the invoice. Copy 1 is sent to the customer. Copy 2 is used to record the sale and is later filed in the accounts receivable department by date. Copy 3 is filed in the billing department by date.

4. The company needs to classify sales to subsidiaries apart from other sales so that the consolidated financial statement eliminations will be accurate. That is, the company wants to avoid the error of understating the elimination of intercompany profit and, therefore, overstating net income and inventory. The control procedure is as follows: A billing supervisor reviews each invoice copy 2 to see whether the billing clerk imprinted sales to the company's four subsidiaries with a big red "9" (the code for intercompany sales). The supervisor does not initial or sign the invoices.

EP 9-6 Control Objectives, Procedures, Assertions, and Tests. LO3, 4, 5, 6 Exhibit EP 9-6 contains an arrangement of examples of transaction errors (lettered a–g) and a set of auditee control procedures and devices (numbered 1–15). You should photocopy Exhibit EP 9-6 to use for completing the requirements of this question.

EXHIBIT EP 9-6

Direction of Control Testing

a. Sales recorded, goods not shipped
b. Goods shipped, sales not recorded
c. Goods shipped to a bad credit risk customer
d. Sales billed at the wrong price or wrong quantity
e. Product line A sales recorded as Product line B
f. January sales recorded in December
Control Procedures
1. Sales order approved for credit
2. Prenumbered shipping document prepared, sequence checked
3. Shipping document quantity compared to sales invoice
4. Prenumbered sales invoices, sequence checked
5. Sales invoice checked to sales order
6. Invoiced prices compared to approved price list
7. General ledger code checked for sales product lines
8. Sales dollar batch totals compared to sales journal
9. Periodic sales total compared to same-period accounts receivable postings
10. Accountants given instructions to date sales on the date of shipment
11. Sales entry date compared to shipping document date
12. Accounts receivable subsidiary totalled and reconciled to accounts receivable control account
13. Intercompany accounts reconciled with subsidiary company records
14. Credit files updated for customer payment history
15. Overdue customer accounts investigated for collection

Required:

a. Opposite the examples of transaction errors lettered a–f in Exhibit EP 9-6, write the name of the control objective organizations wish to achieve to prevent, detect, or correct the error.

b. Opposite each numbered control procedure, place an X in the column that identifies the error(s) the procedure is likely to control by prevention, detection, or correction.

c. For each error/control objective, identify the financial statement assertion most benefited by the control.

d. For each company control procedure numbered 1–15 in Exhibit EP 9-6, write an auditor's control test that could produce evidence on the question of whether the company's control procedure has been installed and is operating effectively.

EP 9-7 Controls and Control Weaknesses in Purchasing System. `LO3, 4, 5, 6, 7`

Part A

The following are internal control procedures found in the purchases and payment process of your auditee, Integrated Measurement Systems Inc.

Required:

For each control procedure:

a. Explain the type of control that is being applied.

b. Identify the control objective(s) that the control procedure meets.

c. Describe in detail one test of controls the auditor could perform to test the effectiveness of the control.

Control 1

Purchase requests (PRs) from operating departments are authorized by the appropriate person in the requesting department.

Control 2

The purchasing clerk verifies that there is a signature on the PR and then issues a prenumbered purchase order (PO) for the items required. The purchasing clerk retains copies of the PR and the PO and files them by PO number.

Control 3

The purchasing manager reviews the PO to see whether the PR is authorized, and, if so, approves it and forwards it to the buyer.

Control 4

The Buyer must select a vendor from a preapproved list for all POs over $5,000. For POs under $5,000, the Buyer can select any vendor.

Control 5

The receiver who accepts the goods into the warehouse verifies that the quantity received matches the bill of lading (BL) and signs on behalf of Integrated Measurement Systems for receipt of the goods listed on the BL. If there is a discrepancy in the quantity received, the receiver does not sign the BL; the BL is sent to the buyer to resolve the problem with the vendor.

Control 6

The purchasing clerk matches the signed BL with the filed copies of the PO and PR.

Part B

The following are internal control weaknesses found in the purchases and payment process of your auditee, Integrated Measurement Systems.

Required:

For each control weakness:

d. Describe the control risk that exists because of the weakness—what could go wrong?

e. Explain whether a monetary financial statement misstatement could result because of the weakness, and, if so, what it would be.

f. Describe in detail the impact the weakness will have on your other audit procedures.

Control Weakness 1

The purchasing clerk does not verify that the PRs are authorized by an appropriate person in the operating department, but only checks that there is a signature on the document.

Control Weakness 2

Access to the warehouse is not controlled and anyone can enter and leave any time.

Control Weakness 3

The receiver does not match the BL to an authorized PO.

EP 9-8 Explain Computer Control Procedures. `LO2, 4` At a meeting of the corporate audit committee attended by the general manager of the products division and you, representing the internal audit department, the following dialogue took place:

Jiang (committee chair): Marks has suggested that the internal audit department conduct an audit of the computer activities of the products division.

Smith (general manager): I don't know much about the technicalities of computers, but the division has some of the best computer people in the company.

Jiang: Do you know whether the internal controls protecting the system are satisfactory?

Smith: I suppose they are. No one has complained. What's so important about controls anyway, as long as the system works?

Jiang turns to you and asks you to explain IT control policies and procedures.

Required:

Address your response to the following points:

a. State the principal objective of achieving control over (*i*) input, (*ii*) processing, and (*iii*) output.

b. Give at least three methods of achieving control over (*i*) source data for input, (*ii*) data processing, and (*iii*) output.

EP 9-9 Testing Computer Processing. `LO3, 4` An experienced auditor remarked that it is only necessary to check the additions and extensions on one invoice generated by an IT-based system, because if the computer program does one invoice correctly it will do them all correctly, so there is no point in testing a statistical sample of invoices.

Required:

a. Comment on whether or not you agree with this statement. Give your reasons.

b. Assume that a company had effective controls over program changes in prior years, but during the current year a new programmer was hired who was not qualified for the job and did not document changes to the programs that were made during the year. Would this fact have an impact on your response for (*a*)?

EP 9-10 Control Tests and Risks of Misstatement. `LO4` The four questions below are taken from an internal control questionnaire. For each question, state (*i*) one control test you could use to find out whether the control technique was really used, and (*ii*) what error or fraud could occur if the question were answered "no," or if you found the control was not effective.

1. Are blank (sales) invoices available only to authorized personnel?
2. Are (sales) invoices checked for the accuracy of quantities billed? prices used? mathematical calculations?
3. Are the duties of the accounts receivable bookkeeper separate from any cash functions?
4. Are customer accounts regularly balanced with the control account?

EP 9-11 Control Risk Assessment, Online Input. `LO4` The Canada Revenue Agency allows e-filing. Registered tax professionals can submit taxpayers' annual income tax returns online over the Internet. The taxpayer's annual return information is automatically entered into the tax department's computer system. No paper forms or receipts need to be submitted, but the taxpayer must retain them because tax department auditors might ask to see them in the future. The tax return and any refund due are processed much more quickly than when paper forms are mailed in. A refund can be electronically deposited to the taxpayer's bank account, sometimes within one week.

Required:

Comment on the control strengths and weaknesses of the e-file system. In the case of weaknesses, provide recommendations on how they can be compensated for.

EP 9-12 Cost Benefit of Control Testing and Combined versus Substantive Audit Approach Decisions. `LO4` Four cases of control procedures used for financial statement items in different businesses are given below.

Required:

a. For each control procedure, evaluate whether there are significant risks in the business that would make this control essential to preventing or detecting the risks of material misstatements in the financial statements, or whether the control is less essential. Explain your evaluations.
b. Discuss whether you would use a combined approach for each item by testing the control, or whether you would choose a substantive approach where you rely only on substantive audit work for the item and do not test the control. Explain your reasoning.

CASES AND CONTROLS

CASE 1
The business processes a high volume of cash sales transactions through retail stores (e.g., Canadian Tire). There is a significant risk that not all sales will be recorded.

CASE 2
The inventory controller performs a monthly variance analysis to ensure production costs are staying within budget. There is a risk that avoidable cost overruns will occur if timely action is not taken when variances from budget occur.

CASE 3
The company's petty cash fund of $200 is kept in a locked box by the receptionist, who must present valid signed receipts for all expenditures to the controller when the fund runs low. The controller authorizes the payables manager to issue a cheque to "cash" to replenish the fund back up to $200. There is a risk that petty cash funds will be misappropriated.

CASE 4
The company uses an Internet-based sales order system. Customers enter order details online and pay online by entering their credit card information. The order entry system automatically checks that order details are correct and the goods are in stock, calculates the price, and verifies the validity of the credit card payment online with the credit card company. After these control routines are run, a shipping order is automatically created that simultaneously creates entries in the accounting system to recognize the revenue and costs of sales.

DISCUSSION CASES

DC 9-1 Backup Procedures, Availability of Data for Audit Tests. `LO1, 2, 3, 4, 5, 6` Whistler Corp. is a new audit engagement for your firm. Whistler backs up all its sales transaction detailed data for each month on a portable external hard drive. The drive is retained offsite for three months and then reused. This system is used because the company only has four drives, which cost over $100 each, and offsite storage charges are on a per-drive basis. The Whistler information system manager considers this to be a cost-effective backup procedure. Following the request of their former auditors, Whistler retains backup drives for December (the year-end) and the following January until the financial statement audit is completed. The audit is usually completed by the end of April.

Required:

a. Discuss the impact of this backup procedure on Whistler's control risk. Suggest alternative feasible approaches Whistler's management could use to improve internal control. Explain fully how your recommendations improve control and reduce risk. How would you communicate such recommendations to management?

b. Discuss the impact Whistler's backup procedure has on your audit approach. Consider any limitations it may impose on audit tests or analytical procedures, or the possibility of your firm's using a combined audit approach. Suggest alternative feasible approaches that may improve your audit scope.

DC 9-2 Control Risk Assessment and Testing—Costs and Benefits. `LO1, 2, 3, 4, 5, 6` The following are narrative descriptions of sales systems and controls for two different businesses.

Avocet Inc.

Avocet is a franchise fast food restaurant business. When customers order food, the counter person presses the appropriate buttons on the cash register. There is a button for each menu item. The point of sale (POS) system retrieves the current item prices from the price files, extends for quantities ordered, and displays the sale total on the cash register screen. A sales entry is also generated in the daily sales register. The customer's payment is then entered and their food order is displayed on a screen in the food preparation area. The POS system generates a cash receipt entry for the cash register and also in the daily cash receipts register. Food preparation staff put together the order and place it in the pickup area behind the front counter. When the food order is filled, the staff clears the order from the system; this generates an entry in the inventory system to remove the food and packaging items sold from the perpetual inventory listing.

A restaurant manager is on duty at all times. The manager circulates between the counter and food services areas, observing that cash received is placed in the register and spot-checking that food orders match with cash sales. If a customer receives an incorrect order, the manager can void the sale entry using a special key in the cash register and a secret password for the POS entries. A corrected order is then input by the usual method, if required. At the close of each day's business, the cash in the register is totalled and agreed to the cash, debit card, and credit card slips collected in the register during the day. Differences of less than $10 are recorded in an account named "Cash over/under." Larger discrepancies will be investigated by scrutinizing the day's entries and interviewing all counter people using the register. The sales and cash information from the POS system is then uploaded to the franchise company head office, where it is consolidated with the reports from all the restaurants in the system. On a weekly basis, the food and packaging inventory on hand in the restaurant is counted and reconciled to the inventory system. The inventory usage is also compared with the sales records for reasonableness.

Bobolink Limited

Bobolink is a new-car dealership. Once a customer has decided to buy a car, the car salesperson fills out a purchase agreement form, including the description of the car, the serial number, and the name and address of the purchaser. The agreed-upon sale price is entered, along with any extras, such as options or extended warranties, any allowance for a used car traded in, additional dealer preparation fees, licensing fees, and various taxes. A second form is used outlining the car purchase financing. The financing can be cash, a bank loan prearranged by the customer, or a lease arranged by Bobolink's financing company. Both forms are reviewed by the customer, and if they are satisfactory, the customer signs. The salesperson then takes the signed forms to the dealership's general manager for review and approval. If payment is by cash, the cash is given to the general manager at this point. Any discrepancies in the payment or paperwork are corrected and must be agreed to by the customer. Once the sales documents are completed, the ownership papers and keys are handed over to the customer, who drives away with the car. The sales documents are faxed to the car manufacturer's sales head office for inventory and warranty purposes, and to the bank or leasing company, if applicable. The sales information is entered by the Bobolink bookkeeper to the financial system and the inventory system. The bookkeeper follows up on collection of the funds from the bank or leasing company, which usually takes two to three days. The sales information is also set up in the dealership management system for purposes of sales incentives and commissions, future service work, and sales follow-up.

Required:

a. Compare and contrast the control risks in these two businesses.

b. Identify input, processing, and output control procedures that exist in each business, including the control objective for each.

c. Comment on whether each business control system relies on prevention of errors, early detection of errors, or later detection and correction. Do you think the control method designed by management in each business is the most effective and efficient system for its particular control risks? Can you recommend any more cost-effective control techniques?

d. Identify control strengths and weaknesses in the two sales systems in relation to the seven control objectives described in the chapter.

e. Assume you are required to test controls in both these audits. Write control tests that address all the control objectives. Also, indicate the financial statement assertion(s) that each control test addresses.

f. Assume that it is your responsibility to decide whether to rely on controls in these two audits. Evaluate the cost-benefit trade-off of testing controls in both businesses. Recommend an audit approach for each, giving your reasons.

DC 9-3 Costs and Benefits of Control. `LO1, 2, 3, 5` The following questions and cases deal with the subject of cost-benefit analysis of internal control. Some important concepts in cost-benefit analysis are as follows.

1. *Measurable benefit.* Benefits or cost savings may be measured directly or may be based on estimates of expected value. An expected loss is an estimate of the amount of a probable loss multiplied by the frequency or probability of the loss-causing event. A measurable benefit can arise from the reduction of an expected loss.

2. *Qualitative benefit.* Some gains or cost savings may not be measurable, such as company public image, reputation for regulatory compliance, customer satisfaction, and employee morale.

3. *Measurable costs.* Controls may have direct costs, such as wages and equipment expenses.

4. *Qualitative cost factors.* Some costs may be indirect, such as lower employee morale created by over-controlled work restrictions.

5. *Marginal analysis.* Each successive control feature may have marginal cost and benefit effects on the control problem.

Case A

Porterhouse Company has numerous bank accounts. Why might management hesitate to spend $20,000 (half of a clerical salary) to assign someone the responsibility of reconciling each account every month for the purpose of catching the banks' accounting errors? Do other good reasons exist to justify spending $20,000 each year to reconcile bank accounts monthly?

Case B

Harper Hoe Company keeps a large inventory of hardware products in a warehouse. Last year, $500,000 was lost to thieves who broke in through windows and doors. Josh Harper figures that installing steel doors with special locks and burglar bars on the windows at a cost of $25,000 would eliminate 90% of the loss. Hiring armed guards to patrol the building 16 hours a day at a current annual cost of $75,000 would eliminate all the loss, according to officials of the Holmes Security Agency. Should Josh arrange for one, both, or neither of the control measures?

Case C

The Merry Cafeteria formerly collected from each customer as he or she reached the end of the food line. A cashier, seated at a cash register, rang up the amount (displayed on a digital screen) and collected money. Management changed the system, and now a clerk at the end of the line operates a calculator/printer machine and gives each customer a paper tape. The machine accumulates a running total internally. The customer presents the tape at the cash register on the way out and pays.

The cafeteria manager justified the direct cost of $30,000 annually for the additional salary and $500 for the new machine by pointing out that she could serve four more people each weekday (Monday through Friday) and 10 more people on Saturday and Sunday. The food line now moves faster and customers are more satisfied. (The average meal tab is $12, and total costs of food and service are considered fixed.) "Besides," she said, "my internal control is better." Evaluate the manager's assertions.

Case D

Assume, in the Merry Cafeteria situation cited above, that the better control of separating cash custody from the end-of-food-line recording function was not cost beneficial, even after taking all measurable benefits into consideration. As an auditor, you believe the cash collection system deficiency is a significant deficiency in internal control, and you have written it as such in your letter concerning reportable conditions, which you delivered to Merry Cafeteria's central administration. The local manager insists on inserting her own opinion on the cost-benefit analysis in the preface to the document that contains your report. Should you, in your report, express any opinion or evaluation on the manager's statement?

DC 9-4 Controls, Fraud Risk. **LO1, 2, 7** The SB Construction Company has two divisions. The president, Su, manages the roofing division. Su has delegated authority and responsibility for management of the modular manufacturing division to Gee. The company has a competent accounting staff and a full-time internal auditor. Unlike Su, however, Gee and his secretary handle all the bids for manufacturing jobs, purchase all the materials without competitive bids, control the physical inventory of materials, contract for shipping, supervise the construction work, bill the customers, approve all bid changes, and collect the payment from customers. With Su's tacit approval, Gee has asked the internal auditor not to interfere with his busy schedule.

Required:

a. Discuss the internal control in this fact situation, and identify fraud risks that could arise.

b. Assume you are the independent external auditor of SB. Explain your responsibilities to report on this situation to SB's management and board of directors.

DC 9-5 Cash Receipts Control. `LO3, 4, 5` Sally's Craft Corner was opened in 20X0 by Sally Moore, a fashion designer employed by Bundy's Department Store. Sally is employed full-time at Bundy's and travels frequently to shows and marts in Vancouver, Montreal, and Toronto. She enjoys crafts, wanted a business of her own, and saw an opportunity in Vancouver. The Corner now sells regularly to about 300 customers, but business only began to pick up in 20X6. The staff includes two salespeople and four office personnel, and Sally herself helps out on weekends.

Sales have grown, as has the Corner's reputation for quality crafts. The history is as follows:

	SALES	DISCOUNTS AND ALLOWANCES	NET SALES
20X2	$164,950	$ 5,000	$159,950
20X3	185,750	5,500	180,250
20X4	176,100	5,200	170,900
20X5	183,800	5,700	178,100
20X6	239,500	9,500	230,000
20X7	294,700	14,800	279,900
20X8	372,300	$22,300	350,000

With an expanding business and a need for inventory, the Corner is now cash poor. Prices are getting higher every month, and Sally is a little worried. The net cash flow is only about $400 per month after allowance of a 3% discount for timely payments on account. So, she has engaged you as auditor and also asks for recommendations you might have about the cash flow situation. The Corner has never been audited.

During your review of internal control, you have learned the following about the four office personnel:

Janet Bundy is the receptionist and also helps customers. She is the daughter of the Bundy Department Store owner and a long-time friend of Sally's. Janet helped Sally start the Corner. They hang out together when Sally is in town. She opens all the mail, answers most of it herself, but turns over payments on account to Sue Kenmore.

Sue Kenmore graduated from high school and started working as a bookkeeper-secretary at the Corner in 20X6. She wants to go to university but cannot afford it right now. She is very quiet in the office, but you have noticed she has some fun with her friends in her new BMW. In the office, she gets the mailed-in payments on account from Janet, takes payments over the counter in the store, checks the calculations of discounts allowed, enters the cash collections in the cash receipts journal, prepares a weekly bank deposit (and mails it), and prepares a list (remittance list) of the payments on account. The list shows amounts received from each customer, discount allowed, and amount to be credited to the customer's account. She is also responsible for approving the discounts and credits for merchandise returned.

Ken Murphy has been the bookkeeper-clerk since 20X2. He also handles other duties. Among them, he receives the remittance list from Sue, posts the customers' accounts in the subsidiary ledger, and gives the remittance list to David Roberts, the bookkeeping supervisor. Ken also prepares and mails customers' monthly statements. Ken is rather dull, interested mostly in hunting on weekends, but is a steady worker. He always comes to work in a beat-up pickup truck—an eyesore in the parking lot.

David Roberts, the bookkeeping supervisor, started working for The Corner in 20X7 after giving up his small practice as a public accountant. He posts the general ledger (using the remittance list as a basis for cash received entries) and prepares monthly financial statements. He also approves and makes all other ledger entries and reconciles the monthly bank statement. He reconciles the customer subsidiary records to the accounts receivable control each month. David is very happy not to have to contend with the pressures he experienced in his practice as a public accountant.

Required:

a. Draw a simple flowchart of the cash collection and bookkeeping procedures.
b. Identify any reportable conditions or material weakness in internal control. Explain any reasons why you might suspect that errors or irregularities may have occurred.
c. Recommend corrective measures you believe necessary and efficient in this business.

DC 9-6 Tests of Controls, Information Technology–Based Sales System. LO4, 6 Garganey Corp. manufactures automobile dashboards and interior components for Big Motors Inc. (BMI). BMI requires that all its suppliers be connected to its computerized procurement and manufacturing system. BMI's production planning system generates components requirements lists, which are then transferred electronically to various suppliers' computers for them to bid on. Garganey's production system calculates the cost of manufacturing the components at the required times, including materials, labour, overtime charges, overhead, and profit. Garganey makes a bid on the order and, if its bid is accepted by BMI, BMI's production schedule for that component is downloaded to Garganey's production system so that the required parts will be manufactured and delivered to BMI's plants at the times they are required in the BMI assembly lines. When the components are completed, Garganey's system generates a shipping instructions document, which is signed by the trucking company that picks up the components and delivers them to BMI. When the components arrive at BMI, they are inspected and, if approved, payment for the order is automatically transferred from BMI's bank account to Garganey's bank account. Any adjustments for quantities short-shipped are deducted from the amount BMI transfers, and an adjustment memo is communicated electronically to Garganey's sales system.

Required:

Discuss the factors an auditor would consider in planning the internal control audit program for Garganey. Using the tests of controls procedures described in the chapter as a starting point, adapt the procedures to be suitable for the IT-based sales system used by Garganey. Describe control testing procedures that will generate evidence about the effectiveness of Garganey's internal controls. Also discuss the pros and cons of choosing a combined audit approach rather than a substantive approach for this situation.

DC 9-7 Flowchart Control Points. LO4, 5, 6 Each number of the flowchart in Exhibit DC 9-7 locates a control point in the labour processing system of your auditee, Alouette Inc.

Required:

a. Make a list of the control points, and, for each point, describe the type of internal control procedure that ought to be specified.
b. Assume that Exhibit DC 9-7 is the system description in Alouette's prior year's audit file. During the current year, the company converted to an electronic security card system. Each employee is issued a security card with a magnetic stripe containing his or her identity code. At the start of the shift the employee swipes his or her security card to enter the factory floor. Using an internal clock, the scanner

generates a start time entry in the system's attendance detail records file. The employee then reports to the floor supervisor to be assigned to a job for his or her shift. The supervisor uses a terminal that displays a real-time list of checked-in employees and enters the job number assignment beside the employee's name. The job costing system automatically creates an open daily job transaction entry. At the end of the shift the employee swipes his or her card to exit the factory floor, and the total shift time is entered to the open job transaction. The daily job transaction entry is then closed and a labour charge entry for the employee's shift is generated in the job costing system and in the payroll file.

You have been assigned to assess controls for the current-year audit. Update Exhibit DC 9-7 to reflect the new employee attendance and job costing systems described above. Identify control points in the new systems, and indicate control procedures that should be used to prevent errors in payroll and job costing.

EXHIBIT DC 9-7

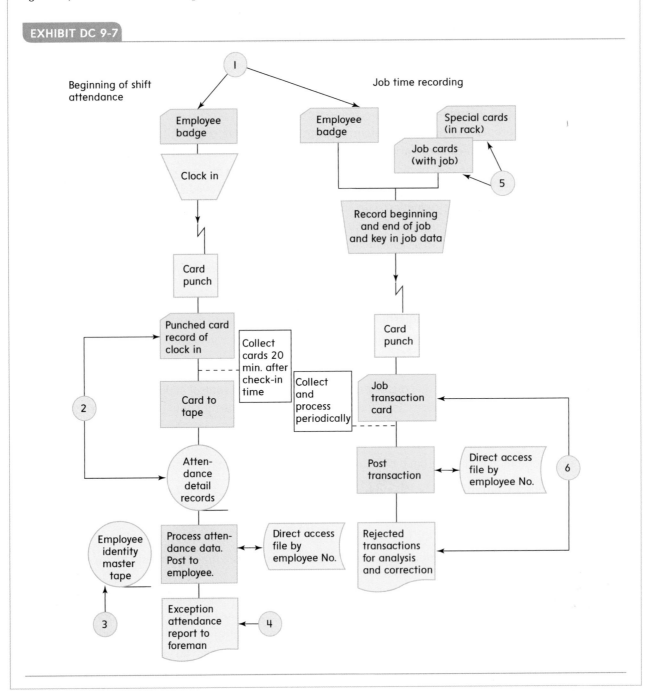

DC 9-8 Audit Approach, Computer Service Organization. `LO2, 4` Eider Equipment Leasing Limited is in the financing lease business. It uses a service organization to compute lease payment schedules. Eider's customers sign standard equipment leases ranging from 3 to 15 years. The details of the leases are summarized and sent to the service organization for generating the schedules. Hard-copy reports from the service organization are delivered to Eider monthly and used by its bookkeeper to generate entries in the company's general ledger system, which is run on a popular accounting software package.

Required:

a. Design two or more appropriate audit approaches for verifying leasing revenues in this auditee.

b. List factors that would indicate which approach will be most efficient and effective.

DC 9-9 Audit Approach Decision, Combined or Substantive. `LO2, 4` Golden Years Inc. owns and operates 20 rental retirement properties. It has a total of 9,000 one-bedroom and 3,000 two-bedroom rental units. Tenants pay rent monthly by giving a cheque to the property manager. The manager deposits the cheques at the bank and sends the deposit information and tenant listing to Golden Years' head office, where the accounting manager enters the information into the sales journal and general ledger. The Accounting Manager reconciles the bank statements monthly.

You are in charge of auditing Golden Years' revenues and receivables for its 20X3 year-end. Golden Years' draft financial statements report rental revenues of $102.6 million, tenant receivables of $400,000, and net income of $5.9 million.

Required:

a. Indicate whether you would use a substantive or combined approach to audit Golden Years' revenues, giving your reasons.

b. Develop an audit program (list of audit procedures) to provide sufficient appropriate evidence that the rental revenues reported in the company's 20X3 financial statements are not materially misstated.

DC 9-10 Management and Auditor Responsibilities Related to Internal Control. `LO1` Bultz & Prime LLP is the external auditor for Bain Corp. You have been assigned to this audit. You are meeting with Chelsea, the Director of Finance, to discuss existing internal controls in order to evaluate them, and she asks you the following:

"As you go through all of our controls, can you please write up a report with any deficiencies you notice? Also, if you and your audit team could come up with some suggestions on how to improve existing controls or add new controls, that would be great! We know you like to rely on controls during your audits, so if you can let us know how to get better, the audit should be a lot easier next year. After you are done with me, you can also go and talk to Mark, the quality control manager for our production facility. He may also be able to use your recommendations for his department."

Required:

Prepare a response to Chelsea to indicate the responsibilities of the external auditors and the responsibilities of Bain Corp.'s management. Ensure that you remain professional in your response and that you adapt your tone to someone who is not familiar with the auditing rules and requirements. Explain to Chelsea why each element you identify is, or is not, the responsibility of the auditor.

Internal Control Assessment Aids for Audit Planning

LO8 Describe the contents and purpose of internal control questionnaires in an auditor's control evaluation.

This appendix provides details on practice aids that auditors can use to assess company-level controls and control activities, a questionnaire for developing narrative-style internal control documentation, and some basic symbols and design rules for creating internal control flowcharts.

INTERNAL CONTROL QUESTIONNAIRE FOR DEVELOPING A NARRATIVE-STYLE DOCUMENTATION OF A CONTROL SYSTEM

Exhibit 9A–1 provides an example of an internal control questionnaire for company-level controls and control activities. Its points apply to all the processes and accounting cycles that will be covered in Chapters 11 through 14 of Part 3 of the text. We will provide separate detailed internal control questionnaires for the controls related to each process in the relevant chapters, after the nature of each business process and accounting cycle has been explained: revenues/receivables/receipts (Chapter 11), purchases/payables/payments (Chapter 12), production and payroll (Chapter 13), and finance and investment (Chapter 14).

This aid can give you a sense of how auditors apply professional judgment to decide on the appropriate approach to obtaining assurance from control and substantive evidence in planning a particular audit engagement.

This questionnaire is designed to assist the auditor in assessing the strength of internal control. Internal control is divided into company-level controls and control activities.

- Company-level controls are the overall control environment, management's risk assessment procedures, information systems and communication, and monitoring.
- Control activities include general and application controls. General controls are policies and procedures that apply to all information systems and business processes. Application controls are those that are specific to each of the main operating processes and their related accounting cycles.

SYMBOLS AND DESIGN RULES FOR DEVELOPING FLOWCHART DOCUMENTATION OF A CONTROL SYSTEM

LO9 Describe the contents of flowcharts and their use to document controls in accounting processes.

Exhibit 9A–2 contains a few simple flowchart symbols. An audit supervisor should be able to understand the chart without consulting a lengthy index of symbols. It should be legible and drawn with a template and ruler or with computer software. The starting point in the system should, if possible, be placed at the upper left-hand corner, with the flow of procedures and documents moving from left to right and from top to bottom, as much as is possible. Narrative explanations should be written on the chart as annotations or be part of a readily available reference key.

The flowchart should communicate all relevant information and evidence about segregation of responsibilities, authorization, and accounting and control procedures in an understandable, visual form. Exhibit 9A–3 shows a partial flowchart representation of the beginning stages of a sales and delivery processing system. The out-connectors shown by the circled A and B indicate continuation on other flowcharts. Ultimately, the flowchart ends by showing entries in accounting journals and inventory ledgers.

EXHIBIT 9A–1

Internal Control Questionnaire for Company-Level Controls and Control Activities

INTERNAL CONTROL QUESTIONNAIRE		
AUDITEE: _____		
F/S PERIOD: _____		

COMPANY-LEVEL CONTROLS	Auditor Responses	Audit File References
CONTROL ENVIRONMENT The control environment refers to management's overall attitude, awareness, and actions concerning the importance of internal control to address the risks of the business and reduce inherent risks and the risk of a material misstatement. 　Consider the following aspects and evidence of strength or weakness: **Tone at the Top** • Do management actions and attitudes show character, integrity, and ethical values? • Are the audit committee and board of directors (or others responsible for governance of the organization) competent, knowledgeable, actively involved, and influential in the organization? • Does management have well-defined policies and objectives that communicate its commitment to integrity and ethical values? **Commitment to Competence** • Does management have sufficient experience to operate the business? • Does management assign authority and responsibility appropriately? • Does management provide accounting and key employees with the resources, training, and information necessary to discharge its duties? • Do management's hiring and promotion policies emphasize competence and trustworthiness? **Management's Operating Style and Philosophy** • Does management encourage a strong control environment? • Does the organizational structure provide a framework for establishing key areas of authority, responsibility, and reporting lines that promote strong internal control at all stages of planning, executing, and reviewing the organization's activities for achieving its objectives? • Do management actions remove or reduce incentives and opportunities for employees to act dishonestly? • Is there a mandatory vacation policy for employees performing key control functions? • Does management implement controls over information systems? • Does management maintain appropriate physical safeguards over cash, investments, inventory, and/or fixed assets? • Does management establish adequate controls over accounting estimates and choice of accounting principles, where applicable?		
		(continued)

Internal Control Questionnaire for Company-Level Controls and Control Activities (*continued*)

COMPANY-LEVEL CONTROLS	Auditor Responses	Audit File References

MANAGEMENT'S RISK ASSESSMENT PROCESS
For financial reporting purposes, management's risk assessment process should identify internal and external events and circumstances that can impair the organization's ability to initiate, record, process, and report financial data that is consistent with the assertions management makes in its financial statements.
 	
Consider the following aspects:
• Has management established policies and assigned responsibility to personnel for identifying, evaluating, and mitigating risks?
• Does management have an ongoing process to identify risk and ensure exposure to such risks is minimized? Risks include
  – changes in business and regulatory operating environment
  – new personnel
  – changes in information systems
  – rapid change in operations
  – new technology
  – new business models, products, or activities, including financial instruments/derivatives
  – organizational restructuring
  – foreign expansion
  – new accounting standards
• Does management independently evaluate the organization's internal control environment to assess its effectiveness?		

INFORMATION AND COMMUNICATIONS
High-quality management information is an essential component of internal control. Creating and communicating information is relevant to operating decisions and to financial reporting objectives. The auditor is concerned mainly with the financial reporting information system, consisting of the procedures and records established to initiate, record, process, and report transactions, events, and conditions and to maintain accountability for the related assets, liabilities, and equity.
 	
Consider the following aspects:
• Does management have documented policies and procedures to develop, operate, and maintain information systems, related business processes, and accounting cycles that produce reliable and timely financial information?
• Has management implemented an information system that is well designed to achieve the following financial reporting objectives?
  – Identify and record all valid transactions related to the organization in their proper reporting period.
  – Capture sufficient detail to permit proper classification, measurement, and presentation of transactions in the financial statements and note disclosures in accordance with GAAP or other appropriate basis of accounting.
• Are appropriate lines of authority and reporting clearly established?
• Does management gather information from and communicate information to appropriate people on a timely basis?
• Is there a communication process available for people to report suspected improprieties? For example, has management established an effective whistle-blower program as it relates to financial reporting?
• Is there a disaster recovery plan in place to ensure minimum disruption should management information, accounting records, or other important data be destroyed, damaged, or stolen?		

MONITORING
Consider the following aspects:
• Has management established effective monitoring procedures?
• Does management have a business plan that is monitored against actual results?
• Does management monitor compliance with internal control policies and procedures?
• Does management investigate variances and take proper and timely corrective action?
 	
Control activities are the policies and procedures that ensure actions are taken to address risks that threaten the achievement of the entity's objectives.
    Control activities are part of the information system, can be manual or IT based, are directed toward the control objectives, and are applied at various organizational and functional levels.
    This questionnaire divides control activities questions into general controls and application controls. General controls tend to affect many or all of the underlying accounting processes, while application controls relate to each specific accounting process.
		(continued)

EXHIBIT 9A-1

Internal Control Questionnaire for Company-Level Controls and Control Activities (*continued*)

COMPANY-LEVEL CONTROLS	Auditor Responses	Audit File References
General Controls General controls are pervasive policies and procedures that tend to affect to most or all processes in the information system and most or all organizational levels. Consider the following: • Are there policies and procedures in place to – prevent unauthorized access or changes to programs and data? – ensure the security and privacy of data? – control and maintain key systems? – protect assets susceptible to misappropriation? • Is management's approach to IT planning and new systems development adequate to ensure new systems and systems changes protect the integrity of data and processing? In particular, note procedures that ensure the following: completeness, accuracy, and authorization of data and processing; the existence of adequate management trails; and the protection of the continuity of IT operations by backup procedures and a formal disaster plan. • Are appropriate procedures in place for software and hardware upgrades and other systems maintenance? • Are day-to-day operations adequately controlled by IT support personnel to ensure data integrity? • Are access controls adequate? Consider whether internal access is monitored across the information system such that appropriate personnel have access only to files they need to do their jobs, and unauthorized access is prohibited. • For IT systems and applications run over the Internet or other telecommunications systems, is external access security adequately protected by firewalls, virus protection software, or other IT security features?		
Auditor's conclusion on the company-level and general controls: _____ _____	Prepared by _____ _____	Date _____
Application Controls Application controls relate to recording, processing, and reporting information. They will be specific to the business processes and related accounting cycles that generate financial information. Recording includes identifying and capturing the relevant information for transactions or events. Processing includes calculation, measurement, valuation, and summarization, whether performed by IT-based or manual procedures. Reporting relates to the preparation of financial reports, electronic or printed, that management uses to measure and review the entity's financial performance and reporting to stakeholders. For each accounting cycle, a separate detailed questionnaire should be completed that assesses the following aspects of information processing: • Are data integrity controls adequate? Identify and assess controls over data input to and processed in the accounting cycle that ensure data and processing are valid, complete, and accurate. Consider functions such as edit and validation checks, programmed reasonability checks, dollar limits, sequence numbering, internal confirmation of transaction data transferred from database files to the application, reconciliation, and other relevant control features. • Are access and authorization controls adequate; e.g., are access points for data entry and inquiry (terminal, desktop, laptop, hand-held device, etc.) set up to allow only designated functions to be performed and only authorized personnel to access data, processing, and output? Based on the application control assessment, the auditor will develop a detailed plan setting out the planned audit approach, including decisions on whether to test controls as a component of audit evidence in addition to substantive evidence. Refer to the detailed internal control questionnaires for each business process/accounting cycle provided in Chapters 11–14. This is where the auditor will document control assessments and their conclusion on whether to test controls in the overall audit approach.		*(continued)*

EXHIBIT 9A–2

Standard Flowchart Symbols

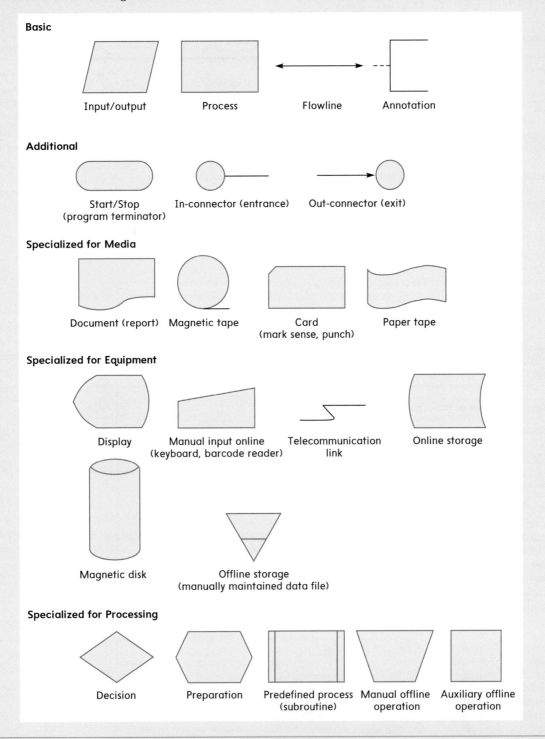

Basic

Input/output   Process   Flowline   Annotation

Additional

Start/Stop
(program terminator)   In-connector (entrance)   Out-connector (exit)

Specialized for Media

Document (report)   Magnetic tape   Card
(mark sense, punch)   Paper tape

Specialized for Equipment

Display   Manual input online
(keyboard, barcode reader)   Telecommunication
link   Online storage

Magnetic disk   Offline storage
(manually maintained data file)

Specialized for Processing

Decision   Preparation   Predefined process
(subroutine)   Manual offline
operation   Auxiliary offline
operation

In Exhibit 9A–3, you can see some characteristics of both flowchart construction and this accounting system.[7] Minimizing the number of flow lines that cross each other is helpful for following the chart. Reading down each department's column shows that initiation authority for transactions (both credit approval and sales invoice preparation) and custody of assets are separated. All documents have an intermediate or final resting place in a file (some of these files are in the flowcharts connected to A and B), thus giving auditors information about where to find audit evidence later.

EXHIBIT 9A–3

Example of a Flowchart for the Revenue Process: Credit Approval and Revenue Processing, Shipment and Delivery

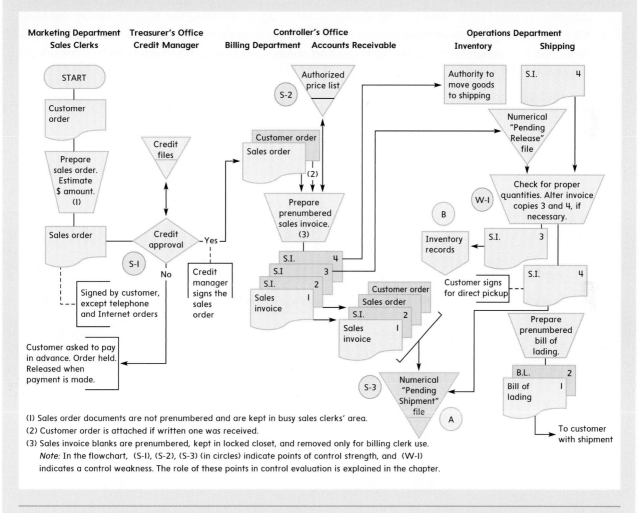

(1) Sales order documents are not prenumbered and are kept in busy sales clerks' area.

(2) Customer order is attached if written one was received.

(3) Sales invoice blanks are prenumbered, kept in locked closet, and removed only for billing clerk use.

Note: In the flowchart, (S-I), (S-2), (S-3) (in circles) indicate points of control strength, and (W-I) indicates a control weakness. The role of these points in control evaluation is explained in the chapter.

APPENDIX 9B Understanding Information Systems and Technology for Risk and Control Assessment (on Connect)

ENDNOTES

1 CAS 315.

2 See Exhibit 9–5 for the related control objectives.

3 See the internal control framework presented in Chapter 7, Exhibit 7–1.

4 Other detailed examples of flowcharts and processing tables (an alternative system documentation format) are provided in Appendix 11B for the revenues/receivables/receipts accounting process.

5 CAS 260 and CAS 265.

6 CAS 260, paragraph 9; CAS 265, paragraphs 9–10.

7 Accounting firms have various methods for constructing flowcharts. The illustrations in this book take the approach of describing an accounting subsystem completely. Some accounting firms use more efficient methods of charting only the documents, information flows, and controls considered important for the audit.

CHAPTER 10

Audit Sampling

In this chapter, we review the general topic of audit sampling, which relies heavily on the concepts of materiality and risk—audit risk, inherent risk, control risk, and detection risk. Audit sampling is not an audit procedure in the same class as the procedures explained in previous chapters. Instead, it is a method of organizing the application of audit procedures, as well as a method of organizing the auditor's decision-making process. Sampling concepts, thus, serve as a useful decision aid for auditors and helps justify the audit opinion. Sampling concepts have taken on a greater importance in auditing standards, as now they are covered in their own Canadian Auditing Standard, CAS 530. This is because audit sampling concepts clarify audit reasoning and introduce more rigour to the audit process. But complications can arise because different accounting firms use different statistical methods, and the different models create their own distinct concepts. In this chapter, we introduce the simplest statistical model, monetary-unit sampling (MUS), which does not have the complications of other models.

Statistical sampling is the more rigorous and formal application of sampling. However, only about one in six audits use statistical sampling of one form or another. These audits tend to be concentrated in the larger public accounting firms.

Nevertheless, what makes knowledge of statistical auditing valuable is that it clarifies the logic of the audit evidence-gathering process by using more-precise concepts. Specifically, statistical auditing makes clearer the meaning of specific types of risks in auditing and some of the materiality concepts introduced in Chapter 5. In addition, auditing uses a different approach in statistics that allows a more straightforward alignment with audit objectives as represented by the concepts of audit assurance and audit risk. This is important, because many view the audit risk concept as the "engine room of the audit."[1] This chapter thus deals with the conceptual foundations of auditing that underlie the audit evidence-gathering process that you have covered in Chapters 5 to 9. In this and later chapters, we make extensive reference to AuG-41, an audit guideline in the *CPA Canada Handbook* at the time of writing. However, this guideline is described as "temporary." It is, however, such a valuable learning tool that we rely on it extensively in this text. AuG-41 helps illustrate the evolution of auditor thinking and the understanding of the existing permanent standards. The same applies to other references to "temporary" *Handbook* sections.

LEARNING OBJECTIVES

After completing this chapter, you will be able to do the following:

LO1   Explain the role of professional judgment in audit sampling decisions.

LO2   Distinguish audit sampling work from non-sampling work.

LO3   Compare and contrast statistical and non-statistical sampling.

LO4   Differentiate between effectiveness risk, efficiency risk, sampling risk, and non-sampling risk.

LO5   Develop a simple audit program to test a client's internal control procedures.

(a) Specify objectives, deviation conditions, populations, and sampling units.

(b) Demonstrate some basic audit sampling calculations.

(c) Evaluate evidence from control testing.

LO6   Develop a simple audit program for an account balance, considering the influences of risk and tolerable misstatement.

(a) Specify objectives and a population of data.

(b) Determine sample size and select sample units.

(c) Evaluate monetary error evidence from a balance audit sample.

LO7   (Appendix 10A) Demonstrate that you can work with statistical sampling tables.

LO8   (Appendix 10B) Demonstrate that you can apply statistical sampling concepts for tests of controls and tests of balances using the audit risk model.

CHAPTER APPENDICES

APPENDIX 10A   Statistical Sampling Tables

APPENDIX 10B   More-Advanced Statistical Sampling Concepts for Tests of Controls and Tests of Balances (on Connect)

EcoPak

EcoPak Inc.

Donna and Caleb have been invited to sit in EcoPak's boardroom to do their interim field work. They are planning to do the tests up to the end of September now, and to finish up later in February when they come back to do the year-end work. As they are meeting with the accounts receivable manager to coordinate how they will do their testing, Nina pops her head in and says, "Hi Donna. Hi Caleb. How are things going on the audit trail?" Donna explains that they are just starting their systems work and getting set up to test the volume credit notes.

"Oh, that is so interesting," Nina says. "You know, it's really been fun and challenging to be a CFO in a growing manufacturing business like EcoPak. But sometimes, I really miss the challenges of being an auditor out in the field, visiting different clients all year round, figuring out all their business risks, their systems and processes, and how to get the evidence to form an opinion on the financial statements. I am really interested to know what you are planning to do to test our volume credit notes because, to be honest, though I review the report for reasonability, there are so many variables at play that I find it hard to know what to expect the amount to be from month to month. And after what we just dealt with in purchasing, I realize that these types of non-routine processes are particularly vulnerable to all kinds of errors and fraud!"

So, Donna gives a general outline to Nina of the test steps she is planning to use in her volume credit notes testing. Donna plans to use a judgmental sampling approach. Her sample will include the two largest credit notes for each of the six largest customers as key items. Then she will take a random sample from the rest of the population of credit notes issued. She will use the audit software of her audit firm, Meyer & Gustav (M&G), to obtain her own list of the credit note transactions from EcoPak's system and use the list to identify her sample items and to do some other tests, such as verifying the totals, checking the numerical sequencing, and looking for any large or unusual items or patterns.

For each volume credit note sample item, Donna will vouch the credit note back to the monthly sales volume reports the clerk has used to determine the eligibility in accordance with the customer contracts, ensure the appropriate level was reached and the discount correctly calculated according to the contract, and then check that each credit issued has been approved by the manager. She will next trace each credit note forward to ensure it is correctly recorded in the sales and accounts receivable accounts in the general ledger. She will also take a small sample of credit notes from the clerk's file of credit note copies and trace back to customer accounts receivable ledgers to make sure they are recorded completely. If there are any discrepancies or unusual findings, she will follow up by discussions with the audit team and further inquiries and document inspections, if required.

"That sounds very comprehensive, Donna! But I guess once you get going, it will go quickly," Nina says. "Oh yes, our interim testing will go pretty quickly, Nina. We have lots of other things to look at! But you will probably be really interested in the approach Caleb has come up with to assess the reasonability of the year-end sales and volume credit notes. It might be something that will help you with your monitoring." When Nina hears about Caleb's analytical procedure, she finds it very powerful and agrees that it is a technique that she can use to make her own monitoring more robust.

The Essentials of Audit Sampling

In our coverage of the audit process so far we have looked at a variety of procedures that auditors perform to obtain evidence to obtain the high level of assurance required to support an audit opinion on financial statements. These procedures were explained in Chapter 8 and are summarized for each step of the audit process in Exhibit 10–1. At the *risk assessment* and *conclusion and reporting* steps of the audit process, auditors rely mainly on inquiry, analysis, and observation procedures. These procedures provide important input to auditors' judgments in these steps of the audit.

In the *response to assessed risk* step, auditors perform specific and detailed procedures to gather persuasive evidence regarding whether there are material misstatements in the financial statements. In particular, if auditors plan to rely on internal control effectiveness, they will perform tests of controls. They will also perform substantive tests of the details of balances to gain direct assurance regarding the financial statements numbers. Recall that these two types of tests differ because they have different objectives: tests of control aim to assess control effectiveness, while substantive tests of detail aim to detect monetary misstatements in accounting numbers. For both these types of tests, auditors will use evidence-gathering techniques such as inspection, confirmation, and reperformance/recalculation. In many cases, these types of procedures will involve examining classes of transactions and account balances made up of a large population of items that are similar in nature. For example, the revenue transaction stream will be made up of a large volume of sales invoices that were issued during the year. The inventory balance will be made up of a large volume of goods involved in the business.

When auditors do tests of high-volume populations of this kind, they usually use sampling techniques, since it is not feasible to test 100% of a large volume of items. Based on statistical theory, we know that by testing a randomly drawn sample that is representative of the whole population, we can form a conclusion about the whole population with a high degree of confidence. These statistical principles are the basis of audit sampling. In practice, auditors often apply sampling techniques in a judgmental way, given the subjective nature of the audit

EXHIBIT 10–1

(Summary from Chapter 8) Types of Evidence Procedures Used in the Steps of the Audit Process

STEPS OF THE AUDIT PROCESS AND AUDITOR'S OBJECTIVES	TYPES OF AUDIT EVIDENCE-GATHERING PROCEDURES USED
RISK ASSESSMENT STEP	
Understanding the auditee and its risks	Inquiries of auditee personnel, including study of prior-audit working paper information Inquiries of external parties, including industry and other research sources
Assessing the risk of material misstatement (inherent and control risks)	Inquiry of auditee personnel Analysis of draft financial statements, including comparisons to prior years Observation, including operation of accounting information system and internal control
RISK RESPONSE STEP	
Testing control effectiveness: • Obtain indirect assurance regarding risk of material misstatements of monetary amounts in financial statements; assess control risk.	Inquiry of auditee personnel Observation of controls performed by auditee personnel Recalculation/reperformance of controls
Substantive testing of details of transactions and account balances: • Obtain direct evidence regarding material misstatement of monetary amounts in financial statements.	Inspections of documents, records, and assets Observation, including scrutiny External confirmation Recalculation/reperformance
Dual-purpose tests of controls and substantive details of transactions and balances: • Obtain evidence regarding both control effectiveness and material misstatement of monetary amounts in financial statements.	Inquiry of auditee personnel Observation of controls performed by auditee personnel Recalculation/reperformance of controls and recording Inspections of documents and records
Substantive analytical procedures	Analysis of relations to other financial and non-financial information Comparison of actual and expected values
CONCLUDING AND REPORTING STEP	
Overall analysis of financial statements and disclosures: • Assess reasonability of overall financial statement amounts, presentation, and related disclosures to ensure fair presentation.	Analysis of relations to other financial and non-financial information Analysis of impact of uncorrected misstatements on ratios and key performance indicators

process and the concept of reasonable assurance. In some cases, however, statistical sampling methods can be applied quite rigorously in performing audit tests.

CAS 530, Audit Sampling, provides useful guidance for auditors for both judgmental and statistical sampling applications. The most important concepts of CAS 530 are set out in the definitions (in paragraph 5); these are the key concepts of classical sampling: audit sampling, population, sampling risk, non-sampling risk, statistical sampling, and stratification. We will discuss these essential concepts next, and several more advanced concepts from CAS 530 are briefly noted at the end.

Audit sampling refers to applying audit procedures to less than 100% of items in a population of audit relevance, such as a class of transactions or an account balance. Every item in the population must have a chance of selection so that the auditor has a reasonable basis for drawing conclusions about the entire population based on the audited sample of items. A population is defined as the entire set of data from which sample items are selected and about which the auditor wants to draw a conclusion.

In practice, auditors can select items from a population in several ways, e.g.,

1. Selecting all items (100% examination)
2. Selecting specific items
3. Audit sampling

Only audit sampling (item 3) allows the auditor to provide evidence on the remainder of a population. Selecting all the items is not really sampling, since everything will be checked. Specific item selection provides evidence only on the items selected, and thus the auditor can logically reach a conclusion only about the selected items. What is unique about audit sampling is that the auditor can use inductive logic to reach a conclusion about items in the part of the population that was not tested. The essence of audit sampling is, first, how auditors can apply this logic, and second, its risks and benefits for auditors.

There are several methods of audit sample selection; the choice depends on the auditor's purpose or objective in selecting the sample. Representative selection is required if the auditor's goal is to reach a conclusion about all items in a population (selected as well as unselected items). Representative sampling can be achieved by randomly selecting items (e.g., using a random number generator as the basis for picking sample items based on a characteristic such as invoice numbers so that every item has an equal chance of being selected), or systematically selecting items (e.g., choosing every 25th item in a population, such as the cash payment transactions journal), or judgmentally selecting items (e.g., flipping through the pages of a long inventory report and arbitrarily stopping on various pages and pointing to an item on each page without following any particular pattern).

Other selection methods may be used that are not considered representative, such as scanning a list of accounts payable balances and picking out the largest numbers or suppliers with the highest volume of purchases, or selecting blocks of data such as 2 weeks out of a 52-week sales journal. Non-representative selection can be used if the auditor's goal is to reach a conclusion about selected items only.

Stratification is a useful technique for selecting samples when the population contains items that vary considerably in value. For example, if the inventory listing contains many low-value items, but also some medium- and a few very high-value items, it may not be representative to base the sample selection on the types of items, since this would tend to pick mostly low-value items. A more representative sampling approach can be achieved by dividing this population into subpopulations, each of which is a group of sampling units that have similar monetary value. The statistical sampling model we use in this book, MUS, automatically accomplishes this with systematic selection. A variation of this approach for a population that contains some individually material items is to divide the population into the material items (which will be subject to 100% examination) and the representative items that will be randomly sampled. MUS automatically accomplishes this as well. Higher-risk items might also be drawn out for 100% examination, for example, very old or disputed outstanding sales invoices. This is a qualitative aspect of sampling and requires professional judgment, as with all sampling methods.

While sampling has many benefits for obtaining reasonable assurance on a timely basis, two kinds of risk are created when auditors sample: sampling risk and non-sampling risk. Sampling risk is the possibility that the auditor's conclusion based on examining a sample of items will be different from the conclusion that would be reached if the entire population were examined. Sampling risk can lead to two types of incorrect conclusions; these are summarized below for tests of control and tests of details.

TYPES OF INCORRECT CONCLUSIONS	TESTS OF CONTROL	TESTS OF DETAILS
Incorrect conclusions that reduce audit effectiveness	Controls are more effective than they actually are.	A material misstatement does not exist when in fact it does.
Incorrect conclusions that reduce audit efficiency	Controls are less effective than they actually are.	A material misstatement exists when in fact it does not.

As you can see, an auditor is primarily concerned with incorrect conclusions that affect audit *effectiveness*, because they are likely to lead to an inappropriate audit opinion. Incorrect conclusions that affect audit *efficiency* arise because these situations often result in doing extra work to determine that the initial conclusions were incorrect. These are not as great a concern as those affecting audit effectiveness, but it is still important to minimize them so valuable time is not wasted.

In essence, sampling risk is like bad luck. Even in a carefully performed sampling application, we still might draw a sample that contains only items that were correct even though the rest of the population was loaded with errors, or we might pick a sample that includes every error in the population while the rest is completely correct.

In contrast, non-sampling risk can be viewed as "bad auditing." It is the possibility that the auditor will make an improper assessment of inherent and/or control risk, or fail to apply audit procedures carefully, or use inappropriate/irrelevant procedures, and generally all other risk of making an incorrect audit conclusion other than sampling risk. Non-sampling risk must be addressed by the quality control policies and procedures in an auditing firm, and it relates closely to the concept of *due care* discussed earlier in the book.

Auditors can use statistical or non-statistical sampling methods. When auditors apply rigorous statistical sampling methods, their approach to sampling will have the following characteristics:

(i) Random selection of the sample items

(ii) The use of probability theory to evaluate sample results, including measurement of sampling risk

Any sampling approach that does not have characteristics (i) and (ii) is considered non-statistical sampling, or judgmental sampling. Non-statistical sampling approaches can be enhanced by using random selection techniques, and as long as the selection method is representative, the findings can be extrapolated to aid in forming a conclusion about the whole population.

Performing sample-based audit procedures involves planning the procedures, collecting the evidence, and evaluating the results to reach a conclusion, as outlined in the table below for the case of non-statistical sampling. (When statistical sampling is used, sampling risk and extrapolated likely misstatement can be calculated; in non-statistical sampling, these are assessed based on the auditor's experience and judgment.)

TESTS OF CONTROL (NON-STATISTICAL SAMPLING)	TESTS OF DETAILS (NON-STATISTICAL SAMPLING)
Plan the procedures: • Specify the audit objectives (assess control effectiveness in relation to significant control objectives). • Define control deviation conditions. • Define the population. • Choose an audit sampling method.	Plan the procedures: • Specify the audit objectives (obtain evidence in relation to the assessed risk of material misstatement at the assertion level). • Specify the performance materiality. • Define the population. • Choose an audit sampling method.
Evidence collection: • Determine the sample size. • Select the sample. • Perform the test of controls procedures.	Evidence collection: • Determine the sample size. • Select the sample. • Perform substantive tests of details procedures.
Evaluate the evidence and conclude: • Calculate the sample deviation rate (SDR). • Determine the rate of deviations in the sample. • Consider that the actual deviation rate for the population may differ due to sampling risk. Make a judgment as to the acceptability of the level of sampling risk. • Compare the SDR to the tolerable deviation rate (TDR); TDR is based on auditor judgment; controls are not expected to be perfect; some level of deviations can be tolerated as long as it's too low to lead to material misstatement.	Evaluate the evidence and conclude: • Determine the amount of known misstatement—the total amount of misstatements actually uncovered by the procedures. • Determine the likely misstatement—based on projecting the misstatement found in the sample to the population using, e.g., the average difference method (or the dollar-unit sampling [DUS] projection method for statistical sampling). • Consider sampling risks, using professional judgment and experience.

(continued)

- Follow up on all deviations uncovered in testing—determine whether deviations are pervasive, deliberate, misunderstandings, or related to financial statement balances.
- Draw final conclusions—if the control risk appears high, the auditor must decide whether to do additional substantive procedures or extend control procedures in the hopes of determining that the actual risk is lower.

- Follow up on all differences uncovered to determine any misunderstanding of generally accepted accounting principles (GAAP), simple mistakes, intentional irregularities suggesting fraud, or management override of controls.
- Evaluate the misstatement—known misstatements and likely misstatements are combined and compared to materiality.
- Sampling risk gives rise to further "possible misstatements"—misstatements that may exist and remain undetected in units not sampled (can be calculated when statistical methods are used).

An example is given in Exhibit 10–2 for stratifying a population in an audit sample for a test of details procedure, and for extrapolating misstatements uncovered in performing the procedure.

Projecting the Known Misstatement to the Population

Say the procedures discover a $600 known misstatement in one of the six stratum 1 items, and $900 in total known misstatements in the remaining 90 sample items. To make a conclusion about the population, the known misstatement in the sample is projected to the population. The sample must be representative, because, if it is not, a projection can produce a misleading number.

As an extreme example, suppose an auditor takes the stratum 1 group of six accounts as being representative of the population. Projecting the $100 average misstatement ($600/6) to 1,506 accounts ($100 × 1,506) would project a total misstatement of $150,600, compared with the recorded accounts receivable total of $400,000. This projection is neither reasonable nor appropriate. Nothing is wrong with the calculation method. The non-representative "sample" is the culprit in this absurd result.

The total known misstatement of $900 in the remaining 90 sample items can be extrapolated to the population; this will be appropriate since the sample is representative. Using the average difference method yields a projected misstatement, or likely misstatement, of $15,000 (i.e., $900/90 × 1,500 = $15,000). Based on the overall material level for the financial statements, auditors would consider whether this size of likely misstatement is significant enough propose a significant adjustment.

EXHIBIT 10–2

Stratification Example—Selecting Sample Sizes

The stratification below subdivides the population into a first stratum of six individually significant accounts and four other strata, each with approximately one-fourth ($75,000) of the remaining dollar balance. This is a typical situation where there are more accounts of smaller value.

The example allocates 90 items to the last four strata. This is referred to as *stratified sampling*. When each stratum gets one-fourth of the sample size, the sample is skewed toward the higher-value accounts: the second stratum has 23 out of 80 sample items, and the fifth stratum has 23 out of 910 items.

STRATUM	BOOK VALUE	NUMBER	AMOUNT	SAMPLE
1	Over $10,000	6	$100,000	6
2	$625–$9,999	80	75,068	23
3	$344–$624	168	75,008	22
4	$165–$343	342	75,412	22
5	$1–$164	910	74,512	23
		1,506	$400,000	96

This stratification deals with a typical situation in which the variability of the account balances and errors in them tend to be larger in the high-value accounts than in the low-value accounts. As a consequence, the sample includes a larger proportion of the high-value accounts (23/80) and a smaller proportion of the low-value accounts (23/910). In addition to size or variability, stratification can be based on other qualitative characteristics the auditor considers important, such as individual, location, date, or product.

Other advanced concepts, which involve considerable auditor judgment, are defined in CAS 530 as tolerable misstatement (closely related to the performance materiality concept), tolerable rate of deviation (like a materiality level for tests of controls, this is the threshold deviation rate—you can think of this as the amount of control deviations that would lead to a material misstatement—the auditor needs to evaluate all deviations quantitatively and qualitatively), and anomaly (a misstatement that is considered so unusual that, in the auditor's judgment, it should not be projected to the rest of the population; identifying an anomaly is a qualitative judgment auditors make and is somewhat controversial since it essentially provides an excuse for the auditor not to demand an adjustment).

Summary of CAS 530: The Canadian Auditing Standards on Audit Sampling

CAS 500 is largely a summary of introductory audit concepts covered in earlier chapters. However, CAS 500 complements CAS 530 by identifying ways of selecting items from a population relevant for auditors (CAS 500.A52):

1. Selecting all items (100% exam)
2. Selecting specific items
3. Audit sampling

CAS 530 (audit sampling) reviews the basic concepts of sampling. It is the first audit standard devoted to sampling topics and indicates the increasing importance of this topic in auditing. The reason for its increasing importance is that it introduces a more rigorous logic to audit judgment and it helps quantify audit risks and uncertainties. In essence, it helps quantify the fundamental concept of information risk to make it more meaningful. Statistical sampling in particular introduces formal models to audit reasoning that can help justify basic decisions on the adequacy of audit testing, and the information risk remaining after completing the audit. See Appendix 10B, Part IV (available on Connect), for a brief history of the audit risk model and how it was influenced by statistical sampling developments in auditing. The audit risk model and related concepts are considered by many to be the most important concepts of auditing from the 20th century.

From the above list you should note that only audit sampling (item 3) allows the auditor to provide evidence on the remainder of a population. Specific item selection provides evidence only on the items selected and thus the auditor can logically reach a conclusion only about the selected items. What is unique about sampling is that the auditor can logically reach a conclusion about items in the population that are not tested using inductive logic. In this chapter we thus focus on the characteristics of reasoning with this logic and the risks and rewards it creates for auditors.

The most important concepts of CAS 530 are the definition of *key classic sampling concepts* in paragraph 5: audit sampling, population, sampling risk, non-sampling risk, statistical sampling, and anomaly to identify unusual misstatements. Let's start with the anomalies concept. Anomalies are a qualitative judgment auditors make about how representative a detected misstatement might be in the population. Specifically, anomalies are misstatements that might be considered so unusual that in the auditor's judgment they should not be projected to the rest of the population. You should view anomalies as qualitative features of misstatements that allow the auditor to not consider the anomaly in the quantitative calculations discussed in the rest of this chapter. Some consider anomalies to be a controversial concept; nevertheless they are in CAS 530. We review the main reasoning concepts that need to be satisfied to support these types of conclusions.

Other concepts covered in CAS 530 are stratification, tolerable misstatements, and tolerable rates of deviation (materiality for tests of controls is called the threshold rate—you can think of this as the amount of control deviations that would lead to a material [tolerable] misstatement). The auditor needs to evaluate all deviations quantitatively and qualitatively.

There are several methods of selecting samples. In parentheses are indicated the possible goals or objectives an auditor might have with each selection technique. Representative means that the auditor's goal is to reach a conclusion about all items in a population (selected as well as unselected items), whereas non-representative means the auditor's goal is to reach a conclusion about selected items only. Note how everything depends on the auditor's purpose or objective in selecting the sample (testing).

The first two selection methods below are suitable for statistical sampling, as we clarify further on:

- Random sampling (representative)
- Systematic sampling (representative)
- Haphazard (judgmental) sampling (representative or non-representative, depending on auditor objectives in selecting the sample or performing the test)
- Block sampling (non-representative)

There are two key features of statistical sampling:

1. **Random sampling** is selection of items when each item has a predictable chance of selection (this predictable amount is what the formulas are based on and allows prediction of sampling risks). The goal is to obtain a *representative sample* of the population.

2. **Statistical evaluation of results** is based on the sampling probability distribution, which is based on some probability model using a predictable chance of selection.

Two types of sampling risk apply to all sampling, statistical and non-statistical:

1. **Effectiveness risk**, from CAS 530.05(c), is the risk of concluding from a sample or test that a material misstatement does not exist when in fact it does (this is also frequently referred to as a Type II error risk in your statistics courses).

2. **Efficiency risk**, from CAS 530.05(c), is the risk of concluding from a sample or test that a material misstatement exists when in fact it does not (this is also frequently referred to as a Type I error risk in your statistics courses).

By CAS 530.14 and CAS 539.A14, auditors must project sample misstatements to the entire population, but this may not be sufficient for deciding on an adjusting entry (specifically, the effectiveness risk may still be too high even for the adjusted amount because the sample size with the detected number of misstatements has too high an effectiveness risk associated with it).

In CAS 530.A3, tolerable misstatement = overall materiality or performance materiality or lower (we show below that with our formulas you can simply use overall materiality as long as that is sufficient to meet user needs for the account or population in question). More specifically, with our formulas below, the planned precision is the tolerable misstatement. Essentially the auditor decides what is tolerable after taking into account materiality. To simplify things in this text we set planned precision to equal materiality, and in Appendix 10B we explain the consequences of this decision.

CAS 530.A6 states that the auditor must clearly define what is a misstatement, both qualitative and quantitative. This is a key audit judgment in sampling.

CAS 530.A13 allows haphazard selection, but some research has shown that it can cause problems due to judgmental biases (these biases are a form of non-sampling error leading to non-sampling risk). Auditors are supposed to control non-sampling errors with proper training, supervision, and public accounting firm quality controls.

By CAS 530.A21–A23 (same as AuG-41), decisions can be based on projected misstatements (this is for non-statistical evaluation). If the results are not acceptable, then the auditor can test alternative controls in the case of control testing, or modify related substantive procedures (using the audit risk model). More details are given in the rest of this chapter and Appendix 10B.

CAS 530, Appendix 1, says that stratification introduces efficiencies. One form of stratification is monetary unit sampling (MUS). Dollar unit sampling (DUS) is one type of MUS. In Canada we use dollars as our currency, so we sometimes refer to DUS, but the same formulas can be applied to any monetary units. MUS also results from having a different perspective on an accounting population, thereby illustrating how a different perspective can have an effect on the audit reasoning process. The formulas below are based on the rate of monetary units, however defined. But once you have settled on the currency, you multiply the currency units (such as dollars, yuan, or euros) by the monetary rate to get the valuation in terms of the currency. In this book we work with Canadian dollars.

CAS 530, Appendices 2 and 3, list factors that influence sample size, which we will see illustrated with MUS below.

CAS 530, Appendix 4, includes the following:

1. Random selection: The objective is to get a representative sample of the population.

2. Systematic selection: This is frequently implemented by adding items through a population. You need to subdivide the population into equal-length intervals called sampling intervals and then randomly select (using the random number table or @RAND function in Microsoft Excel) an item from the first sampling interval. Then add the sampling interval amount to the random number selected, adding your way through the population—this process means you will select one item from each sampling interval, guaranteeing uniform coverage of the population. See Appendix 10B for more details on systematic selection.

3. MUS: MUS, when combined with systematic and random selection, is a very effective way of sampling in continuous online audit environments with electronic evidence. This is one reason MUS dominates in audit practice.

4. Haphazard sampling (unstructured sampling, also referred to as judgmental sampling—the dangers of this approach are emphasized in some research): This is the most widely used approach in practice. Judgmental sampling can also mean something more than haphazard sampling, like the block sampling described in the next line.

5. Block sampling: This is a type of convenience testing, but it is usually not very representative. For example, you may select a block or group of transactions of a particular subperiod or in a particular file, such as testing all transactions during a single month. It may be convenient but usually not very representative of all transactions (such as for a year).

Review Checkpoints

10-1   Why do auditors use the sampling concept as part of their testing procedure?

10-2   What is the essential difference between representative and non-representative testing?

10-3   What is the fundamental difference between statistical and non-statistical sampling?

10-4   Which sampling risk is the most important in auditing and why?

10-5   How do auditors control sampling risk?

10-6   What is non-sampling risk?

10-7   How do auditors control non-sampling risk?

10-8   How do sampling risks relate to the overall audit objective of providing assurance on information?

Introduction to Audit Sampling

LO1   Explain the role of professional judgment in audit sampling decisions.

Audit sampling is the application of an audit procedure to less than 100% of the items within an account balance population or class of transactions in order to evaluate some characteristic of the group.[2] The goal of audit sampling is to get a representative result for an account population or class of transactions. Testing is synonymous with sampling.[3] Sampling was part of the explanation of a control test, which was defined as (1) identifying the data population from which to select a sample of items and (2) describing an action to produce relevant evidence. It is important to understand some sampling theory because it helps explain some of the most important principles of auditing, such as the risk-based approach to auditing. Probability and sampling theory provide the foundations for much of the logic of auditing, including deciding when sufficient evidence has been gathered to support the audit opinion. Sampling theory is the basis of the audit risk model. Just like in your economics course when, for example, you see how the demand equals supply relationship works through equilibrium equations, you can use math to clarify audit and accounting concepts. For example, the basic audit risk model helps clarify the relationship between risk of material misstatement and detection risk. In the more-advanced parts of this book, we probe a little further with math models to deepen your understanding of how risks work in auditing and financial reporting. This chapter begins that process.

This is an important chapter for understanding the logic of auditing. For example, the most fundamental risk concepts in auditing are the effectiveness and efficiency risks, and we relate them to the audit risk model. All risks discussed here are a form of either effectiveness risk or efficiency risk. But the differences in the way these risks behave, and their relative importance for the audit, have a carry-over effect to the other risks based on them. Hence, we treat the distinction between effectiveness and efficiency risk as fundamental. We keep the technical details at a minimum. Supporting details are provided in Appendix 10B.

To understand the definition of audit sampling, you must keep the following definitions in mind. **Audit procedures** are the general audit techniques of Chapter 8 (recalculation/reperformance, observation, confirmation, inquiry, inspection, and analysis). An **account balance** is a control account made up of many constituent items; for example, an accounts receivable control account represents the sum of customers' accounts. A **class of transactions** refers to a group of transactions with common characteristics, such as cash receipts or cash disbursements, but not necessarily added together as an account balance in generally accepted accounting principles (GAAP) financial statements. A **population** is the set of all the elements that

---

audit sampling:
testing less than 100% of a population (items in an account balance or class of transactions) to form a conclusion about some characteristic of the balance or class of transactions

audit procedures:
the general audit techniques of recalculation/reperformance, observation, confirmation, inquiry, inspection, and analysis

account balance:
a control account made up of many constituent items

class of transactions:
groups of accounting entries that have the same source or purpose; credit sales, cash sales, and cash receipts are three different classes

population:
the set of all the elements that constitute an account balance or class of transactions

constitute an account balance or class of transactions; each of the elements within it is a **population unit**. When an auditor selects a sample of the population, each element selected is called a **sampling unit** (e.g., a customer's account, an inventory item, a debt issue, a cash receipt, a cancelled cheque). A **sample** is a set of such sampling units. Specifically, audit sampling is less than 100% examination of items in a population for the purpose of getting a representative result of the population (CAS 530.05). An important professional judgment is how to define a population or class relative to audit objectives.

How Risk and Materiality Are Used in Audit Sampling

Materiality and risk are key concepts in statistical sampling and auditing. This is indicated in CAS 530 by quotations such as the following:

> The determination of an appropriate sample on a representative basis may be made using either statistical or non-statistical methods. Whether statistical or non-statistical methods are used, their common purpose is to enable the auditor to reach a conclusion about an entire set of data by examining only a part of it. Statistical sampling methods allow the auditor to express in mathematical terms the uncertainty he or she is willing to accept and the conclusions of his or her test. The use of statistical methods does not eliminate the need for the auditor to exercise judgment. For example, the auditor has to determine the degree of audit risk he or she is willing to accept and make a judgment as to materiality.

The following box shows how the auditor's professional judgment is applied when deciding how much audit work is required and how the audit finding will be interpreted.

Professional Judgment and the Extent of Audit Testing

Auditing standards have noted that decisions concerning materiality and audit risk are the most significant made in the course of an audit because they form the basis for determining the extent of the auditing procedures to be undertaken (also see CAS 320.06). This illustrates that professional judgment is critical to the appropriate application of audit sampling.

To better understand this, imagine that the audit is a purely scientific endeavour in which the management assertions are hypotheses that have to be either supported (verified) or contradicted by the evidence. An analogy, but not one to be taken too literally, is to think of auditor opinions as being similar to a media opinion poll.

For example, an opinion poll in *The Toronto Star* reported that mayoral candidate M. L. led with 51% of the decided vote over candidate B. H., who had 46% support. This poll was the result of surveying 400 Toronto residents. A sample of this size is considered accurate to within 5 percentage points, 19 times out of 20. In other words, because of the uncertainties associated with the representativeness of the sample of 400, the best the statistician can conclude about M. L.'s prospects is that there is a 95% confidence level that his actual support is in the range 51% ± 5% = 46–56%. The width of this band around M. L.'s best point estimate of 51% is referred to as *sampling precision*, which is related to materiality. The confidence level is most relevant to the auditor when it is related to the assurance level desired from the test. For some statistical models, this alignment with assurance is true only when the statistical test is designed a certain way, as discussed later in this chapter.

Conceptually, an auditor would like conclusions on the financial statements similar to those of a pollster on populations of voters. For example, after audit testing, the auditor may like to conclude that a client's net income number is

(continued)

population unit:
each element of a population

sampling unit:
a unit used for testing a client's population, for example, a customer's account, an inventory item, a debt issue, or a cash receipt

sample:
a set of sampling units

$200,000 ± $10,000, 19 times out of 20. The auditor could make this kind of declaration if the appropriate statistical samples were drawn from all the accounting components that make up net income. In this statistical sampling framework, the degree of accuracy or precision of the sample is related to materiality, that is, the ±$10,000 (or ±5% in the *Star* poll). Audit assurance is the statistical confidence, that is, 19 times out of 20, which is equal to 95%. Thus, if an auditor's report were interpreted purely statistically, "in all material respects" means that the difference between the audit estimate (audit value, or AV) based on audit testing and the reported amount (book value, or BV) is less than material. The level of audit assurance is captured by the words "in our opinion" in the auditor's report. Under this view, the standard audit report indicates, therefore, that there is a high level of assurance that there are no material factual misstatements in the financial statements. We can also look at the complement of assurance, audit risk, discussed in CAS 200, and interpret the standard audit report to mean there is a low level of risk that there are material misstatements in the financial statements after the audit.

Using a statistical sampling framework, the audit report decision will be based on a sufficient amount of testing so that the confidence interval around the auditor's best estimate audit value will both include book value *and* be smaller than materiality; that is, the auditor will have achieved the planned level of assurance from the testing. For example, assume the auditor has done enough testing of a client with a reported net income of $198,000 to conclude with 95% confidence (assurance) that GAAP income is in the interval $198,000 ± $10,000. If materiality is set at 8% of reported income, it equals 0.08 × $198,000 = $15,840. As the achieved precision of $10,000 is less than materiality of $15,840, the auditor can conclude with at least 95% assurance that there is no material error in the reported net income of $198,000.

To reach such a conclusion, the auditor will have to plan the testing so that achieved precision is no larger than materiality. If BV − AV is greater than materiality, the auditor has not obtained the 95% assurance from testing and will have to either do more audit work or insist on an adjustment. Both options involve considerable professional judgment. However, statistical sampling has at least clarified the quantitative issues. Hopefully, this illustrates that statistical sampling does not eliminate professional judgment. But it can aid professional judgment and provide quantitative guidance.

Sampling and the Extent of Auditing

Three aspects of auditing procedures are important—nature, timing, and extent. Nature of audit procedures refers to the six general techniques (recalculation/reperformance, confirmation, inquiry, inspection, observation, and analysis). Timing considers when procedures are performed. More will be said about timing later in this chapter. Audit sampling is concerned primarily with matters of extent—the amount of work done when the procedures are performed. In the context of auditing standards, nature and timing relate most closely to the appropriateness of the evidence, while extent relates most closely to its sufficiency (sample size). Since client files, such as inventory and accounts receivable, can contain thousands of accounting records, it is uneconomical to test them exhaustively, and auditors consider the concept of testing carefully.

Testing is a means of gaining assurance that the amount of error in large files is not material. Statistical sampling is the formal theory supporting the concept of testing, but courts approved it long before statistical theories were introduced to auditing. The majority of testing in auditing was once done on a judgmental basis, but as accounting populations grew, auditors realized that statistical sample sizes could be much smaller than intuition would suggest. For this reason, statistical sampling became increasingly popular in the second half of the 20th century. While both testing methods are equally acceptable by auditing standards, the focus here is on statistics, as the theory underlying it formalizes the reasoning used in pure judgmental (haphazard) testing. Statistical sampling in auditing helps make more precise the key concepts of risk and materiality in auditing. Another advantage of statistical auditing is that it forces auditors to clarify their thinking in planning the audit. For example, statistical auditing forces auditors to define a population more precisely because the statistical conclusion applies only to the part of the population that was statistically sampled. This increased rigour can be useful when justifying the audit work in court, to regulators, and to accountability boards. However, statistical sampling tends to be more time-consuming and requires more training. Hence, definite trade-offs must be made. This is another example of why professional judgment is needed.

The two types of audit programs introduced in Chapter 8 are summarized below. Note that both of these can be performed on a statistical or non-statistical basis.

Two Kinds of Audit Programs: Two Purposes for Audit Sampling

INTERNAL CONTROL PROGRAM	BALANCE AUDIT PROGRAM
Purpose	**Purpose**
Obtain evidence about client's control objective compliance, including	Obtain evidence about client's financial statement assertions, including
Validity	Existence (Occurrence)
Completeness	Completeness
Authorization	Ownership (Rights and obligations)
Accuracy	Valuation
Classification	Presentation and disclosure
Proper period	
Sample	**Sample**
Usually from a class of transactions (population), such as	Usually from items in an asset or liability balance (population), such as
Cash receipts	Accounts receivable
Cash disbursements	Loans receivable
Purchases (inventory additions)	Inventory
Inventory issues	Small tool fixed assets
Sales on credit	Depositors' savings accounts
Expense details	Accounts payable
Welfare payments (eligibility)	Unexpired magazine subscriptions

Review Checkpoints

10-9   Define the following terms: *audit sampling*, *population*, *population unit*, and *sample*.

10-10   What role does professional judgment play in audit decisions regarding materiality, risk, and sampling?

10-11   How does audit assurance relate to audit risk?

10-12   How does sampling relate to forming an audit opinion on financial statements?

Inclusions and Exclusions Related to Audit Sampling

LO2   Distinguish audit sampling work from non-sampling work.

Look again at the audit sampling definition, specifically the statement "to form a conclusion about some characteristic of the balance or class of transactions." This means that an audit procedure is considered audit sampling only if the auditor's objective is to reach a conclusion about the entire account balance or transaction class (the population) on the basis of the evidence obtained from the sample. If the entire population is audited, or if it is only done to gain general familiarity, the work is not considered audit sampling.

Perhaps the distinction between audit sampling and other methods can be seen when considered against the following procedures that are *not* considered audit sampling:

- Complete (100%) audit of all the elements in a balance or class
- Analytical procedures that are overall comparisons, ratio calculations, and the like
- A walk-through—following one or a few transactions through the accounting and control systems to obtain a general understanding of the client's systems
- Methods such as inquiry of employees, obtaining written representations, obtaining inquiry responses via an internal control questionnaire, scanning accounting records for unusual items, and observing personnel and procedures[4]
- Selecting specific items because of their high or key value or some other characteristic of special interest, such as suspected fraud (CAS 530)

Several procedures are typically used in audit sampling applications: recalculation, physical observation of tangible assets, confirmation, and document examination. These procedures are most often applied to the audit of the details of transactions and balances.

Review Checkpoints

10-13 Give examples of auditing procedures that are not sampling applications.

10-14 List audit procedures likely to be applied on a sample basis.

Why Auditors Sample

LO3   Compare and contrast statistical and non-statistical sampling.

Auditors use audit sampling when (1) the nature and materiality of the balance or class does not demand a 100% audit, (2) a decision must be made about the balance or class, and (3) the time and cost to audit 100% of the population would be too great. The latter point is based on the concept of diminishing returns to testing that is illustrated in Appendix 10B. The two sampling designs used are statistical and non-statistical sampling. Exhibit 10–3 provides an overview of the different choices auditors can make about the extent of their testing.

Statistical Sampling

Statistical sampling uses the laws of probability for selecting and evaluating a sample from a population for the purpose of reaching a conclusion about the population. The essential points of this definition are that (1) a statistical sample is selected at random and (2) statistical calculations are used to measure and express the results. Both conditions are necessary for a method to be considered statistical sampling rather than non-statistical sampling.

statistical sampling:
audit sampling that uses the laws of probability to select and evaluate a sample from a population for the purpose of reaching a conclusion about the population

EXHIBIT 10–3

Extent of Audit Testing

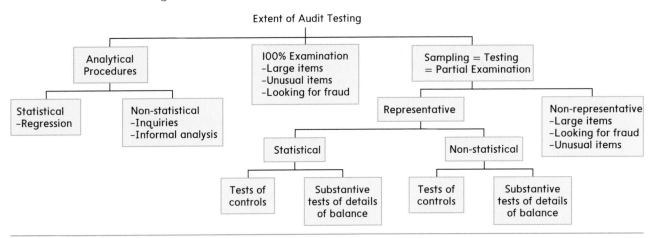

A **random sample** is chosen so that each population item has a predictable probability of being selected in the sample (CAS 530.05). You cannot use statistical calculations with a non-random sample. The mathematical laws of probability don't apply to non-random samples, and basing such calculations on a non-random sample could be misleading.

Any appropriate sample size may be considered statistical sampling. Appropriate in this context means consistent with a statistical sampling model, such as MUS, chosen by the auditor. The model can then be used to calculate the sample size, which indicates the sufficiency of audit work based on risk and materiality objectives. A statistical sampling approach can thus facilitate professional judgments on sufficiency and appropriateness of evidence, as outlined in Exhibit 8–6. A sampling method is statistical by virtue of random selection of the sample coupled with statistical calculation of the results (CAS 530.05).

Use of Statistical Sampling

Use statistical sampling when

- Random numbers can be associated with population items.
- Objective results that can be defended mathematically are desired.
- The auditor has insufficient knowledge about the population to justify a non-statistical sample.
- A representative (random) sample is required.
- Staff are adequately trained in statistical auditing.

Statistical sampling is advantageous because it

- Requires a precise and definite approach to the audit problem.
- Incorporates evaluation showing a direct relation between the sample results and the entire population under audit.
- Requires auditors to specify, and even quantify, particular judgments on risk and materiality.
- Does not eliminate or reduce auditors' professional judgment.
- Allows more objective control of audit risks.
- Results in better planning and documentation when properly implemented (but can be more time-consuming and costly because of the greater formalism required).

random sample:
a set of sampling units so chosen that each population item has an equal likelihood of being selected in the sample

Non-statistical Sampling

Non-statistical (judgmental) sampling is audit sampling in which auditors do not use statistical calculations to express the results. Sample selection can be random sampling or some other selection technique. Auditors are fond of saying that non-statistical sampling involves "consideration of sampling risk in evaluating an audit sample without using statistical theory to measure that risk." In this context, consideration means giving sampling risk some thoughtful attention without directly knowing or measuring its magnitude. Do not confuse sampling and non-sampling risk with statistical and non-statistical sampling. They are not the same, as is further explained in the next learning objective.

Use of Non-statistical Sampling

Use non-statistical sampling when

- Association of population items with random numbers is difficult and expensive.
- Strictly defensible results based on mathematics are not necessary.
- The auditor's knowledge about the population justifies a non-statistical sample with expectation of a reasonable conclusion about the population.
- A representative (random) sample is not required, for example, when an efficient non-statistical sample of large items leaves an immaterial amount unaudited.
- The population is known to be diverse, with some segments especially error prone.

Non-statistical sampling is advantageous because

- It permits a less rigidly defined approach to unique problems that might not fit into a statistical method.
- It permits the auditors to reapply evaluation judgments based on factors in addition to the sample evidence.
- It permits auditors to be less than definite about and omit quantification of particular judgments on risk and materiality.
- It permits auditors to assert standards of subjective judgment. (Thus, the alternative name is judgment sampling.)

Effectiveness Risk, Efficiency Risk, Sampling Risk, and Non-sampling Risk[5]

LO4   Differentiate between effectiveness risk, efficiency risk, sampling risk, and non-sampling risk.

Even when procedures are performed on a sample basis and sufficient evidence is obtained, a conclusion about the population characteristic can still be wrong. For example, suppose an auditor selected 100 sales invoices for audit and found no errors or irregularities in any of them. To conclude from this that there is no significant incidence of errors and irregularities in the entire population of sales invoices might be wrong. How, you ask? The sample might not reflect the actual condition of the population. No matter how randomly or carefully the sample was selected, it might not be a good representation of the extent of errors and irregularities actually in the population.

Review Checkpoints

10-15   Give three reasons why auditors may choose to use sampling.

10-16   What three choices are available to the auditor for deciding on the extent of audit procedures?

10-17   Are testing, partial examination, and sampling the same thing? Explain your response.

non-statistical (judgmental) sampling:
choosing items in a population for audit testing and evaluating the findings based on the auditor's own knowledge and experience rather than statistical methods

10-18   Distinguish between statistical and non-statistical sampling.

10-19   Differentiate between representative and non-representative testing. What client factors determine which is most appropriate in planning audit procedures?

10-20   What is the difference between a statistical representative test and a non-statistical representative test?

10-21   Why can a non-representative test not be done statistically?

Sampling risk is the probability that an auditor's conclusion based on a sample might be different from a conclusion based on an audit of the entire population. If an auditor with more time went through all the invoices and found multiple errors, your sample-based decision would be proved wrong. Apparently, your sample did not represent the population very well. Sampling risk expresses the probability of a wrong decision based on sample evidence, and it is a fact in both statistical and non-statistical sampling methods. With statistical sampling, you can both measure and control sampling risk by auditing sufficiently large samples. With non-statistical sampling, you can "consider" sampling risk without measuring it, something that requires experience and expertise. Other special aspects of sampling risk are discussed later, in the sections on auditing control compliance and account balances.

Two types of sampling risk are efficiency and effectiveness risk. These risks apply to all audit procedures, whether statistical or not, but they are best introduced in a statistical context. **Efficiency risk (type I error risk)** is the risk that the auditor concludes that the population is worse in terms of errors than it really is. **Effectiveness risk (type II error risk)** is the risk that the auditor concludes that the population is better than it really is. Now, which risk covers the situation of the auditor's failing to detect a material misstatement? If you said effectiveness risk you are correct. Effectiveness risk covers the situation where the auditor concludes the population is better (i.e., immaterial misstatements) than it actually is (i.e., material misstatements). Auditors have developed more-specific risk terms for various types of testing, but they are all either efficiency- or effectiveness-type risks. Effectiveness and efficiency risks are the most fundamental risk concepts in auditing. Keep this basic classification in mind to help you better follow the subsequent terminology.

Note also that efficiency and effectiveness risks are very general in that they apply to both statistical and non-statistical sampling. The profession has developed a proliferation of risk terms, but most of these relate to different sources of efficiency- and effectiveness-type errors at different stages of the audit process. For example, we have already noted that all the risks of the audit risk model, including risk of material misstatement, relate to effectiveness-type errors. You can see this just by looking at the definition of effectiveness risk and then comparing it with the definition of the other risks in the audit risk model. Thus, the efficiency and effectiveness risk distinction is the most fundamental categorization of risks in auditing.

We conclude this section with summaries of statistical versus non-statistical sampling and non-sampling risks. The efficiency and effectiveness risk distinction applies to all of these situations, because the distinction applies to any audit situation where immaterial or material misstatements are possible. Since the auditor does not know which state, material or immaterial misstatement, is the true state (if the auditor did know for sure then he or she

sampling risk:
the probability that an auditor's conclusion based on a sample might be different from the conclusion based on an examination of the entire population

efficiency risk (type I error risk):
the risk that the auditor will incorrectly reject an account balance that is not materially misstated; a type of sampling risk

effectiveness risk (type II error risk):
the risk that the auditor will incorrectly accept an account balance that is materially misstated; it can result in audit failure and so is considered to be a more serious problem for the audit than incorrect rejection; a type of sampling risk

would not need to perform audit procedures), these efficiency and effectiveness risk distinctions apply to all of the following summaries. The importance of effectiveness risk for auditing can be seen by noting that an audit deficiency of Chapter 4 can only occur when effectiveness risk is unacceptably high. This occurs when not enough evidence has been gathered (to control effectiveness risk at acceptable levels), or, after gathering the evidence, the risk of undetected material misstatements is too high (because of the small number of errors found in testing).

Non-sampling risk includes the possibility of making a wrong decision, which exists in both statistical and non-statistical sampling. Non-sampling risk's problem is that it cannot be measured. Auditors control it and believe they have reduced it to a negligible level through adequate planning and supervision of the audit, by having policies and procedures for quality control of their auditing practices, and by having internal monitoring and external peer review of their own quality control systems. Auditors are also more open to criticism and fault-finding when erroneous audit decisions result from non-sampling risk. External critics (judges, juries, peer reviewers) have few grounds for criticizing auditors who fall victim to sampling risk, provided that an audit sampling application is planned and executed reasonably well.

Non-sampling risk is all risk other than sampling risk. The audit risk (AR) model given in Chapter 6 is necessary to understanding the breadth of this definition:

$$\text{Risk Model: } AR = IR \times CR \times DR$$

Non-sampling risk can arise from any of the following:

- *Misjudging the inherent risk (IR).* An auditor who mistakenly believes that few material errors or irregularities occur will tend to do less work and, therefore, may fail to detect problems.
- *Misjudging the control risk (CR).* An auditor who is too optimistic about the ability of controls to prevent, detect, and correct errors and irregularities will tend to do less work, with the same results as misjudging the inherent risk.
- *Poor choice of procedures and mistakes in execution—related to detection risk (DR).* Auditors can select procedures inappropriate for the objective (e.g., confirming recorded accounts receivable when the objective is to find unrecorded accounts receivable), fail to recognize errors or irregularities when vouching supporting documents, or sign off on procedures when the work was not actually done.

Examples of Non-sampling Risk

Performing inappropriate procedures: The auditor based the evaluation of inventory obsolescence on forecast sales without adequately evaluating the reasonableness of the forecast assumptions.

Failure to consider test results appropriately: The auditor did not adequately investigate discrepancies in inventory counts and pricing, failing to note misstatements.

Neglecting the importance of analytical review: The auditor might have discovered the client's failure to eliminate intercompany profits if year-to-year product mix, gross profit, and recorded eliminations had been analyzed.

Failure to maintain control over audit procedures: The auditor's lax attitude permitted client employees to tamper with records selected for confirmation.

Lack of professional skepticism: The auditor accepted the client's unsupported verbal representations instead of gathering independent evidence to support management's assertions.

Accounting risk: These are risks related to forecasting the future (risk of forecast errors), typically affecting the measurement or valuation assertions. Accounting risk cannot be eliminated by gathering more evidence, as it is related to auditee business risks not affected by audit procedures. The accounting risk concept helps in identifying deficiencies of accounting estimates that result in misleading financial reporting. Accounting risk and its control are discussed in Chapter 19, Part II (available on Connect).

non-sampling risk:
the possibility of making a wrong decision, which exists in both statistical and non-statistical sampling

EXHIBIT 10–4

Summary of Risks in Audit Testing (Categorized by Type of Test)

RISK	TESTS OF CONTROLS	SUBSTANTIVE TESTS OF BALANCE
Audit risk (AR)	Control risk (CR) component of AR	Risk of incorrect acceptance (RIA) or analytical procedures risk (APR) component of AR
Sampling risk	Risk of selecting a non-representative sample in tests of controls	Risk of selecting a non-representative sample in substantive tests
Efficiency risk	Controlled indirectly via tests of controls	Controlled indirectly via substantive tests
Effectiveness risk	Controlled directly via value for CR	Controlled directly via values for RIA and APR
Non-sampling risk	All other risks associated with testing of controls	All other risks associated with substantive testing

The various risks in auditing are summarized in Exhibit 10–4 by the two broad categories of audit tests. This is the more traditional way of organizing audit risks, as it is based on the two major categories of audit procedures. Exhibit 10–4 focuses on effectiveness risk, efficiency risk, sampling risk, and non-sampling risk associated with gathering evidence. If the effectiveness risks are at unacceptably high levels, then an audit deficiency occurs. This can result in report reservations, as discussed in Chapter 4.

Exhibit 10–5 organizes risk by the primary concepts of efficiency and effectiveness risk. The exhibit thus classifies risks by their relative importance (effectiveness versus efficiency). Note that the importance is reflected by the fact that all risks in the audit risk model fall in the effectiveness risk column. This exhibit summarizes much of the rest of the risk discussion in this chapter.

Sampling Methods and Applications

Audit sampling concerns the amount of work performed and the sufficiency of audit evidence obtained. Its terminology includes many new concepts and definitions. The ones presented in earlier chapters, however, are general and apply to all phases of audit sampling. Knowing them allows you to "speak the language."

Auditors design audit samples to (1) evaluate control effectiveness in assessing control risk and (2) audit account balances in gathering direct evidence about financial statement assertions. These two parts will be covered in the next sections of the chapter. Each design is organized in terms of planning, performing, and evaluating audit sampling.

EXHIBIT 10–5

Summary of Risks in Audit Testing (Now Categorized by Efficiency and Effectiveness Risk Types)

RISK	EFFICIENCY RISK	EFFECTIVENESS RISK
Audit risk (AR)	Not represented in AR model	AR and its control risk (CR), risk of incorrect acceptance (RIA), and analytical procedures risk (APR) components
Sampling risk	Statistical risk of incorrectly rejecting a population or class of transactions	Statistical risk of incorrectly accepting a population or class of transactions
Non-sampling risk	Judgmental risk of incorrectly rejecting a population or class of transactions	Judgmental risk of incorrectly accepting a population or class of transactions
Tests of controls risks	Risk of assessing CR too high (under-reliance on controls)	Risk of assessing CR too low (Over-reliance on controls)
Substantive procedures risks: Detection risk and its components RIA and APR	Risk of incorrect rejection (RIR)	RIA

This chapter is presented in general terms, along the same lines as CAS 530, but with some basic formulas to clarify relationships. The chapter also reconciles with *CPA Canada Handbook* section 5300, the auditing guideline "Applying the Concept of Materiality," and the American Institute of Certified Public Accountants (AICPA) audit and accounting guide titled "Auditing Sampling." (5300 and the AuG are replaced by CAS, but retained in the CPA Canada standards collection on a temporary basis for reference.)

Review Checkpoints

10-22   What is non-sampling risk? Give some examples.

10-23   Define sampling risk.

10-24   Does sampling risk always exist in both statistical and non-statistical sampling? Explain your response.

10-25   Can sampling risk be avoided? Explain.

10-26   Can non-sampling risk be avoided? Explain.

10-27   Are auditors more likely to be sued successfully for sampling risk or for non-sampling risk?

10-28   What two types of audit programs are ordinarily used as written plans for audit procedures?

10-29   What are control tests? What purpose do they serve?

Test of Controls for Assessing Control Risk

LO5   Develop a simple audit program to test a client's internal control procedures.

Auditors must assess control risk to determine the nature, timing, and extent of other audit procedures. Final evaluations of internal control are based on evidence obtained in the review and testing phases of an evaluation. It is difficult to describe control risk assessments, as they depend entirely on judgments made under the circumstances of each specific situation. For example, an auditor might learn that a company requires the bookkeeper to match a shipping order with each sales invoice before recording a sale, as a control against the recording of fictitious sales. Now, suppose this control test shows a number of invoices without supporting shipping orders, possibly causing sales to be overstated. More-extensive work on accounts receivable using confirmation, inquiries, and analytical review related to collectability would deal with this control deficiency. This shows how control testing provides only indirect evidence of the monetary accuracy of the accounts. Failure to have a matching shipping order only increases the probability of a monetary misstatement but does not guarantee a misstatement; the shipping orders might have been misplaced and the recorded sales invoice might still be correct. Only further substantive work, such as direct confirmation with the customer, would provide convincing evidence of a misstatement.

This example related a specific control (matching sales invoices with shipping orders) to a specific set of audit procedures directed toward a possible problem (overstatement of sales and receivables). Generally, auditors reach judgments about control risk, as shown in Exhibit 10–6. Some situations call for a non-quantitative expression and some for a quantitative expression. The quantitative ranges overlap, communicating that auditors cannot put exact numbers on these kinds of evaluations.

Sampling Steps for Tests of Control

LO5a   Specify objectives, deviation conditions, populations, and sampling units.

Audit sampling is a structured, formal approach and plan for conducting control. The seven-step framework helps auditors plan, perform, and evaluate control test results. It also helps auditors accomplish an eighth

EXHIBIT 10–6

Auditor's Assessment of Control Risk

EVALUATION OF INTERNAL CONTROL	JUDGMENT EXPRESSION OF CONTROL RISK	
	NON-QUANTITATIVE	QUANTITATIVE
Excellent control, both as specified and in compliance	Low (1)	10%–30%
Good control, but lacks something in specification or compliance	Moderate (2)	20%–70%
Deficient control, either in specification or compliance or both	High (3)	60%–95%
Little or no control	Maximum	100%

If combining inherent and control risk evaluation is easier, then "low," "moderate," and "high" mean the following, respectively:
1. Low combined inherent and control risk
2. Moderate combined inherent and control risk
3. High combined inherent and control risk

step—careful documentation of the work and reasoning—by showing each of the seven areas to be described in the working papers. The first seven steps are as follows:

1. Specify the audit objectives.

2. Define the deviation conditions.

3. Define the population.

4. Determine the sample size.

5. Select the sample.

6. Perform the control tests.

7. Evaluate the evidence.

Plan the Procedures

The first three steps are the phase of **problem recognition**. When a client describes the control system, the implicit assertion is, "These controls work; people comply with the control procedures and achieve the control objectives." The auditors' question (problem) is, "Is it so? Are the validity and other control objectives achieved satisfactorily?"

Testing of controls is always directed toward producing evidence of the client's performance of its own control procedures. Thus, auditors' procedures should produce evidence about the client's achievement of the seven control objectives.

Specify the Audit Objectives

An example of a validity control procedure is the client's procedure of requiring a shipping order to be matched with a sales invoice before a valid sale is recorded. The specific objective of an auditor's test of controls audit procedure could be, "Determine whether recorded sales invoices are supported by matched shipping orders." The audit procedure itself would be, "Select a sample of recorded sales invoices and vouch them to supporting shipping orders."

The matching of sales invoices to shipping orders is a *key control* and important here. Auditors should identify and audit only the key controls. Incidental controls are not relied on to reduce control risk, and auditing them for compliance just wastes time.

problem recognition:
the first three steps of the sampling method

Define the Deviation Conditions

The terms *deviation, error, occurrence,* and *exception* are synonyms in test of controls sampling. They all refer to departure from a prescribed internal control procedure; for example, an invoice is recorded with no supporting shipping order (bill of lading). Deviation conditions need to be defined at the outset so that the auditors will know a deviation when they see one. As an assistant accountant, you would prefer to be instructed to "select a sample of recorded sales invoices, vouch them to supporting shipping orders, and document cases where the shipping order is missing," rather than, "check recorded sales invoices for mistakes." The latter instruction does not clearly define the deviation conditions and can increase non-sampling risk.

This example is oversimplified, but this vouching procedure for compliance evidence might be used to obtain evidence about several control objectives at the same time. The invoice can be compared with the shipping order for evidence of actual shipment (validity) and reviewed for credit approval (authorization); prices can be compared with the price list (authorization and accuracy); and quantity billed can be compared with quantity shipped (accuracy), recalculated (arithmetic accuracy), compared for correspondence of shipment date and record date (proper period), and traced to postings in the general ledger and subsidiary accounts (accounting).

Exhibit 10–7 shows some deviation conditions laid out in a working paper designed to record the control testing results for a sample of sales invoices.

Test of controls audit sampling is also called **attribute sampling**—sampling in which auditors look for the presence or absence of a control condition. In response to the audit question, "For each sales invoice in the

---

EXHIBIT 10–7

Test of Controls Audit Documentation

Index _m 10.3_   By _J C_   Date _Nov. 11, 20X2_
                        Review _J.D._   Date _Nov. 15, 20X2_

KINGSTON COMPANY
Test of Controls over Recorded Sales
December 31, 20X2

Invoice number	Date	Amount	Bill of lading	Credit approved	Approved prices	Quantities match	Arithmetic accurate	Dates match	Posted to customer
35000	Mar. 30	$ 3,000							
35050	Mar. 31	$ 800			X				
35100	Apr. 2	$ 1,200					Y		
35150	Apr. 3	$ 1,500			Y				
35200	Apr. 5	$ 400							
35250	Apr. 6	$ 300	X			X	Y	X	
32100	Jan. 3	$ 1,000							
32150	Jan. 4	$ 200							
34850	Mar. 25	Missing	X	X	X	X	X	X	
34900	Mar. 26	$ 100			Y				
34950	Mar. 27	$ 200							
Sample = 200		$98,000							
Uncorrected deviations			4	9	5	6	3	7	0

(handwritten annotations above column headers: validity, authorization, authorization, accuracy, accuracy, validity/proper period/completeness, classification)

(handwritten, right margin: → 7 Internal control Tests)

X = Uncorrected deviation.
Y = Deviation occurred but was detected and corrected later.

(handwritten, left margin: attribute sampling)
(handwritten: 4/200 = 2% sample deviation rate)

---

attribute sampling:
the type of audit sampling in control testing in which auditors look for the presence or absence of a control condition

sample, can a matched shipping order be found?" the answer can be only yes or no. With this definition, auditors can count the number of deviations and use the count when evaluating the evidence. Attribute sampling can also be useful in balance auditing; an example is shown in the box below.

A Balance Audit Application of Attribute Sampling

Attribute control test samples are usually drawn from a class of transactions in order to obtain evidence about compliance with control objectives. Attribute samples may be used for balance audit purposes. This example suggests an attribute sample to obtain evidence about an ownership (rights) financial statement assertion.

Question: A lessor is in the business of leasing autos, large trucks, tractors, and trailers. Is it necessary for the auditors to examine the titles to all the equipment?

Answer: It is not necessary, unless some extraordinary situation or circumstance is brought to light, for the auditors to examine titles to all the equipment. Random test verification of title certificates or proper registration of vehicles should be made.

Source: AICPA Technical Practice Aids, 8330.02.

Define the Population

Specifying the control test (compliance) audit objectives and the deviation conditions usually defines the population, that is, the set of all elements in the balance or class of transactions. In our example, the population consists of all the recorded sales invoices, and each invoice is a population unit. In **classical attribute sampling**, a sampling unit is the same thing as a population unit.[6]

Population definition is important because audit conclusions can only be made about the population the sample was selected from. For example, evidence from a sample of recorded sales invoices cannot be used for a conclusion about completeness. Controls related to the completeness objective (in this case, control over failure to record an invoice for goods shipped) can only be audited by sampling from a population representing goods shipped (the shipping order file) and not by sampling from the population of recorded invoices.

The timing of the audit work complicates population definition. Control tests should ideally be applied to transactions executed throughout the entire period under audit. However, auditors often perform control tests at an interim date—a date some weeks or months before the client's year-end date—when the entire population is not available for audit. Doing the work at an interim date is fine, but auditors cannot ignore the period between the interim date and the year-end. Strategies for control in the period after the interim date are explained later.

The question of how well the **physical representation of the population** corresponds to the population itself also complicates the population definition. The physical representation of the population is the auditor's frame of reference for selecting a sample. It can be a journal listing of recorded sales invoices, a file drawer full of invoice copies, a computer file of invoices, or another physical representation. The sample will actually be selected from the physical representation, so it must be complete and correspond to the actual population. The physical representation of the recorded sales invoices as a list in a journal is fairly easy to visualize. However, an auditor should make sure that periodic listings (e.g., monthly sales journals) are added correctly and posted to the general ledger sales accounts. In our example, a selection of individual sales invoices from the sales journal is known to be from the complete population of recorded sales invoices, but some physical representations are not so easy to assess for the completeness of correspondence to their population.

classical attribute sampling:
sampling in which a sampling unit is the same thing as an invoice or population unit

physical representation of the population:
the auditor's frame of reference for selecting a sample, for example, a journal listing of recorded sales invoices

These issues are not changed much whether the records are in electronic or hard-copy form. Electronic records are usually based on the design of an originating hard copy. Hence sampling an electronic population is not that different from sampling a hard-copy population. Of course, it is much easier to read through and summarize an electronic population, so 100% exams are more common in an information technology (IT) audit environment. However, at some point auditors need to reconcile the electronic records with facts in the real world. It is this more time-consuming reconciliation process with other information that largely makes sampling relevant in an IT audit.

The Procedures

LO5b   Demonstrate some basic audit sampling calculations.

The next three performance steps represent the phase of **evidence collection** of the sampling method. These steps are performed to obtain the evidence.

Determine the Sample Size

Sample size—the number of population units to audit—should be determined thoughtfully. Some auditors operate on the "magic number theory" (e.g., select 30, because that is what we have always used on this audit). But a magic number may not provide enough evidence or it may be too large a sample. Auditors must consider four influences on sample size: sampling risk, tolerable deviation rate, expected population deviation rate, and population size.

Sampling Risk (CAS 530.05)   Effectiveness risk and efficiency risk are the two major categories of sampling risk. Sampling risk is defined as the probability that a conclusion based on the audit of a sample might be different from a conclusion based on an audit of the entire population. In other words, when using evidence from a sample for testing controls, an auditor might decide that (1) control risk is very low when, in fact, it is not (i.e., an effectiveness risk error), or (2) control risk is very high when, in fact, it is not so bad (i.e., an efficiency risk error). The more you know about a population (from a larger sample), the less likely you are to reach a wrong conclusion, or the lower the sampling risk will be of making either of the two decision errors. More will be said about these risks in the section on evaluation.

In terms of our example, the important sampling risk is the probability that the sample will reveal few or no recorded sales invoices without supporting shipping orders when, in fact, the population contains many such deviations. This result would lead to the erroneous conclusion that the control worked well. Auditing a larger sample reduces the probability of finding few deviations when many exist. Thus, sample size varies inversely with the amount of sampling risk an auditor is willing to take. We will illustrate with calculations after covering some more concepts.

Tolerable Deviation Rate (CAS 530.05)   Auditors should have an idea of how rates of deviation in the population correspond to control risk assessments. Perfect control compliance is not necessary, so the question is rather what rate of deviation in the population signals control risk of 10%, 20%, or 30%, and so forth, up to 100%. Suppose an auditor believes that $90,000 of sales invoices could contain control deviations without causing a minimum material misstatement in the sales and accounts receivable balances. If the total gross sales are $8.5 million, this judgment implies a **tolerable deviation rate** of about 1% ($90,000/$8.5 million). Since this 1% rate marks the minimum material misstatement, it indicates a low control risk (say, 0.05), and it justifies a great deal of reliance on internal control in the audit of the sales and accounts receivable balances.

---

evidence collection:
steps 4, 5, and 6 of the sampling method, which are performed to get the evidence

tolerable deviation rate:
the rate of deviation that can exist without causing a minimum material misstatement in a test of controls procedure

However, there can be more than one tolerable deviation rate. Each successively higher rate is associated with a higher control risk. Continuing with our example, higher tolerable deviation rates could be associated with higher control risks as follows:[7]

DEVIATION RATE (%)	CONTROL RISK
1	0.05
2	0.10
4	0.20
6	0.30
8	0.40
10	0.50
12	0.60
14	0.70
16	0.80
18	0.90
20	1.00

Since sample size varies inversely with the tolerable deviation rate, the auditor who wants to assess control risk at 0.05 (tolerable rate = 1%) will need to audit a larger sample of sales transactions than another auditor who is willing to assess control risk at 0.40 (tolerable rate = 8%). The desired control risk level and its tolerable rate are a matter of auditor choice.

The tolerable rate is not a fixed rate until the auditor decides what control risk assessment suits the audit plan, at which point it becomes a decision criterion involved in the sampling application. Some auditors express the tolerable rate as a number (necessary for statistical calculation of sample size), while others do not put a number on it. Appendix 10B contains more explanation about determining various tolerable rates.

Expected Population Deviation Rate (CAS 530, Appendix 2)   Auditors usually know of or suspect some control performance conditions. They could have last year's audit experience with the client or information from a predecessor auditor, which informs them about the client's personnel, working conditions, and general control environment. This knowledge contributes to an **expectation about the population deviation rate**, an estimate of the ratio of the number of expected deviations to population size. If there was a 1% deviation in last year's audit, this year's expected rate could be 1% as well. Auditors can also stipulate a zero expected deviation rate, which will produce a minimum sample size for the audit. The reason for using an expected error rate greater than zero is solely for the purpose of reducing efficiency risk over its range. Some accounting firms as a matter of policy use an expected rate of zero errors in budgeting for an audit. The rationale is that auditees should pay extra if the audit is less efficient as a result of finding some errors.

From a common-sense perspective, the expected rate of deviation must be less than the tolerable rate, as there would be no reason to perform any test of controls if the auditor expected to find more error than the tolerable amount. Also, the closer the expected rate is to the tolerable rate, the larger is the sample needed to reach a conclusion that deviations do not exceed the tolerable rate. Thus, sample size varies directly with the expected deviation rate. Some auditors will express the expected rate as a number (necessary for statistical calculations of sample size), while others will not put a number on it.

expectation about the population deviation rate:
an estimate of the ratio of the number of expected deviations to population size

The simplified approach we use in this chapter to illustrate the calculations does not quantify the expected population deviation—effectively, the expected rate is zero. This expected error rate results in use of the smallest statistical sample sizes possible, consistent with auditor effectiveness risk and materiality objectives. Some auditors use these smallest statistical sample sizes as a guide to the minimal amount of testing even for non-statistical sampling (e.g., see AICPA, "Audit Sampling Guide," May 1, 2008, edition, p. 34). Statistical sample size calculations can, thus, be an important guide in all audit sampling situations (CAS 530). The application case in Appendix 10B shows that the primary purpose of quantifying the expected deviation rate is to control the efficiency risk. Appendix 10B explains how to work with non-zero expected population deviation rates.

Population Size   Common sense probably tells you that samples should be larger for bigger populations (a direct relationship). While your common sense is accurate, practically speaking, the appropriate sample size for a population of 100,000 units may be only two or three sampling units larger than that for a 10,000-unit population. Not much difference! By using the same calculation for both populations, your sample size for the 10,000 population is proportionally bigger, and thus more conservative. The general principle is that if you use the simplified formulas for very large populations, you end up with slightly conservative results. Many practising auditors find this trade-off worthwhile.

The four influences on sample size in this section, and summarized in Exhibit 10–8, are applicable to both statistical and non-statistical sampling.

Calculating Sample Size   The preceding discussion of sample size determinants gives you a general understanding of the four influences on sample size. Next, we consider a simplified way of calculating sample sizes with a brief overview of basic formulas and tables used in statistical auditing.

Some basic formulas provide an overview of the most fundamental mechanics of statistical auditing. Two key points at which the formulas and tables are used in statistical sampling are (1) sample-size planning and (2) sample evaluation. With the commonly used approach of **monetary-unit sampling (MUS)**, the same formula and table can be applied to both tests of controls and substantive tests of balances. MUS is common because it is effective, efficient, and the easiest approach to use. MUS can be used for control tests either with MUS selection or with physical representation of a population of transactions.

EXHIBIT 10–8

Sample-Size Relationships: Test of Controls Auditing

| SAMPLE-SIZE INFLUENCE | PREDETERMINED SAMPLE SIZE WILL BE | | |
	HIGH RATE OR LARGE POPULATION	LOW RATE OR SMALL POPULATION	SAMPLE-SIZE RELATIONSHIP
1. Acceptable sampling risk	Smaller	Larger	Inverse
2. Tolerable deviation rate	Smaller	Larger	Inverse
3. Expected population deviation rate	Larger**	Smaller	Direct
4. Population	Larger*	Smaller*	Direct

*The effect on sample size is quite small for a population of 1,000 or more.
**The effect of this is explained in Appendix 10B. Many auditors do not quantify the expected rate because it relates to the less serious efficiency risk control, not the more serious effectiveness risk, as discussed earlier this chapter.

---

monetary-unit sampling (MUS):
a modified form of attributes sampling that permits auditors to reach conclusions about monetary amounts as well as compliance deviations

We begin by illustrating the use of MUS formulas in sample-size planning for tests of control. The following discussion is based on the R value table given in Appendix 10A and uses the formula $R = nP$; R is the value from the table in Appendix 10A; n is the sample size; and P stands for the precision, or accuracy, desired for the statistical test. Note that this table gives a unique R value for each combination of K (number of errors) and confidence level. Since, as explained in Appendix 10B, MUS uses the negative approach, confidence level = one minus effectiveness risk. Therefore, the auditor controls effectiveness risk with MUS by picking the appropriate confidence level. Selection of the K value influences the efficiency risk. Specifically, the higher the K value used, the lower is the efficiency risk over much of the range of possible immaterial misstatements. With a valid MUS sample size the efficiency risk is always controlled at zero when there are no errors.

For planning audit sample sizes using the basic equation $R = nP$ and solving for n, we get the equation $n = R/P$. This equation for n summarizes the key factors affecting the sufficiency of audit evidence: the relationship between confidence level (R value), materiality (P value), and the extent of audit testing (sample size n). That is, the amount of audit work is directly proportional to the confidence level and inversely proportional to the materiality level used.

For tests of controls and substantive tests, solve for n (as above) in the formula $R = nP$, where $R = {}_{CL}R_K$ is a confidence-level (CL) factor that is unique for each combination of CL and K from the table of values for R given in Appendix 10A. P is based on overall materiality or specific materiality, as discussed in CAS 320 and Chapter 5. With non-MUS models, sometimes the overall or specific materiality is adjusted lower in sample planning, thereby creating the performance materiality concept of CAS 320 and the tolerable misstatement concept of CAS 530.A3. For tests of controls, a further complication is created by the need to link control deviation rates to the adjusted materiality, as discussed above. This is likely why CAS 530.05 introduces the tolerable rate of deviation and distinguishes it from tolerable misstatement. The tolerable rate of deviation is represented as a rate or proportion. The auditor must use professional judgment in specifying K, CL, and planned P. The effects of these various decisions on sample size are summarized in Exhibit 10–8. Using these concepts results in the simplified approach described in this section.

P is the amount, as a rate, that the auditor considers the tolerable rate of deviation for the population being tested. When being set, it has to take into consideration the additive effect of errors in other accounting populations representing other balances or transaction streams. In this stage of sampling, the planned P might be an amount lower than the tolerable rate of deviation so that the auditor can reduce efficiency risk. Firm practice varies: efficiency risk can be indirectly controlled through the *planned K* value, the *planned P* value, or a combination of the two. The most common strategy is to use $K = 0$ and a *planned P* in the range of half to full tolerable rate of deviation, whichever the auditor deems more appropriate in the circumstances. We discuss these options further in Appendix 10B. Here, the calculations are simplified by assuming that planned P is set equal to the tolerable rate of deviation. This results in the smallest sample size possible for the stated confidence level and precision. This smallest sample size is used by many firms as a guide to sufficient sample sizes for all representative sampling, whether statistical or non-statistical (e.g., see AICPA, "Audit Sampling Guide," May 1, 2008, edition, p. 34). These properties are illustrated in the Application Case of Appendix 10B.

In the formula CL = 1 − effectiveness risk, effectiveness risk is the risk that the test will fail to detect a tolerable rate of deviation when it exists—the risk of incorrect acceptance (RIA). Efficiency risk is the risk of concluding that there is a material misstatement when, in fact, the misstatements are immaterial—the risk of incorrect rejection (RIR).

To illustrate the calculations using the table of R values in Appendix 10A, let us assume the auditor wants a confidence level of 95%; uses $K = 0$ to make the sample planning as simple as possible (this results in the smallest sample size for the planned confidence level); and sets planned P so that it equals the tolerable deviation rate, which we assume here is 0.05, so planned $P = 0.05$. Using our formula $n = R/P$ and the table, you should get the following results: $n = 3.0/0.05 = 60$, so that your planned sample size, given these objectives, is 60. We will use this sample size to evaluate the sample results a little further on.

Working with tables based on the above formulas will minimize the use of formulas. For example, the simplified table titled "Table to Determine Sample Sizes for Tests of Control Using the Monetary-Unit Sampling

Approach" in Appendix 10A is constructed using the calculations with formulas in the preceding paragraph. A table is usually based on some formula or algorithm. When using such a table, the auditor only needs to identify the required effectiveness risk ($= 1 - $ CL) and tolerable deviation rate. In constructing the table, the expected error rate is zero ($K = 0$), thereby leading to the smallest sample size possible for the stated confidence level and tolerable rate. This table is restricted to the most common effectiveness risk levels of 0.10 and 0.05 and the most commonly used tolerable deviation rates. Thus, the table is quite small. To figure out the sample size, the auditor looks up the number in the table that is at the intersection of the desired effectiveness risk and tolerable rate. Using a desired effectiveness risk of 0.05 (or, equivalently, a desired confidence level of 0.95) and a tolerable rate for tests of controls of 0.05, the table gives 60 as the desired sample size. The same size sample could have been calculated using the formula. Your instructor will indicate to you which approach is to be used in your course.

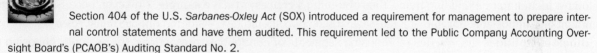

A Note on Testing of Controls for Audits of Internal Control Statements

Section 404 of the U.S. *Sarbanes-Oxley Act* (SOX) introduced a requirement for management to prepare internal control statements and have them audited. This requirement led to the Public Company Accounting Oversight Board's (PCAOB's) Auditing Standard No. 2.

What does testing of controls mean in this new context? First, internal control statements focus on company-level control objectives such as "tone at the top," corporate codes of conduct, and corporate governance in general. Second, the focus is on the design of internal control at a specific point in time. Third, auditors need to utilize an authoritative framework for evaluating the design. For example, the PCAOB requires that the following be considered as part of the framework of suitable internal control criteria for the purpose of reporting on internal control: control environment, risk assessment, control activities, information and communication, and monitoring. This chapter stresses testing of detailed control activities.

Select the Sample

Auditing standards express two requirements for samples: (1) Sampling units must be selected from the population an audit conclusion will apply to, ideally from transactions executed throughout the period under audit, and (2) a sample must be representative of the population it is drawn from. Thus, a sample mirrors the characteristics of the population, but auditors cannot guarantee its representativeness. After all, that is what sampling risk is all about—the probability that the sample might not mirror the population well enough.

Auditors can try to attain representativeness by selecting random samples—each unit in the population has an equal probability of being included in the sample. Intentionally or accidentally excluding a segment of a population can render a sample non-representative. Random samples are often selected by assigning a number to each population unit (sometimes the units are prenumbered forms) and then choosing a selection of random numbers to make up the sample. A printed random number table (one is provided in Appendix 10A) or a computerized random number generator, such as the @RAND function in Microsoft Excel, will generate a list of random numbers. This method is known as **unrestricted random selection**.

Systematic random selection is another popular method. It is especially popular with MUS. To use it, the population size and a predetermined sample size are needed. A random starting place in the physical representation (list of sales invoices recorded in a sales journal, for example) is chosen, and then every Kth unit is selected, where the value for K is population size divided by sample size. For example, if 10,000 invoices, numbered from 32071 to 42070, were issued and you want a sample of 200, first randomly choose a starting place, say invoice

unrestricted random selection:
using a printed random number table or computerized random number generator to obtain a list of random numbers

systematic random selection:
using a predetermined population and sample size and random starting places

35000, and then select every Kth = 10,000 ÷ 200 = 50th invoice. So, the next invoice would be 35050, then 35100, then 35150, and so on. If the end of the list is reached before 200 are selected, cycle back to the sequence beginning invoice, 32071, and continue. Most systematic samples are selected using five or more random starts in the population. MUS can use systematic sampling as just described or work with the dollar value of the transactions processed instead. The population size is then the monetary value of the population. For example, assume the 10,000 invoices had a total value of $10,000,000; then the sampling interval would be $50,000; that is, select every 50,000th dollar. This means finding the invoice associated with that dollar and continuing as previously described.

With sample selection there is a critical distinction between statistical and non-statistical audit sampling. In statistical sampling evaluation, the sample must be random, while in non-statistical plans, auditors sometimes use sample selection methods where randomness and representativeness cannot easily be evaluated. **Haphazard selection** refers to any unsystematic way of selecting sample units, for example, closing your eyes and dipping into a file drawer of sales invoices to pick items. You may pick only the crumpled ones that stick out, and they may be different from most of the other invoices in the drawer. Also, your method cannot be described so that someone can **replicate** it. Some auditors describe haphazard sampling as choosing items without any special reason for including or excluding items, thus obtaining a **representative sample**. However, because it is hard to document and impossible to replicate, haphazard selection should be considered only as a last resort.

Block sampling is the practice of choosing segments of contiguous transactions, for example, choosing the sales invoices processed on randomly chosen days, say February 3, July 17, and September 29. Implicitly, the block-sampling auditor has defined the population unit as a business day (260 to 365 of them in a year) and has selected three—not much of a sample. Block sampling is undesirable because it is hard to get a representative sample of blocks efficiently; having enough blocks means there is a huge number of invoices to audit for compliance.

Some auditors try to get the best of both worlds and use statistical sampling formulas to determine the sample size (as explained above), but combine this with haphazard selection, which is commonly used in auditing. Sample sizes determined using the formulas are frequently much smaller than your intuition would suggest. See the Application Case at the end of this chapter. This helps explain the initial popularity of statistical sampling—it greatly reduced audit work! However, these formulas are valid only with random selection or close approximations to random selection.

Haphazard sampling is intended to be representative of a population, but rigorous random or systematic selection is *not* used. Thus, the probability of selecting a particular item becomes unpredictable. Research by Hall and Herron illustrates one source of such unpredictability: bias due to non-sampling errors.[8] Specifically, judgmental biases arise from items that stand out or draw attention (brightly coloured items, large items, isolated items of inventory or files) or items that are easier to access. When auditors use haphazard sampling they should be trained in de-biasing procedures if they want this type of evidence to be acceptable in court. Otherwise, the auditor must be prepared to non-statistically sample a very large proportion of the population (30% or more). For example, in many practical situations, the auditor would need to test about 10 times as many items as the sample size formulas with true random selection indicate. That is quite a penalty to pay for not using true random selection! This illustrates another advantage of the more formal statistical sampling—potentially smaller amounts of testing can result, as documented by Hall and Herron's article.

haphazard selection:
an unsystematic way of selecting sample units

replicate:
reperform a selection procedure and get the same sample units

representative sample:
a sample that mirrors the characteristics of the population being studied

block sampling:
choosing segments of contiguous transactions; undesirable because it is hard to get a representative sample efficiently

Another practical reason auditors would want to use statistical sampling is that it allows an objective measure of the sampling risk, specifically, the risk of failing to detect a material misstatement (effectiveness risk). Statistical sampling allows calculation of a measurable risk that an auditor is taking in the testing process. The disadvantage of this is the extra training required to use statistical methods properly. Auditors have been deterred by the training costs associated with using statistics, but the Hall and Herron article shows that it is just as important to get training in correctly applying non-statistical representative sampling! Failure to do so puts the auditor at risk of not properly applying audit procedures.

Perform the Control Tests

An internal control program consists of procedures designed to produce evidence about the effectiveness of a client's internal control performance, and now you are ready to obtain the evidence. The control tests are explained in Chapter 8.

Review Checkpoints

10-30   Why can poor controls over the existence of sales result in an overstated accounts receivable balance at year-end?

10-31   In control testing, why is it necessary to define a compliance deviation in advance? Give seven examples of compliance deviations.

10-32   Which judgments must an auditor make when deciding on a sample size?

10-33   Describe the influence of each judgment on sample size.

10-34   Name and describe four sample selection methods.

The Evidence

LO5c   Evaluate evidence from control testing.

The final step is **evidence evaluation** of the sampling method. First, you determined whether each specified key control procedure worked satisfactorily. Then you gathered relevant compliance evidence. Now you need to evaluate the evidence and make justifiable decisions about the control risk.

Evaluate the Evidence

Test of controls audit sampling provides evidence of whether a client's internal control procedures are being followed satisfactorily. Compliance evidence, therefore, is very important for the conclusion about control risk. When auditors evaluate sample-based compliance evidence, there are two sampling risk decision errors they might make: assessing the control risk too low or assessing it too high. The **risk of assessing the control risk too low** is the probability that the compliance evidence in the sample indicates low control risk when the actual (but unknown) degree of compliance justifies a higher control risk assessment. This can lead to failure to do the necessary additional work and threatens the effectiveness of the audit. This is the effectiveness risk for tests of

evidence evaluation:
the final step of the sampling method; to evaluate the evidence and make justifiable decisions about the control risk

risk of assessing the control risk too low:
the probability that the compliance evidence in the sample indicates low control risk when the actual (but unknown) degree of compliance justifies a higher control risk assessment

controls. On the other hand, the **risk of assessing the control risk too high** is the probability that the control test evidence in the sample indicates high control risk when the actual (but unknown) degree of compliance justifies a lower control risk assessment. This is the efficiency risk for tests of controls. Assessing the control risk too high triggers more audit work than was planned and threatens the efficiency of the audit.

Audit efficiency is important, but audit effectiveness is more important. For this reason, auditing standards require only a low risk of assessing the control risk too low, especially when this decision error could cause an auditor to do significantly less work on the related account balances. These risks and decisions are illustrated in Exhibit 10–9. Keeping these risks in mind, evaluating evidence includes calculating the sample deviation rate, comparing it with the tolerable rate, and following up all the deviations discovered.

Superseded Terminology: Overreliance and Underreliance

Several years ago, professional terminology was changed from "reliance on control" to "assessment of control risk." However, old habits die hard, and you will probably still encounter these uses of control terminology:

Overreliance is the result of realizing the risk of assessing control risk too low. If auditors think control risk is low when in fact it is higher, they will over-rely on internal control and restrict other audit procedures when they should actually perform more work. Overreliance is the same as effectiveness risk of tests of controls.

Underreliance is the result of realizing the risk of assessing control risk too high. If auditors think control risk is high when in fact it is lower, they will under-rely on internal control and perform more audit work when less work would suffice. Underreliance risk is the same as efficiency risk of tests of controls.

Calculate the Sample Deviation Rate   The first piece of hard evidence is the sample deviation rate. Suppose an auditor selected 60 recorded sales invoices and vouched them to shipping orders (bills of lading), finding one without shipping orders. The sample deviation rate is $1/60 = 1.7\%$. This is the best single-point estimate of the actual, but unknown, deviation rate in the population. However, you cannot say that the deviation rate in the population is exactly 1.7%. Chances are the sample is not exactly representative; the actual but unknown population deviation rate could be lower or higher.

Judge the Deviation Rate in Relation to the Tolerable Rate and the Risk of Assessing the Control Risk Too Low   Suppose the auditor in the example believed the tolerable rate was 5% (same as in planning above), justifying a control risk assessment of CR = 0.40. In a non-statistical sampling case, this auditor is supposed to think of the sample deviation rate (1.7%) in relation to the tolerable rate (5%), and about the

EXHIBIT 10–9

The Test of Controls Audit Sampling Decision Matrix

ACTUAL STATE OF INTERNAL CONTROLS (ACTUAL POPULATION DEVIATION RATE)	SAMPLE POPULATION DEVIATION RATE	
	LESS THAN TOLERABLE RATE	GREATER THAN TOLERABLE RATE
The deviation rate is less than the tolerable rate, so the control is performed satisfactorily.	Correct decision	Control risk too high decision error (efficiency risk for tests of controls)
The deviation rate is greater than the tolerable rate, so the control is not performed satisfactorily.	Control risk too low decision error (effectiveness risk for tests of controls)	Correct decision

risk of assessing the control risk too high:
the probability that the compliance evidence in the sample indicates high control risk when the actual (but unknown) degree of compliance would justify a lower control risk assessment

risk (of assessing control risk too low) that the actual, but unknown, deviation rate in the population exceeds 8%. The decision in this case depends on the auditor's experience and expertise. The non-statistical auditor might conclude that the population deviation rate is probably 8% because the sample deviation rate of 1.7% is so much lower. The *CPA Canada Handbook* guideline AuG-41, paragraph 42, suggests this logic. AuG-41 does not assume that the auditor is using statistical sampling. However, it must assume that the auditor used a minimal sample size as determined by a statistical formula, because the population is always rejected statistically when the sample size is too small (this happens because efficiency risk is larger than planned, and to get it smaller requires a larger sample). If too small a sample size is selected, the statistical formulas always reject, even if no errors are found.

Sample Evaluation Things are more explainable, in text, with a quantitative model, such as statistical sample evaluation, which explains why statistical sampling is more popular. Sample evaluation essentially involves solving for P in the formula $R = nP$ so that $P = R/n$. When P is calculated in this way it is referred to as *achieved P*, or the *achieved UEL* (upper error limit). Achieved P is calculated after the sample has been taken and the results are known. This means that the number of errors (K) detected by the sample is already known, the confidence level (CL = 1 − effectiveness risk) is known, and the sample size taken is already known. Thus, we can solve for achieved UEL = achieved $P = R/n$, where $R = {}_{CL}R_K$, CL is the specified confidence level, and K is the number of errors *found* in the sample (not the number expected, as in sample-size planning).

The auditor establishes decision criteria by first assigning a number to the risk of assessing the control risk too low, say 5%, and then assigning a number to the tolerable rate, say 5%. A statistical table is then used to calculate a sampling error–adjusted upper limit, which is the sample deviation rate adjusted upward to allow for the idea that the actual population rate could be higher. In this example, the adjusted limit, the UEL, can be calculated as 5%. This is obtained with the MUS formula and table by solving for achieved precision (achieved P) as follows: achieved $P = R/n$ using $K = 1$ (number of errors actually found in the sample) to get the R value with $K = 1$ and 95% CL (effectiveness risk = 0.05), which is $R = 4.75$. Now calculate the achieved $P = R/n = 4.75/60 = 0.08$. The statistical decision rule is based on comparing the 0.08 to tolerable (0.05). This finding means "the probability is more than 5% that the actual but unknown population deviation rate is greater than 5%." The decision criterion was "the actual but unknown population deviation rate needs to be 5% or lower, with 5% risk of assessing the control risk too low." So, the decision criterion is not satisfied, and the control risk assessment (0.40) associated with the 5% tolerable rate cannot be justified.[9]

From a critical thinking perspective, this justification step uses statistical theory to support the conclusion. Many would view such a conclusion as better supported than one based on non-statistical sampling. One of the advantages of statistical auditing is that it makes sample evaluation less ambiguous, as is illustrated next.

The 0.08 is the maximum error at the specified confidence level (0.95). This is then compared with what is material or tolerable. The basic rule is that, if achieved P, or UEL, is greater than material or tolerable, reject the population—otherwise, accept it. Compare this rule with AuG-41, paragraph 42, and note that this MUS rule is less ambiguous. In the case of tests of controls, rejection of the population is equivalent to assessing control risk as high; that is, there is no (or reduced) reliance on controls.

As in sample planning, the use of appropriate tables eliminates the need for the formulas. For example, Appendix 10A has tables titled "Table to Evaluate Sample Results for Tests of Controls." These tables provide for two widely used confidence levels: 95% and 90%, the equivalent to planned effectiveness risk levels of 5% and 10%, respectively. The table values are the interaction of sample sizes (left-hand column) and number of errors. In our illustration, we use 0.05 effectiveness risk (= 1 − 95% CL) and a sample size of 100 to get a UEL of 7% (rounded up) for this confidence level. This conservative UEL of 7% can be interpreted as the maximum error rate at 95% CL. The decision rule is to accept reliance on the controls (or accept the population) if the UEL is less than tolerable; otherwise, reject or reduce reliance (or reject the population error as unacceptable). This result is more conservative (higher UEL) than in the paragraph above, but done with tables, not formulas. You can get a more accurate value of 6.3% by dividing the R value at the top (6.3) by the sample size (100). Your instructor will tell you which approach to use in your course.

Achieved *P* can always be interpreted as the maximum error rate for the specified CL. There are additional complications for substantive testing, but these formulas are the only thing necessary for a conceptual understanding. These formulas or tables of MUS are so simple and so effective that they are now the most widely used in audit practice.

MUS is also so widely used because taking an appropriate sample does not require advance knowledge of the recorded amount of the population, as the other statistical approaches do. This makes MUS particularly appropriate for audits involving continuous, online, real-time reporting of sales and purchases as might be demanded in e-commerce audits. This is further explained in Appendix 10B.

Follow Up All Deviations   The evaluation described so far has been mostly quantitative in nature, involving counts of deviations, deviation rates and tolerable rate, and risk judgment criteria. Qualitative evaluation through determining the nature and cause of the deviations is also necessary. A single deviation can be the tip of the iceberg—a sign of pervasive deficiency. Auditors are obligated by the standard of due audit care to investigate known deviations so that nothing important will be overlooked.

Qualitative evaluation is sometimes called **error analysis** because each deviation from a prescribed control procedure is investigated to determine its nature, cause, and probable effect on financial statements. The analysis is essentially judgmental and involves a decision on whether the deviation is (1) a pervasive error in principle affecting all like transactions or just the one, (2) a deliberate control breakdown or unintentional, (3) a result of misunderstood instructions or careless inattention to control duties, or (4) directly or remotely related to a money amount measurement in the financial statements. Clearly, different qualitative perceptions of the seriousness of a deviation result from error analysis findings.

When the decision criteria are not satisfied and the preliminary conclusion is that the control risk is high, the auditors need to decide what to do next. The deviation follow-up can lead to more account balance audit work by making changes to the nature, timing, and extent of other audit procedures. If you suspect the sampling results overstate the actual population deviation rate (i.e., that efficiency risk is occurring), you can perform the control tests on more sample units in hopes of deciding that the control risk is actually lower. However, when faced with the preliminary "non-reliance" decision, you should never manipulate the quantitative evaluation by raising the tolerable rate or setting the risk of assessing the control risk too low. Supposedly, these two decision criteria were carefully determined in the planning stage, and only new information is a good basis for easing them.

Timing of Test of Controls Audit Procedures

Earlier, you learned that auditors can perform the control testing at an interim date—a date before the client's year-end. When control testing is early, an audit manager must decide what to do about the remaining period (e.g., the period October through December after doing test of controls auditing in September for a December 31 year-end audit).

The decision turns on several factors: (1) the results of the work at interim might, for example, indicate poor control performance and high control risk, (2) inquiries made after interim may show that a particular control procedure has been abandoned or improved, (3) the length of the remaining period may be short enough to forgo additional work or long enough to suggest a need for continuing the test of controls audit, (4) the dollar amounts affected by the control procedure may have been much larger or much smaller than before, (5) evidence obtained about control as a by-product of performing substantive procedures for the remaining period may show enough about control performance that separate work on this is unnecessary, or (6) work performed by the company's internal auditors may be relied on for the remaining period.

error analysis:
qualitative evaluation of control risk

Depending on these circumstances, an auditor can decide to (1) continue the test of controls because knowledge of control performance is necessary to justify restriction of other audit work or (2) stop further test of controls audit work because (a) there is enough evidence derived from other procedures or (b) information shows the control has failed, control risk is high, and other work will not be restricted. Whatever the judgment, audit effectiveness and efficiency should always be uppermost in the auditor's mind.

Review Checkpoints

10-35   In test of controls auditing, why should auditors be more concerned with the risk of assessing the control risk too low than with that of assessing it too high?

10-36   What important decision must be made when test of controls auditing is performed and control risk is evaluated at an interim date several weeks or months before the client's fiscal year-end?

Substantive Procedures for Auditing Account Balances

LO6   Develop a simple audit program for an account balance, considering the influences of risk and tolerable misstatement.

When audit sampling is used for auditing the assertions in account balances, the monetary amount of the population units is the main interest, not the presence or absence of control deviations, as is the case with attribute sampling. **Substantive tests of details auditing** are done to obtain direct evidence about the dollar amounts and disclosures in the financial statements.

Substantive-purpose procedures include analytical procedures and test (audit) of details of transactions and balances. Analytical procedures involve overall comparisons of account balances with prior balances, financial relationships, non-financial information, budgeted or forecast balances, and balances derived from estimates calculated by auditors (refer to the discussion of analytical procedures in Chapter 8). Analytical procedures are not usually applied on a sample basis. So, substantive procedures for auditing details are the normal procedures used in account balance audit sampling.

Risk Model Expansion

Up to now you have worked with a conceptual risk model that included detection risk (DR). Detection risk is actually a combination of two risks: **analytical procedures risk** (APR) is the probability that analytical procedures will fail to detect material errors, and the **risk of incorrect acceptance** (RIA) is the probability that test-of-detail procedures will fail to detect material errors. The two types of procedures are considered independent, so detection risk is DR = APR × RIA, and the expanded risk model is

$$AR = IR \times CR \times APR \times RIA$$

substantive tests of details auditing:
procedures to obtain direct evidence about the dollar amounts and disclosures in the financial statements

analytical procedures risk:
the risk that analytical procedures will fail to detect material misstatements (effectiveness risk associated with analytical procedures risk)

risk of incorrect acceptance:
the decision to accept a balance as being materially accurate when the balance is materially misstated

This model is still a conceptual tool. It can now be used to help you understand some elements of sampling for auditing the details of account balances. First, recognize that auditors exercise professional judgment in assessing the inherent risk (IR), control risk (CR), analytical procedures risk (APR), and audit risk (AR). If these four risks are given, you can then manipulate the model to express the risk of incorrect acceptance:

$$RIA = \frac{AR}{IR \times CR \times APR}$$

With AR, IR, and APR held constant, RIA varies inversely with CR, that is, the higher the assessed CR, the lower the planned RIA, and vice versa. Furthermore, this is also true of the risk of material misstatement (RMM) concept of CAS 530, since $RMM = IR \times CR$.

More about Sampling Risk

Substantive-purpose procedures produce the evidence enabling an auditor to decide whether an account balance is materially in conformity with GAAP. Thus, auditors run the sampling risks of making one of two decision errors. The risk of incorrect acceptance represents the decision to accept a balance as being materially accurate when, in fact (unknown to the auditor), the balance is materially misstated. This is the effectiveness risk for a substantive test. The other decision error risk, the **risk of incorrect rejection**, represents the decision that a balance is materially misstated when, in fact, it is not. This is the efficiency risk for a substantive test. These sampling risk relationships are shown in Exhibit 10–10.

Incorrect Acceptance (Effectiveness Risk)

The risk of incorrect acceptance is considered the more important of the two decision error risks. When an auditor decides an account book balance is materially accurate (hence, needs no adjustment), the audit work on that account is considered finished, the decision is documented in the working papers, and the audit team proceeds to work on other accounts. If the account is, in fact, materially misstated, an unmodified opinion on the financial statements is unwarranted and the effectiveness of the audit is damaged.

Incorrect Rejection (Efficiency Risk)

When an auditor decides an account book balance is materially misstated, more audit work is performed to determine the adjustment. The risk is that the book balance really is a materially accurate representation of the (unknown) actual value, and the audit manager may recommend an unnecessary adjustment.

Incorrect rejection is not as serious as incorrect acceptance. When auditors first begin to think a balance may contain a material misstatement, they try to determine why this occurred. To estimate the amount, more

EXHIBIT 10–10

The Account Balance Audit Sampling Decision Matrix

AUDIT DECISION ALTERNATIVES (BASED ON SAMPLE EVIDENCE)	UNKNOWN ACTUAL ACCOUNT BALANCE IS	
	Materially* accurate	Materially misstated
The book value of the account is materially accurate.	Correct decision	Incorrect acceptance
The book value of the account is materially misstated.	Incorrect rejection	Correct decision

*"Materially" in this context refers to the "material misstatement" assigned to the account balance. It is either the overall materiality or the specific materiality discussed in Chapter 5.

risk of incorrect rejection:
the decision to accept a balance as being materially misstated when it is not

evidence will be sought. The data will be reviewed for a source of systematic error, and the amounts of errors will be analyzed carefully. Client personnel may do a complete analysis to determine a more accurate account balance.

If the initial decision was, in fact, an incorrect rejection, this other work allows the auditors to decide if the recorded amount is really misstated or the sample was not representative. Hence, steps will be taken to determine the amount of error, and there is a chance for the error to be reversed. Incorrect rejection can affect the efficiency of an audit by causing unnecessary work.

Materiality and Tolerable Misstatement

Determining a threshold for the materiality of misstatements in financial statements is a tough problem under any circumstances. Audit sampling for substantive audits of particular account balances adds another wrinkle. Auditors must also decide on an amount of material misstatement—a judgment of the amount of monetary misstatement that may exist in an account balance or class of transactions. As discussed in Chapter 4, this materiality may be the overall materiality or the specific materiality of CAS 320 in Chapter 5. In MUS, these are the only materialities needed, as explained in the discussion case of Appendix 10B. Note that both of these materialities relate directly to user needs. In other words, MUS does not need to consider the complications introduced by the performance materiality concept of CAS 320.09 or the related tolerable misstatement concept of 530.A3 based on performance materiality. These concepts are needed by other statistical models, not MUS. The use of these concepts in CAS 530 illustrates the impact of using the variety of quantitative models that are possible in statistical sampling. It all depends on which one is being used for a particular line item in the financial statements that the population represents.

When you see the word *materiality* or *material* in this book, henceforth, it refers to user-needs materiality. This is a key audit planning judgment. The way we use the term, therefore, is not an artifact of the statistical model. Audit risk, therefore, is the risk that all the audit work on an account balance will not reveal a user-needs material misstatement. This concept is further discussed in Appendix 10B.

In this stage of sampling, the planned P might be an amount lower than the overall or specific materiality of Chapter 5, so that the auditor can reduce efficiency risk. Firm practice varies: efficiency risk can be indirectly controlled through the *planned K* value, the *planned P* value, or a combination of the two. The most common strategy is to use $K = 0$ and a *planned P* in the range of half to full overall or specific materiality, whichever the auditor judges more appropriate in the circumstances. We discuss these options further in Appendix 10B. Here, the calculations are simplified by assuming that planned P is set equal to overall or specific materiality.

Sampling Steps for an Account Balance Audit

Sampling for the audit of account balances is similar to the steps of test of controls audit sampling. An example related to auditing receivables illustrates these steps; test of controls sampling was illustrated with the audit of a control procedure for sales invoices. This work can produce independent evidence of sales overstatement resulting from a breakdown of the control or other causes. The seven-step framework helps auditors plan, perform, and evaluate account balance detail audit work. It also helps auditors accomplish an eighth step—careful documentation of the work—by showing each of the seven areas to be described in the working papers. The first seven steps are as follows:

1. Specify the audit objectives.
2. Define the population.
3. Choose an audit sampling method.
4. Determine the sample size.

5. Select the sample.

6. Perform the substantive-purpose procedures.

7. Evaluate the evidence.

Plan the Procedures

LO6a   Specify objectives and a population of data.

The three planning steps are the problem recognition phase of the sampling method. When a client presents the financial statements, they might make the following assertions: the trade accounts receivable exist (existence) and are *bona fide* obligations owed to the company (ownership); all the accounts receivable are recorded (completeness); they are stated at net realizable value (valuation); and they are properly classified as current assets, presented, and disclosed in conformity with GAAP (presentation). Each assertion represents a hypothesis (problem) to be tested.

Specify the Audit Objectives

When sampling to confirm accounts receivable, the specific objective is to decide whether the client's assertions about existence, rights (ownership), and valuation are materially accurate. This auditing is **hypothesis testing**—the auditors hypothesize that the book value is materially accurate about existence, ownership, and valuation. The evidence will enable them to accept or reject the hypothesis. The audit objective is to determine the monetary misstatement by comparing the recorded balances to the balances found through the evidence.

Define the Population

CAS 530 says that auditors must ensure that the population is appropriate for the specific objectives of the audit procedure, and that it is complete. A population of the recorded accounts receivable balances suits the objective of obtaining evidence about existence, ownership, and valuation. It also suits the related objective of obtaining evidence about sales overstatement. In the case of accounts receivable, each customer's account balance is a population unit. If obtaining evidence about completeness and sales understatement were the objectives, the recorded accounts receivable would be the wrong population.

Ordinarily, the sampling unit is the same as the population unit. Sometimes, however, it is easier to define the sampling unit as a smaller part of a population unit. For example, an auditor may want to audit samples of individual invoices for customers instead of working with each customer's balance.

Since a sample will be drawn from a physical representation of the population (e.g., a printed trial balance or computer file of customers' accounts), the auditors must determine whether it is complete. Re-adding the trial balance and reconciling it to the control account total does this.

Auditing standards (CAS 530) require auditors to use their judgment in deciding if any population units should be removed from the population and audited separately (not sampled) because sampling risk (risk of incorrect acceptance or incorrect rejection) with respect to them is not justified. Suppose, for example, the accounts receivable amounted to $400,000, but six of the customers had balances of $10,000 or more, for a sum of $100,000. The next-largest account balance is less than $10,000. If materiality is $10,000, the six accounts are considered **individually significant items** because each exceeds the material misstatement amount, and they should be removed from the population and audited completely.

---

hypothesis testing:
when auditors hypothesize that the book value is materially accurate regarding existence, ownership, and valuation

individually significant items:
items in account balances that exceed the material misstatement amount; in audit sampling these should be removed from the population and audited completely

In the jargon of audit sampling related to account balances, subdividing the population is known as **stratification**. The total population is subdivided by account balance size. For example, a small number of accounts totalling $75,000 may be the first (large balance) of, say, four strata. The remaining three strata might each contain a total of approximately $75,000 in recorded balances, but each is made up of a successively larger number of customer accounts with successively smaller account balances. Stratification can be used to increase audit efficiency (smaller total sample size). A stratification example appears in the following box, which repeats Exhibit 10–2 for your convenience.

Stratification Example—Selecting Sample Sizes

The stratification below subdivides the population into a first stratum of six individually significant accounts and four other strata, each with approximately one-fourth ($75,000) of the remaining dollar balance. This is a typical situation where there is a greater number of accounts of smaller value.

The example allocates 90 items to the last four strata. This is referred to as *stratified sampling.* When each stratum gets one-fourth of the sample size, the sample is skewed toward the higher-value accounts: the second stratum has 23 out of 80 sample items, and the fifth stratum has 23 out of 910 items.

STRATUM	BOOK VALUE	NUMBER	AMOUNT	SAMPLE
1	Over $10,000	6	$100,000	6
2	$625–$9,999	80	75,068	23
3	$344–$624	168	75,008	22
4	$165–$343	342	75,412	22
5	$1–$164	910	74,512	23
		1,506	$400,000	96

This stratification deals with a normal situation in which the variability of the account balances and errors in them tend to be larger in the high-value accounts than in the low-value accounts. As a consequence, the sample includes a larger proportion of the high-value accounts (23/80) and a smaller proportion of the low-value accounts (23/910). In addition to size or variability, stratification can be based on other qualitative characteristics the auditor considers important, such as individual, location, date, or product.

Choose an Audit Sampling Method

An auditor must decide whether to use statistical or non-statistical sampling methods. If statistical sampling is chosen, another choice needs to be made. In statistical sampling, sampling methods utilizing classical variables in normal distribution theory are available. However, MUS, which uses attribute sampling theory, is used more widely in practice. Some of the technical characteristics of the statistical methods are explained more fully in Appendix 10B.

The calculation examples shown later in this chapter use the MUS method. This calculation is relatively simple and illustrates the important points.

Perform the Procedures

LO6b   Determine sample size and select sample units.

The next three steps represent the evidence-gathering phase of the sampling process. Figuring sample size correctly for account balance auditing is an important aspect of this and requires consideration of several influences.

stratification:
subdividing the population in an audit sample by, for example, account balance size

Figuring a sample size in advance helps guard against underauditing (not obtaining enough evidence) and overauditing (obtaining more evidence than needed). It can also control the cost of the audit. An arbitrary sample size could be used for the accounts receivable confirmation procedures, but if it turned out to be too small, processing more confirmations might be impossible before the audit report deadline. Alternative procedures could become costly and time-consuming. A predetermined sample size is not as important in other situations where the auditors can increase the sample simply by choosing more items from those available in the client's office.

Determine the Sample Size

Whether using statistical or non-statistical sampling methods, auditors first need to establish decision criteria for the risk of incorrect acceptance (effectiveness risk for substantive testing), the risk of incorrect rejection (efficiency risk for substantive testing), and the material misstatement criterion to be used with the substantive test. Also, auditors may want to estimate the expected dollar amount of misstatement. These decision criteria should be determined before any evidence is obtained from a sample.

Risk of Incorrect Acceptance, or Effectiveness Risk of the Substantive Test   The audit risk model can be your guide in assessing this risk. A suitable risk of incorrect acceptance depends on the assessments of inherent risk, control risk, and analytical procedures risk. The risk of incorrect acceptance varies inversely with the combined product of the other risks. The larger the combined product of the other risks, the smaller will be the allowable risk of incorrect acceptance.

Suppose, for example, two different auditors, both believing 0.05 is an acceptable level of audit risk, independently assess the client's control risk and their own analytical procedures and arrive at the following conclusions.

Auditor A believes the inherent risk is high (IR = 1.0), the control risk is moderate (CR = 0.50), and analytical procedures will not be performed (APR = 1.0). Audit procedures need to be planned so that the risk of incorrect acceptance will be about 10%:

$$RIA = \frac{AR}{IR \times CR \times APR} = \frac{0.05}{1.0 \times 0.50 \times 1.0} = 0.10$$

Auditor B believes the inherent risk is high (IR = 1.0), the control risk is very low (CR = 0.20), and analytical procedures will not be performed (APR = 1.0). Audit procedures need to be planned so that the risk of incorrect acceptance will be about 25%:

$$RIA = \frac{AR}{IR \times CR \times APR} = \frac{0.05}{1.0 \times 0.20 \times 1.0} = 0.25$$

Use the model with caution. You can learn from these examples that auditor A's account balance sampling work must provide less risk than auditor B's. Since sample size varies inversely with the risk of incorrect acceptance, auditor A's sample will be larger. In fact, when the control risk is lower, as B's is, the acceptable risk of incorrect acceptance is higher. Thus, auditor B's sample of customers' accounts receivable can be smaller than auditor A's sample.

Risk of Incorrect Rejection, or Efficiency Risk   Like the risk of incorrect acceptance, the risk of incorrect rejection exists in both statistical and non-statistical sampling. It can be controlled, usually by auditing a larger sample, and sample size varies inversely with the risk of incorrect rejection. MUS deals with incorrect rejection (efficiency risk) by increasing sample size above the minimum associated with using $K = 0$ in sample planning. The simplified approach to sample planning we use here sets $K = 0$ so that the sample size is the smallest possible for the stated confidence level and materiality.

Material Misstatement   Material misstatement—which can be either a performance materiality or an overall materiality depending on the auditor's judgment for the line item being tested—must also be considered in both non-statistical and statistical sampling. In statistical sampling, material misstatement must be expressed as a dollar amount or as a proportion of the total recorded amount. The sample size varies inversely with the amount of misstatement considered material. The greater the materiality, the smaller the sample size needed.

Expected Dollar Misstatement   Auditors estimate an **expected dollar misstatement** amount based on last year's audit findings or on other knowledge of the accounting system. Increasing the expectations of dollar misstatement has the effect of increasing the sample size. This is done through reducing the planned precision in planning the sample size. The purpose of doing this is to reduce efficiency risk throughout the range of immaterial misstatements. The more dollar misstatement expected, the larger the sample size should be. So, sample size varies directly with the amount of expected dollar misstatement. The main reason for using expected errors is to control efficiency risk, as discussed earlier in this chapter. See the chapter Application Case for an illustration and Appendix 10B to further understand this technical point.

Variability within the Population   Auditors using non-statistical sampling must take into account the degree of dispersion, or typical skewness, of some accounting populations. **Skewness** is the concentration of a large proportion of the dollar amount in only a small number of the population items. For example, $100,000 (25%) of the total accounts receivable is in 6 customers' accounts, while the remaining $300,000 is in 1,500 customers' accounts.

As a general rule, auditors should be careful about populations whose unit values range widely, say from $1 to $10,000. In this case, for your population to be representative, you would need to take a larger sample than if the range were only from $1 to $500. Sample size should vary directly with the range of population unit values. Populations with high variability should be stratified, as shown in the stratification example above.

When classic statistical sampling methods are used, there must be an estimate of the population **standard deviation**, which is a measure of the population variability. When using MUS, this estimate is not needed, as the unit of selection is each recorded dollar rather than the account balance. Thus, there is no variability in the population of recorded dollars, as each dollar has the same value. (See Appendix 10B for more details.)

MUS sample sizes can be calculated as they are for tests of controls. The same sample planning formula can be applied as long as all monetary amounts are converted to a rate or percentage. Thus, for example, if you have an accounts receivable population with a balance of $10,000,000, you determine materiality to be $300,000. If you wish to plan a sample size for confirming receivables with 95% confidence level, then first convert materiality as a rate by calculating its proportion of the recorded value: $P = 300,000/10,000,000 = 0.03$. This is simply putting materiality in relative terms. Now you can apply the formula as before to calculate the sample size: $n = R/P = 3.0/0.03 = 100$.

As you can see, the calculation of sample sizes under MUS is very similar for both tests of controls and tests of balances. The calculations for both are summarized in Exhibit 10–11.

You can now prove to yourself the efficiency effects of relying on internal controls using the audit risk model. In the above receivables example, assume you desired 95% CL because you planned audit risk at 0.05, and you assessed inherent and control risk at the maximum of 1.0. Hence, you had to get all your assurance from the substantive test using a detection risk (DR) of 0.05. The detection risk is the same as effectiveness risk

---

expected dollar misstatement:
a preliminary estimate of expected monetary misstatements in a total monetary value recorded for a population

skewness:
the concentration of a large proportion of the dollar amount in only a small number of the population items

standard deviation:
a measure of population variability

EXHIBIT 10–11

Sufficiency of Audit Evidence

SUMMARY OF SIMPLIFIED CALCULATIONS OF SAMPLE SIZE		
KEY CONCEPTS	TESTS OF CONTROLS	SUBSTANTIVE TESTS OF BALANCE
Basic formula	$R = nP$	$R = nP$
Assessment of materiality or tolerable error rate	P = tolerable error rate	P = materiality as a proportion of the recorded balance
Assessment of effectiveness risk = 1 − confidence level = 1 − CL	Effectiveness risk is based on control risk from audit risk model	Effectiveness risk is risk of incorrect acceptance of audit risk model
R value	From table use $K = 0$ and desired confidence level.	From table use $K = 0$ and desired confidence level.
Extent of testing = sample size	$n = \frac{{}_{CL}R_K}{P}$	$n = \frac{{}_{CL}R_K}{P}$

or the risk of incorrect acceptance. Now, assume that you assessed control risk below maximum at 0.50 (instead of at maximum at 1.0); then, using the risk model, you can prove to yourself that detection risk is revised to 0.10; that is, you accept more risk (get less assurance) from your substantive testing. This is reflected by the reduced sample size: $n = R/P = 2.31/0.03 = 77$ (always round up to ensure the sample is large enough). You have thus reduced your substantive testing by 23 (100 − 77) as a result of your increased reliance on internal controls. This is a simple example, but it illustrates the basic principle of internal control reliance using the audit risk model.

These influences are summarized in Exhibit 10–12.

EXHIBIT 10–12

Sample-Size Relationships: Audit of Account Balances Using Monetary-Unit Sampling

	PREDETERMINED SAMPLE SIZE WILL BE		
SAMPLE-SIZE INFLUENCE	HIGH RATE OR LARGE AMOUNT	LOW RATE OR SMALL AMOUNT	SAMPLE-SIZE RELATION
1. Risk of incorrect acceptance	Smaller	Larger	Inverse
2. Risk of incorrect rejection*	Smaller	Larger	Inverse
3. Tolerable misstatement	Smaller	Larger	Inverse
4. Expected misstatement*	Larger	Smaller	Direct

*These effects are discussed in Appendix 10B. They are ignored under the simplified approach used here, and many practitioners treat these effects as insignificant.

Select the Sample

As was the case with test of controls audit samples, account balance samples must be representative. The same selection methods as discussed for tests of controls can be used for MUS in substantive testing. Unrestricted random selection and systematic MUS selection will obtain random samples for statistical applications. Appendix 10B outlines unique features of MUS selection in more detail. Haphazard and block selection methods have the same drawbacks as they have in test of controls audit samples.

Perform the Substantive-Purpose Procedures

The basic assertions in a presentation of accounts receivable are that they exist, they are complete (no receivables are unrecorded), the company has the right to collect the money, they are valued properly at net realizable value, and they are presented and disclosed properly in conformity with GAAP. A substantive-purpose audit program consists of account balance–related procedures designed to produce evidence about these assertions. The test procedures listed in the box on the two purposes of sampling above ("Two Kinds of Audit Programs: Two Purposes for Audit Sampling") will obtain the evidence related to the assertions also listed in the box, as further explained below.

The confirmation procedures should be performed for all the sampling units, and other procedures must be performed as necessary for evidence relating to existence, ownership, and valuation. It is important to audit all the sample units, even the hard ones. Auditing just those customers whose balances are easy might bias the sample. Sometimes, however, you will be unable to audit a sample unit; there may be no response to the confirmation requests, sales invoices supporting the balance may not be found, and no payment may have been received after the confirmation date. Auditing standards contain the following guidance in this situation:

- If your evaluation conclusion isn't affected by the misstated balance, then you can let it go. If your evaluation conclusion is to accept the book value, the account should not be big enough to change that. If your evaluation conclusion is already to reject the book value, this account misstatement just reinforces the decision.
- If considering the entire balance to be misstated would change an acceptance decision to a rejection decision, you may need to expand the sample, perform the procedures on the new items (other than confirmation), and reevaluate the results.
- If control risk related to the balance was assessed to be low, you should consider whether this finding contradicts the low control risk assessment.

Review Checkpoints

10-37 Write the expanded risk model. What risk is implied for test of detail risk when IR = 1.0, CR = 0.40, APR = 0.60, AR = 0.048, tolerable misstatement = $10,000, and the estimated standard deviation in the population = $25?

10-38 Explain why control risk is inversely related to the risk of incorrect acceptance.

10-39 Why does the efficiency risk affect audit efficiency and the effectiveness risk affect audit effectiveness?

10-40 When auditing account balances, why is an incorrect acceptance decision considered more serious than an incorrect rejection decision?

10-41 What should be the relationship between tolerable misstatement in the audit of an account balance and the amount of monetary misstatement considered material to the overall financial statements?

10-42 What general set of audit objectives can you use as a frame of reference for specific objectives for the audit of an account balance?

10-43 What audit purpose is served by stratifying an account balance population and by selecting some units from the population for 100% audit verification?

The Evidence

LO6c Evaluate monetary error evidence from a balance audit sample.

The final step represents the evidence evaluation and decision-making phase of the sampling method. Your decisions about existence, ownership, and valuation need to be justifiable by sufficient appropriate quantitative and qualitative evidence. You should be concerned first with the quantitative evaluation of the evidence. Qualitative follow-up is also important and is discussed later.

Evaluate the Evidence

Quantitative evaluation of substantive tests of balances using MUS is the same as that for tests of controls. For example, reject if achieved P is greater than or equal to materiality; otherwise accept the population total recorded amount. The complications arise from possible variability of the misstatements when calculating achieved P. Appendix 10B outlines how to deal with these complications. Exhibit 10–13 summarizes these statistical evaluations.

Auditing standards for this evaluation are not written with a particular approach, such as MUS, in mind. Instead, they deal with general features of quantitative evaluation already captured by the particular approaches of formulas, and we review these general considerations here. The reconciliation to particular calculations with MUS is given in Appendix 10B. These are the basic steps in quantitative evaluation:

- Figure the total amount of actual monetary error, the **known misstatement (identified misstatement)**, found in the sample.
- Project the known misstatement to the population. The projected amount is the **likely misstatement (projected misstatement)**.
- Compare the likely misstatement to the material misstatement for the account and consider (1) the risk of incorrect acceptance—that likely misstatement is calculated to be less than material misstatement even though the actual misstatement in the population is greater, or (2) the risk of incorrect rejection—that likely misstatement is calculated to be greater than material misstatement, even though the actual misstatement in the population is smaller. This decision can be made statistically, thus reducing non-sampling error with the test. Details are given in Appendix 10B.

Amount of Known Misstatement   Hypothetical audit evidence from the sample for the previous stratification example is shown in the box "Stratification Example—Selecting Sample Sizes." In this example, total accounts receivable is $400,000, while $100,000 of the total is in six large balances, which are to be audited separately. The remainder is in 1,500 customer accounts whose balances range from $1 to $9,999. Suppose the audit team selected 90 of these accounts and applied the confirmation or vouching procedures to each of them, and the evidence showed $136 of net overstatement of the recorded amounts. This amount is the known misstatement for this sample of 90 customer accounts.

Project the Known Misstatement to the Population   Let us review the discussion around Exhibit 10–2. To make a decision about the population, the known misstatement in the sample is projected to the population. The sample must be representative, because if it is not, a projection can produce a misleading number. As an extreme example, suppose one of the six large accounts, which were all audited, contained a $600 disputed amount. Investigation showed the customer was right and management agreed, so the $600 is the amount of known misstatement. If an auditor takes this group of six accounts as being representative of the population, projecting the $100 average misstatement ($600/6) to 1,506 accounts ($100 × 1,506) would project a total misstatement of $150,600, compared with the recorded accounts receivable total of $400,000. This projection is neither reasonable nor appropriate. Nothing is wrong with the calculation method. The non-representative "sample" is the culprit in this absurd result.

Consider Sampling Risks   These are risks of making wrong decisions (incorrect acceptance or incorrect rejection) in both non-statistical and statistical sampling. The smaller the sample, the greater both risks are.

known misstatement (identified misstatement):
the total amount of actual monetary error found in a sample or other non-sampling auditing procedures

likely misstatement (projected misstatement):
the projection of a known misstatement identified in a representative sample to the whole population

EXHIBIT 10–13

Evaluating Sample Results

EVALUATING SAMPLE RESULTS*		
KEY CONCEPTS	**TESTS OF CONTROL**	**SUBSTANTIVE TESTS OF BALANCE**
Basic formula	$R = nP$	$R = nP$
Solve for achieved P	$P = \dfrac{R}{n}$	$P = \dfrac{R}{n}$
Basic decision rule	If achieved P > tolerable error rate, then reject; otherwise, accept reliance on control.	If achieved P > materiality, then reject; otherwise, accept the recorded total for the population.
Consequence of decision:		
If accept	Can rely on controls to extent planned at stated confidence level	Can accept client's recorded amount at stated confidence level
If reject	Need to rely on controls less than expected	Need to sample more or insist on an adjustment (adjust to most likely value as indicated by sample mean extrapolated to the population)

*n is known, and R is known based on detected errors, K, and planned confidence level.

Common sense tells you that the less you know about a population because of a small sample, the more risk you run of making a wrong decision.

Auditing guidance suggests you can use your experience and professional judgment to consider the risk. If the projected likely misstatement is considerably less than tolerable misstatement, chances are good that the total actual misstatement in the population will be less than tolerable misstatement. However, when the projected likely misstatement is close to material misstatement, the risk of incorrect acceptance may exceed the acceptable risk that an auditor initially established as a decision criterion (see AuG-41, paragraph 42).

The risk of incorrect rejection is a similar situation. Again, the judgment depends on the size of the sample and the kinds and distribution of misstatements discovered. This judgment can be significantly aided by using statistical theory, as explained in Appendix 10B.

Auditors take the rejection decision seriously and conduct enough additional investigation to determine the amount and adjustment required—extra work that mitigates the risk of incorrect rejection. In the example, if the sample of 90 customers' accounts had shown total misstatement of $900 (yielding the $15,000 projected misstatement using the average difference method), most auditors would consider the evidence insufficient to propose a significant adjustment. (However, correction of the $900 should not by itself be a sufficient action to satisfy the auditors.)

When using non-statistical sampling, auditors use their experience and expertise to take risks into account. Statistical samplers can add statistical calculations to these considerations of sampling risk.

Qualitative Evaluation   The numbers are not enough. Auditors are required to follow up each monetary difference to determine whether it arose from (a) misunderstanding of accounting principles, (b) simple mistakes or carelessness, (c) an intentional irregularity, or (d) management override of an internal control procedure. Auditors also need to relate the differences to their effect on other amounts in the financial statements. For example, overstatements in accounts receivable may indicate overstatement of sales revenue.

Likewise, you should not overlook the information that can be obtained in account balance auditing about the performance of internal control procedures—the dual-purpose characteristic of auditing procedures. Deviations (or absence of deviations) discovered when performing substantive procedures can help confirm or contradict an auditor's previous conclusion about control risk. If many more monetary differences than expected arise, the control risk conclusion may need to be revised and more account balance auditing work done.

Knowledge of the source, nature, and amount of monetary differences is very important in explaining the situation to management and directing additional work to areas where adjustments are needed. The audit work is not complete until the qualitative evaluation and follow-up are done.

Evaluate the Amount of Misstatement The *CPA Canada Handbook* guideline AuG-41 requires the aggregation of known misstatement (identified misstatement in the guideline) and projected likely misstatement (likely aggregate misstatement in the guideline). The aggregation is the sum of (a) known misstatement in the population units identified for 100% audit and (b) the projected likely misstatement for the population sampled. The theory underlying (b) is that the projected likely misstatement is the best single estimate of the amount that would be determined if all the accounts in the sampled population had been audited. You can see the importance of sample representativeness in this regard. This aggregation should be judged in combination with other misstatements found in the audit of other account balances to determine whether the financial statements taken as a whole need to be adjusted and, if so, in what amount.

The evaluation of amounts is not over yet, however. It cannot be said that the projected likely misstatement is the exact amount that would be found if all the units in the population were audited. The problem arises from **sampling error**—the amount by which a projected likely misstatement amount could differ from an actual (unknown) total as a result of the sample not being exactly representative. Of course, auditors are mostly concerned with the possibility that the actual total misstatement might be considerably more than the projected likely misstatement.

This sampling phenomenon gives rise to the concept of **possible misstatement**, or maximum possible misstatement (the third kind, in addition to known and likely misstatement), which is interpreted in AuG-41 as the further misstatement remaining undetected in the units not selected in the sample. Non-statistical auditors use their experience and professional judgment in considering additional possible misstatement. Statistical auditors, however, use statistical calculations to measure possible misstatement.

In Appendix 10B, the basic example shows how to calculate a possible misstatement. For the illustration here, if the possible misstatement is less than the amount considered material ($10,000), then it could be judged as acceptable (assuming no qualitative factors come into play). If the possible misstatement were higher than $10,000, then the evidence would suggest that the misstatement in the account exceeds $10,000. For a more complete discussion of the evaluation of statistical substantive testing of details results, see Appendix 10B.

Timing of Substantive Audit Procedures

Account balances can be audited, at least in part, at an interim date. When this work is done before the company's year-end, auditors must extend the interim-date audit conclusion to the balance sheet date. **Extending the audit conclusion** involves performing substantive-purpose audit procedures on the transactions in the remaining period and on the year-end balance to produce sufficient appropriate evidence for a decision about the year-end balance. It is unreasonable to audit a balance (say, accounts receivable) as of September 30, and then, without further work, accept the December 31 balance.

sampling error:
the amount by which a projected likely misstatement amount could differ from an actual (unknown) total as a result of the sample not being exactly representative

possible misstatement:
the further misstatement remaining undetected in the units not selected in the sample

extending the audit conclusion:
performing substantive-purpose audit procedures on the transactions in the remaining period and on the year-end balance to produce sufficient appropriate evidence for a decision about the year-end balance

If the company's internal control over transactions that produce the balance under audit is not particularly strong, you should time the substantive detail work at year-end instead of at interim. Likewise, if rapidly changing business conditions predispose managers to misstate the accounts (try to slip one by the auditors), the work should be timed at year-end. In most cases, careful scanning of transactions and analytical review comparisons should be performed on transactions that occur after the interim date.

As an example of the process, accounts receivable confirmation can be done at an interim date. Later, efforts must be made to ascertain whether controls continued to be reliable. You must scan the transactions of the remaining period, audit any new large balances, and update work on collectability, especially with analysis of cash received after the year-end.

Audit work is performed at interim for two reasons: (1) to spread the accounting firms' workload so that not all the work on clients is crammed into December and January and (2) to make the work efficient and enable companies to report audited financial results soon after the year-end. Some well-organized companies with well-planned audits report their audited figures as early as five or six days after their fiscal year ends.

Balance Audit Sampling Failure

The company owned surgical instruments that it lent and leased to customers. The auditors decided to audit the existence of the assets by confirming them with the customers who were supposed to be holding and using them. From the population of 880 instruments, the auditors selected eight for confirmation, using a sampling method that purported to produce a representative selection.

Two confirmations were never returned, and the auditors did not follow up on them. One returned confirmation indicated that the customer did not have the instrument in question; the auditors were never able to find it. Nevertheless, the auditors concluded that the $3.5 million recorded amount of the surgical instrument assets was materially accurate.

Judges who heard complaints on the quality of the audit work concluded that it was not performed in accordance with generally accepted auditing standards (GAAS) because the auditors did not gather sufficient evidence concerning the existence and valuation of the surgical instruments. GAAS require auditors to project the sample findings to the population. The auditors did not do so. They never calculated (non-statistical) the fact that $1,368,750 of the asset amount could not be confirmed or found to exist. The sample of eight was woefully inadequate, both in sample size and in the proportionately large number of exceptions reported. There was a wholly insufficient statistical basis for concluding that the account was fairly stated under generally accepted accounting principles (GAAP).

Source: U.S. Securities and Exchange Commission, Administrative Proceeding File No. 3–6579 (Initial Decision, June 1990).

Review Checkpoints

10-44 What kind of evidence evaluation consideration should an auditor give to the dollar amount of a population unit that cannot be audited?

10-45 What are the three basic steps in quantitative evaluation of monetary amount evidence when auditing an account balance?

10-46 The projected likely misstatement may be calculated, yet further misstatement may remain undetected in the population. How can auditors take the further misstatement under consideration when completing the quantitative evaluation of monetary evidence? How is this done by formula?

10-47 What additional considerations are in order when auditors plan to audit account balances at an interim date several weeks or months before the client's fiscal year-end date?

APPLICATION CASE WITH SOLUTION & ANALYSIS

Auditor Accused of Not Doing Sufficient Testing

DISCUSSION CASE

In a famous U.S. Securities and Exchange Commission (SEC) investigation of the 1972 audit of Giant Stores by the accounting firm of Touche Ross (Accounting Series Release No. 153A, 27 June 1979), the SEC accused Touche Ross of, among other things, not doing sufficient testing to detect $300,000 of fictitious advertising credits supposedly granted to Giant Stores by its suppliers. When the credit was recorded, the accounts payable accounts were debited. The advertising manager had prepared a list of 1,100 suppliers to which advertising credits had been granted, and the SEC claimed that the sample size of 24 used by the auditor to test these recorded credits for accuracy was too small to reach a valid conclusion about the material accuracy of the cumulative $300,000 of advertising credits. By manipulating the company's financial records, Giant Stores executives converted a $2.5 million loss for 1972 into a $1.5 million profit. Was the SEC correct in arguing that the auditor did insufficient testing of the advertising credits? Can the auditor justify that 24 items was a sufficient sample size?

SOLUTION & ANALYSIS

Our interest here is in the quantitative aspects of the analysis using the sample size formulas learned here to illustrate how they can be used to defend the auditor's judgment. Without any sampling theory it would be difficult to defend the auditor's conclusion. But with some MUS theory it is relatively easy to do so, as we illustrate here.

Note what the auditor knows with the information given here: the financial statements show a profit of $1.5 million and the auditor's task is to verify its accuracy. (Note that the auditor does not know that this profit is fictitious and the actual loss of $2.5 million is hidden. If the auditor knew these things in advance there would be no need for the audit!) First, the auditor needs to calculate a materiality to use in planning the audit. A common rule of thumb is 5% of net income, so let's use that here since we have very limited information on Giant Stores' financial statements. So, materiality is 0.05 of $1.5 million, or $75,000. Next we must define the relevant population to be tested. It is evident from the SEC accusation that the amount of testing of the $300,000 of advertising credits is a critical issue. This effectively defines the population in terms relevant for applying MUS. Specifically, what is relevant here is the MUS sample size (n) relative to that actually used by the auditor. Under MUS, $n = R/P$, where $P =$ (materiality)/(recorded payables or credits for payables, depending on how the population is defined). For example, by AuG-41, materiality is $0.05 \times$ reported net income of $1.5 million = $75,000, so that $P = \$75,000/\$300,000 = 0.25$. If we use a 95% confidence level, $R = 3.0$, so that $n = 3/0.25 = 12$. The auditor thus picked a sample size twice as large as required by MUS. Note this shows that the SEC may be wrong in saying that 24 items is not a sufficient sample size. Your reasons are those of statistical theory and MUS. What are the SEC's reasons? Is a 95% confidence level reasonable? Is the materiality of $300,000 reasonable? With MUS we can focus on the key judgments necessary to decide on the sufficiency of testing and determine what is sufficient in an objective manner. These are the major advantages of relying on a formal model like MUS to help guide audit judgments and to make them more justifiable. Note especially the importance of auditor judgment in defining the relevant population.

SUMMARY

- Audit sampling was explained in this chapter as an organized method of making decisions. Two kinds of decisions were shown: (1) assessment of control risk and (2) the decision about whether financial statement assertions in an account balance are fairly presented. The method is organized by two kinds of audit programs to guide the work on these two decisions: (1) the internal control program and (2) the balance audit program. The audit sampling itself can be attribute sampling for test of controls and balance audit (variables) sampling for auditing the assertions in an account balance. **LO1, 2, 3**

- Risk in audit decisions was explained in the context of non-sampling and sampling risk, with sampling risk further subdivided into two types of decision errors: (1) assessing control risk too low and incorrect acceptance of a balance and (2) assessing control risk too high and incorrect rejection of an account balance. The first pair damages the effectiveness of audits, and the second pair damages the efficiency of audits. **LO4**

- Audit sampling is a method of organizing the application of audit procedures and a disciplined approach to decision problems. Both types of sampling were explained in basic terms of planning the audit procedures, performing the audit procedures, and evaluating the evidence produced by the audit procedures. The latter process was reinforced with some differences and monetary unit sampling (MUS) projections of misstatement amounts. The mechanics were illustrated in the last section. **LO5, 6**

- Audit programs for test of controls procedures and balance audit procedures were illustrated and integrated with earlier chapters. One of the goals of this chapter was to enable students to understand these procedural programs in the context of audit sampling. The other goal was to clarify the concepts of risk and materiality introduced in the earlier chapters. **LO5, 6**

KEY TERMS

account balance	individually significant items	risk of assessing the control risk too high
analytical procedures risk	known misstatement (identified misstatement)	risk of assessing the control risk too low
attribute sampling	likely misstatement (projected misstatement)	risk of incorrect acceptance
audit procedures	monetary-unit sampling (MUS)	risk of incorrect rejection
audit sampling	non-sampling risk	sample
block sampling	non-statistical (judgmental) sampling	sampling error
class of transactions		sampling risk
classical attribute sampling	physical representation of the population	sampling unit
effectiveness risk (type II error risk)		skewness
efficiency risk (type I error risk)	population	standard deviation
error analysis	population unit	statistical sampling
evidence collection	possible misstatement	stratification
evidence evaluation	problem recognition	substantive tests of details auditing
expectation about the population deviation rate	random sample	systematic random selection
expected dollar misstatement	replicate	tolerable deviation rate
extending the audit conclusion	representative sample	unrestricted random selection
haphazard selection		
hypothesis testing		

MULTIPLE-CHOICE QUESTIONS FOR PRACTICE AND REVIEW

MC 10-1 `LO1` In an audit sampling application, an auditor performs procedures on

a. all the items in a balance and makes a conclusion about the whole balance.
b. less than 100% of the items in a balance and formulates a conclusion about the whole balance.
c. less than 100% of the items in a class of transactions for the purpose of becoming familiar with the client's accounting system.
d. the client's unaudited financial statements as an analysis when planning the audit.

MC 10-2 `LO3` Auditors consider statistical sampling to be characterized by

a. representative sample selection and non-mathematical consideration of the results.
b. carefully biased sample selection and statistical calculation of the results.
c. representative sample selection and statistical calculation of the results.
d. carefully biased sample selection and non-mathematical consideration of the results.

MC 10-3 `LO2` In audit sampling applications, what is sampling risk?

a. A characteristic of statistical sampling applications but not of non-statistical applications
b. The probability that the auditor will fail to recognize erroneous accounting in the client's documentation
c. The probability that accounting errors will arise in transactions and enter the accounting system
d. The probability that an auditor's conclusion based on a sample might be different from the conclusion based on an audit of the entire population

MC 10-4 `LO5` When auditing the client's performance of control for the completeness objective related to recording sales, auditors should draw sample items from which of the following?

a. A sales journal list of recorded sales invoices
b. A file of shipping documents
c. A file of customer order copies
d. A file of receiving reports for inventory additions

MC 10-5 `LO5` Nelson Williams was considering the sample size needed for a selection of sales invoices for the test of controls audit of the LoHo Company's internal controls. He presented the following information for two alternative cases:

	CASE A	CASE B
Acceptable risk of underreliance	High	Low
Acceptable risk of overreliance	High	Low
Tolerable deviation rate	High	Low
Expected population deviation rate	Low	High

Nelson should expect the sample size for Case A to be which of the following?

a. Smaller than the sample size for Case B
b. Larger than the sample size for Case B
c. The same as the sample size for Case B
d. Not determinable relative to the Case B sample size

MC 10-6 `LO6` Nelson next considered the sample size needed for a selection of customers' accounts receivable for the substantive audit of the total accounts receivable. He presented the following information for two alternative cases:

	CASE X	CASE Y
Acceptable risk of incorrect acceptance	Low	High
Acceptable risk of incorrect rejection	Low	High
Tolerable dollar misstatement in the account	Small	Large
Expected dollar misstatement in the account	Large	Small
Estimate of population variability	Large	Small

Nelson should expect the sample size for Case X to be which of the following?

a. Smaller than the sample size for Case Y
b. Larger than the sample size for Case Y
c. The same as the sample size for Case Y
d. Not determinable relative to the Case Y sample size

MC 10-7 `LO6` Which of the following should be considered an audit procedure for obtaining evidence?

a. An audit sampling application in accounts receivable selection
b. Existence and proper valuation of the accounts receivable
c. Sending a written confirmation on a customer's account balance
d. Non-statistical consideration of the amount of difference reported by a customer on a confirmation response

MC 10-8 `LO6` When calculating the total amount of misstatement relevant to the analysis of an account balance, an auditor should add which of the following to the misstatement discovered in individually significant items?

a. The projected likely misstatement and the additional possible misstatement estimate
b. The known misstatement in the sampled items
c. The known misstatement in the sampled items, the projected likely misstatement, and the additional possible misstatement estimate
d. The additional possible misstatement estimate

MC 10-9 `LO6` Eddie audited the LoHo Company's inventory on a sample basis. He audited 120 items from an inventory compilation list and discovered net overstatement of $480. The audited items had a book (recorded) value of $48,000. There were 1,200 inventory items listed, and the total inventory book amount was $490,000. Which of these calculations is (are) correct?

a. Known misstatement of $48,000 using the average difference method
b. Projected likely misstatement of $480 using the sample stratification method
c. Computed upper error limit (UEL) of $49,000 using the taintings method
d. Projected likely misstatement of $4,800 using the average difference method

MC 10-10 `LO6` Stefani audited the client's accounts receivable, but she could not get any good information about customer 102's balance. The customer responded to the confirmation, saying, "Our system does not provide detail for such a response." The sales invoice and shipping document papers have been lost, and the customer has not yet paid. What should Stefani do?

a. Get another customer's account to consider in the sample.

b. Treat customer 102's account as being entirely wrong (overstated) if doing so will not affect her audit conclusion about the receivables taken altogether.

c. Require adjustment of the receivables to write off customer 102's balance.

d. Treat customer 102's account as accurate because there is no evidence saying it is fictitious.

MC 10-11 **LO4** The risk of incorrect acceptance in balance audit sampling and the risk of assessing control risk too low in test of controls sampling both relate to which of the following?

a. Effectiveness of an audit

b. Efficiency of an audit

c. Control risk assessment decisions

d. Evidence about assertions in financial statements

MC 10-12 **LO3** An advantage of statistical sampling is that it helps an auditor

a. eliminate non-sampling risk.

b. reapply evaluation judgments based on factors in addition to the sample evidence.

c. be precise and definite in the approach to an audit problem.

d. omit quantification of risk and materiality judgments.

MC 10-13 **LO4** To determine the sample size for a balance audit sampling application, an auditor should consider the tolerable misstatement, the risk of incorrect acceptance, the risk of incorrect rejection, the population size, plus which one of the following?

a. The expected monetary misstatement in the account

b. The overall materiality for the financial statements taken as a whole

c. The risk of assessing control risk too low

d. The risk of assessing control risk too high

EXERCISES AND PROBLEMS

EP 10-1 Sampling and Non-sampling Audit Work. **LO2, 3** The accounting firm of Mason & Jarr performed the work described in each separate case below. The two partners are worried about properly applying standards regarding audit sampling. They have asked for your advice.

Required:

Write a report addressed to the partners, stating whether they did or did not observe the essential elements of audit sampling standards in each case.

a. Mason selected three purchase orders for raw materials from the LIZ Corporation files, and from there traced each one through the accounting system. He saw the receiving reports, purchasing agent's approvals, receiving clerks' approvals, vendors' invoices (now stamped paid), entry in the cash disbursement records, and cancelled cheques. This work gave him a first-hand familiarity with the cash disbursement system, and he felt confident about understanding related questions in the internal control questionnaire completed later.

b. Jarr observed the inventory-taking at SER Corporation. She had an inventory list of the different inventory descriptions with the quantities taken from the perpetual inventory records. She selected the 200 items with the largest quantities and counted them after the client's shop foreman had completed his count. She decided not to check out the count accuracy on the other 800 items. The shop foreman miscounted in 16 cases. Jarr concluded the rate of miscount was 8%, so as many as 80 of the 1,000 items might be counted wrongly. She asked the foreman to recount everything.

c. CSR Corporation issued seven series of short-term commercial paper notes near the fiscal year-end to finance seasonal operations. Jarr confirmed the obligations under each series with the independent trustee for the holders, studied all seven indenture agreements, and traced the proceeds of each issue to the cash receipts records.

d. At the completion of the EH&R Corporation audit, Mason obtained written representations, as required by auditing standards, from the president, the CFO, and the controller. He did not ask the chief accountant at headquarters or the plant controllers in the three divisions for written representations.

EP 10-2 Test of Controls Audit Procedure Objectives and Control Deviations. `LO5` This exercise asks you to specify control test objectives and define deviations in connection with planning the test of controls audit of Kingston Company's internal controls.

Required:

a. For each control cited below, state the objective of an auditor's test of controls audit procedure.

b. For each control cited below, state the definition of a deviation from the control.

1. The credit department supervisor reviews each customer's order and approves credit by making a notation on the order.

2. The billing department must receive written notice from the shipping department of actual shipment to a customer before a sale is recorded. The sales record date is supposed to be the shipment date.

3. Billing clerks carefully look up the correct catalogue list prices for goods shipped and recheck the amounts billed on invoices for the quantities of goods shipped.

4. Billing clerks review invoices for intercompany sales and mark each one with the code "9" so that they will be posted to intercompany sales accounts.

EP 10-3 Timing of Test of Controls Audit Procedures. `LO5` Auditor Magann was auditing the authorization control over cash disbursements. She selected cash disbursement entries made throughout the year and vouched them to paid invoices and cancelled cheques bearing the initials and signatures of people authorized to approve the disbursements. She performed the work on September 30, up to which date the company had issued cheques numbered from 43921 to 52920. Since 9,000 cheques had been issued in nine months, she reasoned that 3,000 more could be issued in the three months before the December 31 year-end. About 12,000 cheques had been issued last year. She wanted to take one sample of 100 disbursements for the entire year, so she selected 100 random numbers in the sequence 43921 to 55920. She audited the 80 cheques in the sample that were issued before September 30, and she held the other 20 randomly selected cheque numbers for later use. She found no deviations in the sample of 80—a finding that would, in the circumstances, cause her to assign a low (20%) control risk to the probability that the system would permit improper charges to be hidden away in expense and purchase inventory accounts.

Required:

Take the role of Magann and write a memo to the audit manager (dated October 1) describing the audit team's options with respect to evaluating control performance for the remaining period, October through December.

EP 10-4 Evaluation of Quantitative Test of Controls Evidence. `LO5, 8` Assume you audited control compliance in the Kingston Company for the deviations related to a random selection of sales transactions, as shown in Exhibit EP 10-4. For different sample sizes, the number of deviations was as in Exhibit EP 10-4.

Required:

For each deviation and each sample, calculate the rate of deviation in the sample (sample deviation rate).

EXHIBIT EP 10-4

	SAMPLE SIZES									
	30	60	80	90	120	160	220	240	260	300
Missing sales invoice	0	0	0	0	0	0	0	0	0	0
Missing bill of lading	0	0	0	0	0	1	2	2	3	3
No credit approval	0	3	6	8	10	14	17	23	26	31
Wrong prices used	0	0	0	0	2	4	8	9	9	12
Wrong quantity billed	1	2	4	4	4	5	5	5	5	5
Wrong invoice arithmetic	0	0	0	0	1	2	2	2	2	3
Wrong invoice date	0	0	0	0	0	2	2	2	2	2
Posted to wrong account	0	0	0	0	0	0	0	0	0	0

EP 10-5 Stratification Calculation of Projected Likely Misstatement Using the Ratio Method. `LO6` The stratification calculation example in the chapter shows the results of calculating the projected likely misstatement using the difference method. Assume the results shown in Exhibit EP 10-5 were obtained from a stratified sample.

Required:

Apply the ratio calculation method to each stratum to calculate the projected likely misstatement (PLM). What is the PLM for the entire sample?

EXHIBIT EP 10-5

			SAMPLE RESULTS		
STRATUM	POPULATION SIZE	RECORDED AMOUNT	SAMPLE	RECORDED AMOUNT	MISSTATEMENT AMOUNT*
1	6	$100,000	6	$100,000	$ −600
2	80	75,068	23	21,700	−274
3	168	75,008	22	9,476	−66
4	342	75,412	22	4,692	−88
5	910	74,512	23	1,973	23
	1,506	$400,000	96	$137,841	$−1,005

*A negative misstatement indicates overstatement of the book value, and a positive misstatement indicates understatement.

EP 10-6 Determining Risk of Incorrect Acceptance. `LO5, 6` In the dialogue between the Kingston auditors, Fred said, "Our analytical procedures related to receivables didn't show much. The total is down, consistent with the sales decline, so the turnover is up a little. If any misstatement is in the receivables total, it may be too small to be obvious in the ratios."

Jill replied, "That's good news if the problems are immaterial. Too bad we can't say analytical procedures reduce our audit risk. What about internal control?"

Fred responded: "I'd say it's about a 50–50 proposition. Sometimes control seemed to work well; sometimes it didn't. I noticed a few new people doing the invoice processing last week when we were here for a conference. Incidentally, I lump the inherent risk problems and internal control risk problems together when I think about internal control risk. Anyway, firm policy is to plan a sample for a low overall audit risk for the receivables."

Required:

Based on this dialogue information, use the expanded risk model to determine a test of detail risk. Relate this risk to sample size determination.

DISCUSSION CASES

DC 10-1 Projected Likely Misstatement. `LO6` When Marge Simpson, PA, audited the Candle Company inventory, a random sample of inventory types was chosen for physical observation and price testing. The sample size was 80 different types of candles and candle-making inventory. The entire inventory contained 1,740 types, and the amount in the inventory control account was $166,000. Simpson had already decided that a misstatement of as much as $6,000 in the account would not be material. The audit work revealed the following eight errors in the sample of 80.

BOOK VALUE	AUDIT VALUE	ERROR AMOUNT
$600.00	$622.00	$ 22.00
15.50	14.50	(1.00)
65.25	31.50	(33.75)
83.44	53.45	(29.99)
16.78	15.63	(1.15)
78.33	12.50	(65.83)
13.33	14.22	0.89
93.87	39.87	(54.00)
$966.50	$803.67	$(162.83)

Required:

Calculate the projected likely misstatement using the difference method. Discuss the decision choice of accepting or rejecting the $166,000 book value (recorded amount) without adjustment.

DC 10-2 Exercises in Applying the Basic Formula and Using the *R* Value Table in Appendix 10A. `LO5` This case gives auditor judgment and audit sampling results for six populations (see Exhibit DC 10-2). Assume large population sizes.

Required:

a. For each population, did the auditor select a smaller sample size than is indicated by using the tables for determining sample size (assume $K = 0$ in sample size planning)? Explain the effect of selecting either a larger or a smaller size than those determined in the tables.

b. Calculate the sample deviation rate and the achieved P or upper error limit (UEL) for each population.

c. For which of the six populations should the sample results be considered unacceptable? What options are available to the auditor?

d. Why is analysis of the deviations necessary even when the populations are considered acceptable?

e. For the following terms, identify which is an audit decision, which is a non-statistical estimate made by the auditor, which is a sample result, and which is a statistical conclusion about the population.

  1. Estimated population deviation rate
  2. Tolerable deviation rate
  3. Acceptable risk of overreliance on internal control
  4. Actual sample size
  5. Actual number of deviations in the sample
  6. Sample deviation rate
  7. Achieved P or UEL

EXHIBIT DC 10-2

	1	2	3	4	5	6
Tolerable deviation rate or error rate as a percentage (equals materiality for the test)	6	3	8	5	20	15
Acceptable risk of overreliance on internal control in percentage = Effectiveness Risk = 1 − Confidence Level	5	5	10	5	10	10
Actual sample size	100	100	60	100	20	60
Actual number of deviations (errors) in the sample	2	0	1	4	1	8

CRITICAL THINKING

CT 10-1 **LO4** Does non-sampling risk include improper application of GAAP? Discuss.

CT 10-2 **LO4** Do you think the general decision rule "if achieved P > materiality, then reject; otherwise accept the population" should be applied to all estimates in financial reporting whether statistical or not? Discuss.

Statistical Sampling Tables

LO7 Demonstrate that you can work with statistical sampling tables.

R VALUE TABLE

CONFIDENCE LEVELS				K VALUE: NUMBER OF SAMPLE ERRORS	CONFIDENCE LEVELS		
75%	80%	85%	90%		95%	97.5%	99%
R	R	R	R		R	R	R
1.39	1.61	1.90	2.31	0	3.00	3.69	4.51
2.70	3.00	3.38	3.89	1	4.75	5.58	6.64
3.93	4.28	4.73	5.33	2	6.30	7.23	8.41
5.11	5.52	6.02	6.69	3	7.76	8.77	10.05
6.28	6.73	7.27	8.00	4	9.16	10.25	11.61
7.43	7.91	8.50	9.28	5	10.52	11.67	13.11
8.56	9.08	9.71	10.54	6	11.85	13.06	14.58
9.69	10.24	10.90	11.78	7	13.15	14.43	16.00
10.81	11.38	12.08	13.00	8	14.44	15.77	17.41
11.92	12.52	13.25	14.21	9	15.71	17.09	18.79
13.03	13.66	14.42	15.41	10	16.97	18.40	20.15

TABLE OF RANDOM DIGITS

32942	95416	42339	59045	26693	49057	87496	20624	14819
07410	99859	83828	21409	29094	65114	36701	25762	12827
59981	68155	45673	76210	58219	45738	29550	24736	09574
46251	25437	69654	99716	11563	08803	86027	51867	12116
65558	51904	93123	27887	53138	21488	09095	78777	71240
99187	19258	86421	16401	19397	83297	40111	49326	81686
35641	00301	16096	34775	21562	97983	45040	19200	16383
14031	00936	81518	48440	02218	04756	19506	60695	88494
60677	15076	92554	26042	23472	69869	62877	19584	39576
66314	05212	67859	89356	20056	30648	87349	20389	53805
20416	87410	75646	64176	82752	63606	37011	57346	69512
28701	56992	70423	62415	40807	98086	58850	28968	45297
74579	33844	33426	07570	00728	07079	19322	56325	84819
62615	52342	82968	75540	80045	53069	20665	21282	07768

(continued)

93945	06293	22879	08161	01442	75071	21427	94842	26210
75689	76131	96837	67450	44511	50424	82848	41975	71663
02921	16919	35424	93209	52133	87327	95897	65171	20376
14295	34969	14216	03191	61647	30296	66667	10101	63203
05303	91109	82403	40312	62191	67023	90073	83205	71344
57071	90357	12901	08899	91039	67251	28701	03846	94589
78471	57741	13599	84390	32146	00871	09354	22745	65806
89242	79337	59293	47481	07740	43345	25716	70020	54005
14955	59592	97035	80430	87220	06392	79028	57123	52872
42446	41880	37415	47472	04513	49494	08860	08038	43624
18534	22346	54556	17558	73689	14894	05030	19561	56517
39284	33737	42512	86411	23753	29690	26096	81361	93099
33922	37329	89911	55876	28379	81031	22058	21487	54613
78355	54013	50774	30666	61205	42574	47773	36027	27174
08845	99145	94316	88974	29828	97069	90327	61842	29604
01769	71825	55957	98271	02784	66731	40311	88495	18821
17639	38284	59478	90409	21997	56199	30068	82800	69692
05851	58653	99949	63505	40409	85551	90729	64938	52403
42396	40112	11469	03476	03328	84238	26570	51790	42122
13318	14192	98167	75631	74141	22369	36757	89117	54998
60571	54786	26281	01855	30706	66578	32019	65884	58485
09531	81853	59334	70929	03544	18510	89541	13555	21168
72865	16829	86542	00396	20363	13010	69645	49608	54738
56324	31093	77924	28622	83543	28912	15059	80192	83964
78192	21626	91399	07235	07104	73652	64425	85149	75409
64666	34767	97298	92708	01994	53188	78476	07804	62404
82201	75694	02808	65983	74373	66693	13094	74183	73020
15360	73776	40914	85190	54278	99054	62944	47351	89098
68142	67957	70896	37983	20487	95350	16371	03426	13895
19138	31200	30616	14639	44406	44236	57360	81644	94761
28155	03521	36415	78452	92359	81091	56513	88321	97910
87971	29031	51780	27376	81056	86155	55488	50590	74514
58147	68841	53625	02059	75223	16783	19272	61994	71090
18875	52809	70594	41649	32935	26430	82096	01605	65846
75109	56474	74111	31966	29969	70093	98901	84550	25769
35983	03742	76822	12073	59463	84420	15868	99505	11426

Source: The Rand Corporation, *A Million Random Digits with 100,000 Normal Deviates* (Glencoe: Free Press, 1955), p. 102.

TABLE TO DETERMINE SAMPLE SIZES FOR TESTS OF CONTROL USING THE MONETARY-UNIT SAMPLING APPROACH												
TOLERABLE RATE OF DEVIATIONS OR ERRORS												
	0.01	0.02	0.03	0.04	0.05	0.06	0.07	0.08	0.09	0.10	0.15	0.20
EFFECTIVENESS RISK = 0.05	300	150	100	75	60	50	43	38	34	30	20	15
EFFECTIVENESS RISK = 0.10	231	116	77	58	47	39	33	29	26	24	16	12

TABLE TO EVALUATE SAMPLE RESULTS FOR TESTS OF CONTROLS USING THE MONETARY-UNIT SAMPLING APPROACH: COMPUTED UPPER ERROR LIMITS AS A PERCENT (ACHIEVED P'S) FOR CONFIDENCE LEVEL = 95%

Effectiveness Risk = 0.05

R VALUE	3	4.75	6.3	7.76	9.16	10.52	11.85	13.15	14.44	15.71	16.97
Actual Number of Errors Found in the Sample											
Sample Size	0	1	2	3	4	5	6	7	8	9	10
20	15	*	*	*	*	*	*	*	*	*	*
25	12	19	*	*	*	*	*	*	*	*	*
30	10	16	*	*	*	*	*	*	*	*	*
35	9	14	18	*	*	*	*	*	*	*	*
40	8	12	16	20	*	*	*	*	*	*	*
45	7	11	14	18	*	*	*	*	*	*	*
50	6	10	13	16	19	*	*	*	*	*	*
55	6	9	12	15	17	20	*	*	*	*	*
60	5	8	11	13	16	18	20	*	*	*	*
65	5	8	10	12	15	17	19	*	*	*	*
70	5	7	9	12	14	16	17	19	*	*	*
75	4	7	9	11	13	15	16	18	20	*	*
80	4	6	8	10	12	14	15	17	19	20	*
90	4	6	7	9	11	12	14	15	17	18	19
100	3	5	7	8	10	11	12	14	15	16	17
125	3	4	6	7	8	9	10	11	12	13	14
150	2	4	5	6	7	8	8	9	10	11	12
175	2	3	4	5	6	7	7	8	9	9	10
200	2	3	4	4	5	6	6	7	8	8	9
250	2	2	3	4	4	5	5	6	6	7	7
300	1	2	3	3	4	4	4	5	5	6	6

TABLE TO EVALUATE SAMPLE RESULTS FOR TESTS OF CONTROLS USING THE MONETARY-UNIT SAMPLING APPROACH: COMPUTED UPPER ERROR LIMITS AS A PERCENT (ACHIEVED P'S) FOR CONFIDENCE LEVEL = 90%

Effectiveness Risk = 0.10

R VALUES	2.31	3.89	5.33	6.69	8.00	9.28	10.54	11.78	13.00	14.21	15.41
Actual Number of Errors Found in the Sample											
Sample Size	0	1	2	3	4	5	6	7	8	9	10
20	12	20	*	*	*	*	*	*	*	*	*
25	10	16	*	*	*	*	*	*	*	*	*
30	8	13	18	*	*	*	*	*	*	*	*
35	7	12	16	20	*	*	*	*	*	*	*
40	6	10	14	17	20	*	*	*	*	*	*

(continued)

45	6	9	12	15	18	*	*	*	*	*	*
50	5	8	11	14	16	19	*	*	*	*	*
55	5	8	10	13	15	17	20	*	*	*	*
60	4	7	9	12	14	16	18	20	*	*	*
65	4	6	9	11	13	15	17	19	20	*	*
70	4	6	8	10	12	14	16	17	19	*	*
75	4	6	8	9	11	13	15	16	18	19	*
80	3	5	7	9	10	12	14	15	17	18	20
90	3	5	6	8	9	11	12	14	15	16	18
100	3	4	6	7	8	10	11	12	13	15	16
125	2	4	5	6	7	8	9	10	11	12	13
150	2	3	4	5	6	7	8	8	9	10	11
175	2	3	4	4	5	6	7	7	8	9	9
200	2	2	3	4	4	5	6	6	7	8	8
250	1	2	3	3	4	4	5	5	6	6	7
300	1	2	2	3	3	4	4	4	5	5	6

Appendix 10B: More-Advanced Statistical Sampling Concepts for Tests of Controls and Tests of Balances (on Connect)

ENDNOTES

1   E. Turner, "How much is enough?" *CA Magazine*, March 2010, pp. 49–51.

2   CAS 530.05(a).

3   Canadian Institute of Chartered Accountants, *Terminology for Accountants*, 4th edition (CICA, 1992).

4   "Audit sampling," *Audit and Accounting Guide* (AICPA, 1983), pp. 1–3.

5   Effectiveness and efficiency risks are the most fundamental risk concepts in auditing.

6   MUS, however, defines a sampling unit differently as the monetary (dollar) value of the sampling unit. In effect, each recorded dollar is viewed as a sampling unit. This allows wider use of attribute sampling as a substantive test and greatly simplifies formulas that need to be learned with statistical auditing. MUS is explained in detail in Appendix 10B.

7   Accounting firms have different policies for associating tolerable deviation rates with control risk categories. Some start with a minimum rate of 1%, and others start with higher rates.

8   T. Hall and T. Herron, "How reliable is haphazard sampling?" *CPA Journal*, January 2006, pp. 26–27.

9   Changing the example to suppose deviations were found creates a problem for the non-statistical sampler. He or she must think harder about the evidence (a 5.5% sample rate) in relation to the tolerable rate (8%) and acceptable risk. The statistical sampler can measure the UEL at 8.3%, which is greater than the 8% tolerable rate at a 10% risk of overreliance. The control fails the decision criterion test. Appendix 10B contains more information about making these calculations using statistical tables and formulas.

PART 3

Performing the Audit

The Revenues, Receivables, and Receipts Process and Cash Account Balance

This chapter starts with a prelude to Part 3, giving an overview of how the audit planning explained in Part 2 links to performing the audit in the main business processes of a typical organization. The chapter then describes the accounting process related to a business's revenues: accepting customer orders, delivering goods and services to customers, accounting for customer sales and accounts receivable, collecting and depositing cash received from customers, and reconciling bank statements. It then describes the control considerations, typical control tests, and substantive audit programs used in auditing the revenues, receivables, and receipts process. Special technical notes on auditing the existence assertion using confirmations and on auditing bank reconciliations are provided. An Application Case with suggested solution and analysis is given at the end of the chapter to demonstrate the performance of audit procedures in situations where errors or frauds might be discovered in the revenues, receivables, and receipts process.

LEARNING OBJECTIVES

After completing this chapter, you will be able to do the following:

LO1 Describe the revenues, receivables, and receipts process, including typical risks, transactions, account balances, source documents, and controls.

LO2 Describe the auditor's control risk assessment and control tests for auditing control over customer credit approval, delivery, accounts receivable, cash receipts, and bank statements.

LO3 Explain how the auditor's risk assessment procedures and control testing link to the key assertions and audit objectives in designing a substantive audit program for the cash account balance.

LO4 Describe the typical substantive procedures used to address the assessed risk of material misstatement in the main account balances and transactions in the revenues, receivables, and receipts process.

LO5 Explain the importance of the existence assertion for the audit of cash and accounts receivable.

LO6 Identify considerations for using confirmations when auditing cash and accounts receivable.

LO7 Describe the audit of bank statement reconciliations and how auditors identify accounts receivable lapping and suspicious cash transactions.

LO8 (Appendix 11A) Describe the internal control questionnaires used in audit practice.

LO9 (Appendix 11B) Describe the accounting control system documentation approaches used in audit practice.

LO10 (Appendix 11C) Describe the organization and contents of the sections contained in typical audit documentation files.

CHAPTER APPENDICES

APPENDIX 11A Internal Control Questionnaires

APPENDIX 11B System Documentation Examples for the Revenues, Receivables, and Receipts Process

APPENDIX 11C Example of an Audit Engagement File Index (on Connect)

EcoPak

EcoPak Inc.

Caleb and Donna completed their interim audit work on the systems and controls at EcoPak on schedule. Shree has also completed her work on the information technology (IT) systems, finding they are designed well and provide effective controls over authorization of transactions, accuracy, and completeness of processing the data. The audit team's interim work has identified a strong control environment and general controls in the company, since Nina has made a point of ensuring that good processes have been implemented, including appropriate segregation of duties to the extent possible given the size of the company. Nina performs many key reconciliation and review controls procedures and analyzes all the accounts for the year-end to make sure any posting or misclassification errors are corrected prior to preparing the draft financial statements, before the auditors even see them.

One weakness the team noted was that Mike's user ID gives him access to both the inventory and the sales processes, which are considered incompatible functions. Nina explains that they set it up that way because Mike sometimes has to work quite closely with customer relations when a new customized product is being developed: "This was the easiest way for him to get all the information he needs to make sure customers get what they want and the new pricing is appropriate." To fully assess this risk, the team has verified that Mike has no access to any financial accounting processes, so the risk of misstatement is reduced.

The audit team concluded that there are effective control procedures in the sales processing and credit note processing functions that can be relied on as a basis for planning lower extents of substantive work on the sales transactions. Belinda reviewed the files and was satisfied with their work and the reasonableness of their conclusions. She agrees that Mike's access is probably not a big problem, but that it should be mentioned to the board as a management letter recommendation to consider whether a more customized access profile could be implemented to meet Mike's information needs. She does warn the team, however: "You guys are *very* lucky on this audit. Nina is highly qualified and seems to run a tight ship in the accounting area, so it looks like this could be a very clean audit. But even so, don't let your guard down. We need sufficient evidence beyond the fact that management has good controls, and misstatements are always possible!"

The time is now approaching to begin making arrangements with EcoPak's management to visit their business to complete the year-end audit work. Belinda asks Donna to carry on with preparing the substantive audit programs for her review so that she can finalize the assignment of audit staff to the year-end. Since Caleb will be starting with the cash balance audit, Donna prepares that plan first and goes over it with Caleb so he will be ready to go when they get back to the EcoPak offices. Donna uses the firm's template program form as a starting point and then tailors it for EcoPak's business and its processes and for the team's findings to date on its internal control. Based on the results of their control tests, Donna concludes that there are strong controls in place for the existence, completeness, and ownership assertions of the cash balance, so this can be taken into account in the extent of further testing of these assertions. They did not perform control tests specifically related to the valuation and presentation of cash, as it would be more efficient to simply rely on substantive procedures for these assertions. Taking into account their inherent risk assessments and their control findings, Donna designs an audit program for cash, with further procedures to respond to the residual risk of misstatement, applying the audit risk model to determine the residual risk for each assertion. She then turns her attention to tailoring the other substantive programs for the revenues, receivables, and receipts process, and then for the rest of EcoPak's processes. Tariq wants to review the completed planning file early next week before a meeting he has scheduled with Kam, Mike, and Zhang. This means Donna needs to get it to Belinda by Friday morning to give her time to review it first. Once all the reviews are completed, Donna and Caleb head out to EcoPak's offices to complete their field work.

Preview of Part 3: Linking Audit Planning to Performing an Independent Financial Statement Audit

You are about to begin Part 3 of the text, which illustrates how the audit activities, concepts, and tools presented in Part 2 are applied in practice to perform audits. In Part 3, simplified business situations will be used as examples to illustrate the links from planning considerations to actually doing the audit work.

In Chapter 5, we discussed how the auditor's understanding of the auditee's business—its environment, risks, systems, and controls—is the basis for developing an appropriate *overall audit strategy*, which sets out the preliminary decisions on the scope of the audit. As covered in Chapters 4 and 5, the audit scope defines the entity and the financial information that is the subject of the audit opinion. The overall strategy also sets out the audit's timing and the approach to be used to gather sufficient appropriate evidence. As discussed, the strategy involves the following:

- Determining appropriate materiality levels for planning purposes
- Assessing the auditee's industry, legal, and regulatory environment; generally accepted accounting principles (GAAP); and changes in the company's management, information systems, or operations that can affect financial reports

- Identifying material financial statement components and high-risk audit areas
- Determining the audit evidence required to assess internal control effectiveness
- Deciding, on a preliminary basis, whether controls will be tested, what substantive evidence will be required, and what the timing for the procedures will be

Based on the overall strategy, the auditor will communicate to auditee management and those charged with its governance about the resources and cooperation that will be required from auditee personnel, so that arrangements can be made for access to records and personnel at the time planned for performing the interim and final audit work. The audit firm's internal resource needs are also specified in the overall strategy: How many audit staff are required and what experience levels do they need? Are audit staff with special expertise in IT or tax issues required? Will external experts be required for valuation assistance? Will other offices of the audit firm be involved for multi-location businesses, or will the work of other audit firms be used?

Overall audit strategy development also sets out a schedule for *audit team meetings*, timing of the process, and experience levels required for *working paper reviews*. The auditor's assessment of management's internal controls is made at the company level and at the application level (transactions, balances, and disclosures, and the assertions of each). Details of this assessment were covered in Part 2, but this prelude provides a questionnaire guiding the auditor in this assessment for the overall strategy development stage of the audit.

The overall strategy is the basis for the detailed audit plan, which is a set of audit programs designed for all the accounting processes in the auditee's business. A business enterprise can be viewed as being made up of several business processes, each with a related accounting process. This view of a business is useful for an organization's management and its systems development purposes, and it is likely also to be an effective approach in most audit engagements. The accounting processes we will examine in Part 3 are as follows:

- Revenues, receivables, and receipts process (Chapter 11)
- Purchases, payables, and payments process (Chapter 12)
- Payroll and production process (Chapter 13)
- Finance and investment process (Chapter 14)

Even though organizations may differ, generally, these four processes cover the key functions that need to be managed and accounted for in any organization. The **detailed audit plan** for each process includes specific *audit programs* that take effectiveness and efficiency into consideration in (1) specifying the *nature, extent, and timing* of *audit procedures* to assess inherent and control risk at the assertion level and (2) planning further audit procedures that will be done to reduce these risks to an acceptably low level for issuing an audit opinion. The detailed audit plan also covers decisions about managing the audit team: assigning staff with necessary competencies, supervision and review to allow less experienced staff to develop *professional skepticism* and judgment, and the *time budgets* required. Finally, the evidence and knowledge gained from performing audit procedures provide feedback to the audit planning process and may suggest that the current or future overall strategy and audit plan should be modified in terms of the **audit scope**, timing, or extent. The diagram below summarizes this development process for the overall strategy and the detailed audit plan.

detailed audit plan:
an audit planning document outlining the nature, timing, and extent of audit procedures to assess the risk of financial statement misstatement and obtain the necessary audit evidence for each assertion for all significant transactions, balances, and disclosures, including staffing decisions and time budgets

audit scope:
the entity and the financial statements that will be covered by the audit engagement, and the client documents and records to be examined to provide the necessary audit evidence

Relating Audit Planning to Audit Performance

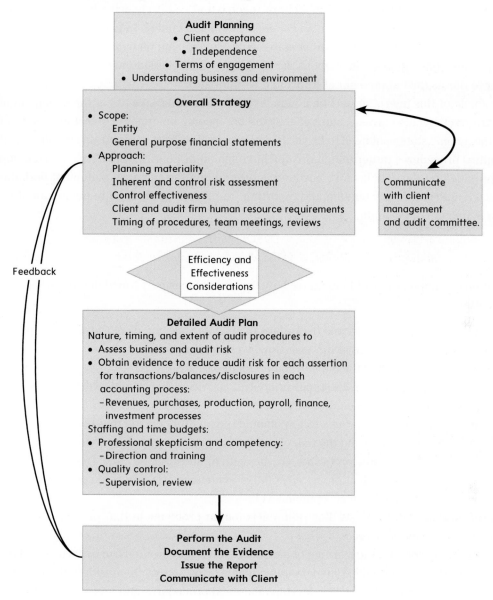

Business Processes and Accounting Cycles: The Big Picture

To keep things as simple as possible, the design and execution of audit programs for each business process will be focused on individually, even though the processes are all interrelated. Exhibit 6–12, "Capturing an Organization's Business Processes in Its Financial Statements," gave a big-picture view of how the processes fit together in an organization. The shares and debt coming into the entity and being invested in capital assets are handled mainly in the finance and investment process (Chapter 14); creation of goods and services involves the purchases, payables, and payments process (Chapter 12) as well as the payroll and production processes (Chapter 13); and generation of revenues is handled in the revenues, receivables, and receipts process (Chapter 11).

The financial statements covered by the auditor's opinion are part of the big-picture approach as well. Exhibit 7–4, "The Financial Reporting Process in an Auditee Company," expanded the picture to show the role of business processes and controls in capturing information about the entity's events and environment into its accounting system, allowing production of a set of general purpose financial statements. The full set of statements—that is, the balance sheet, statement of income and comprehensive income, cash flow statement, and statement of shareholders' equity—are all connected so that a change in one particular statement will flow through to all the related accounts in the other statements. By focusing on balance sheet accounts and changes in them, we are also gaining assurance about the rest of the financial statement accounts that are connected to it. We refer to this as the **balance sheet approach to auditing**.

As an example of this interrelationship, a high level of audit assurance about the change in net assets and shareholder transactions also gives assurance that the net income amount is correct and that only the allocations within the income statement need to be verified as reasonable. This verification can often be done by using mainly analytical procedures rather than more costly vouching or confirmation. This interrelationship reflects the control provided by the double-entry accounting system and the financial statement definitions set out in GAAP. These strengths of the accounting and reporting framework are helpful in pulling all of the audit work together for completion of the audit.

Overview of Chapters 11 through 16

The organization of Chapters 11 to 14 illustrates how the audit plan is performed in the processes. Each chapter follows this pattern:

- An overview of the business risks and the transactions, balances, and disclosures in that process is given.
- Significant risks of misstatement at the assertion level are analyzed.
- An example of the process and the main accounts related to it is given.
- Key control assertions and risks, the types of control activities that would address those risks, and procedures auditors can use to assess controls are covered.
- Examples of alternative controls tests follow, should the auditors decide that reliance on effective controls would be cost effective in reducing the risk of not detecting a material misstatement.
- Examples of substantive audit programs are presented, showing the link from risk assessment at the assertion level, to control evaluation, to substantive evidence gathering that could be used in a particular context to reduce audit risk to an acceptable level.
- An Application Case with analysis illustrating accounting problems in that process and how audit procedures can uncover them is offered.
- A chapter summary reviews the learning objectives covered and provides an overview of the balance sheet approach to analyzing financial statement components. This approach considers the relationships among accounts and how they can be used to develop analytical procedures and assess the impact of the types of misstatements commonly discovered in each process.

Part 3 concludes with two chapters covering issues that the auditor must address to complete the audit and form an audit opinion. Chapter 15 covers audit procedures that gather some final evidence to complete the audit. It presents procedures for auditing revenues and expenses and the cash flow statement. It also discusses the evaluation of potential unrecorded liabilities by obtaining lawyers' confirmation letters, the review of subsequent events, management representation letters, and the management letter. The standards for documenting the audit work in the final audit file are reviewed, and the overall review of evidence is obtained. Chapter 16 explains how auditors apply judgment to assess the misstatements identified and their materiality, propose financial statement adjustments to management, assess the overall financial statement presentation

balance sheet approach to auditing:
using audit analysis of changes in balance sheet accounts as a basis for obtaining preliminary assurance about the related income statement accounts and cash flow information

and disclosure, and form an audit opinion. Based on the opinion formed, the final step is to prepare the appropriate form of audit report to attach to the financial statements.

Note that there are many references in Part 3 to details of generally accepted auditing standards (GAAS) issued in the *CPA Canada Assurance Handbook* as Canadian Auditing Standards (CASs), which are virtually identical to the International Standards on Auditing (ISAs).[1] Since this text is aimed at students who will most likely be auditing under Canadian or international GAAS, the text refers, for the most part, to the auditing and assurance recommendations set out by the standard-setting boards of CPA Canada in the CASs and the International Federation of Accountants (IFAC) in the ISAs. The U.S. auditing standards for private companies have been moving toward harmonization with international GAAS. The American Institute of Certified Public Accountants (AICPA) has a set of clarified auditing standards based on ISAs that came into effect for private companies for periods ending on or after December 15, 2012. However, U.S. pronouncements and standard setting are structured somewhat differently in response to unique U.S. legal, regulatory, and political circumstances, and auditing standards for public companies are set by federal regulation through the Public Company Accounting Oversight Board (PCAOB). This text refers to U.S. standards when they are likely to lead to similar developments in future Canadian or international GAAS. For those who wish to learn more about U.S. GAAS, refer to the PCAOB and AICPA websites for specific details.

The Essentials of Auditing a Business's Revenues, Receivables, and Receipts Process

Revenue creation is the main focus of any organization, and management will have strategies in place to generate revenues as well as business processes to implement the strategies. The accounting process for revenue transactions also involves processing the related accounts receivable account balance and cash receipts transactions. The two routine journal entries in this process are as follows:

Dr Accounts Receivable	Dr Cash
Cr Sales Revenues	Cr Accounts Receivable

Management's main control objectives for revenues relate to the completeness, accuracy, and authorization of revenue transactions, to ensure that all sales are recorded for the proper amounts and credit granting is appropriate. Auditors' main concern is with management's controls over the validity of sales transactions, since recording non-existent revenues would overstate the performance of the business, potentially misleading financial statement users. Auditor control testing in the revenue process is usually required when there is a high volume of revenue transactions, especially when there is a lot of variability in the amounts recorded. Controls over cash receipt transactions are also often tested to ensure they are valid. The results of the auditor's control testing will affect the nature of further substantive audit work to be performed, as well as the sample sizes and timing of further procedures.

Substantive audit procedures that are commonly used in the revenues, receivables, and receipts accounting process are briefly outlined here. For cash, the auditor obtains a confirmation of bank account details at the period-end directly from the bank and reperforms the auditee's reconciliation of bank account balances to general ledger cash account balances. For accounts receivable, a sample of outstanding customer accounts receivable balances is usually confirmed, and cutoff information for cash receipts and sales invoicing are agreed to the cutoff for receivables balances. The auditor also evaluates the adequacy of the auditee's allowance for bad debts, often based on the aged trial balance of customer account balances and a review of historical collection patterns. The substantive verification of sales revenues is often performed by using dual-purpose audit procedures that provide evidence about control effectiveness and substantive evidence that the general ledger amounts are correct. Auditors will test the controls over revenue processing for a sample of revenue transactions recorded in the general ledger and also vouch the same sample of transactions back to supporting sales documents, such as shipping records (packing slips) and customer orders, to provide substantive evidence about the occurrence and the monetary valuation assertions. Similarly, cash receipts can be tested by dual-purpose procedures, vouching credit entries in accounts receivables back to valid cash bank deposits or records of authorized credit notes.

The audit of revenues, receivables, and receipts is focused on the risk of material misstatement related to the existence assertion. This is because overstatements of revenues and related assets pose the greatest threat, due to potential management incentives to overstate these performance-related measures. Also, financial statement users are very interested in these measures to evaluate the success and potential of the business.

Review Checkpoints

11-1   What are the main classes of transactions and related account balances for the revenue process?

11-2   What are management's main control objectives related to the revenue process? Why?

11-3   What are an auditor's main concerns related to revenue transactions? Why?

11-4   In what situations is it most likely that auditors will decide to test controls over revenue transactions?

11-5   What are some common substantive audit procedures for revenues, cash, and accounts receivable?

11-6   Give two examples of dual-purpose tests that can be used in the revenue process.

11-7   What assertion is the auditor most concerned about in auditing the revenues, receivables, and receipts process? Why?

11-8   What is an example of a substantive audit procedure that provides evidence related to the existence of cash? of accounts receivable?

Understanding the Revenues, Receivables, and Receipts Process

LO1   Describe the revenues, receivables, and receipts process, including typical risks, transactions, account balances, source documents, and controls.

Revenue creation is the focus of strategy and business processes for any organization because revenues provide the cash flows that are its lifeblood. The auditor must understand the business's method of generating revenues and the use of them in the operation of the business in order to assess the business risk and the risk that the financial statements are misstated, as discussed in Chapter 6. In a for-profit business, costs incurred must generate enough sales revenue to provide profits to sustain operations and also provide investment returns to owners and creditors. A not-for-profit organization must also generate enough revenues to pay for the activities necessary to achieve its charitable or other purposes.

Assertion-Based Risk Assessment for Revenues, Receivables, and Receipts

To assess risks in the revenue-generating processes, the auditor mainly considers the revenue and cash receipts transactions, as well as the accounts receivable balances. Important presentation and disclosure issues relating to revenues include revenue recognition policies, related party transactions, commitments, and economic dependencies.

At the assertion level, risks related to the existence/occurrence and ownership of revenues may arise if management chooses overly aggressive revenue recognition policies (e.g., Nortel, Xerox), perhaps because of management incentives or pressure to meet performance targets. Complex sales arrangements that involve multiple deliverables with differing rights of return by customers, or complex revenue recognition situations, such as long-term contracts, may also increase the existence and ownership risks, as revenue may be recognized inappropriately. Ownership risks may exist where managers can transfer funds between related entities under their control (e.g., Enron, Hollinger). Completeness risks relate to recordkeeping and custodial controls over cash receipts; these must ensure that all revenues the business earns are received by the company and recorded in full. Fraudulent misappropriation of cash by employees is a key completeness risk in the revenue process. Because substantial flows of funds may be involved in the revenue processes of some businesses (e.g., financial services, banking), **money laundering**—processing monetary profits of crime to cover up their sources and convert them to "clean" cash—is also an ownership risk related to the revenue transactions. Valuation and ownership risks can exist when substantial revenues are generated in foreign countries because of currency exchange risks and potential restrictions on removing money from these countries. Presentation and disclosure risks include revenue recognition policy explanations; reporting significant revenue categories separately; accruals of complex revenue streams, such as royalties or long-term contracts; reporting the extent of barter transactions (e.g., in e-commerce); or disclosing contractual commitments to sell inventory at fixed prices. These are only some examples of risks that may exist in a particular business. You can see how an auditor's in-depth understanding of the auditee's business, the revenue-generating strategy that drives it, and the environment it operates in is critical to a comprehensive assessment of business risks and the possible financial misstatements that these risks can lead to.

This chapter uses simple examples to outline the business processes and related accounting process for recording and controlling revenues, accounts receivable, and cash receipts. It explains the control activities that are important in these processes, how to evaluate and test these controls, and how to design and implement the substantive audit tests that provide evidence that the resulting financial statements are fairly reported. The risk of non-existent or incorrectly valued revenues or receivables can often be addressed by confirmation and analytical procedures. Control tests in the revenue transaction processes may also provide assurance that the controls effectively lower the risk of material misstatement, thereby reducing the amount of assurance required from substantive evidence. Revenue completeness usually relies on controls and control testing; substantive testing alone may not provide sufficient evidence for the completeness assertion for revenues.

Revenues, Receivables, and Receipts Process: Typical Activities

The picture in Exhibit 11–1 presents a skeleton overview of typical activities in the revenues, receivables, and receipts process in a business that sells inventory (a similar process is used in a service business, except that a service is provided to the customers rather than a tangible good).[2] The basic process functions, shown in bold, are as follows: (1) receiving and processing customer orders, (2) credit granting, (3) delivering goods and services to customers, (4) billing customers and accounting for accounts receivable, and (5) collecting and depositing cash received from customers. As you follow the exhibit, you can track some of the elements of the control structure, shown in the green ovals. Control will be strengthened by ensuring that these functions are performed by different people. Further examples of controls related to this process are provided in Appendix 11A, Exhibit 11A–2.

In practice, you would have obtained a detailed organizational chart as part of the audit planning. This chart identifies the specific auditee personnel responsible for the various functions in the process. These are the people you will work with to design and perform your audit work. Your audit documentation for significant processes will be in the form of system narratives, flowcharts, or process tables: these are described next.

money laundering:
engaging in specific financial transactions in order to conceal the identity, source, and/or destination of money resulting from an illegal act, which may involve organized crime, tax evasion, or false accounting

EXHIBIT 11–1

Revenues, Receivables, and Receipts Process: Overview Diagram of Typical Activities

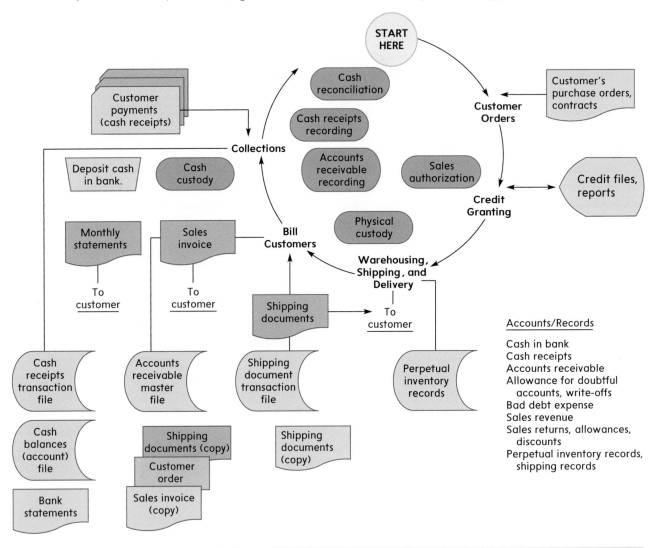

Review Checkpoints

11-9   What is the basic sequence of activities and related accounting in the revenues, receivables, and receipts process?

11-10   What are some risks of material misstatement in the assertions for revenues?

Revenues and Accounts Receivable: Processing and Controls

This section gives a narrative description of a system for processing customer sales orders. Alternative documentation formats, such as a flowchart diagram or a process table, could be used for this description, and examples of these formats are provided in Appendix 11B. At the starting point, company personnel receive the customer's purchase order and create a sales order, entering it into a computer system. The computer system then performs automatic authorization procedures—determining whether the customer is a regular or new customer, approving credit, and checking the availability of inventory. (If inventory is short, a back order is entered.) Once these authorizations are in a computer system, access to the master files for additions, deletions, and other changes must be limited to responsible persons; otherwise, it is possible for errors to occur, e.g., orders processed for fictitious customers, credit approved for bad credit risks, or packing slips created for goods that do not exist in the inventory.

When a customer order passes the authorizations, the system (1) creates a record in the pending order master file, (2) transmits a packing slip to the stockroom and shipping department, and (3) updates the inventory master file to show the commitment (removal) of the inventory. The pending order and the packing slip should be numbered sequentially so that the system can determine if any transactions have not been completed (completeness objective of control). The packing slip is the stockkeeper's authorization to release inventory to the shipping department and the shipping department's authorization to release goods to a trucker or the customer. It may be helpful to think about how these activities are performed in a company you have done business with, such as Amazon.

The company's internal control will feature important types of control activities designed to prevent things from going wrong. The control activities include employee procedures relating to keeping custody of assets and records; properly recording transactions and events; and performing reconciling procedures to check the completeness and integrity of the records by comparison to other summaries, reports, or the actual assets themselves. These control activities, and what could go wrong if they are ineffective or missing, are described in more detail below.

Custody

Physical custody of inventory starts with the stockroom or warehouse. Custody is transferred to the shipping department when the packing slip is authorized. As long as the system works, custody is under proper control. However, if the stockkeeper or the shipping department personnel have the power to change the quantity shown on the packing slip, they can cause errors in the system by billing the customer for too small or too large a quantity. With collusion, this can allow inventory to be stolen, for example, shipping a customer more than it will be billed for, covered up by the alterations in the records. (This is a combination of custody and recording functions, a segregation-of-duties control weakness. A computer record or log of such changes is a control procedure creating an electronic audit trail.)

Custody of the accounts receivable records is with the personnel who have the power to enter those records directly or to enter transactions to alter them (e.g., transfers, returns, allowance credits, write-offs). Ideally, personnel with the ability to enter accounts receivable records do not also have sole authorization over the entries or the ability to perform reconciliations, as this can reduce the probability of catching the person's recording errors, such as omitting part of a sales order from a sales invoice. This kind of combination of authorization and recording responsibility is another example of a control weakness due to a lack of segregation of incompatible duties.

Shipping Employee Caught by Computer!

A customer paid off a shipping department employee to change the quantity on the packing slip and bill of lading to a smaller quantity than was actually shipped. This caused the customer's invoices to be understated. The employee did not know that a computer log recorded all the entries altering the original packing slip record. An alert internal auditor noticed the pattern of "corrections" made by the shipping employee. A trap was laid by initiating fictitious orders for this customer, and the employee was observed making the alterations. This independent review of the transactions was an effective control for detecting the missing sales.

Recording

When delivery or shipment is complete, the shipping personnel enter the completion of the transaction in the system, which (1) produces a bill of lading shipping document, evidence of an actual delivery or shipment; (2) removes the pending order from the inventory recording system; and (3) produces a sales invoice (prenumbered the same as the order and packing slip) that bills the customer for the quantity shipped, according to the bill of lading. Shipping personnel who have the power to enter or alter these transactions or to intercept the invoice that is supposed to be sent to the customer have undesirable combinations of authorization, custody, and recording responsibilities. This is a control weakness because it provides an opportunity for employees to commit a fraud by misappropriating inventory and concealing it in the accounting records. Another authorization in the system is the price list master file containing product unit prices for billing customers. Those with power to alter this file can authorize price changes, which could allow the employee to undercharge a favoured customer and even to get kickbacks as part of a fraud scheme, so this function needs to be segregated from people who record customer receivables and receipts.

Periodic Reconciliation

For accounts receivable, the sum of customers' unpaid balances in the subledger should reconcile with the accounts receivable control account total in the general ledger. Usually, this is an automated procedure, as the computer system updates the subledger and general ledger simultaneously, so any out-of-balance situation suggests a system problem that needs to be investigated. Internal auditors, or employees who are independent of the inventory and receivables recording functions, can perform periodic comparison of the customers' obligations (according to the customers) with the recorded amount by requesting confirmations from the customers. These confirmations are often requested for long-overdue accounts, based on the *aged trial balance*—a list of the customers and their balances—with the balances classified in columns indicating the different age categories (e.g., current, 1–30 days past due, 31–60 days past due, 61–90 days past due, and over 90 days past due). (Refer to the special note on the audit use of confirmations later in this chapter.)

Cash Receipts and Cash Balances: Processing and Controls

There are numerous ways to receive payments: cash and cheques over the counter, via electronic funds transfer, through the mail, and by receipt in a lockbox. In a lockbox arrangement, a fiduciary (e.g., a bank) opens the box, lists the receipts, deposits the money, and sends the remittance advices showing the amount received from each customer to the company. While most companies need little authorization to accept a payment, authorization is important for approving discounts and allowances taken. Receiving cash and approving discounts is another example of incompatible duties that provide an opportunity for employees to defraud the company. A flowchart diagram of a manual system for processing cash receipts is shown in Exhibit 11B–2 in Appendix 11B.

Custody

In many organizations, someone takes the cash and cheques, which gives them custody of the physical cash for a time. Control over this custody can vary: responsibility can be rotated so that one person does not have this custody all the time; there could be teams of two or more people, so they would need to collude to steal money, or there could be arrangements outside the company for actual cash custody (e.g., the lockbox arrangement, or direct deposit to the company's bank account). Since initial custody cannot be avoided, it is good control to prepare a list of the cash receipts as early in the process as possible, and then separate the actual cash from the bookkeeping documents. The cash goes to a cashier or treasurer's office, where a bank deposit is prepared and made. The list goes to the accountants, who record the cash receipts. This list may simply be a stack of the remittance advices received with the customers' payments. Many organizations use electronic payment systems (e.g., for debit and credit cards in stores or over the Internet). These systems reduce the amount of physical cash in custody, relying instead on programmed systems control to ensure the payments transferred are authorized and complete.

Recording

The accountants who record cash receipts and credits to customer accounts should not handle the cash. They should use the remittance list to make entries to the cash and accounts receivable control accounts and to the customers' accounts receivable subsidiary account records. In fact, a good error-checking procedure is to have cash receipts entries and subsidiary account entries made by different people. Then, later, the accounts receivable entries and balances can be compared (reconciled) to determine whether the proper source documents (remittance lists) were used to make error-free accounting entries.

Periodic Reconciliation

Bank account reconciliations should be prepared carefully. Deposit slips are compared with cash remittance lists, and the totals should be traced to the general ledger entries. Likewise, paid cheques should be traced to the cash disbursements listing (journal) and the general ledger. Electronic funds transfers should be traced from the banking system reports to cash receipts, cash payments journals, and general ledger entries. The reconciliation should be done by someone other than the accountant responsible for cash accounting, such as the office manager or administrative assistant. (Refer to the special note on auditing bank reconciliations later in this chapter.)

Review Checkpoints

11-11   What purpose is served by prenumbering sales orders, shipping documents (packing slips and bills of lading), and sales invoices?

11-12   Why is controlled access to computer programs and master files (such as credit files and price lists) important in a control environment?

11-13   Why is it a control weakness if the same employee can authorize inventory transfers and record accounts receivable entries?

11-14   Why should a list of cash remittances be made and sent to the accounting department? Is it easier to send the cash and cheques to the accountants so that they can accurately enter the credits to customers' accounts?

Audit Evidence in Management Reports and Data Files

Management generates a variety of reports to provide important audit evidence for revenues, accounts receivable, and cash receipts. Some examples follow.

Pending Order Master File

The pending order master file contains sales transactions started but not yet completed in the system and thus not recorded as sales and accounts receivable. Old orders may represent shipments actually made, but for some reason the shipping department did not enter the shipping information (or entered an incorrect code that did not match the pending order file). The pending order backlog can be reviewed for evidence relating to the completeness assertion for recorded sales and accounts receivable.

Credit Check Files

The computer system may make automatic credit checks, but up-to-date maintenance of the credit information is very important. Customers' credit status is concerned with possibly uncollectible receivables, which constitute important audit evidence about the valuation assertion. Credit checks on old or incomplete information are not good credit checks. A sample of the files can be tested for current status, or the company's records can be reviewed for evidence of updating operations.

Price List Master File

The computer system may produce customer invoices automatically, but, if the master price list is wrong, the billings will be wrong. The computer file can be compared with an official price source for accuracy and authorization. (As a control, an employee should perform this comparison every time the prices are changed.) Incorrect pricing can lead to revenues and receivables being measured incorrectly, affecting the valuation assertion.

Sales Detail (Sales Journal) File

The sales detail (sales journal) file should contain the detailed sales entries, including the shipping references and dates. It can be scanned for entries without shipping references (fictitious sales) and for matching recording dates with shipment dates (sales recorded before shipment). This file also contains the population of debit entries to the accounts receivable, so this evidence is relevant to the existence/occurrence assertion for revenues and receivables. When there are high volumes of sales entries, these files can be tested with computer-assisted auditing techniques (CAATs). Some examples of CAATs are as follows:

- Auditor-designed analyses of customers or geographic regions assessed as high risk
- Scrutiny for unusually large entries that can indicate fraud or error
- Scrutiny for items in round numbers, same values, or just below some control dollar limit that occur more frequently than expected
- Verification of numerical continuity of invoices and agreement to general ledger entries

Sales Analysis Reports

The auditor can perform analytical procedures on a variety of sales analyses. Sales classified by product line or region constitute information for the business segment disclosures. Those classified by period or by sales employee can show unusually high or low volumes that may need investigation if error is suspected. This information can provide evidence related to completeness and existence, or occurrence, of revenues, and it is also useful for assessing the proper presentation or classification of revenue information in the financial statements, as shown in the following box relating to presentation of quarterly sales figures.

Peaks and Valleys

During the year-end audit, the independent auditors reviewed the weekly sales volume reports classified by region. They noticed that sales volume was very high in region 2 for the last two weeks of March, June, September, and December. The volume was unusually low in the first two weeks of April, July, October, and January. In fact, the peaks far exceeded the volume in all the other six regions. Further investigation revealed that the manager in region 2 was holding open the sales recording at the end of each quarterly reporting period in an attempt to make the quarterly reports look good. The analysis revealed to the auditors that the improper sales cutoff led to overstated sales at quarter-end.

Aged Accounts Receivable Trial Balance

The list of accounts receivable balance details is called the **accounts receivable subsidiary ledger**. The summary of the subsidiary ledger by invoice dates is called the **aged accounts receivable trial balance**. If the general ledger control account total is larger than the sum in the aged trial balance, too bad! A receivable amount not identified with a customer cannot be collected! The trial balance is the population used for confirmation. (See the special notes on the existence assertion and on using confirmations, later in this chapter.) The aging information is used in assessing the allowance for doubtful accounts. (An aged trial balance is shown in Exhibit 11–10.) The credit department uses the aged trial balance for follow-up of overdue and delinquent customer accounts. This is important evidence for assessing the existence, completeness, and valuation assertions for accounts receivable.

Cash Receipts Journal

The cash receipts journal contains all the detail for cash deposits and credits to various accounts and is the population of entries that should be the credits to accounts receivable for customer payments. It also contains any adjusting or correcting entries resulting from the bank account reconciliation. These entries may signal the types of accounting errors or manipulations that happen in the cash receipts accounting and provide evidence relating to existence and completeness of cash and accounts receivable.

Review Checkpoints

11-15   What accounting records and files could an auditor examine to find evidence of unrecorded sales, inadequate credit checks, and incorrect product unit prices?

11-16   Suppose you selected a sample of customers' accounts receivable and wanted to find supporting evidence for the entries in the accounts. Where would you go to vouch the debit entries? What would you expect to find? Where would you go to vouch the credit entries? What would you expect to find? What assertions are you finding evidence about?

Control Risk Assessment

LO2   Describe the auditor's control risk assessment and control tests for auditing control over customer credit approval, delivery, accounts receivable, cash receipts, and bank statements.

Control risk assessment governs the nature, timing, and extent of substantive audit procedures that will be applied in the audit of the accounts and records in the revenues, receivables, and receipts processes (listed in the lower right corner of Exhibit 11–1). These include the following:

- Cash in bank
- Cash receipts

accounts receivable subsidiary ledger:
a detailed listing of outstanding accounts receivable balances by individual customers that adds up to the total balance in the general ledger accounts receivable "control" account; reconciliation of the subsidiary ledger and the control account is an important control procedure and a key audit test

aged accounts receivable trial balance:
a list of all outstanding accounts receivable balances organized by how long they have been outstanding; used to manage collection and assess the accounting requirement to provide an allowance for possible uncollectible accounts

control risk assessment:
a process the auditor uses to understand the client's internal control in order to identify and assess the risks of material misstatement of the financial statements, whether due to fraud or error, and to design and perform further audit procedures

- Accounts receivable
- Allowance for doubtful accounts and write-offs
- Bad debt expense
- Sales revenue
- Sales returns, allowances, and discounts
- Perpetual inventory records and shipping records

Information about the control structure is often gathered though internal control questionnaires, introduced in Chapter 9. A selection of other questionnaires for both general controls and application controls over cash receipts, sales revenues, and accounts receivable is found in Appendix 11A. These questionnaires provide details of desirable control policies and procedures. The questions are organized under headings that identify the important control objectives: environment and general accounting controls, validity, completeness, authorization, accuracy, classification, and proper period recording.

General information about internal controls can also be gathered by a walk-through procedure. Here the auditors take a single example of a transaction and "walk it through" from its initiation to its recording in the accounting records. The revenues, receivables, and receipts process walk-through involves following a sale from the initial customer order through credit approval, delivery of goods or services, and billing; to the entry in the sales journal and subsidiary accounts receivable records; and finally to its subsequent collection and cash deposit. Sample documents are collected, and employees in each department are questioned about their specific duties. Walk-throughs (1) verify or update the auditors' understanding of the auditee's sales/accounts receivable accounting system and control procedures and (2) show whether the controls the auditee reported in the internal control questionnaire are actually in place. The walk-through, combined with inquiries, can contribute evidence about appropriate separation of duties, a basis for assessing control risk to be low. However, a walk-through is too limited in scope to provide sufficient evidence about whether the control procedures were operating effectively during the period under audit. A larger sample of transactions for specific control testing is necessary to provide actual evidence about control effectiveness.

General Control Considerations

Control procedures for proper segregation of responsibilities should be in place and operating. Control activities that should be segregated are indicated in the green ovals in Exhibit 11–1, showing that the authorization of sales and credit should be performed by persons who do not have custody, recording, or reconciliation duties. Custody of inventory and cash is by those who do not directly authorize credit, record the accounting entries, or reconcile the bank account. Recording (accounting) is performed by those who do not authorize sales or credit, handle the inventory or cash, or perform reconciliations. Periodic reconciliations should be performed by employees who do not have authorization, custody, or recording duties related to the same assets. Combinations of two or more of these responsibilities in one person, one office, or one information system may open the door for errors and fraud.

Cash management commonly requires people who handle cash to be insured under a **fidelity bond**—an insurance policy that covers most kinds of cash embezzlement losses. Fidelity bonds do not prevent or detect embezzlement, but failing to carry the insurance exposes the company to complete loss when embezzlement occurs. However, a company must prove its losses before it can collect on them—another good reason for internal controls.

fidelity bond:
a type of insurance policy that covers theft of cash by employees

The control structure includes general controls and also application control activities that provide for detailed control-checking procedures. The following set of procedures should take place:

1. Sales orders entered only with a customer order
2. Credit-check code or manual signature recorded by authorized means
3. Inventory and shipping area access restricted to authorized persons
4. Access to billing programs and blank invoice forms restricted to authorized personnel
5. Sales and accounts receivable recorded only when all supporting shipping documentation is in order (i.e., sales and receivables recorded as of the date the goods were shipped or services were provided, and cash receipts recorded as of the date the payments were received)
6. Customer invoices compared with bills of lading and customer order details to verify that quantities billed match quantities shipped and that the goods were shipped in correct quantities and pricing to proper locations
7. Pending order files reviewed to ensure timely billing and recording
8. Bank statements reconciled in detail, monthly

The "Fictitious Revenue" box below illustrates improper period recording. It is one of a class of widespread financial reporting problems commonly referred to as **revenue recognition problems**. Many of the financial restatements filed with securities regulators by public companies involve revenue recognition, most of these dealing with premature revenue recognition. Since management's motivation is to increase revenues, the risk of fraud in revenue recognition is always high. For this reason, CAS 240 requires auditors to always consider fraud risk to be present in the audit of revenues, and to perform procedures to confirm or dispel this presumption.

Timing is critical to many accounting issues. For example, major retailers that buy in bulk receive discounts from suppliers if they meet sales targets. But how are these rebates accounted for? The prudent practice is to wait until the targets are met. However, companies such as Kmart in the United States and Royal Ahold in the Netherlands, once the world's third-largest food retailer, appear to have booked these payments before they were earned. In 2001/2002, Ahold may have booked the total expected bulk discounts as profit in the first year of a multi-year contract. Its CEO and CFO both resigned in February 2002. Ahold has been referred to as "Europe's Enron." Controls related to proper timing in the recording of transactions are becoming more important in the current environment.

Fictitious Revenue

A Mississauga (Ontario) computer peripheral-equipment company was experiencing slow sales, so the sales manager entered some sales orders for customers who had not ordered anything. The invoices were marked "hold," while the delivery was to one of the company's own warehouses. The rationale was that these customers would buy the equipment eventually, so why not anticipate the orders! (However, it is a good idea not to send them the invoices until they actually make the orders, hence the "hold.") Due to management's override of the controls, the "sales" and "receivables" were recorded in the accounts, and the financial statements contained overstated revenue and assets. The ability of management to override controls is the main reason GAAS require auditors to always get some substantive evidence—auditors cannot rely entirely on testing control effectiveness.

revenue recognition problems:
techniques used by financial statement preparers to manipulate reported revenues resulting in low-quality earnings

Control Tests

An organization should have input, processing, and output control procedures in place and operating in order to prevent, detect, and correct accounting errors. You studied the general control objectives in Chapter 9 (validity, completeness, authorization, accuracy, classification, and proper period cutoff). Exhibit 11–2 puts these in the perspective of the revenue process with examples of specific objectives. Study this exhibit carefully, as it expresses the control objectives in specific examples rather than in the abstract.

EXHIBIT 11–2

Internal Control Objectives: Revenue Process (Sales Revenues)

GENERAL OBJECTIVES	EXAMPLES OF SPECIFIC OBJECTIVES
1. Recorded sales are *valid* and documented.	Customer purchase orders support invoices. Bills of lading or other shipping documentation exist for all invoices. Recorded sales in sales journal are supported by invoices.
2. Valid sales transactions are recorded *completely*, with none omitted.	Invoices, shipping documents, and sales orders are prenumbered and the numerical sequence is checked. Overall comparisons of sales are made periodically by a statistical or product-line analysis.
3. Sales are *authorized* according to company policy.	Credit sales are approved by the credit department. Prices used in preparing invoices are from the authorized price schedule.
4. Sales invoices are *accurately* prepared.	Invoice quantities are compared with shipment and customer order quantities. Prices are checked and mathematical accuracy independently checked after the invoice is prepared.
5. Sales transactions are properly *classified*.	Sales to subsidiaries and affiliates are classified as intercompany sales and receivables. Sales returns and allowances are properly classified.
6. Sales transactions are recorded in the *proper period*.	Sales invoices are recorded on the shipment date.

The last general objective relates to recording sales in the proper period, a problem of timing, a growing concern to the profession. One of the most important audit procedures is **sales cutoff testing**, which gives evidence about whether transactions have been recorded in the proper period, either before or after the period-end date. If revenues and expenses that belong in the current period are recorded after the cutoff date, there is a completeness misstatement (i.e., an understatement) in the current period. If transactions that belong in the next period are recorded too early, there will be an existence/occurrence misstatement in the current period. If the auditee recognizes sales when title passes from seller to buyer—the point when the risks and rewards of ownership are transferred—the date when the shipment or delivery of the auditee's inventory is made is the critical point when the revenue should be recorded. Auditors test sales cutoff by vouching shipping documents for a sample of sales recognized just before the year-end to check that the shipping dates and deliveries were in fact before year-end. This provides evidence of the existence/occurrence of these sales, which is the auditors' main concern. The auditors also test the first sales after year-end to verify that those shipments also occurred after year-end, to get evidence about the completeness assertion for the current period. Note that cutoff errors are a type of **reversing error** (i.e., they have an equal and opposite effect) in the following period. Objective 6 in Exhibit 11–2 refers to shipment date.

sales cutoff testing:
control procedures designed to ensure sales transactions are recorded in the proper period

reversing error:
errors in the current period that will have an equal and opposite effect in the following period

Shipment of inventory is closely tied to the audit of inventory, so we will defer that discussion to Chapter 12. The relationship between all of these illustrates that the processes are not independent of each other, the important point here being that sales cutoff related to proper recording of sales for the period is closely linked to inventory shipments to customers and to the shipping terms (**FOB shipping** or **FOB destination**). The effect of shipping terms on cutoff tests is also explained in Chapter 12.

Some control tests can be used to effectively test procedures in more than one way at the same time. **Two-direction testing**, for instance, audits both control over completeness in one direction and control over validity in the other. Completeness determines if all the sample transactions that occurred were recorded (none omitted), and validity determines if recorded transactions actually occurred (were real). An example of the first direction is examining a sample of shipping documents (from the file of all shipping documents) to determine whether invoices were prepared and recorded. The second direction is determining whether supporting shipping documents exist and verifying the actual shipment. The content of each file is compared with that of the other. This is illustrated in Exhibit 11–3.

EXHIBIT 11–3

Two-Direction Audit Testing

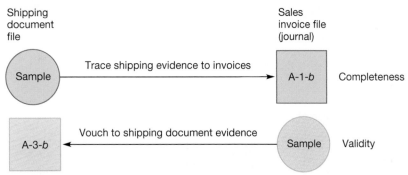

Note: The A-1-*b* and A-3-*b* codes refer to control tests listed in Exhibit 11–4.

Exhibit 11–4 contains a selection of control tests, many of which are steps verifying the content and character of sample documents from one file against the content and character of documents in another file. This process leads to objective evidence about the effectiveness of controls and the reliability of accounting records. These samples are usually attribute samples similar to those you studied in Chapter 10.

Control objectives tested by the audit procedures are also shown in Exhibit 11–4. These test of controls procedures produce evidence that helps auditors determine whether the specific control objectives listed

FOB shipping:
terms of sale indicating that title to goods sold transfers from seller to buyer when the goods are handed over from the seller to the shipping company that will ultimately deliver them to the buyer; can give rise to an amount of inventory-in-transit at year-end that is owned by an auditee company (the buyer) that is not physically on hand at the auditee's premises

FOB destination:
terms of sale indicating that title to goods sold transfers from seller to buyer when the goods reach the buyer's destination; can give rise to an amount of inventory-in-transit at year-end that is owned by an auditee company (the seller) that is not physically on hand at the auditee's premises

two-direction testing:
audit control over both completeness in one direction and validity in the other

in Exhibit 11–2 were achieved. Appendix 11A illustrates internal control questionnaires used in deciding on the extent of the testing in Exhibit 11–4. (This exhibit is very general and not affected by whether manual or IT-based procedures are used to record a transaction.) Exhibits 11–5 and 11–6 will later illustrate two of the substantive audit programs that would be affected by the control testing results illustrated in Exhibit 11–4.

EXHIBIT 11–4

Control Tests for Sales, Cash Receipts, and Receivables*

	CONTROL OBJECTIVE
A. Sales	
1. Select a sample of shipping documents:	
(a) Scan for missing numbers.	Completeness
(b) Trace to related sales invoices.	Completeness
2. Scan sales invoices for missing numbers in the sequence.	Completeness
3. Select a sample of recorded sales invoices (sales journal):	
(a) Perform recalculations to verify arithmetic accuracy.	Accuracy
(b) Vouch to supporting shipping documents. Note dates and quantities.	Validity Accuracy Proper period
(c) Vouch prices to approved price lists.	Authorization
(d) Vouch credit approval.	Authorization
B. Cash Receipts	
1. Select a sample of recorded cash receipts (cash receipts journal):	
(a) Vouch to deposit slip and remittance list.	Validity
(b) Trace to bank statement.	Validity
2. Select a sample of remittance lists (or daily cash reports):	
(a) Trace to cash receipts journal.	Completeness
(b) Trace to bank statement.	Accuracy
C. Accounts Receivable	
1. Select a sample of customers' accounts:	
(a) Vouch debits to supporting sales invoices.	Validity
(b) Vouch credits to supporting cash receipts documents and approved credit memos.	Validity
2. Select a sample of credit memos:	
(a) Review for proper approval.	Authorization
3. Observe mailing of monthly customer statements.	Validity

*Auditors will assess the control environment and general controls over the accounting process at an overall level to ensure proper procedures are performed and the general ledger and subledger processing of sales invoices, credit memos, and cash receipts is accurate and complete.

Summary: Control Risk Assessment

The auditor must evaluate the evidence obtained from an understanding of the internal control structure and from control tests (phases 1 and 2 of the control evaluation, as explained in Chapter 9). The tests set out in Exhibit 11–4 might show that control objectives are being met, and then control risk can be assessed as being low. On the other hand, the tests might reveal weaknesses, such as posting sales without shipping documents, charging customers the wrong prices, or recording credits to customers without supporting credit memos. In that case, control risk will be assessed as high and little reliance can be placed on controls.

If a low control risk is assessed, auditors can rely on the effectiveness of the controls to reduce the risk of material misstatement. In this case, the substantive audit procedures on the account balances can be performed in cost-saving ways. For example, the accounts receivable balances can be confirmed at a date prior to the year-end when more audit staff have time available, and the sample size can be fairly small.

If tests of controls reveal weaknesses, control risk is assessed high and the substantive procedures will need to be more extensive and provide more assurance, to lower the risk of failing to detect material error in the account balances. For example, the confirmation procedure may need to be scheduled on the year-end date with an extensive sample of customer accounts. Descriptions of control deficiencies, weaknesses, and inefficiencies are incorporated in a management letter to auditee management. Significant control deficiencies must also be communicated to those charged with governance.

Standards Check

CAS 265 Communicating Deficiencies in Internal Control to Those Charged with Governance and Management

6. (b) Significant deficiency in internal control—A deficiency or combination of deficiencies in internal control that, in the auditor's professional judgment, is of sufficient importance to merit the attention of those charged with governance. (Ref: Para. A5)

9. The auditor shall communicate in writing significant deficiencies in internal control identified during the audit to those charged with governance on a timely basis. (Ref: Para. A12–A18, A27)

10. The auditor shall also communicate to management at an appropriate level of responsibility on a timely basis (Ref: Para. A19, A27)

    (a) In writing, significant deficiencies in internal control that the auditor has communicated or intends to communicate to those charged with governance, unless it would be inappropriate to communicate directly to management in the circumstances; and (Ref: Para. A14, A20–A21)

    (b) Other deficiencies in internal control identified during the audit that have not been communicated to management by other parties and that, in the auditor's professional judgment, are of sufficient importance to merit management's attention. (Ref: Para. A22–A26)

Source: *CPA Canada Handbook—Assurance*, 2014.

Accounts Receivable Confirmation Findings and Prior Control Assessment

Accounts receivable confirmation is a substantive procedure designed to obtain evidence of the existence and gross amount (valuation) of customers' balances directly from the customer. If such confirmations show numerous exceptions, however, auditors will be concerned with the controls over the details of sales and cash receipts transactions, even if previous control assessment seemed to show little control risk. This indicates a reassessment of control risk that may call for additional substantive procedures.

Review Checkpoints

11-17   What account balances are included in the revenues, receivables, and receipts process?

11-18   What specific control policies and procedures (in addition to separation of duties and responsibilities) should be in place and operating in a control structure governing revenue recognition and cash accounting?

11-19   What is a walk-through of a sales transaction? How can the walk-through procedure complement the use of an internal control questionnaire?

11-20   What are the two important characteristics of a control test? What actions are typically used to perform control tests?

11-21   What is two-direction testing of controls? What are the objectives of two-direction testing in auditing the revenues, receivables, and receipts process?

Example of Linking Risk Assessment to Substantive Audit Procedures for Audit of Cash Account Balance

LO3   Explain how the auditor's risk assessment procedures and control testing link to the key assertions and audit objectives in designing a substantive audit program for the cash account balance.

This section of the chapter presents a detailed exhibit of a substantive audit program, using the EcoPak case. For this exhibit, we choose the cash account balance audit program, since cash is an account that is affected by the revenues, receivables, and receipts process as well as all the other processes. The cash balance audit is usually completed as early as possible in the audit, because knowing that the cash balance is fairly stated is an important foundation for obtaining sufficient appropriate audit evidence overall. Exhibit 11–5 shows how an auditor would respond to a questionnaire by noting the findings from the risk assessments and control testing done to date. These assessments are then the basis for assessing risk, assertion by assertion. Based on the assertion-level risks, the auditor specifies the audit procedures that need to be performed. This is a very challenging exercise in applying professional judgment! The exhibit can give you a realistic idea of how auditors respond to their risk assessments at the assertion level by obtaining reliable evidence that is relevant to the higher-risk assertions in each account balance and transaction stream.

The example program is comprehensive and includes some procedures that might not be performed if the risk of material misstatement for the related assertion is quite low. Many auditors prefer to use comprehensive audit program templates to start off, however, as it can give them another chance to think through their prior decisions about risk and evaluate the costs and benefits of performing audit procedures. Sometimes, a simple and quick procedure can provide good evidence. This is often the case for the cash balance, the account we will be looking at in this exhibit. Auditors find it worthwhile to do a very thorough audit of cash, because most operating transactions run through the cash balance, and because the consequences of missing a big misstatement here would be so devastating to the auditor's reputation (the Parmalat audit failure described in the box after the exhibit is a good example).

So, many auditors will decide to obtain confirmation of every bank account, even those with small balances or minimal activity during the audited period. On the other hand, for more costly, time-consuming procedures, such as confirmation of accounts receivable balances, auditors may decide to limit their extents or not perform the procedure at all if they assess the risk as very low.

Dairy Foods Giant Parmalat Goes Sour—Where Was That $4.9 Billion in Cash?

The accounting calamity at Italian dairy foods giant Parmalat was one of the largest financial frauds in history. In the investigation, Italian prosecutors discovered that managers simply invented assets to offset as much as $16.2 billion in liabilities and falsified accounts over a 15-year period. Some of Parmalat's assets were supposedly held in a $4.9 billion Bank of America account of a Parmalat subsidiary in the Cayman Islands. Auditors first inquired about the Cayman Islands account in December 2002 and received a letter on Bank of America stationery in March 2003 confirming the existence of the account. The letter was apparently a forgery, concocted by someone in Parmalat's Italian headquarters. The very size of the alleged account should have raised a red flag. "Things have been strange at Parmalat since the mid-1980s," says one senior investment banker, who avoided all business with the company. "It smelled bad." As the fast-growing dairy group returned time and again to the corporate debt market—issuing some $8 billion in bonds between 1993 and 2003—analysts, investment bankers, and fund managers all began questioning Parmalat's strange hunger for debt despite its apparent mountain of cash.

For its part, Parmalat's auditor claimed that the "letter" from Bank of America vouching for the cash was a forgery good enough to fool them into approving the falsified accounts. The audit firm claims that it too was the "victim" of a fraud. But investigating magistrates say that, according to former finance officials with Parmalat, the auditor used Parmalat's internal mail to request financial information, rather than dealing with banks or other parties directly. If so, it would mean that the auditors were not going outside of a closed loop of internal communications to independently scrutinize vital transactions.

The Parmalat scandal revealed an alarming lack of transparency at one of Europe's largest and most global companies. Like many companies in Europe, Parmalat is family controlled through a chain of holding companies, making corporate governance and supervision by regulators more difficult. The Parmalat board, consisting overwhelmingly of family members and Parmalat insiders, wasn't prone to raising questions.

Sources: businessweek.com/stories/2004-01-11/how-parmalat-went-sour; businessweek.com/stories/2004-01-25/the-milk-just-keeps-on-spilling-at -parmalat; "Milking Lessons," economist.com/node/2320134.

The audit program starts off with the auditor's risk assessments from the planning stages, and the auditor's conclusions based on performing the control tests (such as those set out in the example in Exhibit 11–4). The control test results allow the auditor to conclude on the control risk level that is appropriate for deciding on the *nature*, *timing*, and *extent* of the substantive procedures that should be performed to reduce the risk of not detecting a material misstatement to an acceptably low level. A detailed audit program such as the one shown in Exhibit 11–5 shows the list of procedures describing the "nature" of each (this refers to the kinds of evidence-gathering methods to be used), the planned "extents" (this could be a sample size, or an indication that all the relevant items will be looked at), and the "timing" (when the auditors plan to perform the procedure, which could be at the period-end date in the case of procedures such as cutoff and counts; during the field work visits for procedures such as those involving analysis, confirmations, and examination of source documents; or at the audit report date for such procedures as obtaining management's final representations about the accounts).

Looking more closely at the responses in Exhibit 11–5, we see that the audit senior, Donna, has recorded the assessments of risk at the assertion level based on the overall risk assessment procedures and control tests performed to date. We assume she concluded that there is a moderate risk of fraud in this account and that risk at the overall financial statements level is also moderate, based on the overall assessment performed earlier in the planning and approved by the engagement partner. The audit file index references (e.g., "522" in red) indicate where the risk-assessment work and conclusions have been documented in the audit file. The index references are based on the audit-file indexing example shown in Appendix 11C (available on Connect).

EXHIBIT 11–5

Example of Substantive Audit Program Responding to Assessed Risk of Material Misstatement

AUDIT PROGRAM				
AUDITEE: ECOPAK INC.				**FILE INDEX:** A-100
FINANCIAL STATEMENT PERIOD: y/e DECEMBER 31, 20X1				
ACCOUNT: CASH BALANCE				
Consider risk assessment findings:	High √	Moderate √	Low √	Provide specific risk description or audit file documentation reference:
	High	Moderate	Low	
What fraud risk level has been assessed related to this account (e.g., theft of assets, unrecorded or fictitious transactions, inappropriate journal entries)?		√		No indicators of fraud have been noted by staff, but cash is vulnerable to fraud so risk is more than low. [Ref: 522]
What is the assessed risk level for this account at the financial statement level (e.g., consider business risks, entity-level control environment, risk assessment and monitoring, general IT controls, management override, going-concern risks, related party transactions)?		√		See overall risk assessment at financial statement level. [520]
What is the assessed inherent risk level at the assertion level for	High	Moderate	Low	[584]
Existence?		√		
Completeness?		√		
Ownership?		√		
Valuation?			√	
Presentation?	√			
If tests of key controls have been conducted, what is the assessed control risk? (Note: If no controls were tested, control risk must be assessed as "high.")	High	Moderate	Low	[585]
Existence			√	
Completeness			√	
Ownership			√	
Valuation	√			
Presentation	√			
Reduce residual detection risk by performing substantive procedures.	High	Moderate	Low	[605]
Existence			√	
Completeness			√	
Ownership			√	
Valuation		√		
Presentation	√			
				(continued)

EXHIBIT 11–5

Example of Substantive Audit Program Responding to Assessed Risk of Material Misstatement *(continued)*

Substantive audit program in response to assessed risks:				
Substantive audit procedures	Assertions for *CASH:* evidence is related to [E, C, O, V, P*]	Timing	Extent (if applicable)	Working paper documentation reference
(Of the procedures listed below, perform those considered necessary to provide sufficient appropriate evidence to address the assessed risks and reduce risk of material misstatement to an acceptable level.)				
1. Prepare a "Lead Sheet" with a list of all cash accounts and current and prior period balances. Tie current balances into period-end general ledger. Agree prior balances to prior period audit file and financial statements, if available.	E, C, V	*Feb. 20X2*	*100%*	*A–1*
2. Analytical procedures: Develop expectations for cash balances and interest income/expense, based on inquiries and your understanding of the business. Inquire about any unusual cash transactions or balances.	E, C, V	*Feb. 20X2*	*N/A*	*A–10*
3. Obtain confirmations from all banks auditee has dealt with (request from banks using standard bank confirmation form).	E, C, O, V, P	*Jan. 20X2*	*100%*	*A–20*
4. Review the bank confirmation for loans, collateral, or guarantees.	P	*Feb. 20X2*	*100%*	*A–20*
5. Obtain auditee-prepared reconciliations of all bank accounts. For each bank account, perform the following:		*Feb. 20X2*		*A–30*
(a) Trace the bank balance on the reconciliation to the bank confirmation.	E, C, O, V		*100%*	*A–30*
(b) Trace the reconciled book balance to the general ledger.	E, C, V		*100%*	*A–30*
(c) Verify a sample of outstanding cheques and outstanding deposits to source documents.	V		*10 largest cheques 100% of deposits*	*A–30*
(d) Recalculate the arithmetic on auditee-prepared bank reconciliations.	V		*100%*	*A–30*
(e) Ensure all differences are explained by valid timing differences or bank errors, or are adjusted by appropriate journal entries.	E, C, O, V, P		*100%*	*A–31*
6. Ask the auditee to request cutoff bank statements for a period after the financial statement date (e.g., two weeks or one month), to be mailed directly to the audit firm; in a low-risk audit, an account detail report directly from the auditee's online banking can be used.	E, C, O, V, P	*Feb. 20X2*	*Reviewed online bank account detail under audit control as of Feb. 6, 20X2.*	*A–40*
(a) Trace deposits in transit on the reconciliation to bank deposits early in the next period.	E		*100%*	*A–40*
(b) Trace outstanding cheques on the reconciliation to cheques cleared in the next period.	C		*10 largest cheques*	*A–40*
				(continued)

EXHIBIT 11–5

Example of Substantive Audit Program Responding to Assessed Risk of Material Misstatement   (*continued*)

(c) Prepare a schedule of interbank transfers for a period of 10 business days before and after the year-end date. Verify that the dates of book entries for these transfers agree with bank entries and reconciliation items, if any, to ensure amounts are only counted in the cash balance once.	E, C	Feb. 20X2	10 days	A-40
(d) If any material outstanding cheques at period-end have not cleared by the end of the audit field work, confirm the related disbursements with the payee.	C	End of field work	100%	n/a (none)
7. If significant amounts of cash are held outside bank accounts at period-end, count cash funds in the presence of an auditee representative.	E, C, O, V	Dec. 31, 20X1	100%	n/a (none)
8. Inquire if any outstanding cheques have been prepared but not mailed at period-end, verifying if these are material and should be reclassified as accounts payable.	E, P	Dec. 31, 20X1	100%	Inquired of Nina, CFO—none (representation letter point 350)
9. Ensure all foreign currency cash balances have been translated to reporting currency at the correct period-end rate.	V	Dec. 31, 20X1	100%	A-1 All bank accounts CDN$
10. Ensure all cash is properly presented on the balance sheet and in the cash flow statement.	P	Mar. 20X2	100%	120
11. Ensure all required disclosures related to cash balances and banking terms are provided in the financial statement notes.	P	Mar. 20X2	100%	120
12. Obtain written management representations on matters such as compensating balance agreements, debt covenants, restrictions on cash, or other disclosure issues.	P	Audit report date		350

AUDITOR'S CONCLUSIONS

Based on my professional judgment, the evidence obtained is sufficient and appropriate to conclude that the risk of material misstatement of the <u>CASH BALANCE</u> is acceptably low.

Prepared by *Donna Ladona*   Date *Feb. 12, 20x2*

Reviewed by *Tariq Khan*   Date *Feb. 14, 20x2*

* E, C, O, V, P = existence, completeness, ownership, valuation, presentation.

For the inherent risk assessments, Donna has concluded that, ignoring controls, there is a moderate inherent risk that cash might be misstated by errors, such as not recording cash EcoPak has paid out (the cash therefore does not exist any more from EcoPak's perspective), not recording cash received (therefore, EcoPak's cash balance is not complete), or not deducting *outstanding cheques* issued from the bank account in the *bank reconciliation* (the cash is now "owned" by the payee on the cheque, not by EcoPak). Assuming EcoPak has only Canadian dollar bank accounts, she has assessed a low inherent risk for valuation. For presentation, she has assessed a high inherent risk, which we can assume is based on such concerns as inaccuracies arising in a manual preparation of the cash flow statement and disclosure of complex banking arrangements, since EcoPak relies quite heavily on bank lines of credit for its operating and financing cash needs. Her reference to file index "584" indicates a working paper where these assessments are explained in more detail.

Turning to Donna's control risk assessments, we can note that—based on testing the identified strengths in controls relating to existence, completeness, and valuation—Donna has concluded that control risk is lower for these assertions, such that further substantive procedures related to those assertions can be fairly limited. However, in the case of valuation and presentation, where controls were not tested, more extensive tests of details and other substantive procedures are performed, since the auditors have no basis for reducing their reliance on substantive evidence. Despite what the actual control risk is in such cases, if they are not tested the auditor simply proceeds on the basis that the control risk is high.

Based on the inherent and control risk assessments, Donna has determined how much *residual detection risk* is left. This *residual risk* must be reduced by the auditors' detection procedures: gathering substantive evidence to bring the risk of material misstatement down to the acceptable level for the audit (i.e., the **planned acceptable audit risk level (acceptable audit risk level))**. In the case of the existence, completeness, and ownership assertions, Donna assessed a moderate inherent risk of material misstatement, and the assessed combined risk of material misstatement was lowered considerably by strong controls (low control risk). This means there is little risk left and only limited substantive procedures are required (in comparison, say, to another audit where these controls were not as effective). For the valuation assertion, inherent risk was assessed to be low, but no controls were tested in relation to it, so some moderate substantive evidence still needs to be obtained to make sure the cash valuation is appropriate. In the case of the presentation assertion, this was assessed with a high inherent risk, and no controls were tested for it, so all the assurance required will need to come from substantive sources. Using her assertion-level risk assessments, Donna is now in a position to identify the procedures required to obtain the required substantive evidence to support her conclusion on EcoPak's year-end cash balance.

Based on the risk assessments, in the detailed substantive program section of Exhibit 11–5, Donna has selected appropriate types of substantive tests and procedures and decided on how extensive the procedures need to be, as well as the optimal time to perform the procedures. This substantive audit program form is also used to summarize the audit findings by providing reference to the audit file pages where the work is documented, and to record the auditor's final conclusion based on the evidence obtained. You can appreciate how the audit program illustrated in Exhibit 11–5 helps the audit firm schedule staff to perform the work; gives the staff assigned to do the work a very helpful set of instructions to follow; and gives the audit manager and partner a concise, efficient way to review the adequacy of the audit work performed.

Substantive Audit Programs for the Revenues, Receivables, and Receipts Process

LO4   Describe the typical substantive procedures used to address the assessed risk of material misstatement in the main account balances and transactions in the revenues, receivables, and receipts process.

This section provides further examples of substantive procedures that are used for other elements of the revenues, receivables, and receipts process of a typical business. These examples are concise lists of basic substantive procedures, along with the related assertions they address. Exhibit 11–6 shows a program for auditing accounts receivable and notes receivable account balances, and Exhibit 11–7 is a program for auditing revenue transactions.

Unlike Exhibit 11–5, the programs illustrated in Exhibits 11–6 and 11–7 are generic; they are not tailored to a specific engagement's risk. It is important to note that the full risk assessment illustrated in Exhibit 11–5 would always be done in each audit program to design an appropriate set of audit procedures linked to the assessed risks at the assertion level in each auditee's specific circumstances.

planned acceptable audit risk level (acceptable audit risk level):
the level of audit risk determined by the auditor at the planning stage to be acceptable based on engagement characteristics, achieved by performing control tests and substantive procedures that lower audit risk to the acceptable level

EXHIBIT 11-6

Audit Program for Accounts and Notes Receivable: Selected Substantive Procedures

AUDITEE: *ECOPAK INC.*		FILE INDEX: *C-100*
FINANCIAL STATEMENT PERIOD: *y/e DECEMBER 31, 20X1*		
ACCOUNT: *ACCOUNTS & NOTES RECEIVABLE BALANCES*		

Substantive audit program in response to assessed risks:

Substantive audit procedures	Assertions for ACCOUNTS & NOTES RECEIVABLE: evidence is related to [E, C, O, V, P*]	Timing	Extent (if applicable)	Working paper documentation reference
(Of the procedures listed below, perform those considered necessary to provide sufficient appropriate evidence to address the assessed risks and reduce the risk of material misstatement to an acceptable level.)				
1. Obtain an aged trial balance of individual customer accounts. Recalculate the total and trace to the general ledger control account.	E, C			
2. Send confirmations to all accounts over $X. Select a random sample of all remaining accounts for confirmation.	E, C, V			
(a) Investigate differences reported by customers.				
(b) Perform alternative procedures on accounts that do not respond to positive confirmation requests.				
(i) Vouch cash receipts after the confirmation date for subsequent payment.				
(ii) Vouch sales invoices and shipping documents.				
3. Evaluate the adequacy of the allowance for doubtful accounts.	V			
(a) Vouch a sample of *current* amounts in the aged trial balance against sales invoices to determine whether amounts aged current should be aged past due.				
(b) Compare the current-year write-off experience to the prior-year allowance.				
(c) Vouch cash receipts after the balance sheet date for collections on past-due accounts.				
(d) Obtain financial statements or credit reports and discuss collections on large past-due accounts with the credit manager.				
(e) Calculate an allowance estimate using prior relations of write-offs and sales, taking under consideration current economic events.				
4. Review the bank confirmations, loan agreements, and minutes of the board for indications of pledged, discounted, or assigned receivables.	O, P			
5. Inspect or obtain confirmation of notes receivable.	E, C, V			
6. Recalculate interest income and trace to the income account.	V			
				(continued)

EXHIBIT 11–6

Audit Program for Accounts and Notes Receivable: Selected Substantive Procedures   *(continued)*

7. Obtain written management representations regarding pledge, discount, or assignment of receivables, and about receivables from officers, directors, affiliates, or other related parties.	E, C, O, V, P			
8. Review the adequacy of control over recording of all charges to customers (completeness) audited in the sales transaction test of controls audit program.	C, V			

AUDITOR'S CONCLUSIONS

Based on my professional judgment, the evidence obtained is sufficient and appropriate to conclude that the risk of material misstatement of the *ACCOUNTS & NOTES RECEIVABLE BALANCES* is acceptably low.

Prepared by _____   Date _____

Reviewed by _____   Date _____

* E, C, O, V, P = existence, completeness, ownership, valuation, presentation.

EXHIBIT 11–7

Audit Program for Sales Revenue Transactions: Selected Substantive Procedures

AUDITEE: *ECOPAK INC.*		**FILE INDEX:** *705*
FINANCIAL STATEMENT PERIOD: *y/e DECEMBER 31, 20X1*		
ACCOUNT: *SALES REVENUES TRANSACTIONS*		

Substantive audit program in response to assessed risks:

Substantive audit procedures	Assertions for REVENUES evidence is related to [E, C, O, V, P*]	Timing	Extent (if applicable)	Working paper documentation reference
(Of the procedures listed below, perform those considered necessary to provide sufficient appropriate evidence to address the assessed risks and reduce the risk of material misstatement to an acceptable level.)				
1. Select a sample of recorded sales invoices and vouch to underlying shipping documents.	E, V, O			
2. Select a sample of shipping documents and trace to sales invoices.	C			
3. Obtain production records of physical quantities sold and calculate an estimate of sales dollars based on average sale prices.	V			
4. Compare revenue dollars and physical quantities with prior-year data and industry economic statistics.	E, C, V			
5. Select a sample of sales invoices prepared a few days before and after the balance sheet date and vouch to supporting documents for evidence of proper cutoff.	E, C			
6. Review accounting policies for revenue recognition and ensure they comply with the company's financial reporting framework and are properly disclosed.	P			

AUDITOR'S CONCLUSIONS

Based on my professional judgment, the evidence obtained is sufficient and appropriate to conclude that the risk of material misstatement of the *REVENUES* is acceptably low.

Prepared by _____   Date _____

Reviewed by _____   Date _____

* E, C, O, V, P = existence, completeness, ownership, valuation, presentation.

The audit of the revenues, receivables, and receipts processes verifies that there is no material misstatement in the balance of accounts receivable and the two transaction streams that run through it—revenues and cash receipts. By focusing on the balance sheet account of the process, we can analyze the accounts receivable balance changes and the financial statement items related to them by studying the continuity of the accounts receivable account over the period being audited.

Analysis of Financial Statement Relationships

A **continuity schedule** is a working paper that shows the movements in the account balances and the other financial statement amounts that should tie in with them. Exhibit 11–8 illustrates a continuity schedule for the accounts receivable balance.

As these relationships illustrate, procedures to audit the revenues, receivables, and receipts allow assessment of whether all components of this system are reported accurately in the financial statements. These relationships also indicate analytical procedures that can detect material misstatements. For example, the ratios measuring collection period or number of days of sales in accounts receivable can indicate non-existent sales revenues or receivables that are not likely to be collected.

EXHIBIT 11–8

Continuity Schedule for the Accounts Receivable Balance

AUDITED AMOUNT	FINANCIAL STATEMENT WHERE AMOUNT IS REPORTED
Opening balance of accounts receivable	Balance sheet (prior-year comparative figures)
Add: Revenues from credit sales	Income statement (component of total revenues)
Deduct: Cash received against accounts receivable	Cash flow statement (direct method)
Deduct: Uncollectible accounts written off	Balance sheet (change in allowance for doubtful accounts)*
Ending balance of accounts receivable	Balance sheet (current-year figures)

*The bad debt expense and the allowance for doubtful accounts balance can be analyzed using the same technique. Question EP 11-7 at the end of the chapter asks you to provide the continuity schedule for the allowance for doubtful accounts and to identify the related financial statement items that it will have to be agreed to in the audit file.

Misstatement Analysis

The financial statement relationships noted in the section above can also be used to analyze the impact of misstatements discovered in the audit. For example, consider the impact if the following cutoff error occurs: a cash receipt that was received on December 31, 20X1, was not recorded until January 2, 20X2. In the continuity schedule in Exhibit 11–8, the cash receipts transaction total deducted from accounts receivable will be too small, leading to an overstatement of accounts receivable (and an understatement of the cash balance).

As another example, consider if a sale on account for $13,000 was recorded on December 31, 20X1, and the auditor's cutoff testing revealed the shipment did not occur until the first week of the following year. In this case, sales revenues in the income statement will be overstated. Also, the amount of revenues added to the accounts receivable balance in Exhibit 11–8 will be overstated by $13,000, leading to an overstatement

---

continuity schedule:
a working paper that shows the movements in an account balance from the beginning to the end of the period under audit; used to analyze the account balance changes and the other financial statement items related to them

in the balance sheet. The misstatement will also affect the inventory and cost of sales—assuming a gross margin of 40%, the inventory and cost of sales will be understated by $7,800. As required by CAS 450, the auditor must accumulate misstatements identified during the audit, other than those that are clearly trivial. A worksheet used for this purpose is illustrated in Exhibit 16–1 of Chapter 16. This sales cutoff error will be carried forward, as well as the related error in inventory cutoff. The accumulated misstatements worksheet shows the impact of all misstatements on the balance sheet and income statement and sets out the debits and credits of proposed adjusting entries to correct them, if management chooses to do so.

Special Note: The Existence Assertion

LO5 Explain the importance of the existence assertion for the audit of cash and accounts receivable.

When considering assertions and obtaining evidence about accounts receivable and other assets, auditors must emphasize the existence and ownership (rights) assertions. (For liability accounts, the emphasis is on the completeness assertion, as will be explained in Chapter 12.) This priority is placed on existence because many audit failures are due to auditors giving a clean audit opinion on financial statements that have overstated assets and revenues and understated expenses. For example, credit sales recorded too early (fictitious sales) result in overstated accounts receivable and overstated sales revenue, and failure to amortize prepaid expenses results in understated expenses and overstated current assets.

Identifying the population of assets to audit for existence and ownership is easy because the company has asserted the assets' existence by putting them on the balance sheet. The audit procedures described in the following sections can be used to obtain evidence about the existence and ownership of accounts receivable and other assets.

Recalculation

Assets that depend largely on calculations are best audited by using recalculation procedures. For example, expired prepaid expenses are recalculated using vouching of basic documents, such as loan agreements (prepaid interest), rent contracts (prepaid rent), and insurance policies (prepaid insurance). Depreciation expenses are recalculated using original acquisition and payment documents and term (useful life) estimates. A bank reconciliation is a special kind of calculation, and it can be audited. (There is a special note on auditing a bank reconciliation later in this chapter.)

Inspection of Physical Assets

Inventories and fixed assets can be inspected and counted (there is more on inventory observation in Chapter 12). Titles to automobiles, land, and buildings can be vouched, sometimes using public records. Petty cash and undeposited receipts can be observed and counted, but the cash in the bank cannot. Securities held as investments can be inspected if documents are held by the auditee.

Confirmation

Letters of confirmation can be sent to banks and customers, asking for a report of the balances owed to the company. Likewise, if securities held as investments are in the custody of banks or brokerage houses, the custodians can be asked to report the names, numbers, and quantity of the securities held for the company. In some cases, inventories held in public warehouses or out on consignment can be confirmed with the other party. (Refer to the special note on confirmations later in this chapter.)

Inquiry

While inquiries to management do not provide convincing evidence about existence and ownership, inquiries should always be made about the company's agreements to maintain compensating cash balances (these restricted cash amounts cannot be classifiable as "cash" among the current assets), the pledge or sale of accounts receivable with recourse in connection with financings, and the pledge of other assets as collateral for loans.

Inspection of Documents: Vouching

Evidence of ownership can be obtained by vouching the title documents for assets. Examination of loan documents may yield evidence of the need to disclose assets pledged as loan collateral.

Inspection of Documents: Scanning

Assets are supposed to have debit balances, and auditors can scan accounts receivables, inventory, and fixed assets for credit balances that usually reflect errors in the recordkeeping, for example, customer overpayments, failure to post purchases of inventory, and depreciation of assets by more than cost. The names of debtors can be scanned for officers, directors, and other related parties, to identify related party balances that need to be reported and disclosed separately in the financial statements.

Analysis

A variety of analytical comparisons may be employed, depending on the circumstances and the nature of the business. Comparisons of asset and revenue balances with recent history may help detect overstatements. Relationships such as receivables turnover, gross margin ratio, and sales-asset ratios can be compared with historical data and industry statistics for evidence of overall reasonableness. Account interrelationships can also be used in analytical review. For example, sales returns and allowances and sales commissions generally vary directly with dollar sales volume, bad debt expense usually varies directly with credit sales volume, and freight expense varies with the physical sales volume. Accounts receivable write-offs should be compared with earlier estimates of doubtful accounts.

Review Checkpoints

11-22   Why is it important to emphasize the existence and ownership (rights) assertions when auditing cash and accounts receivable?

11-23   Which audit procedures are usually the most useful for auditing the existence and ownership (rights) assertions? Give some examples.

Special Note: Using Confirmations

LO6   Identify considerations for using confirmations when auditing cash and accounts receivable.

The confirmation audit procedure was introduced in Chapter 8. This special note gives some details about using confirmations in the audit of cash and accounts receivable. The use of confirmations for cash balances and trade accounts receivable is considered a generally accepted auditing standard.[3] However, auditors may decide not to use them if suitable alternative procedures are available and applicable in particular circumstances. Justifications for the decision not to use confirmations for trade accounts receivable in a particular audit should be documented. Acceptable reasons could be that (1) receivables are not material; (2) confirmations would be ineffective, based on prior years' experience or knowledge that responses could be unreliable; and (3) other substantive test of details procedures provide sufficient appropriate evidence, and the assessed combined level of inherent risk and control risk associated with the financial statement assertions being audited is low.

Standards Check

CAS 505 External Confirmations

External Confirmation Procedures

7. When using external confirmation procedures, the auditor shall maintain control over external confirmation requests, including

    (a) Determining the information to be confirmed or requested; (Ref: Para. A1)

    (b) Selecting the appropriate confirming party; (Ref: Para. A2)

    (c) Designing the confirmation requests, including determining that requests are properly addressed and contain return information for responses to be sent directly to the auditor; and (Ref: Para. A3–A6)

    (d) Sending the requests, including follow-up requests when applicable, to the confirming party. (Ref: Para. A7).

13. If the auditor has determined that a response to a positive confirmation request is necessary to obtain sufficient appropriate audit evidence, alternative audit procedures will not provide the audit evidence the auditor requires. If the auditor does not obtain such confirmation, the auditor shall determine the implications for the audit and the auditor's opinion in accordance with CAS 705. (Ref: Para. A20).

Source: *CPA Canada Handbook—Assurance*, 2014.

Simple Analytical Comparison

The auditors prepared a schedule of the monthly credit sales totals for the current and prior years. They noticed several variations, but one, in November of the current year, stood out in particular. The current-year credit sales were almost twice those of any prior November. Further investigation showed that a computer error had caused the November credit sales to be recorded twice in the control accounts. The accounts receivable and sales revenue were materially overstated as a result.

A Decision Not to Use Accounts Receivable Confirmations

Surepart Manufacturing Company sold all its production to three auto manufacturers and six aftermarket distributors. All nine of these customers were well-known companies that typically paid their accounts in full by the 10th day of the following month. The auditors were able to vouch the cash receipts for the full amount of the accounts receivable in the bank statements and cash receipts records in the month following the Surepart year-end. Confirmation evidence was not considered necessary in these circumstances as the risk of material misstatement was deemed to be very low.

Confirmations of Cash and Loan Balances

The standard bank confirmation form shown in Exhibit 11–9 is used to confirm deposit and loan balances.

The exhibit shows the blank form that would be sent by the auditee to its bank and an illustration of a completed form returned from the bank for the EcoPak case.

A word of caution is in order: while financial institutions may note exceptions to the information typed in a confirmation and may confirm items omitted from it, the auditor should not rely solely on the form to satisfy the completeness assertion, insofar as cash and loan balances are concerned. Officers and employees of financial institutions cannot be expected to search their information systems for balances and loans that may not be immediately evident as assets and liabilities of the auditee company. However, it is a good idea to get bank confirmation of zero balances on accounts the company represents as closed during the year. (If a non-zero balance is confirmed, the auditors have evidence that some asset accounting has been omitted in the company records.)

Bank Confirmation Form

Blank Bank Confirmation Form Sent to EcoPak's Bank:

Bank Confirmation

Areas to be completed by client are marked §, while those to be completed by the financial institution are marked †.

FINANCIAL INSTITUTION § (Name, branch, and full mailing address)

CONFIRMATION DATE §
(All information to be provided as of this date)
(See Bank Confirmation Completion Instructions)

CLIENT (LEGAL NAME) §

The financial institution is authorized to provide the details requested herein to the below-noted firm of accountants

§ _____
Client's authorized signature
Please supply copy of the most recent credit facility agreement (initial if required) §_____

I. LOANS AND OTHER DIRECT AND CONTINGENT LIABILITIES (If balances are nil, please state)

NATURE OF LIABILITY/ CONTINGENT LIABILITY †	INTEREST (Note rate per contract)		DUE DATE †	DATE OF CREDIT FACILITY AGREEMENT †	AMOUNT AND CURRENCY OUTSTANDING †
	RATE †	DATE PAID TO †			

ADDITIONAL CREDIT FACILITY AGREEMENT(S) _____
Note the date(s) of any credit facility agreement(s) not drawn upon and not referenced above † _____

---

2. DEPOSITS/OVERDRAFTS

TYPE OF ACCOUNT §	ACCOUNT NUMBER §	INTEREST RATE §	ISSUE DATE (If applicable) §	MATURITY DATE (If applicable) §	AMOUNT AND CURRENCY (Brackets if Overdraft) †

EXCEPTIONS AND COMMENTS (See Bank Confirmation Completion Instructions)†

STATEMENT OF PROCEDURES PERFORMED BY FINANCIAL INSTITUTION †
The above information was completed in accordance with the Bank Confirmation Completion Instructions.

_____ BRANCH CONTACT _____
Authorized signature of financial institution   Name and telephone number

Please mail this form directly to our public accountant in the enclosed addressed envelope.

Name:
Address:

Telephone:
Fax:

(continued)

EXHIBIT 11–9

Bank Confirmation Form   *(continued)*

Bank Confirmation Form Completed and Returned to Auditor by Bank Official for EcoPak:

Bank Confirmation

Areas to be completed by client are marked §, while those to be completed by the financial institution are marked †

| FINANCIAL INSTITUTION §
(Name, branch, and full mailing address)

WEST COUNTRY BANK
Main Branch
100 King Street
Townville BC
V4E 5F6

CONFIRMATION DATE December 31, 20X1
(All information to be provided as of this date)
(See Bank Confirmation Completion Instructions) | CLIENT (LEGAL NAME) §   ECOPAK INC.
                                        22 Industrial Avenue
                                        Townville BC
                                        V3B 2C1
The financial institution is authorized to provide the details requested
herein to the below-noted firm of accountants

§ _____*Mina Amine*_____
Client's authorized signature
Please supply copy of the most recent credit facility agreement (initial
if required) §_____ |

1. LOANS AND OTHER DIRECT AND CONTINGENT LIABILITIES (If balances are nil, please state)

NATURE OF LIABILITY/ CONTINGENT LIABILITY †	INTEREST (Note rate per contract)		DUE DATE †	DATE OF CREDIT FACILITY AGREEMENT †	AMOUNT AND CURRENCY OUTSTANDING †
	RATE †	DATE PAID TO †			
§2,000,000 Operating Line of Credit Account # 0995-1622	Prime plus 1%		N/A	March 12, 20X1	nil

ADDITIONAL CREDIT FACILITY AGREEMENT(S)_____
Note the date(s) of any credit facility agreement(s) not drawn upon and not referenced above †_____

2. DEPOSITS/OVERDRAFTS

TYPE OF ACCOUNT §	ACCOUNT NUMBER §	INTEREST RATE §	ISSUE DATE (If applicable) §	MATURITY DATE (If applicable) §	AMOUNT AND CURRENCY (Brackets if Overdraft) †
Current	189168461	nil			$368,202.11
Money Market	520153615	variable			$505,000.00
US$ Current	730844022	nil			$1,612.98

EXCEPTIONS AND COMMENTS (See Bank Confirmation Completion Instruction)†

STATEMENT OF PROCEDURES PERFORMED BY FINANCIAL INSTITUTION †
The above information was completed in accordance with the Bank Confirmation Completion Instructions.

_____   BRANCH CONTACT   _____
Authorized signature of financial institution   Name and telephone number

Please mail this form directly to our public accountant in the enclosed addressed envelope.

| Name: Meyer & Gustav, LLP
Address: 200 Avenue Street
        Townville BC
        V7H BJ9

Telephone: 555 666 7777
Fax: 555 666 7778 | SIGNATURE GUARANTEED
West Country Commercial Banking
Townville Commercial Centre
100 King Street, 12th Floor
Townville BC V4E 5F6
_____Manager |

Source: Developed by the Canadian Bankers Association and the Canadian professional accounting bodies.

The auditor should also be alert for evidence of transactions with banks or bank accounts other than those for which there are general ledger accounts. For example, loan documents or cheques written on other banks may come to light during scanning or other document examination procedures. Inquiries of management should be made to assess whether bank confirmations should be obtained from these banks and whether any financial statement impact exists.

Confirmation of Accounts and Notes Receivable

Confirmations provide evidence of existence of accounts and notes receivable. Those to be confirmed should be documented in the working papers with an aged trial balance. A partial aged trial balance is shown in Exhibit 11–10, annotated to show the auditor's work. Accounts for confirmation can be selected at random or in accordance with another plan consistent with the audit objectives. Statistical methods are useful for determining the sample size, and audit software accessing receivables files could be used to select and print the confirmations.

EXHIBIT 11–10

Illustration of Audit Working Paper—Aged Accounts Receivable Trial Balance (Partial)

C-20

ECOPAK INC.
ACCOUNTS RECEIVABLE
December 31, 20X1

Prepared DD
Date Jan. 12, 20X2
Reviewed BP
Date Jan. 17, 20X2

	Aged					Collection	
	Current	30-60 Days	61-90 Days	Over 90 Days	Total	Current	Past Due
Ace Specialties	12,337 X				12,337 X pc u	12,337	
Bakery Supreme	712				712	712	
Charley Cafes	1,486 X	420 X			1,906 X pc	1,486	420
Deli Delites				755	755		
Waffles Unlimited			531 X		531 X pc		531
Zedd's				214	214		214
Balance per books	335,000	30,000	20,000	15,000	400,000 (9)	320,000	25,000
Billing errors	(11,000)		(1,000)		(12,000) (1)		
Adjusted balance	324,000	30,000	19,000	15,000	388,000		

X Traced to accounts receivable subsidiary ledger

pc Positive confirmation mailed Jan. 4. Replies C-230

u No reply to positive confirmation, vouched charges to invoices

9 Traced to general ledger control account

(1) Billing error adjustment explained on working paper C-220

Note: See C-220 for analysis of doubtful accounts and our test of reasonableness.

However, confirmations of accounts, loans, and notes receivable may not produce sufficient appropriate evidence regarding the ownership (rights) assertion. Debtors may not be aware that the auditee has sold its accounts, notes, or loans receivable to financial institutions or to the public (as collateralized securities). Auditors need to perform additional inquiry and details procedures to get evidence of the ownership of the receivables and of the appropriateness of disclosures related to financing transactions secured by receivables. Responses that reveal a dispute over the account or unwillingness to pay may also provide some evidence related to the valuation assertion.

Positive and Negative Confirmations

Confirmations can be either positive or negative. An example of a positive confirmation of accounts receivable that could be used in the EcoPak audit is shown in Exhibit 11–11. It gives the customer the option of confirming its total balance owing, or of selected invoices if its system makes agreeing the total balance infeasible. A variation of the positive confirmation is the blank form, which does not contain the balance; customers are asked to fill it in themselves. The blank positive confirmation may produce better evidence because the recipients need to get the information directly from their own records instead of just signing the form and returning it with no exceptions noted. (However, the effort involved may result in a lower response rate.)

EXHIBIT 11–11

Positive Confirmation Letter

D-23

Eco Pak
Townville

January 12, 20X2

Equality Roasters
Accounts Payable Department
Quarter Road
Campool, BC

Dear Sir or Madam:

In connection with our audit, our auditors, Meyer & Gustav LLP request confirmation of your account with us. Our records show an amount receivable from you of $125,540.55 as at December 31, 20XI.

In the event that your accounting system does not permit confirmation of your entire account balance, please confirm the following items were outstanding and receivable from you at the above date. The amounts listed below represent only a selection of those items making up your total balance.

Date	Invoice Number	Amount
October 12, 20XI	101-100567	$32,430.00
December 15, 20XI	121-100987	$79,100.00

If you agree with (a) the above account balance, or (b) the outstanding item(s) set out above, please complete and sign this letter in the space provided below. If you do not agree with the above information, please provide us with the details of any differences.

An envelope is enclosed for your convenience in returning this letter to the attention of Donna Ladona at Meyer & Gustav LLP, 200 Avenue Street, Townville, BC. Your early attention to this request will be appreciated.

Yours truly,
ECOPAK INC.

Signed _____*Mina Amine*_____

_____ ECOPAK Authorized Officer _____

CONFIRMATION:

a) We confirm that the above balance is correct except as noted below:

It's correct and we have paid the October invoice on January 3, 20X2.

By: J.Java *Joey Java*, Accounts Payable Manager.

_____ Name, signature, and title

b) We confirm that the above invoice(s) was (were) outstanding at [date]:

_____ Name, signature, and title

Exhibit 11–12 shows an example of a negative confirmation form (since EcoPak's auditors are assumed to use only positive confirmations, this example is for a different audit). Note that the positive form asks for a response, while the negative form asks for a response only if something is wrong with the balance. Thus, lack of response to negative confirmations is considered as evidence that nothing is wrong. For this reason, CAS 505 states that evidence from negative confirmations is less reliable than evidence from positive confirmations, and it requires that negative confirmations be used only when the risk of misstatement is low and the auditor has reason to believe the recipients will not disregard the request. For example, in the audit of an investment management business (such as the one illustrated in Exhibit 11–12), if the balance of a client's investment account has been understated, it would be very motivated to respond to the confirmation request to get this error corrected. A customer with an outstanding account payable balance, however, may be less motivated to confirm its liability. So, negative confirmation for accounts receivables is unlikely to provide sufficient appropriate evidence in many audits.

EXHIBIT 11–12

Negative Confirmation Letter

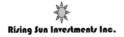

Rising Sun Investments Inc.

January 3, 20X3

Mr. Xavier Riche, President
Riche Family Holdings Inc.
Suite 5808
Magnifia Tower
Toronto, ON

Dear Sir:

Our auditors, Meyer & Gustav LLP, are making their regular audit of our financial statements. Part of this audit includes direct verification of client balances.

PLEASE EXAMINE THE DATA BELOW CAREFULLY AND COMPARE THEM TO YOUR RECORDS OF YOUR INVESTMENT ACCOUNT WITH US.

IF OUR INFORMATION IS NOT IN AGREEMENT WITH YOUR RECORDS, PLEASE STATE ANY DIFFERENCES IN THE SECTION AT THE BOTTOM OF THIS PAGE AND RETURN DIRECTLY TO OUR AUDITORS IN THE RETURN ENVELOPE PROVIDED.

IF THE INFORMATION IS CORRECT, NO REPLY IS REQUIRED.

As of December 31, 20X2, we show the following account balance:

Investment Name	Amount
RSI-High Yield Global Bond Fund	$1,062,003.16

Yours truly,

Signed _____ *Asher Unwin* _____
Rising Sun Investments Inc., Chief Financial Officer

CONFIRMATION:
The above balance does not agree with our records. We show
$1,067,779.50 as of Dec. 31, 20X2.

By: Xavier Riche *Xavier Riche,* President, Riche Family Holdings Inc.
Name, signature, and title

Standards Check

CAS 505 External Confirmations

Negative Confirmations

15. Negative confirmations provide less persuasive audit evidence than positive confirmations. Accordingly, the auditor shall not use negative confirmation requests as the sole substantive audit procedure to address an assessed risk of material misstatement at the assertion level unless all of the following are present: (Ref: Para. A23)

    (a) The auditor has assessed the risk of material misstatement as low and has obtained sufficient appropriate audit evidence regarding the operating effectiveness of controls relevant to the assertion;

    (b) The population of items subject to negative confirmation procedures comprises a large number of small, homogeneous account balances, transactions, or conditions;

    (c) A very low exception rate is expected; and

    (d) The auditor is not aware of circumstances or conditions that would cause recipients of negative confirmation requests to disregard such requests.

Source: *CPA Canada Handbook—Assurance*, 2014.

The positive form is used when individual balances are relatively large or when accounts are in dispute. They may ask for information about either the account balance or specific invoices, depending on knowledge about how customers maintain their accounting records. The negative form is used only when inherent risk and control risk are considered low, when a large number of small balances is involved, and when customers can be expected to consider the confirmations properly.

A special positive confirmation letter may be used for possibly inappropriate **bill-and-hold transactions**. While bill-and-hold sales transactions are not necessarily a GAAP violation when customers have actually requested this arrangement, they have often been associated with financial fraud and should be investigated. The bill-and-hold confirmation is an example of a confirmation request to verify the substance of a transaction from the customer's point of view. It requests confirmation of the customer's agreement to be billed and for the auditee to hold the inventory for the time being, to provide evidence that it is appropriate to recognize the revenue.

Controlling Delivery and Receipt of Confirmations

Delivering confirmations to the intended recipient is a problem that requires auditors' careful attention. Auditors need to control the confirmations, including the addresses to which they are sent, to ensure they were not mailed to company accomplices who will provide false responses. Features of the reply, such as postmarks, fax responses, letterhead, email, telephone, or other characteristics that suggest responses are false should be carefully reviewed. Auditors should follow up electronic and telephone responses by returning the call if the number is known, looking up telephone numbers, or using a directory to determine the respondent's address to verify its origin. Furthermore, with the lack of response to a negative confirmation there is no guarantee that the intended recipient received it, even if the auditor carefully controlled the mailing. Audit firms can use secure third-party confirmation services that will integrate with a firm's electronic working papers and independently authenticate all participants to the confirmation, with a turnaround time of about 24 hours instead of several weeks.[4]

bill-and-hold transactions:
sales that a customer has asked to be billed/invoiced for but does not want to be shipped immediately; require a special audit confirmation of the details of the customer's agreement to ensure revenue recognition is appropriate

The **confirmation response rate** for positive confirmations is the proportion of the number returned to the number sent. This varies depending on whom the confirmations are sought from, but generally the auditor is aiming at a 100% response. Non-responses are tolerated if the amounts can be verified by other audit procedures. The **detection rate for confirmations** is the ratio of the number of misstatements reported to auditors in confirmation responses to the number of actual account misstatements. Experience indicates that negative confirmations tend to have lower detection rates than positive confirmations, and detection rates for misstatements favouring recipients (i.e., an accounts receivable understatement) also tend to be less likely. Overall, positive confirmations are considered to be more effective than negative confirmations, but results depend on the type of recipients, the size of the account, and the type of account being confirmed. Confirmation effectiveness depends on attention to these factors and on prior years' experience with particular accounts.

Second and third requests for positive confirmations should be sent to non-respondents. If there is no response or the response specifies an exception to the auditee's records, alternative substantive procedures should be used to audit the account. These procedures include finding sales invoice copies, shipping documents, and customer orders to verify the existence of sales transactions. They also include finding evidence of customer payments in cash receipts and bank statements.

When random sampling is used, all selected accounts in the sample should be audited rather than substituting an easier-to-audit customer account into the sample as a replacement for one that does not respond to a confirmation request. If the amount cannot be verified by confirmation or alternative procedures, the auditor has to consider that the account balance does not exist.

Confirmation at Dates Other Than Year-End

Confirmation of receivables may be performed at an interim date to help the audit firm spread work throughout the year and avoid the pressures that occur around December 31. Also, the audit can be completed sooner after the year-end date if confirmation has been done earlier. Internal control over transactions affecting receivables is the biggest concern when confirming accounts before the balance sheet date. The following additional procedures should be considered when confirmation is done at an interim date:

1. Obtain a summary of receivables transactions from the interim date to the year-end date.
2. Obtain a year-end trial balance of receivables, compare it with the interim trial balance, and obtain evidence and explanations for large variations.
3. Consider additional confirmations as of the balance sheet date if balances have increased materially or a material new customer balance has been added.

Summary: Confirmations

Confirmations of cash balances, loans, accounts receivable, and notes receivable can provide very reliable audit evidence. Confirmation is usually required to provide sufficient appropriate audit evidence, unless auditors can justify substituting other procedures in a particular audit. The bank confirmation is a standard positive form. Confirmations for accounts and notes receivable can be in positive or negative form, and the positive form may be a blank confirmation.

Auditors must control confirmations to ensure that responses are received from the real debtors and not from persons intercepting the confirmations to give false responses. Responses by email, telephone, fax, or other means not written and signed by a recipient should be followed up. Second and third requests should

confirmation response rate:
the ratio of the number of confirmations returned to the number sent

detection rate for confirmations:
the ratio of the number of misstatements reported to auditors to the number of actual account misstatements

be sent for positive confirmation responses, and non-responding customers should be audited by alternative procedures. Accounts in a sample should not be left unaudited (e.g., "They didn't respond"), and easy-to-audit accounts should not be substituted for hard-to-audit ones in a sample. These techniques might raise the apparent response rate, but they do not increase the persuasiveness of the audit evidence obtained.

Confirmations yield evidence about existence. While the value is also confirmed, the fact that a debtor admits to owing the debt does not mean it can pay. While confirmations can give some clues about collectability of accounts, other procedures must audit this. Also, confirmations of accounts, notes, and loans receivable provide only partial evidence of the ownership (rights) assertion of these financial assets, so other corroborating evidence of ownership must be obtained.

Review Checkpoints

11-24   List the information an auditor should ask for in a standard bank confirmation sent to an auditee's bank.

11-25   Distinguish between positive and negative confirmations. Under what conditions would you expect each type of confirmation to be appropriate?

11-26   Distinguish between confirmation response rate and confirmation detection rate.

11-27   What are some of the justifications for not using confirmations of accounts receivable on a particular audit?

11-28   What special care should be taken with regard to examining the sources of accounts receivable confirmation responses?

Special Note: Audit of Bank Reconciliations

LO7   Describe the audit of bank statement reconciliations and how auditors can identify accounts receivable lapping and suspicious cash transactions.

The company's bank reconciliation is the primary means of valuing cash in the financial statements. The amount of cash in the bank is almost always different from the amount in the books (financial statements), and the reconciliation is performed to explain the difference. A company-prepared bank reconciliation is audited; auditors should not prepare the reconciliation, as this is a company control function.

A bank reconciliation is shown in Exhibit 11–13. The bank balance is confirmed and cross-referenced to the bank confirmation working paper. The reconciliation is recalculated, the outstanding cheques and deposits in transit totals are recalculated, and the book balance is traced to the trial balance (which has been traced to the general ledger). The reconciling items should be vouched to determine whether outstanding cheques were really not paid and that deposits in transit were actually sent to the bank before the reconciliation date. The auditor vouches the bank reconciliation items against a **cutoff bank statement**—a complete bank statement, including all paid cheques and deposit slips for a 10- to 20-day period following the reconciliation date, or the next regular monthly statement, received directly by the auditors. Note that the cash balance audit program in Exhibit 11–5 includes detailed substantive procedures related to auditing the bank reconciliation and Exhibit 11–9 shows the bank confirmation form used in practice.

cutoff bank statement:
a complete bank statement showing paid cheques, deposits, and other bank account transactions for a 10- to 20-day period following the reconciliation date

EXHIBIT 11–13

Bank Reconciliation

A.20

ECOPAK INC.
BANK RECONCILIATION-NORTH COUNTRY BANK
General Account
Dec. 31, 20X1
(Prepared by client)

Prepared *C.C. Jan. 10, 20X3*
Reviewed *J.R.A. Jan. 10, 20X2*

Balance per bank statement   506,100 c

Add:

   Deposit in transit as of Dec. 31, 20X1   51,240 n

Deduct outstanding cheques: 557,340

Date	No.	Payee		
Dec. 10, 20X0	842	Ace Supply Company	500	⨉
Nov. 31, 20X1	1280	Ace Supply Company	1,800	✓
Dec. 15, 20X1	1372	Northwest Lumber Co.	30,760	✓
Dec. 28, 20X1	1412	Gibson & Johnson	7,270	✗
Dec. 30, 20X1	1417	North Country payroll	20,000	✓
Dec. 30, 20X1	1418	Ace Supply Company	2,820	✓
Dec. 30, 20X1	1419	City Utilities	2,030	✓
Dec. 30, 20X1	1420	Howard Coatings Inc.	8,160	✓

Balance per book   73,340

484,000 f   *adjusting JE*

(amount) B   *Send to Cash lead sheet*

new balance f c

Error on ...

Note: Obtained cutoff bank statement Jan. 9, 20X2 (A.23)

∧ f   Footed (recalculated)

c   Confirmed by bank standard bank confirmation (A.22)

n   ~~Vouched~~ Traced to cutoff bank statement, deposit recorded by bank
         on Jan. 3, 20X2. Vouched to ~~duplicate deposit slip validated Jan. 3, 20X2~~   *WP# for cut-off stmt C-?*
                                                                                            CRJ ≤ Dec.31

✓   Vouched to paid cheque cleared with cutoff bank statement   *C-? vouch to CDJ*
                                                                       ≤ Dec.31/xx

✗   Vouched to statement from law firm

⨉   Amount in dispute per controller

Vouching outstanding cheques and deposits in transit is a matter of comparing cheques that cleared in the cutoff bank statement with the list of outstanding cheques, looking for evidence that all cheques written prior to the reconciliation date were on the list of outstanding cheques. The deposits shown in transit should be recorded by the bank in the first business days of the cutoff period. If otherwise, they may have been made up from receipts of the period after the reconciliation date. Other documents should be vouched for large outstanding cheques not cleared in the cutoff period. These procedures are keyed and described by tick marks in Exhibit 11–13.

Accounts Receivable Lapping

When the business receives many payments from customers, cheques listed on a sample of deposit slips (from the reconciliation month and other months) are compared with the detail of customer credits listed on the day's posting to customer accounts receivable (daily remittance list or other record of detail postings) in a detailed audit. This is a test for **accounts receivable lapping**—a manipulation of accounts receivable entries to hide a theft or fraud. For example, an employee steals a payment by collecting from customer A without recording the payment. Before customer A's account becomes past due and attracts the attention of a credit manager, customer B's similar-sized payment is credited to customer A's account. Then, before customer B's account goes past due, a payment from customer C is credited to customer B's account, and so on. This fraud may grow and go on indefinitely. The audit procedure is to look for credits given to customers who did not make payments on the day in question. This requires some careful vouching work, especially when many sales are for similar amounts. An example of this type of comparison is given in Audit 11.1 in the Application Case at the end of this chapter.

Careful Reconciliation

Suppose the cashier who prepares the remittance list stole and converted customer A's cheques for personal use. The cashier knows this will work only until customer A complains that the company has not given it credit for its payments. So, the cashier later puts customer B's cheques in the bank deposit, but shows customer A on the remittance list; thus, the accountants give customer A credit. So far, so good for preventing customer A's complaint, but now customer B needs to be addressed. This "lapping" of customer payments to hide an embezzlement can be detected by a bank reconciliation comparison of the cheques deposited (customer B) with the remittance credit recorded (customer A). Sometimes, the lapping is covered by issuing a credit note for customer B. This illustrates the importance of proper authorization and control of credit notes.

Suspicious Cash Transactions

While examining the bank reconciliation, auditors should be alert for large cash transactions with no apparent business purpose. These may indicate the possibility of **cheque kiting** or management **window dressing** between affiliated companies. Cheque kiting is a scam that involves building up apparent balances in one or more bank accounts based on uncollected (float) cheques drawn against similar accounts in other banks. New technologies and procedures in the banking industry have greatly reduced the float time in clearing cheques between financial institutions, making kiting much more difficult. For example, electronic scans of cheques can process deposits before a kite can be started, and software detecting suspicious transactions can identify an attempted kite. Management may engage in window dressing the balance sheet by transferring large sums of cash between different entities under control close to the period-end. Recording the transfer-out slightly late, or the inflow slightly early, can result in the cash appearing in two places at once. This can inflate current assets and may help conceal a bank covenant violation based on the current ratio.

accounts receivable lapping:
a manipulation of the accounts receivable entries to hide a theft or fraud

cheque kiting:
a scam that involves building up apparent balances in one or more bank accounts based on uncollected (float) cheques drawn against similar accounts in other banks when there is a time lag in clearing items between the banks

window dressing:
in financial reporting, the inappropriate manipulation of account balances by management, usually at the end of a period, to make the financial position or performance reported in the financial statements appear more attractive to users; often involves using accounting policies, journal entries, or actual cash transactions between related parties that have no real business purpose, resulting in artificial embellishment of the company's results or liquidity to obtain some benefit (e.g., salaries and bonuses that depend on how well the company performed)

Professional money managers working for cash-conscious businesses try to have minimal unused balances in their accounts, and their efforts can sometimes look like suspicious transfers. Tight cash flows can motivate window dressing, however, to inflate cash balances deceitfully. This amounts to fraudulent financial reporting. If cash transfers are recorded in the books, negative balances resulting from cheques drawn on insufficient funds will appear. Perpetrators may try to hide inappropriate bank transfers by not recording the deposits and cheques. Such manoeuvres may be detectable in a bank reconciliation audit. Since Cash is the key account and most operating transactions run through it, an inability to obtain sufficient appropriate evidence to audit cash will probably result in a pervasive limitation on the audit scope and an inability to form an audit opinion on the financial statements.

A key audit test for inappropriate window dressing is preparing a **bank transfer schedule** in which all interbank transfers a few days before and after the year-end are traced to the accounting records. This schedule shows each cheque amount, the name of the paying bank (with the book recording date and the cheque clearing date), and the name of the receiving bank (with the book deposit date and the bank clearing date), using information taken from the cancelled cheques and the cleared deposits in the bank statements. The purpose of this schedule is to see that both sides of the transfer transaction are properly recorded in the same period. You may note that this test is similar in design to a cutoff test for transaction processing.

Summary: Bank Reconciliations, Lapping, and Cash Window Dressing

The combination of all the procedures performed on the bank reconciliation provides evidence of existence, valuation, and proper cutoff of the bank cash balances. Auditors use a cutoff bank statement to obtain independent evidence of the proper listing of outstanding cheques and deposits in transit on a bank reconciliation.

Note that if the auditor reperforms the bank reconciliation, it is a substantive procedure, because it yields direct evidence on monetary misstatements. However, if the auditor checks that bank reconciliations are performed on a regular basis, this is a test of controls that provides only indirect evidence of the risk of monetary misstatements.

Additional procedures might detect attempts at lapping accounts receivable collections and inappropriate bank transfers. Auditing the details of customer payments listed in bank deposits in comparison with details of customer payment postings (remittance lists) will show lapping. Preparing schedules of intercompany bank transfers just before and after year-end will detect double counting of amounts that inflates the reported cash balance.

Review Checkpoints

11-29   What is a cutoff bank statement? How is it used by auditors?

11-30   What is lapping? What procedures can auditors employ for its detection?

11-31   What is the purpose of auditing intercompany bank transfers just before and after the year-end?

bank transfer schedule:
an audit analysis summarizing all the transfers between the auditee's bank accounts in the days just before and after the period-end to verify that each amount transferred is included in only one account at the period-end, not double counted

APPLICATION CASE WITH SOLUTION & ANALYSIS

Detecting Misstatements in the Revenues, Receivables, and Receipts Process

INTRODUCTION

This Application Case contains specific examples of tests of controls and substantive audit procedures used to gather evidence in the revenues, receivables, and receipts process. The purpose of substantive audit procedures differs from that of tests of controls in that substantive procedures are designed to provide direct audit evidence about the dollar amounts in account balances, while tests of controls provide audit evidence about the company's performance of its own control procedures. Substantive procedures include tests of details of balances and transactions as well as focused analytical procedures. Substantive procedures must follow the assessment of control risk, as auditors cannot rely exclusively on controls. Dual-purpose procedures can be designed that cover substantive and control testing purposes simultaneously.

In this Application Case, as well as in those of subsequent chapters, each audit case situation describes an error or fraud that occurred, followed by an audit approach analysis that explains the audit objective (assertion), controls relevant in the business process, tests of controls, and substantive procedures that could be considered in an approach to the case. The audit approach section presumes that the auditors do not know everything about the situation. (As a student of the case, you have inside information.) Each audit situation is set up with the following framework.

CASE DESCRIPTION

This offers the background of what happened in the case: the dollar amount of overstated assets and revenue, or understated liabilities, and expenses that resulted; the method or cause of the misstatement (accidental error, intentional irregularity, or fraud attempt); the failure of controls that made it possible; and the amounts involved.

Audit Trail

This is a set of telltale signs of erroneous accounting and missing or altered documents.

SOLUTION & ANALYSIS

Audit Approach

This section contains the following parts: audit objective and controls relevant to the process.

Audit Objective

This refers to the recognition of a financial statement assertion for which evidence needs to be obtained. The assertions are about existence of assets, liabilities, revenues, and expenses; their valuation; their complete inclusion in the account balances; the rights and obligations inherent in them; and their proper presentation and disclosure in the financial statements. (These assertions were introduced in Chapter 6.)

Controls Relevant to the Process

This is a recognition of the control procedures that should be used by an organization to prevent and detect errors and fraud.

Audit Procedures

These are evidence-gathering procedures—tests of controls, dual-purpose procedures, and tests of details of balance.

Audit Results

This is a summary of the auditors' findings and their implications.

In the end-of-chapter review section, similar discussion cases allow you to test your ability to design audit procedures for the detection of errors or fraud.

DISCUSSION CASE

Jack's first year on the audit trail has been an exciting one. He has worked on many audits and gained experience in a wide variety of situations that have helped him develop his professional judgment. While meeting with some new junior audit staff members, Jack describes three very different experiences in auditing the revenues, receivables, and receipts process. The three audit situations he encountered provide a lot of insight into the risk of material misstatements. The first case involved misstatement due to employee embezzlement, the second involved fraudulent financial reporting by management, and the third was an unintentional error by the accounting department.

AUDIT 11.1 The Embezzling Cashier

CASE DESCRIPTION

Cash embezzlement by an employee at a new audit client, Sports Equipment Inc. (SEI), an equipment retailer, caused overstated accounts receivable, overstated customer discounts expense, and understated cash sales. SEI also failed to earn interest income on funds "borrowed." Over a six-year period, D. Bakel, the assistant controller of SEI, built up a $350,000 average balance in a Sport Equipment Company (SEC) account, which earned a total of $67,500 in interest that should have been earned by SEI. By approving the "extra" discounts, Bakel also skimmed 2% of about $1 million in annual sales, for a total of $120,000. Since SEI would have had net income before taxes of about $1.6 million over the six years, Bakel's embezzlement took about 12.5% of the income.

SEI maintained accounts receivable for school boards in the region; its other customers received credit only by using their own credit cards. Bakel was the company cashier, receiving all the incoming payments on school board accounts and credit card accounts, as well as all the other cash and cheques taken over the counter. Bakel prepared the bank deposit (and delivered the deposit to the bank), listing all the cheques and currency; prepared a remittance worksheet (daily cash report) that showed amounts received, discounts allowed on school board accounts, and amounts to credit to the accounts receivable; and reconciled the bank statement. No one else reviewed the deposits or the bank statements except the independent auditors.

Bakel opened the bank account in the name of Sport Equipment Company (SEC), after properly incorporating the company with the government Ministry of Commerce. He took over-the-counter cash and cheques and school board payments from the SEI receipts and deposited them in the SEC account. No one, including the bank, noticed the difference between the rubber stamp endorsements for the two similarly named corporations. Bakel kept the money in the SEC account, earning interest on it, and then wrote SEC cheques to SEI to replace the "borrowed" funds. In the meantime, new SEI receipts were being deposited to SEC. When Bakel deposited SEC cheques in SEI, giving the schools credit, an additional 2% customer discount was approved. Thus, the school boards received proper credit later, but SEC paid in a discounted amount.

Audit Trail

SEI's bank deposits showed fairly small currency deposits as Bakel was nervous about taking too many SEI cheques, so preferred to take cash. As shown in the examples below, the deposit slips listed the SEC cheques Bakel deposited, as the bank tellers usually check this. The remittance worksheet, on the other hand, did not show SEC cheques but rather receipts from school boards and currency, and not many over-the-counter cheques from customers. The transactions became complicated enough that Bakel had to use the computer in the office to keep track of the school boards that needed to get credit. There were no vacations for this hard-working cashier because the discrepancies might be noticed by a substitute employee.

SOLUTION & ANALYSIS

Audit Approach

Audit Objective

The auditor's objective was to obtain evidence determining whether the accounts receivable recorded on the books represented claims against real customers in the gross amounts recorded.

Controls Relevant to the Process

The authorization related to cash receipts, custody of cash, recording of cash transactions, and bank statement reconciliation should be separate duties assigned to different people. Independent review of one or more of these duties should be performed as a supervisory control designed to detect errors and fraud.

Unfortunately, at SEI, Bakel had all these duties. (While recording was not actually performed, Bakel provided the source document—the remittance worksheet that the other accountant used to make the cash and accounts receivable entries.) According to the company president, the only "control" was the diligence of "our long-time, trusted, hard-working assistant controller." Assessing the control risk on this new audit, Jack's audit team identified serious control weaknesses. By thinking like a crook to imagine ways these control weakness could allow Bakel to commit fraud, the auditors discovered the scheme for cash theft and accounts receivable lapping.

Audit Procedures

Dual-Purpose Tests

Since Bakel's "honest and diligent" performance was the "control" of the accounting and control procedures that should have been performed by two or more people, the auditors performed a dual-purpose test of controls and obtained substantive details of cash receipts transactions as they relate to accounts receivable credits. The samples and direction of test procedure are as follows:

(a) Validity direction—Select a sample of customer accounts receivable, and reconcile payment credits to remittance worksheets and bank deposits, including recalculation of discounts allowed according to sales terms (2%), classification (customer name), identification, and correspondence of receipt date to recording date.
(b) Completeness direction—Select a sample of remittance worksheets (or bank deposits), vouch details to bank deposit slips (trace details to remittance worksheets if the sample is bank deposits), and trace forward to complete accounting posting in customer accounts receivable.

Test of Details of Balance

The auditors sent positive confirmations on all 72 school board accounts. Since there was a control risk of incorrect accounting, the accounts receivable confirmation was performed at the year-end date, using positive confirmations. Blank confirmations were used, and the "sample" included all the accounts, since the number was not too large.

Audit Results

The audit tests showed four cases of discrepancy where the responses stated that the boards had paid the balances before the confirmation date. Follow-up procedures on their accounts receivable credit in the next period showed they had received credit in remittance reports, and the bank deposits had shown no cheques from the school boards, but had contained a cheque from SEC. To further investigate, the auditors used the Internet, telephone book, chamber of commerce directory, and a visit to a local Ministry of Commerce office to determine the location and identity of SEC. Further investigation of SEC revealed the connection of Bakel, who was confronted and then confessed.

BANK DEPOSIT SLIP		CASH REMITTANCE REPORT				
		NAME	AMOUNT	DISCOUNT	ACCOUNTS RECEIVABLE	SALES
Jones	25					
Smith	35	Jones	25	0	0	25
Hill Dist.	980	Smith	35	0	0	35
Sport Equip	1,563	Hill Dist.	980	20	1,000	0
Currency	540	Marlin Dist.	480	20	500	0
Deposit	3,143	Waco Dist.	768	32	800	0
		Currency	855	0	0	855
		Totals	3,143	72	2,300	915

AUDIT 11.2 Bill Early, Bill Often!

CASE DESCRIPTION

McGossage Company is a long-time audit client of Jack's firm that has been experiencing profit pressures for two years now. A recessionary economy reduced profits, but the company reported net income decreases that were not as severe as other companies in its industry. In the audit, it was discovered that employees were recording sales too early and failing to account for customer discounts taken, resulting in overstated sales and receivables, understated discounts expense, and overstated net income.

As misstatements go, some of these were on the materiality borderline. Sales were overstated 0.3% and 0.5% in the prior and current year, respectively. Accounts receivable were overstated 4% and 8%. But the combined effect was to overstate the division's net income by 6% and 17%. Selected data are as follows:

	ONE YEAR AGO		CURRENT YEAR	
	REPORTED	ACTUAL	REPORTED	ACTUAL
Sales	$330.0	$329.0	$350.0	$348.0
Discounts expense	1.7	1.8	1.8	2.0
Net income	6.7	6.3	5.4	4.6

In McGossage's grocery products division, sales had been recorded for orders prepared for shipment but not actually shipped until later. Employees backdated the shipping documents. Gross profit on these "sales" was about 30%. Customers took discounts on payments, but the company did not record them, leaving the debit balances in the customers' accounts receivable instead of charging them to discounts and allowances expense. Company accountants were instructed to wait 60 days before recording discounts taken.

The division vice-president and general manager knew about these accounting practices, as did a significant number of the 2,500 employees in the division. The division managers were under orders to achieve profit objectives they considered unrealistic, thus creating pressure on them to misstate the financial results.

Audit Trail

The customers' accounts receivable balances contained amounts due for discounts the customers had already taken. The cash receipts records showed payments received without credit for discounts. Discounts were entered monthly by a special journal entry. The unshipped goods were on the shipping dock at year-end, with papers showing earlier shipping dates.

SOLUTION & ANALYSIS

Audit Approach

Audit Objective

The auditors' objectives were to obtain evidence to determine if sales were recorded in the proper period, if gross accounts receivable represented the amounts due from customers at year-end, and if discounts expenses were recognized in the proper amount in the proper period.

Controls Relevant to the Process

The accounting procedures manual should state that sales are to be recorded on the date of shipment (or when title passes, if later); management overrode this control procedure by having shipping employees date the shipping papers incorrectly. Cash receipts procedures call for discounts to be authorized and recorded when they are taken by customers; management overrode this control procedure by giving instructions to delay the recording.

Audit Procedures

Tests of Controls

Auditors used questionnaires and inquiries to determine the company's accounting policies, as it is possible that employees and managers would conceal these from auditors unless asked directly. Pointed questions about revenue recognition and discount recording policies might elicit revealing answers.

Dual-Purpose Procedures

The auditors selected a sample of cash receipts, examined them for authorization, recalculated the customer discounts, and traced them to accounts receivable input for recording of the proper amount on the proper date. They selected a sample of shipping documents and vouched them to customer orders, and then traced them to invoices and to recording in the amounts receivable input with proper amounts on the proper dates. These tests follow the tracing direction—data representing the beginning of transactions (cash receipts, shipping) are traced through the company's accounting process.

Tests of Details of Balance

The auditors confirmed a sample of customer accounts and used analytical relationships of past years' discount expense to a relevant base (sales, sales volume) to calculate an overall test of the discounts expense. They recorded shipping details including relevant dates for any inventory on the shipping dock at year-end and traced to the sales invoice to check dating.

Audit Results

The managers lied to the auditors about their revenue and expense timing policies. The sample of shipping documents showed no dating discrepancies because the employees had inserted incorrect dates. The analytical procedures on discounts did not show the misstatement because the historical relationships were too erratic to show a deficient number (outlier). However, the sample of cash receipts transactions showed that discounts were not calculated and recorded at time of receipt. Additional inquiry led to discovery of the special journal entries and admission of the recording delay. Two customers in the sample of 65 confirmations responded with exceptions that turned out to be unrecorded discounts. Two other customers in the confirmation sample complained that they did not owe for late invoices on December 31. Follow-up showed the shipments were goods on the shipping dock noticed by auditors during the December 31 inventory taking. The shipping documents were dated December 26. The sales recording had them recorded as "bill and hold" on December 29.

AUDIT 11.3 Thank Goodness It's Friday

CASE DESCRIPTION

In the audit of Alpha Brewery Corporation (Alpha), Jack's audit team found that overstated sales caused net income, retained earnings, current assets, working capital, and total assets to be overstated. Overstated cash collections did not change the total current assets or total assets, but they increased the amount of cash and decreased the amount of accounts receivable by an offsetting amount, affecting the liquidity ratios that Alpha's bank monitors. Alpha recorded sales of $672,000 and gross profit of $268,800 over the January 1–4 period. Cash collections on customers' accounts amounted to $800,000.

Alpha generally has good control policies and procedures related to authorization of transactions for accounting entry, and the accounting manual has instructions for recording sales transactions in the proper accounting period. The company regularly closes the accounting process each Friday at 5 p.m. to prepare weekly management reports. The year-end date (cutoff date) is December 31, and, in 20X0, December 31 was a Monday. However, the accounting was performed through Friday as usual, and the accounts were closed for the year on January 4.

Audit Trail

All the entries were properly dated after December 31, including the sales invoices, cash receipts, and shipping documents. However, the trial balance from which the financial statements were prepared was dated December 31, 20X0, even though the accounts were actually closed on January 4. Nobody noticed the slip of a few days because the Friday closing was normal.

SOLUTION & ANALYSIS

Audit Approach

Audit Objective

The auditors' objectives were to obtain evidence to determine the existence, completeness, and valuation of sales for the year ended December 31, 20X0, and of the cash and accounts receivable as of December 31, 20X0.

Controls Relevant to the Process

The company had in place proper instructions for dating transactions on the actual date they occurred, entering sales and cost of goods sold on the day of shipment, and entering cash receipts on the day received in the company offices. An accounting supervisor should have checked the entries through Friday to make sure the dates corresponded to the actual events and that the accounts for the year were closed with Monday's transactions.

Audit Procedures

Tests of Controls

In this case, the auditors needed to be aware of the company's weekly routine closing and of the possibility that the Monday occurrence of December 31 might cause a problem. Asking the question "Did you cut off the accounting on Monday night this week?" might elicit the "Oh, we forgot!" response. It would be normal to sample transactions around the year-end date to determine if they were recorded in the proper accounting period. To do this, they selected transactions from 10 days before and after the year-end date and inspected the dates on supporting documentation.

Tests of Details of Balance

For sales overstatements, the auditors confirmed a sample of accounts receivable. If the accounts were too large, the auditors expected the debtors to say so, thus leading to detection of sales overstatements. Cash overstatement was audited by examining the bank reconciliation to see whether deposits in transit (the deposits sent late in December) actually cleared the bank early in January. Obviously, the January 4 cash collections could not reach the bank until at least Monday, January 7. That is too long for a December 31 deposit to be in transit to a local bank.

 The completeness of sales recordings was audited by selecting a sample of sales transactions and supporting shipping documents in the early part of the next accounting period (January 20X1). Sales of 20X0 could be incomplete if recording of December shipments had been postponed until January, and this procedure would detect them if the shipping documents were dated properly. The completeness of cash collections and accounts receivable credits was audited by examining the cash deposits early in January for any sign of holding cash without entry until January.

 In this case the existence objective was more significant to discovering the problem than the completeness objective; after all, the January 1–4 sales, shipments, and cash collections did not "exist" in December 20X0.

Audit Results

The test of controls sample from the days before and after December 31 quickly revealed the problem. Company accounting personnel were embarrassed, but there was no intent to misstate the financial statements. This was a simple error. The company readily made the following adjustment:

	DEBIT	CREDIT
Sales	$672,000	
Inventory	403,200	
Accounts receivable	800,000	
Accounts receivable		$672,000
Cost of goods sold		403,200
Cash		800,000

Review Checkpoints

11-32 In the Audit 11.1 case, name one bank reconciliation control procedure that could have revealed signs of embezzlement.

11-33 What feature(s) of a cash receipts internal control system would be expected to prevent the cash receipts journal and recorded cash sales from reflecting more than the amount shown on the daily deposit slip?

11-34 In the Audit 11.2 case, what information might have been obtained from each of the following: inquiries, detailed test of controls procedures, observations, and confirmations?

11-35 With reference to the Audit 11.3 case, how would an understanding of the business and management reporting system have contributed to discovery of the open cash receipts journal cutoff error?

SUMMARY

- The revenues, receivables, and receipts process consists of customer order processing, credit checking, goods shipping, customer billing, accounts receivable accounting, cash receipts collection, and accounting. Companies reduce control risk by having a suitable separation of authorization, custody, recording, and periodic reconciliation duties. Error-checking procedures of comparing customer orders and shipping documents are important for billing customers the right prices for the delivered quantities. Otherwise, many things could go wrong—from sales to fictitious customers or those with bad credit to billings for the wrong quantities at the wrong prices at the wrong time. **LO1**

- Auditors consider environmental and general controls and then assess specific application controls. Internal control questionnaires often used in practice are provided in Appendix 11A to illustrate the nature of the auditor inquiries and observations used to assess control risk. Controls activities may be tested through observation, inspection, and reperformance procedures. Examples of control tests in this process were provided. **LO2**

- Substantive programs are developed by linking the auditor's risk assessments to the risks of material misstatements in revenue transactions, accounts receivable balance, and cash receipts transactions. A detailed example showing the process documenting and linking risk assessments to the design of an audit program of substantive procedures was provided for one example, the cash balance. Similar linking exercises would be used to develop substantive audit procedures in response to the assessed risks at the assertion level for all the significant classes of transactions, account balances, and disclosures. **LO3**

- Generic substantive audit programs were illustrated by providing examples of typical substantive procedures that would be considered, depending on the risks assessed in each particular case. **LO4**

- Three topics were given special technical notes in the chapter. The existence assertion is very important in the audit of cash and receivables assets, as misleading financial statements often include overstated assets and revenue. **LO4**

- Confirmations are very important substantive procedures for obtaining audit evidence about asset existence from outside parties. **LO6**

- Bank reconciliations were shown to be an audit opportunity to recalculate the amount of cash reported in the financial statements and to look for signs of accounts receivable lapping and inappropriate banking transfers that inflated reported cash balances at year-end. **LO7**

This chapter concluded with an application case and suggested solution analysis that told the stories of three audit situations, with one involving a cash embezzlement scheme using the practice of lapping accounts receivable. Cash collection is a critical point for asset control. Many cases of embezzlement occur in this process.

KEY TERMS

accounts receivable lapping	continuity schedule	online input validation
accounts receivable subsidiary ledger	control risk assessment	planned acceptable audit risk level
aged accounts receivable trial balance	cutoff bank statement	(acceptable audit risk level)
audit scope	detailed audit plan	revenue recognition problems
balance sheet approach to auditing	detection rate for confirmations	reversing error
bank transfer schedule	fidelity bond	sales cutoff testing
bill-and-hold transactions	FOB destination	two-direction testing
cheque kiting	FOB shipping	window dressing
confirmation response rate	money laundering	

MULTIPLE-CHOICE QUESTIONS FOR PRACTICE AND REVIEW

MC 11-1 **LO7** Which of the following is the best protection for a company that wishes to prevent the lapping of trade accounts receivable?

- *a.* Segregate duties so that the bookkeeper in charge of the general ledger has no access to incoming mail.
- *b.* Segregate duties so that no employee has access to both cheques from customers and currency from daily cash receipts.
- *c.* Have all customers make payments directly to the company's bank by electronic transfer.
- *d.* Request that customers' payment cheques be made payable to the company and addressed to the treasurer.

MC 11-2 **LO3** Which of the following internal control procedures will most likely prevent the concealment of a cash shortage from the improper write-off of a trade account receivable?

- *a.* Write-offs must be approved by a responsible officer after review of credit department recommendations and supporting evidence.
- *b.* Write-offs must be supported by an aging schedule showing that only receivables overdue several months have been written off.
- *c.* Write-offs must be approved by the cashier who is in a position to know if the receivables have, in fact, been collected.
- *d.* Write-offs must be authorized by company field sales employees who are in a position to determine the financial standing of the customers.

MC 11-3 **LO4** Auditors sometimes use comparisons of ratios as audit evidence. For example, an unexplained decrease in the ratio of gross profit to sales suggests which of the following possibilities?

a. Unrecorded purchases

b. Unrecorded sales

c. Merchandise purchases charged to selling and general expense

d. Fictitious sales

MC 11-4 **LO4** An auditor is auditing sales transactions. One step is to vouch a sample of debit entries from the accounts receivable subsidiary ledger back to the supporting sales invoices. What would the auditor intend to establish by this step?

a. Sales invoices represent bona fide sales.

b. All sales have been recorded.

c. All sales invoices have been properly posted to customer accounts.

d. Debit entries in the accounts receivable subsidiary ledger are properly supported by sales invoices.

MC 11-5 **LO2** If a dishonest bookkeeper is trying to conceal defalcations involving receivables, which of the following accounts would the auditor most likely expect the bookkeeper to charge?

a. Miscellaneous income

b. Petty cash

c. Miscellaneous expense

d. Sales returns

MC 11-6 **LO2** Which of the following would the auditor consider to be an incompatible operation if the cashier receives remittances?

a. The cashier prepares the daily deposit.

b. The cashier makes the daily deposit at a local bank.

c. The cashier posts the receipts to the accounts receivable subsidiary ledger cards.

d. The cashier endorses the cheques.

MC 11-7 **LO4** The audit working papers often include an auditee-prepared aged trial balance of accounts receivable as of the balance sheet date. The aging is best used by the auditor for which of the following?

a. Evaluating internal control over credit sales

b. Testing the accuracy of recorded charge sales

c. Estimating credit losses

d. Verifying the existence of the recorded receivables

MC 11-8 **LO4** Which of the following might be detected by an auditor's cutoff review and examination of sales journal entries for several days prior to the balance sheet date?

a. Lapping year-end accounts receivable

b. Inflating sales for the year

c. Kiting bank balances

d. Misappropriating merchandise

MC 11-9 **LO6** Confirmation of individual accounts receivable balances directly with debtors will, of itself, normally provide evidence concerning which of the following?

a. Collectability of the balances confirmed

b. Ownership of the balances confirmed

c. Existence of the balances confirmed

d. Internal control over balances confirmed

MC 11-10 `LO7` Which of the following is the most effective technique for detecting suspicious cash transactions between intercompany banks?

a. Review the composition of authenticated deposit slips.

b. Review subsequent bank statements.

c. Prepare a schedule of the bank transfers.

d. Prepare a year-end bank reconciliation.

MC 11-11 `LO2` What is the best reason for prenumbering, in sequence, documents such as sales orders, shipping documents, and sales invoices?

a. Enables determination of the accuracy of each document

b. Enables determination of the proper period recording of sales revenue and receivables

c. Allows checking of the numerical sequence for missing documents and unrecorded transactions

d. Enables determination of the validity of recorded transactions

MC 11-12 `LO1` When a sample of customer accounts receivable is selected for the purpose of vouching debits for evidence of existence, the auditors will vouch them to which other items?

a. Sales invoices with shipping documents and customer sales invoices

b. Records of accounts receivable write-offs

c. Cash remittance lists and bank deposit slips

d. Credit files and reports

MC 11-13 `LO5` In the audit of cash and accounts receivable, the main emphasis should be on which assertion?

a. Completeness

b. Existence

c. Obligations

d. Presentation and disclosure

MC 11-14 `LO6` When accounts receivable are confirmed at an interim date, the auditors are not concerned with which of the following?

a. Obtaining a summary of receivables transactions from the interim date to the year-end date

b. Obtaining a year-end trial balance of receivables, comparing it with the interim trial balance, and obtaining evidence and explanations for large variations

c. Sending negative confirmations to all the customers as of the year-end date

d. Considering the necessity for some additional confirmations as of the balance sheet date if balances have increased materially

MC 11-15 `LO6` The negative request form of accounts receivable confirmation is most likely to be acceptable in which case?

	ASSESSED LEVEL OF CONTROL RISK RELATING TO RECEIVABLES IS	NUMBER OF SMALL BALANCES IS	PROPER CONSIDERATION BY THE RECIPIENT IS
a.	Low	Many	Likely
b.	Low	Few	Unlikely
c.	High	Few	Likely
d.	High	Many	Likely

(© 2000, American Institute of CPAs. All Rights Reserved. Adapted by permission.)

MC 11-16 **LO4** When an auditor selects a sample of shipping documents and takes the tracing direction of a test to find the related sales invoice copies, the evidence is relevant for deciding which of the following?

a. If shipments to customers were invoiced
b. If shipments to customers were recorded as sales
c. If recorded sales were shipped
d. If invoiced sales were shipped

(© 2000, American Institute of CPAs. All Rights Reserved. Adapted by permission.)

EXERCISES AND PROBLEMS

EP 11-1 Cash Receipts: Control Objectives and Control Examples. **LO1, 2**

Required:

Prepare a table similar to Exhibit 11–2 on internal control objectives for cash receipts.

EP 11-2 Cash: Substantive Audit Procedures on Bank Reconciliation. **LO3, 5, 7** The following auditee-prepared bank reconciliation is being examined by you during an audit of the financial statements of Cynthia Company.

CYNTHIA COMPANY BANK RECONCILIATION VILLAGE BANK ACCOUNT 2 DECEMBER 31, 20X0		
Balance per bank (*a*):		$18,375.91
Deposits in transit (*b*):		
Dec. 30	$1,471.10	
Dec. 31	2,840.69	4,311.79
Subtotal		22,687.70
Outstanding cheques (*c*):		
837	6,000.00	
1941	671.80	
1966	320.00	
1984	1,855.42	
1985	3,621.22	
1987	2,576.89	
1991	4,420.88	(19,466.21)
Subtotal		3,221.49
NSF cheque returned		
Dec. 29 (*d*):		200.00
Bank charges		5.50
Error: cheque no. 1932		148.10
Customer receivable collected by electronic funds transfer ($3,050 less $50 service fee) (*e*):		(3,025.00)
Balance per books (*f*):		$ 550.09

Required:

Indicate one or more audit procedures that should be performed in gathering evidence in support of each of the items (*a*) through (*f*) above.

(© 2000, American Institute of CPAs. All Rights Reserved. Adapted by permission.)

EP 11-3 Sales Cutoff and Cutoff Bank Statement. `LO2, 5, 7`

Required:

a. You wish to test Houston Corporation's sales cutoff at June 30. Describe the steps you should include in this test.
b. You obtain a July 10 bank statement directly from the bank. Explain how this cutoff bank statement should be used
   1. in your review of the June 30 bank reconciliation, and
   2. to obtain other audit information.

(© 2000, American Institute of CPAs. All Rights Reserved. Adapted by permission.)

EP 11-4 Alternative Accounts Receivable Procedures. `LO1, 5, 6` Several accounts receivable confirmations have been returned with the notation "verification of supplier statements is no longer possible because our data processing system does not accumulate each supplier's invoices."

Required:

What alternative auditing procedures could be used to audit these accounts receivable?

(© 2000, American Institute of CPAs. All Rights Reserved. Adapted by permission.)

EP 11-5 Accounts Receivable Audit Procedures. `LO1, 4, 5` During the audit of the December 31, 20X5, financial statements, the auditor identifies cash amounts received after December 31, 20X5, and traces these amounts to the cash account in the general ledger and to the accounts receivable subledger balances at December 31, 20X5.

Required:

a. What kind of procedure is this? Which financial statement assertion does it provide evidence for? What is that evidence?
b. What records or documents would the auditor need to look at to identify cash amounts received after year-end?

EP 11-6 Accounts Receivable Audit Procedures. `LO4, 6` The auditor is considering confirming zero-balance accounts from the auditee's accounts receivable subledger to provide evidence concerning the completeness assertion for accounts receivables and sales.

Required:

a. What are the advantages and limitations of this procedure?
b. How would the decision to use this procedure relate to the auditor's control assessment? In particular, discuss the kinds of controls the auditee would be expected to have and the procedures the auditor could use to test them.

EP 11-7 Continuity Schedule for Allowance for Doubtful Accounts. `LO4`

Required:

a. Complete the following continuity schedule indicating how the movements in the allowance for doubtful accounts tie into other amounts in the financial statements.

b. Prepare an audit program listing the procedures that can be used to audit the accounts in this system. Demonstrate how your audit program addresses all the relevant assertions.

AUDITED AMOUNT	FINANCIAL STATEMENT WHERE AMOUNT IS REPORTED
Opening balance of allowance for doubtful accounts	
Add:	
Deduct:	
Ending balance of allowance for doubtful accounts	

EP 11-8 Cutoff Bank Statement for Auditing the Bank Reconciliation. `LO7` Velma Inc. is a very modern company that strives to be paperless in all its administrative functions. Velma has arranged with its bank to receive all its banking transaction information online, through the bank's online banking website. Velma's auditor want to get a cutoff bank statement as of January 20, 20X1, to complete the audit of the bank reconciliation.

Required:

a. Explain what a cutoff bank statement is and its purpose in auditing the bank reconciliation.

b. Describe one way that Velma's auditor can obtain a cutoff bank statement if the bank is unable to provide a paper copy.

DISCUSSION CASES

DC 11-1 Internal Control Questionnaire for Book Buy-Back Cash Fund. `LO2` Taylor, a PA, has been engaged to audit the financial statements of University Books Incorporated. University Books maintains a large, revolving cash fund exclusively for the purpose of buying used books from students for cash. The cash fund is active all year because the nearby university offers a large variety of courses with varying start and completion dates throughout the year.

Receipts are prepared for each purchase. Reimbursement vouchers are periodically submitted to replenish the fund.

Required:

Construct an internal control questionnaire to be used in evaluating the system of internal control over University Books' use of the revolving cash fund to buy back books. The internal control questionnaire should be designed to require a Yes or No response to each question. Do not discuss the internal controls over books that are purchased.

(© 2000, American Institute of CPAs. All Rights Reserved. Adapted by permission.)

DC 11-2 Test of Controls Audit Procedures for Cash Receipts. `LO1, 2` You are the in-charge auditor examining the financial statements of the Gutzler Company for the year ended

December 31. During late October, with the help of Gutzler's controller, you completed an internal control questionnaire and prepared the appropriate memoranda describing Gutzler's accounting procedures. Your comments relative to cash receipts are as follows:

> All cash receipts are sent directly to the accounts receivable clerk with no processing by the mail department. This clerk keeps the cash receipts journal, prepares the bank deposit slip in duplicate, posts from the deposit slip to the subsidiary accounts receivable ledger, and mails the deposit to the bank.

> The controller receives the validated deposit slips directly (unopened) from the bank. She also receives the monthly bank statement directly (unopened) from the bank and promptly reconciles it.

> At the end of each month, the accounts receivable clerk notifies the general ledger clerk, by journal voucher, of the monthly totals of the cash receipts journal for posting to the general ledger.

> Each month, the general ledger clerk records the total debits to cash from the cash receipts journal. The clerk also, on occasion, makes debit entries in the general ledger cash account from sources other than the cash receipts journal, for example, funds borrowed from the bank.

Certain standard auditing procedures listed below have already been performed by you in the audit of cash receipts:

- All columns in the cash receipts have been totalled and cross-totalled.
- Postings from the cash receipts journal have been traced to the general ledger.
- Remittance advices and related correspondence have been traced to entries in the cash receipts journal.

Required:

Considering Gutzler's internal control over cash receipts and the standard auditing procedures already performed, list all other auditing procedures that should be performed to obtain sufficient appropriate audit evidence regarding cash receipts control, and give the reasons for each procedure. Do not discuss the procedures for cash disbursements and cash balances. Also, do not discuss the extent to which any of the procedures are to be performed. Assume adequate controls exist to ensure that all sales transactions are recorded. Organize your answer sheet as follows:

Other Audit Procedures	Reason for Other Audit Procedures

(© 2000, American Institute of CPAs. All Rights Reserved. Adapted by permission.)

DC 11-3 Cash Receipts: Weaknesses and Recommendations. `LO2` The Pottstown Art League operates a museum for the benefit and enjoyment of the community. During hours when the museum is open to the public, two volunteer clerks positioned at the entrance collect a $5 admission fee from each non-member patron. Members of the Art League are permitted to enter free of charge on presentation of their membership cards.

At the end of each day, one of the clerks delivers the proceeds to the treasurer. The treasurer counts the cash in the presence of the clerk and places it in a safe. Each Friday afternoon, the treasurer and one of the clerks deliver all cash held in the safe to the bank, and they receive an authenticated deposit slip that provides the basis for the weekly entry in the cash receipts journal.

The board of directors of the Pottstown Art League has identified a need to improve the system of internal control over cash admission fees. The board has determined that the cost of installing turnstiles or sales booths or otherwise altering the physical layout of the museum will greatly exceed any benefits that may be derived. However, the board has agreed that the sale of admission tickets must be an integral part of its improvement efforts.

Required:

The board of directors has requested your assistance. Prepare a report for presentation and discussion at their next board meeting that identifies the weaknesses in the existing system of cash admission fees and suggests recommendations.

(© 2000, American Institute of CPAs. All Rights Reserved. Adapted by permission.)

DC 11-4 Control Weaknesses: Shipping and Billing. **LO2** Ajax Inc. recently implemented a new accounting system to process the shipping, billing, and accounts receivable records more efficiently. During the interim work of Ajax's auditors, an assistant completed the review of the accounting system and the internal controls. The assistant determined the following information concerning the computer systems and the processing and control of shipping notices and customer invoices:

The computer system documentation consists of the following items: program listings, error listings, logs, and database dictionaries. The system and documentation are maintained by the IT administrator. To increase efficiency, batch totals and processing controls are not used in the system.

Ajax ships its products directly from two warehouses, which forward shipping notices to general accounting. There, the billing clerk enters the price of the item and accounts for the numerical sequence of the shipping notices. The billing clerk also manually prepares daily adding machine tapes of the units shipped and the sales amounts. The computer processing output consists of the following:

(a) A three-copy invoice that is forwarded to the billing clerk
(b) A daily sales register showing the aggregate totals of units shipped and sales amounts that the billing clerk compares with the adding machine tapes

The billing clerk mails two copies of each invoice to the customer and retains the third copy in an open invoice file that serves as a detailed accounts receivable record.

Required:

a. Prepare a list of weaknesses in internal control (manual and computer), and for each weakness make one or more recommendations.
b. Suggest how Ajax's computer processing over shipping and billing could be improved through the use of remote terminals to enter shipping notices. Describe appropriate controls for such an online data entry system.

DC 11-5 Bank Reconciliation: Cash Shortage. **LO4, 7** The Patrick Company had poor internal control over its cash transactions. Facts about its cash position at November 30 were as follows:

The cash books showed a balance of $18,901.62, which included undeposited receipts. A credit of $100 on the bank statement did not appear on the books of the company. The balance according to the statement was $15,550.

When you received the cutoff bank statement on December 10, the following cancelled cheques were enclosed: No. 6500 for $116.25, No. 7126 for $150.00, No. 7815 for $253.25, No. 8621 for $190.71, No. 8623 for $206.80, and No. 8632 for $145.28. The only deposit was in the amount of $3,794.41 on December 7.

The cashier handles all incoming cash and makes the bank deposits personally. He also reconciles the monthly bank statement. His November 30 reconciliation is shown below.

Balance, per books, November 30	$18,901.62	
Add: Outstanding cheques:		
8621	$ 190.71	
8623	206.80	
8632	145.28	442.79
		19,344.41
Less: Undeposited receipts		3,794.41
Balance per bank, November 30		15,550.00
Deduct: Unrecorded credit		100.00
True cash, November 30		$15,450.00

Required:

a. You suspect that the cashier has stolen some money. Prepare a schedule showing your estimate of the loss.
b. How did the cashier attempt to conceal the theft?
c. Based only on the information above, name two specific features of internal control that are missing.
d. If the cashier's October 31 reconciliation is known to be in order and you start your audit on December 5, what specific auditing procedures could you perform to discover the theft?

(© 2000, American Institute of CPAs. All Rights Reserved. Adapted by permission.)

DC 11-6 Receivables Audit Procedures. LO3, 4, 6, 7 The ABC Appliance Company, a manufacturer of small electrical appliances, deals exclusively with 20 distributors situated throughout the country. At December 31 (the balance sheet date), receivables from these distributors aggregated $875,000. Total current assets were $1.3 million.

With respect to receivables, the auditors followed the procedures outlined below in the course of the annual audit of financial statements:

1. Reviewed the system of internal control and found it to be exceptionally good.
2. Reconciled the subsidiary and control accounts at year-end.
3. Aged the accounts—none were overdue.
4. Examined detailed sales and collection transactions for February, July, and November.
5. Received positive confirmations of year-end balances.

Required:

Criticize the completeness or incompleteness of the above program, giving reasons for your recommendations concerning the addition or omission of any procedures.

(© 2000, American Institute of CPAs. All Rights Reserved. Adapted by permission.)

DC 11-7 Rent Revenue. `LO4` You were engaged to conduct an audit of the financial statements of Clayton Realty Corporation for the year ending January 31. The examination of the annual rent reconciliation is a vital portion of the audit. The following rent reconciliation was prepared by the controller of Clayton Realty Corporation and was presented to you. You subjected it to various audit procedures:

CLAYTON REALTY CORPORATION RENT RECONCILIATION FOR THE YEAR ENDED JANUARY 31	
Gross apartment rents (Schedule A)	$1,600,800*
Less vacancies (Schedule B)	20,000*
Net apartment rentals	1,580,300
Less unpaid rents (Schedule C)	7,800*
Total	1,572,500
Add prepaid rent collected (Schedule D)	500*
Total cash collected	$1,573,000

Schedules A, B, C, and D are available to you but have not been illustrated. You have conducted an assessment of the control risk and found it to be low. Cash receipts from rental operations are deposited in a special bank account.

Required:

What substantive audit procedures should you employ during the audit in order to substantiate the validity of each of the dollar amounts marked by an asterisk (*)?

(© 2000, American Institute of CPAs. All Rights Reserved. Adapted by permission.)

DC 11-8 Business Risk, Evidence Analysis, Sales Detail. `LO1, 3, 4` Rosella is the senior in charge of the current-year audit of Harrier Limited, a company that designs and manufactures highly sophisticated machines used to make precision plastic parts and instruments. The machines have a high dollar value (ranging from $500,000 to over $1,000,000), and there is a long lead time between receiving a customer's order and specifications and designing the machine, building it, and testing it. Because of these business factors, sales do not tend to follow a regular pattern, but certain constraints exist that can be used to analyze the reasonability of sales for audit purposes. Customer orders are tracked as the "backlog" file, and sales can be expected to follow the backlog after allowing for design, manufacturing, and testing time. This takes between two and three months, on average. Another factor is the physical limitation of the factory and equipment: there are 12 job stations where machines can be built, so a maximum of 12 machines can be in the work-in-process inventory at any one time.

Harrier's shares are privately held by its founder and president and several outside investors, but it issued bonds to the public several years ago and is subject to debt covenants that require it to maintain a current ratio of 1.5 to 1.0 and a debt to equity ratio of 0.5 to 1.0 at each year-end. In addition, no dividends or management bonuses can be paid out unless the net income before taxes is at least $1,000,000. The draft statements for the current year meet all covenants and show a net income before taxes of $1,300,000.

In reviewing the monthly sales for the current year, Rosella notices several anomalies. First, 15 machines were shipped in December, the last month of the current year, while in December of the prior year only 6 were shipped. The average monthly shipment volume is between 5 and 6 machines. Also, the average gross profit on sales in prior years, and in most months, is approximately 40%. The gross profit on the December sales is 75%. The annual sales were $66 million, with $15 million of this occurring in December. The annual gross profit is $33 million, with $11 million of this occurring in December. While scrutinizing the cash records for the first month of the new year to look for unaccrued liabilities, Rosella notices some large amounts paid for travel expenses for employees and for shipments of "spare parts" to customers. Inquiries of the employees reveal that they are engineers and technicians who were required to spend two or three weeks in various cities where the December machine sales were shipped in order to "work out the bugs" and add some parts to these machines.

Required:

a. What are the main business risks in Harrier Limited? What are the risks of financial statement misstatements that Rosella should be aware of?

b. What types of evidence collection procedures were used, and what assertions do they provide evidence about?

c. Analyze the information Rosella obtained and offer reasonable explanations for the sales anomalies noted. What additional inquiries should Rosella make to form an opinion on the operating results reported in Harrier's draft financial statements? What is your conclusion on the draft sales and gross profits amounts, based on your analysis of the facts given?

d. Harrier's revenue recognition policy is to recognize revenue when the machines are shipped and title passes to customers. This point occurs when the machines are loaded on the truck at Harrier's factory. Given this policy, what adjustment (if any) would be required in Harrier's current financial statements given the conclusion you reached in (c) above?

DC 11-9 Negative Confirmations. `LO1, 4, 6, 7` The auditor of a stock brokerage company, Roller Securities Inc., sends out negative confirmations of account details for a sample of about 50% of the stock brokerage's customers, selected at random. Historically, 2–5% of the confirmations have been returned, and the majority of the discrepancies reported have been understatements. Investigation of the discrepancies rarely indicates an error on Roller Securities Inc.'s part. Usually, they are explained by transactions that are in progress or pending over the year-end, by late payments on the customer's part, or by other mistakes in the customer's own records.

Required:

a. Describe the inherent risks and the internal control risks that exist for customer accounts at Roller Securities Inc.

b. Discuss the advantages and disadvantages of using negative confirmations to provide audit evidence about the assertions in this case. Comment on the persuasiveness of the evidence the negative confirmations provide. Do you think it can be sufficient to support the auditor's opinion?

DC 11-10 Substantive Testing for Sales. `LO1, 4` Parts Inc. sells electrical components to large department stores and also has a few cash sales to electricians. Sales invoices are prepared for all sales. Cash sales are recorded to the cash receipts journal, and cash is deposited to the bank each day. All sales to large stores are credit sales and are handled by sales clerks by telephone or email.

The sales clerk takes the customer's request, checks the authorized customer list for credit limits (if it is a credit sale), prepares the sales invoice, and sends one copy to the inventory control department, which sends the ordered goods to the shipping department. For cash sales, the inventory control clerk brings the items sold to the sales counter and the goods are given to the purchaser at the time of sale. For credit sales, the shipping clerk signs the inventory control copy of the sales invoice and then prepares a shipping invoice. A third copy of the sales invoice is forwarded to the accounting department so that a clerk can enter the sale into the sales journal. The shipping invoices are maintained in the shipping department in case a shipment needs to be checked. All goods are shipped FOB shipping point.

Required:

a. Design two audit procedures, in addition to sample selection, that will provide evidence of the occurrence/existence of sales. Identify the procedure (trace, compare, vouch, and so on) and the documents you are using, and explain why these procedures will show whether recorded sales are valid.

b. Design two audit procedures that will provide evidence of the completeness of sales. Identify the procedure (trace, compare, vouch, and so on) and the documents you are using, and explain why these procedures will show whether recorded sales are complete.

(Adapted from External Auditing (AU1), June 2011, with permission of Chartered Professional Accountants of Canada, Toronto, Canada. Any changes to the original material are the sole responsibility of the author (and/or publisher) and have not been reviewed or endorsed by the Chartered Professional Accountants of Canada.)

DC 11-11 Municipal Government, Employee Theft. `LO2, 3, 4` This case is modelled on the Application Case in the chapter.

Case Description: In the audit of a municipal government, the auditors discovered that receivables for property taxes were overstated because the tax assessor stole some taxpayers' payments. J. R. Shelstad had been the tax assessor-collector for 15 years in the Ridge Municipal District, a large metropolitan area. Known as a "good personnel manager," Shelstad pocketed 100–150 counter payments each year, in amounts of $500–$2,500, stealing about $200,000 a year for a total of approximately $2.5 million. The district had assessed about $800–$900 million per year in property tax revenues, so the annual theft was less than 1%. Nevertheless, the taxpayers got mad.

In Shelstad's assessor-collector office, staff processed tax notices on a computer system and generated 180,000 tax notices each October. A summary listing report was printed and used to check "paid" when payments were received. Payments were processed by computer, and a master file of accounts receivable records (tax assessments, payments) was kept on the computer hard drive.

Shelstad often took over the front desk at lunchtime so the teller staff could enjoy lunch together. During these times, Shelstad took tax payments over the counter, gave the taxpayers a counter receipt, and pocketed some of the money, which was never entered in the computer system.

Shelstad eventually resigned when the district's assessor-collector office was eliminated upon the creation of a new region-wide tax agency.

Audit Trail: The computer records showed balances due from many taxpayers who had actually paid their taxes. The book of printed notices was not marked "paid" for many taxpayers who had received counter receipts. These records and the daily cash receipts reports (cash receipts journal) were available at the time the independent auditors performed the most recent annual audit in April. To keep his fraud going and prevent auditors from detecting it, Shelstad persuaded the auditors that the true "receivables" were the delinquencies turned over to the region's legal counsel. Their confirmation sample and other work were based on this population. Thus, confirmations were not sent to fictitious balances that Shelstad knew had been paid. When Shelstad resigned in August, a power surge permanently destroyed the hard drive where the receivables file was stored, and the cash receipts journals could not be found. When the new regional agency managers took over the tax assessment, they noticed that the total of delinquent taxes disclosed in the audited financial statements was much larger than the total turned over to the region's legal counsel for collection and foreclosure.

AUDIT APPROACH ANALYSIS

Audit Objective: The auditors' objective is to obtain evidence determining if the receivables for taxes (delinquent taxes) represent genuine claims collectible from the taxpayers.

Controls Relevant to the Municipal Tax Revenue Process: The municipal system for establishing the initial amounts of taxes receivable was fine. Professional staff appraisers and the independent appraisal review board established the tax base for each property, and the municipal council set the price (tax rate). The computer system authorization for billing was validated on these two inputs.

The cash receipts system was well designed, calling for preparation of a daily cash receipts report (cash receipts journal that served as a source input for computer entry). This report was always reviewed by the "boss," Shelstad.

Unfortunately, Shelstad had the opportunity and power to override the controls and become both cash handler and supervisor. He made the decisions about sending delinquent taxes to the region's legal counsel for collection, but the ones he knew to have been paid but stolen were withheld.

Required:

Describe in detail the audit procedures you would perform in this case. Consider tests of control and substantive tests such as dual-purpose tests of transactions and/or tests of details of balance. In particular, identify the information that could have been obtained from confirmations directed to the real population of delinquent accounts receivable (i.e., including the ones that had been stolen by Shelstad). Which tests do you consider likely to detect Shelstad's theft? Why?

DC 11-12 Audit of Revenue with Accounting for Different Components. `LO1, 3, 4` It is Monday, September 13, 20X1. You, a PA, work at Fife & Richardson LLP, a public accounting firm. Ken Simpson, one of the partners, approaches you mid-morning regarding Brennan & Sons Limited (BSL), a private company client for which you performed the August 31, 20X0, year-end audit.

"It seems there have been substantial changes at BSL this year," Ken explains. "I'm going there tomorrow, and since you will be on the audit again this year, it would be beneficial for you to come. I took the liberty of retrieving information from last year's files so you can refresh your memory about this client (Exhibit DC 11-12–1)."

EXHIBIT DC 11-12–1

Excerpt from Permanent File

Date of incorporation:	October 27, 1982	
Year-end:	August 31	
Ownership:	50 common shares	Harold Thomas
	50 common shares	Kyle Stanton

The next day, you and Ken meet with Jack Wright, the accounting manager at BSL. Jack gives you the internally prepared financial statements (Exhibits DC 11-12–2 and DC 11-12–3). To your surprise, there are also financial statements for two new companies. Jack quickly explains that BSL incorporated two subsidiaries in January 20X1, each with the same year-end as BSL:

Brennan Transport Ltd. (Transport)—100% owned by BSL

Brennan Fuel Tank Installations Inc. (Tanks)—75% owned by BSL

EXHIBIT DC 11-12–2

Internal Financial Statements—Balance Sheets

	BRENNAN & SONS LIMITED BALANCE SHEET AS AT AUGUST 31 (IN THOUSANDS OF DOLLARS)			
	20X0	**20X1**		
	(audited)	(unaudited)		
	BSL	BSL	Transport	Tanks
Assets				
Cash	$ 467	$ 75	$ 67	$ 82
Accounts receivable	970	603	119	–
Inventory	10	500	–	15
	1,447	1,178	186	97
Note receivable	–	431 (note 1)	–	–
Property, plant, & equipment	4,768	13,400	400	80
Investment in subsidiaries	–	2	–	–
Intangible asset	–	–	–	20 (note 2)
	$6,215	$15,011	$586	$197
Liabilities				
Accounts payable	$ 315	$ 813	$128	$166
Note payable	–	–	431 (note 1)	–
Mortgage payable	100	6,500	–	–
	415	7,313	559	166
Shareholders' Equity				
Common stock	1	1	1	1 (note 3)
Retained earnings	5,799	7,697	26	30
	5,800	7,698	27	31
	$6,215	$15,011	$586	$197

Notes:

1. Note receivable/payable for sale of trucks and trailers from BSL to Transport, interest at 8%

2. Training costs for Sean Piper, owner/installer

3. Includes Sean's equity interest

Internal Financial Statements—Income Statements

BRENNAN & SONS LIMITED
INCOME STATEMENT
FOR THE YEAR ENDED AUGUST 31
(IN THOUSANDS OF DOLLARS)

	20X0	20X1		
	(audited) BSL (12 months)	(unaudited) BSL (12 months)	Transport (8 months)	Tanks (8 months)
Revenue				
Scrap metal	$11,000	$10,003	$ –	$ –
Transportation services	900	300 (note 4)	700 (note 4)	–
Fuel tank installations	–	–	–	320
	11,900	10,303	700	320
Cost of sales				
Scrap metal	1,600	1,440	–	–
Transportation services	700	340	550	–
Fuel tank installations	–	–	–	220
Gross margin	9,600	8,523	150	100
General & administration (note 5)	8,491	7,930	90	50
Interest expense	9	120	16	–
Income before other income	1,100	473	44	50
Other income				
Gain on sale of equipment	–	84	–	–
Gain on sale of property	–	2,500	–	–
Interest income	–	16	–	–
Property rental	–	90 (note 6)	–	–
Income before income tax	1,100	3,163	44	50
Income tax	440	1,265	18	20
Net income	$ 660	$ 1,898	$ 26	$ 30

Notes:

4. Transport took over transportation services in January

5. 20X1 General & administration includes amortization

6. $10,000 per month from Transport and $5,000 per month from Tanks for six months

You diligently take notes during the meeting (Exhibit DC 11-12–4). Jack states that BSL will prepare consolidated financial statements for audit based on Canadian GAAP to satisfy the bank's request.

Ken asks that you work on the overall planning for these engagements. As part of your planning, he asks you to discuss the new accounting issues that arise as a result of the changes during the year, and to evaluate their implications for the engagements.

Notes from Your Meeting with Jack Wright

BSL continues to operate the scrap metal business. BSL's management thinks the price of metal is going to go up in the near future and has therefore started stockpiling for the first time. Unfortunately, BSL does not really have an inventory tracking system in place. If, in fact, it turns out that stockpiling is a good way for BSL to make money, it will install a better system. The company did its best to log each of the amounts going into the stockpile as it was added, knowing that an amount for its year-end inventory balance would need to be determined. BSL also used a known engineering formula to come up with an estimate for year-end inventory and tried to measure the different piles of metal as a way of counting what was on hand at August 31, 20X1. The different methods came up with different amounts, so management went with the initial amount based on the log. Jack noted that we would have had a good laugh at the different ways they tried to measure the piles if we'd been there to see it.

As soon as it was incorporated on January 1, 20X1, Transport took over BSL's transportation operations. Transport provides transportation services to BSL and external customers, the same as BSL did. BSL sold the trucks to Transport in late January at fair market value. However, Transport didn't have the funds to buy the equipment, so BSL issued a note receivable at what Jack believed to be the market interest rate.

Tanks installs and maintains pre-engineered, above-ground fuel storage tank systems, a new line of business for BSL. Sean Piper, a good friend of one of BSL's owners, approached BSL last fall with the idea. Sean was willing to take the necessary training to become a certified fuel tank installer, and he wanted 50% ownership in Tanks. The owners of BSL agreed it was a great opportunity but wanted more control. The parties settled on Sean's receiving 25% ownership of Tanks.

As part of the agreement, BSL was required to provide a guarantee pertaining to Tanks' licensing application to the environmental authority, since Tanks was a newly formed corporation. Although other vendors sell the same tanks and installation services separately, Tanks only sells the tank combined with installation and service. The tank is marked up by 20% on the price paid and is sold including installation and a five-year maintenance package for a total of $40,000. One hundred percent of the revenue is recognized when the sales agreement is signed by the customer. The tank is then delivered and installed at the customer's site within two to three weeks of signing. The fuel tanks need to be pressure-tested every year, and the measurement gauge needs to be checked. Tanks will perform the maintenance services for customers for the first five years. Thereafter, Tanks will offer to continue to perform the maintenance for a contract price of $5,000 a year.

Nature of the Business: BSL operates as a scrap metal dealer and processor. It buys used scrap metal from individuals and businesses and then bundles the different metals and sells them in larger quantities at a higher price to bigger recycling businesses. BSL's revenue fluctuates significantly because of the volatility in the market rates for steel and non-ferrous metals. To help control costs, BSL uses its own trucks and trailers to do the pickups. BSL earns additional revenue by providing transportation services to other businesses and by renting out the trucks during slower periods.

As part of BSL's overall strategy, the owners admit a willingness to take risks. They monitor the marketplace and are always on the lookout for new business opportunities. They even found a piece of land on the outskirts of the city that they thought would be great for a dump they considered operating themselves. They decided not to make an offer, but may reconsider in 20X1.

For BSL's 20X0 audit, materiality was set at $70,000.

Required:

Prepare a memo to the audit engagement partner discussing the planning for the BSL audit engagement. Your memo should discuss planning considerations for the audit of the consolidated financial statements, the risk assessments, and materiality decisions for the overall audit strategy. As part of your planning, discuss the new revenue accounting issues that arise as a result of the changes during the year and evaluate their implications for the engagement. [Assume that BSL will use Accounting Standards for Private Enterprises (ASPE) as its financial reporting framework. Given the timing of the case, ASPE can be adopted, and it will meet the bank's requirement for Canadian GAAP.]

(Source: CPA Canada 2010 Uniform Final Exam, adapted.)

DC 11-13 Special Confirmation Procedures for Bill-and-Hold Transactions. LO6 Specialties Papers Inc. (SPI) makes a unique type of paper that is used in specialized biohazard cleanup operations. Since customers cannot predict when they will need large supplies of the paper, they typically purchase a quantity of paper and ask SPI to hold it in its warehouse until they order it to be delivered. Kelly is auditing the revenues of SPI for the first time and notices a number of sales classified as bill and hold. She consults with more-senior auditors in her firm and learns that while bill-and-hold sales transactions are not necessarily a GAAP violation when customers have actually requested this arrangement, they have often been associated with financial fraud and should be investigated. It is the substance rather than the form of the transaction that is important. Kelly realizes she needs to do some GAAP research to get up to speed on this accounting issue. She learns that according to IAS 18, *Revenue,* the following conditions should be met for revenue recognition to be appropriate, including for any bill-and-hold sales arrangements:

(14) Revenue from the sale of goods shall be recognized when all the following conditions have been satisfied:
   (a) the entity has transferred to the buyer the significant risks and rewards of ownership of the goods;
   (b) the entity retains neither continuing managerial involvement to the degree usually associated with ownership nor effective control over the goods sold;
   (c) the amount of revenue can be measured reliably;
   (d) it is probable that the economic benefits associated with the transaction will flow to the entity; and
   (e) the costs incurred or to be incurred in respect of the transaction can be measured reliably.

(15) The assessment of when an entity has transferred the significant risks and rewards of ownership to the buyer requires an examination of the circumstances of the transaction. In most cases, the transfer of the risks and rewards of ownership coincides with the transfer of the legal title or the passing of possession to the buyer. This is the case for most retail sales.

(16) If the entity retains significant risks of ownership, the transaction is not a sale and revenue is not recognized.

Kelly also learns from some auditing research that a special positive confirmation letter is often used for possibly inappropriate bill-and-hold transactions. An example of this confirmation is illustrated in Exhibit DC 11-13.

Required:

a. Discuss how the issues Kelly is addressing in the SPI audit illustrate that auditors must have a good understanding of the auditee, its business, and its products in order to identify the warning signs of revenue recognition misstatements and fraud.

b. Discuss the nature of the special bill-and-hold confirmation, and what evidence it will provide (i.e., is it an example of a confirmation request to verify the contractual substance of a sales transaction from the customer's point of view?).

EXHIBIT DC 11-13

Confirmation Request for a Bill-and-Hold Transaction

[Client Letterhead]

[Date]

[Name and address of customer employee with sufficient authority to commit customer]

Dear [Name]:

Our auditors [public accounting firm name and address] are auditing our financial statements at [balance sheet date]. Please compare the following information with your records and report directly to our auditors whether that information is correct:

We sold you [product description] on [date] for [total sales price] under your purchase order [date and number].

[Product description] has been sold to you on our normal payment terms as described in our invoice [number and date], and those terms have not been modified. There are no written or oral amendments to the terms specified in the purchase order.

At your request we are holding [product description] at your risk on our premises, and title has passed to you.

You requested us to hold [product description] for you because [description of business reason for delayed shipment].

There are no written or oral amendments to the terms specified in the purchase order.

You are obligated to pay us [total sales price] by [payment due date].

Please use the enclosed pre-addressed, postage-paid reply envelope. Because this response is needed for our auditors to complete their audit, we would appreciate a prompt response.

Very truly yours,

[Signature and title of authorized client representative]

If the above information is correct, please confirm. If your understanding of anything described above differs in any respect, please explain.

Date: _____

Signed: _____

Source: © 2000, American Institute of CPAs. All Rights Reserved. Adapted by permission.

Internal Control Questionnaires for the Revenues, Receivables, and Receipts Process

LO8 Describe the internal control questionnaires used in audit practice.

Exhibit 11A–1 provides an example of the type of form that could be used to guide the auditor's assessment of the effectiveness of application controls in the two main classes of transactions and the main account balance in the revenues, receivables, and receipts process. Note that in practice, forms like this can provide only a general starting point, and the actual audit work must always be tailored to the specifics of each engagement.

Exhibit 11A–2 provides a few examples of the types of controls one expects to find in a typical system, such as the one illustrated in Exhibit 11–1 of the chapter.

EXHIBIT 11A–1

Internal Control Questionnaires for the Revenues, Receivables, and Receipts Process

INTERNAL CONTROL QUESTIONNAIRE FOR REVENUES, RECEIVABLES, AND RECEIPTS PROCESS AUDITEE: _____ F/S PERIOD: _____	Auditor Responses	Audit File References
OVERALL COMPANY-LEVEL CONTROL AND GENERAL CONTROL ACTIVITIES ASSESSMENT		

(Refer to responses recorded for questions in Exhibit 9A–1 in Appendix 9A)
Are company-level and general control activities adequate as they apply to the revenues, receivables, and receipts components of the information system?
 	
• Consider the impact of any weakness in company-level and general control activities on the planned audit approach and procedures.
• Assess the potential for weaknesses to result in a material misstatement of the financial information generated from this accounting cycle. If a significant risk of misstatement is assessed, perform procedures to determine the extent of any misstatement.
 	
Consider the adequacy of the following general controls in place in the revenues, receivables, and receipts process to
 	
  – Prevent unauthorized access or changes to programs and data
  – Ensure the security and privacy of data
  – Control and maintain key systems
  – Protect assets susceptible to misappropriation
  – Ensure completeness, accuracy, and authorization of data and processing
  – Ensure that adequate management trails exist
		(continued)

EXHIBIT 11A–1

Internal Control Questionnaires for the Revenues, Receivables, and Receipts Process   (*continued*)

	Auditor Responses	Audit File References
APPLICATION CONTROL ASSESSMENTS		
CASH RECEIPTS TRANSACTIONS APPLICATION CONTROLS		
Environment and General Controls Relevant to This Application		
1. Are receipts deposited daily, intact, and without delay?		
2. Does someone other than the cashier or accounts receivable bookkeeper take the deposits to the bank?		
3. Are the duties of the cashier entirely separate from recordkeeping for notes and accounts receivable? from general ledger recordkeeping? Is the cashier denied access to receivables records or monthly statements?		
4. Does someone reconcile the accounts receivable subsidiary to the control account regularly (to determine whether all entries were made to customers' accounts)?		
5. Are employees with access to cash covered by fidelity insurance against embezzlement losses (also called fidelity bonding of employees)?		
Application Control Assessment		
Validity objective:		
6. Is a bank reconciliation performed monthly by someone who does not have cash custody or recordkeeping responsibility?		
7. Are the cash receipts journal entries compared with the remittance lists and deposit slips regularly?		
Completeness objective:		
8. Does the person who opens the mail make a list of cash received (a remittance list)?		
9. Are currency receipts controlled by mechanical devices? Are machine totals checked by the internal auditor?		
10. Are prenumbered sales invoice or receipt books used? Is the numerical sequence checked for missing documents?		
Authorization objective:		
11. Does a responsible person approve discounts taken by customers on their payments on account?		
Accuracy objective:		
12. Is a regular (e.g., monthly) bank reconciliation performed by the internal auditor or someone other than the employee making the deposits?		
13. Is the remittance list compared with the deposit by someone other than the cashier?		
Classification objective:		
14. Does the accounting manual contain instructions for classifying cash receipts credits?		
Proper period objective:		
15. Does the accounting manual contain instructions for dating cash receipts entries the same day as the date of receipt?		
SALES TRANSACTIONS APPLICATION CONTROLS		
Environment and General Controls Evaluation Relevant to This Application		
1. Is the credit department independent of the marketing department?		
2. Are non-routine sales controlled by the same procedures described below (e.g., sales to employees, cash-on-delivery (COD) sales, disposals of property, cash sales, and scrap sales)?		
3. Are summary journal entries approved before posting?		
Application Control Assessment		
Consider whether the auditee has appropriate policies and procedures in place to meet the following control objectives:		
Validity objective:		
4. Is access to the sales invoicing process restricted to appropriate personnel?		
5. Are prenumbered bills of lading or other shipping documents produced and completed in the shipping department?		(*continued*)

Internal Control Questionnaires for the Revenues, Receivables, and Receipts Process *(continued)*

	Auditor Responses	Audit File References
Completeness objective:		
6. Are sales invoices prenumbered?		
7. Is the sequence checked for missing invoices?		
8. Is the shipping document numerical sequence checked for missing bill of lading numbers?		
Authorization objective:		
9. Are all credit sales approved by the credit department prior to shipment?		
10. Are sales prices and terms based on approved pricing lists and credit policies?		
11. Are returned sales credits and other credits supported by documentation as to receipt, condition, and quantity, and approved by a responsible officer?		
Accuracy objective:		
12. Are shipped quantities compared with invoice quantities?		
13. Are sales invoices checked for error in quantities, prices, extensions and totals, and freight allowances, and against customers' orders?		
14. Is there an overall check on arithmetic accuracy of period sales data by a statistical or product-line analysis?		
15. Are periodic sales data reported directly to general ledger accounting independent of accounts receivable accounting?		
Classification objective:		
16. Does the accounting manual contain instructions for classifying sales, and are employees following these instructions?		
Proper period objective:		
17. Does the accounting manual contain instructions to date sales invoices on the shipment date, and are employees following these instructions?		
ACCOUNTS RECEIVABLE BALANCE APPLICATION CONTROLS		
Environment and General Controls Relevant to This Application		
1. Are customers' subsidiary records maintained by someone who has no access to cash?		
2. Is the cashier denied access to the customers' records and monthly statements?		
3. Does someone regularly reconcile the accounts receivable subsidiary to the control account?		
4. Are delinquent accounts listed periodically for review by someone other than the credit manager?		
5. Are written-off accounts kept in a memo ledger or credit report file for periodic access?		
6. Is the credit department separated from the sales department?		
7. Are notes receivable in the custody of someone other than the cashier or accounts receivable recordkeeper?		
8. Is custody of negotiable collateral in the hands of someone not responsible for handling cash or keeping records?		
Application Control Assessment		
Consider whether the auditee has appropriate policies and procedures in place to meet the following control objectives:		
Validity objective:		
9. Are customers' statements sent to them regularly (e.g., monthly) by the accounts receivable department?		
10. Are direct confirmations of accounts and notes obtained periodically by the internal auditor?		
11. Are differences reported by customers routed to someone outside the accounts receivable department for investigation?		
12. Are returned goods checked against receiving reports?		
Completeness objective:		
(Refer to completeness questions in the sales and cash receipts questionnaires.)		
13. Are credit memo documents prenumbered and the sequence checked for missing documents?		
		(continued)

EXHIBIT 11A–1

Internal Control Questionnaires for the Revenues, Receivables, and Receipts Process *(continued)*

Authorization objective: 14. Is customer credit approved before orders are shipped? 15. Are write-offs, returns, and discounts allowed after the discount date subject to approval by a responsible officer? 16. Are large loans or advances to related parties approved by the directors? *Accuracy objective:* 17. Do the internal auditors periodically confirm customer accounts to determine accuracy? *Classification objective:* 18. Are receivables from officers, directors, and affiliates identified separately in the accounts receivable records? *Proper period objective:* (Refer to proper period objective questions in the sales and cash receipts questionnaires.)		
Auditor's conclusion on the effectiveness of application controls in the revenues, receivables, and receipts process: _____ _____	Prepared by ____ ____	Date ____

EXHIBIT 11A–2

Examples of Controls in a Revenues, Receivables, and Receipts Process, Relating to Exhibit 11–1

- Each system terminal allows access only to designated functions. For example, the terminal at the shipping dock cannot be used to enter initial sales information or to access the payroll database.
- An identification number and a password (issued on an individual-person basis) are required to enter the sales, and for each subsequent command entered to process the transaction. Unauthorized entry attempts are logged and immediately investigated. Further, certain passwords have "read-only" (cannot change any data) authorization. For example, the credit manager can determine the outstanding balance of any account or view online "reports" summarizing overdue accounts receivable but cannot enter credit memos to change the balances.
- All input information is immediately logged to provide restart processing should any terminal become inoperative during the processing.
- A transaction code calls up on the terminals a full-screen "form" that appears to the operator in the same format as the original paper documents. Each clerk must enter the information correctly or the computer will not accept the transaction. This is called **online input validation** and utilizes validation checks such as missing data, check digit, and limit tests.
- All documents prepared by the computer are sequentially numbered, and the number is stored as part of the sales record in the accounts receivable database.
- A daily search of the pending order database is made by the computer system, and sales orders outstanding more than seven days are listed on a report accessible to marketing management.

online input validation:

inputting information correctly or the computer will not accept the transaction; uses validation checks such as missing data, check digit, and limit tests

System Documentation Examples for the Revenues, Receivables, and Receipts Process

LO9 Describe the accounting control system documentation used in audit practice.

This appendix provides examples of systems documentation prepared using flowchart and process table diagram formats. These formats may be use in lieu of, or in addition to, narrative descriptions. Exhibit 11B–1 diagrams an IT-based system for processing customer sales orders and accounts

Sales and Accounts Receivable Processing Flowchart Example: Information Technology–Based System

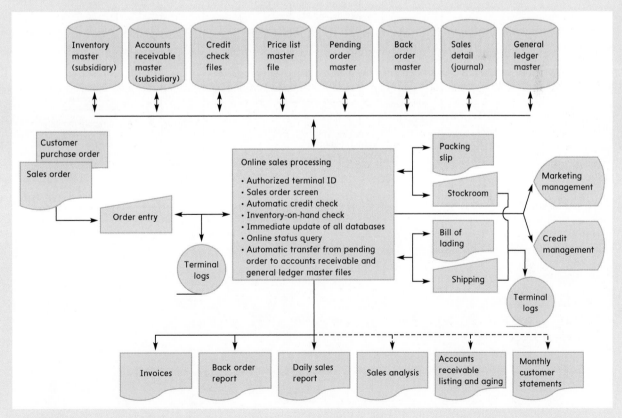

receivable. Exhibit 11B–2 show a manual system of processing cash receipts, and Exhibit 11B–3 shows the same system using an input/process/output table as the documentation format. The narrative descriptions of these systems in the chapter correspond to the activities and records shown in these diagrams.

EXHIBIT 11B–2

Cash Receipts Processing Flowchart Example: Manual System

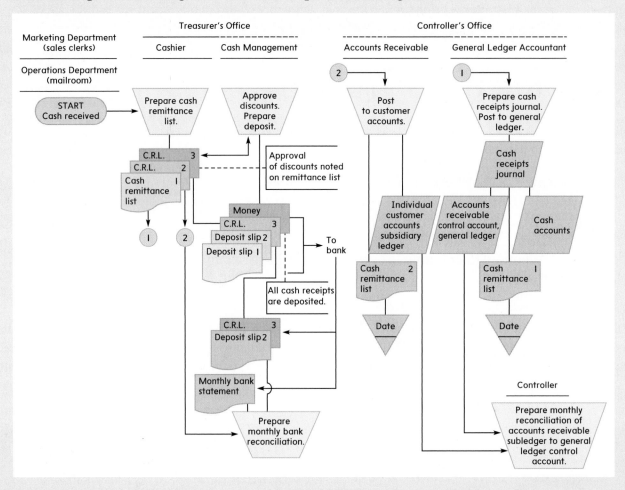

EXHIBIT 11B–3

Cash Receipts Processing Input/Process/Output Table Example: Manual System

INPUT	ACTIVITY	PERFORMED BY	FREQUENCY	OUTPUT
Customer payment collected	List cash receipts by customer and invoice number.	Cashier	Daily	Cash remittance list
Cash remittance list	Approve any discounts taken.	Cash management	Daily	Approved cash remittance list [3 copies]
Approved cash remittance list [1]	Prepare deposit slip for bank.	Cashier	Daily	Deposit slip
Bank deposit slip	Take cash and deposit slip to bank.	Cash management	Daily	Bank-stamped deposit slip
Approved cash remittance list [2]	Post to customer accounts.	Accounts receivable clerk	Daily	Accounts receivable subledger update
Approved cash remittance list [3]	Post to cash receipts journal.	General ledger accountant	Daily	Accounts receivable subledger update
Accounts receivable subledger update	Post total cash receipts to general ledger accounts receivable control account.	General ledger accountant	Daily	General ledger update
Accounts receivable reconciliation	Agree total accounts receivable subledger balance to balance of accounts receivable control account in general ledger.	Controller	Monthly	Reconciliation summary with documented support for all reconciling items
Bank reconciliation	Reconcile cash balance per general ledger to balance per bank statement.	Cash management	Monthly	Reconciliation summary with documented support for all reconciling items

APPENDIX 11C Example of an Audit Engagement File Index (on Connect)

ENDNOTES

1   The only differences between CASs and ISAs are a small number of amendments that are necessary to reflect particular Canadian laws and regulations. These amendments do not affect how an auditor performs a financial statement audit.

2   This picture is not a flowchart. Flowcharts are illustrated in Appendix 11B.

3   CAS 505.

4   B. Fox, "Preventing confirmation fraud," *The Auditor's Report*, Spring 2004, p. 15, www2.aaahq.org/audit/Pubs/ Audrep/04spring/Spring2004.pdf.

CHAPTER 12

The Purchases, Payables, and Payments Process

This chapter summarizes the purchases, payables, and payments business process, which involves the purchase of goods (inventory); services (expenses); and property, plant, and equipment (PPE) (fixed assets), and the expenditure of cash (cash payments) to pay for purchases, as well as the related audit procedures. It then describes the control considerations, typical control tests, and substantive audit programs used in auditing the purchases, payables, and payments business process. The chapter provides special notes on inventory observation, accounts payable completeness, and auditing PPE and intangible assets. The Application Case at the end of the chapter demonstrates the performance of audit procedures in situations where errors or frauds might be discovered in the purchases, payables, and payments process.

LEARNING OBJECTIVES

After completing this chapter, you will be able to do the following:

LO1 Describe the purchases, payables, and payments process, including typical risks, transactions, account balances, source documents, and controls.

LO2 Describe the auditor's control risk assessment and control tests for auditing control over the purchase of inventory, services, and fixed assets, and for the payment of cash.

LO3 Describe the typical substantive procedures used to respond to the assessed risk of material misstatement in the main account balance and transactions in the purchases, payables, and payments process.

LO4 Identify audit considerations for observing the physical inventory count.

LO5 Explain the main auditing procedures used for property, plant, and equipment and intangible assets.

LO6 Explain the importance of the completeness assertion for auditing the accounts payable liabilities, and the procedures used to search for unrecorded liabilities.

LO7 (Appendix 12A) Describe internal control questionnaires used in audit practice for the purchases, payables, and payments process.

CHAPTER APPENDIX

APPENDIX 12A Internal Control Questionnaires for the Purchases, Payables, and Payments Process

EcoPak Inc.

EcoPak will perform a physical count of their inventory on December 31 to coincide with their year-end date. The count will take from 4 p.m. until approximately 11 p.m. This is a crucial, time-sensitive opportunity to collect audit evidence, so Donna takes the following steps to make sure it is done well. First, she discusses the inventory with various people at EcoPak to identify inventory risk factors and internal controls, including cutoff procedures. Next, she calls Nina and obtains EcoPak's inventory count instructions and its procedures for tying the count information into the accounting records to prepare the financial statements. She then develops a plan for M&G to attend the company's inventory count to observe the execution of the count, and to perform the necessary audit procedures, such as performing test counts. She also plans follow-up procedures that will allow the audit team to tie the count information into the final inventory listing that supports the valuation in the financial statements, to allow them to reach a conclusion on whether it is fairly presented. Since it is M&G's first year auditing EcoPak, they assessed the inherent risks in inventory as high and decided to go with a totally substantive approach rather than testing controls. They will reconsider this approach for next year's audit, based on their greater experience with the company's inventory processes.

Donna notes some other key information about the count. The main raw materials items to count are processed biomass fibre, binding solutions, coatings, and ink. These will all be measured by volume, based on engineering specifications. There will also be a stock of finished products prepared for shipments in early January to fill outstanding orders. There are also quantities of a variety of products on hand for samples, prototypes, or any urgent unplanned orders that might arise.

Donna was happy to hear that EcoPak plans to complete all production and shut down the production lines on December 28 to allow for quarterly maintenance and cleaning of the equipment. This will also make the count easier, as there will be no work in process (WIP) or movements of raw materials and finished goods. Experienced production workers will perform the count under Mike's supervision. During the count, the workers will also count the supplies and moulds used in the production process, which are carried as separate inventory categories, and the plant and equipment, which are capitalized. Once the count is finished, Nina will review the count information for completeness and any outstanding issues that need to be addressed before the workers leave for the holidays. The plant and offices will be closed until January 3.

Donna has decided that Caleb will attend the EcoPak count to perform the required audit procedures. Even though he has never observed a count before, Donna feels confident that he understands what the audit team needs to achieve by observing the physical inventory and by doing the audit test counts and other procedures at EcoPak's year-end. So, she has no hesitation in assigning Caleb to do the count on his own.

Donna also asks Caleb to get information for cutoff testing while he is at the count: last cheques issued and last deposits for cash, last shipments for sales and accounts receivable, and last inventory receipts for the inventory and payables. And since this is a new audit, Caleb should also ask the factory manager to show him the various machines and equipment items that are listed in the plant equipment schedule.

Caleb is a bit nervous about attending the count on his own, but he realizes that the most important objective is for a person independent of EcoPak to make observations, perform test counts, and inspect the assets and related documents. He has seen EcoPak's operations and had a tour of the factory during their interim visit, so he feels he has a good knowledge of what he needs to do at the count. "As long as I keep good notes of everything and follow the program, it should be fine," he thinks to himself. Also, Donna has arranged to be available by cell phone in case he has any questions. Donna will not be going to the EcoPak count because she has been assigned to an inventory observation at another client, Jetstream Inc., a large jet turbine manufacturer, where she will need to supervise two assistants. Jetstream is a much more complex audit due to the high value and complicated technical design of its inventory, a large balance of WIP in various stages of completion, and very complex accounting processes. Also, Jetstream is a public company with some financial challenges, so that makes the engagement a lot riskier than EcoPak. Caleb realizes Donna will have a lot of challenges of her own on December 31! And, as it turns out, Caleb is in for quite a complex learning experience himself—he gets quite a surprise just as he is finishing up his day at the count.

When Caleb arrives at the count, the workers are receiving their instructions from Nina, and during the afternoon he observes them following these quite closely. He is provided with the schedules of plant equipment as well as copies of the count sheets the workers are now completing for the raw material, finished goods, and supplies counts. Caleb decides to do the cutoff work first and then turn to the test counts. While he is out on the loading dock noting the last receiving reports numbers for the last materials received, he notes a shipment of 100 crates of ink that the shipper/receiver, Karl, had signed for at 3:55 p.m. The crates were tagged and included in the count, but there was no receiving report issued for them. Caleb goes and finds Karl, who explains that this order arrived just as he was going off to help with the count, so he was going to leave off entering it until after the holiday. Caleb points out that since the inventory is physically on hand, it should be counted and the paperwork showing that it was received should be processed into the accounts payable system. "Yes, I see your point. We have counted and tagged these crates to include them in our count, so I guess we need to set up the amount payable, too." Karl logs into the system and issues the appropriate document, Receiving Report #24-0909, and Caleb records this as the last receipt of inventory. "The gates are locked now, so even if another truck arrives they won't be able to drop anything off. This one really will be the last receipt for this year!" Karl tells Caleb.

As he is getting set to leave the dock, Caleb notices a small shipment of finished product sitting on the loading dock with shipping document #14-1546, dated December 30, for pickup by Kingston Transport attached. When he asks Karl about it, Karl takes a look at the document and says, "Looks like the truck didn't make it in to pick this up last night. Now the gates are closed, so that means this will the first shipment of next year—I'd better make sure accounting knows." So Caleb notes that #14-1545 was the last shipment, and #14-1546 should be the first of next year.

At this point, Mike comes looking for Caleb to tell him the production engineer is about to finish measuring the main vats of processing fibres. "Since that's most of our inventory, I thought it was something you would want to observe for sure!" Caleb heads down to the storage vats area with Mike. On the way, he notices an unlocked room full of spare moulds with three workers busy counting them. Mike explains, "The moulds are really expensive and if one breaks it shuts down the line until we can replace it. So, we keep a good supply of spares in the locked storage. You will probably want to take some tests in there too, after we finish in the vat room. Quite a few dollars are tied up in there."

The Essentials of Auditing a Business's Purchases, Payables, and Payments Process

Businesses have to spend money to make money, and keeping track of payments to various suppliers is a critical management process. Typically there will be a variety of suppliers to pay, and many different types of assets and expenses to pay for. The accounting process for purchasing transactions also involves processing the related accounts payable balance and cash payment transactions (also called "cash disbursements"). The two main journal entries in this process are as follows:

Dr Various asset or expense accounts	Dr Accounts Payable
Cr Accounts Payable	Cr Cash

Management's main control objectives for the purchases, payables, and payments process relate to the validity, accuracy, and authorization of purchases and cash payments. Because the risk of employee fraud involving misappropriation of cash or other company assets is a major concern, strong controls are needed to ensure the company's expenditures are appropriate. Classification is also an important control objective, since there are usually many different reasons to spend money, and some are for expenses with no future benefit, but others that have future benefits need to be classified as assets. Note that purchases of PPE can involve investments of large amounts of money and thus require a separate approval process from the highest level of governance. This may be part of the finance and investment process (discussed in Chapter 14) in many organizations. In this text, we will cover the purchase of PPE as part of the purchasing process here in Chapter 12, because many of the controls and procedures related to expenditures are similar, and junior audit team members are often involved in examining the accounting for PPE.

Auditors' concern is with management's controls over the validity, completeness, authorization, and proper period cutoff for purchasing and payment transactions, to ensure that financial statements include all the liabilities that exist at year-end, and that expenses and assets are correctly classified. Auditor control testing in the purchasing process is usually required, since there tends to be a high volume of transactions affecting various accounts. Controls over cash payment transactions are often tested to ensure only authorized and valid cash payments can be made, since this can provide assurance that control risk is lowered, affecting many other accounts in the audit. The main control tests will trace records of goods and services received (e.g., purchase orders, bills of lading, supplier invoices, new assets) to authorization and recording of payables and payments in the general ledger, and test proper recording of cutoff at period end. The results of the auditor's control testing will affect the nature of further substantive audit work to be performed, as well as the sample sizes and timing of further procedures.

Substantive audit procedures that are commonly used in the purchases, payables, and payments process include reconciliation of bank account balances, analysis of accrual and expense accounts for reasonability, vouching of major expenses and asset purchases (inventory, PPE, and intangible assets) to supporting documents, and examining payments made just after year-end to ensure any related to the current period were accrued.

The audit of the purchases, payables, and payments process focuses on the risk of material misstatement related to the *completeness* assertion, since understatements of liabilities and expenses hide poor financial performance and skew debt-related ratios that creditors monitor to assess the safety of their loans. Misstatements caused by improper capitalization of expenses are also a concern as they result in overstatements of assets and income, which can affect important user decisions and evaluations.

Review Checkpoints

12-1   What are the main classes of transactions and related account balances for the purchases process?

12-2   What are management's main control objectives related to the purchases process? Why?

12-3   What are an auditor's main concerns related to purchasing and payment transactions? Why?

12-4   Why do auditors frequently choose to test controls in the purchases, payables, and payments process?

12-5   What substantive audit procedures are often performed for purchases, payables, and cash payments?

12-6   How do the results of the auditor's control testing affect the plan to perform substantive procedures?

12-7   What assertion is the auditor most concerned about in auditing the purchases, payables, and payments process? Why?

Understanding the Purchases, Payables, and Payments Process

LO1   Describe the purchases, payables, and payments process, including typical risks, transactions, account balances, source documents, and controls.

Purchases of goods and services are a major part of cash outflow in most organizations. For this reason, they will be subject to a fairly high level of management planning and control. Purchases may result in the organization's acquiring assets, for example, inventory, fixed assets (such as PPE), or intangibles (such as patents and customer lists). Some purchases of goods, such as supplies, are expensed, and purchases of services are mainly expensed. Costs of purchasing goods and services may be deferred in some cases, if they relate to producing inventory (see Chapter 13) or internally developed assets, such as buildings and new products (deferred development costs).

Risk Assessment for Purchases, Payables, and Payments

To assess risks in the purchasing-related processes, the auditor focuses on purchasing and cash payment transaction streams and accounts payable balances. Important disclosures relating to purchases include asset capitalization and valuation policies, inventory cost flow assumption policies, contractual commitments, and related party transactions. The auditor's understanding of the auditee's business and environment will point to specific business risks and the related financial misstatement risks that can arise from the auditee's purchases, payables, and payments activities. Some examples of the risks at the assertion level are as follows.

Existence risks could involve inventory being overstated due to double counting or other errors in the year-end physical inventory count. Purchased assets may include improper capitalization of costs to increase reported profits (e.g., WorldCom). Improper cutoff can lead to overstating inventory on hand at period-end if shipments received after period-end are included.

Ownership risks can include inventory held on consignment being recorded as the company's own inventory, in error. In an owner-managed business, some personal expenses of the owner may be run through the company to avoid income taxes.

Completeness risks relate mainly to the possibility of unrecorded liabilities. Goods or services received but not yet paid for at year-end may not have been accrued. Provisions for future costs, such as warranties, may be missing or understated. Improper cutoff can also lead to incomplete recording of liabilities if purchased goods that are still in transit are not accounted for at period-end.

Valuation risks can exist when purchases are denominated in foreign currency; if inventory or property values decline because of market conditions, obsolescence, or improper storage; or if intangible assets are improperly valued. Frauds relating to purchases and payables can arise from collusion between suppliers and employees to overstate purchase transactions payments, for example, via kickback schemes.

Presentation and disclosure risks include not properly presenting separate categories of inventory, PPE, or intangible assets; inadequate capitalization policy notes; and failure to disclose contractual commitments to make future purchases at fixed prices.

As you start to consider assertion-based risks more carefully, you will note that sometimes the same error or problem can affect more than one assertion. For example, if inventory held on consignment is included in the company's own inventory balance, this error affects both the existence and ownership assertions. The great value of the assertions concept to auditors is that it provides a wide net for catching all kinds of things that could have gone wrong in a particular auditee's business to result in material misstatements in its financial statements.

This chapter outlines simple examples of processes for purchasing services, inventory, and fixed assets, as well as the related accounting process and its control activities. The main risk in these processes is incomplete recognition of expenses and liabilities. Control tests in the purchasing processes and physical inspection of inventory and fixed assets address existence, completeness, and valuation assertions, and some substantive evidence for completeness is obtained from examining payments subsequent to year-end. It may be necessary to further inspect documents and use confirmations for more evidence in assessing the ownership assertion.

Purchases, Payables, and Payments Process: Typical Activities

Exhibit 12–1 presents a skeleton overview of the typical activities and transactions involved in the purchases, payables, and payments process, and it also lists the accounts and records typically involved. The basic activities are (1) requesting purchases of goods and services, (2) receiving them, (3) recording costs and liabilities, and (4) paying the bills. The green ovals in the exhibit show the main elements of the control structure: **authorization (procedure)**, **custody**, **recordkeeping (documents and records)**, and **periodic reconciliation (reconciling)**. These control activities are described in the following sections. Further examples of controls related to the illustrated process are provided in Exhibit 12A–2 in Appendix 12A.

The purchases, payables, and payments process involves meeting various departments' identified requirements for goods and services, issuing purchase orders to suppliers, receiving the goods and services, and taking custody of goods received. Accounts payable to suppliers are recorded once the goods have been received or the services have been used, usually at the time the supplier invoice is received. The payables are recorded in a subledger by supplier name and in a control account in the general ledger. Payments involve transferring money (e.g., by cash, cheque, or electronic funds transfer [EFT]) to the supplier, which relieves the liability in both the supplier subledger and the general ledger control account. Frequently, suppliers provide monthly statements of the amount owing, which are reconciled to the subledger balance to ensure the correct amounts are being paid.

The company's control system will feature important types of control activities, including employee procedures relating to keeping custody of assets and records; authorizing purchases and payments; properly recording transactions and events; and reconciling to check the completeness and integrity of the records by comparison to other summaries, reports, or the actual assets themselves. These control activities are described in more detail below.

Authorization

Purchases are requested (requisitioned) by people who know the needs of the organization. A purchasing department finds the best prices and quality and issues a purchase order. Obtaining competitive bids is a good practice because involving several suppliers tends to produce the best prices. It also reduces the risk of frauds involving collusion between suppliers and purchasing department employees, such as inflating purchases to increase sales commissions to the supplier, who then kicks back some of these commissions to the purchasing employee.

authorization (procedure):
a control activity that assigns specific individuals in an organization the responsibility for approving the initiation of transactions on behalf of the organization

custody:
a control activity that identifies the individuals in an organization with the responsibility to hold and safeguard the organization's assets and/or records

recordkeeping (documents and records):
a control activity that involves the preparation of entries and supporting materials in an accounting information system

periodic reconciliation (reconciling):
a control activity that involves regularly comparing reports, summaries, and balances in an accounting information system to the actual assets, or detailed components of accounts, to ensure they agree or indicate any discrepancies, such as a bank reconciliation, supplier reconciliation, inventory count, or agreeing the accounts receivable subledger total to the balance in the general ledger accounts receivable control account

EXHIBIT 12–1

Purchases, Payables, and Payments Process: Overview Diagram of Typical Activities

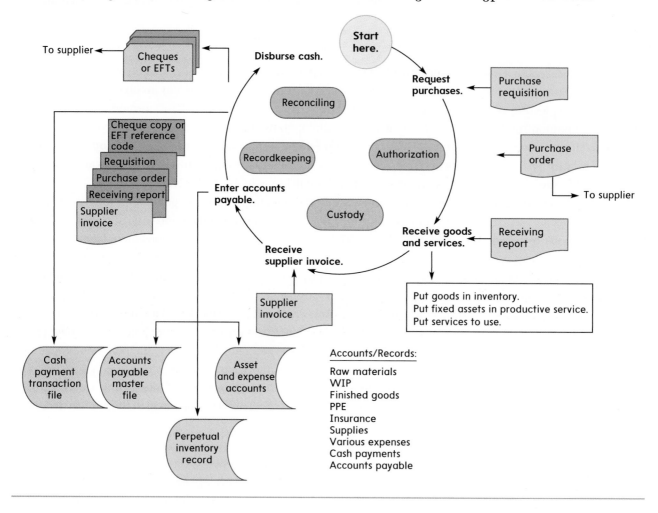

Payments to suppliers are authorized by an accounts payable department employee matching purchase orders, supplier invoices, and internal receiving reports to show there is a valid obligation to pay. Accounts payable obligations are usually recorded when the purchaser receives the goods or services ordered. Cheques are signed by an authorized person. Companies may have a policy requiring two signatures on cheques over a certain amount. Also, a company may have EFT arrangements with suppliers that allow an authorized person to transfer money directly from the company's bank account to the supplier's account. Invoices should be marked "paid" or otherwise stamped to show that they have been processed completely, so that they will not be paid a second time (which would be an existence assertion error).

Custody

The receiving department is responsible for inspecting received goods for quantity and quality (producing a receiving report) and passing them on (e.g., to inventory warehousing, fixed asset installation). Services are accepted by the people responsible for them. For cash in the company's bank accounts, custody belongs to those authorized to sign cheques or transfer funds.

Access to the computerized purchase authorization program, or to blank documents if manual procedures are used—such as purchase orders, receiving reports, and blank cheques—is also a custody issue. If unauthorized persons can access these or have authorization involving them, they can forge a purchase order to a fictitious supplier, forge a receiving report, send a false invoice from a fictitious supplier, and then prepare a company cheque in payment, which is embezzlement.

Recordkeeping

When the purchase order, supplier's invoice, and receiving report are matched, the accounting system will enter the accounts payable with (1) debits to proper inventory, fixed asset, and expense accounts and (2) a credit to accounts payable. When cheques are prepared, entries are made to debit accounts payable and credit cash.

Too Much Trouble

A trucking company self-insured claims of damage to goods in transit, processed claims reports, and paid customers from its own bank accounts. Several persons were authorized to sign cheques. One person thought it "too much trouble" to stamp the claims reports as PAID and said, "That's textbook stuff anyway." Numerous claims were recycled to other cheque signers, and $80,000 in claims was paid in duplicate before the problem was discovered.

Review Checkpoints

12-8   What is a purchase requisition?

12-9   Which assertion is affected if duplicate payments are made from the same supporting documents? How can this type of error be prevented?

Periodic Reconciliation

A periodic reconciliation of existing assets to recorded amounts is not shown in Exhibit 12–1, but it occurs when (1) a physical inventory count compares inventory on hand with perpetual inventory records, (2) a bank account reconciliation compares book cash balances with bank cash balances, (3) an inspection compares fixed assets with detailed fixed asset records, (4) preparation of an accounts payable trial balance compares the detail of accounts payable with the control account in the general ledger, and (5) accounts payable personnel compare suppliers' reports and monthly statements with recorded liabilities.

Audit Evidence in Management Reports

Computer processing of purchases and payments transactions makes it possible for management to generate reports for control purposes, but it can also can provide important audit evidence. Exhibit 12–2 shows how computer processing might do this, and it is discussed in the following section.

Open Purchase Orders

Held in an open purchase order file, purchase orders are open from the time they are issued until the goods and services are received. Generally, no liability exists until the transactions are complete. However, auditors may find evidence of losses on purchase commitments in this file if market prices have fallen below the purchase order price.

Unmatched Receiving Reports

Normally, liabilities should be recorded on the date the goods and services are received and accepted. Sometimes, however, supplier invoices arrive later and the accounts payable department holds the receiving reports, unmatched with invoices, until the information for recording an accounting entry arrives. Auditors can scan the unmatched receiving report file to see if the company has material unrecorded liabilities on the financial statement date. The matching control procedures ensure purchases are valid by verifying that the purchases are real and approved prior to processing the payment.

EXHIBIT 12–2

Management Control Reports Useful for Audit Evidence

MANAGEMENT REPORT	CONTROL PURPOSE	POTENTIAL AUDIT EVIDENCE
Open purchase orders	Completeness of accounts payable	Purchase commitments, valuation of inventory
Unmatched receiving reports	Validity of purchases recorded	Unaccrued liabilities for purchases
Unmatched supplier invoices	Validity of purchases recorded	Unaccrued liabilities for purchases
Accounts payable trial balance	Proper accounting of cash flow management	Existence and completeness of payables
Purchases journal	Completeness and validity of inventory, purchases, and expenses	Analysis of inventory changes and expense reasonability
Inventory reports	Completeness, validity, and valuation of inventory	Analysis of inventory balances, valuation, selection of samples for test counts, and valuation tests
Fixed asset reports	Completeness, validity, and valuation of fixed assets, accumulated depreciation, and depreciation expense	Analysis of changes in fixed asset balances, selection of sample additions for vouching, and recalculation of depreciation expense
Cash payments report	Expenditure reviews by management for validity, authorization	Selection of sample for testing existence, authorization, and proper cutoff of payments

Unmatched Supplier Invoices

Supplier invoices may arrive in the accounts payable department before the receiving process is complete. These invoices are held, unmatched with receiving reports, until there is information that the goods and services were actually received and accepted. Systems failures and human coding errors can cause unmatched invoices and receiving reports to sit around unnoticed when all the information is actually at hand. Auditors can inspect the unmatched invoice file and compare it with the unmatched receiving report file to determine whether liabilities are unrecorded.

Accounts Payable Trial Balance

This trial balance is a list of payable balances, totalling up the outstanding invoices for each supplier. The sum of the supplier balances will agree with the accounts payable control account in the general ledger. Typically, recording to the supplier account and the control account is a simultaneous updating procedure in a computerized accounting system, so differences indicate a system problem. Note that some organizations record payables by individual invoices instead of by supplier names, so the trial balance is a list of unpaid invoices, which still will agree with the control account balance. This type of system is sometimes called an *open invoice system*. The ideal trial balance for audit purposes contains the names of all of an organization's suppliers, even if their balances are zero. The audit "search for unrecorded liabilities" should include the small and zero balances, especially for regular suppliers, because these may be the places where liabilities are unrecorded. Major suppliers will send regular statements of amounts outstanding, and the company usually has a control procedure that reconciles suppliers' statements with accounts payable. Details of these supplier reconciliations can be audited to detect any unrecorded liabilities. All paid and unpaid accounts payable should have supporting documents or computerized records, including a purchase requisition (if any), purchase order (if any), supplier invoice, receiving report (if any), and cheque copy (or notation of cheque number, date, and amount) or EFT reference details, as shown in Exhibit 12–1. Similar records should be available for audit verification in a computerized accounts payable system.

Classify the Debits Correctly

Invoices for expensive repairs were not clearly identified, so the accounts payable accountants entered the $125,000 as capitalized fixed assets instead of as repairs and maintenance expense. This initially understated expenses and overstated pretax income by $125,000 for 1 year, although the incorrectly capitalized expenses were written off as depreciation over the 10-year life of the assets. This spread the misstatement over many years, lowering its materiality.

Thinking Ahead

Lone Moon Brewing purchased bulk aluminum sheets and manufactured its own cans. To ensure a source of raw materials, the company entered into a long-term purchase agreement for three million kilograms of aluminum sheeting at 80 cents per kilogram. At the end of this year, 1.5 million kilograms had been purchased and used, but the market price had fallen to 64 cents per kilogram. Lone Moon was on the hook for a $240,000 (1.5 million kilograms × 16 cents) purchase commitment in excess of current market prices, so the auditors required management to disclose this fact in the company's financial statements.

Purchases Journal

This listing of all purchases may exist as a printed report, or only in a computer transaction file. In either event, it provides raw data for (1) audit analysis of purchasing patterns, which may exhibit characteristics of errors or fraud, and (2) a sample selection of transactions for control tests of supporting documents for validity, authorization, accuracy, classification, and proper period recording. A company may have already performed analyses of purchases, and auditors can use these for analytical evidence, provided the analyses are produced under reliable control conditions.

Inventory Reports (Trial Balance)

A wide variety of inventory reports are useful for analytical evidence. An item-by-item trial balance should agree with a control account (if balances are kept in dollars). Auditors can use this trial balance (1) to scan for unusual conditions (e.g., negative item balances, overstocking, and valuation problems) and (2) as a population for sample selection for a physical inventory observation (audit procedures to obtain evidence about the existence of inventory included in the account). The scanning and sample selection may be computer-audit applications on a computerized inventory report file.

Fixed Asset Reports

These reports are similar to inventory reports because they show the details of fixed assets in control accounts and they can be used for scanning and sample selection as well. A sample selection of fixed assets acquired can be verified against costs shown on purchase invoices. The information for depreciation calculation (cost, useful life, method, and salvage) can be audited by sampling, or a computer application can perform recalculations.

Cash Payments Report

The cash payments process produces a cash payments journal—sometimes printed, sometimes maintained only as a computer file. This journal should contain the date, cheque or EFT reference number, payee, amount, account debited for each cash payment, and a cross-reference to the supplier invoice number or other reason for the payment. A sample can be selected from the population of transactions in the cash payments journal for control tests of supporting documents for validity, authorization, accuracy, classification, and proper period recording of payments.

The Sign of the Credit Balance

Auto Parts & Repair Inc. kept perpetual inventory records and fixed assets records on its computer system. Because of the size of the files (8,000 parts in various locations and 1,500 asset records), the company never printed reports for visual inspection. Auditors ran a computer audit "sign test" on inventory balances and fixed asset net book balances. The test called for a printed report for all balances less than zero. The auditors discovered 320 negative inventory balances caused by failure to record purchases and 125 negative net asset balances caused by depreciating assets more than their cost.

Review Checkpoints

12-10   Where could an auditor look to find evidence of losses on purchase commitments? on unrecorded liabilities to suppliers?

12-11   List the main supporting source documents used in a purchases, payables, and payments process.

12-12   List the management reports that can be used for audit evidence. What information in them can be useful to auditors?

Control Risk Assessment

LO2   Describe the auditor's control risk assessment and control tests for auditing control over the purchase of inventory, services, and fixed assets, and for the payment of cash.

Control risk assessment is important because it governs the nature, timing, and extent of substantive audit procedures that will be applied in the audit of account balances in the purchases, payables, and payments process. These account balances include the following:

- Inventory
- PPE (fixed assets) and intangible assets
- Depreciation and amortization expense
- Accumulated depreciation/amortization
- Accounts and notes payable
- Cash
- Expenses—administrative (supplies, legal fees, audit fees, taxes, insurance), selling (commissions, travel, delivery, advertising), manufacturing (maintenance, freight in, utilities), and so on

General Control Considerations

Control policies for proper segregation of responsibilities should be in place and operating. The green ovals in Exhibit 12–1 show the control activities that should be segregated. Proper segregation means that people with authorization (requisitioning, purchase ordering) responsibilities do not have custody, recording, or reconciliation duties. Custody of inventory, fixed assets, and cash belongs with people who do not directly authorize purchases or cash payments, record the accounting entries, or reconcile physical assets and cash to recorded amounts. Recording (accounting) is done by people who do not authorize transactions, have custody of assets, or perform reconciliations. Simultaneous updating and process controls are in place in the computerized accounting system. Periodic reconciliations are performed by people who do not have authorization, custody, or recording duties related to the same assets. Combinations of two or more of these responsibilities in a single person, office, or computer system may open the door for errors or frauds. An employee who has incompatible duties could make errors that go undetected, or even steal assets from the company and cover it up by making false accounting entries.

Purchase Order Splitting

A school board's purchasing agent had authority to buy supplies in amounts of $1,000 or less without being required to get competitive bids for the best price. The purchasing agent wanted to favour local businesses owned by her friends instead of large chain stores, so she broke up the year's $350,000 supplies order into numerous $900–$950 orders, paying about 12% more to local stores than would have been paid to the large chains. In return, the purchasing agent received very generous discounts and gifts from these local businesses. The auditors discovered this practice by scanning the purchases journal and investigating the frequent small amounts that were being paid to the same payee. They recommended to management that a regular supervisor review of the purchases journal may improve control over authorization of purchases.

In addition, internal controls should provide for detail-checking control procedures. For example, (1) all purchase requisitions and purchase orders are approved by authorized personnel, (2) purchase order master files changes are made by authorized persons only, (3) physical security for inventory warehouses and fixed asset locations (storerooms, fences, locks, etc.) is adequate, (4) accounts payable are recorded only when all the supporting documentation is in order (purchases and payables as of the date goods and services were received and payments on the date the cheques (or EFTs) leave the organization's control), (5) procedures exist to prevent making duplicate payments for the same invoice, and (6) supplier invoices are compared with purchase orders and receiving reports to verify the price and that the quantity billed is the same as the quantity received. The following box offers an example of the consequences of weak management controls—in this case, when authorization controls for contract payments are inadequate in a government department.

Where Tax Dollars Go

The Auditor General of Canada (AGC) had some harsh words for the federal government in an 83-page report released just days before an expected election call. The report criticized the way the government's departments and services spend money and was particularly critical of Human Resources Development Canada (HRDC; now Human Resources and Skills Development Canada [HRSDC]), pointing out its sloppy paperwork, careless spending, and vague job creation figures. HRDC was at the centre of a scandal starting in January 2000 when an internal audit found massive mismanagement in its $1-billion jobs grants program. The AGC's report confirms that finding and condemns poor accountability between the department and its programs, and within HRDC itself. The audit cites breaches of authority, improper payment practices, and limited monitoring of recipient projects' finances and activities. It also found an inadequate process to decide which projects should get money, including examples of some that were not eligible for funding but received it anyway.

Auditor General Sheila Fraser said in a 2002 speech:

"Our audit of HRDC grants and contributions showed what happens when there is no longer a balance between the insistence on performance and controls, and more emphasis is placed on one of these components. Management's priorities were to implement strategic initiatives and improve service. We found that it had not placed enough emphasis on maintaining vital control while it reduced red tape and improved service."

In Alberta, the provincial government's health care monopoly, Alberta Health Services (AHS), spent almost $250 million between 2012 and 2013, nearly half a million a day, on consultants. Consultants were paid to help AHS executives with projects like "buying art," "staff scheduling transformation," and "executive coaching . . . (in) . . . self-discovery . . . ." And in the midst of these scandals, the AHS board insisted on paying out millions in bonuses to its executives. Given that the actual mandate of the taxpayer-funded AHS is to support provision of health services to Albertans, opposition politicians and the press and the public were outraged by the waste of taxpayer funds.

(continued)

The Delhi 2010 Commonwealth Games were a showcase for India's status as an emerging global power, but the headlines were stolen by allegations of corruption and spending irregularities. Venue delays, shoddy construction, and budget overruns tripled the cost of the event to US$6 billion. In 2011, India's national auditor accused the Delhi government of wasteful spending of at least US$29 million during its "ill-conceived and ill-planned" program to beautify the city before the Games. In 2014, Delhi's newly elected chief minister ordered the state anti-corruption bureau to investigate alleged irregularities in a deal by the previous Delhi state government to buy expensive imported street lights before the event, a 310 million rupee ($5.5 million) contract for the lights. Numerous legal cases have also been filed in Delhi courts and outside, relating to disputes in finance, workforce, catering, merchandising, cleaning and waste management, technology, and other functional areas connected to the Games.

Sources: CBC News, "Auditor General delivers stinging rebuke to Ottawa," October 22, 2000, at cbc.ca/news/canada/auditor-general-delivers-stinging-rebuke-to-ottawa-1.230824; Notes for an address by Sheila Fraser, FCA, Auditor General of Canada, to Canada Mortgage and Housing, June 11, 2002, Ottawa, Ontario, at oag-bvg.gc.ca/internet/English/sp_20020611_e_23844.html; Lorne Gunter, "Alberta health minister Fred Horne has to go." at edmontonsun.com/2014/04/10/health-minister-just-doesnt-get-ahs-problems, April 10, 2014; The Sydney Morning Herald, "India launches corruption inquiry into Delhi Commonwealth Games," at smh.com.au/sport/india-launches-corruption-inquiry-into-delhi-commonwealth-games-20140206-325kr.html, February 14, 2014; Press Trust of India, "Commonwealth Games corruption: Organising Committee faces Rs 350 crore worth legal cases," at sports.ndtv.com/othersports/news/215193-commonwealth-games-corruption-organising-committee-faces-rs-350-crore-worth-legal-cases, October 6, 2013.

Information gathering about the control structure often begins with an internal control questionnaire. An example of a questionnaire is provided in Appendix 12A. The questionnaire can be studied for details of desirable control policies and procedures, as it is organized under headings that identify the important control objectives: environment, validity, completeness, authorization, accuracy, classification, and proper period recording.

Review Checkpoints

12-13   What functions should be segregated in the purchases, payables, and payments process?

12-14   What are some controls that might prevent the embezzling of cash by creation of fictitious supplier invoices?

12-15   How could an auditor determine if the purchasing agent had practised purchase order splitting?

Control Tests

An organization should have detailed control procedures in place and operating to prevent or detect and correct accounting errors. You studied the general control objectives in Chapter 9 (validity, completeness, authorization, accuracy, classification, and proper period recording). Exhibit 12–3 demonstrates these in a purchasing activity situation, with examples related to specific purchasing objectives. Study this exhibit carefully.

Auditors can perform tests to determine whether controls said to be in place and operating are actually being performed properly by company personnel. Recall from Chapter 9 that a *control test* consists of (1) identifying the data population from which a sample of items will be selected for audit and (2) describing the action that will produce relevant evidence. The actions involve vouching, tracing, observing, scanning, and recalculating—procedures for obtaining evidence used in a final control risk assessment. If control procedures are not well performed, auditors need to design substantive audit procedures to try to detect whether control failures have produced materially misleading account balances.

Proper timing is very important in the recording of the purchase transaction, and **purchase cutoff** tests provide assurance, as indicated in objective 6 of Exhibit 12–3. In a perpetual inventory system, the inventory

purchase cutoff:
recording purchase transactions in the proper period, including accruals of payments not due until the following period

EXHIBIT 12–3

Internal Control Objectives (Purchases)

GENERAL CONTROL OBJECTIVES	EXAMPLES OF SPECIFIC CONTROL OBJECTIVES
1. Recorded purchases are *valid* and documented.	• Purchases of inventory (or fixed assets) are supported by supplier invoices, receiving reports, purchase orders, and requisitions (or approved capital budget).
2. Valid purchase transactions are recorded and *none omitted*.	• Requisitions, purchase orders, and receiving reports are prenumbered and numerical sequence is checked. • Overall comparisons of purchases are made periodically by statistical or product-line analysis.
3. Purchases are *authorized* according to company policy.	• All purchase orders are supported by requisitions from proper persons (or approved capital budgets). • Purchases are made from approved suppliers only after bids are received and evaluated.
4. Purchase orders are *accurately* prepared.	• Completed purchase order quantities and descriptions are independently compared with requisitions and suppliers' catalogues. • Freight-in is included as part of purchase and added to inventory (or fixed assets) costs.
5. Purchase transactions are properly *classified*.	• Account distributions for invoices are appropriate and reviewed independent of preparation. • Purchases from subsidiaries and affiliates are classified as intercompany purchases and payables. • Purchase returns and allowances are properly classified. • Purchases for repairs and maintenance are segregated from purchases of fixed assets.
6. Purchase transactions are recorded in the *proper period*.	• Perpetual inventory and fixed asset records are updated as of the date goods are received or title of ownership is transferred.

records are kept up to date continuously. In a periodic system, the inventory level is known only at the physical inventory count date. Even in perpetual systems, however, there should be an annual inventory count to reconcile records with actual inventory. The inventory count procedures are described in more detail later in this chapter. Thus, for both types of inventory systems, the inventory cutoff test date is the date the physical inventory is taken and accounting records are adjusted to distinguish between sales and purchases before the cutoff date and those after it.

A **cutoff error** is a failure to assign a transaction to the proper period. For example, the shipping terms *FOB destination* and *FOB shipping* indicate the date that legal title to the inventory is transferred to the purchaser: when goods are received, in the case of FOB destination, and when goods leave the seller's premises, in the case of FOB shipping. Delivery time can thus have a major impact on proper recording of purchases, payables, inventory, sales, and receivables. The appropriate accounting depends on the shipping terms and whether the auditee is the buyer or seller in the transaction. These are major considerations in cutoff procedures related to inventory. Note that the auditee control system's ability to detect and correct cutoff errors justifies the auditor's decision to perform more or fewer cutoff audit procedures.

The auditee may use a cutoff date other than the balance sheet date if controls are strong enough to ensure that transactions between the cutoff and year-end are recorded accurately and completely. In this situation, the auditor verifies both the cutoff and the transactions in the **roll-forward period**, the period between cutoff and year-end, to ensure that the year-end balance is not misstated.

cutoff error:
when transactions are recorded in the wrong period, either by postponing to the next period or accelerating next-period transactions into the current period

roll-forward period:
the period between the cutoff and fiscal year-end, when a cutoff is made before the year-end

---

EXHIBIT 12–4

Control Tests for Purchases, Payments, and Accounts Payable

	CONTROL OBJECTIVE
Consider the control environment	
Observe whether purchasing department personnel understand how to implement control activities assigned to them.	All control objectives
A. Purchases	
1. Select a sample of receiving reports:	
(a) Vouch to related purchase orders and note missing receiving reports (missing numbers).	Authorization Completeness
(b) Trace to inventory record posting of additions.	Completeness
B. Payments and Other Expenses	
1. Select a sample of payment cheque or EFT numbers:	
(a) Scan for missing documents (missing numbers).	Completeness
(b) Vouch supporting documentation for evidence of accurate arithmetic, correct classification, proper approval, and proper date of entry.	Accuracy Classification Authorization Proper period
2. Select a sample of recorded expenses from various accounts and vouch them to (a) cancelled cheques or EFT references and (b) supporting documentation.	Validity Classification
C. Accounts Payable	
1. Select a sample of open accounts payable and vouch to supporting documents of purchase (purchase orders, suppliers' invoices).	Validity
2. Trace debits arising from accounts payable transactions for proper classification.	Classification
3. Select a sample of accounts payable entries recorded after the balance sheet date and vouch to supporting documents for evidence of proper cutoff—evidence that a liability should have been recorded as of the balance sheet date.	Proper period

Exhibit 12–4 shows a selection of tests for controls over purchase, payment, and accounts payable transactions. The samples are usually attribute samples designed along the lines of those studied in Chapter 10. On the right, the exhibit shows the control objectives tested by the audit procedures shown on the left.

Control Tests for Inventory Records

Many organizations have material investments in inventories. In some engagements, auditors need to determine whether they can rely on the accuracy of perpetual inventory records. For example, if inventory is to be physically counted at a date other than year-end, the controls need to be relied on to verify inventory changes in the roll-forward period. Tests of controls over accuracy involve tests of the additions (purchases) to the inventory detail balances and tests of the reductions (issues) of the item balances.

Exhibit 12–5 pictures the two-direction testing of audit samples. The samples of receiving reports and issue slips (or packing slips) meet the completeness direction requirement: everything received recorded as an addition to and everything issued recorded as a reduction of the balance. The sample from the perpetual inventory transaction records meets the validity direction requirement: everything recorded as an addition or reduction is supported by receiving reports and issue documents.

Exhibit 12–6 contains a selection of tests for controls over perpetual inventory records similar to that of Exhibit 12–4. Note that some of these tests are dual-purpose procedures as they also provide

EXHIBIT 12–5

Two-Direction Testing of Audit Samples

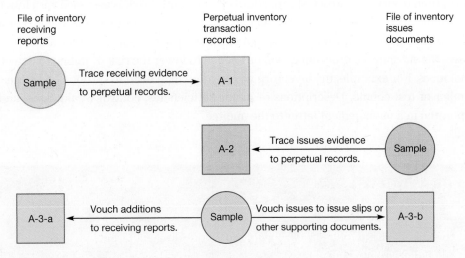

Note: The symbols A-1, A-2, A-3-a, and A-3-b are cross-references to the procedures in Exhibit 12–6.

substantive evidence regarding the inventory balance. As before, the samples are usually attribute samples designed along the lines of those studied in Chapter 10. The control objectives tested are in the column on the right.

EXHIBIT 12–6

Control Tests for Inventory Records

	CONTROL OBJECTIVE
Consider the control environment	
Observe whether inventory department personnel understand and implement control activities assigned to them.	All control objectives
A. Inventory Receipts and Issues	
1. Select a sample of receiving reports and trace to perpetual inventory record entry of receipt.	Authorization Completeness
2. Select a sample of sales invoices, bills of lading or other shipping documents, or production requisitions and trace to perpetual inventory record entry of issue.	Authorization Completeness
3. Select a sample of inventory items from the perpetual records:	
(a) Vouch additions to receiving reports.	Validity
(b) Vouch issues to invoices, bills of lading or other shipping documents, or production requisitions.	Validity
B. Cost of Sales	
1. With the sample of issues in A-2 above:	
(a) Review the accounting summary of quantities and prices for mathematical accuracy.	Accuracy
(b) Trace posting of amounts to the general ledger.	Completeness
2. Obtain a sample of cost of goods sold entries in the general ledger and vouch to supporting summaries of finished goods issues.	Validity
3. Review (recalculate) the appropriateness of standard costs, if used, to price inventory issues and cost of goods sold. Review the disposition of variances from standard costs.	Accuracy

Summary: Control Risk Assessment

The audit manager or senior in charge on the audit evaluates the evidence obtained from an understanding of the internal controls and from the control test procedures. If the control risk is assessed very low, the substantive audit procedures on the account balances can be limited for efficiency. For example, the inventory observation test counts could be done prior to year-end and with a small sample size. On the other hand, if tests of controls reveal weaknesses, the substantive procedures will be needed to lower the risk of failing to detect material error in the account balances. For example, the inventory observation may need to be done on the year-end date and with a large number of test counts. Descriptions of major deficiencies, control weaknesses, and inefficiencies should be incorporated in a management letter to the auditee.

Review Checkpoints

12-16 Describe the two general characteristics of a control test.

12-17 How is the information from the shipping department, receiving department, and warehouse used to update perpetual inventory records?

12-18 In fixed asset management and accounting, which functional responsibilities should be delegated to separate departments or management levels?

Substantive Audit Programs for the Purchases, Payables, and Payments Process

LO3 Describe the typical substantive procedures used to respond to the assessed risk of material misstatement in the main account balances and transactions in the purchases, payables, and payments process.

This section provides examples of substantive procedures that may be considered for auditing the purchases, payables, and payments process. These examples are concise lists of basic substantive procedures, along with the related assertions they address. As discussed in Chapter 11, the risk assessments and results of any control testing are taken into account in selecting the nature, timing, and extent of further substantive procedures. For example, if controls are considered effective, confirmations of supplier account balances are usually not considered necessary. On the other hand, if there are control weaknesses potentially affecting the accuracy and completeness of accounts payable balances, the auditor may decide to confirm outstanding balances with major suppliers. Exhibit 12–7 shows selected substantive procedures for accounts payable and related accounts, such as accrued liabilities and unearned revenues. Exhibit 12–8 shows a generic program for inventory balance and the related expense, cost of sales. Exhibit 12–9 shows a program for PPE and intangible assets, and related depreciation and amortization accounting. The following sections of the chapter present special technical notes that go into more detail on some of the procedures related to assertions that tend to have high risks of material misstatement in many audit situations. Typical procedures used to respond to these risks are discussed in these sections.

EXHIBIT 12–7

Example of Substantive Audit Program Responding to Assessed Risks of Material Misstatement for Accounts Payable and Accrued Liabilities: Selected Substantive Procedures

AUDIT PROGRAM				
AUDITEE: *ECOPAK INC.*			**FILE INDEX:** *BB-100*	
FINANCIAL STATEMENT PERIOD: *y/e DECEMBER 31, 20X1*				
ACCOUNT: *Accounts Payable and Accrued Liabilities*				
Substantive audit program in response to assessed risks at the assertion level:				
Consider risk assessment findings and conclusion on residual detection risk to be reduced by performing substantive procedures. (Of the procedures listed below, perform those considered necessary to provide sufficient appropriate evidence to address the assessed risks and reduce risk of material misstatement to an acceptable level.)				*[Reference to relevant working papers]*
Substantive audit procedures:	Assertions evidence is related to [E, C, O, V, P*]	Timing	Extent	Working paper reference
A. Accounts Payable				
1. Obtain a trial balance of recorded accounts payable as of year-end.				
(a) Recalculate its total and trace the total to the general ledger Accounts Payable control account.	E, C			
(b) Vouch a sample of balances to suppliers' statements.	E, C, O			
(c) Review the trial balance for unusual items, related party payables, or other items and follow up with management inquiries.	E, C			
2. When concerned about the possibility of unrecorded payables, send confirmations to creditors, especially those with small or zero balances and those with whom the company has done significant business.	C			
3. Conduct a search for unrecorded liabilities by examining client reconciliations of suppliers' statements to Accounts Payable control account and payments from the bank accounts made for a period after year-end, and by performing other procedures required to respond to assessed risk.	C			
4. Inquire about terms that justify classifying payables as long term instead of current.	V, P			
5. Obtain written management representations about completeness of Accounts Payable, related party payables, and pledges of assets as collateral for liabilities.	C, O, V, P			
B. Accrued and Other Liabilities, Unearned Revenues				
1. Obtain a schedule of all accrued and other liabilities and unearned revenues. Agree each balance to the general ledger, and compare with prior-period balances.	E, C			
				(continued)

EXHIBIT 12–7

Example of Substantive Audit Program Responding to Assessed Risks of Material Misstatement for Accounts Payable and Accrued Liabilities: Selected Substantive Procedures   (*continued*)

2. Determine the basis for accrual/deferral, discuss the nature of each item with management, recalculate the recorded amounts, and determine whether each item is properly allocated to the current or a future accounting period and properly classified as current or long term.	V, P			
3. Obtain or prepare a continuity schedule showing all significant additions and subtractions from balances during the audited period, and vouch them to supporting documents, such as invoices, contracts, receipts, or calculations. Tie all expense items to revenue and expense audit working papers.	E, C, V			
4. In other audit work on revenues and expenses, be alert to items that should be considered deferred or accrued.	C, P			
5. Scan the expense accounts in the trial balance, and compare with prior year. Investigate unusual differences that may indicate failure to account for a deferral or accrual item.	C, P			
6. For estimated liabilities, such as warranties, determine and evaluate the basis of estimation, recalculate the estimate, and assess its reasonableness. Ensure management's disclosure accounting policy is properly applied.	E, C, V			
7. Obtain written management representations about completeness and appropriate presentation of accrued and other liabilities and deferred revenue.	C, O, V, P			
Misstatement summary: Summarize here all misstatements discovered in executing this program. Carry all forward for accumulation in the Summary of Accumulated Misstatements worksheet (Exhibit 16–1).				

AUDITOR'S CONCLUSIONS

[If the audit program is completed satisfactorily and the audit objectives are met, a conclusion such as the following would be recorded by the auditor performing the work.]

Based on my professional judgment, the evidence obtained is sufficient and appropriate to conclude that the risk of material misstatement of the ACCOUNTS PAYABLE, ACCRUED AND OTHER LIABILITIES: UNEARNED REVENUE *is acceptably low.*

Prepared by _____   Date _____

Reviewed by _____   Date _____

*E, C, O, V, P = existence, completeness, ownership, valuation, presentation.

Review Checkpoints

12-19   In what situations would auditors send confirmation letters to suppliers to audit accounts payable? Why?

12-20   What information would be included in a continuity schedule for an accrued liability?

EXHIBIT 12–8

Example of Substantive Audit Program Responding to Assessed Risks of Material Misstatement for Inventory and Cost of Goods Sold: Selected Substantive Procedures

AUDIT PROGRAM				
AUDITEE: *ECOPAK INC.*			**FILE INDEX:** *D-100*	
FINANCIAL STATEMENT PERIOD: *y/e DECEMBER 31, 20X1*				
ACCOUNT: *Inventory and Cost of Goods Sold*				
Substantive audit program in response to assessed risks:				
Consider risk assessment findings and conclusion on residual detection risk to be reduced by performing substantive procedures. (Of the procedures listed below, perform those considered necessary to provide sufficient appropriate evidence to address the assessed risks and reduce risk of material misstatement to an acceptable level.)				*[Reference to relevant working papers]*
Substantive audit procedures:	Assertions evidence is related to [E, C, O, V, P*]	Timing	Extent	Working paper reference
A. Inventory Balance				
1. Obtain the auditee's final inventory compilation and tie into relevant general ledger accounts and supporting evidence from the observation of the company's physical inventory count, as follows:				
(a) Trace the samples of inventory items audited at the physical inventory count observation to the final inventory compilation.	E, C			
(b) Select a further sample of items from the physical inventory listing and verify existence by finding them in the inventory.	E, C			
(c) Trace other information (items, quantities) recorded from the inventory listing at the count date to the final compilation.	E, C			
(d) Inquire about and make note of any damaged or scrap inventory, or inventory that appears slow moving or obsolete.	V			
2. Scan the inventory compilation for items added from sources other than the physical count and items that appear to be large round numbers or systematic fictitious additions.	E			
3. Select a sample of inventory items from the final compilation. Vouch unit prices to suppliers' invoices or other cost records. Recalculate the multiplication of unit times price.	V			
4. Recalculate the extensions and totalling of the final inventory compilation for arithmetic accuracy.	V			
5. For selected inventory items and categories, determine the replacement cost and the applicability of lower-of-cost-and-market valuation.	V, P			
6. Determine whether obsolete or damaged goods should be written down: (a) Inquire about obsolete, damaged, unsaleable, slow-moving items. (b) Scan the perpetual records for slow-moving items. (c) Ensure obsolete and damaged goods observed during the physical observation have been removed from the final inventory compilation. (d) Compare the listing of obsolete, slow-moving, damaged, or unsaleable inventory from last year's audit to the current inventory compilation.	V			
				(continued)

EXHIBIT 12–8

Example of Substantive Audit Program Responding to Assessed Risks of Material Misstatement for Inventory and Cost of Goods Sold: Selected Substantive Procedures   *(continued)*

7. At year-end (at physical inventory count observation), obtain the numbers of the last shipping and receiving documents for the year. Tie these into the sales, inventory/cost of sales, and accounts payable entries to verify proper cutoff. Note FOB terms in force, and ensure that goods-in-transit is correctly cut off.	E, C			
8. Read bank confirmations, debt agreements, and minutes of the board, and inquire about pledge or assignment of inventory to secure debt.	O, P			
9. Inquire about inventory out on consignment and about inventory on hand that is consigned in from suppliers.	E, C, O			
10. Confirm or inspect inventories held in public warehouses.	E, C, V			
11. Obtain written management representations concerning completeness of inventory; valuation accounting policies; and whether there are any pledges of inventory as collateral, intercompany sales, or other related party transactions.	C, O, V, P			
B. Cost of Sales				
1. Select a sample of recorded cost of sales entries and vouch to supporting documentation.	E, C			
2. Select a sample of basic transaction documents (such as sales invoices, production reports) and determine whether the related cost of goods sold was calculated and recorded properly.	E, C, V			
3. Determine whether the accounting costing method used by the client (such as FIFO, average cost, standard cost) was applied properly.	V, P			
4. Compute the gross margin rate and compare with prior years. Follow up with management on unusual fluctuations.	E, C, V			
5. Compute the ratio of cost elements (such as labour, material) to total cost of goods sold and compare with prior years. Follow up with management on unusual fluctuations.	E, C			
Misstatement summary: Summarize here all misstatements discovered in executing this program. Carry all forward for accumulation in the Summary of Accumulated Misstatements worksheet (Exhibit 16–1).				

AUDITOR'S CONCLUSIONS
[If the audit program is completed satisfactorily and the audit objectives are met, a conclusion such as the following would be recorded by the auditor performing the work.]
Based on my professional judgment, the evidence obtained is sufficient and appropriate to conclude that the risk of material misstatement of the INVENTORY AND COST OF SALES is acceptably low.

Prepared by _____   Date _____

Reviewed by _____   Date _____

*E, C, O, V, P = existence, completeness, ownership, valuation, presentation.

Review Checkpoints

12-21 List key substantive audit procedures used to address the inventory valuation assertion.

12-22 How is information collected during the auditor's attendance at the physical inventory count used in the audit of the inventory balance?

12-23 What cutoff misstatements can arise if the FOB terms for sales shipped are not properly accounted for? What about for inventory received?

EXHIBIT 12–9

Example of Substantive Audit Program Responding to Assessed Risks of Material Misstatement for Property, Plant, and Equipment and Intangible Assets: Selected Substantive Procedures*

AUDIT PROGRAM				
AUDITEE: ECOPAK INC.				**FILE INDEX:** U-100
FINANCIAL STATEMENT PERIOD: y/e DECEMBER 31, 20X1				
ACCOUNT: Property, Plant, & Equipment and Intangible Assets: Depreciation and Amortization Expense				
Substantive audit program in response to assessed risks at the assertion level:				
Consider risk assessment findings and conclusion on residual detection risk to be reduced by performing substantive procedures. (Of the procedures listed below, perform those considered necessary to provide sufficient appropriate evidence to address the assessed risks and reduce risk of material misstatement to an acceptable level.)				*[Reference to relevant working papers]*
Substantive audit procedures:	Assertions evidence is related to [E, C, O, V, P**]	Timing	Extent	Working paper reference
A. Property, Plant, & Equipment (PPE) and Intangible Assets				
1. Summarize and recalculate detailed PPE and intangible asset subsidiary records, and reconcile to general ledger control account(s).	E, C			
2. Select a sample of asset subsidiary records: (a) Perform a physical observation (inspection) of the fixed assets recorded. (b) Inspect title or other ownership legal documents, if any. (c) Inspect supporting documentation (e.g., invoices, contracts, purchase agreements) or obtain written confirmation of acquisition and ownership.	E E, O E, O			
3. Obtain, or prepare, a continuity schedule of the balances, showing asset additions and disposals for the period: (a) Vouch to disposals to documents, indicating proper approval. (b) Vouch costs of additions to invoices, contracts, or other supporting documents. (c) Determine whether all costs of shipment, installation, testing, and the like have been properly capitalized. (d) Vouch proceeds (on dispositions) to cash receipts or other asset records. (e) Recalculate gain or loss on dispositions. (f) Agree amounts to detailed fixed asset records and general ledger control account(s).	C E, V V V, P V, P E, C, V			
4. Observe a physical inventory taking of the fixed assets, and compare with detailed assets records.	E, C			
5. If any property is valued at fair value, examine and verify supporting valuation evidence, such as independent appraisals.	V			
6. Obtain written representations from management regarding ownership, completeness, and any pledging of assets as security for loans and leased assets.	C, O, V, P			
B. Depreciation/Amortization				
1. Analyze amortization expense for overall reasonableness with reference to costs of assets (or fair values if used) and average depreciation rates.	V			*(continued)*

EXHIBIT 12–9

Example of Substantive Audit Program Responding to Assessed Risks of Material Misstatement for Property, Plant, and Equipment and Intangible Assets: Selected Substantive Procedures* (*continued*)

2. Obtain, or prepare, a continuity schedule of accumulated amortization showing beginning balance, current amortization, disposals, and ending balance. Trace to amortization expense and asset disposition analyses. Trace amounts to general ledger account(s).	E, C, P			
3. Recalculate amortization expense and trace to general ledger account(s).	E, C, P			
C. Related Accounts				
1. Analyze insurance for adequacy of coverage.	V, P			
2. Analyze property taxes to determine whether taxes due on assets have been paid or accrued.	O (C for liability)			
3. Select a sample of rental expense entries. Vouch to rent/lease contracts to determine whether any leases qualify for capitalization.	V, P			
4. Select a sample of repair and maintenance expense entries, and vouch them to supporting invoices for evidence of property that should be capitalized.	V			
Misstatement summary: Summarize here all misstatements discovered in executing this program. Carry all forward for accumulation in the Summary of Accumulated Misstatements worksheet (Exhibit 16–1).				

AUDITOR'S CONCLUSIONS
[If the audit program is completed satisfactorily and the audit objectives are met, a conclusion such as the following would be recorded by the auditor performing the work.]
Based on my professional judgment, the evidence obtained is sufficient and appropriate to conclude that the risk of material misstatement of the PROPERTY, PLANT, & EQUIPMENT AND INTANGIBLE ASSETS, AND RELATED DEPRECIATION AND AMORTIZATION EXPENSE is acceptably low.

Prepared by _____   Date _____

Reviewed by _____   Date _____

*The programs illustrated in Exhibits 12–7 to 12–9 are generic and, in practice, will need to be tailored to a specific audit engagement's risk assessments, to design an appropriate set of audit procedures linked to the assessed risks at the assertion level in each auditee's specific circumstances.
**E, C, O, V, P = existence, completeness, ownership, valuation, presentation.

Review Checkpoints

12-24   What assertion(s) are addressed by a physical inspection of PPE?

12-25   What key items on the fixed assets continuity schedule are vouched to supporting documentation?

12-26   What is the main evidence used to audit depreciation expense?

To cap off this general description of an audit program for a purchases, payables, and payments process, note the following analysis approaches used to integrate the audit findings.

Analysis of Financial Statement Relationships

The audit of the purchases, payables, and payments processes results in verifying the balance of accounts payable/accrued liabilities and the two transaction streams that run through it—purchases/expenses and payments.

As an overall analysis technique, we can analyze balance changes and the financial statement items related to them by preparing a continuity schedule. The accrued legal fees balance shown below is one example for the purchases, payables, and payments process. (The relationship between inventory purchases and balance sheet amounts will be analyzed in Chapter 13.)

AUDITED AMOUNT	FINANCIAL STATEMENT WHERE AMOUNT IS REPORTED
Opening balance of accrued liability for legal fees	Balance sheet (component of accrued liabilities in prior-year comparative figures)
Add: New legal services expensed during the year	Income statement expense (e.g., legal services acquired)
Deduct: Cash paid against payables	Cash flow statement (direct method)
Ending balance of accrued liability for legal fees	Balance sheet (component of accrued liabilities in current-year figures)

As these relationships illustrate, our procedures to audit the purchases, payables, and payments process allow us to assess whether all components of this system of related amounts are reported accurately in the financial statements. These relationships also indicate analytical procedures that can detect material misstatements. For example, the ratios that measure inventory turnover or expense-to-revenue ratios exploit these relationships and can indicate non-existent inventory or misstatement in expense accounts and liabilities.

Misstatement Analysis

The financial statement relationships can also be used to analyze the kinds of misstatements that may be uncovered in the audit work. Consider the following situations.

Say the auditors discover by their testing of the payments that a cutoff error has occurred. After the books were closed for the year-end on December 31, one additional cheque was issued that was not recorded. The auditors learned through inquiries that this happened when the CFO had to see the company lawyer on a last-minute issue late on December 31 and asked the payables manager to issue a cheque to pay the lawyer's outstanding bill of $42,000, which had been set up in accounts payable when it was received earlier in the year. (A sharp auditor would also be sure to find out what the "last-minute" legal issue was!) This cutoff error results in the payment amount deducted from the accrued liability balance being too small, making the accrued liability balance too big, that is, overstated. Since the cash part of the transaction was also unrecorded, the cash balance is overstated (this difference will also be picked up in the bank reconciliation audit). This misstatement will be carried forward to the accumulated misstatements worksheet in the audit file, as illustrated in Exhibit 16–1 of Chapter 16.

Consider another type of misstatement related to the expense accounts and accruals. The electricity company billed the company for December based on an estimate of its usage, and this bill was accrued at the year-end. However, on February 3, the electricity company sent a revised bill based on a meter reading, and the actual electricity charges were higher than the accrued amount by $3,700. Since the new bill was received when the audit field work was being performed, it was noted by the auditors in their subsequent payments testing. Inquiries revealed that the company's electricity usage in December was much higher than in the past because it was an exceptionally cold month, and at one point, the loading dock door froze open over a weekend, causing a great deal of power to be wasted. The impact of the error is that too little was added to the accounts payable account, and too little was expensed, so liabilities are understated and net income is overstated. This misstatement will also be carried forward to the accumulated misstatements worksheet (see Exhibit 16–1) for evaluation at the final stage of the audit when the audit partner must assess whether the misstatements uncovered accumulate to a material amount.

The following sections provide more detail on substantive procedures related to some of the key assertions to be audited in account balances and transactions related to the purchases, payables, and payments process. Three special notes are given discussing audit considerations for the observation of the physical inventory count; the valuation of PPE; and the completeness of liabilities. These are areas that often have high assessed risk, warranting a rigorous response.

Special Note: Physical Inventory Observation and Audit of Inventory and Cost of Sales

> **LO4** Identify audit considerations for observing the physical inventory count.

The audit procedures for inventory and related cost of sales accounts can be extensive, as there are many facets of inherent risk and control risk to consider, and the process of obtaining evidence about inventory financial statement assertions can be complex. Inventories are significant assets in many businesses and reflect the unique characteristics of the business's operations. Significant to manufacturing, wholesale, and retail organizations, inventories are also frequently material to the financial statements of service organizations. For some types of businesses, inventories constitute a significant percent of total assets and represent the largest current asset.

A material misstatement in inventory has a pervasive effect on financial statements. It will cause misstatements in current assets, working capital, total assets, cost of sales, gross margin, and net income. While analytical procedures can help indicate inventory presentation problems, physical observation of the auditee's inventory count is the best way to detect inventory misstatements. Canadian Auditing Standards (CAS 501) require that auditors attend the physical inventory counting when inventory is material to the financial statements, to provide evidence of the existence and condition of inventory. While auditors rarely count the entire inventory, management's procedures for recording and controlling the count should be evaluated and observed, inventory inspected, and test counts performed. Later, the final inventory records should be tested to ensure they accurately reflect the evidence the auditor obtained at the physical counting.

Standards Check

CAS 501 Audit Evidence—Specific Considerations for Selected Items

4. If inventory is material to the financial statements, the auditor shall obtain sufficient appropriate audit evidence regarding the existence and condition of inventory by
   (a) Attendance at physical inventory counting, unless impracticable, to (Ref: Para. A1–A3)
      (i) Evaluate management's instructions and procedures for recording and controlling the results of the entity's physical inventory counting; (Ref: Para. A4)
      (ii) Observe the performance of management's count procedures; (Ref: Para. A5)
      (iii) Inspect the inventory; and (Ref: Para. A6)
      (iv) Perform test counts. (Ref: Para. A7–A8)
   (b) Performing audit procedures over the entity's final inventory records to determine whether they accurately reflect actual inventory count results.

Source: *CPA Canada Handbook–Assurance,* 2014.

In some audits, obtaining evidence about an inventory's existence and valuation requires expert knowledge in a field other than accounting or auditing, as described in CAS 620. Often, experts employed by the auditee's management will provide tests and reports for this purpose. An auditee will likely have employees with the expertise required, for example, to assess the assembly stage of highly technical equipment held as WIP inventory, or to calculate the quantity of raw material in containers or stockpiles based on measures of volume and density. Alternatively, if a high risk is assessed, an expert employed by the audit firm or an outside expert engaged by the audit firm to assist the team may be assigned to provide evidence that is considered more independent, and reliable, than that obtained from management's experts. In evaluating the need for an expert, the auditor first considers whether alternative sources of sufficient appropriate evidence are available and more cost effective. For example, an outside expert's report prepared for the auditee but for another purpose may also be relevant and reliable for the auditor's purposes.

Standards Check

CAS 620 Using the Work of an Auditor's Expert

6. For purposes of the CASs, the following terms have the meanings attributed below:
   (a) Auditor's expert—An individual or organization possessing expertise in a field other than accounting or auditing, whose work in that field is used by the auditor to assist the auditor in obtaining sufficient appropriate audit evidence. An auditor's expert may be either an auditor's internal expert (who is a partner or staff, including temporary staff, of the auditor's firm or a network firm), or an auditor's external expert. (Ref: Para. A1–A3)
   (b) Expertise—Skills, knowledge and experience in a particular field.
   (c) Management's expert—An individual or organization possessing expertise in a field other than accounting or auditing, whose work in that field is used by the entity to assist the entity in preparing the financial statements.

Nature, Timing, and Extent of Audit Procedures

8. The nature, timing, and extent of the auditor's procedures with respect to the requirements in paragraphs 9–13 of this CAS will vary depending on the circumstances. In determining the nature, timing, and extent of those procedures, the auditor shall consider matters including (Ref: Para. A10)
   (a) The nature of the matter to which that expert's work relates;
   (b) The risks of material misstatement in the matter to which that expert's work relates;
   (c) The significance of that expert's work in the context of the audit;
   (d) The auditor's knowledge of and experience with previous work performed by that expert; and
   (e) Whether that expert is subject to the auditor's firm's quality control policies and procedures. (Ref: Para. A11–A13)

The Competence, Capabilities, and Objectivity of the Auditor's Expert

9. The auditor shall evaluate whether the auditor's expert has the necessary competence, capabilities, and objectivity for the auditor's purposes. In the case of an auditor's external expert, the evaluation of objectivity shall include inquiry regarding interests and relationships that may create a threat to that expert's objectivity. (Ref: Para. A14–A20)

Obtaining an Understanding of the Field of Expertise of the Auditor's Expert

10. The auditor shall obtain a sufficient understanding of the field of expertise of the auditor's expert to enable the auditor to (Ref: Para. A21–A22)
    (a) Determine the nature, scope, and objectives of that expert's work for the auditor's purposes; and
    (b) Evaluate the adequacy of that work for the auditor's purposes.

Source: *CPA Canada Handbook—Assurance*, 2014.

Take note of the following details related to auditors' observation of physical inventory taking. The first task is to review the auditee's inventory-taking instructions. The instructions should include the following:

- Names of auditee personnel responsible for the count
- Dates, times, and locations of inventory taking
- Names of auditee personnel who will participate in the inventory taking
- Instructions for recording accurate descriptions of inventory items, for count and double count, and for measuring or translating physical quantities (such as counting by measures of litres, barrels, metres, dozens)
- Instructions for making notes of obsolete or worn items

- Instructions for the use of tags, cards, count sheets, or other media devices, and for their collection and control
- Plans for shutting down plant operations or for taking inventory after store closing hours, and plans for having goods in proper places (such as on store shelves instead of on the floor, or in a warehouse rather than in transit to a job)
- Plans for counting or controlling movement of goods in receiving and shipping areas if those operations are not shut down during the count
- Instructions for recording cutoff information, such as document numbers and details relating to last shipments and last receipts of inventory at period-end
- Instructions for compilation of the count information (such as computer processing of scanned codes, or manual input of tags or count sheets) into final inventory listings or summaries
- Instructions for pricing the inventory items
- Instructions for review and approval of the inventory count and notations of obsolescence or other matters by supervisory personnel

These instructions characterize a well-planned counting operation. As the plan is carried out, the independent auditors should be present to hear the count instructions being given to the auditee's count teams and to observe the instructions being followed.

Many physical inventories are counted at year-end when the auditor is present to observe. The auditor can perform *two-direction testing* by (1) selecting inventory items from a perpetual inventory master file and going to the location to obtain a test count, which produces evidence for the existence assertion, and (2) selecting inventory from locations on the warehouse floor, obtaining a test count, and tracing the count to the final inventory compilation, which produces evidence for the completeness assertion. If the company does not have perpetual records and a file to test for existence, the auditor must be careful to obtain a record of all the counts and to use it for the existence-direction tests.

However, other situations, as described below, frequently occur.

Physical Inventory Not Taken on Period-End Date

Auditees sometimes count the inventory on a date other than the balance sheet date. The auditor observes this count, following the same procedures as for a period-end count. For the period between the count date and the balance sheet date, additional roll-forward or rollback auditing procedures must be performed on inventory purchase (increasing) and issue (decreasing) transactions during that period. The inventory on the count date is

---

Standards Check

CAS 501 Audit Evidence—Specific Considerations for Selected Items

5. If physical inventory counting is conducted at a date other than the date of the financial statements, the auditor shall, in addition to the procedures required by paragraph 4, perform audit procedures to obtain audit evidence about whether changes in inventory between the count date and the date of the financial statements are properly recorded. (Ref: Para. A9–A11)

A11. Relevant matters for consideration when designing audit procedures to obtain audit evidence about whether changes in inventory amounts between the count date, or dates, and the final inventory records are properly recorded include
   - Whether the perpetual inventory records are properly adjusted.
   - Reliability of the entity's perpetual inventory records.
   - Reasons for significant differences between the information obtained during the physical count and the perpetual inventory records.

Source: *CPA Canada Handbook—Assurance,* 2014.

reconciled to the period-end inventory by appropriate addition or subtraction of the receiving and issue transactions that have occurred in the roll-forward or rollback period.

Cyclical Inventory Counting

Some companies count inventory on a cyclical basis but never take a complete count on a single date. Businesses that count inventory this way claim that they have accurate perpetual records and that they carry out the counting as a means of testing the records and maintaining their accuracy. In these cases, the auditors must understand management's counting plan and evaluate its appropriateness, and they should attend and perform tests whenever the value of inventory to be counted is material. They must be present during some counting operations to evaluate the counting plans and their execution. The procedures listed above for an annual count are used, test counts are made, and the audit team forms a conclusion concerning the accuracy (control) of perpetual records.

Auditors Not Present at Auditee's Inventory Count

It might happen on a first audit that the audit firm is appointed after the beginning inventory has already been counted. The auditors should still review the auditee's plan for the already completed count. Some test counts of current inventory should be made and traced to current records to form a conclusion about the reliability of perpetual records. If the actual count was recent, intervening transaction activity may be tested and reconciled back to the beginning inventory.

However, it may be very difficult to reconcile more than a few months' transactions to an unobserved beginning inventory. Auditors may use the interrelationships between sales activity, physical volume, price variation, standard costs, and gross profit margins to form a conclusion about the reasonableness of the beginning inventory. This must be done very carefully, and, if the auditors cannot satisfy themselves as to the beginning inventory balance, a modification in the auditor's report is normally called for (CAS 510).

Standards Check

CAS 501 Audit Evidence—Specific Considerations for Selected Items

6. If the auditor is unable to attend physical inventory counting due to unforeseen circumstances, the auditor shall make or observe some physical counts on an alternative date, and perform audit procedures on intervening transactions.

7. If attendance at physical inventory counting is impracticable, the auditor shall perform alternative audit procedures to obtain sufficient appropriate audit evidence regarding the existence and condition of inventory. If it is not possible to do so, the auditor shall modify the opinion in the auditor's report in accordance with CAS 705. (Ref: Para. A12–A14)

Source: *CPA Canada Handbook—Assurance*, 2014.

Inventories Located off the Auditee's Premises

The auditors must determine the locations and values of inventories that are located off the auditee's premises, perhaps in the custody of consignees or in public warehouses. If amounts are material and control is not exceptionally strong, the audit team may visit these locations and conduct onsite test counts. However, if amounts are not material or related evidence (periodic reports, cash receipts, receivables records, shipping records) is adequate and control risk is low, then direct confirmation with the inventory custodian may be sufficient appropriate evidence of existence (CAS 501).

INVENTORY COUNT AND MEASUREMENT CHALLENGES	
EXAMPLES	**CHALLENGES**
Lumber	Identifying quality or grade
Piles of sugar, coal, scrap steel	Need for geometric computations, aerial photos
Items weighed on scales	Accuracy of scales
Bulk materials (oil, grain, chemicals, liquids in storage tanks)	Dipping measuring rods into tanks Sample for assay or chemical analysis
Diamonds, jewellery	Identification and quality determination Need for an expert
Pulp wood	Quantity measurement estimation Need for aerial photos
Livestock	Movement not controllable (count critters' legs and divide by four—two for chickens)

Source: Adapted from CICA, Audit of Inventories, *Auditing Procedure Study* (1986), p. 28.

Summary: Inventory Observation

The physical observation procedures are designed to audit for existence and completeness (physical quantities) and also to provide support for audit valuation procedures (e.g., recalculation of appropriate FIFO, weighted average, specific item, or other pricing at cost, and evaluation of lower-of-cost-and-net-realizable-value write-down of obsolete or damaged inventory). After the observation is complete, auditors should have sufficient appropriate evidence of physical quantities and valuations to ensure the inventory compilation includes goods (a) owned, on hand, and counted; (b) owned but not on hand (consigned out or stored in outside warehouses); and (c) in transit (purchased and recorded but not yet received, or shipped FOB destination but not yet delivered to customers). The inventory compilation should exclude goods (a) in the perpetual records but not owned; (b) on hand, already sold, but not yet delivered; and (c) on hand but not owned (consigned in).

Review Checkpoints

12-27   In the review of an auditee's inventory-taking instructions, what characteristics are the auditors looking for?

12-28   Explain two-direction sampling in the context of inventory test counts.

12-29   What procedures are followed to audit inventory when the physical inventory is taken on a cyclical basis or on a statistical plan but never as a complete count on a single date?

Special Note: Audit of Property, Plant, and Equipment and Intangible Assets

LO5   Explain the main auditing procedures used for property, plant, and equipment and intangible assets.

PPE and intangible assets are the long-term assets used in an entity's operations. To be considered assets, they must be controlled by the entity and be expected to provide future economic benefits to it. PPE include land, buildings, equipment, vehicles, computers, leasehold improvements, and other physical types of assets. PPE are also called "fixed assets." Intangible assets are identifiable non-monetary assets, such as patents, licences, copyrights, trademarks, application software, development costs, and customer lists, that do not have a physical substance. The risks, controls, and audit procedures required to respond to the risks in the assertions of PPE and intangible assets are outlined in this section.

Risks and Controls

Generally, the existence, completeness, and ownership assertions for PPE are likely to have a low assessed risk of misstatement and will be fairly straightforward to verify, since reliable evidence that is relevant to these assertions is usually available, as is introduced below. Since acquisitions of PPE tend to be infrequent, non-routine, high-value transactions, they will have senior management approval requirements. Due to their special nature, PPE purchase transactions may be processed separately from the main purchasing process, but for study purposes we include the audit of PPE in this chapter. For intangible assets, the existence assertion tends to have a high risk, as it can be complex to determine whether a particular expenditure meets the definition of an intangible asset under generally accepted accounting principles (GAAP) (e.g., *CPA Canada Accounting Handbook*, Part II, section 3064, or IFRS/IAS 38).

Valuation can be a very high risk assertion and challenging to verify, as there are many allocations and estimates involved. Presentation can also be a challenging assertion to verify when complex assets are acquired with multiple components that need to be classified separately, or as bundled purchases of different types of assets. PPE and intangible assets with definite lives are initially recorded at their acquisition costs and then amortized to expense over their expected useful lives. Intangible assets with indefinite lives are not amortized but are tested periodically for value impairment. Due to these assets' long lives, a number of valuation changes can occur over time. Thus, there is a high degree of complexity involved in applying GAAP for subsequent measurement, amortization, and recording of impairment losses.

Recall that the valuation assertion mainly concerns whether the monetary amount included in financial statements complies with the applicable financial reporting principles. For example, under International Financial Reporting Standards (IFRS) (IAS 16 and IAS 38), management can choose the traditional cost model or a revaluation model based on fair value estimates, indicating the complexity of valuation for PPE and intangible assets. Also, if market conditions or production technologies change over time, an asset's value may become impaired, requiring a write-down to be recorded. A further complexity arises if the company has an obligation to restore the property to its original condition at the end of its useful life, to remove any environmental damage created during its operation, for example, for mining or oil extraction. In this case an asset retirement obligation must be estimated based on the present value of the expected future costs, and this amount is included in the value of the depreciable PPE. Overall, the accounting choices available within GAAP, and the subjective kinds of information used, can open the door for management bias in coming up with estimates. Also, the amounts invested in these long-lived operating assets can be quite large. These factors can often lead to the risk of material misstatement for the valuation assertion being high for PPE and intangible assets. As discussed earlier on the subject of auditing the valuation of unusual types of inventory, auditors may also need to rely on experts in asset valuation, engineering, or other sciences for evidence related to complex types of PPE and intangibles.

The main presentation issues are to ensure that management's accounting policies for PPE are appropriate and fully disclosed, and that the categories and appropriate monetary values of PPE elements are presented in the balance sheet and notes in accordance with the applicable financial reporting framework. Disclosures are required of the details and assumptions of the various valuation tests and models used. Auditors need to verify that these are in accordance with GAAP, and more important, that these GAAP methods match what management actually used to come up with its numbers. Much of this information involves estimates, and Chapter 19 (available on Connect) elaborates on the audit considerations related to obtaining reasonable assurance on accounting estimates, which can bear a high level of accounting risk. The box below provides examples of accounting policy disclosures for PPE and intangibles from various Canadian public companies' audited financial statements, to give you a sense of the complexity and estimations involved.

Examples of Public Companies' Accounting Policy Notes for Property, Plant, and Equipment and Intangible Assets

Note 2: Summary of Significant Accounting Policies

2(g) Property, plant, and equipment

Production equipment, office equipment, and computer software and equipment are stated at cost less accumulated depreciation and accumulated impairment losses. Depreciation of these assets, on the same basis as other property assets, commences when the assets are ready for their intended use.

Pre-production costs relating to installations of major new production equipment are expensed in the period in which they occurred.

Depreciation is recognized so as to write off the cost of assets less their residual values over their useful lives, using the straight-line method. The estimated useful lives, residual values, and depreciation method are reviewed at each year-end, with the effect of any changes in estimate accounted for on a prospective basis.

ASSET	BASIS	PERIOD
Buildings	Straight-line	20–40 years
Equipment	Straight-line	4–20 years
Production equipment	Straight-line	10–20 years
Office equipment	Straight-line	5 years
Computer software and equipment	Straight-line	3 years

Leasehold improvements are amortized on a straight-line basis over the lesser of the terms of the leases or their useful lives.

Effective January 1, 20X0, the Company revised the estimated useful life of its production equipment from 10 and 15 years to 20 years. The changes in estimates, which were applied prospectively, resulted in a reduction in depreciation of $2,126,000 ($2,017,000) for the year ended December 31, 20X1 (20X0).

When parts of an item of plant and equipment have different useful lives, they are accounted for as separate items (major components). The cost of replacing a component of an item of plant and equipment is recognized in the carrying amount of the item if it is probable that the future economic benefits of the item will occur and its cost can be measured reliably. The costs of day-to-day maintenance of plant and equipment are recognized directly in the statement of income.

An item of property, plant, and equipment is de-recognized upon disposal, or when no future economic benefits are expected to arise from the continued use of the asset. The gain or loss arising on the disposal or retirement of an item of property, plant, and equipment is determined as the difference between the sales proceeds and the carrying amount of the asset and is recognized in profit or loss.

When the Company has a legal right or constructive obligation to restore a site on which an asset is located either through make-good provisions in lease agreements or decommissioning of environmental risks, the present value of the estimated costs of dismantling and removing the asset and restoring the site are included in the carrying value of the asset with a corresponding increase to provisions. Borrowing costs directly attributable to the acquisition, construction, or production of qualifying property, plant, and equipment that takes an extended period of time to be placed into service are added to the cost of the assets, until such time as the assets are substantially ready for their intended use.

2(h) Assets under finance lease

Assets held under finance leases are depreciated over their expected useful lives on the same basis as owned assets or, where shorter, the term of the relevant lease.

2(i) Impairment

At each reporting date, or sooner if there is an indication that an asset may be impaired, the Company reviews the carrying amounts of its assets to determine whether there is any indication that those assets have suffered an impairment loss. If any such indication exists, the recoverable amount of the asset is estimated in order to determine the extent of the impairment loss (if any).

The recoverable amount is the higher of fair value less costs to sell and value in use. In assessing value in use, the estimated future cash flows are discounted to their present value using a pretax discount rate that reflects current market

(continued)

assessments of the time value of money and the risks specific to the assets for which the estimates of future cash flows have not been adjusted. If the recoverable amount of the assets is estimated to be less than their carrying amount, the carrying amount is reduced to the recoverable amount.

An impairment loss is recognized immediately in profit or loss.

Where an impairment loss subsequently reverses, the carrying amount of the assets is increased to the revised estimate of its recoverable amount, but such that the increased carrying amount does not exceed the carrying amount that would have been determined had no impairment loss been recognized for the asset in prior years. A reversal of an impairment loss is recognized immediately in profit or loss.

2(j) Grants and investment tax credits

Grants and investment tax credits are accounted for using the cost reduction method and are amortized to earnings as a reduction of depreciation, using the same rates as those used to depreciate the related property, plant, and equipment.

2(k) Intangible assets

Intangible assets consist primarily of customer relationships and client lists, application software, and favourable leases. They are recorded at cost less accumulated amortization and impairment losses and amortized on a straight-line basis, over the estimated useful lives as follows:

Patents	Between 2 and 17 years
Customer relationships and client lists	Between 2 and 30 years
Application software	Between 3 and 10 years
Favourable leases	Term of the lease
Other	Between 2 and 20 years

Expenditure on research activities is recognized as an expense in the period in which it is incurred.

The main financial controls of concern in this area relate to authorization of acquisitions, proper classification of assets and expenses, accuracy of the depreciation calculations and recording, and application of appropriate revaluation or impairment testing procedures. In larger organizations with many different types of fixed assets, the information system will likely have a specialized subledger module for keeping the details and integrating the summary data with the general ledger system. In smaller entities, the details may be kept in a separate schedule, often a spreadsheet, which is used to update general ledger balances through manual journal entries. A further complication is that the tax values of assets can differ from their accounting values when companies choose depreciation accounting policies that differ from those prescribed for income tax purposes (i.e., capital cost allowance, or CCA). Such differences necessitate a separate tax-based schedule of asset values and also give rise to deferred tax balances for accounting purposes in some financial reporting frameworks (which also need to be audited!).

Currently, most companies continue to use the cost basis for capital assets, and that will be the main focus of the following discussion. Generally, the assets are initially recorded at cost and then the cost is allocated by depreciation (or amortization) expense to periods of use over the life of the assets. Depreciation and amortization allocation approaches are designed to allocate costs systematically to the accounting periods in which their benefits are consumed, which results in a smoother income measure. While these allocations are estimates, approaches used have been well accepted for many decades. Still, these are important and often material estimates, and like all management estimates, the risk of management bias must always be kept in mind by auditors. Be on the lookout for questionable changes to useful lives or depreciation methods, improper cost capitalization, idle assets still on the books, or estimates based on unreasonable assumptions. See, for example, item 2(g) in the box above; the auditors need to determine if this is a reasonable change.

Exhibit 12–10 shows a typical continuity schedule used to keep track of details underlying the valuation of PPE and intangible assets. Often, management will prepare this type of schedule for its own control purposes,

EXHIBIT 12–10

Example of Continuity Schedule Working Paper for Property, Plant, and Equipment and Intangible Assets

AUDITEE:	EcoPak Inc.	FILE INDEX:	W-10
FINANCIAL STATEMENT PERIOD:	y/e December 31, 20X1		

Prepared by	Reviewed by
O.S.	D.E.
Date Mar 11, 20X2	Date Mar. 20, 20X2

LONG-LIVED ASSETS CONTINUITY SCHEDULE

ASSET CATEGORY	W/P REF.	COST Balance Dec. 31, 20X0	Additions	Disposals	Balance Dec. 31, 20X1	ACC. DEPR/AMORT. Balance Dec. 31, 20X0	Depreciation/ Amortization	Disposals	Impairment	Balance Dec. 31, 20X1	NET BOOK VALUE Dec. 31, 20X1	NET BOOK VALUE Dec. 31, 20X0	
PROPERTY, PLANT, & EQUIPMENT													
LAND	W-20	250,650	0	0	250,650	0	0	0	0	0	250,650	250,650	[t]
BUILDING	W-20	760,321	0	0	760,321	608,257	30,413	0	0	638,670	121,651	152,064	[t]
PRODUCTION MACHINERY - LINE 1	W-30	2,950,550	0	500,563	2,449,987	1,475,275	244,999	250,282	579,995	2,049,987	400,000	1,475,275	[t]
PRODUCTION MACHINERY - LINE 2	W-30	148,808	2,980,311	0	3,129,119	0	312,912	0	0	312,912	2,816,207	148,808	[t]
COMPUTER EQUIPMENT	W-30	88,501	22,544	15,000	96,045	59,738	21,130	15,000	0	65,868	30,177	28,763	[t]
TOTALS		4,198,830	3,002,855	515,563	6,686,122	2,143,270	609,453	265,282	579,995	3,067,437	3,618,685	2,055,560	[t]
INTANGIBLE ASSETS													
PATENT	W-10	40,260	0	0	40,260	2,368	2,368	0	0	4,736	35,524	37,892	[t]
PRODUCTION SOFTWARE	W-20	0	165,892	0	165,892	0	16,178	0	0	16,178	149,714	0	[t]
CUSTOMER RELATED SOFTWARE	W-20	111,996	0	0	111,996	47,998	190,393	0	0	238,391	(126,395)	63,998	[t]
TOTALS		152,256	165,892	0	318,148	50,367	208,940	0	0	259,306	58,842	101,889	[t]
		[a] [tb]	[e]	[f]	[c]	[a] [tb]	[g] *	[f]	[h]	[d]	[d]	[a] [tb]	

AUDIT VERIFICATION SUMMARY: Based on the Audit Programs filed at W-100 and V-100 [g]

[a] Agreed to prior year's financial statement audit file.

[tb] Agreed to prior-year financial statements.

[c] Agreed to general ledger account balance.

[d] Footed: Recalculated totals and cross totals - all are correct.

[e] Additions verified on W-31 and V-21 by vouching a sample of additions to valid supporting payments and proper account allocations.
- Conclusion is that amounts are valid, complete, accurate, authorized, and properly classified.

[f] Disposals verified on W-32, by vouching amounts to documentation of sale or scrap, recalculation of cost and accumulated depreciation amounts removed from the accounts, and inquiries of management regarding reasons.
- Conclusion is disposal amounts are valid, complete, accurate, authorized, and properly classified.

[g] Depreciation and amortization calculations verified on W-40 and V-30 by recalculation, agreeing rates and methods to stated management accounting policies, and assessing reasonability based on asset types and industry practices.

*There is a misstatement in the amortization expense for the addition to production software. The bookkeeper recorded $17,000 because the software was put into operation in November. However, the CFO notes their usual policy is to record no amortization in first year of use. This $17,000 overstatement carried forward to the Summary of Accumulated Misstatements for management decision on correcting journal entry. See W/P# 335.
- Except for the error in amortization calculation, my conclusion is depreciation and amortization expenses are reasonable.

[h] Impairment testing reviewed on W-50—the value-in-use of the old production line has declined and it is being phased out as the new line is more efficient. Impairment testing discussed with management. Only production line I found to be potentially impaired. Management's estimation methods and assumptions reviewed. Estimation method and assumptions discussed and assessed with G&M's valuation expert, P. Enge, and found to be reasonable.
- Conclusion is impairment value estimate appears to be within a reasonable range and is not materially misstated. No other assets found to be impaired.

[t] Audited balances carried forward to final financial statement and notes worksheet at 120.

and the auditors can use it as a working paper on which to summarize their verification work and conclusions. An example of the audit work related to impairment testing and recognized impairment losses is shown in item [h] of the Audit Verification Summary at the bottom of Exhibit 12–10.

Examples of the main audit procedures applied to PPE and intangible assets are set out in the audit program in Exhibit 12–9. Note that the analytical procedures involve study of industry trends, business strategy, changes in products or production methods, and changes in sales volumes, as these can have an impact on the recoverability of the company's investments in its long-term operating assets. Control tests are generally performed in the underlying purchases, payments, and payments cycle, though controls specific to these account balances may also be identified and considered for reliance, particularly when there are many different individual assets to keep track of. Substantive procedures include physical inspection and inspection of documents, recalculation, and use of experts regarding valuation if it is complex and specialized. Inquiry is an important source of evidence for evaluating completeness, as well as aspects of valuation that may relate to management's intended use of various operating assets, but corroborating documentation-based evidence is also crucial.

Summary

The special note outlines some standard procedures used to obtain evidence about the existence, completeness, and ownership assertions, as well as the cost allocation aspect of the valuation assertions for PPE. The fair value aspect of valuation assertion risk relating to complexity of components; fair value option under IFRS IAS 16; and estimation bias, which is difficult to debate due to subjectivity of the allocations, are challenging issues the auditing profession is currently grappling with.

Review Checkpoints

12-30   Explain why the valuation assertion often has a high risk of misstatement for PPE and intangible assets.

12-31   What is the purpose of a continuity schedule for PPE and intangibles in audit working papers?

Special Note: The Completeness Assertion for Liabilities

LO6   Explain the importance of the completeness assertion for auditing the accounts payable liabilities, and the procedures used to search for unrecorded liabilities.

When considering assertions and obtaining evidence about accounts payable and other liabilities, auditors must emphasize the completeness assertion. In contrast, for asset accounts the emphasis is on the existence and ownership assertions. This is necessary because companies are typically less concerned about timely recording of expenses and liabilities than they are about timely recording of revenues and assets. Also, management may have incentives to understate liabilities and expenses to show more favourable performance or financial position than is really the case. Of course, GAAP fair presentation requires timely accrual of liabilities and their associated expenses.

Evidence verifying the completeness assertion is more difficult to find than for the existence assertion. Auditors cannot rely entirely on a management assertion of completeness, even with a favourable assessment of control risk. Substantive procedures, tests of details, or analytical procedures should also provide corroborating evidence. The **search for unrecorded liabilities** is a set of procedures designed to yield audit evidence of

search for unrecorded liabilities:
a set of procedures for inspecting documents and records in the period following the audit client's balance sheet date designed to yield audit evidence of liabilities relating to the current period that were omitted, thus violating the completeness assertion

liabilities that were not recorded in the reporting period. This search should normally be performed up to the audit report date in the period following the auditee's balance sheet date.

The following list of procedures is useful in the search for unrecorded liabilities. The audit objective is to search all the places where there might be evidence of them, and if none are revealed, it is reasonable to conclude that all material liabilities were recorded.

Trade payables	• Study the accounts payable trial balance for dates showing fewer payables than are usually recorded near the year-end, evidence that invoices aren't being recorded. • Confirm accounts payable with suppliers, especially regular suppliers showing small or zero balances in the year-end accounts payable. (Suppliers' monthly statements controlled by the auditors may also be used.) Verify supplier addresses so confirmations will not be misdirected—perhaps deliberately. • List the unmatched supplier invoices. From the unmatched receiving report file and receiving reports prepared after year-end, determine when the goods were received. Determine which invoices, if any, should be recorded. • Trace the unmatched receiving reports to accounts payable entries, and determine if any recorded in the next accounting period need to be reported in the current accounting period under audit. • Vouch a sample of payments from the accounting period following the balance sheet date against supporting documents (invoice, receiving report) to determine if the related liabilities were recorded in the proper accounting period. Select the sample from the post-year-end cutoff bank statement to audit the cash balance. • Scan the open purchase order file at year-end for purchase commitments at fixed prices. From current prices, determine if any adjustments for loss and liability are needed due to unrecorded losses on forward purchase contracts.
Accrued liabilities	• A checklist of accrued expenses will help determine whether the company has been conscientious in expense and liability accruals, including accruals for wages, interest, utilities, sales and excise taxes, payroll taxes, income taxes, real property taxes, rent, sales commissions, royalties and warranties, and guarantee expense.
Taxes payable	• Inspect Canada Revenue Agency notices of assessment, which may contain evidence of income or other taxes in dispute that may need to be recorded as liabilities.
Unearned revenues	• When auditing the details of sales revenue, the terms of sale will help determine if any amounts should be deferred as unearned revenue. (Initial information is gained by inquiries to management about terms of sale, such as customers' rights of cancellation or return.)
Contingent liabilities	• Review responses from the auditee's lawyers to requests for information about pending or threatened litigation and about unasserted claims and assessments. These may indicate a need for contingent liability accruals or disclosures. (CAS 501 requires that inquiry letters prepared by the auditee be sent to the auditee's lawyers, requesting a response directly to the auditors.) • A schedule of casualty insurance on fixed assets is used to determine the adequacy of insurance in relation to asset market values. Inadequate insurance and self-insurance create risks that should be disclosed in the notes to the financial statements.
Long-term debt	• Trace liabilities reported by financial institutions to the accounts. (See the bank confirmation.) Since a bank may not report all auditee liabilities to auditors, other corroborating evidence for possible unrecorded debts should also be obtained. • Review terms of any debt due within one year but classified long term because the company plans to refinance it on a long-term basis. This cannot be based on management's intent; debtholders or financial institutions must have shown in writing a willingness to refinance the debt before it can be classified long term.
General analysis	• Apply analytical procedures appropriate in the circumstances. In general, accounts payable volume and period-end balances should increase when the company increases physical production volume or engages in inventory stockpiling. Some liabilities may be related to other activities; for example, sales taxes are functionally related to sales dollar totals, payroll taxes to payroll totals, excise taxes to sales dollars, and volume and income taxes to income. • Confirm life insurance policies with insurance companies to ask whether the company has any loans against the cash value of the insurance. Also request the names of the beneficiaries of the policies. If a party other than the company benefits from the insurance, inquire about the business purpose of making insurance proceeds payable to other parties. The other party may be a creditor on unrecorded loans.

Review Checkpoints

12-32 Describe the purpose of and give examples of audit procedures in the search for unrecorded liabilities.

12-33 Explain the difference in approach between confirmation of accounts receivable and confirmation of accounts payable.

12-34 In substantive auditing, why is the emphasis on the completeness assertion for liabilities instead of on the existence assertion, as in the audit of assets?

APPLICATION CASE WITH SOLUTION & ANALYSIS

Detecting Misstatements in the Purchases, Payables, and Payments Process

INTRODUCTION

In this Application Case, we will demonstrate tests of controls and substantive audit procedures in the evidence-gathering process related to purchases, payables, and payments. The case situation for each audit presented parallels the framework shown in Chapter 11's Application Case. It provides context for the auditing decisions, rather than presenting a list of detection procedures in the abstract. Lists of a selection of control tests are found in Appendix 12A, and selected detailed substantive procedures for payables and payments processes are found in the examples of substantive audit programs provided in the chapter.

DISCUSSION CASE

As Jack told the new junior auditors his stories about revenue-related misstatements, Syed, one of the audit firm's senior partners, joined in the conversation: "You really have had an interesting first year, Jack! Most people don't see two frauds and a material cutoff error in their first year on the audit trail. Next year you will move on to auditing more complex areas, such as accounts payable and inventory. So, let me tell you some of the stories I have seen over many years in auditing. In some ways, fraud and other misstatements are even more likely in the purchases, payables, and payments process than in revenues. This is not only because there are complex accounts involved but also because the main business purpose of the auditee's purchasing process is to move cash out of the organization. That means errors often result in cash outflows. Also, it can be easier to subvert the process fraudulently, and harder for management controls and auditors to detect it. One thing you will notice early on is that well-managed organizations tend to have the strongest controls in this part of their accounting system. But here are four stories of misstatements that I or my colleagues have experienced in practice. The first one involves an employee fraud in the cash payment process, the second is a supplier overcharging situation, the third is an inventory valuation scam by employees, and the fourth is a misstatement due to management's misestimating forecasts used to calculate amortization expense."

AUDIT 12.1 Copying Money

CASE DESCRIPTION

Argus Productions Inc. (Argus) is a motion picture and commercial production company. Improper expenditures for copy services were charged to production costs by an employee, Welby, who had the power to perform incompatible functions in the purchases, payables, and payments process. Because of his authority at Argus, over a period of five years, Welby was able to conduct a fraud that brought him $475,000 in false and inflated billings. (During this period, Argus's net income was understated a modest amount because copying costs were capitalized as part of production costs and then amortized over a two- to three-year period.)

Argus management had assigned Welby authority and responsibility for obtaining copies of scripts used in production. Established procedures permitted Welby to arrange for outside script-copying services, receive the copies, and approve the bills for payment. In effect, Welby was both the purchasing department and the receiving department for this particular service. To a certain extent, Welby was also the accounting department because he approved the bills for payment and coded them for assignment to projects. Welby did not make the actual accounting entries or sign the cheques.

Welby set up a fictitious company under the registered name of Quickprint Company with himself as the incorporator and shareholder. The company had a post office box number, letterhead stationery, and nicely printed invoices, but no printing equipment. Copy services were subcontracted by Quickprint to real printing businesses, which billed Quickprint. Welby then wrote Quickprint invoices to Argus, billing the production company at the legitimate shop's rate, but for a few extra copies each time. Welby also submitted Quickprint bills to Argus for fictitious copying jobs on scripts for movies and commercials that never went into production. As the owner of Quickprint, Welby endorsed Argus's cheques and deposited the money in the fake copy company's bank account, paid the legitimate printing bills of the subcontractors, and took the rest for personal use.

Audit Trail

Argus's production cost files contained all the Quickprint bills, sorted under the names of the movie and commercial production projects. Welby even created files for proposed films that never went into full production and, thus, should not have had script-copying costs. There were no copying service bills from any shop other than Quickprint.

SOLUTION & ANALYSIS

Audit Approach

Audit Objective

The auditors' objective was to obtain evidence of the valid existence (occurrence) and valuation of copying charges capitalized as film production costs.

Controls Relevant to the Purchasing Process

Authority to request copies and authority for purchasing should be assigned to different employees. The accounting, including the coding of cost assignments to production projects, should also be performed by someone else. A managerial review of production results might cause the excess costs to be noticed.

The request for a particular number of copies of a script should come from someone who knows the number needed. This person should act as the receiving department, signing off on the requested number of copies and the payment. This procedure would prevent waste and excess cost, especially if the requesting person were held responsible for the project's profitability.

Purchasing is always done by a company agent—Welby, in this case. Purchasing agents generally have authority to look for the best service at the best price, with or without bids from competitors. A requirement to obtain bids is usually a good idea, but legitimate purchasing is often done with sole-source suppliers, without bidding. The accounting department should be responsible for coding invoices to the projects, thus making it possible to detect costs charged to projects that are not actually in production. Someone with managerial responsibility should review project costs and the purchasing practices. However, this is an expensive use of executive time. It was not spent in the Argus case, with unfortunate results.

Audit Procedures

Tests of Controls

While gaining their understanding of the control structure at Argus, auditors learned about all the trust and responsibility vested in Welby. The embezzlement was for about $95,000 per year, and total copying costs under Welby were around $1 million—inflating a cost by more than 10% might attract unwanted attention. (Note that the materiality concept even applies to the decisions of fraudsters!)

Company-level controls were very weak, especially in the combination of duties performed by Welby and in the lack of managerial review. For all practical purposes, there were no application controls to test, since the weak company-level controls meant they would not be effective anyway. A test of proper classification to see whether Welby had approved the copying cost invoices and coded them to active projects might have uncovered Welby's payments for copying scripts of movies that never went into production, had these costs been verified against a valid list of authorized projects. Unfortunately, Welby also produced an "authorized production listing" that included the fictitious projects, which the auditors accepted.

Dual-Purpose Procedures

Vouching costs charged to projects against supporting source documents for a sample of movie project files tests the validity of capitalized costs. Tracing a sample of payments to the project cost records is a test of completeness and proper classification of capitalized costs, and, if traced to the approved list of productions, it tests authorization. Since Welby had used convincing falsified documents, these audit procedures might not indicate any control exceptions. This case also illustrates the effect and limitations in audit effectiveness of materiality levels; Welby deliberately kept this fraud below the radar.

Tests of Details of Balance

Substantive procedures are directed toward obtaining evidence about the existence of film projects, the completeness of the costs charged to them, the ownership of copyrights, the valuation of the capitalized project costs, and the proper allocation and disclosure of amortization methods. These key substantive procedures are the same as the test of controls procedures; thus, when performed at the year-end date on the capitalized cost balances, they can be considered as dual-purpose audit procedures.

Any of the procedures described as test of controls procedures should show evidence of projects that had never gone into production. Auditors should be careful to obtain a list of actual projects before they begin the procedures. Chances are high that the discovery of bad project codes with copying cost would reveal a pattern of Quickprint bills.

Knowing that controls over copying costs are weak, auditors could be tipped off to the possibility of a Welby–Quickprint connection. Efforts to locate Quickprint should be made. Inquiry with the provincial Ministry of Commerce for names of the Quickprint incorporators would reveal Welby's connection. The audit findings could then be turned over to a trained investigator to arrange an interview with and confrontation of Welby.

Audit Results

In this case, the manager of production, who was worried about profitability, requested that the internal auditors review project costs. They performed the procedures described above on 100% of the transactions and, thus, noticed the dummy projects and the Quickprint bills, investigated the ownership of Quickprint, and discovered Welby's association. First efforts to locate Quickprint's shop by telephone, chamber of commerce, or other city directories failed. They were careful not to direct any mail to the post office box for fear of alerting the then-unknown parties involved. Through a ruse at the post office, a sly internal auditor had already learned that Welby had rented the box, but they did not know if anyone else was involved. Alerted, the internal auditors gathered all the Quickprint bills and determined, with witnesses, the total charged for non-existent projects. Welby was interviewed by Argus managers and readily confessed.

AUDIT 12.2 Receiving the Missing Oil

CASE DESCRIPTION

Johnson Chemical began a new contract with Madden Oil Distributors to supply fuel oil for the plant generators on a cost-plus contract, for a price of $0.45 per litre. Madden delivered the oil weekly in a 20,000-litre tank truck to Johnson's storage tanks. Because of short shipments by Madden, Johnson's fuel oil supplies inventory and fuel expense were inflated. During the first year, Madden shorted Johnson on quantity by 160,000 litres (loss = 160,000 × $0.45 = $72,000) and charged 5 cents per litre more than competitors (loss = 940,000 litres × $0.05 = $47,000) for a total overcharge of $119,000—not to mention the inferior sludge mix occasionally delivered.

Johnson's receiving employees observed the pumping and recorded the quantity on a receiving report, which was forwarded to the accounts payable department and held pending arrival of Madden's invoice. The quantities received were then compared with the quantities billed by Madden, before the invoice was approved for payment and a cheque prepared for signature by the controller. Since it was a cost-plus contract, Madden's billing price was not checked against any standard price. The receiving employees were rather easily fooled by Madden's driver. He mixed sludge with the oil, but the receiving employees did not take samples to check for quality. He called out Johnson's storage tank content falsely at the beginning (e.g., 4,000 litres on hand when 8,000 were actually in the tank), and the receiving employees did not check the gauge themselves. The tank truck was not weighed at entry and exit to determine the amount delivered. During the winter months, when fuel oil use was high, Madden ran in extra trucks more than once a week, but pumped nothing when the receiving employees were not looking. Quantities "received" and paid during the first year of the contract (in litres) were as follows:

Jan.	124,000	May	72,000	Sept.	84,000
Feb.	112,000	June	56,000	Oct.	92,000
Mar.	92,000	July	60,000	Nov.	132,000
Apr.	76,000	Aug.	56,000	Dec.	144,000

Audit Trail

The receiving reports all agreed with the quantities billed by Madden. Each invoice had a receiving report attached in the Johnson accounts payable files. Even though Madden had many trucks, the same driver always came to the Johnson plant, as evidenced by his signature on the reports (along with the receiving employees' initials). At $0.45 per litre, Madden charged $495,000 for 1,100,000 litres of fuel for the year. The previous year, Johnson paid a total of $360,000 for 900,000 litres, but nobody made a complete comparison with last year's quantity and cost.

SOLUTION & ANALYSIS

Audit Approach

Audit Objective

The auditors' objective was to obtain evidence that all fuel oil billed and paid was actually received in the quality expected, at a fair price.

Controls Relevant to the Process

Receiving employees should be given the tools and techniques they need to do a good job. Scales at the plant entrance could weigh the trucks in and out, determining the amount of fuel delivered. (Mass per litre is a well-known measure.) Sampling for simple chemical analysis would give evidence of the quality of the oil. Receiving employees should be instructed on the importance of their job, to encourage conscientiousness. They should have been instructed to read the storage tank gauges themselves instead of relying on Madden's driver. Lacking these tools and instructions, they were easy marks for the wily driver.

Audit Procedures

Tests of Controls

The information from the "understanding the control structure" phase needs to be very detailed if it is to alert the auditors to the poor receiving practices. Procedures include inquiring with the receiving employees to learn about their practices and work habits. The control procedure supposedly in place was the receiving report on the oil delivered. A control test procedure would be to take a sample of Madden's bills and compare quantities billed with quantities received while verifying the price billed against the contract. Because of the deception by Madden's driver, this would not have shown anything unusual, unless perhaps the auditor became suspicious of the fact that the same driver made all the deliveries.

Tests of Details of Balance

The balances in question are the fuel oil supply inventory and the fuel expense. The inventory is easily audited by reading the tank storage gauge for the quantity. The price is found in Madden's invoices. However, a lower-of-cost-and-market test requires knowledge of market prices for the oil. Since Johnson Chemical apparently has no documentation of competing prices, the auditor will need to research with other oil distributors to get the prices. Presumably, the auditors would learn that the price is approximately $0.40 per litre. The expense balance can be audited like a cost of goods sold amount. With knowledge of the beginning fuel inventory, the quantity "purchased," and the quantity in the ending inventory, the fuel oil expense quantity can be calculated. This expense quantity can be priced at Madden's price per litre.

Substantive Analytical Procedures

Analytical procedures applied to the expense revealed the larger quantities used and the unusual pattern of deliveries, leading to suspicions of Madden and the driver. Aware of the current year's higher expense and the evidence of a lower market price, the auditors obtained the fuel oil delivery records from the prior year. They are shown in the table below. (The numbers in parentheses are the additional litres delivered in the current year.)

Jan.	112,000 (12,000)	May	52,000 (20,000)	Sept.	60,000 (24,000)
Feb.	96,000 (16,000)	June	44,000 (12,000)	Oct.	80,000 (12,000)
Mar.	80,000 (12,000)	July	40,000 (20,000)	Nov.	112,000 (20,000)
Apr.	68,000 (8,000)	Aug.	36,000 (20,000)	Dec.	120,000 (24,000)

Audit Results

Having found a consistent pattern of greater "use" in the current year, with no operational explanation for it, the auditors took to the field. With the cooperation of the receiving employees, the auditors read the storage tank measure before the Madden driver arrived. They hid in an adjoining building to watch (and film) the driver call out an incorrect reading, pump the oil, sign the receiving report, and depart. Then they took samples. These observations were repeated for three weeks. They saw short deliveries, tested inferior products, and built a case against Madden and the driver. Johnson recovered the overcharges from Madden and, of course, immediately switched to a different fuel supplier!

AUDIT 12.3 Retread Tires

CASE DESCRIPTION

Ritter Tire Wholesale Company had a high-volume truck and passenger car tire business in Hamilton, Ontario (area population 500,000). J. Lock, the chief accountant, was a long-time trusted employee who had supervisory responsibility over the purchasing agent as well as general accounting duties. Lock had worked several years as a purchasing agent before moving into the accounting job. Lock carried out a fraudulent scheme for three years, diverting tires that cost Ritter $2.5 million, which Lock then sold for $2.9 million. Inventory and income were overstated by Lock's substitution of the new-tire inventory with lower-quality retread tires, which he valued at new-tire prices. (Lock's cost for retread tires was approximately $500,000.)

Lock often prepared the purchase orders, and the manufacturers were directed to deliver the tires to a warehouse in Milton (a town of 60,000, about 30 kilometres north of Hamilton). Ritter Tire received the manufacturers' invoices, which Lock approved for payment. Lock and an accomplice (his brother-in-law) sold the tires from the Milton warehouse and pocketed the money. At night, Lock moved cheaper retread tires into the Ritter warehouse so the space would not be empty. As chief accountant, Lock could override controls (e.g., approving invoices for payment without a receiving report), and T. Ritter (president) never knew the difference because the cheques presented for her signature were not accompanied by the supporting documents.

Audit Trail

Ritter Tire's files were well organized. Each cheque copy had supporting documents attached (invoice, receiving report, purchase order), except for the misdirected tire purchases, which had no receiving reports. These purchase orders were all signed by Lock, and the shipping destination on them was the Milton address. There were no purchase requisition documents because "requisitions" were in the form of verbal requests from salespeople. There was no paper evidence of the retread tires because Lock simply bought them elsewhere and moved them in at night when nobody was around.

SOLUTION & ANALYSIS

Audit Approach

Audit Objective

The auditors' objective was to obtain evidence of the existence and valuation of the inventory. (President Ritter engaged external auditors for the first time in the third year of Lock's scheme, after experiencing a severe cash squeeze.)

Controls Relevant to the Process

Competent personnel should perform the purchasing function. Lock and the other purchasing agents were competent and experienced. They prepared purchase orders, required by manufacturers for shipment, authorizing the purchase of tires. A receiving department prepared a receiving report, after counting and inspecting each shipment, by filling in the "quantity column" on a copy of the purchase order. (A common receiving report is a "blind" purchase order that has all the purchase information except the quantity, which the receiving department fills in after an independent inspection and count.) Receiving personnel made notes if the tires showed blemishes or damage. As chief accountant, Lock approved invoices from the manufacturers for payment after comparing the quantities with the receiving report and the prices with the purchase order. The cheques for payment were produced on the computerized accounting system when Lock entered the invoice payable in the system. The computer software did not void transactions without a receiving report reference because many expenses legitimately had no receiving reports. The key weaknesses in the control structure are that (1) no one on the accounting staff has the opportunity to notice missing receiving reports for invoices that should have had them, and (2) Ritter has no supporting documents when cheques are signed. Lock is a trusted employee.

Audit Procedures

Tests of Controls

Because the control procedures for cross-checking the supporting documents were said to be in place, the external auditors could test these controls by the following procedure.

Select a sample of purchases (manufacturers' invoices payable entered in the computer system), and do the following:

1. Study the related purchase order for (a) valid manufacturer name and address; (b) date; (c) delivery address; (d) unit price, with reference to catalogue or price list; (e) correct arithmetic; and (f) approval signature.
2. Compare purchase order information with the manufacturers' invoice.
3. Compare the purchase order and invoice with the receiving report for (a) date, (b) quantity and condition, (c) approval signature, and (d) location.

Tests of Details of Balance

Ritter Tire did not maintain perpetual inventory records, so the inventory was a periodic system—an inventory figure calculated from the annual physical inventory count and costing compilation. The basic audit procedure was to observe the count by taking a sample from different locations on the warehouse floor, recounting the employees' count, controlling the count sheets, and inspecting the tires for quality and condition (related to proper valuation). The auditors kept their own copy of all the count sheets with their test count notes and notes identifying tires as "new" or "retread." (They took many test counts in the physical inventory sample as a result of the test of controls work, described following.)

Audit Results

Forty manufacturers' invoices were selected at random for the test of controls procedure. The auditors were good. They had reviewed the business operations, and Ritter had said nothing about having operations or a warehouse in Milton, although a manufacturer might have been instructed to "drop-ship" tires to a customer there. The auditors noticed three missing receiving reports, all of them with purchase orders signed by Lock and requesting delivery to the same Milton address. They asked Lock about the missing receiving reports, and got this response: "It happens sometimes. I'll find them for you tomorrow." When Lock produced the receiving reports, the auditors noticed these were in a current numerical sequence (although dated much earlier), filled out with the same pen, and signed with an illegible scrawl not matching any of the other receiving reports they had seen.

The auditors knew the difference between new and retread tires when they saw them, and confirmed their observations with employees taking the physical inventory count. When Lock priced the inventory, new-tire prices were used, and the auditors knew the difference.

Ritter took the circumstantial evidence to a trained investigator who interviewed the manufacturers and obtained information about the Milton location. The case against Lock led to criminal theft charges and conviction.

AUDIT 12.4 Amortize the Drum Slowly

CASE DESCRIPTION

Candid Production Company was a major producer of theatrical movies. The company usually had 15 to 20 films in release at theatres across the nation and in foreign countries. Movies also generated revenue through video/DVD licences and product sales (T-shirts, toys, etc.). Over a four-year period, Candid's net asset value (unamortized cost of films) was overstated through taking too little amortization expense: Candid Productions postponed recognition of a $20 million amortization expense, thus inflating assets and income. Movie production costs are capitalized as assets and then amortized to expense as revenue is received from theatre ticket and DVD sales and from other sources of revenue. The amortization depends on the total revenue forecast and the current-year revenue amount. As the success or failure of a movie unfolds at the box office, revenue estimates are revised. (The accounting amortization is similar to depletion of a mineral resource, which depends on estimates of recoverable minerals and current production.)

Candid Production was not too candid: Its recent film, *Bang the Drum Slowly*, was forecast to produce $50 million total revenue over six years, while early box office returns showed only $10 million in the first eight months in the theatres. Revenue usually declines rapidly after initial openings, and DVD and other revenues depend on the box office success of a film. Accounting "control" with respect to film-cost amortization depends on the revenue forecasts, and the revision of them. In this case, these were overly optimistic, showing the expense recognition and overstating assets and income.

Audit Trail

Revenue forecasts are based on many factors, including facts and assumptions about number of theatres, ticket prices, receipt-sharing agreements, domestic and foreign reviews, and moviegoer tastes. Several publications track the box office records of movies. You can see them on entertainment websites, in newspapers, and in the industry trade publications. Of course, the production companies themselves are the major source of the information, and company records do show the revenue realized from each movie. Revenue forecasts can be checked against actual results, and the company's history of forecasting accuracy can be determined by comparing actuals with forecasts over many films and many years.

SOLUTION & ANALYSIS

Audit Approach

Audit Objective

The auditors' objective was to obtain evidence determining if revenue forecasts provide a sufficient basis for calculating film-cost amortization and net asset value of films.

Controls Relevant to the Process

Revenue forecasts need to be prepared by a systematic and methodical process that documents both the facts and the underlying assumptions of the forecast. Forecasts should break down the revenue estimate by years, and the accounting system should produce comparable actual revenue data so that forecast accuracy can be assessed after the fact. Forecast revisions should be prepared with as much detail and documentation as original forecasts.

Audit Procedures

Tests of Controls

The general procedures and methods used by personnel responsible for revenue forecasts should be studied (inquiries and review of documentation), including their sources of information—both internal and external. Procedures for review of mechanical aspects (arithmetic) should be tested by recalculating the final estimates for a sample of finished forecasts. Specific procedures for forecast revision should be studied in the same way. Reviewing the accuracy of the forecasts of other movies against actual revenues helps in a circumstantial way, but past accuracy on different film experiences may not be directly helpful to forecasting for a new, unique product.

Tests of Details of Balance

The audit of amortization expense concentrates on the content of the forecast itself. The forecasts used in the amortization calculation should be studied to distinguish underlying reasonable expectations from hypothetical assumptions. A hypothetical assumption states a condition that is not necessarily expected to occur, but it is nonetheless used to prepare an estimate—an if-then statement. For example, "If *Bang the Drum Slowly* sells 15 million tickets in the first 12 months of release, then domestic revenue and product sales will be $40 million, and foreign revenue can eventually reach $10 million." Auditors need to assess the reasonableness of the 15-million-ticket assumption. It helps to have some early actual data from the film's release in hand before the financial statements need to be finished and distributed. For actual data, industry publications ought to be reviewed, with special attention paid to competing films and critics' reviews (yes, even movie reviews can be useful as audit evidence!).

Audit Results

The auditors were not skeptical enough about the revenue forecasts, and they did not weigh unfavourable actual-to-forecast history comparisons heavily enough. Apparently, they let themselves be convinced by exuberant company executives that the movies were comparable with the blockbuster *Guardians of the Galaxy*. The audit of forecasts and estimates used in accounting determinations are very difficult to arrive at, especially when company personnel have incentives to hype the numbers, seemingly with conviction. The postponed amortization expense finally came home to roost in big write-offs when the company management changed.

Review Checkpoints

12-35 Give some examples of receiving departments in the audit application cases above.

12-36 In Audits 12.1 and 12.3, frauds involving fictitious people, businesses, and locations occurred. Where can auditors obtain information showing whether people, businesses, and locations are real or not?

12-37 How can analysis be used to discover excess costs? (See Audit 12.2.)

12-38 How can analysis be used to discover understated expenses? (See Audit 12.4.)

12-39   Why must auditors understand the physical characteristics of inventoried assets?

12-40   Why is professional skepticism important for auditors? Give two case examples.

12-41   What evidence could the verbal inquiry audit procedure produce in Audits 12.1, 12.2, and 12.3?

SUMMARY

- The purchases, payables, and payments process consists of purchase requisitioning, purchase ordering, receiving goods and services, recording suppliers' invoices, accounting for accounts payable, and making payments of cash. Companies reduce control risk by having a suitable separation of authorization, custody, recording, and periodic reconciliation duties. Error-checking procedures of comparing purchase orders and receiving reports with supplier invoices are important for recording proper amounts of accounts payable liabilities. Supervisory control is provided by separating the duties of preparing cash payment cheques and actually signing them. Otherwise, many things could go wrong, ranging from processing false purchase orders to failing to record liabilities for goods and services received. **LO1**

- Auditors assess the auditee's controls over the purchases, payables, and payments process by evaluating whether the general and environmental controls and application controls effectively reduce the risk of material misstatement in purchasing transactions, accounts payable and other liability balances, and cash payments transactions. They test any key controls that they decide to rely on to reduce substantive testing. **LO2**

- Substantive programs are developed by linking the auditor's risk assessments to the risks of material misstatements in purchasing transactions, accounts payable and other liability balances, and cash payments transactions. The chapter provided examples of typical substantive procedures that would be considered, depending on the risks assessed in each particular case. **LO3**

- Three topics had special technical notes in the chapter, covering some important assertion-based risks and audit approaches. The physical inventory observation audit work was a special section because actual contact with inventories (and fixed assets, for that matter) provides auditors with direct eyewitness evidence of important tangible assets. **LO4** The valuation assertion for property, plant, and equipment (PPE) and intangible assets was discussed in detail, as this is often high risk due to the complexity and subjectivity of the estimates involved in accounting for long-lived assets over the years of use. **LO5** The completeness assertion is very important in the audit of liabilities because misleading financial statements often contain unrecorded liabilities and expenses. The search for unrecorded liabilities is an important set of audit procedures used on all audits. **LO6**

Cash payment is a critical point for asset control. Many cases of embezzlement occur in this process. Illustrative application cases in the chapter told of some embezzlement schemes involving payment of fictitious charges to dummy companies set up by employees. Suggested solutions analyzing these cases give examples of how auditors approached the different situations, and the procedures they used to find the problems.

KEY TERMS

authorization (procedure)

custody

cutoff error

periodic reconciliation (reconciling)

purchase cutoff

recordkeeping (documents and records)

roll-forward period

search for unrecorded liabilities

MULTIPLE-CHOICE QUESTIONS FOR PRACTICE AND REVIEW

MC 12-1 **LO1** When verifying debits to the perpetual inventory records of a non-manufacturing company, an auditor would be most interested in examining a sample of which of these purchasing documents?

a. Approvals
b. Requisitions
c. Invoices
d. Orders

MC 12-2 **LO2** Which of the following is an internal control weakness for a company whose inventory of supplies consists of a large number of individual items?

a. Supplies of relatively little value are expensed when purchased.
b. The cycle basis is used for physical counts.
c. The warehouse manager is responsible for maintenance of perpetual inventory records.
d. Perpetual inventory records are maintained only for items of significant value.

MC 12-3 **LO2** To protect against the preparation of improper or inaccurate cash payments, which effective internal control procedure would be required for all cheques?

a. Signed by an officer after necessary supporting evidence has been examined
b. Reviewed by a senior officer before mailing
c. Sequentially numbered and accounted for by internal auditors
d. Perforated or otherwise effectively cancelled when they are returned with the bank statement

MC 12-4 **LO4** An auditee's purchasing system ends with the recording of a liability and its eventual payment. Which of the following best describes the auditor's primary concern with respect to liabilities resulting from the purchasing system?

a. Accounts payable are not materially understated.
b. Authority to incur liabilities is restricted to one designated person.
c. Acquisition of materials is not made from one supplier or one group of suppliers.
d. Commitments for all purchases are made only after established competitive bidding procedures are followed.

MC 12-5 **LO2** Which of the following is an internal control procedure that would prevent a paid supplier invoice from being presented for payment a second time?

a. Invoices should be prepared by individuals who are responsible for signing payment cheques.
b. Disbursement cheques should be approved by at least two responsible management officials.
c. The date on a supplier invoice should be within a few days of the date it is presented for payment.
d. The official signing the cheque should compare it with the supplier invoice details and stamp "paid" on the invoice.

MC 12-6 **LO3** Which of the following procedures would best detect the theft of valuable items from an inventory that consists of hundreds of different items selling for $1 to $10 and a few items selling for hundreds of dollars?

a. Maintain a perpetual inventory of only the more valuable items with frequent periodic verification of the validity of the perpetual inventory record.
b. Have an independent audit firm prepare an internal control report on the effectiveness of the administrative and accounting controls over inventory.

c. Have separate warehouse space for the more valuable items with frequent periodic physical counts and comparison with perpetual inventory records.

d. Trace items from the physical inventory count to the detailed year-end inventory compilation list.

MC 12-7 **LO2** Budd, the purchasing agent of Lake Hardware Wholesalers, has a relative who owns a retail hardware store. Budd arranged for hardware to be delivered by Lake's suppliers/manufacturers to the relative's retail store on a COD basis, thereby enabling his relative to buy at Lake's wholesale prices. Budd was probably able to accomplish this because of Lake's poor internal control over which of the items listed?

a. Payment cheques

b. Cash receipts

c. Perpetual inventory records

d. Purchase orders

MC 12-8 **LO4** Which of the following is the best audit procedure for determining the existence of unrecorded liabilities?

a. Examine confirmation requests by creditors whose accounts appear on a subsidiary trial balance of accounts payable.

b. Examine a sample of cash payments in the period subsequent to the year-end.

c. Examine a sample of invoices a few days prior to and subsequent to the year-end to ascertain whether they have been properly recorded.

d. Examine unusual relationships between monthly accounts payable and recorded purchases.

MC 12-9 **LO2** When evaluating inventory controls with respect to segregation of duties, which of the following would an auditor be least likely to do?

a. Inspect documents.

b. Make inquiries.

c. Observe procedures.

d. Consider policy and procedure manuals.

MC 12-10 **LO5** An auditor will usually trace the details of the test counts made during the observation of the physical inventory taking for a final inventory compilation. If the sample for the physical observation test counts was chosen from the final inventory schedule, this audit procedure is undertaken to provide evidence that items physically present and observed by the auditor at the time of the physical inventory count are which of the following?

a. Owned by the auditee

b. Not obsolete

c. Physically present at the time of the preparation of the final inventory schedule

d. Included in the final inventory schedule

MC 12-11 **LO5** An auditor will usually trace the details of the test counts made during the observation of the physical inventory taking for a final inventory compilation. If the sample for the physical observation test counts was chosen from the inventory in the physical location, this audit procedure is undertaken to provide evidence that items physically present and observed by the auditor at the time of the physical inventory count are which of the following?

a. Owned by the auditee

b. Not obsolete

c. Physically present at the time of the preparation of the final inventory schedule

d. Included in the final inventory schedule

MC 12-12 `LO4` Which of the following procedures is least likely to be performed before the balance sheet date?

a. Observation of inventory

b. Review of internal control over cash payments

c. Search for unrecorded liabilities

d. Confirmation of receivables

MC 12-13 `LO5` The physical count of inventory of a retailer was higher than shown by the perpetual records. Which of the following could explain the difference?

a. Inventory items had been counted but the tags placed on the items had not been taken off the items and added to the inventory accumulation sheets.

b. Credit memos for several items returned by customers had not been recorded.

c. No journal entry had been made on the retailer's books for several items returned to its suppliers.

d. An item purchased FOB shipping had not arrived at the date of the inventory count and was not reflected in the perpetual records.

MC 12-14 `LO5` From the auditor's point of view, inventory counts are more acceptable prior to the year-end under which of the following circumstances?

a. Internal control is weak.

b. Accurate perpetual inventory records are maintained.

c. Inventory is slow moving.

d. Significant amounts of inventory are held on a consignment basis.

MC 12-15 `LO1` To determine whether accounts payable are complete, an auditor performs a test to verify that all merchandise received is recorded. Which of the following is the population for this test?

a. Suppliers' invoices

b. Purchase orders

c. Receiving reports

d. Cancelled cheques

MC 12-16 `LO2` Which of the following internal control procedures most likely addresses the completeness assertion for inventory?

a. The WIP account is periodically reconciled with subsidiary inventory records.

b. Employees responsible for the custody of finished goods do not perform the receiving function.

c. Receiving reports are prenumbered and the numbering sequence is checked periodically.

d. There is a separation of duties between the payroll department and inventory accounting personnel.

MC 12-17 `LO6` Which of the following is an auditor's objective related to the valuation assertion for the auditee's PPE and intangible assets?

a. Obtain evidence that the auditee has legal rights to its patents.

b. Obtain evidence that the auditee has legal title to the building included in its PPE.

c. Evaluate management's estimate of impairment of its manufacturing equipment.

d. Verify that the auditee's depreciation policies are accurately described in the notes to the financial statements.

EXERCISES AND PROBLEMS

EP 12-1 Liabilities: Authorization Control. `LO1, 2` The essential characteristic of the liabilities control system is to separate the authorization and approval to initiate a transaction from the responsibility for recordkeeping.

Required:

What would constitute the authorization for accounts payable recording? What documentary evidence could auditors examine as evidence of this authorization?

EP 12-2 Cash Payment Transactions: Completeness Control. `LO1, 2` The use of prenumbered documents is an important feature for control to ensure that all valid transactions are recorded and none are omitted.

Required:

How could auditors gather evidence that the control for completeness of cash payments was being used properly by a company?

EP 12-3 Automated Transactions: Authorization Control. `LO1, 2` Two automated transactions can be produced in a computerized accounting system: (1) cheque printing and signature and (2) purchase order at a preprogrammed stock reorder point.

Required:

Assume management is uncomfortable with the computer system automatically creating transactions and would like to add manual controls to authorize the transactions prior to the transaction being processed. How could management delay these transactions until they were reviewed and authorized?

EP 12-4 Liabilities: Insurance Coverage. `LO1`

Required:

Why should auditors be concerned with the adequacy of casualty insurance coverage of an auditee's physical property?

EP 12-5 Inventory: Inquiry-Based Evidence. `LO3, 5`

Required:

What evidence regarding inventories and cost of sales can the auditor typically obtain from inquiry?

EP 12-6 Assessing Specific Risks: Property, Plant, and Equipment. `LO6` Auditors plan their audit procedures to respond to the assessed risks of material misstatements in the financial statements by gathering evidence about management's assertions. Risk assessment involves considering what could go wrong that would lead to a material misstatement for each major account area.

Required:

List 9 or 10 examples of considerations of what could go wrong to indicate the risk of misstatement in PPE and related accounts.

EP 12-7 Repair and Maintenance Auditing. `LO6`

Required:

Why should the repairs and maintenance expense account be audited at the same time as the PPE accounts?

EP 12-8 Property, Plant, and Equipment: Audit Procedures. **LO6** Audit procedures may be classified as follows:

Recalculation/reperformance

Observation

Confirmation

Inquiry

Inspection of documents (vouching, tracing, scanning)

Inspection of physical assets

Analysis

Required:

Describe how each procedure may be used to gather evidence on fixed assets and which broad financial statement assertion(s) (existence, completeness, ownership [rights], valuation [allocation], and presentation and disclosure) are being addressed by the use of the procedure.

EP 12-9 Accounts Payable Internal Control Questionnaire Items: Control Objectives, Test of Controls Procedures, and Possible Errors or Fraud. **LO1, 2** Listed below is a selection of items from the internal control questionnaire on payables in Appendix 12A.

1. Are invoices, receiving reports, and purchase orders reviewed by the cheque signer?
2. Are cheques dated in the cash payments journal with the date of the cheque?
3. Are the quantity and quality of goods received determined at the time of receipt by receiving personnel independent of the purchasing department?
4. Are suppliers' invoices matched against purchase orders and receiving reports before a liability is recorded?

Required:

For each item:

a. Identify the control objective to which it applies.
b. Specify one test of controls audit procedure an auditor could use to determine whether the control was operating effectively.
c. Using your business experience, your logic, your imagination, or all three, give an example of an error or fraud that could occur if the control were absent or ineffective.

EP 12-10 Inventory Count, Measurement. **LO1, 5** Consider the following examples of inventories in various businesses:

1. Pharmaceuticals in a drug company
2. Fine chemical compounds in a biotechnology company
3. Software in an information technology development company
4. New condominium office units in a commercial real estate developer
5. Fine art works in an interior design business

Required:

For each item, indicate the challenges auditors would face in trying to count and measure the inventory, and suggest an approach to obtain sufficient appropriate audit evidence.

EP 12-11 Inventory, Analysis of Gross Margin. **LO3** Li was assigned to work on the audit of A1 Clothing Ltd. because she has been auditing similar companies for three years and is considered to be knowledgeable about the clothing retailing industry in Canada. Her employer, Bing PAs, audited A1 in 20X5 for the first time and had difficulty verifying the opening inventory number. This year, in 20X6, Li has the audited ending balance from 20X5, so she does not expect any problems with the inventory account. However, while doing the preliminary work for the audit, she calculated the gross profit margin and was surprised by her findings. Li thinks the gross margin indicates that the ending inventory for 20X5 may be incorrect.

	20X5	20X6
Sales of clothing	$10,000,000	$9,000,000
Cost of goods sold	7,000,000	5,500,000
Inventory	1,800,000	6,200,000

Required

Explain whether you agree with Li. Support your answer with at least three points.

(Adapted from External Auditing (AU1), June 2011, with permission of Chartered Professional Accountants of Canada, Toronto, Canada. Any changes to the original material are the sole responsibility of the author (and/or publisher) and have not been reviewed or endorsed by Chartered Professional Accountants of Canada.)

EP 12-12 Inventory, Impact of Cutoff Error. **LO3** You are performing the audit of the CXX Limited (CXX) financial statements for its year ended September 30, 20X0. CXX is a private company and operates a grocery distribution business in the Greater Toronto Area. CXX's audited financial statements are used mainly by its bank, which has made a large operating loan to CXX. The bank requires CXX to maintain a quick ratio of at least 1.2, based on its year-end financial statements; otherwise, the bank can require CXX to repay the loan in full immediately.

CXX's accounting policy is to value its inventory based on the FIFO cost flow assumption. On September 30, 20X0, CXX received a large truckload of pomegranate juice from California Fruit Inc. Since these goods were in CXX's warehouse at year-end, they were included in the year-end physical inventory count. During your audit you discovered that the company's accountant did not record this purchase in the accounts payable balance until October 10, 20X0, when an invoice was received from the supplier, California Fruit, in the amount of $65,000.

Before correcting this error, CXX's draft financial statements show inventory of $900,000, total current assets of $1,500,000, accounts payable of $250,000, and total current liabilities of $450,000.

Required:

a. Explain how the accounts in the CXX September 30, 20X0, financial statements will be affected by this error. In your explanation, identify the assertion(s) violated by this error.
b. Give one example of an audit procedure that would have discovered this error. Explain clearly how this procedure could discover the error.
c. What is the impact of this error on CXX's quick ratio? Show calculations.
  Note: Quick ratio = Current assets excluding inventory/Current liabilities.
d. Would you consider this error to be material? Justify your response.

EP 12-13 Property, Plant, and Equipment Audit Evidence and Assertions. **LO3, 6** Alvin is auditing Demure Fashions Inc., a chain of women's clothing stores. Demure operates six stores in shopping malls across the Toronto area and has been an audit client of Alvin's firm for several years. Alvin has been assigned the audit of Demure's store fixtures account. This year the audit partner has instructed Alvin that detection risk for the store fixtures account must be reduced to a very low level because Demure is negotiating new financing that will use the store fixtures as collateral.

Demure's chief accountant has given Alvin a detailed list of all the store fixtures (shelving, clothing display racks, and sales counters) included in Demure's general ledger account. The accounting policy is to record store fixtures at cost, with depreciation recognized using the straight-line method.

On the company's year-end date, January 2, 20X1, Alvin visited all six of the stores, looked at the fixtures in place, and compared them to the descriptions on the list. In eight cases he could not locate the listed fixture and asked the store manager where it was. In every case, the manager said the fixture unit had been placed in storage because it was broken and in need of repair. In one new store, Alvin found nine new clothing racks that were not included on the list. The store manager told him these racks had been purchased a few days before year-end.

Required:

a. Identify three types of audit evidence Alvin has obtained, and explain which assertion(s) this evidence is relevant to.

b. Of the evidence Alvin obtained, which do you think is the most reliable? Why?

c. The procedures described above do not address the valuation assertion for PPE. Explain why these procedures do not address this assertion. Describe one additional procedure Alvin should perform to provide relevant evidence regarding the valuation assertion.

EP 12-14 Audit of Electronics Inventory. `LO1, 2` During his examination of the inventories and related accounts of Consumer Electronics Inc., a manufacturer and distributor of small appliances, an auditor encountered the following:

a. Several trucks loaded with finished goods were parked at the shipping dock. The contents of the trucks were excluded from the physical inventory.

b. The finished goods inventory included high volumes of several products, and many of their cartons were old and covered with dust. In response to the auditor's questions, the plant manager stated that there was no problem as "all of these goods will eventually be sold, although some price incentives may be necessary."

c. While reviewing the complex calculations used to develop the unit production costs of items in finished goods, the auditor noted that the costs of the company's electrical engineering department had been treated as period expenses in previous years but were included in manufacturing overhead in the current year.

d. The company installed a new perpetual inventory system during the year. The auditor noted that many of the company's recorded year-end quantities differed from the actual physical inventory counts. Partly because of these problems, the company took a complete physical inventory at year-end.

Required:

Describe the additional audit procedures (if any) that the auditor should perform to obtain sufficient appropriate evidence in each of the preceding situations.

(Adapted from External Auditing (AU1), June 2011, with permission of Chartered Professional Accountants of Canada, Toronto, Canada. Any changes to the original material are the sole responsibility of the author (and/or publisher) and have not been reviewed or endorsed by Chartered Professional Accountants of Canada.)

DISCUSSION CASES

DC 12-1 Purchasing Control Procedures. `LO1, 2` Long, PA, has been engaged to examine and report on the financial statements of Maylou Corporation. During the review phase of the study of Maylou's system of internal control over purchases, Long was given the following document flowchart for purchases (see Exhibit DC 12-1).

Required:

Identify the procedures relating to purchase requisitions and purchase orders that Long would expect to find if Maylou's system of internal control over purchases is effective. For example, purchase orders are prepared only after properly considering the time to order and quantity to order. Do not comment on the effectiveness of the flow of documents as presented in the flowchart or on separation of duties.

(© 2000, American Institute of CPAs. All Rights Reserved. Adapted by permission.)

EXHIBIT DC 12-1

Maylou Corporation—Document Flowchart for Purchases

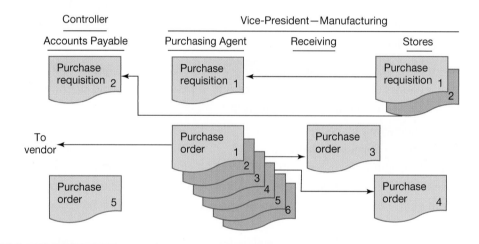

DC 12-2 Control Tests for Cash Disbursements. `LO1, 2` The Runge Controls Corporation manufactures and markets electrical control systems: temperature controls, machine controls, burglar alarms, and the like. Electrical and semiconductor parts are acquired from outside suppliers, and systems are assembled in Runge's plant. The company incurs other administrative and operating expenditures. Liabilities for goods and services purchased are entered in an accounts payable journal, at which time the debits are classified to the asset and expense accounts they apply to. The company has specified control procedures for approving supplier invoices for payment, for signing cheques, for keeping records, and for reconciling the chequing accounts. The procedures appear to be well specified and well placed in operation. You are the senior auditor on the engagement, and you need to specify a program (list) of control tests to audit the effectiveness of the controls over cash payments.

Required:

Using the six general internal control objectives discussed in Chapter 9, specify two or more control tests to audit the effectiveness of typical control procedures. (*Hint:* From one sample of recorded cash payments,

CONTROL OBJECTIVE	SPECIFIC CONTROL OBJECTIVE FOR CASH DISBURSEMENTS TRANSACTIONS	TEST OF CONTROLS PROGRAM
Completeness	All valid cash payments are recorded and none are omitted.	Determine the numerical sequence of cheques issued during the period and scan the sequence for missing numbers. (Scan the accounts payable records for amounts that appear to be too long outstanding, indicating liabilities for which payment may have been made but not recorded properly.)

you can specify control tests related to several objectives. See Exhibit 12–4 for examples of control test procedures over cash payments.) Organize your list according to the example shown below for the completeness objective.

DC 12-3 Unrecorded Liabilities Procedures. LO3, 4 You were in the final stages of your audit of the financial statements of Ozine Corporation for the year ended December 31, 20X2, when you were consulted by the corporation's president. The president believes there is no point in your examining the 20X3 accounts payable records and testing data in support of 20X3 entries. He explained that (1) bills pertaining to 20X2 that were received too late to be included in the December accounts payable were recorded as of the year-end by the corporation by journal entry, (2) the internal auditor made tests after the year-end, and (3) he would provide you with a letter certifying that there were no unrecorded liabilities.

Required:
a. Should your procedures for unrecorded liabilities be affected by the fact that the auditee made a journal entry to record 20X2 bills that were received later? Explain.
b. Should your test for unrecorded liabilities be affected by the fact that a letter is obtained in which a responsible management official certifies that to the best of his knowledge all liabilities have been recorded? Explain.
c. Should your test for unrecorded liabilities be eliminated or reduced because of the internal audit work? Explain.
d. What sources, in addition to the 20X3 accounts payable records, should you consider to locate possible unrecorded liabilities?

(© 2000, American Institute of CPAs. All Rights Reserved. Adapted by permission.)

DC 12-4 Accounts Payable Confirmations. LO3, 4 Clark and his partner, Kent, both PAs, are planning their audit program for the audit of accounts payable on the LeClair Corporation's annual audit. Saturday afternoon, they reviewed the thick file of last year's working papers, and both of them remembered all too well the six days they spent last year on accounts payable.

Last year, Clark had suggested that they mail confirmations to 100 of LeClair's suppliers. The company regularly purchases from about 1,000 suppliers, and these account payable balances fluctuate widely, depending on the volume of purchases and the terms LeClair's purchasing agent is able to negotiate. Clark's sample of 100 was designed to include accounts with large balances. In fact, the 100 accounts confirmed last year covered 80% of the total accounts payable.

Both Clark and Kent spent many hours tracking down minor differences reported in confirmation responses. Non-responding accounts were investigated by comparing LeClair's balance with monthly statements received from suppliers. Ultimately, they determined that the accounts payable balance was not materially misstated.

Required:

a. Identify the accounts payable audit objectives that the auditors must consider in determining the audit procedures to be performed.
b. Identify situations when the auditors should use accounts payable confirmations, and discuss whether they are required to use them.
c. Discuss why the use of large dollar balances as the basis for selecting accounts payable for confirmation may not be the most efficient approach, and indicate a more efficient sample selection procedure that could be followed when choosing accounts payable for confirmation.

DC 12-5 Inventory Count Observation: Planning and Substantive Audit Procedures. `LO3, 5` Cindy Li is the partner in charge of the audit of Blue Distributing Corporation, a wholesaler that owns one warehouse containing 80% of its inventory. Cindy is reviewing the working papers that were prepared to support the firm's opinion on Blue's financial statements. Cindy wants to be certain that essential audit procedures are well documented in the working papers.

Required:

a. What evidence should Cindy expect to find that the audit observation of the auditee's physical count of inventory was well planned and that assistants were properly supervised?
b. What substantive audit procedures should Cindy find in the working papers that document management's assertions about existence and completeness of inventory quantities at the end of the year? (Refer to Exhibit 12–8 for procedures.)

(© 2000, American Institute of CPAs. All Rights Reserved. Adapted by permission.)

DC 12-6 Sales/Inventory Cutoff. `LO3, 5` Your auditee took a complete physical inventory count under your observation as of December 15 and adjusted the inventory control account (perpetual inventory method) to agree with the physical inventory. Based on the count adjustments as of December 15, and after review of the transactions recorded from December 16 to December 31, you are almost ready to accept the inventory balance as fairly stated.

However, your review of the sales cutoff as of December 15 and December 31 disclosed the following items not previously considered:

COST	SALES PRICE	SHIPPED	DATE BILLED	CREDITED TO INVENTORY CONTROL
$28,400	$36,900	Dec. 14	Dec. 16	Dec. 16
39,100	50,200	Dec. 10	Dec. 19	Dec. 10
18,900	21,300	Jan. 2	Dec. 31	Dec. 31

Required:

What adjusting journal entries, if any, would you make for each of these items? Explain why each adjustment is necessary.

(© 2000, American Institute of CPAs. All Rights Reserved. Adapted by permission.)

DC 12-7 Inventory Count Observation: Planning and Substantive Audit Procedures. `LO3, 5` SCI makes clothes under its own labels, and also makes clothes to order under the labels of several large retailers. The large retailers usually order goods to be manufactured and held by SCI until the time comes when they are ready to put them in their stores. These large retailers pay SCI 50% of the invoice cost when SCI notifies them that the goods have been manufactured and are available, and they pay the balance when the goods are shipped to their stores. To postpone tax, SCI recognizes revenue on the retail sales when the goods are shipped. SCI's inventory is a highly material amount, making up about 55% of its total assets. Materiality has been set at $300,000 for the purpose of planning and performing the SCI audit.

Required:

a. Describe in detail the testing you would perform during the inventory count, and describe the audit objective(s) of each test.

b. Provide three different ways of stratifying the selection of inventory items for sampling. Explain why you would stratify the inventory in each listed way.

c. During the inventory count, a truck arrives at the warehouse to pick up a rush customer order, and the sales manager commands all the employees to stop working on the count and load the truck. What risks does this event give rise to, and how would these risks affect your audit procedures?

d. One of the inventory items you selected to test count is a quantity of 5,000 silk dresses at a cost of $80 each. The employees are unable to locate this inventory, so the sales manager is called over to help. He orders you to select a different item to test. When you explain that you must verify the item you have selected, he accuses you of stealing the inventory and threatens to call the police unless you leave immediately. Discuss your professional responsibilities in this situation and what actions you would take.

DC 12-8 Inventory Procedures Using Generalized Audit Software. `LO3, 5` You are conducting an audit of the financial statements of a wholesale cosmetics distributor with an inventory consisting of thousands of individual items. The distributor keeps its inventory in its own distribution centre and in two public warehouses. A perpetual inventory database is maintained on a computer system and updated at the end of each business day. Each individual record of the perpetual inventory database contains the following data:

- Item number
- Location of item
- Description of item
- Quantity on hand
- Cost per item
- Date of last purchase
- Date of last sale
- Quantity sold during year

You are planning to observe the distributor's physical count of inventories as of a given date. You will have available a computer file, provided by the auditee, of the above items taken from their database as of the date of the physical count. Your firm has a generalized audit software package that can upload and analyze the auditee's computer data files.

Required:

List the basic inventory auditing procedures and, for each, describe how the use of the general purpose audit software package and the perpetual inventory database might be helpful to the auditor in performing such auditing procedures. (See Exhibit 12–8 for substantive audit procedures for inventory.)

Organize your answer as follows:

Basic inventory auditing procedures	How general purpose audit software and the inventory file data might be helpful

(© 2000, American Institute of CPAs. All Rights Reserved. Adapted by permission.)

DC 12-9 Manufacturing Equipment and Accumulated Depreciation. `LO3, 6` For the audit of the financial statements of the Louis Manufacturing Company for its year ended December 31, you have been assigned the audit of the fixed assets accounts (Manufacturing Equipment, Manufacturing Equipment—Accumulated Depreciation, and Repairs to Manufacturing Equipment). Your review of Louis's policies and procedures has disclosed the following relevant information:

1. The Manufacturing Equipment account includes the net invoice price plus related freight and installation costs for all of the equipment in Louis's manufacturing plant.
2. The Manufacturing Equipment—Accumulated Depreciation accounts are supported by a subsidiary ledger, which shows the cost and accumulated depreciation for each piece of equipment.
3. An annual budget for capital expenditures of $5,000 or more is prepared by the executive committee and approved by the board of directors. Capital expenditures over $5,000 that are not included in this budget must be approved by the board of directors, and variations of 20% or more must be explained to the board. Approval by the supervisor of production is required for capital expenditures under $5,000.
4. Company employees handle installation, removal, repair, and rebuilding of the machinery. Work orders are prepared for these activities and are subject to the same budgetary control as other expenditures. Work orders are not required for external expenditures.

Required:

a. Prepare a list of the major specific objectives (assertions) for your audit of the Manufacturing Equipment, Manufacturing Equipment—Accumulated Depreciation, and Repairs of Manufacturing Equipment accounts. Do not include in this listing the auditing procedures designed to accomplish these objectives.
b. Prepare an audit program applicable to the current-year additions to the Manufacturing Equipment account.

(© 2000, American Institute of CPAs. All Rights Reserved. Adapted by permission.)

DC 12-10 Peacock Company: Incomplete Flowchart of Inventory and Purchasing Control Procedures. `LO1, 2` Peacock Company is a wholesaler of soft goods. The inventory comprises approximately 3,500 different items. The company employs a computerized batch processing system to maintain its perpetual inventory records. The system is run each weekend so that inventory reports are available on Monday morning for management use. The system has been functioning satisfactorily for the past 10 years, providing the company with accurate records and timely reports.

The preparation of purchase orders has been automated as a part of the inventory system to ensure that the company will maintain enough inventory to meet customer demand. When an item of inventory falls below a predetermined level, a record of the inventory items is written. This record is used in conjunction with the supplier file to prepare the purchase orders.

Exception reports are prepared during the update of the inventory and the preparation of the purchase orders. These reports list any errors or exceptions identified during the processing. In addition, the system provides for management approval of all purchase orders exceeding a specified amount. Any exceptions or items requiring management approval are handled by supplemental runs on Monday morning and are combined with the weekend results.

EXHIBIT DC 12-10

Peacock Company: Inventory and Purchase Order Procedure

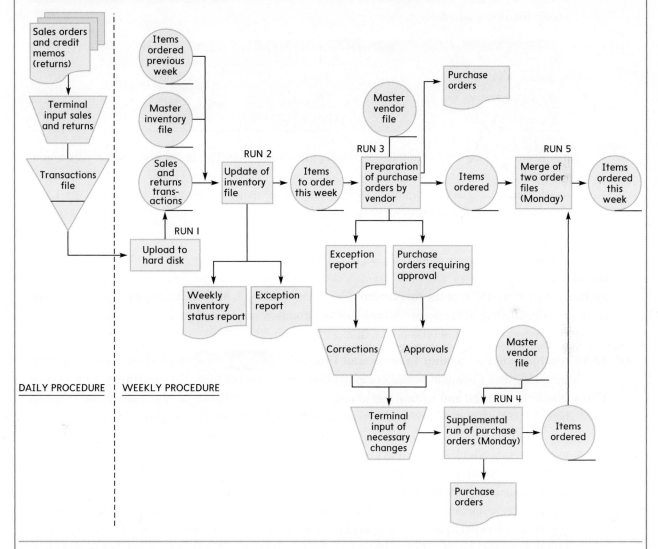

Required:

a. The illustrated system flowchart (see Exhibit DC 12-10) of Peacock Company's inventory and purchase order system was prepared, but several steps that are important to the successful operations of the system are omitted from the chart. Describe the steps that have been omitted, and indicate where the omissions have occurred. Do not redraw the flowchart.

b. In order for Peacock's inventory/purchase order system to function properly, control procedures should be included in the system. Describe the type of control procedures Peacock Company should use in its system to ensure proper functioning, and indicate where these procedures would be placed in the system.

(© 2000, American Institute of CPAs. All Rights Reserved. Adapted by permission.)

DC 12-11 Inventory Evidence and Long-Term Purchase Contracts. `LO3` During the audit of Mason Company Inc. for the calendar year 20X2, you noticed that the company produces aluminum cans at the rate of about 40 million units annually. On the plant tour, you noticed a large stockpile of raw aluminum in storage. Your inventory observation and pricing procedures showed this stockpile to be the raw materials inventory of 400 tonnes valued at $240,000 (average cost). Inquiry with the production chief yielded the information that 400 tonnes was about a four-month supply of raw materials. Suppose you learn that Mason had executed a non-cancellable long-term purchase contract with All Purpose Aluminum Company to purchase raw materials on the following schedule:

DELIVERY DATE	QUANTITY (TONNES)	TOTAL PRICE
January 30, 20X3	500	$300,000
June 30, 20X3	700	420,000
December 30, 20X3	1,000	500,000

Because of recent economic conditions, principally a decline in the demand for raw aluminum and a consequent oversupply, the price stood at $400 per tonne (1 tonne = 1,000 kilograms) as of January 15, 20X3. Commodities experts predict that this low price will prevail for 12–15 months or until there is a general economic recovery.

Required:

a. Describe the procedures you would employ to gather evidence about this contract (including its initial discovery).

b. As Mason's auditor, which of the facts given in the case would you have to discover for yourself based on your understanding of the auditee's business, environment, and risks?

c. Discuss the effect this contract has on the financial statements.

DC 12-12 Analysis of Purchasing Process and Controls. `LO1, 2` Integrated Measurement Systems Inc. (IMS) is a Canadian public company that manufactures high-end measuring devices used primarily in the oil and natural gas industries. In 20X3, it had sales of $100 million and earnings before income tax of $5 million. The company has a December 31 year-end.

Ted Pollock, IMS's CEO, is a proponent of strong corporate governance. He has spent the last year strengthening IMS's internal control environment. He believes that organizations that demonstrate good corporate governance practices will be perceived favourably by the markets. Ted wants to make a presentation to IMS's audit committee supporting the position that throughout the year the company's internal controls functioned in accordance with the company's control objectives. Depending on the reaction of the audit committee, Ted would like to make the presentation an annual event. IMS has hired your professional services firm to assist Ted in preparing the content of his presentation.

Your firm is currently assessing the purchasing process. Accordingly, IMS has provided you with relevant material and access to the company's resources (Exhibit DC 12-12–1). As part of the analysis of this process, IMS has asked you to

1. Identify the existing key internal controls within the purchasing process

2. Describe the procedures that IMS could use to test the controls

3. Identify the internal control weaknesses within the purchasing process, and recommend improvements

EXHIBIT DC 12-12-1

Purchasing Process Documentation Updated November 20X3

The purchasing process has four major components, namely:

1. Vendor prequalification
2. Purchase of goods and/or services
3. Receipt of goods
4. Settlement

Process description

The purchasing process begins when there is a requirement for goods or services. A manually completed purchase request form is sent from the operating department (e.g., Sales, Marketing, Manufacturing) to the purchasing department. The purchasing clerk numbers these documents and reviews each purchase request form to verify that a signature is present.

Purchase request forms must be authorized by the signature of a person with the appropriate level of authority. The amount of the expenditure determines the level of authority required, and the expenditure authorization levels are organized in tiers. Because there are so many possible combinations of departments and authorization levels, the operating departments are responsible for ensuring that their purchase request forms are signed by individuals with the appropriate level of authority. This requirement eliminates the need for the purchasing clerk to check the specifics of their signatures.

The purchasing clerk sends the purchase requests to the purchasing manager for review and approval.

The approved purchase request is then sent to the buyer, who sources the purchase. If the amount is below $5,000, selection of the supplier is left up to the buyer. For purchases in excess of $5,000 but less than $25,000, a supplier from the Prequalification Listing is selected, again at the discretion of the buyer. For purchases in excess of $25,000, a formal bidding process is performed. However, at the discretion of the buyer, the bidding process can be waived if it is deemed to be cost inefficient.

Upon selection of the supplier, the buyer inputs the purchase request information into a purchase order form. The purchase order is forwarded to the purchasing manager for review, and a photocopy is made and filed, in numerical order, with the appropriate photocopy of the purchase request. The original purchase order is then sent back to the buyer, who delivers it to the supplier.

All goods are received in the warehouse. All employees have access to the warehouse. The goods are checked against the packaging slip and are examined for damage and so on. If the goods are acceptable, the bill of lading is signed off by the receiver. A copy of the signed bill of lading is then forwarded to the purchasing clerk, who matches it to the file copy of the purchase request and purchase order. If there are differences in the details (over/under shipment, wrong product, etc.), the bill of lading is forwarded to the buyer for resolution with the supplier. If no problems are noted, copies of the three documents are sent to the payables group for settlement.

The receiver, Janet Smith (who was hired six months ago), sends the goods to the user department that made the original purchase request along with a photocopy of the bill of lading. The user department agrees the quantities noted by the receiver and files the bill of lading. User departments have noted that, recently, the number of manual adjustments to the quantities shipped versus received has been increasing.

Any unmatched purchase requests and purchase orders that remain outstanding for over 90 days are returned by the purchasing clerk to the user department that originally ordered the goods on the assumption that the goods have been received. It is then the responsibility of the user department to follow up and forward the paperwork to the payables group for settlement.

If a signed bill of lading for which there is no source documentation (i.e., no purchase request or purchase order exists) is forwarded to the purchasing clerk, the purchasing clerk follows up with the buyer to understand the nature of the receipt. At the same time, a copy of the bill of lading is also sent to the payables group.

It is now the first week of March 20X4. The partner responsible for the IMS audit engagement provides you with her notes from a meeting with Ted (Exhibit DC 12-12–2). You have been asked by the partner to prepare the analysis of IMS's purchasing process, addressing the three requirements, and to identify any additional issues and make any observations that would be relevant to the engagement.

Required:

Prepare an analysis of IMS's purchasing process, addressing the three requirements requested by the IMS CEO, in a report format suitable for the CEO's use.

(© 2000, American Institute of CPAs. All Rights Reserved. Adapted by permission.)

EXHIBIT DC 12-12-2

Meeting Notes Received from Partner

I met today with the CEO of IMS, Ted Pollock, for the purpose of discussing his needs. He provided the following information:

- IMS's corporate governance framework: IMS has adopted an approach to establishing a strong corporate governance framework that includes

  1. Documentation of the existing processes and controls
  2. Identification of the key controls in the process
  3. Evaluation and testing of the internal controls and implementation of improvements

- Control objectives that relate to the purchasing process:

  1. Proper approval of all transactions
  2. Safeguarding of company assets
  3. Prevention and detection of errors and irregularities
  4. Accuracy and completeness of books and records
  5. Appropriate use of information

DC 12-13 Purchasing Defalcation in a Manufacturing Company. `LO1, 2, 3` On January 11, at the beginning of your annual audit of the Grover Manufacturing Company's financial statements for the year just ended December 31, the company president confides to you that an employee is living on a scale in excess of that which his salary would support.

The employee has been a buyer in the purchasing department for six years and has charge of purchasing all raw materials and supplies. He is authorized to sign purchase orders for amounts up to $2,000. Purchase orders in excess of $2,000 require the countersignature of the general purchasing agent.

The president understands that the usual audit of financial statements is not designed to disclose immaterial fraud or conflicts of interest, although such events may be discovered. The president authorizes you, however, to expand your regular audit procedures and to apply additional audit procedures to determine whether there is any evidence that the buyer has been misappropriating company funds or has been engaged in activities that are a conflict of interest.

Required:

List the audit procedures that you would apply to the company records and documents in an attempt to do the following:

1. Discover evidence within the purchasing department of defalcations being committed by the buyer. Give the purpose of each audit procedure.
2. Provide leads about possible collusion between the buyer and suppliers. Give the purpose of each audit procedure.

DC 12-14 Inventory Assertions, Risk Assessment, Audit Procedures. `LO3, 5`

Required:

Refer to the case facts given in Chapter 11, DC 11-12, and answer the following questions:

a. What is your assessment of the risk of material misstatement at the assertion level for the BSL inventory? Make reference to case facts to support your conclusions.
b. Describe the substantive procedures you would include in your audit program for verifying the quantity and the pricing of BSL's inventory. Explain how these procedures respond to the risks you have assessed in (a).
c. Identify three CASs that would apply to auditing BSL's inventory, and outline the requirements that are relevant.

DC 12-15 Repairs Expense, Error Adjustment. `LO3, 6` You are the auditor of Bittern Inc. Bittern's long-standing policy is to capitalize all repairs and maintenance payments that exceed $10,000, without assessing the nature of the expenditure. Many of Bittern's buildings and equipment are aging, and repairs are becoming frequent and more expensive. You have concerns that a material amount of building repairs and maintenance expense is being capitalized, so you undertake a detailed examination of all the building asset additions during the current year. Your analysis indicates that approximately $400,000 of repairs expense has been capitalized as buildings in the current year. Materiality for the audit is $500,000. In the prior year's audit, the staff noted approximately $100,000 of repairs expenses had been capitalized, but no adjustment was recorded. The estimated useful life of Bittern's buildings is 25 years, and the average remaining useful life of their buildings is approximately 8 years.

Required:

a. Describe the impact of the above error on the current-year financial statements and the impact it will have on future periods' financial statements when the error reverses, if it is not adjusted.

b. Describe the impact the unadjusted error from the prior year will have on the current year's financial statements.

c. State whether you would require Bittern to adjust for this error, and support your conclusion. If you require an adjustment, provide the required journal entry.

d. What recommendation would you include in the management letter relating to the situation above?

DC 12-16 Mining Properties, Using Work of Experts. `LO3, 6` White Ice Mines Inc. is a mining company. During 20X4, White Ice acquired a diamond mine located in the far north for $800 million from Albatross Inc. The purchase price is based on the mine's inventory of extracted diamonds, with an appraised value of $300 million, plus diamond reserves estimated in the range of $600 million to over $2 billion. White Ice raised $100 million of the funds to acquire the mine by issuing public shares on the Canadian Adventure Exchange, with the remainder being lent by a consortium of three major Canadian banks. Shortly after the initial public offering (IPO), a shareholder resolution was passed requiring White Ice to appoint new auditors from one of the large national auditing firms. The previous auditor was a small firm that was also the auditor for Albatross for many years. The new auditor of White Ice is examining the existence, valuation, and ownership assertions for its mining assets for the year ended December 31, 20X4. White Ice informs the auditor that its mining specialists provided the appraisals for use in preparing the prospectus for their IPO of shares, and to satisfy the due diligence inquiries of the three banks. The new auditor has determined that it will be necessary to rely on an independent expert to provide a valuation report to support the audit opinion.

Required:

a. Refer to CAS 620 (Using the Work of an Auditor's Expert), and develop an audit program for verifying White Ice's diamond mine investment.

b. White Ice's management is concerned that using another expert will drive up the audit cost. The managers (some of whom previously worked for a mining company called Bre-X) suggest it would be more efficient for the auditor to rely on the expert's reports already provided for the IPO and the bank financing. As the new auditor, how would you respond to this suggestion? You may want to refer to CAS 550 (Related Parties) for guidance.

DC 12-17 Purchasing Process; Property, Plant, and Equipment; and Information Technology General Controls. LO1, 2, 5 Grafite International Inc. (Grafite) is a manufacturer of various components used in the electricity distribution industry. It has factories across the country, and its customer base includes a variety of municipal and provincial electricity distributors. You are an audit senior with Grafite's external auditors, Eden & Choi, Licensed Public Accountants. You are currently familiarizing yourself with Grafite's operations to plan the audit of Grafite's financial statement for its September 30, 20X5, year-end.

In the past six months Grafite has made significant changes to some of its manufacturing processes and as a result has purchased new equipment. Because of the changes, Grafite has a lot of equipment that is no longer being used. Purchase requisitions for all new equipment have been authorized by production managers. Since all their attention has been focused on starting up the new equipment, little has been done about the old, unused equipment.

You have learned that Grafite has also made some changes in its purchasing department to cut costs. Two purchasing department employees were laid off. As a result, supplier statement reconciliations are no longer being performed; these used to be performed monthly by one of the laid-off purchasing department employees. Also, updates to supplier details in the purchase ledger master file can now be made by anyone in the purchasing department who has time to do it, not just by the manager.

Required:

a. Identify and explain the impact of three internal controls weaknesses in Grafite's purchasing process. Recommend a control procedure Grafite should implement to address each of these weaknesses.
b. Explain the impact of these deficiencies on your planned audit program for PPE.
c. Describe four substantive audit procedures you would perform for PPE at your year-end audit to determine whether PPE is materially misstated.

DC 12-18 Cash Payments Fraud: Medical Benefits Claims. LO1, 2, 3 This case uses the same framework as the Application Case in the chapter.

Case Description Beta Magnetic, a large company, experienced a fraud in the cash payments processed for employees' supplementary medical benefit claims. Fictitious benefit claims were paid by the company, which self-insured up to $50,000 per employee for supplementary benefits costs (such as physiotherapy and acupuncture) not covered by other medical and benefits coverage plans. The expense account that included legitimate and false charges was "employee supplementary medical benefits."

As manager of the claims payment department, Martha Lee was considered one of Beta Magnetic's best employees. She never missed a day of work in 10 years, and her department had one of the company's best efficiency ratings. Controls were considered good, including the verification by a claims processor that (1) the patient was a Beta employee, (2) treatments were covered by the company-sponsored plan, (3) the charges were within approved guidelines and not covered by another plan, (4) the cumulative claims for the employee did not exceed $50,000 (if over $50,000, a claim was submitted to an insurance company), and (5) the calculation for payment was correct. After verification processing, claims were sent to the claims payment department to pay the medical practitioner directly. No payments ever went directly to employees. Martha prepared false claims on real employees, forging the signature of various claims processors, adding her own review approval, naming bogus medical practitioners who would be paid by the payment department. The payments were mailed to various post office box addresses and to her husband's business address.

Nobody ever verified claims information with the employee. The employees received no reports of medical benefits paid on their behalf. While the department had performance reports by claims processors, these reports did not show claim-by-claim details. No one verified the credentials of the medical practitioners. Over the last seven years, Martha and her husband stole $3.5 million, and, until the last, no one noticed anything unusual about the total amount of claims paid.

Audit Trail The falsified claim forms were in Beta's files, containing all the fictitious data on employee names, processor signatures, medical practitioners' bills, and phony medical practitioners' addresses. The cancelled cheques, "endorsed" by the doctors, were returned by the bank and kept in Beta's files. Martha and her husband were somewhat clever: They deposited the cheques in various banks in accounts opened in the names and identification of the "medical practitioners."

Martha did not make any mistakes in covering the paper trail. She drew the attention of an auditor who saw her take her 24 claims-processing employees out to an annual staff appreciation luncheon in a fleet of stretch limousines.

Audit Approach Analysis The auditor's objective is to obtain evidence determining whether employee medical benefits "existed" in the sense of being valid claims paid to valid medical practitioners.

Controls relevant to the process are good as far as they go. The claims processors used internal data in their work—employee files for identification and treatment descriptions submitted by medical practitioners with comparisons to plan provisions and mathematical calculations. This work amounted to all the approval necessary for the claims payment department to prepare a cheque. There were no controls that connected the claims data with outside sources, such as employee acknowledgment or investigation of medical practitioners.

Required:

Describe in detail the audit procedures you would perform in this case. Consider tests of control and substantive tests, such as dual-purpose tests of transactions and/or tests of details of balance. Which tests do you consider likely to detect Martha's theft? Why?

Internal Control Questionnaires for the Purchases, Payables, and Payments Process

LO7 Describe internal control questionnaires used in audit practice for the purchases, payables, and payments process.

Exhibit 12A–1 is an example of the type of form that could be used to guide the auditor's assessment of the effectiveness of application controls in the main classes of transactions and the main account balances related to the purchases, payables, and payments process. Note that, in practice, forms like this can provide only a general starting point, and the actual audit work must always be tailored to the specifics of each engagement.

EXHIBIT 12A–1

Internal Control Questionnaire for the Purchases, Payables, and Payments Process

INTERNAL CONTROL QUESTIONNAIRE FOR PURCHASES, PAYABLES, AND PAYMENTS PROCESS AUDITEE:_____ F/S PERIOD:_____	Auditor Responses	Audit File References
OVERALL COMPANY-LEVEL CONTROL AND CONTROL ACTIVITIES ASSESSMENT		

(Refer to responses recorded for questions in Exhibit 9A–1 in Appendix 9A.)
1. Are company-level and general control activities adequate as they apply to the purchases, payables, and payments components of the information system?
   • Consider the impact of any weakness in company-level and general control activities on the planned audit approach and procedures.
   • Assess the potential for weaknesses to result in a material misstatement of the financial information generated from this accounting process. If a significant risk of misstatement is assessed, perform procedures to determine the extent of any misstatement.
2. Consider the adequacy of the following general controls in place in the purchases, payables, and payments process to
   • Prevent unauthorized access or changes to programs and data
   • Ensure the security and privacy of data
   • Control and maintain key systems
   • Protect assets susceptible to misappropriation
   • Ensure completeness, accuracy, and authorization of data and processing
   • Ensure that adequate management trails exist		

(continued)

Internal Control Questionnaire for the Purchases, Payables, and Payments Process *(continued)*

	Auditor Responses	Audit File References
APPLICATION CONTROL ASSESSMENTS		
PURCHASING AND ACCOUNTS PAYABLE APPLICATION CONTROLS		

Environment and general controls relevant to this application:

1. Is the purchasing department independent of the accounting department, receiving department, and shipping department?
2. Are receiving report copies transmitted to inventory custodians? to purchasing? to the accounting department?
3. Is the accounts payable detail ledger balanced periodically with the general ledger control account to ensure system processing integrity?

Application Control Assessments:

Consider whether the auditee has appropriate policies and procedures in place to meet the following control objectives:

Validity objective:

4. Are suppliers' invoices matched against purchase orders and receiving reports before a liability is recorded?

Completeness objective:

5. Are the purchase order forms prenumbered, and is the numerical sequence checked for missing documents?
6. Are receiving report forms prenumbered, and is the numerical sequence checked for missing documents?
7. Is the accounts payable department notified of goods returned to suppliers?
8. Are unmatched receiving reports reviewed frequently and investigated for proper recording?

Authorization objective:

9. Are competitive bids received and reviewed for certain items?
10. Are all purchases made only on the basis of approved purchase requisitions?
11. Are purchases made for employees authorized through the regular purchases procedures?
12. Are purchase prices approved by a responsible purchasing officer?
13. Are all purchases, whether for inventory or expense, routed through the purchasing department for approval?
14. Are shipping documents authorized and prepared for goods returned to suppliers?
15. Are invoices approved for payment by a responsible officer?

Accuracy objective:

16. Are the quantity and quality of goods received determined at the time of receipt by receiving personnel independent of the purchasing department?
17. Are suppliers' monthly statements reconciled with individual accounts payable accounts?
18. In the accounts payable department, are invoices checked against purchase orders and receiving reports for quantities, prices, and terms?

Classification objective:

19. Do the chart of accounts and accounting manual give instructions for classifying debit entries when purchases are recorded?
20. Are account distributions recorded for supplier invoices and independently verified prior to being entered in the accounts payable system?

Proper period objective:

21. Does the accounting manual give instructions to date purchase/payable entries on the date of receipt of goods?

(continued)

EXHIBIT 12A–1

Internal Control Questionnaire for the Purchases, Payables, and Payments Process   (*continued*)

CASH DISBURSEMENTS PROCESSING APPLICATION CONTROLS Environment and general controls relevant to this application: 1. Are persons with cash custody or cheque-signing or EFT authority denied access to accounting journals, ledgers, and bank reconciliations? 2. Is access to blank cheques or EFT functions denied to unauthorized persons? 3. Are all payments except petty cash made by cheque? 4. Are cheque signers prohibited from drawing cheques to cash? 5. Is signing blank cheques prohibited? 6. Are voided cheques mutilated and retained for inspection? 7. Is the bank reconciliation reviewed by an accounting official with no conflicting cash receipts, cash payments, or recordkeeping responsibilities? 8. If the organization has internal auditors, do they periodically conduct a surprise audit of bank reconciliations? Application Control Assessments: Consider whether the auditee has appropriate policies and procedures in place to meet the following control objectives: *Validity objective:* 9. Are invoices, receiving reports, and purchase orders reviewed by the cheque signer? 10. Are the supporting documents stamped "paid" (to prevent duplicate payment) before being returned to accounts payable for filing? 11. Are cheques mailed directly by the signer and not returned to the accounts payable department for mailing? *Completeness objective:* 12. Are blank cheques prenumbered, and is the numerical sequence checked for missing documents? *Authorization objective:* 13. Do cheques require signatures by two approved officers? If cheques are machine-signed, is there dual control over the machine signature process? If EFTs are used, are approved signatures required to release funds? *Accuracy objective:* 14. Are bank accounts reconciled by personnel independent of cash custody or recordkeeping, and appropriate reconciliation adjustments independently verified? *Classification objective:* 15. Do the chart of accounts and accounting manual give instructions for determining debit classifications of payments not charged to accounts payable? 16. Is the distribution of charges double-checked periodically by an official? Is the budget used to check on gross misclassification errors? 17. Are special payments (e.g., payroll and dividends) made from separate bank accounts? *Proper period objective:* 18. Are cheques dated in the cash payments journal with the date of the cheque?		
INVENTORY TRANSACTION PROCESSING CONTROLS Environment and general controls relevant to this application: 1. Are perpetual inventory records kept for raw materials? supplies? WIP? finished goods? 2. Are perpetual records subsidiary to general ledger control accounts? 3. Do the perpetual records show quantities only? quantities and prices? 4. Are inventory records maintained by someone other than the inventory stores custodian? 5. Are merchandise or materials on consignment (not the property of the company) physically segregated from goods owned by the company?		*(continued)*

EXHIBIT 12A–1

Internal Control Questionnaire for the Purchases, Payables, and Payments Process   (*continued*)

	Auditor Responses	Audit File References
6. Is there a periodic review for overstocked, slow-moving, or obsolete inventory? Have any adjustments been made during the year? 7. Are perpetual inventory records kept in dollars periodically reconciled to general ledger control accounts? Application Control Assessments: Consider whether the auditee has appropriate policies and procedures in place to meet the following control objectives: *Validity objective:* 8. Are additions to inventory quantity records made only on receipt of a receiving report copy? 9. Do inventory custodians notify the records department of additions to inventory? *Completeness objective:* 10. Are reductions of inventory record quantities made only on receipt of inventory issuance documents? 11. Do inventory custodians notify the inventory records department of reductions of inventory? *Authorization objective:* Refer to question 8 above (additions). Refer to question 10 above (reductions). *Accuracy objective:* 12. If standard costs have been used for inventory pricing, have they been reviewed for current applicability? *Classification objective:* 13. Are periodic counts of physical inventory made to correct errors in the individual perpetual records? *Proper period objective:* 14. Does the accounting manual give instructions to record inventory additions on the date of the receiving report? 15. Does the accounting manual give instructions to record inventory issues on the issuance date?		
PROPERTY, PLANT, AND EQUIPMENT ASSETS AND RELATED TRANSACTIONS PROCESSING APPLICATION CONTROLS Environment and general controls relevant to this application: 1. Are detailed property records maintained for the various fixed assets? Application Control Assessments: Consider whether the auditee has appropriate policies and procedures in place to meet the following control objectives: *Validity objective:* 2. Is the accounting department notified of actions of disposal, dismantling, or idling of a productive asset? for terminating a lease or rental? 3. Are fixed assets inspected periodically and physically counted? *Completeness objective:* 4. Is casualty insurance carried? Is the coverage analyzed periodically? When was the last analysis? 5. Are property tax assessments periodically analyzed? When was the last analysis? *Authorization objective:* 6. Are capital expenditure and leasing proposals prepared for review and approval by the board of directors or by responsible officers? 7. When actual expenditures exceed authorized amounts, is the excess approved?		*(continued)*

EXHIBIT 12A–1

Internal Control Questionnaire for the Purchases, Payables, and Payments Process   (*continued*)

Accuracy objective: 8. Is there a uniform policy for assigning depreciation rates, useful lives, and salvage values? 9. Are depreciation calculations checked by internal auditors or other officials? *Classification objective:* 10. Does the accounting manual contain policies for capitalization of assets and for expensing repair and maintenance? 11. Are subsidiary fixed assets records periodically reconciled to the general ledger accounts? 12. Are memorandum records of leased assets maintained? *Proper period objective:* 13. Does the accounting manual give instructions for recording fixed asset additions on a proper date of acquisition?		
Auditor's conclusion on the effectiveness of general and application controls in the purchases, payables, and payments process: _____	Prepared by _____	Date _____

Exhibit 12A–2 provides examples of the types of controls one expects to find in a typical system, such as the one illustrated in Exhibit 12–1 of the chapter.

EXHIBIT 12A–2

Examples of Purchases and Payables Controls Relating to Exhibit 12–1

- Each terminal or user access identification allows performance of only designated functions. For example, the receiving clerk's terminal or user ID cannot accept a purchase order entry.
- An identification number and password (used on an individual basis) is required to enter the non-automatic purchase orders, suppliers' invoices, and receiving report information. Further, certain passwords have "read-only" authorization. These are issued to personnel authorized to determine the status of various records, such as an unpaid invoice, but not authorized to enter data.
- All input is immediately logged to provide restart processing should the system become inoperative during the processing.
- The transaction codes call up a full-screen "form," and each clerk must enter the information correctly (online input validation) or the computer will not accept the data.
- All printed documents are computer numbered, and the number is stored as part of the record. Further, all records in the open databases have the supplier's code number as the primary search and matching field key. Of course, status searches could be made by another field. For example, the inventory number can be the search key to determine the status of a purchase of an item in short supply.
- A daily search of the open databases is made. Purchases outstanding for more than 10 days and the missing "document" records are summarized on a report that is investigated to assess reasons for the delay.
- For suppliers with EFT arrangements, funds transfers are initiated by the payables clerk and summarized on an EFT daily report. The daily EFT report is reviewed and approved by a designated person in the treasurer's office. If cheques are prepared to process payment, the cheque signature is printed, using a signature plate that is installed on the computer printer only when cheques are printed. A designated person in the treasurer's office maintains custody of this signature plate and must take it to the computer room to be installed when cheques are printed. This person also has the combination to the separate document storage room where the blank cheque stock is kept and is present at all cheque printing runs. The printed cheques are taken immediately from the computer room for mailing.

CHAPTER 13

Payroll and Production Processes

This chapter provides an overview of the payroll process by which employees are compensated, and an overview of the production process by which raw materials, labour, and overhead are converted into finished goods and services. The production process is integrated with the payroll process, as labour cost information from payroll is allocated to the cost of finished goods and services. Our coverage presents these related processes in two sections: Section I covers the payroll process, which will be present in every organization with employees, and Section II covers the production process of a manufacturing business, including inventory valuation, amortization, and cost of goods sold. Application cases demonstrate the application of audit procedures in situations where errors or frauds might be discovered.

LEARNING OBJECTIVES

After completing this chapter, you will be able to do the following:

LO1 Describe the key risks of misstatement in the payroll and production processes.

LO2 Describe the payroll process: typical transactions, account balances, source documents, and controls.

LO3 Describe control tests for auditing control over hiring, firing, and payment of employees in the payroll process.

LO4 Give examples of the typical substantive procedures used to address the assessed risk of material misstatement in the main accounts in the payroll process.

LO5 Describe the production process: typical transactions, account balances, source documents, and controls.

LO6 Describe control tests for auditing control over conversion of materials and labour in the production process.

LO7 Describe the typical substantive procedures used to address the assessed risk of material misstatement in the main accounts in the production process.

LO8 (Appendix 13A) Describe the internal control questionnaires used in audit practice for the payroll and production processes.

CHAPTER APPENDICES

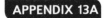

APPENDIX 13A   Internal Control Questionnaires for the Payroll and Production Processes

EcoPak Inc.

Caleb's evening at the EcoPak inventory count is going well. By 6 p.m. he has inspected 100% of the items on the property, plant, and equipment (PPE) schedule. Caleb learns from Nina that the moulds installed in the machines are considered part of the production equipment, whereas the spare moulds are included in inventory. He makes note of this in the file so that he can follow up at the next team meeting on whether this accounting policy results in a fair presentation of these assets. By 8 p.m. he has completed fairly extensive tests (floor-to-list and list-to-floor counts) of the finished goods and spare moulds inventories. He has also checked a number of the EcoPak employees' counts and recorded additional information from their final count sheets for follow-up later.

He closely observed the measurement process for the vats of raw materials and was able to verify the readings and measures that the engineers used in their volume calculations. The raw material inventory consists of large vats of processed fibre, a goopy substance that is mixed with binding agent solutions, left to cure for several days, and then aerated and sprayed into moulds that shape the material into coffee cups, cutlery, and so on. The aerating spray process is EcoPak's own patented technology. Based on review of Nina's preliminary inventory balances, he notes that while the volume of the raw material is very large, its dollar value is actually considerably less than materiality. So, he decides he has done enough on that balance.

The spare moulds, however, reflect a balance that is several times materiality, so he makes sure he has a lot of reliable evidence about their quantities and condition. He notes a number of moulds at the back of the storage area that are very dusty and is told by the production manager that they are for a product that EcoPak never gets orders for any more. "But that item was once used by one of our best customers, so we should keep them on hand in case they ever decide to go back to that type of package." Caleb makes a note to discuss the valuation of this part of the spare moulds inventory with Donna.

At about 9 p.m., it looks like Caleb is close to being finished (and in good time to ring in the New Year with his friends). Just as he gets to the very back of the plant for a look at the last area, he becomes aware of a lot of vibration and noise from the back production line—it is running a job! But Nina told him that production would be shut down. Mike confirms to Caleb that it was not possible to keep the lines completely shut down—an urgent order that needed to be completed by January 3 came in the night before, and they had to get it going right away. Mike comments, "I guess this kind of messed up Nina's nice neat plan for the count, and I am sorry about that. But business comes first. Kam's been working on this account for two years, and now they are finally giving us a chance! If we meet this deadline, this could turn into a huge new account that will increase our sales by a good 30% and allow us to expand our new cutlery production line, which is currently underutilized. That will make us the industry leader in biodegradable disposable cutlery. This could be the big breakthrough for EcoPak!"

When Nina finds out, she's annoyed, but quickly agrees that the order is too important to the company's success to turn down just to make the accounting job easier. "Still, Mike," she says, "you could have told me sooner—you know I need to know what's going on!" She gives Caleb a quick estimate of the dollar value likely to be involved—about 50% of their performance materiality.

Caleb is really unsure about what to do, so he calls Donna. Donna is having some issues of her own at the turbine work-in-process (WIP) inventory count but explains how to assess the situation. "Get a copy of the bill of materials for the job being processed. Then, ask the production manager for a timetable that we can use to assess the percentage of completion at year-end. Have him show you where they are in the process right now, and make lots of notes. It's good you could get a handle on the expected dollar amount likely to be involved; that will help a lot."

At around 10 p.m., Mike and Nina are satisfied with the count information the employees have provided. As Nina brings out some ginger ale and cake to celebrate with them, Mike also hands each worker a $500 cash bonus. "I got a cheque for $5,000 made out to 'Cash' from Nina yesterday, so I could give my guys and gals a nice reward for handling the count today." Mike explains. Caleb had noted this as one of the last cheques of the year to follow up for cutoff, so now he knows what it was for—payroll. As he makes a note to see how it got accounted for, Mike calls out, "Hey Caleb, I guess I should have gotten a cash bonus to give you, too? After all, you found a couple of errors and helped us get the count done successfully!" Caleb explains that he is just doing his job and it would not be appropriate to take that kind of payment, since it might look like he lacks independence. Nina smiles, "I know . . . it's kind of too bad, but that's the right answer, Caleb!" At 10:30 p.m., Caleb enters 6.5 hours in the inventory on his time sheet for the week and heads out for a well-deserved couple of days off.

The Essentials of Auditing the Payroll Process and the Production Costing Process

The payroll process supports the human resources function in an organization, generating the payments to hourly and salaried employees, and capturing these costs in the accounting system. Accruals for payroll costs are often required at a period-end since the payroll dates may not always occur on the date that the accounting period ends. The main entry in the payroll accounting process is as follows:

Dr Wages & Salaries Expenses
Cr Cash, or Wages and Salaries Accruals
Cr Employee withholdings due to governments

For payroll, management's main control objectives are the authorization and validity of payroll payments, to ensure only real employees are paid, and only for the work they have done. The accuracy of calculating payroll withholdings that must be remitted to the government is another important control objective. Since the process involves a high volume of small payments to individuals, there is a risk of employee fraud. Segregation of duties, authorization of input data, and review of output (the payroll register summarizing the employee payment details) are key management control activities for payroll. Many organizations outsource the payroll processing to outside payroll specialist services, since this ensures segregation of the payments from the authorization of payroll amounts, as well as accuracy of processing. Auditors' main concern is with management's controls over validity, accuracy, and authorization, and they often test controls over payroll processing by using dual-purpose tests of the payroll reports. By establishing the reliability of the payroll summary reports, auditors can use substantive procedures such as analysis of reasonableness of annual payroll expense details and recalculation of year-end accruals to provide relevant substantive evidence that the amounts are not materially misstated.

This chapter also looks at the production accounting process, by which businesses accumulate the costs of manufacturing an inventory of products to sell, or the costs related to generating the services that they provide. The production process captures information about the costs of the main revenue-generating activities of the business, so it produces a lot of critical strategy-related information for managing the business's activities. The payroll costs related to the labour component of production will be allocated into the production cost accounting process; these two processes are integrated in the information system.

Focusing on inventory production, the main control risks management needs to address are the validity and completeness of inventory quantities and the accuracy of cost data. Physical counts and reconciliation of the count quantities to the perpetual records are important. Also important are good cutoff procedures for inventory purchasing, for manufacturing cost allocations (labour, material, and overhead costs), and for shipment of sales. Since manufacturing inventory is often a high-volume, complex accounting process, control testing by auditors is often a good approach so that the various management reports related to inventory can be relied upon to do analysis and other substantive detail tests of samples of inventory items.

The main substantive auditing procedures related to manufacturing inventory are to attend and perform tests of the physical inventory count, to test the pricing data supporting the inventory's cost, to test the allocation of costs to WIP and finished goods, and to perform market value tests to verify the net realizable value. Auditors always test the cutoffs between inventory and purchasing/production, and between inventory and sales/shipping. Inquiry, inspection of documents, and analysis regarding FOB terms and revenue recognition policies are used to determine when ownership of inventories transfers to or from the auditee. Analytical procedures such as gross margin analysis and analysis of trends in sales, often using detailed management reports, are useful for assessing risks of material misstatements in inventory existence, completeness, and valuation assertions. Manufacturing inventory tends to be a fairly complex account to audit, so it is typically assigned to more-experienced audit team members.

Review Checkpoints

13-1 What are the main classes of transactions and related account balances for the payroll process?

13-2 What are the main risks for payroll, and management's main control objectives and control activities related to the payroll process? Why?

13-3 What are an auditor's main concerns related to payroll transactions? Why?

13-4 In what situations is it most likely that auditors will decide to test controls over payroll transactions?

13-5 What are some common substantive audit procedures for payroll? What financial statement assertions do these procedures provide evidence about?

13-6 What is the management purpose for information generated about costs of producing manufactured inventory, or services that are sold to customers?

13-7 What are the main classes of transactions and related account balances for the production process?

13-8 What are the main risks for production of manufactured inventory, and management's main control objectives related to the process? Why?

13-9 What are an auditor's main concerns related to production cost transactions? Why?

13-10 In what situations is it most likely that auditors will decide to test controls over the production process?

13-11 What are some common substantive audit procedures for inventory and the production process? What financial statement assertions do these procedures provide evidence about?

Risk Assessment for the Payroll and Production Processes

LO1 Describe the key risks of misstatement in the payroll and production processes.

For auditors, the payroll process is significant in virtually every organization that has employees. For businesses involved in manufacturing goods, it is also important for auditors to understand the production process. Risk considerations are explained for each of these processes.

Payroll Process

Payroll is the payments to hourly wage workers and salaried employees. Payments to employees involved in production are usually transferred to the cost of inventory (or self-constructed assets, internally generated intangible assets, etc.). Other wages and salaries are expensed in the current period. Payments to employees are the main transaction stream in the payroll process, and the main balances related to the process are relatively small year-end accruals for payroll liabilities. Ownership is the key assertion at risk here; the process involves small payments to individuals, so it is vulnerable to employee fraud. The major control risks are payments to fictitious employees (sometimes called "ghosts" on the payroll) and for more hours than are actually worked. The classification control objective is also important in the payroll process to ensure payroll costs are correctly allocated to inventory and appropriate classes of expenditures in the financial statements.

The assessment of payroll system control has to consider that the many transactions in this cycle add up to a large dollar amount, even though they result in small balance sheet account amounts at year-end. Because of this, reviews of control effectiveness and dual-purpose tests of controls and transaction details are used in many audit engagements, and the substantive audit procedures devoted to auditing the payroll-related, year-end balances can be more limited.

Risk assessment involves ensuring that payroll processing duties are well segregated and that independent reviews and approvals are effective. Substantive evidence is available from reconciling to government income tax reports and analysis of reasonableness of payroll expenses and accruals.

Production Process

Businesses produce many different types of tangible assets for sale or internal use. While each business will generate its revenues by a unique value-adding strategy, all will have similar production cost accounting processes that capture relevant costs and allocate them to asset accounts. In a manufacturing business, the main function of production cost accounting is allocation of material, labour, and overhead costs to the inventory items being produced. Service businesses, in contrast, bill customers for performing a specific job, such as a haircut or snowplowing, when the service is completed. Therefore, their productive activities are not inventoried. Professional service firms, such as lawyers and accountants, usually earn revenues based on the time spent on the assigned work; it could be hours, days, or weeks. For billing the customer, they have accounting systems that track hours spent on each job, giving them an intangible "inventory" of WIP showing hours worked that have not yet been billed. If a company wants to report direct costs of providing services, allocation of various costs such as salaries and supplies will be required and classification control procedures should be in place.

The production accounting process discussed in this chapter generates important information for management decisions on setting product and service selling prices, product-line profitability, producing or contracting production out, and production volume. The process also generates the reported balance sheet value of inventory or other assets. The flexibility and judgment involved in these costing processes lead to a risk of misstatement that the auditor has to assess. The inherent risk in this process also tends to be high because the information is complex and the transaction volumes involved can be large. This text focuses mainly on manufacturing businesses, while other types of production businesses have the same basic accounting requirements but with differing specific activities and costs.

Transaction streams in the production process are allocations from various material and overhead purchases, using accounts discussed in Chapter 12. Allocations are also made for labour costs, a payroll expenditure discussed later in this chapter. The main balances are finished inventory and WIP. **Cost of goods sold**

cost of goods sold:
costs such as materials, labour, overhead, freight, and so on, that are necessary to get goods to the stage when they can be sold; calculated as the beginning inventory, plus costs added during the period, less the ending inventory; offset against sales revenues, it indicates the gross profit or gross margin on sales on which analytical expectations can be based

expense is calculated from the changes in inventory, purchases, and other allocated costs, and from adjustments that result from reconciling booked quantities to a physical count of the inventory. The main disclosure is the inventory valuation policy, including lower-of-cost-and-market policy.

The risks for inventory relate to two aspects: physical quantities and valuation (or pricing). If the production process is the business's main activity, management should have strong controls over existence and completeness related to inventory quantities. Physical counts and reconciliation to booked quantities are very effective control procedures that auditors test substantively. Existence and completeness risks in inventory as well as related accounts receivable and payable balances are affected by cutoff errors. The valuation risk is affected by controls over pricing procedures for purchases and other manufacturing costs, and by the possibility that market values can fall below cost. Analytical procedures, often using detailed management reports, are useful for assessing risks related to the existence, completeness, and valuation assertions. Ownership risks relate to transfer of title to inventory, as it may not happen at the same time as the physical transfer. Ownership is assessed by inquiries, and by examining documents and inventory movements subsequent to year-end. Presentation risks include disclosure of inventory pledged as collateral, descriptions of accounting policies, and details of write-downs and reversals, as illustrated in the following box.

Example of Manufacturing Company Inventory Financial Statement Disclosures

Note 3 Significant Accounting Policies

(i) Inventories:

Inventories are stated at the lower of cost and net realizable value. The cost of inventories is based on the first-in, first-out principle and includes expenditures incurred in acquiring the inventories and bringing them to their existing location and condition. In the case of manufactured inventories, cost includes an appropriate share of variable and fixed overheads based on normal operating capacity. Any excess, unallocated, fixed overhead costs are expensed as incurred. Net realizable value is the estimated selling price in the ordinary course of business, less the estimated costs of completion and selling expenses.

13. Inventories:

	20X2	20X1	20X0
Raw materials	122,584	124,138	123,570
Work-in-process	13,753	12,266	9,619
Finished goods	137,367	135,757	133,230
Spare parts	4,314	3,914	3,393
	278,018	276,075	269,812

During 20X2, the Company recorded, within cost of sales, inventory write-downs for slow-moving and obsolete inventory of $16,080 (20X1: $21,539) and reversals of previously written-down items of $5,688 (20X1: $11,366).

Review Checkpoint

13-12   List the main risks auditors are concerned with in assessing risk in the payroll and production processes of a typical manufacturing business.

Section I: Understanding the Payroll Process

LO2   Describe the payroll process: typical transactions, account balances, source documents, and controls.

Every company has a payroll process. It may include payrolls for manufacturing labour, research scientists, administrative personnel, or all of these. Subsidiary operations, partnerships, and joint ventures may consider *management fees* charged by a parent company or general partner as payroll. Payroll can take different forms. Personnel management and the payroll accounting cycle include transactions affecting the wage and salary accounts as well as those affecting pension benefits, deferred compensation contracts, stock option plans, employee benefits (such as health insurance), payroll taxes, and related liabilities for these costs. It is very important that auditors verify the payroll system's compliance with local, provincial, and federal laws regarding deductions, overtime rules (e.g., after 8 hours in a day or 40 hours in a week), minimum wage rates, and so on. Failures to comply can lead to large liabilities. Many companies find it cost effective to use an outside payroll service organization to process and distribute payroll directly to employees' bank accounts because income taxes, rates, and calculations change frequently, and service organizations are better able to keep up to date with these changes.

Exhibit 13–1 is a skeleton diagram of a payroll process. It starts with hiring (and firing) people, moves on to determining employee wage rates and deductions, recording attendance and work (timekeeping), and payment

EXHIBIT 13–1

Payroll Process

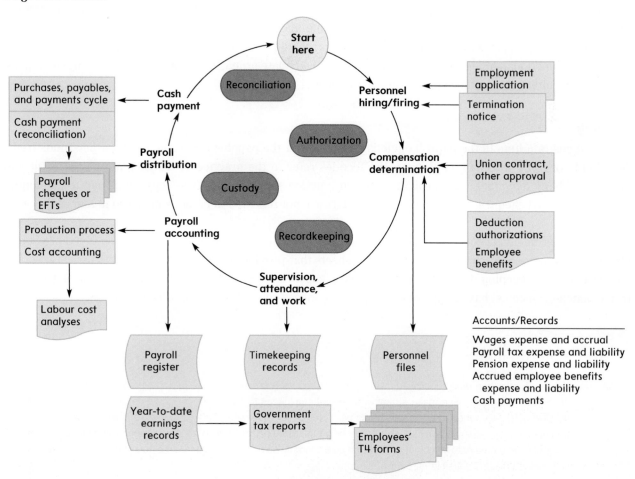

of wages and salaries, and ends with preparation of governmental (tax) and internal reports. One of these internal reports is a report of labour cost to the cost accounting department, which links the payroll cycle with cost accounting in the production cycle.

Five functional responsibilities should be performed by separate people or departments. They are as follows:

1. Personnel Management (Human Resources)—hiring and firing

2. Supervision—approval of work time

3. Timekeeping and Cost Accounting—payroll preparation and cost accounting

4. Payroll Accounting—cheque preparation and related payroll reports (this is often outsourced to a payroll processing service organization, which may be affiliated with the company's bank)

5. Payroll Distribution—actual custody of cheques and distribution to employees by cash, cheque, or direct bank deposit (outside payroll processing services typically include processing direct deposits to employees)

The elements that follow are part of the payroll control structure.

Authorization

A department (such as Human Resources) with authority to add new employees to the payroll, delete terminated employees, obtain authorizations for deductions (e.g., insurance, charitable donations, withholding-tax exemptions), and transmit authority for pay rate changes to the payroll department should be independent of the other functions. The supervision function should include authorization power. All pay base data (hours, job number, absences, time off allowed for emergencies, and the like) should be approved by an employee's immediate supervisor. Authorization is also a feature of the timekeeping and cost accounting functions. The data that pay is based on (e.g., hours, piece-rate volume, and incentives) should be accumulated independent of other functions. Many of the functional duties and responsibilities described relate primarily to non-salaried (hourly) employees. For salaried employees, no timekeeping data are collected.

Custody

The main custody item in the payroll cycle is possession of the paycheques, cash, or electronic funds transfer (EFT) codes used to pay employees. (EFT codes refer to the practice of transferring pay directly into employees' bank accounts.) A payroll distribution function should control the delivery of pay to employees so that unclaimed cheques, cash, or incomplete EFTs are not returned to persons involved in any of the other functions.

There are elements of custody of important documents in the supervision and timekeeping functions. Supervisors usually have access to time cards or time sheets that provide the basis for payment to hourly workers. Likewise, the timekeeping devices (e.g., time clocks, supervisory approval of time cards or time sheets, electronic punch-in systems) have a type of custody of employees' time-base for payroll calculations.

Approval of Fictitious Overtime

A supervisor at Austin Stoneworks discovered that she could approve overtime hours even though an employee had not worked 40 regular-time hours. She made a deal with several employees to alter their work time cards and split the extra payments. Over a 12-year period, the supervisor and her accomplices embezzled $107,000 in excess payments.

The employees' time cards were not reviewed after being approved by the supervisor. The company's payroll computer program did not have a valid data combination test that paid overtime only after 40 regular-time hours were paid. These two control weaknesses made it possible for employees to misappropriate Austin's cash.

Recordkeeping

The *payroll accounting* function prepares individual paycheques, pay envelopes, or EFTs using rate and deduction information supplied by the human resources function and base data supplied by the timekeeping-supervision function. Those in charge of the authorization and custody functions should not also prepare the payroll, as they might be tempted to pay fictitious employees.

In many companies, payroll processing is outsourced to specialized service organizations (ADP, Ceridian, etc.). This outsourcing is cost effective since keeping an in-house payroll program up to date with current tax and social insurance deductions rates requires a lot of programming time. This outsourcing also adds an element of segregation of duties since the payments are generated outside the company's accounting system. The input and output aspects of the process must still be controlled within the company, however.

Payroll accounting maintains individual year-to-date earnings records and prepares the provincial and federal tax reports (income tax and Canada or Quebec Pension Plan [CPP, QPP] withholding, employment insurance [EI] reports, and annual T4 forms). The payroll tax returns (e.g., the federal T4 summary reporting income taxes, EI, and pension withholdings from employees for the year) are useful records for audit recalculation and overall testing (analytical) procedures. They should correspond to company records and financial statement amounts. When an outside payroll processing service is used, it will usually provide the detailed journal entries to record each payroll as well as the year-end T4 forms and summaries.

Periodic Reconciliation

The payroll bank account can be reconciled as any other bank account, and the transactions can also be reconciled to recorded wage cost and expense. Some companies send each supervisor a copy of the payroll register showing the employees paid under their authority and responsibility. The supervisor gets a chance to re-approve the payroll after it is completed. This provides an opportunity to notice whether any persons not approved have been paid and charged to the supervisor's accountability.

The payroll report sent to cost accounting can be reconciled to the labour records, charging labour cost to production. The cost accounting function should determine whether the labour paid is the same as the labour cost used in the cost accounting calculations.

Not Enough Control, No Feedback, Bye-Bye Money

Homer had been in payroll accounting for a long time. He knew it was not uncommon to pay a terminated employee severance benefits and partial pay after termination; Homer received the termination notices and the data for the final paycheques. But Homer also knew how to keep the terminated employee on the payroll for another week, pay a full week's compensation, change the EFT code, and take the money for himself. The only things he could not change were the personnel department's copy of the termination notices, the payroll register, and the individual employee pay records used for withholding tax.

Fortunately for Homer, nobody reconciled the cost accounting labour charges to the payroll. The supervisors did not get a copy of the payroll register for post-payment approval, so they did not have any opportunity to notice the extra week. Nobody ever reviewed the payroll with reference to the termination notices. Former employees never complained about more pay and withholding reported on their T4s since the difference in the totals was fairly small.

Homer and his wife, Marge, retired comfortably to a villa in Spain on a nest egg that had grown to $850,000. After Homer retired, the company experienced an unexpected decrease in labour costs and higher profits. The lack of independent reviews of payroll register details by the supervisors who would have known the details of when employees left was a serious control weakness that allowed a lot of the company's money to end up in Homer's hands.

Audit Evidence in Management Reports and Files

Payroll systems produce numerous reports. Some are internal reports and bookkeeping records. Others are government tax reports.

Personnel Files

The department responsible for payroll (e.g., Human Resources) keeps individual employee files. The contents usually include an employment application, background investigation report, notice of hiring, job classification with pay rate authorization, and authorizations for deductions (e.g., health benefits, life insurance, retirement contribution, union dues, and income tax exemptions). When employees retire, quit, or are otherwise terminated, appropriate notices of termination are filed. These files contain the raw data for important pension and post-retirement benefit accounting involving an employee's age, tenure with the company, wage record, and other information used in actuarial calculations.

A personnel file should establish the reality of a person's existence and employment. The background investigation report (prior employment, references, social insurance number validity check, credentials investigation, and perhaps a private investigator's report) is important for employees in sensitive positions such as accounting, finance, and asset custody. Capable personnel are a primary system control. Errors and frauds perpetrated by people who falsify their credentials (identification, education, prior experience, criminal record, and the like) abound. A fidelity bond for employees through an insurance company offers some protection from this risk.

Timekeeping Records

For employees paid by the hour or on various incentive systems, records of time, production, piecework, or other measures are the basis of their pay. These records are collected in a variety of ways. Old-fashioned time clocks still accept employee time cards and imprint the time when work started and ended. More sophisticated systems use card readers to perform the same function. Production employees may clock in for various jobs or production processes in a system that assigns labour costs to various stages of production.

Timekeeping records should be approved by supervisors to show that employees actually worked the hours (or produced the output) reported to the payroll department. A supervisor's signature or initials should be on the documents used by the payroll department as the basis for periodic pay. In computerized payroll systems, this approval comes in the form of the supervisory passwords used to input data.

Payroll Register

The payroll register typically contains a record for each employee, showing the gross regular pay, gross overtime pay, income tax withheld, EI and CPP or QPP withheld, other deductions, and net pay, as illustrated in Exhibit 13–2.

EXHIBIT 13–2

Example of a Payroll Register for EcoPak

				ECOPAK INC.			Page		1
				Summary Payroll Register			Date		25/6/X7
							Period		11/04/X7
Company – Home . . 00100							Payroll ID		001
Employee Number	Employee Name	Hours	Wages	Benefits	Gross Pay	Deductions	Taxes	Net Pay	Cheque Number
12–001	Lee, Kam	40.00	2,038.46	583.05	2,038.46	101.92	465.37	1,471.17	171504
12–002	Parker, Michel	40.00	1,692.31	139.79	1,692.31	63.12	410.12	1,219.07	171505
12–003	Kolomov, Igor	40.00	2,615.38	490.39	2,955.38	143.12	927.76	1,884.50	171506
12–023	Merker, Anna	40.00	1,361.54	315.78	1,538.54	66.81	322.84	1,148.89	171507
13–001	Parker, Naomi	40.00	1,826.92	403.80	2,064.42	103.70	513.65	1,447.07	171508
13–024	Cameron, Daniel	40.00	1,591.35	370.65	1,798.23	107.83	407.85	1,282.55	171509
14–005	Tsipras, Alexis	40.00	1,909.20	444.78	2,157.88	128.86	489.42	1,539.06	171510
ETC.									

When the company processes its own payroll, the net pay amount is usually transferred from the company's main operating bank account to a special payroll **imprest bank account (imprest fund)**.

To illustrate the details of payroll bookkeeping, the journal entry for the transfer of net payroll, for example, is as follows:

Payroll Bank Account 25,774
    General Bank Account 25,774

When an outside payroll processing service is used, a cheque or bank transfer for the net payroll is usually issued from the operating bank account to the payroll organization. The payroll service organization then processes the distributions to individual employees' bank accounts, so a separate payroll bank account is not required. The payroll amounts are accumulated to create the payroll posting to the general ledger, as in this example:

Wages clearing account 40,265
    Employee income taxes payable account 7,982
    Employee CPP account 3,080
    EI premium payable account 2,100
    Life insurance premium payable account 1,329
    Payroll bank account 25,774

The payroll register is the primary original record for payroll accounting. It contains the implicit assertions that the employees are real company personnel (existence assertion), that they worked the time or production they were paid for (rights/ownership assertion), that the amount of the pay is calculated properly (valuation assertion), and that all the employees were paid (completeness assertion). The presentation and disclosure assertion depends on the labour cost analysis explained below.

Payroll department records also include the cancelled cheques containing the employees' endorsements, or a similar electronic record for direct deposits.

imprest bank account (imprest fund):
an account or fund used by a business for small, routine expenditure items that is restored to a fixed amount periodically; used for payroll bank accounts and petty cash funds

Labour Cost Analysis

The cost accounting department can receive its information in more than one way. Systems may independently report time and production work data from the production floor directly to the cost accounting department. Cost accounting departments may receive labour cost data from the payroll department. When the information is received independently, it can be reconciled in quantity (time) or amount (dollars) with a report from the payroll department. This reconciliation makes sure that the cost accounting department is using actual payroll data and that the payroll department is paying only for work performed.

The cost accounting department (or a similar accounting function) is responsible for the cost distribution—the most important part of the payroll presentation and disclosure assertion. The cost distribution assigns payroll to the accounts where it belongs for internal and external reporting. As an illustration of the accounting, using its input data, the cost accounting department may make a distribution entry such as the following:

Production job A	14,364
Production job B	3,999
Production process A	10,338
Selling expense	8,961
General and administrative expense	2,603
Wages clearing account	40,265

Payroll data flow from the hiring process, through the timekeeping function, into the payroll department, to the cost accounting department, and, finally, to the accounting entries that record the payroll for inventory cost determination and financial statement presentation. The same data are used for various government and tax reports.

Government and Tax Reports

Provincial and federal income and pension plan laws introduce complications into payroll systems. Several reports are produced that auditors can use in tests of controls and substantive tests of the balances produced by accumulating payroll transactions in year-to-date (YTD) records.

Year-to-Date Earnings Records

The YTD earnings records are the cumulative subsidiary records of each employee's gross pay, deductions, and net pay. Each time a periodic payroll is produced, the YTD earnings records are updated with the new information. The YTD earnings records are a subsidiary ledger of the wages and salaries cost and expense in the financial statements. Theoretically, like any subsidiary and control account relationship, their sum (e.g., the gross pay amounts) should be equal to the costs and expenses in the financial statements. The trouble with this reconciliation idea is that there are usually many payroll cost/expense accounts in a company's chart of accounts. The production wages may be scattered in several different accounts, such as inventory (WIP and finished goods) and selling, general, and administrative expenses.

The YTD records do, however, provide the data for periodic governmental and tax forms. They can usually be reconciled to the tax reports. Companies in financial difficulty have been known to try to postpone payment of employee taxes, EI, and CPP or QPP withheld. However, the consequences can be serious. The Canada Revenue Agency (CRA) can and will padlock the business and seize the assets for non-payment. After all, the withheld taxes belong to the employee's accounts with the government, and the employers are obligated to pay over the amounts withheld from employees along with a matching share for the CPP and EI.

Employee Income Tax Reports

In Canada, the T4 slip is the annual report of gross salaries and wages as well as the income tax, pension plan, and employment insurance withheld. Copies are filed with the CRA or Quebec Ministry of Finance, and copies are sent to employees for preparing their income tax returns. The T4 contains the YTD accumulations for the employee, along with their address and social insurance number. In certain procedures (described later), auditors can use the name, address, social insurance number, and dollar amounts to obtain evidence about the existence of employees. The T4 can be reconciled to the payroll tax reports.

Beware the "Clearing Account"

Clearing accounts (also called "suspense accounts") are temporary storage places for transactions awaiting final accounting. Like the wages clearing account illustrated in the entries above, all clearing accounts should have zero balances after the accounting is completed.

A balance in a clearing account means that some amounts have not been classified properly in the accounting records. If the wages clearing account has a debit balance, some labour cost has not been properly classified in the expense accounts or cost accounting classifications. If the wages clearing account has a credit balance, the cost accountant has assigned more labour cost to expense accounts and cost accounting classifications than the amount actually paid.

Review Checkpoints

13-17 What important information can be found in employees' personnel files?

13-18 What is important about background checks using the employment applications submitted by prospective employees?

13-19 What payroll documentation supports the validity and accuracy of payroll transactions?

13-20 Which government tax returns can be reconciled in total with employees' YTD earnings records? reconciled in total but not in detail?

13-21 What is the purpose of examining endorsements on the back of payroll cheques?

Control Risk Assessment

LO3 Describe control tests for auditing control over hiring, firing, and payment of employees in the payroll process.

The major risks in the payroll process are as follows:

- Paying fictitious "employees" (employees that do not exist, invalid transactions)
- Overpaying for time or production (inaccurate transactions, improper valuation)
- Accounting for costs and expenses incorrectly (incorrect classification, improper or inconsistent presentation and disclosure)

The assessment of payroll system control risk is significant because there are so many transactions in this process, yet they result in small amounts in balance sheet accounts at year-end. Therefore, auditors often decide to use a combined audit approach, testing controls and transaction details using dual-purpose tests to lower assessed control risk so that less-substantive testing is required.

General Control Considerations

Control procedures for proper segregation of responsibilities should be in place and operating. From Exhibit 13–1, you can see that proper segregation involves authorization (human resources department hiring and firing, pay rate, and deduction authorizations) by persons who do not have payroll preparation, paycheque distribution, or reconciliation duties. Payroll distribution (custody) is in the hands of those who neither authorize employees' pay rates or time, nor prepare the payroll cheques. Recordkeeping is performed by payroll and cost accounting personnel who do not make authorizations or distribute pay. Combinations of two or more of the duties of authorization, payroll preparation and recordkeeping, and payroll distribution in one person, office, or computerized system may open the door for errors and fraud.

In addition, the control structure should provide for detail-checking procedures: (1) periodic comparison of the payroll register with the human resources department files to check for hiring authorizations and terminated employees not deleted, (2) periodic rechecking of wage rate and deduction authorizations, (3) reconciliation of time and production paid to cost accounting calculations, (4) reconciliation of YTD earnings records with tax returns, and (5) payroll bank account reconciliation.

Some companies have in-house information technology (IT) systems to gather payroll data, calculate payroll amounts, print cheques, and transfer electronic deposits. Their complexity varies, however, from simply writing payroll cheques to an integrated system preparing management reports and cost analyses based on payroll and cost distribution inputs. Payroll accounting is frequently contracted out to specialized service organizations. Regardless of the technology, the basic management and control functions of ensuring a flow of data to the payroll department should be in place. Computer audit techniques, such as test data, can be used to audit general controls that may be embedded in a computerized payroll system, and penetration tests can be used to verify effectiveness of general controls over security and authorized access. Outside payroll service organizations are typically well known and reputable global operations, and in this case auditors can generally take the reports received from them as having been processed under strong accuracy and completeness controls. Validity, authorization, classification, and proper period control objectives must still be addressed by controls within the company's own payroll process, regardless of whether in-house or outsourced processing is used.

Internal Control Questionnaire

Information about the payroll process control structure is often gathered initially through an internal control questionnaire. Exhibit 13A–1 in Appendix 13A shows details of desirable policies and procedures for the control environment and the important control objectives—validity, completeness, authorization, accuracy, classification, and proper period recording.

Control Tests

An organization should have detailed control procedures in place and operating to prevent, detect, and correct accounting errors. The general control objectives were covered in Chapter 9. Exhibit 13–3 puts these in the perspective of the payroll functions with examples of specific objectives.

Auditors can perform control tests to determine whether controls that are said to be in place and operating are actually being performed properly by company personnel. Exhibit 13–4 contains a selection of procedures for testing controls over payroll, together with the control objective each tests. The samples are usually attribute samples designed along the lines discussed in Chapter 10.

Covert Surveillance

Covert surveillance sounds like spy work, and it does include certain elements of that.

Auditors can test controls over employees' clocking in for work shifts by personally observing the process—observing whether anybody clocks in with two time cards or with two or more electronic entries, or leaves the premises after clocking in.

Auditors need to be careful not to make themselves obvious. Standing around in a manufacturing plant at 6 a.m. in a business suit is as good as printing "Beware of Auditor" on your forehead. People will then be on their best behaviour, and you will observe nothing unusual.

Find an unobtrusive observation post. Stay out of sight. Keep detailed records of what you see; even take a video, if permitted. Get a knowledgeable and trustworthy office employee to accompany you to interpret various activities. Perform an observation that has a chance of producing evidence of improper behaviour.

EXHIBIT 13–3

Control Objectives (Payroll Process)

GENERAL OBJECTIVES	EXAMPLES OF SPECIFIC CONTROL ACTIVITIES
1. Recorded payroll transactions are *valid* and documented.	Payroll accounting is separated from personnel and timekeeping. Time cards are approved by the supervisor. Payroll files are periodically compared with personnel files.
2. Valid payroll transactions are *recorded completely,* and none are omitted.	Employees' complaints about paycheques are investigated and resolved (written records are maintained and reviewed by internal auditors).
3. Payroll names, rates, hours, and deductions are *authorized.*	Names of new hires or terminations are reported immediately in writing to payroll by the personnel department. Authorizations for deductions are kept on file. The pay rate is authorized by union contract, agreement, or written policy and approved by a personnel officer.
4. Payroll computations contain *accurate* gross pay, deductions, and net pay.	Payroll computations are checked by a person independent of preparation. Totals of payroll register are reconciled to totals of payroll distribution by cost accounting. If an outside payroll processing service is used, reports are reviewed for reasonableness before updating the general ledger accounts.
5. Payroll transactions are *classified* correctly as direct or indirect labour or other expenses.	Employee classification is reviewed periodically. Overall charges to indirect labour are periodically compared with direct labour and total product costs.
6. Payroll costs and expenses are recorded in the *proper period.*	Month-end accruals are reviewed by internal auditors. Payroll is computed, paid, and booked in a timely manner.

Two Directions of Control Tests

The control tests in Exhibit 13–4 are designed to test the payroll accounting in two directions. One is the completeness direction, which matches personnel file content to payroll department files and the payroll register. The procedures trace the human resources department authorizations to the payroll department files—procedure A-1-c in Exhibits 13–4 and 13–5. The other direction of the test is validity. The control performance of interest here is the preparation of the payroll register. Exhibit 13–5 shows that the sample for this test is from the completed payroll registers. The individual payroll calculations are vouched to the personnel files (procedure B-1-a).

Generalized audit software can be used to test controls in the payroll process. Files are matched (e.g., personnel master file and payroll master file), and unmatched records and differences in common fields can be printed out. Statistical samples of files can be printed for vouching to union contracts or other authorizations. Statistical samples can be selected for recalculation by the software or printed out as working papers for tracing and vouching, using the procedures in Exhibit 13–4.

The tests of controls and transaction details are evidence of the reliability of internal management reports and analyses. In turn, reliance on these reports and analyses, along with other analytical relationships, is a major portion of the substantive audit of payroll, compensation costs, and labour costs assigned to inventory and costs of goods sold.

The test of controls procedures are designed to produce evidence of the following items:

- Adequacy of personnel files, especially the authorizations of pay rate and deductions used in calculating pay
- Accuracy of the periodic payrolls recorded in accounts and in employees' cumulative wage records; the procedures tend to centre on the periodic payroll registers
- Accuracy of cost accounting distributions and management reports (the cost accounting for labour costs must be reasonably accurate because good management reports contribute to cost control; the auditor who relies on the cost accounting system must determine whether it contains and transmits accurate information)

EXHIBIT 13–4

Control Tests for Payroll

	CONTROL OBJECTIVE
A. Personnel Files and Compensation Documents	
1. Select a sample of personnel files:	
(a) Review personnel files for complete information on employment date, authority to add to payroll, job classification, wage rate, and authorized deductions.	Authorization Classification Authorization
(b) Trace pay rate to union or other contracts or other rate authorization. Trace salaries to directors' minutes for authorization.	Authorization
(c) Trace pay rate and deduction information to payroll department files used in payroll preparation.	Completeness
2. Obtain copies of pension plans, stock options, profit sharing, and bonus plans. Review and extract relevant portions that relate to payroll deductions, fringe benefit expenses, accrued liabilities, and financial statement disclosure.	Validity Completeness
3. Trace management compensation schemes to minutes to verify board of directors' approval.	Authorization Accuracy
B. Payroll	
1. Select a sample of payroll register entries:	
(a) Vouch employee identification, pay rate, and deductions to personnel files or other authorizations.	Authorization
(b) Vouch hours worked to time-clock records and supervisor's approval.	Validity Authorization
(c) Recalculate gross pay, deductions, and net pay.	Accuracy
(d) Recalculate a selection of periodic payrolls.	Accuracy
(e) Vouch to cancelled payroll cheque. Examine employees' endorsement or payroll distribution report details.	Accuracy Validity
2. Select a sample of time-clock entries or other records of hours worked. Note supervisor's approval and trace to periodic payroll registers.	Authorization Completeness
3. Trace a sample of employees' payroll entries to individual payroll records maintained for tax reporting purposes. Reconcile total of employees' payroll records with payrolls paid for the year.	Completeness Accuracy
4. Review computer-printed error messages for evidence of the use of check digits; valid codes; limit tests; and other input, processing, and output application controls. Investigate correction and resolution of errors.	Accuracy
5. Trace payroll information to management reports and to general ledger account postings.	Accuracy
6. If applicable, obtain control of a periodic payroll and conduct a surprise distribution of paycheques.	Validity
C. Cost Distribution Reports	
1. Select a sample of cost accounting analyses of payroll:	
(a) Reconcile periodic totals with payroll payments for the same periods.	Completeness
(b) Vouch to time records.	Validity
2. Trace cost accounting labour cost distributions to management reports and postings in general ledger and subsidiary account(s).	Classification
3. Select a sample of labour cost items in (a) ledger accounts and/or (b) management reports. Vouch to supporting cost accounting analyses.	Validity

EXHIBIT 13–5

Two-Direction Test of Payroll Controls

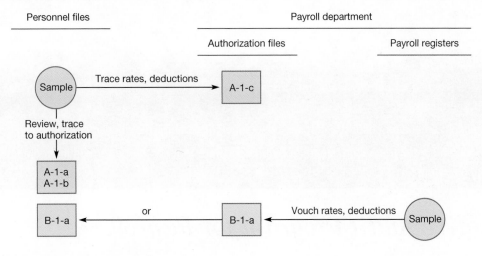

Note: The A-1-a, etc., codes refer to control tests listed in Exhibit 13–4.

Overt Surveillance

Surprise Payroll Distribution

In organizations that distribute paycheques by hand, auditors may perform a surprise observation of a payroll distribution in connection with tests for overstatement. This involves taking control of paycheques and accompanying a company representative as the distribution takes place. The auditor ensures that each employee is identified and that only one cheque is given to each individual. Unclaimed cheques are controlled, and in this manner the auditor hopes to detect any fictitious persons on the payroll. Auditors need to be extremely careful to notice any duplication of employee identification or instance of one person attempting to pick up two or more cheques.

Summary: Control Risk Assessment

The audit manager or senior accountant in charge of the audit should evaluate the evidence obtained from an understanding of the internal control structure and from the test of controls audit procedures. If the control risk is assessed very low, the substantive audit procedures on the account balances can be limited. For example, it may be appropriate to rely on management reports generated by the payroll system.

On the other hand, if tests of controls reveal weaknesses, improper segregation of duties, inaccurate cost reports, inaccurate tax returns, or lax human resources policies, then substantive procedures will need to be designed to lower the risk of failing to detect material error in the financial statements. However, the irregularities of paying fictitious employees and overpaying for fraudulent time records do not normally misstate the financial statements, as long as the improper payments are expensed. (The losses are expensed, as they should be!) The misstatement is failing to distinguish "payroll fraud losses" from legitimate wages expense and cost of goods sold and then disclose them, but such losses would probably be immaterial in a single year's financial statements, anyway. While it is not a central part of their work of detecting material misstatements in financial statements, auditors nevertheless do perform procedures that may find payroll fraud.

Review Checkpoints

13-22 What are common errors and fraud in the payroll process? Which control characteristics are auditors looking for to prevent or detect these errors and fraud?

13-23 Why is it unwise for an auditor to stand by the plant gate and time clock to observe employees checking in for work shifts?

13-24 How can an auditor determine whether the amount of labour cost charged to production was actually paid to employees?

13-25 Why might an auditor conduct a surprise observation of a payroll distribution? What should be observed?

13-26 Describe a control test using generalized audit software that can be performed in a computerized payroll system.

Substantive Audit Program for Payroll

LO4 Give examples of the typical substantive procedures used to address the assessed risk of material misstatement in the main accounts in the payroll process.

Exhibit 13–6 provides a template audit program for obtaining substantive evidence in relation to payroll expenses and balances. The program outlines the substantive procedures typically used to audit the payroll process. Analytical procedures are often a key source of evidence. Substantive evidence is obtained through examination of transactions and resulting account balances.

EXHIBIT 13–6

Example of Substantive Audit Program Responding to Assessed Risk of Material Misstatement for Payroll Expenses and Balances: Selected Substantive Procedures

SUBSTANTIVE AUDIT PROGRAM				
AUDITEE: ECOPAK INC.			**FILE INDEX:** 730	
FINANCIAL STATEMENT PERIOD: y/e DECEMBER 31, 20X1				
ACCOUNT: Payroll expenses and balances				
Substantive audit program in response to assessed risks:				
Consider risk assessment findings and conclusion on residual detection risk to be reduced by performing substantive procedures. (Of the procedures listed below, perform those considered necessary to provide sufficient appropriate evidence to address the assessed risks and reduce the risk of material misstatement to an acceptable level.)				*[Reference to relevant working papers]*
SUBSTANTIVE AUDIT PROCEDURES	Assertions evidence is related to [E, C, O, V, P*]	Timing	Extent	Working paper reference
Analytical procedures 1. Develop expectations for payroll expenses based on understanding the entity, including production volumes, new product lines, labour union agreements, prior period's payroll expenses, industry changes, etc.				
2. Perform the following analysis, and obtain satisfactory explanations from management for relationships observed: (a) Significant changes or trends in payroll expenses compared with prior period(s) and/or budgets in total and as a percentage of sales (b) Payroll expenses compared with related accrued liabilities (c) Average annual wage in comparison with work force, minimum wage rates, etc.	E, C, V			*(continued)*

EXHIBIT 13–6

Example of Substantive Audit Program Responding to Assessed Risk of Material Misstatement for Payroll Expenses and Balances: Selected Substantive Procedures   *(continued)*

(d) Payroll expenses compared with non-financial information such as production volume, facility size, manufacturing process times, product-line changes				
(e) Payroll and benefits by employee type or class by comparing with prior period and budgets (e.g., benefits as a percentage of total payroll, average salary per employee).				
(f) Reasonableness of average hourly rates and average salary per employee when compared with normal rates or salary classes				
3. Consider management responses to inquiries about	E, C, V			
(a) Changes to payroll policies and procedures, noting any changes from prior periods.				
(b) Any salary or rate increases, significant increases in staffing, and/or changes to the benefit plan or regulations.				
Conclude whether these are consistent with the payroll expenses and balances reported for the current period.				
Tests of details of transactions and balances	E, V, O			
4. For payroll and benefits:				
(a) Scan the payroll journal for the period for large and unusual items, and ascertain the propriety of such items.				
(b) Ask responsible payroll personnel about any instances of fictitious employees, employees with unusual contract terms or conditions, or unrecorded transactions.				
5. For high assessed risk of misstatement of payroll and benefits:				
Select a sample of employee payroll payments from the payroll journal and perform the following:	E, C, V			
(a) Trace employee's name, job category, and employee number to authorized personnel records.				
(b) Agree pay rate to authorized wage, union contract, or other authorized record.				
(c) Agree hours worked to clock card or other time record.				
(d) Inquire of employee's supervisor regarding the person's job description, and assess reasonableness of their pay rate.				
(e) Agree hours worked to labour cost allocated to inventory cost accounting records.	P			
(f) Recalculate gross and net pay using employee TD1 and current tax withholding tables for income tax withheld and CPP and EI deduction rates, and by examining authorization forms for other payroll deductions, such as company pension plan or group insurance.				
6. If the period-end is close to the calendar year-end, compare the total payroll costs to the T4 summary. Investigate and document any significant differences.	E, C, V			
7. Examine paid and endorsed payroll cheques, or payroll bank account debit entry details, of selected employees and trace to data in the payroll journal.	O			
Misstatement summary:				
Summarize here all misstatements discovered in executing this program. Carry all forward for accumulation in the Summary of Accumulated Misstatements worksheet (Exhibit 16–1).				
AUDITOR'S CONCLUSIONS [If the audit program is completed satisfactorily and the audit objectives are met, a conclusion such as the following would be recorded by the auditor performing the work.] *Based on my professional judgment, the evidence obtained is sufficient and appropriate to conclude that the risk of material misstatement of the PAYROLL EXPENSES AND BALANCES is acceptably low.* Prepared by _____ Date _____ Reviewed by _____ Date _____				

* E, C, O, V, P = existence, completeness, ownership, valuation, presentation.

Review Checkpoints

13-27   Describe analytical procedures that can be used for payroll transactions and balances.

13-28   Explain how government forms and reports can be used in the audit of payroll transactions and balances.

To cap off this general description of an audit program for a payroll process, note the following analysis approaches used to integrate the audit findings.

Analysis of Financial Statement Relationships

The audit of the payroll process verifies the balances of various payroll liabilities and wages/salary expense. As an overall analysis technique, we can analyze balance changes and the financial statement items related to them by preparing a continuity schedule. The accrued salaries payable balance is used as an example for the payroll process:

AUDITED AMOUNT	FINANCIAL STATEMENT WHERE AMOUNT IS REPORTED
Opening balance of salaries payable	Balance sheet (prior-year comparative figure)
Deduct: Payment of salaries (from the first payroll processed in new period)	Cash flow statement (direct method)
Add: Calculated accrual required at the end of the current period	Income statement salary expense
Ending balance of salaries payable	Balance sheet (current-year figure)

Analytical procedures that use these relationships include various expense ratios and accrual reasonableness tests. Misstatements in the existence, completeness, and valuation assertions for personnel-related expenses may result in unexplained fluctuations in these relationships.

Misstatement Analysis

Consider the following misstatement that might be discovered in an audit. The auditors examined the payroll process and learned that the company payroll had been paid up to December 30, prior to its year-end of December 31. Since the company shut down for December 31, the payroll accountant decided that it was not necessary to accrue the last day's payroll, which amounts to $2,500. The auditors did not agree; whether the offices were closed is not relevant because the employees were still being paid for that day, and the financial statements are dated December 31. This error means the accrued payroll liability and the payroll expense for the year are both understated. (The account analysis for this accrued liability will follow the same format as the one given for legal expenses and accrual at the end of Chapter 12.) This amount of misstatement, taken alone, is immaterial, but it is not trivial, so it must be carried forward and added to the summary of accumulated misstatements (see Exhibit 16–1) for evaluation in forming the audit opinion at the end of the audit.

Section II: Understanding the Production Process

LO5   Describe the production process: typical transactions, account balances, source documents, and controls.

Exhibit 13–7 is a skeleton diagram showing the activities and accounting involved in a production process. These begin with production planning, including inventory planning and management. Production planning can

EXHIBIT 13–7

Production Process

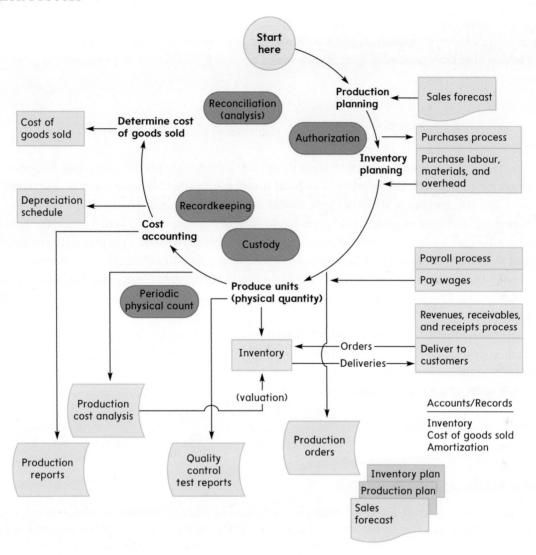

involve the use of a sophisticated, computerized long-range plan with just-in-time (JIT) inventory management, or it can be done by a simple ad hoc method ("Hey, Joe, we got an order today. Go make 10 units!"). Most businesses try to estimate or forecast sales levels and seasonal effects, and they plan facilities and production schedules to meet forecast customer demand. As shown in Exhibit 13–1, the production cycle interacts with the purchasing process (see Chapter 12) and the payroll process (discussed in Section I of this chapter) for the acquisition of fixed assets, materials, supplies, overhead, and labour.

The physical output of a production process is the inventory (from raw materials to WIP to finished goods). Inventory auditing and physical inventory taking were explained in Chapter 12, and Exhibit 11–1 in Chapter 11 showed the connection of inventory to the revenue process in terms of orders and deliveries.

Most of the transactions in a production cycle are cost accounting allocations, unit cost determinations, and standard cost calculations. These are internal transactions, produced entirely within the company's accounting system. Exhibit 13–7 shows the elements of depreciation cost calculation, cost of goods sold determination, and job cost analysis as examples.

The audit of inventory consists of two phases: verifying the physical units and testing the unit costs. Physically observing the inventory count, including any equivalent units calculations for WIP, is the main procedure for verifying physical units. The unit costing of inventory (also referred to as *price tests*) for purchased inventory, such as the inventory of retailers, was partly covered in Chapter 12. In the cost-testing procedures for produced or manufactured inventory, the cost allocations and computations are much more complex (as you may have noticed in your management accounting courses). For example, in process costing the following formula is used:

$$\text{Unit Cost of Production} = \frac{\text{Production Costs}}{\text{Equivalent Units of Production}}$$

Once the unit costs of production are known, the total inventory production costs for reporting purposes are unit cost times number of units. The total inventory production cost must be allocated between cost of sales (on the income statement) and inventory (on the balance sheet). This allocation of costs between inventory and cost of goods sold includes proper allocation of any cost variances. This is necessary because a budget system is a control system, and for external reporting purposes the actual costs, not the standard or budgeted costs, must be disclosed. This allocation will affect the cost amounts the auditor uses in inventory valuation tests that assess whether recorded inventory costs are lower than market-based net realizable values. The box below shows how errors can arise in allocating standard overhead costs to inventory.

Valuation of manufactured inventory, manufactured cost of goods sold, and any self-constructed PPE assets is based on these internal cost allocations. Therefore, the appropriateness of such cost allocations is a critical part of the audit of the valuation assertion of inventory and fixed assets.

As you follow Exhibit 13–7, you can track the elements of the control structure below.

Overhead Allocation Analysis

The cost accounting department at Pointed Publications Inc. routinely allocated overhead to book-printing runs at the standard rate of 40% of materials and labour cost. The debit was initially to the finished books inventory, while the credit went to an "overhead allocated" account that was offset against other entries in the cost of goods sold calculation, which included all the actual overhead incurred. During the year, 10 million books were produced and $40 million of overhead was allocated to them. The auditors noticed that actual overhead expenditures were $32 million, and 3 million books remained in the ending inventory.

This finding resulted in the conclusion that the inventory was overstated by $2.4 million, and the cost of goods sold was understated by $2.4 million.

	COMPANY ALLOCATION (USING STANDARD OVERHEAD RATE)	AUDITOR ANALYSIS (USING ACTUAL OVERHEAD)
Books produced	10.00 million	10.00 million
Labour and material cost	$100.00 million	$100.00 million
Overhead allocated	$ 40.00 million	$ 32.00 million
Cost per book	$ 14.00 million	$ 13.20 million

(continued)

	COMPANY ALLOCATION (USING STANDARD OVERHEAD RATE)	AUDITOR ANALYSIS (USING ACTUAL OVERHEAD)
Cost of goods sold		
Labour and materials cost	$100 million	$100.0 million
Overhead allocated to books	40 million	
Overhead incurred	32 million	32.0 million
Overhead credited to cost	(40 million)	
Ending inventory	(42 million)	(39.6 million)
Total cost of goods sold	$ 90 million	$ 92.4 million
Cost of goods sold per company		$ 90.0 million
Difference (understated)		$ 2.4 million

Audit Conclusion: Cost of sales is understated by $2.4 million. Difference is carried forward to accumulated misstatements summary worksheet in audit file documentation.

Authorization

Production authorization starts with production planning, which is usually based on a sales forecast. Production planning interacts with inventory planning to generate production orders. These production orders specify the materials and labour required, as well as the timing for the start and end of production. Managers in the sales/marketing and production departments usually sign off their approval on plans and production orders. Since sales volume and inventory requirements change with economic conditions and company success or failure, these plans and approvals are dynamic; they are amended according to changing needs. Authorization can also include plans and approvals for subcontracting work to other companies. The process of taking bids and executing contracts can be a part of the planning-authorization system.

The production order usually includes a *bill of materials* (a specification of the materials authorized for the production). The materials requisitions are prepared based on the authorization of the bill of materials, and these requisitions become the authorization for the inventory custodian to release raw materials and supplies to the production personnel. They then become the inventory recordkeeper's authorizations to update the raw materials inventory files to record reductions in the raw materials inventory.

Later, when production is complete, the production reports, the physical inventory units, and the quality control test reports for the physical units are the authorizations for the finished goods inventory custodian to place the units in the finished goods inventory. These same documents are the inventory recordkeeper's authorization to update the inventory record files with the additions.

Custody

Supervisors and workers have physical custody of materials, equipment, and labour while production work is performed. They requisition materials from the raw materials inventory, assign people to jobs, and control the pace of work. In a sense, they have custody of a moving inventory. The WIP (an inventory category) is "moving" and changing form in the process of being transformed from raw materials into finished goods.

Control over this custody is more difficult than control over a closed warehouse full of raw materials or finished goods. It can be exercised by holding supervisors and workers accountable for the use of materials specified in the production orders, the timely completion of production, and the quality of the finished goods. This accountability can be achieved with good cost accounting, cost analysis, and quality control testing.

Recordkeeping (Cost Accounting)

When production is completed, production orders and the related records of material and labour used are forwarded to the cost accounting department. Since these accounting documents may come from the production personnel, effective separation depends on the department's receiving independent notices from other places, especially notifications of materials issued from the inventory custodian and of the labour costs assigned by the payroll department.

The cost accounting department calculates the cost per unit, standard cost, and variances. It may also determine the allocation of overhead to production in general, to production orders, and to finished units. Depending on the design of the company's accounting system, these costs are used in inventory valuation and, ultimately, in determining the cost of goods sold. Often, this department is responsible for calculating the depreciation of production assets and the amortization of intangibles.

Periodic Reconciliation

Periodic reconciliation compares actual assets and liabilities with amounts recorded in the company accounts (e.g., the physical count of inventory with the perpetual inventory records, vendors' monthly statements with the recorded accounts payable). Exhibit 13–7 shows the periodic reconciliation of physical inventory to recorded amounts. The features and audit considerations of this reconciliation were covered in Chapter 12. The WIP inventory can also be observed, although the "count" of partially completed units is subjective. It can be costed based on the labour, materials, and overhead used at its stage of completion.

Most other periodic reconciliations in the production cycle are analyses of internal information. After all, other than physical inventory, no external transactions or physical units are unique to production and cost accounting. The analyses include costing the production orders, comparing the cost with prior experience or with standard costs, and determining **lower-of-cost-and-net-realizable-value (LCNRV)** valuations. In a sense, the LCNRV calculations are a reconciliation of product cost to the external market price of product units.

Review Checkpoints

13-29   What functions are normally associated with the production process? Why is an understanding of the production process, including the related data processing and cost accounting, important to auditors evaluating the control structure as part of their assessment of control risk?

13-30   Describe a walk-through of a production transaction from production orders to entry in the finished goods perpetual inventory records. What document copies would be collected? what controls noted? what duties separated?

13-31   Describe how the separation of (1) authorization of production transactions, (2) recording of these transactions, and (3) physical custody of inventories can be specified among the production, inventory, and cost accounting departments.

13-32   What features of the cost accounting system would be expected to prevent the omission of recording materials used in production?

---

lower-of-cost-and-net-realizable-value (LCNRV):
an accounting rule that requires inventory to be reported at its cost, or, if the amount that could be obtained by selling it net of any selling costs is less than its cost, at that lower amount; the lower amount is achieved by recording a write-down

Audit Evidence in Management Reports and Files

Most production accounting systems produce timely reports that managers use to supervise and control production. Auditors use them as supporting evidence for assertions about WIP and finished goods inventories and about cost of goods sold.

Sales Forecast

Several aspects of business planning, notably the planning of production and inventory levels, are based on management's sales forecasts. If the auditors want to use the forecast for substantive audit decisions, assurance about its reasonableness needs to be obtained, particularly about assumptions built into it. In addition, the mechanical accuracy of the forecast should be verified.

Because much of the year under audit will have passed when the audit work begins, the forecasts can help the auditor to understand the nature and volume of production orders and the level of materials inventory on hand. Forecasts for the following year are used in valuing the inventory (e.g., LCNRV if the forecast indicates slow-moving and potentially obsolete inventory). If a write-down from cost to market value is required, this increases the amount of cost of goods sold that is shown in the financial statements. Special care must be taken when using forecasts with inventory valuation, because an overly optimistic forecast can lead to a failure to write down inventory.

The SALY Forecast

The auditors were reviewing the inventory items that had not been issued for 30 days or more to assess whether any items need to be written down because their market values were lower than cost. The production manager showed them the SALY forecast that indicated a continuing need for the materials in products that were expected to have reasonable demand. The auditors agreed that the forecasts supported the prediction of future sales of products at prices that would cover the cost of the slow-moving material items.

Unfortunately, they neglected to ask the meaning of SALY in the designation of the forecast. They did not learn that it means "same as last year." It is not a forecast at all. The products did not sell at the prices expected, and the company experienced losses the following year that should have been charged to cost of goods sold earlier. Auditors can often use management reports to design various analytical procedures, but if those reports are not reliable, the auditors' analysis findings are not going to provide very reliable evidence either!

Production Plans and Reports

Management's plan for the amount and timing of production provides general information to the auditors, but the production orders and inventory plan associated with it are even more important. These carry the information about requirements for raw materials, labour, and overhead, including the requisitions for purchase and use of materials and labour. These documents are the initial authorizations for control of the inventory and production.

Production reports record the completion of production quantities. When coupled with the related cost accounting reports, they are the company's record of the cost of goods placed in the finished goods inventory. In most cases, auditors will audit the cost reports as part of determining the cost valuation of inventory and cost of goods sold.

Amortization Schedule

The cost accounting department may prepare the schedule of the depreciation (amortization) of production assets. Depreciation on productive assets is usually included as a component of manufacturing overhead cost. Company accountants may prepare similar schedules for the company's other (non-production) fixed assets. These often list a large number of different assets and involve large dollar amounts of asset cost and calculated depreciation expense. An illustration of a depreciation schedule for non-current assets (PPE and intangible assets) was presented in Chapter 12, in Exhibit 12–10. The depreciation schedule is audited by assessing the reasonableness of the company's depreciation methods and estimates of useful life and residual values, by recalculating the depreciation expense, and by vouching supporting documents for additions and disposals. When the schedule covers hundreds of assets and numerous additions and disposals, auditors can (a) use computer auditing methods to recalculate the depreciation expense and (b) use sampling to choose additions and disposals for tests of controls and substantive audits. The beginning balances of assets and accumulated amortization should be traced to the prior-year audit's working papers. This schedule can be made into an audit working paper and placed in the auditor's files for future reference, as was illustrated in Exhibit 12–10.

Review Checkpoints

13-33   When auditors want to use an auditee's sales forecast for general familiarity with the production process or for evaluation of slow-moving inventory, what kind of work should be done on the forecast?

13-34   If the actual sales for the year are substantially lower than the sales forecast at the beginning of the year, what potential valuation problems may arise in the production accounts?

13-35   What production documentation supports the valuation of manufactured finished goods inventory?

13-36   What items in an auditee's production asset and amortization schedule can auditors use for designing audit procedures? Describe these audit procedures.

Control Risk Assessment

LO6   Describe control tests for auditing control over conversion of materials and labour in the production process.

Control risk assessment is important because it governs the nature, timing, and extent of substantive audit procedures that will be applied in the audit of account balances in the production accounting process. These account balances include the following:

- Inventory—raw materials, WIP, finished goods
- Cost of goods sold
- Depreciation—depreciation expense, accumulated depreciation

Several aspects of auditing purchased inventories and physical quantities are covered in Chapter 12. With respect to inventory valuation, this chapter points out the cost accounting function and its role in determining the cost valuation of manufactured finished goods.

General Control Considerations

Control procedures for proper segregation of responsibilities should be in place and operating. From Exhibit 13–7, you can see that proper segregation involves authorization (production planning and inventory planning) by those who do not have custody, recording, or cost accounting and reconciliation duties. Custody of inventories (raw materials, WIP, and finished goods) is in the hands of people who do not (a) authorize the amount or timing of production or the purchase of materials and labour, (b) perform the cost accounting recordkeeping, or (c) prepare cost analyses (reconciliations). Cost accounting (a recording function) is performed by those who do not authorize production or have custody of assets in the process of production. However, you will usually find that the cost accountants prepare various analyses and reconciliations directly related to production activities. Combinations of two or more of the duties of authorization, custody, and cost accounting in one person, one office, or one computerized system may open the door for errors or fraud.

In addition, the control structure includes the following detail-checking procedures:

1. Production orders contain a list of materials and their quantities, and they are approved by a production planner/scheduler.

2. Materials requisitions are (a) compared, in the cost accounting department, with the list of materials on the production order and (b) approved by the production operator and the materials inventory stockkeeper.

3. Job labour time records are signed by production supervisors, and the cost accounting department reconciles the amounts with the labour report from the payroll department.

4. Production reports of finished units are signed by the production supervisor and finished goods inventory custodian and then forwarded to cost accounting.

These control operations track the raw materials and labour through the production process. With each internal transaction, the responsibility and accountability for assets are passed to the next person or location.

Many companies have complex systems for managing production and material flows. These information systems are customized, because production processes vary considerably for different products and factories. Even within the same company, different information systems may be used to manage different products or different locations. Some parts of the production process and accounting may be done manually, while others are automated. JIT manufacturing and supply chain management systems have expanded in many companies with the availability of electronic data interchange and other information technologies. Auditors need to be familiar with the components and functions of these systems and their implications for auditing. Paper source documents and authorization signatures may not exist for automated functions. Even though the information system and technology may be complex and specific to the entity, auditors should make sure the basic management and control functions of ensuring the flow of labour and materials to production and controlling waste are in place.

Internal Control Questionnaires

Information about the production process control structure is often initially gathered by completing an internal control questionnaire. Exhibit 13A–1 in Appendix 13A is an example of an internal control questionnaire, and it can be studied for details of desirable control policies and procedures. The internal control questionnaire lists control activities found in the manual aspects of a production cost accounting system. The automated aspects that have no paper trail must be assessed to see whether each control objective is met through application controls or other verification procedures, for example, input/output checks.

Control Tests

An organization should have functioning control activities that prevent, detect, and correct accounting errors. You studied the general control objectives in Chapter 9 (validity, completeness, authorization, accuracy, classification, and proper period recording). Exhibit 13–8 puts these in the perspective of production activity, with examples of specific control objectives. Study this exhibit carefully, as it expresses the control objectives in examples specific to production.

Auditors perform control tests to determine whether controls said to be in place and operating are actually being performed properly by company personnel. Recall that a control test consists of (1) identification of the data population from which a sample of items will be selected for audit and (2) an expression of the action that will be taken to produce relevant evidence, such as vouching, tracing, observing, scanning, or recalculating.

Exhibit 13–9 contains a selection of control tests for auditing controls over the accumulation of costs for WIP inventory. This is the "inventory" of things in the production process. Upon completion, the accumulated costs become the cost valuation of the finished goods inventory. The exhibit presumes that there are production cost reports, which are updated as production takes place; labour reports assigning labour cost to the job; reports of materials used and materials requisitions charging raw materials to the production order; and

EXHIBIT 13–8

Control Objectives (Production Process)

GENERAL OBJECTIVES	EXAMPLES OF SPECIFIC CONTROL ACTIVITIES
1. Recorded production transactions are *valid* and documented.	Cost accounting is separated from production, payroll, and inventory control. Material use reports are compared with raw material stores issue slips. Labour use reports are compared with job time tickets.
2. Valid production transactions are *recorded completely* and none omitted.	All documents are prenumbered and numerical sequence is reviewed.
3. Production transactions are *authorized*.	Material use and labour use are prepared by the foreperson and approved by the production supervisor.
4. Production job cost transactions computations contain *accurate* figures.	Job cost sheet entries are reviewed by a person independent of preparation. Costs of inventory used and labour used are reviewed periodically. Open job cost sheets are periodically reconciled to the WIP inventory accounts
5. Labour and materials are *classified* correctly as direct or indirect.	The production supervisor is required to account for all material and labour used as direct or indirect.
6. Production transactions are recorded in the *proper period*.	Production reports of material and labour used are prepared weekly and transmitted to cost accounting. Job cost sheets are posted weekly and summary journal entries of WIP and work completed are prepared monthly.

EXHIBIT 13–9

Control Tests for Work-in-Process Inventory

	CONTROL OBJECTIVE
1. Reconcile the open production cost reports to the WIP inventory control account.	Completeness
2. Select a sample of open and closed production cost reports:	
(a) Recalculate all costs entered.	Accuracy
(b) Vouch labour costs to labour reports.	Validity
(c) Compare materials-used reports with bills of materials and materials requisitions, and company labour reports with summary of payroll.	Accuracy
(d) Vouch material costs to issue slips and materials-used reports.	Validity
(e) Vouch overhead charges to overhead analysis schedules.	Accuracy
(f) Trace selected overhead amounts from analysis schedules to cost allocations and to invoices or accounts payable vouchers.	Validity
3. Select a sample of issue slips from the raw materials stores file:	
(a) Determine if a matching requisition is available for every issue slip.	Completeness
(b) Trace materials-used reports into production cost reports.	Completeness
4. Select a sample of time clock or other records of hours worked from the payroll file. Trace to job time tickets, labour reports, and production cost reports.	Completeness
5. Select a sample of production orders:	
(a) Determine whether the production order was authorized.	Authorization
(b) Match to the bill of materials and labour hour needs.	Completeness
(c) Trace the bill of materials to material requisitions, material issue slips, materials-used reports, and production cost reports.	Completeness
(d) Trace labour hour needs to labour reports and production cost reports.	Completeness

overhead allocation calculations. Some or all of these documents may be in the form of computer records. The samples are usually attribute samples designed along the lines of those studied in Chapter 10. On the right-hand side, Exhibit 13–9 shows the control objectives tested by the audit procedures listed.

Two Directions of the Test of Controls Procedures

The procedures listed in Exhibit 13–9 are designed to test the production accounting in two directions, the first being the completeness direction, testing whether all production ordered to be started is recorded. Exhibit 13–10 shows that the sample for this testing direction is taken from the population of production orders found in the production planning department. The cost accumulation is traced forward into the production cost reports in the cost accounting department. The procedures keyed in the boxes (5-a, b, c, d) are cross-references to the procedures in Exhibit 13–9. Potentially, these procedures will find any scheduled production that has been cancelled because of technical or quality problems, which means there should be some writing off or scrapping of partially completed production units.

The other direction of the test is validity, which is concerned with the proper recording of WIP and finished goods in the general ledger. Exhibit 13–11, which is a sample for this test, is from the production reports (quantity and cost) recorded in the inventory accounts. This sample references production cost reports filed in the cost accounting department. From these basic records, the recorded costs can be recalculated, vouched to labour reports, compared with the payroll, and vouched to records of material used and overhead incurred. The procedures keyed in the boxes (2-a, b, c, d, e, f) are cross-references to the procedures in Exhibit 13–9. These procedures might reveal that there is improper valuation of the recorded inventory cost.

Summary: Control Risk Assessment

The audit manager or senior in charge of the audit should evaluate the evidence obtained from an understanding of the internal control structure and from the test of controls audit procedures. If the control risk is assessed very low, the substantive audit procedures on the account balances can be limited in cost-saving ways. For example, the inventory valuation substantive tests can be limited in scope (i.e., smaller sample sizes), and there can be more confidence that the overall analytical procedures will be able to detect material misstatements not otherwise evident in the accounting details.

EXHIBIT 13–10

Test of Production Cost Controls: Completeness Direction

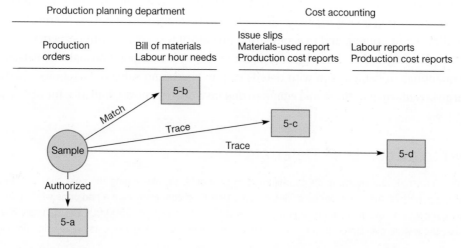

Note: The 5-a, etc., codes refer to control tests listed in Exhibit 13–9.

EXHIBIT 13–11

Test of Production Cost Controls: Validity Direction

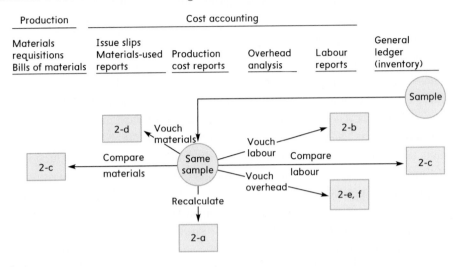

Note: The 2-a, etc., codes refer to control tests listed in Exhibit 13–9.

On the other hand, if tests of controls reveal weaknesses, amortization calculation errors, and cost accumulation errors, the substantive procedures must be designed to lower the risk of failing to detect material error in the inventory and cost of goods sold account balances. For example, the amortization cost may have to be completely recalculated and reviewed again by the auditors, valuation calculations may need to be performed for a large number of the inventoried production reports, and contract terms related to cost overruns may need to be investigated to determine if they should be carried as assets (e.g., as inventory or unbilled receivables) or written off. Descriptions of major control deficiencies, control weaknesses, and inefficiencies may need to be communicated to the auditee management and those charged with governance.

Since inventory production accounting often involves processing high volumes of transactions and keeping track of items in different locations, computer assisted audit testing can be efficient. Computerized components of the production information system may range from simple batch systems, which automate data processing, to transaction-driven integrated systems, which capture the production progress electronically from devices on the production line. Computer audit techniques, such as test data, may be used to audit controls in such systems. For tests of details of transactions and balances, auditor-created or auditor-tested software for verifying all (or a sample) of the inventory transaction processing can include (a) selecting items for test counting based on auditor-determined criteria, (b) sorting inventory items by location to facilitate observations, (c) recalculating extensions on inventory quantities and pricing, and (d) comparing inventory test counts with perpetual records. Audit software can also perform analytical review procedures, for example, identifying unusual fluctuations in current and prior inventory quantities in comparison with details of purchases and sales transactions, spotting negative or unreasonably large inventory quantities, and summarizing inventory turnover statistics for obsolescence analysis.

Improper Production Loss Deferrals

Alton Corporation incurred cost overruns on its shipbuilding contracts. By classifying the cost overruns as an asset for financial reporting purposes, Alton postponed writing off an $18 million cost overrun. If it had been written off in the proper period, the company would have reported a large loss instead of a net income of $500,000 for the year. The auditors did not discover that there were overstated asset values, since they relied on management estimates and production reports

(continued)

that concealed the cost overruns. When Alton wrote off the $18 million two years later by restating its financial statements, its shareholders requested that the auditors be replaced.

International Technologies Corporation (ITC) experienced cost overruns on fixed price contracts, claims for price escalation, and kickback arrangements with suppliers. ITC recorded and reported these costs as "unbilled receivables," using the account to misrepresent the cost overruns as escalation payments due from the customer, while the contract did not provide for any such payment. ITC used the unbilled receivables account as a hiding place for improper and questionable payments on the contracts so it could show them as legitimate reimbursable contract costs in order to avoid (a) writing them off as expense and (b) showing the true nature of the items. ITC also buried uncollectible contract costs, which indicated losses on fixed price contracts, in other unrelated contracts that were still profitable. When ITC's auditor uncovered the materially overstated assets, it required a write-down. This revealed that ITC was insolvent, and it was acquired by another technology company that quickly fired ITC's management.

Review Checkpoints

13-37 What primary functions should be segregated in the production process?

13-38 How does the production order document or record provide a control over the quantity of materials used in production?

13-39 Where might an auditor find accounting records of cost overruns on contracts? improper charges? improperly capitalized inventory?

13-40 Evaluate the following statement made by an auditing student: "I do not understand cost accounting; therefore, I want to get a job with an auditing firm where I will only have to know financial accounting."

13-41 Which population of documents or records would an auditor sample to determine whether (a) all authorized production was completed and placed in inventory or written off as scrap and (b) finished goods inventory was actually produced and properly costed?

Substantive Audit Program for the Production Process

LO7 Describe the typical substantive procedures used to address the assessed risk of material misstatement in the main accounts in the production process.

Exhibit 13–12 shows a list of typical substantive procedures used to obtain evidence related to production transactions, and their impact on the financial statements. It provides a template substantive audit program for the production process. As always, the auditor's risk assessments are used to adapt the template to respond to the risks present in a particular audit engagement.

Review Checkpoints

13-42 Explain how the auditor's risk assessment affects the design of the substantive audit program.

13-43 In the audit of inventory, what is the purpose of the analytical procedure that compares gross profit margin by month for the last two fiscal periods?

13-44 What substantive tests of details of transactions and balances are used to verify the pricing of manufactured inventory items? Which assertion do these procedures mainly address?

EXHIBIT 13–12

Example of Substantive Audit Program Responding to Assessed Risk of Material Misstatement for Production Costing: Selected Procedures

SUBSTANTIVE AUDIT PROGRAM				
AUDITEE: *ECOPAK INC.*				**FILE INDEX:** *720*
FINANCIAL STATEMENT PERIOD: *y/e DECEMBER 31, 20X1*				
PROCESS: *Inventory production costing*				
Substantive audit program in response to assessed risks at the assertion level:				
Consider risk assessment findings and conclusion on residual detection risk to be reduced by performing substantive procedures. (Of the procedures listed below, perform those considered necessary to provide sufficient appropriate evidence to address the assessed risks and reduce risk of material misstatement to an acceptable level.)				*[Reference to relevant working papers]*
SUBSTANTIVE AUDIT PROCEDURES	Assertions evidence is related to [E, C, O, V, P*]	Timing	Extent	Working paper reference

Analytical procedures
1. Perform the following analysis and obtain satisfactory explanations from management for relationships observed:
  (a) Compare gross profit margin (i.e., as a percentage of sales) by product and compare with prior periods.
  (b) Compare gross profit margin by product with the standard markup.
  (c) Compare gross profit margin by month for the last two fiscal periods. Note any differences in the gross profit margin in the months before and after the period-end.
	E, C, V			

Tests of details of transactions and balances
1. Select the significant items contained in the inventory balance and perform the following procedures:
  (a) Raw material:
    Agree cost to suppliers' invoices, shipping charges, and customs brokers' charges.
  (b) WIP and finished goods:
    Review cost elements and costing calculations by product for accuracy and reasonableness.
    Compare labour rates used with the payroll records.
  (c) Overhead applied to inventory:
    Assess the reasonableness of overhead rates used by comparing amounts applied with actual overhead in the accounting records.
	V, O
	
	V
	
	V			

2. Ensure inventory costs in a foreign currency have been translated at the period-end exchange rate.	V			
3. Assess reasonableness of accounting policies chosen by the entity in relation to common practice in the industry, consistency with previous periods, and impact on net income.	P			
4. Obtain evidence of current market prices of raw materials and finished goods, and expected costs of selling these, to determine whether net realizable value (NRV) exceeds their carrying costs. If not, a write-down to NRV is required for fair presentation.	V, P			
				(continued)

Example of Substantive Audit Program Responding to Assessed Risk of Material Misstatement for Production Costing: Selected Procedures *(continued)*

Misstatement summary: Summarize here all misstatements discovered in executing this program. Carry all forward for accumulation in the Summary of Accumulated Misstatements worksheet (see Exhibit 16–1).	
AUDITOR'S CONCLUSIONS [If the audit program is completed satisfactorily and the audit objectives are met, a conclusion such as the following would be recorded by the auditor performing the work.] *Based on my professional judgment, the evidence obtained is sufficient and appropriate to conclude that the risk of material misstatement of the* <u>INVENTORY PRODUCTION COSTING</u> *is acceptably low.* Prepared by _____ Date _____ Reviewed by _____ Date _____	

* E, C, O, V, P = existence, completeness, ownership, valuation, presentation.

To link this general description of an audit program for a production process to the approaches used to integrate the audit findings and form a conclusion, note the following analyses.

Analysis of Financial Statement Relationships

The audit of the production process verifies the balances of inventory and cost of goods sold. To integrate the findings from a balance sheet perspective, we can analyze balance changes and the financial statement items related to them by preparing a continuity schedule. The finished goods inventory balance is used as an example for the production process:

AUDITED AMOUNT	FINANCIAL STATEMENT WHERE AMOUNT IS REPORTED
Opening balance of finished goods inventory	Balance sheet (prior-year comparative figure)
Add: Purchases of materials during the year Labour costs allocated Overhead costs allocated	Cash flow statement (direct method)
Deduct: Costs allocated to WIP inventory	Balance sheet (current-year balance of WIP inventory, usually in inventory detail note)
Deduct: Cost of goods sold	Income statement expense
Ending balance of finished goods inventory	Balance sheet (current-year figure before any valuation adjustment, if required)

Analytical procedures that use these relationships include inventory turnover ratios and gross margin analyses. Misstatements in the existence, completeness, and valuation assertions for inventory may result in unexplained fluctuations in these relationships.

Misstatement Analysis

Consider the following misstatement that might be discovered in an audit. At the end of the prior year, the auditor of a machine parts manufacturer made note of a quantity of inventory that appeared to be slow moving. At that time, management asserted that the inventory was a special part that was occasionally needed by some customers, so it would eventually be sold. Accordingly, the auditors accepted that a write-down was not needed at that time. At the end of the current year, however, this same inventory of parts is still on hand and still has not been written down. When the auditors dig further and interview the sales manager, she informs them that the last customer that would have used this part had changed its process earlier in the year, so there may be no market for this type of part any more. The cost recorded for the inventory is $21,000, and the auditor concludes that this cost is not likely to be recoverable; thus it should have been written off through cost of sales. Note that in the analysis above, this error understates cost of sales amount deducted, leaving the inventory balance too high (overstated). This misstatement will be carried forward to the summary of accumulated misstatements (see Exhibit 16–1) for evaluation in forming the audit opinion at the end of the audit.

APPLICATION CASE WITH SOLUTION & ANALYSIS

Detecting Misstatements in the Payroll and Production Processes

INTRODUCTION

In this application case, we will demonstrate tests of controls and substantive audit procedures in the evidence-gathering process related to the payroll and production processes. The case situation for each audit presented parallels the framework shown in Chapter 11's application case. The case situation provides context for the auditing decisions, rather than presenting a list of detection procedures in the abstract. Lists of detailed procedures, a selection of control tests, and detailed substantive procedures for payroll and production are found in the chapter discussions above.

DISCUSSION CASE

In his second year as an auditor, Jack is assigned to audit the payroll and inventory in Kromax Inc., a large manufacturing company. After the initial audit team meeting and his review of the prior years' audit files, Jack is starting to design his detailed audit programs for this year. Kromax is publicly traded and has been experiencing very poor profit results this year. Jack wants to make sure his procedures will address the risks of material misstatement, which may be higher this year than in the past, but he finds that many aspects of the payroll and manufacturing production processes are unfamiliar. Jack gets an opportunity to meet over lunch with Syed, one of his firm's senior partners. He knows Syed is always willing to help out less-experienced auditors by sharing stories about interesting audit situations. When Jack asks him specifically about audits where the auditors detected misstatements due to errors or frauds in payroll or production, Syed relates the following audit stories showing errors in cost of sales recording and payroll embezzlement through payment of fictitious employees.

AUDIT 13.1 Ghosts on the Payroll

CASE DESCRIPTION

Maybelle was responsible for preparing personnel files for new hires, approving wages, verifying time cards, and distributing payroll cheques for the BlueBonnet Company. She embezzled funds by "hiring" fictitious employees, faking their records, and issuing cheques to them through the payroll system. She deposited some cheques in several personal bank accounts and cashed others, endorsing all of them with the names of the fictitious employees as well as her own. Maybelle stole $160,000 by creating these "ghosts," usually 3 to 5 of 112 people on the payroll, and paying them an average of $456 per week for three years.

Sometimes, the ghosts quit and were later replaced by others. But she stole "only" about 2% of the payroll funds during the period.

Audit Trail

Payroll creates a large paper trail with individual earnings records; T4 tax forms; payroll deductions for taxes, insurance, and pension plans; and payroll tax reports. Maybelle mailed all the T4 forms to the same post office box.

SOLUTION & ANALYSIS

Audit Approach

Audit Objective

The auditor's objective is to obtain evidence of the existence and validity of payroll transactions.

Controls Relevant to the Process

Different people should be responsible for hiring (preparing personnel files), approving wages, and distributing payroll cheques. These controls relate to the authorization and ownership objectives. "Thinking like a crook" in their fraud risk assessment led the audit team to suspect that Maybelle could put people on the payroll and obtain their cheques.

Audit Procedures

Tests of Controls

Audit for transaction authorization and validity. Random sampling may not work because of the small number of ghosts. Look for the obvious. Select several weeks' cheque blocks, account for numerical sequence (to see whether any cheques have been removed), and examine cancelled cheques for two endorsements.

Tests of Details of Balance

There may be no "balance" to audit other than the accumulated total of payroll transactions, and the total may not appear out of line with history because the fraud is small in relation to total payroll and has been going on for years. Scan cancelled payroll cheque endorsement details and trace these to personnel files. Observe a payroll distribution on a surprise basis, noting any employees who do not collect their cheques, and follow up by examining prior cancelled cheques for these missing employees. Scan personnel files for common addresses.

Audit Results

Both the surprise distribution observation and the scan for common addresses provided the names of two to three exceptions. These led to prior cancelled cheques (which Maybelle had not removed and the bank reconciler had not noticed) that carried Maybelle's own name as endorser. When confronted, she confessed.

AUDIT 13.2 Unbundled before Its Time

CASE DESCRIPTION

Western Corporation assembled and sold computer systems. A systems production order consisted of hardware and peripheral equipment specifications and software specifications with associated performance criteria. Western brought in new auditors who discovered that items in production were being treated as finished goods "sold" before actual completion, which caused understated inventory, overstated cost of goods sold, overstated revenue, and overstated income. Western was routinely recording the hardware component of contracts too soon, recognizing revenue and cost of goods sold that should have been postponed until later when the customer accepted the entire system. In the last three years, the resulting income overstatements amounted to 12%, 15%, and 19% of the reported operating income before taxes.

Customer contracts always required that the unit be assembled to specifications, with hardware and software installation and testing, before accepting the finished installation and paying for the entire package. Order completion usually took three to eight months. About 200 to 250 production orders were charged to cost of goods sold each year. For internal accounting purposes, Western "unbundled" production orders into the hardware and software components of the customer orders so that production processing and cost accounting were performed as if the two were independent orders. When the hardware was installed and tested (with or without customer acceptance), Western recorded part of the contract price as sales revenue and the related cost of goods sold. The amount "due from customers" was carried in an asset account entitled "unbilled contract revenue," and no billing statement was sent to the customer at that time.

When the software component was completed, installed, tested, and accepted, the remainder of the contract price was recorded as revenue, the cost of the software was recorded as cost of goods sold, and a billing statement was sent to the customer. The "unbilled contract revenue," which now matched the customer's obligation, was moved to accounts receivable. While the two order components were in process (prior to installation at the customer's location), accumulated costs were carried in a WIP inventory account.

Audit Trail

Customer orders and contracts contained all the terms relating to technical specifications, acceptance testing, and the timing of the customer's obligation to pay. Copies of the technical specification sections of the contracts were attached to both the hardware and software production orders prepared and authorized in the production planning department. During production, installation, and testing, each of these orders was the basis of the production cost accumulation and subsidiary record of the WIP inventory. At the end, the production reports along with the accumulated costs became the production cost report and supporting documentation for the cost of goods sold entry.

SOLUTION & ANALYSIS
Audit Approach
Audit Objective

The auditors' objective is to obtain evidence of the actual occurrence of cost of goods sold transactions, thereby yielding evidence of the completeness of recorded inventory.

Controls Relevant to the Process

The major control lies in the production planning department approval of orders identifying a total unit of production (in this case, the hardware and software components combined). Nothing is wrong with approving separate orders for efficiency of production, but they should be cross-referenced so that both production personnel and the cost accounting department see them as separate components of the same order unit.

Audit Procedures
Tests of Controls

Even though the company generated a large amount of revenue, it had relatively few production orders (200–250). A sample of completed production orders should be taken and vouched to the customer orders and contracts. This is done to determine the validity of the production orders in relation to customer orders and whether the cost of goods sold was recorded in the proper period. (Audit of accuracy and completeness of the cost accumulation can also be carried out on this sample, making it a dual-purpose test, as further described below.)

Even though the auditors can read the customer contracts, inquiries should be made about the company's standard procedures for the timing of revenue and cost of goods sold recognition to determine what is actually being done in practice.

Tests of Details of Balance

The sample of completed production orders can also be used in a dual-purpose test of the cost of goods sold balance. For the balance audit, the primary points are the existence and completeness of the dollar amounts accumulated as the cost of the contracts and the proper cutoff for recording the cost. The existence of the "unbilled contract revenue" asset account in the general ledger should raise a red flag. Such an account always means that management has estimated a revenue amount that has not been determined according to contract or billed to the customer according to contract terms. Even though the revenue is "unbilled," the related cost of goods sold should still be in the cost of goods sold account. While accounting theory and practice permit recognizing unbilled revenue in certain cases (e.g., percentage of completion for construction contracts), there have been abuses.

Audit Results

When the company decided to issue shares to the public, a new audit firm was engaged. The new auditor team performed the dual-purpose procedures already outlined, made the suggested inquiries, and investigated the unbilled contract revenue account. They learned about management's unbundling policy and insisted that it be changed so that revenue was recognized only when all the terms of the contract were met. (The investigation yielded the information about prior years' overstatements of revenue, cost of goods sold, and income.) Part of the reason for insisting on the change of policy was the finding that Western did not have a very good record of quality control and customer acceptance of software installation. Customer acceptance was often delayed several months while systems engineers debugged software. On several occasions Western solved the problems by purchasing complete software packages from other developers.

Review Checkpoints

13-45 How can an auditor find out whether payroll control procedures were followed by company personnel?

13-46 In a production situation similar to the Audit 13.2 case, what substantive audit work should be done on a sample of completed production orders (cost reports) recorded as cost of goods sold?

SUMMARY

- The payroll and production processes produce information about costs of manufactured inventory and employee salaries. These tend to be highly automated processes where transaction volumes are high. The main risk in the payroll process relates to making unauthorized payments. Risks in the production process arise mainly related to the valuation of inventory, for example, if there are errors in allocating material, labour, and overhead costs to production. Well-designed information systems and controls are very important to control risks in both these processes. Payroll and production information systems produce many internal documents, reports, and files that are sources of audit information. These systems mostly involve evidence made up of internal documentation, with relatively little external documentary evidence. Aside from physical inventory, the accounts in the payroll and production processes are intangible: they cannot be observed, inspected, touched, or counted in any meaningful way. **LO1**

- The payroll process consists of hiring, rate authorization, attendance and work supervision, payroll processing, and paycheque distribution. Key controls in the payroll process are the segregation of approval and payments functions, proper documentation and recording of payroll transactions, and periodic reconciliations of total payroll amounts. **LO2**

- Auditors often use analysis and dual-purpose testing to provide evidence about control effectiveness and substantive evidence about the existence, completeness, valuation, and ownership assertions related to payroll. **LO3**

- The extent and nature of further substantive testing depend on the auditor's risk assessment. Typical substantive procedures in the payroll process relate to vouching payments to supporting documents, such as time cards and approved pay rates, and verifying that payments were received by legitimate employees. An example of an audit program for a payroll process showing a selection of typical substantive procedures was provided. **LO4**

- The production process involves production planning; inventory planning; acquisition of labour, materials, and overhead (purchases, payables, and payment process); custody of assets while work is in process and when finished products are stored in inventory; and cost accounting. Payroll is also an important part of the production process for manufacturing businesses where management and control of labour costs are important. Companies reduce control risk in the production process by separating authorization, custody, recording, and periodic reconciliation duties. Error-checking procedures of analyzing production orders and finished production cost reports are important for proper determination of inventory values and proper valuation of cost of goods sold. Without these procedures, many things could go wrong, ranging from overvaluing the inventory to understating costs of production by deferring costs that should be expensed. **LO5**

- Most audit procedures for the production process are analytical and dual-purpose procedures related to inventory and costs of sales, testing both the company's control procedures and the existence, valuation, and completeness assertions made by accumulating the results of numerous labour and overhead transactions. **LO6**

- The extent and nature of further substantive testing depends on the auditor's risk assessment. Typical substantive procedures in the production process relate to testing the underlying costing of the period-end inventory balance, and the transactions underlying the costs of sales expense for the period. An example of an audit program for a production process showing a selection of typical substantive procedures was provided. **LO7**

Payroll accounting is critical to expenditure control, as embezzlement often occurs during this process. Cost accounting is a central feature of the production process, and reports can be manipulated. Chapter application cases provided examples of these along with procedures for detecting them.

KEY TERMS

cost of goods sold	imprest bank account (imprest fund)	lower-of-cost-and-net-realizable-value (LCNRV)

MULTIPLE-CHOICE QUESTIONS FOR PRACTICE AND REVIEW

MC 13-1 `LO1` Why is the ownership assertion a key risk in the payroll process?

a. The year-end accruals are small so they may be incomplete.
b. Payroll duties cannot easily be segregated in most businesses.
c. Evidence from government income tax reports is often audited.
d. The payroll process involves a high volume of small payments to individuals.

MC 13-2 `LO2` Effective internal control over the payroll function should include procedures that segregate the duties of making salary payments to employees and which of the following procedures?

a. Controlling employment insurance claims
b. Maintaining employee personnel records
c. Approving employee fringe benefits
d. Hiring new employees

MC 13-3 `LO4` Which of the following is the best way for an auditor to obtain evidence about whether every name on a company's payroll is that of a legitimate employee currently on the job?

a. Examine personnel records for accuracy and completeness.
b. Examine employees' names listed on payroll tax returns for agreement with payroll accounting records.
c. Ask to meet, in person, randomly selected employees from the payroll register.
d. Control the mailing of annual T4 tax forms to employee addresses in their personnel files.

MC 13-4 `LO3` It would be appropriate for the payroll accounting department to be responsible for which of the following functions?

a. Approval of employee time records
b. Maintenance of records of employment, discharges, and pay increases
c. Preparation of periodic government reports of employees' earnings and withholding taxes
d. Temporary retention of unclaimed employee paycheques

MC 13-5 `LO3` To minimize the opportunities for fraud, unclaimed payroll payments should be handled by which of the following procedures?

a. Deposited in a safe deposit box
b. Held by the payroll custodian
c. Deposited in a special bank account
d. Held by the controller

MC 13-6 `LO6` In testing an automated payroll system, an auditor would be least likely to use test data to test controls related to which of the following?

a. Missing employee numbers
b. Proper signature approval of overtime by supervisors
c. Time tickets with invalid job numbers
d. Agreement of hours per clock card with hours on time tickets

MC 13-7 `LO7` Analytical procedures applied to management's production cost reports provide evidence for which assertion(s)?

a. Existence, completeness, and valuation
b. Ownership
c. Physical inspection of quantities
d. Presentation

MC 13-8 `LO7` When an auditor tests a company's cost accounting system, what are the auditor's procedures designed primarily to determine?

a. Quantities on hand have been computed based on acceptable cost accounting techniques that reasonably approximate actual quantities on hand.
b. Physical inventories are in substantial agreement with book inventories.
c. The system is in accordance with GAAP and is functioning as planned.
d. Costs have been properly assigned to finished goods, WIP, and cost of goods sold.

MC 13-9 `LO7` The auditor tests the quantities of materials charged to WIP by vouching these quantities to which one of the following?

a. Cost ledgers
b. Perpetual inventory records
c. Receiving reports
d. Material requisition

MC 13-10 `LO5` Which effective auditee internal control procedure prevents discrepancies between the cost accounting for labour cost and the payroll paid?

a. Reconciliation of totals on production job time tickets with job reports by the employees responsible for the specific jobs
b. Verification of agreement of production job time tickets with employee time cards by a payroll department employee
c. Preparation of payroll transaction journal entries by an employee who reports to the personnel department director
d. Custody of pay rate authorization forms by the supervisor of the payroll department

(© 2000, American Institute of CPAs. All Rights Reserved. Adapted by permission.)

EXERCISES AND PROBLEMS

EP 13-1 Internal Control Questionnaire Items: Misstatements That Could Occur from Control Weaknesses. `LO5, 6` Refer to the internal control questionnaire on a payroll system (Exhibit 13A–1 in Appendix 13A) and assume the answer to each question is "no."

Required:

Prepare a table matching each question to an error or fraud that could occur because of the absence of the control. Your column headings should be as follows:

Question	Possible Error or Fraud Due to Weakness

EP 13-2 Internal Control Questionnaire Items: Control Objectives, Control Tests, and Possible Misstatements. `LO1, 5, 6` Listed below is a selection of items from the payroll processing internal control questionnaire in Exhibit 13A–1.

1. Are names of terminated employees reported in writing to the payroll department?
2. Are authorizations for deductions, signed by the employees, on file?
3. Is the timekeeping department (function) independent of the payroll department?
4. Are timekeeping and cost accounting records (such as hours, dollars) reconciled with payroll department calculations of hours and wages?

Required:

For each question:

a. Identify the control objective to which the question applies.
b. Specify one test of controls audit procedure an auditor could use to determine whether the control was operating effectively (see Exhibit 13–4 for procedures).
c. Using your business experience, your logic, and/or your imagination, give an example of a misstatement caused by error or fraud that could occur if the control were absent or ineffective.

EP 13-3 Major Risks in the Payroll Process. `LO5, 6`

Required:

Prepare a schedule of the major risks in the payroll process. Identify the control objectives and financial statement assertions related to each. Lay out a three-column schedule as follows:

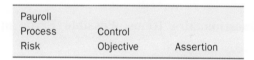

Payroll Process Risk	Control Objective	Assertion

EP 13-4 Payroll Processed by a Service Organization. `LO6` Assume that you are the audit senior conducting a review of the payroll system of a new auditee. While you are in the process of interviewing the payroll department manager, she makes the following statement: "We don't need many controls since our payroll is done outside the company by Automated Data Processing, a service organization."

Required:

Evaluate the payroll department manager's statement, and describe how a service organization affects an auditors' review of controls. You may want to refer to Chapter 9.

EP 13-5 Payroll Tests of Controls. `LO5, 6` The diagram in Exhibit EP 13-5 describes several payroll test of controls procedures. It shows the direction of the tests, leading from samples of time cards, payrolls, and cumulative year-to-date earnings records to blank squares.

Required:

For each blank square in Exhibit EP 13-5, write a payroll test of controls procedure and describe the evidence it can produce. (*Hint:* Refer to Exhibit 13–5.)

Diagram of Payroll Test of Controls

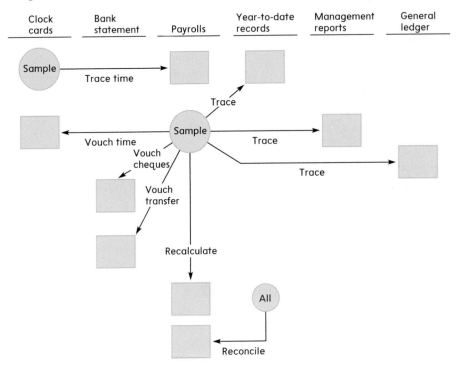

EP 13-6 Internal Control Questionnaire Items: Possible Error or Fraud Due to Weakness.
LO2, 3

Required:

Refer to the internal control questionnaire for the production process (Appendix 13A, Exhibit 13A–2), and assume the answer to each question is "no." Prepare a table matching questions to errors that could occur because of the absence of the control. Your column headings should be as follows:

Question	Possible Error or Fraud Due to Weakness

EP 13-7 Controls Tests Related to Controls and Objectives. **LO1, 2, 3** Each of the following controls test procedures may be performed during the audit of the controls in the production process.

Required:

For each procedure (*a*) identify the internal control procedure (strength) being tested, and (*b*) identify the internal control objective(s) being addressed.

1. Balance and reconcile detailed production cost sheets to the WIP inventory control account.
2. Scan closed production cost sheets for missing numbers in the sequence.
3. Vouch a sample of open and closed production cost sheet entries to (*i*) labour reports and (*ii*) issue slips and materials-used reports.

4. Locate the material issue forms. Are they prenumbered? kept in a secure location? available to unauthorized persons?

5. Select several summary journal entries in the WIP inventory: (*i*) vouch to weekly labour and material reports and to production cost sheets, and (*ii*) trace to control account.

6. Select a sample of the material issue slips in the production department file. Examine for the following:

   (*i*) Issue date/materials-used report date
   (*ii*) Production order number
   (*iii*) Supervisor's signature or initials
   (*iv*) Name and number of material
   (*v*) Raw material stores clerk's signature or initials
   (*vi*) Matching material requisition in raw material stores file, noting date of requisition

7. Determine by inquiry and inspection if cost clerks review dates on report of units completed for accounting in the proper period.

EP 13-8 Cost Accounting Test of Controls. `LO1, 2` The diagram in Exhibit EP 13-8 describes several cost accounting test of controls procedures. It shows the direction of the tests, leading from samples of cost accounting analyses, management reports, and the general ledger to blank squares.

Required:

For each blank square in Exhibit EP 13-8, write a cost accounting test of controls procedure and describe the evidence it can produce. (*Hint:* Refer to Exhibit 13–10.)

EXHIBIT EP 13-8

Diagram of Cost Accounting Test of Controls

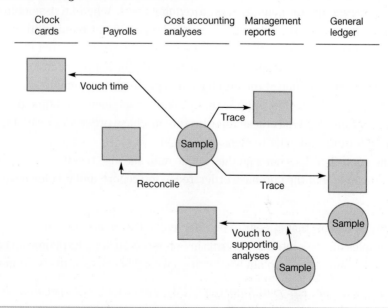

EP 13-9 **Work-in-Process Inventory, Tests of Control.** LO2 Assume an auditor finds the following errors while performing tests of controls for WIP inventory in a custom machinery manufacturing business.

Required:

For each finding, state which control objective is affected, what control deficiency is indicated, and what further investigation (if any) should be undertaken by the auditor.

a. Budgeted labour hours are 30% lower than actual labour costs and production cost reports.
b. Of 20 time-clock entries examined for July 14, 3 do not appear on the daily labour report or production cost report for that day.
c. Weekly labour cost reports do not agree with the weekly payroll summary.
d. The open production report used to cost WIP inventory contains costs of materials for which no matching amount and description are found on the materials-used reports and no material issue slip is on file in the material storage department.

EP 13-10 **Strengths and Weaknesses of Inventory Production Controls.** LO2 Peterson Electronics manufactures radio equipment. Its manufacturing plant and warehouse are located in the same building. When parts are received at the warehouse, the receiver compares the type of goods and quantity to a copy of the purchase order available online. If the quantity received differs from the quantity on the purchase order, the receiver adjusts the purchase order amount online. When the goods are checked by the receiver, she emails the accounting department, recording the type of goods, quantity, and date received. The accounting department uses the email to create a receiver's report, and the purchase order is then printed and filed in the accounting department. The online system allows the company to reduce paper, as a hard copy is not needed until the goods are actually received. The company's order-entry and tracking system automatically assigns the next number in a series to the purchase order just before printing.

After the receipt of inventory has been recorded, the parts are physically moved to the warehousing area, which is located in a locked-up area at the end of the plant. There is a stores department in a separate area for supplies, such as gloves, wire, and adhesives, all of which are used in significant quantities on a regular basis. When an assembly line worker requires supplies, the supervisor fills out a serially prenumbered requisition card, signs it, and gives it to the worker, who then takes it to the stores department to obtain the needed items. Each supervisor has a stock of requisition cards. When the supplier's invoice is received by the purchasing department, one of the purchasing department staff emails the accounting department, noting the invoice amount, supplier name, date of shipment, and type of goods. The accounting department then matches these items to the purchase order and receiving report and prepares a cheque for the controller to sign.

The controller does not sign the cheque until she also receives an email from the accounting staff indicating that the purchase order, receiving report, and invoice have been matched.

Required

a. List four internal controls that appear to be effective in Peterson's system.
b. List three examples of weak internal controls in Peterson's system. Explain why each of your examples would be a weak control; i.e., explain what can go wrong because of the weakness.

(Adapted from External Auditing (AU1), June 2011, with permission of Chartered Professional Accountants of Canada, Toronto, Canada. Any changes to the original material are the sole responsibility of the author (and/or publisher) and have not been reviewed or endorsed by Chartered Professional Accountants of Canada.)

DISCUSSION CASES

DC 13-1 Controls and Substantive Testing in Wages Payroll. `LO2, 3, 4` You are the audit senior on the engagement team that is performing the audit of MR Roboto Inc.'s financial statements for its December 31, 20X5, year-end. Your firm has audited MR Roboto for the past three years. You are now reviewing the company's payroll process and controls, in order to start designing your audit programs.

MR Roboto operates a nuclear waste processing and storage operation in a remote region of Ontario. The process is mainly automated, but the company has a small workforce of 40 employees who monitor the processing plant and the storage areas. The facility is staffed 24 hours a day, seven days a week. There are also 15 employees who work in the company's administration. The payroll accounting process includes some automated and some manual procedures. You have documented the description of the plant employee payroll process and its internal controls, as follows.

The plant employees work seven-hour shifts and are paid based on hours worked. There are four shifts per day to allow overlap of employees during shift changes, since the plant processes must be monitored at all times. Employees are assigned an employee number when they are hired and are required to clock in and out by swiping their employee identification cards at the plant entrance. The time-clock data is linked into the computerized payroll system, which processes the payroll and produces a weekly report of hours worked. There is no monitoring of employees' clocking in/out process. One of the audit team members observed an employee clocking in with two employee swipe cards. When the employee noticed the auditor watching, he explained that the other employee will be working on the shift " . . . but he just stopped on the way in to pick up the coffee and donuts for our shift change meeting."

The payroll system calculates the weekly cash wages to be paid to each employee, based on their hourly rates, by taking the information from the payroll system's hours worked report, multiplying it by the appropriate hourly wage rates, and calculating the appropriate tax deductions. The plant employees are paid in cash because the location of the plant is remote and there is no bank within hundreds of kilometres. These calculations are not checked by anyone, as they are generated by the payroll system.

Each Friday, the payroll department prepares the pay packets and physically hands these out to the plant employees who are on day shifts. Every employee must present his or her employee identification card to receive the pay packet. For employees on the night shifts, the pay packets are distributed by the night supervisor. If any packets are not claimed, the night supervisor keeps them and returns them to the payroll department on the next business day.

During your inquires, the CFO informs you that early in the current year, the government income tax department assessed the tax withholdings of MR Roboto and determined that too little tax had been deducted. The error occurred because the company had failed to update the system to the current year's tax rates. MR Roboto's CFO is asking why your audit of last year's financial statements did not discover this error.

Required:

a. Identify three control weaknesses in the payroll system of MR Roboto. Explain the possible implications of each weakness, and provide a recommendation to address it.

b. Describe the substantive procedures you would perform to verify the valuation and completeness of MR Roboto's payroll expenses.

c. Explain the responsibilities of management and auditors of MR Roboto in relation to compliance with laws and regulations under CAS 250, "Consideration of Laws and Regulations in an Audit of Financial Statements."

DC 13-2 Control Tests, Evaluation of Possible Diversion of Payroll Funds. [LO5, 6, 7] The Generous Loan Company has 100 branch loan offices. Each office has a manager and four or five subordinates who are employed by the manager. Branch managers prepare the weekly payroll, including their own salaries, and pay employees from cash on hand. Employees sign the payroll sheet signifying receipt of their salary. Hours worked by hourly personnel are inserted in the payroll register sheet from time cards prepared by the employees and approved by the manager.

The weekly payroll register sheets are sent to the head office along with other accounting statements and reports. The head office compiles employee earnings records and prepares all federal and provincial salary reports from the weekly payroll sheets.

Salaries are established by head office job-evaluation schedules. Salary adjustments, promotions, and transfers of full-time employees are approved by a head office salary committee based on the recommendations of branch managers and area supervisors. Branch managers advise the salary committee of new full-time employees and terminated employees. Part-time and temporary employees are hired without advising the salary committee.

Required:

a. Prepare a payroll audit program to be used in the head office to audit the branch office payrolls of the Generous Loan Company. See Exhibit 13–4 for sample audit procedures.
b. Based on your review of the payroll system, how might funds for payroll be diverted fraudulently?

(© 2000, American Institute of CPAs. All Rights Reserved. Adapted by permission.)

DC 13-3 Croyden Factory Inc.: Evaluation of Flowchart for Payroll Control Weaknesses. [LO5, 6]
A PA's audit working papers contain a narrative description of a segment of the Croyden Factory Inc. payroll system and an accompanying flowchart (Exhibit DC 13-3) as follows:

The internal control system, with respect to the personnel department, is well functioning and is not included in the accompanying flowchart.

At the beginning of each workweek, payroll clerk No. 1 reviews the payroll department files to determine the employment status of factory employees. Clerk No. 1 then prepares time cards and distributes them as each individual arrives at work. This payroll clerk, who is also responsible for custody of the cheque signature stamp machine, verifies the identity of each payee before delivering signed cheques to the supervisor.

At the end of each workweek, the supervisor distributes payroll cheques for the preceding workweek. Concurrent with this activity, the supervisor reviews the current week's employee time cards, notes the regular and overtime hours worked on a summary form, and initials the time cards. The supervisor then delivers all time cards and unclaimed payroll cheques to payroll clerk No. 2.

Required:

a. Based on the narrative and accompanying flowchart, what are the weaknesses in the system of internal control?
b. Based on the narrative and accompanying flowchart, what inquiries should be made with respect to clarifying the existence of possible additional weaknesses in the system of internal control?

Note: Do not discuss the internal control system of the personnel department.

(© 2000, American Institute of CPAs. All Rights Reserved. Adapted by permission.)

EXHIBIT DC 13-3

Croyden Inc. Factory Payroll System

Factory employee	Factory supervisor	Personnel	Payroll clerk No. I	Payroll clerk No. 2	Bookkeeping

Flowchart contents:

START (Factory supervisor)

Payroll update and withholding — Copy, Copy, Copy

A (Payroll clerk No. 2)

Clock time cards E F → Regular and overtime hours computed and noted on clock cards → Employment status wage rate and authorized payroll deductions checked → Gross and net payroll computed; Payroll register prepared

Factory employee:
- Clock time cards E → Time clock punched in and out daily → Clock cards submitted for approval weekly
- Clock time cards F → Time clock punched in and out daily → Clock cards E F → Clock cards reviewed and initialled; summary of regular and overtime hours prepared → Clock time cards / Summary of regular and overtime hours (D) → Delivered to payroll clerk No. 2

Personnel: File reviewed Weekly clock cards prepared → A

Payroll clerk No. I:
- Clock time cards E F → D
- Payroll register I 2 → D
- Payroll register I → D
- Column totals cross-footed → Sequentially numbered payroll cheques prepared → Payroll cheques Supervisor Employees

Identity of payee verified; cheques signature stamped → Cheques delivered to factory supervisor

Regular and overtime hours verified

Gross pay, net pay, and numerical sequence of cheques verified

Payroll cheques Supervisor Employees → Payroll cheques distributed → A

File sequence
A = alphabetic
File sequence
A = alphabetic by employee name
B = date (end of week)

DC 13-4 Vane Corporation: Control Weaknesses in Computerized Payroll System. **LO6** The Vane Corporation is a manufacturing concern that has been in business for the past 18 years. During this period, the company has grown from a very small family-owned operation to a medium-size company with several departments. Despite this growth, many procedures employed by Vane have been in effect since the business was started.

Vane's current payroll process is semi-automated. The payroll operation involves each worker picking up a weekly time card on Monday morning and writing in his or her name and identification number. These blank cards are kept near the factory entrance. Workers fill in their daily arrival and departure times each day on the card. Each Monday, the factory supervisor collects the time cards for the previous week and sends them to data processing.

In data processing, the time cards are entered into the computerized payroll system. The system updates the payroll records and prints out the paycheques. The cheques are written on the regular chequing account; imprinted by a signature plate with the treasurer's signature; and sent to the factory supervisors, who distribute them to the workers or hold them for absent workers to pick up later. Supervisors notify data processing of new employees, terminations, changes in hourly pay rates, or any other changes affecting payroll.

The workers also complete a job time ticket for each individual job they work on each day. These are collected daily and sent to cost accounting, where they are used to prepare a cost distribution analysis.

Further analysis of the payroll function reveals the following:

1. A worker's gross wages never exceed $1,000 per week.
2. Raises never exceed 55 cents per hour for the factory workers.
3. No more than 20 hours of overtime are allowed each week.
4. The factory employs 150 workers in 10 departments.

The payroll function had not been operating smoothly for some time, but even more problems have surfaced since the payroll was computerized. The factory supervisors would like a weekly report indicating worker tardiness, absenteeism, and idle time so that they can determine the amount of productive time lost and the reasons for the lost time. The following errors and inconsistencies have been encountered the past few pay periods:

1. A worker's paycheque was not processed properly because he had transposed two digits in his identification number on his time card.
2. A worker was issued a cheque for $4,531.80 when it should have been $453.18.
3. One worker's paycheque was not written, and this error was not detected until the paycheques for that department were distributed by the supervisor.
4. Some of the payroll register records were accidentally erased from the system when a data processing clerk tried to reorganize and rename the files in the hard drive. Data processing attempted to re-establish the destroyed portion from original source documents and other records.
5. One worker received a much larger paycheque than he should have. A clerk had keyed 84 instead of 48 for hours worked.
6. Several paycheques issued were not included in the totals posted to the payroll journal entry to the general ledger accounts. This was not detected for several pay periods.
7. In processing non-routine changes, a data processing clerk included a pay rate increase for one of his friends in the factory. By chance, this was discovered by another employee.

Required:

Identify the control weaknesses in Vane's payroll procedures and in the computer processing as it is now conducted. Recommend the necessary changes to correct the system. Arrange your answer in the following columnar format:

Control weaknesses	Recommendations
1.	1.

DC 13-5 Payroll Process: False Claims for Hours Worked. `LO1, 5, 6, 7` This case follows the framework of the Application Case and Analysis in the chapter.

Case Description The case involves overpayment of wages to employees making false claims for hours worked. A temporary personnel agency assigned Nurse Jane to work at Municipal Hospital. The personnel agency paid Nurse Jane and then billed Municipal Hospital for the wages and benefits. Supporting documents were submitted with the personnel agency's bills.

Nurse Jane claimed payroll hours on agency time cards, which showed approval signatures of a hospital nursing shift supervisor. This shift supervisor had been terminated by the hospital several months prior to the periods covered by the time cards in question. Nurse Jane worked one or two days per week but submitted time cards for a full 40-hour work week.

Nurse Jane's wages and benefits were billed to the hospital at $22 per hour. False time cards charging about 24 extra hours per week cost the hospital $528 per week. Nurse Jane was assigned to Municipal Hospital for 15 weeks during the year, so she caused overcharges of about $7,900. She then told three of her crooked friends about the procedure, and they overcharged the hospital another $24,000.

Audit Trail Each hospital work station keeps ward shift logs, which are sign-in sheets showing nurses on duty at all times. Nurses sign in and sign out when going on and off duty. Municipal Hospital maintains personnel records showing, among other things, the period of employment of its own nurses, supervisors, and other employees.

Audit Approach Analysis

Audit Objective The auditor's objective is to obtain evidence determining whether wages were paid to valid employees for actual time worked at the authorized pay rate.

Controls Relevant to the Process Control procedures in the payroll process should include a hiring authorization for putting employees on the payroll. For temporary employees, this authorization includes contracts for nursing time, conditions of employment, and terms, including the contract reimbursement rate. Control records of attendance and work should be kept (ward shift log). Supervisors should approve time cards or other records used by the payroll department to prepare paycheques.

In this case, the contract with the personnel agency provided that approved time cards had to be submitted as supporting documentation for the agency billings.

Required:

Describe in detail the audit procedures you would perform in this case. Consider tests of control and substantive tests, such as dual-purpose tests of transactions and/or tests of details of balance. Which tests do you consider likely to detect the overpayment of hourly wages? Why?

DC 13-6 Control over Department Labour Cost in a Job Cost System. `LO1, 2, 3` The Brown Printing Company accounts for the services it performs on a job cost basis. Most jobs take a week or less to complete and involve two or more of Brown's five operating departments. Actual costs are accumulated by job. To ensure timely billing, however, the company prepares sales invoices based on cost estimates.

Recently, several printing jobs have incurred losses. To avoid future losses, management has decided to focus on cost control at the department level. Since labour is a major element of cost, management proposes a department labour cost report. This report will originate in the payroll department as part of the biweekly payroll and then go to an accounting clerk for comparison with total labour cost estimates by department. If the actual total department labour costs in a payroll are not much more than the estimated total department labour cost during that period, the accounting clerk will send the report to the department supervisor. If the accounting clerk concludes that a significant variance exists, the report will be sent to the assistant controller. The assistant controller will investigate the cause when time is available and recommend corrective action to the production manager.

Required:

Evaluate the proposal:

a. Give at least three common aspects of control the department labour cost report proposal complies with. Give an example from the case to support each aspect cited.

b. Give at least three common aspects of control the department labour cost report proposal does not comply with. Give an example from the case to support each aspect cited.

(© 2000, American Institute of CPAs. All Rights Reserved. Adapted by permission.)

DC 13-7 Audit of Manufacturing Property, Plant, and Equipment and Depreciation Allocated to Inventory. `LO4` Bart's Company has prepared the fixed asset and depreciation schedule shown in Exhibit DC 13-7. The following information is available:

- The land was purchased eight years ago when Building 1 was erected. The location was then remote but is now bordered by a major freeway. The appraised value is $35 million.
- Building 1 has an estimated useful life of 35 years and no residual value.
- Building 2 was built by a local contractor this year. It also has an estimated useful life of 35 years and no residual value. The company occupied it on May 1 this year.
- Equipment A was purchased January 1 six years ago, when the estimated useful life was eight years with no residual value. It was sold on May 1 for $500,000.
- The computer system was placed in operation as soon as Equipment A was sold. It is estimated to be in use for six years with no residual value at the end.
- The company estimated the useful life of the press at 20 years with no residual value.
- Truck 1 was sold during the year for $1,000.
- Truck 2 was purchased on July 1. The company expects to use it for five years and then sell it for $2,000.
- All amortization is calculated by the straight-line method using months of service.

Required:

a. Audit the depreciation calculations. Are there any errors? Put the errors in the form of an adjusting journal entry, assuming 90% of the depreciation on the buildings and the press has been charged to cost of goods sold and 10% is still capitalized in the inventory, and the other depreciation expense is classified as general and administrative expense.

b. List two audit procedures for auditing the fixed asset additions.

c. What will an auditor expect to find in the Gain and Loss on Sale of Assets account? What amount of cash flow from investing activities will be in the cash flow statement?

EXHIBIT DC 13-7

Property, Plant, and Equipment Continuity Schedule

	PROPERTY, PLANT, AND EQUIPMENT ASSETS AND DEPRECIATION							
	ASSET COST (000S)				ACCUMULATED DEPRECIATION (000S)			
DESCRIPTION	BEGINNING BALANCE	ADDED	SOLD	ENDING BALANCE	BEGINNING BALANCE	ADDED	SOLD	ENDING BALANCE
Land	10,000			10,000				
Building 1	30,000			30,000	6,857	857		7,714
Building 2		42,000		42,000		800		800
Equipment	5,000		5,000	0	3,750	208	3,958	0
Computer system		3,500		3,500	583			583
Press	1,500			1,500	300	150		450
Truck 1	15		15	0	15		15	0
Truck 2		22		22		2		2
Total	46,515	45,522	5,015	87,022	10,922	2,600	3,973	9,549

DC 13-8 Inventory Costing Errors, Standard Manufacturing Costs. LO1, 2, 3, 4 Thermox Inc. manufactures heating elements and devices. One of its main raw material components is steel tubing. During the current year, Thermox's new raw material buyer began purchasing steel tubing from a U.S. supplier. The buyer found this supplier's prices to be considerably lower than those of the previous Canadian suppliers.

Thermox's cost accounting department uses standard manufacturing costs to determine its inventory cost and cost of goods sold. In her audit of the reasonableness of the standard costs, the audit senior is vouching the raw materials components list to supplier invoices and supporting documents. She notes several steel tubing purchases in March that were invoiced in U.S. dollars (a U.S. dollar at this time was worth about $1.25 Canadian). However, the U.S. dollar amount, not the Canadian dollar amount, is used in the standard costing formula. Steel tubing constitutes 70% of Thermox's standard manufacturing cost. The audit senior extends her vouching and discovers that all steel tubing purchases from March to the December year-end were from the same U.S. supplier and were invoiced in U.S. dollars.

The audit senior then examines the U.S. supplier's monthly statements of account and discovers that Thermox's accounts payable department has been paying the U.S. steel tubing invoices in Canadian dollars. Thus Thermox has been short-paying the U.S. supplier by about 25%. Because of this related error, no significant cost variances appeared for raw materials, which would have alerted Thermox management to the problem.

Required:

a. What impact will this error have on Thermox's year-end inventory balance and its cost of sales if standard costs are used and no variances are adjusted? What impact will this error have on accounts payable? State any assumptions you make.

b. What records will the audit senior need to examine, and what tests and analyses will she need to perform to assess the magnitude of the error in inventory, cost of goods sold, and accounts payable?

c. What control deficiency would allow this type of error to occur, and what kind of control procedure(s) could be implemented to prevent this type of error?

DC 13-9 Audit of Real Estate Inventory.   LO1, 2, 3, 4   Desai Developments Limited (DDL) is in the business of buying undeveloped land in the regions outside Calgary and holding it until it has development permits and market conditions are favourable for development. DDL began operations 12 years ago. Once a property is ready for development, DDL contracts with various construction companies to build the houses. DDL handles all the promotions and sales of the houses once they are completed.

Because of recent changes in environmental laws and zoning restrictions, some of the sites DDL originally purchased for subdivisions can no longer be used for this purpose. However, golf courses are still permissible on these sites because they can preserve wetlands and forests. DDL is, therefore, now undertaking a new business model that involves developing and operating golf courses. DDL will also sell off the outer edges of the golf course properties as building lots for large "estate lot" homes, which are still permitted because they have a lower impact on the environment.

The president of DDL, Mira Desai, owns 51% of the DDL common shares. Her relatives hold the remainder. DDL has also financed its operation by bank mortgages on the land. Mira now wants to issue preferred shares in DDL to private investors and use the proceeds to pay back the bank mortgages and fund the golf course developments. The plan is for the preferred shares to be non-voting, to pay a 6% non-cumulative dividend per year, and to provide the preferred shareholder with a lifelong membership in one of the golf courses. She has found several investors who are interested in the preferred shares, but DDL will need to provide prospective investors with DDL's 20X5 financial statements prepared in accordance with GAAP.

Mira is considering engaging your audit firm to provide an audit opinion on DDL's GAAP financial statements. Up until now, DDL has only prepared unaudited financial statements primarily for tax purposes and has always used accounting methods that result in paying the minimum amount of tax. In discussions with Mira, and from reviewing DDL's most recent annual financial statements (for the year ended December 31, 20X5), you learn the following:

1. DDL currently owns four properties that have been approved for golf course development. It has finalized the plans and will start development in the spring of 20X6. DDL owns five other properties that may be suitable for future golf course developments.

2. DDL owns another eight properties approved for residential subdivisions. Recently DDL received an offer from another property development company, Atim Corp., to purchase all eight of these properties for $50 million. The mortgages on these properties are $45 million. Mira is interested in exiting from the subdivision development to allow DDL to focus on the golf course business. She is considering making a counteroffer in which DDL would form a 50–50 joint venture with Atim Corp. DDL would contribute the properties to this joint venture entity and Atim would contribute the cash and management skills to construct and sell the subdivision homes.

3. DDL has capitalized the purchase price of the land, legal fees relating to the purchase, and land transfer taxes. All other costs related to the properties, such as property taxes, interest, earth-moving costs, and fees for architectural and landscaping plans, have all been expensed to maximize tax deductions.

4. DDL's net income from the subdivision business has varied widely over the years, with profits in years when housing developments are completed and sold, and losses in other years. Revenue is recognized when each house is sold. The average subdivision development takes about 18 months to complete. A golf course development will take about two years because of the extensive landscaping and planting required.

5. The golf course development costs can be partly financed by selling the estate lots around the golf course site to the custom-home builders. As part of its agreement with these construction

companies, DDL will handle the sales promotions and marketing of the houses for a 10% commission on selling prices.

6. To date, DDL has completed five housing subdivision developments. The first development, completed about 10 years ago, has recently been in the news because methane and other noxious gases have been seeping into basements. Environmental assessments have determined that the subdivision was built on what was a landfill site in the 1950s. It was never properly sealed off prior to redevelopment and is now releasing gases that are dangerous to people. Environmental consultants estimate it will cost up to $2 million to remediate the properties so the houses will be safe to live in. The current owners of these homes have started legal action against DDL. DDL's lawyers believe that the company that sold DDL the land had fraudulently withheld relevant information about the prior use of the land, so that DDL will not be liable for the remediation costs.

7. DDL received a government loan of $6 million in early 20X5, under a program aimed at helping developers cope with the impact of the changes in environmental regulations. The entire loan is forgivable if DDL produces a commercially viable golf course by the end of 20X7. Half of the government loan amount was recorded as revenue in 20X5 because, in DDL management's view, the golf course development is 50% complete.

8. Late in 20X5, DLL rented earth-moving equipment to start the golf course development work. The equipment lease agreement has a 10-year term and required a $200,000 payment at the start of the term, with payments of $200,000 thereafter at the start of each of the next nine years. The equipment could have been purchased for $1,265,650 in cash and has an expected useful life of 10 years. The relevant borrowing rate for assessing this lease is 12% per year.

Required:

a. Prepare a report outlining the considerations your firm would have to make before accepting the audit of DDL.

b. Assuming your firm accepts the engagement, prepare a detailed and complete audit plan that addresses the accounting and other information items noted previously. Also, suggest any other information that you would want for planning the audit.

DC 13-10 Risk Assessments and Responses for Manufacturing Inventory. `LO4` Sun-House Solar Inc. (SHS) is a medium-size private company that develops solar energy systems for sale and installation in private residences. It is privately owned, with the majority of the shares held by the company's president, Yong Shu. SHS started up five years ago. Its first two years were mostly involved in research and development. Over the past three years, SHS has been very successful and its customer sales and installations have grown continuously. SHS's main raw material is silicone, which it purchases on the world market so that it can keep a one-year supply on hand at its factory in Woodbridge. It also has some purchase commitments for silicone at prices far above the current spot price, which it would only use if there was a huge increase in the price of silicone on the world market.

Shu has engaged your audit firm to do the current year's audit because she plans to obtain $20 million in financing to allow further commercialization of the SHS systems. The plan is to turn SHS into a public company and issue shares on the Toronto Stock Exchange. Your firm has accepted the engagement and assigned you to prepare the audit plan. You have obtained the preliminary general ledger trial balance from the SHS chief financial officer. The CFO is a qualified professional accountant with 15 years' experience as a financial officer in various public companies before joining SHS two years ago.

The following is a summary of the accounts that appear in this trial balance as at year-end:

ACCOUNT	BALANCE DR/(CR)
Cash	$101,209
Accounts receivable	85,019
Allowance for bad debts	(15,000)
Inventory, finished goods	100,550
Inventory, work in process	44,666
Inventory, unassembled solar panels	67,890
Inventory, raw materials	834,445
Property, plant, and equipment	3,700,990
Accumulated amortization, property, plant, and equipment	(901,108)
Patents, at cost	1,010,000
Accounts payable	(198,009)
Warranty provision	(30,000)
Shareholder loan, non–interest bearing	(5,400,000)
Share capital, common shares	1,000
Retained earnings	1,261,558
Revenue	(4,812,202)
Cost of goods sold	1,666,502
General and administrative expenses	802,500
Research and development expenses	190,000
Other expenses	1,489,990

Required:

a. Identify three factors your audit firm would have to consider in order to accept the SHS audit engagement for the current year, and explain how each factor affects the acceptance decision.

b. What materiality levels would you use for planning this audit? Show your calculations and justify your decisions.

   You can assume your audit firm's policy is that performance materiality should be 70% of the materiality level for financial statements as a whole, unless specific information indicates a different value should be used.

c. What audit risk level would you want to achieve for this engagement? Describe your choice in terms of one of these levels: highest, medium, lowest. Explain the factors that support your decision.

d. Identify and explain three business risk factors in SHS that you would need to understand in order to assess the risk of material misstatement in its financial statements.

e. Based on the business risk analysis for SHS, your audit manager is concerned the SHS finished goods inventory account balance has high risks of material misstatement. Your manager has asked you to assess the risk of material misstatement at the assertion level for this account. Use the level high, medium, or low to describe your assessments. Explain the factors that support your assessments.

f. Outline a substantive audit program that responds to the risks at the assertion level that you have assessed, above, for SHS's inventory.

Internal Control Questionnaires for the Payroll and Production Processes

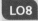 **LO8** Describe the internal control questionnaires used in audit practice for the payroll and production processes.

Exhibits 13A–1 and 13A–2 are examples of the type of form that could be used to guide the auditor's assessment of the effectiveness of application controls in the main classes of transactions and the main account balances related to the payroll and production processes. Note that in practice, forms like this can provide only a general starting point, and the actual audit work must always be tailored to the specifics of each engagement.

EXHIBIT 13A–1

Internal Control Questionnaire: Payroll Process

INTERNAL CONTROL QUESTIONNAIRE FOR PAYROLL ACCOUNTING PROCESS AUDITEE: _____ F/S PERIOD: _____	Auditor Responses	Audit File References
PROCESS: Payroll		
OVERALL COMPANY-LEVEL CONTROL AND CONTROL ACTIVITIES ASSESSMENT (Refer to responses recorded for questions in Exhibit 9A–1 in Appendix 9A.)		
APPLICATION CONTROL ASSESSMENTS *PAYROLL APPLICATION CONTROLS* **Environment and General Controls Relevant to This Application:** 1. Are all employees paid by cheque or direct deposit to their bank accounts? 2. If a special payroll bank account is used, is the payroll bank account reconciled by someone who does not prepare, sign, or deliver paycheques? 3. Are payroll cheques signed by persons who neither prepare cheques nor keep cash funds or accounting records? 4. If an outside payroll processing service is used, is the list of employees paid by the service reviewed by the employees' supervisor or someone else who cannot add or make changes to the employee payroll list submitted to the processing service? 5. Are payroll department personnel rotated in their duties? required to take vacations? bonded? 6. Is the timekeeping department (function) independent of the payroll department?		*(continued)*

EXHIBIT 13A–1

Internal Control Questionnaire: Payroll Process   (*continued*)

Application Control Assessments:
Consider whether the auditee has appropriate policies and procedures in place to meet the following control objectives:

Validity objective:
   7. Are names of terminated employees reported in writing to the payroll department?
   8. Is the payroll periodically compared with personnel files?
   9. Are cheques distributed by someone other than the employee's immediate supervisor?
  10. Are unclaimed wages controlled by a responsible officer?
  11. Do internal auditors conduct occasional surprise distributions of paycheques, or for direct deposit payroll do they conduct random verification of the existence of a sample of current employees who are included on the payroll register?

Completeness objective:
  12. Are names of newly hired employees reported in writing to the payroll department?
  13. Are blank payroll cheques prenumbered and the numerical sequence checked for missing documents?

Authorization objective:
  14. Are all wage rates determined by contract or approved by a personnel officer?
  15. Are authorizations for deductions, signed by the employees, on file?
  16. Are time cards or piecework reports prepared by the employee approved by his or her supervisor?
  17. Is a secure time clock and time recording system used to record hours worked by each employee?
  18. Is the payroll register sheet signed by the employee preparing it and approved prior to payment?

Accuracy objective:
  19. Are timekeeping and cost accounting records (such as hours, dollars) reconciled with payroll department calculations of hours and wages?
  20. Are payrolls audited periodically by internal auditors?

Classification objective:
  21. Do payroll accounting personnel have instructions for classifying payroll debit entries?
  22. Are payroll records reconciled with government tax reports (e.g., T4 summary)?

Proper period objective:
  23. Are monthly, quarterly, and annual wage accruals reviewed by an accounting officer?

Auditor's conclusion on the effectiveness of application controls in the payroll accounting process: _____ _____	Prepared by ____ ____	Date ____ ____

EXHIBIT 13A–2

Internal Control Questionnaire: Production Process

INTERNAL CONTROL QUESTIONNAIRE FOR PRODUCTION ACCOUNTING PROCESS AUDITEE: _____ F/S PERIOD: _____	Auditor Responses	Audit File References
PROCESS: Inventory production costing		
OVERALL COMPANY-LEVEL CONTROL AND CONTROL ACTIVITIES ASSESSMENT (Refer to responses recorded for questions in Exhibit 9A–1 in Appendix 9A.)		
APPLICATION CONTROL ASSESSMENTS *PRODUCTION APPLICATION CONTROLS* **Environment and General Controls Relevant to This Application** 1. Are access controls properly designed to restrict access to production initiation documents and functions to authorized personnel? Consider production system user identity assignments and access to blank production order forms, materials and labour requisitions forms, and finished goods inventory issue forms. 2. Are physical access controls in place to ensure only authorized personnel have custody of materials, WIP, and finished goods? 3. Is production cost accounting segregated from factory production functions? 4. Are summary journal entries reviewed and approved by an accounting supervisor? **Application Control Assessment** Consider whether the auditee has appropriate policies and procedures in place to meet the following control objectives: *Validity objective:* 5. Are material requisitions and job time tickets reviewed by the production supervisor after factory personnel prepare them? 6. Are the weekly direct labour and materials-used reports reviewed by the production supervisor after factory personnel prepare them? *Completeness objective:* 7. Are production orders, materials and labour requisitions, job time tickets, and inventory issue slips prenumbered and the numerical sequence checked for missing documents? *Authorization objective:* 8. Are authorizations of production orders and materials and labour requisitions independently verified? *Accuracy objective:* 9. Are differences between inventory issue slips and materials-used reports recorded and reported to the cost accounting supervisor? 10. Are differences between job time tickets and the labour report recorded and reported to the cost accounting supervisor? 11. Are standard costs used? If so, are they reviewed and revised periodically? 12. Are differences between reports of units completed and finished goods entries recorded and reported to the cost accounting supervisor? *Classification objective:* 13. Does the accounting manual give instructions for proper classification of cost accounting transactions? *Proper period objective:* 14. Does the accounting manual give instructions to date cost entries on the date of use? Does an accounting supervisor review monthly, quarterly, and year-end cost accruals?		
Auditor's conclusion on the effectiveness of application controls in the production accounting process: _____ _____	Prepared by ____ ____	Date ____ ____

The Finance and Investment Process

In essence, the finance and investment process is how a company plans for capital requirements and raises the money by borrowing, selling shares, and entering into acquisitions and joint ventures. Dividend, interest, and income tax payments are part of the related accounting cycle. This cycle also includes the accounting for investments in marketable securities, joint ventures and partnerships, and subsidiaries. The finance portion of the process deals with acquiring money to fund the company's activities. The investment portion deals with investing money in revenue-generating assets and other long-term investments. The process has become much more complex through the use of sophisticated financial engineering that is used to manage client financial and business risk. Auditors have to make sure that these complex risks are properly disclosed in financial reporting.

LEARNING OBJECTIVES

After completing this chapter, you will be able to do the following:

LO1 Describe the finance and investment process: risk assessment, typical transactions, source documents, controls, and account balances.

LO2 List control tests for auditing control over debt, owners' equity, and investment transactions.

LO3 List the typical substantive procedures used to respond to the assessed risk of material misstatement in the main account balance, and in transactions in the finance and investment process.

LO4 Describe the most common fraud problems in the finance and investment process.

LO5 (Appendix 14A) List the risk management and control activities with derivative securities.

LO6 (Appendix 14B) Describe generally accepted accounting principles for private enterprises.

CHAPTER APPENDICES

APPENDIX 14A Derivative Securities—An Example of Risks That Management and Auditors Face (on Connect)

APPENDIX 14B Generally Accepted Accounting Principles for Private Enterprises (on Connect)

EcoPak Inc.

The EcoPak audit team is reaching the final days of its field work. Today, Donna is auditing EcoPak's long-term debt and shareholders' equity balances and transactions. She has started by reviewing the draft financial statements and the minutes of the board of directors meetings to identify important items that need to appear in the financial statements and notes. She notices that a new $2 million operating line of credit was arranged with EcoPak's bank to finance the purchase of new production equipment in April. This line is secured by the new equipment and bears interest at the prime rate plus 2.5%. The previous credit line of $1 million is still in place as well; it is secured by the inventory and accounts receivable and bears interest of prime plus 1%. Donna reviews the legal documents to ensure the details of these liabilities will be correctly presented and disclosed in the notes to the financial statement. She also notes the minutes recording the board's approval of the loan increase. She ensures she has read all the minutes for all the meetings held up to today, to make sure there are no other new debts or other items approved that are not recorded in the financial statements.

To verify the interest expense, Donna applies an analytical procedure—taking the monthly average loan balances from the bank statements and applying the applicable average interest charge for each month, she develops an expectation that is within $400 of the amount that is recorded in the draft financial statements, so she concludes that the interest expense amount is reasonable.

Turning to the shareholders' equity, Donna notes that there are no changes in the number of common shares outstanding during the year. Kam, Mike, and Nina each hold 100 common shares. Inspection of the minutes of the December 15 board meeting shows the approval of a common share dividend of $300,000 to be distributed on January 15 of the next year to the shareholders of record on December 15. The same meeting also shows board approval of the issue of 30 new common shares to Zhang upon conversion of 10% of her convertible preferred share holding, to take effect on January 15 of the next year.

Donna knows that Nina has not yet finished drafting the financial statement notes but is not sure why the dividend payable does not appear in the draft balance sheet. She meets with Nina first thing the next day to discuss the dividend payable and also the disclosure of the issuing of new common shares.

"The dividend payable is included in accrued liabilities for now. It's the first dividend we've ever paid, and I didn't have another account set up for it yet in the general ledger, so I just stuck it in there to save time. When you review the rest of my final journal entries you will see it—it's GJ #12-15-1, making a debit to retained earnings and a credit to accrued liabilities. But you are right that it needs to go on a separate line, and I will make sure it is presented that way in the next draft of the statements. And yes, absolutely, the new common shares that were issued to Zhang after year-end ought to be disclosed in the notes as a subsequent event. I hope to finish drafting up those notes by tomorrow and will email them to you in draft form as soon as I'm done. Thanks for pointing these issues out, Donna. Are you getting near the end of the field work by now?"

"Pretty near," Donna replies, "We should be able to finish the last few procedures tomorrow or the next day at the latest. Then you can have your boardroom back!"

The Essentials of Auditing the Finance and Investment Process

The finance and investment process contains a wide variety of accounts—share capital, dividends, long-term debt, interest expense, tax expenses and future income taxes, financial instruments, derivatives, equity method investments, related gains and losses, consolidated subsidiaries, goodwill, and other intangibles. These accounts involve some of the most technically complex accounting standards. They create most of the difficult judgments for financial reporting. For example, the decision to use hedge accounting with derivatives involves consideration of whether five difficult to assess conditions are met (IAS 39, para. 88).

Transactions in these accounts are generally controlled by senior officials. Therefore, internal control is centred on the integrity and accounting knowledge of these officials. The procedural controls over details of transactions are not very effective because senior managers can override them and order their own desired accounting presentations. As a consequence, auditors' work on the assessment of control risk is directed toward the senior managers, the board of directors and their authorizations, and the design of finance and investment deals. The corporate governance controls introduced in Appendix 6B (available on Connect) are particularly important for this process.

Substantive programs are developed by linking the auditor's risk assessments to the risks of material misstatements in the financing and investing transactions. This chapter provides examples of typical substantive procedures that would be considered, depending on the risks assessed in each particular case.

Fraud and clever accounting in the finance and investment cycle get directed most often toward producing misleading financial statements. While theft and embezzlement can occur, the accounts in this cycle have frequently been the ones manipulated and misvalued so that financial positions and results of operations look better than the company's reality. Off-balance-sheet financing and investment transactions with related parties are explained in this chapter as areas easily targeted for fraudulent financial reporting.

As a result of the risks and complexities of the accounting issues associated with the finance and investment process, much time can be spent with the audit committee and internal auditors (discussed in Appendix 6B) on auditing this process.

Review Checkpoint

14-1 Why is the finance and investment cycle particularly important for auditors?

Understanding the Finance and Investment Process

LO1   Describe the finance and investment process: risk assessment, typical transactions, source documents, controls, and account balances.

The finance and investment process involves the client company's legal structure, how it raises capital from shareholders and creditors, its intercorporate investments, and related parties. Each entity will have its own mix of these components. Understanding these important aspects of the corporate structure and their implications for financial statement misstatement risks requires the input of the most experienced audit team members. The corporate governance controls introduced in Appendix 6B are relevant to this risk assessment and are discussed in more detail in this chapter.

The account balances in the finance and investment process include those for financial instruments, such as long-term investments and debt, share capital, and contributed surplus. Dividend and interest payments are regular transactions. Disclosure requirements in the finance and investment process are extensive and include accounting policies for intercorporate investments; valuation bases of derivatives and other financial instruments; hedging activities using derivatives and other financial instruments; continuity of financial instrument balances and share capital; detailed terms, interest rates, and repayment dates of debt; and details of any contingent liabilities.

The estimates required in fair value accounting of financial instruments may have helped cause the global credit crisis, as shown in the Chapter 1 box titled "Accounting Blamed for Global Credit Crisis." That article indicates how increasingly crucial the finance and investment process is to both individual auditees and the entire economy.

Paul Krugman, the 2008 winner of the Nobel Prize in economics, attributes the 2008/2009 economic crisis to widespread fraud on Wall Street: frauds carried out through the finance and investment process and based on risky gambles using other peoples' money. The following box contains what Krugman had to say shortly after he accepted the Nobel Prize.

The Madoff Economy

The revelation that Bernard Madoff—brilliant investor (or so almost everyone thought), philanthropist, pillar of the community—was a phony has shocked the world, and understandably so. The scale of his alleged $50 billion Ponzi scheme is hard to comprehend.

Yet surely I'm not the only person to ask the obvious question: How different, really, is Mr. Madoff's tale from the story of the investment industry as a whole?

The financial services industry has claimed an ever-growing share of the nation's income over the past generation, making the people who run the industry incredibly rich. Yet, at this point, it looks as if much of the industry has been destroying value, not creating it. And it's not just a matter of money: the vast riches achieved by those who managed other people's money have had a corrupting effect on our society as a whole.

Let's start with those pay checks. Last year, the average salary of employees in "securities, commodity contracts, and investments" was more than four times the average salary in the rest of the economy. Earning a million dollars was nothing special and even incomes of $20 million or more were fairly common. The incomes of the richest Americans have exploded over the past generation, even as wages of ordinary workers have stagnated; high pay on Wall Street was a major cause of that divergence.

But surely those financial superstars must have been earning their millions, right? No, not necessarily. The pay system on Wall Street lavishly rewards the appearance of profit, even if that appearance later turns out to have been an illusion.

Consider the hypothetical example of a money manager who leverages up his clients' money with lots of debt, then invests the bulked-up total in high-yielding but risky assets, such as dubious mortgage-backed securities. For a while—say, as long as a housing bubble continues to inflate—he (it's almost always a he) will make big profits and receive big bonuses. Then, when the bubble bursts and his investments turn into toxic waste, his investors will lose big—but he'll keep those bonuses.

O.K., maybe my example wasn't hypothetical after all.

So, how different is what Wall Street in general did from the Madoff affair? Well, Mr. Madoff allegedly skipped a few steps, simply stealing his clients' money rather than collecting big fees while exposing investors to risks they didn't understand. And, while Mr. Madoff was apparently a self-conscious fraud, many people on Wall Street believed their own hype. Still, the end result was the same (except for the house arrest): the money managers got rich; the investors saw their money disappear.

We're talking about a lot of money here. In recent years the finance sector accounted for 8% of America's GDP, up from less than 5% a generation earlier. If that extra 3% was money for nothing—and it probably was—we're talking about $400 billion a year in waste, fraud, and abuse.

But the costs of America's Ponzi era surely went beyond the direct waste of dollars and cents.

Meanwhile, how much has our nation's future been damaged by the magnetic pull of quick personal wealth, which for years has drawn many of our best and brightest young people into investment banking, at the expense of science, public service, and just about everything else?

Most of all, the vast riches being earned—or maybe that should be "earned"—in our bloated financial industry undermined our sense of reality and degraded our judgment.

(continued)

Think of the way almost everyone important missed the warning signs of an impending crisis. How was that possible? How, for example, could Alan Greenspan have declared, just a few years ago, that "the financial system as a whole has become more resilient"—thanks to derivatives, no less? The answer, I believe, is that there's an innate tendency on the part of even the elite to idolize men who are making a lot of money, and to assume that they know what they're doing.

After all, that's why so many people trusted Mr. Madoff.

Now, as we survey the wreckage and try to understand how things can have gone so wrong, so fast, the answer is actually quite simple: What we're looking at now are the consequences of a world gone Madoff.

Source: Paul Krugman, Op-Ed Columnist, "The Madoff economy," *The New York Times*, Editorial Section, December 19, 2008, page A45, nytimes.com/2008/12/19/opinion/19krugman.html?_r=0.

We discuss the Madoff fraud and Ponzi schemes via financial reporting in more detail in Chapter 21 (available on Connect). For now, we note that Krugman's view is consistent with the observation of the Public Company Accounting Oversight Board (PCAOB), as early as 2005, that "Financial engineering, in general, involves structuring a transaction to achieve a desired accounting that is not consistent with the economics of the transaction." The PCAOB, thus, seems to view financial engineering via derivatives and other financial instruments of the finance and investment process as primarily a tool to create deceptive accounting.[1]

The credit crisis that started on Wall Street in 2007 spread globally and to the broader capital markets. Throughout 2007–2009, there was a cascading series of failures of financial institutions and government intervention, with secondary effects on markets and individual corporations, which eventually impacted the global economy. The events led to calls for accounting and auditing changes. Many came to question why those "fake profits" were so widespread and why auditing and accounting practices had allowed them to exist.

This brief summary of recent events illustrates why reporting of the finance and investment process is becoming increasingly important, and why this process is more and more regarded as a risky part of the audit of financial statements. With this background, we begin the detailed study of this process.

The International Financial Reporting Standards (IFRS) apply to accounts within the finance and investment process: measurement and recognition of financial instruments and derivatives at fair values, comprehensive income reporting, and consolidation of variable-interest enterprises. There are differences between the risks in public companies and those "without public accountability." In particular, the latter group in Canada has the option to use Accounting Standards for Private Enterprises (ASPE), which means they can use simpler accounting principles, such as cost basis for financial assets or taxes-payable basis for income taxes (see Appendix 14B). Like Canada, other countries that have adopted IFRS for public companies allow similar exceptions for smaller, private entities. For example, the accounting for equity of small private companies is much simpler than that for large public companies. This makes the audits of small private firms simpler as well. The complexities reviewed here may not apply to smaller audit engagements. Your instructor will direct you on the expectations in your course.

Risk Assessment for the Finance and Investment Process

At the assertion level, the main risks are completeness of debt, valuation of financial instruments, disclosures of risks relating to financial instruments and derivatives, and presentation and disclosure of intercorporate investments. Controls in the finance and investment process involve the highest level of management, and auditors usually use substantive procedures to assess presentation and verify changes and balances. Since these are long-term (financing/investing) or permanent (shares issued) items in the financial statements, it is important to include copies of all legal documents relating to loans, partnerships, leases, joint venture investments, and other long-term legal arrangements in audit documentation. These legal documents must be retained in permanent audit files so auditors can check that the contracts are properly accounted for and disclosed in future audits. The same goes for **articles of incorporation** (which set out authorized classes of shares, their features, shareholder rights, etc.) and records of issuing shares approved by the board of directors in the minutes.

It is also important for auditors to document management's rationale and procedures for accounting estimates and the audit procedures used to verify them, to help future auditors both assess the methods and apply them consistently if there is no reason to change them. Note that changing economic and business conditions are risk factors and may indicate that estimation methods should be changed as well.

Finance and Investment Process—Typical Activities

The finance and investment process relates to a large number of accounts and records: tangible or intangible assets; liabilities; deferred credits; shareholders' equity; gains and losses; expenses; and related taxes such as income tax, goods and services tax (GST) or harmonized sales tax (HST), and provincial sales tax (PST). The major accounts and records are listed in Exhibit 14–1 and include some of the more complicated topics in accounting: equity method accounting for investments, consolidation accounting, goodwill, income taxes, and financial instruments, to name a few. We will not explain the accounting for these balances and transactions, but instead concentrate on a few important aspects of auditing them. Exhibit 14–1 shows a skeleton outline of the finance

EXHIBIT 14–1

Finance and Investment Process

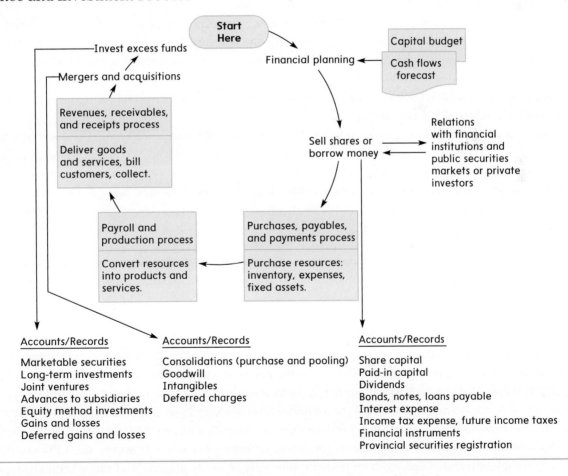

Accounts/Records

Marketable securities
Long-term investments
Joint ventures
Advances to subsidiaries
Equity method investments
Gains and losses
Deferred gains and losses

Accounts/Records

Consolidations (purchase and pooling)
Goodwill
Intangibles
Deferred charges

Accounts/Records

Share capital
Paid-in capital
Dividends
Bonds, notes, loans payable
Interest expense
Income tax expense, future income taxes
Financial instruments
Provincial securities registration

articles of incorporation:
a corporation's legal documents that set out its purpose, for example, classes of shares that can be issued

and investment process, the main functions of which are (1) financial planning and raising capital; (2) interacting with the processes of (i) purchases, payables, and payments; (ii) production and payroll; (iii) revenues, receivables, and receipts; and (3) entering into mergers, acquisitions, and other investments.

Good Corporate Governance: A Key Control for the Finance and Investment Process

Corporate governance was introduced to you in Appendix 6B. The role of boards of directors (or their equivalent) is crucial to good governance. The responsibilities of boards of directors are determined by the organization's legal and administrative framework.[2] This view considers the directors to be stewards of the organization and, as such, to be responsible for overseeing the conduct of the business and monitoring management, while giving all major issues affecting the business and affairs of the organization proper consideration. The contributions by the board of directors to internal control are given as follows:

- *Approving and monitoring mission, vision, and strategy:* endeavouring to see that the organization has the right approach in order to both add to shareholder and/or stakeholder value and improve its chances of viability and success
- *Approving and monitoring the organization's ethical values:* acting as guardian of the organization's values, and as its conscience
- *Monitoring management control:* overviewing the systems whereby the CEO and senior management exercise their power and influence over the rest of the organization
- *Evaluating senior management:* evaluating the competence and integrity of the CEO and other members of senior management, as it is primarily through them that the board exercises its power and influence
- *Overseeing external communications:* responsibility for the organization's communication of information to and from external parties
- *Assessing the board's effectiveness:* evaluating how well the board discharges its roles and responsibilities as part of the organization's overall control

These make up a comprehensive, idealized role for the board, one that might not be fully realized in practice. Nevertheless, this guideline is an authoritative source on good corporate governance practices with respect to control of management activities, especially as they relate to the finance and investment process. These elements of board control, especially the last four, are a useful benchmark in auditor evaluation of internal controls in this cycle.

Debt and Shareholders' Equity Capital

Transactions in debt and shareholders' equity capital are typically few in number but large in monetary amount. They are handled by the highest levels of management, and the control-related duties and responsibilities reflect this high-level attention.

Authorization

Financial planning starts with the CFO's cash flow forecast. It informs the board of directors and management of the business plans, the prospects for cash inflows, and the needs for cash outflows. The forecast is usually integrated with the capital budget, which contains the plans for asset purchases and business acquisitions. A capital budget approved by the board of directors is the authorization for major asset acquisitions and investments.

Sales of share capital and debt financing transactions are usually authorized by the board of directors. All the directors must sign registration documents for public securities offerings. However, the CFO usually has authority to complete transactions, such as periodic renewals of notes payable and other ordinary types of financing transactions, without specific board approval of each transaction. Auditors should expect to find the authorizing signatures of the CEO, the CFO, the board of directors, and perhaps other high-ranking officers on financing documents.

Many financing transactions are **off the balance sheet**. Companies can enter into obligations and commitments that are not required to be recorded in the accounts. Examples are various business and financing options such as leases, endorsements on discounted notes or on other companies' obligations, letters of credit, guarantees, repurchase or remarketing agreements, commitments to purchase at fixed prices, commitments to sell at fixed prices, and certain kinds of stock options. Many of these were discussed in previous chapters as part of the assessment of the risk of material misstatement related to the disclosure assertion.

Custody

In large companies, banks and trust companies serve as registrars and transfer agents of share certificates. A registrar keeps the shareholder list and, from time to time, determines the shareholders eligible to receive dividends (shareholders of record on a dividend record date) and those entitled to vote at the annual meeting. A transfer agent handles the exchange of shares, cancelling the shares surrendered by sellers and issuing new certificates to buyers. The same bank or trust company might provide both services.

Small companies often keep their own shareholder records. A share certificate book looks like a chequebook, with perforated stubs for recording the number of shares, the owner's name and other identification, and the date of issue. Actual unissued share certificates are attached to the stubs, like unused cheques in a chequebook. The missing certificates have been sent to the share owners. Custody of the share certificate book is important because the unissued certificates are like money or collateral. Share certificates can be improperly sold to buyers, who think they are genuinely issued, or can be used as collateral with unsuspecting lenders.

Lenders have custody of **debt instruments** (e.g., leases, bonds, notes, and loans payable). A CFO may have copies, but they are just records. However, when a company repurchases its debt instruments, these enter the custody of trustees or company officials, usually the CFO. Until they are cancelled and destroyed, they can be misused by improperly reselling them to unsuspecting investors.

Recordkeeping

The accounting department and the CFO or controller keep records of notes, loans, and bonds payable. Recordkeeping procedures are similar to those used to account for vendor accounts payable: payment notices from lenders are compared with the accounting records, due dates are monitored, interest payments are set up for payment on due dates, and accruals for unpaid interest are made on financial reporting dates. If the company has only a few debt instruments outstanding, no subsidiary records of these are needed. All the information is in the general ledger accounts. (Companies with a large number of bonds, loans, and notes may keep control and subsidiary accounts, as is done for accounts receivable.) As all or some of the notes become due, the CFO and the controller have the necessary information to properly classify current and long-term amounts.

The functions of authorization, custody, and reconciliation for another class of credit balances, calculated liabilities and credits, are not easy to describe. These include lease obligations, future income taxes, pension and post-retirement benefit liabilities, and foreign currency translation gains and losses. They are accounting creations, calculated according to accounting rules and using basic data from company plans and operations, and management usually enjoys considerable discretion in structuring them. These accounting calculations often involve significant accounting estimates by management. Auditors should consider whether company accountants have been realistic in these calculated liabilities and are following generally accepted accounting principles (GAAP), paying careful attention to how these estimates may affect decisions of financial statement users.

---

off the balance sheet:
refers to how certain obligations and commitments do not have to be reported on the balance sheet, such as purchase commitments and operating leases

debt instruments:
legally documented obligations between a borrower and a lender, such as bonds payable, leases, or mortgages payable

Periodic Reconciliation

The share certificate book should be periodically inspected to ensure that only certificates in the possession of actual owners are outstanding. If necessary, company officials can confirm this with the holders of record. Reports with similar information can be obtained from registrars and transfer agents to verify that the numbers of outstanding shares agree. (Without this reconciliation, counterfeit shares handled by the transfer agent and recorded by the registrar might go unnoticed.)

A trustee with duties and responsibilities similar to those of registrars and transfer agents can handle ownership of bonds. Confirmations and reports from bond trustees can be reconciled to the company's records.

Investments and Intangibles

A company may have many or only a few investments, and these may include a large variety or a limited set of investment types. Intangible assets may be in the form of purchased assets (e.g., patents, trademarks) or accounting allocations (e.g., goodwill, deferred costs). A manufacturing or service company is the context for the sections following, and investments and intangibles may be fairly incidental in these businesses. Financial institutions (banks, trust companies), investment companies, mutual funds, insurance companies, and the like have more elaborate systems for managing their investments and intangibles.

An important type of investment is the financial instrument, which IFRS 9 defines as "any contract that gives rise to a financial asset of one entity and a financial liability or equity instrument of another entity." The definition encompasses a wide range of financial instruments, from simple loans and deposits to complex derivatives, structured products, and some commodity contracts. Financial instruments can vary greatly in terms of their complexity, due to the high volume of individual cash flows and complex formulas for determining cash flows that arise from the uncertainty or variability of future cash flows. The main reason for using financial instruments is to reduce exposures to business risks, for example, changes in exchange rates, interest rates, and commodity prices, or a combination of these risks. On the other hand, the inherent complexities of some financial instruments may also result in increased risk. Thus, the extent of an entity's use of financial instruments and the degree of complexity of the instruments are important determinants of the necessary level of sophistication of the entity's internal control. For example, smaller entities may use less structured products and simple processes and procedures to achieve their objectives.

Authorization

All investment policies and major individual investment transactions should be approved by the board of directors, executive committee, or its investment committee. However, there is a great deal of variety between companies in the nature and amount of transactions that must have specific high-level approval. Often, it is the role of those charged with governance to set the tone regarding and approve and oversee the extent of use of

The Little Lease that Could

The Quick-Fly commuter airline was struggling. According to its existing debt covenants, it could not incur any more long-term liabilities. The company needed a new airplane to expand its services, so it "rented" one. The CFO pointed out that the deal for the $12 million airplane was a non-cancellable operating lease because (1) Quick-Fly does not automatically own the plane at the end of the lease; (2) the purchase option of $1,500,000 is no bargain; (3) the lease term of 133 months is 74%, not 75%, of the plane's estimated 15-year economic life; and (4) the present value of the lease payments of $154,330 per month, discounted at the company's latest borrowing rate of 14%, is $10.4 million, which is less than the 90% of fair value (0.90 × $12 million = $10.8 million) criterion in paragraph 3065.06 of the *CPA Canada Handbook*.

The CFO did not record a long-term lease obligation (liability). Do you agree with this accounting conclusion?

financial instruments, while it is management's role to manage and monitor the entity's exposures to those risks. The board of directors is always closely involved in major acquisitions, mergers, and share buyback plans.

Custody

Custody of investments and other intangible assets varies. Some investments, such as shares and bonds, are represented by actual negotiable certificates that may be kept in a brokerage account in a "house name" (the brokerage company). In that case, custody rests with the company official who is authorized to order the buy, sell, and delivery transactions. The certificates may also be in the possession of the owner (client company), in which case they should be in a safe or a bank safety deposit box. Only high-ranking officers (e.g., CFO, CEO, president, chair of the board) should have combinations and keys.

Other kinds of investments, such as joint ventures and partnerships, do not have formal negotiable certificates, and custody may instead take the form of management responsibility. The venture and partnership agreements that are evidence of these investments are usually merely filed with other important documents, as they are not readily negotiable. Management's supervision and monitoring of the operations are the true custody.

Authorization: Here Today, Gone Tomorrow

The treasurer of Travum County had many responsibilities as CFO. She invested several million dollars of county funds with a California-based investment money manager. Soon thereafter, news stories of the money manager's expensive personal lifestyle and questionable handling of clients' funds began to circulate, indicating that clients could lose much of their investments. At the same time, news stories about the treasurer's own credit card spending habits were published locally, indicating that she had obtained a personal credit card by using the county's name.

Although no county funds were lost and no improper credit card bills were paid, the county commissioners temporarily suspended the treasurer's authority to choose investment vehicles for county funds.

Having custody of most intangibles works in theory but is messy in practice. There are legal documents and contracts for financial instrument transactions, patents, trademarks, copyrights, and similar legal intangibles. These are seldom negotiable and are usually kept in ordinary company files. Company managers may be assigned responsibility to protect exclusive rights granted by various intangibles. Accounts like goodwill, deferred charges, and pension obligations are intangibles created by accountants' estimates and calculations. They have no physical substance, but they are "in the custody" of the accountants who calculate them.

Recordkeeping

Purchases of share and bond investments require authorization by the board of directors or other responsible officials. Because a higher level of approval is required for these, the cheque for the investment is signed by a higher-ranking finance officer, such as the CFO or treasurer. If the company has few investments, no subsidiary records are maintained and all information is kept in the general ledger accounts. If the company has many investments, a control account and subsidiary ledger may be maintained.

The recordkeeping for the maintenance of some investment and intangible accounts over time can be complicated. This is the place where complex accounting standards for equity method accounting, consolidations, goodwill, intangibles amortization and valuation, deferred costs, future income taxes, pension and post-retirement benefit liabilities, and various financial instruments enter the picture. High-level accountants who prepare financial statements get involved with the accounting rules and management estimates required. The accounting for these balances is influenced by management plans and estimates of future events and interpretations of the accounting standards. These decisions are risk areas for overstatement of assets, understatement of liabilities, and understatement of expenses because managers can exercise considerable discretion and auditors seldom have hard evidence confirming or refuting these management assessments.

Periodic Reconciliation

Inspection and count of negotiable securities certificates is the most significant reconciliation opportunity in the investments and intangibles accounts. Certificates on hand are inventoried, inspected, and compared with the information recorded in the accounts. (Written confirmations are requested for securities held by brokerage firms.)

A securities "inventory count" should include a record of the name of the company represented by the certificate, the interest rate for bonds, the dividend rate for preferred shares, the due date for bonds, the serial numbers on the certificates, the face value of bonds, the number or face amount of bonds and shares, and notes on the name of the owner shown on the face of the certificate or on the endorsements on the back (should be the client company). This reconciliation should happen reasonably often and not wait until the independent auditors' annual visit. A securities count in a financial institution holding thousands of shares in multimillion-dollar asset accounts is a major undertaking.

The auditors should record the same information in the audit working papers when performing the securities inspection and count. If a security certificate has been pledged as collateral for a loan and is in the hands of a creditor, it can be confirmed or inspected only through a visit to the creditor. The fact that it has been pledged as collateral may be an important disclosure note. Securities counts and reconciliations are important because companies do sometimes try to substitute others' securities for missing ones. If securities have been sold and replaced without any accounting entries, the serial numbers will show that the certificates recorded in the accounts are not the same as the ones on hand.

Review Checkpoints

14-2 When management carefully crafts a lease agreement to barely fail the tests for lease capitalization and liability recognition, should the auditor insist on capitalization anyway?

14-3 What would constitute the authorization for loans payable? What documentation is evidence of this authorization?

14-4 Give five examples of off-balance-sheet information. Why should auditors be concerned with such items?

14-5 What features of a client's share capital are important in the audit?

14-6 What information about share capital could be confirmed with outside parties? How could auditors corroborate this information?

14-7 How can auditors verify the names of the issuers, number of shares held, certificate numbers, maturity value, and interest and dividend rates in an audit of investment securities?

14-8 Describe the procedures and documentation of a controlled count of a client's investment securities.

14-9 What information should be included in a working paper for the audit of investment securities?

Control Risk Assessment

LO2 List control tests for auditing control over debt, owners' equity, and investment transactions.

In the finance and investment process, auditors inquire about and look for control procedures, such as authorization, custody, recordkeeping, and periodic reconciliation. They especially look for information about the level of management involved in these functions. Samples of transactions are not normally part of the control risk assessment work, as they can be in the other operations processes covered in Chapters 11–13. Because finance and investment transactions are usually individually material, each transaction is audited in detail. The extent of substantive audit work on finance and investment cycle accounts is not reduced by relying on controls, but lack of controls can mean significant amounts of extended procedures because the risk of material misstatement from improper financing and investing transactions is high.

General Control Considerations

There should be control procedures for handling of responsibilities. Policies on this will vary greatly between companies, but the discussion related to Exhibit 14–1 indicates that these responsibilities are basically in the hands of senior management officials.

Segregation of incompatible duties does not really apply in the financing and investing functions. It is hard to have a strict segregation of functional responsibilities when the same principal officers authorize, execute, and control finance and investment activities. It is not realistic for a CEO to authorize investments but not have access to shareholder records, securities certificates, and the like. Real segregation of duties is found in middle management and lower ranks but is hard to create and enforce in upper-level management. A company should have compensating control procedures in place.

One compensating control could be involvement of two or more people in each important functional responsibility. Or, alternatively, oversight or review can be substituted. For example, if the board of directors authorized the purchase of securities or creation of a partnership, the CFO or the CEO could carry out the transactions, have custody of certificates and agreements, manage the partnership or the portfolio of securities, oversee the recordkeeping, and make the decisions about valuations and accounting (authorizing the journal entries). These are rather normal management activities, and they combine several responsibilities. The compensating control could be periodic reports to the board of directors, oversight by the investment committee of the board, and a periodic reconciliation of securities certificates in a portfolio with the amounts and descriptions recorded in the accounts by internal auditors. The external auditors' review of the minutes of board of directors meetings described in Chapter 16 is a particularly important procedure for this process.

Control over Accounting Estimates

An accounting estimate amount shows the approximate effect of past business transactions or events on the present status of an asset or liability. Accounting estimates are common in financial statement reporting. Examples are allowance for doubtful receivables, loss provisions, and valuation of stock options using a mathematical model. Accounting estimates can have a significant or pervasive effect on reported results, either individually or when considered in the aggregate.[3] They are included in basic financial statements because (1) the measurement of some values is uncertain, usually depending upon the outcome of future events, or (2) relevant data cannot be accumulated on a timely, cost-effective basis. Some examples of accounting estimates in the finance and investment process are shown in the following box.

Finance and Investment Process Estimates

Financial instruments: valuation of securities, classification into trading versus investment portfolios, probability of a correlated hedge, sales of securities with puts and calls

Accruals: compensation in stock option plans, actuarial assumptions in pension costs

Leases: initial direct costs, executory costs, residual values, capitalization interest rate

Rates: imputed interest rates on receivables and payables

Other: losses and net realizable value on segment disposal and business restructuring, fair values in non-monetary exchanges

Management is responsible for making estimates and should have a process and control structure designed to reduce the likelihood of their material misstatement. The following are some items that this control structure should involve:

- Management communication of the need for proper accounting estimates
- Accumulation of relevant, sufficient, and reliable data for estimates
- Preparation of estimates by qualified personnel
- Adequate review and approval by appropriate levels of authority
- Comparison of estimates with subsequent results to assess the reliability of the estimation
- Assessment by management of the consistency between accounting estimates and company operational plans

Auditors' test of controls of estimation procedures involve inquiries about the process. They might ask who prepares estimates, when they are prepared, what data are used, who reviews and approves the estimates, and if the estimates are being compared with subsequent actual events. Auditors will also study data documentation, comparisons of prior estimates with subsequent actual experience, and intercompany correspondence concerning estimates and operational plans. Much of the audit test of controls of estimates has a bearing on the substantive quality of the estimation process and on the estimate itself. Further substantive audit procedures include recalculating the mathematical estimate; developing an auditor's own independent estimate based on reasonable alternative assumptions; and comparing the estimate to subsequent events, to the extent they are known before the end of the field work.

CAS 540 adopts a risk-based approach to the audit of accounting estimates, including fair value accounting estimates. It addresses matters such as the auditor's evaluation of the effect of estimation uncertainty on risk assessments, management's estimation methods, the reasonableness of management assumptions, and the adequacy of disclosures. CAS 540 defines an accounting estimate as an approximation of a monetary amount in the absence of a precise means of measurement. Estimation uncertainty is the likelihood that the accounting estimates and related disclosures are not accurate.

Accounting estimates will have relatively high estimation uncertainty when they are based on significant assumptions and subjective judgment. Examples are fair value accounting estimates for derivative financial instruments not publicly traded and fair value accounting estimates based on a highly specialized client-developed model, or for which there are assumptions or inputs that cannot be observed in the marketplace. When accounting estimates give rise to significant risks, the auditor should also evaluate how adequately the estimation uncertainty is disclosed in the financial statements. In some cases, the estimation uncertainty may be so great that the recognition criteria in the applicable financial reporting framework are not met and the accounting estimate cannot be made. In such situations, critical thinking involving integration of accounting and auditing theories is used to come up with appropriate reporting solutions. Conceivably, such reporting situations may also present new opportunities for management fraud. The earlier "Madoff Economy" box illustrates the extent to which estimation uncertainties have spread to the financial services sector. The importance of estimation uncertainties has grown enormously in financial reporting over the past few decades. For this reason, Chapter 19 (available on Connect) discusses in more detail the audit issues associated with increased estimation uncertainties in financial reporting.

Control Risk Assessment for Notes and Loans Payable

From the preceding discussion, you can tell that test of controls audit procedures take a variety of forms—inquiries, observations, study of documentation, comparison with related data (such as tax returns), and detailed audit of some transactions. The detailed audit of transactions, however, is a small part of the test of controls because finance and investment transactions are generally small in number, while their amounts are large. However, some companies have numerous debt financing transactions, and in such cases a more detailed control risk assessment can be done that includes selecting a sample of transactions for control risk assessment evidence.

An internal control questionnaire for notes and loans payable is found in Exhibit 14–2. It illustrates typical questions about the control objectives. These inquiries give auditors insights into the review and approval procedures for major financing transactions, the accounting system for them, and the error-checking review procedures.

Internal Control Questionnaire: Notes and Loans Payable Application

Environment and General Controls Relevant to This Application

1. Are records kept by someone who cannot sign notes or cheques?

Application Control Assessment

Validity objective:

2. Are paid notes cancelled and stamped "paid" and filed?

Completeness objective:

3. Is all borrowing authorization by the directors checked to determine whether all notes payable are recorded?

Authorization objective:

4. Are direct borrowings on notes payable authorized by the directors, the treasurer, or the CFO?

5. Are two or more authorized signatures required on notes?

Accuracy objective:

6. Are bank due notices compared with records of unpaid liabilities?

Classification objective:

7. Is sufficient information available in the accounts to enable financial statement preparers to classify current and long-term debt properly?

Accounting objective:

8. Is the subsidiary ledger of notes payable periodically reconciled with the general ledger control account(s)?

Proper period objective:

9. Are interest payments and accruals monitored for due dates and financial statement dates?

Auditors can select a sample of notes payable transactions for detail test of controls, provided that the population of notes is large enough to justify it. Exhibit 14–3 lists a selection of these procedures, with the relevant control objectives noted on the right.

Control Risk Assessment for Derivatives and Related Financial Instruments

Derivative financial instruments can have a significant impact on audit procedures because they are complex and common. Accounting standards also require that these instruments be accounted for at fair value and that other information about them be in financial statement notes.

Control Tests for Notes and Loans Payable

	CONTROL OBJECTIVE
1. Read directors' and finance committee's minutes for authorization of financing transactions (such as short-term notes payable, bond offerings).	Authorization
2. Select a sample of paid notes:	
(a) Recalculate interest expense for the period under audit.	Accuracy
(b) Trace interest expense to the general ledger account.	Completeness
(c) Vouch payment to cancelled cheques.	Validity
3. Select a sample of notes payable:	
(a) Vouch to authorization by directors or finance committee.	Authorization
(b) Vouch cash receipt to bank statement.	Validity

In many cases, derivative financial instruments can reduce a company's exposures to risks, such as changes in exchange rates, interest rates, and commodity prices. On the other hand, the nature of activities involving derivative financial instruments, and derivative financial instruments themselves, may also result in increased business risk in some companies. This both increases and presents new inherent risk factors for the auditor to consider in terms of the values of derivative financial instruments. Their values are volatile and large, and unexpected decreases in their fair values can result in large losses to report in the income statement. The complexity of derivative activities increases the risk that management may not fully understand how to manage them, thus exposing the company to the risk of large losses.

There are various sources of guidance in the audit of derivatives. CPA Canada's IAPN 1000 describes derivatives and the relevant accounting standards that apply as guidance for auditors of companies where derivative financial instruments are used. It sets out managements' and auditors' responsibilities and describes the risks and audit risk assessment in detail. IAPN 1000 also describes internal control considerations specific to derivatives activities, including the control environment and control systems required to meet the control objectives. The following control objectives relate specifically to derivative financial instruments:

- Transactions are executed in accordance with approved policies.
- Information, including fair value information, is recorded on a timely basis; is complete and accurate; and has been properly classified, described, and disclosed.
- Misstatements in the processing of accounting information are prevented or detected in a timely manner.
- Activities are monitored regularly to recognize and measure events affecting related financial statement assertions.
- Changes in the fair value are appropriately accounted for and disclosed to the right people from both an operational and a control viewpoint. Valuation may be a part of ongoing monitoring activities.
- Control systems for those instruments designated as hedges should assure that these meet the criteria for hedge accounting, both at their inception and regularly thereafter.

AuG-39 also deals with transaction records used for derivative financial instruments (database, register, or subsidiary ledger) and suggests the audit procedures of checking the transaction records for accuracy and independently confirming the derivative transactions with counterparties. The auditor needs to assess whether there are appropriate controls over input, processing, and maintenance of the transaction records because these will often be used to provide accounting information for disclosures in the financial statements and other risk management uses, such as exposure reports for comparison with company risk policy limits. Further detailed guidance in AuG-39 covers control testing, obtaining management representations, and communicating with those charged with governance relating to derivatives positions and trading.

Audit of derivative financial instruments is also covered in IAPN 1000 (International) and SAS No. 92 (American Institute of Certified Public Accountants [AICPA]). These list the following as key control procedures for derivatives:

- Derivatives activities are monitored by independent control staff.
- Approval (oral, at least) from members of senior management who are independent of derivatives activities is obtained by derivatives personnel prior to exceeding limits.
- Exceeding of limits and divergences from approved derivatives strategies are properly addressed by senior management.
- Accurate transmittals of derivatives positions are made to the risk measurement systems.
- Reconciliations are performed to ensure data integrity across a full range of derivatives.
- Constraints are designed and activities are monitored, identifying excesses justified by traders, risk managers, and senior management.
- Regular review of the identifying controls and financial results of the derivatives activities are performed by senior management, an independent group, or an individual that management designates, to determine

whether controls are being effectively implemented in the entity's business objectives and whether strategies are being achieved.

- Limits are reviewed in the context of changes and strategy, risk tolerance of the entity, and conditions.

Risk Factors of Derivatives

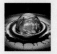

The following are examples of unique, inherent risk factors associated with derivatives:

- Many derivatives are not recognized in the financial statements. As a result, there is an increased risk that derivatives and related fees, premiums, commissions, receivables, and payables will not be captured and recorded by control systems.
- Because derivatives are financial instruments whose values are derived from underlying market rates or indexes, their values change as these rates or indexes change. Increasing volatility of interest rates, commodity prices, and foreign currency rates may cause widely fluctuating derivative values.
- Entities use derivatives (a) to manage risk (that is, to hedge) and (b) to speculate. Derivatives used for hedging purposes must be accounted for differently than those used to speculate.

Audit Considerations for Derivatives

The following are steps that the auditor might consider taking when auditing an entity involved with derivative financial instruments.

- Obtain an understanding of the nature and extent of the use of derivatives to determine whether they may have a significant effect on the audit or on the financial statements.
- Make preliminary decisions on the materiality of derivatives and the level of inherent risk during the planning stage of the audit.
- Ensure that audit staff who will be performing audit procedures on derivatives have an appropriate level of knowledge and experience.
- Consider whether it is necessary to use the work of a specialist (see "Using the work of an auditor's expert," CAS 620 of the *CPA Canada Handbook*, for guidance).
- Consider the extent to which it is appropriate to use the work of internal audit (see CAS 610, "Using the work of internal auditors").
- Obtain an understanding of the control-environment factors affecting derivative activities (see IAPN 1000 and CAS 315, Appendix 2, of the *CPA Canada Handbook* for examples).

Source: "Auditing derivative financial instruments, studies and standards alert," *CA Magazine,* January/February 1995, p. 66.

When applicable, auditors design tests of the preceding controls for derivatives to determine the extent of substantive tests needed. Key substantive procedures for derivatives include confirmations with issuers, brokers, or counterparties; physical inspection of derivatives contracts; inspection of underlying agreements and other supporting documentation in paper or electronic form; review of minutes of the board of directors' meetings; and confirmation of quoted prices from broker dealers or from derivatives exchanges. For more background on the unique risks represented by derivatives activities, see the sample letter later in the chapter, which illustrates the important substantive procedure of a confirmation request detailing outstanding derivative instruments for a client. In addition, Appendix 14A more fully discusses the risks and controls associated with derivative securities. Auditors increasingly need to be aware of these relatively new risk management practices and their effect on financial reporting.

Summary: Control Risk Assessment

The audit manager or senior accountant in charge of the audit should evaluate the evidence gathered through understanding the internal control structure and from test of controls procedures. These procedures can take many forms because management systems for finance and investment accounts vary between clients. There is always a risk that high-level company executives will not act in the best interests of the company, its owners, or

An Estimated Valuation Based on Future Development

 Gulf & Western Industries (G&W) sold 450,000 shares of Pan American stock from its investment port-folio to Resorts International (Resorts). Resorts paid $8 million plus 250,000 shares of its unregistered common stock. G&W recorded the sale proceeds as $14,167,500, valuing the unregistered Resorts shares at $6,167,500, which was approximately 67% of the market price of Resorts shares at the time ($36.82 per share). G&W reported a gain of $3,365,000 on the sale.

Four years later, Resorts shares fell to $2.63. G&W sold its 250,000 shares back to Resorts in exchange for 1,100 acres of undeveloped land on Grand Bahamas Island. For its records, Resorts got a broker-dealer's opinion that its 250,000 shares were worth $460,000. For property tax assessment purposes, the Bahamian government valued the undeveloped land at $525,000.

G&W valued the land on its books at $6,167,500, which was the previous valuation of the Resorts shares. The justification was an appraisal of $6,300,000 based on the estimated value of the 1,100 acres when ultimately developed (i.e., built into an operating resort and residential community). However, G&W also reported a loss of $5,527,000 in its tax return (effectively valuing the land at $640,500). The Securities and Exchange Commission (SEC) accused G&W of failing to report a loss of $5.7 million in its financial statements. Do you think the loss should have appeared in the G&W income statement?

Source: I. Kellog, *How to Find Negligence and Misrepresentation in Financial Statements* (New York: Shepard's/McGraw-Hill, 1983), p. 279.

its creditors. This risk can be particularly well hidden by the complexity of transactions in finance and investment activities and can result in fraudulent financial reporting. For this reason, control risk assessment must be tailored for each company's specific circumstances.

Some control considerations can be generalized. There are common features characterizing control over management's production of accounting estimates. Detail testing through samples of transactions can produce evidence about compliance with control policies and procedures as well, for instance, when there are numerous notes payable transactions.

In general, substantive audit procedures on finance and investment accounts are not limited in extent. It is very common for auditors to perform substantive audit procedures on 100% of these transactions and balances, as there are not many transactions, and the audit cost for complete coverage is not high. But control deficiencies and unusual or complicated transactions might cause auditors to adjust the nature and timing of audit procedures. Complicated financial instruments, pension plans, exotic equity securities, related party transactions, and non-monetary exchanges of investment assets call for procedures designed to find evidence of error and fraud. The next section deals with some of the finance and investment process assertions, and it has some cases for your review.

Review Checkpoints

14-10 What is a compensating control for the finance and investment process? Give some examples for finance and investment accounts.

14-11 What are some of the specific, relevant aspects of management's control over the production of accounting estimates? What are some inquiries auditors can make?

14-12 When a company has produced an estimate of an investment valuation based on a non-monetary exchange, what source of comparative information can an auditor use?

14-13 If a company does not monitor notes and loans payable for due dates and interest payment dates in relation to financial statement dates, what misstatements can appear in the financial statements?

14-14 Generally, how much emphasis is placed on adequate internal control in the audit of each of long-term debt, share capital, contributed surplus, and retained earnings?

Substantive Audit Programs for the Finance and Investment Process

Assertions, Substantive Procedures, and Audit Cases for Finance and Investment Accounts

LO3 List the typical substantive procedures used to respond to the assessed risk of material misstatement in the main account balance, and in transactions in the finance and investment process.

Exhibit 14–4 gives an illustrative audit program for owners' equity.

Audit Program for Owners' Equity

1. Obtain an analysis of owners' equity transactions. Trace additions and reductions to the general ledger.
   (a) Vouch additions to directors' minutes and cash receipts.
   (b) Vouch reductions to directors' minutes and other supporting documents.

2. Read the directors' minutes for owners' equity authorization. Trace to entries in the accounts. Determine whether related disclosures are adequate.

3. Confirm outstanding common and preferred shares with share registrar agent.

4. Vouch stock option and profit-sharing plan disclosures to contracts and plan documents.

5. Vouch treasury stock transactions to cash receipts and cash disbursement records and to directors' authorization. Inspect treasury stock certificates.

6. When the company keeps its own share records, perform the following:
   (a) Inspect the share record stubs for certificate numbers and number of shares.
   (b) Inspect the unissued certificates.
   (c) Obtain written client representations about the number of shares issued and outstanding.

As discussed above, the main control over financial reporting of the auditee's finance and investment activities comes from the highest level of management and those charged with governance. Also, there often are a few quite sizable transactions and balances in the financing and investing process. Consequently, auditors tend to seek out reliable substantive evidence for any transactions, supplementing the important management representations they obtain regarding these accounts. The long-term debt and shareholders' equity balances in this part of the balance sheet mainly report the financial position of the equity- and debtholders of the firm. Since these are the main users of the entity's financial statements, it is important that this information be perfectly accurate, and that fully informative disclosures of the details of the investors' and creditors' positions regarding the company are provided. For example, there should be a recalculation of interest expense by the auditor as evidence that the liabilities and expenses are accurately recorded.

Exhibits 14–5 and 14–6 provide examples of working papers for substantive audit programs that would be used in a typical company for the account balances, transactions, and disclosures in the finance and investment process. These include the owners' equity accounts; loans and long-term debts payable; and investments of various types, such as short-term holdings of debt or shares, investments in other companies for significant influence, and investments in controlled subsidiaries. After the working papers, there is a discussion of the audit logic behind each program.

EXHIBIT 14–5

Example of Substantive Audit Program for Owners' Equity Account Responding to Assessed Risk of Material Misstatement: Selected Substantive Procedures

SUBSTANTIVE AUDIT PROGRAM		
AUDITEE *ECOPAK INC.*		**FILE INDEX:** *UU-100*
FINANCIAL STATEMENT PERIOD: *y/e DECEMBER 31, 20X1*		
ACCOUNT: *Owners' Equity*		

Substantive audit program in response to assessed risks at the assertion level:				
Consider risk assessment findings and conclusion on residual risk of material misstatement to be reduced by performing substantive procedures. (Of the procedures listed below, perform those considered necessary to provide sufficient appropriate evidence to address the assessed risks and reduce risk of material misstatement to an acceptable level.)				*[Reference to relevant working papers]*
Substantive audit procedures	Assertions evidence is related to [E, C, O, V, P*]	Timing	Extent	Working paper reference
1. Obtain an analysis of owners' equity transactions. Trace additions and reductions to the general ledger. (a) Vouch additions to directors' minutes and cash receipts. (b) Vouch reductions to directors' minutes and other supporting documents.	E, C, V			
2. Read the directors' minutes for owners' equity authorization. Trace to entries in the accounts. Determine whether related disclosures are adequate.	E, C, O, P			
3. Confirm outstanding common and preferred shares with share registrar agent.	E, C, O			
4. Vouch stock option and profit-sharing plan disclosures to contracts and plan documents.	P			
5. Vouch treasury stock transactions to cash receipts and cash disbursement records and to directors' authorization. Inspect treasury stock certificates.	P			
6. When the company keeps its own share records: (a) Inspect the share record stubs for certificate numbers and number of shares. (b) Inspect the unissued certificates. (c) Obtain written client representations about the number of shares issued and outstanding.	E, C, O, V			

AUDITOR'S CONCLUSIONS:
Based on my professional judgment, the evidence obtained is sufficient and appropriate to conclude that the risk of material misstatement of the <u>OWNERS' EQUITY</u> *is acceptably low.*

Prepared by _____   Date _____
Prepared by _____   Date _____

* E, C, O, V, P = existence, completeness, ownership, valuation, presentation.

EXHIBIT 14–6

Example of Substantive Audit Program for Notes and Loans Payable and Long-Term Debt Account Responding to Assessed Risk of Material Misstatement: Selected Substantive Procedures

SUBSTANTIVE AUDIT PROGRAM					
AUDITEE *ECOPAK INC.*				FILE INDEX: *KK-100*	
FINANCIAL STATEMENT PERIOD: *y/e DECEMBER 31, 20X1*					
ACCOUNT *Notes and Loans Payable and Long-Term Debt*					

Substantive audit program in response to assessed risks at the assertion level:

Consider risk assessment findings and conclusion on residual risk of material misstatement to be reduced by performing substantive procedures. (Of the procedures listed below, perform those considered necessary to provide sufficient appropriate evidence to address the assessed risks and reduce risk of material misstatement to an acceptable level.)				*[Reference to relevant working papers]*
Substantive audit procedures	Assertions evidence is related to [E, C, O, V, P*]	Timing	Extent	Working paper reference
1. Obtain a schedule of notes payable and other long-term debt (including capitalized lease obligations) showing beginning balances, new notes, repayments, and ending balances. Trace to general ledger accounts.	E, C, V			
2. Confirm liabilities with creditor: amount, interest rate, due date, collateral, and other terms. Some of these confirmations may be standard bank confirmations.	E, C, O, V, P			
3. Review the standard bank confirmation for evidence of assets pledged as collateral and for unrecorded obligations.	C, P			
4. Read loan agreements for terms and conditions that need to be disclosed and for pledge of assets as collateral.	C, V, P			
5. Recalculate the current portion of long-term debt and trace to the trial balance, classified as a current liability.	V, P			
6. Study lease agreements for indications of need to capitalize leases. Recalculate the capital and operating lease amounts for required disclosures.	E, C, O, V, P			
7. Recalculate interest expense on debts and trace to the interest expense and accrued interest accounts.	E, C, O, V, P			
8. Obtain written representations from management concerning notes payable, collateral agreements, and restrictive covenants.	C, P			

AUDITOR'S CONCLUSIONS:
Based on my professional judgment, the evidence obtained is sufficient and appropriate to conclude that the risk of material misstatement of the NOTES AND LOANS PAYABLE AND LONG-TERM DEBT *is acceptably low.*

Prepared by _____   Date _____
Prepared by _____   Date _____

* E, C, O, V, P = existence, completeness, ownership, valuation, presentation.

Substantive Audit Programs—Exhibits of Working Papers

Owners' Equity

Management makes assertions about the existence, completeness, rights and obligations, valuation and presentation, and disclosure of owners' equity. Typical specific assertions include the following:

1. The number of shares shown as issued is, in fact, issued.

2. No other shares (including options, warrants, and the like) have been issued and not recorded or reflected in the accounts and disclosures.

3. The accounting is proper for options, warrants, and other share issue plans, and related disclosures are adequate.

4. The valuation of shares issued for non-cash consideration is proper, in conformity with accounting principles.

5. All owners' equity transactions have been authorized by the board of directors.

An illustrative program of substantive audit procedures for owners' equity can be found in Exhibit 14–4, above. Some key substantive procedures are discussed below.

Inspection of Documentation   Owners' equity transactions are usually well documented in board of directors meeting minutes, proxy statements, and securities offering registration statements. Transactions can be vouched to these documents, and the cash proceeds can be traced to the bank accounts.

Confirmation   Share capital may be subject to confirmation when independent registrars and transfer agents are employed. Agents are responsible for knowing the number of shares authorized and issued and for keeping lists of shareholders' names. The basic information about share capital—such as number of shares, classes of shares, preferred dividend rates, conversion terms, dividend payments, shares held in the company name, expiration dates and terms of warrants, and share dividends and splits—can be confirmed with them. Auditors corroborate many of these things by inspection and reading of share certificates, charter authorizations, directors' minutes, and registration statements. However, when there are no independent agents, most audit evidence is gathered by vouching share record documents (such as certificate book stubs). When circumstances call for extended procedures, information on outstanding shares is confirmed directly with the holders.

Long-Term Liabilities and Related Accounts

Exhibit 14–6 shows an example of a substantive program for long-term liabilities. The primary audit concern with the verification of long-term liabilities is that all liabilities are recorded and that the interest expense is properly paid or accrued. This makes the completeness assertion paramount. During procedures in all areas, auditors are alert to the possibility of unrecorded liabilities. For example, when fixed assets are acquired during the year under audit, auditors should inquire about the source of funds for financing the new asset.

Management makes assertions about existence, completeness, rights and obligations, valuation and presentation, and disclosure. Typical specific assertions relating to long-term liabilities are as follows:

1. All material long-term liabilities are recorded.

2. Liabilities are properly classified according to their current or long-term status. The current portion of long-term debt is properly valued and classified.

3. New long-term liabilities and debt extinguishments are properly authorized.

4. Terms, conditions, and restrictions relating to non-current debt are adequately disclosed.

5. Disclosures of maturities for the next five years and the capital and operating lease disclosures are accurate and adequate.

6. All important contingencies are either accrued in the accounts or disclosed in footnotes.
    Exhibit 14–7 illustrates some substantive audit procedures for notes and loans payable and for long-term debt. Below are some key audit procedures.

EXHIBIT 14–7

Audit Program for Notes and Loans Payable and Long-Term Debt

1. Obtain a schedule of notes payable and other long-term debt (including capitalized lease obligations) showing beginning balances, new notes, repayments, and ending balances. Trace to general ledger accounts.

2. Confirm liabilities with creditor: amount, interest rate, due date, collateral, and other terms. Some of these confirmations may be standard bank confirmations.

3. Review the standard bank confirmation for evidence of assets pledged as collateral and for unrecorded obligations.

4. Read loan agreements for terms and conditions that need to be disclosed and for pledge of assets as collateral.

5. Recalculate the current portion of long-term debt and trace to the trial balance, classified as a current liability.

6. Study lease agreements for indications of need to capitalize leases. Recalculate the capital and operating lease amounts for required disclosures.

7. Recalculate interest expense on debts and trace to the interest expense and accrued interest accounts.

8. Obtain written representations from management concerning notes payable, collateral agreements, and restrictive covenants.

Confirmation When auditing long-term liabilities, auditors usually obtain independent written confirmations for notes, loans, and bonds payable. In the case of loans payable to banks, the standard bank confirmation may be used. The amount and terms of bonds payable, mortgages payable, and other formal debt instruments can be confirmed by requests to holders or a trustee. The confirmation request should include questions not only about amount, interest rate, and due date but also about collateral, restrictive covenants, and other items of agreement between lender and borrower. Confirmation requests should be sent to lenders the company has done business with in the recent past, even if no liability balance is shown at the confirmation date. This is part of the search for unrecorded liabilities. (Chapter 12 has more on this search.)

Many of the auditor's procedures for financial instruments can be used to address a number of assertions. For example, procedures to address the existence of an account balance at period-end will also address the occurrence of a class of transactions, and may also assist in establishing proper cutoff. This is because financial instruments arise from legal contracts and, by verifying the accuracy of the recording of the transaction, the auditor can also verify its existence, obtain evidence to support the occurrence and rights and obligations assertions, and confirm that transactions are recorded in the correct accounting period.

For financial instruments, there should be external confirmation of trades, bank accounts, and custodian payments. This can be done by direct confirmation with the counterparty (including the use of bank confirmations), where a reply is sent directly to the auditor. Alternatively, this information may be obtained from the counterparty's systems through a data feed. Where this is done, controls to prevent tampering with the computer systems through which the information is transmitted may be considered by the auditor in evaluating the reliability of the evidence from the confirmation. If confirmations are not received, the auditor may be able to obtain evidence by reviewing contracts and testing relevant controls. External confirmations, however, often do not provide adequate audit evidence with respect to the valuation assertion, though they may assist in identifying any side agreements (IAPN 1000).

Off-Balance-Sheet Financing

Confirmation and inquiry procedures are used to obtain responses on a class of items loosely termed *off-balance-sheet information*. These items include terms of loan agreements, leases, endorsements, guarantees, and insurance policies (whether issued by a client insurance company or owned by the client). Among these items is the difficult-to-define set of "commitments and contingencies" that often poses evidence-gathering problems. Some common types of commitments are shown in Exhibit 14–8.

EXHIBIT 14-8

Off-Balance-Sheet Commitments

TYPE OF COMMITMENT	TYPICAL PROCEDURES AND SOURCES OF EVIDENCE	ASSERTION
1. Repurchase or remarketing agreements	1. Vouching of contracts, confirmation by customer, inquiry of client management	1. Existence
2. Commitments to purchase at fixed prices	2. Vouching of open purchase orders, inquiry of purchasing personnel, confirmation by supplier	2. Existence/ occurrence
3. Commitments to sell at fixed prices	3. Vouching of sales contracts, inquiry of sales personnel, confirmation by customer	3. Existence/valuation
4. Loan commitments	4. Vouching of open commitment file, inquiry of loan officers	4. Existence/valuation
5. Lease commitments	5. Vouching of lease agreement, confirmation with lessor or lessee	5. Existence/valuation/ ownership

Footnote disclosure should be considered for the types of commitments shown in this exhibit. Some of them can be estimated and valued, allowing them to be recorded in the accounts and shown in the financial statements themselves (e.g., fixed price purchase commitments and losses on fixed price sales commitments).

Analytical relationships are used to help verify interest expense, which is generally related item by item to interest-bearing liabilities. Interest expense amounts can be recalculated for long-term liability transactions (including those that have been retired during the year). The amount of debt, the interest rate, and the time period are used to determine whether the interest expense and accrued interest are properly recorded. The audit results are compared with the recorded interest expense and accrued interest accounts to detect (1) greater expense than audit calculations show, indicating some interest paid on an unknown debt, possibly an unrecorded liability; (2) lesser expense than audit calculations show, indicating misclassification, failure to accrue interest, or an interest payment default; or (3) interest expense equal to audit calculations. The first two possibilities raise questions for further study, while the third shows a correct correlation between debt and debt-related expense.

A current controversy involving use of off-balance-sheet debt concerns the litigation against the bankrupt Lehman Brothers investment bank (whose failure was the catalyst for the 2008 financial crisis) and its auditors. The basic fact issues of this case are outlined in the box below. The box illustrates the huge (and potentially misleading) financial statement impact that off-balance-sheet accounting rules can have. The rules have since been modified, indicating that there should be better, broader principles underlying the detailed rules. The Lehman case is further explored in Discussion Case DC 14-10 at the end of this chapter.

Lehman Brothers: Causes of Bankruptcy

Prior to its collapse in 2008, Lehman Brothers employed a typical investment banking strategy of a high-risk, high-leverage model. Lehman's balance sheet at the time showed approximately $700 billion in longer-term assets, with only $25 billion in short-term liabilities. In order to stay afloat, Lehman was borrowing hundreds of millions of dollars per day. Investor confidence is key to the success of this strategy.

At the same time, since 2007 Lehman had also been heavily invested in the subprime real estate market, thinking that they could "buy low and sell high."

However, when Bear Sterns collapsed in March of 2008, investor confidence began to erode. Lehman incurred a $2.8 billion loss in the second quarter of 2008 due to large asset write-downs. In the face of the changing financial climate, Lehman attempted to show a positive liquidity position despite its decreasing profitability. Lehman claimed to have significantly reduced its net leverage ratio to below 12.5. How? By engaging in the accounting policy of "REPO 105."

(continued)

An ordinary repurchase (REPO) transaction is designed to facilitate short-term financing over the span of a few days. In 2007, there was $12 trillion worth of these loans in the market at any given time. Shown below is this transaction, whose goal is to reduce leverage (debt) on the balance sheet.

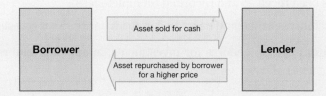

Under IAS 39/FASB No. 125, the accounting treatment for REPO is as follows:

- Balance Sheet—The asset stays on the books of the borrower as this is *not* a sale. A corresponding liability is created.
- Income Statement—The spread ("repo interest") is treated as payment of interest.

Lehman engaged in REPO deals just before quarter-end, at which time they ensured that the fair market value of the asset was 105% greater than the amount of cash received. This allowed Lehman to recognize the transactions as a sale rather than as a liability, despite the fact that they bought the asset back within 7–10 days. Using the REPO 105 loophole allowed Lehman to record the transactions as shown on the right, rather than as a conventional REPO transaction, at left.

Regular REPO	REPO 105
Journal Entry	Journal Entry
Dr. Cash	Dr. Cash
Cr. Liability	Cr. Sales

The impact on Lehman's financial statements was that tens of billions of dollars was borrowed without recording a liability. Cash from these transactions was used to pay down other liabilities, which in turn reduced the total liabilities, total assets, and leveraging ratios. Lehman then borrowed from other sources to pay back this debt after quarter-end. Through this process, Lehman was able to hide $50 billion of liabilities from investors, reducing its leverage ratio by 13% (from 13.9 to 12.1) in the second quarter of 2008.

Deferred Credits: Calculated Balances

Existence and valuation of several types of deferred credits are calculated. Examples are (1) deferred profit on instalment sales involving the gross margin and the sale amount; (2) future income taxes and investment credits involving tax book timing differences, tax rates, and amortization methods; and (3) deferred contract revenue involving contract provisions for prepayment, percentage-of-completion revenue recognition methods, or other terms unique to a contract. Auditors can check the calculations for accuracy.

Investments and Intangibles

A company might have a wide variety of investments and relationships with affiliates. Investment accounting for these may be by the cost or equity method, either without consolidation or with full consolidation, depending on the size and influence represented by the investment. Purchase method consolidations usually create problems of accounting for the fair value of acquired assets and the related goodwill. Specific assertions are typical of a variety of investment account balances:

1. Investment securities are on hand or are held in safekeeping by a trustee (existence).
2. Investment cost does not exceed market value (valuation).
3. Significant-influence investments are accounted for by the equity method (valuation).
4. Purchased goodwill is properly valued (valuation).

5. Capitalized intangible costs relate to intangibles acquired in exchange transactions (valuation).

6. Research and development costs are properly classified (presentation).

7. Amortization is properly calculated (valuation).

8. Investment income has been received and recorded (completeness).

9. Investments are adequately classified and described in the balance sheet (presentation).

A program of substantive audit procedures for investments, intangibles, and related accounts is shown in Exhibit 14–9.

EXHIBIT 14–9

Example of Substantive Audit Program for Investments and Related Accounts Responding to Assessed Risk of Material Misstatement: Selected Substantive Procedures

SUBSTANTIVE AUDIT PROGRAM				
AUDITEE *ECOPAK INC.*				FILE INDEX: *B-100*
FINANCIAL STATEMENT PERIOD: *y/e DECEMBER 31, 20X1*				
ACCOUNT: *Investments and related accounts*				
Substantive audit program in response to assessed risks at the assertion level:				
Consider risk assessment findings and conclusion on residual risk of material misstatement to be reduced by performing substantive procedures. (Of the procedures listed below, perform those considered necessary to provide sufficient appropriate evidence to address the assessed risks and reduce risk of material misstatement to an acceptable level.)				*[Reference to relevant working papers]*
Substantive audit procedures	Assertions evidence is related to [E, C, O, V, P*]	Timing	Extent	Working paper reference
1. Obtain a schedule of all investments, including purchase and disposition information for the period. Reconcile with investment accounts in the general ledger.	E, C			
2. Inspect or confirm with a trustee or broker the name, number, identification, interest rate, and face amount (if applicable) of securities held as investments.	E, C, O, V, P			
3. Vouch the cost of recorded investments to brokers' reports, contracts, cancelled cheques, and other supporting documentation.	V			
4. Vouch recorded sales to brokers' reports and bank deposit slips, and recalculate gain or loss on disposition.	E, C, V			
5. Recalculate interest income and look up dividend income in a dividend reporting service (such as Moody's or Standard & Poor's annual dividend record).	E, C, V			
6. Obtain market values of investments, and determine whether the appropriate valuation method has been applied as required by the auditee's financial reporting framework. Determine whether any write-down or write-off is necessary. Scan transactions soon after the client's year-end to see if any investments were sold at a loss. Recalculate the unrealized gains and losses required for marketable equity securities disclosures.	V			
7. Read loan agreements and minutes of the board, and inquire of management about pledge of investments as security for loans.	P			
8. Obtain written representations from the client concerning pledge of investment assets as collateral.	P			

EXHIBIT 14-9

Example of Substantive Audit Program for Investments and Related Accounts Responding to Assessed Risk of Material Misstatement: Selected Substantive Procedures *(continued)*

9. Obtain audited financial statements of joint ventures, investee companies (equity method of accounting), subsidiary companies, and other entities in which an investment interest is held. Evaluate indications of significant controlling influence. Determine proper balance sheet classification. Determine appropriate consolidation policy in conformity with accounting principles.	E, C, O, V, P			
10. Review acquisition documents for proper calculation of purchased goodwill.	E, C, V			
11. Inquire of management about legal status of patents, leases, copyrights, and other intangibles.	E, C, V			
12. Review documentation of new patents, copyrights, leaseholds, and franchise agreements	E, C, O			
13. Vouch recorded costs of intangibles to supporting documentation and cancelled cheque(s).	V			
14. Select a sample of recorded research and development expenses. Vouch to supporting documents for evidence of proper classification.	P			
15. Recalculate amortization of copyrights, patents, and other intangibles.	E, C, V			

AUDITOR'S CONCLUSIONS

Based on my professional judgment, the evidence obtained is sufficient and appropriate to conclude that the risk of material misstatement of the <u>INVESTMENTS AND RELATED ACCOUNTS</u> *is acceptably low.*

Prepared by _____   Date _____
Prepared by _____   Date _____

* E, C, O, V, P = existence, completeness, ownership, valuation, presentation.

Unlike the current assets accounts, which typically include many small transactions, the non-current investment accounts usually consist of a few large entries. This difference has internal control and substantive audit procedure implications, and auditors will concentrate on the authorization of transactions, since each transaction is likely to be material in itself and the authorization will give significant information about the proper classification and accounting method. The controls are usually not reviewed, tested, or evaluated at an interim date but are included in year-end procedures when the transactions and their authorizations are audited. The following box shows a few of the trouble spots in audits of investments and intangibles.

Trouble Spots in Audits of Investments and Intangibles

- Valuation of investments at cost or market and classification as held-to-maturity or financial assets held for trading or available for sale
- Determination of significant-influence relationship for equity method investments
- Proper determination of goodwill in consolidations
- Capitalization and continuing valuation of intangibles
- Realistic distinctions of research, feasibility, and production milestones for capitalization of development costs
- Adequate disclosure of restrictions, pledges, or liens related to investment assets

An increasing problem area identified by regulators such as the PCAOB and the Canadian Public Accountability Board (CPAB) is the audit of accounting estimates, especially fair value estimates. Fair value accounting is used for many investments in financial instruments. A more detailed review of the problem that arises for audit of derivatives and other financial instruments is discussed in Appendix 14A.

Confirmation Written confirmation obtained from outside parties is fairly limited for investments, intangibles, and related income and expense accounts. Securities held by trustees or brokers should be confirmed, and the confirmation should request the same descriptive information the auditor looks for in the physical count (described earlier in this chapter). CPA Canada recommends that the sample letter below be used for confirming information related to derivative instruments.

Request for Statement Detailing Outstanding Derivative Instruments
[Auditee letterhead]

[Date]

[Financial institution official responsible for account]
[Financial institution name]
[Financial institution address]

Dear [financial institution official responsible for account]:

In connection with their audit of our financial statements for the year ended March 31, 20X9, our auditors, PA & Co., have requested a statement summarizing all derivative financial instruments entered into by the company and outstanding at March 11, 20X9. Derivative financial instruments include futures, foreign exchange contracts, forward rate agreements, interest rate swaps, and options contracts, or other financial instruments with similar characteristics.

In your response, please include the following information for each instrument:

1. The principal, stated, face, or other similar amount (sometimes also referred to as the notional amount) on which future payments are based
2. The date of maturity, expiration, or execution
3. Any early settlement options, including the period in which, or date at which, the options may be exercised and the exercise price or range of prices
4. Any options to convert the instrument into, or exchange it for, another financial instrument or some other asset or liability, including the period in which, or date at which, the options may be exercised, and the conversion or exchange ratio(s)
5. The amount and timing of scheduled future cash receipts or payments of the principal amount of the instrument, including instalment repayments and any sinking fund or similar requirements
6. The stated rate or amount of interest, dividend, or other periodic return on principal and the timing of payments
7. Any collateral held or pledged
8. The currency of the cash flows if these are other than Canadian funds
9. Where the instrument provides for an exchange, information noted in 1 to 8 above for the instrument to be acquired in the exchange
10. Any condition of the instrument or an associated covenant that, if contravened, would significantly alter any of the other terms

Please mail the above-noted information directly to our auditors in the enclosed addressed envelope. Should you wish to discuss any details of this confirmation request with our auditors, please contact (name of audit staff member) at staff@auditfirm.com, or 111-222-3333, or by fax at 111-222-3334.

Yours truly,

[Authorized signatory of the auditee company management]

Inquiries about Intangibles Auditors query company counsel about any lawsuits or defects relating to patents, copyrights, trademarks, or trade names as a specific request in the inquiry letter to the law firm. (Chapter 15 contains more information about this inquiry letter.)

Income from Intangibles Royalty income from patent licences received is confirmed. This income amount is usually audited by examining licence agreements and vouching the licensee's reports and related cash payment.

Inspection Investment property is inspected in the same way as the fixed assets are. The principal goal is to determine the actual existence and condition of the property. Official documents of patents, copyrights, and trademark rights can be inspected to see that they are, in fact, in the name of the client.

Documentation Vouching Investment costs should be vouched to brokers' reports, monthly statements, or other documentary evidence of cost. At the same time, the amounts of sales are traced to gain or loss accounts, and the amounts of sales prices and proceeds are vouched to the brokers' statements. Auditors should determine what method of cost-out assignment was used (i.e., FIFO, specific identification, or average cost) and whether it is consistent with prior years' transactions. The cost of real and personal property can likewise be vouched to invoices or other documents of purchase, and title documents (such as on land or buildings) may be inspected.

Market valuation of securities may be required. Depending on the financial reporting framework it uses and the nature of the items, a company may need to record financial assets and liabilities at their fair values at year-end. The auditor will need to obtain evidence of market values or recent sales of investments to verify these fair values. The most reliable data for valuation of a financial instrument is the market value in an actively traded, liquid, competitive market. A less-reliable estimate of the value of a financial instrument is to use a discounted cash flow model. Auditors must use the fair value hierarchies specified by the applicable GAAP, with level 1 of the IFRS hierarchy for fair value estimates representing the least level of estimation uncertainty and levels 2 and 3 representing increasing levels of measurement uncertainty. In CAS 540, what are referred to as *estimation uncertainties* are synonymous with what IFRS refer to as measurement uncertainties.

Models can be used when price cannot be directly observed in a market. Judgment is needed to decide if a market is inactive. Models should reflect the assumptions of market participants, including assumptions about risk. Management is expected to document its valuation policies and model used to value a particular financial instrument, including the rationale for the model(s) used, the selection of assumptions in the valuation methodology, and the entity's consideration of whether adjustments for measurement uncertainty are necessary. These aspects of dealing with estimates are considered an advanced audit topic and are covered in more detail in Chapter 19. Most entities use third-party pricing sources when valuing securities either as a primary source or as a source of corroboration for their own valuations. These third-party pricing sources generally fall into two categories:

- Pricing services, including consensus pricing services
- Brokers providing broker quotes

The reliability of this evidence depends very much on the source, and this has proved to be a major problem area in audits, according to recent CPAB reports. For example, some third-party pricing sources make more information available about their process, such as methodology, assumptions, and data at the asset level. In contrast, most brokers provide only limited information about inputs and assumptions used in developing a quote. Some third-party pricing sources have more experience in only certain types of financial instruments. A quoted price from the broker who sold the financial instrument to the entity or from one having a close relationship with the entity being audited may not be reliable. Auditors must consider the reliability of the estimates in these different situations.

Obtaining prices from multiple third-party pricing services may provide useful information about measurement uncertainty for financial instruments. A wide range of prices may indicate higher measurement uncertainty and may suggest that the financial instrument is sensitive to small changes in data and assumptions. A narrow range may suggest lower measurement uncertainty and less sensitivity to changes in data and assumptions. An auditor may feel that he or she is unable to get an understanding of the process used to generate the price, including controls over the reliability of the process, or the auditor may not have access to the model, assumptions, and other inputs used. In such cases, the auditor may decide to undertake development of a point estimate or a range to evaluate management's point estimate in responding to assessed risk. Further consideration of these issues is an advanced topic, covered in Chapter 19, which discusses the concepts and principles auditors should consider in developing and using point estimates or ranges of estimates for financial reporting.

Valuation in the areas of research and development (R&D) and deferred development costs is done by extensive vouching. Evidence should determine whether costs are properly classified as assets or as R&D expense. A sample of recorded amounts is selected, and the purchase orders, receiving reports, payroll records, authorization notices, and management reports are compared with them. Some R&D costs may resemble non-R&D costs (e.g., supplies, payroll costs), so auditors must be alert for costs that appear to relate to other operations.

External Documentation Auditors use quoted market values of securities to calculate market values. If quoted market values are not available, financial statements for investments are analyzed for evidence of basic value. If the financial statements are unaudited, the evidence indicated by them is considered to be extremely weak.

Income amounts can be verified by consulting published dividend records for dividends actually declared and paid during a period (e.g., Moody's and Standard & Poor's dividend records). Since auditors know the holding period of securities, dividend income can be calculated and compared with the amount in the account. Any difference could indicate a cutoff error, misclassification, defalcation, or failure to record a dividend receivable. Applying interest rates to bond or note investments produces a calculated interest income figure (making allowance for amortization of premium or discount, if applicable).

Equity Method Investments

When equity method accounting is used for investments, auditors need the audited financial statements of the investee company. Inability to obtain these from a closely held investee may indicate that the auditee investor does not have the significant influence over the investee company that is required for use of equity method accounting. These statements are used to recalculate the auditee's share of income to recognize in the accounts and to audit the disclosure of investees' assets, liabilities, and income disclosed in notes (a disclosure recommended when investments accounted for by the equity method are material).

Depreciation and Amortization Recalculation   Depreciation or amortization expense owes its existence to a calculation, and recalculation based on audited costs and rates is sufficient appropriate audit evidence. The term *depreciation* is commonly used when referring to amortization of tangible (fixed) assets.

The appraisals, judgments, and allocations within merger and acquisition transactions that are used to assign portions of the purchase price to tangible assets, intangible assets, liabilities, and goodwill should be reviewed. Inspection of transaction documentation is ideal, but verbal inquiries may help auditors understand the circumstances of a merger.

Questions about lawsuits challenging patents, copyrights, or trade names may indicate problem areas for further investigation. Likewise, questions about research and development successes and failures may alert the audit team to problems of valuation of intangible assets and related amortization expense. Responses to questions about licensing of patents can be used in the audit of related royalty revenue accounts.

Inquiries about Management Intentions   Inquiries should deal with the nature of investments and the reasons for holding them. Management's expressed intention that a marketable security investment be considered a long-term investment may be the only evidence for classifying it as long term and not as a current asset. That classification will affect the accounting treatment of market values and the unrealized gains and losses on investments.

Review Checkpoints

14-15   What are some of the typical assertions found in owners' equity descriptions and account balances?

14-16   How can confirmations be used in auditing shareholder capital accounts? notes payable? loans and bonds payable?

14-17   What are some of the typical assertions found in long-term liability accounts?

14-18   What procedures do auditors employ to obtain evidence of the cost of investments? investment gains and losses? investment income?

14-19   Why are auditors interested in substantial investment losses occurring early in the period following year-end?

14-20   What is the concept of "substance versus form" in relation to financing and investment transactions and balances? (Refer to the off-balance-sheet and application cases in the chapter.)

14-21   What are some of the trouble spots for auditors in the audits of investments and intangibles?

APPLICATION CASE WITH SOLUTION & ANALYSIS

Detecting Misstatements in the Finance and Investment Process

INTRODUCTION

At the point in the chapter, we present an application case that contains specific examples of tests of controls and substantive audit procedures used to gather evidence in the finance and investment process. The case situation for each audit presented parallels the framework shown in Chapter 11's application case. Each case situation provides context for the auditing decisions, rather than presenting a list of detection procedures in the abstract. If you would like to review lists of detailed procedures, a selection of control tests and detail substantive procedures for cash and accounts receivable is found in Appendix 11A.

DISCUSSION CASE

While preparing to audit the investments and financing process of one of the firm's larger clients, Jack does some research work to become more knowledgeable about the risks in these areas. He finds news stories about four audits where misstatements occurred. These cases involved improper issue of securities, misstatement of tax loss carryforwards, misuse of related party transactions to keep liabilities off the balance sheet, and an example of non-consolidation of a controlled company to conceal losses.

AUDIT 14.1 Unregistered Sale of Securities

CASE DESCRIPTION

The Bliss Solar Heating Company (Bliss) sold investment contracts to the public in the form of limited partnership interests. These "securities" sales should have been under a public registration filing with the provincial securities regulator, but they were not. Under the terms of the deal, these investors purchased solar hot water heating systems for residential and commercial use from Bliss and then entered into arrangements to lease the equipment to Nationwide Corporation, which, in turn, rented the equipment to end users. The limited partnerships were, in effect, financing conduits for obtaining investors' money to pay for Bliss's equipment. The investors' return of capital and profit depended on Nationwide's business success and ability to pay under the lease terms. The amounts involved are not known, but all the money put up by the limited partnership investors was at risk and largely not disclosed to the investors.

Audit Trail

Bliss published false and misleading financial statements, which used a non-GAAP revenue recognition method and failed to disclose cost of goods sold. Bliss overstated Nationwide's record of equipment installation and failed to disclose that Nationwide had little cash flow from end users (resulting from rent-free periods and other inducements). Bliss knew, but failed to disclose to prospective investors, that a number of previous investors had filed petitions with the federal tax court to contest Canada Revenue Agency's disallowance of the tax credits and benefits claimed in connection with their investments in Bliss's tax-sheltered equipment lease partnerships.

SOLUTION & ANALYSIS

Audit Approach

Audit Objective

The auditor's objective is to obtain evidence determining whether capital fundraising methods comply with provincial securities laws and whether financial statements and other disclosures are misleading.

Controls Relevant to the Process

Management should employ experts—lawyers, underwriters, and accountants—who can determine whether securities and investment contract sales require registration.

Audit Procedures

Tests of Controls

Auditors should learn about the business backgrounds and securities-industry expertise of the senior managers, study the authorization of the fundraising method in the minutes of the board of directors meetings, obtain and study opinions of lawyers and underwriters about the legality of the fundraising methods, and inquire about management's interaction with the provincial securities regulator in any presale clearance. (The securities regulator will give advice about the necessity for registration.)

Tests of Details of Balance

Auditors should study the offering documents and literature used in the sale of securities to determine whether financial information is being used properly. In this case, the close relationship with Nationwide and the experience of earlier partnerships give reasons for extended procedures to obtain evidence about the representations concerning Nationwide's business success (in this case, lack of success).

Audit Results

The auditors gave unqualified reports on Bliss's materially misstated financial statements. They apparently did not question the legality of the sales of the limited partnership interests as a means of raising capital, nor did they perform procedures to verify representations made concerning Bliss or Nationwide finances. Two partners in the audit firm were enjoined for violations of the securities laws. They resigned from practice before the provincial securities regulator and were ordered not to perform any assurance services for companies making filings with the securities regulator. They were later expelled from the Chartered Professional Accountants of Ontario (CPA Ontario) for failure to cooperate with the disciplinary committee in its investigation of alleged professional ethics violations.

AUDIT 14.2 Tax Loss Carryforwards

CASE DESCRIPTION

 Etna Life & Casualty Insurance Company had losses in its taxable income operations in 2001 and 2002. Confident that future taxable income would absorb the losses, the company booked and reported a future income tax asset for the tax loss carryforward. The provincial securities regulator maintained that the company understated its tax expense and overstated its assets. Utilization of the loss carryforward was not "more likely than not to be realized," as required by the then-effective *CICA Handbook*, paragraph 3465.24.

Etna forecast several more years of taxable losses (aside from its non-taxable income from tax-exempt investments) followed by years of taxable income, which would eventually offset the losses and allow the company to utilize the benefit of the losses carried forward to offset against future taxable income. The company maintained there was no reasonable doubt that the forecasts would be achieved.

At first, the carryforward tax benefit was $25 million, soon growing to over $200 million, then forecast to become an estimated $1 billion before the losses would be reversed and absorbed by the forecast future taxable income. In 2003, the first full year in which these forecasts had an impact, Etna's net income was 35% lower than it had been in 2001, instead of just 6% lower, as a result of the carryforward benefit recognized.

Audit Trail

The amounts of tax loss were clearly evident in the accounts and Etna made no attempt to hide the facts. The portfolio of taxable investments and all sources of taxable income and deductions were well known to the company accountants, management, and independent auditors.

SOLUTION & ANALYSIS

Audit Approach

Audit Objective

The auditor's objective is to obtain evidence determining whether realization of the benefits of the tax loss carryforward are "more likely than not to be realized."

Controls Relevant to the Process

The relevant control in this case concerns the assumptions and mathematics underlying the forecasts that justify recording the tax loss carryforward benefit. These forecasts are the basis for an accounting estimate of "more likely than not."

Audit Procedures

Tests of Controls

Auditors should make inquiries and determine the following. Who prepared the forecasts? When were they prepared? What data were used? Who reviewed and approved the forecast? Is there any way to test the accuracy of the forecast with actual experience?

Tests of Details of Balance

Aside from auditing the assumptions underlying the forecasts and recalculating the compilation, the test of balances amounted to careful consideration of whether the forecast, or any forecast, could meet the test required by accounting standards. The decision was a judgment of whether the test of "more likely than not to be realized" was met.

The auditors should obtain information about other situations in which recognition of tax loss carryforward benefits was allowed in financial statements. Other companies have booked and reported such benefits when gains from sales of property were realized before the financial statement was issued and when the loss was from discontinuing a business line, leaving these businesses with long profit histories.

Audit Results

The provincial securities regulator was tipped off to Etna's accounting recognition of the tax loss carryforward benefit by a story in *Financial Post* magazine, which described the accounting treatment. Etna's defence was based on the forecasts. The securities regulator countered that the forecasts did not provide assurance beyond any reasonable doubt that future taxable income would be (1) sufficient to offset the loss carryforward and (2) earned during the prescribed carryforward period, as prescribed by the *CPA Canada Handbook*. For this reason, the securities regulator concluded that the "virtually certain realization" was not established. The securities regulator won the argument. Etna revised its previously issued quarterly financial statements, and the company abandoned the attempt to report the tax benefit.

AUDIT 14.3 Off-Balance-Sheet Inventory Financing

CASE DESCRIPTION

Verity Distillery Company used the "product repurchase" ploy to convert its inventory to cash, failing to disclose the obligation to repurchase it later. Related party transactions were not disclosed. To do this, Verity's president formed Veritas Corporation, making himself and two other Verity officers the sole shareholders. The president arranged to sell $40 million of Verity's inventory of whiskey, still in the aging process, to Veritas, showing no gain or loss on the transaction. The officers negotiated a 36-month loan with a major bank to get the money Veritas needed for the purchase, pledging the inventory as collateral. Verity pledged to repurchase the inventory for $54.4 million, which amounted to the original $40 million plus 12% interest for three years.

The $40 million purchased 40% of Verity's normal inventory, and the company's cash balance was increased by 50%. While the current asset total was not changed, the inventory ratios (e.g., inventory turnover, days' sales in inventory) were materially altered. Long-term liabilities were understated by not recording the liability. The ploy was actually a secured loan with inventory pledged as collateral, but this reality was neither recorded nor disclosed. The total effect would be to keep debt off the books, avoid recording interest expense, and record inventory later at a higher cost. Subsequent sale of the whiskey at market prices would not affect the ultimate income results, but the unrecorded interest expense would be buried in the cost of goods sold. The net income in the year the "sale" was made was not changed, but the normal relationship of gross margin to sales was distorted by the zero-profit transaction.

Audit Trail

The contract of sale was in the files, specifying the name of the purchasing company, the $40 million amount, and the cash consideration. Nothing mentioned the relationship between Veritas and the officers. Nothing mentioned the repurchase obligation. However, the sale amount was unusually large.

SOLUTION & ANALYSIS
Audit Approach
Audit Objective

The auditors' objective is to obtain evidence determining whether all liabilities are recorded. Be alert to undisclosed related party transactions.

Controls Relevant to the Process

The relevant control in this case rests with the integrity and accounting knowledge of the senior officials who arranged the transaction. Authorization in the board minutes might detail the arrangements, but, if they wanted to hide it from the auditors, they would also suppress the telltale information in the board minutes.

	BEFORE TRANSACTION	RECORDED TRANSACTION	SHOULD HAVE RECORDED
Assets	$530	$530	$570
Liabilities	390	390	430
Shareholders' equity	140	140	140
Debt/equity ratio	2.79	2.79	3.07

Audit Procedures
Tests of Controls

Inquiries should be made about large and unusual financing transactions, although this may not elicit a response because the event is a sales transaction, according to Verity. Other audit work on controls in the revenues, receivables, and receipts process may turn up the large sale. Fortunately, this one stands out.

Tests of Details of Balance

Analytical procedures to compare monthly or seasonal sales will probably identify the sale as large and unusual, which should lead to an examination of the sales contract. Auditors should discuss the business purpose of the transaction with knowledgeable officials. If being this close to discovery does not bring out an admission of the loan and repurchase arrangement, the auditors should investigate further. Even if the "customer" name is not a giveaway, a quick inquiry for corporation records at the relevant provincial ministry (online in some databases) will show the names of the officers, exposing the nature of the deal. Veritas's financial statements should be requested.

Audit Results

The auditors found the related party relationship between the officers and Veritas. Confronted, the president admitted the attempt to make the cash position and the debt/equity ratio look better than it was. The financial statements were adjusted to reflect the "should have recorded" set of figures shown previously.

AUDIT 14.4 A Consolidation by Any Other Name

CASE DESCRIPTION

 Digilog Inc. formed a company named DBS International (DBSI) and controlled it but did not consolidate its financial position and results of operations in the Digilog financial statements. Digilog income was overstated, and assets and liabilities were understated.

Digilog formed DBSI to market Digilog's computer equipment but kept it separate to avoid the adverse impact of reporting expected startup losses in Digilog's financial statements. Instead of owning shares in DBSI, Digilog financed the company with loans convertible at will into 90% of DBSI's stock. (Otherwise, the share ownership was not in Digilog's name.) Since Digilog did not control DBSI (control is defined as 50% or more ownership), DBSI was not consolidated, and the initial losses were not reported in Digilog's financial statements. (See *CPA Canada Handbook*, section 1591, for the usual presumptions concerning the level of ownership leading to control.) Several hundred thousand dollars of losses in the first two years of DBSI operations were not consolidated. Ultimately, the venture became profitable and was absorbed into Digilog.

Audit Trail

DBSI's formation was not a secret. It was authorized and the incorporation papers were available. Loan documents showing the terms of Digilog's loans to DBSI were in the files.

SOLUTION & ANALYSIS
Audit Approach
Audit Objective

The auditor's objective is to obtain evidence determining whether proper accounting methods (cost, equity, and consolidation) were used for investments.

Controls Relevant to the Process

The relevant control in this case rests with the integrity and accounting knowledge of the senior officials who arranged the transaction. Proper documentation of authorization as well as financing and operating transactions between the two corporations should be in the companies' files.

Audit Procedures

Tests of Controls

Inquiries should be made about large and unusual financing transactions. Minutes of the board of directors meetings should be studied to find related authorizations. These authorizations and supporting papers signal the accounting issues and interpretations of GAAP required under the circumstances.

Tests of Details of Balance

The central issue in this case is the interpretation of accounting standards regarding required consolidation. Existence, completeness, valuation, and ownership were not problematic audit issues. Unless these are extenuating factors as per *CPA Canada Handbook*, section 1591, accounting standards require consolidation of subsidiaries over 50% owned and prohibit consolidation of subsidiaries less than 50% owned. Digilog's purpose in financing DBSI with loans instead of direct share ownership was to skirt the 50% ownership criterion, thus keeping the DBSI losses out of the Digilog consolidated financial statements. The "test of the balance" (decision of whether to require consolidation) amounted to an interpretation of the substance versus form of ownership through convertible notes instead of direct shareholding.

Audit Results

Digilog, with concurrence of its independent audit firm, adopted the narrow interpretation of ownership. Since Digilog did not "own" DBSI stock, DBSI was not "controlled," and its assets, liabilities, and results of operations were not consolidated. The regulator disagreed and acted on the position that the convertible feature of the loans and the business purpose of the DBSI formation were enough to attribute control to Digilog. The company was enjoined from activities resulting in violations of certain reporting and anti-fraud provisions of the *Provincial Securities Act* and was required to amend its financial statements for the years in question. The regulator also took action against the audit firm partner in charge of the Digilog audit.

Other Aspects of Clever Accounting and Fraud

LO4   Describe the most common fraud problems in the finance and investment process.

 Clever accounting and fraud that affect the fair presentation of material equity accounts, investments, and intangibles must be considered. Improper accounting presentations are engineered more frequently by senior officials than by middle management or those of lower ranks. Top management personnel who deal with the transactions involved in investments, long-term debt, and shareholders' equity are not subject to the kind of control that lower-level employees experience, and they are often able to override detailed procedural controls.

Long-Term Liabilities and Owners' Equity

The clever accounting and fraud connected with liability and owners' equity accounts differ significantly from those associated with asset and revenue accounts. Few employees are tempted to steal a liability, although fictitious liabilities may be created as a means of misdirecting cash payments into the hands of an officer. Auditors should be alert for such fictions in the same sense that they are alert to the possibility of having fictitious accounts receivable. The area of liabilities and owners' equity also contains possibilities for company fraud against outsiders. This class of fraud is most often accomplished through material misrepresentations or omissions in financial statements and related disclosures.

Officers and employees can use share or bond instruments improperly. Unissued shares or bonds and treasury stock may be used as collateral for personal loans. Even though the company may not be damaged or suffer loss by this action (unless the employee defaults and the securities are seized), the practice is unauthorized and is contrary to company interests. Employees could gain access to shareholder lists and unissued coupons, using them for improper payments of dividends and interest on securities that are not outstanding.

Proper custodial control of securities (either by limited-access vaults or an independent disbursing agent) prevents most such occurrences. Reconciling authorized dividend and interest payments to actual payments detects unauthorized payments. If the company did not perform this checking procedure, auditors should include it in their own analytical recalculation procedures. Many liability, equity, and off-balance-sheet transactions are outside the reach of the normal internal control procedures that can operate effectively over ordinary transactions (such as purchases and sales) processed by clerks and machines. Auditors are justified in performing extensive substantive auditing of long-term liability, equity, and other high-level managed transactions and agreements, as control depends in large part on the integrity and accounting knowledge of management.

Income tax evasion and fraud result from actions of managers. Evasion and fraud may be accomplished by (1) simple omission of income, (2) unlawful deductions (such as contributions to political campaigns, capital cost allowance on non-existent assets, or capital cost allowance in excess of cost), or (3) sham transactions for the sole purpose of avoiding taxation. Auditors should be able to detect errors of the first two categories if the actual income and expense data have been sufficiently audited in the financial statements. The last category, **contrived sham transactions**, is harder to detect because a dishonest management can skilfully disguise them. Some of the fraud awareness procedures outlined in Chapter 21 (available on Connect) may be useful and effective.

Financial statements may be materially misstated through omission or understatement of liabilities and by failure to disclose technical defaults on loan agreement restrictions. These restrictions or debt covenants are very important to the viability of the client because if they are violated, creditors can force the client into bankruptcy. Auditor knowledge of these restrictions and comparison with the client's current financial condition pinpoint audit risk areas and help assess the going-concern assumption. The procedures for search for unrecorded liabilities may be used to discover such omissions and understatements (Chapter 12). If auditors discover that loan agreement terms have been violated, they should bring the information to the client's attention and insist on proper disclosure in notes to the financial statements. In both situations (liability understatement and loan default disclosure), management's actions, reactions, and willingness to adjust the financial figures and to make adverse disclosures are important insights for auditors' evaluation of managerial integrity, something that has an important bearing on the auditors' perceptions of risk for the audit engagement as a whole.

Misstatements in the financial statements can arise from error or fraud. According to CAS 240, the term *error* refers to an *unintentional* misstatement in financial statements, including the omission of an amount or a disclosure, or an incorrect accounting estimate arising from oversight or misinterpretation of facts. The term *fraud* refers to an *intentional* act by one or more individuals to misstate the financial statements to deceive users and obtain an unjust or illegal advantage. Although fraud is a broad legal concept, the auditor is only concerned with fraud that causes a material misstatement in the financial statements. Auditors do not make legal determinations of fraud.

Intent is difficult to prove, but if the auditor identifies a possible bias on the part of management in making accounting estimates, the auditor should consider whether there is a risk of material misstatement due to fraud.[4] For example, is it possible that the cumulative effect of bias in management's accounting estimates is designed to smooth earnings over two or more accounting periods, or to achieve a designated earnings level to deceive financial statement users? The audit needs to be performed with professional skepticism, meaning the auditor

contrived sham transactions:
fictitious transactions created for illegal purposes, such as evading taxes

(a) should be aware of factors that increase the risk of misstatement and (b) should be sensitized to evidence that contradicts the assumption of management's good faith.

If enough red flags are present, the auditor will assess a higher inherent risk, resulting in the following actions:

- Obtain more reliable evidence.
- Expand the extent of audit procedures performed.
- Apply audit procedures closer to or as of the balance sheet date.
- Require more extensive supervision of assistants, and/or assistants with more experience and training.

In essence, if the auditor suspects that the financial statements are misstated, he or she should perform procedures to confirm or dispel that suspicion. Generally, however, the auditor is less likely to detect material misstatements arising from fraud because of the deliberate concealment involved. When the auditor does obtain evidence of a non-trivial misstatement or fraud, he or she should inform the appropriate level of management, and the audit committee or board of directors should be informed.[5]

A company, its individual managers, and the auditors might easily violate securities regulations. Chapter 2 covers the general framework of regulation by provincial securities commissions. Auditors must know the provisions of the securities laws so that they can identify both situations that constitute obvious fraud and transactions that may be subject to the law. Having recognized or raised questions about a securities transaction, auditors should submit the facts to competent legal counsel for an opinion. Auditors are not expected to be legal experts, but they have the duty to recognize obvious instances of impropriety and to pursue investigations with the aid of legal experts.

Similarly, auditors should assist clients in observing securities commission rules and regulations on matters of timely disclosure. Timely disclosure rules are phrased as management's duties, and auditors are not required to carry out any specific procedures or to make any specific disclosures. The regulations require management to disseminate any material information, favourable or unfavourable, so that investors can incorporate it in their decision making. Announcements and disclosures must be made very soon after information becomes known. If situations arise during the year when the independent auditors are not present, they cannot be held responsible or liable. However, auditors may learn of the information inadvertently or the client may come to the auditor for advice. In such cases, auditors should advise their clients according to the requirements of law and regulations.

Auditors are currently pressured to discover more information about off-balance-sheet contingencies and commitments and to discover the facts of management involvement with other parties to transactions. Auditors' knowledge of the things that are not in accounting records depends in large part on information that management and its legal counsel reveal. Nevertheless, certain investigative procedures are available (see Chapters 7 and 21). The expectation for auditors to discover more information is a part of the public pressure on them to take more responsibility for fraud detection.

Investments and Intangibles

Theft, diversion, and unauthorized use of investment securities can occur in several ways. If safekeeping controls are weak, securities can simply be stolen, in which case it is a police problem rather than an auditing problem. Diversions, such as using securities as collateral during the year, returning them for a count, and then giving them back to the creditor without disclosure to the auditor, are more common. If safekeeping methods require entry signatures (as for a safety deposit box), auditors may be able to detect the in-and-out movement. The best chance of discovery is creditor confirmation of the collateral arrangement. In a similar manner, securities may be removed by an officer, sold, and then repurchased before the auditors' count. The auditors' record of the certificate numbers should reveal this change, since the returned certificates (and their serial numbers) will not be the same as the ones removed. The rapid growth in use of derivative securities as investments and hedges has created new and unique problems for auditors, not the least of which is lack of familiarity with these financial instruments. Appendix 14A provides an overview of the problems in this area.

Cash receipts from interest, royalties on patent licences, dividends, and sales proceeds may be stolen. The accounting records may or may not be manipulated to cover the theft. In general, this kind of defalcation should be prevented by cash receipts control; however, since these receipts are usually irregular and infrequent, the cash control system may not be as effective as it is for regular receipts on trade accounts. If the income accounts are not manipulated to hide stolen receipts, auditors will find less income in the account than their audit calculations tell them should be there based on other records. If sales of securities are not recorded, auditors will notice that securities are missing when they try to inspect or confirm them. If the income accounts have been manipulated to hide stolen receipts, vouching of cash receipts will detect the theft, or vouching may reveal some offsetting debit buried in some other account.

Accounting values may be manipulated in a number of ways: purchases of assets at inflated prices, leases with affiliates, acquisitions of patents for shares given to an inventor or promoter, sales to affiliates, and fallacious decisions about amortization. Business history has recorded several cases of non-arm's-length transactions with promoters, officers, directors, and controlled companies (even "dummy" companies) designed to drain the company's resources and fool the auditors.

In one case, a company sold assets to a dummy purchaser set up by a director to bolster sagging income. The auditors did not know that the purchaser was a shell. All the documents of sale looked to be in order, and cash sales proceeds had been deposited. The auditors were not informed of a secret agreement by the seller to repurchase the assets at a later time. This situation illustrates a devious manipulation. All transactions with persons closely associated with the company (related parties) should be audited carefully with reference to market values, particularly when a non-monetary transaction is involved (such as shares exchanged for patent rights). Sales and lease-back and straight lease transactions with insiders should likewise be audited carefully.

Finally, with the increasing use of accounting estimates in financial statements, including the increasing use of fair value accounting, auditors need to be concerned with unethical or fraudulent estimates. This is a relatively new concern in financial reporting but one that is taking increasing prominence with the issuance of CAS 540. We devote a separate chapter (Chapter 19) to the special problems associated with the audit of accounting estimates.

Analysis of Financial Statement Relationships

The audit of the finance and investment process verifies that there is no material misstatement in the balance of long-term investments and liabilities (financial instruments) and share capital or in the transaction streams that are related to them, dividends and interest. The following table summarizes the relationships that can be used as a basis for a misstatements analysis of the share capital account.

AUDITED AMOUNT	FINANCIAL STATEMENT WHERE AMOUNT IS REPORTED
Opening balance of share capital	Balance Sheet (prior-year comparative figures)
Add:	
Proceeds of shares issued during the year	Statement of Shareholders' Equity and Cash Flow Statement (financing activity)
Deduct:	
Reductions for shares redeemed during the year	Statement of Shareholders' Equity and Cash Flow Statement (financing activity)
Ending balance of share capital	Balance Sheet (current-year figures)

Misstatement Analysis

As an example of a type of misstatement that might be discovered in the finance and investment process, consider a situation where the auditor discovers the auditee has obtained new long-term debt during the year with a total balance of $250,000. Inspection of the loan contract reveals that $50,000 of the total is due for repayment during the following year, but the accountant has failed to set that amount out in the current liabilities section of the balance sheet in preparing the financial statements. This is a misclassification type of misstatement that affects two amounts within the balance sheet, such that it has no income impact. But it has a significant impact on current liabilities, the current ratio, and other information that may have an impact on users, so it should be accumulated as a misstatement for overall analysis at the end of the audit (see Exhibit 16–1 in Chapter 16).

Review Checkpoints

14-22   What is the single most significant control consideration in connection with clever accounting and fraud in finance and investment accounts?

14-23   Which is more likely to exist in the finance and investment cycle accounts: (1) fraud against the company or (2) fraud by the company in financial or tax reporting? Explain.

14-24   What should an auditor do when violation of securities laws is suspected?

14-25   What is the danger for auditors when company officials engage in undisclosed related party transactions?

SUMMARY

- The finance and investment process contains a wide variety of accounts—share capital, dividends, long-term debt, interest expense, tax expenses and future income taxes, financial instruments, derivatives, equity method investments, related gains and losses, consolidated subsidiaries, goodwill, and other intangibles. These accounts involve some of the most technically complex accounting standards. They create most of the difficult judgments for financial reporting.   **LO1**

- Transactions in these accounts are generally controlled by senior officials. Therefore, internal control is centred on the integrity and accounting knowledge of these officials. The procedural controls over details of transactions are not very effective because senior managers can override them and order their own desired accounting presentations. As a consequence, auditors' work on the assessment of control risk is directed toward the senior managers, the board of directors and their authorizations, and the design of finance and investment deals.   **LO2**

- Substantive programs are developed by linking the auditor's risk assessments to the risks of material misstatements in the financing and investing transactions. The chapter provided examples of typical substantive procedures that would be considered, depending on the risks assessed in each particular case.   **LO3**

- Fraud and clever accounting in the finance and investment cycle get directed most often to producing misleading financial statements. While theft and embezzlement can occur, the accounts in this cycle have frequently been the ones manipulated and misvalued so that financial positions and results of operations look better than the company's reality. Off-balance-sheet financing and investment transactions with related parties are explained as areas easily targeted for fraudulent financial reporting.   **LO4**

This chapter ends the book's coverage of audit applications for various processes and their related accounts. Chapters 15 and 16 contain several topics involved in putting the finishing touches on an audit.

KEY TERMS

articles of incorporation	debt instruments	off the balance sheet
contrived sham transactions		

MULTIPLE-CHOICE QUESTIONS FOR PRACTICE AND REVIEW

MC 14-1 **LO3** Jones was engaged to examine the financial statements of Gamma Corporation for the year ended June 30, 20X3. Having completed an examination of the investment securities, which of the following is her best method of verifying the accuracy of recorded dividend income?

a. Tracing recorded dividend income to cash receipts records and validated deposit slips
b. Utilizing analytical review techniques and statistical sampling
c. Comparing recorded dividends with amounts appearing on federal tax returns
d. Comparing recorded dividends with a standard financial reporting service's record of dividends

MC 14-2 **LO1** When a large amount of negotiable securities is held by the client, planning by the auditor is necessary to guard against which of the following?

a. Unauthorized negotiation of the securities before they are counted
b. Unrecorded sales of securities after they are counted
c. Substitution of securities already counted for other securities that should be on hand but are not
d. Substitution of authentic securities with counterfeit securities

MC 14-3 **LO3** Which of the following is the most important consideration of an auditor when examining the shareholders' equity section of a client's balance sheet?

a. Changes in the share capital account are verified by an independent share transfer agent.
b. Stock dividends and stock splits during the year under audit were approved by the shareholders.
c. Stock dividends are capitalized at par or stated value on the dividend declaration date.
d. Entries in the share capital account can be traced to resolutions in the minutes of the board of directors meetings.

MC 14-4 **LO3** If the auditor discovers that the carrying amount of a client's available-for-sale financial assets is greater than its market value at the balance sheet date, what should the auditor insist on?

a. The approximate market values of the investments are shown in parentheses on the face of the balance sheet.
b. The investments are classified as long term for balance sheet purposes with full disclosure in the footnotes.
c. The decline in value is recognized in the financial statements.
d. The liability section of the balance sheet separately shows a charge equal to the amount of the loss.

MC 14-5 **LO3** Which of the following is the primary reason for preparing a reconciliation between interest-bearing obligations outstanding during the year and interest expense in the financial statements?

a. Evaluating internal control over securities
b. Determining the validity of prepaid interest expense

c. Ascertaining the reasonableness of imputed interest

d. Detecting unrecorded liabilities

MC 14-6 **LO3** Why should the auditor insist that a representative of the client be present during the inspection and count of securities?

a. To lend authority to the auditor's directives

b. To detect forged securities

c. To coordinate the return of all securities to proper locations

d. To acknowledge the receipt of securities returned

MC 14-7 **LO2** When independent share transfer agents are not employed and the corporation issues its own shares and maintains share records, how should cancelled share certificates be handled?

a. Defaced to prevent reissuance and attached to their corresponding stubs

b. Not defaced, but segregated from other share certificates and retained in a cancelled certificates file

c. Destroyed to prevent fraudulent reissuance

d. Defaced and sent to the federal finance minister

MC 14-8 **LO3** When a client company does not maintain its own share capital records, the auditor should obtain written confirmation from the transfer agent and registrar concerning which of the following?

a. Restrictions on the payment of dividends

b. The number of shares issued and outstanding

c. Guarantees of preferred share liquidation value

d. The number of shares subject to agreements to repurchase

MC 14-9 **LO3** Which item of all corporate share capital transactions should ultimately be traced?

a. Minutes of the board of directors meetings

b. Cash receipts journal

c. Cash disbursements journal

d. Numbered share certificates

MC 14-10 **LO3** A corporate balance sheet indicates that one of the corporate assets is a patent. Where will an auditor most likely be able to obtain a written representation of this patent from?

a. Patent lawyer

b. Regional patent office

c. Patent inventor

d. Patent owner

MC 14-11 **LO2** An audit program for the examination of the retained earnings account should include a step that requires verification of which of the following?

a. Market value used to charge retained earnings to account for a two-for-one share split

b. Approval of the adjustment to the beginning balance as a result of a write-down of accounts receivable

c. Authorization for both cash and share dividends

d. Gain or loss resulting from disposition of available-for-sale financial assets

EXERCISES AND PROBLEMS

EP 14-1 Internal Control Questionnaire for Equity Investments. `LO1, 2` Cassandra Corporation, a manufacturing company, periodically invests large sums in marketable equity securities. The investment policy is established by the investment committee of the board of directors. The treasurer is responsible for carrying out the committee's directives. All securities are held by Cassandra's brokerage company.

Your internal control questionnaire with respect to Cassandra's investments in equity securities contains the following three questions:

1. Is investment policy established by the investment committee of the board of directors?
2. Is the treasurer solely responsible for carrying out the investment committee's directive?
3. Are all securities stored in a bank safety deposit box?

Required:

a. What is the purpose of the above three questions?
b. What additional questions should your internal control questionnaire include concerning the company's investment in marketable equity securities? (*Hint:* Prepare questions to cover the control objectives—validity, completeness, authorization, accuracy, classification, and proper period.)

(© 2000, American Institute of CPAs. All Rights Reserved. Adapted by permission.)

EP 14-2 Long-Term Investment Securities. `LO3` You are auditing the financial statements of Bass Corporation for the year ended December 31, and you are about to begin an audit of the non-current investment securities. Bass's records indicate that the company owns various bearer bonds, as well as 25% of the outstanding common shares of Commercial Industrial Inc. You are satisfied with the evidence supporting the presumption of significant influence over Commercial. The various securities are at two locations as follows:

1. Recently acquired securities are in the company's safe in the custody of the treasurer.
2. All other securities are in a bank safety deposit box. All securities in Bass's portfolio are actively traded in a broad market.

Required:

a. Assuming that the system of internal control over securities is satisfactory, what are the objectives (specific assertions) for the audit of the non-current securities?
b. What audit procedures should you undertake with respect to the audit of Bass's investment securities?

(© 2000, American Institute of CPAs. All Rights Reserved. Adapted by permission.)

EP 14-3 Securities Examination and Count. `LO3` You are in charge of the audit of the financial statements of the Demot Corporation for the year ended December 31. The corporation has had the policy of investing its surplus funds in marketable securities. Its share and bond certificates are kept in a safety deposit box in a local bank. Only the president and the treasurer of the corporation have access to the box.

You were unable to obtain access to the safety deposit box on December 31 because neither the president nor the treasurer was available. Your assistant will accompany the treasurer to the bank on January 11 to examine the securities, but he has never examined securities that were being kept in a safety deposit box and requires instructions. The inspection should only take an hour.

Required:

a. List the instructions you would give for examining the share and bond certificates in the safety deposit box. Include the details of the securities to be examined and the reasons for examining these details.

b. Your assistant reports that the treasurer had entered the box on January 4 to remove an old photograph of the corporation's original building. The photograph was lent to the local chamber of commerce. List the additional audit procedures required because of the treasurer's action.

(© 2000, American Institute of CPAs. All Rights Reserved. Adapted by permission.)

EP 14-4 Securities Procedures. `LO3` You were engaged to examine the financial statements of Ronlyn Corporation for the year ended June 30. On May 1, the corporation borrowed $500,000 from the bank to finance plant expansion. However, because of unexpected difficulties in acquiring the building site, the expansion had not begun as planned. To make use of the borrowed funds, management decided to invest in shares and bonds; on May 16 the $500,000 was invested in securities.

Required:

In your audit of investments, how would you

a. Audit the recorded dividend or interest income?

b. Determine market value?

c. Establish the authority for security purchases?

(© 2000, American Institute of CPAs. All Rights Reserved. Adapted by permission.)

EP 14-5 Research and Development. `LO3` The Hertle Engineering Company depends on new product development to maintain its position in the market for drilling tool equipment. The company conducts an extensive R&D program and has charged all R&D costs to current operations in accordance with *CPA Canada Handbook* requirements.

The company began Project Able in January 20X1 with the goal of patenting a revolutionary drilling bit design. Work continued until October 20X2, when the company applied for a patent. Costs were charged to the R&D expense account in both years, except for the cost of a computer program that engineers plan to use in Project Baker, scheduled to start in December 20X2. The computer program was purchased from Computeering Inc. in January 20X1 for $45,000.

Required:

a. Give an audit program for the audit of R&D costs on Project Able. Assume that you are auditing the company for the first time at December 31, 20X2.

b. What evidence would you require for the audit of the computer program that has been capitalized as an intangible asset? As of December 31, 20X2, this account has a balance of $40,000 (cost less $5,000 amortized as a part of Project Able).

(© 2000, American Institute of CPAs. All Rights Reserved. Adapted by permission.)

EP 14-6 Intangibles. `LO1, 2` Sorenson Manufacturing was incorporated on January 3, 20X1. The corporation's financial statements for its first year's operations were not examined by a PA. You have been engaged to audit the financial statements for the year ended December 31, 20X2, and your examination is substantially completed.

A partial trial balance of the company's accounts is given in Exhibit EP 14-6:

CHAPTER 14 The Finance and Investment Process 799

EXHIBIT EP 14-6

Sorenson Manufacturing Corporation Partial Trial Balance at December 31, 20X2

	TRIAL BALANCE	
	DEBIT	CREDIT
Cash	$11,000	
Accounts receivable	42,500	
Allowance for doubtful accounts		$ 500
Inventories	38,500	
Machinery	75,000	
Equipment	29,000	
Accumulated amortization		10,000
Patents	85,000	
Leasehold improvements	26,000	
Prepaid expenses	10,500	
Goodwill	24,000	

The following information relates to accounts that may yet require adjustment:

1. Patents for Sorenson's manufacturing process were purchased January 2, 20X2, at a cost of $68,000. An additional $17,000 was spent in December 20X2 to improve machinery covered by the patents and charged to the patents account. The patents had a remaining legal term of 17 years.

2. The balance in the goodwill account includes $24,000 paid December 30, 20X1, for an advertising program estimated to increase Sorenson's sales over a period of four years following the disbursement.

3. The leasehold improvement account includes (1) the $15,000 cost of improvements, with a total estimated useful life of 12 years, which Sorenson, as tenant, made to leased premises in January 20X1; (2) movable assembly line equipment costing $8,500, which was installed in the leased premises in December 20X2; and (3) real estate taxes of $2,500 paid by Sorenson, which, under the terms of the lease, should have been paid by the landlord. Sorenson paid its rent in full during 20X2. A 10-year non-renewable lease was signed January 3, 20X1, for the leased building that Sorenson used in manufacturing operations. No amortization of the leasehold improvements has been recorded.

Required:

Prepare adjusting entries as necessary.

(© 2000, American Institute of CPAs. All Rights Reserved. Adapted by permission.)

EP 14-7 Long-Term Note. **LO3** You were engaged to examine the financial statements of Ronlyn Corporation for the year ended June 30. On May 1 the corporation borrowed $500,000 from the bank to finance plant expansion. The long-term note agreement provided for the annual payment of principal and interest over five years. The existing plant was pledged as security for the loan.

Due to unexpected difficulties in acquiring the building site, the plant expansion had not begun as planned. To make use of the borrowed funds, on May 16, management invested the $500,000 in securities.

Required:

a. What are the audit objectives for examining long-term debt?

b. Prepare an audit program for the examination of the long-term note agreement between Ronlyn and the bank.

(© 2000, American Institute of CPAs. All Rights Reserved. Adapted by permission.)

EP 14-8 Long-Term Financing Agreement. **LO3** You have been engaged to audit the financial statements of Broadwall Corporation for the year ended December 31, 20X2. During the year, Broadwall obtained a long-term loan from a local bank pursuant to the following financing agreement:

1. The loan was to be secured by the company's inventory and accounts receivable.
2. The company was to maintain a debt-to-equity ratio not to exceed 2:1.
3. The company was not to pay dividends without permission from the bank.
4. Monthly instalment payments were to commence July 1, 20X2.

In addition, the company also borrowed, on a short-term basis, substantial amounts from the president of the company just prior to the year-end.

Required:

a. For the purposes of your audit of the financial statements of Broadwall Corporation, what procedures should you employ in examining the described loans? Do not discuss internal control.

b. What financial statement disclosures should you expect to find with respect to the loan from the president?

EP 14-9 Bond Indenture Covenants. **LO3** The following covenants are extracted from the indenture of a bond issue. Failure to comply with its terms in any respect automatically advances the due date of the loan to the date of non-compliance (the regular due date is 20 years hence).

Required:

Give any audit steps or reporting requirements you believe should be taken or recognized in connection with each of the following from the indenture:

1. The debtor company shall endeavour to maintain a working capital ratio of 2:1 at all times, and, in any fiscal year following a failure to maintain said ratio, the company shall restrict compensation of officers to a total of $500,000. Officers for this purpose shall include chair of the board of directors, president, all vice-presidents, secretary, and treasurer.
2. The debtor company shall keep all property that is security for this debt insured against loss by fire to the extent of 100% of its actual value. Policies of insurance comprising this protection shall be filed with the trustee.
3. The debtor company shall pay all taxes legally assessed against property that is security for this debt within the time provided by law for payment without penalty, and shall deposit receipted tax bills or equally acceptable evidence of payment of same with the trustee.
4. A sinking fund shall be deposited with the trustee by semiannual payments of $300,000, from which the trustee shall, at his or her discretion, purchase bonds of this issue.

(© 2000, American Institute of CPAs. All Rights Reserved. Adapted by permission.)

EP 14-10 Shareholders' Equity. **LO1, 3** You are a PA examining the financial statements of Pate Corporation for the year ended December 31. The financial statements and records of Pate Corporation have not been audited by a PA in prior years.

Pate Corporation was founded in 1992. The corporation has 10 shareholders and serves as its own registrar and transfer agent. There are no capital share subscription contracts in effect.

The shareholders' equity section of the balance sheet at December 31 follows:

Shareholders' equity:	
Share capital—10,000 no par value shares authorized; 5,000 shares issued and outstanding	$ 50,000
Contributed capital	32,580
Retained earnings	47,320
Total shareholders' equity	$129,900

Required:

a. Prepare the detailed audit program for the examination of the three accounts of the shareholders' equity section of the balance sheet. Organize the audit program under broad financial statement assertions. (Do not include in the audit program the audit of the results of the current year's operations.)

b. After all other figures on the balance sheet have been audited, it may appear that the retained earnings figure is a balancing figure and requires no further audit work. Why don't auditors audit retained earnings as they do the other figures on the balance sheet? Discuss.

(© 2000, American Institute of CPAs. All Rights Reserved. Adapted by permission.)

DISCUSSION CASES

DC 14-1 Intercompany and Interpersonal Investment Relations. **LO3** You have been engaged to audit the financial statements of Hardy Hardware Distributors Inc. as of December 31. In your review of the corporate non-financial records, you have found that Hardy Hardware owns 15% of the outstanding voting common shares of Hardy Products Corporation. Upon further investigation, you learn that Hardy Products Corporation manufactures a line of hardware goods, 90% of which are sold to Hardy Hardware.

James L. Hardy, president of Hardy Hardware, has supplied you with objective evidence that he personally owns 30% of the Hardy Products voting shares and that the remaining 70% is owned by Janice L. Hardy, his sister and president of Hardy Products. James also owns 20% of the voting common shares of Hardy Hardware Distributors. Another 20% is held by an estate of which James and Janice are beneficiaries, and the remaining 60% is publicly held.

Hardy Hardware has consistently reported operating profits greater than the industry average. Hardy Products Corporation, however, has a net return on sales of only 1%. The Hardy Products investment has always been reported at cost, and no dividends have been paid by the company. During the course of your conversations with the Hardy siblings, you learn that you were appointed as auditor because the siblings had a heated disagreement with the former auditor over the issues of accounting for the Hardy Products investment and the prices at which goods have been sold to Hardy Hardware.

Required:

a. Identify the issues in this situation as they relate to (1) conflicts of interest and (2) controlling influences among individuals and corporations.

b. Should the investment in Hardy Products Corporation be accounted for using the equity method?

c. What evidence should the auditor seek with regard to the prices paid by Hardy Hardware for products purchased from Hardy Products Corporation?

d. What information would you consider necessary for adequate disclosure in the financial statements of Hardy Hardware Distributors?

Instructions for Discussion Cases DC 14-2 and DC 14-3

These cases are designed like the ones in the Application Cases. They give the problem, the method, the audit trail, and the amount. Your assignment is to write the audit approach analysis portion of the case, organized around these sections:

Audit objectives: Express the objective in terms of the facts supposedly asserted in financial records, accounts, and statements. (Refer to the discussion of assertions in Chapter 5.)

Control procedures relevant to the process: Write a brief explanation of control considerations, especially the kinds of manipulations that may arise from the situation described in the case.

Tests of controls: Write some procedures for getting evidence about existing controls, especially procedures that could discover management manipulations. If there are no controls to test, then there are no procedures to perform; go to the next section. A "procedure" should instruct someone about the source(s) of evidence to tap and the work to do.

Tests of details of balance: Write some procedures for getting evidence about the existence, completeness, valuation, ownership, and presentation or disclosure assertions identified in your objective section above.

Audit results: Write a short statement about what you expect to discover with your procedures.

DC 14-2 Related Party Transaction "Goodwill." LO3

Problem: Gulwest Industries, a public company, used a contrived amount of goodwill to overstate assets and disguise a loss on discontinued operations. The company had decided to discontinue its unprofitable line of business of manufacturing sporting ammunition. They had capitalized the startup cost of the business, and, with its discontinuance, the $7 million deferred cost should have been written off. Instead, Gulwest formed a new corporation named Amron and transferred the sporting ammunition assets (including the $7 million deferred cost) to it in exchange for all the Amron shares. In the Gulwest accounts, the Amron investment was carried at $12.4 million, which was the book value of the assets transferred (including the $7 million deferred cost).

Gulwest and a different public company (Big Industrial) agreed to create another company (BigShot Ammunition). Gulwest transferred all the Amron assets to BigShot in exchange for (1) common and preferred shares of Big, valued at $2 million, and (2) a note from BigShot in the amount of $3.4 million. Big Industrial thus acquired 100% of the shares of BigShot. Gulwest management reasoned that it had "given" Amron shares valued at $12.4 million to receive shares and notes valued at $5.4 million, so the difference must be goodwill. Thus, the Gulwest accounts carried amounts for Big Industrial shares ($2 million), BigShot note receivable ($3.4 million), and goodwill ($7 million).

Audit trail: Gulwest directors included in the minutes an analysis of the sporting ammunition business's lack of profitability. The minutes showed approval of a plan to dispose of the business, but they did not use the words "discontinue the business." The minutes also showed approval of the creation of Amron, the deal with Big Industrial along with the formation of BigShot, and the acceptance of Big's shares and Bigshot's note in connection with the final exchange and merger.

Amount: As explained above, Gulwest avoided reporting a write-off of $7 million by overstating the value of the assets given in exchange for the Big Industrial shares and the BigShot Ammunition note.

DC 14-3 Related Party Transaction Valuation. `LO3` Follow the instructions preceding Discussion Case DC 14-2. Write the audit approach section of this case.

In Plane View

Problem: Whiz Corporation overstated the value of shares given in exchange for an airplane and, thereby, understated its loss on disposition of the shares. Income was overstated. Whiz owned 160,000 Wing Company shares, carried on the books as an investment in the amount of $6,250,000. Whiz bought a used airplane from Wing, giving in exchange (1) $480,000 cash and (2) the 160,000 Wing shares. Even though the quoted market value of the Wing shares was $2,520,000, Whiz valued the airplane received at $3,750,000, indicating a share valuation of $3,270,000. Thus, Whiz recognized a loss on disposition of the Wing shares in the amount of $2,980,000.

Whiz justified the airplane valuation with another transaction. On the same day it was purchased, Whiz sold the airplane to the Mexican subsidiary of one of its subsidiary companies (two layers down; but Whiz owned 100% of the first subsidiary, which in turn owned 100% of the Mexican subsidiary). The Mexican subsidiary paid Whiz with US$25,000 cash and a promissory note for US$3,725,000 (market rate of interest).

Audit trail: The transaction was within the authority of the CEO, and company policy did not require a separate approval by the board of directors. A contract of sale and correspondence with Wing detailing the terms of the transaction were in the files. Likewise, a contract of sale to the Mexican subsidiary, along with a copy of the deposit slip and a memorandum of the promissory note, were on file. The note itself was kept in the company vault. None of the Wing papers cited a specific price for the airplane.

Amount: Whiz overvalued the Wing shares and justified this with a related party transaction with its own subsidiary company. The loss on the disposition of the Wing shares was understated by $750,000.

DC 14-4 Audit of Long-Term Debt. `LO3` In Note 12 of its December 2001 consolidated financial statements, Bell Canada reported long-term debt outstanding totalling $9.075 billion. This amount is made up of 35 separate debentures, with maturity dates ranging from 2001 to 2054, in amounts ranging from $125 million to $700 million, with interest rates ranging from 2.7% to 11.45%. The income statement for the year reports interest expense on this long-term debt of $725 million.[6]

Required:

List the assertions relating to Bell Canada's long-term debt and interest expense. Describe the audit procedures that you would perform to verify the debt and interest expense for 2001.

DC 14-5 Long-Term Debt Working Paper Review. `LO3` The long-term debt working paper in Exhibit DC 14-5 was prepared by client personnel and audited by AA, an audit staff assistant, during the calendar year 20X2 audit of Canadian Widgets Inc., a continuing audit client. You are the engagement supervisor, and your assignment is to review this working paper thoroughly.

Required:

Identify and prepare a list explaining the deficiencies that should be discovered in the supervisory review of the long-term debt working paper.

(© 2000, American Institute of CPAs. All Rights Reserved. Adapted by permission.)

EXHIBIT DC 14–5

CANADIAN WIDGETS INC.
Working Papers December 31, 20X2

Index	KI	
	Initials	Date
Prepared by	AA	Mar. 22, 20X2
Approved by		

Lender	Interest Rate	Payment Terms	Collateral	Balance Dec. 31, 20X1	20X2 Borrowings	20X2 Reductions	Balance Dec. 31, 20X2	Interest paid to	Accrued Interest Payable Dec. 31, 20X2	Comments
First Commercial Bank	12%	Interest only on 25th of month, principal due in full Jan. 1, 20X6, no prepayment penalty	Inventories	$ 50,000 ✓	$300,000 A Jan. 31, 20X2	$100,000 Jun. 30, 20X2	$ 250,000 CX ⊕	Dec. 25, 20X2	$2,500 NR	Dividend of $80,000 paid Sep. 2, 20X2 (W/P N-3) violates a provision of the debt agreement, which thereby permits lender to demand immediate payment; lender has refused to waive this violation.
Lender's Capital Corp.	Prime plus 1%	Interest only on last day of month, principal due in full Mar. 5, 20X4	2nd Mortgage on Park St. Building	100,000 ✓	50,000 A	—	200,000 C	Dec. 31, 20X2	—	
Gigantic Building & Loan Assoc.	12%	$5,000 principal plus interest due on 5th of month, due in full Dec. 31, 20X3	1st Mortgage on Park St. Building	720,000 ✓	—	60,000	660,000 C	Dec. 5, 20X2	5,642 R	Prime rate was 8% to 9% during the year.
J. Lott, majority shareholder	0%	Due in full Dec. 13, 20X5	Unsecured	300,000 ✓	—	100,000 N	200,000 C	—	—	Reclassification entry for current portion proposed (See RJE-3) Borrowed additional $100,000 from J. Lott on Jan. 7, 20X3.
				$1,170,000 F	$350,000 F	$260,000 F	$1,310,000 T/B F		$8,142 T/B F	

Interest costs for long-term debt

Interest expense for year	$ 281,333 T/B
Average loan balance outstanding	$1,406,667 R

Five-year maturities (for disclosure purposes)

Year-end		
Dec. 31, 20X3	$	60,000
Dec. 31, 20X4		260,000
Dec. 31, 20X5		310,000
Dec. 31, 20X6		60,000
Dec. 31, 20X7		360,000
Thereafter		360,000
		$1,310,000 F

Tick-mark legend
F   Re-added, foots correctly
C   Confirmed without exception, W/P K-2
CX Confirmed with exception, W/P K-3
NR Does not recompute correctly
A   Agreed to loan agreement, validated bank deposit ticket, and board of directors authorization, W/P W-7
⊘   Agreed to cancelled cheques and lender's monthly statements
N   Agreed to cash disbursements journal and cancelled cheques dated Dec. 31, 20X2, clearing Jan. 8, 20X3
T/B Traced to working trial balance
✓   Agreed to Dec. 31, 20X1 working papers
R   Agreed interest rate, term, and collateral to copy of note and loan agreement
⊕   Agreed to cancelled cheques and board of director's authorization, W/P W-7

Overall Conclusions
Long-term debt, accrued interest payable, and interest expense are correct and complete at Dec. 31, 20X2.

DC 14-6 Audit of Pension Expense. **LO3** Clark, PA, has been engaged to perform the audit of Kent Ltd.'s financial statements for the current year. Clark is about to commence auditing Kent's employee pension expense. Her preliminary inquiries concerning Kent's pension plan lead her to believe that some of the actuarial computations and assumptions are so complex that they are beyond the competence ordinarily required of an auditor. Clark is considering engaging Lane, an actuary, to assist with this portion of the audit.

Required:

a. What are Clark's responsibilities with respect to the findings of Lane, if she wishes to rely on those findings?
b. Distinguish between the circumstances where it is and is not appropriate for Clark to refer to Lane in the auditor's report.

> *(Adapted from External Auditing (AU1), June 2011, with permission of Chartered Professional Accountants of Canada, Toronto, Canada. Any changes to the original material are the sole responsibility of the author (and/or publisher) and have not been reviewed or endorsed by the Chartered Professional Accountants of Canada.)*

DC 14-7 Board of Directors, Control Role. **LO2**

Required:

What is the role of the company's board of directors in controlling management's activities? Why is this particularly important in the finance and investment cycle? How does the board exercise this control, and how can the auditor evaluate the board's effectiveness?

DC 14-8 Derivative Instruments, Controls, and Audit Procedures. **LO2, 3** Barrick Gold, a Canadian public corporation, has operations in six main countries. Barrick produces and sells gold, its primary product, as well as by-products such as silver and copper. These activities expose Barrick to a variety of market risks, such as changes in commodity prices, foreign currency exchange rates, and interest rates. Barrick has a risk management program that seeks to reduce the potentially adverse effects of volatility in these markets on its operating results. It uses derivative instruments to mitigate significant unanticipated earnings and cash flow fluctuations that may arise. These instruments include spot deferred sales contracts, options contracts, interest rate swaps, and foreign currency forward exchange contracts. Barrick's derivatives activities are subject to the management, direction, and control of its finance committee as part of its oversight of Barrick's investment activities and treasury function. The finance committee, comprising five members of Barrick's board of directors, including its CEO, approves corporate policy on risk management objectives, provides guidance on derivative instrument use, reviews internal procedures relating to internal control and valuation of derivative instruments, monitors derivatives activities, and reports to the board. Implementation of these policies is delegated to Barrick's treasury function.[7]

Required:

a. Identify the control risks in Barrick's derivatives activities and the key controls indicated in the above description. Provide a brief description of specific control procedures that are likely used by Barrick's treasury function to implement the risk management policies.
b. Describe audit procedures that could be used to test these controls and substantive tests for derivatives activities at Barrick.

DC 14-9 Audit of Finance Transactions: Internet Business. **LO1, 3** City Search Inc. (CSI) is a technology company providing local search engine services in the Greater Toronto Area (GTA).

CSI combines online search capability with a print directory (City Pages) focusing specifically on GTA websites. Consumers use the search engine and print directory to locate local businesses. Businesses use the search engine and print directory to attract potential customers to their places of business through paid advertisements. CSI began operations in March 20X3 and launched its first sales campaign for print and online search advertisements in June 20X3. Since that time, over 600,000 copies of the City Pages have been distributed to businesses and residences.

The original financing to start CSI came from several wealthy investors who purchased common shares. Additional common shares were issued to the public in late 20X4. These shares initially sold for $2.40, but, during 20X5, the share price fell to less than $1.00. The decline in price is mainly because two of the original investors sold large blocks of shares for whatever they could get as the business was not proving to be as successful as they expected. In early 20X5, the CSI board of directors hired a new president, Bill Dorado, to aggressively promote the CSI directory as a superior directory for local shopping and entertainment searches, and to find innovative ways to increase revenues and CSI's share price.

Businesses that are clients of CSI pay an advertising fee for print and online directory listings that include the business name, address, phone number, type of products/services offered, and website link. CSI will also create a website for clients for a one-time fee that varies depending on the number of pages, links, and type of content the client wants. CSI clients can also purchase banner advertising that pops up when users browse through the online directory. Clients sign a contract for the ad frequency they require and are billed monthly. Clients can also purchase additional advertising features, such as moving graphics; audio; and a special patented "bull's-eye target" (BT) feature, which concentrates the client's ads in directory locations they choose. For example, a home-decorating service can sign up for BT service that will cause their ads to be shown whenever users are searching for home products businesses.

In February 20X6, CSI entered into an agreement with Flogg Investments Inc. (FII) in which FII agreed to sell newly issued common shares of the company for total gross proceeds of up to $8 million. The proceeds raised from the new common shares will be used by CSI to support its growth initiatives and for working capital and general corporate purposes, including repayment of loans from shareholders that amounted to approximately $4 million as of December 31, 20X5.

Your firm was recently engaged to audit CSI's 20X5 financial statements. The previous auditors that reported on the 20X3 and 20X4 financial statements have resigned. In communicating with the predecessor auditors, you find out that they resigned due to a change in circumstances that led to their firm's partners not being independent of CSI. To date, CSI has provided the audit partner of your firm, who is in charge of the audit, with preliminary financial statements (prior to audit) for its most recent year-end, December 31, 20X5. You are assigned to plan the audit. From reviewing these preliminary financial statements and talking to Bill Dorado, you have learned the following:

1. CSI recognizes revenue on a straight-line basis as each service is provided over the terms of its individual client contracts. The contracts range in length from three months to four years, with the majority lasting for two years. Revenues from contracts ranging from one to four years are deferred and amortized as each service is provided. Upfront direct costs associated with these revenues, including the production costs and selling commissions, are deferred and amortized over the life of each client contract on a straight-line basis. Adjustments are made to deferred revenue and deferred production costs for cancellations at the time they are made. Cancellations are permitted if clients relocate outside the GTA or close their business. CSI

management estimates the future value of contracts in progress and compares this value with deferred production costs to ensure these costs are fully recoverable.

2. CSI's revenue is generated mainly through the sale of advertising to local businesses, many of which are small and medium-size enterprises (up to 50 employees). In the ordinary course of operations, CSI may extend credit to these advertisers for advertising purchases on a case-by-case basis, a practice that is common in the industry. CSI management evaluates the collectability of its trade receivables from its clients, based upon a combination of factors, including aging of receivables, on a periodic basis, and records a general allowance for doubtful accounts and bad debt expense. When management becomes aware of a client's inability to meet its financial obligations to CSI (such as in the case of bankruptcy or significant deterioration in the client's financial position and payment experience), a specific bad debt provision is recorded to reduce the client's related trade receivable to its estimated net realizable value.

3. CSI is a registered member of three barter networks serving the GTA marketplace. CSI sells its services and purchases goods and services through these networks. The full market value of a contract sale settled through a barter network is recorded in accounts receivable and deferred revenue at the time of the sale. Revenues are recognized in income on a straight-line basis over the term of the contract. Receivables are reduced when a good or service purchased through a barter network has been received. The president believes this bartering arrangement was an astute business move that "saves us tons of cash and increases revenues at the same time."

4. CSI has signed contracts with two well-known, local retail chains that want to start direct online retailing and have paid CSI $13.5 million to develop all their online shopping systems, including customer relations management and payment processing. CSI has never completed this type of system before but has the technical expertise from developing its own systems. CSI expects the contract to be completed by the end of 20X6. CSI recorded $6.5 million of the $13.5 million as revenues in 20X5, deferring the rest to be reported when the work is completed.

5. The president and several top CSI executives have received options to purchase common shares at a fixed price of $1 per share. None of the options have been exercised yet.

6. The BT technology was patented by CSI in early 20X4. In late 20X4, the BT patent was sold for $7 million to LivePatents Inc., which is owned by one of the original CSI investors, who is also a board member of CSI. CSI repurchased the patent in early 20X5 for $10 million, by paying $7 million in cash and issuing a loan payable to LivePatents Inc. for the remainder. The patent is shown on CSI's balance sheet at its cost of $10 million and is being amortized over 17 years.

7. Internal search engine development costs are recorded at cost. The company provides for amortization of these costs at the following annual rates:

- Directory research and design costs—30% declining-balance basis
- Internal directory design costs—30% declining-balance basis

Required:

Prepare a detailed and complete audit plan that addresses the accounting and other information items noted in this case. Also, suggest any other information that you would want to obtain for planning the audit.

DC 14-10 Critical Thinking Regarding Accounting Rules, Fairness of Presentation, and the Lehman Bros. Investment Bank Reporting before Its Failure. LO4 As indicated in the box in this chapter, Lehman attempted to structure end-of-quarter transactions as sales of financial instruments when in substance it turned out be temporary borrowing of cash. This allowed it to hide up to $50 billion of debt in some quarters. The auditor claimed this was in accordance with GAAP. In a lawsuit filed by New York's Attorney General in December 2010, the official claim is that the auditor knowingly committed fraud and conspired with Lehman Brothers to reclassify tens of billions of dollars on the balance sheet. This was the first time the *Martin Act* (New York's more stringent securities regulation, which served as a model for the SEC Acts) had been used against auditors. On March 22, 2012, the auditor was unsuccessful in moving the case from New York's state court to federal court.

Discuss in class whether Lehman's financial statements were in conformity with U.S. GAAP (refer to FASB's SFAS 140: Accounting for Transfers and Servicing of Financial Assets and Extinguishments of Liabilities). Did the financial statements present fairly?

APPENDIX 14A Derivative Securities—An Example of Risks That Management and Auditors Face (on Connect)

APPENDIX 14B Generally Accepted Accounting Principles for Private Enterprises (on Connect)

ENDNOTES

1   PCAOB, *Review of Existing Standards—Principles of Reporting*, Background Paper: Standing Advisory Group Meeting, October 5–6, 2005, p. 7, pcaobus.org/News/Events/Documents/10052005_SAGMeeting/Principles_of_Reporting.pdf.

2   *Guidance for Directors on Governance Processes for Control*, CICA, Toronto, Canada, 1996.

3   CAS 540.

4   *CPA Canada Handbook*, paragraph 5135.081.

5   *CPA Canada Handbook*, section 5135.

6   Bell Canada, 2001 Consolidated Financial Statements.

7   Barrick Gold Corporation, 2001 Consolidated Financial Statements.

Completing the Audit Work

In this chapter, we will complete the final evidence-gathering work, tying up the loose ends of the audit. The chapter covers the issues, techniques, procedures, and documents that are considered in completing an audit of financial statements. The audit of the flow accounts that are reported in the income statement, the cash flow statement, and the statement of retained earnings can only be completed once all the period's transactions have been completed at the period-end. The audit procedures related to revenue and expense accounts are covered in the first part of the chapter.

Other audit procedures relate to the year-end amounts on the balance sheet. The audit of many of these amounts has already been covered in Chapters 11 through 14. However, there are procedures—such as audit for subsequent events, contingencies, commitments or contractual obligations, overall evaluation of audit results, overall analysis of the financial statements, and presentation and disclosure issues—that still need to be considered after the balances have been audited but before forming a conclusion on whether the financial statements are fairly stated. These and related issues are covered in the second part of this chapter.

At the completion of the audit, the audit engagement partner must provide an opinion that is properly supported by the audit evidence, which must all be documented in the audit files. The application of professional judgment in assessing the adequacy of the audit work and the fairness of the overall financial statement presentation, forming the audit opinion, and writing the appropriate audit report are topics covered in Chapter 16.

LEARNING OBJECTIVES

After completing this chapter, you will be able to do the following:

LO1 Describe the balance sheet account groups that the major revenue and expense accounts are associated with, as well as the substantive analytical procedures applied to audit revenues and expenses.

LO2 Outline the overall analytical procedures to be performed at the final stage of the audit, including analysis of the income statement, cash flow statement, financial statement presentation, and disclosures.

LO3 Explain the procedures used at the audit completion stage to identify any contingencies and contractual commitments, including the use of lawyers' letters.

LO4 Given a set of facts and circumstances, classify a subsequent event by type and proper treatment in the financial statements, and outline the implications of the timing of discovery of the event for the auditor's report.

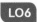

LO5 Explain why written management representations are obtained and what items are generally included in the representation letter, including identification of related parties.

LO6 Outline the procedures used to complete the documentation of the audit engagement.

EcoPak Inc.

Donna and Belinda have pulled together the audit files, and most of the work has been done and documented. One of the last procedures required is to obtain a response from the company's lawyers to the legal inquiry letter regarding any legal claims. Nina has sent off the letter to EcoPak's law firm, Rotie, Cicery and Associates LLP and given a copy to Donna. EcoPak's letter states that "there are no claims or possible claims with respect to which the law firm's advice or representation has been sought and which are outstanding," and it instructs the law firm to respond directly to the M&G audit firm.

When the lawyer who handles EcoPak, Charles Rotie, receives the inquiry letter, he immediately realizes there is a problem. He has done a good deal of work preparing a defence for EcoPak against a possible claim. Several customers of a fast food company that uses EcoPak food packages claim they were made ill by toxic content from either the food or the packaging. Their lawyer has been in touch with lawyers for both the fast food chain and EcoPak as packaging supplier to discuss the case they are pulling together in support of the customers' claim. Charles arranges a conference call with Nina and Kam to discuss his response to the letter of inquiry.

"As you know, I have been advising you on a possible claim regarding the three customers of Fast & Good Inc. who believe the food and/or your packaging may have caused them some serious illness. This possible claim was not included in your inquiry letter, so it won't be mentioned in my response letter, to maintain the confidentiality of our lawyer–client communications. However, in these circumstances, it is important for me to advise you that you do have a responsibility to inform your auditors of the possible claim and to ensure that your financial statements contain all disclosures and adjustments necessary for fair presentation. The work I have done so far indicates it is unlikely the claim will proceed against EcoPak as we can quite easily show this same EcoPak product has been used safely many thousands of times in identical applications with no ill effects, and the particular batch that the packages in question came from has had no other incidence of this type of problem."

On the last day of the field work, the engagement partner and manager, Tariq and Belinda, have arranged to meet with Nina and Kam at the EcoPak offices to go over the final draft of the financial statements and discuss any remaining outstanding issues, including the written representations that Nina and Kam will be asked to provide in a letter dated as of the upcoming board meeting at which the financial statements will be approved. Donna attends the meeting as well and is surprised to find the atmosphere in the meeting room extremely tense and unfriendly. Nina seems like a different person from the one she has gotten to know while working on the audit.

Once Tariq gets through all the points he wants to raise, he asks if there are any issues Nina or Kam wishes to add, and if they will be able to sign the representations that Tariq has drafted. Nina points to one line in the representation letter and says, "We will need to alter this line about us not being aware of any legal claims against the company. Our lawyer has advised us that even though this is a remote possibility, and could never add up to more than a very small amount, there is a possible legal claim against us that we should let you know about. But we are not going to accrue or even disclose the matter—in our view it is a ridiculous claim that should not be given the time of day, let alone a disclosure in our financial statements! I am not going to let something so stupid jeopardize our debt covenants or our opportunity to make an IPO next year."

Donna is quite upset by the all this emotion and animosity from Nina, but she is very impressed with how Tariq is able to calm everything down. "No need to jump to any conclusions now, Nina," he replies. "If the claim is remote and not likely to amount to a material amount, the treatment you are suggesting, no accrual or disclosure, may well be acceptable under GAAP. But as independent auditors, you understand that we will need to have more of the details, and it would be preferable if your lawyer could provide them, so we can meet our responsibility to base our conclusion on sufficient appropriate evidence."

Once the secret is out, Donna feels the air clear quickly, and the good relations with Nina and Kam return. Nina agrees to contact Charles and give him permission to respond to the inquiry with all the details of the possible claim he has been working on. After the meeting, Donna and Caleb pack up their things to head back to their own office. As they are saying goodbye to Nina, she says to them, "Thanks to you both for your efficient work and being so considerate of my staff's time. I know a few more questions will probably come up as you tie up all the loose ends to complete the audit documentation files, so don't hesitate to call me if I can help. Take care!"

The Essentials of Completing the Audit Work

So far in our coverage of the financial statement audit process, we have looked at the evidence-gathering programs auditors perform related to the auditee's main accounting processes. As the engagement gets nearer to its end, auditors must address some final matters to complete their work. First, they must analyze the income statement to ensure it fairly presents the categories of revenue and expenses and is consistent with the evidence they obtained from auditing all the major balance sheet accounts and transactions. Additional substantive procedures may be required on specific income statement items that were not yet examined sufficiently. The auditors must also review the rest of the financial statements: the cash flow statement, statement of changes in equity, and note disclosures. To complete the audit, auditors also look for evidence regarding any unrecorded liabilities, additional contingencies, commitments, and subsequent events that should be reflected in the financial statements. Since all of these matters can be material to financial statement users, management is responsible for incorporating them into the financial statements and disclosures to fairly present the financial condition, performance, and cash flows of the business for the period, in accordance with generally accepted accounting principles (GAAP). The final evidence to be gathered is management's written representations regarding the fair presentation of the financial statements. The auditors will also perform a final overall analysis of the financial statements to make sure the whole set is presented appropriately and is consistent with the evidence obtained and documented in the audit files. This final analysis is usually done by the engagement partner.

These last procedures are done as late as possible in the engagement, so they are as up to date as possible when the auditor dates and issues the auditor's report. The audit report date is critical because it indicates to users the point up to which the auditors have searched for evidence about the fair presentation of the financial statements. While the above completion procedures are always required by generally accepted auditing standards (GAAS), note that others may also be considered necessary in a particular audit, in the auditor's judgment. The essentials of these completion procedures are as follows.

The auditor must analyze the income statement to ensure that it is consistent with the evidence obtained in auditing the main accounting processes and properly classified into relevant descriptive income categories: revenue, expense, gain, or loss. Note that the main audit procedures have provided evidence on the period-end balance sheet numbers and changes in them over the period. This change in the net assets (net assets = assets − liabilities) ties into the bottom line on the statement of income because of the mathematical articulation of the financial statements (i.e., change in net assets ± transactions with shareholders = income for the period). So if the change in net assets is materially correct, and changes in the shareholders' accounts are correct, the only misstatements that can exist in the income statement will be due to misclassifying the income elements. Misclassifications affect the fairness of presentation because they can prevent financial statement readers from understanding the composition and trends in the main drivers of the company's financial performance. Similarly, since the cash balance and change in it for the period will have been audited thoroughly, the auditor must now analyze the cash flow statement components to ensure the classification into financing, investing, and operating cash flow categories is fairly presented. The major items presented in the cash flow statement, such as additions to property, plant, and equipment (PPE); repayments of long-term debt; and dividends paid, will also tie into the auditor's analysis of the change in the related balance sheet account (PPE, long-term debt, and retained earnings, respectively).

Contingencies are matters that may have a material impact, but only if some future event occurs. An example is when the company is being sued, but the law court's judgment has not been decided yet. GAAP require contingent liability amounts that are measurable and will probably become payable to be recognized as provisions in the balance sheet. If there is less probability that the contingency will occur or if the amount cannot be measured with reasonable certainty, contingencies still require disclosure in the financial statement notes. *Commitments* are contracts that bind the company to make transactions under fixed terms in the future, which may end up not to be in the company's favour. An example is a commitment to sell goods for a fixed price for the next two years—even if the market price of the goods goes up, the company is stuck with the fixed price. Since commitments affect future cash flows, information about them has to be provided in the notes to help users predict performance.

Subsequent events are events that occur after the financial statement period, but before the financial statements are authorized and issued. These events could either reduce some uncertainty about amounts reported in the financial statements or indicate important changes that could have a material effect on the company in the future. The auditor must consider whether such events are significant enough to require inclusion in the financial statements. If a subsequent event affects the financial position at the period-end, adjustment is required. For example, say a large, highly material note receivable from a customer was expected to be collected when due, so no allowance was set up in the financial statements for the year ended on December 31, 20X1. If the auditee learns in January 20X2 that the customer went bankrupt in December 20X1, that note receivable should be written off in the 20X1 year-end financial statements. The new information relates to conditions that existed at the 20X1 year-end, so it is relevant to include in the financial statements. If the bankruptcy didn't occur until January 20X2, it would be a different situation, since at the 20X1 year-end the financial statements were not misstated; they reflect the facts as of that date. But since the note receivable is material, there should be a disclosure in the 20X1 financial statement notes. The note will give users important information for better understanding the impact of this event on the future financial condition and performance of the auditee. Other examples of events that occur after year-end but require disclosure in the year-end notes are new issue of common shares or a large amount of long-term debt—these affect the future financial condition and the equity interests of the current shareholders, so fair presentation requires that they be informed, even though these events did not directly affect the financial statement balances at the year-end.

To seek evidence about whether any contingencies, commitments, or material subsequent events have not been picked up through the regular payables and financing accounting processes, auditors use investigation procedures such as confirmation with the auditee's lawyers, scanning of transactions and bank records after the year-end, inquiries of management, inspection of contracts and minutes of directors' meetings, and review of current events that may be relevant to the auditee's business. Auditors perform these procedures as late as possible during the audit engagement because they are responsible for searching for evidence that is relevant to the fair presentation of the financial statements up until the date of their auditor's report.

Finally, auditors must obtain specific *written representations* from management to confirm that all the information it has provided to the auditors during the engagement has been accurate and complete and that it is not aware of any matters that have not been properly reported in the financial statements. These written representations by themselves do not provide sufficient appropriate audit evidence because they are essentially just inquiry-based evidence. Still, the representations are necessary to support the other audit evidence obtained and are required by CAS 580.

Once the evidence-gathering procedures are completed, senior audit team members review the files to ensure that all the planning, evidence obtained, audit judgments, and conclusions recorded there are complete and clearly documented. This body of evidence supports the last step in the audit process, in which the audit engagement partner takes final responsibility for forming an opinion and issuing the auditor's report. This involves reviewing the documentation to ensure that sufficient and appropriate evidence has been obtained to achieve reasonable assurance that the financial statements are not materially misstated (i.e., the scope of the audit has not been restricted in any significant way). It also involves evaluating the nature and extent of all the misstatements discovered by the audit to conclude whether the financial statements fairly present the financial position, performance, cash flows, and supplementary information required to comply with GAAP (i.e., the financial statements are not materially misstated in any aspect). This final judgment in forming the audit opinion will be discussed in Chapter 16.

Review Checkpoints

15-1   What are the main evidence-gathering procedures that are left until the last part of the engagement? Why are these procedures done as late as possible in the engagement?

15-2   What is the purpose of the auditor's evaluation of the income statement?

15-3   What is the purpose of the auditor's review of the complete set of financial statements that management has prepared for audit?

15-4   How does the analysis of the income statement link to the audit of the balance sheet accounts and the changes in them over the period?

15-5   How can misclassifications within the income statement affect fair presentation, even if the bottom-line net income is not misstated?

15-6   What is the auditor's main goal in analyzing the cash flow statement?

15-7   Give examples of important items in a cash flow statement that will tie into balance sheet account analyses.

15-8   What are contingencies? How are they presented in financial statements to comply with GAAP? Why?

15-9   What are commitments? How are they presented in financial statements to comply with GAAP? Why?

15-10   What are subsequent events? Distinguish two main types.

15-11   Which type of subsequent event requires adjustment to the period-end financial statements under GAAP? Give an example, and explain why this presentation is required by GAAP.

15-12   Which type of subsequent event is not adjusted for in the period-end financial statements under GAAP but requires disclosure in the notes? Give an example, and explain why this presentation is required by GAAP.

15-13   What kinds of procedures do auditors use to get evidence related to contingencies, commitments, and subsequent events? When during the audit engagement process do auditors perform these procedures? Why?

15-14   What are written representations? Why do auditors require them from management?

15-15   What kind of evidence is provided by written representations by management? Explain how this evidence is necessary, but not sufficient, according to GAAS.

15-16   What is contained in a set of completed audit files?

The Completion Stage of the Audit

The completion stage of the audit can be viewed as the nexus of all the audit work and judgments involved in reaching a final conclusion on whether the financial statements are fairly presented. All members of the audit team are involved in this final stage, but especially so the most experienced members, such as the audit **engagement partner**, who makes the final decision on the audit opinion. The activities and decisions at the completion stage are advanced topics in auditing, but in this introductory text, we present them to finish the story of how the audit work supports the ultimate and public product of the audit engagement, the auditor's report. Many of the procedures and decisions we will discuss occur concurrently. Exhibit 15–1 provides an overview, showing these activities as a framework for the discussion in this and the next chapter.

EXHIBIT 15–1

Audit Completion Activities and Judgments

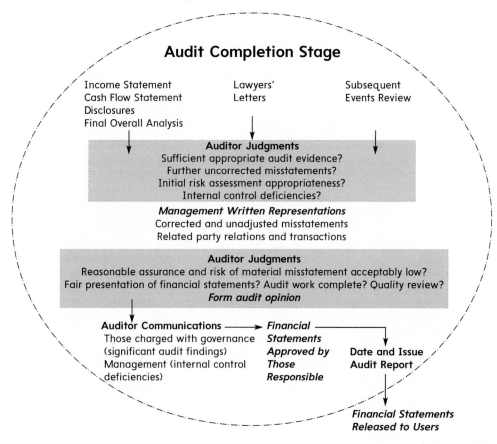

Completing the Audit of Revenues and Expenses

LO1 Describe the balance sheet account groups that the major revenue and expense accounts are associated with, as well as the substantive analytical procedures applied to audit revenues and expenses.

As the field work nears its end, the major revenue and expense accounts will have been audited in connection with related balance sheet accounts. Next, auditors need to consider other revenue and expense accounts. The broad financial statement assertions are the basis for specific assertions and audit objectives for these accounts. Those typical to the revenue and expense accounts are as follows:

1. Revenue accounts represent all the valid transactions recorded correctly in the proper account, amount, and period.

engagement partner:
one of the most experienced members of the audit team, who makes the final decision on the audit opinion

2. Revenue recognition policies are in accordance with established accounting principles and are consistent with the underlying economic substance of the earnings process.

3. Expense accounts represent all the valid expense transactions recorded correctly in the proper account, amount, and period.

4. Revenues, expenses, and cost of goods sold, as well as extraordinary, unusual, or infrequent transactions, are adequately classified and disclosed.

Revenue

The following types of revenue and related topics will have been audited, either in whole or in part, prior to the completion stage of the engagement:

REVENUE AND RELATED TOPICS	RELATED ACCOUNT GROUPS
Sales and sales returns	Receivables
Lease revenue	Fixed assets and receivables
Franchise revenue	Receivables and intangibles
Dividends and interest	Receivables and investments
Gain or loss on asset disposals	Fixed assets, receivables, and investments
Rental revenue	Receivables and investments
Royalty and licence revenue	Receivables and investments
Long-term sales commitments	Revenue and receivables
Product-line reporting	Revenue and receivables
Accounting policy disclosure	Revenue and receivables

The working papers' cross-references to the revenue accounts in the trial balance should reflect the extent to which the revenue items have already been audited with the related accounts, and revenues not audited completely should be evident. By reviewing the trial balance cross-references, auditors will verify that all revenue and gain or loss accounts and their amounts are listed.

Analytical procedures can be used as substantive procedures to compare the revenue accounts and amounts with prior-year data and with multiple-year trends to look for unusual fluctuations. Comparisons with budgets, internal monthly reports and forecasts, and relevant non-financial data will determine whether any events need explanation or analysis. The explanations will then be verified by further audit procedures. For example, if management explains that the sales dollar increase is a consequence of a price increase, the auditor can corroborate that by referencing price lists used in the audit tests of sales transactions.

All miscellaneous or other revenue accounts and all clearing accounts with credit balances are analyzed by identifying each important item and amount in the account, followed by document vouching and inquiry to determine whether amounts should be classified elsewhere. All clearing accounts should be eliminated and the amounts classified as revenue, deferred revenue, liabilities, deposits, or contra-assets. Miscellaneous revenue and clearing accounts can harbour accounting errors, since accountants use them for unusual items they are not sure how to record, for example, proceeds from sale of assets, insurance premium refunds, and insurance proceeds.

Exhibit 15–2 shows selected procedures that would be part of an audit program for revenues and expenses. The audit program in Exhibit 15–2 also includes procedures for assessing the reasonability of sales taxes collected or collectible (e.g., HST/GST or PST). Because these taxes apply to many of the revenue and expense items, they are best audited in this program.

EXHIBIT 15–2

Example of an Audit Program for Revenues and Expenses: Selected Procedures

REVENUES

1. Obtain auditee's monthly analyses of sales, cost of goods sold, and gross profit by product line, department, division, or location.
   (a) Trace amounts to the general ledger.
   (b) Compare the analyses with prior years, and seek explanations for significant variations.
   (c) Determine one or more standard markup percentages and calculate expected gross profits. Inquire for explanations of significant variations compared with actual results.

2. Coordinate procedures for audit of revenue with evidence obtained in other audit programs:

Sales and sales returns	Sales control	Gain, loss on asset disposals	Fixed assets
	Cash receipts control		Investments
	Accounts receivable	Rental revenue	Accounts receivable
Lease revenue	Capital assets		Investments
	Accounts receivable	Royalty and licence revenue	Accounts receivable
Franchise revenue	Accounts receivable		Intangibles
	Intangibles	Long-term sales commitments	Accounts receivable
Dividends and interest	Accounts receivable		Inventory
	Investments		

3. Scan the revenue accounts for large or unusual items and for debit entries. Inquire as to the nature of any such items. Vouch to supporting documentation.

4. Obtain written management representations about terms of sales, completeness of recorded sales transactions, rights of return, consignments, classification of crowdfunding receipts (equity or revenue?), and unusual or infrequent transactions.

EXPENSES

5. Obtain schedules of expense accounts comparing the current year with one or more prior years.
   (a) Trace amounts to the general ledger.
   (b) Compare the current expenses to prior years, and seek explanations for significant variations.
   (c) Be alert to significant variations that could indicate failure to defer or accrue expenses.

6. Compare the current expenses with the company budget, if any. Inquire for and investigate explanations of significant variances.

7. Coordinate procedures for audit of expenses with evidence obtained in other audit programs:

Purchases, cost of goods sold	Acquisition control	Bad debt expense	Accounts receivable
	Cash disbursement control	Depreciation expense	Fixed assets
	Inventory	Property taxes, insurance	Prepaids and accruals
Inventory valuation losses	Inventory		Fixed assets
Warranty and guarantee expense	Inventory	Lease and rental expense	Fixed assets
	Prepaids and accruals	Repairs and maintenance	Fixed assets
	Accounts payable	Interest expense	Long-term liabilities
Royalty and licence expense	Inventory	Pension and retirement benefits	Liabilities
Marketing and product research	Investments	Payroll and compensation	Payroll control
and development	Intangibles		Payroll control
Investment value losses	Investments	Sales commissions	Payroll control
Rental property expenses	Investments		
Amortization of intangibles	Intangibles		

8. Prepare analyses of sensitive expense accounts, such as legal and professional fees, travel and entertainment, repairs and maintenance, taxes, and others unique to the company. Vouch significant items therein to supporting invoices, contracts, reimbursement forms, tax notices, and the like for proper support and documentation.

9. Scan the expense accounts for large or unusual items and for credit entries. Inquire as to the nature of any such items. Vouch to supporting documentation.

10. Obtain written management representations about long-term purchase commitments, contingencies, completeness of recorded expenses, and unusual or infrequent transactions.

(continued)

EXHIBIT 15–2

Example of an Audit Program for Revenues and Expenses: Selected Procedures *(continued)*

SALES TAXES

11. Obtain an understanding of the sales tax legislation the auditee company must follow (e.g., HST/GST, PST).

12. Review the trial balance income statement accounts to identify all revenue and expense accounts that would attract HST/GST or other sales taxes.

13. Obtain or prepare a summary of the client's sales tax return filings (e.g., monthly, quarterly, or annual HST/GST filings for CRA) showing all remittances or refunds for the audited period.

14. Identify any adjustments necessary, such as the capitalization or disposal of assets, inventory adjustments, or zero-rated supplies.

15. For HST/GST, recalculate the HST/GST receivable and payable and reconcile to summary of client filings to determine reasonability. If there are any unexplained differences, discuss with management to resolve them.

16. Agree the HST/GST remittances/refunds information to the continuity schedule for related balance sheet HST/GST recoverable/payable account(s).

Expenses

Most major expense items will have been audited in connection with other account groupings, but minor expenses may still be unaudited. As a brief review, the following major expenses may have been audited in whole or in part as the audit nears its end:

EXPENSES	RELATED ACCOUNT GROUPS
Purchases and cost of goods sold	Inventories
Inventory valuation losses	Inventories
Warranty and guarantee expenses	Inventories and liabilities
Royalty and licence expenses	Inventories and liabilities
Marketing and product research and development	Investments and intangibles
Investment value losses	Investments and intangibles
Rental property expenses	Investments and intangibles
Amortization of intangibles	Investments and intangibles
Bad debt expenses	Receivables
Amortization expenses	Fixed assets
Property taxes and insurance expenses	Fixed assets and liabilities
Lease and rental expenses	Fixed assets
Repairs and maintenance expenses	Fixed assets and liabilities
Legal and professional fees	Liabilities
Interest expense	Liabilities
Pension and retirement benefits	Liabilities and payroll
Payroll and compensation costs	Payroll
Sales commissions	Payroll

As with the revenue accounts mentioned in the previous section, if audit work is complete for expense accounts, there will be cross-referencing from the working papers to the trial balance. Some significant expenses may not have been audited completely (such as property tax expense), and some finishing-touch vouching of supporting documents may be required.

Minor expenses, such as office supplies, telephone, utilities, and similar accounts, are not audited until late in the engagement. Generally, the dollar amounts in these individual accounts are not material, and there is little relative risk that they will result in misleading financial statements. Auditors usually audit these kinds of accounts with substantive analytical procedures, such as comparing the balances with those of one or more prior periods. The dollar amounts are reviewed for unusual changes (or lack thereof, if reasons for change are known). Comparing balances and inquiring to get reasonable explanations may be enough to decide whether the amounts are fairly presented.

On the other hand, the questions may suggest a risk of misstatement. If more evidence is needed, auditors may vouch some expenses to supporting documents (invoices, cancelled cheques, correspondence with professional advisors). If the auditors performed tests of controls on a sample of expenditure transactions in the purchases, payables, and payments process audit program, some of these expense transactions were selected for testing auditee compliance with control objectives (validity, completeness, authorization, accuracy, classification, and proper period). This evidence should be used. Analytical comparisons with budgets, internal reports and forecasts, and relevant non-financial data may also be made. Management may have already explained any variations from the budget, or the auditors may need to investigate variations.

All miscellaneous or other expense accounts and clearing accounts with debit balances should be analyzed by listing each important item on a working paper and vouching it to supporting documents. These may include abandonments of property, items not deductible for tax purposes, and payments that should be classified in other expense accounts. Clearing accounts should be analyzed and the contents classified by type or source and accounted for properly.

Advertising, travel and entertainment expense, and charitable donations accounts are analyzed in detail because they are particularly sensitive to management policy violations and income tax consequences. They must be documented carefully if they are to stand a Canada Revenue Agency (CRA) auditor's examination. Questionable items may have an impact on the income tax expense and liability. Minor embezzlements or falsification can be detected by careful auditors; however, a detailed audit of expense account payments may be of greater interest to the efficiency-minded internal auditor than to the independent auditor. The independent auditors are concerned that the paid-out amount is fairly presented, regardless of whether employees overstated their expenses. Evidence of expense account falsification may be presented to management, but the overpayments are still an expense of the business and need to be included in its financial statements.

Review Checkpoints

15-17   Certain revenue and expense accounts are usually audited in conjunction with related balance sheet accounts. List the most likely related balance sheet accounts for these revenue and expense accounts: lease revenue, franchise revenue, royalty and licence revenue, amortization expense, repairs and maintenance expense, and interest expense.

15-18   Why are many of the revenue and expense accounts audited by analytical procedures only?

15-19   What procedures can be applied to audit minor expense accounts?

Overall Analytical Procedures

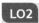 Outline the overall analytical procedures to be performed at the final stage of the audit, including analysis of the income statement, cash flow statement, financial statement presentation, and disclosures.

Analytical procedures are used at these three points during the audit:

1. For risk assessment at the planning stage (discussed in Chapter 6)

2. As a substantive test procedure (discussed in Chapters 8, 11–14)

3. During the overall evaluation of the financial statements at the end of the audit

Canadian Auditing Standards (CASs) require the auditor to design and perform **overall analytical procedures** at the completion stage of the audit to help form a conclusion about whether the financial statements are a fair representation of what the auditors learned in the course of the audit (CAS 520). Using analytical procedures to assess the reasonableness of reported results after most of the audit work has been performed is an effective means of obtaining assurance.

Standards Check

CAS 520 Analytical Procedures

Analytical Procedures That Assist When Forming an Overall Conclusion
6. The auditor shall design and perform analytical procedures near the end of the audit that assist the auditor when forming an overall conclusion as to whether the financial statements are consistent with the auditor's understanding of the entity. (Ref: Para. A17–A19)

Source: *CPA Canada Handbook–Assurance,* 2014.

The results of overall analytical procedures on the final draft financial statements help the auditor reach reasonable conclusions to base the auditor's opinion on. The procedures are similar to those for risk assessment, for example, comparing financial and non-financial data and examining ratios and trends for unexpected relationships. However, by performing this analysis at a late stage in the audit, the auditors have the benefit of considerable knowledge about the auditee's business and a better basis on which to form expectations about the financial statement relationships, increasing their chances of noticing something out of line. This analysis can be sharper and more focused on finding potential misstatements than the preliminary risk assessment was. It may identify a risk of material misstatement not recognized at the early stage, in which case the planned audit procedures are revised to address this new risk. The final analysis procedures are a very important over-arching element of forming an audit opinion and will be referred to again as we consider different steps in finalizing the audit report in Chapter 16.

The cash flow statement is prepared after the balance sheet and income statement are finalized, so it is audited at the completion stage of the audit. Verifying the cash flow statement explains the major changes

overall analytical procedures:
analysis designed and performed near the end of an audit engagement to assist the auditor in forming an overall conclusion about whether the financial statements are consistent with the auditor's understanding of the auditee's business and with the audit evidence obtained

in balance sheet accounts and thus provides analytical evidence that the financial statement relations are properly presented. It also bridges the balance sheet and income statement by explaining the relationship between net income and operating cash flow when the indirect method is used. These alternative presentations of the financial performance and changes in financial position should be evaluated by the auditors in relation to their knowledge of the year's activity. For example, a large financing inflow from new debt should match up with disclosure about the new loan. Also, many items of the cash flow will tie into audits of other balances; for example, cash flows for both additions to and proceeds from disposal of fixed assets should tie in to audit working paper information on fixed assets.

Auditors also verify the information presented in the statement of changes in retained earnings and shareholders' equity at this stage to ascertain that account classifications, aggregations, and summarizations are comparable to those of the prior year in an assessment of the consistency of the financial reporting and the overall adequacy of disclosures. Certain other tests done in the completion procedures of the engagement, such as the search for contingent liabilities, commitments, and guarantees, will result in information that requires disclosure but no amounts recognized on the balance sheet. Auditors may use a checklist to ensure all disclosures required by GAAP are considered. An example of such a checklist is shown in the box that follows. Remember that checklists like this are useful starting points for auditors, but they need to be tailored to the circumstances of each audit engagement—they are not a substitute for the auditor's judgments about what is relevant in a particular situation.

FINANCIAL STATEMENT PRESENTATION AND DISCLOSURE CHECKLIST

AUDITEE: ECOPAK INC.		**FILE INDEX:** 315	
FINANCIAL STATEMENT PERIOD: y/e DECEMBER 31, 20x1			
This checklist is to be used to assess whether the financial statements and the notes include all required disclosures for fair presentation.	Disclosure assertions [ORO, C, CU, AV*]	Response	File reference
Consider the following: Do the notes include, where relevant, all specific disclosure requirements as per GAAP** or applicable financial reporting framework, such as the following? • a statement of compliance with GAAP (e.g., IFRS or ASPE) • a summary of significant accounting policies applied, explaining the measurement basis used in preparing the financial statements, and all other accounting policies relevant to understanding the financial statements • information about significant judgments management made • information about major sources of estimation uncertainty and assumptions that could result in material adjustments to carrying values of assets and liabilities in the next financial period Is supporting information for significant financial statement items included in the notes, correctly cross-referenced, and in the order in which each item is presented, including • contingent liabilities, commitments, guarantees? • related party transactions? • details of significant income and cash flow statement components? • any income statement components that are unusual and not expected to occur frequently? • non-financial information about risk management and capital management objectives and policies? • impaired assets? • discontinued operations?			

(continued)

	Disclosure assertions [ORO, C, CU, AV*]	Response	File reference
Is other information required for fair presentation disclosed, such as • going-concern uncertainties? • accounting changes? • dividends declared after period-end but before financial statements are issued, and cumulative preferred dividends not recognized? • restatements? Is the comparative information provided appropriate? Do all events, transactions, and other information presented and disclosed in the financial statements pertain to the entity? Are the disclosures complete, based on the audit findings?			

AUDITOR'S CONCLUSION

Based on my professional judgment, the evidence related to the appropriateness and completeness of overall financial statement presentation and disclosures supports the conclusion that the financial statements are fairly presented in accordance with the applicable financial reporting framework:

_____

_____

_____

Prepared by _____   Date _____

Reviewed by _____   Date _____

Notes:

* CAS 315, paragraph A111(c), sets out special assertions related to presentation and disclosure that reflect their purpose in augmenting the financial statements for users by providing further details and interpretations, as follows:

    (i) Occurrence and rights and obligations—disclosed events, transactions, and other matters have occurred and pertain to the entity. [ORO]

    (ii) Completeness—all disclosures that should have been included in the financial statements have been included. [C]

    (iii) Classification and understandability—financial information is appropriately presented and described, and disclosures are clearly expressed. [CU]

    (iv) Accuracy and valuation—financial and other information is disclosed fairly and at appropriate amounts. [AV]

** International Financial Reporting Standards (IFRS) and Accounting Standards for Private Enterprises (ASPE) are sets of GAAP. For IFRS, IAS 1 provides requirements for presentation and disclosure in financial statements. For ASPE, *CPA Canada Handbook—Accounting,* Part II, section 1400, provides disclosure requirements.

Unusual Transactions

Significant audit evidence and reporting problems can arise if management transactions artificially create earnings. Generally, these transactions will run through a complicated structure of subsidiaries, affiliates, and related parties, and they involve large amounts of revenue. While transactions may not be concealed, there might be certain guarantees that management has not revealed to the auditors. The transactions may be carefully designed and timed to provide the most favourable income result.

It is difficult to characterize these **unusual transactions** because they vary so widely. Controversies have arisen in the past over revenue recognized on bundled sales of hardware, software, and technology

unusual transactions:

a term used to describe a variety of transactions that may be artificially created to manipulate financial statements, especially earnings, and that tend to be complex and difficult for auditors to understand and verify services; on the construction percentage-of-completion method; on sales of assets at inflated prices to management-controlled dummy corporations; on sales of real estate to independent parties with whom the seller later associates for development of the property (making guarantees on indemnification for losses); and on disclosure of revenues by source. Often transactions are designed to exploit weaknesses or loopholes in the current accounting standards, the "gaps in GAAP." These revenue issues pose a combination of evidence-gathering and reporting-disclosure problems. Three illustrations of such problems are given in the box that follows.

Unusual Revenue Transactions

Merger

National Fried Chicken Inc., a large fast-food franchiser, began negotiations in August to purchase Provincial Hot Dog Company, a smaller convenience food chain. At August 1, 20X6, Provincial's net worth was $7 million, and National proposed to pay $8 million cash for all the outstanding shares. In June 20X7, the merger was consummated and National paid $8 million, even though Provincial's net worth had dropped to $6 million by that time. Consistent with prior years, Provincial lost $1 million in the 10 months ended June 1, 20X7, after showing a net profit of $1.5 million for June and July 20X7. At June 1, 20X7, the fair value of Provincial's net assets was $6 million, and National accounted for the acquisition as a purchase, recording $2 million in goodwill. National proposed to show in consolidated financial statements the $1.5 million of post-acquisition income.

Audit Resolution. The auditors discovered that the purchase price was basically set at 16 times expected earnings and that management had carefully chosen the consummation date in order to maximize goodwill (and reportable net income in fiscal 20X7). The auditors required that $1 million of goodwill be treated as a goodwill impairment in the year ended July 31, 20X7, so that bottom-line income would be $500,000.

Real Estate Deal

In August, a company sold three real estate properties to BMC for $5,399,000 and recognized profit of $550,000. The agreement covering the sale committed the company to use its best efforts to obtain permanent financing and to pay underwriting costs for BMC. The agreement also provided BMC with an absolute guarantee against loss from ownership and a commitment by the company to complete construction of the properties.

Audit Resolution. The auditors determined that the terms of this agreement made the recognition of profit improper because the company had not shifted the risk of loss to BMC.

Real Estate Development, Strings Attached

In December 20X6, Black Company sold one half of a tract of undeveloped land to Red Company in an apparent arm's-length transaction. The portion sold had a book value of $1.5 million, and Red Company paid $2.5 million in cash. Red Company planned to build and sell apartment houses on the acquired land. In January 20X7, Black and Red formed a new joint venture to develop the entire tract. The two companies formed a partnership, each contributing its one half of the total tract of land. They agreed to share equally in future capital requirements and profits or losses.

Audit Resolution. The auditor discovered that Black and Red were both controlled by the same person. The $1 million profit from the sale was not recognized as income in Black's 20X6 financial statements, and Black's investment in the joint venture was valued at $1.5 million.

Review Checkpoints

15-20   How might unusual revenue transactions cause significant audit evidence and reporting problems?

15-21   How are analytical procedures used for overall evaluation of the financial statements at the final stage of the audit? How does the use of analysis at this stage differ from its use at the risk assessment stage? at the substantive evidence–gathering stage?

15-22   What procedures can be used to verify the accuracy of the information presented in the cash flow statement?

Sequencing of Audit Events

At this point, it is helpful to note the sequencing of audit events. Based on the organization of the audit, some audit work might be done at an interim period some time before the balance sheet date, followed by completion of the work at later dates. Interim audit work is done months before the balance sheet date, with auditors working at the auditee's offices for a time, leaving, and then returning at the exact balance sheet date for certain procedures, such as cutoff tests, and then returning again after the balance sheet date for the year-end field work. At the year-end visit, the auditor will have the first draft of management's unaudited financial statements (or trial balance) prepared by the auditee personnel. The audit team can then start where the interim work left off, completing the work on control risk assessment and audit of balances. Certain procedures, however, such as lawyers' letters, written management representation letters, and subsequent events reviews, discussed below, are always left to the final stages of the audit work. Often, they will be completed back at the audit firm's office after the field work visit has finished. These written communications are dated as close as possible to the audit report date because the auditors are responsible until that date for determining whether important events occurring after the balance sheet date are properly entered in the accounts or disclosed in the financial statement notes.

Procedures to Detect Contingencies and Claims

LO3 Explain the procedures used at the audit completion stage to identify any contingencies and contractual commitments, including the use of lawyers' letters.

Fair presentation of the financial statements requires that appropriate recognition and measurement policies be applied so that users get enough information about the nature, timing, and extent of future obligations. **Contingent liabilities** are possible obligations of a company that will be confirmed only if some future event occurs, where whether it occurs is not totally within the company's control. A contingent liability is not recognized as a *provision* in the balance sheet unless its amount can be estimated reliably and it is probable that the future event giving rise to it will occur, but its existence must be disclosed in the notes. **Contingencies** can also give rise to possible assets; *contingent assets* would be disclosed if they are probably going to be received by the entity, but are never recognized as assets in the balance sheet until the future event confirms their existence.

    Commitments are contracts that establish both rights and obligations for each of the contracting parties. When neither party has performed any of the obligations, the contract is called an *executory contract*; these are not recognized as liabilities because no obligation exists yet. However, significant commitments should still be disclosed because they provide important information for users about the timing and extent of future cash flows. An exceptional situation to consider is when an executory contract is considered to be an *onerous contract* because it imposes unavoidable costs on the company that exceed the expected benefits. If a contract is onerous, a liability exists and must be recognized.

contingent liabilities:
possible obligations of a company that will be confirmed only if some future event occurs; if probable to occur and measurable they are recognized as a *provision* in the balance sheet unless their amount can be estimated reliably and it is probable that the future event giving rise to them will occur, but their existence must be disclosed in the notes

contingencies:
existing situations involving uncertainty about one or more future events that when resolved may confirm an increase or decrease in an asset or liability; assessed at the completion stage of an audit to determine whether fairly presented in the balance sheet and/or notes

commitments:
contracts that establish both rights and obligations for each of the contracting parties relating to the amounts and timing of future cash flows; assessed at the completion stage of an audit to determine whether fairly presented in the balance sheet and/or notes

The main audit procedures performed to get evidence about contingencies and commitments are inspecting contracts and legal correspondence, reviewing minutes of directors' meetings, obtaining lawyer's letters from the auditee's lawyers confirming any outstanding claims against the auditee, and obtaining written management representations regarding contingencies and commitments. The lawyer's letter provides the most reliable evidence for these items and is discussed in detail next.

Communication with Auditee's Lawyer

The **lawyer's confirmation letter** is one of the most important audit confirmations. CAS 501 requires auditors to perform procedures identifying litigation and claims against the auditee, and where there is a risk of material misstatement, auditors must communicate directly with the auditee's legal counsel. This is done by an inquiry letter from management to the lawyer, with a copy of the lawyer's response going directly from the lawyer to the auditor. The objective is to provide audit evidence about any potentially material litigation or claims against the auditee, to determine if management's estimates of the possible costs of these are reasonable, and to assess whether there are any unrecorded liabilities that should be reported in the financial statements. Exhibit 15–3 is an example of an inquiry letter. The auditor asks management to send inquiry letters to all lawyers who performed work for the auditee during the period under audit. This request informs the lawyer that their client, the auditee, is waiving the privilege of confidentiality of communications between lawyer and client, permitting the lawyer to give information to the auditors.

As implied by the letter in Exhibit 15–3, questions about contingencies, litigations, claims, and assessments should be directed to both legal counsel and management because an auditor has the right to expect to be informed by management about all material contingent liabilities. Audit procedures useful in this regard include the following:

- Inquire and discuss with management the policies and procedures for identifying, evaluating, and accounting for litigation, claims, and assessments.
- Obtain from management a description and evaluation of litigation, claims, and assessments.
- Examine documents in the auditee's possession concerning litigation, claims, and assessments, including correspondence and invoices from lawyers.
- Obtain assurance from management that it has disclosed all material unasserted claims that the lawyer has advised them might result in litigation.
- Read minutes of meetings of shareholders, directors, and appropriate committees. Read contracts, loan agreements, leases, and correspondence from taxing or other governmental agencies.
- Obtain information concerning guarantees from bank confirmations.

The inquiry letter is an effective means of learning about material contingencies. Even so, a devious or forgetful management or a careless lawyer may fail to tell the auditor of some important factor or development. Auditors have to be alert and sensitive to all possible contingencies so that they can ask the right questions at the right time. Auditors have a natural tendency to look out for adverse contingencies, but potentially favourable events should also be investigated and disclosed (such as the contingency of litigation for damages when the auditee is the plaintiff). If management or its lawyers fail to provide adequate information about lawsuit contingencies, the auditor should consider whether this represents a scope limitation on the audit. A serious audit scope limitation requires a qualification in the audit report or a disclaimer of opinion.

Auditors face other challenges when it comes to using lawyers' responses to audit the presentation and disclosure of contingencies. The box after Exhibit 15–3 illustrates the kind of wording lawyers use in their letters.

lawyer's confirmation letter:
an inquiry letter sent from the auditee's management to the auditee's lawyer, with a copy of the lawyer's response going directly from the lawyer to the auditor to provide audit evidence about any potentially material litigation or claims involving the auditee; obtained at the completion stage of the audit to assess whether all claims are fairly presented in the balance sheet and/or notes

EXHIBIT 15–3

Sample Lawyer Letter*

(Version for use when there are claims or possible claims to be listed)

[On client letterhead]

[To law firm]

[Date]

Dear Sir(s) or Madam(s):

In connection with the preparation and audit of our financial statements for the fiscal period ended [date] [which include the accounts of the following entities**], we have made the following evaluations of claims and possible claims with respect to which your firm's advice or representation has been sought:

Description	Evaluation
[name of entity, name of other party, nature, amount claimed, and current status]	[Indicate likelihood of loss (or gain) and estimated amount of ultimate loss (or gain), if any, or indicate that likelihood is not determinable or amount is not reasonably estimable.]

Would you please advise us, as of [effective date of response], on the following points:

(a) Are the claims and possible claims properly described?

(b) Do you consider that our evaluations are reasonable?

(c) Are you aware of any claims not listed above that are outstanding? If so, please include in your response letter the names of the parties and the amount claimed.

This inquiry is made in accordance with the Joint Policy Statement of January 1978 approved by The Canadian Bar Association and the Auditing and Assurance Standards Board of CPA Canada.

Please address your reply, marked "Privileged and Confidential," to this company and send a signed copy of the reply directly to our auditor, [name and address of auditor].

Yours truly,

c.c. [name of auditor]

---

* The letter should be appropriately modified if the client advises that certain matters have been excluded in accordance with paragraph 12 of the Joint Policy Statement.

** Delete if inapplicable. If applicable, refer to paragraph 11 regarding signing of the inquiry letter.

Source: © *CPA Canada Handbook*, CAS 501.

Interpreting the Lawyers' Letter

Lawyers take great care in forming responses to auditees' requests for information to be transmitted to auditors. This care causes problems of interpretation for auditors. The difficulty arises over lawyers' desire to preserve lawyer–client confidentiality yet cooperate with auditors and the financial reporting process that seeks full disclosure.

The Canadian Bar Association policy statement observes that "[i]t is in the public interest that the confidentiality of lawyer–client communications be maintained." Accordingly, any *possible* claims omitted from the inquiry letter will not be referred to by the law firm in its response letter.[1]

However, the policy statement does require the law firm to specify in its response any *identified* claim that has been omitted from the client's inquiry letter. It notes that it is in the public interest that financial statements contain all disclosures and adjustments necessary for fair presentation; thus, the law firm should discuss any omitted possible claims with the client to ensure the client is informed of its responsibility to inform its auditor of such matters.

Consequently, lawyers' responses to auditors may contain vague and ambiguous wording. Auditors need to determine whether a contingency is "likely, unlikely, or not determinable."[2] Although there are no comparable Canadian guidelines, in the United States the following lawyer responses can be properly interpreted to mean "remote," even though the word is not used:

- We are of the opinion that this action will not result in any liability to the company.
- It is our opinion that the possible liability to the company in this proceeding is nominal in amount.

(continued)

- We believe the company will be able to defend this action successfully. We believe that the plaintiff's case against this company is without merit.
- Based on the facts known to us, after a full investigation, it is our opinion that no liability will be established against the company in these suits.

However, auditors should view the following response phrases as unclear, or providing no information, about the probable, reasonably possible, or remote likelihood of an unfavourable outcome for a litigation contingency:[3,4]

- We believe the plaintiff will have serious problems establishing the company's liability; nevertheless, if the plaintiff is successful, the damage award may be substantial.
- It is our opinion that the company will be able to assert meritorious defences. ["Meritorious," in lawyer language, apparently means that the judge will not summarily throw out the defences.]
- We believe the lawsuit can be settled for less than the damages claimed.
- We are unable to express an opinion on the merits of the litigation, but the company believes there is absolutely no merit.
- In our opinion the company has a substantial chance of prevailing. ["Substantial chance," "reasonable opportunity," and similar phrases indicate uncertainty of success in a defence.]

Source: Adapted from *CPA Canada Assurance Handbook—CAS 501*, Appendix, "Joint Policy Statement Concerning Communications with Law Firms," paragraphs 13–15; PCAOB AU Section 9337, *Inquiry of a Client's Lawyer Concerning Litigation, Claims, and Assessments: Auditing Interpretations of Section 337* (available at pcaobus.org/Standards/Auditing/Pages/AU9337.aspx)

Exhibit 15–4 shows an example of a lawyer's response letter.

EXHIBIT 15–4

Sample Lawyer's Response Letter

[On law firm letterhead]

Privileged and Confidential

[To auditee]

[Date—as close as possible to audit report date]

Dear Sir(s) or Madam(s):

In connection with the preparation and audit of your financial statements for fiscal period ended [date], in response to your inquiries regarding the following claim and possible claim with respect to which our firm's advice of representation has been sought:

Description	Evaluation
A product liability claim has been made by a customer who was permanently injured while using a product purchased from the company.	Likelihood is not determinable and amount of claim is not likely to be significant.

We advise that, as of [effective date of response], the above claim is properly described, and the evaluation of the likelihood of loss and amount of claim are reasonable.

We further advise that we have not been engaged to act as legal council in relation to any claims not listed above.

This response is made in accordance with the Joint Policy Statement of January 1978 approved by The Canadian Bar Association and the Auditing and Assurance Standards Board of CPA Canada.

As requested, a signed copy of the reply has been sent directly to your auditor, [name and address of auditor].

Yours truly,

Lawyer representing auditee in the claim

c.c. [name of auditor]

Source: Based on © *CPA Canada Assurance Handbook—CAS 501* Appendix, schedule A.

Review Checkpoints

15-23   The following was included in a letter auditors received from the auditee's lawyers, in response to a letter sent to them that was similar to Exhibit 15–4: "Several agreements and contracts to which the company is a party are not covered by this response since we have not advised or been consulted in their regard." How might the auditor's report be affected by that statement in the letter regarding a pending lawsuit against the auditee? Explain.

15-24   In addition to the lawyer's letter, what other procedures can be used to gather evidence regarding contingencies?

15-25   Why might companies and auditors experience difficulty making appropriate disclosures about litigation contingencies? (Consider the scenario in the EcoPak case at the beginning of this chapter as an exampe.)

Events Subsequent to the Balance Sheet Date

LO4   Given a set of facts and circumstances, classify a subsequent event by type and proper treatment in the financial statements, and outline the implications of the timing of discovery of the event for the auditor's report.

Material events that occur after the balance sheet date may require adjustments to and/or disclosures in the financial statements. Auditors (and management) are responsible for gathering evidence on these subsequent events and evaluating how they should be reflected in the financial statements (CAS 560). Their impact on the audit report depends on whether they are discovered before or after the audit report date. This section first describes the two different types of subsequent events that can occur and then considers how the timing of discovery affects how the auditor addresses them in the audit report.

Standards Check

CAS 560 Subsequent Events

Events Occurring between the Date of the Financial Statements and the Date of the Auditor's Report

5.   The auditor shall perform audit procedures designed to obtain sufficient appropriate audit evidence that all events occurring between the date of the financial statements and the date of the auditor's report that require adjustment of, or disclosure in, the financial statements have been identified. The auditor is not, however, expected to perform additional audit procedures on matters to which previously applied audit procedures have provided satisfactory conclusions. (Ref: Para. A6)

Source: *CPA Canada Handbook—Assurance*, 2014.

Two Types of Subsequent Events

Subsequent events are events, favourable or unfavourable, that occur between the financial statement date and the date when the financial statements are authorized and issued to users. **Material subsequent events** can be classified into two different types, based on how each type should be treated in the financial statements.

> **material subsequent events:**
> two types of events that are discovered after the year-end date, one type being events that existed at year-end that actually have a material impact on the year-end financial statements and the second being events did not happen until after the year-end but are judged to be materially relevant to users of the year-end financial statement data

The first type are those events that provide evidence about conditions that existed at year-end but are coming to light after the year-end date; these actually affect year-end financial statement numbers so they require adjustment of the dollar amounts of one or more financial statement line items (along with the addition of any related explanatory disclosure required in the notes). We will refer to this type as **subsequent event requiring adjustment in financial statement numbers**. The second type are events that relate to conditions that arose after year-end, and since they did not exist at year-end, they should not be reflected in the year-end financial statement numbers. But if they provide important information for users because the event may have an important impact on the entity in the future, these events need to be disclosed in the notes to those statements. Users need to know about it when they make decisions and predictions based on the year-end numbers. We will refer to the second type as **subsequent event requiring disclosure but not adjustment**.

Subsequent Event Type Requiring Adjustment in Financial Statement Numbers

A subsequent event that provides new information regarding financial conditions that existed at the date of the balance sheet affects the numbers in it. Amounts in the financial statements for the period under audit need to be changed as a result. An example of this is if shortly after year-end, the company made a large sale of inventory at prices below the carrying value of the inventory recorded in the financial statements. Since this fact existed at the financial statement date it should be reflected there, by writing the year-end inventory down to its net realizable value (which is now known with certainty) and recording a loss. The following are other examples of this type of subsequent event:

- A loss on uncollectible trade accounts receivable resulting from the bankruptcy of a major customer (the customer's deteriorating financial condition existed prior to the balance sheet date)
- Litigation settled for an amount different than was estimated (the litigation took place prior to the balance sheet date)

Subsequent Event Type Requiring Financial Statement Disclosure Only, Not Adjustment

Subsequent events that relate to the period after the balance sheet date do not require adjustment of financial statement line items. Recall that the auditor's responsibility for adequate disclosure runs to the audit report date. Consequently, even for events that arise after the balance sheet date, auditors consider their importance to users and whether fair presentation of the financial statements requires their disclosure. This type of subsequent event may be significant enough that disclosure is necessary to keep the financial statements from being misleading. Disclosure is normally in the form of a narrative note. An example of this type is a material decline in the fair value of investments between the year-end and the date of issuing the financial statements. Since this decline relates to the period after year-end, it is not appropriate to reflect at the financial statement date, but it is important information for users nonetheless. Other examples of this second type of subsequent event are as follows:

- A major acquisition or sale of a business unit after the financial statement date
- Destruction of a major operating asset by a fire after the financial statement date
- Significant decrease in net realizable value of inventory after the balance sheet date

subsequent event requiring adjustment in financial statement numbers:
the type of material subsequent event that requires adjustment of the dollar amounts of one or more financial statement line items along with any related additional explanatory note disclosure

subsequent event requiring disclosure but not adjustment:
the type of material subsequent event that happened after year-end and should not be reflected in the year-end financial statement numbers but needs to be disclosed in the notes to those financial statements because it is likely to be materially relevant to decisions and predictions based on those financial statements

- Big changes in foreign currency exchange rates or tax rate after year-end that will have a material impact on future financial statements
- Loss on an uncollectible trade receivable resulting from a customer's fire or flood loss subsequent to the balance sheet date (in contrast to a customer's slow decline into bankruptcy, cited above as a subsequent event type requiring adjustment in financial statement numbers)
- Issue of bonds payable or share capital after year-end
- Settlement of litigation when the event giving rise to the claim took place subsequent to the balance sheet date
- Loss of plant or inventories as a result of fire or flood subsequent to year-end

Occasionally a subsequent event is so significant that the best disclosure is to present **pro forma financial data**—an additional note disclosure presenting the financial statements "as if" the event had occurred on the date of the balance sheet.[5]

Retroactive recognition of the effect of stock dividends and splits is an exception covered in the box below. The issue here is timely and informative communication to financial statement users; the stock dividend or split will have been completed by the time the financial statements reach users, and to report financial data as if they had not occurred might be considered misleading.

Subsequent Event Stock Split

On February 15, the company approved a two-for-one stock split to be effective on that date. The fiscal year-end was the previous December 31, and the financial statements as of December 31 showed 50 million shares authorized, 10 million shares issued and outstanding, and earnings per share of $3.

Audit Resolution. Note disclosure was made of the split and of the relevant dates. The equity section of the balance sheet showed 100 million shares authorized and 20 million shares issued and outstanding. The income statement reported earnings per share of $1.50. Earnings per share of prior years were adjusted accordingly. The note disclosed comparative earnings per share on the pre-dividend shares.

Subsequent Events and the Audit Report

Subsequent events are taken into account in finalizing the audit report and in some cases can affect the audit report dating. This is discussed in Chapter 16 with the topic of dating the audit report.

Audit Program for the Subsequent Period

An example of an audit program to search for subsequent events is given in Exhibit 15–5. Some audit procedures in the period subsequent to the balance sheet date may include those in the audit program for determining cutoff and proper valuation of balances as of the balance sheet date (panel A in Exhibit 15–5). However, procedures specifically designed for gathering evidence about the two types of subsequent events are different and separate from the rest of the audit program (panel B in Exhibit 15–5).

pro forma financial data:
the presentation of financial statements as if a subsequent event had occurred on the date of the balance sheet; perhaps the best way to show the effect of a business purchase or other merger

EXHIBIT 15–5

Auditing Procedures for the Period Subsequent to the Balance Sheet Date

A. **Procedures performed in connection with other audit programs**
   1. Use a cutoff bank statement to
      (a) Examine cheques paid after year-end that are, or should have been, listed on the bank reconciliation.
      (b) Examine bank posting of deposits in transit listed on the bank reconciliation.
   2. Vouch collections on accounts receivable in the month following year-end for evidence of existence and collectability of the year-end balances.
   3. Trace cash disbursements of the month after year-end to accounts payable for evidence of any liabilities unrecorded at year-end.
   4. Vouch write-downs of fixed assets after year-end evidence that such valuation problems existed at the year-end date.
   5. Vouch sales of investment securities, write-downs, or write-offs in the months after the audit date for evidence of valuation at the year-end date.
   6. Vouch and trace sales transactions in the month after year-end for evidence of proper sales and cost of sales cutoff.

B. **Additional auditing procedures for subsequent events**
   1. Obtain the latest available interim financial statements and
      (a) Compare them with the financial statements being reported on, and make any other comparisons considered appropriate in the circumstances. Investigate any unusual fluctuations
      (b) Inquire of officers and other executives responsible for financial and accounting matters about whether the interim statements have been prepared on the same basis as that used for the statements under examination. Assess the impact of any changes on comparability
   2. Scan the accounting records for the subsequent event period (such as general ledger, general journal entries, sales journal, purchases journal, cash receipts journal, and cash disbursements journal), and investigate any unusual transactions or entries.
   3. Inquire of and discuss with officers and other executives responsible for financial and accounting matters (limited where appropriate to major locations)
      (a) Whether any substantial contingent liabilities or commitments existed at the date of the balance sheet being reported on or at the date of inquiry
      (b) Whether there was any significant change in the share capital, long-term debt, or working capital to the date of inquiry
      (c) The current status of items in the financial statements being reported on that were accounted for on the basis of tentative, preliminary, or inconclusive data
      (d) Whether any unusual adjustments have been made during the period from the balance sheet date to the date of inquiry
   4. Read the available minutes of meetings of shareholders, directors, and appropriate committees; inquire about matters dealt with at meetings for which minutes are not available.
   5. Request that the client send a letter to legal counsel inquiring about outstanding claims, possible claims, and management's evaluation, with the reply to be sent directly to the auditor.
   6. Obtain written representations, dated as of the date of the auditor's report, from appropriate officials, generally the CEO and CFO, about whether any events occurred subsequent to the date of the financial statements that, in the officer's opinion, would require adjustment or disclosure in these statements.
   7. Make such additional inquiries or perform such procedures as considered necessary and appropriate to dispose of questions that arise in carrying out the foregoing procedures, inquiries, and discussions.

Summary of Subsequent Events in an Audit

Auditing standards for subsequent events consider two types of events: (1) events that occurred or conditions that existed on or before the audit report date that would have caused the auditor to amend the audit report, and (2) events and conditions that arise after the balance sheet date but that are nonetheless important for understanding the financial statements. Auditors may learn of a subsequent event at different times: before the audit report date, after the audit report date but before the financial statements are released to users, or after the audited financial statements have been released. It is most important to remember that auditors have an active, procedural responsibility for discovering both types of subsequent events up to the audit report date and for ensuring that they are properly reported in the financial statements, but they are not required to perform procedures after the audit report date. However, because they are associated with financial statements upon which they have given an audit opinion, auditors still have responsibilities after the audited financial statements have been released, whenever they become aware of new relevant facts or omitted audit procedures. These issues are summarized in the timeline in Exhibit 15–6 and are further discussed in Chapter 16, where we will cover the independent auditor's report.

Auditor Responsibilities for Subsequent Events Review in the Audit Process

DATE OF FINANCIAL STATEMENTS	DATES WHEN AUDITORS PERFORM AND COMPLETE THEIR FIELD WORK	DATE OF FINANCIAL STATEMENTS' APPROVAL BY DIRECTORS (THOSE WITH AUTHORITY)	DATE OF AUDITOR'S REPORT	DATE OF RELEASE OF AUDITED FINANCIAL STATEMENTS TO USERS	DATES WHEN FINANCIAL STATEMENTS ARE IN CIRCULATION
Example: December 31, 20X1	*Example:* December 20X1 to February 20, 20X2	*Example:* February 21, 20X2	*Example:* February 21, 20X2	*Example:* February 28, 20X2	*Example:* February 28, 20X2, and later
	Auditors are required to perform procedures to search for evidence of subsequent events (CAS 580). Most subsequent event procedures will be performed near the date of the auditor's report.			Auditors have no responsibility to actively search for evidence of subsequent events after the audit report date but must respond to any new facts about subsequent events that come to their attention (CAS 560; see also Appendix 16B).	

Review Checkpoints

15-26 What are the two types of subsequent events? How are they treated differently in the financial statements?

15-27 What treatment is given stock dividends and splits occurring after the balance sheet date but before the audit report is issued? Explain.

Management's Written Representations

LO5 Explain why written management representations are obtained and what items are generally included in the representation letter, including identification of related parties.

Management responds to numerous auditor inquiries during the course of an audit. These representations are very important components of audit evidence, but they are not sufficient by themselves. As much as possible, auditors should corroborate management representations with evidence from additional procedures.

Auditors should also obtain **written representations** from management on matters of audit importance (CAS 580). These representations exist as a letter on the auditee's letterhead, addressed to the auditor, signed by responsible officers (normally the CEO, CFO, and other appropriate managers), and dated as of the date of the auditor's report. The letter, referred to as the **management representation letter**, covers events and representations running beyond the balance sheet date up to the audit report date.

In most cases, the written management representations are related to the assertions in the financial statements but provide more detailed information. They are not sufficient evidence for auditors and not a good defence against criticism for failing to perform audit procedures independently. ("Management told us in writing that the inventory costing method was FIFO and adequate allowance for obsolescence was provided" is not a good excuse for failing to get the evidence from the records and other sources!) However, in some cases these

written representations:
written statements by management and, where appropriate, those charged with governance, provided to the auditor to confirm certain matters or to support other audit evidence in addition to the representations contained in the financial statements, the assertions therein, or supporting books and records, obtained at the final point in the audit prior to issuing an opinion

management representation letter:
written statements by management provided to the auditor to confirm certain matters or to support other audit evidence as required by CAS 580

are the only evidence about important matters of management intent, for example, (1) "We will discontinue the parachute manufacturing business, wind down the operations, and sell the remaining assets" (i.e., accounting for discontinued operations), and (2) "We will exercise our option to refinance the maturing debt on a long-term basis" (i.e., classifying maturing debt as long term).

A primary purpose of the management representation letter is to impress upon management its responsibility for the financial statements. It may also establish an auditor's defences against questions of management integrity: a management lie to the auditors will be captured in writing in the letter. Auditors draft the management representation letter to be prepared on the auditee's letterhead for signature by company representatives. This draft is reviewed with senior auditee personnel and then finalized.

Auditing standards indicate that the following written representations must be obtained in all audits:[6]

- That management has fulfilled its responsibility for the preparation and presentation of the financial statements in accordance with the applicable financial reporting framework, as set out in the terms of the audit engagement
- That management has provided the auditor with all relevant information to conduct the audit engagement, as agreed in the terms of engagement
- That all transactions have been recorded and are reflected in the financial statements

The auditor may consider it necessary to get other written representations in some circumstances. These other representations could include the following:

- Appropriate selection and application of accounting policies
- Appropriate recognition, measurement, presentation, or disclosure of the financial statements
- Plans or intentions that may affect the carrying value or classification of assets and liabilities
- Liabilities, both actual and contingent
- Title to, or control over, assets, liens, or encumbrances on assets, and assets pledged as collateral
- Aspects of laws, regulations, and contractual agreements that may affect the financial statements, including non-compliance

In situations of fraud risk or known frauds, going-concern uncertainty, correction of material misstatements uncovered in the audit, material estimates, related parties, and subsequent events, other written representations may be required. Several other representations may be relevant in particular businesses or industries, for example, environmental liabilities; derivative financial instruments; the appropriateness of accounting policies for complex

Standards Check

CAS 580 Written Representations

Written Representations about Management's Responsibilities

Preparation of the Financial Statements

10. The auditor shall request management to provide a written representation that it has fulfilled its responsibility for the preparation of the financial statements in accordance with the applicable financial reporting framework, including, where relevant, their fair presentation, as set out in the terms of the audit engagement. (Ref: Para. A7–A9, A14, A22)

Information Provided and Completeness of Transactions

11. The auditor shall request management to provide a written representation that
    (a) It has provided the auditor with all relevant information and access as agreed in the terms of the audit engagement; and
    (b) All transactions have been recorded and are reflected in the financial statements. (Ref: Para. A7–A9, A14, A22)

Description of Management's Responsibilities in the Written Representations

12. Management's responsibilities shall be described in the written representations required by paragraphs 10 and 11 in the manner in which these responsibilities are described in the terms of the audit engagement.

Source: *CPA Canada Handbook—Assurance*, 2014.

areas of accounting; and areas involving management's judgment and estimates, such as revenue recognition, fair value measurements, transfers of receivables, hedging relationships, and consolidation of variable interest entities.

The representation letter provides management with a summary of the uncorrected financial statement misstatements found by the auditor during the audit, and it obtains management's representation of its belief that these are immaterial to the financial statements—a summary of such items is included in or attached to the letter. Management representations are also required for auditors involved with prospectuses[7] and for review engagements.[8] An example of a written representation letter is shown in Exhibit 15–7.

Audit of Related Party Transactions

A representation letter answers these key questions: Has the auditee identified all its **related parties** to the auditor? Has the auditee been involved in any related party transactions (see Exhibit 15–7)? Auditors are responsible for obtaining reasonable assurance that related parties have been identified and that there is appropriate disclosure with such parties in the financial statements.[9] Related parties exist when one party either has the ability to exercise control or joint control, directly or indirectly, or has significant influence over the other. Parties are related when they are subject to common control, joint control, or common significant influence. Related parties could include management and immediate family members. Related party transactions are particularly important in Canada because of the high concentration of corporate ownership.

The problem with related party transactions is that since they are not **arm's length**, they may not reflect the normal terms of trade that occur with most transactions with external parties. Related party accounting is one of the few areas of substantive difference between IFRS and ASPE in the *CPA Canada Handbook*. While ASPE provide measurement and disclosure standards for related party transactions, IFRS (IAS 24) only requires disclosures. The auditor's main problem is identifying these transactions. Management inquiry is the main procedure (as in the management representation obtained in Exhibit 15–7), but others include reading the minutes of meetings of shareholders, directors, and executive and audit committees, as well as acquiring a general knowledge of the auditee's business.[10]

Unusual transactions might point to undisclosed relationships, so being skeptical about these during an audit is critical. The team discussions provide a good opportunity to ensure that the audit team is aware of related party relationships and transactions that could leave the financial statements susceptible to fraud or error. Some indications of the existence of undisclosed related parties are as follows:

- Abnormal terms of trade, such as unusually high or low selling prices, interest rates, and repayment terms
- Large, unusual transactions, particularly those recognized at or near the balance sheet date
- Transactions that lack an apparent business reason, or where the legal form of the transactions seems to conceal its actual economic substance

In addition to the auditor's business risk assessment, the following further procedures can help to identify the existence of related party transactions:[11]

- Review prior-year working papers for related party transactions.
- Review the entity's procedures for identifying related parties.
- Obtain written representation from management concerning identification and adequacy of related party disclosures.

related parties:
a term used to describe a situation in which one party has the ability to exercise, directly or indirectly, control, joint control or significant influence over another and hence they may not deal with each other at arm's length; in an audit includes the auditee's management and immediate family members

arm's length:
a situation in which two people, or entities, are both independent and acting in their own best interest in their dealings with each other because neither has undue influence over the other

EXHIBIT 15-7

Illustrative Written Representation Letter

[Auditee Letterhead]

[To Auditor]   [Date]

This representation letter is provided in connection with your audit of the financial statements of ABC Company for the year ended December 31, 20X0, for the purpose of expressing an opinion as to whether the financial statements are presented fairly, in all material respects, in accordance with International Financial Reporting Standards.

We confirm the following:

Financial Statements

- We have fulfilled our responsibilities for the preparation and presentation of the financial statements as set out in the terms of the audit engagement dated [insert date], and, in particular, the financial statements are fairly presented in accordance with International Financial Reporting Standards.
- Significant assumptions used by us in making accounting estimates, including those measured at fair value, are reasonable.
- Related party relationships and transactions have been appropriately accounted for and disclosed in accordance with the requirements of International Financial Reporting Standards. We have disclosed to you all parties that can be considered to be related parties for the purpose of financial reporting under International Financial Reporting Standards.
- All events subsequent to the date of the financial statements and for which International Financial Reporting Standards require adjustment or disclosure have been adjusted or disclosed.
- The effects of uncorrected misstatements are immaterial, both individually and in the aggregate, to the financial statements as a whole. A list of the uncorrected misstatements is attached to the representation letter.
- [Any other matters that the auditor may consider appropriate, such as whether financial statements have been appropriately recognized, measured, presented, or disclosed:
  - Plans or intentions that may affect the carrying value or classification of assets and liabilities
  - Liabilities, both actual and contingent
  - Title to, or control over, assets, and the liens or encumbrances on assets, and assets pledged as collateral
  - Aspects of laws, regulations, and contractual agreements that may affect the financial statements, including non-compliance
  - A going-concern uncertainty, if any]

Information Provided

- We have provided you with
  - All information, such as records and documentation, and other matters that are relevant to the preparation and presentation of the financial statements
  - Additional information that you have requested from us
  - Unrestricted access to those within the entity
- All transactions have been recorded in the accounting records and are reflected in the financial statements.
- We have disclosed to you the results of our assessment of the risk that the financial statements may be materially misstated as a result of fraud.
- We have disclosed to you all information in relation to fraud or suspected fraud that we are aware of and that affects the entity and involves
  - Management
  - Employees who have significant roles in internal control
  - Others where the fraud could have a material effect on the financial statements
- We have disclosed to you all information in relation to allegations of fraud, or suspected fraud, affecting the entity's financial statements communicated by employees, former employees, analysts, regulators, or others.
- We have disclosed to you all known actual or possible non-compliance with laws and regulations whose effects should be considered when preparing financial statements.
- We have disclosed to you the identity of the entity's related parties and all the related party relationships and transactions of which we are aware.
- [Any other matters that the auditor may consider necessary]

[signed]   [signed]

Auditee CEO   Auditee CFO

Source: Adapted from CAS 580.

Having identified related party transactions, the auditor can perform the following substantive procedures:

- Confirm the terms and amounts of the transactions with the related parties.
- Inspect evidence in possession of the related party.
- Confirm or discuss information with persons associated with the transactions, such as banks, lawyers, guarantors, and agents.

CAS 550 also requires the auditor to communicate significant matters identified during the audit that concern related party transactions or relationships to those charged with governance.

The box below illustrates how related party transactions can be used to significantly alter the financial statements. The illustration is based on an actual Canadian company trading on NASDAQ and the TSX.

Turning Expenses into Revenues

CB is a major biotechnology company in Canada that did not like the effect that expensing research and development (R&D) had on its earnings. So, CB proceeded to create a related entity, CC, to which it made a capital contribution of $100 million. A series of share exchanges involving shares of both companies had the net effect of a debit to retained earnings and a credit to cash for $100 million on CB's financial statements. An agreement was then reached in which CC paid CB a fee in exchange for a technology licence. CC used the $100 million it had received from CB to repay CB for CB's R&D costs. CB accounted for the amounts received from CC as revenue.

In the words of CB's chairman of the board, "This initiative will enable us to leverage our investment in R&D and pursue the ongoing development of exciting new products, without unduly affecting the company's baseline earnings."

Review Checkpoints

15-28   What is the purpose of a management representation letter?

15-29   What representations would you request that management make in the representation letter with respect to related parties? receivables? inventories? minutes of meetings? subsequent events?

15-30   Why are written management representations and lawyers' letters obtained at the final stage of the audit and dated as close as possible to the audit report date?

15-31   How can related party transactions affect the financial statements?

Audit Documentation Working Paper Review

LO6   Outline the procedures used to complete the documentation of the audit engagement.

A typical audit team includes the engagement partner, audit manager, onsite supervisor, one or more audit staff members, and any experts required. Soon after completion, each audit documentation working paper is reviewed by the audit supervisor, and sometimes by the audit manager, to ensure that all necessary procedures were performed with due professional care, and that all procedures performed are adequately documented with clear tickmark notations and conclusions indicated. To wrap up the audit field work, the supervisor or manager makes a final review of all the working papers, which may be recorded using paper, electronic, or other media. This final review ensures that all accounts on the trial balance have a **working paper reference index**, the sign that audit work

working paper reference index:
a table of contents listing all the index numbers used to identify sections of the audit working paper files

has been finished on that account, and that all procedures in the audit program are "signed off" with a date and initials. Any outstanding work or issues are summarized at this point for the manager's and partner's attention, usually in a working paper called the "to-do list."

The manager and engagement partner's review comes next, and it focuses more on the overall scope of the audit. The manager and engagement partner are very involved with the planning of the audit and may perform some of the field work on difficult areas, but they are usually not involved in preparing the detailed working papers. Even though the working papers are reviewed by the onsite supervisor, the partner who is going to sign the audit report should review them as well, since he or she has the final responsibility for ensuring sufficient appropriate audit evidence has been obtained and documented. Additions to the to-do lists, citing omissions or deficiencies, are prepared during these reviews and must be cleared by the audit staff before the final work is completed.

Treatment of the to-do lists varies among audit firms. Some prefer to destroy the lists after the work is performed and documented in the working papers as a "cleanup" of notes relating to loose ends. Other firms keep the lists as signed off, and cross-reference them for the work performed, believing the lists are evidence of careful review and completion of the audit. Sometimes, retained to-do lists backfire on auditors by showing questions raised but not resolved.

Under CSQC-1, audit firms must have quality control procedures in place to determine, for each audit engagement, whether an **engagement quality review** needs to be completed before issuing the audit report. This is a second-partner review of the working paper documentation and the financial statements, including notes. It must be performed by a partner not responsible for the client relationship to ensure that the quality of audit work and reporting is in keeping with the quality standards of the audit firm (the specific requirements are set out in CAS 220). Engagement quality reviews are automatically required for listed public entities, and the firm's quality control policies must also consider whether one should be required in other situations, such as for a first-time audit or an engagement that is considered very risky. Considering all the professional judgments that have been made in completing the audit to this stage, these reviews allow the files to be reviewed with a fresh set of eyes by someone very experienced and competent. This can increase the chance that any questionable or erroneous judgments will be scrutinized and resolved, indicating how the quality control mechanism can be very effective in improving the quality of audit outcomes.

The completed working paper files are assembled for secure, long-term storage. Those retained in electronic files must have data integrity controls in place. Usually, the files are completed within 60 days of the audit report date and are retained for at least five years. When field work is complete, the final audit time reports for billing purposes and audit staff performance evaluation reports are prepared by the audit supervisor.

A completion checklist is often used in practice, to help ensure nothing is overlooked. An example of this type of practice form is provided in Appendix 16A.

Review Checkpoints

15-32   What is the purpose of to-do lists in the audit documentation? What is a good reason for keeping the to-do lists in the audit working paper files?

15-33   Describe an engagement quality review. Who performs it, and what is its purpose?

engagement quality review:
the review of working papers and financial statements by a partner not responsible for client relations; ensures that the quality of the audit work is in keeping with the standards of the audit firm

APPLICATION CASE WITH SOLUTION & ANALYSIS

When in Doubt, Defer!

DISCUSSION CASE

Jack is now starting his third year of auditing and is accumulating some valuable experience. One day, he has lunch with a former classmate, Stella, who now works for the securities market regulator as an inspector. They are discussing some of the ways auditors get in trouble. Stella tells him about a case her boss worked on a few years ago. "This really showed me why, even when all the staff does a good job, audits just can't work if the partner isn't independent," Stella said. As he listens to this case, Jack thinks about some similar issues partners on his audits had to fight their way through to make sure the financial statements ended up being fairly presented. He realizes that it takes a lot of integrity to provide a high-quality audit result.

CASE DESCRIPTION

SaCom manufactured electronic and other equipment for private customers and government military defence contracts. The company was deferring costs under the headings of work in process, military contract claims, and R&D test equipment, thus overstating assets, understating cost of goods sold, and overstating income. Disclosure of the auditor's fees was manipulated and understated. SaCom reported net income of about $5,420,000 for the year, an overstatement of approximately 50%.

To achieve better reported profit, near the end of the year, the company used a journal entry to remove $1,700,000 from cost of goods sold and to defer it as tooling, leasehold improvements, and contract award and acquisition costs. The company capitalized certain expenditures as R&D test equipment ($1,400,000) and claims for reimbursement on defence contracts ($3,780,000).

In connection with a public offering of securities, the firm doing the audit billed SaCom $225,000 for professional fees. The underwriters objected, so the auditors agreed to forgive $170,000 of the fees while SaCom agreed to pay higher fees the following year (150% of standard billing rates). SaCom disclosed audit fees in the registration statement in the amount of $55,000. This amount was paid from the proceeds of the offering.

Audit Trail

The $1,700,000 deferred costs were primarily labour costs, and the company altered the labour time records to be able to provide substantiating documentation. The auditors discovered the alterations by noticing that the jobs were left with labour costs that were too small, in light of the work performed. The R&D test equipment cost had already been charged to cost of goods sold with no indication of a reason for deferral when originally recorded. Deferral was accomplished with an adjusting journal entry. The company did not have documentation for the adjusting entry, except for an estimate of labour cost (44% of all labour cost in a subsidiary was capitalized during the period). The claim for reimbursement on defence contracts did not have documentation specifically identifying the costs as being related to the contract. (Auditors know that defence department auditors insist on documentation and justification before approving such a claim.) The audit fee arrangement was known to the audit firm, and it was recorded in an internal memorandum.

SOLUTION & ANALYSIS
Audit Approach
Audit Objective

The auditors' objective is to obtain evidence of the existence of production costs capitalized as tooling, leasehold improvements, contract award and acquisition costs, R&D test equipment, and claims for reimbursement on defence contracts.

Controls Relevant to the Process

The major control lies in the procedures for documenting the validity of cost deferral journal entries.

Audit Procedures

Tests of Controls

The procedure is to select a sample of journal entries, suspect ones in this case, and vouch them to supporting documentation and authorization. Experience has shown that non-standard adjusting journal entries are the source of accounting errors and fraud more often than standard accounting for regular transactions. This makes adjusting journal entries a ripe field for control and substantive testing.

Tests of Details of Balance

The account balances created by the deferral journal entries can be audited in a dual-purpose procedure by auditing the supporting documentation. These balances were created entirely by the journal entries, and their "existence" as legitimate assets, deferrals, and reimbursement claims depends on the believability of the supporting explanations. In connection with the defence contract claim, auditors can obtain evidence of its existence by reviewing the extensive documentation required by government contract auditors. (As a separate matter, the auditors could search for unrecorded liabilities, but they already knew about the deferred accounting fees.)

Audit Results

By performing the procedures outlined, the audit team discovered all the questionable accounting. However, the partners in the auditing firm insisted on rendering unqualified opinions on the SaCom financial statements, without adjustment. One partner owned 300 shares of the company's stock in the name of a relative (without the consent or knowledge of the relative). Another audit partner later arranged a bank loan to the company to get $225,000 to pay past-due audit fees. This partner and another, along with their spouses, guaranteed the loan. (When the bank later disclosed the guarantee in a bank confirmation, the confirmation was removed from the audit working paper file and destroyed.)

Regulatory Actions against the Auditors

The securities market regulator investigated the auditors' conduct in the SaCom audit and, among other things, barred the audit firm for a period (about six months) from accepting new audit clients, and it also barred the partners involved in the SaCom audit work from involvement with new audit clients for various periods of time. The partners had violated several rules of professional conduct and were therefore subject to disciplinary action by their provincial institute (see Chapter 3 for discussion of rules of professional conduct).

Review Checkpoints

15-34 What red flag is raised when a company has an unbilled contract revenue account in its general ledger?

15-35 Why should auditors always select the auditee's adjusting journal entries made in the closing process for detailed audit?

SUMMARY

This chapter covered several aspects of completing an audit.

- As the work draws to a close, several income and expense accounts may still need to be audited. This work is largely done through analytical comparisons of these balances with those of prior years and with current expectations. While large and significant revenues and expenses have usually already been audited in connection with the audit of other accounts in the process, at this stage in the audit it is a good idea to step back and review large and unusual revenue and expense transactions recorded near the end of the year. Often, these have been the vehicles for income statement manipulation. Some examples were given in the chapter. **LO1**

- Analytical procedures performed at the end of the audit were explained in terms of their role of allowing the most senior members of the audit team, usually the engagement partner, to ensure the financial statements reflect the evidence and knowledge obtained in the course of performing the audit. **LO2**

- Information from lawyers is especially important in evidence about litigation contingencies and their disclosure, according to *CPA Canada Handbook* section 3290 and IAS 37. The most important topic, preparing and obtaining the lawyer's letter as confirmation regarding any outstanding claims and contingencies, was discussed. A special box described particular problems in interpreting lawyers' letters. **LO3**

- Subsequent events were explained in detail, including the two types of subsequent events that can affect financial statements, and the auditor's procedural responsibility for events following the balance sheet date. **LO4**

- Management's written representations provide key evidence regarding many important details and assertions, and without them the audit scope is considered limited. Several requirements for the management representation letter were specified in the chapter. **LO5**

- The chapter ended with coverage of the final file review process and the compilation of a file of audit documentation for review and retention by the audit firm, to be available for inspection or for the auditors' defence in the case of a lawsuit. These are firm-level and engagement-level requirements that exist to increase the quality of audits, as set out in CSQC-1 and CAS 220. These files are the documentary basis for forming the audit opinion, to be covered next. **LO6**

Forming the audit opinion based on the audit findings will be covered in detail in the next chapter, which explains the application of professional judgment to achieve the final objective and focal point of the whole financial statement audit engagement, and its only public result—the auditor's report.

KEY TERMS

arm's length

commitments

contingencies

contingent liabilities

engagement partner

engagement quality review

lawyer's confirmation letter

management representation letter

material subsequent events

overall analytical procedures

pro forma financial data

related parties

subsequent event requiring
    adjustment in financial statement
    numbers

subsequent event requiring disclosure
    but not adjustment

unusual transactions

written representations

working paper reference index

MULTIPLE-CHOICE QUESTIONS FOR PRACTICE AND REVIEW

MC 15-1 **LO1** When auditing the year-end balance of interest-bearing notes payable, which account are the auditors most likely to audit at the same time?

a. Interest income

b. Interest expense

c. Amortization of intangible assets

d. Royalty revenue

MC 15-2 **LO5** What is the main purpose of a written management representation letter?

a. Shift responsibility for financial statements from the management to the auditor.

b. Provide a substitute source of evidence for detail procedures auditors would otherwise perform.

c. Provide management a place to make assertions about the quantity and valuation of the physical inventory.

d. Obtain management's acknowledgement of its ultimate responsibility for the financial statements and disclosures.

MC 15-3 **LO3** Which of these procedures or sources is not likely to provide evidence about contingencies?

a. Scan expense accounts for credit entries.

b. Obtain a representation letter from the auditee's lawyer.

c. Read the minutes of the board of directors meetings.

d. Examine terms of sale in sales contracts.

MC 15-4 **LO4** The auditors learned of a subsequent event that involves information about a condition that existed at the balance sheet date. Which of the following subsequent events is of the type that requires the company to adjust its December 31 financial statements?

a. Sale of an issue of new shares for $500,000 on January 30

b. A $10,000 settlement of a damage lawsuit for a customer's injury sustained February 15

c. A February $100,000 settlement of litigation that had been estimated at $12,000 in the December 31 financial statements

d. Storm damage of $1 million to the company's buildings on March 1

MC 15-5 **LO6** Until when do auditors have a responsibility to perform procedures to find subsequent events?

a. The year-end balance sheet date

b. The audit report date

c. The date the audited financial statements are delivered to the users

d. The end of audit field work

MC 15-6 **LO2** Which of the following procedures is part of the audit completion work?

a. Risk assessment

b. Control testing

c. Overall evaluation of the financial statements

d. Preparation of the cash flow statement

MC 15-7 `LO6` Which of the following is not required by CASs?

a. Management representation letter
b. Lawyer's letter
c. Management letter
d. Engagement letter

EXERCISES AND PROBLEMS

EP 15-1 Management Representation Letter. `LO5` In connection with your audit, you request that management provide you with a letter containing certain representations, such as the following:

1. The auditee has satisfactory title to all assets.
2. No contingent or unrecorded liabilities exist except as disclosed in the letter.
3. No shares of the company's stock are reserved for options, warrants, or other rights.
4. The company is not obligated to repurchase any of its outstanding shares under any circumstances.

Required:

a. Explain why you believe a letter of representation should be provided to you.
b. In what way, if any, do these management representations affect your audit procedures and responsibilities?

(© 2000, American Institute of CPAs. All Rights Reserved. Adapted by permission.)

EP 15-2 Engagement and Management Representation Letters. `LO5` The two major written understandings between an auditor and management, in connection with an audit of financial statements, are the engagement letter and the management representation letter.

Required:

a.   i. What are the objectives of the engagement letter?
    ii. Who should prepare and sign the engagement letter?
   iii. When should the engagement letter be sent?
    iv. Why should the engagement letter be renewed periodically?

b.   i. What are the objectives of the management representation letter?
    ii. Who should sign the management representation letter?
   iii. When should the management representation letter be obtained?
    iv. Why should the management representation letter be prepared for each examination?

(© 2000, American Institute of CPAs. All Rights Reserved. Adapted by permission.)

EP 15-3 Lawyer's Letters. `LO3` Auditors are required to obtain representation letters from the auditee's lawyer to elicit information on claims and possible claims that may affect the financial statements.

Required:

a. Discuss the audit evidence provided by a lawyer's letter. Explain which assertions and financial statement amounts the lawyer's letter relates to.

b. What other evidence may be available to an auditor that can corroborate the completeness of the claims the auditee has listed in the lawyer's letter?

c. What should be the effective date of the lawyer's letter? Why?

EP 15-4 Management Representation Letters.   LO5   Refer to the example of a management representation letter in Exhibit 15–7.

Required:

a. What are the assumptions about the audit engagement in this management representation letter?

b. Which of the representations in the example letter need to be provided regardless of their materiality?

c. If an event subsequent to the date of the balance sheet has been disclosed in the financial statements, what modification would be made to the example letter?

d. If management has received a communication regarding an allegation of fraud or suspected fraud, what modification would be made to the example letter?

EP 15-5 Procedures for Identifying Contingent Liabilities.   LO3   In 20X0, Jay Inc. and Vee Ltd., both Canadian manufacturing companies, decided to form a joint venture to build and operate a manufacturing plant in Asia. Their joint venture would have lower operating costs and faster access to Asian markets. Your audit client, Jay, borrowed $4,000,000 and arranged for further long-term debt from its banker, Manufacturing Bank of Canada. Jay is currently being sued because it cancelled a purchase agreement it had with another company, Boilers Inc., to purchase some equipment.

Required:

Prepare four audit procedures, in addition to obtaining a representation from the auditee management and communicating with the company's law firm, to identify the contingent liabilities, if any, of Jay. Do not include any analytical procedures in your list.

> *(Adapted from External Auditing (AU1), September 2010, with permission of Chartered Professional Accountants of Canada, Toronto, Canada. Any changes to the original material are the sole responsibility of the author (and/or publisher) and have not been reviewed or endorsed by the Chartered Professional Accountants of Canada.)*

EP 15-6 Business Processes, Financial Statement Articulation, and XBRL Application.   LO1, 2, 6   The final review stage of the audit involves taking an overall view of the financial statements and assessing how fairly they reflect the underlying economic events and conditions that occurred in the entity. This exercise involves pulling together difference aspects of the text material that help auditors take this overall integrated view, and considering the case of a real company's financial statements.

Required:

a. Obtain an example of a current set of financial statements from the database of public company documents available at SEDAR.com. For each of the items included in the entity's business processes in Exhibit 6–12, identify which financial statement it will appear in and all the other financial statement items to which it is related.

b. Using the file index system illustration in Appendix 11C (available on Connect), provide an index of what a typical audit file for your example company financial statements would be likely to contain.

c. XBRL is an Internet-based technology for presenting financial data on web pages and exchanging it over the Internet with other users' systems. Companies are increasingly being required to provide their financial statements in XBRL format. Information on the underlying structure of XBRL and how it works can be found at the website XBRL.org. Further research can be done at other websites for reference, for example, sec.gov/edgar.shtml (EDGAR online). Describe how each financial statement item you identified in (a) above could be defined/tagged in XBRL to appear in the financial statements. If the financial data item has been audited, can XBRL allow the auditor's assurance to be communicated to users at the same time as the data? How?

DISCUSSION CASES

DC 15-1 Management Representation Letter Omissions. **LO5** During the audit of the annual financial statements of Amis Manufacturing Inc., the company's president, Vance Molar, and Wendy Dweebins, the engagement partner, reviewed matters that were supposed to be included in a management representation letter. Upon receipt of the following representation letter, Wendy contacted Vance to state that it was incomplete.

To John & Wayne, Public Accountants:

In connection with your examination of the balance sheet of Amis Manufacturing Inc. as of December 31, 20X2, and the related statements of income, retained earnings, and cash flows for the year then ended, for the purpose of expressing an opinion on whether the financial statements present fairly the financial position, results of operations, and cash flows of Amis Manufacturing Inc., in conformity with generally accepted accounting principles, we confirm, to the best of our knowledge and belief, the following representations made to you during your audit. The following were not present:

- Plans or intentions that may materially affect the carrying value or classification of assets or liabilities
- Communications from regulatory agencies concerning non-compliance with, or deficiencies in, financial reporting practices
- Agreements to repurchase assets previously sold
- Violations or possible violations of laws or regulations whose effects should be considered for disclosure in the financial statements or as a basis for recording a loss contingency
- Unasserted claims or assessments that our lawyer has advised are probable and that must be disclosed in accordance with Canadian GAAP
- Capital stock purchase options or agreements or capital stock reserved for options, warrants, conversions, or other requirements
- Compensating balance or other arrangements involving restrictions on cash balances

Vance Molar, President

Amis Manufacturing Inc.

March 14, 20X3

Required:

Identify the other matters that Molar's representation letter should specifically confirm.

(© 2000, American Institute of CPAs. All Rights Reserved. Adapted by permission.)

DC 15-2 Subsequent Events Procedures. **LO4** You are in the process of winding up the field work on Top Stove Corporation, a company that manufactures and sells kerosene space-heating stoves. To date, there has been every indication that the financial statements of the company present fairly the position of the company at December 31 and the results of its operations for the year then ended. Top Stove had total assets at December 31 of $4 million and a net profit for the year (after deducting federal and provincial income taxes) of $285,000. The principal records of the company are a general ledger, cash receipts record, accounts payable register, sales register, cheque register, and general journal. Financial statements are prepared monthly. Your field work will be completed on February 20, and you expect the company's board to meet and approve the final financial statements on March 12.

Required:

a. Write a brief statement about the purpose and period to be covered in a review of subsequent events.
b. Outline the program you would follow to determine what transactions involving material amounts, if any, have occurred since the balance sheet date.

(© 2000, American Institute of CPAs. All Rights Reserved. Adapted by permission.)

DC 15-3 Subsequent Events: Cases. **LO4** The following events occurred in independent cases, but in each instance the event happened after the close of the fiscal year under audit but before the financial statements were authorized for issue, which is also the audit report data. For each case, state what impact, if any, you would expect on the financial statements (and notes). The balance sheet date in each instance is December 31, 20X1.

1. On December 31, the commodities handled by the company had been traded in the open market for $1.40 per kilogram. This price had prevailed for two weeks, following an official market report that predicted vastly enlarged supplies; however, no purchases were made at $1.40. The price throughout the preceding year, and several prior years, had been about $2. On January 18, 20X2, the price returned to $2, following disclosure of an error in the official calculations of the prior December—correction of which destroyed the expectations of excessive supplies. Inventory at December 31, 20X1, had been valued on a lower-of-cost-and-net-realizable-value basis, using the prevailing price known at that time, $1.40.

2. On February 1, 20X2, the board of directors adopted a resolution accepting an investment banker's offer to guarantee the marketing of $100 million of preferred shares.

3. On January 22, 20X2, one of the auditee's three major plants burned down, a $50 million loss that was covered to $40 million by insurance.

4. The auditee in this case is an open-end-type investment company. In January, 20X2, new management took control. By February 20X2 it had sold 90% of the investments carried at December 31, 20X1, and had purchased substantially more speculative ones.

5. This company has a wholly owned but not consolidated subsidiary producing oil in a foreign country. A serious rebellion began in that country on January 18, 20X2, and continued beyond the completion of your audit work. There has been extensive coverage of the fighting here.

6. The auditee, Comtois Corp., sells property management software systems. Shortly before its December 31, 20X1, year-end, Comtois's president finalized a large sale to a provincial ministry. The contract has been completed and all the terms agreed to by the assistant deputy minister, but the minister herself is the only one authorized to sign the contract because of the large dollar amount involved. As of the date Comtois's board authorized the financial statements to be issued, March 3, 20X2, Comtois has not yet received the signed contract because the minister has not been available. The president wants to recognize the revenue in Comtois's 20X1 fiscal year anyway so that the salespeople and managers involved can be paid a bonus this year based

on it. The auditee's stated accounting policy for revenue recognition on these types of sales, established five years earlier, is to recognize revenue when the sales contract is signed.

7. During its fiscal year ending December 31, 20X1, Noriker Inc. issued common shares to its vice-president of marketing. At the date of issuing these shares, the company also provided the vice-president with a non-interest-bearing loan of $50,000 to purchase the shares. While reviewing the minutes of all the Noriker board of directors meetings during the audit fieldwork, Noriker's auditor notes that in a meeting on February 12, 20X2, the Noriker board agreed to forgive this loan, effective on that day.

(© 2000, American Institute of CPAs. All Rights Reserved. Adapted by permission.)

DC 15-4 Subsequent Events: Cases. `LO4` In connection with your examination of the financial statements of Olars Manufacturing Corp. for the year ended December 31, your post–balance sheet audit procedures disclosed the following items:

1. January 3: The provincial government approved construction of an expressway. The plan will result in the expropriation of land owned by Olars Manufacturing Corp. Construction will begin late next year. No estimate of the expropriation award is available.

2. January 4: The funds for a $25,000 loan to the corporation made by Ms. Olars on July 15 were obtained by her with a loan on her personal life insurance policy. The loan was recorded in the loan payable to officers account. Ms. Olars's source of the funds was not disclosed in the company records. The corporation pays the premiums on the life insurance policy, and Mr. Olars, husband of the president, is the owner and beneficiary of the policy.

3. January 7: The mineral content of a shipment of ore en route on December 31 was determined to be 72%. The shipment was recorded at year-end at an estimated content of 50% by a debit to raw material inventory and a credit to accounts payable in the amount of $20,600. The final liability to the vendor is based on the actual mineral content of the shipment.

4. January 15: A series of personal disagreements have arisen between Ms. Olars, the president, and Ms. Tweedy, her sister-in-law, the treasurer. Ms. Tweedy resigned, effective immediately, under an agreement whereby the corporation would purchase her 10% share ownership at book value as of December 31. Payment is to be made in two equal amounts in cash on April 1 and October 1. In December the treasurer had obtained a divorce from Ms. Olars's brother.

5. January 31: As a result of reduced sales, production was curtailed in mid-January and some workers were laid off. On February 5 all the remaining workers went on strike. To date, the strike is unsettled.

6. February 10: A contract was signed whereby Mammoth Enterprises purchased from Olars Manufacturing all of the latter's capital assets (including rights to receive the proceeds of any property expropriation), inventories, and rights to conduct business under the name "Olars Manufacturing Division." The transfer's effective date will be March 1. The sale price was $500,000, subject to adjustment after a physical inventory count. Important factors contributing to the decision to enter into the contract were the policy of the board of directors of Mammoth Industries to diversify the firm's activities and the report of a survey conducted by an independent market appraisal firm, which revealed a declining market for Olars's products.

Required:

Assume that the above items came to your attention prior to completion of your audit work on February 15. For each of the above items:

a. Give the audit procedures, if any, that would have brought the item to your attention. Indicate other sources of information that may have revealed the item.

b. Discuss the disclosure that you would recommend for the item, listing all details. Indicate those, if any, that should not be disclosed. Give your reasons for recommending or not recommending their disclosure.

(© 2000, American Institute of CPAs. All Rights Reserved. Adapted by permission.)

DC 15-5 Lawyer's Letters. `LO3` The controller of Kim Engineering Ltd. (KEL) sent a legal representation letter to KEL's law firm at the request of the company's auditors. The controller told the auditors that there are no ongoing lawsuits. The lawyers replied to the letter, agreeing that there were no outstanding or possible claims of which they have knowledge, or for which their advice has been sought.

However, the controller was not aware that the board of directors had sought legal advice from a second law firm regarding a harassment lawsuit. Due to the nature of the matter, the board of directors did not want anyone to know about the possible claim. There are no records of it outside of the president's office, but the auditor noticed it when reviewing the minutes of the board of directors meetings. The auditor, therefore, requested that a letter be sent to the second law firm as well.

One of the members of the board of directors is Yung, who started the company 20 years ago, but is now retired from any duties other than being a director. When the company first started, Yung performed almost all of the duties herself, but over the years, her duties have been assigned to other people. For example, only the controller or the president of the company can sign cheques on behalf of the company, and the controller's authority is limited to $15,000. Any cheque request must be supported by an authorized purchase requisition, and any request over $15,000 must be authorized by the president. The accounting manager does all of the bank reconciliations himself, but his assistant enters the journal entries according to the accounting manager's instructions.

Required:

a. Indicate what the effect will be on the audit if the auditor receives no response from the second law firm.
b. If the second law firm replies and provides information to the auditor, indicate how the auditor should treat this information for financial statement purposes.
c. State whether the control risk is high or low, and support your decision with *four* points.

(Adapted from External Auditing (AU1), September 2010, with permission of Chartered Professional Accountants of Canada, Toronto, Canada. Any changes to the original material are the sole responsibility of the author (and/or publisher) and have not been reviewed or endorsed by the Chartered Professional Accountants of Canada.)

DC 15-6 Subsequent Events, Pro Forma Disclosures. `LO4, 6` Assume that you are the financial statement auditor in the following independent cases, and you are completing your audit in February 20X2.

1. During January 20X2, the company's management decided to sell rental real estate properties that accounted for approximately 40% of its total revenues in 20X1.
2. The company's main factory was closed for six weeks in January and February of 20X2 because of ice storm damage. The factory resumed full operations in late February.
3. One of the company's factories was destroyed by a fire in January. The plant was old and will not be replaced, as production can be taken up by excess capacity in other plants.
4. In late February, the company's board of directors agreed to settle an outstanding claim by paying $15 million to former employees. The employees suffered health problems related to asbestos exposure during the years of their employment. A contingent liability was disclosed but not accrued as of December 31, 20X1, because of the uncertainty surrounding the outcome of the lawsuit.
5. For the past four years, the company has made 90% of its revenues and profits from sales of specialty cable to computer manufacturers. Early in 20X2, it has become apparent that there is massive overcapacity in this industry, and demand for the product has fallen to almost zero. It is not expected to recover for several years, and may never recover if alternative technologies developed in the meantime make the product unnecessary.

Required:

For each of these subsequent events, indicate if you would require the auditee company to adjust its December 20X1 year-end financial statements, disclose the event in the 20X1 financial statements, and/ or provide pro forma financial information in the 20X1 financial statements. Give reasons to support your responses, and state any assumptions you make.

DC 15-7 Franchising Revenues. LO1, 6 You are an auditor with ZZ, a public accounting firm. Your firm has just accepted a new engagement to audit the annual financial statements of Chestnut Limited, a medium-size restaurant business. Chestnut operates a chain of specialty fast food restaurants. Most of the restaurants are franchised, and Chestnut receives franchise fees based on the franchisee store's net sales revenues.

Chestnut receives 4% of net sales as a base franchise fee, 1% as an advertising fee, and 0.5% as an administration fee for processing franchisee accounting information and issuing reports in standard format. Franchisee sales information is uploaded daily to Chestnut's central accounting system, where it is input into the franchise reporting system to generate daily, monthly, and year-end management reports.

Required:

Assume you are an audit manager reviewing the audit work on the franchise revenues that has been documented by the staff during their field work at Chestnut. What procedures do you expect are included in their audit work? State any assumptions you make.

DC 15-8 Revenues, General Journal Entries. LO1, 2, 6 Town & Country Cable Inc. (TCC) is a cable television provider serving customers in small towns and rural areas. Its shares are privately held, but it issued a 20-year bond eight years ago to the public. The bond contains restrictive covenants, which include requirements for TCC to maintain a current ratio of at least 2:1 at each fiscal year-end, and a ratio of operating cash flows to current liabilities of at least 1:0. If the covenants are violated, the bondholders have the right to demand repayment, raise the interest rate, and/or liquidate the company. In recent years, TCC has seen very little growth from new customer installations because most people are now choosing wireless service instead of cable. At the same time, TCC's existing installed customer base has been shrinking because many have switched to wireless for more content and lower cost. As a result of these changes in its operating environment, TCC has been close to violating its restrictive covenants in the past two years.

Petra is the senior on the current-year audit. While scrutinizing a 300-page printout of the general journal entries for the year for material entries and seeing nothing but small adjustments for payroll and purchasing discounts, Petra is about to sign off on the procedure. Then she notices 10 journal entries in a row in the middle of November that debit account #22000 (current accrued liabilities) and credit account #54400 (other operating income). The entries are all for different immaterial amounts, but all are to the same two accounts, and all have the same explanatory note: "To adjust accrued liabilities as per instructions memo of Nov. 2." On further investigation, Petra finds 40 more entries to these accounts with the same explanation. The entries are all for different, immaterial amounts but add up to a large, material amount. The accountant who made these general journal entries is no longer employed by TCC, and no one else in the accounting department knows anything about the "memo of November 2."

Required:

a. What is professional skepticism in auditing? Do the circumstances in this scenario make you skeptical?

b. Provide and evaluate three possible explanations for the auditor's findings in the TCC audit. Explain how the auditor could determine whether these entries result in a material misstatement of TCC's financial statements.

c. If these entries do result in financial statements that are materially misstated, what other procedures in the audit may also have revealed these entries?

DC 15-9 Revenue, Audit Procedures. **LO1, 6** While performing analytical procedures as part of his audit of the revenue and expense accounts at Galloway Inc., the auditor notes that Galloway's sales revenues in the current year have increased by 20% over the prior year. Galloway manufactures and sells business forms and has seen declining sales over the past few years as its customers have been changing to paperless, online process methods. In fact, in the prior year's audit there was concern about Galloway's ability to meet its long-term debt covenants, which require at least a 2:1 current ratio and pretax earnings that are at least 10 times long-term debt interest charges. To meet these debt covenant restrictions, no bonuses were paid to management in the prior year. When the auditor discussed the current-year sales figures with the sales manager, she informed him that Galloway had increased its prices by 50% in the third quarter of the current year to offset the lower sales volumes. Management had determined that Galloway's remaining customers were restricted to using paper-based documentation for various business reasons and thus would accept higher prices. During this interview, the chief accountant was passing by and, overhearing the topic, made the following comments: "Note that the accounts receivable balance is also much higher than last year, which is totally consistent with the higher sales. This should tie together your analysis, so your audit work on sales and accounts receivable must now be complete. We are looking forward to having our boardroom back when you auditors finally finish the job and leave!"

Required:

Discuss the nature and the persuasiveness of the audit evidence the auditor is gathering in the above scenario. What additional evidence would you recommend he obtain to support his conclusion on the sales revenue figure? How would you recommend this audit work be documented in the audit files?

ENDNOTES

1   *CPA Canada Assurance Handbook*—CAS 501, Appendix, "Joint Policy Statement Concerning Communications with Law Firms," paragraph 14.

2   Ibid., paragraphs 13 and 15.

3   Adapted from AU 9337.

4   *CPA Canada Assurance Handbook*—Other Canadian Standards, section 8200.

5   This type of pro forma disclosure is usually provided in a note to the historic financial statements. For this type of event, *pro forma financial statements* can help users see how the financial statements would have looked with the event included, even though it is not appropriate to include it in the historic financial statement amounts reported under GAAP. For example, in addition to historic financial statements, pro forma financial data may be the best way to show the effect of a business purchase or other merger, or the sale of a major portion of assets.

6   CAS 580.

7   *CPA Canada Handbook—Assurance*, 2014, "Other Canadian Standards," section 7150.

8   *CPA Canada Handbook—Assurance*, 2014, "Other Canadian Standards," section 8200.

9   CAS 550.

10   CAS 550, CAS 315.

11   CAS 550.

CHAPTER 16

Applying Professional Judgment to Form the Audit Opinion and Issue the Audit Report

At the completion of the audit, the auditor is required to provide an opinion that is properly supported by the audit evidence and findings reflected in the audit files. The misstatements uncovered in the audit must be analyzed and assessed against the materiality level. Professional judgment must be applied by auditors in forming a conclusion on whether the financial statements are not materially misstated and are fairly presented, and on whether the audit evidence obtained is sufficient and appropriate to support the opinion. An audit report must be issued that presents the appropriate form of opinion. These and related issues are covered in this chapter.

LEARNING OBJECTIVES

After completing this chapter, you will be able to do the following:

LO1 Describe the role of professional judgment in achieving the overall objectives of the independent auditor in conducting an audit of financial statements as set out in CAS 200.

LO2 Explain how accumulated misstatements are evaluated at the conclusion of an audit to form an opinion on the fair presentation of general purpose financial statements.

LO3 Describe the different forms of audit opinion, explain the decisions underlying the auditor's choice of form, and explain how the date of the audit report is determined.

LO4 Explain the purpose of emphasis of matter and other matter paragraphs in an audit report.

LO5 Summarize the auditor's communications throughout and at the conclusion of the engagement.

LO6   (Appendix 16A) Familiarize yourself with a checklist form used in practice to ensure all audit work has been properly completed at the end of the engagement.

LO7   (Appendix 16B) Explain how subsequent events can lead to dual dating of an audit report, and list the auditor's responsibilities when relevant facts become known after the audit report has been issued.

CHAPTER APPENDICES

APPENDIX 16A   Audit Completion Checklist

APPENDIX 16B   The Impact of Subsequent Events on Audit Reports

EcoPak Inc.

EcoPak's board meeting with its auditors to approve the annual financial statements has been scheduled for February 28. Tariq has reviewed all the files and has asked his partner Phyllis to do an engagement quality review, since it is a new audit engagement and the company has plans to do an IPO in the near future. M&G's policy is to have an audit team meeting after these reviews are completed to prepare the audit engagement partner for this board meeting and to finalize the auditor communication with those charged with governance.

Tariq has concluded that the scope of the audit has been acceptable, and that the financial statements comply with generally accepted accounting principles (GAAP; International Financial Reporting Standards [IFRS]) and include all the disclosures needed to achieve fair presentation. All the misstatements identified by the audit were adjusted, though their overall impact on income was much less than materiality. Two misclassification misstatements were addressed appropriately in the final version of the financial statements. Several control issues that arose during the audit have been noted for inclusion in the management letter. Tariq has discussed these points with Nina, and she has agreed they should be reported to the board at the upcoming meeting.

Prior to the board meeting, Nina also informed Tariq about a recent development. A venture capital firm is interested in investing in EcoPak shares, a substantial investment that would allow EcoPak to greatly reduce its bank debt and give it a much stronger balance sheet. The venture capitalists want to see the audited financial statements and will likely base their offer on a multiple of last year's earnings before interest, taxes, and depreciation/amortization (EBITDA). Tariq realizes that being aware of this specific financial statement user affects the risk profile of the engagement and perhaps would have lowered the overall materiality level they selected at the initial planning stage. However, he notes that they had already selected a relatively low performance materiality level due to its being a first-time audit, so they are probably fine even with this major change in the type of users who will be making decisions based on the financial statements.

At the February 28 board meeting, Tariq informs the board that M&G plans to issue an unmodified opinion in the audit report and that it will also include an other matter (OM) paragraph noting that the prior year's financial statements were audited by a different firm, as is standard practice for M&G and other auditing firms. EcoPak's board and management affirm to Tariq that in their view all the required financial statements and disclosures have been included. The board passes a resolution stating that it has taken full responsibility for the financial statements' fair presentation in accordance with IFRS, and this resolution is duly recorded in the minutes. Nina and Kam provide Tariq with a signed letter containing all the representations he has recommended. After the meeting ends, Tariq issues and signs the audit report with a date of February 28.

The Essentials of Applying Professional Judgment to Form the Audit Opinion and Issue the Audit Report

As we started into this book's explanation of the financial statement audit process, we noted that the auditor's overall objective in a financial statement audit is to form an opinion on whether management has fairly presented the financial statements and to communicate that opinion to the intended users of the financial statements in the auditor's report. We saw that financial statement users expect the risk of being misled or deceived by the information to be reduced when an independent auditor provides an opinion that the financial statements are fairly presented.

An auditor must use professional judgment to form this opinion. To apply professional judgment, auditors use their education and professional training, and the knowledge and experience they have gained in their professional work. Judgment involves making decisions, identifying a problem, considering different possible actions, and choosing the best course of action. The choice involves thinking critically about the relevant facts in the situation, the people potentially affected by the decision, and the consequences of the choice. To identify relevant facts, an auditor must keep an attitude of professional skepticism—thinking about the possibilities and being alert to situations that might suggest something is wrong in the financial statements. Things that go wrong in financial statements are referred to as *material misstatements* in generally accepted auditing standards (GAAS) terms.

We saw that there are two aspects covered by the opinion given in the audit report, the *scope of the audit* and the conclusion on whether the financial statements are *fairly presented* according to GAAP.

The engagement partner reviews the audit file documentation to determine whether the scope of the work performed was adequate to provide sufficient appropriate audit evidence related to all material assertions in the financial statements. If the scope was acceptable, no modification is required to the description of the scope of the work supporting the audit opinion. If there are limitations of the scope of the auditors' work, the auditor needs to reflect this problem in the report. If the impact of the area the auditors were unable to examine is isolated, so that it is not likely to have a pervasive impact on the financial statements, a *qualified audit opinion* is issued. In this report, the restriction(s) on the scope of the auditors' work is (are) explained in the paragraph that discusses the auditor's responsibilities, and the opinion is modified to carve out the accounts that could not be adequately verified because of the *scope limitation*. For example, if the auditor was unable to observe and test the physical inventory count due to a hurricane, the accounts to be excluded from the audit opinion are inventory, costs of sales, profit, and retained earnings. If the impact of the scope restriction is extensive and the inability to perform required audit procedures could affect many aspects of the financial statements, the auditor will not be able to issue any kind of opinion. An example is when the company's accounting records are all lost in a fire, so there are no documents available for the auditors to inspect. In this situation auditors issue what is called a *disclaimer of opinion*: they state that they are unable to provide any opinion because they could not get sufficient appropriate evidence about many important aspects of the financial statements.

The other aspect covered in the audit report is that the financial statements have been fairly presented and comply with GAAP; they are not materially misstated. The causes of misstatements are accidental errors in preparing financial statements, or deliberate attempts to mislead the users, which are called fraud. But between innocent errors at one end of the spectrum, and blatant fraud at the other, is a range of grey areas where a lot of subjectivity exists in the financial statements themselves. Auditor objectivity and skepticism are essential for deciding whether a grey area reflects some degree of management bias. Management will often want to influence user perceptions of the reported results in a certain direction, but at what point does the bias cross a line and become unfairly manipulative and potentially misleading to users? The most challenging part of the audit is identifying and obtaining evidence that gives the auditor a reasonable basis for reaching conclusions that the financial statement information is, or is not, fairly presented; i.e., it has not crossed that line between being acceptable and being manipulated with the intent to be misleading. These conclusions must be defensible to others with similar professional skills, so auditors must keep their own thought processes objective. They can't allow their conclusions to be influenced by management's biased presentation of the facts. Most people in management positions will not deliberately mislead others, but they may not be aware that their own perceptions of reality are skewed in a certain direction—generally toward seeing the company's performance in the most positive light possible. This makes it very important for auditors to maintain their objectivity. Using a skeptical perspective and a disciplined, logical thought process to build up evidence to support their conclusions is the best way to succeed in providing an appropriate opinion on the financial statements.

Forthcoming audit reporting standards will require the auditor of a listed company (i.e., a public company) to provide a list of key audit matters (KAMs) as part of the audit report. At the time of writing, these requirements have been issued as International Standards on Auditing (ISAs) to take effect by the end of 2016 and are being considered for issue in Canada, likely to come into effect at a later date than the ISAs. KAMs are those issues that auditors considered to be the most significant judgments made during the audit. Making these issues transparent to financial statement users is a way to show the more subjective or disputed aspects of accounting that auditors and management had to resolve to ensure the financial statements are fairly presented.

The end result of the audit-gathering efforts is a list of misstatements that were identified in performing the procedures and have not yet been corrected by management. As the audit proceeds and errors are uncovered, the auditor reports them to management as proposed adjusting entries. In private companies, when auditors report known misstatements to management, it is common for management to make the adjustments to improve the accuracy of the financial statements. In public companies, the situation can be different, since public companies will often issue a press release to report the earnings number to the market as soon as possible, but this will be before the full audited financial statements are ready to be issued. In these cases, management may not be willing to make adjustments that would change the earnings number already publicly announced.

As a result, there can be cases where unadjusted errors will remain in the financial statements, and the auditors must assess whether these errors accumulate to an amount that exceeds the materiality level they have set for the financial statements as a whole. If the misstatements accumulate to a total that is less than the auditors' materiality level, the auditors can issue a clean audit opinion, with no modifications. If they accumulate to more than the auditors' materiality level, management will have to adjust for at least enough to bring the accumulated total below materiality; otherwise the auditor will need to issue a modified opinion.

If a modified opinion is required, but the impact of the unadjusted misstatements can be isolated and does not pervasively affect the financial statements, a qualified opinion is used that explains the impact of the misstatement. For example, if management failed to record an impairment loss on intangible assets, the misstatement would affect the value of intangible assets, impairment loss and profit on the income statement, and retained earnings. If the impact of the misstatements is pervasive, affecting many aspects of the financial statements, the auditor may need to issue an adverse opinion, which states the auditor's belief that the financial statements are not fairly presented. An example that might result in an adverse opinion is if management refuses to consolidate large and material subsidiary companies—this affects all the accounts in the financial statements.

Even when the audit indicates that the monetary misstatements have not accumulated to a material level, the auditor must also be concerned with the potential for likely misstatements, unrealistic estimates, disclosure inadequacy, and other qualitative considerations affecting the fair presentation of the financial statements. On this basis, the auditor will form an opinion on whether the financial statements are fairly presented. However, these other considerations may lead the auditor to believe there are additional important matters to communicate to users, even when it is appropriate to give a clean opinion on the fairness of presentation of the financial statements. Auditors may provide additional information in the audit report by including emphasis of matter (EOM) paragraphs or OM paragraphs (and in future, for listed companies, KAMs will be required).

An EOM paragraph is used to draw readers' attention to important information that is presented or disclosed in the financial statements. The most common use is when the financial statements include a note about a going-concern uncertainty—the EOM in the auditors' report will advise readers that this important note is present so they will be more likely to take it into account in assessing the company's financial position. (Note, however, that when the new KAMs requirements are applied in practice, a matter reported as a KAM would not also be reported in an EOM paragraph.) An OM paragraph refers to a matter that the auditor believes will help users understand the audit, the auditor's responsibilities, or the auditor's report. An OM does not relate to matters that are presented or disclosed in the financial statements. An example is reporting that the comparative financial statements were audited by a different audit firm.

Note that clean, unmodified opinions are by far the most common. Since the main reason for the audit is to provide assurance to users that information risk is low, management has incentives to correct misstatements to avoid the consequence of users believing the information risk is high. If they believe the information risk is high, users will lower the value they place on the company and be less likely to invest in or lend money to it. Also, securities law requires public companies to obtain clean audit reports—otherwise their shares will be de-listed from the stock market—a very negative consequence! However, the institutional factors that favour clean audit opinions can also be reasons to move toward more customized auditor commentaries in future audit reporting standard developments that can expand the insights and information value of clean audit opinions.

Once the judgment is made, the audit report can be finalized. The final event that has to occur before the auditors' report can be dated, signed, and provided to the company is for those charged with governance to take responsibility for the final financial statements. This normally occurs at an annual board of directors meeting at which the financial statements are presented, the auditor has an opportunity to address the board and take any questions the directors may have, and a motion to approve the audited annual financial statements is approved. The date of this approval is the date the auditor puts on the audit report. As discussed earlier, auditors are not responsible for considering new events and evidence that come to their attention after this date with regard to this set of financial statements, though relevant and significant events would be noted in terms of their impact on the next period's financial statements. If, however, material information comes to light that existed during the time of the audit work and that the auditors should have discovered, they do have an obligation to consider the impact it would have had on the financial statements and on their report. If users may have been misled as a result of the overlooked information and any adjustments that should have been made to the financial statements, and/or to the auditor's report, the auditors need to take steps to make sure users receive this new information.

A final point regarding completing the audit engagement and issuing the report is to summarize the various points of communication between auditors and those charged with governance and/or management (sometimes those charged with governance and management are the same group; sometimes there is a separate board or audit committee charged with governance that oversees the management group). Two earlier points where correspondence with those charged with governance was required were the engagement letter once the engagement was accepted, and a summary of the main planning decisions as the field work stage of the audit is beginning. At the end of the audit, the main correspondence required is a report of significant audit findings and a letter summarizing any internal control weaknesses the auditor found. Significant audit findings include matters such as the summary of unadjusted misstatements, the nature of the misstatements identified, any disagreements with management regarding significant estimates or disclosures, and any significant control deficiencies that have been reported to management (these would be reported to and discussed with management as soon as possible after auditors discovered them, and then to those charged with governance once management has responded to them).

The financial statement audit process now is completed. Congratulations on making it to the finish line!

Review Checkpoints

16-1   What is a person using when they apply professional judgment in an audit engagement?

16-2   What is involved in exercising professional judgment?

16-3   How does an auditor identify facts that are relevant to determining whether there are misstatements in the financial statements being audited?

16-4   What two aspects of the audit engagement are expressed in the auditor's report?

16-5   Why does the engagement partner review all the audit documentation as a starting point in forming an opinion on whether the financial statements are fairly presented?

16-6   What does it mean if the auditor gives a qualified opinion because of a scope limitation? Give an example of when this situation might arise.

16-7   What impact does a scope limitation on obtaining evidence about the ending inventory have on the auditor's opinion?

16-8   What would cause the auditor to need to issue a disclaimer of opinion?

16-9   What is implied by stating an opinion that the financial statements fairly present a company's financial position at period-end and its performance and cash flows for the period then ended?

16-10   What are two causes of misstatements?

16-11   Is it possible that a misstatement cannot be clearly categorized as being due to error or to fraud? Explain your position.

16-12   If the auditor believes that management has reported revenues and assets too aggressively (i.e., overstated them), does this mean management is dishonest? Explain your response.

16-13   What is the role of objectivity in conducting an audit that complies with GAAS?

16-14   How is professional skepticism related to objectivity?

16-15   What are KAMs in an audit report?

16-16   Why might management of a public company be reluctant to adjust misstatements that auditors discovered? How might this situation be different in a private company? Why?

16-17   What kind of audit opinion is appropriate if the intangible asset balance has not been prepared in accordance with GAAP because the value of the assets is very unlikely to be realized, and this is the only misstatement in the financial statements? What information would the auditor include in the report, and what type of opinion would be given?

16-18   What conditions would result in an auditor issuing an adverse opinion? What is the message being communicated to readers by an adverse audit opinion?

16-19   What other aspects of financial reporting are relevant to forming an audit opinion on financial statements, besides the monetary misstatements uncovered in the audit work?

16-20   If an auditor decides an unmodified opinion is appropriate, why would there be a need to add additional information to the auditor's report?

16-21   What is an EOM paragraph? When and why would it be used?

16-22   What is an OM paragraph? When and why would it be used?

16-23   When would KAMs be included in an audit report? How might these matters affect users of audited financial statements?

16-24 Why are clean unmodified opinions by far the most common form of audit report?

16-25 What determines the date that auditors put on their report? What is the significance of this date to the auditors? to the financial statement users?

16-26 If auditors discover matters after the audit report date that would have changed the financial statements, and/or their audit report on those statements, what do they need to do?

16-27 What are two main areas of audit findings that auditors communicate to those charged with governance at the conclusion of the audit?

16-28 What do audit team members do to celebrate the successful completion of the audit?

Applying Professional Judgment to Form the Audit Opinion

LO1 Describe the role of professional judgment in achieving the overall objectives of the independent auditor in conducting an audit of financial statements as set out in CAS 200.

Throughout our discussion of the audit process to this point in the text, we have seen many examples of the panoply of decisions auditors need to make. For example, should the engagement be accepted at all, what is material to users, what are the risks of material misstatement, what audit procedures are required to respond to these risks to provide assurance that the financial statements are not materially misstated, is the evidence we have sufficient and appropriate to provide reasonable/high assurance regarding a material misstatement, and what does the evidence indicate? In making these decisions, auditors need to apply their professional judgment. This section provides a brief discussion of the role of professional judgment in meeting the auditor's overall objectives, as set out in CAS 200. Forming the audit opinion is the culmination of these professional judgments.

What are the auditor's overall objectives in conducting a financial statement audit in accordance with CASs? CAS 200 sets these out as follows:[1]

11. (a) To obtain reasonable assurance about whether the financial statements as a whole are free from material misstatement, whether due to fraud or error, thereby enabling the auditor to express an opinion on whether the financial statements are prepared, in all material respects, in accordance with an applicable financial reporting framework; and

11. (b) To report on the financial statements, and communicate as required by the CASs, in accordance with the auditor's findings.

12. In all cases, when reasonable assurance cannot be obtained and a qualified opinion in the auditor's report is insufficient in the circumstances for purposes of reporting to the intended users of the financial statements, the CASs require that the auditor disclaim an opinion or withdraw (or resign) from the engagement . . . .

As introduced in Chapter 2, CAS 200 provides a framework of the key principles that guide the conduct of a financial statement audit in accordance with GAAS. It explains the nature and scope of an audit engagement that will achieve the above objectives. By defining the scope, authority, and structure of the CASs, it establishes the general responsibilities of an independent auditor that are applicable in all audits, including the obligation to comply with the CASs. Now that you have covered most of the audit process leading up to achieving the overall objectives, it would be very useful to reread CAS 200 and apply the perspectives you have gained in the context of the auditor's ultimate responsibility—forming the audit opinion.

CAS 200 Overall Objectives of the Independent Auditor and the Conduct of an Audit in Accordance with Canadian Auditing Standards

3. The purpose of an audit is to enhance the degree of confidence of intended users in the financial statements. This is achieved by the expression of an opinion by the auditor on whether the financial statements are prepared, in all material respects, in accordance with an applicable financial reporting framework. In the case of most general purpose frameworks, that opinion is on whether the financial statements are presented fairly, in all material respects, or give a true and fair view in accordance with the framework. An audit conducted in accordance with CASs and relevant ethical requirements enables the auditor to form that opinion.

5. As the basis for the auditor's opinion, CASs require the auditor to obtain reasonable assurance about whether the financial statements as a whole are free from material misstatement, whether due to fraud or error. Reasonable assurance is a high level of assurance. It is obtained when the auditor has obtained sufficient appropriate audit evidence to reduce audit risk (that is, the risk that the auditor expresses an inappropriate opinion when the financial statements are materially misstated) to an acceptably low level. However, reasonable assurance is not an absolute level of assurance, because there are inherent limitations of an audit which result in most of the audit evidence on which the auditor draws conclusions and bases the auditor's opinion being persuasive rather than conclusive. (Ref: Para. A28–A52)

Objectives Stated in Individual CASs

21. To achieve the overall objectives of the auditor, the auditor shall use the objectives stated in relevant CASs in planning and performing the audit, having regard to the interrelationships among the CASs, to (Ref: Para. A67–A69)

   (a) Determine whether any audit procedures in addition to those required by the CASs are necessary in pursuance of the objectives stated in the CASs; and (Ref: Para. A70)

   (b) Evaluate whether sufficient appropriate audit evidence has been obtained. (Ref: Para. A71)

Failure to Achieve an Objective

24. If an objective in a relevant CAS cannot be achieved, the auditor shall evaluate whether this prevents the auditor from achieving the overall objectives of the auditor and thereby requires the auditor, in accordance with the CASs, to modify the auditor's opinion or withdraw from the engagement (where withdrawal is possible under applicable law or regulation). Failure to achieve an objective represents a significant matter requiring documentation in accordance with CAS 230. (Ref: Para. A75–A76)

Source: *CPA Canada Handbook—Assurance*, 2014.

To achieve the overall objective of an audit, the auditor needs to formulate and report an audit opinion on the financial statements. To reach this goal, auditors need to exercise professional judgment and maintain professional skepticism throughout the planning and performance of the audit. Professional judgment is defined as the application of relevant training, knowledge, and experience within the context provided by auditing, accounting, and ethical standards, in making informed decisions about the courses of action that are appropriate in the circumstances of the audit engagement. Professional skepticism refers to an auditor attitude that includes a questioning mind, being alert to conditions that may indicate possible misstatement due to error or fraud, and a critical assessment of audit evidence (CAS 200, paragraphs 15 and 16)

At the conclusion of the audit process, the engagement partner must form an opinion on the auditee's financial statements and prepare an appropriate audit report. Throughout the text to this point, we have seen many situations where the auditors have been required to use their judgment to decide on materiality levels, assess risk, design appropriate procedures responding to the risk, and draw conclusions about potential misstatements based on their findings. Auditor judgments include evaluating the auditee management's judgments in applying accounting policies, making accounting estimates, and preparing the financial statements and notes, by considering such issues as the following:[2]

- Is there documentation of the relevant accounting standards and other applicable sources that were considered by management and the auditor?

- Are the judgments based on facts and circumstances that are clearly documented?
- Are any assumptions used justified and documented by management? Did the auditor challenge them and subject them to audit procedures?
- Were ranges of probable outcomes considered and documented by management? Were these evaluated for reasonability by the auditor? If not reasonable, what additional procedures did the auditor perform to support an opinion?
- Did the auditor consult, and is this documented?

All decisions and conclusions need to be well documented so that an experienced auditor can understand the significant professional judgments that have been made. It is not enough for the auditor just to say a decision was "based on my professional judgment"; the documentation must clearly show the facts and circumstances— or sufficient appropriate audit evidence—and explain how these support the decision.

Given the complexity of many audit engagements, and the tendency of people (even auditors!) to succumb to biases or shortcuts in their thinking, audit practice has developed requirements for consultation. These can take the form of one-on-one meetings with experts (who may be internal or external to the firm, whichever is required) and audit team meetings. Auditors must have the necessary competencies to achieve reasonable judgments, and consultations facilitate this as audit team members with appropriate knowledge, seniority, experience and full information can exchange relevant facts and perspectives. These meetings play an important role in the application of professional judgment at all stages in the audit. As a general rule, the less experienced the practitioner or engagement team, and the less knowledge they have of the specific industry or accounting topic, the greater their need for consultation. The greater the matter's complexity, materiality, and risk, the greater is the need for consultation.

Documentation of consultations is key, both for ensuring all sides to the consultation acknowledge the issues discussed and resulting conclusions and for demonstrating to subsequent reviewers or inspectors that necessary consultations took place.

Based on facts and circumstances known by the auditor up to the date of the report, consultation assists in making informed and reasonable judgments.

Review Checkpoints

16-29   What is the overall objective of an audit of an organization's financial statements, and how does an auditor achieve this objective?

16-30   What judgments are made by the auditee's management in preparing its financial statements?

16-31   How does consultation facilitate good professional judgment at the conclusion of the audit?

Overall Evaluation of Audit Evidence and Misstatements

LO2   Explain how accumulated misstatements are evaluated at the conclusion of an audit to form an opinion on the fair presentation of general purpose financial statements.

Once the audit team's evidence-gathering work is completed and documented, the engagement partner reviews the files to make a final evaluation of the adequacy of the work. Judgment is applied to evaluate whether the evidence documented adequately addresses the risks identified and to note the effect of identified and likely misstatements that could cause the financial statements not to be fairly presented in accordance with GAAP (the applicable fair presentation framework) or to be misleading to users. The box below relates a story in which an auditor was not satisfied with the evidence the firm was able to collect and had to resign. The story also delves into challenges auditors and regulators are facing in the current international business environment.

TSX-Listed Chinese Forestry Company's Auditor Resigns

Sino-Forest Corp. reported that Ernst & Young LLP resigned as the company's auditor in April 2012, in yet another setback for the scandal-plagued Chinese timber company. The accounting firm refused to sign off on the Mississauga-based and Hong Kong–headquartered company's financial results, after a $50 million internal investigation was unable to resolve key questions surrounding Sino-Forest's relationships and dealings with its business partners. In its resignation letter, Ernst & Young noted that Sino-Forest "remained unable to satisfactorily address outstanding issues in relation to its 2011 financial statements."

Sino-Forest's downward spiral began in June 2011, when U.S. short seller Muddy Waters LLC accused it of fraudulently exaggerating the size of its forestry assets. According to documents released by the committee of directors investigating fraud allegations against the TSX-listed firm, several executives of Sino-Forest, including its former CEO and its co-founder, had financial ties to the parent company of a key supplier of forestry assets. Those links raise questions about whether Sino-Forest bought and sold Chinese forest land at fair market value, as they would have if all the deals were with arm's-length parties. The Chinese timber firm's collapse sent shock waves through the investment community and focused attention on its audit firm, Ernst & Young LLP. Ernst & Young was Sino-Forest's long-time auditor, signing off on the company's financial statements for years. It came under the spotlight when Sino-Forest was accused of fraud and was named in multiple class action lawsuits related to the company's collapse.

Around the same time, Canada's audit regulator, the Canadian Public Accountability Board (CPAB), released results of a three-month review of work done by Canadian audit firms with Chinese clients, saying their work has been a "disappointment." "...a lot of things that we felt were fundamental auditing processes and procedures were just not applied," CPAB chief executive officer Brian Hunt said in an interview. The findings include misapplied fundamental audit procedures, notably around cash confirmations, as well as a failure of the auditors to have a sufficient understanding of the entity and its environment. CPAB found a lack of professional skepticism when auditors were confronted with evidence that should have raised red flags regarding potential fraud risk. CPAB called its report "a wakeup call" for Canada's auditing profession to improve its work in foreign jurisdictions, and it has demanded accounting firms fix deficiencies in their audits of 12 China-based companies whose shares trade on Canadian stock exchanges.

In March 2012, the Ontario Securities Commission (OSC), Canada's most powerful securities regulator, issued a report on its review of Canadian stock listings by companies with most of their operations in China and other emerging markets. That report found weak links at every stage of the listing process, including the role played by auditors. The OSC's review of emerging-market issuers stemmed from the allegations against Sino-Forest.

Sources: Euan Rocha and Jennifer Kwan, "Sino-Forest auditor resigns; shares being delisted," April 5, 2012, reuters.com/article/2012/04/05/sinoforest-auditor-idUSL2E8F52PG20120405; Peter Koven, "Sino-Forest auditor Ernst & Young resigns," *Postmedia News*, April 5, 2012, business.financialpost.com/investing/sino-forest-auditor-ernst-young-resigns; Peter Koven, "Sino-Forest defends opaque procedures in lawsuit against shortseller," April 5, 2012, business.financialpost.com/news/fp-street/sino-forest-defends-opaque-procedures-in-lawsuit-against-shortseller; Andy Hoffman, "Sino-Forest executives linked to key timber supplier," Asia-Pacific Reporter, *The Globe and Mail*, December 11, 2011, theglobeandmail.com/globe-investor/sino-forest-executives-linked-to-key-timber-supplier/article2267389/; Andy Hoffman "Sino-Forest auditor Ernst & Young resigns," Asia-Pacific Reporter, *The Globe and Mail*, April 5, 2012, theglobeandmail.com/globe-investor/sino-forest-auditor-ernst-young-resigns/article4098734/; Janet McFarland, "Canadian audits of China firms had major gaps: regulator," *The Globe and Mail*, February 21, 2012, theglobeandmail.com/globe-investor/canadian-audits-of-china-firms-had-major-gaps-regulator/article2344920/; "News and opinion on accounting in China: Canadian regulators and Chinese companies," China Accounting Blog, chinaaccountingblog.com/weblog/canadian-regulators-and.html.

As discussed in Chapter 15, the engagement partner would also perform final analytical procedures at this stage to check whether the results corroborate the audit findings or suggest additional risks that may not have been addressed. As you can appreciate from your study of the audit process, an audit team learns a lot more about the entity and the events of the audited period after performing their work than they could know at the planning stage. If at any point in the audit the findings suggest materiality or risk assessments should be revised, auditors must determine if it is necessary to go back and perform additional procedures to respond to the revised materiality or assessed risk. The final evaluation stage is the last chance for the team to get it right, so this is an important decision for the audit partner. In practice, auditors may use audit completion checklists as an aid to help ensure all the key matters have been addressed and considered to conclude the audit work. An example of this type of practice aid is provided in Appendix 16A.

Standards Check

CAS 200 Overall Objectives of the Independent Auditor and the Conduct of an Audit in Accordance with Canadian Auditing Standards

A20. Professional skepticism is necessary to the critical assessment of audit evidence. This includes questioning contradictory audit evidence and the reliability of documents and responses to inquiries and other information obtained from management and those charged with governance. It also includes consideration of the sufficiency and appropriateness of audit evidence obtained in the light of the circumstances, for example, in the case where fraud risk factors exist and a single document, of a nature that is susceptible to fraud, is the sole supporting evidence for a material financial statement amount.

A22. The auditor cannot be expected to disregard past experience of the honesty and integrity of the entity's management and those charged with governance. Nevertheless, a belief that management and those charged with governance are honest and have integrity does not relieve the auditor of the need to maintain professional skepticism or allow the auditor to be satisfied with less-than-persuasive audit evidence when obtaining reasonable assurance.

Source: *CPA Canada Handbook—Assurance*, 2014.

Once the partner is satisfied with the adequacy of the evidence, any remaining uncorrected misstatements must be discussed with the auditee management and any necessary adjustments approved by them. The audit standards require that all identified and likely misstatements, other than those that are clearly **trivial misstatements**, must be accumulated in a **summary of misstatements** and discussed with management. Note that the threshold amount to be used to assess what is "clearly trivial" needs to be decided and documented early in the planning so it will be applied consistently by everyone working on the engagement. In the case of identified, known misstatements, management will often approve appropriate journal entries to correct them. For various reasons, however, some adjustments may be **passed adjustments (waived adjustments)**, which means the auditor agrees with the auditee management that they will remain as **unadjusted (uncorrected) misstatements**. The auditing standards require that any such uncorrected misstatements be quantitatively and qualitatively immaterial.

Since identified misstatements are matters on which there is usually general agreement, you may wonder why management would not simply correct them all in the interests of more accurate presentation. However,

trivial misstatements:
misstatements that are considered to be so small and insignificant that auditors can disregard accumulating or reporting them to management; the threshold level for what amount is considered trivial must be set at the planning stage of the audit

summary of misstatements:
an audit file schedule that lists all the identified and likely misstatements uncovered in the audit procedures and analyzes their impact on fair presentation of the financial statements

passed adjustments (waived adjustments):
unadjusted misstatements discovered by an auditor that management decides not to correct but auditors can accept since they are not material to fair presentation of the financial statements

unadjusted (uncorrected) misstatements:
errors in financial statements that are discovered by the auditor but management decides not to correct, due to cost-benefit or other considerations

there are practical considerations that make this a cost-benefit decision. Recall from your study of the double-entry accounting model what happens when we change one number—at least one other number has to change somewhere to keep the balance. In the case of income misstatements, not only will the bottom line change, but something on the balance sheet will also have to change. Also, the income tax will change. There may also be bonuses, dividends, or other payments that are based on a percentage of income; these will also change. And in some cases, management may have issued a press release showing their earnings long before the audit is completed and then may find it would raise questions if a different number appeared in the audited reports, even if the difference is not material. In some cases, management may not agree that the misstatement exists. For all these reasons, it is quite common for some identified misstatements to be left unadjusted. In the case of an unadjusted income misstatement, its impact remains in the opening retained earnings balance carried forward to the next period, and it will reverse (i.e., have the opposite impact on income) in the next and/or future periods.

Auditing research shows that the ultimate decisions regarding adjustment of misstatements result from **auditor–client negotiations** at the final stages of the audit.[3] Management may be reluctant to adjust the financial statements in certain situations, such as when the adjustments change income and an earnings announcement has already been published in the press. The audit scandals discussed throughout the book can be viewed as situations where the auditors did not negotiate successfully and management prevailed. Obviously, there was a high cost to firms like Arthur Andersen for allowing materially misstated financial statements to be released to the public.

Exhibit 16–1 is a summary worksheet ("scoresheet") showing the misstatements accumulated in the various sections of the audit files. Exhibit 16–1 illustrates a working paper used to summarize all the misstatements uncovered in an audit, indicate different areas where they arose, and address their impact on the financial statements. If the accumulated total of the misstatements exceeds materiality, some action is required to correct them. Otherwise, the financial statements are materially misstated. Note that the misstatements in Exhibit 16–1 are carried forward from the examples in the "Misstatement Analysis" sections of Chapters 11 through 14. Take particular note of those misstatements that affect both the balance sheet and the income statement. These errors are of concern since many key user decisions are based on the income measure. Other types of errors involve misclassifications within the balance sheet or income statement. While such errors do not affect the income measure, they are also a concern because they may distort important ratios that users rely on, for example, debt covenants requiring a minimum current ratio to be maintained.

Ideally, management would correct every misstatement, and this would make an audit partner's job much easier! But, as discussed above, management often has reasons to resist adjusting certain errors, and if the resulting overall misstatement of the financial statements is less than materiality, an audit partner does not have a strong negotiating position to insist on further adjustments because the audit standards essentially require adjustment of material levels of misstatement.

Up to this point, we have dealt with identified monetary, quantitative misstatements, but the audit partner must also be concerned with the potential for likely misstatements, unrealistic estimates, disclosure inadequacy, and other qualitative considerations affecting the fair presentation of the financial statements. On this basis, the auditor will form an opinion on whether the financial statements are fairly presented. The auditor must reach a conclusion on whether the audit has provided reasonable assurance that the risk of material misstatement is acceptably low. While such assessments depend on the specific context of each audit engagement, an important point to appreciate here is that the partner really needs to exercise good judgment in a very complex and risky assessment. This takes experience and strong moral reasoning, and in some cases, sheer courage to fight for what the auditor thinks is the right thing to do. This is why it typically takes 10 or more years of audit experience at increasing levels of responsibility before an auditor is considered capable of being an engagement partner.

auditor–client negotiations:
discussions between auditor and management, usually at the end of an audit engagement, concerning decisions on whether or not to adjust the financial statements for identified and likely misstatements discovered by the auditor

EXHIBIT 16–1

Example of Working Paper for Accumulated Misstatements

AUDITEE: *EcoPak Inc.* FINANCIAL STATEMENT PERIOD: *y/e December 31, 20X1*	SUMMARY OF ACCUMULATED MISSTATEMENTS	FILE INDEX: *335*

F/S MATERIALITY: *10,000*

Prepared by: *D.L.* Date: *Mar. 15, 20X2*
Reviewed by: *T.K.* Date: *Mar. 16, 20X2*

Description of Misstatement W/P REF.	AMOUNT OF OVERSTATEMENT (UNDERSTATEMENT) OF FINANCIAL STATEMENTS			PROPOSED ADJUSTING ENTRIES				
	ASSETS DEC. 31, 20X0	LIABILITIES	PRETAX INCOME	ACCOUNTS	INCOME STATEMENT Debit	Credit	BALANCE SHEET Debit	Credit
1. Unrecorded cash disbursements (Ch. 12) *BB-1*	42,000	42,000		ACCOUNTS PAYABLE CASH			42,000	42,000
2. Improper sales cutoff (Ch. 11) *705*	13,000 (7,800)	13,000	13,000 (7,800)	SALES ACCOUNTS RECEIVABLE INVENTORY COST OF SALES (60%)	13,000 7,800	7,800	7,800	13,000
3. Inventory write-off (Ch. 13) *D-1*	21,000		21,000	COST OF SALES INVENTORY	21,000			21,000
4. Under-accrued electricity bill (Ch. 12) *BB-1*		(3,700)	3,700	UTILITIES EXPENSE ACCOUNTS PAYABLE	3,700			3,700
5. Omitted accrual for last day's payroll (Ch. 13) *730*		(2,500)	2,500	PAYROLL EXPENSE ACCRUED LIABILITIES	2,500			2,500
6. Software amortization calculation error for first year of use (Ch. 12) *U-1*	(17,000)		(17,000)	ACCUMULATED AMORTIZATION AMORTIZATION EXPENSE		17,000	17,000	
7. Current portion of long-term debt misclassified as long-term liability (Ch. 14) *U-1*		50,000 (50,000)		LONG-TERM DEBT CURRENT PORTION LONG-TERM DEBT			50,000	50,000
8. Income tax impact of the above net income over-statement ($15,400*40%)	(6,160)		(6,160)	INCOME TAXES PAYABLE INCOME TAX EXPENSE		6,160	6,160	
	45,040	35,800	9,240		40,200	30,960	122,960	132,200

SUMMARY OF F/S IMPACT:

NET INCOME CHANGE	(9,240)
CURRENT ASSETS CHANGE	(62,040)
CURRENT LIABILITIES CHANGE	14,200
WORKING CAPITAL CHANGE	(76,240)

Note that Exhibit 16–1 is based only on identified factual misstatements (e.g., it does not consider likely misstatements extrapolated from audit sampling applications). In this method, the uncorrected misstatements are aggregated in various ways to see if they total to a material amount. For example, if materiality is based on net income and is assessed to be 5% of recorded net income, the auditor must aggregate all misstatements affecting net income. This can be based on either (1) changes in net assets (assets less liabilities) or the equivalent or (2) revenues less expenses. Given the nature of the double-entry system, either approach should yield the same number. In this exhibit's example, the net effect of uncorrected identified misstatements on net income is computed as follows:

Misstatements in net income = Misstatements in changes in net assets = Misstatements in changes in assets − Misstatements in changes in liabilities

Using the values in this exhibit,

42,000(A) + 13,000(A) + 21,000(A) − 7,800(A) − 17,000(A) − 6,160(A) − [+ 42,000(L) − 3,700(L) − 2,500(L) + 50,000(L) − 50,000(L)] = $9,240

= misstatements in revenues − misstatements in expenses

= 13,000(R) − [6,160(E) + 7,800(E) − 21,000(E) − 3,700(E) − 2,500(E) + 17,000(E)] = $9,240

= total net misstatements in net income (overstatement; i.e., to eliminate all the misstatements, auditee's proposed net income must be reduced by $9,240).

This total of $9,240 is then compared with the predetermined overall materiality. If $9,240 is less than material, the auditor may conclude that further adjustments are not necessary. In the exhibit, we assume the materiality is $10,000, so if management decided

(continued)

EXHIBIT 16–1

Example of Working Paper for Accumulated Misstatements   (*continued*)

not to make the adjusting entries for the misstatements that affect income, the auditor could find this acceptable. The misclassification of the current portion of long-term debt is material and, even though it does not affect income, it needs to be corrected. An implication of not correcting the income misstatements is that in the following year (in the case of current assets or liabilities, or over the life of the asset for amortization) they will reverse, that is, have the opposite impact on income. When adjustments are passed, as is possible when their total is less than materiality, auditors still need to keep track of these reversals because they could push the total level of misstatement in the current year over the limit.

This analysis, in summary, is based on uncorrected, identified misstatements only, and it is perfectly appropriate in cases where the auditor tests 100% of the transactions. This level of testing is likely done for cash, capital assets, non-current liabilities, and shareholders' equity. For accounts such as inventory, receivables, and payables, which can represent large populations of individual items, the auditor may wish to use sampling theory concepts to include likely and possible misstatement in the assessment of whether the misstatements are material. Adjustments and decision making based on sampling situations are covered in Appendix 10B.

Auditee Approval of Adjusting Entries and Financial Statement Disclosure

The financial statements, including adjustments to the draft version, are the responsibility of management. Some adjusting entries identified in the audit may be approved by management as they are dealt with during the ongoing field work, and others may be approved at the final wrap-up.

Exhibit 16–1 summarizes the misstatements accumulated in the various sections of the audit files. It is the basis for the auditor's end-of-audit proposed adjusting journal entries. Auditors evaluate the uncorrected misstatements to see how these will affect the financial statements and to help decide which ones must be adjusted to support an unmodified ("clean") audit opinion and which ones may be passed. A passed adjustment is one the auditors decide not to insist on because the uncorrected misstatement does not materially affect the financial position and results of operations. In private companies, when auditors report these to management, it is common for management to make the adjustments to improve the accuracy of the financial statements. In public companies the situation can be different, since public companies often issue a press release to report the earnings number to the market as soon as possible, but before the full audited financial statements are ready to be issued. In these cases, adjustments below the overall materiality level are more likely to be passed by the auditor, because management may not be willing to make adjustments if it changes the earnings number already publicly announced.

The proposed adjustments shown in Exhibit 16–1 are those required to correct the misstatements noted in the misstatement analysis sections of Chapters 11 through 14. They are (1) recording cheques written and mailed but not in the books, (2) reversing recorded sales for goods shipped after the balance sheet date and reversing the 60% cost of goods sold, (3) writing off obsolete and damaged inventory, (4) recording the understated expense found in the search for unrecorded liabilities, (5) recording the understated payroll expense found in the audit of payroll, (6) correcting an amortization calculation error, (7) reclassifying the current portion of long-term debt, and (8) recording a tax refund asset for overpaid income taxes based on the overstated income number (could be a debit to tax liability if all the taxes for the year had not already been paid). Summary effects on income, current assets, current liabilities, and working capital are shown at the bottom of the worksheet. These help auditors assess the potential impact of the adjustments on financial statement users, for example, on lenders who are monitoring working capital ratio limits in debt covenants.

The adjusting entries shown in Exhibit 16–1 are labelled "proposed" because they are still subject to management's approval. A final list of all approved adjusting entries is given to the auditee accounting staff so that formal entries can be made, bringing the accounting records into balance with the financial statements.

The auditee must also approve all disclosure in the notes. Any additional disclosures auditors consider necessary are usually drafted as proposed notes. They must be considered carefully before being presented to management for its decision on whether to accept them as company disclosures.

Evaluation of Misstatements' Materiality

The accumulated audit evidence is the main basis for deciding if the amount of uncorrected misstatement is material. Chapter 5 explained how the audit is planned with the objective of detecting misstatements that are material, either individually or in aggregate, to the financial statements as a whole. Recall that the auditor considers materiality at the planning stage, while performing the audit, and at the final evaluation stage, when forming the audit opinion. The auditor uses professional judgment to determine a materiality level for planning and performing the audit, basing this on the amount of misstatement that would probably influence decisions of a person relying on the financial statements to make business and economic decisions. At the final evaluation stage, the auditor considers individual and aggregate misstatements discovered, their nature and cause, whether they indicate a possibility of further misstatements, and how they quantitatively and qualitatively affect the financial statements.

Misstatements have various causes, such as arithmetical mistakes (e.g., an addition error in a physical inventory count), use of inappropriate accounting principles, incorrect application of accounting principles, and disagreements about valuation or other estimates. They may occur accidentally or through misunderstanding, be the result of embezzlement, or be deliberate misrepresentations. As discussed in Chapter 5, a key qualitative factor in the auditor's assessment is evidence of deliberate misstatements intended to improve or defer earnings in order to achieve management's goals. These goals, such as obtaining an earnings-based bonus, may not be aligned with those of the company's capital providers, which are usually the most important users of the audited financial statements.

Exhibit 16–2 (which is based on AuG-41)[4] illustrates four possible outcomes of an audit and explains how professional judgment is applied in each case to determine the impact on the audit opinion. For evaluating whether the financial statements as a whole are materially misstated, uncorrected misstatements can be classified into three main categories: known, likely, and further possible. In the terminology of AuG-41, a known misstatement (identified misstatement) is a factual misstatement actually identified during the audit, so there is no uncertainty about its existence. A likely misstatement (projected misstatement) is one that probably exists based on audit evidence examined, for example, the projected effect of a misstatement identified in representative samples or management accounting estimates or of policy choices that the auditor considers unreasonable. A **further possible misstatement** is one that could exist over and above the total of known and likely misstatements because of the fundamental limitations of auditing, for example, sampling and non-sampling risks (as discussed in Chapter 10), forecasting uncertainties in accounting estimates, and minimum review accounts (those subjected to minimal verification because they have a very low assessed risk of misstatement). The amount of possible misstatement cannot be precisely quantified, but the auditor must exercise professional judgment in addressing this possibility, particularly when the total approaches materiality,

further possible misstatement:
a misstatement that could exist over and above the total of known and likely misstatements because of the limitations of the testing concept of auditing

EXHIBIT 16–2

Relating Misstatements to Materiality to Form the Audit Opinion

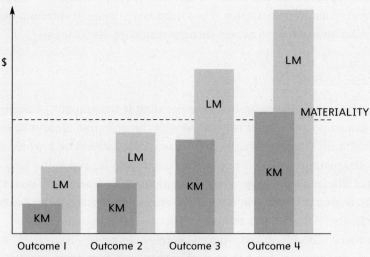

KM: Known misstatements in aggregate
LM: Likely misstatements in aggregate

Explanations of Outcomes

This chart shows some possible outcomes when auditors evaluate the accumulated misstatements they found in the audit and compare them to the materiality level set for the financial statements as a whole. As discussed in Chapter 5, this level is the auditors' judgment of the maximum amount of misstatement that could have accumulated in financial statements that will still be accurate enough for users to rely on. The level is initially set in the planning stage of the audit, but it may be adjusted as the audit proceeds if relevant information comes to the auditors' attention that suggests a different level is appropriate. Here we summarize the main implications of these outcomes.

Outcome 1: This outcome is frequently encountered in practice when auditees agree to correct most known misstatements. The level of known and likely aggregate misstatement is well below materiality, so the auditor may consider it very unlikely that the maximum possible misstatement would be quantitatively material. This supports giving an unmodified opinion on the financial statements. If, however, the auditor is skeptical about why management is not correcting the known misstatements the audit has revealed, these misstatements could be considered to be material for qualitative reasons. Essentially, these can be viewed as "intentional" misstatements, since management could have eliminated them.

Outcome 2: Here the sum of known and likely misstatements is close to, but below, materiality. This indicates that the auditor's best estimate is that financial statements are not materially misstated. The auditor must still assess how likely it is that additional, undetected misstatements exist that might cause the financial statements to be materially misstated. In this case, the auditor might propose that some or all known misstatements be corrected to bring the level of misstatement well below materiality so that an unmodified opinion could be given. The auditor might also consider performing additional auditing procedures to reduce the assessment of likely and further possible misstatements. Ultimately, the auditor will have to consider qualitative factors and exercise professional judgment in deciding whether an unmodified opinion is appropriate.

Outcome 3: Here the known misstatements are less than materiality but, when combined with likely misstatements, the level exceeds materiality. In this case, the auditor's best estimate is that the financial statements are materially misstated. The auditor would want management to correct some or all of the known misstatements. In practice it may be difficult for management to correct the likely misstatements since they are estimated by the auditors by extrapolating the errors found in sampling applications. If adjusting the known misstatements reduces the levels to sufficiently below materiality, an unmodified opinion can be given, subject also to consideration of qualitative factors. If the sum is still too high, auditors can perform additional testing—if this finds few or no additional errors, a lower amount of likely misstatement is present. If, on the other hand, further testing finds more known misstatements, the financial statements are likely to be materially misstated, so a qualified opinion is required.

Outcome 4: Here the level of known misstatements exceeds materiality. In this case a qualified opinion is required, since the audit evidence indicates the financial statements are materially misstated. Even if management will correct the known misstatements, the likely misstatements will probably still exceed materiality and prevent giving an unmodified opinion. As discussed in outcome 3, the auditors may consider further testing to verify their assessment of the level of likely misstatement. Again, the final decision is subject to consideration of qualitative factors.

or when misstatements are due to general control breakdowns rather than isolated instances. The relationship between the known and likely misstatements and materiality is important because it determines the nature of the auditor's opinion on the financial statements.[5]

Complications in audit evaluation can arise from measurements involving **management estimates**. Auditors are supposed to keep track of the differences between management estimates and the most **reasonable estimates** supported by audit evidence. They also identify estimates with high risk due to **forecast error** and assess whether these are fairly presented under the circumstances. In areas where GAAP are evolving, such as fair valuation of financial instruments (as discussed in Chapter 14), the accounting standards might not provide detailed implementation guidance, so the auditor needs to exercise judgment, guided by general principles and reporting objectives, to assess fair presentation. As will be discussed in Chapter 19, Part II (available on Connect), calibration techniques can be applied to different levels of aggregation within the financial statements, combined with probability management techniques using stochastic modelling methods such as the Monte Carlo method with calibrated estimates from "subject matter experts." There are increasingly sophisticated company- and industry-based data that auditors can use with probability management, and this is likely to be a source of audit innovation in the future. Of course, much depends on how the profession deals with the basic problems of accounting for uncertainty, as will be discussed in Chapter 19, Part II.

Auditors are also supposed to evaluate the estimate differences as a group for indications of a systematic bias (CAS 540, paragraphs 21 and A125) and examine the combination of differences and other likely misstatements found by other audit procedures. Accumulated uncorrected misstatements (passed adjustments) from prior periods may also have an impact because they may reverse and affect the materiality of the current year's misstatements (CAS 450, paragraph 11[b]).

Overall evaluation also connects materiality to assertions. Materiality is defined as the amount of misstatements from all sources that would affect a user decision. Thus, materiality may also presume that users mainly care that the aggregate misstatement for all assertions is less than material, rather than which particular assertions were affected. Again, review Exhibit 16–1 and consider the assertions affected by the misstatements: completeness, valuation, existence, and presentation.

Review Checkpoints

16-32 Why are auditors' drafts of adjusting entries and note disclosures near the end of the audit always labelled "proposed"?

16-33 What are uncorrected misstatements, and what role do they play in forming the audit opinion on the financial statements?

16-34 Outline the auditor's considerations at the end of the audit to form the opinion, especially referring to those requiring professional judgment.

management estimates:
financial statement numbers that management develops based on the probability of future financial events using forecasting models and assumptions

reasonable estimates:
management estimates that an auditor assesses to be supported by reliable evidence and not biased

forecast error:
the difference between the future financial information as estimated by management and the actual financial outcome that is realized

Writing an Audit Opinion on the Financial Statements

Forms of Audit Opinion

LO3   Describe the different forms of audit opinion, explain the decisions underlying the auditor's choice of form, and explain how the date of the audit report is determined.

To form an opinion on whether the **financial statements** are presented fairly in all material respects and in accordance with GAAP, the auditor must make a number of professional judgments as set out in CAS 700. The forms of opinion were discussed in Chapter 4, and the process auditors must use to decide which is the appropriate form of opinion is set out in Exhibit 4–7. We will now revisit this decision in the context of having completed the audit work. The first decision is whether the audit team has obtained sufficient appropriate audit evidence providing reasonable assurance that the financial statements as a whole are free from material misstatement due to fraud or error. Chapter 15 focused on the completion of the audit work and review of the audit file documentation by senior members of the audit team to determine whether the scope of work completed was adequate to support an audit opinion. As discussed in Chapter 4, any deficiency in the scope of the audit can lead to a modified opinion if the scope limitation effects can be isolated or to a disclaimer if the effects could have a pervasive impact on the financial statements overall. Opinion formation also includes deciding if any uncorrected misstatements are material, either individually or in aggregate. If there is a material level of misstatement that can be isolated in specific items in the financial statements, a qualified opinion can be provided, but if the misstatements are pervasive to the financial statements, an adverse opinion is called for.

Under CAS 200 the auditor must also decide whether the **applicable financial reporting framework** chosen by management is acceptable. Note that this decision needs to be made at the engagement acceptance stage, but for study purposes we have left this complexity to the final step in the audit process. **Acceptable financial reporting frameworks** can be either **special purpose financial reporting frameworks** or **general purpose financial reporting frameworks** and either type can also be classified

financial statements:
the structured representation of historical financial information, including related notes and summary of significant accounting policies, intended to communicate an entity's economic resources or obligations at a point in time or the changes therein for a period of time in accordance with a financial reporting framework; usually refers to a complete set of financial statements as determined by the requirements of the applicable financial reporting framework

applicable financial reporting framework:
the financial reporting framework adopted by management and/or those charged with governance in the preparation of the financial statements that is acceptable in view of the nature of the entity and the objective of the financial statements, or that is required by law or regulation

acceptable financial reporting frameworks:
a basis of preparing an entity's financial statements that an auditor has determined is acceptable because it provides appropriate criteria against which the financial statements can be audited; financial reporting standards promulgated for certain types of entities by recognized/authorized accounting standard-setting organizations are presumed to be acceptable for general purpose financial statements prepared by such entities

special purpose financial reporting frameworks:
financial reporting frameworks used to prepare financial statements tailored to meet the financial information needs stipulated by a particular user or user group

general purpose financial reporting frameworks:
financial reporting frameworks used to prepare financial statements designed to meet the common financial information needs of a wide range of users

as a **fair presentation framework** or a **compliance framework**. These categories of **financial reporting framework** are summarized in the four categories in the following box.

Four Categories of Acceptable Financial Reporting Frameworks

	General Purpose Financial Statements	Special Purpose Financial Statements
Fair Presentation Framework	1	2
Compliance Framework	3	4

Source: CAAA 2008 Audit Education Update.

The most common reporting framework in Canada is the general purpose, fair presentation type of framework, since Canadian GAAP (e.g., IFRS, ASPE) are considered to provide fair presentation for general purpose reporting. The importance of the fair presentation framework is that auditors can use the words *present fairly* only for fair reporting frameworks. This difference in wording can be appreciated by studying the two wording examples in the box below.

Key Difference in Auditor's Standard Opinion Wording—General Purpose Financial Statements

FAIR PRESENTATION FRAMEWORKS	COMPLIANCE FRAMEWORKS
"...the financial statements present fairly, in all material respects, the...in accordance with (the applicable fair presentation financial reporting framework—generally this is IFRS for public companies, or Canadian accounting standards for private enterprises)." (CAS 700)	"...the financial statements have been prepared, in all material respects, in accordance with (applicable acceptable general purpose framework)..." (CAS 700)

Source: CAAA 2008 Audit Education Update.

fair presentation framework:
a financial reporting framework that requires financial statements to be prepared in compliance with the framework and that acknowledges explicitly or implicitly that, to achieve fair presentation of the financial statements, it may be necessary for management to provide disclosures beyond those specifically required by the framework or acknowledges explicitly that it may be necessary for management to depart from a requirement of the framework to achieve fair presentation of the financial statements in those extremely rare situations where this is necessary; referred to as GAAP if used for general purpose financial statements; includes IFRS and ASPE

compliance framework:
a financial reporting framework that requires financial statements to be prepared in compliance with the requirements of the framework but does not contain the acknowledgments required for fair presentation

financial reporting framework:
a set of criteria that provides a basis for preparing an entity's financial statements; may be general purpose or special purpose

What exactly is a "fair" framework? CAS 200 and CAS 700 together state that the following requirements need to be met for a fair presentation framework:

(i) The framework acknowledges explicitly or implicitly that, to achieve fair presentation of the financial statements, it may be necessary for management to provide disclosures beyond the specific requirements of the framework (CAS 200, para. 13, and CAS 700, para. 7 (b)(i)); or

(ii) The framework acknowledges explicitly that, in extremely rare circumstances, it may be necessary for management to depart from a specific requirement of the framework to achieve fair presentation of the financial statements (CAS 200, para. 13, and CAS 700, para. 7 (b)(ii)).

(iii) A fair presentation framework (as opposed to a "compliance" framework) "embodies sufficiently broad principles *that can serve as a basis* for developing and applying accounting policies that are consistent with the underlying requirements of the framework" (CAS 200, paragraph A6, and CAS 700, paragraph 14) (emphasis added).

These three criteria for fair presentation reporting suggest principles-based reasoning for accounting, following the same logic as principles-based reasoning in professional ethics, as discussed in Appendix 3A (available on Connect). In principles-based reasoning, if there is a conflict between a more detailed accounting standard and a more general principle, then the general principle has precedence and can override the detailed rule. This is how the auditor can logically justify deviating from detailed accounting standards in a fair presentation framework. Such conflict should be rare, however, since the detailed rules are supposed to provide more-detailed guidance in the application of a principle. That is, usually the principle and rule should be consistent. Probably the most common example of an inconsistency is when an accounting estimate results in significant or unacceptably high accounting risk, as will be discussed in Chapter 19, Part II.

To assess fair presentation, the audit engagement partner considers the results of the final overall financial statement analysis and assesses whether the overall presentation, structure, and content of the financial statements and notes represent the underlying transactions and events fairly, from the perspective of users (CAS 520).

The auditor must be satisfied that the information presented in the financial statements is relevant, reliable, comparable, and understandable. Fair presentation also requires the financial statements to adequately disclose the significant accounting policies applied so that users can understand the effect of transactions and events on the information. The auditor assesses whether the terminology used and the titles of financial statements are appropriate and understandable. The final analysis considers the qualitative aspects of the accounting used, including indications of management bias in selecting accounting policies and making accounting estimates. The accounting risk concept is intended to help auditors guide reasonableness of forecasts in accounting estimates. For example, if management's assumption leads to an unacceptably high accounting risk estimate, the auditor may question the reasonableness of that assumption. An adjustment to the estimate, note disclosure of the questionable assumption(s), or note disclosure of the estimation uncertainties may be necessary for fair presentation.[6] Such adjustments and additional disclosures are what differentiate fair presentation reporting from compliance reporting. Compliance reporting is discussed in Chapter 21 (available on Connect). Examples of compliance reporting are cash basis reporting and tax basis financial reporting.

The trend in auditing is to replace qualitative analysis with more objective quantitative analysis or models. This parallels trends in other fields, such as finance. Prime examples are the audit risk model and risk-based auditing generally, which are greatly influenced by statistical sampling theory. Different qualitative misstatements may require different concepts of risk, such as accounting risk or fraud risk, which are discussed in Chapter 19, Part II, and Chapter 21, respectively.

Summary

When the auditor concludes that the financial statements are presented fairly in all material respects in accordance with GAAP, an unmodified opinion can be expressed. If, based on the audit evidence, the auditor concludes that the financial statements are not free from material misstatement (GAAP departure), or is unable to obtain sufficient appropriate audit evidence to conclude that the financial statements are free from material misstatement (scope limitation), the auditor must give a modified opinion in the auditor's report in accordance with CAS 705. Modified opinions were described in detail in Chapter 4.

Review Checkpoints

16-35   Under what circumstances is an auditor required to give a modified audit opinion? List four types of modified audit opinions that would be given and the circumstances that would give rise to each. Under what circumstances can an auditor express an unmodified opinion on financial statements?

16-36   List the four types of financial reporting frameworks for financial statements set out in CAS 200. What requirements must be met for a financial reporting framework to be considered to provide fair presentation? How would IFRS and ASPE be classified in terms of fair presentation? Why are these two frameworks widely used in practice?

16-37   Describe the three requirements that need to be met for a financial reporting framework to be considered a fair presentation framework.

Date of Opinion

Since the auditor's opinion is provided on financial statements that are the responsibility of management, the auditor is not in a position to conclude that sufficient appropriate audit evidence has been obtained until evidence is obtained that management has prepared all the financial statements and related note disclosures required by the applicable financial reporting framework and has accepted responsibility for them.

Standards Check

CAS 700 Forming an Opinion and Reporting on Financial Statements

41.   The auditor's report shall be dated no earlier than the date on which the auditor has obtained sufficient appropriate audit evidence on which to base the auditor's opinion on the financial statements, including evidence that (Ref: Para. A38–A41)

(a) All the statements that make up the financial statements, including the related notes, have been prepared; and

(b) Those with the recognized authority have asserted that they have taken responsibility for those financial statements.

Source: *CPA Canada Handbook—Assurance*, 2014.

The evidence of this acceptance having occurred results from a formal decision of the board, those charged with governance, or management to accept the final financial statements. Typically, the auditor attends this meeting and obtain a copy of the minutes showing the decision as documentation. The date of this meeting is the audit report date, and the auditor is responsible for searching for evidence in relation to the fair presentation of the financial statements up to this date.

Chapter 15 discussed subsequent events that can in some situations give rise to information being included in financial statements that came to light after the audit report date but before the financial statements were issued to users. Such situations can result in a need to put dual dates on an audit report, as explained in Appendix 16B.

Significant Matter Paragraphs: Additional Information in the Audit Report

LO4   Explain the purpose of emphasis of matter and other matter paragraphs in an audit report.

Sometimes auditors opt to add additional information in the audit report. There are two types of additions possible under CAS 706: emphasis of matter (EOM) paragraphs and other matter (OM) paragraphs. These are used to enrich the information content beyond the standard unmodified report wording. Under CAS 706, the EOM paragraph can be used for a broad range of issues. One or more EOM paragraphs can be added to the audit report regarding something in the financial statements that the auditor believes readers should consider important or useful, even when the auditor intends to write an unmodified opinion paragraph. For example, EOM paragraphs are required when a material uncertainty regarding the going-concern assumption is properly disclosed (as further discussed in Chapter 19, available on Connect), and an unmodified opinion is given. Indeed, the matter emphasized is not supposed to be mentioned in the opinion sentence. The following box contains an illustration of such an EOM paragraph related to a significant uncertainty affecting the financial statements.

Example of an Emphasis of Matter Paragraph

Without qualifying our opinion, we draw attention to Note X to the financial statements. The Company is the defendant in a lawsuit alleging infringement of certain patent rights and claiming royalties and punitive damages. The Company has filed a counter action, and preliminary hearings and discovery proceedings on both actions are in progress. The ultimate outcome of the matter cannot currently be determined and no provision for any liability that may result has been made in the financial statements.

Source: CAS 706, *CPA Canada Handbook—Assurance*, 2014.

OM paragraphs are distinguished from EOM paragraphs by the nature of information they include. EOM paragraphs refer only to information presented or disclosed in the financial statements, whereas OM paragraphs relate to information that is not presented or disclosed in the financial statements, but that the auditor considers necessary to communicate to users because it is relevant to their understanding of the audit, the auditor's responsibilities, or the auditor's report. For example, OM paragraphs can be used to inform financial statement readers that the comparative year financial statements were audited by a different audit firm, or that other information in a document containing the audited financial statements (such as Management Discussion and Analysis in an annual report) contains information that is materially inconsistent with information in the audited financial statements.

EOM and OM paragraphs can be viewed as other ways in which the CASs attempt to make operational the fair presentation concept. Note that EOM and OM paragraphs are not modified opinions. If the final evaluation discussed above results in the conclusion that there are deficiencies in either the audit evidence obtained or the fair presentation of the financial statements, the types of modifications discussed in Chapter 4, and above, come into play.

Evolution of the Audit Report

CAS 700, in force at the time of writing, requires a form of audit report that has been used in Canada since 2011. The International Standards on Auditing (ISA 700) report on which it is modelled came into effect in 2007. Compared to the previous format, the 2011 format primarily expanded the description of the auditor's responsibilities and work performed from half a paragraph to three full paragraphs. Despite this change, wide-ranging discussions and research continue to consider ways to improve the report further. Many commenters felt that the public concerns and criticisms of the previous version still had not been addressed by this expanded description, because essentially it was still highly standardized (i.e., boilerplate) wording. It was believed that financial statement users wanted more specific information about the reporting entity and the audit that was performed.

As was introduced in Appendix 4A of Chapter 4, in January 2015 the International Auditing and Assurance Standards Board (IAASB) issued broad-ranging revisions to the audit-reporting requirements in the ISAs, as well as a new standard, ISA 701, *Communicating Key Audit Matters in the Independent Auditor's Report*. These revised auditing standards, and a new standard for reporting **key audit matters**, have been issued in respond to the criticisms and concerns being raised about boilerplate audit reporting. The new ISA requirements take effect for audited financial statements for fiscal periods ending on or after December 15, 2016. These new standards are expected to be introduced in Canada but may have a later effective date. Any modifications required to reflect the Canadian legal and regulatory environment are expected to be minor.

The box below discusses these revised ISA audit reporting standards, which are in the process of being adopted as CASs at the time of writing.

Evolution of Audit Reporting—Auditors to Report Key Audit Matters for Audits of Listed Company Financial Statements

Prior to the issue of the new international auditing standards in January 2015, the long-standing view of the auditing profession was that audit reporting should be highly standardized to best serve the public interest. This view was embodied in ISA 700, paragraph 4 (prior to the 2015 revisions), which stated, "This ISA promotes consistency in the auditor's report. Consistency in the auditor's report, when the audit has been conducted in accordance with ISAs, promotes credibility in the global marketplace by making more readily identifiable those audits that have been conducted in accordance with globally recognized standards. It also helps to promote the user's understanding and to identify unusual circumstances when they occur" (ISA 700, para. 4, 2014 version).

Academic and professional research, however, raised concerns about the relevance and understandability of standardized audit reports, which are often perceived by users as boilerplate reports that communicate little valuable information. Many of the recommendations coming out of this research pointed to breaking away from highly standardized wording to allow more flexibility and more detailed information to be reported by the independent auditor.

In response to these criticisms and perceived deficiencies, in January 2015 the IAASB issued revised audit reporting standards. ISA 700, paragraph 4 (revised in 2015), now states, "The requirements of this ISA are aimed at addressing an appropriate balance between the need for consistency and comparability in auditor reporting globally and the need to increase the value of auditor reporting by making the information provided in the auditor's report more relevant to users. This ISA promotes consistency in the auditor's report, but recognizes the need for flexibility to accommodate particular circumstances of individual jurisdictions. Consistency in the auditor's report ... [the rest is unchanged]."

The most profound of these revisions is the new ISA 701, *Communicating Key Audit Matters in the Independent Auditor's Report*. ISA 701's requirement for auditors to communicate KAMs is intended to provide more transparency to financial statement users about the audit that was performed. KAMs are defined as those matters that, in the auditor's professional judgment, were most significant in performing the audit for the current year. It is expected that communicating KAMs will also help intended users understand the entity and the areas of significant management judgment in the audited financial statements, and may also provide a basis for users to further engage with management and those charged with governance about issues related to the entity, its audited financial statements, or the audit that was performed.

(continued)

key audit matters:
those issues that, in the auditor's professional judgment, were most significant in the financial statement audit of the current period and are important information to communicate to financial statement users in the auditor's report, selected from the issues communicated with those charged with governance at the end of the audit

ISA 701 applies to audits of complete sets of general purpose financial statements for listed (i.e., publicly traded) entities, as well as other circumstances when the auditor decides it is appropriate to communicate KAMs in the auditor's report.

Auditors are supposed to select from all the matters communicated to those charged with governance, those particular matters that required significant auditor attention in performing the audit. Determining which are the key matters is based on factors such as whether the matter related to

- an area of higher assessed risk of material misstatement
- unusual changes in the entity or unusual transactions in the current period
- important auditor judgments relating to management judgments such as valuation estimates with high levels of uncertainty (i.e., high accounting risk)
- any major events that occurred during the period that had a big impact on performing the audit, and
- any other matter that required significant auditor attention during the current audit

These new audit reporting standards were the result of many years of research and extensive public discussion and comment. How they are implemented in practice once they come into force will be of great interest to financial statement preparers, users, researchers, and students.

Review Checkpoints

16-38   Explain the difference between EOM and OM paragraphs. Distinguish these two from a KAM (in ISA 701).

16-39   Give an example of a situation that would be reported in an EOM paragraph in an audit report containing an unmodified opinion.

Auditor Communications

LO5   Summarize the auditor's communications throughout and at the conclusion of the engagement.

Throughout the audit, the engagement partner and team members communicate continuously with the auditee's management, those charged with governance, and the auditee's personnel. Most of this communication is oral, and some involves written correspondence. This section outlines the key formal **auditor communications** that are required.

Summary of Audit Correspondence

Many types of formal correspondence have been mentioned in this text. Since we are now at the final stage of the audit, having completed the work and formed the audit opinion, this is a good place to summarize these correspondence items and when they typically occur. Exhibit 16–3 summarizes the audit correspondence that is used. Refer also to the detailed flow diagram on the inside cover, which shows the communications that auditors are required to make throughout the audit process.

auditor communications:
all the correspondence auditors use with auditee personnel, officers, and third parties to conduct the audit; communication with management and those charged with governance includes the engagement letter, summary of planning, internal control deficiencies ("management letter"), management representation letter, and significant audit findings summary; communication with third parties includes confirmation letters from creditors, debtors, and lawyers

EXHIBIT 16–3

Audit Correspondence

TYPE	FROM	TO	TIMING	PURPOSE
Engagement letter (acceptance)	Auditor (auditee)	Auditee (auditor)	Before engagement	To establish the terms of the engagement
Summary of audit planning decisions	Auditor	Auditee	At start of engagement field work	To inform the client of the planned scope, timing, and materiality decisions affecting the performance of the audit
Internal control deficiencies	Auditor	Auditee	Interim or after audit, when deficiencies are discovered	To advise management (and those charged with governance if weaknesses are material) of control weaknesses that have come to the auditor's attention
Confirmations (replies)	Auditee (third parties)	Third parties (auditor)	Throughout the audit	To obtain independent audit evidence from external parties
Lawyer's letter (reply)	Auditee in-house lawyer or management	Lawyer (auditor)	Near end of audit	To obtain independent audit evidence from the auditee's lawyers regarding possible contingencies or claims against the company
Management representation letter	Auditee management	Auditor	Audit report date	To obtain necessary evidence regarding management's information relevant to the financial statements
Significant audit findings summary	Auditor	Directors, those charged with governance	Planning, during audit, and after audit report	To inform and advise those charged with governance of the key auditor decisions and findings throughout the engagement

Communications with Those Charged with Governance (Audit Committees or Equivalent)

Once the auditor has concluded the audit work, the audit files are reviewed and complete, and a decision is made on the appropriate form of audit opinion, it is time for the auditor to communicate with those charged with governance regarding the significant audit findings and the planned audit report. Those charged with governance are responsible for ensuring that the organization is accountable to its stakeholders. The organization's financial statements are a key component of this accountability obligation, and those charged with governance must take responsibility for them before the auditor can issue his or her audit report. This section will review all the communications occurring throughout the audit and then discuss those carried out at the completion of the audit.

The two main communications occurring at the end report significant audit findings to those charged with governance (CAS 260) and internal control weaknesses discovered during the audit to management (CAS 265). If the control deficiencies are significant, they are also reported in writing to those charged with governance (CAS 265). Excerpts from an example of an internal control deficiencies letter to management can be found in Discussion Case DC 16-6, Exhibit DC 16-6–2, at the end of the chapter. Exhibit 16–4 provides an example of a letter to those charged with governance, reporting the findings of the audit of a private real estate investment company.

The communication with those charged with governance is an opportunity for the auditors to present issues that, if they are insightful and well supported by facts and circumstances encountered during the audit, can be very helpful to those responsible for directing an organization. In many organizations, those charged with governance are a separate committee of board members, the audit committee, formed specifically to oversee the presentation of the audited financial statements, and in other organizations they are the board of directors itself.

EXHIBIT 16-4

Example of Auditor Communication of Significant Audit Findings: Letter from Auditor to Those Charged with Governance, per CAS 260 and CAS 265

May 17, 2012

The Board of Directors
Richmond Limited
1600 90th Street
Cogito, Ontario

Dear Sirs or Madams:

We have been engaged to audit the financial statements of Richmond Limited ("the company") for the year ending December 31, 20X1.

Canadian generally accepted auditing standards for audit engagements require that we communicate with you regarding certain matters relating to the audit. These matters are as follows:

Responsibilities

Our responsibility is to form and express an opinion on the financial statements that have been prepared by the company's management with the oversight of those charged with governance. An audit does not relieve management or those charged with governance of their responsibilities.

Planning

During the course of the audit, we provided management with an overview of the planned scope and timing of the audit. The level of materiality, which is the amount of cumulative misstatement at which the statements would be viewed by users as misleading, was set at $75,000.

Comments Regarding Internal Control

1. There are currently no identifiable controls over revenue completeness at the Little Hotel. We recommend that this situation be reviewed and appropriate controls implemented.
2. During the audits of Home-away Corp., we encountered problems with receivables collection, accounting estimates, and general audit documentation that were not encountered in other files. We recommend that the control and reporting structures of this company be evaluated with a view to making improvements in these areas.

Other Audit Findings

1. A Phase II environmental assessment was done with respect to the possible sale of the LaCroix Mall property and concluded that annual visual inspection of asphalt and soil conditions at the site was an appropriate course of action. The consultants were also of the view that the property could be financed by most major lenders under these conditions. The potential buyer has asked for certification by the Ministry of the Environment before they will complete the purchase, which would cost roughly $70,000. Since the company does not have to sell the property and could continue to operate it in normal fashion, which is expected to more than recover the property's cost, there appears to be no impairment to the value of the property at this time. We agree with management's view that this issue is not of sufficient significance to disclose in the financial statements at this time.
2. We have made some recommendations to Your Home Rentals Ltd. with respect to clarifying the treatment of Harmonized Sales Tax in several of its residential real estate joint venture agreements to clarify the HST treatment of various non-arm's-length transactions. There is considerable complexity in this area of HST. While some progress has been made on these matters, there remains a lack of a comprehensive approach to this issue.

Independence

We are required to identify and report to you relationships between the company and ourselves that, in our professional judgment, may reasonably be thought to bear on our independence and objectivity.

In determining which relationships to report, the standards require us to consider relevant rules and related interpretations prescribed by the professional ethics codes and applicable legislation, covering such matters as

(a) Holding a financial interest, either directly or indirectly, in a client
(b) Holding a position, either directly or indirectly, that gives the right or responsibility to exert significant influence over the financial or accounting policies of a client
(c) Personal or business relationships of immediate family, close relatives, partners, or retired partners, either directly or indirectly, with a client
(d) Economic dependence on a client
(e) Provision of services in addition to the audit engagement

(continued)

EXHIBIT 16–4

Example of Auditor Communication of Significant Audit Findings: Letter from Auditor to Those Charged with Governance, per CAS 260 and CAS 265   (*continued*)

We are not aware of any relationships between the company and ourselves that, in our professional judgment, may reasonably be thought to bear on our independence and objectivity, which have occurred to date.

Use of Report

This report is intended solely for the use of the board of directors, management, and others charged with governance of the company and should not be used for any other purposes.
We are available to discuss the matters contained in this letter at any time.

Yours truly,

Meyer & Gustav
Public Accountants, LLP

The following discussion will assume an audit committee, and similar requirements follow for other types of governance structures. The auditor and management should, in advance, review the information to be covered with the audit committee. On some matters (e.g., company operations), management should report and the auditor then comment. On other matters, such as audit findings, the auditor should report and management then comment. Both should be present in meetings with those charged with governance to discuss these reports, which may be written or oral. When the auditor communicates in writing with an audit committee, the report should indicate that it is intended solely for use by the audit committee. In some instances, the auditor may identify matters to discuss without the presence of management.

The auditor should keep notes of these audit committee discussions, which should be compared with the audit committee minutes of the meeting. Any inconsistencies must be resolved with the audit committee or board of directors. The auditor should also communicate all matters affecting approval of the annual financial statements to the board of directors prior to such approval. Normally, the auditor works within the audit committee's regular cycle of meetings.

The audit committee's expectations need to be clarified and put in writing. The most important matters arising from the audit of financial statements that should be communicated to the audit committee are as follows:

1. Auditor responsibility under GAAS
2. Planning of the current audit
3. Material weaknesses in internal controls
4. Illegal acts
5. Fraud
6. Significant accounting principles and policies selected by management
7. Management judgments and accounting estimates
8. Misstatements, adjusted and uncorrected
9. Other information in annual reports (e.g., narrative information)
10. Disagreements with management
11. Consultation with other accountants by management
12. Significant findings of the audit
13. Difficulties encountered in performing the audit (e.g., unreasonable delays in obtaining information from management)

14. Effects of new developments in accounting standards, or of legislative or regulatory requirements, on the auditee's financial reporting

15. Use of experts

16. Audit and non-audit services that the auditor is providing to the auditee

17. Summary of the audit approach

If the auditor considers that an audit committee's response to the matters communicated is seriously inappropriate, he or she may need to communicate directly with the board of directors or even have an obligation to report to outside regulatory authorities. For example, the "well-being reporting requirement" under federal financial institutions legislation may require the auditor to report to the Superintendent of Financial Institutions "any significant weaknesses in internal control which have the potential to jeopardize the financial institution's ability to continue as a going concern."[7] Because auditee confidentiality is an issue, the auditor should seek legal advice about the best manner of reporting to outside authorities.

Review Checkpoints

16-40 What is the purpose of the auditor's communication with those charged with governance at the completion of the audit? What are some important matters that this communication should include?

16-41 Why must the auditor communicate significant findings with those charged with governance prior to dating the audit report?

16-42 What information would the auditor communicate to management and to those charged with governance regarding internal control deficiencies discovered during the audit?

APPLICATION CASE WITH SOLUTION & ANALYSIS

Final Overall Analysis Uncovers Unusual Related Party Transactions

DISCUSSION CASE

In his third year as an auditor, Jack assists an audit partner in completing the final analytical procedures and working paper review for a new audit of a group of mining companies. The audit file shows that in 20X9 Alta Gold Company, a public "shell" corporation, was purchased for $1,000 by the Blues brothers.

Operating under the corporate names of Diamond King and Pacific Gold, the brothers had also purchased numerous mining claims in auctions conducted by the Ministry of Natural Resources. They invested a total of $40,000 in 300 claims between the two companies. A series of transactions followed.

(a) Diamond King sold limited partnership interests in its 175 Northwest Territories diamond claims to local investors, raising $20 million to begin mining production.

(b) Pacific Gold then traded its 125 British Columbia gold mining claims for all the Diamond King assets and partnership interests, valuing the diamond claims at $20 million. Diamond King valued the gold claims received at $20 million as the fair value in the exchange.

(c) The brothers then put $3 million obtained from dividends into Alta Gold, and, with the aid of a $15 million bank loan, Alta Gold purchased half of the Diamond King gold claims for $18 million.

(d) The Blues brothers then arranged for Alta Gold to obtain another bank loan of $38 million to purchase the remainder of Diamond King's assets and all of Pacific Gold's mining claims. They paid off the Diamond King limited partners.

(e) At the end of 20X9, Alta Gold had cash of $16 million and mining assets valued at $58 million, with liabilities on bank loans of $53 million.

Alta Gold had in its files the partnership offering documents, receipts, and other papers showing partners' investment of $20 million in the Diamond King limited partnerships. The company also had Pacific Gold and Diamond King contracts for the exchange of mining claims. The $20 million value of the exchange was justified in light of the limited partners' investments.

One appraisal report in the files showed that there was no basis for valuing the exchange of Diamond King claims other than the price limited partner investors had been willing to pay. A second appraiser reported a probable value of $20 million for the exchange, based on proven production elsewhere, but no geological data on the actual claims had been obtained. The $18 million paid by Alta Gold to Diamond King had similar appraisal reports.

Audit Trail

The transactions occurred over a period of 10 months. The Blues brothers had $37 million cash in Diamond King and Pacific Gold, as well as the $16 million in Alta. All of the cash was borrowed from a bank that had granted the loan to Alta Gold with the mining claims and production as security. The mining claims that had cost $40,000 were now in Alta's balance sheet at $58 million; the $53 million in loans from the bank was secured by 300 mining claim papers.

SOLUTION & ANALYSIS

Audit Approach

Audit Objective

The auditors' objective is to obtain evidence of the existence, valuation, and rights (ownership) in the mining claim assets. The review of the working papers indicated a number of audit issues and outstanding procedures still to be done.

Controls Relevant to the Process

The audit file documentation assessing of internal controls relevant to accounting for mining property investments indicated that Alta Gold, Pacific Gold, and Diamond King had no control structure. All transactions were engineered by the Blues brothers, including the hiring of friendly appraisers. The only control that might have been effective was the process for granting the bank loan, but the bank failed to exercise appropriate procedures to evaluate the risk in the loans to Alta Gold.

Another effective control could have been engagement of competent, independent appraisers. Since the auditors will use (or try to use) the appraisers' reports, the procedures involve investigating the reputation, engagement terms, and independence of the appraisers. The auditors can use local business references, local financial institutions with lists of approved appraisers, membership directories of the professional appraisal associations, and interviews with the appraisers themselves.

Audit Procedures

Test of Details of Balance

The procedures for auditing the asset values include tracing and analyzing the path of each transaction. This includes obtaining knowledge of the owners and managers of the several companies and the identities of the limited partner investors. If the Blues brothers have not disclosed their connection with the other companies (and perhaps with the limited partners), the auditors need to inquire at the government's commerce department offices to discover the identities of the players in this flip game. Numerous complicated pre-merger transactions in small corporations and shells often signal manipulated valuations. Loan applications and supporting papers should be examined to determine the representations made by Alta Gold when obtaining the bank loans. These papers may reveal some contradictory or exaggerated information. Ownership of the mining claims might be confirmed with the government's resource department auctioneers or found in the local deed records (spread all over the Northwest Territories and British Columbia).

Audit Results

Based on their final file review and analysis, Jack and the partner find that the audit staff assigned had documented the many transactions and loans, but they had not been able to unravel the complicated exchanges and they never questioned the relationship of Alta Gold to Diamond King and Pacific Gold. They never investigated and discovered the Blues brothers' involvement in the other side of the exchanges and the purchase transactions. They accepted the appraisers' reports as competent and independent but had not adequately supported these conclusions. The audit partners realize that the audit is far from complete. Attempting to contact the Blues brothers, the only directors of all the corporations, to communicate the findings at this point of the audit, it is learned that both have left the country on extended trips and cannot be contacted. Further investigation reveals the identities of the various related parties in the flips. The audit cannot be completed, and the initial decision to accept this new engagement is deemed not appropriate based on the facts learned subsequently. Jack's audit firm withdraws from the engagement without issuing a report (a close call; the bank that lent the $53 million was not so lucky). The audit firm begins an investigation to find out how the inappropriate acceptance decision was made so it can implement necessary improvements to its quality control procedures.

Review Checkpoint

16-43   What impact can related party transactions have in some cases of asset valuation?

SUMMARY

This chapter ended this text's adventures in auditing with a review of the professional judgments applied to form the audit opinion at the completion of the engagement. This closes the circle that began back in Chapter 4, which explained the write-up of the audit report itself. Chapter 4 introduced the audit report to show you the final objective and focal point of the whole financial statement audit engagement. Chapters 5 through 16 have elaborated on how auditors achieve this ultimate objective—assessment of audit evidence and findings to form the auditor's opinion.

- The many professional judgments made in the process of achieving the overall objectives of the independent auditor were outlined in the context of CAS 200. **LO1**

- The chapter described how misstatements identified over the course of the audit are accumulated for evaluation in comparison to materiality. The nature of various types of misstatements and their impact on evaluating whether there is a material misstatement at the overall financial statement level were discussed. **LO2**

- At the conclusion of an audit, the engagement partner evaluates the sufficiency and appropriateness of the evidence documented in the audit files to determine whether the scope of the audit supports a clean opinion. The evaluation of fair presentation involves not only considering the nature and size of misstatements but also qualitative considerations of whether the presentation and disclosures achieve fair presentation. Different types of applicable financial reporting frameworks, and the reporting appropriate for a fair presentation framework, were explained. **LO3**

- The purpose of emphasis of matter (EOM) and other matter (OM) paragraphs was outlined, that is, to provide additional information in an audit report, separately from the decision on the form of opinion. EOM paragraphs expand on information that is contained in the financial statements, and OM paragraphs relate to issues that are not in the financial statements but that the auditor believes are important for users to be aware of. **LO4**

- The auditor's communications throughout and at the conclusion of the engagement were summarized. Auditor correspondence was listed, and the end-of-audit communications with those charged with governance were detailed. **LO5**

The next chapter (available on Connect) will discuss other types of engagements that are common in public practice, and the remaining chapters (also available on Connect) will present a variety of advanced issues in the public accounting profession.

KEY TERMS

acceptable financial reporting frameworks

applicable financial reporting framework

auditor–client negotiations

auditor communications

compliance framework

dual dating

fair presentation framework

financial reporting framework

financial statements

forecast error

further possible misstatement

general purpose financial reporting frameworks

key audit matters

management estimates

passed adjustments (waived adjustments)

reasonable estimates

special purpose financial reporting frameworks

summary of misstatements

trivial misstatements

unadjusted (uncorrected) misstatements

MULTIPLE-CHOICE QUESTIONS FOR PRACTICE AND REVIEW

MC 16-1 **LO1** What does a person use when they apply professional judgment in an audit engagement?

a. Loyalty to the client management

b. Their education and professional training in finance

c. The knowledge and experience they have gained in their professional work as auditors

d. Strict adherence to professional ethics codes

MC 16-2 **LO1** Auditor objectivity and skepticism are critical to concluding whether financial statements are fairly presented because

a. accidental errors can occur in preparing financial statements and can always be distinguished from deliberate fraudulent misstatements.

b. when there are deliberate attempts to mislead financial statement users, auditors must charge management with fraud.

c. they must decide whether grey areas where a lot of subjectivity exists in the financial statements reflect management bias.

d. management will always be biased and try to manipulate the financial statements in their favour.

MC 16-3 `LO2` Managers of private companies are more likely than managers of public companies to correct misstatements the auditors discover because

a. accuracy is more important in private companies than public companies.

b. public company managers will be fired if they make errors in the financial statements.

c. private companies are not required to comply with IFRS.

d. public companies often issue press releases reporting their earnings before the full financial statements are issued and do not want to announce changes to the reported earnings.

MC 16-4 `LO3` Two aspects that affect the form of opinion in an auditor's report are

a. the need to issue a modified report or an adverse report.

b. the scope of the auditor's work and the fairness of presentation of the financial statements in accordance with GAAP.

c. the knowledge and experience the auditors have gained in their professional work.

d. the scope of the financial reporting framework and the fairness of the audit evidence obtained.

MC 16-5 `LO3` Unmodified audit opinions are most common because

a. auditors want to retain the client's business in future.

b. public companies are required to get qualified audit reports with unmodified opinions.

c. auditors exercise judgment to eliminate most modifications.

d. company management benefits from unmodified opinions because they reduce the information risk faced by the financial statement users.

MC 16-6 `LO3` The "subsequent discovery of facts that existed at the balance sheet date" refers to knowledge obtained after which date?

a. The date the audit report was delivered to the auditee

b. The audit report date

c. The company's year-end balance sheet date

d. The date interim audit work was complete

MC 16-7 `LO4` An EOM paragraph is used

a. to provide additional information that is not presented or disclosed in management's financial statements.

b. so that public companies can always receive unmodified audit opinions.

c. to describe the auditor's exercise of judgment during the performance of the audit.

d. when the company has disclosed a material uncertainty about its ability to continue as a going concern.

MC 16-8 `LO5` The auditor is required to communicate with those charged with governance, usually an audit committee, regarding the significant audit findings and the planned form of audit report prior to their approval of the financial statements because

a. the auditor is responsible for presenting financial statements that comply with GAAP.

b. the findings of the audit are an important factor for those charged with governance in deciding whether the financial statements are acceptable for their approval.

c. all non-trivial control deficiencies must be reported to a level of management above the level responsible for the control.

d. auditors will have information about the financial statements to which those charged with governance do not have access.

EXERCISES AND PROBLEMS

EP 16-1 Misstatements, Adjustments. `LO2` For the following findings, indicate the income statement and balance sheet accounts that are affected and whether these accounts are over- or understated, and provide an adjusting entry to correct the misstatement, if required. Assume a December 31 year-end.

Required:

a. Outstanding cheques totalling $44,000 were deducted from the cash balance on December 23 but deliberately not mailed out to avoid a bank overdraft over the holidays. The cheques were in payment of various raw material supplier accounts.

b. Sales of $79,000 were recorded on goods that were shipped after year-end and included in the year-end inventory count. The cost of these goods is $53,000.

c. A lawyer's bill for services rendered in November was not paid or accrued.

d. The allowance for bad debts has a credit balance of $80,000. The accounts receivable balance is $150,000, and a reasonable estimate is that all but $10,000 of this will be collected.

e. As of December 31 the company has recognized $250,000 of revenue on a $750,000 contract to construct a bridge. The construction work has not yet started, but $40,000 of building materials for the job was received and expensed as contract costs. At this point, the company has not been able to estimate the total costs of construction.

EP 16-2 Professional Judgment. `LO1` Professional judgment is essential to auditors and the quality of audits.

Required:

a. Explain professional judgment in the context of an audit, giving three examples of situations in the audit process that require use of it.

b. The GAAS from the *CPA Canada Handbook* include specific standards intended to enhance the quality and value of audits. Identify three requirements in CASs that relate to general, examination, and reporting standards, and explain how each one can help junior auditors develop their professional judgment.

EP 16-3 Auditor Communication with Entity and Liability. `LO5` Requirements set out in the auditing standard CAS 260 require an auditor to communicate certain issues and information to those charged with governance of the auditee entity as a financial statement audit proceeds.

Required:

Review the requirements in CAS 260, and discuss how they may affect the risk of an auditor's being liable to the auditee entity. Contrast this with the impact, if any, on the auditor's liability to shareholders (as discussed in Chapter 3). For an analytical perspective, consider the auditor's exposure to both sides as resulting from the three-party accountability relationship (discussed in Chapter 3). Provide your conclusion on whether this CAS requirement reduces auditor liability risk from either of these sides.

EP 16-4 Form of Opinion, Misleading Financial Statements. `LO3` At the end of her audit of Jolie Angelique Inc., Emma concludes that there are material misstatements affecting many accounts, with the result that the financial statements as a whole are misleading. The company's management refuses to adjust the financial statements, however.

Required:

a. List the four forms of modified audit opinions set out in CAS 705.
b. Explain which form of audit opinion would be appropriate in this situation.

EP 16-5 Form of Opinion, Emphasis of Matter Paragraph for Going-Concern Uncertainty. `LO4` Courtney Heart is completing the audit of Profile Framing Ltd. The framing business is seasonal and very competitive. She discovers that a major long-term debt in the draft financial statements is actually due for repayment two months after the close of the financial year. The company president is negotiating with Profile's bank to renew the debt for a further two-year term and has been in to see two other banks about arranging new loans. The president has been keeping a close eye on cash flow and negotiating with suppliers about payment terms and extensions of credit. The cash flow for the current year has declined considerably since the year before, and the operating cash flow is negative due to pressure to reduce prices to compete with a discount framing chain that has been opening shops close to Profile's. With the busy holiday gift season approaching, Profile needs to purchase inventory, but it has no cash and its suppliers have all refused to provide any more goods except on a cash-only delivery basis.

Required:

a. Discuss the liquidity and solvency issues faced by Profile. How do these issues affect Profile's financial statements? Consider the disclosures that should be made regarding its financial condition.
b. Assuming Courtney is satisfied that Profile's financial statements adequately disclosed the financial uncertainties it is facing, describe the form of opinion and the EOM paragraph she will include in her audit report.

DISCUSSION CASES

DC 16-1 Warranty Provision Audit Issues. `LO1, 3` Breton Inc. manufactures industrial lighting fixtures with two main product lines: interior and exterior fixtures. The fixtures are sold with a one-year warranty on parts and labour. During 20X0, Breton's engineering group undertook a five-year review of its warranty claims history and costs and established that an appropriate accounting policy for warranty costs is to accrue 3% of annual sales for exterior fixtures and 2% of annual sales for interior fixtures. PA, Breton's auditor, has used this analysis as the basis for evaluating the provision for estimated warranty cost at year-end for the past two years' audits. During 20X3, Breton's competition increased as light fixtures from China entered the market, selling for prices 40–50% lower. To maintain its customer base, Breton's senior management decided to promote the higher quality of Breton's products and expanded Breton warranty coverage to two years to support these quality claims. However, to keep costs in line, there were no changes to materials used or production methods. PA is now assessing the 20X3 year-end provision for estimated warranty costs and learns that there is no plan to change the approach for developing the estimate. Breton salespeople receive commissions of 1% of gross sales. Senior managers, including the CFO, receive bonuses only if the company's pretax profit exceeds $300,000.

Required:

a. Discuss the implications of the changes in Breton's competitive environment and business strategy for the audit of its warranty liability estimate. Do you think it is fairly presented?

b. If you were the CFO, what arguments would you make to support not changing the method used to estimate warranty liability for the current year?

c. What actions do you recommend PA take in this case?

DC 16-2 Fixed Asset Dispositions, Accounting Misstatements. **LO2** During the current year, Karabakh Ltd. sold off all the heating and air conditioning equipment in one of its buildings because it was being converted from an assembly plant to a warehouse. The equipment was sold to a neighbouring business, which paid $400,000. The equipment was about 10 years old, originally cost $1 million, and was approximately 90% depreciated. Karabakh's bookkeeper recorded the sale as follows:

dr Cash	400,000	
cr Sales revenue		400,000

Required:

a. What impact does the misstatement have on Karabakh's financial statements? Outline which accounts will be affected and the dollar amounts of these effects.

b. Assume this transaction is material to Karabakh's financial statements. What procedures would allow the Karabakh auditor to find this bookkeeping error?

c. Propose a draft adjusting journal entry to correct the entry.

DC 16-3 Going-Concern Uncertainty and Audit Reporting. **LO1, 2, 3, 4** The auditors of the CRX Inc. financial statements for the year ended December 31, 20X7, have decided that there is substantial doubt that CRX can continue to exist as a going concern because the company has experienced significant operating losses since 20X5 and has had to get permission from its lenders to postpone its debt payment requirements. CRX's management has agreed to describe the problems in the president's message to the shareholders in their annual report but has decided not to reflect this situation in the notes to the financial statements.

Required:

Discuss fully the type of audit opinion to be issued in this situation, including a description of any information that would be necessary to the standard audit report. Describe what change(s) would be necessary for CRX to obtain an unmodified audit opinion in this case.

DC 16-4 Scope Limitation and Audit Reporting. **LO3** Yue is auditing the accounts receivable for Slawson & Slawson, LLP, a large law partnership. The managing partner of the law firm has prohibited the auditor from confirming any of the law firm's accounts receivable. The lawyers are concerned that their clients would consider it a breach of confidentiality for the auditor to know they had engaged the lawyer's services and would not understand that the auditor is also operating under strict professional rules that require confidentiality. The accounts receivable balance is highly material. Yue is not able to satisfy himself as to the receivable balance by alternative means.

Required:

a. Describe the type and format of audit report that should be issued in this case.

b. Explain the type of evidence that Yue was trying to obtain by confirming the law firm's accounts receivable balances, and then explain the assertion(s) and the specific audit objectives that this evidence relates to.

c. Why do you think it was not possible to obtain this evidence by alternative means?

DC 16-5 Subsequent Discovery of Facts and Audit Reporting. `LO3, 4` Refer to the Application Case at the end of the chapter. Assume that instead of withdrawing from the engagement, the auditors in this case had issued a clean audit report on all the companies in the case for the 20X9 year-end. They used the appraisals and other representations from the Blues brothers as evidence that the mining properties were correctly valued and the financial statements were fairly presented. One month after the audited financial statements were issued to shareholders, the auditors contacted the companies' accountant about their unpaid fees and learned that the companies had run out of cash and ceased operations. It is suspected that the Blues brothers took all the cash that the bank had lent to the companies and fled the country.

Required:

What are the auditors' responsibilities in this situation?

DC 16-6 Management Letter Issues, Internal Audit. `LO5` Goal Products Limited (GPL) is the official manufacturer and distributor of soccer balls for the North American League of Soccer (NALS), a professional soccer association. GPL was founded 15 years ago and became a Canadian publicly traded company on July 1, 20X1. GPL has one plant in Canada, and it has one in the United States that is operated through a subsidiary of GPL.

It is now October 20, 20X3. You, PA, were recently hired as the manager of financial reporting for GPL. In your first week, you must review the first draft of the quarterly reporting package and provide comments to the financial reporting team on any issues you note. As you start your review you receive an email from the CFO, Joey Bonaducci (Exhibit DC 16-6–1).

Required:

a. Take on the role of PA in the case, and comment on the general process being used by GPL to prepare the responses to the external auditor's management letter and bring them to the audit committee.

b. In the role of PA in the case, assess the adequacy of the internal auditor's work and responses. State your conclusions on whether Sandra's responses will be satisfactory to the external auditor.

c. Take the role of the external auditor in the case. Discuss what impact the weaknesses, if not addressed, will have on planning the audit engagement for next year.

(Adapted from CPAC UFE, Paper III, Simulation 1, 2009, with permission of Chartered Professional Accountants of Canada, Toronto, Canada. Any changes to the original material are the sole responsibility of the author (and/or publisher) and have not been reviewed or endorsed by the Chartered Professional Accountants of Canada.)

EXHIBIT DC 16-6–1

Email from Joey Bonaducci

Hi PA,

Before you start reviewing the quarterly reporting packages, we need to prepare a response to the management letter we received from the external auditors for the year ended June 30, 20X3, for presentation at the next audit committee meeting next week.

Sandra Dee, who is responsible for GPL's internal audit work among her many other duties, has looked into the issues and prepared our responses (Exhibit DC 16-6–2). Please review the draft report prepared by Sandra, and make sure the auditors will be satisfied with our response.

Joey B.

Auditor's Management Letter Excerpts and GPL's Internal Audit Department Responses

PA, I'm sure you will agree with my conclusions once you read the details below. Let me know, though, if you think we need to implement any new controls.

Based on the procedures I performed and those performed by the external auditors at year-end, and the fact that they did not note any material differences, our existing controls are considered adequate.

Sandra Dee, GPL Internal Audit Manager

MANAGEMENT LETTER ISSUE	ISSUE RAISED BY EXTERNAL AUDITOR	INTERNAL AUDIT TESTING AND RESPONSE
Capital asset software	We identified several deficiencies in our review and evaluation of amortization processes. A software program calculates an amortization amount on a monthly basis, which is then recorded as a journal entry directly to the general ledger. However, the program has not been reviewed to ensure additions and deletions are recorded properly and amortization policies are applied appropriately. Due to recent staffing changes, current staff members have inadequate knowledge of the software. As a result, the software is no longer tracking the detailed cost build-up of individual assets for acquisitions. Only the final costs of assets are known. Also, there is no process for completing a reasonability check of the balances.	I performed my own test of reasonability. There were minimal acquisitions during the year ended June 30, 20X3. Any variances resulted from differences between the amortization rates used in the system and those used in my reasonability tests. The variances were immaterial.
Sales contract monitoring	We identified deficiencies in management's sales contract process again this year. There is no monitoring process to ensure sales contracts are adequately authorized and non-standard contracts are reviewed and approved by authorized personnel. As a result, not all contracts were approved or reviewed, and in some cases no final versions of contracts could be found.	I performed a test of details on a few of our current contracts, and everything was fine.
Sales contract monitoring	In addition, there is a lack of segregation of duties. The person maintaining the contract files is also responsible for making deposits and doing bank reconciliations. Since there are insufficient controls for contract approval and modification, this person could modify contracts and deposits to disguise fraud.	Unfortunately, the accounting department is short staffed. Nothing can be done to address the segregation of duties issue.
Internal audit	Only one person within the organization is responsible for the internal audit procedures, and that person does not possess a recognized designation. Also, that person spends a significant amount of time performing other duties, so has little time to dedicate to internal audit responsibilities.	Well, yes, I am very busy. But I have always been able to fit all my assigned duties into the work week.
Consolidation procedures	The Canadian and U.S. companies are consolidated using a large spreadsheet that is maintained solely by the accounting manager. Modifications have been made to the spreadsheet, and as a result, small differences are recorded in retained earnings. No formal process is in place to verify the accuracy of the spreadsheet.	I examined the spreadsheet last year, and it was fine. We have always adjusted for the differences because they are not material enough for us to spend more time on them.

Audit Completion Checklist

LO6 Familiarize yourself with a checklist form used in practice to ensure all audit work has been properly completed at the end of the engagement.

This appendix illustrates a practice aid that can be used at the end of an audit to ensure that the important issues have all been considered and addressed in completing the engagement and issuing the appropriate audit opinion and report.

Checklist—Audit completion

Entity _____   Period ended _____

PSC = Procedure successfully completed
F/S = Financial statements

TCWG = Those charged with governance
FSA = Financial statement area (balances, transactions, disclosures, etc.)

PART 1—AUDIT COMPLETION CHECKLIST	CAS REF.	W/P REF.	PSC? (Y/N) (INITIALS)	SUMMARIZE EXCEPTIONS OR DIFFICULTIES ENCOUNTERED
PRELIMINARY ACTIVITIES				
1. Have we documented our conclusions (Forms 405 and 410) with respect to (a) Acceptance/continuance of the engagement? (b) Compliance with relevant ethical requirements such as independence? (c) The resolution of any issues identified in (a) and (b) above?	220			
2. Are the following communications on file: (a) Terms of engagement (engagement letter)? (b) Where applicable, the planned scope and timing of the audit? (c) Where applicable, a letter of instructions to a component auditor or to the auditor's expert? (d) For listed entities, an independence letter?	210 260 600/620 260			
PLANNING AND RISK ASSESSMENT				
3. Have revisions to overall and performance materiality been documented? (Form 420)	320			
4. Have matters raised in audit team discussions been appropriately reflected in the overall strategy and audit plans? (Forms 430 and 436)	300			

(continued)

Checklist—Audit completion *(continued)*

PART 1 — AUDIT COMPLETION CHECKLIST	CAS REF.	W/P REF.	PSC? (Y/N) (INITIALS)	SUMMARIZE EXCEPTIONS OR DIFFICULTIES ENCOUNTERED
5. Have all the planned risk assessment procedures been performed and results documented (Form 426)?	300			
6. Have the risks of material misstatement in the F/S (fraud and error) been documented and assessed at: (a) The F/S level (pervasive risks and controls)? (b) The assertion level (specific risks and controls by FSA)?	315			
7. Have the assessed risks in step 6 above been updated to reflect any changes required as a result of the audit procedures performed?	315			
8. Have significant control deficiencies been communicated in writing to TCWG?	265			
RESPONDING TO RISK				
9. Has the overall response (Form 605) to assessed risks at the F/S level been implemented and results documented?	330			
10. Has the response to significant risks been implemented and results documented?	330			
11. Have the planned further audit procedures been performed and results documented?	330			
12. Have working papers been signed off and dated by the preparer and reviewer?	230			
13. Have file review notes been removed after the questions have been cleared?	—			
14. Have actual audit hours been compared to budget and variances explained?	—			
15. Is file documentation sufficient that an experienced auditor, having no previous connection with the engagement, could understand • The nature, timing and extent of the audit procedures performed? • The results of the audit procedures and the evidence obtained? • Significant findings or issues arising and conclusions reached?	230			
FINANCIAL STATEMENTS				
16. Do the F/S agree with the entity's underlying accounting records (i.e., entity's subledgers and general ledger)?	330			
17. Are the F/S and notes accurately cross-referenced?				
18. Are the accounting policies and assumptions used in preparation of the financial statements consistent with the financial statement disclosures?				

(continued)

Checklist—Audit completion   (*continued*)

PART 1—AUDIT COMPLETION CHECKLIST	CAS REF.	W/P REF.	PSC? (Y/N) (INITIALS)	SUMMARIZE EXCEPTIONS OR DIFFICULTIES ENCOUNTERED
19. Do the F/S contain all the necessary disclosures required by the applicable financial reporting framework (FRF900 series)?				
20. Were analytical procedures performed at or near the end of the audit and any inconsistencies with file documentation identified and addressed?	520			
REPORTING				
21. Identified misstatements: (a) Has management been asked to correct all identified misstatements (other than clearly trivial) (Form 335) and reasons obtained/considered for any misstatements not corrected? (b) Where applicable, have TCWG been informed of misstatements remaining uncorrected by management and asked to correct them? If so, were reasons obtained/considered for any misstatements not corrected by TCWG?	450			
22. Have subsequent events that may require adjustment of, or disclosure in, the F/S been identified and addressed?	560			
23. Have discussions of significant audit matters with management and TCWG been documented with details of the decisions made?	230			
24. Has there been adequate two-way communication between us and TCWG for the purpose of the audit? If not, were the reasons evaluated and appropriate action taken?	260			
25. Has the auditor's report been appropriately worded and dated? The date can be no earlier than approval of final F/S by the recognized authority (i.e., board of directors or owner/manager).	700			
26. Are the following documents on file: • Signed management representation letter (dated on or before date of audit report)? • Letter to management and TCWG outlining significant audit findings?	580 260			
27. Where applicable, has the Engagement Quality Control Reviewer signed off on the file *before* the audit report was dated?	CSQC 1 220			
28. Has other information (such as an annual report) related to the F/S been read to ensure consistency?	720			

Prepared by _____ Date _____ Reviewed by _____ Date _____

(continued)

Checklist—Audit completion   *(continued)*

PART 2—PARTNER/PRACTITIONER CONCLUSION

	Comments

1. I have maintained my independence throughout the engagement.

2. I ensured the need for professional skepticism was communicated to the engagement team and that appropriate communication took place regarding information/conditions that may indicate risks of material misstatement due to fraud or error.

3. I am satisfied that the risk assessment and further audit procedures performed were sufficient and appropriate to reduce audit risk to an acceptably low level.

4. I have reviewed, signed off, and dated
   - All audit working papers not reviewed and signed off by others.
   - Sufficient working papers to be satisfied with the adequacy of our audit.

5. I have reviewed the audit completion documents, which adequately document significant findings and issues identified during the audit and how they were resolved.

6. I am satisfied that subject to any exceptions referred to in our audit report,
   - Our audit was conducted in accordance with generally accepted auditing standards and no restrictions in scope were imposed on us.
   - The audit evidence obtained is sufficient and appropriate to provide a basis for our audit opinion.
   - The F/S are presented fairly in all material respects, in accordance with the applicable financial reporting framework.

7. I am satisfied that our audit report is appropriately worded.

Engagement Partner/Practitioner _____ Date _____

Source: Canadian Professional Engagement Manual 2014—Forms.

APPENDIX 16B

The Impact of Subsequent Events on Audit Reports

LO7 Explain how subsequent events can lead to dual dating of an audit report, and list the auditor's responsibilities when relevant facts become known after the audit report has been issued.

Subsequent Events and the Audit Report

To understand the impact of subsequent events on finalizing the audit report, consider the three possible scenarios listed in the box below and the responsibilities that follow from them. These three situations and their different impact on the audit and audit report are illustrated in a timeline format in Exhibit 16B–1.

TIMING OF SUBSEQUENT EVENT	IMPACT ON AUDIT AND REPORT
1. Events that occurred between the date of the financial statements and the date of the auditor's report	Auditors are responsible for actively searching for these to ensure they are properly reflected in the financial statements if required. Procedures to search for subsequent events that are relevant to the assertions in the financial statements are included in every audit program.
2. Facts the auditor learns of after the date of the auditor's report but before the date the financial statements are issued	Auditors are responsible for making sure these are properly reflected in the financial statements. If it is appropriate to amend the financial statements, the auditor carries out the procedures necessary on the amendment and amends the audit by including an additional date restricted to that amendment. Dual dating is used because the original date applies to everything except the subsequent event, as the auditor is not required to extend the search for other possible subsequent events up to the second date. Only the subsequent events are audited up to the second date, so both dates are included.
3. Facts the auditor becomes aware of after the financial statements and audit report have been issued to users.	This should be a rare occurrence if audits are performed diligently. But if information does come to light that could or should have been known at the time the financial statements and audit report were issued, the following determinations are required. If the auditors would have amended the auditor's report had the facts been known, they must determine with management whether financial statements need amendment. If so, and management amends, the auditor must extend procedures and issue a new audit report that emphasizes reasons for amended financial statements. If management does not amend, the auditor takes steps to prevent users from relying on the audit report.

EXHIBIT 16B–1

Timeline for Auditor's Subsequent Events Responsibilities

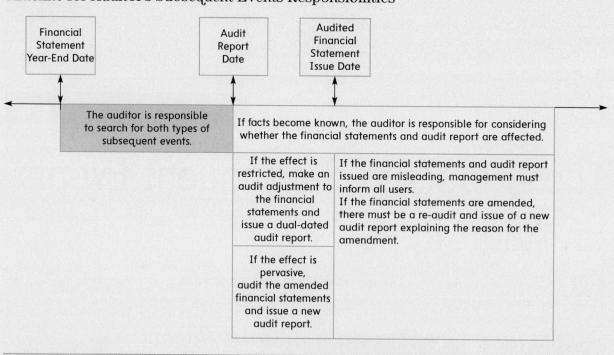

Dual Dating in the Audit Report

Dual dating refers to instances of dating the audit report as of the date that financial statements are approved by the auditee's responsible parties (e.g., the company's board of directors) and attaching an additional later date to disclosure of a significant subsequent event of the type that requires financial statements to be amended. Sometimes, after completion of the audit but before issuance of the report, a significant event comes to the audit team's attention. The purpose of dual dating is twofold: (1) to provide a means of inserting important information learned after the audit report date into the financial statement note disclosures, and (2) to inform users that the auditor takes full responsibility for discovering subsequent events only up to the audit report date and for the specifically identified later event. However, responsibility is not taken for other events that may have occurred after the audit report date. Dual dating is used to cut off the subsequent event procedural responsibility at the earlier date. An example of dual dating wording is as follows: "[Date of auditor's report], except as to Note Y, which is as of [date of completion of audit procedures restricted to amendment described in Note Y]" (CAS 560, paragraph A12).

Facts Become Known after the Financial Statements Are Issued

While auditors are under no obligation to continue audit procedures past the report date, if they happen to learn later of relevant facts, they have an obligation to determine if the information is reliable and if the facts existed at the date of the report. They must then determine with management whether financial statements need amendment, and if so whether management is willing to issue restated financial statements. When these conditions are affirmed and the auditors believe that people are relying on the report, steps should be taken to withdraw the first report, perform the additional procedures required, issue a new report, and inform anyone currently relying on the financial statements. Basically, the decisions relate to the importance and impact of the information, the cooperation of the auditee in taking necessary action, and the actions to be taken. The auditee's cooperation facilitates all of this, but the auditors have a duty to notify the public of an earlier, potentially misleading audit report, even if the auditee does not cooperate.

Standards Check

CAS 560 Subsequent Events

Facts Which Become Known to the Auditor after the Financial Statements Have Been Issued

17. If management does not take the necessary steps to ensure that anyone in receipt of the previously issued financial statements is informed of the situation and does not amend the financial statements in circumstances where the auditor believes they need to be amended, the auditor shall notify management and, unless all of those charged with governance are involved in managing the entity, those charged with governance, that the auditor will seek to prevent future reliance on the auditor's report. If, despite such notification, management or those charged with governance do not take these necessary steps, the auditor shall take appropriate action to seek to prevent reliance on the auditor's report. (Ref: Para. A18)

A18. Where the auditor believes that management, or those charged with governance, have failed to take the necessary steps to prevent reliance on the auditor's report on financial statements previously issued by the entity despite the auditor's prior notification that the auditor will take action to seek to prevent such reliance, the auditor's course of action depends upon the auditor's legal rights and obligations. Consequently, the auditor may consider it appropriate to seek legal advice.

Source: *CPA Canada Handbook—Assurance*, 2014.

dual dating:
refers to instances of dating the audit report as of the date that financial statements are approved by the auditee's responsible parties; includes an additional date indicating that the auditor's procedures on subsequent events are restricted solely to the amendment of the financial statements described in the relevant note to the financial statements, which outlines the effects of the subsequent event or events causing that amendment

Review Checkpoints

16B-1   What is the purpose of dual dating an audit report?

16B-2   What is a subsequent event? What is the difference between a subsequent event that occurs between the balance sheet date and the audit report date and the discovery after the audit report date of facts that existed at the report date? Describe the auditor's responsibility for each.

16B-3   If, subsequent to issuing a report, the auditor discovers information that existed at the report date and materially affects the financial statements, what actions should the auditor take if the auditee consents to disclose the information? What action should be taken if the auditee (including the board of directors) refuses to make disclosure?

16B-5   After the audit report has been issued, someone discovers that the auditee had a material, unrecorded bank loan outstanding at year-end. There was no confirmation requested from that bank, as the auditors were not aware of the auditee's relation with that bank. What steps should an auditor take in this situation?

ENDNOTES

1   *CPA Canada Handbook—Assurance*, 2014.

2   Adapted from Paul Lohnes, "CPAB Presentation on Professional Judgment," to CICA-SME, February 2008.

3   For example, see S. A. McCracken, S. Salterio and M. Gibbins, "Auditor-client management relationships and roles in financial reporting negotiations," *Accounting, Organizations and Society*, May–July 2008, pp. 362–383; and M. Gibbins, S. A. McCracken, and S. Salterio, "The chief financial officer's perspective on negotiations with auditor on financial reporting issues," *Contemporary Accounting Research*, Summer 2007.

4   The approach described here is based on guidelines and concepts that were provided in *CPA Canada Handbook*, AuG-41: Applying the concept of materiality.

5   Adjustments based on likely and possible misstatements are covered in Appendix 10B and are less common in practice. The likely and further possible misstatements are auditor estimates, so it may be difficult for the auditor to make a defensible argument that they should be adjusted, and for the auditee to agree to adjust them.

6   T. B. Bell and J. B. Griffin, "Commentary on auditing high-uncertainty fair value estimates," *Auditing: A Journal of Practice & Theory*, February 2012, pp. 147–155; B. E. Christensen, S. M. Glover, and D. A. Wood. "Extreme estimation uncertainty in fair value estimates: Implications for audit assurance," *Auditing: A Journal of Practice & Theory*, February 2012, pp. 127–146.

7   As described in the *CPA Canada Handbook*, Assurance and Related Services Guideline, AuG-17, "Transactions or conditions reportable under the 'well-being reporting requirement' in federal financial institutions legislation."

PART 4

Advanced Issues in Professional Public Accounting Practice

The five chapters in Part 4 (Chapters 17–21) are available on Connect. They are designed to stand alone, or they can be integrated with the preceding chapters as part of a first course in auditing. The material in Part 4 could also be combined with some of the earlier chapters and some readings, such as those indicated in the text, as the basis for a second, advanced, audit course. Such a course could focus, for example, on auditor problems and judgments in evaluating the quality of financial reporting.

Chapter 17 deals with other assurance and some non-assurance services offered by public accounting firms. Chapter 18 covers the more detailed aspects of professional ethics, expanding on the coverage in Chapter 3. Chapter 19 is devoted to the increasingly important topic of the audit of accounting estimates. The chapter has two parts. Part I clarifies the difficult concepts of CAS 540 using the idea of accounting risk associated with the point estimate concept of CAS 540. Part II deals with the more complex issues of estimation uncertainty associated with reasonable ranges of CAS 540. Recent research and increasing concerns expressed by regulators indicate that this is considered an important and growing problem area of the current audit environment. Estimation uncertainty is analyzed and integrated with the IFRS conceptual framework for financial reporting with the help of the accounting risk concept. This integration guides auditor judgments with respect to appropriate financial reporting. New analytical tools have been added in the form of accounting analytics that use market information and Monte Carlo simulations to help verify accounting estimates. These tools help make operational critical thinking about the ethicality of accounting estimates. Chapter 20 covers auditor legal liability issues in more detail, extending the coverage of this topic beyond the introductory level of Chapter 3. Finally, Chapter 21 covers the conceptual framework for assurance engagements and some specialized assurance engagements. The second half of Chapter 21 covers fraud awareness auditing in more detail. It provides a deeper understanding of the skeptical mindset and specialized procedures needed to more effectively detect frauds. This chapter has benefited from our association with the Association of Certified Fraud Examiners.

KEY TERMS

acceptable financial reporting frameworks a basis of preparing an entity's financial statements that an auditor has determined is acceptable because it provides appropriate criteria against which the financial statements can be audited; financial reporting standards promulgated for certain types of entities by recognized/authorized accounting standard-setting organizations are presumed to be acceptable for general purpose financial statements prepared by such entities (*Chapter 16*)

account balance a control account made up of many constituent items (*Chapter 10*)

accountability relationship a relationship in which at least one of the parties needs to be able to justify its actions or claims to another party in the relationship (*Chapter 1*)

accounting the process of recording, classifying, and summarizing into financial statements a company's transactions that create assets, liabilities, equities, revenues, and expenses (*Chapter 1*)

accounting deficiency reservation a reservation based on a known GAAP departure (*Chapter 4*)

accounting measurement uncertainties similar to estimation uncertainty, which is defined in CAS 540.07 as "the susceptibility of an accounting estimate and related disclosures to an inherent lack of precision in its measurement," except that accounting measurement uncertainties apply to all accounting measurements, not just accounting estimates (*Chapter 4*)

accounting process transactions streams and related account balances used to capture financial data about a business process in the accounting information system; also referred to as an *accounting cycle* (*Chapter 6*)

accounting risk (account level) the part of information risk due to incorrectly predicting events, especially in accounting estimates (*Chapter 1*)

accounts receivable lapping a manipulation of the accounts receivable entries to hide a theft or fraud (*Chapter 11*)

accounts receivable subsidiary ledger a detailed listing of outstanding accounts receivable balances by individual customers that adds up to the total balance in the general ledger accounts receivable "control" account; reconciliation of the subsidiary ledger and the control account is an important control procedure and a key audit test (*Chapter 11*)

accuracy a management control objective of ensuring that monetary transaction amounts are calculated correctly during data input, processing, and output (*Chapter 9*)

acting in the public interest acting in the interests of the users of the financial statements; also, more generally, fulfilling the social role expected of the professional accountant (*Chapter 1*)

adverse opinion an auditor's declaration that financial statements are not in accordance with GAAP (*Chapter 2*)

aged accounts receivable trial balance a list of all outstanding accounts receivable balances organized by how long they have been outstanding; used to manage collection and assess the accounting requirement to provide an allowance for possible uncollectible accounts (*Chapter 11*)

analysis audit procedures that involve identifying the components of financial information and evaluating financial information by studying plausible relationships among both financial and non-financial data to identify fluctuations or relationships that are inconsistent with other relevant information or that differ from expected values by a significant amount and need to be investigated in order to assess risk of material misstatement, obtain substantive evidence, or form an overall opinion at the end of the audit (*Chapter 8*)

analytical procedures specific methods and tests used by an auditor to perform analysis on client financial information to better understand it, by using techniques such as breaking a complex item down into finer aspects and comparing it to other items (*Chapter 5*)

analytical procedures risk the risk that analytical procedures will fail to detect material misstatements (effectiveness risk associated with analytical procedures risk) (*Chapter 10*)

anchoring preconceived notions about control risk that auditors carry over when they perform an audit on a client year after year, a potential pitfall if conditions have changed (*Chapter 6*)

applicable financial reporting framework the financial reporting framework adopted by management and/or those charged with governance in the preparation of the financial statements that is acceptable in view of the nature of the entity and the objective of

the financial statements, or that is required by law or regulation (*Chapter 16*)

application controls control procedures performed at the application level relating to data input, processing, and output in an accounting information system (*Chapter 7*)

arm's length a situation in which two people, or entities, are both independent and acting in their own best interest in their dealings with each other because neither has undue influence over the other (*Chapter 15*)

articles of incorporation a corporation's legal documents that set out its purpose, for example, classes of shares that can be issued (*Chapter 14*)

assertions claims that management makes in financial statements that the auditor needs to verify or refute by obtaining relevant audit evidence (*Chapter 6*)

associated with financial statements any involvement of a public accountant with financial statements issued by a client (*Chapter 4*)

association a term used within the profession to indicate a public accountant's involvement with an enterprise or with information issued by that enterprise (*Chapter 4*)

assurance engagement an engagement in which the auditor adds either reasonable (high) or moderate (negative) levels of assurance (*Chapter 1*)

attention directing refers to the main purpose of analytical procedures when they are performed for risk assessment procedures early in the audit engagement, which is to focus the auditor's assessment on unusual changes or conditions (*Chapter 5*)

attest engagement a type of assurance engagement in which a public accountant is hired to perform procedures and issue a report resulting from those procedures that affirms the validity of an assertion; also known as an attestation engagement (*Chapter 1*)

attribute sampling the type of audit sampling in control testing in which auditors look for the presence or absence of a control condition (*Chapter 10*)

audit approach decision an auditor's choice of whether to use a combined audit approach that includes testing internal control effectiveness or a substantive audit approach that obtains all the evidence from substantive sources (*Chapter 8*)

audit committees groups that monitor management's financial reporting responsibilities, including meeting with the external auditors and dealing with various audit and accounting matters that may arise (*Chapter 2*)

audit deficiency reservation a reservation based on insufficient audit evidence (scope restriction) (*Chapter 4*)

audit evidence all the information used by an auditor to form the conclusions on which the auditor's opinion is based, obtained from performing audit procedures or from other sources; see *evidence*

Audit Guidelines (AuGs) the part of the *CPA Canada Handbook* that provides procedural guidance on implementing generally accepted auditing standards (*Chapter 2*)

audit objectives the auditor's goals in relation to obtaining audit evidence that verifies or refutes management's financial statement assertions (*Chapter 6*)

audit of internal control over financial reporting the engagement that results in an audit report on the effectiveness of a client's internal control over financial reporting (*Chapter 17*)

audit plan a document containing all the detailed audit programs listing the procedures to be performed in response to the assessed risk of material misstatement on an audit, guided by the decisions made in the overall audit strategy (*Chapter 2*)

audit procedures the general audit techniques of recalculation/reperformance, observation, confirmation, inquiry, inspection, and analysis (*Chapter 10*)

audit program a document listing the specific detailed audit procedures to be performed in each accounting process to gather sufficient appropriate evidence through control tests, analytical procedures, and other tests of balances to address the audit objectives set out in the program; includes the risk assessment program, the internal control program, and the balance audit program (*Chapter 2*)

audit quality management policies and procedures auditors and audit firms apply to ensure audits are done in accordance with professional auditing standards and are effective (*Chapter 5*)

audit risk (account level) the probability that an auditor will fail to find a material misstatement that exists in an account balance (*Chapter 1*)

audit risk (financial statement level) the probability that an auditor will fail to express a reservation of opinion on financial statements that are materially misstated, lowered to an acceptable level by an auditor obtaining reasonable assurance by performing evidence-gathering procedures (*Chapter 6*)

audit risk model a simplified model that conceptualizes audit risk as the product of two elements, the risk of material misstatement and the detection risk, that are assumed to independently determine its level (*Chapter 6*)

audit sampling testing less than 100% of a population (items in an account balance or class of transactions) to form a conclusion about some characteristic of the balance or class of transactions (*Chapter 10*)

audit scope the entity and the financial statements that will be covered by the audit engagement, and the client documents and records to be examined to provide the necessary audit evidence (*Chapter 11*)

audit societies the term coined by Michael Power for societies in which there is extensive examination by auditors of economic and other politically important activities (*Chapter 1*)

auditee the entity (company, proprietorship, organization, department, etc.) being audited; usually it refers to the entity whose financial statements are being audited (*Chapter 1*)

auditing the verification of information by someone other than the one providing that information (*Chapter 1*)

auditing standards the subset of assurance standards dealing with "high" or "reasonable" levels of assurance in assurance engagements (*Chapter 1*)

auditor–client negotiations discussions between auditor and management, usually at the end of an audit engagement, concerning decisions on whether or not to adjust the financial statements for identified and likely misstatements discovered by the auditor (*Chapter 16*)

auditor communications all the correspondence auditors use with auditee personnel, officers, and third parties to conduct the audit; communication with management and those charged with governance includes the engagement letter, summary of planning, internal control deficiencies ("management letter"), management representation letter, and significant audit findings summary; communication with third parties includes confirmation letters from creditors, debtors, and lawyers (*Chapter 16*)

auditor's risk from taking the engagement the possibility that negative consequences will arise for an auditor's professional practice as a result of taking on a particular audit engagement, such as damage to reputation, litigation, or financial loss (*Chapter 5*)

authorization a management control objective of ensuring that transactions are approved before they are recorded (*Chapter 9*)

authorization (procedure) a control activity that assigns specific individuals in an organization the responsibility for approving the initiation of transactions on behalf of the organization (*Chapter 12*)

balance audit program a list of the substantive procedures for gathering direct evidence on the assertions (i.e., existence, completeness, valuation, ownership, presentation) about dollar amounts in the account balances (*Chapter 8*)

balance sheet approach to auditing using audit analysis of changes in balance sheet accounts as a basis for obtaining preliminary assurance about the related income statement accounts and cash flow information (*Chapter 11*)

bank transfer schedule an audit analysis summarizing all the transfers between the auditee's bank accounts in the days just before and after the period-end to verify that each amount transferred is included in only one account at the period-end, not double counted (*Chapter 11*)

bill-and-hold transactions sales that a customer has asked to be billed/invoiced for but does not want to be shipped immediately; require a special audit confirmation of the details of the customer's agreement to ensure revenue recognition is appropriate (*Chapter 11*)

block sampling choosing segments of contiguous transactions; undesirable because it is hard to get a representative sample efficiently (*Chapter 10*)

bridge working paper audit documentation that connects (bridges) the control evaluation to subsequent audit procedures by summarizing the major control strengths and weaknesses, listing test of control procedures for auditing the control strengths, and suggesting substantive audit procedures to be performed to respond to the weaknesses (*Chapter 9*)

business risk the probability that significant conditions, events, circumstances, or actions might arise that will adversely affect the entity's ability to achieve its objectives and execute its strategies (*Chapter 1*)

business risk–based audit approach (risk-based audit approach) the requirement for the auditor to understand the client's business risks and strategy in order to assess the risks of material misstatement in the financial statements and design appropriate audit procedures in response to those risks (*Chapter 6*)

Canadian Auditing Standards (CAS) the audit standards in Canada using the equivalent International Standards on Auditing (ISAs) and the same numbering system as the ISAs; the subset of assurance standards dealing with "high" or "reasonable" levels of assurance in assurance engagements (*Chapter 1*)

Canadian Coalition for Good Governance a group of the largest pension and mutual funds, whose purpose is to monitor executives and boards of directors to see whether they comply with good corporate governance and financial reporting practices (*Chapter 2*)

Canadian Public Accountability Board (CPAB) the board organized to monitor the auditors of public companies in Canada (*Chapter 2*)

Canadian Securities Administrators (CSA) the organization of Canadian provincial securities market administrators and regulators (*Chapter 3*)

certified internal auditors persons who have met the Institute of Internal Auditors' criteria for professional certified internal auditor credentials (*Chapter 21*)

Chartered Professional Accountants of Canada (CPA Canada) the professional body of chartered professional accountants in Canada (*Chapter 1*)

cheque kiting a scam that involves building up apparent balances in one or more bank accounts based on uncollected (float) cheques drawn against similar accounts in other banks when there is a time lag in clearing items between the banks (*Chapter 11*)

class of transactions groups of accounting entries that have the same source or purpose; credit sales, cash sales, and cash receipts are three different classes (*Chapter 10*)

classical attribute sampling sampling in which a sampling unit is the same thing as an invoice or population unit (*Chapter 10*)

classification a management control objective of ensuring that transactions are recorded in the correct accounts in the accounting information system, including general ledger accounts, subledger accounts, and journals (*Chapter 9*)

clean opinion the highest level of assurance, with an opinion sentence that reads, "In our opinion, the accompanying financial statements present fairly, in all material respects . . ." (*Chapter 4*)

client the person or company who retains the auditor and pays the fee (*Chapter 1*)

combined audit approach an approach to performing an audit that involves obtaining assurance from reliance on internal controls based on testing their effectiveness, combined with assurance from substantive procedures (*Chapter 9*)

commission a percentage fee charged for professional services for executing a transaction or performing some other business activity (*Chapter 18*)

commitments contracts that establish both rights and obligations for each of the

contracting parties relating to the amounts and timing of future cash flows; assessed at the completion stage of an audit to determine whether fairly presented in the balance sheet and/or notes (*Chapter 15*)

communication the procedures and channels used to process and share information among people in an organization to enhance understanding and effectiveness, including accounting policies, control activities, and people's roles and responsibilities (*Chapter 7*)

company-level controls internal control framework components that permeate the organization and affect the quality of its financial reporting and disclosures, consisting of the control environment; the entity's risk assessment process; the information system, including the related business processes, relevant to financial reporting and communication; and monitoring of controls (*Chapter 7*)

compensating control an alternative, effective control that achieves the same purpose as a missing control, such that the missing control is not considered to be a control deficiency that needs to be communicated to management or those charged with governance (*Chapter 9*)

completeness a management control objective of ensuring that valid transactions are not missing from the accounting records (*Chapter 9*)

compliance auditing when an audit engagement is being done for the sole purpose of reporting on compliance with laws, regulations, or rules (*Chapter 21*)

compliance framework a financial reporting framework that requires financial statements to be prepared in compliance with the requirements of the framework but does not contain the acknowledgments required for fair presentation (*Chapter 16*)

comprehensive governmental auditing auditing that goes beyond an audit of financial reports to include economy, efficiency, and effectiveness audits (*Chapter 1*)

confirmation an audit procedure by which auditors obtain evidence in the form of a direct written response to the auditor from a third party (the confirming party), in paper form, or by electronic or other medium; usually the evidence is related to certain account balances or other information such as terms of agreements or transactions with third parties; also called external confirmation (*Chapter 8*)

confirmation response rate the ratio of the number of confirmations returned to the number sent (*Chapter 11*)

conflict of interest a situation faced by a professional accountant in which there may be a divergence between the interests of two (or more) parties (e.g., clients) for whom the

professional accountant undertakes a professional activity, or between the interests of the professional accountant and the interests of such parties, that could create a threat to the professional accountant's objectivity or other fundamental ethical principles (*Chapter 1*)

consequentialism a moral theory that the choice of action is made based solely on the consequences, that is, that it maximizes utility; note that economics and business are based on this theory (*Chapter 3*)

contingencies existing situations involving uncertainty about one or more future events that when resolved may confirm an increase or decrease in an asset or liability; assessed at the completion stage of an audit to determine whether fairly presented in the balance sheet and/or notes (*Chapter 15*)

contingent liabilities possible obligations of a company that will be confirmed only if some future event occurs; if probable to occur and measurable they are recognized as a *provision* in the balance sheet unless their amount can be estimated reliably and it is probable that the future event giving rise to them will occur, but their existence must be disclosed in the notes (*Chapter 15*)

continuity schedule a working paper that shows the movements in an account balance from the beginning to the end of the period under audit; used to analyze the account balance changes and the other financial statement items related to them (*Chapter 11*)

contrived sham transactions fictitious transactions created for illegal purposes, such as evading taxes (*Chapter 14*)

control activities specific company procedures designed to control processes, transactions, and applications that affect accounting information; consisting of general control activities and application-based control activities (*Chapter 7*)

control environment the attitudes, operating styles, capabilities, and actions of an organization's governance and management functions in relation to the organization's internal control that can provide the resources, policies, and discipline to establish a "tone at the top" that is conducive to the organization meeting its strategic objectives, providing reliable internal and external financial reporting, and operating efficiently and ethically; considered to be the foundation for all other components of internal control (i.e., control activities, management's risk assessment process, information system and communication, monitoring) (*Chapter 7*)

control framework (internal control framework, internal control structure) a model used to present the different elements of an organization's internal control structure and how they fit together, useful to auditors for documenting their understanding of an auditee's internal control over financial reporting; the control framework developed by COSO is commonly used by auditors because it is recommended by generally accepted auditing standards (*Chapter 7*)

control risk the risk that the client's internal controls will not prevent or detect a material misstatement (*Chapter 6*)

control risk assessment a process the auditor uses to understand the client's internal control in order to identify and assess the risks of material misstatement of the financial statements, whether due to fraud or error, and to design and perform further audit procedures (*Chapter 11*)

control strengths specific features of effective controls that would prevent, detect, or correct material misstatements (*Chapter 9*)

control testing (compliance testing) performing procedures to assess whether controls are operating effectively (*Chapter 6*)

control weaknesses the lack of effective controls in particular areas that would allow material errors to get by undetected (*Chapter 9*)

controls relevant to the audit elements of an auditee's internal control that directly or indirectly affect the risk of material misstatement of the financial statements being audited (*Chapter 9*)

corporate governance the ways in which the suppliers of capital to corporations assure themselves of getting a return on their investment; more generally, under the corporate social responsibility view, corporate governance is the system set up to hold a corporation accountable to employees, communities, the environment, and similar broader social concerns, in addition to being accountable to the capital providers (*Chapter 2*)

COSO (Committee of Sponsoring Organizations of the Treadway Commission) an organization that investigated corporate fraud and developed a control framework that has become the standard for the design of controls by companies and evaluation of controls by auditors; the COSO control framework is cited by the Public Company Accounting Oversight Board in its auditing standards on internal control as an acceptable framework against which control design and effectiveness should be evaluated (*Chapter 17*)

cost of goods sold costs such as materials, labour, overhead, freight, and so on, that are necessary to get goods to the stage when they can be sold; calculated as the beginning inventory, plus costs added during the period, less the ending inventory; offset against sales revenues, it indicates the gross profit or gross margin on sales on which analytical expectations can be based (*Chapter 13*)

critical thinking the process of justifying one's conclusion or decision by providing good or acceptable reasons (*Chapter 3*)

critical thinking framework principles and concepts to help structure your thinking for more ethical reporting so that your conclusions will be better justified (*Chapter 3*)

current file the administrative and evidence audit working papers that relate to the audit work for the year being audited (*Chapter 8*)

custody a control activity that identifies the individuals in an organization with the responsibility to hold and safeguard the organization's assets and/or records (*Chapter 12*)

cutoff bank statement a complete bank statement showing paid cheques, deposits, and other bank account transactions for a 10- to 20-day period following the reconciliation date (*Chapter 11*)

cutoff error when transactions are recorded in the wrong period, either by postponing to the next period or accelerating next-period transactions into the current period (*Chapter 12*)

dangling debit (or credit) a false or erroneous debit (or credit) balance that exists because one or more accounts are misstated (*Chapter 5*)

debt instruments legally documented obligations between a borrower and a lender, such as bonds payable, leases, or mortgages payable (*Chapter 14*)

defalcation fraud in which an employee takes assets (money or property) from an organization for personal gain; may be due to corruption or asset misappropriation (*Chapter 7*)

deontological (Kantian) ethics the moral theory that an action is right if it is based on a sense of duty or obligation (*Chapter 3*)

detailed audit plan an audit planning document outlining the nature, timing, and extent of audit procedures to assess the risk of financial statement misstatement and obtain the necessary audit evidence for each assertion for all significant transactions, balances, and disclosures, including staffing decisions and time budgets (*Chapter 11*)

detection rate for confirmations the ratio of the number of misstatements reported to auditors to the number of actual account misstatements (*Chapter 11*)

detection risk the risk that the auditor's procedures will fail to find a material misstatement that exists in the accounts (*Chapter 6*)

detective controls control procedures designed to detect any error or fraud that has occurred in the accounting information system; must also be accompanied by appropriate procedures designed to effectively

correct any errrors; see *preventive controls* (*Chapter 7*)

direct reporting engagement a type of assurance engagement in which the assertions are implied and not written down in some form (*Chapter 1*)

direction of the test a description of the nature of an audit test procedure in terms of whether it involves vouching from the accounting records back to source documents ("grave to cradle") or tracing from the source documents up to the accounting records ("cradle to grave") (*Chapter 9*)

disclaimer of opinion an auditor's declaration that no opinion is given on financial statements and the reasons this is so, usually due to a scope limitation; also called a denial of opinion (*Chapter 2*)

dual dating refers to instances of dating the audit report as of the date that financial statements are approved by the auditee's responsible parties; includes an additional date indicating that the auditor's procedures on subsequent events are restricted solely to the amendment of the financial statements described in the relevant note to the financial statements, which outlines the effects of the subsequent event or events causing that amendment (*Chapter 16*)

dual-purpose audit procedure an auditing procedure designed to provide both control effectiveness evidence and substantive evidence from the same sample of items; can increase efficiency in obtaining audit evidence (*Chapter 9*)

e-commerce any trade that takes place by electronic means (*Chapter 6*)

effectiveness risk (type II error risk) the risk that the auditor will incorrectly accept an account balance that is materially misstated; it can result in audit failure and so is considered to be a more serious problem for the audit than incorrect rejection; a type of sampling risk (*Chapter 10*)

efficiency risk (type I error risk) the risk that the auditor will incorrectly reject an account balance that is not materially misstated; a type of sampling risk (*Chapter 10*)

embezzlement fraud involving employees or non-employees wrongfully taking money or property entrusted to their care, custody, and control; often accompanied by false accounting entries and other forms of lying and cover-up (*Chapter 7*)

employee fraud the use of dishonest means to take money or other property from an employer (*Chapter 7*)

engagement letter a document that sets out the terms of the engagement forming a contract between the auditor and the client when a new audit engagement is accepted (*Chapter 5*)

engagement partner   one of the most experienced members of the audit team, who makes the final decision on the audit opinion (*Chapter 15*)

engagement quality review   the review of working papers and financial statements by a partner not responsible for client relations; ensures that the quality of the audit work is in keeping with the standards of the audit firm (*Chapter 15*)

enterprise resource planning systems (ERPs)   information systems in which inputs and outputs from many or all the business processes are processed in an integrated manner, so the accounting component of the information system will be closely related to many other functional areas, such as sales, inventory, human resources, and cash management (*Chapter 6*)

entity's risk assessment process   management's process for identifying business risks that could affect financial reporting objectives and for deciding on actions to address and minimize these risks; understanding this process helps auditors assess the risk that the financial statements could be materially misstated; see *management's risk assessment process* (*Chapter 6*)

error analysis   qualitative evaluation of control risk (*Chapter 10*)

errors   in financial statement auditing, unintentional misstatements or omissions of amounts or disclosures in financial statements (*Chapter 7*)

ethical dilemma   a problem that arises when a reason to act in a certain way is offset by a reason to not act in that way (*Chapter 3*)

ethical reporting principle   a principle proposed to represent the main concerns of third-party users of financial statements (*Appendix 1B*)

evidence   anything that provides proof of an assertion, or helps to form a conclusion or judgment; see *audit evidence*

evidence collection   steps 4, 5, and 6 of the sampling method, which are performed to get the evidence (*Chapter 10*)

evidence evaluation   the final step of the sampling method; to evaluate the evidence and make justifiable decisions about the control risk (*Chapter 10*)

evidence-gathering procedures   the activities auditors perform to obtain independent proof in relating the financial statements to the assertions in order to meet the audit objectives (*Chapter 6*)

expectation about the population deviation rate   an estimate of the ratio of the number of expected deviations to population size (*Chapter 10*)

expectations gap   the difference that can arise between what the public expects of the auditor's social role and what the professional standards and practices deliver (*Chapter 1*)

expected dollar misstatement   a preliminary estimate of expected monetary misstatements in a total monetary value recorded for a population (*Chapter 10*)

expenditure analysis   comparing the suspect's spending with known income (*Chapter 21*)

extending the audit conclusion   performing substantive-purpose audit procedures on the transactions in the remaining period and on the year-end balance to produce sufficient appropriate evidence for a decision about the year-end balance (*Chapter 10*)

extent and selection of audit procedures   the amount of audit work planned, such as sample size for an audit test and the method for selecting sample items (*Chapter 8*)

external auditors   auditors who are outsiders and independent of the entity being audited (*Chapter 1*)

fair presentation framework   a financial reporting framework that requires financial statements to be prepared in compliance with the framework and that acknowledges explicitly or implicitly that, to achieve fair presentation of the financial statements, it may be necessary for management to provide disclosures beyond those specifically required by the framework or acknowledges explicitly that it may be necessary for management to depart from a requirement of the framework to achieve fair presentation of the financial statements in those extremely rare situations where this is necessary; referred to as GAAP if used for general purpose financial statements; includes IFRS and ASPE (*Chapter 16*)

fidelity bond   a type of insurance policy that covers theft of cash by employees (*Chapter 11*)

financial reporting   the broad-based process of providing statements of financial position (balance sheets), statements of results of operations (income statements), statements of results of changes in financial position (cash flow statements), and accompanying disclosure notes (footnotes) to outside decision makers who have no internal source of information such as the management of the company has (*Chapter 1*)

financial reporting framework   a set of criteria that provides a basis for preparing an entity's financial statements; may be general purpose or special purpose (*Chapter 16*)

financial statement closing process   the final adjusting journal entries and other procedures management oversees at the final stage of preparing financial statements (*Chapter 9*)

financial statements   the structured representation of historical financial information, including related notes and summary of significant accounting policies, intended to communicate an entity's economic resources or obligations at a point in time or the changes therein for a period of time in accordance with a financial reporting framework; usually refers to a complete set of financial statements as determined by the requirements of the applicable financial reporting framework (*Chapter 16*)

FOB destination   terms of sale indicating that title to goods sold transfers from seller to buyer when the goods reach the buyer's destination; can give rise to an amount of inventory-in-transit at year-end that is owned by an auditee company (the seller) that is not physically on hand at the auditee's premises (*Chapter 11*)

FOB shipping   terms of sale indicating that title to goods sold transfers from seller to buyer when the goods are handed over from the seller to the shipping company that will ultimately deliver them to the buyer; can give rise to an amount of inventory-in-transit at year-end that is owned by an auditee company (the buyer) that is not physically on hand at the auditee's premises (*Chapter 11*)

forecast error   the difference between the future financial information as estimated by management and the actual financial outcome that is realized (*Chapter 16*)

forensic accounting   the application of accounting and auditing skills to legal problems, both civil and criminal (*Chapter 1*)

fraud   in financial statement auditing, an intentional act by one or more individuals (the fraudsters) among management, those charged with governance, employees, or third parties, involving the use of deception to obtain an unjust or illegal advantage over someone (the victim) (*Chapter 1*)

fraud audit questioning (FAQ)   a non-accusatory method of asking key questions during a regular audit to give personnel an opportunity to supply information about possible misdeeds (*Chapter 21*)

fraud auditing   a proactive approach to detect financial frauds using accounting records and information, analytical relationships, and an awareness of fraud perpetration and concealment efforts (*Chapter 1*)

fraud by management incompetence   a false claim by management of its capabilities used to conceal deceptive financial reporting by making it look unintended (*Appendix 1B*)

fraud incentive   when management is under pressure, from sources outside or inside the entity, to achieve an expected (perhaps unrealistic) earnings target or financial outcome, particularly as the consequences to management for failing to meet financial goals can be significant; also, when individuals are tempted to misappropriate assets because, for example, they are living beyond their means (*Chapter 7*)

fraud opportunity   when an individual believes internal control can be overridden to allow a fraud to be perpetrated, for example, when the individual is in a position of trust or has knowledge of specific deficiencies in internal control (*Chapter 7*)

fraud rationalization   when individuals possess an attitude, character, or set of ethical values allowing them to knowingly and intentionally commit a dishonest act, or when otherwise honest individuals are in an environment that puts sufficient pressure on them to commit a fraudulent act (*Chapter 7*)

fraud risk   in financial statement auditing, the possibility that fraud has resulted in intentional misstatement in the financial statements; two types of intentional misstatements are relevant to the auditor: those resulting from fraudulent financial reporting and those resulting from misappropriation of assets (*Chapter 7*)

fraud triangle   a model of the three factors that make fraud likely: incentive, opportunity, and rationalization (or similar concepts) (*Chapter 6*)

fraudulent financial reporting   intentional manipulation of reported financial results (by manipulation of accounting records or supporting documents, misrepresentation or omission of significant information, or intentional misapplication of accounting principles) to portray a misstated economic picture of the firm by which the perpetrator seeks an increase in personal wealth through a rise in stock price or compensation (*Chapter 7*)

further possible misstatement   a misstatement that could exist over and above the total of known and likely misstatements because of the limitations of the testing concept of auditing (*Chapter 16*)

general controls   organizational features that have a pervasive impact on accounting processes and applications and the effectiveness of application-level control procedures (*Chapter 7*)

general purpose financial reporting frameworks   financial reporting frameworks used to prepare financial statements designed to meet the common financial information needs of a wide range of users (*Chapter 16*)

generally accepted accounting principles (GAAP)   those accounting methods that have been established in a particular jurisdiction through formal recognition by a standard-setting body, or by authoritative support or precedent, such as the accounting recommendations of the *CPA Canada Handbook* (*Chapter 1*)

generally accepted auditing standards (GAAS)   those auditing recommendations that have been established in a particular jurisdiction by formal recognition by a standard-setting body, or by authoritative support or precedent such as the auditing and assurance recommendations of the *CPA Canada Handbook* (*Chapter 2*)

haphazard selection   an unsystematic way of selecting sample units (*Chapter 10*)

highly effective audit   an audit designed to have a very high chance of detecting material misstatements in the financial statements, which is a major goal of the auditor's control evaluation process (*Chapter 9*)

horizontal analysis   the analytical procedure of comparing changes of financial statement numbers and ratios across two or more years (*Chapter 5*)

hypothesis testing   when auditors hypothesize that the book value is materially accurate regarding existence, ownership, and valuation (*Chapter 10*)

illegal act   in financial statement auditing, non-compliance with a domestic or foreign statutory law or government regulation attributable to the entity under audit, or to management or employees acting on the entity's behalf; this does not include personal misconduct by the entity's management or employees unrelated to the entity's business activities (*Chapter 7*)

imperatives   universal principles assumed by monistic moral theories (*Chapter 3*)

implied warranty concept   holds that the auditor is responsible once it can be proved that the audited financial statement is wrong, so the issue of whether the auditor is negligent is irrelevant (*Appendix 1B*)

imprest bank account (imprest fund)   an account or fund used by a business for small, routine expenditure items that is restored to a fixed amount periodically; used for payroll bank accounts and petty cash funds (*Chapter 13*)

individually significant items   items in account balances that exceed the material misstatement amount; in audit sampling these should be removed from the population and audited completely (*Chapter 10*)

information hypothesis   holds that audit services are demanded to reduce the information risk to users of financial statements (*Appendix 1B*)

information risk   the possible failure of financial statements to appropriately reflect the economic substance of business activities (*Chapter 1*)

information system   a set of interrelated functions that collect, process, store, and distribute information in an organization; in relation to financial reporting, the manual and technology-based procedures and records used in the accounting system to capture and report an organization's transactions, events, and conditions to maintain accountability for the related assets, liabilities, and equity and ensure information required to be disclosed is appropriately reported in the financial statements (*Chapter 7*)

information technology (IT)   the hardware and software needed to process data (*Chapter 1*)

inherent risk   the probability that material misstatements could have occurred (*Chapter 6*)

initial public offering (IPO)   first-time offering of a corporation's shares to the public (*Chapter 2*)

inquiry   audit procedures that involve asking knowledgeable persons within the auditee organization or outside for relevant financial and/or non-financial information; may provide the auditor with information not available otherwise, provide corroboration for other audit evidence obtained, or provide conflicting information that requires additional audit investigation; includes written representations from management that are obtained at the end of an audit engagement (*Chapter 8*)

inspection   audit procedures that involve examining an auditee's records or documents, whether internal or external, in paper form, electronic form, or other media, or physically examining an asset; provides evidence of, for example, the existence of an asset, the occurrence of a transaction, or the appropriate application of GAAP to the item; inspection of documents takes the form of vouching, tracing, and scanning; also called inspection of documents, physical inspection (*Chapter 8*)

insurance hypothesis   predicts that auditors are demanded so that they may be sued if there is a business failure or investor losses due to inaccuracies in the financial statements (*Appendix 1B*)

interim audit work   covers procedures performed several weeks or months before the balance sheet date (*Chapter 5*)

interim date   a date before the end of the period under audit when some of the audit procedures might be performed, such as control evaluation and testing (*Chapter 2*)

internal auditing   verification work performed by company employees who are trained in auditing procedures; mainly used for internal control purposes, but external auditors can rely on internal audit work if certain criteria are met (*Chapter 1*)

internal control   the system of policies and procedures needed to maintain adherence to a company's objectives; especially, the accuracy of recordkeeping and safeguarding of assets (*Chapter 2*)

internal control program   an audit planning document summarizing the auditor's understanding of internal control and the control testing procedures to be performed to assess control risk and control effectiveness; sometimes called the interim audit program (*Chapter 8*)

internal control questionnaire   a checklist used by auditors to gather evidence about the auditee's control environment and its general and application control activities (*Chapter 9*)

International Federation of Accountants (IFAC)   an organization dedicated to developing international auditing standards (*Chapter 1*)

international harmonization   international convergence of national accounting and auditing standards with IFRS and ISAs, including going concern, fraud, and the audit risk model (*Chapter 1*)

International Standards on Auditing (ISAs)   the auditing standards of the International Federation of Accountants (*Chapter 1*)

key audit matters   those issues that, in the auditor's professional judgment, were most significant in the financial statement audit of the current period and are important information to communicate to financial statement users in the auditor's report, selected from the issues communicated with those charged with governance at the end of the audit (*Chapter 16*)

known misstatement (identified misstatement)   the total amount of actual monetary error found in a sample or other non-sampling auditing procedures (*Chapter 10*)

lawyer's confirmation letter   an inquiry letter sent from the auditee's management to the auditee's lawyer, with a copy of the lawyer's response going directly from the lawyer to the auditor to provide audit evidence about any potentially material litigation or claims involving the auditee; obtained at the completion stage of the audit to assess whether all claims are fairly presented in the balance sheet and/or notes (*Chapter 15*)

legal responsibilities   auditor responsibilities imposed by the legal system (*Chapter 3*)

levels of assurance   the amount of credibility provided by accountants and auditors (*Chapter 4*)

likely misstatement (projected misstatement)   the projection of a known misstatement identified in a representative sample to the whole population (*Chapter 10*)

limited liability partnership (LLP) a company whose partners' liability is limited to the capital they have invested in the business (*Chapter 1*)

lower-of-cost-and-net-realizable-value (LCNRV)   an accounting rule that requires inventory to be reported at its cost, or, if the amount that could be obtained by selling it net of any selling costs is less than its cost, at that lower amount; the lower amount is achieved by recording a write-down (*Chapter 13*)

management discussion and analysis (MD&A)   a section of the annual report that includes management's analysis of past operating and financial results; can also include forward-looking information; the financial statement auditor reviews the information to ensure there is nothing that is inconsistent with the audited financial statements, but the MD&A itself is not audited (*Chapter 21*)

management estimates   financial statement numbers that management develops based on the probability of future financial events using forecasting models and assumptions (*Chapter 16*)

management letter (management control letter)   a written communication to management of control deficiencies uncovered by the auditor (*Chapter 9*)

management override of controls   when management uses its authority and responsibility for the organization's internal control as a means to ignore or circumvent controls; often a facilitator of fraudulent financial reporting (*Chapter 9*)

management representation letter written statements by management provided to the auditor to confirm certain matters or to support other audit evidence as required by CAS 580; see *written representations* (*Chapter 15*)

management's draft financial statements the set of financial statements an auditor receives from the auditee's management at the start of the year-end audit work, containing the management assertions (claims) that will be subject to verification by the auditor (*Chapter 5*)

management's risk assessment process the methods used by an organization's management to identify the risks to be managed, including those that can lead to misstated financial information, and to determine appropriate actions; see entity's risk assessment process (*Chapter 7*)

material subsequent events   two types of events that are discovered after the year-end date, one type being events that existed at year-end that actually have a material impact on the year-end financial statements and the second being events did not happen until after the year-end but are judged to be materially relevant to users of the year-end financial statement data; see *subsequent event requiring adjustment in financial statement numbers* (*Chapter 15*)

materiality   an audit concept related to an auditor's judgment about matters, such as errors or omissions in the preparation and presentation of financial statements, that could reasonably be expected to influence economic decisions of people using those financial statements, i.e., matters that would be material to those decisions (*Chapter 1*)

materiality for the financial statements as a whole (overall materiality)   an auditor's judgment regarding what is the largest amount of uncorrected monetary misstatement that might exist in financial statements that still fairly presents the auditee's financial position and results of operations under an acceptable financial reporting framework (*Chapter 5*)

minutes   formal written records of key events and decisions made in a formal meeting, such as a corporate board meeting (*Chapter 5*)

misappropriation of assets   the theft or misuse of an organization's assets (a type of defalcation) (*Chapter 7*)

mitigating factors   elements of financial flexibility (saleability of assets, lines of credit, debt extension, dividend elimination) available as survival strategies in circumstances of going-concern uncertainty, which may reduce the financial difficulty problems (*Chapter 19, Part I*)

modified opinion report   an audit report that contains an opinion paragraph that does not give the positive assurance that everything in the financial statements conforms with GAAP; includes qualified opinion, adverse opinion, and disclaimer of opinion reports (*Chapter 2*)

monetary-unit sampling (MUS)   a modified form of attributes sampling that permits auditors to reach conclusions about monetary amounts as well as compliance deviations (*Chapter 10*)

money laundering   engaging in specific financial transactions in order to conceal the identity, source, and/or destination of money resulting from an illegal act, which may involve organized crime, tax evasion, or false accounting (*Chapter 11*)

monistic theories   ethical theories that assume universal principles apply regardless of the specific facts of a situation (*Chapter 3*)

monitoring   management's ongoing process for reviewing and assessing whether the control procedures in place are adequate to address control risks and are operating effectively as intended, and determining areas that need improvement (*Chapter 7*)

monitoring hypothesis   based on the principal-agent framework of economic theory, holds that utility-maximizing agents (the managers) have the incentive to contract for mechanisms to monitor their opportunistic behaviour and will demand audits (monitoring) whenever the cost of monitoring is less than the agents' loss without the monitoring (*Appendix 1B*)

moral imagination   the part of ethical reasoning where one has the ability to imagine others' feelings about the consequences of a decision (*Chapter 3*)

moral responsibilities   the rules and principles conforming to broad social norms of behaviour (*Chapter 3*)

nature of audit procedures   the six general techniques of an account balance audit program: recalculation/reperformance, confirmation, inquiry, inspection, observation, and analysis (*Chapter 8*)

nature, timing, and extent   the aspects that fully describe a specific audit procedure in an audit program, which indicate the evidence techniques the procedure uses and its objective related to financial statement assertions or control effectiveness; when during the engagement it will be performed; and the sampling approach, sample size, and basis of selecting sample items (*Chapter 9*)

negative assurance (moderate assurance)   a statement that, having carried out a professional engagement, nothing has come to the public accountant's attention that would give reason to believe that matters under consideration do not meet specified suitable criteria (*Chapter 4*)

negligence-based concept   holds that auditor negligence needs to be proved in court to support claims against auditors (*Appendix 1B*)

no assurance   the public accountant provides zero assurance credibility because there is no independent verification of the data provided by the client; for example, compilation engagement (*Chapter 4*)

non-excludability   a product of audited financial statements by which the auditor is unable to prevent any user from consuming the good (*Appendix 1B*)

non-rival consumption   a product of audited financial statements by which one person's consumption of a good does not prevent another person from consuming it (*Appendix 1B*)

non-sampling risk   the possibility of making a wrong decision, which exists in both statistical and non-statistical sampling (*Chapter 10*)

non-statistical (judgmental) sampling   choosing items in a population for audit testing and evaluating the findings based on the auditor's own knowledge and experience rather than statistical methods (*Chapter 10*)

observation   an audit procedure that consists of looking at a process or procedure being performed by others, for example, the auditor's observation of inventory counting by the entity's personnel, or of the performance of control activities (*Chapter 8*)

off the balance sheet   refers to how certain obligations and commitments do not have to be reported on the balance sheet, such as purchase commitments and operating leases (*Chapter 14*)

online input validation   inputting information correctly or the computer will not accept the transaction; uses validation checks such as missing data, check digit, and limit tests (*Chapter 11*)

operational auditing (performance auditing or management auditing)   auditors' study of business operations for the purpose of making recommendations about economic and efficient use of resources, effective achievement of business objectives, and compliance with company policies (*Chapter 1*)

overall analytical procedures   analysis designed and performed near the end of an audit engagement to assist the auditor in forming an overall conclusion about whether the financial statements are consistent with the auditor's understanding of the auditee's business and with the audit evidence obtained (*Chapter 15*)

overall audit strategy   an audit planning document that sets the scope, timing, and direction of the audit, and that guides the development of the audit plan, including the reporting objectives; the nature, timing, and extent of resources necessary to perform the engagement; and the nature of the communications required (*Chapter 5*)

passed adjustments (waived adjustments)   unadjusted misstatements discovered by an auditor that management decides not to correct but auditors can accept since they are not material to fair presentation of the financial statements; see *uncorrected misstatements* (*Chapter 16*)

peer review   a study of a firm's quality control policies and procedures, followed by a report on a firm's quality of audit practice; usually done as a special engagement by another audit firm hired for the task by the firm reviewed (*Appendix 2B*)

performance materiality   an amount set by the auditor at less than materiality for the financial statements as a whole, to reduce to an appropriately low level the probability that the aggregate of uncorrected and undetected misstatements exceeds materiality for the financial statements as a whole (*Chapter 5*)

periodic reconciliation (reconciling)   a control activity that involves regularly comparing reports, summaries, and balances in an accounting information system to the actual assets, or detailed components of accounts, to ensure they agree or indicate any discrepancies, such as a bank reconciliation, supplier reconciliation, inventory count, or agreeing the accounts receivable subledger total to the balance in the general ledger accounts receivable control account (*Chapter 12*)

permanent file   audit working papers that are of continuing interest from year to year, including the client company's articles of incorporation, shareholder agreements, major contracts, and minutes (*Chapter 8*)

pervasive materiality   departures from generally accepted accounting principles that are so significant that they overshadow the financial statements or affect numerous accounts and financial statement relationships (*Chapter 4*)

physical representation of the population   the auditor's frame of reference for selecting a sample, for example, a journal listing of recorded sales invoices (*Chapter 10*)

planned acceptable audit risk level (acceptable audit risk level)   the level of audit risk determined by the auditor at the planning stage to be acceptable based on engagement characteristics, achieved by performing control tests and substantive procedures that lower audit risk to the acceptable level (*Chapter 11*)

planning memorandum   audit documentation where all planning activities are recorded and summarized; usually includes the overall audit strategy, the audit plan, and detailed audit programs (*Chapter 8*)

pluralistic theories   ethical theories that assume that there are no universal principles and that the best approach is to use the principles that are most relevant in a particular case (*Chapter 3*)

population   the set of all the elements that constitute an account balance or class of transactions (*Chapter 10*)

population unit   each element of a population (*Chapter 10*)

positive assurance   a high, but not absolute, level of assurance; also referred to as reasonable assurance in the context of audit reporting (*Chapter 4*)

possible misstatement   the further misstatement remaining undetected in the units not selected in the sample (*Chapter 10*)

practice inspection   the system of reviewing and evaluating practice units' audit files and other documentation by an independent external party (*Appendix 2B*)

pre-audit risk management activities   procedures auditors perform before accepting an audit engagement to comply with professional standards and ensure the client and the engagement do not pose an unacceptably high risk of audit failure (*Chapter 5*)

predecessor   the auditor that held the engagement previously, before a new successor auditor took on the engagement (*Chapter 5*)

present fairly (fairly present)   in financial reporting, that management's financial statements achieve the properties of being a faithful representation of the economic realities they purport to portray, and of not being misleading to users (*Chapter 5*)

preventive controls   control procedures designed primarily to ensure that error or fraud does not occur in the first place in the accounting information system; see *detective controls* (*Chapter 7*)

primary beneficiaries   third parties for whose primary benefit the audit or other accounting service is performed (*Chapter 20*)

pro forma financial data   the presentation of financial statements as if a subsequent event had occurred on the date of the balance sheet; perhaps the best way to show the effect of a business purchase or other merger (*Chapter 15*)

problem recognition   the first three steps of the sampling method (*Chapter 10*)

procedures   to obtain direct evidence about the dollar amounts and disclosures in the financial statements (*Chapter 10*)

professional judgment   the application of relevant training, knowledge, and experience, within the context provided by auditing, accounting, and ethical standards, in making informed decisions about the courses of action that are appropriate under the circumstances of the audit engagement (*Chapter 1*)

professional responsibilities   the rules and principles for the proper conduct of an auditor in his or her work; necessary to obtain the respect and confidence of the public, achieve order within the profession, and provide a means of self-policing the profession; also known as *professional ethics* (*Chapter 3*)

professional skepticism   an auditor's tendency to question management representations and look for corroborating evidence before accepting these representations (*Chapter 1*)

proper period cutoff   a management control objective of ensuring that transactions occurring near a period-end are recorded in the period in which they correctly belong according to the company's financial reporting framework (e.g., generally accepted accounting principles) (*Chapter 9*)

proportionate liability   a legal liability regime where a party found to be partly liable is only responsible for paying a part of the damages in proportion to their share of the blame (*Chapter 3*)

prospectus   the set of financial statements and disclosures distributed to all purchasers in an offering registered under Securities Law (*Chapter 2*)

providing assurance   the adding of credibility to financial information by objective intermediaries (*Chapter 1*)

public accountant (PA)   an individual doing audit work with a public accounting firm; includes Chartered Professional Accountants (CPAs) (*Chapter 1*)

Public Company Accounting Oversight Board (PCAOB)   a five-member board created through the Sarbanes-Oxley Act (SOX) to oversee the auditors of public companies in the United States (*Chapter 2*)

public good   a good that has the properties of non-rival consumption and non-excludability (*Appendix 1B*)

public sector   activities of all levels of government (*Chapter 1*)

purchase cutoff   recording purchase transactions in the proper period, including accruals of payments not due until the following period (*Chapter 12*)

qualified reports   audit reports that contain an opinion paragraph that does not give the positive assurance that everything in the financial statements is in conformity with generally accepted accounting principles; see *modified opinion reports* (*Chapter 4*)

quality inspection   an examination and evaluation of the quality of the overall practice (*Appendix 2B*)

quality of earnings   the extent to which the reported earnings number represents actual economic performance, rather than selective accounting policy choices or management manipulation (*Chapter 6*)

random sample   a set of sampling units so chosen that each population item has an equal likelihood of being selected in the sample (*Chapter 10*)

reasonable estimates   management estimates that an auditor assesses to be supported by reliable evidence and not biased (*Chapter 16*)

recalculation   an audit procedure that involves redoing computations already performed by auditee personnel to determine if the result is accurate; may be done manually or electronically (*Chapter 8*)

recordkeeping (documents and records)   a control activity that involves the preparation of entries and supporting materials in an accounting information system (*Chapter 12*)

related parties   a term used to describe a situation in which one party has the ability to exercise, directly or indirectly, control, joint control, or significant influence over another and hence they may not deal with each other at arm's length; in an audit includes the auditee's management and immediate family members (*Chapter 15*)

reliance letter   a document that accountants sign showing that they have been notified that a particular recipient of the financial statements and audit report intends to rely upon them for particular purposes (*Chapter 3*)

reperformance   an audit procedure in which the auditor executes a procedure that is part of the auditee's internal control to obtain evidence about the effectiveness of controls or the accuracy of the auditor's understanding of the auditee's information system (*Chapter 8*)

replicate   reperform a selection procedure and get the same sample units (*Chapter 10*)

reportable matters   significant deficiencies in the design or operation of the company's internal control structure, which could adversely affect its ability to report financial data in conformity with generally accepted accounting principles (*Chapter 17*)

representational faithfulness   when information presented in an entity's financial statements closely corresponds to the actual underlying transactions and events affecting it, conveying their economic substance rather than simply their legal form (*Chapter 5*)

representative sample   a sample that mirrors the characteristics of the population being studied (*Chapter 10*)

reservations   major variations on the standard audit report (*Chapter 4*)

revenue recognition problems   techniques used by financial statement preparers to manipulate reported revenues resulting in low-quality earnings (*Chapter 11*)

reversing error   errors in the current period that will have an equal and opposite effect in the following period (*Chapter 11*)

risk assessment program   an audit planning document listing the specific procedures for gaining understanding of the auditee's business transaction processing systems and controls, as well as for assessing the inherent risks and the control risk for the assertions in financial account balances and transaction streams (*Chapter 8*)

risk-based reasoning (RBR)   reasoning using the following decision rule: if an actual estimation uncertainty associated with a recorded amount is greater than an acceptable level, then reject the recorded amount; otherwise, accept it (*Chapter 19, Part I*)

risk of assessing the control risk too high   the probability that the compliance evidence in the sample indicates high control risk when the actual (but unknown) degree of compliance would justify a lower control risk assessment (*Chapter 10*)

risk of assessing the control risk too low   the probability that the compliance evidence in the sample indicates low control risk when the actual (but unknown) degree of compliance justifies a higher control risk assessment (*Chapter 10*)

risk of incorrect acceptance   the decision to accept a balance as being materially accurate when the balance is materially misstated (*Chapter 10*)

risk of incorrect rejection   the decision to accept a balance as being materially misstated when it is not (*Chapter 10*)

risk of material misstatement   the auditor's assessment of the probability that the financial statements are materially misstated prior to being audited; assessed at the level of the financial statements overall, based on pervasive factors such as fraud, going concern, or other significant business-level risks, to develop the overall audit strategy; and also assessed as the combined inherent and control risk at the assertion level for developing a detailed audit plan and specific procedures (*Chapter 6*)

risk of material misstatement at the financial statement level   the auditor's assessment, based on pervasive factors such as fraud, going concern, or other significant business-level risks, of the probability that errors or fraud have affected the financial statements overall such that financial statement users may be misled (*Chapter 5*)

roll-forward period the period between the cutoff and fiscal year-end, when a cutoff is made before the year-end (*Chapter 12*)

sales cutoff testing control procedures designed to ensure sales transactions are recorded in the proper period (*Chapter 11*)

sample a set of sampling units (*Chapter 10*)

sampling error the amount by which a projected likely misstatement amount could differ from an actual (unknown) total as a result of the sample not being exactly representative (*Chapter 10*)

sampling risk the probability that an auditor's conclusion based on a sample might be different from the conclusion based on an examination of the entire population (*Chapter 10*)

sampling unit a unit used for testing a client's population, for example, a customer's account, an inventory item, a debt issue, or a cash receipt (*Chapter 10*)

scanning an audit procedure in which the auditor quickly reviews a whole report, account, journal, or other listing in the auditee's records to look for any unusual items that require further investigation (*Chapter 8*)

scope limitation a condition where auditors are unable to obtain sufficient appropriate evidence (*Chapter 4*)

search for unrecorded liabilities a set of procedures for inspecting documents and records in the period following the audit client's balance sheet date designed to yield audit evidence of liabilities relating to the current period that were omitted, thus violating the completeness assertion (*Chapter 12*)

Securities and Exchange Commission (SEC) the main U.S. government agency regulating the securities markets in the United States (*Chapter 2*)

self-regulation a situation where the government gives a professional group the power to monitor and discipline its members (*Chapter 2*)

significant control deficiency an identified control deficiency or combination of deficiencies that the auditor believes exposes the entity to a serious risk of material misstatement (*Chapter 9*)

significant risks identified and assessed risks of material misstatement that, in the auditor's judgment, require special audit consideration (*Chapter 5*)

skewness the concentration of a large proportion of the dollar amount in only a small number of the population items (*Chapter 10*)

special purpose financial reporting frameworks financial reporting frameworks used to prepare financial statements tailored to meet the financial information needs stipulated by a particular user or user group (*Chapter 16*)

specific materiality the materiality level(s) to be applied to those particular classes of transactions, account balances, or disclosures for which misstatements of lesser amounts than materiality for the financial statements as a whole could reasonably be expected to influence the economic decisions of users taken on the basis of the financial statements (*Chapter 5*)

specific performance materiality the amount(s) set by the auditor at less than the specific materiality level(s) to reduce to an appropriately low level the probability that the aggregate of uncorrected and undetected misstatements exceeds specific materiality (*Chapter 5*)

standard deviation a measure of population variability (*Chapter 10*)

statistical sampling audit sampling that uses the laws of probability to select and evaluate a sample from a population for the purpose of reaching a conclusion about the population (*Chapter 10*)

stratification subdividing the population in an audit sample by, for example, account balance size (*Chapter 10*)

subsequent event requiring adjustment in financial statement numbers the type of material subsequent event that requires adjustment of the dollar amounts of one or more financial statement line items along with any related additional explanatory note disclosure (*Chapter 15*)

subsequent event requiring disclosure but not adjustment the type of material subsequent event that happened after year-end and should not be reflected in the year-end financial statement numbers but needs to be disclosed in the notes to those financial statements because it is likely to be materially relevant to decisions and predictions based on those financial statements (*Chapter 15*)

substantive audit approach an approach to performing an audit that involves obtaining assurance only from substantive procedures, with no reliance on internal control effectiveness (*Chapter 9*)

substantive audit procedures designed to detect material misstatements at the assertion level; comprising tests of details (classes of transactions, account balances, and disclosures) and substantive analytical procedures (*Chapter 6*)

substantive tests of details auditing procedures to obtain direct evidence about the dollar amounts and disclosures in the financial statements (*Chapter 10*)

successor a new auditor who takes over the engagement from the predecessor (*Chapter 5*)

sufficient appropriate audit evidence information obtained by an auditor in relation to one or more audit objectives (assertions) that is adequately persuasive to support a logical conclusion; "sufficiency" generally refers to the quantity (sample size) and independence of the evidential matter in relation to the level of risk of material misstatement; "appropriateness" generally refers to the level of reliability of the evidential matter and its relevance to the audit objective (*Chapter 8*)

summary of misstatements an audit file schedule that lists all the identified and likely misstatements uncovered in the audit procedures and analyzes their impact on fair presentation of the financial statements (*Chapter 16*)

systematic random selection using a predetermined population and sample size and random starting places (*Chapter 10*)

those charged with governance person(s) or organization(s) (may include management) responsible for overseeing the strategic directions of the entity and obligations related to the accountability of the entity; includes overseeing the financial reporting process (*Chapter 5*)

three-party accountability an accountability relationship in which there are three distinct parties (individuals): an asserter, an assurer, and a user of the asserted information (*Chapter 1*)

timing of audit procedures when the planned audit procedures are to be performed, either before, at, or after period-end (*Chapter 8*)

tolerable deviation rate the rate of deviation that can exist without causing a minimum material misstatement in a test of controls procedure (*Chapter 10*)

tort legal action covering civil complaints other than breach of contract; normally initiated by users of financial statements (*Chapter 3*)

tracing an audit procedure that involves examining documents based on the selection of evidence in supporting documents of transactions or other events and then following the information forward through the accounting processing system to find whether it has been included in the auditee's general ledger accounts; sometimes referred to as "cradle to grave" testing (*Chapter 8*)

trivial misstatements misstatements that are considered to be so small and insignificant that auditors can disregard accumulating or reporting them to management; the threshold level for what amount is considered trivial must be set at the planning stage of the audit (*Chapter 16*)

two-direction testing   audit control over both completeness in one direction and validity in the other (*Chapter 11*)

unadjusted (uncorrected) misstatements errors in financial statements that are discovered by the auditor but management decides not to correct, due to cost-benefit or other considerations; see *passed adjustments, waived adjustments* (*Chapter 16*)

unaudited—see Notice to Reader   a note the accountant places on each page of financial statements in performing write-up or compilation work (*Chapter 17*)

unmodified opinion report   an audit report in which the auditor is not calling attention to anything wrong with the audit work or the financial statements (*Chapter 2*)

unrestricted random sample   a sample obtained by means of unrestricted random selection (*Appendix 10B*)

unrestricted random selection   using a printed random number table or computerized random number generator to obtain a list of random numbers (*Chapter 10*)

unusual transactions   a term used to describe a variety of transactions that may be artificially created to manipulate financial statements, especially earnings, and that tend to be complex and difficult for auditors to understand and verify (*Chapter 15*)

utilitarianism   a moral theory that the right choice is the one that results in the greatest good for the greatest number of people (*Chapter 3*)

validity   a management control objective of ensuring that the recorded transactions are ones that should be recorded, that is, that they exist (*Chapter 9*)

value-for-money (VFM) audit   an audit concept from the public sector that incorporates audits of economy, efficiency, and effectiveness (*Chapter 1*)

vertical analysis   the analytical procedure of comparing all financial statement items with a common base, for example, total assets or total sales (*Chapter 5*)

vouching   an audit procedure that involves examining documents based on the selection of transactions, entries, or balances that appear in the auditee's general ledger accounts and seeking evidence that supports the validity of the item; sometimes referred to as "grave to cradle" testing (*Chapter 8*)

walk-through procedure   an audit procedure that follows one or more transactions through an accounting process to confirm that the documents, procedures, and work flows documented in the auditor's system description narrative or flowcharts are accurate (*Chapter 9*)

white-collar crime   misdeeds committed by business and government professionals, typically non-violent (*Chapter 7*)

window dressing   in financial reporting, the inappropriate manipulation of account balances by management, usually at the end of a period, to make the financial position or performance reported in the financial statements appear more attractive to users; often involves using accounting policies, journal entries, or actual cash transactions between related parties that have no real business purpose, resulting in artificial embellishment of the company's results or liquidity to obtain some benefit (e.g., salaries and bonuses that depend on how well the company performed) (*Chapter 11*)

working paper reference index   a table of contents listing all the index numbers used to identify sections of the audit working paper files (*Chapter 15*)

written representations   written statements by management and, where appropriate, those charged with governance, provided to the auditor to confirm certain matters or to support other audit evidence in addition to the representations contained in the financial statements, the assertions therein, or supporting books and records, obtained at the final point in the audit prior to issuing an opinion; see *management representation letter* (*Chapter 15*)

year-end audit work   audit procedures performed at and shortly after the balance sheet date (*Chapter 5*)

INDEX

A

AADBA statements, 900, 902
AbitibiBowater Inc., 194
absolute size, 209
acceptable audit risk level, 579
acceptable financial reporting frameworks, 866–868
account balance, 503
account balance audit (audit sampling example)
  audit plan, 529–530
  evidence collection, 531–535
  evidence evaluation, 535–538
  steps of, 529–530
accountability relationship, 7
accounting, 9–11. *See also* public accounting
accounting contingency, 151–152
accounting control activities. *See* control activities
accounting credibility, 135
accounting deficiency reservation, 143
accounting estimates. *See also* accounting judgments; estimation uncertainties
  accounting measurement uncertainties, 151, 152
  accounting risk, 868, 962–965
  audit opinion, 142
  AuG-41, 965–966
  CAS 540, 960
  Cockburn analysis, 966–968
  finance/investment process, 767–768
  financial statement materiality, 205–206
  fraud risk, 339
  future events forecasting, 962–964
  going-concern assumption, 957–959
  governance responsibility paragraph, 139
  information risk, 1006–1007
  key audit matters paragraph, 138
  Libor, 963
  range. *See* range
  risk of material forecasting errors, 962–965
  risk-based reasoning. *See* risk-based reasoning (RBR)
accounting information system. *See* information system
accounting judgments. *See also* accounting estimates
  critical and good-faith thought process, 954–955
  definition, 948–949
  documentation, 955–957
  going-concern assumption, 957
accounting measurement uncertainties, 151
accounting processes
  business processes, 284
  definition, 280
  example, 282–283
  financial statements and, 284
  types of, 280–281

accounting risk
  audit risk vs., 977
  calculation illustrations, 981–982
  concepts, 1007
  definition, 962
  future events forecasting, 962–964
  information risk. *See* information risk
  RBR benchmarks, 985–990
  reasonable range, 977–982
accounting risk (account level)
  accounting estimates, 868
  adequate disclosure, 60
  definition, 20
  non-sampling risk, 511
Accounting Standards Oversight Council, 934
accounts payable trial balance, 638
accounts receivable. *See* revenues
accounts receivable lapping, 594–595, 596
accounts receivable subsidiary ledger, 567
accumulated misstatements. *See also* known misstatement; misstatements
  adjusting entries, 862–863
  audit opinion and, 857–859, 863–865
  auditor–client negotiations, 860
  correction of, 859–860
  materiality evaluation, 863–865
  passed (waived) adjustments, 859
  professional judgment, 863–865
  summary of misstatements, 859
  trivial misstatements, 859
  unadjusted misstatements, 859
  working paper file, 860–862
accuracy
  assertions, 267, 441
  control objectives, 439
  definition, 440
  internal control questionnaire, 449
  purchases, 645
  revenues, 572
acting in the public interest, 7, 94
Adams Committee, 897
Adelphia Communications, 42
adequate disclosure, 60
adverse opinion. *See also* audit opinion
  audit report reservation, 143
  definition, 60–61, 128
  pervasive materiality, 145–146
advertising, 927–928
Advisory Committee on Improvements to Financial Reporting (CIFiR), 954–957
aged accounts receivable trial balance, 567, 588
agency theory, 8–9
Agostino, Dominic, 1087
Alberta Health Services (AHS), 641
allocation, 260, 267
Altman Z-score, 958

American Bankers Association, 18
American Institute of Certified Public Accountants (AICPA), 907
American Institute of CPAs (AICPA), 30
American International Group Inc., 18
amortization recalculation, 784
amortization schedule, 723–724
analysis. *See also* analytical procedures
  analytical procedures and, 372–373
  audit evidence, 363, 365–366
  audit program, 390
  definition, 196, 372
  evidence and, 373–374
  relevance of evidence, 383
  reliability, 373
  types of evidence, 367
  working paper software, 397
analytical procedures. *See also* analysis
  analysis and, 372–373
  attention directing, 199–203
  audit completion stage, 819–823
  CAS 315, 196
  CAS 520, 196, 373, 819
  definition, 196–197
  evidence and, 364, 366, 373–374
  management's draft financial statements, 199
  overall procedures, 819
  preliminary procedures, 196–203, 273
  relevance of evidence, 383
  reliability of audit evidence, 383
  representational faithfulness, 199
  revenue existence assertion, 584
  types of, 197–198, 200
analytical procedures risk, 527–528
anchoring, 273, 952
anchoring and adjustment heuristic, 951
annual reports services, 1072
anomalies, 500
another appropriate disclosed basis of accounting (AADBA), 900, 902
anti-fraud, 1037
applicable financial reporting framework, 866
application controls
  company-level controls, 322
  control activities, 442, 447
  control assessment, 426
  definition, 326
  internal control questionnaire, 448–449
  procedures, 442–443, 447
appropriateness, 382–384, 386. *See also* sufficient appropriate audit evidence
Ariad Pharmaceuticals Inc., 1032
arm's length, 833
Arthur Andersen, 42–44, 94, 392
articles of incorporation, 760–761

OVERVIEW OF THE AUDIT PROCESS AS

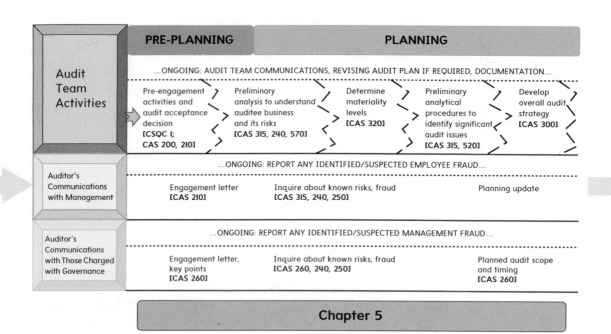

Chapter 5

The previous year's audit experience is used to plan for next year.

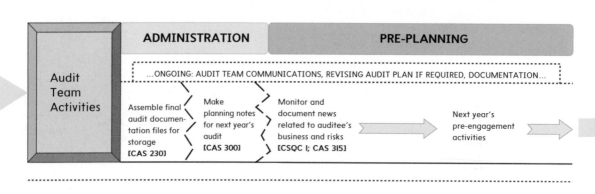